# Comprehensive Gynecology

## 7th Edition


**Roger A. Lobo, MD**
*Professor, Obstetrics and Gynecology*
*Division of Reproductive Endocrinology*
*Columbia University*
*New York, New York*

**David M. Gershenson, MD**
*Professor*
*Gynecologic Oncology and Reproductive Medicine*
*University of Texas MD Anderson Cancer Center*
*Houston, Texas*

**Gretchen M. Lentz, MD**
*Professor, Obstetrics and Gynecology*
*Adjunct Professor, Urology*
*Division Director, Urogynecology*
*Urogynecology and Female Urology Clinic*
*University of Washington Medical Center*
*Seattle, Washington*

**Fidel A. Valea, MD**
*Professor and Vice-Chair of Education*
*Residency Program Director*
*Fellowship Director, Division of Gynecologic Oncology*
*Department of Obstetrics and Gynecology*
*Duke University School of Medicine*
*Durham, North Carolina*




ELSEVIER

ELSEVIER

1600 John F. Kennedy Blvd.
Ste 1800
Philadelphia, PA 19103-2899

**Comprehensive Gynecology** ISBN: 978-0-323-32287-4


**Library of Congress Cataloging-in-Publication Data**
Lobo, Roger A., editor. | Gershenson, David M. (David Marc), 1946- , editor. | Lentz, Gretchen M., editor. | Valea, Fidel A., editor.
Comprehensive gynecology / [edited by] Roger A. Lobo, David M. Gershenson, Gretchen M. Lentz, Fidel A. Valea.
7 edition. | Philadelphia : Elsevier, [2017] | Preceded by Comprehensive gynecology / [edited by] Gretchen M. Lentz ... [et al.].
6th ed. c2012. | Includes bibliographical references and index.
LCCN 2015038440 | ISBN 9780323322874 (hardcover : alk. paper) | MESH: Genital Diseases, Female. | Genital Neoplasms, Female.
LCC RG101 | NLM WP 140 | DDC
618.1--dc23 LC record available at http://lccn.loc.gov/2015038440

*Executive Content Strategist:* Kate Dimock
*Senior Content Development Specialist:* Rae Robertson
*Publishing Services Manager:* Patricia Tannian
*Project Manager:* Stephanie Turza
*Design Direction:* Brian Salisbury

Printed in the United States of America

Last digit is the print number: 9 8 7 6 5 4

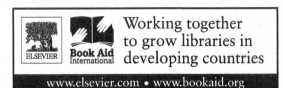

# Comprehensive Gynecology

# Contributors


**Arnold Advincula, MD**
Levine Family Professor of Obstetrics and Gynecology at Columbia University Medical Center
Vice Chair of Women's Health and Chief of Gynecology
Department of Obstetrics and Gynecology
Columbia University
New York, New York

**Ellen S. Baker, MD**
Department of Gynecologic Oncology
University of Texas MD Anderson Cancer Center
Houston, Texas

**Jamie N. Bakkum-Gamez, MD**
Associate Professor of Obstetrics and Gynecology
Mayo Clinic
Rochester, Minnesota

**Diane C. Bodurka, MD**
Professor and Vice President Medical Education
Gynecologic Oncology and Reproductive Medicine
University of Texas MD Anderson Cancer Center
Houston, Texas

**Geneviève Bouchard-Fortier, MD, SM**
Department of Gynecologic Oncology
University of Toronto
Toronto, Ontario, Canada

**Sarah M. Carlson, MD**
Department of Obstetrics and Gynecology
Einstein Medical Center
Philadelphia, Pennsylvania

**Janet Choi, MD**
Medical Director
Colorado Center for Reproductive Medicine
New York, New York

**Leslie Clark, MD**
Clinical Fellow
Division of Gynecologic Oncology
University of North Carolina
Chapel Hill, North Carolina

**Robert L. Coleman, MD**
Professor and Deputy Chair
Department of Gynecologic Oncology and Reproductive Medicine
University of Texas MD Anderson Cancer Center
Houston, Texas

**Allan Covens, MD**
Chair, Department of Gynecologic Oncology
University of Toronto;
Head, Department of Gynecologic Oncology
Sunnybrook Health Sciences Centre
Toronto, Ontario, Canada

**Deborah S. Cowley, MD**
Professor, Psychiatry and Behavioral Sciences
University of Washington
Seattle, Washington

**Mary Segars Dolan, MD**
Associate Professor of Gynecology and Obstetrics
Emory University School of Medicine
Atlanta, Georgia

**Sarah K. Dotters-Katz, MD**
Clinical Instructor and Fellow
Obstetrics and Gynecology
University of North Carolina
Chapel Hill, North Carolina

**Nataki C. Douglas, MD, PhD**
Assistant Professor
Obstetrics and Gynecology
Columbia University Medical Center
New York, New York

**Sean C. Dowdy, MD**
Professor of Obstetrics and Gynecology
Mayo Clinic
Rochester, Minnesota

**Linda O. Eckert, MD**
Professor, Obstetrics and Gynecology
University of Washington
Seattle, Washington

**Jonathan R. Foote, MD**
Fellow, Division of Gynecologic Oncology
Department of Obstetrics and Gynecology
Duke University Medical Center
Durham, North Carolina

**Michael Frumovitz, MD**
Associate Professor and Fellowship Director
Gynecologic Oncology and Reproductive Medicine
University of Texas MD Anderson Cancer Center
Houston, Texas

**Carolyn Gardella, MD**
Associate Professor, Obstetrics and Gynecology
University of Washington;
Gynecology Service Chief of Surgery
Veterans Administration Puget Sound
Seattle, Washington

**Paola Alvarez Gehrig, MD**
Professor and Chief
Division of Gynecologic Oncology
University of North Carolina
Chapel Hill, North Carolina

**David M. Gershenson, MD**
Professor
Gynecologic Oncology and Reproductive Medicine
University of Texas MD Anderson Cancer Center
Houston, Texas

**Jennifer Bushman Gilner, MD, PhD**
Fellow, Clinical Associate
Obstetrics and Gynecology
Duke University
Chapel Hill, North Carolina

**Jay Goldberg, MD**
Professor
Department of Obstetrics and Gynecology
Einstein Medical Center;
Director
Philadelphia Fibroid Center
Philadelphia, Pennsylvania

**Laura J. Havrilesky, MD**
Department of Obstetrics and Gynecology
Division of Gynecologic Oncology
Duke University Medical Center
Durham, North Carolina

**Cherie Hill, MD**
Assistant Professor of Gynecology and Obstetrics
Emory University School of Medicine
Atlanta, Georgia

**Anuja Jhingran, MD**
Professor
Department of Radiation Oncology
University of Texas MD Anderson Cancer Center
Houston, Texas

**James M. Kelley III, JD**
Shareholder and Partner
Elk and Elk Co. Ltd.
Cleveland, Ohio

**Sanaz Keyhan, MD**
Clinical Instructor
Department of Obstetrics and Gynecology
Duke University School of Medicine
Durham, North Carolina

**Rosanne M. Kho, MD**
Associate Professor
Director, Benign Gynecologic Surgery
Cleveland Clinic
Cleveland, Ohio

**Anna C. Kirby, MD**
Department of Obstetrics and Gynecology
University of Washington
Seattle, Washington

**Mukta Krane, MD**
Associate Professor of Surgery
Department of Surgery
Division of General Surgery
University of Washington Medical Center
Seattle, Washington

**Jeffrey A. Kuller, MD**
Professor of Obstetrics and Gynecology
Division of Maternal-Fetal Medicine
Duke University Medical Center
Durham, North Carolina

**Eduardo Lara-Torre, MD**
Interim Chair and Vice-Chair for Academic Affairs
Residency Program Director of Obstetrics and Gynecology
Department of Obstetrics and Gynecology
Carilion Clinic;
Associate Professor of Obstetrics and Gynecology and Pediatrics
Virginia Tech Carilion School of Medicine and Research Institute
Roanoke, Virginia

**Gretchen M. Lentz, MD**
Professor, Obstetrics and Gynecology
Adjunct Professor, Urology
Division Director, Urogynecology
Urogynecology and Female Urology Clinic, University of Washington Medical Center
Seattle, Washington

**Roger A. Lobo, MD**
Professor, Obstetrics and Gynecology
Division of Reproductive Endocrinology
Columbia University
New York, New York

**Karen H. Lu, MD**
Chair and Professor
Gynecologic Oncology and Reproductive Medicine
University of Texas MD Anderson Cancer Center
Houston, Texas

**Vicki Mendiratta, MD**
Associate Professor
Obstetrics and Gynecology
University of Washington
Seattle, Washington

**Larissa A. Meyer, MD**
Assistant Professor
Gynecologic Oncology and Reproductive Medicine
University of Texas MD Anderson Cancer Center
Houston, Texas

**Lisa Muasher, MD**
Associate Residency Program Director
Department of Obstetrics and Gynecology
Duke University School of Medicine
Durham, North Carolina

**Suheil J. Muasher, MD**
Professor of Obstetrics and Gynecology
Duke University School of Medicine
Durham, North Carolina

**James W. Orr, Jr., MD**
Florida Gynecologic Oncology, 21st Century Oncology
Medical Director, Regional Cancer Center
Lee Memorial Health Systems
Fort Myers, Florida

**Thomas M. Price, MD**
Associate Professor of Obstetrics and Gynecology
Duke University
Durham, North Carolina

**Beth W. Rackow, MD**
Assistant Professor, Obstetrics and Gynecology
Division of Reproductive Endocrinology
Columbia University
New York, New York

**Pedro T. Ramirez, MD**
Professor
Department of Gynecologic Oncology and Reproductive Medicine
University of Texas MD Anderson Cancer Center
Houston, Texas

**Katherine Rivlin, MD**
Department of Family Planning and Obstetrics-Gynecology
Columbia University Medical Center
New York, New York

**David T. Rock, MD**
Fellowship Director, Society of Gynecologic Oncology Breast Fellowship
Regional Breast Care, 21st Century Oncology
Regional Cancer Center
Lee Memorial Health Systems
Fort Myers, Florida

**Timothy Ryntz, MD**
Assistant Professor
Obstetrics and Gynecology
Columbia University School of Medicine
New York, New York

**Mila Pontremoli Salcedo, MD**
Professor
Department of Gynecology and Obstetrics
Federal University of Health Sciences/Irmandade Santa Casa de Misericordia/Porto Alegre
Rio Grande do Sul, Brazil;
Visiting Scientist
Department of Gynecologic Oncology and Reproductive Medicine
University of Texas MD Anderson Cancer Center
Houston, Texas

**Samith Sandadi, MD**
Breast Fellow, Society of Gynecologic Oncology
Florida Gynecologic Oncology, 21st Century Oncology
Regional Cancer Center
Lee Memorial Health Systems
Fort Myers, Florida

**Kathleen M. Schmeler, MD**
Department of Gynecologic Oncology
University of Texas MD Anderson Cancer Center
Houston, Texas

**Judith Ann Smith, PharmD**
Associate Professor
Obstetrics, Gynecology, and Reproductive Sciences
UTHealth—University of Texas Medical School at Houston
Houston, Texas

**Pamela T. Soliman, MD**
Associate Professor
Gynecologic Oncology and Reproductive Medicine
University of Texas MD Anderson Cancer Center
Houston, Texas

**Anil K. Sood, MD**
Professor and Vice Chair
Gynecologic Oncology and Reproductive Medicine
University of Texas MD Anderson Cancer Center
Houston, Texas

**Premal H. Thaker, MD**
Associate Professor, Gynecologic Oncology
Obstetrics and Gynecology
Washington University School of Medicine
St. Louis, Missouri

**Mireille Truong, MD**
Assistant Professor
Department of Obstetrics and Gynecology
Virginia Commonwealth University
Richmond, Virginia

**Fidel A. Valea, MD**
Professor and Vice-Chair of Education
Residency Program Director
Fellowship Director, Division of Gynecologic Oncology
Department of Obstetrics and Gynecology
Duke University School of Medicine
Durham, North Carolina

**Carolyn Westhoff, MD**
Sarah Billinghurst Solomon Professor of Reproductive Health
Columbia University Medical Center
New York, New York

# Preface

*Try to learn something about everything and everything about something.*
**Thomas Huxley**

*Comprehensive Gynecology* is now in its seventh edition, and it is humbling to note that it has almost been 30 years since the first edition was published in 1987.

The current editors are indebted to our mentors who pioneered the original work. The contributions of Drs. William Droegemueller, Authur L Herbst, Daniel R. Mishell, Jr., and Morton A. Stenchever were monumental and provided the impetus for our following in their footsteps. We are also saddened by the fact that in 2015, we lost Mort, who is now in a better place. Also, as we close out this edition, we have just learned that we have also lost our esteemed mentor, Dan Mishell, who passed away in May 2016. Both men have contributed so much to the field, and to us personally, and have done so much to improve the lives of women.

In line with the quote above from Huxley, the British biologist and philosopher, we continue to attempt to be *comprehensive.* We want the reader to be comfortable with all aspects of gynecology; some readers will wish to be more expert in certain subspecialty areas such as urogynecology, oncology, or reproductive endocrinology.

In this edition we are privileged to welcome Fidel Valea as one of the editors, taking over the duties from Vern L. Katz, who elected to retire. We would like to thank Vern once again for his contributions.

Rather than adding new chapters, we have split some in two to provide better focus on the subject areas, and also organized the chapters to provide better flow. We have added several co-authors, continuing the trend we established with the previous edition. This is a major departure from the early editions, where the four editors wrote all of the chapters. We feel adding additional talent to the authorship provides a more comprehensive and validated approach to the dissemination of knowledge in gynecology.

In this edition, we have provided the most important references in the body of the chapter, allowing the reader to have immediate access to the source, rather than having to search for the reference. However, we have maintained a full bibliography for many chapters, available online.

In this edition we have also provided video content to make this a more visual experience for the reader. New and better illustrations have also been added to assist in visual learning. The cover is also a departure from our previous editions and speaks to our wish to impart a visual experience and emphasize contemporary techniques of minimally invasive procedures for gynecological surgery.

Nearly every chapter has maintained key points of importance, which have been bundled together in an online synopsis of the entire book. This will allow rapid assessment of the content of each chapter for more in-depth reading of areas of greater interest as well as provide key learning facts in all areas of gynecology.

We hope readers will enjoy this edition and learn as much as they can from this ever-evolving field in order to provide better health care for women.

We would like to give a big thanks to our editors, Kate Dimock, and particularly Rae Robertson, who have stewarded us through this process.

We would also like to give a big thank you, with great appreciation and love, to our families, without whose support and encouragement this project could not have been accomplished.

*Roger A. Lobo, MD*
*David M. Gershenson, MD*
*Gretchen M. Lentz, MD*
*Fidel A. Valea, MD*

# Contents

Part I BASIC SCIENCE

# 1

# Fertilization and Embryogenesis

## Meiosis, Fertilization, Implantation, Embryonic Development, Sexual Differentiation

*Thomas M. Price*

Several areas of medical investigation have brought increased attention to the processes of fertilization and embryonic development, including teratology, stem cell research, immunogenetics, and assisted reproductive technology. The preimplantation, implantation, and embryonic stages of development in the human can now be studied because of the development of newer techniques and areas of research. This chapter considers the processes of oocyte meiosis, fertilization and early cleavage, implantation, development of the genitourinary system, and sex differentiation.

## OOCYTE AND MEIOSIS

The oocyte is a unique and extremely specialized cell. The primordial germ cells in both males and females are large eosinophilic cells derived from endoderm in the wall of the yolk sac. These 700 to 1300 cells migrate to the germinal ridge by way of the dorsal mesentery of the hindgut by ameboid action by 5 to 6 weeks. Oogenesis begins with the replication of the diploid oogonia through mitosis to produce primary oocytes, reaching a peak number of 600,000 (95% prediction interval: 70,000-5,000,000) at 18 to 22 weeks of gestation. Through apoptosis the numbers decline to about 360,000 (95% prediction interval: 42,000 to 3,000,000) at menarche (Wallace, 2010). As can be seen, there is a large variance among individuals and a direct correlation between the number of fetal oocytes and the age of menopause. Accelerated apoptosis is seen in Turner syndrome resulting in few oocytes at birth (Modi, 2003).

The meiotic process actually begins at 10 to 12 weeks' gestation and is the mechanism by which diploid organisms reduce their gametes to a haploid state so that they can recombine again during fertilization to become diploid organisms. In humans, this process reduces 46 chromosomes to 23 chromosome structures in the gamete. The haploid gamete contains only one chromosome for each homologous pair of chromosomes, so it has either the maternal or paternal chromosome for each pair, but not both. Meiosis is also the mechanism by which genetic exchange is completed through chiasma formation and crossing over (recombination) between homologous chromosome pairs. Two meiotic cell divisions are required to produce haploid gametes. In the human female, oogonia enter meiosis in "waves" (Fig. 1.1)— that is, not all oogonia enter meiosis at the same time. Meiosis initiation is dependent on mesonephric-produced retinoic acid (Childs, 2011).

Oocytes in the first substage of prophase, leptotene, are found in the human fetal ovary as early as 10 weeks' gestation. With increasing gestational age, greater proportions of oocytes in later stages of meiosis may be observed, and by the end of the second trimester of pregnancy, the majority of oocytes in the fetal ovary have cytologic characteristics that are consistent with the diplotene/dictyotene substages of prophase I of meiosis I (the stage at which the oocytes are arrested until ovulation) (Fig. 1.2).

Meiosis is preceded by interphase I during which DNA replication occurs, thus transforming the diploid oogonia with a DNA content of $2N$ to an oocyte with a DNA content of $4N$. Meiosis is defined in two stages. The first, known as the reduction division (division I, or meiosis I) initiates in the fetal ovary but is then arrested and completed at the time of ovulation.

Meiosis I starts with prophase I (prophase includes leptotene, zygotene, pachytene, and diplotene), which occurs exclusively during fetal life and sets the stage for genetic exchange that ensures genetic variation in our species (Fig. 1.3). Leptotene is

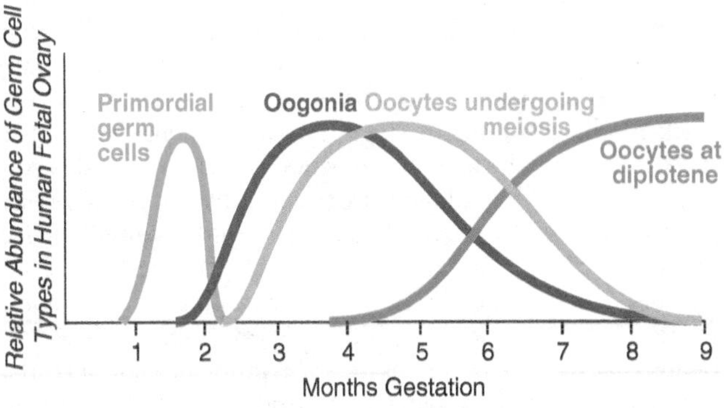


**Figure 1.1** Diagrammatic representation of the different meiotic cell types and their proportions in the ovary during fetal life. (Courtesy of Edith Cheng, MD.)

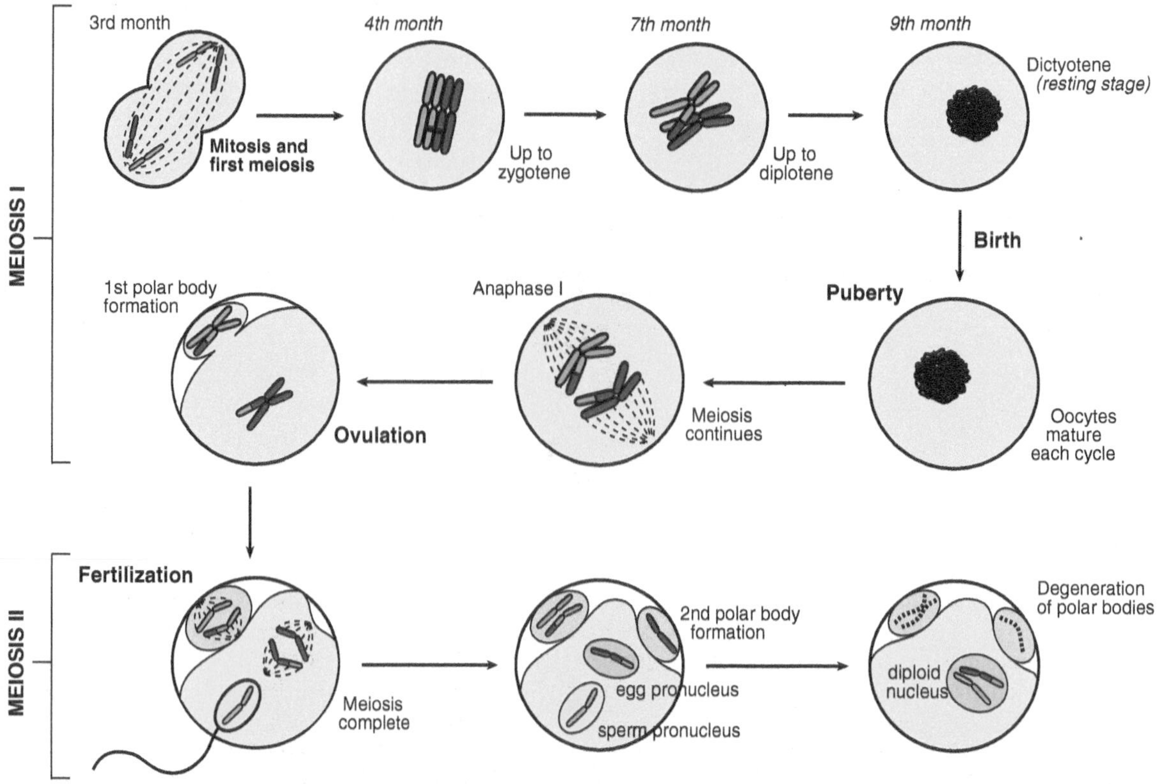


**Figure 1.2** Diagram of oocyte meiosis. For simplicity, only one pair of chromosomes is depicted. Prophase stages of the first meiotic division occur in the female during fetal life. The meiotic process is arrested at the diplotene stage ("first meiotic arrest"), and the oocyte enters the dictyotene stages. Meiosis I resumes at puberty and is completed at the time of ovulation. The second meiotic division takes place over several hours in the oviduct only after sperm penetration. (Courtesy of Edith Cheng, MD.)

proportionately the most abundant of all the prophase I substages in the early gestations. Cells in this meiotic phase are characterized by a large nucleus with fine, diffuse, string-like chromatin evenly distributed within the nucleus (Fig. 1.3, *A*). Chromatin of homologous pairs occupies "domains" and does not occur as distinct linear strands of chromosomes. The zygotene substage is defined by the initiation of pairing, which is characterized by the striking appearance of the synaptonemal complex formation in some of the chromosomes (Fig. 1.3, *B*). There is cytologic evidence of chromosome condensation and linearization, and the chromatin is seen as a fine, string-like structure. The pachytene substage is the most easily recognizable period of the prophase and is characterized by clearly defined chromosomes that appear as continuous ribbons of thick beadlike chromatin (Fig. 1.3, *C*). By definition, this is the substage in which all homologues have paired. In this substage, the paired homologues are structurally composed of four closely opposed chromatids and are known as a *tetrad.* The frequency of oocytes in pachytene increases with gestational age and peaks in the mid-second trimester of pregnancy (at about 20 to 25 weeks' gestation). The diplotene substage is a stage of desynapsis that occurs as the synaptonemal complex dissolves and the two homologous chromosomes pull away from each other. However, these bivalents, which are composed of a maternally and a paternally derived chromosome, are held together at the centromere and at sites of chiasma formation

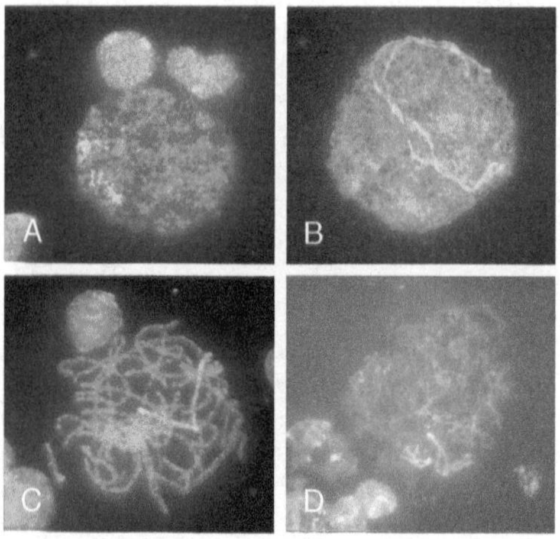


**Figure 1.3** Fetal ovary with fluorescent in situ hybridization. The first three images are meiotic cells from a 21-week fetal ovary. **A,** Fluorescent in situ hybridization (FISH) with a whole chromosome probe for chromosome X was completed to visualize the pairing characteristics of the X chromosome during leptotene. **B,** Zygotene. **C,** Pachytene. **D,** Image of a meiotic cell from a 34-week fetal ovary that underwent dual FISH with probes for chromosomes 13 *(green signal)* and 21 *(red signal)* to illustrate the pairing characteristics of this substage of prophase in meiosis I. (Courtesy of Edith Cheng, MD.)

that represent sites where crossing over has occurred (Fig. 1.3, *D*). In general, chiasma formation occurs only between chromatids of homologous pairs and not between sister chromatids. Usually, one to three chiasmata occur for each chromosome arm. Oocytes at this stage of prophase I constitute the majority of third-trimester fetal and newborn ovaries. Diplotene merges with diakinesis, the last substage of meiosis I, and is a stage of transition to metaphase, lasting many years in humans (Speed, 1985).

With puberty, folliculogenesis occurs with progression of the follicle, consisting of the oocyte and granulosa cells from primordial to antral characterized by granulosa cell proliferation, development of gonadotropin receptors, and expression of enzymes for sex steroid production (Baerwald, 2012). It takes approximately 85 days for a follicle to mature to the point of ovulation. There is no change in the chromosome stage during folliculogenesis.

Meiosis I resumes with the surge of luteinizing hormone prior to ovulation completing metaphase, anaphase, and telophase. The result is two daughter cells, which are diploid (2*N*) in DNA content but contain 23 chromosome structures, each containing two closely held sister chromatids. One daughter cell, the oocyte, receives the majority of the cytoplasm, and the other becomes the first polar body. The polar body is located in the perivitelline space between the surface of the oocyte (oolemma) and the zona pellucida (ZP).

Meiosis II is rapid with the oocyte advancing immediately to metaphase II where the sister chromatids for each chromosome are aligned at the equatorial plate, held together by spindle fibers at the centromere. With sperm penetration, meiosis II is completed with extrusion of the second polar yielding a haploid oocyte (1*N*), entered by a haploid (1*N*) sperm (Fig. 1.4).

## FERTILIZATION AND EARLY CLEAVAGE

In most mammals, including humans, the egg is released from the ovary in the metaphase II stage (Fig. 1.5). When the egg enters the fallopian tube, it is surrounded by a cumulus of granulosa cells (cumulus oophorus) and intimately surrounded by a clear zona pellucida (ZP). Within the zona pellucida are both the egg and the first polar body. Meanwhile, spermatozoa are transported through the cervical mucus and the uterus and into the fallopian tubes.

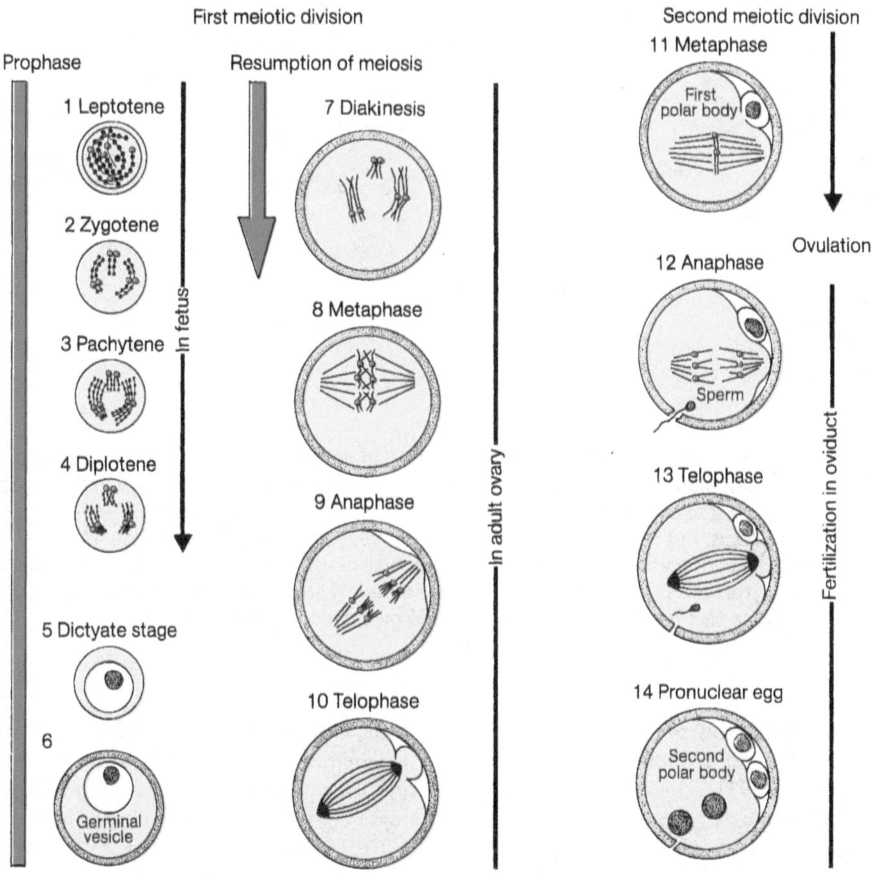


**Figure 1.4** Diagram of oocyte meiosis. For simplicity, only three pairs of chromosomes are depicted (1 to 4). Prophase stages of the first meiotic division, which occur in most mammals during fetal life. The meiotic process is arrested at the diplotene stage ("first meiotic arrest"), and the oocyte enters the dictyate stages (5 to 6). When meiosis is resumed, the first maturation division is completed (7 to 11). Ovulation occurs usually at the metaphase II stage (11), and the second meiotic division (12 to 14) takes place in the oviduct only after sperm penetration. (From Tsafriri A. Oocyte maturation in mammals. In: Jones RE, ed. *The Vertebrate Ovary*. New York: Plenum; 1978.)

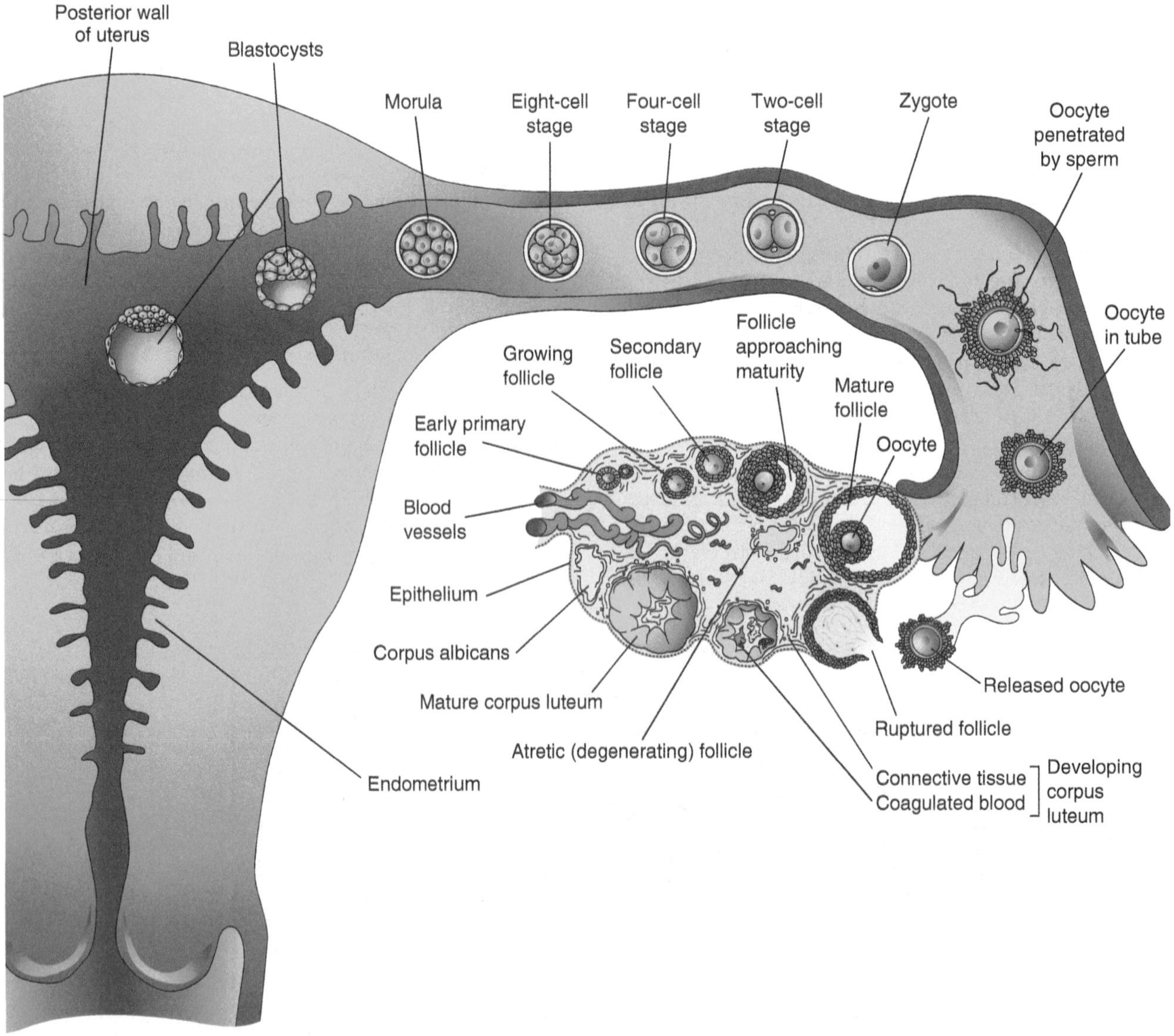


**Figure 1.5** Summary of the ovarian cycle, fertilization, and human development during the first week. Stage 1 of development begins with fertilization in the uterine tube and ends when the zygote forms. Stage 2 (days 2 to 3) comprises the early stages of cleavage (from 2 to about 32 cells, the morula). Stage 3 (days 4 to 5) consists of the free (unattached) blastocyst. Stage 4 (days 5 to 6) is represented by the blastocyst attaching to the posterior wall of the uterus, the usual site of implantation. The blastocysts have been sectioned to show their internal structure. (From Moore KL, Persaud TVN. *The Developing Human: Clinically Oriented Embryology.* 7th ed. Philadelphia: WB Saunders; 2003.)

Although 20 million to 200 million sperm may enter the vagina during intercourse, only 1 in 25,000 will make it to the fallopian tubes (Williams, 1993). This journey involves processes of capacitation, chemotaxis, hyperactivated motility, and acrosome reaction (Fig. 1.6). Capacitation precedes all other changes and involves initial removal of cholesterol from the plasma membrane altering the permeability and fluidity. This allows the influx of calcium and bicarbonate with many downstream effects such as increased cyclic adenosine monophosphate (cAMP), protein tyrosine phosphorylation, and activation of protein kinases (Aitken, 2013). A function of capacitation is to allow localization of protein complexes in the head of the sperm, which will subsequently bind the ZP. Chemotaxis is shown by a greater number of sperm in the ampullary portion of the fallopian tube containing a cumulus-oocyte-complex (COC) compared with the side lacking a COC. In vitro, follicular fluid acts as a chemoattractant, possibly due to progesterone, but the exact responsible constituent(s) of the fluid continues to be debated (Eisenbach, 1999). Hyperactivated motility involves increased vigorous movement of the sperm in order to penetrate the cumulus (granulosa) cells surrounding the oocyte and is most likely due to progesterone. A major action of progesterone is to increase calcium influx into the sperm with multiple downstream effects. Likely, the

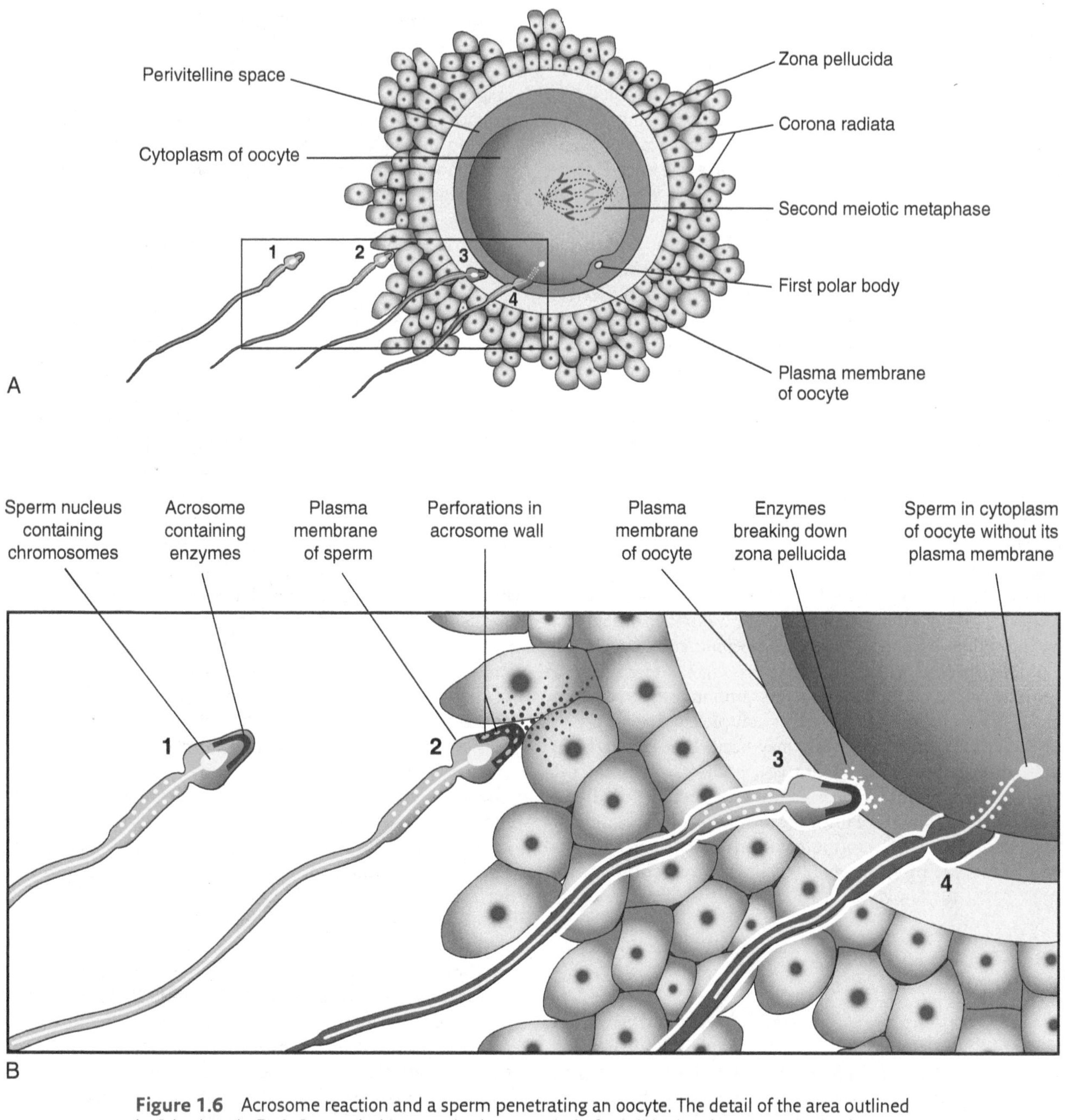


**Figure 1.6** Acrosome reaction and a sperm penetrating an oocyte. The detail of the area outlined in **A** is given in **B**. *1*, Sperm during capacitation, a period of conditioning that occurs in the female reproductive tract.*2*, Sperm undergoing the acrosome reaction, during which perforations form in the acrosome. *3*, Sperm digesting a path through the zona pellucida by the action of enzymes released from the acrosome. *4*, Sperm after entering the cytoplasm of the oocyte. Note that the plasma membranes of the sperm and oocyte have fused and that the head and tail of the sperm enter the oocyte, leaving the sperm's plasma membrane attached to the oocyte's plasma membrane. (From Moore KL, Persaud TVN. *The Developing Human: Clinically Oriented Embryology*. 7th ed. Philadelphia: WB Saunders; 2003.)

progesterone concentration increases as the sperm approaches the egg, resulting in more aggressive motility. When the egg is reached, receptor complexes on the outer most plasma membrane bind to specific ZP glycoprotein receptors (primarily ZP 3). These interactions are very species specific. Human sperm can only bind to the ZP of human, baboon, and gibbon oocytes. Binding results in fenestrations forming between the plasma membrane and the underlying acrosome membrane releasing enzymes including acrosin (a serine protease) to locally degrade the ZP (Chiu, 2014).

As many sperm may initially bind the ZP, a mechanism must be in place to prevent fertilization by more than one sperm (polyspermia). With initial binding of the sperm membrane to the oolemma, a calcium-dependent release of cortical granules occurs. Cortical granules are vesicles containing protein made during oogenesis and located in the periphery of the cell. Contents are released into the perivitelline space and function to modify ZP proteins and enlarge the perivitelline space to prevent sperm entry (Talbot, 2003). With sperm entry, the oocyte completes its second meiotic division, casting off the second polar body into the perivitelline space.

The majority of a single sperm enters the oocyte, and this is indeed the case during intracytoplasmic sperm injection (ICSI) for infertility. Only the centrioles and the nucleus survive, whereas mitochondria in the midpiece and tail are destroyed. The sperm centrioles interact with α-tubulin from the oocyte to form a microtubule network for migration of pronuclei and subsequent separation of chromosomes during the first mitosis (Schatten, 2009). Thus mitochondria are of maternal origin, whereas centrioles are paternal.

Early cell division (cleavage) is not synchronous and varies in time (Fig. 1.7). Time intervals from two pronuclei to two-cell, two-cell to three-cell, three-cell to four-cell, and four-cell to five-cell are 26 hours, 12 hours, 0.8 hours, and 14 hours, respectively, as determined with time-lapse photography during in vitro fertilization (IVF) (Meseguer, 2011). A significant number of fertilized oocytes do not complete cleavage for a number of reasons, including failure of appropriate chromosome arrangement on the spindle, specific gene defects that prevent the formation of the spindle, and environmental factors. Importantly, teratogens acting at this point are usually either completely destructive or cause little or no effect. Twinning may occur by the separation of the two cells produced by cleavage, each of which has the potential to develop into a separate embryo (Hall, 2003). Twinning may occur at any stage until the formation of the blastocyst (blast), because each cell is totipotent. Both genetic and environmental factors are probably involved in the causation of twinning.

### MORULA AND BLASTULA STAGE: EARLY DIFFERENTIATION

After fertilization, the *zygote* (the term for a fertilized egg) has a diameter of 83 to 105 μm and undergoes rapid mitotic division to reach the next stage of approximately 16 cells called a *morula*. After 4 to 5 days traversing the fallopian tube, the embryo arrives into the uterine cavity at the blast stage. The blast is characterized by a cavity (blastocoele) and differentiation of cells into the trophectoderm (TE), which will ultimately produce the fetal membranes and placenta and the inner cell mass (ICM), which will produce the fetus. During IVF, the blast forms 5 days after fertilization with a diameter of 155 to 265 μm consisting of about 40 TE cells and 20 ICM cells. In the human, implantation generally takes place 3 days after the embryo enters the uterus. The development of the blast with the separation of the ICM from the developing TE together make up the first stage of differentiation in the embryo. Differentiation within the ICM proceeds fairly rapidly, and if separation of cells and twinning occur at this point, the twins may be conjoined in some fashion.

Advances in assisted reproductive technology and genetics now provide practitioners assess to the early embryo for preimplantation genetic diagnosis (PGD) of single-gene disorders or preimplantation genetic screening (PGS) for chromosome abnormalities (Fig. 1.8). This technique involves removal of up to 20 TE cells from the day 5 blast for analysis. For PGD of single-gene disorders, DNA is extracted from the cells and the mutation analyzed by polymerase chain reaction (PCR) amplification or single nucleotide polymorphism (SNP) microarray. For PGS of chromosomal defects such as aneuploidy or structural rearrangements, analysis of DNA is performed with comparative genomic hybridization (CGH)-array (Fiorentino, 2014) or partial genomic sequencing (next-generation sequencing).

## IMPLANTATION

Implantation consists of apposition, attachment, and invasion. This complex process has much redundancy and involves multiple factors including ovarian hormones, cytokines, transcription factors, growth factors, and extracellular matrix proteins (ECMs) (Table 1.1). Both the endometrium and the embryo produce these factors. Communication between the embryo and the endometrium is key. Implantation occurs 7 to 10 days after ovulation corresponding to cycle days 21 to 24 of an idyllic 28-day cycle with ovulation on day 14. During apposition the human embryo is oriented with the ICM and polar TE (TE next to the ICM) adjacent to the endometrium.

For attachment to the endometrium, the embryonic cells must first be expelled from the surrounding ZP in the process of "hatching." Hatching involves rupture of the ZP in one small area as opposed to a general dissolution of the entire ZP. This may involve hydrostatic pressure from inside the ZP and from zonalytic proteases produced by the TE and endometrium. These cysteine proteases, named *cathepsins*, are essential for hatching. Attachment of the embryonic cells to the endometrial cells involves cell adhesion proteins, integrins, and ECM proteins such as fibronectin, laminin, and collagen. Integrins are cell surface proteins, which bind extracellular matrix proteins and are expressed on both the luminal epithelium and TE.

Invasion of the TE cells next occurs by penetrating between the luminal epithelial cells, through the basement membrane and into the stroma of the endometrium. These initial TE cells form the extravillous trophoblasts (EVTs), which invade down to the inner third of the myometrium for anchoring and into the spiral arteries for remodeling. During spiral artery remodeling, endovascular EVT disorganize and partially replace the smooth muscle wall and the vascular endothelial cells. Proliferation of endovascular EVT leads to plugging and obstruction of the decidual spiral arteries resulting in a decrease in blood flow and oxygen tension. Low oxygen promotes the proliferation and transformation of cytotrophoblast to syncytiotrophoblast. Prior to 8 weeks' gestation, nutrition to the embryo is derived from endometrial gland secretion and plasma seeping through the obstructed spiral arteries into the intervillous space. With continued remodeling of the spiral arteries, patency is reestablished and maternal blood cells enter the intervillous space at around 9 weeks' gestation with a rise in oxygen tension. Lack of adequate EVT invasion and spiral artery remodeling is a key feature in preeclampsia, intrauterine growth restriction, and stillbirth (Brosens, 2002).

The idea of low oxygen tension during early embryo development has been explored with IVF. With a limited number of

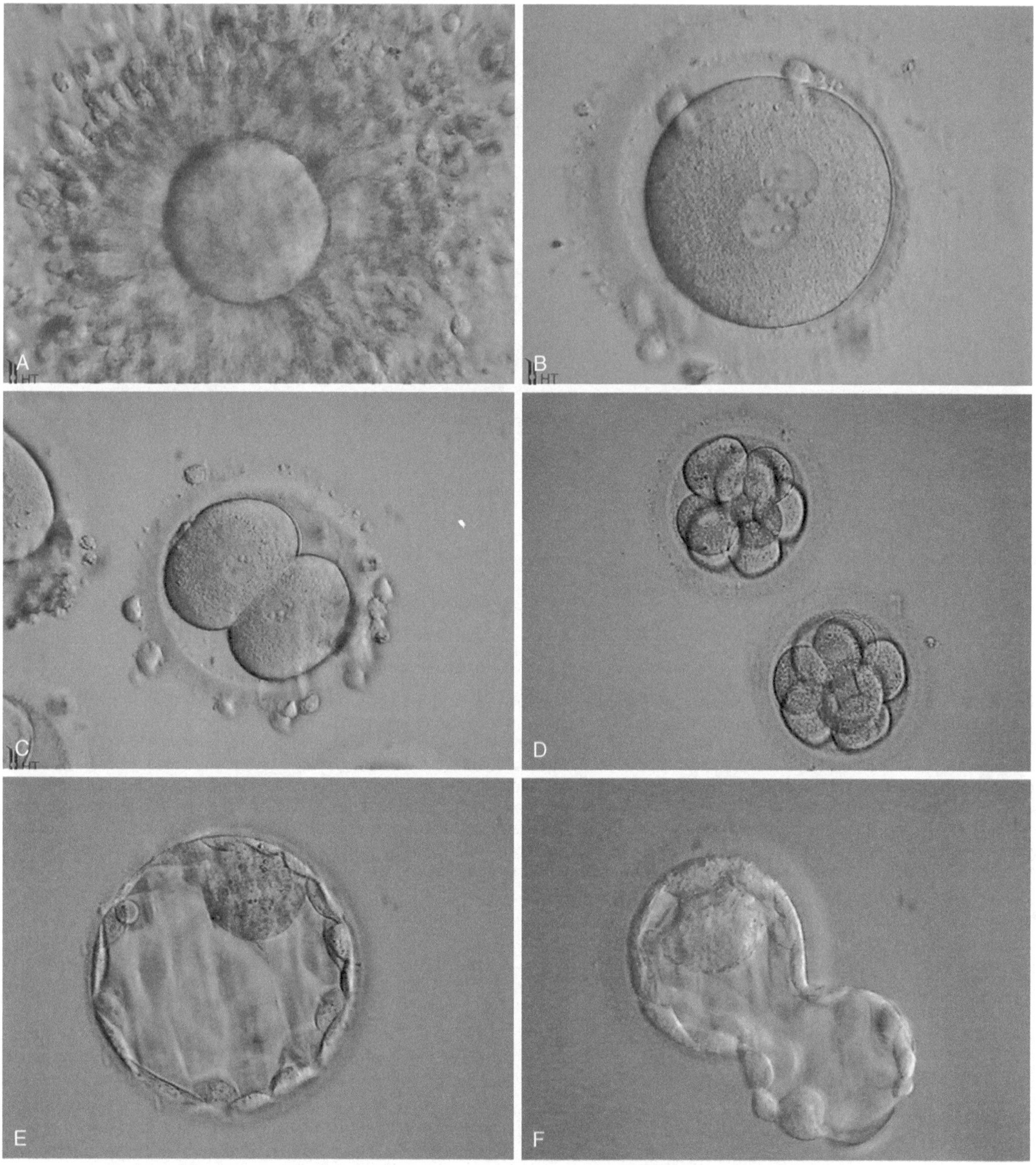


**Figure 1.7** Six photomicrographs of fresh, unmounted human eggs and embryos. **A,** Recently retrieved human oocyte surrounded by cumulus cells. **B,** Fertilized oocyte demonstrating male and female pronuclei and both polar bodies at approximately 11 and 12 o'clock position. **C,** Two-cell zygote with scattered cumulus cells remaining attached to the zone pellucida. **D,** Eight-cell zygotes. **E,** Blastocyst with the inner cell mass seen at 12 o'clock. **F,** A hatching blastocyst in which a portion of the trophectoderm has extruded from the zona pellucida at the 4 o'clock position. (Courtesy of Douglas Raburn, PhD.)

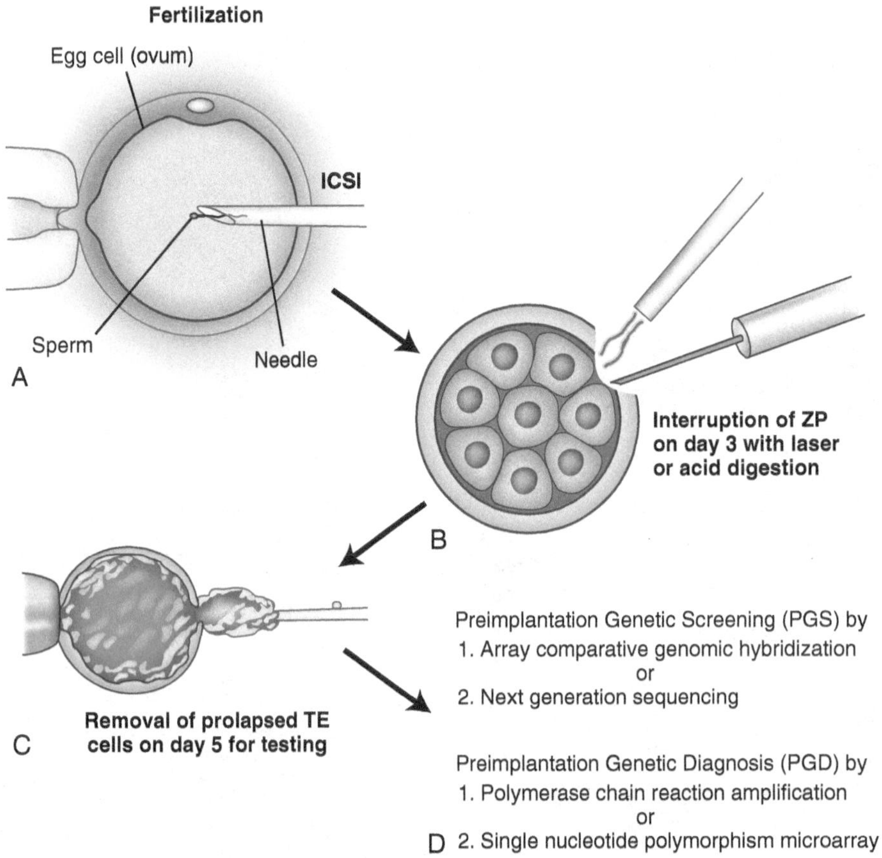


**Figure 1.8** Schematic of preimplantation testing. **A,** Commonly the oocyte is fertilized with a single sperm using the technique of intracytoplasmic sperm injection (ICSI). This precludes the possibility of contamination from sperm remaining attached to the outside of the embryo during embryo biopsy. **B,** On day 3 of culture, when the embryo has cleaved to about eight cells, a small opening is made in the zona pellucida (ZP) with either a laser or brief exposure to an acid solution. **C,** By day 5 of culture, the embryo has progressed to the blastocyst stage and a portion of the trophectoderm (TE) cells have prolapsed out the opening in the zona pellucida. These cells are removed for subsequent DNA isolation. **D,** DNA from trophectoderm cells is used to determine chromosome number, insertions, and deletions for preimplantation genetic screening (PGS) using techniques of array comparative genomic hybridization (aCGH) or next-generation sequencing (NGS). DNA may also be used to detect single-gene abnormalities for different diseases using single nucleotide polymorphism (SNP) microarray or polymerase chain reaction (PCR) amplification in the process of preimplantation genetic diagnosis (PGD).

**Table 1.1** Events of Implantation

| Event | Days after Ovulation |
|---|---|
| Zona pellucida disappears | 4-5 |
| Blastocyst attaches to epithelial surface of endometrium | 6 |
| Trophoblast erodes into endometrial stroma | 7 |
| Trophoblast differentiates into cytotrophoblastic and syncytial trophoblastic layers | 7-8 |
| Lacunae appear around trophoblast | 8-9 |
| Blastocyst burrows beneath endometrial surface | 9-10 |
| Lacunar network forms | 10-11 |
| Trophoblast invades endometrial sinusoids, establishing a uteroplacental circulation | 11-12 |
| Endometrial epithelium completely covers blastocyst | 12-13 |
| Strong decidual reaction occurs in stroma | 13-14 |

trials, culturing embryos in 5% oxygen as opposed to 20% oxygen results in a modest increase in the implantation rate (Bontekoe, 2012).

Villous trophoblast form finger-like projections extending into the intervillous space and thus surrounded by maternal blood. Syncytiotrophoblast form the outer layer with an underlying layer of precursor cytotrophoblast surrounding matrix containing capillaries, fibroblasts, and macrophages. Cytotrophoblasts become less numerous as pregnancy progresses.

Blood levels of the pregnancy hormone human chorionic gonadotropin (hCG) can be detected within 48 hours of implantation. Regular hCG is produced by the syncytiotrophoblast of placental villi. Blood levels peak at 56 to 68 days, reach a nadir at 18 weeks, and then remain fairly constant until delivery. Gonadotropin-releasing hormone (GnRH) produced in the cytotrophoblast and syncytiotrophoblast induces expression of hCG. In spontaneous pregnancies hCG can be detected 9 days following follicle rupture observed by ultrasound. In IVF pregnancies, the hormone can be found 8 days after embryo transfer. hCG levels rise, exponentially up to 8 weeks from the last menstrual period, but the doubling time increases as the level increases. For example, in a conception cycle with ovulation on cycle day 14, the doubling time from cycle days 25 to 37 for hCG is 1.6 days and from days 38 to 44 it is 2.3 days (Zegers-Hochschild, 1994). The doubling time is independent of the number of gestations, although the absolute hCG level is higher for multiple pregnancies.

The classic action of regular hCG is maintenance of the corpus luteum (CL) by binding the luteinizing hormone (LH) receptor for continued estrogen and progesterone production. Yet other identified actions include promotion of angiogenesis in the uterus, myometrial relaxation, inhibition of immune interaction at the utero-placental interface, stimulation of fetal testosterone production, and mediation of hyperemesis through receptors in the brain.

Hyperglycosylated hCG (H-hCG) is produced by the EVT. H-hCG is key in promoting angiogenesis and cell invasion and correspondingly is found in the early first trimester. The protein does not activate the LH receptor and does not preserve CL function. Instead it appears to function via the transforming growth factor beta (TGF-β) receptor (Berndt, 2013). Low levels of H-hCG indicate poor EVT development and are associated with spontaneous abortion and early preeclampsia (Fournier, 2015).

## DECIDUALIZATION

Progesterone is responsible for "decidualization" of the endometrium. This refers to morphologic and functional changes in stromal cells. In humans, stromal cells close to the spiral arteries undergo progesterone-induced decidual changes in the late secretory phase, and this process progresses throughout the stroma with implantation and hCG production. A pregnancy within the uterus is not required and decidualization is a common finding with ectopic pregnancies. Decidual cells show morphologic changes of increased size with increased glycogen and lipid accumulation (Maruyama, 2008). With pregnancy the endometrium is now referred to as the *decidua*, separated into areas of the decidua basalis or placentalis, which interacts with the TE (area of mature placenta), the decidua vera or parietalis (decidua distant from the implantation site), and the decidua capsularis (surrounding the embryo on the side opposite the placenta).

Another classic histologic change seen in early pregnancy is the Arias-Stella reaction (Fig. 1.9). This occurs in the glandular cells with a hallmark of nuclear enlargement. These cells may be misinterpreted as atypical or malignant. In the presence of hCG, the Arias-Stella reaction may be seen in extrauterine tissues such as endometriosis, vaginal adenosis, paraovarian cysts, and mucinous cystadenomas (Arias-Stella, 2002).

Morphologically luminal epithelial cells develop extensions of the plasma membrane called *pinopods* (also called *uterodomes*) during the window of receptivity. Pinopods function to release key proteins including leukemia inhibitory factor (LIF) through exocytosis and apocrine secretion (Kabir-Salmani, 2005).

Downstream effects of progesterone-dependent decidualization have not been completely elucidated, but loss-of-function studies show the necessity of transcription factors including CCAAT/enhancer binding protein Beta (C/EBPβ), Homeobox A10 (Hoxa10), Forkhead/winged helix protein (Fox01), and chicken ovalbumin upstream promoter (COUP-TFII).

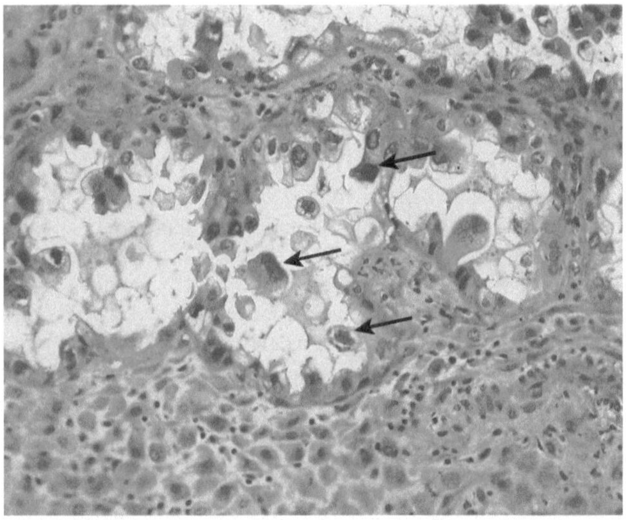

**Figure 1.9** Photomicrograph of the Arias-Stella reaction. hCG action results in nuclear enlargement in endometrial glandular cells *(arrows)* resulting in visual characteristics of malignant cells. Magnification, ×200. (Courtesy of Rex Bentley, MD.)

A functional progesterone receptor requires interaction with "chaperone" proteins. In mice, one of these proteins, named *FK506 binding protein 52 (FKBP52)*, is expressed in the endometrium during the window of receptivity, and a loss of function mutation disrupts decidualization.

LIF is a cytokine produced by endometrial glandular cells around the time of implantation. LIF acts on EVT to increase the fibronectin production necessary for embryo attachment and invasion. Mice lacking expression of LIF (knockout) have both failure of decidualization and implantation (Chen, 2000).

Indian hedgehog (Ihh) protein is a morphogen produced by luminal epithelial cells under the control of progesterone. Morphogens are signaling proteins that diffuse throughout the decidua yielding a concentration gradient. Signaling is dependent on the concentration in a given area. *Ihh* knockout mice fail to decidualize or implant (Ramathal, 2010).

## EMBRYO-ENDOMETRIAL COMMUNICATION

Implantation involves molecular interactions between the embryo and the adjacent endometrium. For example, the embryo produces heparin-binding epidermal growth factor-like growth factor (HB-EGF), which is both found on the cell membrane and is released from the cell (soluble). HB-EGF induces expression of itself in the adjacent endometrial cells (auto-induction loop). HB-EGF on the endometrial cells then acts to attach the embryo via EGF receptors expressed on the embryo (Lim, 2009). Additionally, the soluble HB-EGF from the embryo induces expression of cyclooxygenase to increase prostacyclin ($PGI_2$) in the endometrium resulting in enhanced endometrial vascular permeability to help with embryo invasion (Kim, 1999).

## IMMUNOLOGY OF IMPLANTATION

The paternal contribution to the embryo results in the mother being exposed to allogenic cells. Although villous trophoblasts do not express major human leukocyte antigens (HLA), the EVTs express HLA-C, E, and G, which may be recognized by the maternal immune system. Thus the maternal immune system must be locally suppressed to prevent rejection.

The majority of immune cells in the decidua are uterine natural killer (uNK) cells. These cells are present in the secretory endometrium, under the control of progesterone, and increase in number with pregnancy to form an infiltrate around the invading EVT. These cells start to dissipate in the second trimester. uNK cells are not cytotoxic to trophoblast cells and in fact appear to be supportive. A low number of uNK cells in the decidua of early pregnancy is associated with poor invasion of the EVT. Cytokines such as interferon gamma and angiogenic factors secreted by uNK cells are key to proper EVT development and function.

T-helper (Th) cells are also found in the decidua and are functionally classified as Th1 (cellular immunity), Th2 (humoral immunity), Th3 (production of transforming growth factor-beta for immunosuppression), and Tr1 (production of interleukin 10 for immunosuppression) (Saito, 2007). In early pregnancy, there is an increase in the percentage of decidual Th2 and Th3 cells.

T-regulatory cells (Tregs) function in antigen recognition for future immune tolerance. Mice lacking Treg cells experience abortion when mated with an allogenic male but not when mated with a syngenic male (Darasse-Jèze, 2006). These cells are key in developing tolerance to male antigens. Development of immunity to specific paternal antigens may explain observations including lower preeclampsia rates in women exposed to their partner's semen prior to pregnancy compared with women conceiving with donor insemination (Salha, 1999), and the lower preeclampsia rate in the second pregnancy with the same partner as opposed to a new partner.

### *EARLY ORGANOGENESIS IN THE EMBRYONIC PERIOD*

During the third week after fertilization, the primitive streak forms in the caudal portion of the embryonic disk, and the embryonic disk begins to grow and change from a circular to a pear-shaped configuration. At that point the epithelium superiorly is considered ectoderm and will eventually give rise to the developing central nervous system, and the epithelium facing downward toward the yolk sac is endoderm. During this week the neuroplate develops with its associated notochordal process. By the sixteenth day after conception the third primitive germ layer, the intraembryonic mesoderm, begins to form between the ectoderm and endoderm. Early mesoderm migrates cranially, passing on either side of the notochordal process to meet in front in the formation of the cardiogenic area. The heart soon develops from this area. Later in the third week, extraembryonic mesoderm joins with the yolk sac and the developing amnion to contribute to the developing membranes.

An intraembryonic mesoderm develops on each side of the notochord and neural tube to form longitudinal columns, the paraxial mesoderm. Each paraxial column thins laterally into the lateral plate mesoderm, which is continuous with the extraembryonic mesoderm of the yolk sac and the amnion. The lateral plate mesoderm is separated from the paraxial mesoderm by a continuous tract of mesoderm called the *intermediate mesoderm*. By the twentieth day, paraxial mesoderm begins to divide into paired linear bodies known as *somites*. About 38 pairs of somites form during the next 10 days. Eventually a total of 42 to 44 pairs will develop, and these will give rise to body musculature (O'Rahilly, 1979).

Angiogenesis, or blood vessel formation, can be seen in the extraembryonic mesoderm of the yolk sac by day 15 or 16. Embryonic vessels can be seen about 2 days later and develop when mesenchymal cells known as *angioblasts* aggregate to form masses and cords called *blood islands*. Spaces then appear within these islands, and the angioblasts arrange themselves around these spaces to form primitive endothelium. Isolated vessels form channels and then grow into adjacent areas by endothelial budding. Primitive blood cells develop from endothelial cells as the vessels develop on the yolk sac and allantois. However, blood formation does not begin within the embryo until the second month of gestation, occurring first in the developing liver and later in the spleen, bone marrow, and lymph nodes. Separate mesenchymal cells surrounding the primitive endothelial vessels differentiate into muscular and connective tissue elements. The primitive heart forms in a similar manner from mesenchymal cells in the cardiogenic area. Paired endothelial channels, called *heart tubes*, develop by the end of the third week and fuse to form the primitive heart. By the twenty-first day, this primitive heart has linked up with blood vessels of the embryo, forming a primitive cardiovascular system. Blood circulation starts about this time, and the cardiovascular system becomes the first functioning organ system within the embryo (Clark, 1987). All the organ systems form between the fourth week and seventh week of gestation.

A teratogenic event that takes place during the embryonic period gives rise to a constellation of malformations related to the organ systems that are actively developing at that particular time. Thus cardiovascular malformations tend to occur because of teratogenic events early in the embryonic period, whereas genitourinary abnormalities tend to result from later events. Teratogenic effects before implantation often cause loss of the embryo but not malformations. The effects of a particular teratogen depend on the individual's genetic makeup, other environmental factors in play at the time, the embryonic developmental stage during which the teratogenic exposure occurred, and in some cases the dose of the teratogen and the duration of exposure. Some teratogens in and of themselves are actually harmless, but their metabolites cause the damage. Teratogens may be chemical substances and their by-products, or they may be physical phenomena, such as temperature elevation and irradiation. The embryo is most sensitive to teratogens during organogenesis of the embryonic period from 18 to 56 days postconception. Prior to day 18, exposure is most likely to result in either embryo death with miscarriage or no effect, as the majority of cells are pluripotent (Polifka, 2002). Teratogen exposure after the embryonic period of development may injure or kill the embryo or cause developmental and growth retardation but usually will not be responsible for specific malformations. The period of embryonic development is said to be complete at 56 days (8 weeks) from fertilization or 70 days (10 weeks) from the last menstrual period followed by the fetal stage.

## DEVELOPMENT OF THE GENITOURINARY SYSTEM

The development of the genital organs is intimately involved with the development of the renal system.

### *RENAL DEVELOPMENT*

Nephrogenic cords develop from the intermediate mesoderm as early as the 2-mm embryo stage, beginning in the more cephalad portions of the embryo. Three sets of excretory ducts and tubules develop bilaterally (Little, 2010). The first, the pronephros, with its pronephric ducts, forms in the most cranial portion of the embryo at about the beginning of the fourth week after conception. The tubules associated with the duct probably have no excretory function in the human, but the caudal end will form the adrenal gland. Late in the fourth week, a second set of tubules, the mesonephric tubules, and their accompanying mesonephric ducts begin to develop. These are associated with tufts of capillaries, or glomeruli, and tubules for excretory purposes. Thus the mesonephros functions as a fetal kidney, producing urine for about 2 or 3 weeks. As new tubules develop, those derived from the more cephalad tubules degenerate. Usually about 40 mesonephric tubules function on either side of the embryo at any given time. The gonads arise from the central region of the mesonephros. The metanephros, or permanent kidney, begins its development early in the fifth week of gestation and starts to function late in the seventh or early in the eighth week. The metanephros develops both from the metanephrogenic mass of mesoderm, which is the most caudal portion of the nephrogenic cord, and from its duct system, which is derived from the metanephric diverticulum (ureteric bud). It is a cranially growing outpouching of the mesonephric duct close to where it enters the cloaca. The metanephric duct system gives rise to the ureter, the renal pelvis, the calyces, and the collecting tubules of the adult kidney. A critical process in the development of the kidney requires that the cranially growing metanephric diverticulum meets and fuses with the metanephrogenic mass of mesoderm so that formation of the kidney can take place. Originally the metanephric kidney is a pelvic organ, but by differential growth it becomes located in the lumbar region (Moritz, 1999).

The fetus produces urine starting at 8 weeks' gestation (Underwood, 2005). Starting in the second trimester, fetal urine is a major contributor to amniotic fluid volume. The fetus may swallow the amniotic fluid and recirculate it through the digestive system. Congenital abnormalities that impair normal development or function of the fetal kidneys generally result in little or no amniotic fluid (oligohydramnios or anhydramnios), whereas structural abnormalities of the gastrointestinal tract or neuromuscular conditions that prevent the fetus from swallowing can lead to excess amniotic fluid (polyhydramnios).

### *BLADDER AND URETHRA*

The embryonic cloaca is divided by the urorectal septum into a dorsal rectum and a ventral urogenital sinus. The urogenital sinus, in turn, is divided into three parts: the cranial portion (the vesicourethral canal), which is continuous with the allantois; a middle pelvic portion; and a caudal urogenital sinus portion, which is covered externally by the urogenital membrane. The epithelium of the developing bladder is derived from the endoderm of the vesicourethral canal. The muscular layers and serosa of the bladder develop from adjacent splanchnic mesenchyme. As the bladder develops, the caudal portion of the mesonephric ducts is incorporated into its dorsal wall. The portion of the mesonephric duct distal to the points where the metanephric duct is taken up into the bladder becomes the trigone of the bladder. Although this portion is mesoderm in origin, it is probably epithelialized eventually by endodermal epithelium from the urogenital sinus. In this way the ureters, derived from the metanephric duct, come to open directly into the bladder.

In the male the mesonephric ducts open into the urethra as the ejaculatory ducts. Also in the male, mesenchymal tissue surrounding the developing urethra where it exits the bladder develops into the prostate gland, through which the ejaculatory ducts traverse. Figure 1.10 demonstrates graphically the development of the male and female urinary systems.

The epithelium of the female urethra is derived from endoderm of the vesicourethral canal. The urethral sphincter develops from a mesenchymal condensation around the urethra after the division of the cloaca in the 12- to 15-mm embryo. Following the opening of the anal membrane at the 20- to 30-mm stage, the puborectalis muscle appears. At 15 weeks' gestation, striated muscle can be seen, and a smooth muscle layer thickens at the level of the developing bladder neck, forming the inner part of the urethral musculature. Thus the urethral sphincter is composed of both central smooth muscle and peripheral striated muscle. The sphincter develops primarily in the anterior wall of the urethra in a horseshoe or omega shape (Matsuno, 1984).

## MOLECULAR BASIS OF SEX DIFFERENTIATION

Genetic sex is determined at the time of conception. A Y chromosome is necessary for the development of the testes, and the testes are responsible for the organization of the sexual duct system into a male configuration and for the suppression of the paramesonephric (müllerian) system of the female. In the absence of a Y chromosome or in the absence of a gonad, development will be female in nature. Male differentiation is determined by expression of the *SRY* gene found on the short arm of the Y chromosome. SRY protein is a transcription factor and expression is unique to the Sertoli cell of the developing testis. SRY induces expression of another transcription factor, SOX9, which is also obligatory for male sex differentiation. A loss of function mutation of either SRY or SOX9 results in XY sex reversal, in which genetic males are phenotypic females. Several genes regulate SRY/SOX9 expression including Wilms' tumor suppressor 1 (Wt1) and steroidogenic factor 1 (Sf1). WT1 is a transcription factor expressed in both urinary tract and gonadal tissue. A loss of function mutation results in glomerulosclerosis and gonadal dysgenesis. Sf1 encodes a nuclear receptor necessary for steroidogenesis, gonadal differentiation, and adrenal formation. A loss of function mutation is associated with adrenal failure and XY sex reversal (Ozisik, 2003).

Although ovarian formation can only occur in the absence of *SRY/SOX9*, there are unique genes necessary for development. *FoxL2* encodes a transcription factor necessary for granulosa cell expansion. A loss of function mutation causes ovarian failure with other associated abnormalities found in blepharophimosis-ptosis-epicanthus inversus syndrome (BPES) (De Baere, 2001). *BMP15,* located on the X chromosome, and *GDF9* on chromosome 5 encode growth factors expressed in oocytes required for granulosa cell proliferation. A heterozygous loss of function mutation results in ovarian failure (Di Pasquale, 2004).

The understanding of the molecular basis of sex determination continues to expand with more than 25 genes so far identified in the process (Wilhelm, 2007).

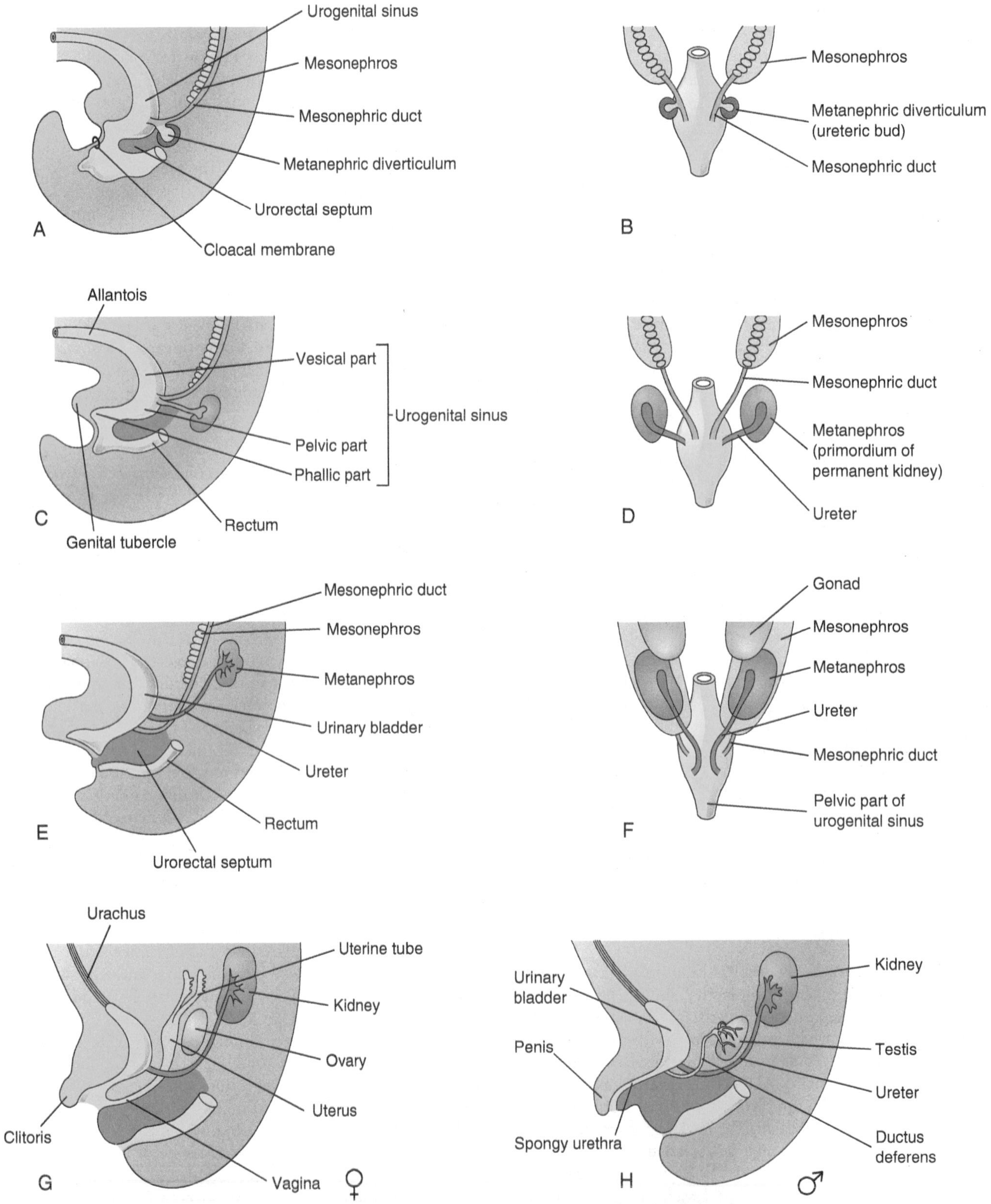


**Figure 1.10** Diagrams showing division of the cloaca into the urogenital sinus and rectum; absorption of the mesonephric ducts; development of the urinary bladder, urethra, and urachus; and changes in the location of the ureters. **A,** Lateral view of the caudal half of a 5-week embryo. **B, D,** and **F,** Dorsal views. **C, E, G,** and **H,** Lateral views. The stages shown in **G** and **H** are reached by the twelfth week. (From Moore KL, Persaud TVN. *The Developing Human: Clinically Oriented Embryology.* 7th ed. Philadelphia: WB Saunders; 2003.)

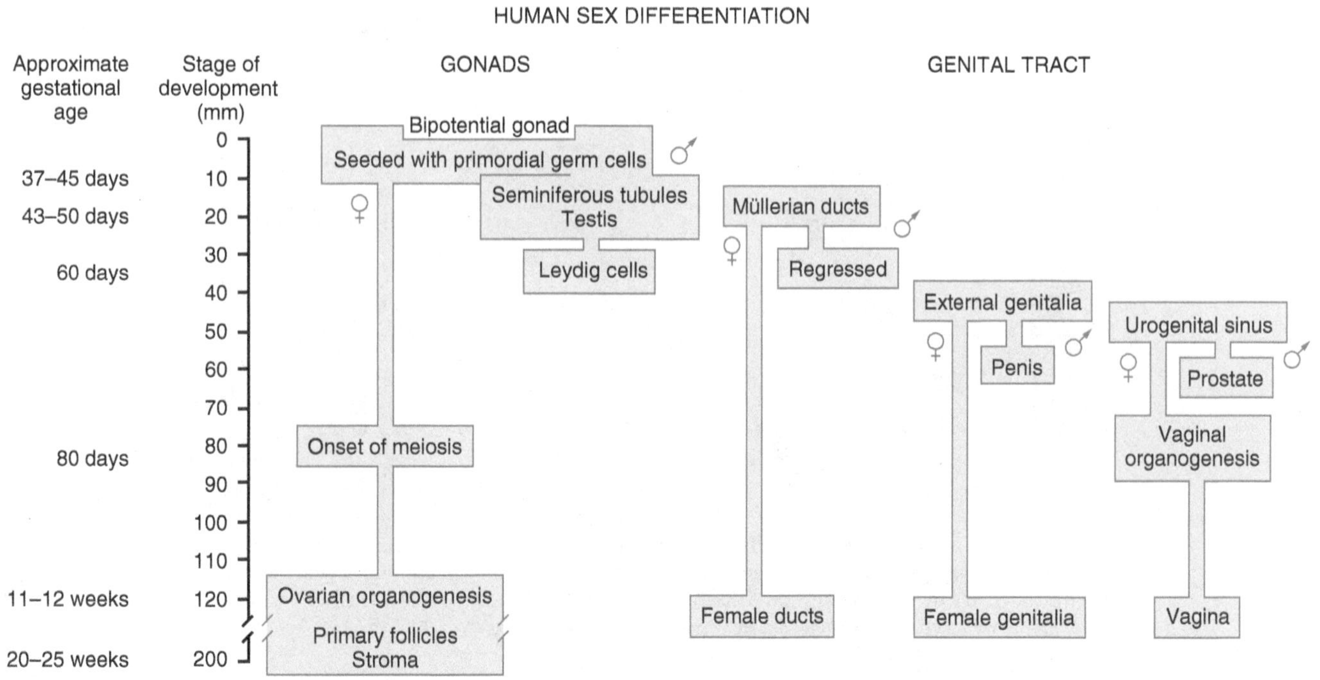


**Figure 1.11** Development of sexual differentiation in the human. Note the lag from male to female development. (Modified from Grumbach MM, Hughes IA, Conte FA. Disorders of sex differentiation. In: Larsen PR, Kronenberg HM, Melmed S, et al, eds. *Williams Textbook of Endocrinology.* 10th ed. Philadelphia: WB Saunders: 2003:870.)

## GENITAL DEVELOPMENT

Male gonadal development precedes female development (Fig. 1.11). During the fifth week after conception, coelomic epithelium, later known as *germinal epithelium*, thickens in the area of the medial aspect of the mesonephros. As germinal epithelial cells proliferate, they invade the underlying mesenchyme, producing a prominence known as the *gonadal ridge*. In the sixth week the primordial germ cells, which have formed at about week 4 in the wall of the yolk sac, migrate up the dorsal mesentery of the hindgut and enter the undifferentiated gonad. The somatic cells of the primitive gonadal ridge then differentiate into interstitial cells (Leydig cells) and Sertoli cells. As they do so, the primordial germ cells and Sertoli cells become enclosed within seminiferous tubules, and the interstitial cells remain outside these tubules. Sertoli cells are encased in the seminiferous tubules in the seventh and eighth weeks. In the eighth week, Leydig cells differentiate and begin to produce testosterone. At this point the mesonephric (wolffian) duct differentiates into the vas deferens, epididymis, and seminal vesicles, whereas the paramesonephric duct (müllerian duct) is suppressed because of the secretion and action of anti-müllerian hormone (AMH), also known as *müllerian inhibitory substance* (MIS), by Sertoli cells.

Primary sex cords, meanwhile, have condensed and extended to the medullary portion of the developing testes. They branch and join to form the rete testis. The testis therefore is primarily a medullary organ, and eventually the rete testis connects with the tubules of the mesonephric system and joins the developing epididymal duct.

Development of the ovary occurs at about the eleventh or twelfth week, although the primordial germ cells have migrated several weeks earlier to the germinal ridge (Fig. 1.12). Two functional X chromosomes are necessary for optimal development of the ovary. Deletion of either the short arm or the long arm of a single X chromosome precludes normal ovarian function, with the former being associated with Turner syndrome (Simpson, 1999). The processes of gonadal development are schematically summarized in Figure 1.13.

## GENITAL DUCT SYSTEM

Early in embryonic life, two sets of paired genital ducts develop in each sex: the mesonephric (wolffian) ducts and the paramesonephric (müllerian) ducts. The mesonephric duct development precedes the paramesonephric duct development. The paramesonephric ducts develop on each side of the mesonephric ducts from the evaginations of the coelomic epithelium. The more cephalad ends of the ducts open directly into the peritoneal cavity, and the distal ends grow caudally, fusing in the lower midline to form the uterovaginal primordium. This tubular structure joins the dorsal wall of the urogenital sinus and produces an elevation, the müllerian tubercle. The mesonephric ducts enter the urogenital sinus on either side of the tubercle.

## MALE GENITAL DUCTS

Seminiferous tubules are produced in the fetal testes during the seventh and eighth weeks after conception. During the eighth week, interstitial (Leydig) cells differentiate and begin to produce testosterone. Male internal genital development is mainly dependent on testosterone, whereas external genitalia are dependent on 5α-dihydrotestosterone (DHT). Testosterone produced

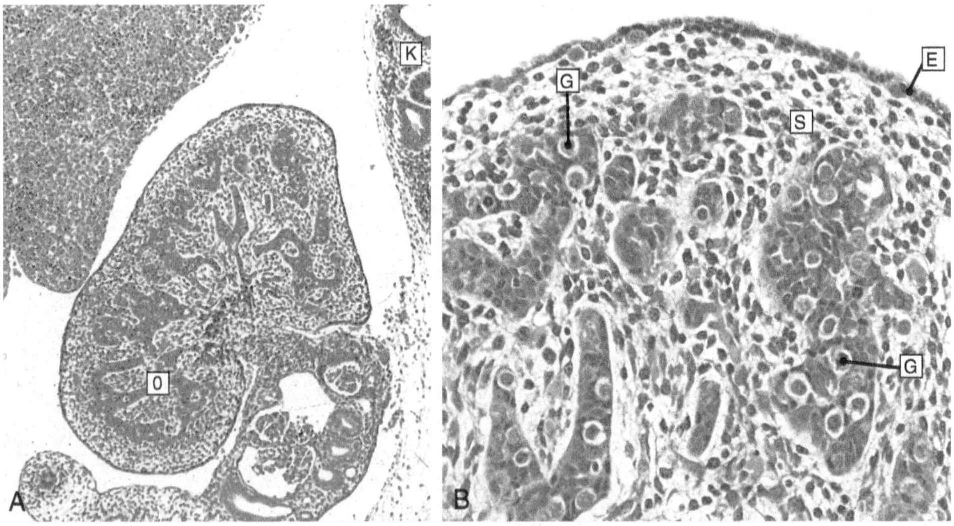


**Figure 1.12** Ovary in embryo. **A,** The developing ovary *(O)* in a 9-week-old fetus is shown close to the developing kidney *(K)*. **B,** At this stage of development, the columns of primordial germ cells *(G)* are embedded in a mesenchymal stroma *(S)* covered by a layer of cuboidal surface cells *(E)*. (From Stevens A, Lowe J. *Human Histology.* 3rd ed. Philadelphia: Elsevier Mosby; 2005:357.)

by the Leydig cells stimulates growth and development of the wolffian duct structures of vas deferens, epididymis, and seminal vesicles. DHT formed in target tissues by the enzyme type 2 5α-reductase is responsible for formation of the prostate, scrotum, and penis (Thigpen, 1993).

Maternal hCG production may be key to male genital development. The maximum serum level of hCG at approximately 8 weeks postconception or 10 menstrual weeks correlates with the timing of male genital formation, and the highest fetal testosterone levels are seen at 11 to 17 weeks with a subsequent decline (Reyes, 1974). hCG acting via the LH receptor is responsible for stimulating Leydig cell testosterone production.

The bulbourethral glands, which are small structures that develop from outgrowths of endodermal tissue from the membranous portion of the urethra, incorporate stroma from the adjacent mesenchyme. The most distal portion of the paramesonephric duct remains, in the male, as the appendix of the testes. The most proximal end of the paramesonephric duct remains as a small outpouching within the body of the prostate gland, known as the prostatic utricle. Rarely, the prostatic utricle is developed to the point where it will excrete a small amount of blood and cause hematuria in adult life (Schuhrke, 1978).

## FEMALE GENITAL DUCTS

In the absence of AMH, the mesonephric ducts regress, and the paramesonephric ducts develop into the female genital tract. This process begins at about 6 weeks and proceeds in a cephalad to caudal fashion. The more cephalad portions of the paramesonephric ducts, which open directly into the peritoneal cavity, form the fallopian tubes. The fused portion, or uterovaginal primordium, gives rise to the epithelium and glands of the uterus and cervix. Endometrial stroma and myometrium are derived from adjacent mesenchyme. Failure of development of the paramesonephric ducts leads to agenesis of the cervix and the uterus referred to as *müllerian agenesis* or Mayer-Rokitansky-Kuster-Hauser syndrome (Langman, 1982). Failure of fusion of the caudal portion of these ducts may lead to a variety of uterine anomalies, including complete duplication of the uterus and cervix or partial duplication of a variety of types, which are outlined in Chapter 11. Peritoneal reflections in the area adjacent to the fusion of the two paramesonephric ducts give rise to the formation of the broad ligaments. Mesenchymal tissue here develops into the parametrium.

Pietryga and Wózniak studied the development of uterine ligaments, documenting the development of the round ligament at the eighth week, the cardinal ligaments at the tenth week, and the broad ligament at week 19. From weeks 8 to 17, the round ligament is connected to the uterine tube (Pietryga, 1992). Beginning at week 18 it comes to arise from the edge of the uterus.

The vagina develops from paired solid outgrowths of endoderm of the urogenital sinus—the sinovaginal bulbs. These grow caudally as a solid core toward the end of the uterovaginal primordium. This core constitutes the fibromuscular portion of the vagina. The sinovaginal bulbs then canalize to form the vagina. Abnormalities in this process may lead to either transverse or horizontal vaginal septa. The junction of the sinovaginal bulbs with the urogenital sinus remains as the vaginal plate, which forms the hymen. This remains imperforate until late in embryonic life, although occasionally, perforation does not take place completely (imperforate hymen). Failure of the sinovaginal bulbs to form leads to agenesis of the vagina (Griffin, 1976).

Auxiliary genital glands in the female form from buds that grow out of the urethra. The buds derive contributions from the surrounding mesenchyme and form the urethral glands and the paraurethral glands (Skene glands). These glands correspond to the prostate gland in males. Similar outgrowths of the urogenital sinus form the vestibular glands (Bartholin glands), which are homologous to the bulbourethral glands in the male. The remnants of the mesonephric duct in the female include a small structure called the *appendix vesiculosa*, a few

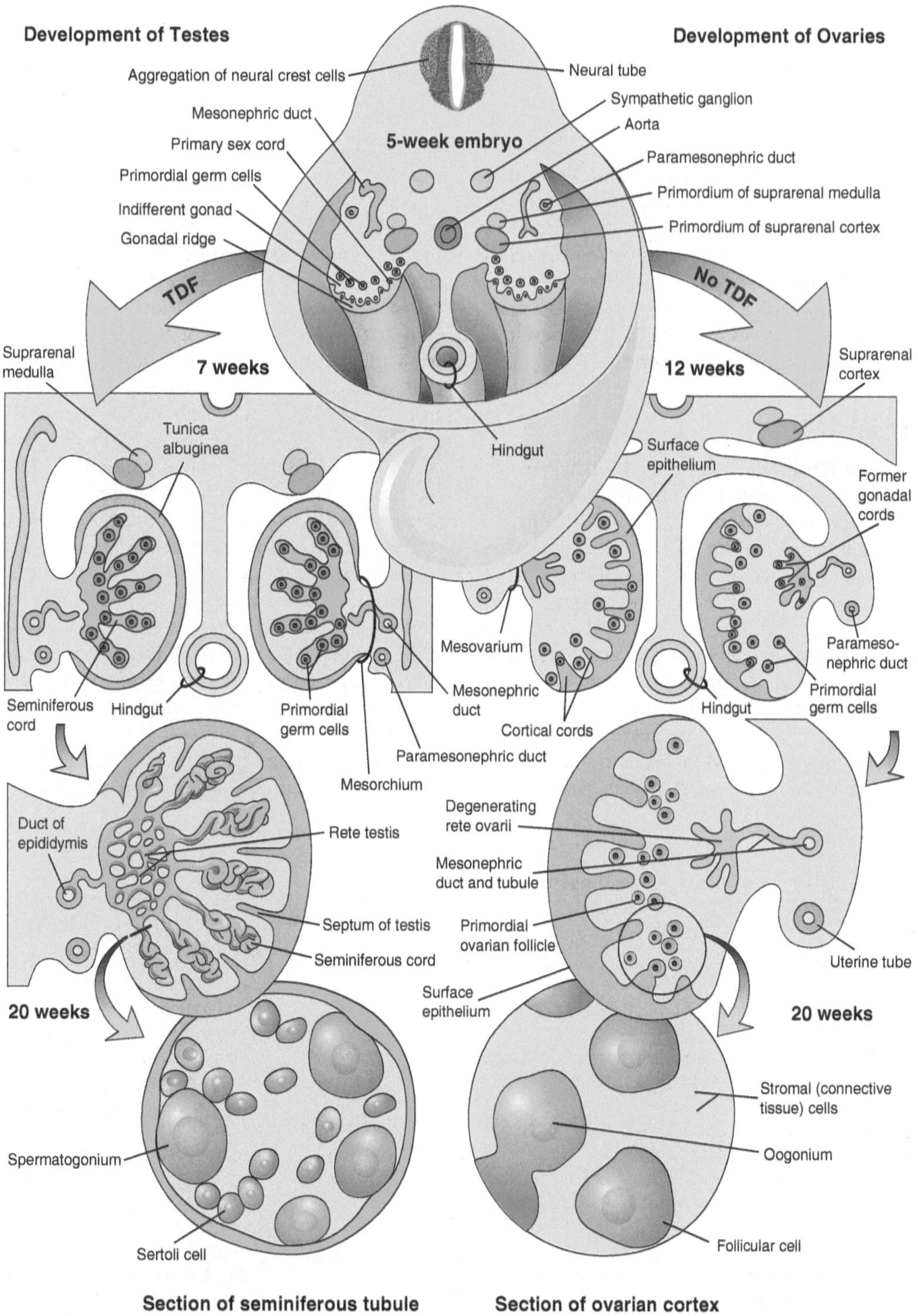


**Figure 1.13** Schematic illustration showing differentiation of the indifferent gonads of a 5-week embryo *(top)* into ovaries or testes. Left side shows the development of testes resulting from the effects of the testis-determining factor (TDF), also called the *SRY gene*, located on the Y chromosome. Note that the gonadal cords become seminiferous cords, the primordium of the seminiferous tubules. The parts of the gonadal cords that enter the medulla of the testis form the rete testis. In the section of the testis at the bottom left, observe that there are two kinds of cells: spermatogonia derived from the primordial germ cells and sustentacular (Sertoli) cells derived from mesenchyme. The right side shows the development of ovaries in the absence of TDF. Cortical cords have extended from the surface epithelium of the gonad, and primordial cells have entered them. They are the primordia of the oogonia. Follicular cells are derived from the surface epithelium of the ovary. (From Moore KL, Persaud TVN. *The Developing Human: Clinically Oriented Embryology*. 7th ed. Philadelphia: WB Saunders; 2003.)

blind tubules in the broad ligaments (the epoophoron), and a few blind tubules adjacent to the uterus (collectively called the *paroöphoron*). Remnants of the mesonephric duct system are often present in the broad ligaments or may be present adjacent to the uterus or the vagina as Gartner duct cysts (Deppisch, 1975). The epoophoron or paroöphoron may develop into cysts. Cysts of the epoophoron are known as *paraovarian cysts* (Chapter 18). Remnants of the paramesonephric duct in the female may be seen as a small, blind cystic structure attached by a pedicle to the distal end of the fallopian tube—the hydatid of Morgagni. Table 1.2 categorizes the adult derivatives and residual remnants of the urogenital structures in both the male and the female. Figure 1.14 outlines schematically the development of the internal sexual organs in both sexes.

## EXTERNAL GENITALIA

In the fourth week after fertilization, the genital tubercle develops at the ventral tip of the cloacal membrane. Two sets of lateral bodies—the labioscrotal swellings and urogenital folds—develop soon after on either side of the cloacal membrane. The genital tubercle then elongates to form a phallus in both males and females. By the end of the sixth week, the cloacal membrane is joined by the urorectal septum. The septum separates the cloaca into the urogenital sinus ventrally and the anal canal and rectum dorsally (Hynes, 2004). The point on the cloacal membrane where the urorectal septum fuses becomes the location of the perineal body in later development. The cloacal membrane is then divided into the ventral urogenital membrane and the dorsal anal membrane. These membranes then open, yielding the vulva and the anal canal. Failure of the anal membrane to open gives rise to an imperforate anus. With the opening of the urogenital membrane, a urethral groove forms on the undersurface of the phallus, completing the undifferentiated portion of external genital development. Differences between male and female embryos can be noted as early as the ninth week, but the distinct final forms are not noted until 12 weeks' gestation (Fig. 1.15).

The phallus grows in length to form a penis, and the urogenital folds are pulled forward to form the lateral walls of the urethral groove on the undersurface of the penis. These folds then fuse to form the penile urethra. Defects in fusion of various amounts give rise to various degrees of hypospadias. The skin at the distal margin of the penis grows over the glans to form the prepuce (foreskin). The vascular portion of the penis (corpora cavernosa penis and corpus cavernosum urethrae) arises from the mesenchymal tissue of the phallus. Finally, the labioscrotal swellings grow toward each other and fuse in the midline to form the scrotum. Later in embryonic life, usually at about the twenty-eighth week, the testes descend through the inguinal canal guided by the gubernaculum (Frey, 1984).

Feminization of the undifferentiated external genitalia occurs in the absence of androgen stimulation. The embryonic phallus does not demonstrate rapid growth and becomes the clitoris. Urogenital folds do not fuse except in front of the anus. The unfused urogenital folds form the labia minora. The labioscrotal folds fuse posteriorly in the area of the perineal body but laterally remain as the labia majora. Beyond 12 weeks' gestation, the labioscrotal folds will not fuse if the fetus is exposed to androgens, though masculinization may occur in other organs of the external genitalia such as growth of the clitoris. The labioscrotal

**Table 1.2** Male and Female Derivatives of Embryonic Urogenital Structures

| | Derivatives | |
|---|---|---|
| **Embryonic Structure** | **Male** | **Female** |
| Labioscrotal swellings | Scrotum | Labia majora |
| Urogenital folds | Ventral portion of penis | Labia minora |
| Phallus | Penis | Clitoris |
| | Glans, corpora cavernosa penis, and corpus spongiosum | Glans, corpora cavernosa, bulb of the vestibule |
| Urogenital sinus | Urinary bladder | Urinary bladder |
| | Prostate gland | Urethral and paraurethral glands |
| | Prostatic utricle | Vagina |
| | Bulbourethral glands | Greater vestibular glands |
| | Seminal colliculus | Hymen |
| Paramesonephric duct | Appendix of testes | Hydatid of Morgagni |
| | | Uterus and cervix |
| | | Fallopian tubes |
| Mesonephric duct | Appendix of epididymis | Appendix vesiculosis |
| | Ductus of epididymis | Duct of epoophoron |
| | Ductus deferens | Gartner duct |
| | Ejaculatory duct and seminal vesicle | — |
| Metanephric duct | Ureters, renal pelvis, calyces, and collecting system | Ureter, renal pelvis, calyces, and collecting system |
| Mesonephric tubules | Ductuli efferentes | Epoophoron |
| | Paradidymis | Paroöphoron |
| Undifferentiated gonad | Testis | Ovary |
| Cortex | Seminiferous tubules | Ovarian follicles |
| Medulla | — | Medulla |
| | Rete testis | Rete ovarii |
| Gubernaculum | Gubernaculum testis | Round ligament of uterus |

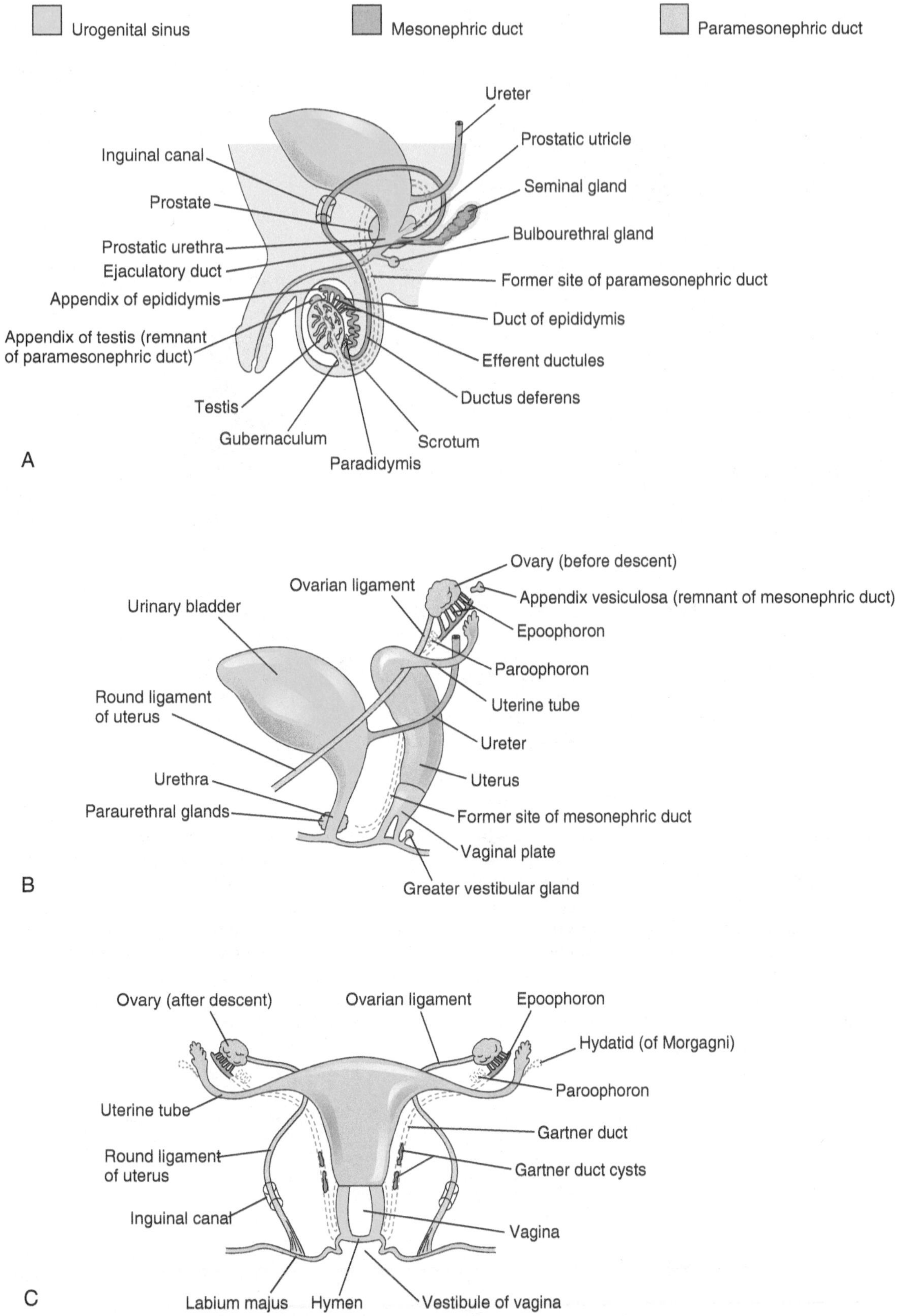


**Figure 1.14** Schematic drawings illustrating development of the male and female reproductive systems from the genital ducts and urogenital sinus. Vestigial structures are also shown. **A,** Reproductive system in a newborn male. **B,** Female reproductive system in a 12-week fetus. **C,** Reproductive system in a newborn female. (From Moore KL, Persaud TVN. *The Developing Human: Clinically Oriented Embryology.* 7th ed. Philadelphia: WB Saunders; 2003.)

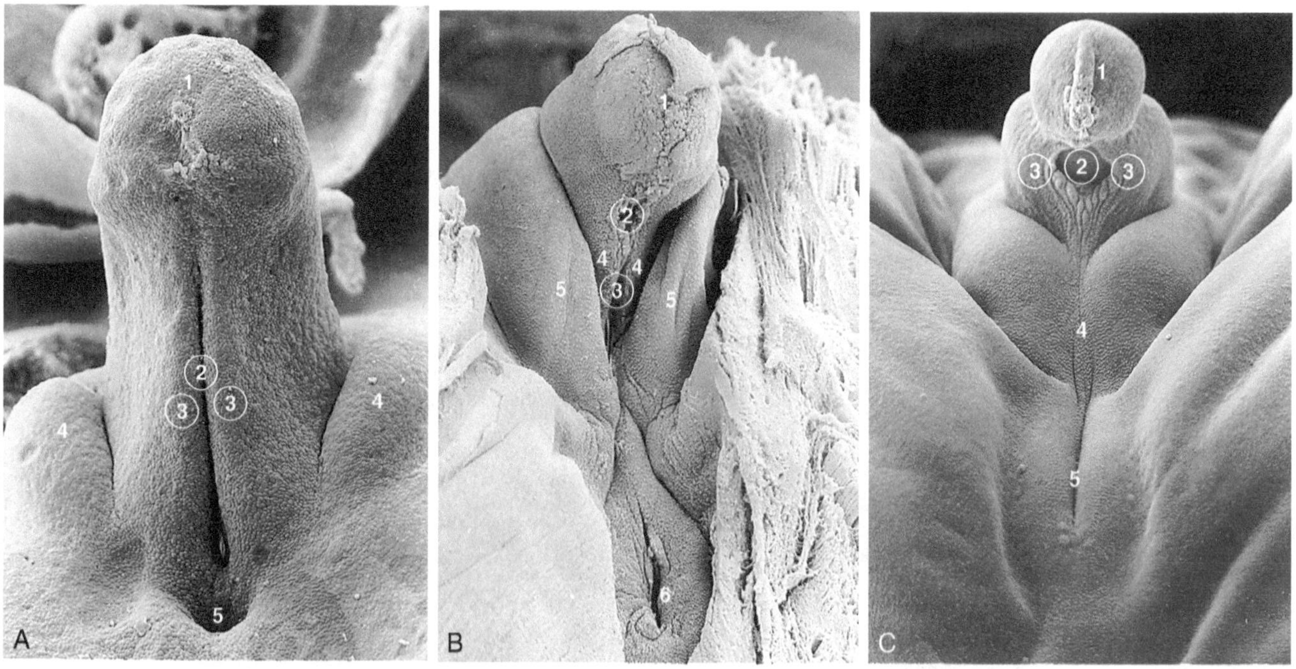


**Figure 1.15** Scanning electron micrographs (SEMs) of the developing male external genitalia. **A,** SEM of the perineum during the indifferent state of a 17-mm, 7-week embryo (×100). *1,* Developing glans of penis with the ectodermal cord. *2,* Urethral groove continuous with the urogenital sinus. *3,* Urogenital folds. *4,* Labioscrotal swellings. *5,* Anus. **B,** External genitalia of a 7.2-cm, 10-week female fetus (×45). *1,* Glans of clitoris. *2,* External urethral orifice. *3,* Opening into urogenital sinus. *4,* Urogenital folds (labia minora). *5,* Labioscrotal swelling (labia majora). *6,* Anus. **C,** SEM of the external genitalia of a 5.5-cm, 10-week male fetus (×40). *1,* Glans of penis with ectodermal cord. *2,* Remains of urethral groove. *3,* Urogenital folds in the process of closing. *4,* Labioscrotal swelling fusing to form the raphe of the scrotum. *5,* Anus. (From Moore KL, Persaud TVN. *The Developing Human: Clinically Oriented Embryology.* 7th ed. Philadelphia: WB Saunders; 2003.)

folds fuse anteriorly to form the mons pubis. A portion of the urogenital sinus between the level of the hymen and the labia develops into the vestibule of the vagina, into which the urethra, the vagina, and the ducts of Bartholin glands enter. Female external genitalia are intensely estrogen receptor–positive compared with the genitalia of the male. These receptors may be seen primarily in the stroma of the labia minora and in the periphery of the glans and interprepuce (Kalloo, 1993). The presence of such receptors suggests that there may be a direct role of maternal estrogens in the development of female external genitalia.

Virilization, masculinization, of a female (karyotype XX) fetus may occur from exposure to androgens, either from the mother or through fetal androgens as a result of genetic deficiencies in the steroid biosynthetic pathway such as occurs in congenital adrenal hyperplasia.

The ovaries do not descend into the labioscrotal folds. A structure similar to the gubernaculum develops in the inguinal canal, giving rise to the round ligaments, which suspend the uterus in the adult. Figure 1.16 summarizes the development of the external genitalia in each sex.

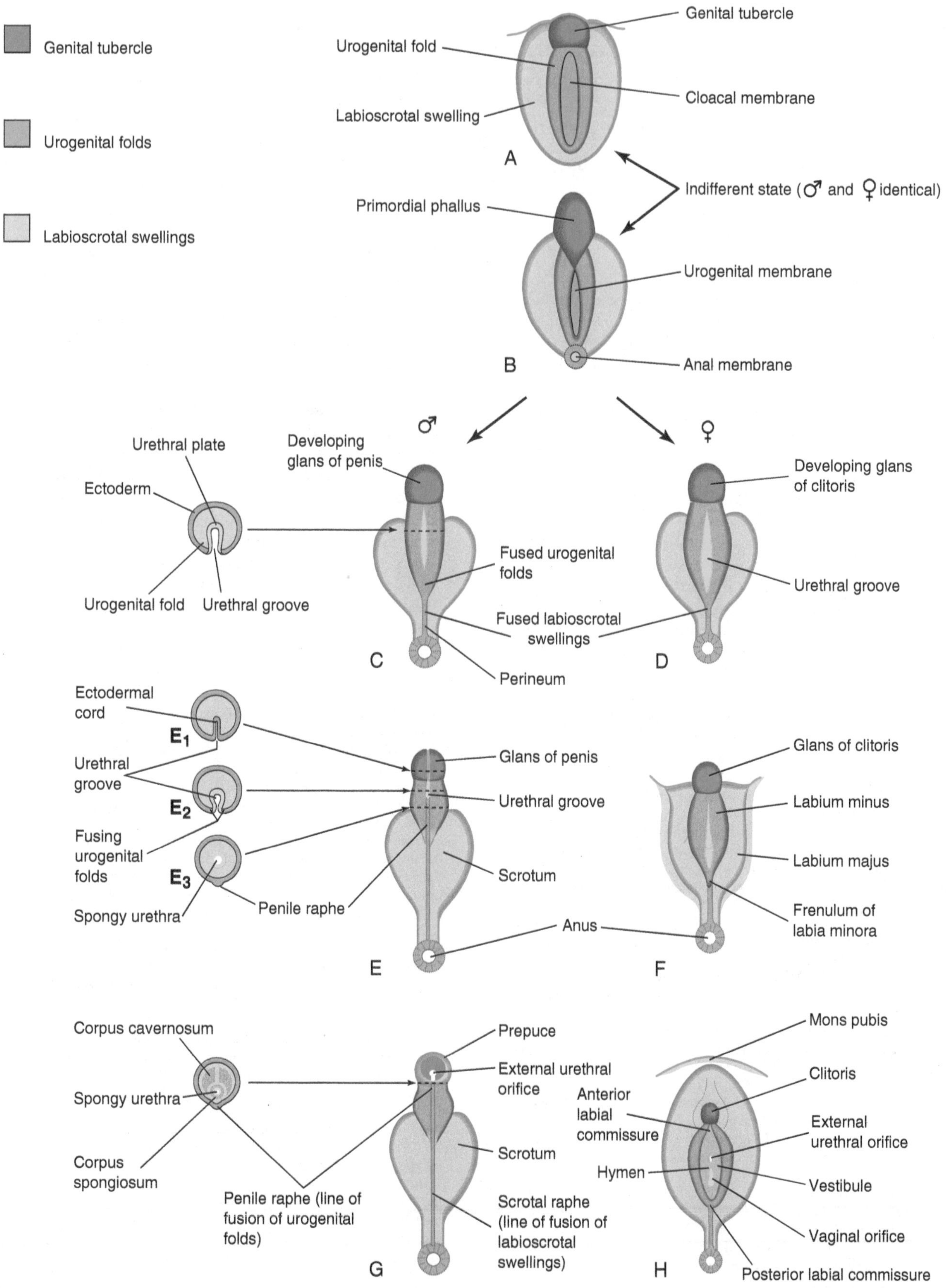


**Figure 1.16** Development of the external genitalia. **A** and **B,** Diagrams illustrating the appearance of the genitalia during the indifferent state (fourth to seventh weeks). **C, E,** and **G,** Stages in the development of male external genitalia at 9, 11, and 12 weeks, respectively. To the left are schematic transverse sections of the developing penis, illustrating formation of the spongy urethra. **D, F,** and **H,** Stages in the development of female genitalia at 9, 11, and 12 weeks, respectively. (From Moore KL, Persaud TVN. *The Developing Human: Clinically Oriented Embryology.* 7th ed. Philadelphia: WB Saunders; 2003.)

## KEY POINTS

- Oocyte meiosis is arrested at the prophase I from the fetal period until the time of ovulation.
- Fertilization occurs in the ampulla of the fallopian tube before the second polar body is cast off.
- After fertilization, first cell division leading to the two-cell embryo takes about 26 hours.
- The human embryo enters the uterus somewhere between 4 and 5 days after conception at the blastocyst stages of development.
- Implantation occurs when trophoblastic cells contact endometrium and burrow beneath the surface. This generally takes place 3 days after the embryo enters the uterus.
- Twinning due to embryo splitting may occur at any time until the formation of the blastocyst, after which time each cell is no longer pluripotent.
- The earliest fetal epithelium to develop is the ectoderm, the second is the endoderm, and the third is the mesoderm.
- hCG is secreted by the syncytiotrophoblast at about the time of implantation. It doubles in quantity every 1.2 to 2 days until 7 to 9 weeks' gestation.
- Angiogenesis is seen by day 15 or 16. Embryonic heart function begins in the third week of gestation.
- Organogenesis is complete by postconception day 56.
- The mesonephric duct system gives rise in the male to the epididymis, vas deferens, and seminal vesicles. Remnants of the mesonephric duct system in the female remain as parovarian cysts and the Gartner duct.
- The paramesonephric duct system develops in the female to give rise to the fallopian tube, uterus, and cervix. Remnants give rise to the hydatid of Morgagni at the end of the fallopian tubes. Remnants in the male remain as the appendix of the testes and prostatic utricle. This duct system is suppressed in the male by the action of AMH.
- The vagina develops from the sinovaginal bulbs, which are outgrowths of the urogenital sinus. Failure of these bulbs to form leads to agenesis of the vagina.
- The adult kidney develops from the metanephros, and its collecting system (ureter and calyceal system) develops from the metanephric (ureteric) bud from the mesonephric duct.
- The urinary bladder develops from the urogenital sinus.
- The *SRY* gene on the Y chromosome is responsible for the development of testes. Without the presence of this gene, the gonadal development is ovarian. With the absence of Sertoli cells, AMH is not produced, the paramesonephric duct system develops into a phenotypic female configuration, and the mesonephric duct system is suppressed.
- The genital tubercle elongates to form the penis in the male and the clitoris in the female.
- Two functional X chromosomes are necessary for optimal development of the ovary.

## KEY REFERENCES


Aitken RJ, Nixon B. Sperm capacitation: a distant landscape glimpsed but unexplored. *Mol Hum Reprod*. 2013;19(12):785–793.

Arias-Stella J. The Arias-Stella reaction: facts and fancies four decades after. *Adv Anat Pathol*. 2002;9(1):12–23.

Baerwald AR, Adams GP, Pierson RA. Ovarian antral folliculogenesis during the human menstrual cycle: a review. *Hum Reprod Update*. 2012;18(1):73–91.

Berndt S, Blacher S, Munaut C, et al. Hyperglycosylated human chorionic gonadotropin stimulates angiogenesis through TGF-β receptor activation. *FASEB J*. 2013;27(4):1309–1321.

Bontekoe S, Mantikou E, van Wely M, et al. Low oxygen concentrations for embryo culture in assisted reproductive technologies. *Cochrane Database Syst Rev*. 2012;11: CD008950.

Brosens JJ, Pijnenborg R, Brosens IA. The myometrial junctional zone spiral arteries in normal and abnormal pregnancies: a review of the literature. *Am J Obstet Gynecol*. 2002;187(5):1416–1423.

Chen J, Cheng J, Shatzer T, et al. Leukemia inhibitory factor can substitute for nidatory estrogen and is essential to inducing a receptive uterus for implantation but is not essential for subsequent embryogenesis. *Endocrinology*. 2000;141(12):4365–4372.

Childs AJ, Cowan G, Kinnell HL, et al. Retinoic acid signalling and the control of meiotic entry in the human fetal gonad. *PLoS One*. 2011;6(6):e20249.

Chiu P, Lam K, Wong R, et al. The identity of zona pellucida receptor on spermatozoa: an unresolved issue in developmental biology. *Semin Cell Dev Biol*. 2014;30:86–95.

Clark E. Mechanisms in the pathogenesis of congenital cardiac malformations. In: Pierpont M, Moller J, eds. *The Genetics of Cardiovascular Disease*. New York: Springer; 1987:3–11.

Darasse-Jèze G, Klatzmann D, Charlotte F, et al. CD4+CD25+ regulatory/suppressor T cells prevent allogeneic fetus rejection in mice. *Immunol Lett*. 2006;102(1):106–109.

De Baere E, Dixon MJ, Small KW, et al. Spectrum of FOXL2 gene mutations in blepharophimosis-ptosis-epicanthus inversus (BPES) families demonstrates a genotype–phenotype correlation. *Hum Mol Genet*. 2001;10(15):1591–1600.

Deppisch LM. Cysts of the vagina: classification and clinical correlations. *Obstet Gynecol*. 1975;45(6):632–637.

Di Pasquale E, Beck-Peccoz P, Persani L. Hypergonadotropic ovarian failure associated with an inherited mutation of human bone morphogenetic protein-15 (BMP15) gene. *Am J Hum Genet*. 2004;75(1):106–111.

Eisenbach M, Tur-Kaspa I. Do human eggs attract spermatozoa? *Bioassays*. 1999;21(3):203–210.

Fiorentino F, Bono S, Biricik A, et al. Application of next-generation sequencing technology for comprehensive aneuploidy screening of blastocysts in clinical preimplantation genetic screening cycles. *Hum Reprod*. 2014;29(12):2802–2813.

Fournier T, Guibourdenche J, Evain-Brion D. Review: hCGs: different sources of production, different glycoforms and functions. *Placenta*. 2015;36(Suppl 1):S60–S65.

Frey HL, Rajfer J. Role of the gubernaculum and intraabdominal pressure in the process of testicular descent. *J Urol*. 1984;131(3):574–579.

Griffin JE, Edwards C, Madden JD, et al. Congenital absence of the vagina. The Mayer-Rokitansky-Kuster-Hauser syndrome. *Ann Intern Med*. 1976;85(2):224–236.

Hall JG. *Twinning*. *Lancet*. 2003;362(9385):735–743.

Hynes PJ, Fraher JP. The development of the male genitourinary system. I. The origin of the urorectal septum and the formation of the perineum. *Br J Plast Surg*. 2004;57(1):27–36.

Kabir-Salmani M, Nikzad H, Shiokawa S, et al. Secretory role for human uterodomes (pinopods): secretion of LIF. *Mol Hum Reprod*. 2005;11(8):553–559.

Kalloo NB, Gearhart JP, Barrack ER. Sexually dimorphic expression of estrogen receptors, but not of androgen receptors in human fetal external genitalia. *J Clin Endocrinol Metab*. 1993;77(3):692–698.

Kim JJ, Wang J, Bambra C, et al. Expression of cyclooxygenase-1 and -2 in the baboon endometrium during the menstrual cycle and pregnancy. *Endocrinology*. 1999;140(6):2672–2678.

Langman J, Wilson D. Embryology and congenital malformations of the female genital tract. In: Blaustein A, ed. *Pathology of the Female Genital Tract*. New York: Springer; 1982:1–12.

Lim HJ, Dey SK. HB-EGF: a unique mediator of embryo-uterine interactions during implantation. *Exp Cell Res*. 2009;315(4):619–626.

Little M, Georgas K, Pennisi D, et al. Kidney Development. *Organogenesis in Development.* 2010:193–229.
Maruyama T, Yoshimura Y. Molecular and cellular mechanisms for differentiation and regeneration of the uterine endometrium. *Endocr J.* 2008;55(5):795–810.
Matsuno T, Tokunaka S, Koyanagi T. Muscular development of the urinary tract. *J Urol.* 1984;132(1):148–152.
Meseguer M, Herrero J, Tejera A, et al. The use of morphokinetics as a predictor of embryo implantation. *Hum Reprod.* 2011;26(10):2658–2671.
Modi DN, Sane S, Bhartiya D. Accelerated germ cell apoptosis in sex chromosome aneuploid fetal human gonads. *Mol Hum Reprod.* 2003;9(4):219–225.
Moritz K, Wintour E. Functional development of the meso- and metanephros. *Pediatr Nephrol.* 1999;13(2):171–178.
O'Rahilly R, Meyer D. The timing and sequence of events in the development of the human vertebral column during the embryonic period proper. *Anat Embryol (Berl).* 1979;157(2):167–176.
Ozisik G, Achermann JC, Meeks JJ, et al. SF1 in the development of the adrenal gland and gonads. *Horm Res.* 2003;59(Suppl 1):94–98.
Pietryga E, Wózniak W. The development of the uterine ligaments in human fetuses. *Folia Morphol (Warsz).* 1992;51(2):181–193.
Polifka JE, Friedman JM. Medical genetics: 1. Clinical teratology in the age of genomics. *CMAJ.* 2002;167(3):265–273.
Ramathal CY, Bagchi IC, Taylor RN, et al. Endometrial decidualization: of mice and men. *Sem Reprod Med.* 2010;28(1):17–26.
Reyes FI, Boroditsky RS, Winter JS, et al. Studies on human sexual development. II. Fetal and maternal serum gonadotropin and sex steroid concentrations. *J Clin Endocrinol Metab.* 1974;38(4):612–617.
Saito S, Shiozaki A, Sasaki Y, et al. Regulatory T cells and regulatory natural killer (NK) cells play important roles in feto-maternal tolerance. *Semin Immunopathol.* 2007;29(2):115–122.
Salha O, Sharma V, Dada T, et al. The influence of donated gametes on the incidence of hypertensive disorders of pregnancy. *Hum Reprod.* 1999;14(9):2268–2273.
Schatten H, Sun Q. The role of centrosomes in mammalian fertilization and its significance for ICSI. *Mol Hum Reprod.* 2009;15(9):531–538.
Schuhrke TD, Kaplan GW. Prostatic utricle cysts (Müllerian duct cysts). *J Urol.* 1978;119(6):765–767.
Simpson JL, Rajkovic A. Ovarian differentiation and gonadal failure. *Am J Med Genet.* 1999;89(4):186–200.
Speed RM. The prophase stages in human foetal oocytes studied by light and electron microscopy. *Hum Genet.* 1985;69(1):69–75.
Talbot P, Dandekar P. Perivitelline space: does it play a role in blocking polyspermy in mammals? *Microsc Res Tech.* 2003;61(4):349–357.
Thigpen AE, Silver RI, Guileyardo JM, et al. Tissue distribution and ontogeny of steroid 5 alpha-reductase isozyme expression. *J Clin Invest.* 1993;92(2):903–910.
Underwood MA, Gilbert WM, Sherman MP. Amniotic fluid: not just fetal urine anymore. *J Perinatol.* 2005;25(5):341–348.
Wallace WH, Kelsey TW. Human ovarian reserve from conception to the menopause. *PLoS One.* 2010;5(1):e8772.
Wilhelm D, Palmer S, Koopman P. Sex determination and gonaldal development in mammals. *Physiol Rev.* 2007;87(1):1–28.
Williams M, Hill CJ, Scudamore I, et al. Physiology: sperm numbers and distribution within the human Fallopian tube around ovulation. *Hum Reprod.* 1993;8(12):2019–2026.
Zegers-Hochschild F, Altieri E, Fabres C, et al. Predicitive value of human chorionic gonadotropin in the outcome of early pregnancy after in-vitro fertilization and spontaneous conception. *Hum Reprod.* 1994;9(8):1550–1555.

# 2
# Reproductive Genetics

*Jennifer Bushman Gilner, Jeffrey A. Kuller, Fidel A. Valea*

## GENETIC BASIS OF DISEASE

Medical research and medical care have been profoundly influenced by the advancement of science that succeeded in sequencing the human genome, allowing scientists to concentrate on translating this genomic text to meaningful prose. As the code is deciphered with increasing resolution, it is apparent that virtually all human diseases have an underlying genetic component, although the conversion from *genotype* to ultimate clinical *phenotype* is not always easily understood.

The overarching goals of medical care have not changed: diagnose, treat, and focus on disease prevention. The new promise of medicine in the postgenomic era is to individualize these goals, such that lifestyle interventions, screening modalities, and pharmaceuticals can be tailored to each person based on his or her unique genomic sequence. These goals have begun to materialize, through examples such as detailed breast cancer screening for women in families with known *BRCA1* or *BRCA2* mutations, or tailored chemotherapeutic regimens based on molecular testing of an individual tumor. Furthermore, there is unprecedented public accessibility of the technology for genomic screening or application of genetic information to medical treatment. Since completion of the Human Genome Project in April 2003, technology has advanced at an extraordinary pace to allow *high-throughput* data generation at increasingly reasonable cost. High-throughput methods involve automation of experiments or assays to allow for simultaneous large-scale repetition. Over the first post-genomic decade, the time to prepare and sequence a complete human genome plummeted from 13 years to a matter of 3 to 4 days, and the cost dropped from just under $30 million to around $1000 (Topol, 2014).

As a result, genetics is a field that all health care professionals need a basic level of familiarity with, not just the subspecialists. Genetics, genomics, and the technology to interpret the information are now an integral part of mainstream medicine (Table 2.1). The obstetrician/gynecologist is often the first-line provider in helping patients navigate this complicated landscape. This chapter focuses on developing a basic understanding of genetic makeup, heritability, and the most commonly used tools for detecting genetic disorders in patients or their offspring.

## BUILDING BLOCKS OF GENETICS

### MOLECULAR BUILDING BLOCKS

Genetic information is encoded in *deoxyribonucleic acid (DNA)* in the nucleus of each cell of the body. DNA molecules are made up of two complementary linear sequences of nucleotides intertwined together as a double helix. The backbone of the linear DNA molecule is composed of a phosphate and a pentose sugar (deoxyribose) to which is attached a nitrogen base. Four such bases are found in a DNA molecule: two purines (adenine [A] and guanine [G]) and two pyrimidines (thymine [T] and cytosine [C]). Purine and pyrimidine occur in equal amounts; A is always paired with T in the two strands of the double helix, and G is always paired with C. The order of bases along the molecule is the genetic *sequence*, and the complete sequence of all 6 billion bases in an individual cell nucleus (3 billion paired bases, arranged in linear antisense strands) makes up the *human genome*.

The Central Dogma published by Francis Crick in 1970 remains at the heart of molecular biology (Crick, 1970). The DNA is transcribed to a complementary *ribonucleic acid (RNA)* molecule (messenger RNA), which may be modified by regulatory sequences or three-dimensional (3D) structure. Three-base *codons* are read and translated to amino acids that are linked to form a protein with some function within the cell or organism (Fig. 2.1). The traditional concept of a *gene* refers to a unit of DNA sequence that codes for production of a protein. Surprisingly, with completion of the Human Genome Project, this gene-centric view of biology turned out to be only the tip of the iceberg in understanding the complex manner in which the genetic sequence translates to human life. Of the 3 billion base pairs that make up the genome, only about 1.5% of the assembled sequence codes for proteins. This coding portion, or *exome* contains about 20,000 to 25,000 genes, which is only a fraction of previous estimates that were predicated on gene number correlating with complexity of the species (Gerstein, 2007). There is now significant interest in the remaining 98.5% of the genome, in how it carries out the blueprint of life. There is a growing field of discovery in the regulatory function of specialized noncoding RNA molecules, called *microRNA (miRNA)*, which appear to be the gatekeepers of many biologic processes (Pritchard, 2012).

Table 2.1 Publicly Available Online Resources for Human Genomic Information

| | | |
|---|---|---|
| **General Reference** | | |
| National Human Genome Research Institute (NHGRI) | | www.genome.gov |
| **Sequence Databases** | | |
| GenBank: collection of all publicly available DNA sequences | National Institutes of Health (NIH) | www.ncbi.nlm.nih.gov/genbank |
| SNPedia: wiki investigating human genetics | River Road Bio, LLC (Cariaso, 2012) | www.SNPedia.com |
| HapMap: multi-ethnic project to catalog SNP haplotypes | Scientists and funding agencies from Japan, the United Kingdom, Canada, China, Nigeria, and the United States | hapmap.ncbi.nlm.nih.gov |
| ENCyclopedia Of DNA Elements (ENCODE) | International consortium to annotation functional elements in the genome (Birney, 2007) | www.encodeproject.org |
| Database of Genomic Variants | The Centre for Applied Genomics, Toronto, Canada (MacDonald, 2014) | dgv.tdag.ca |
| **Genotype/Phenotype Correlation** | | |
| Online Mendelian Inheritance in Man (OMIM) | McKusick-Nathans Institute of Genetic Medicine, Johns Hopkins University School of Medicine (Amberger, 2015) | omim.org |
| Genome-Wide Association Study (GWAS) Central | (Beck, 2014) | www.gwascentral.org |
| **Genome Browsers** | | |
| Ensembl | Wellcome Trust Sanger Institute/European Bioinformatics Institute | www.ensembl.org |
| University of California Santa Cruz (UCSC) Genome Bioinformatics | University of California at Santa Cruz | genome.ucsc.edu |
| NCBI | National Center for Biotechnology Information | www.ncbi.nlm.nih.gov/genome |

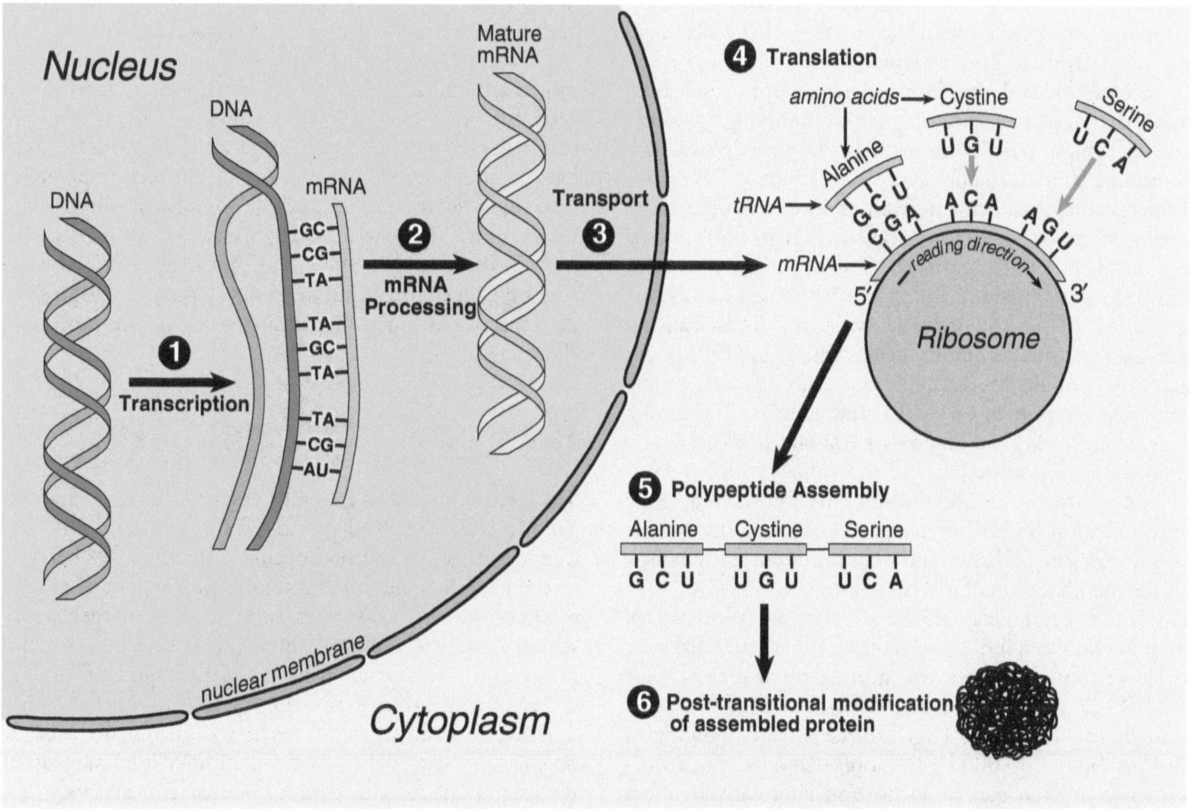


Figure 2.1 Schematic representation of polypeptide production from genetic message to final product. (Courtesy of Edith Cheng, MD.)

## MITOSIS/MEIOSIS

The full genome consists of two copies of the total DNA sequence, packaged into two homologous sets of 23 separate *chromosomes* (22 autosome pairs and 1 allosome, or sex chromosome pair). During cell division, an exact replica of this biologic blueprint is passed to each daughter cell through the process of mitosis. The formation of gametes requires even distribution of the chromosomes to the progeny through the process of meiosis, as described in Chapter 1. Upon fertilization, the zygote regains a full diploid complement of genetic material, equally derived from each parent. This process of replicating, packaging, and passing on genetic material from generation to generation forms the basis of heredity. Furthermore, errors in these processes can cause sequence changes or rearrangement of larger portions of DNA, introducing genetic variation or pathology, depending on the location of the change.

## GENOMIC VARIATION

### Genetic Variation

On April 14, 2003, the Human Genome Project was declared complete, with successful sequencing of the full human genome. Initial interpretation of the sequence result claimed 99.9% similarity between healthy individuals at the DNA sequence level, leaving only 0.1% of the genome sequence to account for individual differences in phenotype (Lee, 2007). Each alternative form of genetic code at any given *locus* is referred to as an *allele*. An individual inherits two alleles of every genetic locus, one from each parent. If both inherited alleles are made up of the same sequence, the individual is *homozygous* for the given locus. If the alleles are different, the individual is *heterozygous*. The allelic options at any given genetic locus derive from single nucleotide substitutions within the DNA sequence. Population sampling has demonstrated that among healthy individuals, the genetic sequence differs at around 10 million points (out of 3.2 billion DNA base pairs). These naturally occurring differences are called *single nucleotide polymorphisms*, or SNPs. To be classified as an SNP, two or more versions of nucleotide sequence must be present in at least 1% of the general population. The term *SNP* is used to describe genetic variation of healthy individuals, as no disease-causing nucleotide change is this common. An example of an SNP known to mediate susceptibility to disease is the delta 32 allele of the beta-chemokine receptor 5, or CCR5. Individuals carrying one copy of the delta 32 allele are somewhat resistant to infection by HIV, the virus that causes AIDS, and individuals with two copies (delta 32 homozygotes, ~1% of whites) are almost completely immune to infection by HIV (Huang, 1996). Thus the genetic variant is not the cause of disease (HIV) but is importantly associated with the manifestation of disease in humans.

In addition to individual sequence variation, comparative genome studies between individual sequences have revealed a far more pervasive form of genetic variation, termed *copy number variants (CNV)* (Iafrate, 2004; Sebat, 2004). These are structural variants, made up of relatively large DNA segments (ranging in size from 1000 bp to 500,000 bp or more) that appear in a variable number at a given genetic locus, and cumulatively affect 360 million nucleotides, or about 12% of the human genome (Redon, 2006). A CNV can be either benign or pathogenic, and a large proportion of identified CNV have as yet unknown significance.

Thus, although SNPs introduce genetic variation at the level of individual base substitutions, CNVs represent variation in the "dose" of a relatively large DNA segment. The collection of genetic sequence variants (SNPs) or CNVs within an individual forms a sort of biologic landscape that will influence how that person experiences or responds to external influences such as challenge from an invading pathogen or ultraviolet ray exposure from the sun. Thus understanding genetic variation in the form of SNPs and CNVs and their biologic influence can reveal a predisposition toward disease, variable susceptibility to infections, or diverse responses to pharmaceuticals as well as side effects from the same compounds. In other words, genetic variation is at the core of our collective goal of "individualized medicine," in which preventive strategies or "designer drugs" can be tailored to an individual based on one's genomic information.

### Epigenetic Variation

There are forms of genetic variation that do not involve a change in nucleotide sequence. Instead, persistent alterations in three-dimensional DNA structure can change the expression pattern of a gene. Covalent modification of histones to alter *chromatin* structure and the covalent addition of methyl groups to cytosine residues in the DNA are the most commonly seen three-dimensional DNA alterations. These patterns of *epigenetic* modification of genes are replicated through successive cell divisions despite unchanged DNA sequence and have the potential to be heritable (Portela, 2010).

Two well-studied mechanisms of epigenetic modification influencing disease phenotype include genomic imprinting and CpG island methylation patterns. Genomic imprinting is a process by which hypermethylation of a specific parental allele causes that allele of the gene to be silenced, and disease may arise if the remaining allele is abnormal. Variable methylation of CpG islands in cancer cells can promote tumorigenesis through loss of proliferative supervision of the cell. Epigenetics is a growing field for understanding complex genotype-phenotype interactions. Epigenetic mechanisms such as methylation have been shown to play a role in multiple other human disease types beyond cancer, including neurodevelopmental disorders, neurodegenerative and neurologic diseases, and autoimmune diseases (Portela, 2010).

## GENETIC PATHOLOGY

The term *mutation* is generally reserved for new changes in the genetic code that lead to altered function and clinical consequences. A gene mutation occurs when there has been a change in the genetic code. The mutation may involve changing a single base, known as a *point mutation*, or a larger segment, in which bases are removed, duplicated, or inserted. Mutations occur as a result of environmental damage to DNA, through errors during DNA replication or repair, and through uneven crossing over and genetic exchange during meiosis. The loss or gain of bases in a protein-coding region may disrupt the reading frame of the triplet codons. Alternatively, a change in base sequence in a noncoding region of DNA may alter the ability of regulatory proteins or RNA molecules to bind to the DNA. Point mutations within the gene could result in an amino acid substitution, leading to different products with altered functions. Figure 2.2 demonstrates such an occurrence for sickle cell anemia caused by the substitution of a single base at a single point. In contrast to sickle cell anemia where there is only one mutation, the cystic fibrosis transmembrane conductance regulator *(CFTR)* gene is an example of a gene for which more than 1000 mutations or alleles have been described to date. Some genes also have regions that are more prone to mutational events (hot spots).

## SINGLE GENE DISORDERS

Disease-causing genetic alterations are categorized by patterns of familial segregation. Any evaluation of the segregation pattern of a trait or disease in a family requires the development of a three-generation *pedigree* (Fig. 2.3). This graphic representation of family history data assists in determining the transmission

| Hemoglobin-Binding Protein | DNA Triplet Codons | | | Amino Acid |
|---|---|---|---|---|
| HgbA (normal) | CTT | CTC | ➡ | Glutamic acid |
| HgbS | CAT | CAC | ➡ | Valine |
| HgbC | TTT | TTC | ➡ | Lysine |

**Figure 2.2** A single base pair substitution in the same DNA triplet codon for glutamic acid at amino acid position 6 for normal hemoglobin results in hemoglobin S (valine in sickle cell disease) or hemoglobin C (lysine in HgbC disease). (Courtesy of Edith Cheng, MD.)

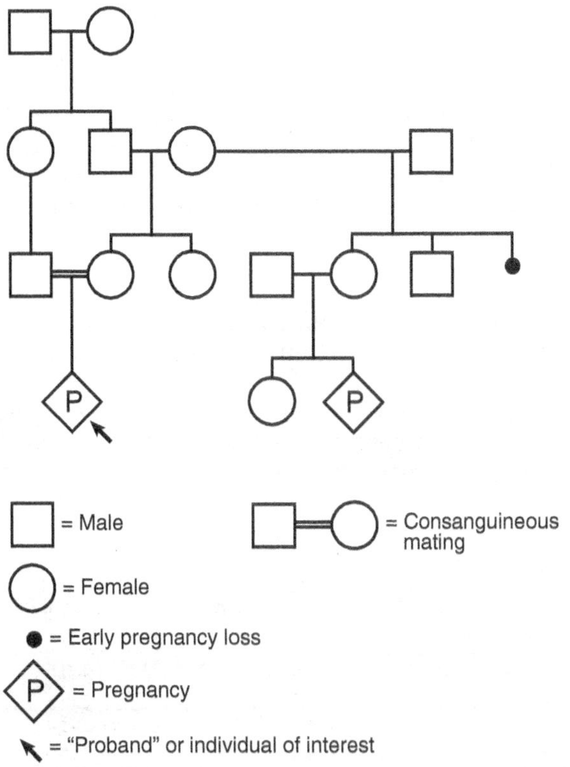


**Figure 2.3** Standard figures and nomenclature for a pedigree. (Courtesy of Edith Cheng, MD.)

pattern of the gene, as well as predicting the risk of recurrence. In some conditions, the pattern of transmission and the constellation of clinical characteristics of affected individuals in the pedigree provide the diagnosis, which otherwise would not be evident if only one individual were evaluated.

### *Mendelian Inheritance Patterns*

#### Autosomal Dominant

In an autosomal dominant mode of inheritance, only one copy of the mutated gene is required for expression of the trait, and the individual is said to be heterozygous for the trait. There are more than 4000 known autosomal dominant conditions, and most occur in the heterozygous form in affected individuals. With a few exceptions, autosomal dominant conditions occurring in the homozygous form (two copies of the affected gene) are rare, the phenotype is more severe, and they are often lethal. An example is achondroplasia, in which two copies of the mutated gene result in a lethal condition.

The general characteristics of autosomal dominant inheritance are illustrated in Figure 2.4 and summarized as follows:

1. Every affected individual has an affected parent (unless this is a new mutation—to be discussed later). The inheritance pattern is vertical.
2. If reproductively fit, the affected person has a 50% risk of transmitting the gene with each pregnancy.
3. The sexes are affected equally.
4. There is father-to-son transmission.
5. An individual who does not carry the mutation will have no risk of transmission to his or her offspring.

Three additional properties associated with, but not exclusive to, autosomal dominant traits are variable *expressivity*, *penetrance*, and new mutations. Variable expressivity describes the severity of the phenotype in individuals who have the mutation. Some autosomal dominant conditions have a clear clinical demarcation between affected and unaffected individuals. However, some conditions express the clinical consequences of the mutation in varying degrees among members of the same family and between different families. These differences in expression are modified by age, sex of the affected individual, the individual's genetic background, and the environment. Variable expression of a condition can lead to difficulties in diagnosis and interpretation of inheritance pattern. Penetrance refers to the probability that a gene will have any clinical manifestation at all in a person

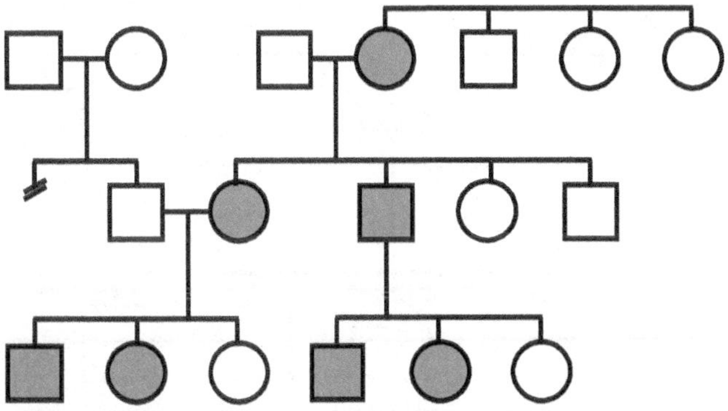

**Figure 2.4** Example of autosomal dominant inheritance. (Courtesy of Edith Cheng, MD.)

known to have the mutation. A condition is 100% penetrant if all individuals with the mutation have any clinical feature of the disease (no matter how minor). A number of autosomal dominant conditions are the result of new mutations. For example, about 70% of achondroplasia cases occur as new mutations. Because this condition has 100% penetrance, the recurrence risk in subsequent pregnancies in the normal parents of an affected child is extremely low, but the risk to the offspring of the affected is 50%. If an autosomal dominant condition is associated with poor reproductive fitness, then the likelihood that the cases occurred because of new mutation is greater.

### Autosomal Recessive

Autosomal recessive conditions are rare and require the affected individual to have two copies of the mutant allele (homozygous) in order to manifest the condition. In the heterozygote carrier, the product of the normal allele is generally able to compensate for the mutant allele and prevent occurrence of the disease. Figure 2.5 is a typical pedigree illustrating autosomal recessive inheritance. The following general statements can be made about an autosomal recessive trait:

1. The characteristic will occur equally in both sexes.
2. For an offspring to be at risk, both parents must have at least one copy of the mutation.
3. If both parents are heterozygous (carriers) for the condition, on average 25% of the offspring will be homozygous for the mutation and manifest the condition, and 50% will be carriers and unaffected. The remaining 25% will not have inherited the mutation at all, will be unaffected, and will not be at risk of transmitting the mutation to any offspring.
4. Consanguinity is often present in families demonstrating rare autosomal recessive conditions.

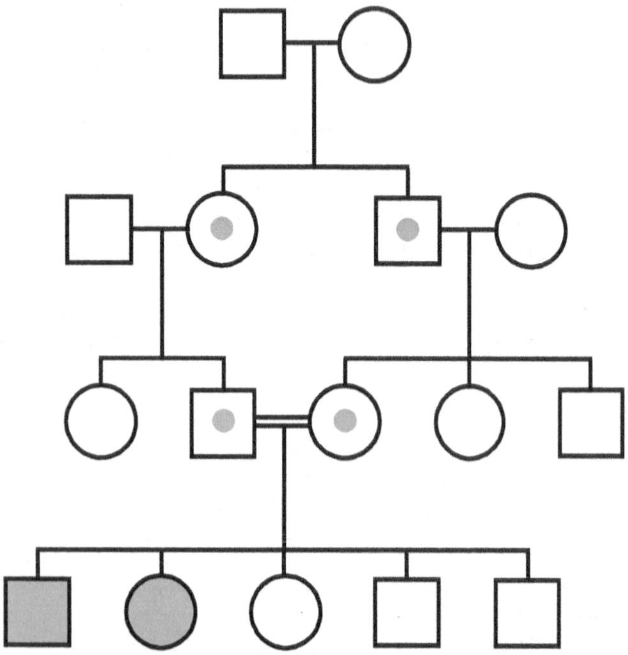

**Figure 2.5** Pedigree illustrating autosomal recessive inheritance. Here the parents of the affected children are first cousins, as denoted by the double line connecting them. (Courtesy of Edith Cheng, MD.)

5. If the disease is relatively rare, it will be clustered among the siblings and will not be seen among other family members such as ancestors, cousins, aunts, and uncles.

Because autosomal recessive conditions require two copies of the mutant allele, and because most matings are not consanguineous, counseling couples about the risk for an autosomal recessive condition requires knowledge of the carrier frequency of the condition in the general population. Cystic fibrosis exemplifies the importance of knowing the population in which screening/counseling is being provided (Table 2.2). Depending on the ethnic group of the mother and father, the risk for a child having cystic fibrosis could be as high as 1 in 1936 ($1/22 \times 1/22 \times 1/4$) if they are Northern European white or considerably less so if they are of Asian descent.

### X-linked Trait

The human X chromosome is quite large, containing about 160 million base pairs, or about 5% of the nuclear DNA. Of the 500 genes that have been mapped to the X chromosome, 70% are known to be associated with disease phenotypes. Diseases caused by genes on the X chromosome are said to be X linked, and most are recessive. In contrast, the Y chromosome is quite small, about 70 million base pairs, and contains only a few genes.

The expression of genes located on the X chromosome demonstrate a unique characteristic known as dosage compensation, a concept which was described by Mary Lyon in the 1960s to explain the equalization of X-linked gene products in males and females (Lyon, 1961). Achievement of dosage compensation is through the principles of X inactivation, also known as the *Lyon hypothesis*. The tenets of the Lyon hypothesis are as follows:

1. One X chromosome in each cell is randomly inactivated in the early female embryo (soon after fertilization).
2. The inactivation process is random: either the paternally or maternally derived X chromosome is chosen. The female is thus a mosaic for genes located on the X chromosome.
3. All descendants of the cell will have the same inactive X chromosome.

The Lyon hypothesis is supported by clinical evidence derived from animal and human observations of traits located on the X chromosome, such as the calico cat pattern of red and black patches of fur on female cats but not on male cats. In humans, males and females have equal quantities of the enzyme glucose-6-phosphate dehydrogenase (G6PD), which is encoded by a gene on the X chromosome. The mechanism for X inactivation

**Table 2.2** Carrier Frequencies for Cystic Fibrosis in Different Populations

| Ethnicity | Chance of Being Carrier | Chance Both Carriers* |
|---|---|---|
| European descent | 1 in 29 | 1 in 841 |
| Hispanic American | 1 in 46 | 1 in 2116 |
| African American | 1 in 65 | 1 in 4225 |
| Asian American | 1 in 90 | 1 in 8100 |

*The chance for an affected child being born to these couples is the chance that both are carriers times ¼.

is unknown at this time but clearly requires the presence of the X inactivation center, which has been mapped to the proximal end of the long arm of the X chromosome (Xq). This center contains an unusual gene called the *X-inactive specific transcript (XIST)*, which seems to control X inactivation, a process that cannot occur in its absence.

The principles of the Lyon hypothesis remain true for the majority of genes located on the X chromosome. The silencing of these genes appears to occur as a function of DNA methylation at the promoter regions of these genes. However, several regions remain genetically active on both chromosomes. They include the pseudoautosomal regions located at the tips of the long and short arms, which are the regions that contain the genes for steroid sulfatase, the Xg blood group, and Kallman syndrome (hypogonadism and anosmia). The pseudoautosomal region on the short arm shares extensive homology with the Y chromosome and is the region involved in the pairing of the X and Y chromosome at meiosis.

Another exception to the Lyon hypothesis is that one X chromosome is nonrandomly, preferentially inactivated. This is observed for most cases of *translocations* between an X chromosome and an autosome. If the translocation is balanced, the structurally normal X chromosome is preferentially inactivated. If the translocation is unbalanced, then the structurally normal X chromosome is always active. These nonrandom patterns of inactivation are an attempt to minimize the clinical consequences of the chromosomal rearrangement. Studies can be done to look at patterns of inactivation, as in the case of prenatal diagnosis, to predict the clinical consequences of a de novo X/autosome translocation in the fetus.

Random inactivation confers a mosaic state for the carrier female. The normal allele is able to compensate for the abnormal allele (as in autosomal recessive traits), and carrier females of X-linked recessive conditions usually do not have clinical manifestations of the disease. Occasionally, however, there is skewed or less than 50-50 chance of inactivation such that the X chromosome carrying the normal allele is inactivated more frequently. In such cases, carrier females display some features of the condition and are referred to as *manifesting heterozygotes*. Manifesting heterozygotes have been described for hemophilia A, Duchenne muscular dystrophy, ornithine transcarbamylase deficiency, and X-linked color blindness. Genetic counseling of recurrence risks for an X-linked recessive condition depends on the sex of the affected parent and of the offspring. Figure 2.6 is a pedigree illustrating X-linked recessive inheritance, the characteristics of which are the following:

1. Affected individuals are usually males unless X-chromosome activation is skewed in the carrier female or the female is homozygous for the trait.
2. The affected males in a kindred are related through females.
3. The gene is not transmitted from father to son.
4. All daughters of affected males will be carriers.
5. Daughters of carrier females have a 50% chance of being carriers; sons of carrier females have a 50% chance of being affected.

### X-linked Dominant Inheritance

The major feature of X-linked dominant inheritance is that all heterozygotes, both male and female, manifest the condition. Although the pedigree may resemble autosomal dominant inheritance, the distinguishing feature is that affected males never have affected sons, and all daughters of affected males are affected. There are usually more affected females than males, and the majority of the females are heterozygotes. Examples of diseases with this mode of inheritance are hypophosphatemic rickets and Rett syndrome.

## *Non-Mendelian Inheritance Patterns (Complex Traits)*

### Trinucleotide-Repeat Disorders: Unstable Mutations

In the early 1990s a new class of genetic conditions was recognized as being due to unstable dynamic mutations in a gene. In classic genetic inheritance, the diseases and their inheritance patterns are due to mutations that are passed on from generation to generation in a stable form. That is, all affected members in a family have the identical inherited mutation. In 1991, however, a number of reports began to describe a new class of genetic condition in which the gene mutation was dynamic and would change with different affected individuals within a family. The most common group of disorders is known as *triplet*, or *trinucleotide repeat, disorders*. More than a dozen diseases are now known to be associated with unstable trinucleotide repeats (Table 2.3) (Cummings, 2000).

These conditions are characterized by an expansion of variable size, within the affected gene, of a segment of DNA that contains a repeat of three nucleotides such as CAGCAGCAG (CAG)*n*, or CCGCCG (CCG)*n*. These triplet repeats are unstable in that they tend to expand as the gene is passed on from generation to generation. The molecular mechanism is most likely misalignment at the time of meiosis. The result of increasing triplet expansion is progressively earlier onset or more severe manifestation of disease with each successive generation. This phenomenon is known as *anticipation*.

The commonality of this group of genetic conditions stops at the shared molecular mechanism. Each disease, otherwise, has its own features. Some, such as myotonic dystrophy, are inherited in an autosomal dominant pattern, but others, such as Friedrich ataxia, are autosomal recessive conditions. The susceptibility of the triplet repeat to expand also may depend on the parent of origin: paternal in Huntington disease and exclusively maternal in fragile X syndrome.

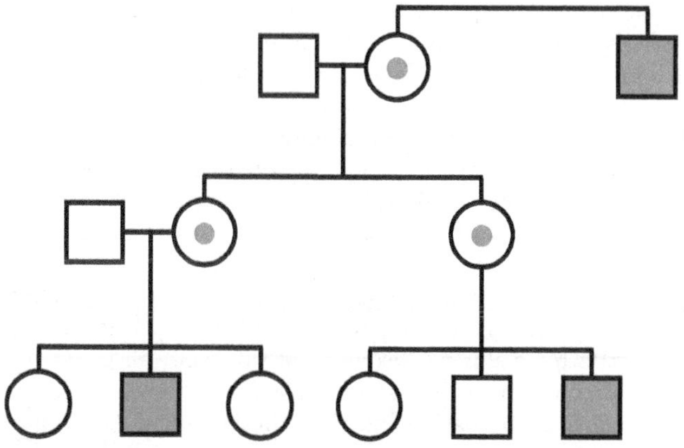

**Figure 2.6** Pedigree illustrating X-linked recessive condition. (Courtesy of Edith Cheng, MD.)

Table 2.3 Some Commonly Known Disorders Associated with Unstable Triplet Repeats

| Disease | Inheritance Pattern | Triplet Repeat | Location of Expansion | Repeat Number | | |
|---|---|---|---|---|---|---|
| | | | | Normal | Unstable | Affected |
| Huntington disease | Autosomal dominant | CAG | Exon coding region | <36 | 29-35 | >35 |
| Fragile X | X-linked | CGG | 5′ untranslated region | <55 | 56-200 | >200 |
| Myotonic dystrophy | Autosomal dominant | GTG | 3′ untranslated region | <35 | 50-100 | >100 |
| Spinal cerebellar ataxias* | Autosomal dominant | CAG | Exon | <40 | Different for each subtype | >40 |
| Friedrich ataxia | Autosomal recessive | GAA | Intron of gene | <33 | 34-65 | >65 |

*Spinal cerebellar ataxias are a heterogeneous group of conditions, all of which appear to be associated with a CAG repeat. Each subtype has its own specific range of normal, unstable, and affected repeat sizes.

## Fragile X Syndrome

Fragile X syndrome, a disease within the unstable triplet group, is the most common heritable form of moderate mental retardation and is second to Down syndrome among the causes of mental retardation in males. In women, a mild carrier state may present as premature menopause. The gene is located on the X chromosome at Xq27.3 and causes a pattern of abnormalities, including mental retardation and characteristic facial features. Disease frequency is approximately 1 in 4000 male births. The condition is due to an expansion of the triplet repeat CGG located in the untranslated region of the first exon of the gene called *FMR1* (fragile X mental retardation 1). The triplet expansion blocks normal function of the *FMR1* gene, thus causing the syndrome.

Normal individuals have about 8 to 50 copies of the CGG triplet, whereas affected individuals have from 200 to more than 1000 copies. Individuals with an intermediate number of copies (52 to 200) are known as *premutation carriers*; this level of "expansion" renders the triplet-repeat segment unstable. These carriers are generally unaffected but are at risk for having affected children or descendants if the premutation expands in successive generations. The premutation, however, can be passed on without expanding.

Long-term follow-up of premutation carriers has revealed that these individuals are not necessarily "unaffected." Premature ovarian failure has been associated with female premutation carriers, and in men, a syndrome of atypical adult-onset ataxia (FXTAS) has now been described (Hagerman, 2004).

Although the unstable triplet is transmitted in an X-linked pattern, the probabilities of the different phenotypes are far from traditional X-linked inheritance. Understanding of this feature of the fragile X syndrome is crucial to genetic counseling and assessing recurrence risks. The possible outcomes of the offspring of a premutation carrier female are the following:

1. Male offspring—three possibilities:
   a. Unaffected by not having inherited the X chromosome with the premutation.
   b. Unaffected by inheriting the X chromosome with the premutation, which did *not* expand (about 20% of the time); this male, however, is at risk for passing the premutation to his daughters, who in turn will be at risk for having affected children. Therefore, for this male, his grandchildren will be at risk for the fragile X syndrome.
   c. Affected by having inherited the abnormal X chromosome, in which the premutation also expanded to a full mutation.
2. Female offspring—four possibilities:
   a. Unaffected by not having inherited the X chromosome with the premutation.
   b. Unaffected by inheriting the X chromosome with the premutation that did *not* expand.
   c. Unaffected, but inherited the X chromosome with an expansion—about 50% of females with the expansion appear to be clinically unaffected.
   d. Affected by inheriting the X chromosome with an expansion.

## Genomic Imprinting and Uniparental Disomy

Genomic imprinting and uniparental disomy refers to the differential activation or expression of genes depending on the parent of origin. In contrast to Mendel's hypothesis that the phenotype of a gene is no different if inherited from the mother or the father, we now understand that there is a group of diseases in which the parent of origin of a gene or chromosome plays a role in the phenotype of the affected individual. The best-studied example of this mechanism is Prader-Willi syndrome (PWS) and Angelman syndrome (AS). Both diseases arise from loss of function of the same gene on chromosome 15, but two different disease phenotypes arise depending on which parental allele is affected. PWS is characterized by obesity, hyperphagia, small hands and feet, hypogonadism, and mental retardation (Jones, 2006). In about 70% of cases, cytogenetic deletion of the proximal arm of the paternally inherited chromosome 15 is observable (15q11-q13). In contrast, the same deletion of the maternally inherited chromosome 15 results in the Angelman phenotype of severe mental retardation, short stature, spasticity, and seizures (Jones, 2006). Interestingly, 30% of subjects with PWS do not have a cytogenetic deletion but rather inherit two intact chromosomes 15 from the mother. No genetic information on chromosome 15 is inherited from the father. This is referred to as *maternal uniparental disomy*. Individuals with Angelman syndrome without a cytogenetic deletion have two copies of the paternally derived chromosome 15 and no chromosome 15 from the mother, a condition termed *paternal uniparental disomy*. These findings indicate that for the region of 15q11-q13, the expression of the PWS phenotype is brought on by the absence of a paternal contribution of the genes in this region. Likewise, the expression of Angelman syndrome is due to the absence of the maternal contribution of genes located at 15q11-q13. The genes in this region are said to be "imprinted" because their parent of origin has been "marked."

Many regions of the human genome have now demonstrated evidence of imprinting. Knowledge of diseases that occur as a result of imprinting has implications in prenatal diagnosis, especially when *mosaicism* is encountered.

### Germline Mosaicism

Mosaicism is defined as the presence of two or more genetically different cell lines in the same individual or tissue derived from a single zygote. All females, because of X inactivation, are mosaics for genes on the X chromosome. Mosaicism, however, is not necessarily evenly or randomly distributed throughout the body. In other words, using the entire body as the whole organism, an individual is mosaic either because different organs or tissues have genetically different cells, but each organ or tissue has the same cell line, or because the genetically different cell lines are dispersed throughout many tissues in the body. The distinction between these two types of mosaicism is particularly important in making a prenatal diagnosis in cases in which mosaicism is identified in amniotic fluid cells. For instance, one cannot be confident that a fetus identified as being mosaic trisomy 21 would necessarily have a less severe mental retardation phenotype because of mosaicism. The brain cells could be all full trisomy 21, but the cells of the skin could all be normal diploid. In germline mosaicism, the implication is that the mutation is present in only one parent and arose during embryogenesis in all or some of the germ line cells but few or none of the somatic cells of the embryo. This concept was developed to explain recurrence of a genetic condition in a sibship (usually autosomal dominant) in which incorrect diagnosis, autosomal recessive inheritance, reduced penetrance, or variable expression could not be the reason for the recurrence. The best example of germline mosaicism is osteogenesis imperfecta type II (lethal form). At the molecular level, the mutation causing the condition is dominant—that is, only one copy of the abnormal gene is necessary to cause this perinatal lethal condition. Yet there are families in which multiple affected pregnancies are seen in the same couple or one parent has recurrences with different partners. If the spontaneous mutation rate for an autosomal dominant mutation is 1 chance in $10^5$, then the probability of two independent spontaneous mutations for the same lethal autosomal dominant condition is $(1/10^5)^2$, a highly unlikely event. Germline mosaicism is now well documented for about 6% of cases of osteogenesis imperfecta type II (Zlotogora, 1998). Unfortunately, the exact recurrence risk is difficult to assess because the proportion of gametes containing the mutation is unknowable.

### Mitochondrial Inheritance: Maternal Inheritance

Most inherited conditions occur as a result of mutations in the DNA of the nucleus (nuclear genome). However, mitochondria have their own DNA molecules, which contain a small fraction of genes whose product are vital to the function of the cell. Mitochondrial DNA (mtDNA), which was completely sequenced in 1981, is small, about 16.5 kilobase pairs (kbp), and is packaged as a circular chromosome located in the mitochondria. A growing number of conditions resulting from abnormalities of the mitochondria have now been identified. Because the mitochondrial apparatus and its function are under the control of both nuclear and mitochondrial genes, many diseases affecting the mitochondria do not follow the typical Mendelian pattern of inheritance. Each human cell contains a population of several hundred or more mitochondria in its cytoplasm. Most of the subunits that make up the mitochondrial apparatus are encoded by the nuclear genome.

Because the primary function of the mitochondria is to provide energy in the form of adenosine triphosphate (ATP) for the cell, mutations that affect the genes that code for oxidative phosphorylation will likely result in cell dysfunction and death. The organs most affected would be those that depend heavily on mitochondria. The diseases that result are generally neuromuscular in nature, such as encephalopathies, myopathies, ataxias, and retinal degeneration, but the mutations have *pleiotropic* effects, meaning multiple different clinical traits are caused by a single gene defect (Johns, 1995).

The most significant characteristic of mitochondrial diseases caused by mutations in mtDNA is that they are all maternally inherited. This is because the cytoplasm of the ovum is abundant with mitochondria, but the sperm contain very few mitochondria. Therefore an individual's mitochondria (and mtDNA) are essentially all inherited from the mother. If the mother has an mtDNA mutation, then all of her children will inherit that mutation. When a mutation arises in the DNA of a mitochondrion in the cytoplasm of the ovum, it is at first one mutation in one mitochondrion. However, as replication and division of this mutated mitochondrion occur, they become randomly distributed among the normal mitochondria and between the daughter cells. One daughter cell by chance may contain a large population of mitochondria with the mutation, but the other has none or very little. Fertilization of the egg with a large proportion of mitochondria containing the mutation would result in an offspring that is at risk for manifesting a mitochondrial disease. Leber hereditary optic neuropathy (LHON) is a well-known mitochondrial disease in which rapid, bilateral loss of central vision occurs as a result of a mutation in mitochondrial DNA. Males and females are affected equally, and all affected individuals are related through maternal lineage.

A second feature of mitochondrial diseases is that of variable expression. Within each cell and tissue, there is a threshold for energy production below which the cells will degenerate and die. Organ systems with large energy requirements will be most susceptible to mitochondrial abnormalities. Thus, if there is an mtDNA mutation, the severity of the mitochondrial disease will depend on the proportion of mitochondria with the mutation that the individual inherited from his or her mother and the susceptibility of different tissues to altered ATP metabolism.

In contrast, abnormalities of mitochondrial function caused by mutations of genes encoded in the nuclear genome will exhibit traditional Mendelian inheritance patterns; autosomal dominant, autosomal recessive and X-linked patterns of mitochondrial disorders have been observed. A few mitochondrial diseases occur as sporadic somatic mutations and have little or no recurrence risk. Table 2.4 lists some of the currently known diseases of mitochondrial function and their inheritance patterns.

## *Multifactorial Inheritance*

Multifactorial inheritance is defined as traits or characteristics produced by the action of several genes, with or without the interplay of environmental factors. A number of structural abnormalities occurring as isolated defects and not part of a syndrome, such as cleft lip with or without cleft palate, open neural tube defect (including anencephaly and spina bifida), and

Table 2.4 Features of Some Disorders of Mitochondrial Function

| Disease | Features | Genetics | Inheritance Pattern |
|---|---|---|---|
| Barth syndrome | Dilated cardiomyopathy, cyclic neutropenia, skeletal myopathy, growth deficiency, abnormal mitochondria | Nuclear DNA encoding mitochondrial protein tafazzin (*TAZ* gene) | X linked |
| Friedreich ataxia | Limb movement abnormalities, dysarthria, absent tendon reflexes | Nuclear DNA encoding mitochondrial protein frataxin (*FXN* gene, triplet repeat) | Autosomal recessive |
| Leber hereditary optic neuropathy (LHON) | Blindness, rapid optic nerve death in young adulthood | Mitochondrial DNA | Maternal |
| Leigh disease (subacute necrotizing encephalomyelopathy) | Infant onset progressive psychomotor regression following viral illness, hypotonia, peripheral neuropathy, lactic acidosis | Many genes:<br>20%-25% mitochondrial DNA (includes neuropathy, ataxia, and retinitis pigmentosa [NARP])<br>75%-80% nuclear DNA | Mitochondrial DNA: maternal<br>Nuclear DNA: autosomal recessive or X linked |
| MERRF | Myotonic epilepsy, ragged red fibers in muscle, ataxia, sensorineural deafness | Mitochondrial DNA | Maternal |
| MELAS | Mitochondrial encephalopathy, lactic acidosis, strokelike episodes, sensorineural deafness | Mitochondrial DNA | Maternal |
| MIDD | Maternally inherited diabetes and deafness | Mitochondrial DNA | Maternal |
| MNGIE | Mitochondrial neurogastrointestinal encephalopathy, childhood-onset gastrointestinal dysmotility, peripheral neuropathy | Nuclear DNA (*TYMP* gene) causes destabilization of mitochondrial DNA | Autosomal recessive |

cardiac defects, are examples of such conditions. When both parents are normal and an affected child is produced, the chance of recurrence is generally between 2% and 5% for any given pregnancy. Because the underlying mechanisms by which the genes and the environment interact to cause these conditions are largely unknown, genetic counseling of recurrence risks must measure the observed recurrence risks in collections of families to generate a population-based empiric risk. These risk rates, however, are modified by many factors including ethnicity, the sex of the carrier parent, the sex of the affected parent and at-risk offspring, the presence of the defect in one or both parents, the number of affected family members, and consanguineous parentage (Kuller, 1996).

## CHROMOSOMAL ABNORMALITIES

In general, genetic replication machinery of the cell is astonishingly accurate, and there are many repair mechanisms the cell uses to maintain fidelity of DNA copies. Thus the incidence of any given single gene disorder, even in high prevalence populations, is relatively low. In contrast, the distribution of genetic material during cell division by mitosis or meiosis is far more prone to mistakes, so that on a population level the risk of chromosome level genetic rearrangements occurs at least 100 times more frequently than single gene disorders. Consider the rate of 1 in 2500 for white babies affected by cystic fibrosis (the most common inherited disease in this population), compared with the estimation that an abnormal chromosome complement occurs in up to 4% of clinically recognized pregnancies (Creasy, 2014).

A variety of chromosome abnormalities may occur during meiosis or mitosis (see Chapter 1) leading to an abnormal *karyotype*, or chromosome complement visible under light microscopy. Chromosome abnormalities fall into several general categories, and many clinical conditions are associated with each type.

### Numerical Chromosomal Abnormalities

Two terms are used in the description of numerical chromosomal abnormalities: *aneuploidy* refers to an extra or missing chromosome, such as in trisomy 21 (Down syndrome) or monosomy X (Turner syndrome), respectively; *polyploidy* refers to numerical chromosome abnormalities in which there is an addition of an entire complement of haploid chromosomes, such as in triploidy, in which three haploid sets occur (69, XXX or XXY or XYY). Numerical or aneuploid chromosome abnormalities involve either autosomes or sex chromosomes. Most occur as the result of *nondisjunction* during meiosis or mitosis in which homologous chromosome pairs fail to disjoin. The result in meiosis is that one daughter cell receives two copies of the homologues and the other receives none. Fertilization with a gamete containing a normal chromosome complement will result in a zygote that is either trisomic or monosomic (Fig. 2.7).

The majority of trisomic conceptions are nonviable, and autosomal trisomies have been seen in abortus material in all but chromosomes 1 and 17. However, trisomies 21, 18, 13, and 22 can result in live births and are associated with advanced maternal age (Fig. 2.8). Trisomy 13 (Patau syndrome) occurs in approximately 1/10,000 live births. The syndrome is characterized by prenatal growth restriction and multiple severe structural defects involving the midline (holoprosencephaly, cleft lip/palate,

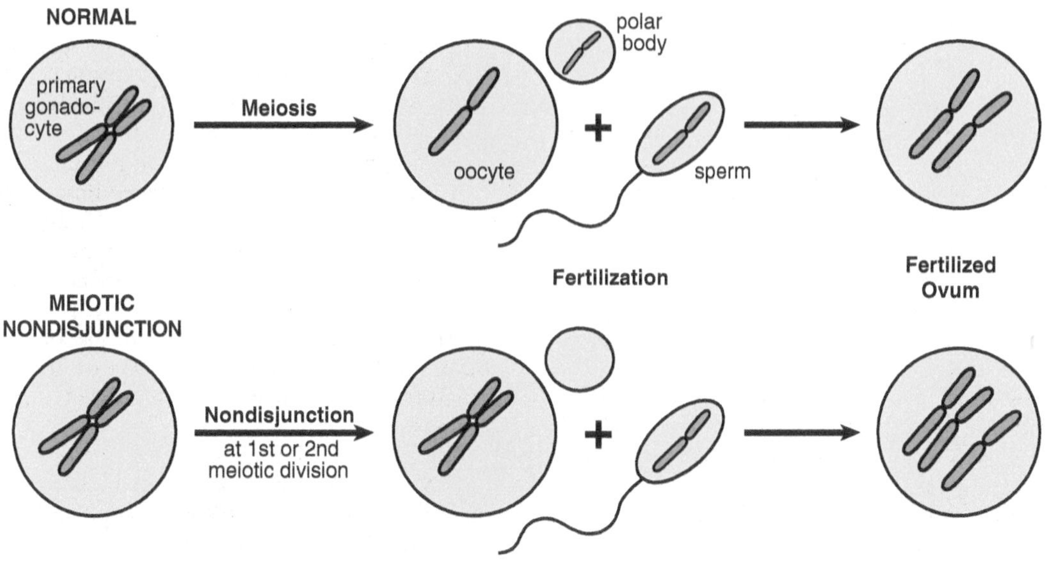


**Figure 2.7** Graphic representation of meiotic nondisjunction. (Courtesy of Edith Cheng, MD.)

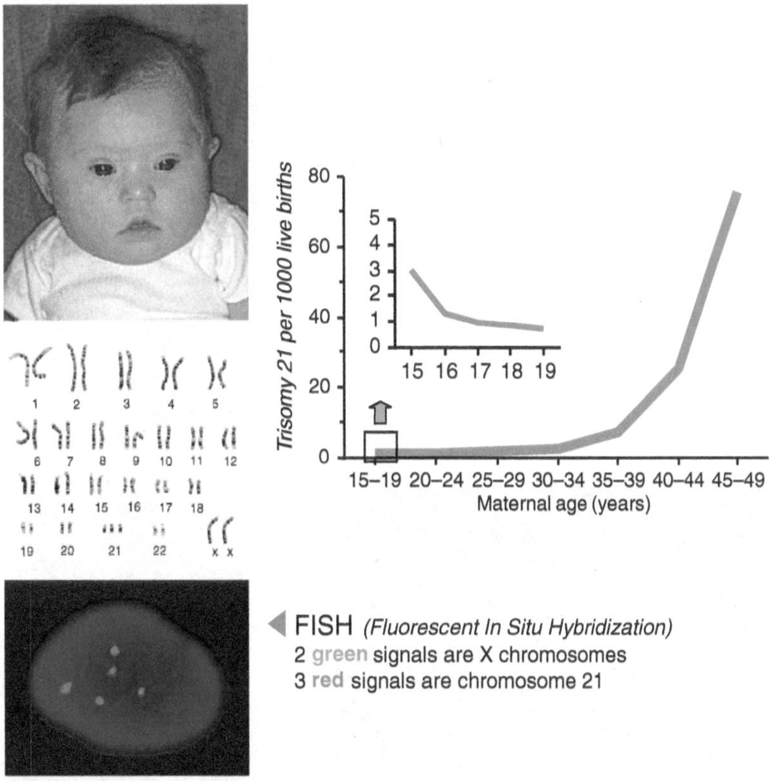


**Figure 2.8** Trisomy 21 infant with karyotype demonstrating three separate chromosomes 21. Interphase fluorescent in situ hybridization (FISH) illustration of screening for trisomy 21. Graph illustrating the maternal age association and increasing risk for aneuploidy. Note that there is an increased risk at the peripubertal ages as well. (Courtesy of Edith Cheng, MD.)

cardiac defects), and postaxial polydactyly. Trisomy 18 (Edwards syndrome) is found in 1/6000 live births and is associated with prenatal growth restriction, rocker bottom feet, and cardiac and renal defects. Trisomy 21 is the most common viable autosomal trisomy and has an incidence of 1/800 live births. The majority (95%) of individuals with Down syndrome have complete trisomy 21—that is, three separate copies of chromosome 21 because of maternal nondisjunction. However, about 2% to 3% of individuals with clinical Down syndrome have a structural rearrangement (Robertsonian translocation—to be discussed in the next section), and another 1% to 3% are mosaic for trisomy 21 (Jones, 2006). Trisomy 22 has been seen in a few live-born individuals and is associated with severe neurologic impairment. Monosomic states involving autosomes are extremely rare and generally lethal.

Sex chromosome aneuploidy usually occurs in the trisomic state. Monosomy Y is lethal and has never been seen in a clinical situation or even in an abortus. In contrast, monosomy of the X chromosome (known as *Turner syndrome*) is the most common chromosomal abnormality found in first trimester abortuses. Because most 45,X conceptions are lethal, the actual incidence of live female births is about 1/5000. At birth, Turner syndrome is characterized by lymphedema, hypotonia, and webbed neck. Girls with Turner syndrome have short stature, a broad chest with widely spaced nipples, cubitus valgus (widened carrying angle of the arms), and gonadal dysgenesis resulting in a lack of secondary sex characteristics, amenorrhea, and infertility (Fig. 2.9). Other features include congenital heart disease (coarctation of the aorta is the most common), kidney disease, and hypertension in later life. Intelligence is generally normal although spatial perception abnormalities are common (Jones, 2006). Hormonal supplementation during puberty allows girls with Turner syndrome to develop secondary sex characteristics.

Unlike autosomal trisomies in which the majority are maternally derived, the 45,X karyotype occurs through paternal nondisjunction and is not associated with advanced maternal or paternal age. There is no increased recurrence for 45,X, which accounts for 50% of women with Turner syndrome. Another 30% to 40% of individuals are mosaic for the 45,X cell line and another cell line (usually 46,XX) because of postzygotic nondisjunction during mitosis. The clinical features of these women will vary depending on the proportion of normal 46,XX cell lines present. However, females who are mosaic with a 45,X/46,XY karyotype are at an increased risk for gonadoblastoma. Therefore women suspected of having Turner syndrome should have a chromosomal analysis, not only for diagnosis but for exclusion of mosaicism for a 46,XY cell line. The remaining 10% to 20% of individuals with Turner syndrome have a structural abnormality of the X chromosome (Table 2.5).

Other trisomies involving the sex chromosomes are seen in 47,XXX, 47,XXY (Klinefelter syndrome), and 47,XYY karyotypes. The incidence of 47,XXX is approximately 1/1000 live female births and is due to maternal nondisjunction associated with increasing maternal age. Most women are phenotypically normal with the exception of possible mild developmental delay; fertility is normal and there may be a slightly increased risk for offspring with aneuploidy involving the sex chromosomes and

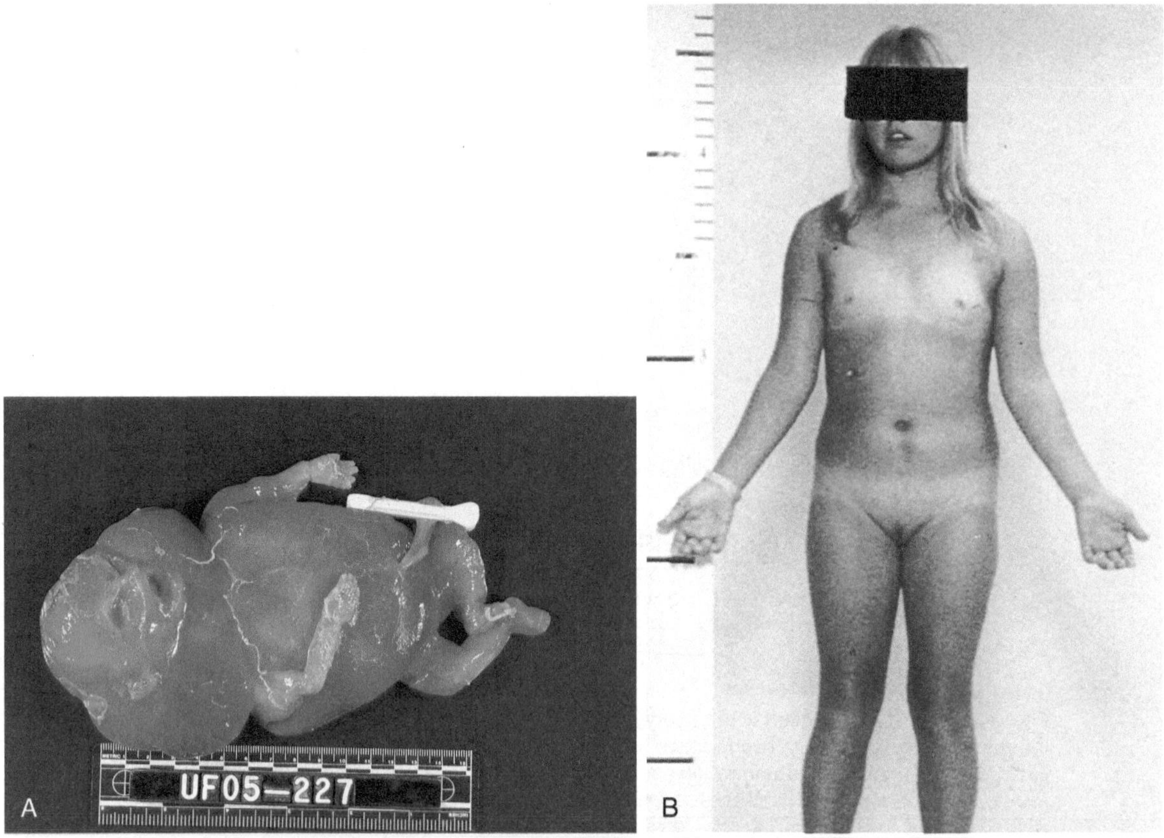


**Figure 2.9** **A**, Photo of a 20-week fetus with Turner syndrome, 45,X. This fetus was diagnosed during a routine 20-week ultrasound for anatomy and growth and was found to have a large cystic hygroma and hydrops. The autopsy revealed a complex cardiac defect, abnormal kidneys, streaked ovaries, and malrotation of the gut with the appendix in the left lower quadrant. **B**, A 17-year-old woman with Turner syndrome. Note the short stature, poor sexual development, and increased carrying angles at elbows. Subject also has webbing of the neck. (**A**, Courtesy of Drs. W. Tony Parks and Corrine Fligner, Department of Pathology, University of Washington.)

autosomes. Klinefelter syndrome, 47,XXY, is a common sex chromosome abnormality associated with maternal age and occurs in 1/1000 live male births. Clinical features include tall gynecoid stature, gynecomastia (with an increased risk for breast cancer), and testicular atrophy. Mental retardation is not a typical feature, but affected individuals may have IQ scores that are lower than those of their siblings. Nondisjunction during spermatogenesis involving the Y chromosome leads to 47,XYY. These males may be taller than average, but they are otherwise phenotypically normal. Contrary to previous and outdated observational studies, this sex chromosome aneuploidy is not associated with an increased disposition to violent crime. However, behavioral problems such as attention deficit disorder may be observed.

Nondisjunctional events during mitosis in the early embryo (after fertilization) will produce individuals with cell populations containing different chromosome numbers. This condition, known as *mosaicism*, may involve the autosomes or the sex chromosomes. The actual phenotype depends on the proportion of aneuploid and euploid cells in the embryo and in the specific organs or tissues involved.

Table 2.5 Karyotypes Discovered in Subjects with Phenotypic Characteristics of Turner Syndrome

| Karyotype | Error |
|---|---|
| 45,X | Deletion X |
| 45,Xi(Xq) | Deletion Xp, Isochromosome Xq |
| 45,X,Xq | Deletion Xp |
| 45,X/46,XX | Mosaicism |
| 45,X/46,XX/47,XXX | Mosaicism |
| 45,X/46,XY | Mosaicism |
| 45,X/46,XY/47,XYY | Mosaicism |
| 45,XringX | Ring chromosome |
| 46,XX | Phenotype with normal karyotype |

### *Structural Chromosome Abnormalities*

Chromosome breaks and rearrangements may lead to no obvious phenotypic consequences (genetically balanced), loss or gain of chromosomal material (genetically imbalanced) that produces abnormalities, or abnormalities resulting from the interruption of a critical gene at the breakpoint site on the chromosome. Types of structural rearrangements include *translocations* (reciprocal and Robertsonian), insertions, *inversions*, *isochromosomes*, duplications, and deletions. The rate of formation of balanced rearrangements is generally very low, $1.6 \times 10^{-4}$, although some chromosomal segments (hot spots) are more prone to breakage than others.

#### Balanced Reciprocal Translocations

Translocations occur as a result of a mutual and physical exchange of chromosome (genetic) material between nonhomologous chromosomes, or chromosomes that are not part of an identical matched pair. There are two main types of translocations, reciprocal and Robertsonian. Balanced reciprocal translocations are found in about 1/11,000 newborns. Figure 2.10 is an example of a hypothetical balanced translocation between the short arms (p arm) of two chromosomes. The carrier of a reciprocal balanced translocation is usually phenotypically normal. However, the carrier is at an increased risk for producing offspring who are chromosomally abnormal. The viability of the genetically unbalanced gametes is highly dependent on the location and amount of involved DNA. In general, however, the recurrence for an unbalanced conception is 3% to 5% for male carriers and 10%

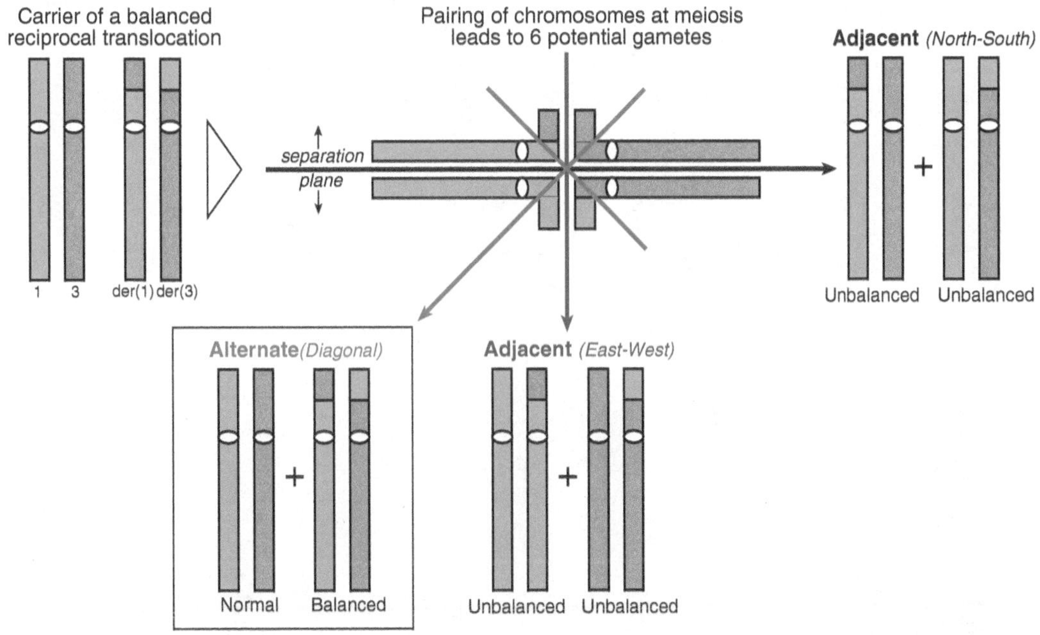


**Figure 2.10** Schematic representation of segregation patterns of a diploid gamete with a reciprocal balanced translocation. Here, exchanges have occurred between the short arms of chromosomes 1 and 3. The two pairs of chromosomes pair in a quadriradial fashion. There are three potential axes in which the cell can divide. Only two of the six potential gametes will be genetically balanced. (Courtesy of Edith Cheng, MD.)

to 15% for female carriers of reciprocal balanced translocations. Recurrence risks depend on the chromosomes involved and the size of the translocated segments.

A second and important type of translocation is the Robertsonian translocation. This is a structural rearrangement between the acrocentric chromosomes: chromosome pairs 13, 14, 15, 21, and 22. These chromosomes have a centromere that is severely offset from the center such that the short arm (p arm) contains minimal genetic material, which can be lost with little or no functional consequence. In this structural rearrangement, the short arms (p arms) of two nonhomologous chromosomes are lost, and the long arms fuse at the *centromere*, forming a single chromosome structure. Figure 2.11 is an example of a Robertsonian translocation involving chromosomes 14 and 21. The phenotypically normal carrier of a Robertsonian translocation has 45 chromosomes in each cell because the two acrocentric chromosomes involved in the translocation have formed into one chromosome structure. This Robertsonian translocation carrier is genetically balanced—that is, he or she has two copies of each chromosome. However, the gametes are at risk to be unbalanced.

One important exception in translocation Down syndrome is that associated with a 21q21q translocation. Here, the chromosome structure is composed of two chromosomes 21. Although this chromosome rearrangement is extremely rare, this translocation confers a 100% risk that the carrier will have abnormal gametes and 100% of viable gametes will result in a conception with Down syndrome. The only other possible outcome is monosomy 21, a complement that is miscarried early.

Chromosome inversions occur when two breaks occur on a chromosome followed by a 180-degree turn of the segment and reinsertion at its original breakpoints. If the centromere is included in the inverted segment, it is called a *pericentric inversion*. If the centromere is not involved, then the inversion is called a *paracentric inversion*. Chromosome inversions are generally considered balanced and usually do not confer an abnormal phenotype unless one of the breakpoints disrupts a critical gene. Inversions, however, do interfere with pairing at meiosis and can result in gametes with chromosome abnormalities.

Isochromosomes occur as a result of the chromosome dividing along the horizontal axis rather than the longitudinal axis at the centromere. The result is a chromosome that has two copies of one arm (p or q) and no copies of the other. Isochromosomes involving autosomes are generally lethal because the resultant conception will be both trisomic and monosomic for genetic information. However, an isochromosome involving the long arm of the X chromosome (iso Xq) is compatible with life.

Finally, deletions and duplications of chromosome segments arise from unequal crossing over at meiosis or from crossing over during pairing of inversions or reciprocal translocations. Breaks resulting in loss of chromosome material at the tip are called *terminal deletions*, and loss of chromosome material between two breaks within a chromosome is called an *interstitial deletion*. There are several well-documented terminal deletion syndromes, including cri du chat (5p-) syndrome, characterized by microcephaly, profound mental retardation, growth retardation, a unique facial appearance, and a distinctive catlike cry.

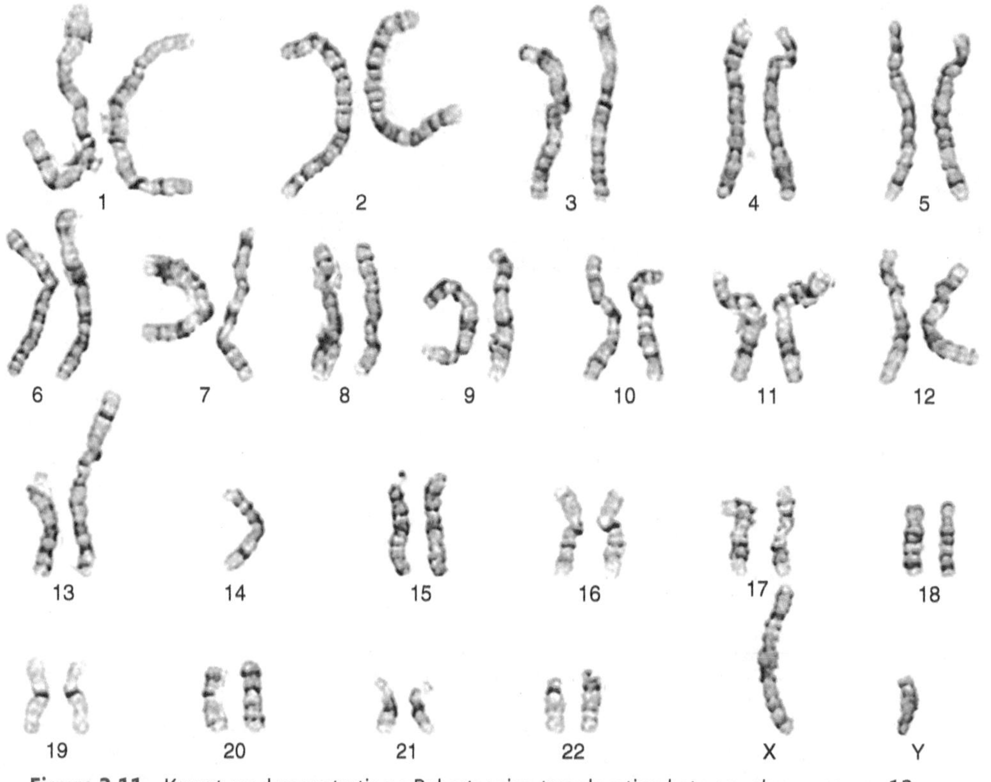


**Figure 2.11** Karyotype demonstrating a Robertsonian translocation between chromosomes 13 and 14. Notice that there are only 45 chromosome structures, but this male is genetically diploid. (Courtesy of Edith Cheng, MD.)

For each of the previously described structural chromosome rearrangements, counseling and prognosis in the prenatal diagnostic setting are critically dependent on comparison to parental karyotypes. Phenotype correlations, particularly with balanced translocations and inversions, may be highly variable and dependent on whether the chromosomal break points disrupt critical genes. If the rearrangement found in a fetal sample is inherited from one of the parents, there is a higher likelihood of a normal phenotype, whereas de novo structural rearrangements have an increased risk of microscopic missing genetic material with phenotypic consequences.

### Microdeletion/Duplication or Contiguous Gene Syndromes

The discussion in the previous section described only phenotypes that were associated with chromosome abnormalities visible with traditional cytogenetic techniques and light microscopy that imply involvement of large segments of chromosomes containing a large number (hundreds) of genes. High-resolution chromosome banding and advances in molecular cytogenetic technology have revealed a new class of chromosome syndromes known as *microdeletions*. These are contiguous gene syndromes in which the involved chromosome region(s) are submicroscopic and so small that a molecular cytogenetic technique such as targeted fluorescent in situ hybridization (FISH), or some form of sequence analysis, is necessary to localize the affected region. Table 2.6 lists some of the more commonly recognized syndromes, most of which are due to deletions; however, some duplication syndromes have now been identified. The phenotypes of these conditions are due to the absence (or duplication) of multiple contiguous genes within the involved region. Fine mapping of the breakpoints in some of these conditions has implicated unequal or abnormal recombination between low-copy repetitive DNA sequences in the area of the deleted or duplicated regions. The discovery of microdeletion/duplication or contiguous gene syndromes has been important in clinical genetics and genetic counseling in that it finally provides a diagnosis, recurrence risk, and prenatal diagnosis for a large group of syndromes that previously had no cytogenetic confirmation. Moreover, these "naturally occurring" sequestered small regions of contiguous genes have provided a powerful tool for developmental geneticists to decipher the critical genes for normal human development. For example, the 22q11 region appears to be rich in genes responsible for specific congenital heart defects and craniofacial anomalies. Importantly, microdeletions/duplications have no age-associated risk of occurrence (Wapner, 2012).

## CHROMOSOME ABNORMALITIES AND PREGNANCY OUTCOME

The incidence and types of chromosome abnormalities differ among spontaneous abortions, stillbirths, and live births. Experience from pregnancies achieved by assisted reproductive technology indicates that 15% of fertilized ova fail to divide. Another 15% fail to implant, and 25% to 30% are aborted spontaneously prior to formation of villi. Of the roughly 40% of fertilized ova that survive the first missed menstrual period, as many as one fourth are aborted spontaneously, so only about 30% to 35% of fertilized ova actually result in live-born infants. Chromosome and lethal genetic abnormalities play a major role in early losses (Zinaman, 1996). This topic is discussed further in Chapter 16. In continuing pregnancies, chromosome abnormalities occur in 1 out of every 154 live births (0.6% overall incidence). The breakdown by type of abnormality is as follows: 22% autosomal trisomy (most commonly trisomy 21, followed by a much lower incidence of trisomy 18 and trisomy 13), 37% sex chromosome aneuploidy, and 41% structural abnormalities (including translocations, insertions, inversions, isochromosomes, duplications, and deletions). Trisomy 21 is the most commonly occurring singular genetic abnormality in live births, occurring at a rate of 1 in 830 live births (0.1%) (Creasy, 2014).

# PERINATAL GENETICS

There is currently available technology to detect a wide range of the previously described genetic and biochemical abnormalities in a developing fetus. As a result, the indications to pursue screening or diagnostic testing for a patient who is pregnant or considering pregnancy include each of the following: known family history of a specific disease, family history suggestive of hereditary neurodevelopmental or cognitive disorders, ethnic background with increased carrier frequency of certain diseases, personal history of miscarriage or infertility, increased risk of aneuploidy related to maternal age, or simply population-based screening risk.

## GENETIC TESTING

Although genetic assessment in some form has become commonplace, it is critically important that providers and patients carefully consider the objectives and potential results of the individual testing options when selecting a test. In the case of aneuploidy screening, the assayed markers only pertain to a *subset*

**Table 2.6** Common Microdeletion/Contiguous Gene Syndromes

| | | Chromosome | | |
|---|---|---|---|---|
| **Syndrome** | **Incidence** | **Location** | **Abnormality** | **Size (Mb)** |
| Sotos | Rare | 5q35 | Deletion | 2.2 |
| Smith-Magenis | 1/25,000 | 17p11.2 | Deletion and duplication | 4 |
| Williams-Beuren | 1/20,000-1/50,000 | 7q11.23 | Deletion | 1.5-1.8 |
| Charcot-Marie-Tooth Type Ia / HNPP | 1/10,000 | 17p12 | Duplication and deletion | 1.5 |
| DiGeorge/velocardiofacial | 1/4,000 | 22q11.21-q11.23 | Deletion | 1.5 |
| Cat's eye | Rare | 22q11 | Duplication | 3 |
| der(22) Emanuel | Rare | | Duplication | 3 |
| Neurofibromatosis | 1/40,000-1/80,000 | 17q11 | Deletion | 1.5 |

of genetic material (usually the most common trisomies, affecting chromosomes 21, 13, 18, and possibly sex chromosomes), and abnormal results require follow up before any diagnosis can be made. Measuring the value of screening tests is traditionally based on sensitivity (detection rate), false-positive rate, and positive predictive value within a population. The predictive value of these tests, or the chance that a positive or negative result is a true positive or true negative, is highly dependent on the prevalence of the disease in the population.

Testing for a specific disease may be warranted by family history or ethnic background, and prenatal diagnosis may potentially allow interventions before the disease would have been detected in the child clinically (Table 2.7). In some rare cases, diagnosis in utero may allow the opportunity to preclude irreversible changes in early development. However, the provider must relay the *scope* and *accuracy* of available testing modalities. For instance, a test that detects a phenotypic manifestation of disease (such as biochemical screening of hexosaminidase activity to assess for Tay-Sachs) is more sensitive for detecting an affected fetus than a genetic sequence panel that may include only a subset of the disease-causing mutations. Alternatively, combination testing "panels" may be available that allow assessment for multiple diseases at once, but all tests are based on the same molecular methods, such as DNA sequence or SNP analysis, so sensitivity of detection for specific diseases may be sacrificed. The increasing availability of these "expanded carrier screening panels" has prompted the American College of Obstetricians and Gynecologists to issue guidelines for patient consent prior to offering expanded screening (Edwards, 2015):

1. Carrier screening of any nature is voluntary, and it is reasonable to accept or decline.
2. Results of genetic testing are confidential and protected in health insurance and employment by the Genetic Information Non-Discrimination Act of 2008.
3. Conditions included on expanded carrier screening panels vary in severity. Many are associated with significant adverse outcomes such as cognitive impairment, decreased life expectancy, and need for medical or surgical intervention.
4. Pregnancy risk assessment depends on accurate knowledge of paternity. If the biologic father is not available for carrier screening, accurate risk assessment for recessive conditions is not possible.
5. A negative screen does not eliminate risk to offspring.
6. Because expanded carrier screening includes a large number of disorders, it is common to identify carriers for one or more conditions. In most cases, being a carrier of an autosomal recessive condition has no clinical consequences for the individual carrier. If each partner is identified as a carrier of a different autosomal recessive condition, offspring are not likely to be affected.
7. In some instances, individuals may learn that they have two pathogenic variants for a condition (homozygous or compound heterozygous) and thus learn through carrier screening that they have an autosomal recessive condition that could affect their personal health. Some expanded screening panels screen for selected autosomal dominant and X-linked conditions, and likewise individuals may learn that they have one of these conditions that might affect their health. Referral to an appropriate specialist for medical management and genetic counseling is indicated in such circumstances to review the inheritance patterns, recurrence risks, and clinical features.

### Genetic Counseling and Risk Assessment

Ordering and sending a genetic test is simple, but the counseling time to ensure appropriate interpretation of the results (positive or negative) is crucial and often time consuming. The role of the care providers (genetic counselors and physicians) is to conduct nondirectional counseling of screening and diagnostic options to provide prospective parents with information to optimize pregnancy outcomes based on their personal values and preferences.

All patients considering genetic screening or testing should have the opportunity to meet with providers who can perform formal pedigrees, conduct patient education and counseling on advantages and disadvantages of testing, and discuss the availability of screening and invasive diagnostic testing when needed.

**Table 2.7** Common Autosomal Recessive Disorders in Ethnic Groups: Carrier Screening Recommended

| Ethnic Group | Genetic Disorder | Carrier Frequency in Ethnic Group | Frequency of Carrier Couples | Screening Test Available? | Detection Rate (%) |
|---|---|---|---|---|---|
| African ancestry | Sickle cell disease (HbS and C) | HbS, 1:10<br>HBC, 1 :20 | 1:130 | Hb electrophoresis | 100 |
| | Sickle cell S-β-thalassemia | | | MCV, Hb electrophoresis | |
| | α-Thalassemia | | | MCV, DNA | |
| Ashkenazi Jews (and Jews of unknown descent) | Tay-Sachs disease | 1:30 | 1:150 | Hexosaminidase A level | 98 |
| | Canavan disease | 1:40 | 1:1600 | DNA mutation | |
| | Familial dysautonomia | 1/32 | 1:32 | DNA mutation | 99 |
| Chinese | α-Thalassemia | | 1:625 | MCV | |
| French Canadian, Cajun | Tay-Sachs disease | | | Hexosaminidase A level | |
| Mediterranean (Italian/Greek/Turks/Spaniards) | β-Thalassemia | | 1:900 | MCV | |
| All patients seeking preconception counseling (especially whites of European origin) | Cystic fibrosis | 1:25-29 | 1:625 | DNA mutation | 80* |

*Hb*, Hemoglobin; *MCV*, mean corpuscular volume.
*Depends on ethnic group: 70% for southern European descent, 90% for northern European descent.
From Creasy RK, Resnik R, Greene MF, et al. *Creasy and Resnik's Maternal-Fetal Medicine Principles and Practice*. 7th ed. Philadelphia: Elsevier; 2014.

Before screening or testing, the patient needs to understand the options that may ensue from a positive test result.

### Biochemical and Sonographic Screening

Multiple screening options are available for detecting fetuses at risk for the most common aneuploidy syndromes, namely trisomies 21, 18, and 13. The choice of test will depend on the gestational age at presentation, number of fetuses, previous obstetric history, family history, availability of sonologists or sonographers certified to detect or measure test parameters, and options or preferences for pregnancy termination.

First trimester screening typically consists of serum measurement of pregnancy-associated plasma protein A (PAPP-A) and either free or total beta human chorionic gonadotropin (βhCG) combined with sonographic measurement of a fluid collection at the back of the fetal neck called the *nuchal translucency* (the three measurements together are called "combined first trimester screening"). Nuchal translucency measurements are validated for the specific gestational age window from $10^{4/7}$weeks to $13^{6/7}$ weeks as determined by crown-rump length, and guidelines for measurement are standardized, which must be followed for the test to maintain published detection rates. A nuchal translucency measurement less than 3 mm is considered normal (Malone, 2005). The primary advantage of first trimester screening is earlier results, which allow for greater privacy and broader options of diagnostic testing and reproductive choices.

Second trimester biochemical screening for aneuploidy (available between about 15 and 20 weeks' gestation) combines measurement of maternal serum alpha-fetoprotein (msAFP), human chorionic gonadotropin (hCG), and unconjugated estriol (to make up the "triple screen"), and it may include inhibin A (called a "quad screen"). There are various iterations of screening, which combine elements of both first and second trimester screening measurements, and performance statistics of these methods depend on the specific analytes included, whether the measurements are independent of one another, and the timing of risk calculation. The most favorable performance statistics are achieved with the "integrated screening" approach, which combines first trimester PAPP-A and nuchal translucency with quad markers in the second trimester, and results are not reported until all measurements are obtained. This method has a Down syndrome detection rate of 94% to 96% with a false-positive rate of 5%, but the advantage of an early result is lost if first trimester screening results are withheld until second trimester screening results have been obtained (Malone, 2005).

Abnormal results of some of the individual elements assayed in aneuploidy screening are also predictive of adverse pregnancy outcomes. For example, abnormal biochemical markers on both first and second trimester screens have been associated with fetal growth restriction, intrauterine fetal demise, preterm delivery, Smith-Lemli-Opitz syndrome (low estriol), and oligohydramnios—albeit with low predictive value (Smith, 2006). Maternal serum AFP (msAFP) is very useful for detection of neural tube defects when measured between 16 and 18 weeks' gestation; the American College of Obstetricians and Gynecologists (ACOG) recommendations include msAFP alone (not in conjunction with the quad screen) as an adjunct test for women who choose first trimester screening for aneuploidy (ACOG, 2007).

### Cell-Free DNA Analysis Noninvasive Prenatal Testing

Early attempts at noninvasive genetically based prenatal screening were focused on isolation of intact fetal cells within the maternal circulation. To date, this technology has been unsuitable for clinical application due to multiple technologic obstacles such as limited numbers of fetal cells, unreliable recovery of fetal cells, and evidence that the cells persist long after pregnancy, thus complicating specificity in the setting of subsequent pregnancies (Bianchi, 2002).

In contrast, the development of methods to identify fetally derived cell-free DNA in maternal plasma has been more successful (Lo, 1997). The initial application of technology to assess cell-free fetal DNA was focused on single-gene disorders for which the abnormal DNA sequence was known in the family, or for determination of fetal gender in cases of families carrying traits for X-linked recessive diseases.

The advent of next-generation sequencing, a high-throughput method of sequencing millions of DNA fragments simultaneously in parallel, rapidly expanded the amount of data that can be gathered from fetal DNA in maternal plasma in a time frame amenable to prenatal screening applications. As a result, cell-free DNA tests to screen for fetal aneuploidy moved quickly through development and into clinical use by 2011 in the United States and Asia, followed by Canada and Europe in 2012. The performance statistics for Down syndrome detection in a high-risk population are far better than any other available methods (Table 2.8); however, the supplementary predictive value of nuchal translucency measurement or biochemical testing is lost (Gil, 2015). There are several available platforms for cell-free fetal DNA analysis; providers should be familiar with whether a chosen assay is designed to detect all chromosomes or only selected chromosomal regions. Furthermore, there is active debate over how to interpret results that are insufficient or results that are discrepant from confirmatory invasive testing. Causes of discrepant results include low fetal fraction of DNA, confined placental mosaicism, true fetal mosaicism, maternal sex chromosome abnormality, organ transplant, co-twin demise, maternal chromosome deletion, maternal tumor, and lab error. Inadequate fetal fraction

**Table 2.8** Screening Test Performance: Prenatal Screening for Down Syndrome

| Test | Detection Rate | False-Positive Rate | PPV (High-Risk) Tri21 Prevalence 1:100 | PPV (Low-Risk) Tri21 Prevalence 1:500 |
|---|---|---|---|---|
| Combined First Tri (NT, PAPP-A, hCG) | 80% | 3% | 21% | 5% |
| Quad (AFP, hCG, inhibin A, estriol) | 60% | 3% | 17% | 4% |
| Sequential screen (Combined First Tri plus Quad) | 97% | 3% | 24% | 6% |
| Cell-free DNA (all methods combined, [Gil, 2015]) | 99.2% | 0.09% | 91.3% | 67.8% |

has been repeatedly demonstrated in a higher proportion of women with elevated body mass index (BMI), and average fetal fraction varies between ethnic groups. Interestingly, the aneuploidy rate is much higher in samples with inadequate fetal fraction than in the general population, suggesting that "no readout" results should be considered a form of positive screen (Norton, 2015).

Current guidelines from multiple U.S. and international professional societies recommend the use of cell-free DNA screening be limited to women with increased risk of fetal aneuploidy. This includes women of advanced maternal age (>35 years at delivery); women with ultrasound findings indicating increased risk of trisomy 13, 18, or 21; prior pregnancy history of a fetus with trisomy 13, 18, or 21; biochemical screening result positive for increased risk of aneuploidy; or known parental balanced Robertsonian translocation with increased risk of trisomy 13 or 21. The relatively lower contribution of Down syndrome to all congenital anomalies in a low-risk cohort argues for the use of a screening tool with a broader scope. Nonetheless, cell-free fetal DNA screening is an area of active research and development, and detection capabilities for a wider range of microdeletion/duplication syndromes may be routine in the near future (Wapner, 2014).

There are promising data on testing applications for accurate detection of fetal microdeletion syndromes such as 22q11.2 (DiGeorge), deletion 5p (cri du chat), and 1p36 (Noonan) using an SNP-based noninvasive prenatal testing (NIPT) approach (Wapner, 2015). Microdeletions are a significant cause of neurocognitive abnormalities, and, importantly, they have no age associated risk, so younger patients have a much higher likelihood of having a child with a clinically significant microdeletion than of having a child with trisomy 21. Thus validation of microdeletion testing from cfDNA samples will significantly expand the utility of NIPT in the general population.

## DIAGNOSTIC TECHNIQUES FOR GENETIC ABNORMALITIES

### Invasive Prenatal Diagnostic Tests

For the goal of prenatal *diagnosis*, the most commonly employed forms of genetic testing are chorionic villus sampling and amniocentesis to obtain cellular samples from pregnancy tissue for cytogenetic analysis.

In the early days of prenatal diagnosis, invasive testing options were offered to women with a high age-related risk of aneuploidy. However, current ACOG recommendations are that all women, regardless of age or risk, be offered biochemical or ultrasound screening and invasive testing (ACOG, 2007). The decision to pursue invasive testing must incorporate considerations of level of risk that the fetus is affected, level of risk associated with the procedure, and the patient's personal impression of the impact of having an affected child. Of note, the risks involved with invasive testing may be much lower than estimates that have been previously quoted since the advent of invasive testing in the 1970s. Results of a meta-analysis that included only contemporary large studies (published after the year 2000, reporting greater than 1000 procedures) demonstrated no significant difference in the risk of miscarriage prior to 24 weeks' gestation for women undergoing amniocentesis or chorionic villus sampling (CVS) compared with those who do not have invasive testing (Akolekar, 2015). Procedure-related risk of miscarriage for amniocentesis was 0.1%, and for CVS it was 0.2%.

Nevertheless, rates of performance of these invasive procedures are significantly declining as screening tests with higher detection rates and lower false-positive rates have become available (i.e., cell-free DNA screening). It is important to note that the range of abnormalities that can be detected is far greater with invasive testing than with any available noninvasive screening tests.

CVS can be performed early in pregnancy (9 to 12 weeks' gestation), in which a biopsy of cytotrophoblast tissue is obtained via ultrasound-guided transabdominal or transcervical route. The patient should be aware of a small rate (1.1%) of indicated follow-up testing to resolve issues from maternal cell contamination or placental mosaicism, but overall cytogenetic diagnosis is successful in 99.7% of those tested (Ledbetter, 1990).

Amniocentesis, generally performed after 15 completed weeks of pregnancy, involves ultrasound-guided transabdominal collection of amniotic fluid containing sloughed fetal cells from skin, gastrointestinal tract, amnion and genitourinary tract.

The predominant use for CVS or amniocentesis samples is cytogenetic analysis. Cells can be analyzed directly or after cell culture for about a week to synchronize cells in metaphase for chromosomal Giemsa staining, or G-banding. With this type of staining, each chromosome has a unique pattern. The stained chromosomes are visualized under light microscopy, and large deletions or rearrangements can be detected (resolution on the order of 5 million to 10 million base pairs, or Mb). Higher resolution or more specific testing for known disease-causing chromosome regions such as 22q11 requires molecular cytogenetic technology. The most widely used procedure is fluorescent in situ hybridization (FISH). FISH takes advantage of the complimentary nature of DNA. In this approach, denatured DNA sequences labeled with a fluorescent dye are hybridized onto denatured chromosomes that have been immobilized onto a slide. The chromosomes are then viewed with a wavelength of light that excites the fluorescent dye (Fig. 2.12). FISH is a powerful tool to confirm or diagnose syndromes that are due to microdeletions of segments of chromosome material (Fig. 2.13).

At the individual gene level, disease-specific testing for families that carry known genetic mutations may be performed on cells from either of these invasive methods using polymerase chain reaction (PCR)–based methods (discussed later). An updated list of relatively common genetic conditions for which DNA-based prenatal diagnosis is available is kept on the Genetic Testing Registry website (www.ncbi.nlm.nih.gov/gtr).

Another powerful diagnostic and investigational tool for human chromosome analysis directly expanded from FISH technology is comparative genome hybridization (CGH). CGH is used to measure differences in copy number or dosage of a particular chromosome segment. Its initial application was in the study of gene dosage in normal and cancer cell lines (Fig. 2.14). This technology has since come into widespread use due to automated platforms allowing for assessment of thousands or even millions of DNA molecules at once and rapidly decreasing cost (see Chromosomal Microarray, presented later).

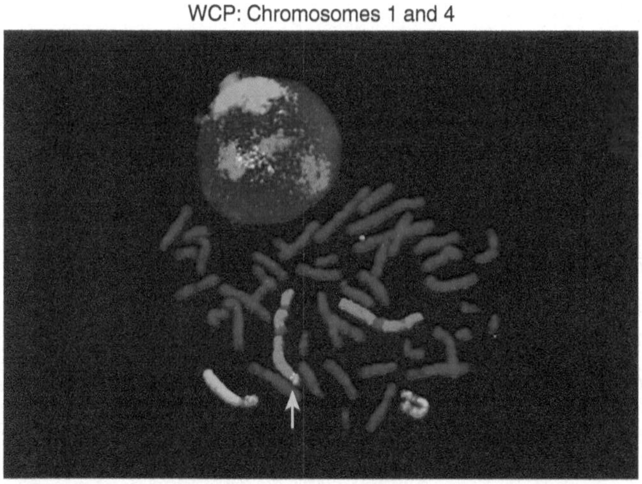


**Figure 2.12** Example of fluorescent in situ hybridization (FISH) with whole-chromosome DNA (whole-chromosome paint [WCP]) from chromosomes 1 (red signal) and 4 (green signal) hybridized onto a metaphase nucleus containing all 46 chromosomes. This FISH study revealed a translocation of a piece of material from chromosome 4 onto chromosome 1. (Courtesy of Lisa Shaffer, PhD, Washington State University.)

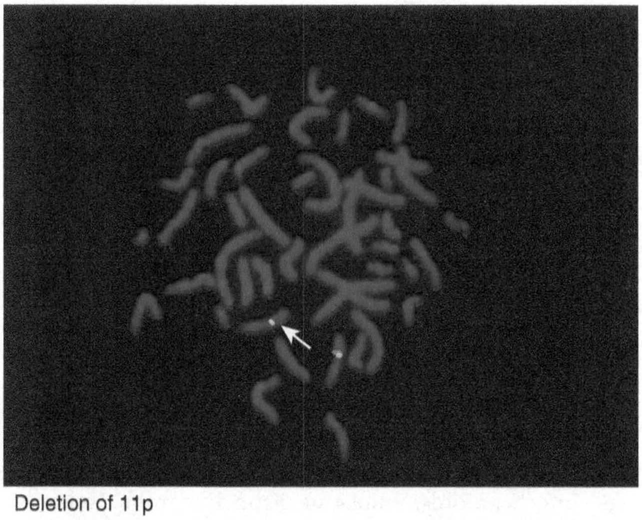


**Figure 2.13** Example of FISH technology in the diagnosis of microdeletion syndromes. Here, standard karyotyping appears to be normal. However, using FISH microdeletion probes, this child was discovered to have a submicroscopic deletion *(arrow)* of the terminal section of the long arm of chromosome 1. The other chromosome containing the red signal is the normal chromosome. (Courtesy of Lisa Shaffer, PhD, Washington State University.)

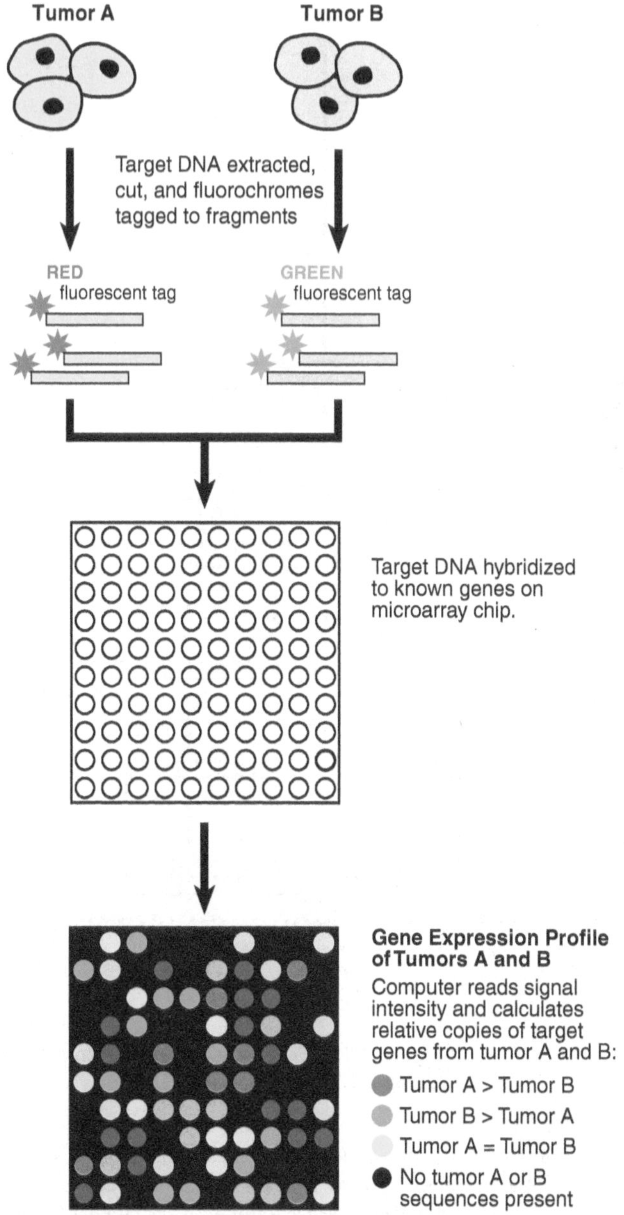


**Figure 2.14** Schematic example of how microarray technology can be used to study or compare gene expression patterns from different sources. Here it is used to compare the gene expression profiles of two different tumors. However, one can easily substitute DNA from two individuals with diabetes. (Courtesy of Edith Cheng, MD.)

### *Molecular Genetic Analysis Techniques*

#### Polymerase Chain Reaction, Southern Blot, Restriction Fragment Length Polymorphism, Linkage

The use of polymerase chain reaction (PCR) permits rapid amplification of a sequence of DNA or multiple different sequences simultaneously for analysis. This is essentially a form of cloning, because PCR can selectively amplify a single sequence of DNA or RNA several billion-fold in only a few hours. By taking advantage of the double-stranded complementary pairing characteristics of DNA, the PCR reaction separates (denatures) the two strands and uses each strand as a template to synthesize two more copies (Fig. 2.15). Target sequences of DNA flanked by primers undergo repeated cycles of heat penetration, hybridization with primers, and DNA synthesis, resulting in an exponential amplification of the target DNA sequence. The amplified DNA sequences can then be "cut" by bacterial enzymes, called *restriction endonucleases*, which recognize and cut specific nucleotide sequences (restriction sites) in the double-stranded DNA molecule. Each enzyme recognizes a unique sequence of nucleotides, usually a palindrome of four to eight base pairs (bp) in length. Because of this sequence specificity, the pattern of DNA fragments resulting from restriction endonuclease digestion will

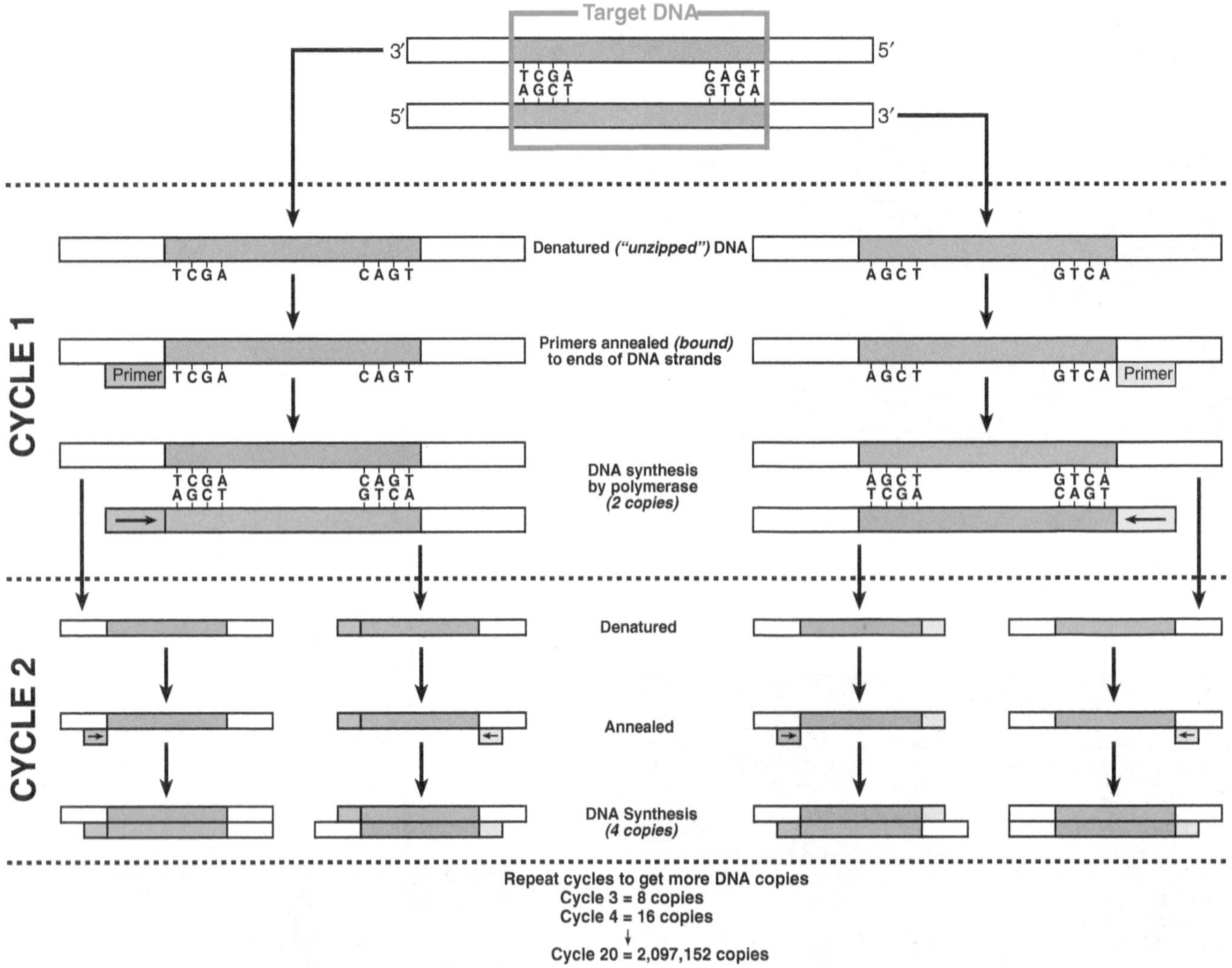


**Figure 2.15** Schematic representation of the polymerase chain reaction (PCR). (Courtesy of Edith Cheng, MD.)

be unique to each gene sequence. The resulting fragments are separated by gel electrophoresis, transferred (blotted) onto a membrane, and hybridized with a radioactively labeled probe with known sequence. This method, known as *Southern blotting*, permits identification of specific DNA fragments of interest and, in some cases, the number of copies of the fragment. Figure 2.16 is an example of how Southern blotting is used to detect the sickle cell gene. Mutations within a gene or near a gene can also alter the recognition sites of restriction endonucleases, which will generate an altered length of DNA fragment containing the gene of interest. These restriction fragment length polymorphisms (RFLPs) can be used to follow the transmission of a gene in a family.

When "direct testing" is not possible, as is the case when the disease-causing gene has not been isolated, when the gene is too large to sequence, or when a mutation cannot be directly found, indirect testing using linkage analysis is the alternative strategy. The simplest explanation for this concept is that DNA markers located (or tightly linked) to the presumptive disease-causing gene/mutation are used as road maps to identify the travel or passage of the gene from an affected parent to an at-risk offspring. This strategy requires that the affected individual has markers that are informative—in other words, unique or distinctive from markers of the nonaffected individual. Multiple family members, both affected and unaffected, must have DNA available for linkage analysis in order for this approach to be informative. The "markers" are often RFLPs. Figure 2.17 uses autosomal dominant breast cancer as an example of how linkage studies are used to predict the inheritance of a gene for which direct mutational analysis is not possible.

### *Chromosomal Microarray*

Chromosomal microarray is a high-throughput technique to detect relative "dose" of genetic material by comparison to a reference standard. A microarray generally consists of a thin slice of glass or silicon about the size of a postage stamp on which threads of synthetic nucleic acids are arrayed. Sample probes are added to the chip, and matches are read by an electronic scanner. The resolution of chromosomal microarray is on the order of 10 to 400 kb, or more than 100-fold greater resolution than traditional G-banding karyotyping.

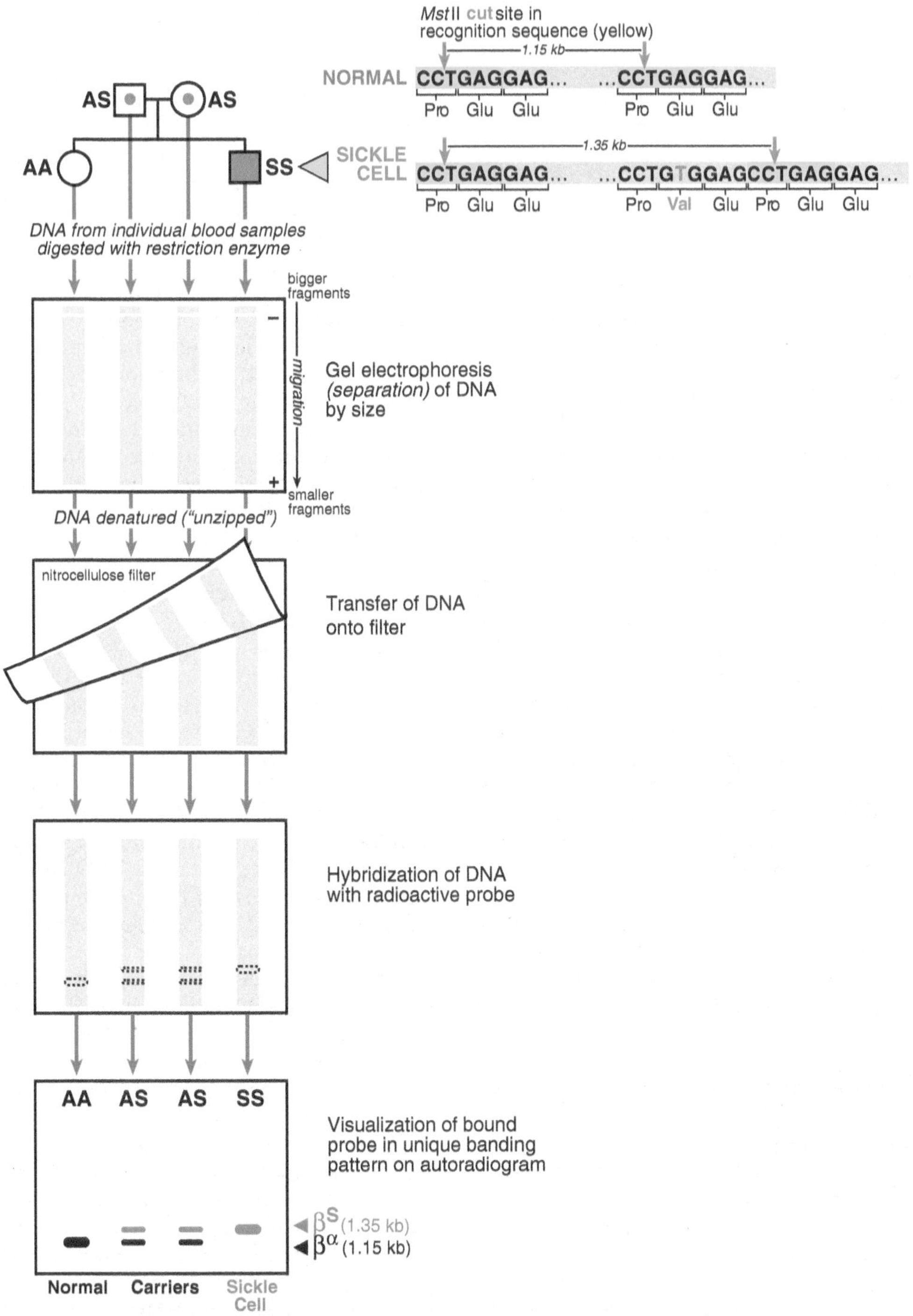


**Figure 2.16** Schematic representation of the Southern blot procedure—in this case, for diagnosis of sickle cell disease. Genomic DNA from the carrier parents, an unaffected daughter, and the affected son is extracted from a sample of peripheral blood. The DNA samples are digested with restriction enzymes and fragmented into smaller pieces. In this case, the restriction enzyme MstII is used specifically because it recognizes the normal sequences that encompass the codons for glutamic acid at position 6 of the hemoglobin A polypeptide. The DNA fragments are separated based on size by gel electrophoresis, then they are transferred (blotted) onto a nitrocellulose filter. The DNA of the filter paper is then hybridized with a specifically labeled DNA probe containing the sequences of interest. The fluorescent or radioactive probe is visualized as bands at sites where the genomic DNA has hybridized with the labeled DNA. (Courtesy of Edith Cheng, MD.)

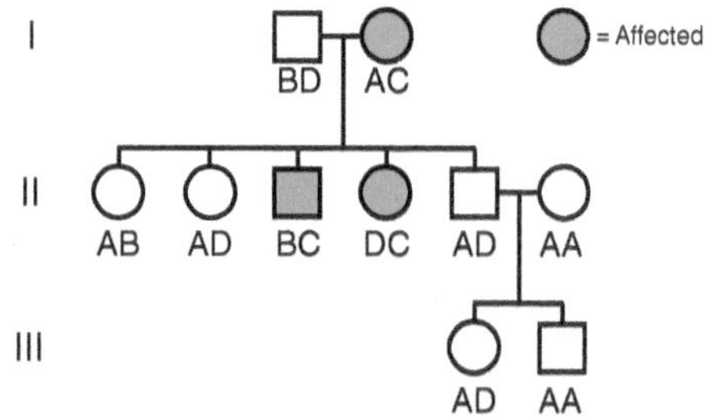


**Figure 2.17** Hypothetical autosomal dominant condition illustrating the principle of indirect mutational analysis. Genetic markers A, B, C, and D are used. In this pedigree, it appears that the condition segregates (travels) with marker C. Therefore the male and female in generation III, who did not inherit marker C, are not expected to manifest the condition. (Courtesy of Edith Cheng, MD.)

There are two general platforms in common use for genome assessment. The first is a form of comparative genomic hybridization, or "array CGH." In brief, two genomic libraries are mixed and hybridized to a panel of reference sequences such that relative "doses" of hybridized sequence can be quantitated. Using this platform, a patient's genome is compared with a normal control, and readout is expressed by comparative intensity between the patient and the control (Snijders, 2001).

The second popular platform is an SNP array. In an SNP array, probes are chosen from DNA locations known to vary by a single base pair. A patient's DNA is hybridized to the array (note this platform does not require a normal standard), and readout is by absolute intensity of signal from bound DNA fragments. This method can detect more abnormalities than just copy number, such as uniparental disomy, determine zygosity, parent of origin for a given mutation, and maternal cell contamination (Beaudet, 2008).

In neonatal and pediatric studies, microarray results have revealed underlying genetic etiologies for 15% to 20% of cases with previously unexplained developmental delay, intellectual disability, or congenital anomalies. Only about 3% of these cases would have been diagnosed by traditional karyotype (Miller, 2010).

In contrast to neonatal studies, which have the advantage of correlating genomic findings with complete physical exam and behavioral phenotype, prenatal applications are limited to phenotypic findings that can be detected by ultrasound. Several studies have demonstrated the incremental diagnostic utility of chromosomal microarray analysis in the setting of a fetus with one or more anomalies on ultrasound but normal karyotype. A prospective National Institute of Child Health and Human Development (NICHD) study identified clinically relevant copy number variants by microarray in 6% of anomalous fetuses with a normal karyotype (Wapner, 2012). Furthermore, the likelihood of identifying either pathogenic CNV or CNV of uncertain significance was more likely in fetuses with multiple anomalies, whereas for isolated findings, the greatest yield was in cardiac and renal anomalies (Donnelly, 2014). Chromosomal microarray is considered the first-line test of an individual with unexplained birth defects or mental retardation, or in unexplained stillbirth (Hillman, 2015).

Clinicians and genetic counselors must continue to exercise reasonable caution when interpreting results of microarray findings. Accurate genotype-phenotype correlations will require ongoing expansion of CNV databases. Many CNV may have dose-dependent phenotypic effects or may be modified by the presence of other genotypic variants.

Traditionally, screening modalities focused on diseases that significantly affect quality of life and have a fetal, neonatal, or early childhood onset and well-defined phenotype. In the post-genome era with high-throughput microarray technology, the identification of molecular alterations in DNA may reveal previously unrecognized genetic variants associated with disease. Yet variant recognition currently outstrips our ability to interpret these alterations. Previously unreported and relatively rare variants with unknown phenotypes will be identified, which requires skilled counseling and interpretation to help patients decide what to do with this information. Informing patients of variants of uncertain significance may generate significant anxiety and negative anticipation. Learning that one's fetus has an abnormality with unquantifiable risks of consequences naturally fosters apprehension, may lead to ambiguity about continuing the pregnancy, and has the potential to cast a shadow of worry in the parents' minds throughout the life of the child.

### *Preimplantation Genetic Diagnosis and Preimplantation Genetic Screening*

Preimplantation genetic diagnosis (PGD) refers to single cell extraction and genetic analysis from either an embryo or the polar body from an oocyte during the process of in vitro fertilization (see also Chapter 1). Initial impetus was to decrease the chances of propagating known genetic disorders in a family. The earliest application was in the setting of a patient known to carry an X-linked recessive gene, so only female embryos (by definition unaffected by the disease of interest) were transferred to the uterus. Since that time, PGD also has become readily available for diagnosis of translocations, single-gene disorders, and inherited mutations that are known to cause cancer susceptibility syndromes.

In contrast to disease-causing genetic abnormalities, there have been numerous studies attempting to use chromosomal aneuploidy screening of a single preimplantation cell (preimplantation genetic screening [PGS]) to improve assisted reproductive technology outcomes. All of the initial studies were based on FISH analysis of the single preimplantation cell, and none of these were able to demonstrate improved live birth rates following selection of embryos designated euploid by this method, thus ACOG did not recommend PGS for management of recurrent miscarriage or recurrent implantation failures (ACOG, 2009). More recently, however, SNP and PCR-based screening methods have been developed and are shown to be more comprehensive and accurate than FISH-based methods for aneuploidy diagnosis in embryo biopsy. A randomized trial using PGS to transfer a single euploid embryo demonstrated improved pregnancy rates compared with untested blastocyst transfer while decreasing the incidence of multiple pregnancies (Forman, 2013).

### *Sequencing*

Sequencing determines the complete nucleotide sequence, or specific order of nucleotides in a gene. By listing the full code, variations from an accepted "normal" (reference or consensus sequence) may be discovered. This has the potential to uncover pathogenic variants as well as benign variants and, given our limited understanding of how the genome is translated, will certainly identify variants of uncertain significance to clinical phenotype.

Clinical use of sequence data from the whole exome (protein-coding region of DNA), or ultimately the whole genome, is considered the next frontier in genetic diagnostic techniques. Whole-exome sequencing continues to raise the bar of expectation for molecular diagnosis with genetic analysis methods. The first large series of clinically applied whole exome analysis touted a 25% molecular diagnosis rate among all patients referred for phenotypes suggesting potential genetic component, and among patients in the study with a neurologic phenotype, molecular diagnosis was as high as 33% (Yang, 2013).

Goals of this magnitude have come within reach through development of *next-generation sequencing.* The original technique of sequencing, called *Sanger sequencing,* involves synthesizing multiple copies of DNA that is complementary to a single-stranded template of interest using nucleotide-specific chain terminators. This generates synthesized fragments of varying length that can be arranged by size, and the reactions containing each terminating base (A, T, G, or C) are kept separated. Then, by "reading" the terminating base of the synthesized copies from smallest to largest, the sequence of the original single-stranded template is revealed. This molecular method was revolutionary, but very time consuming, labor intensive, and limited to relatively short DNA sequences. The quest to uncover the sequence of all 3 billion bases in the human genome propelled extraordinary improvements in scale, speed, and data management. Next-generation sequencing involves preparation of a full DNA library (no longer one small segment at a time) by amplifying (making many copies) and fragmenting the DNA source of interest (genomic DNA, coding DNA). The DNA library now consists of thousands or even millions of small overlapping DNA copy fragments, which are physically bound to a solid surface (platform specific, often beads or glass slides). The fragments are loaded into specialized multiplex machines for parallel sequencing; in other words, the sequence of every fragment on the surface can be assayed simultaneously. Individual sequence reads are subsequently aligned (recall the expected overlap due to random fragmentation of many identical copies of DNA) using various bioinformatics platforms for comparison to a reference sequence. The full set of aligned reads reveals the entire sequence of the starting DNA product. Thus next-generation sequencing can apply the concept of Sanger sequencing to an entire genome with results produced in matter of hours.

At present, the practical clinical application of sequencing is to search one or many genes (or the whole genome) for a causative mutation in the setting of a recognized abnormal phenotype. Particularly in pediatric literature, sequencing has been reported to identify the genetic cause in cases of rare malformation syndromes and previously unexplained neurodevelopmental morbidity. Sequencing can be useful in prenatal counseling or diagnosis if the specific mutation can be identified for a previous child affected by a genetic disorder. Consider, for example, a family with a child diagnosed with cystic fibrosis, but only one parent has one of the known CF mutations. Sequencing of the CF gene in the *proband,* or first affected child, may reveal the previously unrecognized causative mutation in that family.

Data generated from sequencing methods are vast. The primary limitation of both whole-exome sequencing (WES) and whole-genome sequencing (WGS) is that accurate interpretation lags behind the ability to generate sequence data because sequencing is high throughput, but there are currently no similar high-throughput assays of function to assess putative pathologic sequence findings. There is enough natural variation in the human genome that any putative finding requires rigorous validation at the level of sequence, molecular function, and interaction within the full biologic system.

There are many interrogation tools to assess protein-coding portions of the genome. However, the comprehension of the remaining 98.5% of DNA sequence is relatively nascent, with no current way to assay functional loss or gain from these regions (Goldstein, 2013).

## GENETICS OF REPRODUCTIVE MALIGNANCIES

All cancer is genetic. However, most cancer is not inherited. For a normal cell line to be transformed into a malignant cell line, several genetic mutations in that somatic cell line must occur that alter cell growth and differentiation. All cells have mechanisms to either repair a mutation or inhibit growth and replication if errors in DNA occur. Thus before malignancy can arise, most cancer cells have to "escape" those repair functions. The first mutations must occur in either DNA repair genes or genes that suppress growth of abnormal cells (the genes that maintain the integrity of the genome). Subsequent mutations are then passed on to daughter cells. Increasing cell replications occur, and as mutations build up, some will allow the cell line to grow abnormally and often confer biologic advantages over surrounding normal cells. When "enough" DNA change occurs, the resulting abnormal cells are capable of metastasizing, thereby usurping resources of vital organs and, without treatment, eventually may lead to death. This process of multiple sequential mutations is called the "multistep process of cancer." In 5% to 10% of families with cancer, there is a germline (inherited) mutation that predisposes certain tissues to begin to move through the multistep series of mutations more easily. More than 50 inherited cancer syndromes have been described, although the majority of these are inherited through highly penetrant mutations in a dominant fashion. These inherited cancer genes do not cause cancer; rather they allow cancer to "happen more easily." Inherited cancer syndromes that affect female organs are listed in (Table 2.9).

Carefully regulated cellular processes, such as differentiation, proliferation, and programmed cell death, are altered in cancer cells. The stages of carcinogenesis are termed *initiation* (single initial proliferative cell), *promotion* (acquired selective growth advantage), *progression* (tumor characteristics become irreversible), and *metastasis* (process by which cells are displaced). Types of genes and genetic mechanisms involved in malignancy may be grouped into four categories: oncogenes, tumor suppressor genes, DNA repair genes, and epigenetic mechanisms.

Oncogenes (gain of function) behave as growth-promoting genes, and they act in a genetically dominant manner. In other words, only one abnormal copy of the gene will produce a clinically relevant phenotype due to increased gene function. They originate from normal cellular genes called proto-oncogenes. The proto-oncogenes have normal functions within a cell to

**Table 2.9** Inherited Cancer Syndromes Affecting Gynecologic Organ Systems

| Body Part | Cancer Syndrome | Gene Name/ Location |
|---|---|---|
| Breast | Inherited breast-ovarian cancer (autosomal dominant; tumor suppressor gene, involved in the maintenance of genomic stability) | *BRCA1*, 17q21 |
| | Inherited breast-ovarian cancer (autosomal dominant; tumor suppressor gene, involved in the maintenance of genomic stability) | *BRCA2*, 13q12.3 |
| | Li-Fraumeni (autosomal dominant; regulates the cell-cycle arrest that is required to permit repair of DNA damage) | *p53*, 17p13.1 |
| | Cowden | *PTEN*, 10q23.31 |
| | Peutz-Jeghers | *LKB1*, 19p13.3 |
| | p16$^{INK4a}$ | *CDKN2A*, 9p21.3 |
| | p14$^{arf}$ | *CDKN2A*, 9p21.3 |
| Endometrium | Chordoma | |
| | Cowden | |
| | Lynch syndrome (HNPCC) | |
| | Peutz-Jeghers | |
| Fallopian tube | Inherited breast-ovarian cancer | *BRCA1* |
| | Inherited breast-ovarian cancer | *BRCA2* |
| Ovarian | Basal cell nevus | |
| | Inherited breast-ovarian cancer | *BRCA1* |
| | Inherited breast-ovarian cancer | *BRCA2* |
| | Lynch syndrome (HNPCC) | |
| | Peutz-Jeghers | |
| Vulva | Fanconi | |

*HNPCC*, Hereditary nonpolyposis colorectal cancer.

control and enhance cell growth. Oncogene activation (through mutation) can lead to either increased expression of proteins or changes in structure and function of a proto-oncogene's product. For example, the HER 2/neu receptor may be overexpressed by an oncogene. Only a few inherited cancer syndromes involve oncogenes. Examples include the *RET*, *CDK4*, and *KIT* oncogenes. The *RET* oncogene is the underlying cause of multiple endocrine neoplasia (MEN type 2). These individuals have an increased risk to develop endocrine tumors.

Tumor suppressor genes restrain cell growth in damaged cells; therefore loss of the tumor suppressor gene through mutation leads to increased cell proliferation of abnormal cells and cancer development. They account for the majority of autosomal dominant cancer syndromes. Some examples include *BRCA1* and *BRCA2* genes, and the *p53* gene (Li-Fraumeni syndrome). Tumor suppressor genes are dominantly inherited. However, on the cellular level, they are recessive. In other words, a cell must have two genetic hits (one hit to each copy of the gene in question) before the cell can head down the multistep process to cancer. The first hit is inherited, and the second hit is acquired.

DNA repair genes identify and mend DNA replication errors made during replication. When they are nonfunctional, replication errors can lead to cancer development. Lynch syndrome (hereditary nonpolyposis colorectal cancer [HNPCC]) has at least four mismatch repair genes (*MLH1*, *MSH2*, *MSH6*, and *PMS2*) that predispose an individual to colon cancer and uterine cancer. One could imagine these genes as editors that find and correct spelling errors. Loss of their function allows mutations to accumulate and leads the daughter cells down the path of the multistep process of cancer. There are other genes that concentrate on repairing DNA sequences that were damaged by an external source such as radiation. Some examples include Fanconi anemia, Bloom syndrome, ataxia-telangiectasia, and xeroderma pigmentosum. These are the few cancer syndromes that follow an autosomal recessive pattern of inheritance.

Epigenetic mechanisms, as discussed previously, involve alterations in patterns of DNA methylation or DNA packaging (3D structure determined by histone interaction and nucleosome positioning). Cancer cells are frequently characterized by global loss of DNA methylation with paradoxical hypermethylation at CpG islands of certain promoters. Coupled with aberrant packaging that may expose inappropriate genetic areas to allow transcription, the overall consequence is abnormal gene expression, either increased or decreased. One can use this clinically to try and identify the 3% to 5% of patients with endometrial cancer that have Lynch syndrome. Lynch syndrome differs from other hereditary cancer syndromes in that the actual tumor tissue can be screened for Lynch syndrome using immunohistochemistry (IHC) for the four mismatch repair proteins (MLH1, MSH2, MSH6, PMS2), microsatellite instability (MSI) analysis, and MLH1 hypermethylation testing. Positive tests will require confirmatory diagnostic testing, but they help guide germline genetic testing. In an attempt to identify Lynch syndrome in women with endometrial cancer, the Society of Gynecologic Oncology Clinical Practice Statement on Screening for Lynch Syndrome in Endometrial Cancer recommends that all women who are diagnosed with endometrial cancer should undergo systematic clinical screening for Lynch syndrome (review of personal and family history) or molecular screening. Molecular screening of endometrial cancers for Lynch syndrome is the preferred strategy when resources are available (SGO, 2014).

When considering a family history of cancer, one should first obtain a complete history, including who has and who has not had cancer in the family. This information will help determine to which group the family likely belongs: *average risk* (sporadic—somatic cell changes), *moderate risk* (common exposures—somatic cell changes or low penetrance genes), or *high risk* (inherited cancer genes—germline mutations). For certain cancer syndromes, computer models are available to help determine the chance a family has an inherited cancer syndrome. It is important to note that taking a detailed family history involves more than asking who has had cancer. One important factor to be cognizant of is the difference between primary cancers, recurrences, and metastatic disease. Patients rarely understand the subtleties of these important distinctions and inadvertently report inaccurate information. It is common for a woman to tell her physician about a family member who was treated for uterine cancer. Upon detailed history taking the physician finds that the woman had a procedure for cervical dysplasia. This type of information is critical to sort this out in order to provide a risk estimate. Once it is determined to which group the person belongs, then an estimation of that person's risk to develop cancer can be determined, and, finally, an individualized cancer screening recommendations can be agreed upon. Generally, at-risk patients should be referred to genetic counselors or medical geneticists with particular expertise in cancer genetics.

## CANCER GENOME SEQUENCING

With the advent of next-generation sequencing there are several commercial entities providing fast and relatively inexpensive tumor DNA sequencing that has not only revolutionized the genetic research on cancer but also created potentially new therapeutic opportunities as well. Tumor specimens can be tested for a "panel" of genes with a known association to cancer and specifically looking for genetic mutations that are "actionable" mutations, in that pharmacologic agents exist, that target these mutations. Different tumor types can have genetic features in common, making them treatable with the same drugs aimed at the genetic defect. Consider Herceptin, the first cancer drug approved for use with a DNA test to determine who should receive it (now there is also a protein-based test). The U.S. Food and Drug Administration (FDA) cleared it in 1998 to target breast cancers that overexpress the *HER2* gene, a change that drives the cancer cells to multiply. The same mutation has been found in gastric, ovarian, and other cancers. As a result of testing, the drug was approved in 2010 to treat patients with gastric cancers that overexpress the *HER2* gene. The potential application of the next-generation sequencing technology is vast but still needs to be subject to scientific scrutiny before it replaces more standard treatment options.

## ETHICAL CONSIDERATIONS OF GENETIC DIAGNOSIS

Commonly identified "pitfalls" of identifying genetic anomalies that lead to formidable counseling challenges include variants of unknown significance (VOUS), identification of adult-onset disease or parental presymptomatic disorders, revelation of nonpaternity, unsuspected consanguinity, findings linked to diseases with variable expressivity, or microdeletions involving a gene linked to cancer development or progression. There are also growing concerns that complete sequence data may lead to overstated associations of disease with findings of genetic variation.

Prenatal genetic discovery, whether through cell-free DNA screening or direct analysis techniques such as chromosomal microarray or whole-exome sequencing, may have especially precarious consequences. There is a relative paucity of information when basing disease prediction on genetic information alone. Due to variations in strength of association with a given phenotype, differences in penetrance, and potential influence of other genetic or environmental factors on disease phenotype, the weight of the evidence for the reported finding must be carefully considered before irrevocable action such as pregnancy termination or fetal treatment is undertaken. The potential impact even goes beyond the possibility of pregnancy termination. Consider the effect of incidental findings such as Mendelian diseases with adult-onset symptoms, or inherited mutations of cancer-associated genes. This raises the risk of labeling the unborn child as well as the parents or extended family with a predestined illness. Furthermore, these findings may cause considerable unfounded anxiety throughout pregnancy and into childhood, depending on the strength of disease association.

At the outset of the Human Genome Project in 1990, the National Human Genome Research Institute established the Ethical, Legal, and Social Implications (ELSI) Program, a component of the extramural genomics research program of the National Institutes of Health (NIH) (McEwen, 2014). This program has focused on four high-priority areas: the use and interpretation of genetic information, clinical integration of genetic technology, issues surrounding genetics research, and public and professional education about these issues. Research such as the programs funded under ELSI are essential to establish basic guidelines; however, the uses and influence of genetic/genomic diagnosis are vast, and ultimately the individual provider must assume responsibility for pursuing and interpreting the information conscientiously.

## *KEY POINTS*

- Virtually all human diseases have an underlying genetic component. All health care professionals need a basic level of familiarity with genetics and genomics, as this is an integral part of mainstream medicine.
- Genetic variation between healthy individuals exists in the form of SNPs and CNVs providing different "doses" of a large repeated DNA sequence at a given genetic locus, or alterations in three-dimensional DNA structures called *epigenetic modification.*
- Naturally occurring variations in genetic sequence, such as SNPs, may mediate an individual's susceptibility to disease or responsiveness to a particular medication.
- The human genome contains about 3 billion base pairs, of which only about 1.5% makes up the exome, or protein-coding portion. The remaining 98.5% of the human genetic sequence encodes biologically active nucleic acid molecules, which are an active area of molecular biology research.
- Genetic pathology can arise from alteration in the sequence of a gene, changes in the normal amount of a gene product, or sequence changes in regulatory regions, which prevent the cell from expressing the intended gene product.
- When a heterozygous individual who has an autosomal dominant trait mates with a normal individual, 50% of their offspring will have the trait.
- When two individuals who carry an autosomal recessive trait mate, 25% of their offspring will demonstrate the trait and 50% will be carriers.
- X-linked recessive characteristics are transmitted from maternal carriers to male offspring and will affect 50% of the male offspring.

*Continued*

## KEY POINTS—cont'd

- The mechanism of trinucleotide repeat disorders is DNA misalignment during meiosis, which leads to unstable dynamic expansion of the number of three-nucleotide repeats within the gene as it is passed from generation to generation, causing progressively more severe manifestations of disease.
- Prader-Willi and Angelman syndromes demonstrate the concept that certain regions of genetic material are imprinted and depend on dose and inheritance from two separate gametes for normal function.
- The phenotype and severity of disorders that affect the mitochondria are determined by the source of the genetic material (nuclear or mitochondrial DNA), the proportion of affected mitochondria inherited by the cell, as well as the threshold for energy production needed in the affected cell.
- In general, if a couple produces an offspring with a multifactorial defect and the problem has never occurred in the family, it can be expected to be repeated in 2% to 5% of subsequent pregnancies.
- Individuals who carry balanced rearrangements of genetic material are phenotypically normal, but their gametes are at risk for unbalanced genetic content, which may lead to infertility or recurrent pregnancy loss.
- Nondisjunctional events have been described in every autosome except chromosomes 1 and 17. Live births can result from nondisjunctional events involving chromosomes 21, 18, 13, or 22, and these occur more commonly with advancing maternal age.
- There are screening and diagnostic tests available for prenatal diagnosis of a large number of genetic diseases and syndromes. Indications for testing may include family history of a specific disease or recurrent clinical phenotype, ethnic background with increased carrier frequency of a certain disease, poor obstetric outcome history, increased maternal age, or population-based prevalence risk.
- In genetic counseling, the role of the care providers (genetic counselors and physicians) is to conduct nondirectional counseling of screening and diagnostic options in order to provide prospective parents with information to optimize pregnancy outcomes based on their personal values and preferences. Before screening or testing, the patient needs to understand the options that may ensue from a positive test result.
- Genetic screening based on cell-free fetal DNA is currently recommended only for women with increased risk of fetal aneuploidy.
- Definitive diagnosis of a genetic disease in the prenatal period requires tissue diagnosis obtained through invasive testing methods such as preimplantation genetic diagnosis, chorionic villus sampling, or amniocentesis.
- With next-generation sequencing, it is possible to determine the complete sequence data for an individual exome (protein-coding region) or genome (complete genetic material). However, accurate interpretation of these data is limited by unknown function of natural genetic variation and noncoding DNA regions, which make up the majority of the sequence.
- All cancer is genetic. However, most cancer is not inherited. For a normal cell line to be transformed into a malignant cell line, several genetic mutations in that somatic cell line must occur that alter cell growth and differentiation.
- In 5% to 10% of families with cancer, there is a germline (inherited) mutation that predisposes certain tissues to become malignant.
- Types of genes and genetic mechanisms involved in malignancy may be grouped into four categories: oncogenes, tumor suppressor genes, DNA repair genes, and epigenetic mechanisms of aberrant DNA packaging.
- Oncogenes (gain of function) behave as growth-promoting genes, and they act in a genetically dominant manner. In other words, only one abnormal copy of the gene will produce a clinically relevant phenotype due to increased gene function.
- Tumor suppressor genes restrain cell growth in damaged cells; therefore loss of the tumor suppressor gene through mutation leads to increased cell proliferation of abnormal cells and cancer development. They account for the majority of autosomal dominant cancer syndromes.
- DNA repair genes identify and mend DNA replication errors made during replication. When they are nonfunctional, replication errors can lead to cancer development.
- Epigenetic mechanisms involve alterations in patterns of DNA methylation or DNA packaging (3D structure determined by histone interaction and nucleosome positioning).
- Lynch syndrome has a prevalence of 3% to 5% in all patients with newly diagnosed endometrial cancer.
- In patients with endometrial cancer, the actual tumor tissue can be screened for Lynch syndrome using IHC for the four mismatch repair proteins (MLH1, MSH2, MSH6, and PMS2), MSI analysis, and MLH1 hypermethylation testing.

## KEY REFERENCES

Akolekar R, Beta J, Picciarelli G, et al. Procedure-related risk of miscarriage following amniocentesis and chorionic villus sampling: a systematic review and meta-analysis. *Ultrasound Obstet Gynecol.* 2015;45(1):16–26.

Amberger JS, Bocchini CA, Schiettecatte F, et al. OMIM.org: Online Mendelian Inheritance in Man (OMIM®), an online catalog of human genes and genetic disorders. *Nucleic Acids Res.* 2015;43(database issue):D789–798.

American College of Obstetricians and Gynecologists (ACOG). ACOG Committee Opinion No. 430: preimplantation genetic screening for aneuploidy. *Obstet Gynecol.* 2009;113(3):766–767.

American College of Obstetricians and Gynecologists (ACOG). ACOG Practice Bulletin No. 77: screening for fetal chromosomal abnormalities. *Obstet Gynecol.* 2007;109(1):217–227.

Beaudet AL, Belmont JW. Array-based DNA diagnostics: let the revolution begin. *Annu Rev Med.* 2008;59:113–129.

Beck T, Hastings RK, Gollapudi S, et al. GWAS Central: a comprehensive resource for the comparison and interrogation of genome-wide association studies. *Eur J Hum Genet.* 2014;22(7):949–952.

Bianchi DW, Simpson JL, Jackson LG, et al. Fetal gender and aneuploidy detection using fetal cells in maternal blood: analysis of NIFTY I data. National Institute of Child Health and Development Fetal Cell Isolation Study. *Prenat Diagn.* 2002;22(7):609–615.

Birney E, Stamatoyannopoulos JA, Dutta A, et al. Identification and analysis of functional elements in 1% of the human genome by the ENCODE pilot project. *Nature.* 2007;447(7146):799–816.

Cariaso M, Lennon G. SNPedia: a wiki supporting personal genome annotation, interpretation and analysis. *Nucleic Acids Res.* 2012;40(Database issue): D1308–1312.

Creasy RK, Resnik R, Greene MF, et al. *Creasy and Resnik's Maternal-Fetal Medicine Principles and Practice.* 7th edition. Philadelphia: Elsevier; 2014.

Crick F. Central dogma of molecular biology. *Nature.* 1970;227(5258): 561–563.

Cummings CJ, Zoghbi HY. Fourteen and counting: unraveling trinucleotide repeat diseases. *Hum Mol Genet.* 2000;9(6):909–916.

Donnelly JC, Platt LD, Rebarber A, et al. Association of copy number variants with specific ultrasonographically detected fetal anomalies. *Obstet Gynecol.* 2014;124(1):83–90.

Edwards JG, Feldman G, Goldberg J, et al. Expanded carrier screening in reproductive medicine-points to consider: a joint statement of the American College of Medical Genetics and Genomics, American College of Obstetricians and Gynecologists, National Society of Genetic Counselors, Perinatal Quality Foundation, and Society for Maternal-Fetal Medicine. *Obstet Gynecol.* 2015;125(3):653–662.

Forman EJ, Hong KH, Ferry KM, et al. In vitro fertilization with single euploid blastocyst transfer: a randomized controlled trial. *Fertil Steril.* 2013;100(1):100–107 e101.

Gerstein MB, Bruce C, Rozowsky JS, et al. What is a gene, post-ENCODE? History and updated definition. *Genome Res.* 2007;17(6):669–681.

Gil MM, Quezada MS, Revello R, et al. Analysis of cell-free DNA in maternal blood in screening for fetal aneuploidies: updated meta-analysis. *Ultrasound Obstet Gynecol.* 2015;45(3):249–266.

Goldstein DB, Allen A, Keebler J, et al. Sequencing studies in human genetics: design and interpretation. *Nat Rev Genet.* 2013;14(7):460–470.

Hagerman PJ, Hagerman RJ. The fragile-X premutation: a maturing perspective. *Am J Hum Genet.* 2004;74(5):805–816.

Hillman SC, Willams D, Carss KJ, et al. Prenatal exome sequencing for fetuses with structural abnormalities: the next step. *Ultrasound Obstet Gynecol.* 2015; 45(1):4–9.

Huang Y, Paxton WA, Wolinsky SM, et al. The role of a mutant CCR5 allele in HIV-1 transmission and disease progression. *Nat Med.* 1996;2(11):1240–1243.

Iafrate AJ, Feuk L, Rivera MN, et al. Detection of large-scale variation in the human genome. *Nat Genet.* 2004;36(9):949–951.

Johns DR. Seminars in medicine of the Beth Israel Hospital, Boston. Mitochondrial DNA and disease. *N Engl J Med.* 1995;333(10):638–644.

Jones KL, Smith DW. *Smith's Recognizable Patterns of Human Malformation.* 6th ed. Philadelphia: Saunders; 2006.

Kuller JA, Chescheir N, Cefalo RC. *Prenatal Diagnosis & Reproductive Genetics.* St. Louis: Mosby; 1996.

Ledbetter DH, Martin AO, Verlinsky Y, et al. Cytogenetic results of chorionic villus sampling: high success rate and diagnostic accuracy in the United States collaborative study. *Am J Obstet Gynecol.* 1990;162(2):495–501.

Lee C, Iafrate AJ, Brothman AR. Copy number variations and clinical cytogenetic diagnosis of constitutional disorders. *Nat Genet.* 2007;39(7 Suppl):S48–S54.

Lo YM, Corbetta N, Chamberlain PF, et al. Presence of fetal DNA in maternal plasma and serum. *Lancet.* 1997;350(9076):485–487.

Lyon MF. Gene action in the X-chromosome of the mouse (Mus musculus L.). *Nature.* 1961;190:372–373.

MacDonald JR, Ziman R, Yuen RK, et al. The Database of Genomic Variants: a curated collection of structural variation in the human genome. *Nucleic Acids Res.* 2014;42(Database issue):D986–992.

Malone FD, Canick JA, Ball RH, et al. First-trimester or second-trimester screening, or both, for Down's syndrome. *N Engl J Med.* 2005;353(19): 2001–2011.

McEwen JE, Boyer JT, Sun KY, et al. The Ethical, Legal, and Social Implications Program of the National Human Genome Research Institute: reflections on an ongoing experiment. *Annu Rev Genomics Hum Genet.* 2014;15:481–505.

Miller DT, Adam MP, Aradhya S, et al. Consensus statement: chromosomal microarray is a first-tier clinical diagnostic test for individuals with developmental disabilities or congenital anomalies. *Am J Hum Genet.* 2010; 86(5):749–764.

Norton ME, Jacobsson B, Swamy GK, et al. Cell-free DNA analysis for noninvasive examination of trisomy. *N Engl J Med.* 2015;372(17):1589–1597.

Portela A, Esteller M. Epigenetic modifications and human disease. *Nat Biotechnol.* 2010;28(10):1057–1068.

Pritchard CC, Cheng HH, Tewari M. MicroRNA profiling: approaches and considerations. *Nat Rev Genet.* 2012;13(5):358–369.

Redon R, Ishikawa S, Fitch KR, et al. Global variation in copy number in the human genome. *Nature.* 2006;444(7118):444–454.

Sebat J, Lakshmi B, Troge J, et al. Large-scale copy number polymorphism in the human genome. *Science.* 2004;305(5683):525–528.

Society of Gynecologic Oncology (SGO). *SGO Clinical practice statement: screening for Lynch syndrome in endometrial cancer*; March 2014. Available at https://www.sgo.org/clinical-practice/guidelines/screening-for-lynch-syndrome-in-endometrial-cancer/.

Smith GC, Shah I, Crossley JA, et al. Pregnancy-associated plasma protein A and alpha-fetoprotein and prediction of adverse perinatal outcome. *Obstet Gynecol.* 2006;107(1):161–166.

Snijders AM, Nowak N, Segraves R, et al. Assembly of microarrays for genome-wide measurement of DNA copy number. *Nat Genet.* 2001;29(3): 263–264.

Topol EJ. Individualized medicine from prewomb to tomb. *Cell.* 2014;157(1): 241–253.

Wapner RJ, Babiarz JE, Levy B, et al. Expanding the scope of noninvasive prenatal testing: detection of fetal microdeletion syndromes. *Am J Obstet Gynecol.* 2015;212(3):332 e331–339.

Wapner RJ, Levy B. The impact of new genomic technologies in reproductive medicine. *Discov Med.* 2014;17(96):313–318.

Wapner RJ, Martin CL, Levy B, et al. Chromosomal microarray versus karyotyping for prenatal diagnosis. *N Engl J Med.* 2012;367(23):2175–2184.

Yang Y, Muzny DM, Reid JG, et al. Clinical whole-exome sequencing for the diagnosis of mendelian disorders. *N Engl J Med.* 2013;369(16):1502–1511.

Zinaman MJ, Clegg ED, Brown CC, et al. Estimates of human fertility and pregnancy loss. *Fertil Steril.* 1996;65(3):503–509.

Zlotogora J. Germ line mosaicism. *Hum Genet.* 1998;102(4):381–386.

# 3
# Reproductive Anatomy
## Gross and Microscopic, Clinical Correlations

*Fidel A. Valea*

The organs of the female reproductive tract are classically divided into the external and the internal genitalia. The external genital organs are present in the perineal area and include the mons pubis, clitoris, urinary meatus, labia majora, labia minora, vestibule, Bartholin glands, and periurethral glands. The internal genital organs are located in the true pelvis and include the vagina, uterus, cervix, oviducts, ovaries, and surrounding supporting structures. This chapter integrates the basic anatomy of the female pelvis with clinical situations.

Embryologically, the urinary, reproductive, and gastrointestinal tracts develop in close proximity. This relationship continues throughout a woman's life span. In the adult, the reproductive organs are in intimate contact with the lower urinary tract and large intestines. Because of the anatomic proximity of the genital and urinary systems, altered pathophysiology in one organ often produces symptoms in an adjacent organ. The gynecologic surgeon should master the intricacy of these anatomic relationships to avoid surgical complications. The clinician must also appreciate that wide individual differences in anatomic detail exist among patients. Understanding these variations is one of the greatest challenges of clinical medicine.

This chapter focuses on the norms of human anatomy; it does not duplicate the completeness of an anatomic text or surgical atlas.

## EXTERNAL GENITALIA

### Vulva

The *vulva,* or *pudendum,* is a collective term for the external genital organs that are visible in the perineal area. The vulva consists of the following: the mons pubis, labia majora, labia minora, hymen, clitoris, vestibule, urethra, Skene glands, Bartholin glands, and vestibular bulbs (Fig. 3.1).

The boundaries of the vulva extend from the mons pubis anteriorly to the rectum posteriorly and from one lateral genitocrural fold to the other. The entire vulvar area is covered by keratinized, stratified squamous epithelium. The skin becomes thicker, more pigmented, and more keratinized as the distance from the vagina increases.

### MONS PUBIS

The mons pubis is a fatty, rounded eminence that develops hair after puberty. It is directly anterior and superior to the symphysis pubis. The hair pattern, or escutcheon, of most women is triangular. Genetic and racial differences produce a variety of normal hair patterns, with approximately one in four women having a modified escutcheon that has a diamond (male-like) pattern.

### LABIA MAJORA

The labia majora are two large, longitudinal, cutaneous folds of adipose and fibrous tissue. Each labium majus is approximately 7 to 8 cm in length and 2 to 3 cm in width. The labia extend from the mons pubis anteriorly to become lost in the skin between the vagina and the anus in the area of the posterior fourchette. The skin of the outer convex surface of the labia majora is pigmented and covered with hair follicles. The thin skin of the inner surface does not have hair follicles but has many sebaceous glands. Histologically the labia majora have both sweat and sebaceous glands (Fig. 3.2). The apocrine glands are similar to those of the breast and axillary areas. The size of the labia is related to fat content. Usually the labia atrophy after menopause. The labia majora are homologous to the scrotum in the male. The clinical significance of the hair-bearing areas of the vulva is that conditions that involve the skin, such as vulvar intraepithelial neoplasia (VIN), may be found as deep as 3 mm below the surface as it can involve the skin down the hair shafts. That is not the case in the non–hair-bearing areas, such as the labia minora, where the full thickness of the epidermis is usually no more than 1 mm. Hence, treatment of the non–hair-bearing areas would not have to be any deeper than 1 mm to be effective, whereas treatment of the hair-bearing areas would have to be at least 3 mm in depth to cover the potentially deeper skin down the hair shafts.

### LABIA MINORA

The labia minora, or nymphae, are two small, red cutaneous folds that are situated between the labia majora and the vaginal orifice. They are more delicate, shorter, and thinner than the labia majora. Anteriorly, they divide at the clitoris to form superiorly the prepuce and inferiorly the frenulum of the clitoris. Histologically they are composed of dense connective tissue with

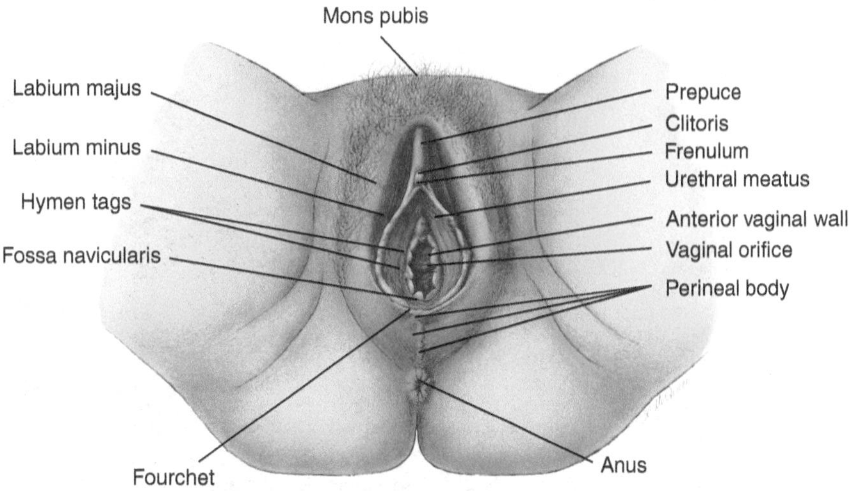


**Figure 3.1** The structures of the external genitalia that are collectively called the *vulva*. (Modified from Pritchard JA, MacDonald PC, Gant NF. *Williams' Obstetrics*. 17th ed. New York: Appleton-Century-Crofts; 1985:8.)

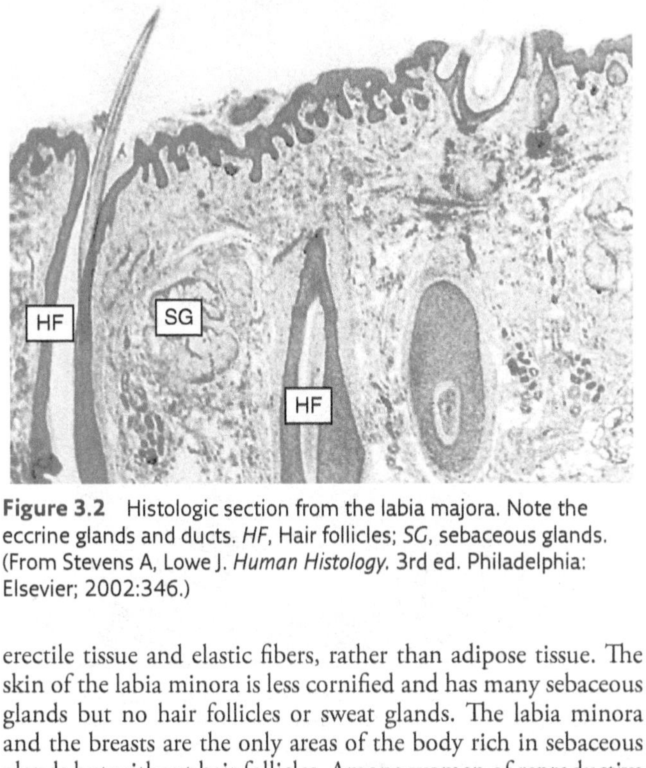


**Figure 3.2** Histologic section from the labia majora. Note the eccrine glands and ducts. *HF*, Hair follicles; *SG*, sebaceous glands. (From Stevens A, Lowe J. *Human Histology*. 3rd ed. Philadelphia: Elsevier; 2002:346.)

erectile tissue and elastic fibers, rather than adipose tissue. The skin of the labia minora is less cornified and has many sebaceous glands but no hair follicles or sweat glands. The labia minora and the breasts are the only areas of the body rich in sebaceous glands but without hair follicles. Among women of reproductive age, there is considerable variation in the size of the labia minora. They are relatively more prominent in children and postmenopausal women. The labia minora are homologous to the penile urethra and part of the skin of the penis in males.

## HYMEN

The hymen is a thin, usually perforated membrane at the entrance of the vagina. There are many variations in the structure and shape of the hymen. The hymen histologically is covered by stratified squamous epithelium on both sides and consists of fibrous tissue with a few small blood vessels. Small tags, or nodules, of firm fibrous material, termed *carunculae myrtiformes,* are the remnants of the hymen identified in adult females.

## CLITORIS

The clitoris is a short, cylindric, erectile organ at the superior portion of the vestibule. The normal adult glans clitoris has a width less than 1 cm, with an average length of 1.5 to 2 cm. Previous childbearing may influence the size of the clitoris, but age, weight, and oral contraceptive use do not change the anatomic dimensions. Usually, only the glans is visible, with the body of the clitoris positioned beneath the skin surface. The clitoris consists of a base of two crura, which attach to the periosteum of the symphysis pubis. The body has two cylindric corpora cavernosa composed of thin-walled, vascular channels that function as erectile tissue (Fig. 3.3). The distal one third of the clitoris is the glans, which has many nerve endings. The clitoris is the female homologue of the penis in the male.

## VESTIBULE

The vestibule is the lowest portion of the embryonic urogenital sinus. It is the cleft distal to the vagina between the labia minora that is visualized when the labia are held apart. The vestibule extends from the clitoris to the posterior fourchette. The orifices of the urethra and vagina and the ducts from Bartholin glands open into the vestibule. Within the area of the vestibule are the remnants of the hymen and numerous small mucinous glands.

## URETHRA

The urethra is a membranous conduit for urine from the urinary bladder to the vestibule. The female urethra measures 3.5 to 5 cm in length. The mucosa of the proximal two thirds of the urethra is composed of stratified transitional epithelium, whereas the distal one third is stratified squamous epithelium. The distal orifice is 4 to 6 mm in diameter, and the mucosal edges grossly appear everted.

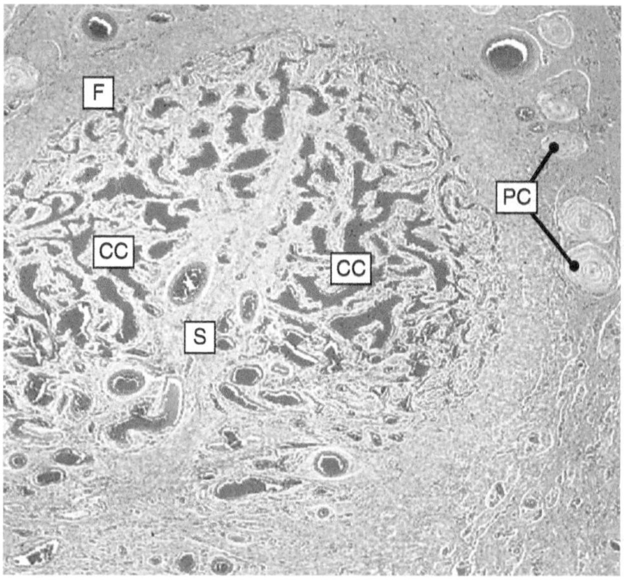


**Figure 3.3** A histologic section of the clitoris. Note the two corpus cavernosa *(CC)*, the septum *(S)*, and the fibrous-collagenous sheath *(F)*. Multiple nerve endings may be seen surrounding the clitoris. *PC*, Pacinian touch corpuscles. (From Stevens A, Lowe J. *Human Histology.* 3rd ed. Philadelphia: Elsevier; 2002:346.)

## SKENE GLANDS

Skene glands, or paraurethral glands, are branched, tubular glands that are adjacent to the distal urethra. Usually Skene ducts run parallel to the long axis of the urethra for approximately 1 cm before opening into the distal urethra. Sometimes the ducts open into the area just outside the urethral orifice. Skene glands are the largest of the paraurethral glands; however, many smaller glands empty into the urethra. Skene glands are homologous to the prostate in the male.

## BARTHOLIN GLANDS

Bartholin glands are vulvovaginal glands that are located immediately beneath the fascia at about 4 and 8 o'clock, respectively, on the posterolateral aspect of the vaginal orifice. Each lobulated, racemose gland is about the size of a pea. Histologically the gland is composed of cuboidal epithelium (Fig. 3.4). The duct from each gland is lined by transitional epithelium and is approximately 2 cm in length. Bartholin ducts open into a groove between the hymen and the labia minora. Bartholin glands are homologous to Cowper glands in the male.

## VESTIBULAR BULBS

The vestibular bulbs are two elongated masses of erectile tissue situated on either side of the vaginal orifice. Each bulb is immediately below the bulbocavernosus muscle. The distal ends of the vestibular bulbs are adjacent to Bartholin glands. They are homologous to the bulb of the penis in the male.

# CLINICAL CORRELATIONS

The skin of the vulvar region is subject to both local and general dermatologic conditions. The intertriginous areas of the vulva remain moist, and obese women are particularly susceptible to chronic infection. The vulvar skin of a postmenopausal woman is sensitive to topical cortisone and testosterone but insensitive to topical estrogen. The most common large cystic structure of the vulva is a Bartholin duct cyst (Fig. 3.5). This condition may become painful if the cyst develops into an acute abscess. Chronic infections of the periurethral glands may result in one or more urethral diverticula. The most common symptoms of a urethral diverticulum are similar to the symptoms of a lower urinary tract infection: urinary frequency, urgency, and dysuria.

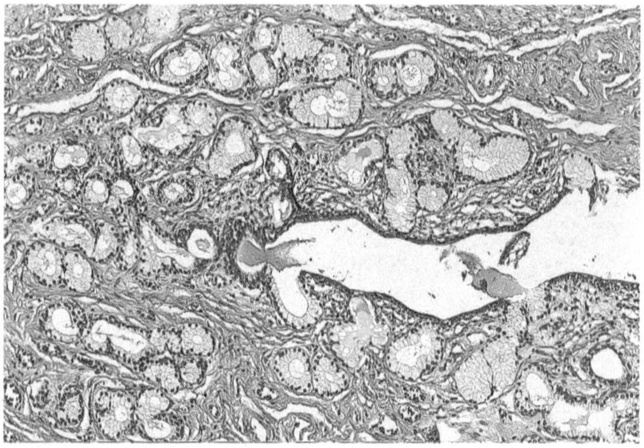

**Figure 3.4** A histologic section of a Bartholin gland. Note the multiple alveoli draining into a central duct. (From Shea CR, Stevens A, Dalziel KL, Robboy SJ. Vulva. In: Robboy SJ, Anderson MC, Russell P, eds. *Pathology of the Female Reproductive Tract.* Edinburgh: Churchill Livingstone; 2002:36.)

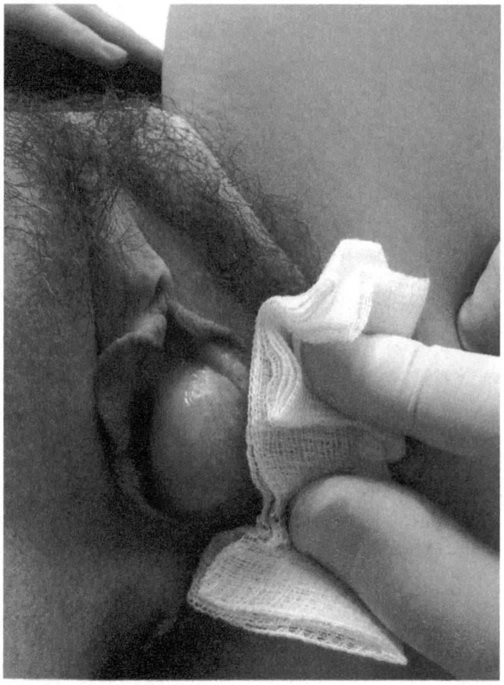

**Figure 3.5** Photograph of left Bartholin duct cyst. (From Di Donato V, Bellati F, Casorelli A, et al. $CO_2$ laser treatment for Bartholin gland abscess: ultrasound evaluation of risk recurrence. *J Minim Invasive Gynecol.* 2013;20[3]:346-352.)

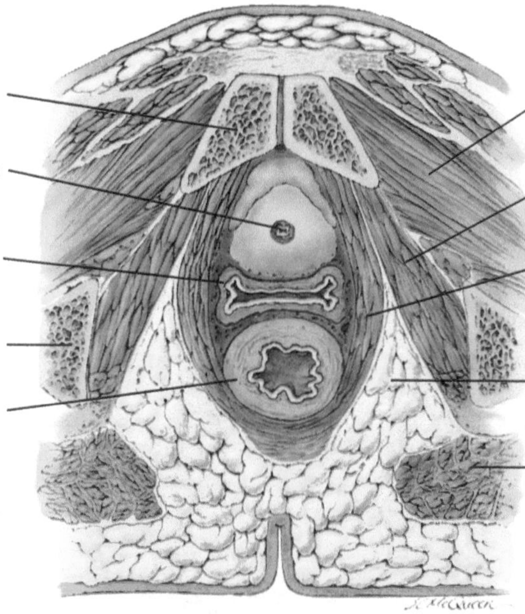


**Figure 3.6** A schematic drawing of a cross section of the female pelvis, demonstrating the H shape of the vagina. Note the surrounding levator ani muscle. (Modified from Pritchard JA, MacDonald PC, Gant NF. *Williams' Obstetrics.* 17th ed. New York: Appleton-Century-Crofts; 1985:12.)

Vulvar trauma such as straddle injuries frequently results in large hematomas or profuse external hemorrhage. The richness of the vascular supply and the absence of valves in vulvar veins contribute to this complication. The abundant vascularity of the region promotes rapid healing, with an associated low incidence of wound infection in episiotomies or obstetric tears of the vulva. The subcutaneous fatty tissue of the labia majora and mons pubis are in continuity with the fatty tissue of the anterior abdominal wall. Infections in this space such as cellulites and necrotizing fasciitis are poorly contained and may extend cephalad in rapid fashion.

## INTERNAL GENITALIA

### VAGINA

The vagina is a thin-walled, distensible, fibromuscular tube that extends from the vestibule of the vulva to the uterus. The potential space of the vagina is larger in the middle and upper thirds. The walls of the vagina are normally in apposition and flattened in the anteroposterior diameter. Thus the vagina has the appearance of the letter H in cross section (Fig. 3.6).

The axis of the upper portion of the vagina lies fairly close to the horizontal plane when a woman is standing, with the upper portion of the vagina curving toward the hollow of the sacrum. In most women an angle of at least 90 degrees is formed between the axis of the vagina and the axis of the uterus (Fig. 3.7). The vagina is held in position by the surrounding endopelvic fascia and ligaments.

The lower third of the vagina is in close relationship with the urogenital and pelvic diaphragms. The middle third of the vagina is suspended by the lower portion of the cardinal ligaments and supported by the levator ani muscles. The upper third is suspended by the upper portions of the cardinal ligaments and the parametria. The vagina of reproductive-age women has numerous transverse folds, vaginal rugae. They help provide accordion-like distensibility and are more prominent in the lower third of the vagina. The cervix extends into the upper part of the vagina. The spaces between the cervix and attachment of the vagina are called *fornices.* The posterior fornix is considerably larger than the anterior fornix; thus the anterior vaginal length is approximately 6 to 9 cm in comparison with a posterior vaginal length of 8 to 12 cm. Vaginal length is increased slightly by a woman's weight and height. Age, conversely, leads to a shortening of vaginal length. A study by Tan and colleagues noted a decrease of 0.08 cm per 10 years. Menopause leads to further shortening.

Histologically the vagina is composed of four distinct layers. The mucosa consists of a stratified, nonkeratinized squamous epithelium (Fig. 3.8). If the environment of the vaginal mucosa is modified, as in uterine prolapse, then the epithelium may become keratinized. The squamous epithelium is similar microscopically to the exocervix, although the vagina has larger and more frequent papillae that extend into the connective tissue. The normal vagina does not have glands. The next layer is the lamina propria, or tunica. It is composed of fibrous connective tissue. Throughout this layer of collagen and elastic tissue is a rich supply of vascular and lymphatic channels. The density of the connective tissue in the endopelvic fascia varies throughout the longitudinal axis of the vagina. The muscular layer has many interlacing fibers. However, an inner circular layer and an outer longitudinal layer can be identified. The fourth layer consists of cellular areolar connective tissue containing a large plexus of blood vessels.

The vascular system of the vagina is generously supplied with an extensive anastomotic network throughout its length. The vaginal artery originates either directly from the uterine artery or as a branch of the internal iliac artery arising posterior to the origin of the uterine and inferior vesical arteries.

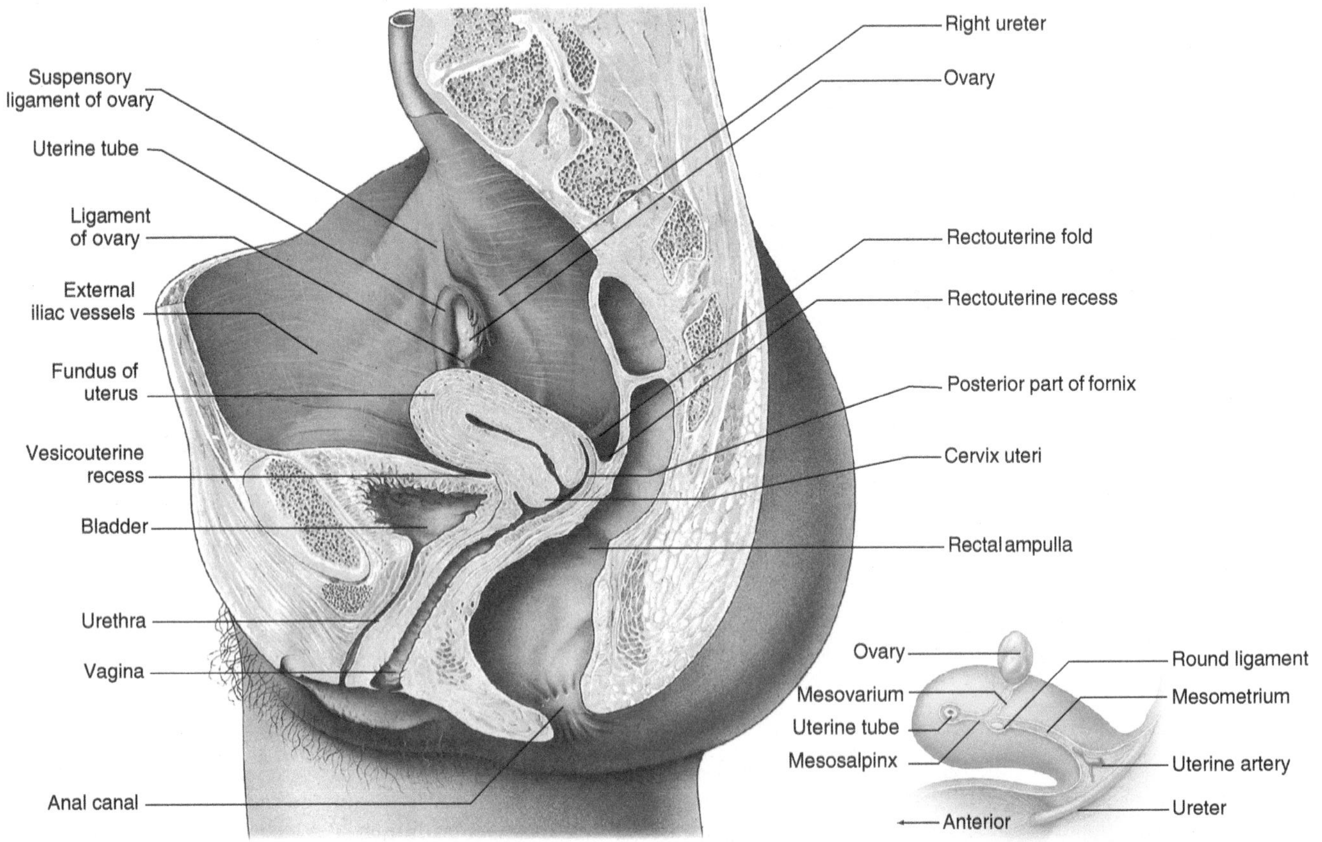


**Figure 3.7** A median sagittal section through the pelvis. The peritoneum is shaded blue. Note the proximal vagina at a diagonal axis and in a near 90-degree juxtaposition to the uterus. In this woman, the uterus is anteflexed. (From Standring S, ed. *Gray's Anatomy.* 39th ed. Edinburgh: Churchill Livingstone; 2005:1321.)

The vaginal arteries may be multiple arteries on each side of the pelvis. There is an anastomosis with the cervical branch of the uterine artery to form the azygos arteries. Branches of the internal pudendal, inferior vesical, and middle hemorrhoidal arteries also contribute to the interconnecting network and the longitudinal azygos arteries.

The venous drainage is complex and accompanies the arterial system. Below the pelvic floor, the principal venous drainage occurs via the pudendal veins. The vaginal, uterine, and vesical veins, as well as those around the rectosigmoid, all provide venous drainage of the venous plexuses surrounding the middle and upper vagina.

The nerve supply of the vagina comes from the autonomic nervous system's vaginal plexus, and sensory fibers come from the pudendal nerve. Pain fibers enter the spinal cord in sacral segments two to four. There is a paucity of free nerve endings in the upper two thirds of the vagina.

The lymphatic drainage is characterized by its wide distribution and frequent crossovers between the right and left sides of the pelvis. In general the primary lymphatic drainage of the upper third of the vagina is to the external iliac nodes, the middle third of the vagina drains to the common and internal iliac nodes, and the lower third has a complex and variable distribution, including the common iliac, superficial inguinal, and perirectal nodes.

## CLINICAL CORRELATIONS

In clinical practice, anatomic descriptions of pelvic organs are derived from Latin roots, such as the word *vagina*, which is derived from the Latin word for sheath. In contrast, the names for surgical procedures of pelvic organs are derived from Greek roots. *Colpectomy, colporrhaphy,* and *colposcopy* are derived from *kolpos* (fold), the Greek word for the *vagina,* or *hysterectomy* (Greek) versus *uterus* (Latin).

Clinicians should consider the H shape of the vagina when they insert a speculum and inspect the walls of the vagina. The posterior fornix is an important surgical landmark, because it provides direct access to the cul-de-sac of Douglas. The distal course of the ureter is an essential consideration in vaginal surgery. Ureteral injury can result from vaginally placed sutures to obtain hemostasis with vaginal lacerations. The anatomic proximity and interrelationships of the vascular and lymphatic networks of the bladder and vagina are such that inflammation of one organ can produce symptoms in the other. For example, vaginitis sometimes produces urinary tract symptoms such as frequency and dysuria.

The Gartner duct cyst, a cystic dilation of the embryonic mesonephros (Fig. 3.9), is usually present on the lateral wall of the vagina. However, in the lower third of the vagina these cysts are present anteriorly and may be difficult to distinguish from a large urethral diverticulum.

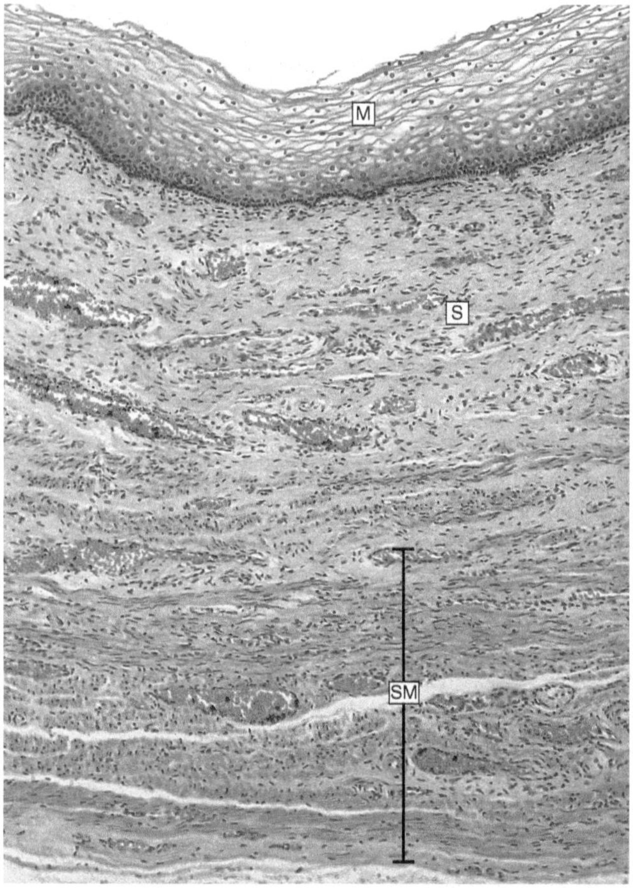


**Figure 3.8** Histologic section of the vaginal squamous epithelium *(M)*. Submucosa *(S)* is well vascularized (lamina propria). *SM*, Smooth muscle. (From Stevens A, Lowe J. *Human Histology.* 3rd ed. Philadelphia: Elsevier; 2002:347.)

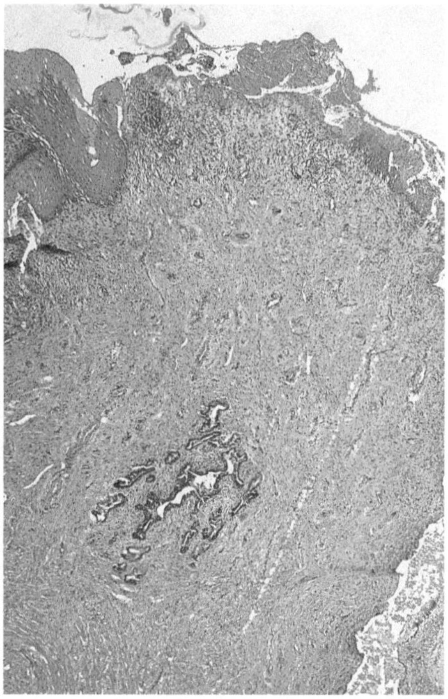

**Figure 3.9** Mesonephric duct remnant in the vaginal wall. (From Robboy SJ, Anderson MC, Russell P, eds. *Pathology of the Female Reproductive Tract.* Edinburgh: Churchill Livingstone; 2002:77.)

An interesting phenomenon is the source of vaginal lubrication during intercourse. For years there was speculation on how an organ without glands is able to "secrete" fluid. Vaginal lubrication occurs from a transudate produced by engorgement of the vascular plexuses that encircle the vagina. This richness of vascularization allows many drugs to readily enter the systemic circulation when placed in the vagina. Medications that are absorbed vaginally go directly into the systemic circulation, bypassing the liver and its metabolism on the first round through the circulation.

The anatomic relationship between the long axis of the vagina and other pelvic organs may be altered by pelvic relaxation resulting primarily from the trauma of childbirth. Atrophy or weakness of the endopelvic fascia and muscles surrounding the vagina may result in the development of a cystocele, rectocele, or enterocele, all possibly contributing to a vaginal vault prolapse. One of many popular operations for vaginal vault prolapse is fixation of the vaginal apex to the sacrospinous ligament. A rare complication of this operation is massive hemorrhage, usually from the arterial or venous branches of the inferior gluteal or pudendal vasculature.

## *CERVIX*

The lower, narrow portion of the uterus is the cervix. The word *cervix* originates from the Latin word for *neck.* The Greek word for *neck* is *trachelos,* and when the cervix is removed, the surgical procedure is termed *trachelectomy.* The cervix may vary in shape from cylindric to conical. It consists of predominantly fibrous tissue in contrast to the primarily muscular corpus of the uterus.

The vagina is attached obliquely around the middle of the cervix; this attachment divides the cervix into an upper, supravaginal portion and a lower segment in the vagina called the *portio vaginalis* (Fig. 3.10). The supravaginal segment is covered by peritoneum posteriorly and is surrounded by loose, fatty connective tissue—the parametrium—anteriorly and laterally.

The canal of the cervix is fusiform, with the widest diameter in the middle. The length and width of the endocervical canal varies; it is usually 2.5 to 3 cm in length and 7 to 8 mm at its widest point. The width of the canal varies with the parity of the woman and changing hormonal levels. The cervical length increases in pregnancy, with maximal length in the second trimester. The cervical canal opens into the vagina at the external os of the cervix. In the majority of women, the external os is in contact with the posterior vaginal wall. The external os is small and round in nulliparous women. The os is wider and gaping following vaginal delivery. Often lateral or stellate scars are residual marks of previous cervical lacerations.

The mucous lining of the endocervical canal of nulliparous women is arranged in longitudinal folds, called plicae palmatae, with secondary branching folds, the arbor vitae (Fig. 3.11). These folds, which form a herringbone pattern, disappear following vaginal delivery.

A single layer of columnar epithelium lines the endocervical canal and the underlying glandular structures. This specialized epithelium secretes mucus, which facilitates sperm transport.

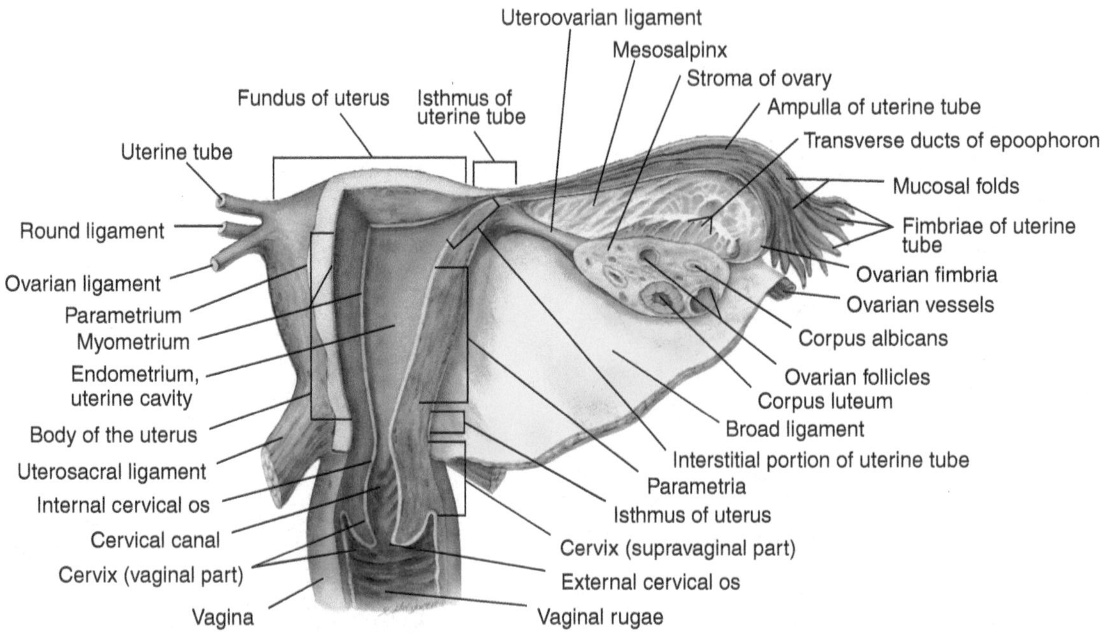


**Figure 3.10** A schematic drawing of a posterior view of the cervix, uterus, fallopian tube, and ovary. Note that the cervix is divided by the vaginal attachment into an external portio segment and a supravaginal segment. Note that the uterus is composed of the dome-shaped fundus, the muscular body, and the narrow isthmus. Note the fimbria ovarica, or ovarian fimbria, attaching the oviduct to the ovary. (Modified from Clemente CD. *Anatomy: A Regional Atlas of the Human Body.* 3rd ed. Baltimore-Munich: Urban & Schwarzenberg; 1987.)

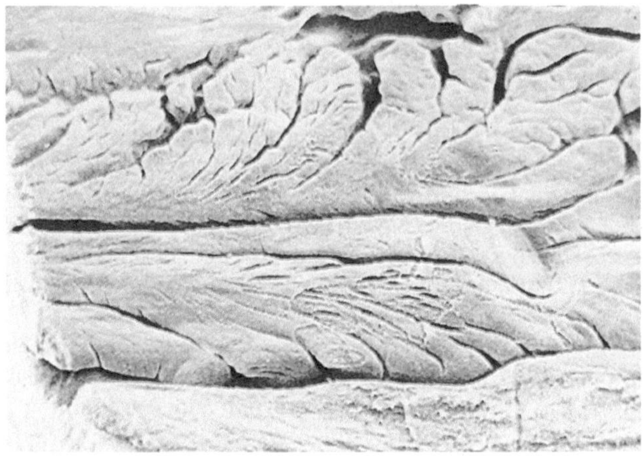

**Figure 3.11** An electron micrograph of the endocervical canal, demonstrating the arbor vitae. These folds and crypts provide a reservoir for sperm. (From Singer A, Jordan JA. The anatomy of the cervix. In Jordan JA, Singer A, eds. *The Cervix.* Philadelphia: WB Saunders; 1976:18.)

An abrupt transformation usually is seen at the junction of the columnar epithelium of the endocervix and the nonkeratinized stratified squamous epithelium of the portio vaginalis (Fig. 3.12). The stratified squamous epithelium of the exocervix is identical to the lining of the vagina.

The dense, fibromuscular cervical stroma is composed primarily of collagenous connective tissue and mucopolysaccharide ground substance. The collagen framework and ground substance are sensitive to hormonal effects. The connective tissue contains approximately 15% smooth muscle cells and a small

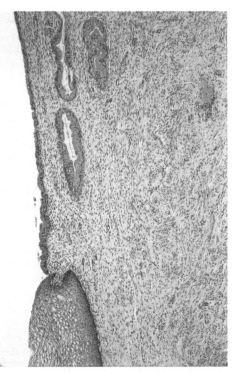

**Figure 3.12** A histologic section through the squamocolumnar junction of the cervix. Note the abrupt transformation from squamous to columnar epithelium. (From Standring S, ed. *Gray's Anatomy.* 39th ed. Edinburgh: Churchill Livingstone; 2005:1335.)

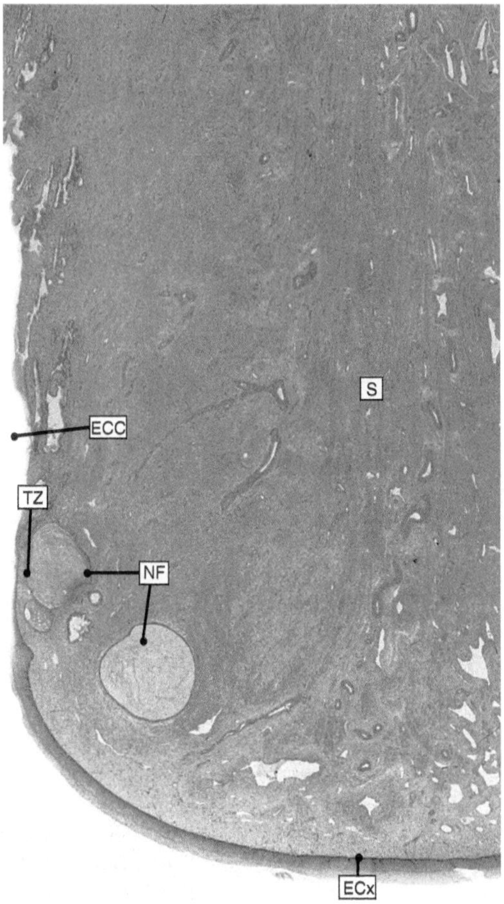


**Figure 3.13** A low-power histologic section of the cervix. The stroma *(S)* has a small amount of smooth muscle. The ectocervix *(ECx)* is covered in stratified squamous epithelium. The endocervix *(ECC)* is lined by tall columnar cells. *NF*, Nabothian follicles, a normal finding; *TZ*, transformation zone. (From Stevens A, Lowe J. *Human Histology*. 3rd ed. Philadelphia: Elsevier; 2002:349.)

amount of elastic tissue (Fig. 3.13). However, there are few muscle fibers in the distal portions of the cervix.

It is not surprising that the cervical and uterine vascular supplies are interrelated. The arterial supply of the cervix arises from the descending branch of the uterine artery. The cervical arteries run on the lateral side of the cervix and form the coronary artery, which encircles the cervix. The azygos arteries run longitudinally in the middle of the anterior and posterior aspects of the cervix and the vagina. There are numerous anastomoses between these vessels and the vaginal and middle hemorrhoidal arteries. The venous drainage accompanies these arteries. The lymphatic drainage of the cervix is complex, involving multiple chains of nodes. The principal regional lymph nodes are the obturator, common iliac, internal iliac, external iliac, and visceral nodes of the parametria. Other possible lymphatic drainage includes the following chains of nodes: superior and inferior gluteal, sacral, rectal, lumbar, aortic, and visceral nodes over the posterior surface of the urinary bladder. The stroma of the endocervix is rich in free nerve endings. Pain fibers accompany the parasympathetic fibers to the second, third, and fourth sacral segments.

## CLINICAL CORRELATIONS

The major arterial supply to the cervix is located on the lateral cervical walls at the 3 and 9 o'clock positions, respectively. Therefore a deep figure-of-eight suture through the vaginal mucosa and cervical stroma at 3 and 9 o'clock helps to reduce blood loss during procedures such as cone biopsy. If the gynecologist is overzealous in placing such a hemostatic suture high in the vaginal fornix, it is possible to compromise the course of the distal ureter just before it enters the bladder.

The transformation zone of the cervix is an important anatomic landmark for clinicians. This area encompasses the transition from stratified squamous epithelium to columnar epithelium. Most cervical dysplasia develops within this transformation zone. The position of a woman's transformation zone, in relation to the long axis of the cervix, depends on her age and hormonal status. When the female is young the transformation zone is located further out on the cervical portio: this is called an *ectropion*. This is a normal finding, especially during pregnancy. As a woman ages, the transformation zone migrates higher up the endocervical canal.

The endocervix is rich in free nerve endings. Occasionally, women experience a vasovagal response during transcervical instrumentation of the uterine cavity. Serial cardiac monitoring during insertion of intrauterine devices demonstrates a reflex bradycardia in some women. The sensory innervation of the exocervix is not as concentrated or sophisticated as that of the endocervix or external skin. Therefore usually the exocervix may be cauterized by either cold or heat without major discomfort to the patient.

The lymphatic drainage of the cervix is fairly organized as described earlier. Similar to other disease sites, sentinel lymph node (SLN) mapping and biopsy for cervical cancer is replacing the more traditional full lymphadenectomies in favor of fewer complications, specifically lymphedema. Sentinel lymph node mapping in cervical cancer was first described in 1999 by Echt and coworkers when they injected 13 patients who had early stage cervical cancer with a blue dye, lymphazurin, and identified SLNs in 15% (Echt, 1999). This technique has been refined over the years and is now performed using near-infrared fluorescence imaging and indocyanine green (ICG) with detection of SLNs in 85% to 90% of cases.

## UTERUS

The uterus is a thick-walled, hollow, muscular organ located centrally in the female pelvis. Adjacent to the uterus are the urinary bladder anteriorly, the rectum posteriorly, and the broad ligaments laterally (Figs. 3.7 and 3.14). The uterus is globular and slightly flattened anteriorly; it has the general configuration of an inverted pear. The short area of constriction in the lower uterine segment is termed the *isthmus* (Fig. 3.15). The dome-shaped top of the uterus is termed the *fundus*. The lower edge of the fundus is described by an imaginary line drawn between the site of entrance of each oviduct. The size and weight of the normal uterus depend on previous pregnancies and the hormonal status of the individual. The uterus of a nulliparous woman is approximately 8 cm long, 5 cm wide, and 2.5 cm thick and weighs 40 to 50 g. In contrast, in a multiparous woman, each measurement is approximately 1.2 cm larger, and normal

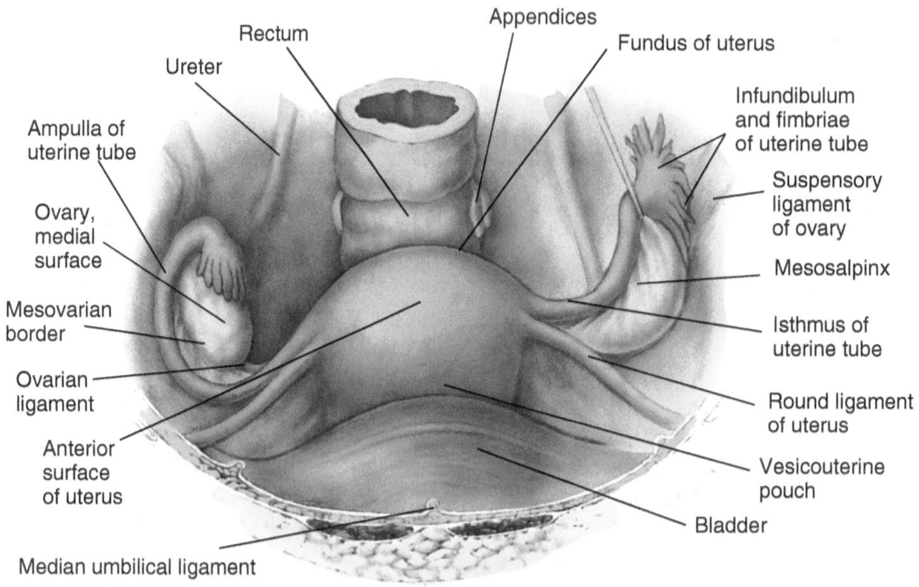


**Figure 3.14** The organs of the female pelvis. The uterus is surrounded by the bladder anteriorly, the rectum posteriorly, and the folds of the broad ligaments laterally. (Modified from Clemente CD. *Anatomy: A Regional Atlas of the Human Body.* 3rd ed. Baltimore-Munich: Urban & Schwarzenberg; 1987.)

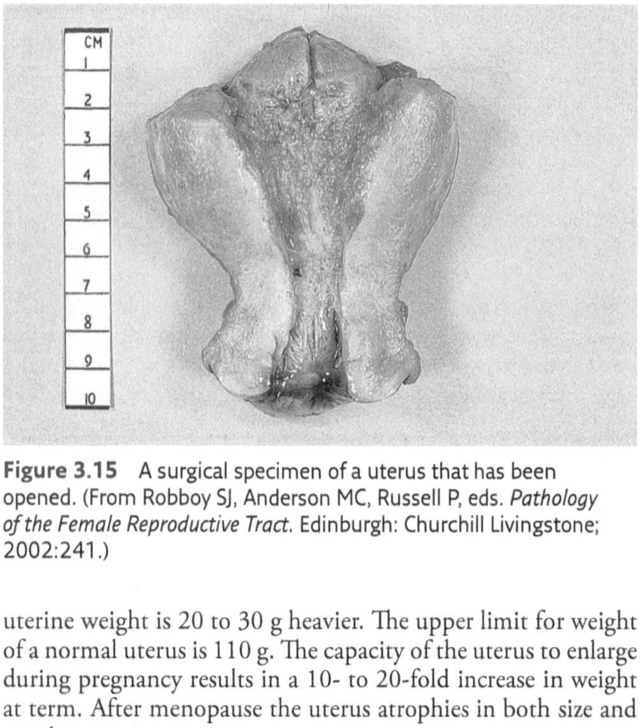


**Figure 3.15** A surgical specimen of a uterus that has been opened. (From Robboy SJ, Anderson MC, Russell P, eds. *Pathology of the Female Reproductive Tract.* Edinburgh: Churchill Livingstone; 2002:241.)

uterine weight is 20 to 30 g heavier. The upper limit for weight of a normal uterus is 110 g. The capacity of the uterus to enlarge during pregnancy results in a 10- to 20-fold increase in weight at term. After menopause the uterus atrophies in both size and weight.

The cavity of the uterus is flattened and triangular. The oviducts enter the uterine cavity at the superolateral aspects of the cavity in the areas designated the cornua. In the majority of women, the long axis of the uterus is both anteverted in respect to the long axis of the vagina and anteflexed in relation to the long axis of the cervix. However, a retroflexed uterus is a normal variant found in approximately 25% of women.

The uterus has three layers, similar to other hollow abdominal and pelvic organs. The thin, external serosal layer makes up the visceral peritoneum. The peritoneum is firmly attached to the uterus in all areas except anteriorly at the level of the internal os of the cervix, where it is only loosely attached. The wide middle muscular layer is composed of three indistinct layers of smooth muscle. The outer longitudinal layer is contiguous with the muscle layers of the oviduct and vagina. The middle layer has interlacing oblique, spiral bundles of smooth muscle and large venous plexuses. The inner muscular layer is also longitudinal. The endometrium is a reddish mucous membrane that varies from 1 to 6 mm in thickness, depending on hormonal stimulation (Fig. 3.16). The uterine glands are tubular and composed of tall columnar epithelium. The cells of the endometrial stroma resemble embryonic connective tissue with scant cytoplasm and large nuclei (Fig. 3.17). The endometrium may be divided into an inner stratum basale and an outer stratum functionale. The stratum functionale may be further subdivided into an inner compact stratum and a more superficial spongy stratum. Only the stratum functionale responds to fluctuating hormonal levels.

The uterine and ovarian arteries provide the arterial blood supply of the uterus. The uterine arteries are large branches of the hypogastric arteries, whereas the ovarian arteries originate directly from the aorta. The veins of the pelvic organs accompany the arteries. Therefore venous drainage from the fundus goes to the ovarian veins and blood from the corpus exits via the uterine veins into the iliac veins. The lymphatic drainage of the uterus is complex. The lymphatics from the fundus and the body of the uterus go to the aortic, lumbar, or pelvic nodes surrounding the iliac vessels, especially the internal iliac nodes. However, it is possible for metastatic disease from the uterus to be found in the superior inguinal nodes transported via lymphatics in the round ligament, or directly spread to the paraaortic nodes. Surprisingly, the lymphatic drainage of the uterus is not that different from the lymphatic drainage of the cervix.

In contrast to other pelvic organs, the afferent sensory nerve fibers from the uterus are in close proximity to the sympathetic nerves. Afferent nerve fibers from the uterus enter the spinal

| Day of Cycle | | Before 14 | 15-16 | 17 | 18 | 19-22 | 23 | 24-25 | 26-27 | 28+ |
|---|---|---|---|---|---|---|---|---|---|---|
| Post-ovulatory day | | - | 1-2 | 3 | 4 | 5-8 | 9 | 10-11 | 12-13 | 14+ |
| Cycle phases | | Proliferative | 'Interval' | Early secretory | | Mid-secretory | | | Late secretory | Menstrual |
| Key feature | | Mitoses | Mitoses and subnuclear vacuoles | Maximum subnuclear vacuoles | Subnuclear vacuoles present | Stromal edema | Focal decidua around spiral arteries | Patchy decidua | Extensive decidua | Stromal crumbling |
| Microscopic features of functional zone | Stroma | Loose stroma. Mitoses | Same as proliferative | Loose stroma, scanty mitoses | Loose stroma | Stromal edema | Focal decidua around spiral arteries. Edema prominent | Decidua throughout stroma. Some edema | Extensive decidua. Prominent granulated lymphocytes | Stromal crumbling. Hemorrhage |
| | Glands | Straight to tightly coiled tubules. Mitoses | Some subnuclear vacuoles, otherwise as proliferative | Extensive subnuclear vacuoles | Dilated glands. Some subnuclear vacuoles | Dilated glands with irregular outline. Luminal secretion | | "sawtooth" glands | Prominent "sawtooth" glands | Disrupted glands. Secretory exhaustion. Regenerating epithelium |
| Appearances | | 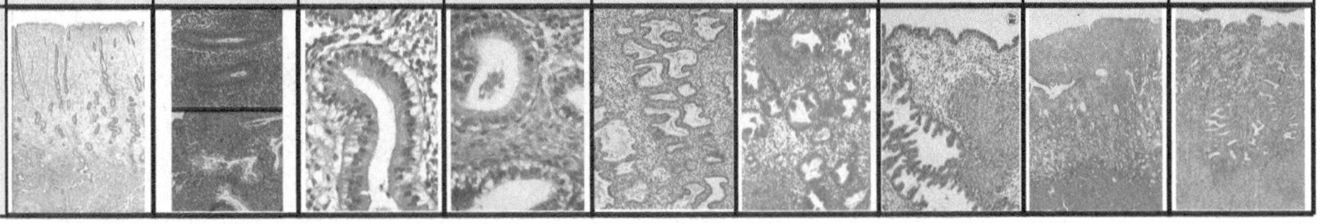 | | | | | | | | |

**Figure 3.16** The endometrium is responsive to the hormonal changes of the menstrual cycle. Glands and stroma change activity and thus histologic appearance throughout the cycle. (From Robboy SJ, Anderson MC, Russell P, eds. *Pathology of the Female Reproductive Tract*. Edinburgh: Churchill Livingstone; 2002:248.)

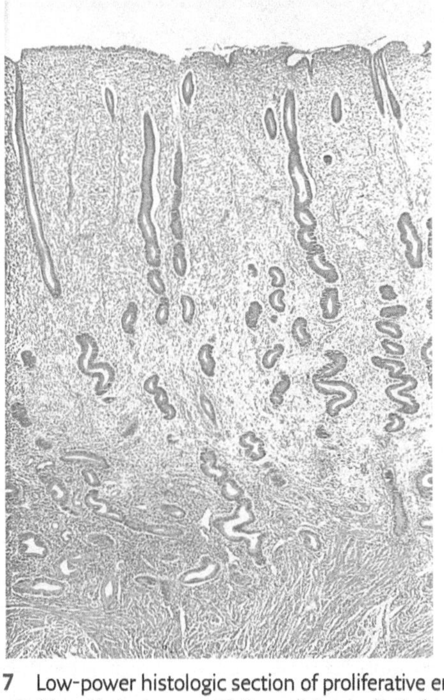

**Figure 3.17** Low-power histologic section of proliferative endometrium. (From Robboy SJ, Anderson MC, Russell P, eds. *Pathology of the Female Reproductive Tract*. Edinburgh: Churchill Livingstone; 2002:248.)

cord at the eleventh and twelfth thoracic segments. The sympathetic nerve supply to the uterus comes from the hypogastric and ovarian plexus. The parasympathetic fibers are largely derived from the pelvic nerve and from the second, third, and fourth sacral segments.

## CLINICAL CORRELATIONS

Removal of the uterus is termed *hysterectomy*, which is derived from the Greek word *hystera*, meaning *womb*. The symptoms of primary dysmenorrhea are treated successfully in most women by prostaglandin synthetase inhibition. Usually a woman's pain is controlled by oral medication. However, it is possible to alleviate uterine pain by cutting the sensory nerves that accompany the sympathetic nerves. This operation is termed a *presacral neurectomy*. During the operation, the gynecologist must be careful to avoid injuring the ureters and also careful to control hemorrhage from vessels in the retroperitoneal space.

The position of the fundus of the uterus in relation to the long axis of the vagina is quite variable. Not only are there differences among individual women, but also in the same woman differences occur secondary to normal activity. In some women the uterus is anteflexed or anteverted, whereas in others the normal position is retroflexed or retroverted. In the 1930s and 1940s, a retroflexed uterus was believed to be one of the primary causes of pelvic pain. To alleviate this condition, many women underwent an anterior uterine suspension. Modern gynecologists have abandoned the suspension operation as a treatment for pelvic pain.

The arterial blood supply enters the uterus on its lateral margins. This relationship allows morcellation of an enlarged uterus to facilitate removal of multiple myomas without appreciably increasing blood loss during vaginal hysterectomy.

Methods of transcervical female sterilization, designed to occlude the tubal ostia at the uterine cornua, are effective and commonly used (Essure). Prior to the application of this method, procedures that blindly injected caustic solutions into the uterine cornua had a high failure rate. Individual differences

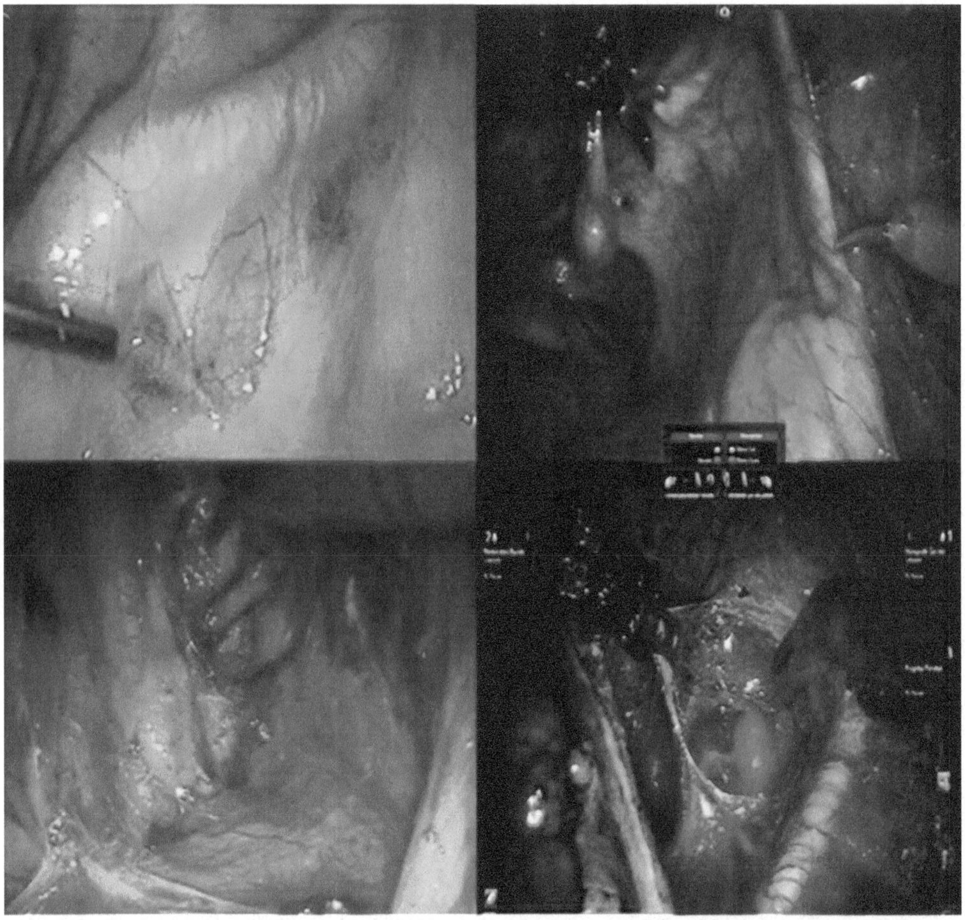

**Figure 3.18** Intraoperative view of sentinel lymph node mapping with isosulfan blue dye on the left and indocyanine green on the right. (From Sinno AK, Fader AN, Roche KL, et al. A comparison of colorimetric versus fluorometric sentinel lymph node mapping during robotic surgery for endometrial cancer. *Gynecol Oncol.* 2014;134[2]:281-286.)

in the size and shape of the uterine cavity and muscular spasm of this region are the primary reasons that sufficient amounts of the caustic chemicals did not reach the fallopian tubes in up to 20% of patients.

Similar to the lymphatic drainage of the cervix, the lymphatic drainage of the uterus has also been studied. Sentinel lymph nodes can also be found on either side of the pelvis/paraaortic areas in 85% to 90% of cases using near-infrared fluorescence imaging and indocyanine green (ICG) (Abu-Rustum, 2014) (Fig. 3.18).

## OVIDUCTS

The paired uterine tubes, more commonly referred to as the *fallopian tubes* or *oviducts,* extend outward from the superolateral portion of the uterus and end by curling around the ovary. The oviducts are also referred to using the prefix *salpingo-,* from the Greek *salpinx,* meaning a tube. The tubes are contained in a free edge of the superior portion of the broad ligament. The mesentery of the tubes, the mesosalpinx, contains the blood supply and nerves. The uterine tubes connect the cornua of the uterine cavity and the peritoneal cavity. The ostia into the endometrial cavity are 1.5 mm in diameter, whereas the ostia into the abdominal cavity are approximately 3 mm in diameter.

The oviducts are between 10 and 14 cm in length and slightly less than 1 cm in external diameter. Each tube is divided into four anatomic sections. The uterine intramural, or interstitial, segment is 1 to 2 cm in length and is surrounded by myometrium. The isthmic segment begins as the tube exits the uterus and is approximately 4 cm in length. This segment is narrow, 1 to 2 mm in inside diameter, and straight. The isthmic segment has the most highly developed musculature. The ampullary segment is 4 to 6 cm in length and approximately 6 mm in inside diameter. It is wider and more tortuous in its course than other segments. Fertilization normally occurs in the ampullary portion of the tube. The infundibulum is the distal trumpet-shaped portion of the oviduct. From 20 to 25 irregular finger-like projections, termed *fimbriae,* surround the abdominal ostia of the tube. One of the largest fimbriae is attached to the ovary, the fimbria ovarica.

The tube contains numerous longitudinal folds, called *plicae,* of mucosa and underlying stroma. Plicae are most prominent in the ampullary segment (Fig. 3.19). The mucosa of the oviduct has three different cell types. Columnar ciliated epithelial cells are most prominent near the ovarian end of the tube and overall compose 25% of the mucosal cells (Fig. 3.20). Secretory cells, also columnar in shape, compose 60% of the epithelial lining and are more prominent in the isthmic segment. Narrow peg cells are

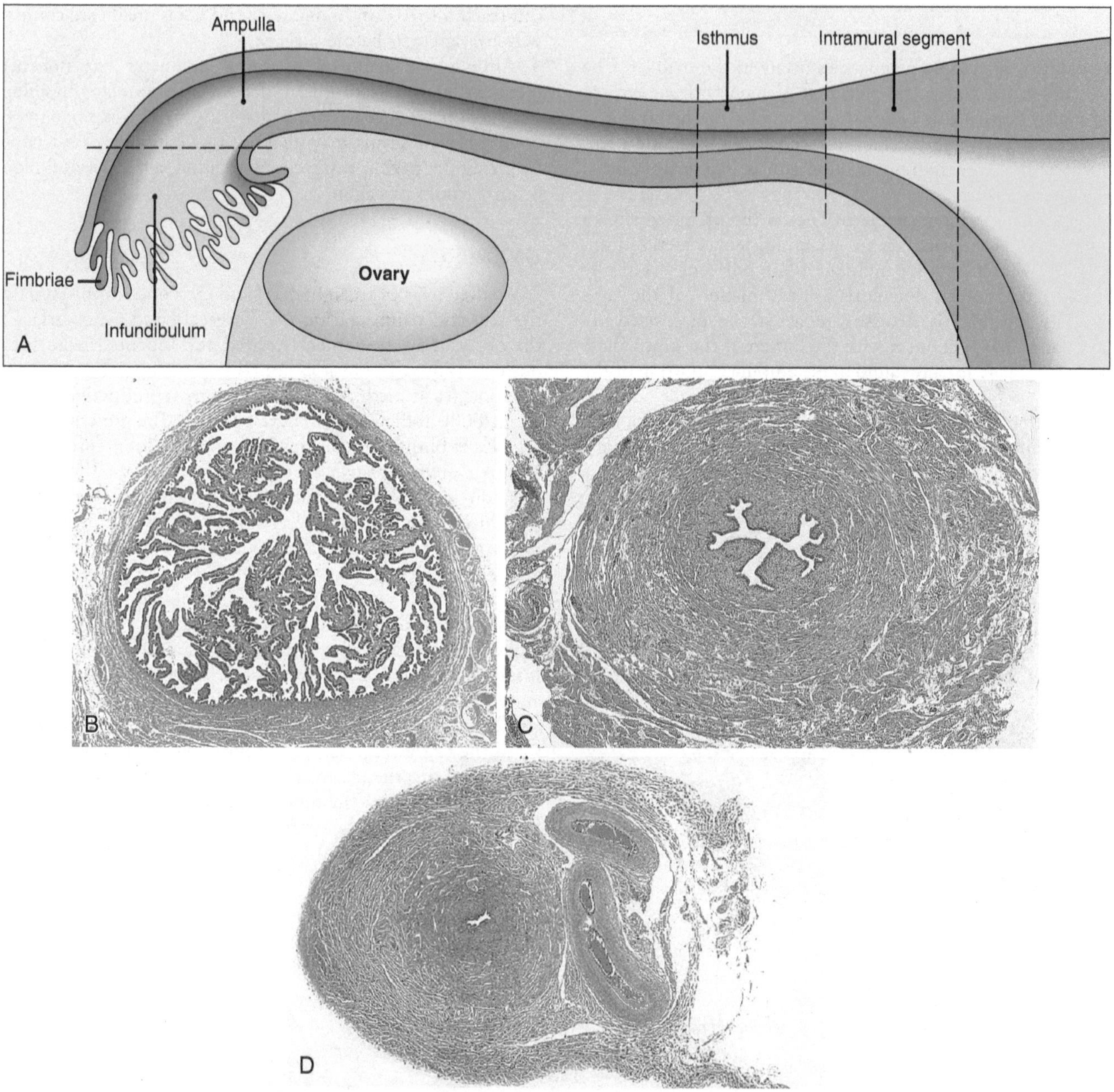


**Figure 3.19** The fallopian tube. **A**, Schematic representation. Note that the intramural segment is within the uterine body. **B**, Low-power histologic section from the ampulla. **C**, Section from the isthmus of the tube. **D**, Section from the isthmus. Note the thick muscular wall. (**A**, **B**, and **D**, From Stevens A, Lowe J. *Human Histology.* 3rd ed. Philadelphia: Elsevier; 2002:354; **C**, From Robboy SJ, Anderson MC, Russell P, eds. *Pathology of the Female Reproductive Tract.* Edinburgh: Churchill Livingstone; 2002:416.)

found between secretory and ciliated cells and are believed to be a morphologic variant of secretory cells. The stroma of the mucosa is sparse. However, there is a thick lamina propria with vascular channels between the epithelium and muscular layers. The smooth muscle of the tube is arranged into inner circular and outer longitudinal layers. Between the peritoneal surface of the tube and the muscular layer is an adventitial layer that contains blood vessels and nerves.

The arterial blood supply to the oviducts is derived from terminal branches of the uterine and ovarian arteries. The arteries anastomose in the mesosalpinx. Blood from the uterine artery supplies the medial two thirds of each tube. The venous drainage runs parallel to the arterial supply. The lymphatic system is separate and distinct from the lymphatic drainage of the uterus. Lymphatic drainage includes the internal iliac nodes and the aortic nodes surrounding the aorta and the inferior vena cava at the level of the renal vessels. The tubes are innervated by both sympathetic and parasympathetic nerves from the uterine and ovarian plexuses. Sensory nerves are related to spinal cord segments T11, T12, and L1.

## CLINICAL CORRELATIONS

The majority of ectopic pregnancies occur in the oviduct. The acute abdominal and pelvic pain that women with an ectopic pregnancy experience is believed to be caused by hemorrhage. The most catastrophic bleeding associated with ectopic pregnancy occurs when the implantation site is in the intramural segment of the tube.

The isthmic segment of the oviduct is the preferred site to apply an occlusive device, such as a clip, for female sterilization. The right oviduct and appendix are often adjacent. Clinically it may be difficult to differentiate inflammation of the tube from acute appendicitis. Accessory tubal ostia are discovered frequently and always connect with the lumen of the tube. These accessory ostia are usually found in the ampullary portion of the tube.

The wide mesosalpinx of the ampullary segment of the tube allows torsion of the tube, which occasionally results in ischemic atrophy of the ampullary segment. Paratubal or paraovarian cysts can reach 5 to 10 cm in diameter and occasionally are confused with ovarian cysts before surgery.

Although a definitive anatomic sphincter has not been identified at the uterotubal junction, a temporary physiologic obstruction has been identified during hysterosalpingography. Sometimes clinicians may alleviate this temporary obstruction by giving the patient intravenous sedation, a paracervical block, or intravenous glucagon.

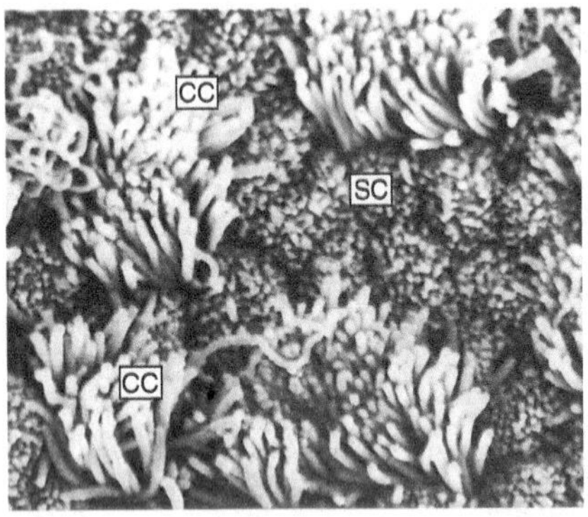


**Figure 3.20** Electron micrograph of the tubal mucosa from the ampulla. *CC*, Ciliated cells; *SC*, secretory cells. (From Stevens A, Lowe J. *Human Histology.* 3rd ed. Philadelphia: Elsevier; 2002:354.)

### *OVARIES*

The paired ovaries are light gray, and each one is approximately the size and configuration of a large almond. The surface of the ovary of adult women is pitted and indented from previous ovulations. The ovaries contain approximately 1 to 2 million oocytes at birth. During a woman's reproductive lifetime, about 8000 follicles begin development. The growth of many follicles is blunted in various stages of development; however, approximately 300 ova eventually are released. The size and position of the ovary depend on the woman's age and parity. During the reproductive years, ovaries weigh 3 to 6 g and measure approximately 1.5 cm × 2.5 cm × 4 cm. As a woman ages, the ovaries become smaller and firmer in consistency. The long axis of the ovary is vertical in a nulliparous woman who is standing, and the ovary rests in a depression of peritoneum named the ovarian fossa. Immediately adjacent to the ovarian fossa are the external iliac vessels, the ureter, and the obturator vessels and nerves.

Three prominent ligaments determine the anatomic mobility of the ovary (Fig. 3.21). The posterior portion of the broad ligament forms the mesovarium, which attaches to the anterior border of the ovary. The mesovarium contains the arterial anastomotic branches of the ovarian and uterine arteries, a plexus of veins, and the lateral end of the ovarian ligament. The ovarian ligament is a narrow, short, fibrous band that extends from the

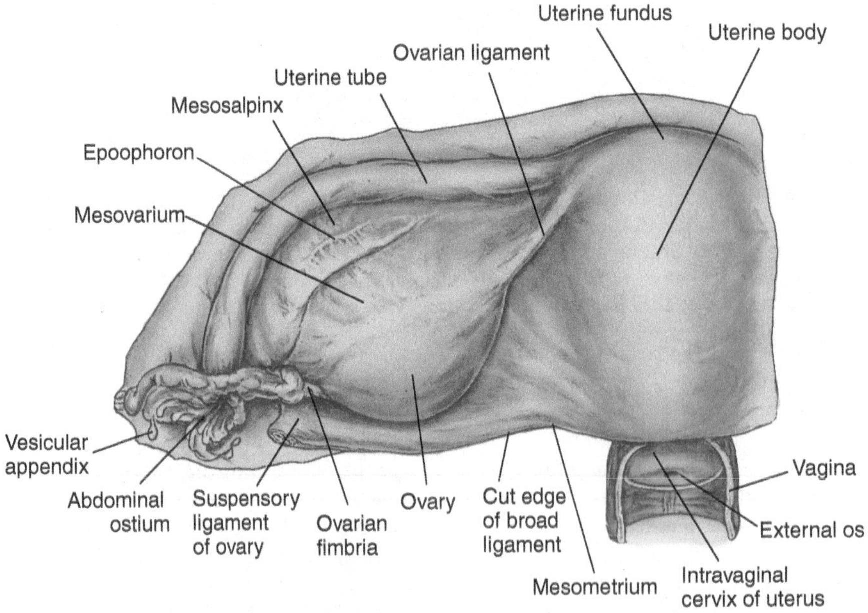


**Figure 3.21** The posterior aspect of the broad ligament—spread out to demonstrate the ovary. (From Standring S, ed. *Gray's Anatomy.* 39th ed. Edinburgh: Churchill Livingstone; 2005:1322.)

lower pole of the ovary to the uterus. The infundibulopelvic ligament, or suspensory ligament of the ovary, forms the superior and lateral aspect of the broad ligament. This ligament contains the ovarian artery, ovarian veins, and accompanying nerves. It attaches the upper pole of the ovary to the lateral pelvic wall.

The ovary is subdivided histologically into an outer cortex and an inner medulla (Fig. 3.22). The ovarian surface is covered by a single layer of cuboidal epithelium, termed the *germinal epithelium*. This term is a misnomer because the cells are similar to those of the coelomic mesothelium, which forms the peritoneum, and because the germinal epithelium is not related to the histogenesis of graafian follicles. If the ovary is transected, numerous transparent, fluid-filled cysts are noted throughout the cortex. Microscopically these are graafian follicles in various stages of development, active or regressing corpus luteum, and atretic follicles. The stroma of the cortex is composed primarily of closely packed cells around the follicles. These specialized connective tissue cells form the theca. The medulla contains the ovarian vascular supply and a loose stroma. The specialized polyhedral hilar cells are similar to the interstitial cells of the testis.

Each of the ovarian arteries arises directly from the aorta just below the renal arteries. They descend in the retroperitoneal space, cross anterior to the psoas muscles and internal iliac vessels, and enter the infundibulopelvic ligaments, reaching the mesovarium in the broad ligament. The ovarian blood supply enters through the hilum of the ovary. The venous drainage of the ovary collects in the pampiniform plexus and consolidates into several large veins as it leaves the hilum of the ovary. The ovarian veins accompany the ovarian arteries, with the left ovarian vein draining into the left renal vein, whereas the right ovarian vein connects directly with the inferior vena cava.

The lymphatic drainage of the ovaries is primarily to the aortic nodes adjacent to the great vessels at the level of the renal veins. Metastatic disease from the ovary occasionally takes a shorter course to the iliac nodes. The autonomic and sensory nerve fibers accompany the ovarian vasculature in the infundibulopelvic ligament. They connect with the ovarian, hypogastric, and aortic plexuses.

## CLINICAL CORRELATIONS

The size of the "normal" ovary during the reproductive years and the postmenopausal period is important in clinical practice. Before menopause a normal ovary may be up to 5 cm in length. Thus a small physiologic cyst may cause an ovary to be 6 to 7 cm in diameter. In contrast, the normal atrophic postmenopausal ovary usually cannot be palpated during pelvic examination.

It is important to emphasize that the ovaries and surrounding peritoneum are not devoid of pain and pressure receptors. Therefore it is not unusual for a woman during a routine pelvic examination to experience discomfort when normal ovaries are palpated bimanually.

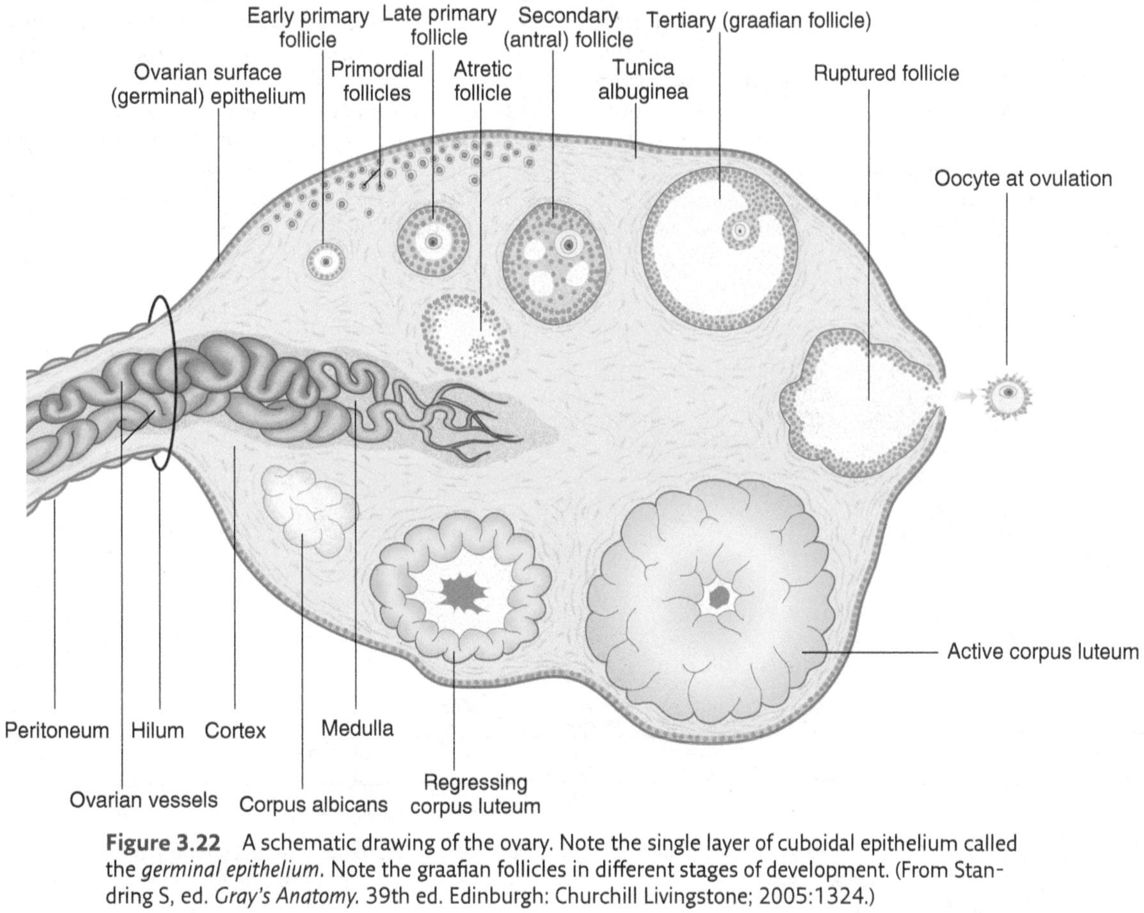


**Figure 3.22** A schematic drawing of the ovary. Note the single layer of cuboidal epithelium called the *germinal epithelium*. Note the graafian follicles in different stages of development. (From Standring S, ed. *Gray's Anatomy*. 39th ed. Edinburgh: Churchill Livingstone; 2005:1324.)

Attempts have been made to alleviate chronic pelvic pain by performing an ovarian denervation operation by cutting and ligating the infundibulopelvic ligaments. This operation has been abandoned because of the high incidence of cystic degeneration of the ovaries, which resulted from the interruption of their primary blood supply that was associated with the neurectomy procedure.

The close anatomic proximity of the ovary, ovarian fossa, and ureter is emphasized in surgery to treat severe endometriosis or pelvic inflammatory disease. It is important to identify the course of the ureter to facilitate removal of all of the ovarian capsule that is adherent to the peritoneum and surrounding structures so as to avoid immediate ureteral injury and residual retroperitoneal ovarian remnants in the future. Prophylactic oophorectomy is performed at the time of pelvic operations in many peri- and postmenopausal women. Sometimes bilateral oophorectomy is technically more difficult when associated with a vaginal procedure in contrast to an abdominal or laparoscopic hysterectomy. Vaginal removal of the ovaries may be facilitated by identifying the anatomic landmarks, similar to the abdominal approach, and separately clamping the round ligaments and infundibulopelvic ligaments.

## VASCULAR SYSTEM OF THE PELVIS

Several generalizations should be made in describing the network of arteries that bring blood to the female reproductive organs. The arteries are paired, bilateral, and have multiple collaterals (Fig. 3.23). The arteries enter their respective organs laterally and then unite with anastomotic vessels from the other side of the pelvis near the midline. There is a long-standing teaching generalization that the pelvic reproductive viscera lie within a loosely woven basket of large veins with numerous interconnecting venous plexuses. The arteries thread their way through this interwoven mesh of veins to reach the pelvic reproductive organs, giving off numerous branching arcades to provide a rich blood supply.

### ARTERIES

#### *Inferior Mesenteric Artery*

The inferior mesenteric artery, a single artery, arises from the aorta approximately 3 cm above the aortic bifurcation. It supplies part of the transverse, descending and sigmoid colon, as well as the rectum, and terminates as the superior hemorrhoidal artery. The inferior mesenteric artery is occasionally torn during node dissections performed in staging operations for gynecologic cancer. Because of the rich collateral circulation from the middle and inferior hemorrhoidal arteries, as well as the marginal artery of Drummond, the inferior mesenteric artery can be ligated without compromise of the distal portion of the colon.

#### *Ovarian Artery*

The ovarian arteries originate from the aorta just below the renal vessels. Each one courses in the retroperitoneal space, crosses anterior to the ureter, and enters the infundibulopelvic ligament. As the artery travels medially in the mesovarium, numerous small branches supply the ovary and oviduct. The ovarian artery unites with the ascending branch of the uterine artery in the mesovarium just under the suspensory ligament of the ovary.

#### *Common Iliac Artery*

The bifurcation of the aorta occurs at the level of the fourth lumbar vertebra, forming the two common iliac arteries. Each common iliac artery is approximately 5 cm in length before the vessel divides into the external iliac and hypogastric arteries.

#### *Hypogastric Artery (Internal Iliac Artery)*

The hypogastric arteries are short vessels, approximately 3 to 4 cm in length. Throughout their course they are in close proximity to the ureters, which are anterior, and to the hypogastric veins, which are posterior. Most commonly (variations are frequent),

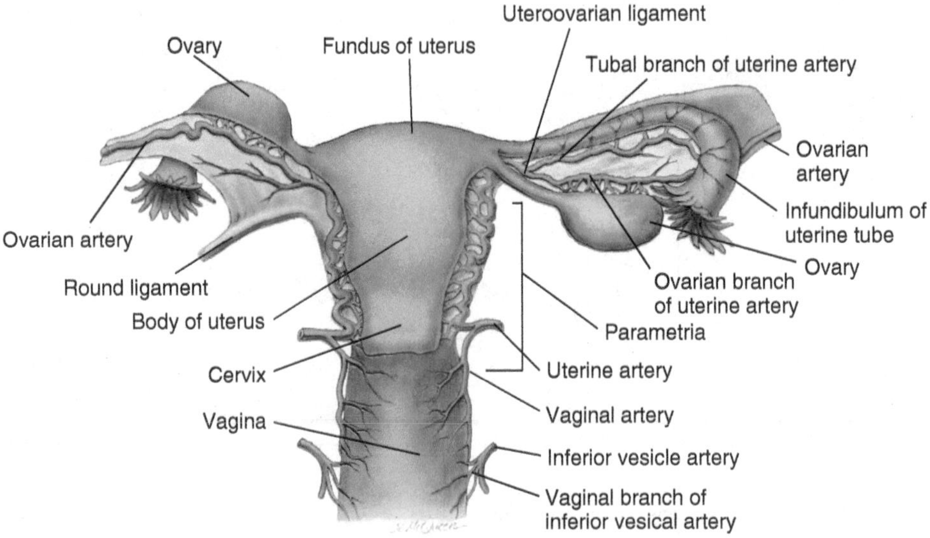


**Figure 3.23** The arteries of the reproductive organs. Note the paired arteries entering laterally and freely anastomosing with each other. (Modified from Clemente CD. *Anatomy: A Regional Atlas of the Human Body.* 3rd ed. Baltimore-Munich: Urban & Schwarzenberg; 1987.)

each hypogastric artery branches into an anterior and a posterior division (or trunk). The branching is usually 2 cm from the common iliac. The posterior trunk gives off three parietal branches: the iliolumbar, lateral sacral, and superior gluteal arteries. The anterior trunk has nine branches. The three parietal branches are the obturator, internal pudendal, and inferior gluteal arteries. The six visceral branches include the umbilical, middle vesical, inferior vesical, middle hemorrhoidal, uterine, and vaginal arteries. The superior vesical artery usually arises from the umbilical artery. The individual branches of the hypogastric artery may vary from one woman to another.

#### *Uterine Artery*

The uterine artery arises from the anterior division of the hypogastric artery and courses medially toward the isthmus of the uterus. Approximately 2 cm lateral to the endocervix, it crosses over the ureter and reaches the lateral side of the uterus. The ascending branch of the uterine artery courses in the broad ligament, running a tortuous route to finally anastomose with the ovarian artery in the mesovarium (Fig. 3.24). Through its circuitous route in the parametrium, the uterine artery gives off numerous branches that unite with arcuate arteries from the other side. This series of arcuate arteries develops radial branches that supply the myometrium and the basalis layer of the endometrium. The arcuate arteries also form the spiral arteries of the functional layer of the endometrium. The descending branch of the uterine artery produces branches that supply both the cervix and the vagina. In each case the vessels enter the organ laterally and anastomose freely with vessels from the other side.

### *VAGINAL ARTERY*

The vaginal artery may arise either from the anterior trunk of the hypogastric artery or from the uterine artery. It supplies blood to the vagina, bladder, and rectum. There are extensive anastomoses with the vaginal branches of the uterine artery to form the azygos arteries of the cervix and vagina.

#### *Internal Pudendal Artery*

This artery is the terminal branch of the hypogastric artery and supplies branches to the rectum, labia, clitoris, and perineum.

### *VEINS*

The venous drainage of the pelvis begins in small sinusoids that drain to numerous venous plexuses contained within or immediately adjacent to the pelvic organs. Invariably there are numerous anastomoses between the parietal and visceral branches of the venous system. In general the veins of the female pelvis and perineum are thin walled and have few valves.

The veins that drain the pelvic plexuses follow the course of the arterial supply. Their names are similar to those of the accompanying arteries. Often multiple veins run alongside a single artery. One special exception is the venous drainage of the ovaries. The left ovarian vein empties into the left renal vein, whereas the right ovarian vein connects directly with the inferior vena cava.

## CLINICAL CORRELATIONS

Although the external iliac artery and its branches do not supply blood directly to the pelvic viscera, they are important landmarks in surgical anatomy. The fact that the external iliac artery gives rise to the obturator artery in 15% to 20% of women must be considered in radical cancer operations with associated node dissections of the obturator fossa. The external iliac artery also gives rise to the inferior epigastric artery. The inferior epigastric artery should be avoided when performing laparoscopic operative procedures.

In certain clinical situations associated with profuse hemorrhage from the female pelvis, hypogastric artery ligation is performed. Because of the extensive collateral circulation, this operation does not produce hypoxia of the pelvic viscera but reduces hemorrhage by decreasing the arterial pulse pressure.

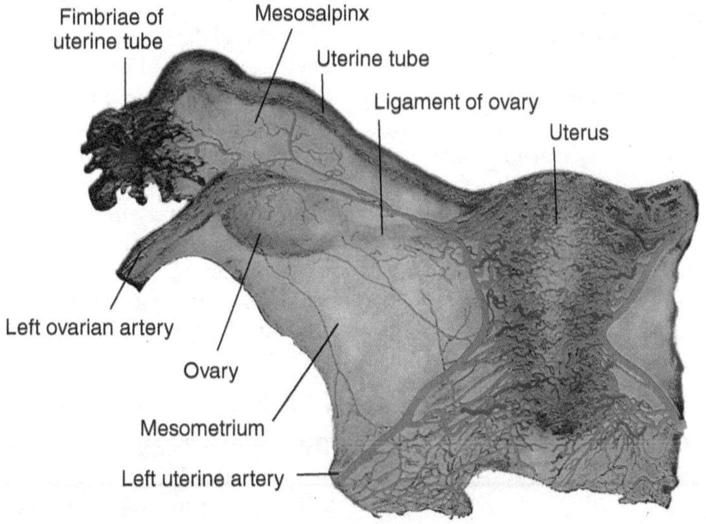


**Figure 3.24** A photograph of an injected specimen demonstrating the rich anastomoses of the uterine and ovarian arteries. (From Warwick R, Williams PL. *Gray's Anatomy*. 35th ed. Edinburgh: Churchill Livingstone; 1973:1361.)

**Box 3.1 Collateral Arterial Circulation of the Pelvis**

**Branches from Aorta**

*Ovarian artery*—anastomoses freely with uterine artery

*Inferior mesenteric artery*—continues as superior hemorrhoidal artery to anastomose with middle and inferior hemorrhoidal arteries from hypogastric and internal pudendal

*Lumbar and vertebral arteries*—anastomose with iliolumbar artery of hypogastric

*Middle sacral artery*—anastomoses with lateral sacral artery of hypogastric

**Branches from External Iliac Artery**

*Deep iliac circumflex artery*—anastomoses with iliolumbar and superior gluteal of hypogastric

*Inferior epigastric artery*—gives origin to obturator artery in 25% of cases, providing additional anastomoses of external iliac with medial femoral circumflex and communicating pelvic branches

**Branches from Femoral Artery**

*Medial femoral circumflex artery*—anastomoses with obturator and inferior gluteal arteries from hypogastric

*Lateral femoral circumflex artery*—anastomoses with superior gluteal and iliolumbar arteries from hypogastric

From Mattingly RF, Thompson JD. *Te Linde's Operative Gynecology.* 6th ed. Philadelphia: JB Lippincott; 1985.

The extent of collateral circulation after hypogastric artery ligation depends on the site of ligation and may be divided into three groups (Box 3.1).

In cases of intractable pelvic hemorrhage, it may be necessary to supplement the effects of bilateral hypogastric artery ligation with ligation of the anastomotic sites between the ovarian and uterine vessels. Ligation of the terminal end of the ovarian artery (utero-ovarian ligament) preserves the direct blood supply to the ovaries and minimizes the fear of subsequent cystic degeneration of the ovaries that may occur after ligation of the vessels in the infundibulopelvic ligaments. Arterial embolization provides an alternative approach to ligation. A catheter is advanced under fluoroscopic visualization, and small particulate material is injected to produce hemostasis in the bleeding vessels. This less invasive technique, when appropriate, may preserve fertility. A rare condition that presents an interesting challenge to the clinician is a congenital arteriovenous (A-V) malformation in the female pelvis. Most of these A-V fistulas are treated with preoperative embolism and subsequent operative ligation.

One of the treatments for repetitive embolization arising from thrombosis is the placement of a vascular umbrella into the inferior vena cava. Collateral circulation exists between the portal venous system of the gastrointestinal tract and the systemic venous circulation through anastomosis in the pelvis, especially in the hemorrhoidal plexus. The pelvic veins also anastomose with the presacral and lumbar veins. Thus though rare, patients may develop trophoblastic emboli to the brain without the trophoblast being filtered by the capillary system in the lungs.

## LYMPHATIC SYSTEM

### EXTERNAL ILIAC NODES

The external iliac nodes are immediately adjacent to the external iliac artery and vein (Figs. 3.25 and 3.26). There are two distinct groups, one situated lateral to the vessels and the other posterior to the psoas muscle. The distal portion of the posterior group is enclosed in the femoral sheath. Most of the lymphatic channels to this group of nodes originate from the vulva, but there are also channels from the cervix and lower portion of the uterus. The external iliac nodes receive secondary drainage from the femoral and internal iliac nodes.

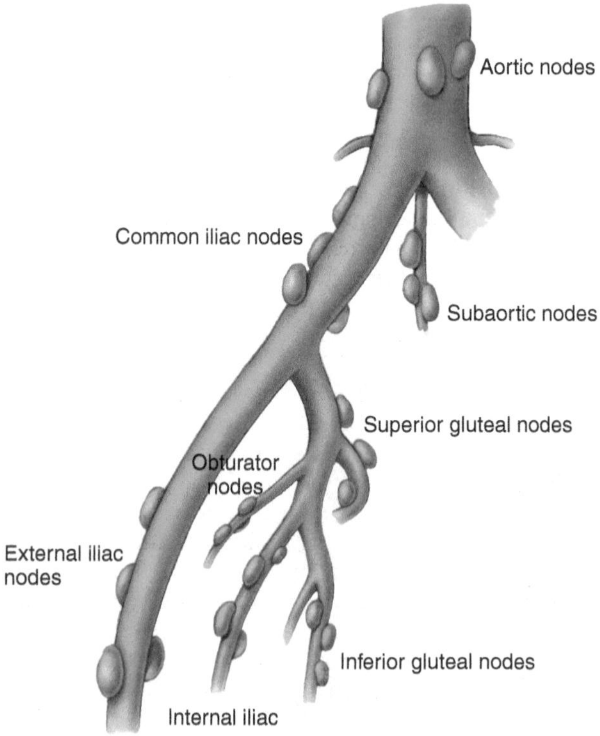


**Figure 3.25** Schematic view of the pelvic lymph nodes. (From Plentl AA, Friedman EA. *Lymphatic System of the Female Genitalia.* Philadelphia: WB Saunders; 1971:13.)

### INTERNAL ILIAC NODES

The internal iliac nodes are found in an anatomic triangle whose sides are composed of the external iliac artery, the hypogastric artery, and the pelvic sidewall. Included in this clinically important area are nodes with special designation, including the nodes of the femoral ring, the obturator nodes, and the nodes adjacent to the external iliac vessels. This rich collection of nodes receives channels from every internal pelvic organ and the vulva, including the clitoris and urethra. The sentinel lymph nodes from the cervix and uterus are frequently found within the internal iliac chain of nodes, most commonly, inferior and medial to the bifurcation of iliac vein.

### COMMON ILIAC NODES

The common iliac nodes are a group of nodes located adjacent to the vessels that bear their name and are between the external iliac and aortic chains. Most of these nodes are found lateral to the vessels. To remove this chain, it is necessary to dissect the common iliac vessels away from their attachments to the psoas muscle, as well as the genitofemoral nerve, which is commonly encased

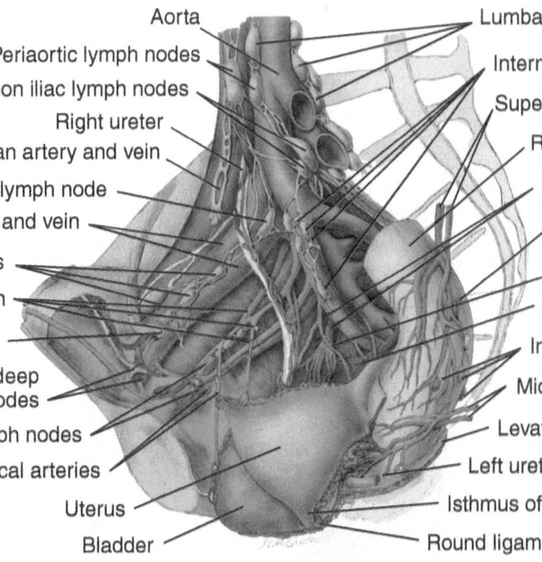


**Figure 3.26** A lateral view of the female pelvis demonstrating the extensive lymphatic network. Note that most of the lymphatic channels follow the courses of the major vessels. (Modified from Clemente CD. *Anatomy: A Regional Atlas of the Human Body.* 3rd ed. Baltimore-Munich: Urban & Schwarzenberg; 1987.)

in lymph nodes. This group receives lymphatics from the cervix, uterus, ovary, and the upper portion of the vagina. Secondary lymphatic drainage from the internal iliac, external iliac, superior gluteal, and inferior gluteal nodes flows to the common iliac nodes.

### *INFERIOR GLUTEAL NODES*

A small group of lymph nodes, the inferior gluteal nodes, are located in anatomic proximity to the ischial spines and are adjacent to the sacral plexus of nodes. It is difficult to remove these nodes surgically. The nodes receive lymphatics from the cervix, the lower portion of the vagina, and Bartholin glands. This group of nodes secondarily drains to the internal iliac, common iliac, superior gluteal, and subaortic nodes.

### *SUPERIOR GLUTEAL NODES*

The superior gluteal nodes are a group of nodes found near the origin of the superior gluteal artery and adjacent to the medial and posterior aspects of the hypogastric vessels. The superior gluteal nodes receive primary lymphatic drainage from the cervix and the vagina. Efferent lymphatics from this chain drain to the common iliac, sacral, or subaortic nodes.

### *SACRAL NODES*

The sacral nodes are found over the middle of the sacrum in a space bounded laterally by the sacral foramina. These nodes receive lymphatic drainage from both the cervix and the vagina. Secondary drainage from these nodes runs in a cephalad direction to the subaortic nodes.

### *SUBAORTIC NODES*

The subaortic nodes are arranged in a chain and are located below the bifurcation of the aorta, immediately anterior to the most caudal portion of the inferior vena cava and over the fifth lumbar vertebra. The primary drainage to this chain of nodes is from the cervix, with a few lymphatics from the vagina. This group is the first secondary chain to receive the efferent lymphatics as lymph flow progresses in a cephalad direction from the majority of other pelvic nodes.

### *AORTIC NODES*

The many aortic nodes are immediately adjacent to the aorta on both its anterior and lateral aspects, predominantly in the furrow between the aorta and inferior vena cava. Primary lymphatics drain from all the major pelvic organs, including the cervix, uterus, oviducts, and especially the ovaries. The aortic chain receives secondary drainage from the pelvic nodes. In general, primary afferent lymphatics drain into the nodes over the anterior aspects of the aorta, whereas secondary efferent drainage from other pelvic nodes is found in those nodes situated lateral and posterior to the aorta.

### *RECTAL NODES*

The rectal nodes are found subfascially and in the loose connective tissue surrounding the rectum. Primary drainage from the cervix flows to the superior rectal nodes, and drainage from the vagina appears in the rectal nodes in the anorectal region. Secondary drainage from the rectal nodes goes to the subaortic and aortic groups.

### *PARAUTERINE NODES*

The number of lymph nodes in the group of parauterine nodes is small; most frequently there is a single node immediately lateral to each side of the cervix and adjacent to the pelvic course of the ureter. Though anatomists frequently do not comment about the parauterine nodes, the group receives special attention in radical surgical operations to treat uterine or cervical malignancy.

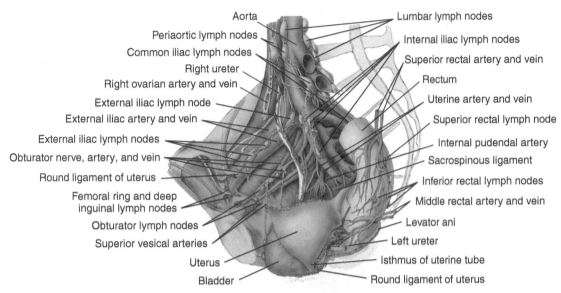

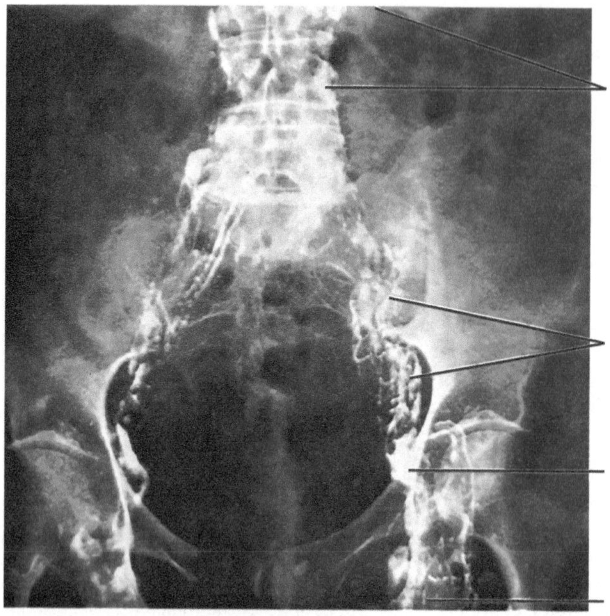


**Figure 3.27** A lymphangiogram of the pelvis and lumbar areas. This radiograph shows the course of the lymphatics from the deep femoral nodes into the iliac nodes. Note the extensive network of nodes in the inguinal region. (From Clemente CD. *A Regional Atlas of the Human Body.* 3rd ed. Baltimore-Munich: Urban & Schwarzenberg; 1987.)

Primary drainage to this node originates in the vagina, cervix, and uterus. Secondary drainage from this node is to the internal iliac nodes on the same side of the pelvis.

### SUPERFICIAL FEMORAL NODES

The superficial femoral nodes are a group of nodes found in the loose, fatty connective tissue of the femoral triangle between the superficial and deep fascial layers. These lymph nodes receive lymphatic drainage from the external genitalia of the vulvar region, the gluteal region, and the entire leg, including the foot. Efferent lymphatics from this group of nodes penetrate the fascia lata to enter the deep femoral nodes (Fig. 3.27).

### DEEP FEMORAL NODES

The deep femoral nodes are located in the femoral sheath, adjacent to both the femoral artery and the vein within the femoral triangle. The femoral triangle is the anatomic space lying immediately distal to the fold of the groin. The boundaries of the femoral triangle are the sartorius and adductor longus muscles and the inguinal ligament. Each space contains, from medial to lateral, the femoral vein, artery, and nerve. This chain receives the primary lymphatics for the lower extremity and receives secondary efferent lymphatics from the superficial lymph nodes and thus the vulva. This group of lymph nodes is in direct continuity with the iliac and internal iliac chains.

## CLINICAL CORRELATIONS

A precise knowledge of pelvic lymphatics is important for the gynecologic oncologist who is surgically determining the extent of spread of a pelvic malignancy. Aortic and pelvic lymphadenectomy operations require precise knowledge of normal anatomy and possible anomalies in both the urinary and vascular systems. The fact that most lymphatic metastatic spread from ovarian carcinoma occurs in a cephalad direction should be emphasized. This explains the importance of sampling paraaortic nodes in staging operations for some ovarian and uterine malignancy. In carcinoma of the vulva, lymphatic drainage is usually unilateral for cancers that are clearly lateral to the midline but may drain to either side with midline or near midline lesions of the pelvis (Coleman, 2013). Thus bilateral node sampling is important for midline lesions, although most vulvar cancers less than 4 cm in size can be managed with SLN mapping and biopsy; limiting the extent of nodal dissection and hopefully limiting morbidity as well. Frequently, the SLN from vulvar cancer surgery can be found just inferior and lateral to the pubic tubercle (Fig. 3.28).

Pelvic hemorrhage, usually from venous bleeding, is the most common acute complication of a lymph node dissection because most pelvic lymph nodes are in anatomic proximity to major pelvic vessels. Lymphocysts in the retroperitoneal space are the most common chronic complication associated with radical node dissections.

For many years it was believed that all the superficial femoral nodes drained to a sentinel node called the *Cloquet node.* The Cloquet node, by the present classification system, would be one of the most distal and medial of the nodes in the external iliac chain. The Cloquet node is only of historical interest, because the assumption is neither anatomically nor clinically correct.

## INNERVATION OF THE PELVIS

### INTERNAL GENITALIA

The innervation of the internal genital organs is supplied primarily by the autonomic nervous system. The sympathetic

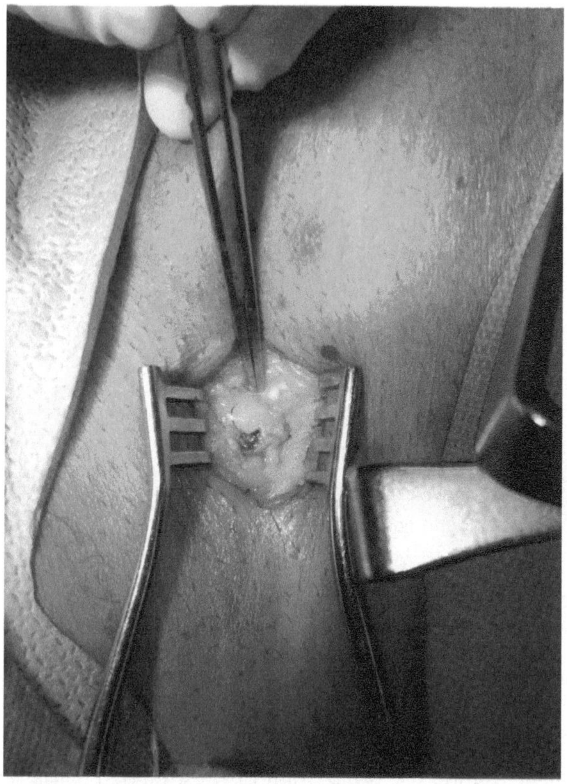

**Figure 3.28** Photo of blue vulvar sentinel lymph node with blue lymphatic channel leading to the node. (Courtesy of Fidel A. Valea, MD.)

portion of the autonomic nervous system originates in the thoracic and lumbar portions of the spinal cord, and sympathetic ganglia are located adjacent to the central nervous system. In contrast, the parasympathetic portion originates in cranial nerves and the middle three sacral segments of the cord, and the ganglia are located near the visceral organs. Although the fibers of both subdivisions of the autonomic nervous system frequently are intermingled in the same peripheral nerves, their physiologic actions are usually directly antagonistic. As a broad generalization, sympathetic fibers in the female pelvis produce muscular contractions and vasoconstriction, whereas parasympathetic fibers cause the opposite effect on muscles and vasodilation.

The semantics of pelvic innervation are confusing and imprecise. A *plexus* is a mixture of preganglionic and postganglionic fibers; small, inconsistently placed ganglia; and afferent (sensory) fibers. Throughout both the anatomic and surgical literature, a plexus may also be termed a *nerve*. For example, the superior hypogastric plexus is also called the *presacral nerve*.

Although autonomic nerve fibers enter the pelvis by several routes, most are contained in the superior hypogastric plexus, which is a caudal extension of the aortic and inferior mesenteric plexuses. The superior hypogastric plexus is found in the retroperitoneal connective tissue. It extends from the fourth lumbar vertebra to the hollow over the sacrum. In its lower portion the plexus divides to form the two hypogastric nerves, which run laterally and inferiorly. These nerves fan out to form the inferior hypogastric plexus in the area just below the bifurcation of the common iliac arteries. The nerve trunks descend farther into the base of the broad ligament, where they join with parasympathetic fibers to form the pelvic plexus. Both motor fibers and accompanying sensory fibers reach the pelvic plexus from S2, S3, and S4 via the pelvic nerves, or nervi erigentes. The pelvic plexus is found adjacent to the coccygeus muscle and sacrospinous ligaments. This "complex" is richly vascularized. The motor fibers to the levator ani (levator ani nerve) arise from the S2 to S4 nerve roots (primarily S3 and S4), traversing perpendicular to the muscle bundles and branching out to innervate the muscle fibers. The levator ani nerve does not innervate the anal sphincter, but the nerve is responsible for pelvic floor support. The pudendal nerve fibers also originate from the sacral plexus, with nerve fibers from S2 to S4. From the pelvic plexus, secondary plexuses are adjacent to all pelvic viscera, namely, the rectum, anus, urinary bladder, vagina, and Frankenhäuser plexus in the uterosacral ligaments. The Frankenhäuser plexus is extensive and contains both myelinated and nonmyelinated fibers passing primarily to the uterus and cervix, with a few fibers passing to the urinary bladder and vagina. The ovarian plexus, like the blood supply to the ovaries, is not part of the hypogastric system. The ovarian plexus is a downward extension of the aortic and renal plexuses.

It is impossible to separate afferent, sensory fibers from pelvic organs into morphologically independent tracts. Most fibers accompany the vascular system from the organ and then enter plexuses of the autonomic nervous system before eventually entering white rami communicates to the cell bodies in dorsal root ganglia of the spinal column. The major sensory fibers from the uterus accompany the sympathetic nerves, which enter the nerve roots of the spinal cord in segments T11 and T12. Thus referred uterine pain is often located in the lower abdomen. In contrast, afferents from the cervix enter the spinal cord in nerve roots of S2, S3, and S4. Referred pain from cervical inflammation and uterine irritation is characterized as low back pain in the lumbosacral region.

## EXTERNAL GENITALIA

The pudendal nerve and its branches supply the majority of both motor and sensory fibers to the muscles and skin of the vulvar region. The pudendal nerve arises from the second, third, and fourth sacral roots. It has an interesting course in which it initially leaves the pelvis via the greater sciatic foramen. Next, it crosses beneath the ischial spine, running on the medial side of the internal pudendal artery. The pudendal nerve then reenters the pelvic cavity and travels in Alcock canal, which runs along the lateral aspects of the ischial rectal fossa. As the nerve reaches the urogenital diaphragm, it divides into three branches: the inferior hemorrhoidal, the deep perineal, and the superficial perineal (Fig. 3.29). The dorsal nerve of the clitoris is a terminal branch of the deep perineal nerve.

The skin of the anus, clitoris, and medial and inferior aspects of the vulva is supplied primarily by distal branches of the pudendal nerve. The vulvar region receives additional sensory fibers from three nerves. The anterior branch of the ilioinguinal nerve sends fibers to the mons pubis and the upper part of the labia majora. The genital femoral nerve supplies fibers to the

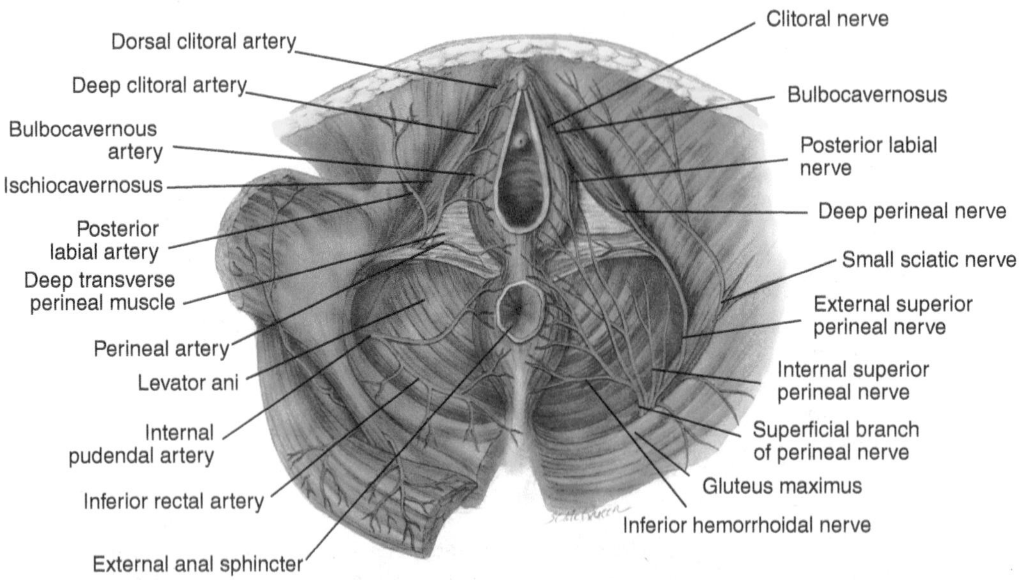


**Figure 3.29** A posterior view of the female perineum demonstrating the pudendal nerve emerging externally. The nerve divides into three segments as it passes out of the pelvis: the inferior hemorrhoidal nerve and the deep and superficial perineal nerves. The clitoral nerve is the terminal branch of the deep perineal nerve. (Modified from Mattingly RF, Thompson JD. *Te Linde's Operative Gynecology.* 6th ed. Philadelphia: JB Lippincott; 1985:49.)

labia majora, and the posterior femoral cutaneous nerve supplies fibers to the inferoposterior aspects of the vulva.

## CLINICAL CORRELATIONS

An unusual but troublesome postoperative complication of gynecologic surgery is injury to the femoral nerve. During abdominal hysterectomy, the femoral nerve may be compromised by pressure from the lateral blade of a self-retaining retractor in the area adjacent to where the femoral nerve penetrates the psoas muscle. During vaginal surgery, the femoral nerve may be injured from exaggerated hyperflexion of the legs in the lithotomy position, because hyperflexion produces stretching and compression of the femoral nerve as it courses under the inguinal ligament.

Because of the low density of nerve endings in the upper two thirds of the vagina, women are sometimes unable to determine the presence of a foreign body in this area. This explains how a "forgotten tampon" may remain unnoticed for several days in the upper part of the vagina until its presence results in a symptomatic discharge, abnormal bleeding, or odor. Infrequent but serious complications of pudendal nerve block are hematomas from trauma to the pudendal vessels and intravascular injection of anesthetic agents. The vessels or nerves are in close anatomic proximity to the ischial spine.

The fallopian tube is one of the most sensitive of the pelvic organs when crushed, cut, or distended, a fact that is appreciated in performing tubal ligations with the patient under local anesthesia. Damage to the obturator nerve during radical pelvic operations does not affect the pelvis directly. Although the nerve has an extensive pelvic course, its motor fibers supply the adductors of the thigh, and its sensory fibers innervate skin over the medial aspects of the thigh. Stitches placed during sacrospinous ligament fixation for pelvic support may interfere with neural roots S2 to S4 and the muscle pudendal and levator ani nerves.

## DIAPHRAGMS AND LIGAMENTS

### *PELVIC DIAPHRAGM*

The pelvic diaphragm is a wide but thin muscular layer of tissue that forms the inferior border of the abdominopelvic cavity. Composed of a broad, funnel-shaped sling of fascia and muscle, it extends from the symphysis pubis to the coccyx and from one lateral sidewall to the other. The primary muscles of the pelvic diaphragm are the levator ani and the coccygeus (Fig. 3.30). This structure is the evolutionary remnant of the tail-wagging muscles in lower animals. The *endopelvic fascia* is another term often used interchangeably with the *pelvic diaphragm*. The *pelvic diaphragm* and *endopelvic fascia* are terms used to characterize the connective tissue, the support for the pelvis, and the pelvic floor. The pelvic diaphragm is composed of collagen, elastic tissue, and muscle.

The muscles of the pelvic diaphragm are interwoven for strength, and a continuous muscle layer encircles the terminal portions of the urethra, vagina, and rectum. The levator ani muscles constitute the greatest bulk of the pelvic diaphragm and are divided into three components, which are named after their origin and insertion: pubococcygeus, puborectalis, and iliococcygeus. Studies using magnetic resonance imaging (MRI) and three-dimensional ultrasound validate the change in terminology from pubococcygeus muscle to a more accurate name—the *pubovisceral muscle.* This grouping of the intermediate component of the levator ani muscle lies posterior to the pubic bone and may be visualized as pubovaginalis, puboanalis, and puboperinealis muscle bundles. These three bundles constitute the pubovisceralis. Cadaveric dissection has also validated the imaging studies. The puborectalis component of the levator ani

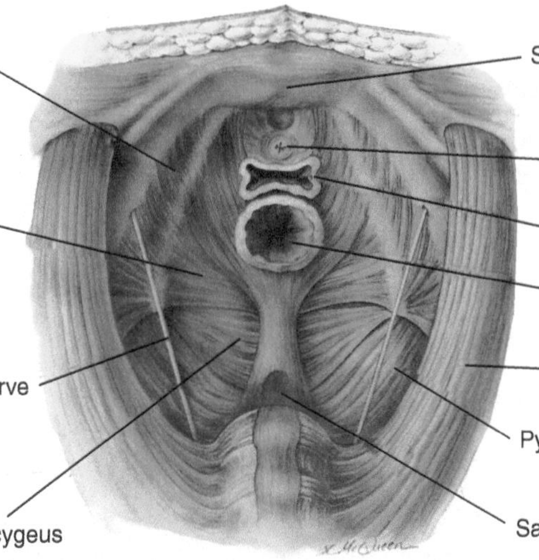


**Figure 3.30** A superior view of the pelvic diaphragm and the pelvic floor. The primary muscles that compose this funnel-shaped sling are the coccygeus and the levator ani. (Modified from Mattingly RF, Thompson JD. *Te Linde's Operative Gynecology.* 6th ed. Philadelphia: Lippincott; 1985:41.)

muscle is dorsal to the rectum and helps form the sling supporting the rectum. The coccygeus is a triangular muscle that occupies the area between the ischial spine and the coccyx.

The paired levator ani muscles act as a single muscle and functionally are important in the control of urination, in parturition, and in maintaining fecal continence. The pelvic diaphragm is important in supporting both abdominal and pelvic viscera and facilitates equal distribution of intraabdominal pressure during activities such as coughing.

## UROGENITAL DIAPHRAGM

The urogenital diaphragm, also called the *triangular ligament,* is a strong, muscular membrane that occupies the area between the symphysis pubis and ischial tuberosities (Fig. 3.31) and stretches across the triangular anterior portion of the pelvic outlet. The urogenital diaphragm is external and inferior to the pelvic diaphragm. Anteriorly, the urethra is suspended from the pubic bone by continuations of the fascial layers of the urogenital diaphragm. The free edge of the diaphragm is strengthened by the superficial transverse perineal muscle. Posteriorly, the urogenital diaphragm inserts into the central point of the perineum. Situated farther posteriorly is the ischiorectal fossa. Located more superficially are the bulbocavernosus and ischiocavernosus muscles.

The urogenital diaphragm has two layers that enfold and cover the striated, deep transverse perineal muscle. This muscle surrounds both the vagina and the urethra, which pierce the diaphragm. The pudendal vessels and nerves, the external sphincter of the membranous urethra, and the dorsal nerve to the clitoris are also found within the urogenital diaphragm. The deep transverse perineal muscle is innervated by branches of the pudendal nerve. The major function of the urogenital diaphragm is to support the urethra and maintain the urethrovesical junction.

## LIGAMENTS

The pelvic ligaments are not classic ligaments but are thickenings of retroperitoneal fascia and consist primarily of blood and lymphatic vessels, nerves, and fatty connective tissue. Anatomists call the retroperitoneal fascia *subserous fascia,* whereas surgeons refer to this fascial layer as *endopelvic fascia.* The connective tissue is denser immediately adjacent to the lateral walls of the cervix and the vagina.

### Broad Ligaments

The broad ligaments are a thin, mesenteric-like double reflection of peritoneum stretching from the lateral pelvic sidewalls to the uterus (Fig. 3.32). They become contiguous with the uterine serosa, and thus the uterus is contained within two folds of peritoneum. These peritoneal folds enclose the loose, fatty connective tissue termed the *parametrium.* The broad ligaments afford minor support to the uterus but are conduits for important anatomic structures. Within the broad ligaments are found the following structures: oviducts; ovarian and round ligaments; ureters; ovarian and uterine arteries and veins; parametrial tissue; embryonic remnants of the mesonephric duct, Wolffian body, and secondary two ligaments; the mesovarium; and the mesosalpinx. The round ligament is composed of fibrous tissue and muscle fibers. It attaches to the superoanterior aspect of the uterus, anterior and caudal to the oviduct, and runs via the broad ligament to the lateral pelvic wall. It, too, offers little support to the uterus. The round ligament crosses the external iliac vessels and enters the inguinal canal, ending by inserting into the labia majora in a fanlike fashion. In the fetus a small, finger-like projection of the peritoneum, known as *Nuck canal,* accompanies the round ligament into the inguinal canal. Generally, the canal is obliterated in the adult woman.

### Cardinal Ligaments

The cardinal, or Mackenrodt, ligaments extend from the lateral aspects of the upper part of the cervix and the vagina to the pelvic wall. They are a thickened condensation of the subserosal fascia and parametria between the interior portion of the two folds of peritoneum. The cardinal ligaments form the base of the broad ligaments, laterally attaching to the fascia

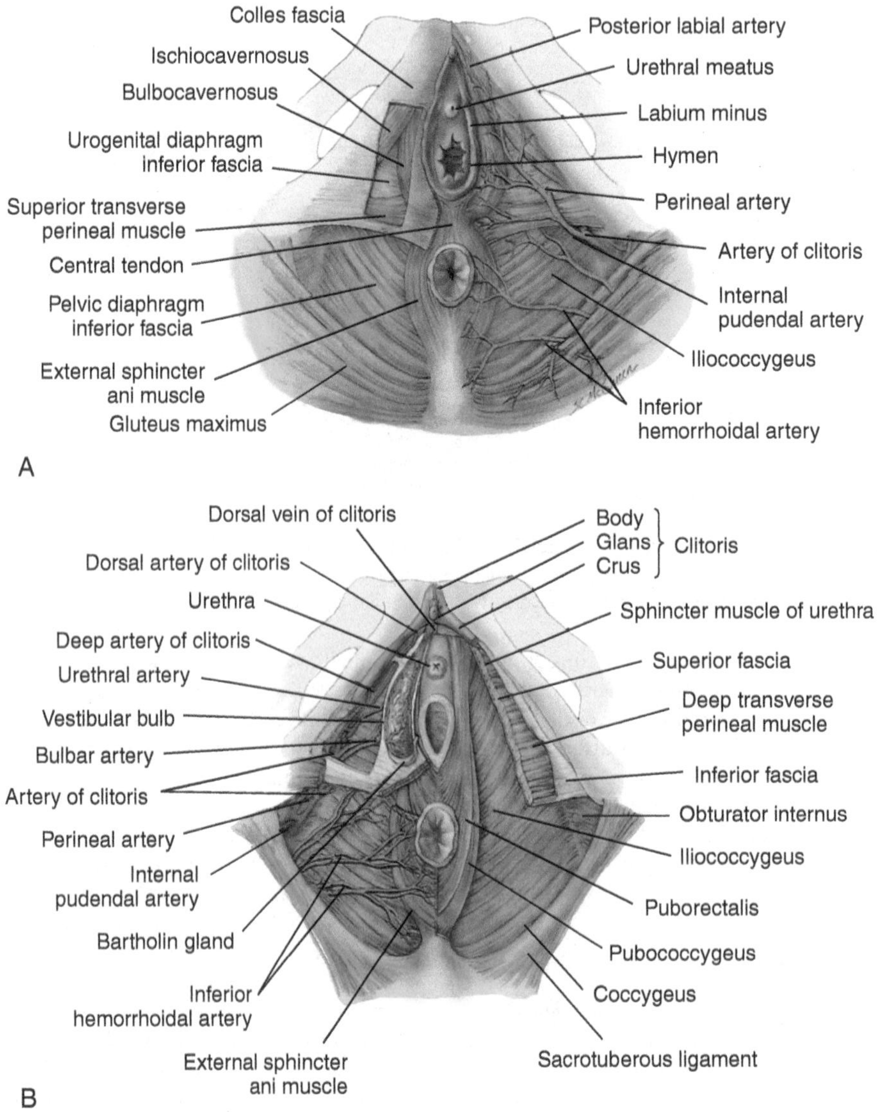


**Figure 3.31** **A,** Schematic views of the perineum demonstrating superficial structures. Note the two layers of the urogenital diaphragm enfolding the deep transverse perineal muscle. **B,** Schematic views of the perineum demonstrating superficial structures and deeper structures. (Modified from Pritchard JA, MacDonald PC, Gant NF. *Williams' Obstetrics*. 17th ed. New York: Appleton-Century-Crofts; 1985:14.)

over the pelvic diaphragm and medially merging with fibers of the endopelvic fascia. Within these ligaments are found blood vessels and smooth muscle. The cardinal ligaments help to maintain the anatomic position of the cervix and the upper part of the vagina and provide the major support of the uterus and cervix.

### *Uterosacral Ligaments*

The uterosacral ligaments extend from the upper portion of the cervix posteriorly to the third sacral vertebra. They are thickened near the cervix and then run a curved course around each side of the rectum and subsequently thin out posteriorly. The external surface of the uterosacral ligaments is formed by an inferoposterior fold of peritoneum at the base of the broad ligaments. The middle of the uterosacral ligaments is composed primarily of nerve bundles. The uterosacral ligaments serve a role in the anatomic support of the cervix.

## CLINICAL CORRELATIONS

The posterior fibers of the levator ani muscles encircle the rectum at its junction with the anal canal, thereby producing an abrupt angle that reinforces fecal continence. Surgical repair of a displacement or tear of the rectovaginal fascia and levator ani muscles resulting from childbirth is important during posterior colporrhaphy. Normal position of the female pelvic organs in the pelvis depends on mechanical support from both fascia and muscles. Vaginal delivery sometimes results in dysfunction of the anal sphincter. The etiology of this problem may be direct

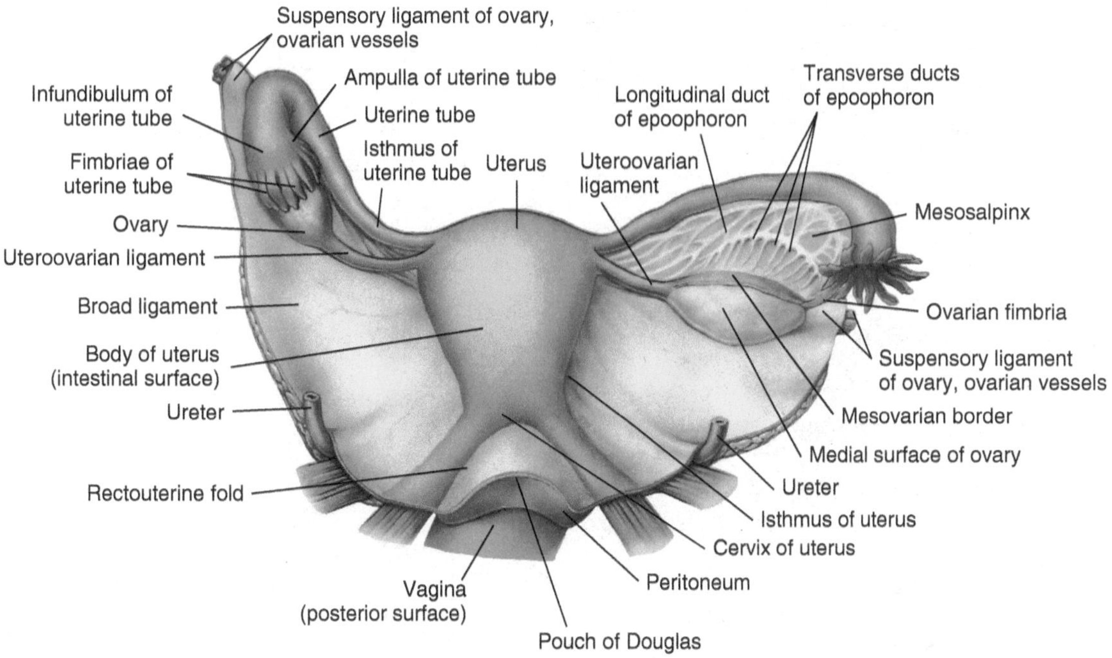


**Figure 3.32** A schematic drawing of the broad ligament, posterior view. Note the many structures contained within the broad ligament. Note the posterior aspect of the rectouterine fold, called the cul-de-sac, or pouch, of Douglas. (Modified from Clemente CD. *Anatomy: A Regional Atlas of the Human Body.* 3rd ed. Baltimore-Munich: Urban & Schwarzenberg; 1987.)

injury to the striated muscles of the pelvic floor or damage to the pudendal and presacral nerves (levator ani nerves) during labor and delivery.

The round ligament is an important surgical landmark in making the initial incision into the parietal peritoneum to gain access to the retroperitoneal space. Direct visualization of the retroperitoneal course of the ureter is an important step in many pelvic operations, including dissections in women with endometriosis, pelvic inflammatory disease, large adnexal masses, broad ligament masses, and pelvic malignancies. A cyst of the Nuck canal may be confused with an indirect inguinal hernia. When a large amount of fluid is placed in the abdominal cavity, postoperative bilateral labial edema may develop in some women because of patency of the canal of Nuck.

During pelvic surgery, traction on the uterus makes the uterosacral and cardinal ligaments more prominent. There is a free space approximately 2 to 4 cm below the superior edge of the broad ligament. In this free space there are no blood vessels, and the two sides of the broad ligament are in close proximity. Often gynecologic surgeons utilize this area to facilitate clamping of the anastomosis between the uterine and ovarian arteries.

## NONGENITAL PELVIC ORGANS

### *URETERS*

The ureters are whitish, muscular tubes, 28 to 34 cm in length, extending from the renal pelvis to the urinary bladder. The ureter is divided into abdominal and pelvic segments. The diameters vary. The abdominal segment is approximately 8 to 10 mm in diameter. The pelvic segment is approximately 4 to 6 mm. A congenital anomaly of a double, or bifid, ureter occurs in 1% to 4% of females. Ectopic ureteral orifices may occur in either the urethra or the vagina. The abdominal portion of the right ureter is lateral to the inferior vena cava. The course of the left ureter is similar to its counterpart on the right side in that it runs downward and medially along the anterior surface of the psoas major muscle.

The iliopectineal line serves as the marker for the pelvic portion of the ureter. The ureters run along the common iliac artery and then cross over the iliac vessels as they enter the pelvis (Fig. 3.33). There is a slight variation between the two sides of the female pelvis. The right ureter tends to cross at the bifurcation of the common iliac artery, whereas usually the left ureter crosses 1 to 2 cm above the bifurcation.

The ureters follow the descending, convex curvature of the posterolateral pelvic wall toward the perineum. Throughout its course, the ureter is retroperitoneal in location. The ureter can be found on the medial leaf of the parietal peritoneum and in close proximity to the ovarian, uterine, obturator, and superior vesical arteries (Fig. 3.34). The uterine artery lies on the anterolateral surface of the ureter for 2.5 to 3 cm. At approximately the level of the ischial spine, the ureter changes its course and runs forward and medially from the uterosacral ligaments to the base of the broad ligament. There the ureter enters into the cardinal ligaments. In this location the ureter is approximately 1 to 2 cm lateral to the uterine cervix and is surrounded by a plexus of veins. A cross-sectional study by Hurd and colleagues, using computed tomography of women with normal anatomy, evaluated the distance from the ureter to the lateral aspect of the cervix. The measurement of the closest distance in any individual woman was (median of all subjects) 2.3 cm ± 0.8 cm (Hurd, 2001). However, the authors noted that in 12% of women, the ureter was less than 0.5 cm from the cervix (Fig. 3.35). This finding emphasizes the caution needed in surgery

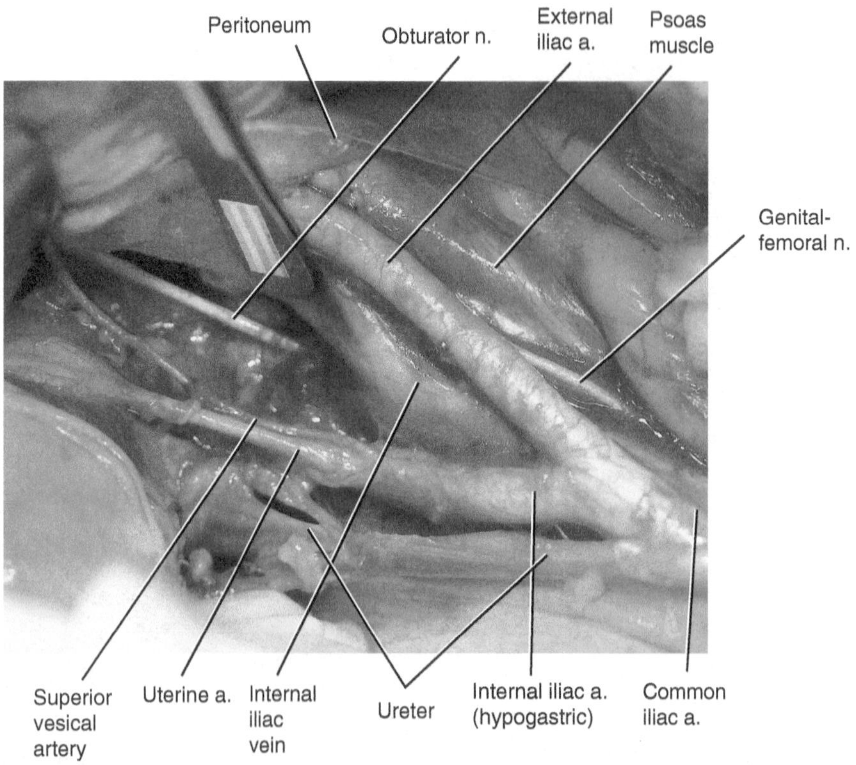


**Figure 3.33** Photograph taken during a dissection of the lateral pelvic wall at the time of a radical hysterectomy. Note the ureter coursing over the common iliac artery in close proximity to the bifurcation. The ureter then drops under and very close to the uterine artery. The retractor is lifting the internal iliac vein. (Courtesy of Deborah Jean Dotters, MD, Eugene, OR.)

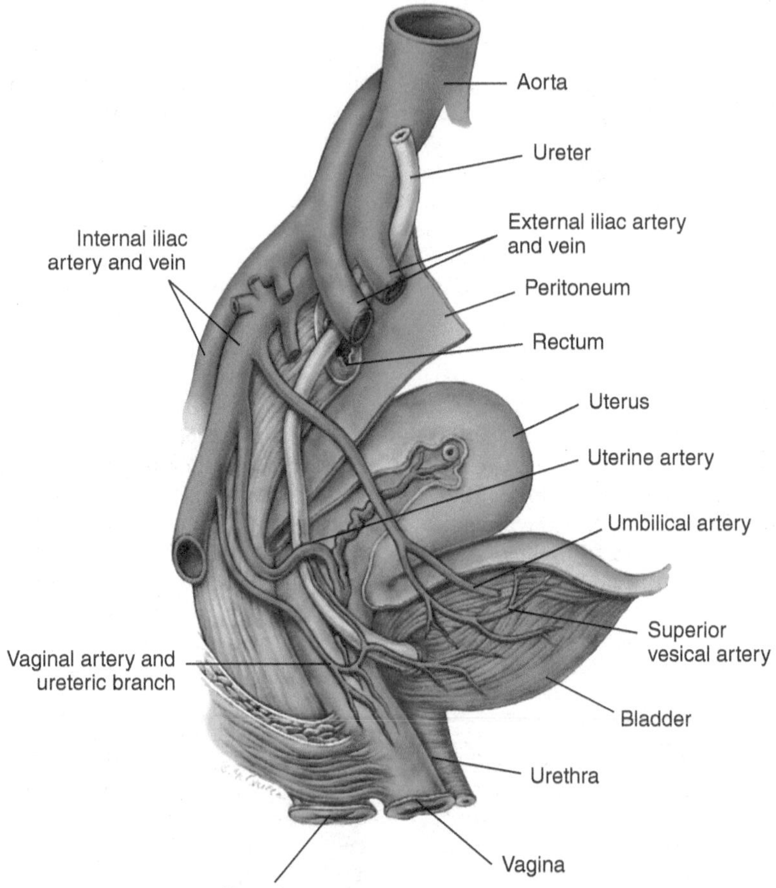


**Figure 3.34** A schematic drawing of the female pelvis, lateral view, demonstrating the ureter's relation to the major arteries. Note the uterine artery crossing over the ureter. (From Buchsbaum HJ, Schmidt JD. *Gynecologic and Obstetric Urology.* Philadelphia: WB Saunders; 1978:24.)

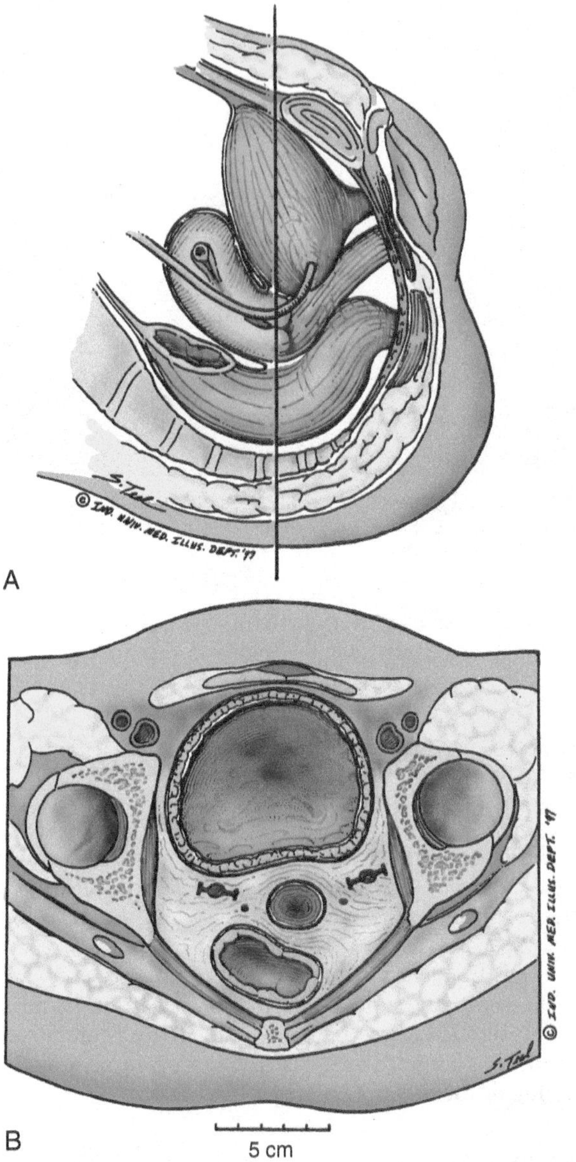


**Figure 3.35** Average location of the ureters in relation to the cervix. **A,** Sagittal view representing the plane from the computed tomography cut noted in **B.** The most proximal point from the ureter to the cervix. Bars represent standard deviation. (From Hurd WW, Chee SS, Gallagher KL, et al. Location of the ureters in relation to the uterine cervix by computed tomography. *Am J Obstet Gynecol.* 2001;184:338.)

to prevent ureteral injury. This close proximity also underscores the fact that ureteral injury may be unavoidable in some women. The ureter then runs upward (ventral) and medially in the vesical uterine ligaments to obliquely pierce the bladder wall. Just before entering the base of the bladder, the ureter is in immediate contact with the anterior vaginal wall and the inferolateral aspect of the space of Retzius.

The ureter has a rich arterial supply with numerous anastomoses from many small vessels that form a longitudinal plexus in the adventitia of the ureter, commonly referred to as the *Waldeyer sheath.* The parent vessels that send branches to this arterial plexus surrounding the ureter include the renal, ovarian, common iliac, hypogastric, uterine, vaginal, vesical, middle hemorrhoidal, and superior gluteal arteries. The ureter is resistant to injury resulting from devascularization unless the surgeon strips the adventitia from the muscular conduit. In general, the blood supply of the abdominal ureter comes from medial sources and the blood supply of the pelvic ureter originates from lateral sources.

## URINARY BLADDER

The urinary bladder is a hollow muscular organ that lies between the symphysis pubis and the uterus. The size and shape of the bladder vary with the volume of urine it contains. Similarly, the anatomic proximity to other pelvic organs depends on whether the bladder is full or empty. The superior surface of the bladder is the only surface covered by peritoneum. The inferior portion is immediately adjacent to the uterus. The urachus is a fibrous cord extending from the apex of the bladder to the umbilicus. The urachus, which is the adult remnant of the embryonic allantois, is occasionally patent for part of its length. The base of the bladder lies directly adjacent to the endopelvic fascia over the anterior vaginal wall. The bladder neck and connecting urethra are attached to the symphysis pubis by fibrous ligaments. The prevesical or retropubic space of Retzius is the area lying between the bladder and symphysis pubis and is bounded laterally by the obliterated hypogastric arteries. This space extends from the fascia covering the pelvic diaphragm to the umbilicus between the peritoneum and transversalis fascia.

The mucosa of the anterior surface of the bladder is light red and has numerous folds. The inferoposterior surface delineated by the two ureteral orifices and the urethral orifice is the trigone. The trigone is a darker red than the rest of the bladder mucosa and is free of folds. When the bladder is empty, the ureteral orifices are approximately 2.5 cm apart. This distance increases to 5 cm when the bladder is distended. The muscular wall of the bladder, the detrusor muscles, is arranged in three layers. The arterial supply of the bladder originates from branches of the hypogastric artery: the superior vesical, inferior vesical, and middle hemorrhoidal arteries. The nerve supply to the bladder includes sympathetic and parasympathetic fibers, with the external sphincter supplied by the pudendal nerve.

## RECTUM

The rectum is the terminal 12 to 14 cm of the large intestine. The rectum begins over the second or third sacral vertebra, where the sigmoid colon no longer has a mesentery. After the large intestine loses its mesentery, its anatomic posterior wall is in close proximity to the curvature of the sacrum. Anteriorly, peritoneum covers the upper and middle thirds of the rectum. The lowest one third is below the peritoneal reflection and is in close proximity to the posterior wall of the vagina. The rectum empties into the anal canal, which is 2 to 4 cm in length. The anal canal is fixed by the surrounding levator ani musculature of the pelvic diaphragm (see Fig. 3.5). The external sphincter of the anal canal is a circular band of striated muscle. Studies of the cross-sectional anatomy of the external anal sphincter by both ultrasound and magnetic resonance imaging have identified two distinct layers of the external anal sphincter. With MRI with three-dimensional reconstruction, Hsu and colleagues noted three separate components to the external sphincter: a main muscle body, a separate encircling subcutaneous band of muscles, and bilateral wing-shaped muscle bands that attach near the ischiopubis (Hsu, 2005). They are a subcutaneous and a deep layer. The rectum, unlike other areas of the large intestine, does not have teniae coli or appendices epiploicae. The arterial supply of the rectum is rich, originating from five arteries: the superior hemorrhoidal artery, which is a continuation of the inferior mesenteric, the two middle hemorrhoidal arteries, and the two inferior hemorrhoidal arteries. Approximately 10% of carcinomas of the large bowel occur within the rectum. Therefore during rectal examination special emphasis to palpate the entire circumference of the rectum, not just the area of the rectovaginal septum, is an important part of screening for colon cancer.

## CLINICAL CORRELATIONS

The anatomic proximity of the ureters, urinary bladder, and rectum to the female reproductive organs is a major consideration in most gynecologic operations. Surgical compromise of the ureter may occur during clamping or ligating of the infundibulopelvic vessels, clamping or ligating of the cardinal ligaments, or wide suturing in the endopelvic fascia during an anterior repair, even with apparent normal anatomy and utmost surgical care. Particular attention to the proximity of the distal ureter to the anterior vagina is very important. Operative injuries to the bladder or ureter occur in approximately 1 out of 100 major gynecologic operations. Bladder injuries are approximately five times more common than ureteral injuries. Two of the classic ways to differentiate a ureter from a pelvic vessel are (1) visualization of peristalsis after stimulation by a surgical instrument and (2) visualization of Auerbach plexuses, which are numerous, wavy, small vessels that anastomose over the surface of the ureter. Injury to the ureter or bladder during urethropexy operations for genuine stress incontinence is common. Therefore many surgeons routinely inject indigo carmine and either open the bladder or perform cystoscopy near the end of the operative procedure.

For years, gynecologic teachers have referred to the area in the base of the broad ligament near the cervix where the uterine artery crosses the ureter as the area where "water flows under the bridge."

The urinary bladder, if properly drained, will heal rapidly after a surgical insult if the blood supply to the bladder wall is not compromised. This capacity allows the gynecologist to use suprapubic cystostomy tube without fear of fistula formation.

There are many different surgical techniques for the repair of urinary stress incontinence. They usually involve either suspension of the periurethral tissues or bladder neck itself. Occasionally, these surgical procedures are complicated by a significant amount of postoperative venous bleeding. A subfascial hematoma may extend as high as the umbilicus in the space of Retzius. One of the most common causes of female urinary incontinence is defective connective tissue, especially in the periurethral connective tissue, the pubourethral ligaments, and pubococcygeus muscles.

Rectal injury may occur during vaginal hysterectomy with associated posterior colporrhaphy. In the middle third of the vagina, the distance between vaginal and rectal mucosa is only a few millimeters, and usually the connective tissue is densely adherent and should be separated by sharp dissection. The rectum bulges anteriorly into the vagina in this area, producing a further challenge during the operative procedure.

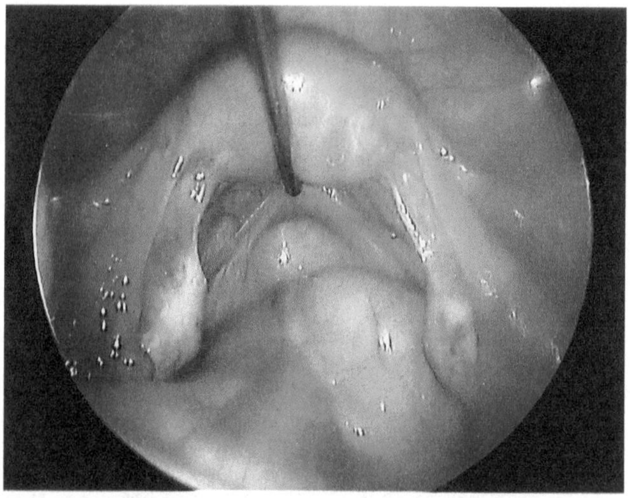

**Figure 3.36** Laparoscopic visualization of a normal pelvis. The probe is elevating the uterus to expose the cul-de-sac of Douglas. (Courtesy of Burke Beller.)

## OTHER STRUCTURES

### CUL-DE-SAC OF DOUGLAS

The cul-de-sac of Douglas is a deep pouch formed by the most caudal extent of the parietal peritoneum. The cul-de-sac is a potential space and is also called the *rectouterine pouch* or *fold* (Figs. 3.32 and 3.36). It is anterior to the rectum, separating the uterus from the large intestine. The parietal peritoneum of the cul-de-sac covers the cervix and upper part of the posterior vaginal wall then reflects to cover the anterior wall of the rectum. The pouch is bounded on the lateral sides by the peritoneal folds covering the uterosacral ligaments.

### PARAMETRIA

The parametria are the coats of extraperitoneal fatty and fibrous connective tissues adjacent to the uterus. The parametria lie between the leaves of the broad ligament and in the contiguous area anteriorly between the cervix and bladder. This connective tissue is thicker and denser adjacent to the cervix and vagina, where it becomes part of the connective tissue of the pelvic floor. The parametria may also thicken in response to radiation, pelvic cancer, infection, or endometriosis.

### PARAVESICAL AND PARARECTAL SPACES

The paravesical and pararectal spaces are actually potential spaces that become true spaces when developed by the surgeon. Development of these spaces is useful in pelvic lymph node dissection and in radical pelvic surgery because it makes the anatomic landmarks so clear. The paravesical space is bordered medially by the bladder and upper vagina and is contiguous with, but lateral to, the space of Retzius. Laterally, it is bordered by the obturator fossa and the external iliac vessels. Inferiorly it is bordered by the pubic ramus, and superiorly it is bordered by by the cardinal ligament.

The pararectal space is developed by dissecting the adventitial tissue within the broad ligament, between the ureter (medially), and the internal iliac vessels (laterally). More deeply, the medial border is the rectum. Superiorly, the pararectal space is limited by the sacral hollow. Inferiorly, it is limited by the cardinal ligament, containing the uterine artery. The paravesical and pararectal spaces are actually potential spaces that become true spaces when developed by the surgeon. Development of these spaces is useful in pelvic lymph node dissection and in radical pelvic surgery because the anatomic landmarks become so clear.

## CLINICAL CORRELATIONS

The parametria and cul-de-sac of Douglas are important anatomic landmarks in advanced pelvic infection and neoplasia. Intrauterine infection, cervical carcinoma, and endometrial carcinoma may penetrate the endocervical stroma or the myometrium and secondarily may invade the loose connective tissue of the parametria.

The pouch of Douglas is easily accessible in performing transvaginal surgical procedures. Posterior colpotomy is frequently chosen for drainage of a pelvic abscess occurring in the cul-de-sac of Douglas.

When the paravesical and pararectal spaces have been developed and the uterus is held on traction medially, the pelvic anatomy, including the ureter, internal and external iliac vessels, obturator fossa, and the cardinal ligament, with the uterine artery crossing the ureter, can be clearly and readily identified.

Many women with uterine prolapse have an associated enterocele, which is a hernia that protrudes between the uterosacral ligaments. Occasionally the cul-de-sac of Douglas is obliterated by the inflammatory process associated with either endometriosis or advanced malignancy.

## *ACKNOWLEDGEMENT*

I would like to thank Dr. Vern Katz for his contributions to this chapter in the previous edition.

## *KEY POINTS*

- The labia majora are homologous to the scrotum in the male. The labia minora are homologous to the penile urethra and a portion of the skin of the penis in males.
- The clitoris is the female homologue of the penis in the male. Skene glands are homologous to the prostate gland in the male.
- The average length of the clitoris is 1.5 to 2 cm. Clinically, in determining clitoromegaly width is more important and should be less than 1 cm, for it is difficult to actually measure the length of the clitoris.
- The female urethra measures 3.5 to 5 cm in length. The mucosa of the proximal two thirds of the urethra is composed of stratified transitional epithelium, and the distal one third is stratified squamous epithelium.
- When a woman is standing, the axis of the upper portion of the vagina lies close to the horizontal plane, with the upper portion of the vagina curving toward the hollow of the sacrum.
- The vaginal length increases with weight and height, and it decreases with age.
- The lower third of the vagina is in close anatomic relationship to the urogenital and pelvic diaphragms.
- The middle third of the vagina is supported by the levator ani muscles and the lower portion of the cardinal ligaments.
- The primary lymphatic drainage of the upper third of the vagina is to the external iliac nodes, the middle third of the vagina drains to the common and internal iliac nodes, and the lower third has a wide lymphatic distribution, including the common iliac, superficial inguinal, and perirectal nodes.
- Descriptive terms for pelvic organs are derived from the Latin root, whereas terms relating to surgical procedures are derived from the Greek root.
- The length and width of the endocervical canal vary. The width of the canal varies with the parity of the woman and changing hormonal levels. It is usually 2.5 to 3 cm in length and 7 to 8 mm at its widest point.
- The fibromuscular cervical stroma is composed primarily of collagenous connective tissue and ground substance. The connective tissue contains approximately 15% smooth muscle cells and a small amount of elastic tissue.
- The major arterial supply to the cervix is located in the lateral cervical walls at the 3 and 9 o'clock positions.
- The pain fibers from the cervix accompany the parasympathetic fibers to the second, third, and fourth sacral segments.
- The transformation zone of the cervix encompasses the border of the squamous epithelium and columnar epithelium. The location of the transformation zone changes on the cervix depending on a woman's hormonal status.
- The uterus of a nulliparous woman is approximately 8 cm long, 5 cm wide, and 2.5 cm thick and weighs 40 to 50 g. In contrast, in a multiparous woman each measurement is approximately 1.2 cm larger and normal uterine weight is 20 to 30 g heavier. The maximal weight of a normal uterus is 110 g.
- In the majority of women, the long axis of the uterus is both anteverted in respect to the long axis of the vagina and anteflexed in relation to the long axis of the cervix. However, a retroflexed uterus is a normal variant found in approximately 25% of women.
- The uterine and ovarian arteries provide the arterial blood supply of the uterus. The uterine arteries are large branches of the anterior division of the hypogastric arteries, whereas the ovarian arteries originate directly from the aorta.

*Continued*

## KEY POINTS—cont'd

- Afferent nerve fibers from the uterus enter the spinal cord at the eleventh and twelfth thoracic segments.
- The oviducts are 10 to 14 cm in length and are composed of four anatomic sections. Closest to the uterine cavity is the interstitial segment, followed by the narrow isthmic segment, then the wider ampullary segment, and distally the trumpet-shaped infundibular segment.
- The right oviduct and appendix are often anatomically adjacent. Clinically it may be difficult to differentiate inflammation of the upper portion of the genital tract and acute appendicitis.
- During the reproductive years, the ovaries measure approximately 1.5 cm × 2.5 cm × 4 cm.
- The ovary in nulliparous women rests in a depression of peritoneum named the *fossa ovarica.* Immediately adjacent to the ovarian fossa are the external iliac vessels, the ureter, and the obturator vessels and nerves.
- Three prominent ligaments determine the anatomic mobility of the ovary: the mesovarian, the ovarian ligament, and the infundibulopelvic ligament.
- The arterial supply of the pelvis is paired, bilateral, and has multiple collaterals and numerous anastomoses.
- The extent of collateral circulation after hypogastric artery ligation depends on the site of ligation and may be divided into three groups: branches from the aorta, branches from the external iliac arteries, and branches from the femoral arteries.
- The internal iliac nodes are found in an anatomic triangle whose sides are composed of the external iliac artery, the hypogastric artery, and the pelvic sidewall. This rich collection of nodes receives channels from every internal pelvic organ and the vulva, including the clitoris and urethra.
- The femoral triangle is the anatomic space lying immediately distal to the fold of the groin. The boundaries of the femoral triangle are the sartorius and adductor longus muscles and the inguinal ligament.
- The pudendal nerve and its branches supply the majority of both motor and sensory fibers to the muscles and skin of the vulvar region.
- The femoral nerve may be compromised by pressure on the psoas muscle during abdominal surgery and by hyperflexion of the leg during vaginal surgery.
- The pelvic diaphragm is important in supporting both abdominal and pelvic viscera and facilitates equal distribution of intraabdominal pressure during activities such as coughing. The levator ani muscles constitute the greatest bulk of the pelvic diaphragm.
- The major function of the urogenital diaphragm is to support the urethra and maintain the urethrovesical junction.
- Contained within the broad ligaments are the following structures: oviducts, ovarian and round ligaments, ureters, ovarian and uterine arteries and veins, parametrial tissue, embryonic remnants of the mesonephric duct and Wolffian body, and two secondary ligaments.
- The cardinal ligaments provide the major support to the uterus.
- A congenital anomaly of a double, or bifid, ureter occurs in 1% to 4% of females.
- When the urinary bladder is empty, the ureteral orifices are approximately 2.5 cm apart. This distance increases to 5 cm when the bladder is distended.
- The distal ureter enters into the cardinal ligament. In this location the ureter is approximately 1 to 2 cm lateral to the uterine cervix and is surrounded by a plexus of veins. In approximately 12% of women, the cervix will be less than 0.5 cm from the cervix.
- Two ways of distinguishing the ureter from pelvic vessels are (1) identification of peristalsis after stimulation with a surgical instrument and (2) identification of Auerbach plexuses.
- Surgical compromise of the ureters may occur during clamping or ligating of the infundibulopelvic vessels, clamping or ligating of the cardinal ligaments, or wide suturing in the endopelvic fascia during an anterior repair.
- The following three important axioms should be in the forefront of decision making during difficult gynecologic surgery: (1) do not assume that the anatomy of the left and right side of the pelvis are invariably identical mirror images; (2) during difficult operations with multiple adhesions, operate from known anatomic areas into the unknown; and (3) from the sage advice of a distinguished Canadian gynecologist, Dr. Henry McDuff: "If the disease be rampant and the anatomy obscure, and the plans of dissection not pristine and pure, do not be afraid, nor faint of heart, try the retroperitoneum, it's a great place to start."

## KEY REFERENCES

Abu-Rustum N. Sentinel lymph node mapping for endometrial cancer: a modern approach to surgical staging. *J Natl Compr Canc Netw.* 2014;12:288-297.

Coleman RL, Ali S, Levenback CF, et al. Is bilateral lymphadenectomy for midline squamous carcinoma of the vulva always necessary? An analysis from Gynecologic Oncology Group (GOG) 173. *Gynecol Oncol.* 2013;128(2):155-159.

Echt ML, Finan MA, Hoffman MS, et al. Detection of sentinel lymph nodes with lymphazurin in cervical, uterine and vulvar malignancies. *South Med J.* 1999;92(2):204-208.

Hsu Y, Fenner DE, Weadock WJ, et al. Magnetic resonance imaging and 3-dimensional analysis of external anal sphincter anatomy. *Obstet Gynecol.* 2005;106(6):1259-1265.

Hurd WW, Chee SS, Gallagher KI, et al. Location of the ureters in relation to the uterine cervix by computed tomography. *Am J Obstet Gynecol.* 2001;184:336.

Suggested Readings can be found on ExpertConsult.com.

# 4

# Reproductive Endocrinology

## Neuroendocrinology, Gonadotropins, Sex Steroids, Prostaglandins, Ovulation, Menstruation, Hormone Assay

*Nataki C. Douglas, Roger A. Lobo*

The endocrine regulation of the reproductive system is very complex. Much information has been obtained since the 1980s, and new information is constantly becoming available. It would be impossible to include all of the findings in a single chapter. Thus this chapter presents only the basic information required to understand this complex topic. More detailed and in-depth information is found in the several books that have been dedicated to this subject.

Successful function of the reproductive system requires the involvement of several organs, none of which acts independently. This chapter discusses the physiology of the hypothalamic-pituitary-ovarian (HPO) axis. For ease of understanding, each organ will be discussed first as an individual unit; information will include the central nervous system control of gonadotropin-releasing hormone (GnRH), the primary neurohormone controlling the whole reproductive endocrine axis, the GnRH action on the anterior pituitary and the resultant secretion of the gonadotropins, the gonadotropins action on the ovaries and the release of gonadal steroids, and finally the action of these sex steroids on the uterus and cervix. Although it is fair to state that the HPO axis is driven by the hypothalamus and its release of GnRH, it is important to point out that normal function of the hypothalamic-pituitary-ovarian endocrine axis requires a remarkable information flow and coordination between each of these organs, as exemplified by the existing inhibitory and stimulatory feedback loops. Their relevance will become obvious in the discussion of the menstrual cycle, which will close the chapter.

## HYPOTHALAMUS AND GnRH

The reproductive process begins in the brain, through the activation of the initial hormonal signal that will release gonadotropins from the pituitary gland. This hormone released by the hypothalamus is **gonadotropin-releasing hormone (GnRH)**, a decapeptide (10 amino acids) (Fig. 4.1). The *GnRH* gene (situated on the short arm of chromosome 8) encodes for a 92 amino acids precursor molecule, composed of a signal peptide sequence, the GnRH sequence itself, a posttranscriptional processing signal (3 amino acids long), and a 56-amino acid peptide known as GnRH-associated peptide (GAP). (Several forms of the GnRH decapeptide have been identified, the principal of which is GnRH-2, which differs from GnRH by 3 amino acids. It is found in several areas of the body, where it may subserve functions unrelated to those of GnRH. Its role in fertility, if any, remains to be determined.)

### *ANATOMY*

#### *Relationship of the Olfactory and GnRH Systems in Early Fetal Life*

Surprisingly, GnRH-synthesizing neurons do not originate within the brain, like the majority of all neurons. Rather, GnRH neurons derive from progenitor cells in the embryonic olfactory placode where they develop. In a particular journey unique for a neuron, GnRH neurons migrate toward the brain during early fetal life to reach the locations that they will occupy during adult life. This migration of GnRH neurons over long distances and through changing molecular environments suggests that numerous factors, local and possibly external, influence this process at its different stages. Such factors play critical roles, such as mediating the adhesion of GnRH neurons to changing surfaces along their voyage, promoting cytoskeleton remodeling, or modulating axonal guidance.

Functional connections between GnRH neurons and the hypophyseal portal system that will transport GnRH to the anterior pituitary gland are established by about 16 weeks of fetal life. Migration failure of GnRH neurons and the resultant lack of the establishment of functional connections are characteristic of patients with **Kallmann syndrome,** who show hypogonadotropic hypogonadism accompanied by anosmia (Tsai, 2006). In the 19-week old fetus with X-linked Kallmann syndrome, the GnRH neurons accompanying the olfactory nerves have been shown to be arrested in their voyage within the meninges, and therefore contact with the brain and the hypophyseal portal system is not established.

#### *GnRH Neuronal System*

In the adult, neurons producing GnRH are present in several hypothalamic nuclei as well as other parts of the brain. However, the majority of GnRH neurons controlling the HPO axis are

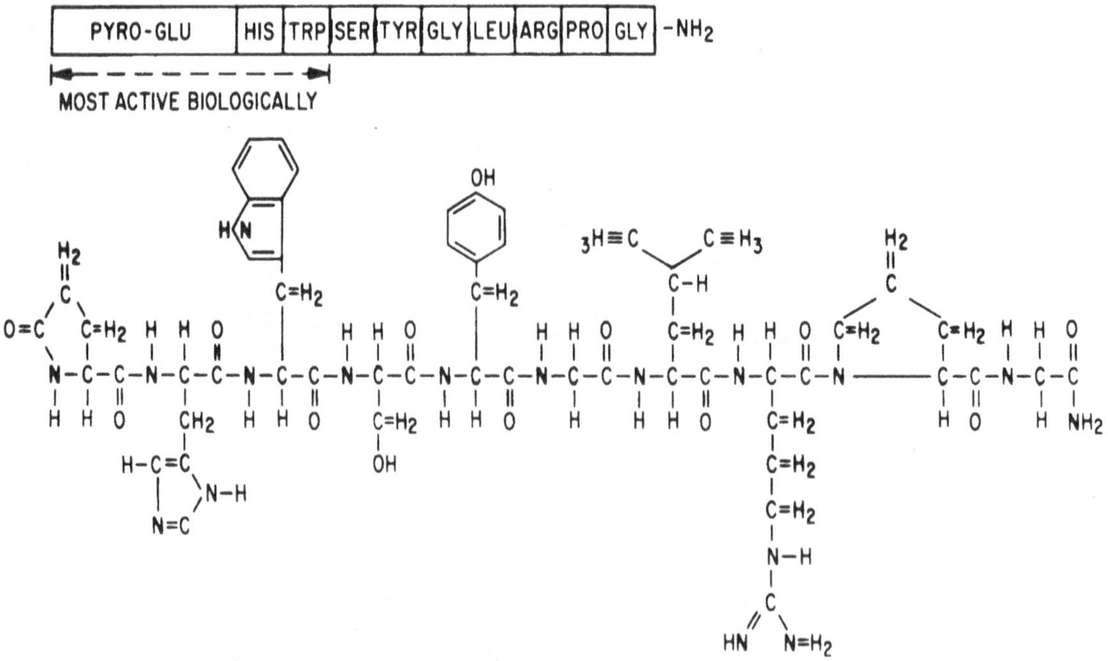


**Figure 4.1** The 10-amino acid sequence of gonadotropin-releasing hormone (GnRH). (From Klerzky OA, Lobo RA. Reproductive neuroendocrinology. In: Mishell DR, Davajan V, Lobo RA, eds. *Infertility, Contraception and Reproductive Endocrinology.* 3rd ed. Cambridge, MA: Blackwell Scientific; 1991.)

located within the anterior hypothalamus and primarily within the medial basal hypothalamus, with the greatest number in the primate within the **arcuate nucleus.** The 92 amino acid GnRH precursor is released into the axons of these neurons and cleaved during transport to yield GnRH and GAP. (The biologic function of GAP or fragments thereof remains to be clarified.)

A substantial number of GnRH axons terminate within the external zone of the **median eminence** (infundibulum) where GnRH is released. This area is the site of an important capillary plexus, with a fenestrated epithelium similar to that of peripheral capillaries, which allows passage of large molecules. (These capillaries differ from brain capillaries, which are not fenestrated. Thus the median eminence is viewed as an area outside the blood-brain barrier.) This pathway is the most relevant one in regard to the control of the pituitary-ovarian axis (Fig. 4.2, *A*). Another substantial projection of GnRH axons is through circumventricular organs, the major of which is the organum vasculosum of the lamina terminalis (OVLT). These areas are also outside the blood-brain barrier. (The function of GnRH release into these areas remains somewhat unknown. One role may be to enable the release of GnRH into cerebrospinal fluid [CSF], perhaps to facilitate actions of GnRH in other areas of the brain. GnRH levels have been found to be elevated in CSF as opposed to being minimal in peripheral blood.) Another possible route of GnRH release may involve specialized ependymal cells, referred to as **tanycytes.** These have been found to extend from the lumen of the third ventricle to the external zone of the median eminence.

### *Transport of GnRH to the Anterior Pituitary*

The capillary plexus of the external median eminence, into which GnRH is released, collects into several **hypophyseal portal vessels,** which descend along the pituitary stalk to terminate within another capillary plexus (hence the term *portal*) within the anterior lobe of the pituitary (see Fig. 4.2, *B*). (Unlike the posterior lobe of the pituitary, also referred to as the neurohypophysis, the anterior lobe has no direct blood supply and receives all of its vascularization from this portal system.) The vascular arrangement whereby GnRH as well as other neurohormones reach the anterior pituitary is very important to the proper function of the endocrine system: it allows for the rapid (within minutes) and undiluted transport of relatively small amounts of neurohormones to the pituitary. This is especially crucial to GnRH, because this neurohormone has a short half-life of about 2 to 4 minutes (it is rapidly degraded by peptidases in blood; as a consequence, GnRH is not measurable in peripheral blood) and because of its pulsatile mode of release (discussed later).

## *PHYSIOLOGY*

### *GnRH Pulse Generator*

Studies have shown that GnRH is characteristically released intermittently, in a pulsatile fashion. Hence comes the concept of the **GnRH pulse generator** responsible for the pulsatile release of the hormone. GnRH pulses occur at about hourly intervals (Fig. 4.3). The rising edge of each GnRH pulse is abrupt, such that GnRH can increase by a factor of 50 within 1 minute. Each GnRH pulse is preceded by an increase in multiunit activity within the area of the arcuate nucleus.

### *Mechanisms Responsible for GnRH Pulsatility*

The cellular basis and the mechanisms that determine the timing of the increase in multiunit activity resulting in pulsatile GnRH activity are still under study. First, there is a growing consensus that pulsatile activity originates from an inherent pace-making activity of the GnRH neuron itself: in vitro data have shown that

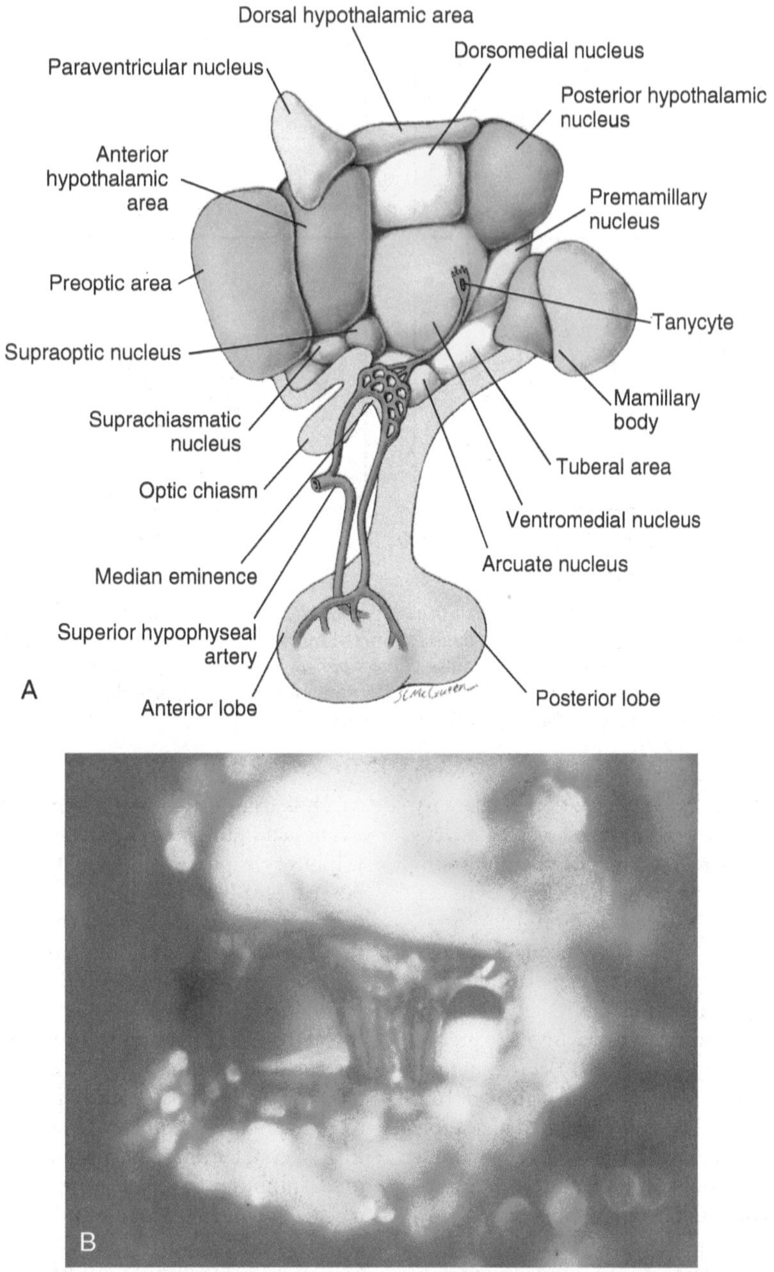


**Figure 4.2** **A,** Nuclear organization of the hypothalamus, shown diagrammatically in a sagittal plane as viewed from the third ventricle. Rostral area is to the left and caudal area is to the right. Fast transport of GnRH pulses released into the median eminence from axons originating from GnRH neurons in the arcuate nucleus occurs through the portal vessels derived from the capillary plexus in the median eminence. **B,** The pituitary stalk and several individual hypophyseal portal veins transporting hypothalamic neurohormones to the anterior pituitary in a nonhuman primate. (**A,** Modified from Moore RY. Neuroendocrine mechanisms: cells and systems. In: Yen SSC, Jaffe R, eds. *Reproductive Endocrinology: Physiology, Pathophysiology and Clinical Management.* Philadelphia: WB Saunders; 1986. **B,** Courtesy of Drs. Peter Carmel and Michel Ferin.)

individual neurons have the capacity of spontaneous oscillations in activity. In this case, such activity would also require a synchronized action from enough neurons to provide a discrete GnRH pulse. Intercommunication between GnRH neurons may occur through gap junctions between such neurons, which have been demonstrated, and through synaptic forms of interaction between cells. Second, evidence has identified a key role of **kisspeptin** (KISS1), a product of the *KISS1* gene, and its receptor (GPR54 or KISS1R) in the regulation of GnRH release (Skorupskaite, 2014). Kiss1 neurons have been found to directly innervate and stimulate GnRH neurons. In humans, mutations or targeted deletions of *KISS1* or of its receptor cause hypogonadotropic hypogonadism. Patients with these mutations, however, do not have anosmia, unlike those with Kallmann syndrome, suggesting that

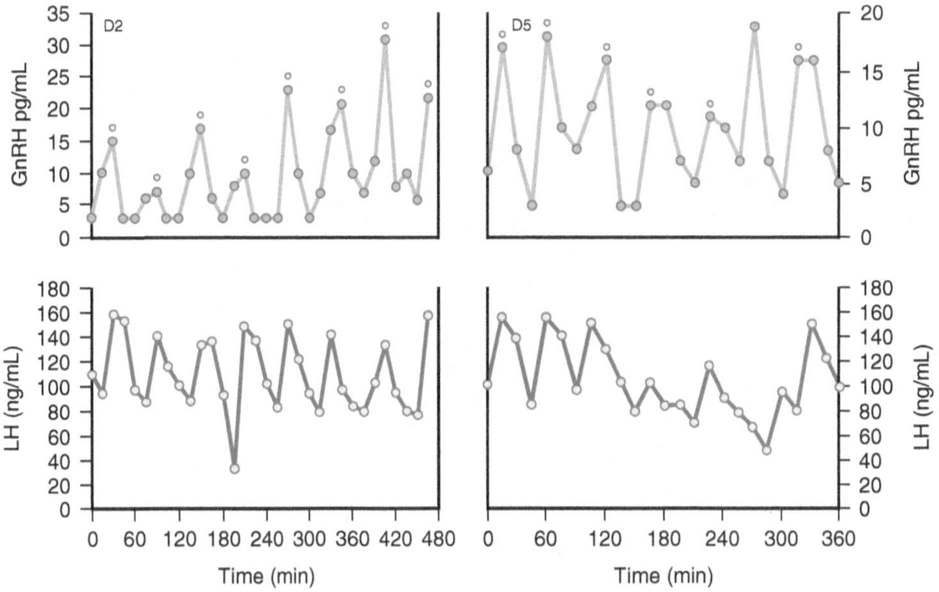


**Figure 4.3** GnRH release by the hypothalamus is pulsatile. Shown in the upper panel are hourly GnRH pulses over an 8-hour period in an ovariectomized monkey in the absence of ovarian steroid modulation. Note the concordance of LH pulses *(lower panel).* (From Xia L, Van Vugt D, Alston EJ, et al. A surge of gonadotropin-releasing hormone accompanies the estradiol-induced gonadotropin surge in the rhesus monkey. *Endocrinology.* 1992;131:2812.)

there are no major deficits in the embryonic migration of olfactory or GnRH neurons. KISS1 neurons within the arcuate nucleus (rodents) and infundibular nucleus (humans) express the estrogen, progesterone, and androgen receptors, and KISS1 signaling in the brain is implicated in mediating sex steroid feedback loops, especially during the preovulatory GnRH/luteinizing hormone (LH) surge. Kisspeptin has been used to induce egg maturation in women undergoing in vitro fertilization therapy, with subsequent fertilization of the mature eggs, embryo transfer into the uterus, and successful human pregnancy (Jayasena, 2014). There is the potential for routine use of kisspeptin to induce ovulation during fertility treatment cycles. KISS1 has also been shown to play a role in the initiation of puberty. A subpopulation of kisspeptin neurons in the human infundibular nucleus co-express neuropeptides neurokinin B and dynorphin (opioid inhibitor) (Skorupskaite, 2014). These kisspeptin-neurokinin-dynorphin (KNDy) neurons express neurokinin B and dynorphin receptors as well as estrogen and progesterone receptors. KNDy neurons coordinate inputs, including sex steroid feedback, to regulate pulsatile kisspeptin secretion. The interaction of KISS1 neurons with other neurotransmitter systems is currently being studied.

### *Modulatory Influences on GnRH Pulsatility*

The foremost modulatory influence on the frequency and amplitude of GnRH pulses is exerted by the ovarian steroid hormones through their feedback loop actions. In general, estradiol is known to decrease GnRH pulse amplitude, whereas progesterone decreases GnRH pulse frequency (see the discussion presented later for details).

Numerous other studies suggest that the spontaneous activity of the GnRH pulse generator may also be modulated by a variety of additional stimulatory and inhibitory afferent neural signals. Stimulatory inputs to GnRH release may originate from neurons using the biogenic amine neuroepinephrine (NE), the amino acid glutamate, and the peptide neuropeptide Y (NPY). Inhibitory inputs may come from amino acid gamma aminobutyric acid (GABA), the biogenic amine dopamine (DA), the endogenous opioid β-endorphin, and the neurosecretory peptide corticotropin-releasing hormone (CRH) neurons. These systems may affect the GnRH pulse generator either *tonally* or *conditionally*.

In the first category, we find, for example, NE as a potential tonal stimulator and GABA as a tonal inhibitor of GnRH release. Administration of α-adrenergic blockers has been shown to reduce pulse frequency in animals, in accord with the postulated tonal stimulatory role for NE. The role of GABA as a tonal inhibitor may be more prominent during the prepubertal period, at which time a diminishing inhibitory GABA tone may activate puberty and the resumption of GnRH pulsatile release. Glutamate's role is more uncertain, although it also is suspected in the initiation of pulses at puberty. Dopamine infusions in women are associated with a decrease in circulating LH and prolactin (dopamine is also known as the prolactin-inhibitory neurohormone). The effect on LH is thought to be mediated through GnRH because, in patients with hypothalamic amenorrhea in whom there appears to be an excess of dopaminergic tone, administration of a dopamine blocker may return the LH pulse frequency to normal. It should also be remembered that specific effects of neurotransmitters on GnRH neurons may be altered by the administration of certain drugs, which may interfere with the proper synthesis, binding, storage, or receptor function of these neurotransmitters. Thus upon treatment with such drugs (for example, methyl dopa, reserpine, tricyclic antidepressants such as propranolol, phentolamine, haloperidol, and cyproheptadine, selective serotonin reuptake inhibitors [SSRIs], or serotonin-norepinephrine reuptake inhibitors

[SNRIs]), patients may develop disorders such as oligomenorrhea or galactorrhea, the result of alterations in GnRH secretion or hyperprolactinemia. Other studies also suggest that hypothalamic prostaglandins may also modulate the release of GnRH; for instance, the midcycle surge of LH (see Menstrual Cycle, presented later in the chapter) can be abolished in animals by the administration of aspirin or indomethacin, which block the synthesis of prostaglandins. Clinical studies have also shown that inhibition of prostaglandin at midcycle may disrupt ovulation.

In the second category, other systems may affect the GnRH system only *conditionally*—that is, under specific hormonal or physiologic conditions. One example is the endogenous opioid **β-endorphin**, which exerts an inhibitory action on GnRH pulsatile activity that depends largely on the endogenous endocrine milieu. This is related to the fact that ovarian hormones control the release of brain β-endorphin within the brain, which is lowest in the absence of estradiol, such as in the ovariectomized nonhuman primate, and highest in the presence of both estradiol and progesterone, such as during the luteal phase of the menstrual cycle. Experimental administration of the opiate antagonist, naloxone, during the luteal phase increases GnRH/LH pulse frequency, significantly suggesting the reversal of an inhibitory action under the endocrine milieu that characterizes the luteal phase. No effect on LH pulsatility follows naloxone injection in postmenopausal or ovariectomized women, unless they are replaced with an estrogen-progesterone therapy. Another example is corticotropin-releasing hormone (CRH), the main neuropeptide controlling the adrenal endocrine axis, which is released in greater amounts during stress. In this condition, increased CRH release negatively affects the GnRH pulse generator, which results in a decrease in GnRH pulse frequency. This action is indirect through the release of β-endorphin and is prevented by the administration of the opiate antagonist naloxone, as demonstrated in studies in nonhuman primates and in patients with hypothalamic amenorrhea, many of whom have elevated levels of cortisol.

### Metabolic Influences and GnRH Release

There is good clinical evidence linking energy homeostasis and reproductive function in the human. A functional reproductive system requires an accurate integration of energy balance, and a significant imbalance may lead to reproductive dysfunction and amenorrhea. Nutritional deprivation and abnormal eating habits are known to interfere with the normal reproductive process. Anorexia nervosa is a well-known and extreme example of how alteration in food intake can result in the suppression of the menstrual cycle. Obesity also may contribute to menstrual disorders.

Growing evidence indicates that complex and extensively integrated physiologic mechanisms connect an active reproductive axis to the metabolic state. The brain, and in particular the hypothalamus and the GnRH pulse generator, function as the center for the integrative metabolic response process. The nature of the afferent signals that provide information about energy metabolism to the reproductive axis is presently under intense study, and data have shown possible roles for several energy-related proteins.

One such example is leptin, an anorexigenic protein that is the product of the *ob* gene and that is primarily produced by adipocytes (Ahima, 2000). Leptin levels are reduced when body fat stores are decreased by fasting. Besides conveying metabolic information to several parts of the brain through its own receptors, leptin also appears to function as one of the metabolic cues regulating the GnRH pulse generator. High leptin levels are interpreted as conducive to reproduction, and the administration of leptin stimulates the secretion of GnRH and of the gonadotropins, with the effects most pronounced in individuals showing signs of reproductive impairment. Peripheral injections of leptin can prevent the reduction in GnRH/gonadotropins and the disturbances in cyclicity that accompany caloric reduction. *Ob/ob* mice, which are leptin deficient because of a mutated leptin gene, besides exhibiting a pronounced obesity, show a complete failure to display normal estrous cycles because of absent GnRH secretion. The latter can be reversed by leptin administration. Evidence suggests a role for kisspeptin in modulating metabolic leptin signals on the hypothalamus and pituitary (Skorupskaite, 2014). Forty percent of kisspeptin neurons in the mouse arcuate nucleus express leptin. Leptin-deficient mice show decreased expression of *Kiss1* mRNA. However, leptin administration only partially restores *Kiss1* mRNA levels, indicating that other mediators are involved in inhibiting kisspeptin signaling in leptin deficiency (Smith, 2006). Another example is the orexigenic peptide, neuropeptide Y (NPY), which is synthesized in the arcuate nucleus. During fasting, expression of *NPY* mRNA increases in this nucleus and intracerebroventricular injection of NPY stimulates food intake. NPY has been shown to affect pulsatile GnRH/LH activity in the nonhuman primate, but this occurs in two apparently contradictory modes, one excitatory and one inhibitory. It was shown in the ovariectomized monkey and rodent that a pulsatile intracerebroventricular infusion of NPY stimulates GnRH release, whereas a continuous infusion clearly decreases the pulsatile electric activity of GnRH neurons as well as pulsatile LH release. In accord with this observation of an inhibitory effect of NPY is that whereas fasting decreases LH secretion in normal mice, fasting mice lacking NPY Y1R have a higher pituitary LH content than wild-type ones. What these data suggest is that although a supportive effect of NPY on the GnRH pulse generator may occur within a limited window of normalcy (i.e., within a normal background of basic and pulsatile NPY release), in physiopathologic situations (i.e., in circumstances mimicking increased endogenous NPY activity such as in undernutrition) an inhibitory effect of NPY on the GnRH pulse generator can be observed. Evidence suggests that kisspeptin neurons can sense and convey information about energy status to GnRH neurons. In rodents, hypothalamic levels of *Kiss1* mRNA are reduced in metabolic conditions, such as undernutrition, uncontrolled diabetes, and immune/inflammatory challenge, which are associated with suppressed gonadotropins. Administration of kisspeptin in rodent models with disrupted metabolism and energy reserves restores gonadotropin secretion, suggesting a potentially important central role of Kiss1 neurons in the regulation of reproduction by metabolic factors (Skorupskaite, 2014).

Overall, in regard to the reproductive system, the GnRH pulse generator actually acts as the link that connects the environment, the internal milieu, and the reproductive axis. Its overall activity most probably reflects the summation of simultaneous stimulatory and inhibitory inputs. It is evident that events, disorders, or drug administration may tip the physiologic balance, cause disruption or cessation of GnRH pulse activity, and lead to disruptions of the menstrual cycle and to reproductive disorders such as oligomenorrhea and hypothalamic amenorrhea.

## ANTERIOR PITUITARY GLAND AND THE GONADOTROPINS

### ANATOMY

The anterior pituitary (also referred to as the **adenohypophysis**) derives from the *Rathke pouch,* a depression in the roof of the developing mouth in front of the buccopharyngeal membrane. It originates at about the third week of life. Origin of the adenohypophysis contrasts with that of the posterior pituitary, the neurohypophysis, which develops as a direct extension of the brain. It should also be noted that whereas the neurohypophysis receives a direct arterial blood supply from the hypophyseal arteries, the only vascularization to the adenohypophysis is through the hypothalamic-hypophyseal portal system (into which GnRH and several other neuropeptides are secreted) (discussed earlier).

The gonadotropes are the specialized cells within the adenohypophysis that produce the **gonadotropins.** Upon stimulation of the gonadotropes by GnRH, two gonadotropins are released into the general circulation and regulate endocrine function in the ovaries and testes.

**Prolactin** is not a gonadotropin, but it is also secreted by the anterior pituitary gland and has important effects on reproduction function. For example, elevations in prolactin can inhibit GnRH release and result in anovulation and hypoestrogenic amenorrhea. This inhibition is thought to be the result of inhibition of kisspeptin-1, which stimulates GnRH release (Bernard, 2015). Prolactin is covered in depth in Chapter 39.

### PHYSIOLOGY

#### GnRH Receptor

Pulses of GnRH released by the GnRH neurons in the arcuate nucleus reach the gonadotropes in the anterior pituitary via the hypophyseal portal circulation. These GnRH pulses then act on GnRH receptors (**GnRH-R**) on the gonadotropes to stimulate both the synthesis and release of both gonadotropins, LH and follicle-stimulating hormone (FSH). Females with GnRH-R mutations typically present with incomplete or absent pubertal development and primary amenorrhea. Although reproductive function is compromised, conception may be successfully obtained following gonadotropin treatment.

On the cell membranes of the gonadotrope, GnRH interacts with high-affinity GnRH receptors. The gene encoding the GnRH-R is located on chromosome 4q13.2-13.3, spanning 18.9 kb. This receptor belongs to a large family of G protein-coupled receptors. These contain seven transmembrane helices connected by six alternating intracellular and extracellular loops, with the amino-terminus located on the extracellular side. In contrast to other protein receptors (see Fig. 4.9, presented later in the chapter), the GnRH-R lacks a carboxy-terminus located on the intracellular site.

##### Activation of the GnRH Receptor

GnRH activation of the receptor requires the release of constraining intramolecular bonds, which maintain the receptor in an inactive configuration. Once activated, the GnRH receptor stimulates cellular production of specific membrane-associated lipid-like diacylglycerols, which, acting as a second messenger, activate several cellular proteins. Among these are the enzyme **protein kinase C (PKC)** and **extracellular signal-regulated kinase (ERK)**, a member of the **mitogen- activated protein kinase (MAPK)** cascade. Phosphorylated ERK activates transcription factors, the result being gene transcription of gonadotropin subunits and the synthesis of both gonadotropins.

Binding of GnRH to its receptor also rapidly mobilizes transient intracellular calcium, which triggers a burst of exocytosis to rapidly release LH and FSH. It also provokes a rapid influx of $Ca^{++}$ into the cell from the extracellular pool, which in turn activates calmodulin, a calcium-binding protein, maintaining gonadotropin release. Diacylglycerols amplify the action of $Ca^{++}$-calmodulin, thereby synergistically enhancing the release of gonadotropins. Administration of a calmodulin antagonist has been shown to decrease GnRH-stimulated gonadotropin release.

##### Estrogens and the GnRH Receptor

Pulsatile GnRH increases *GnRH-R* gene expression and the number of GnRH-R on the gonadotrope's cell surface. The number of GnRH-R also varies with the hormonal environment, with highest number of receptors expressed when high concentrations of estrogens are present. This leads to an increase in the overall $Ca2^{++}$ response and a significantly amplified gonadotropin response to a GnRH pulse. This action explains the variations in the gonadotropin response to GnRH at various times of the menstrual cycle: GnRH pulses of similar amplitude elicit greater gonadotropin responses during the late follicular phase and luteal phase when estradiol levels are highest, but the responses are lower during the early follicular phase when estradiol levels are lowest (Fig. 4.4).

##### GnRH Pulse Frequency and Gonadotropin Release

It is also important to note that varying frequencies of the GnRH pulse signal regulate gonadotropin subunit gene transcription differentially. Overall, a low GnRH pulse frequency favors FSH synthesis, whereas a high GnRH pulse frequency favors LH synthesis. This is well demonstrated experimentally where changing a pulsatile infusion from a high- to a low-pulse frequency results in a matter of days in an increase in the FSH:LH ratio (Fig. 4.5). This phenomenon may play a role during the luteal phase of the menstrual cycle and in the changing FSH:LH ratio that occurs during the passage from one menstrual cycle to another (see Luteal Phase, discussed later). It is also reflected in patients known to have a high GnRH pulse frequency, such as in women with polycystic ovary syndrome, in which a high proportion of patients have a characteristically elevated LH:FSH ratio.

##### GnRH Receptor Desensitization

Gonadotropin release following a GnRH pulse is rapid: within minutes, both FSH and LH are released. It is important to recognize that the pulsatile release mode of GnRH is essential for the maintenance and control of normal gonadotropin secretion.

In contrast to the response to the normal pulsatile mode of GnRH release, sustained exposure of the GnRH-R to constant GnRH concentrations drastically reduces the response of the gonadotrope to subsequent stimulation with GnRH. This phenomenon is referred to as ***homologous desensitization*** or ***downregulation*** of the receptor, which denotes a reduction

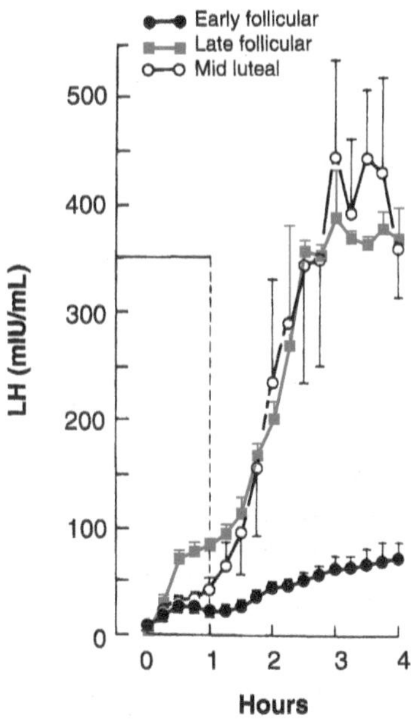


**Figure 4.4** GnRH pulses of similar amplitude elicit greater overall gonadotropin responses during the late follicular phase and luteal phase when estradiol levels are highest, but they elicit lower responses during the early follicular phase when estradiol levels are lowest. Note also a greater early response in the late follicular phase, denoting greater LH reserves under the effect of estradiol. (From Hoff JD, Lasley BL, Wang CF, Yen SSC. The two pools of pituitary gonadotropins: regulation during the menstrual cycle. *J Clin Endocrinol Metab.* 1977;44:302.)

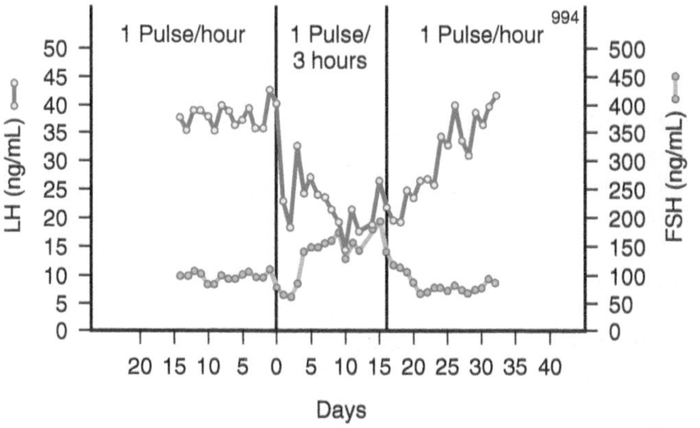


**Figure 4.5** Increase in the FSH:LH ratio following a decrease in the GnRH pulse frequency (from 1 pulse/hour; *left and right panels*) to 1 pulse/3 hour *(center panel)*. Experiment was performed in a monkey lacking endogenous GnRH and infused with GnRH. (From Wildt L, Hausler A, Marshall G, et al. Frequency and amplitude of gonadotropin-releasing hormone stimulation and gonadotropin secretion in the rhesus monkey. *Endocrinology.* 1981;109:376.)

in the ability of GnRH to elicit gonadotropin release after prior continuous exposure to GnRH. This phenomenon is well illustrated in a classic experiment performed by Knobil and collaborators in ovariectomized monkeys lacking endogenous GnRH secretion following lesion of the arcuate nucleus (Fig. 4.6). As illustrated, 6-minute duration pulses administered once an hour restored normal LH levels in these animals. In contrast, when a continuous mode of GnRH infusion was

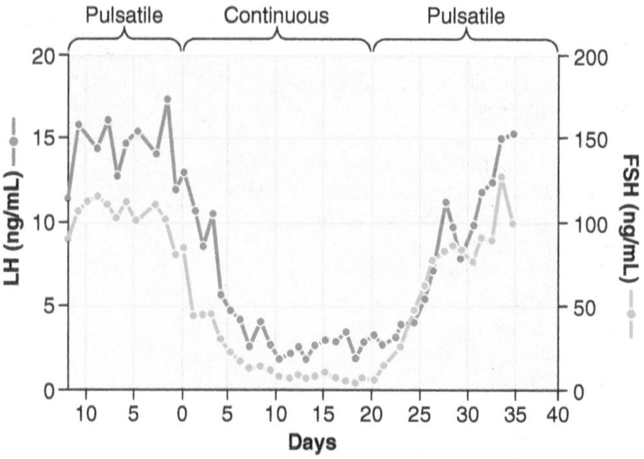


**Figure 4.6** GnRH release in a pulsatile mode is required for a normal pituitary gonadotropin response. An experiment was performed in a monkey lacking endogenous GnRH and infused with hourly pulses of GnRH *(left and right portions)* or with a continuous GnRH infusion *(center portion)*. (From Belchetz PE, Plant TM, Nakai Y, et al. Hypophyseal responses to continuous and intermittent delivery of hypothalamic gonadotropin-releasing hormone. *Science.* 1978;202:631-633.)

substituted to the pulsatile mode, there occurs a profound inhibition of LH concentrations. This reflects desensitization of the GnRH receptor. This phenomenon, which takes a few days to be established, may reflect a loss of active cell surface receptors and be maintained by a loss of functional $Ca^{++}$ channels. However, the mechanism of desensitization is still under investigation, and additional intermediary changes remain to be characterized.

## GnRH Analogues and the GnRH Receptor

The GnRH half-life in the peripheral circulation is very short as peptidases rapidly degrade naturally occurring GnRH by cleaving the decapeptide molecule at the $Gly^6$ to $Leu^7$ and at the $Pro^9$ to $Gly^{10}$ bonds. However, by substituting amino acid 6 in the natural GnRH molecule with a d-amino or replacing amino acid 10 with a N-ethylamide (Na-CH2-CH3) or Aza-Gly (NHNHCO) moiety, gonadotropin-releasing hormone analogues (GnRH analogues) were synthesized and shown to have acquired a greater resistance to enzymatic proteolysis and hence a longer half-life (hours versus 2 to 4 minutes). Following administration of these **GnRH agonists**, there is an initial stimulation of gonadotropin release (flare), followed by the process of desensitization blocking the releasing effect on the gonadotropins. This observation has led to the clinical application of the functional desensitization property of **GnRH analogues (agonists)** having been used to induce a "medical castration" state by shutting down the pituitary-gonadal axis in a variety of clinical conditions. In contrast to GnRH agonists, **GnRH antagonists** act by competing with GnRH for receptor sites and thereby never activating a stimulatory signal. Many of these result from the substitution of amino acids at the 2 or 3 position. Thus GnRH antagonists have the advantage over the GnRH agonists of a rapidly decreasing LH and FSH release, without the flare. Clinical applications for both GnRH agonists and antagonists are listed in Box 4.1.

**Box 4.1 Clinical Applications of GnRH and Its Agonists**

Activation of pituitary-gonadal function (GnRH)
Delayed puberty
Cryptorchidism
Functional hypothalamic amenorrhea
Hypogonadotropic hypogonadism (Kallmann syndrome)
Pituitary-gonadal inhibition (agonists)
Precocious puberty
Hormone-dependent tumors
Endometriosis
Uterine leiomyoma
Breast cancer
Prostatic cancer
Suppression of ovarian function in polycystic ovary syndrome and in vitro fertilization
Premenstrual syndrome
Abnormal uterine bleeding including clotting disorders
Contraception
Suppression of spermatogenesis
Ovulation inhibition

### *Gonadotropins*

There are two distinct gonadotropins: **luteinizing hormone (LH)** and **follicle-stimulating hormone (FSH)**. (A third gonadotropin, chorionic gonadotropin [hCG], is produced in the primate by the placenta.)

#### Structure

LH and FSH are glycoproteins of high molecular weight. They are heterodimers, containing two monomeric units (**subunits**). Both LH and FSH have a similar α-subunit, the structure (92 amino acids) of which is highly conserved. (The same α-subunit is also shared with hCG and thyroid-stimulating hormone [TSH].) However, β-subunits have different structures consisting of different amino acids and carbohydrates. These LH and FSH subunits are each encoded by a separate gene. (The hCG subunits are also different and encoded by six genes.)

The α- and β-subunits are joined by disulfide bonds, which are essential to maintain biologic activity. Reducing agents break the disulfides bounds and reduce or remove the biologic activity of the gonadotropin. Highly purified free subunits have little if any biologic activity relative to that of the intact hormone. However, it is the β-subunit that confers the specific biologic activity of each hormone. For instance, LH has a β-subunit of 121 amino acids, a structure that is responsible for the specificity of the interaction with the LH receptor. LH and FSH also differ in the composition of their sugar moieties. The different composition of several different oligosaccharides affects bioactivity and speed of degradation of each gonadotropin. For example, the biologic half-life of LH is 20 minutes, much shorter than that of FSH (3 to 4 hours). (The half-life of hCG is 24 hours.)

Although both gonadotropins act synergistically in the female, FSH acts primarily on the granulosa cells of the ovarian follicles to stimulate follicular growth, whereas LH acts primarily on the theca cells of these follicles as well as on the luteal cells to stimulate ovarian steroid hormone production (see the following discussion).

# OVARIES

## ANATOMY

### *Ovarian Gametogenesis (Oogenesis)*

Oogenesis begins in fetal life when the *primordial* germ cells, or **oogonia**, migrate to the genital ridge. The number of oogonia increases dramatically from about 600,000 by the second month of fetal life to a maximum of about 7 million by the sixth to seventh month. The oogonia then begin meiotic division (they are now referred to as **primary oocytes**) until they reach the diplotene stage of the prophase (the germinal vesicular stage), in which they will remain until stimulation by gonadotropins in adulthood during the menstrual cycle (discussed later). However, by a process of apoptosis and atresia of the enveloping follicle, which starts prenatally and persists throughout childhood, the number of primary oocytes declines drastically from about 2 to 4 million at birth to become 90% depleted by puberty. Further depletion of the pool occurs throughout adulthood, so by age 37, only about 25,000 and by age 50 only about 1000 oocytes remain.

The traditional dogma that mammals have fixed, nonrenewable oocyte stores established prior to birth has been challenged. Some studies suggest that adult mammalian ovaries possess pluripotent germline stem cells (GSCs) that can differentiate into oocytes, as well as other cell types. Nonmammalian organisms, such as *Drosophila,* do possess ovarian GSCs. Whereas the existence of spermatogonial cells in the adult human testis that give rise to pluripotent GSCs is well accepted, there is considerable evidence that disputes the existence of mammalian adult ovarian GSCs. At this point, there is not sufficient evidence to prove that mammalian oogenesis occurs after birth (Hanna, 2014).

### *Ovarian Folliculogenesis*

The primary oocyte is surrounded by a single layer of granulosa cells in a unit referred to as the **primordial follicle**. Even in the absence of stimulation by gonadotropins, some primordial follicles will develop into **primary** (or preantral) **follicles**, at which stage multiple layers of granulosa cells surround them. Development of follicles to this stage appears to be relatively independent of pituitary control but is probably influenced by intraovarian, nonsteroidal processes that remain to be understood. Development to this stage occurs during the nonovulatory stages of childhood, pregnancy, oral contraceptive use, as well as during ovulatory cycles.

With formation of an antrum (cavity), the follicle, now referred to as a **secondary** or **antral follicle**, enters the final stages of folliculogenesis characterized by the transition from intraovarian regulation to a major control by the hypothalamic-pituitary unit. This requires the presence of the characteristic increase in FSH that occurs in the early menstrual cycle (see Menstrual Cycle, presented later).

The development process from primary follicle (preantral follicle) to secondary or antral follicle, and to a mature preovulatory follicle, the latter during the follicular phase of the cycle, takes about 1 year to complete (Fig. 4.7). Only about 400 follicles complete this process, whereas the majority of follicles undergo programmed cell death. Although little is known about factors controlling growth during the earlier stages, more is known

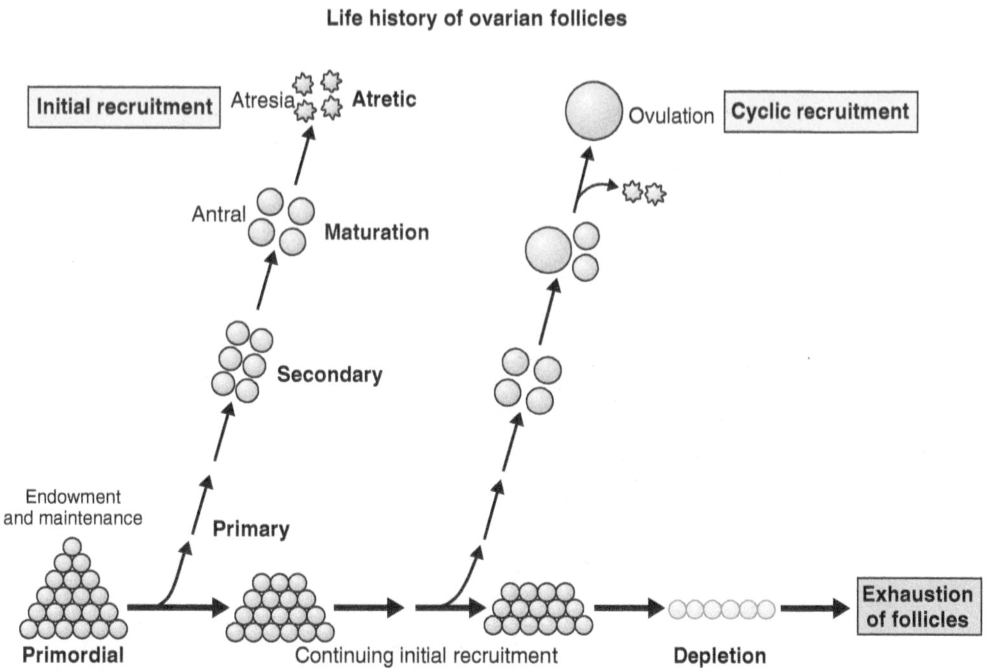


**Figure 4.7** Life history of ovarian follicles: endowment, maintenance, initial recruitment, maturation, atresia or cyclic recruitment, ovulation, and exhaustion. A fixed number of primordial follicles are endowed during early life, and most of them are maintained in a resting state. Growth of some of these dormant follicles is initiated before and throughout reproductive life (initial recruitment). Follicles develop through primordial, primary, and secondary stages before acquiring an antral cavity. At the antral stage, most follicles undergo atresia; however, under the optimal gonadotropin stimulation that occurs after puberty, a few of them are rescued (cyclic recruitment) to reach the preovulatory stage. Eventually, depletion of the pool of resting follicles leads to ovarian follicle exhaustion and senescence. (From McGee EA, Hsueh AJW. Initial and cyclic recruitment of ovarian follicles. *Endocrine Rev.* 2000;21:200-214.)

about the final stage of folliculogenesis during the follicular phase of the menstrual cycle (discussed later).

## *PHYSIOLOGY*

### *Gonadotropin Receptors*

Although the two gonadotropins act synergistically in the female, FSH acts primarily on the granulosa cells of the maturing antral follicle to stimulate follicular growth, whereas LH acts primarily on the theca cells of these follicles to induce steroidogenesis. Binding to and activation of their respective receptors at the cell surface membrane represent the necessary first step in the hormonal function of both FSH and LH.

Gonadotropin receptors are transmembrane G protein-coupled receptors, which possess seven membrane-spanning domains (Fig. 4.8). It is believed that the receptor molecule exists in a conformational equilibrium between active and inactive states, which is shifted by binding of LH or FSH. Upon binding to the gonadotropin, the receptor shifts conformation and mechanically activates the G protein, which detaches from the receptor and activates cyclic adenosine monophosphate (AMP) dependent protein kinases. These protein kinases are present as tetramers with two regulatory units and two catalytic units. Upon binding of cyclic AMP (cAMP) to the regulatory units, the catalytic units are released and initiate the phosphorylation of proteins, which bind to

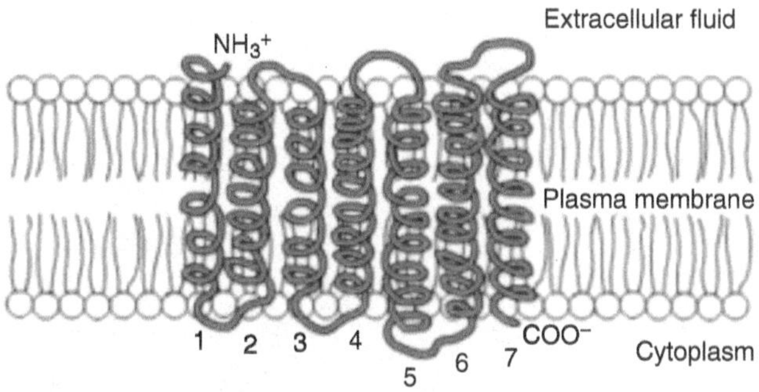


**Figure 4.8** The seven transmembrane α-helix structure of a G protein-coupled receptor, such as that for LH or hCG. (The structure for the GnRH receptor is similar, except that the GnRH-R lacks a carboxy terminus on the intracellular site; see the preceding text.) (From trans-membrane helix of G-protein coupled FSH receptor; from Wikipedia.)

DNA in the cell nucleus, resulting in the activation of genes and leading to the physiologic action (Fig. 4.9).

### *Ovarian Steroids: Biosynthesis*

One primary function of the ovary is the secretion of ovarian steroids, which occurs following binding of both FSH and LH to their respective receptors. The ovary secretes three primary hormones: **estradiol** (the primary estrogen), **progesterone**, and

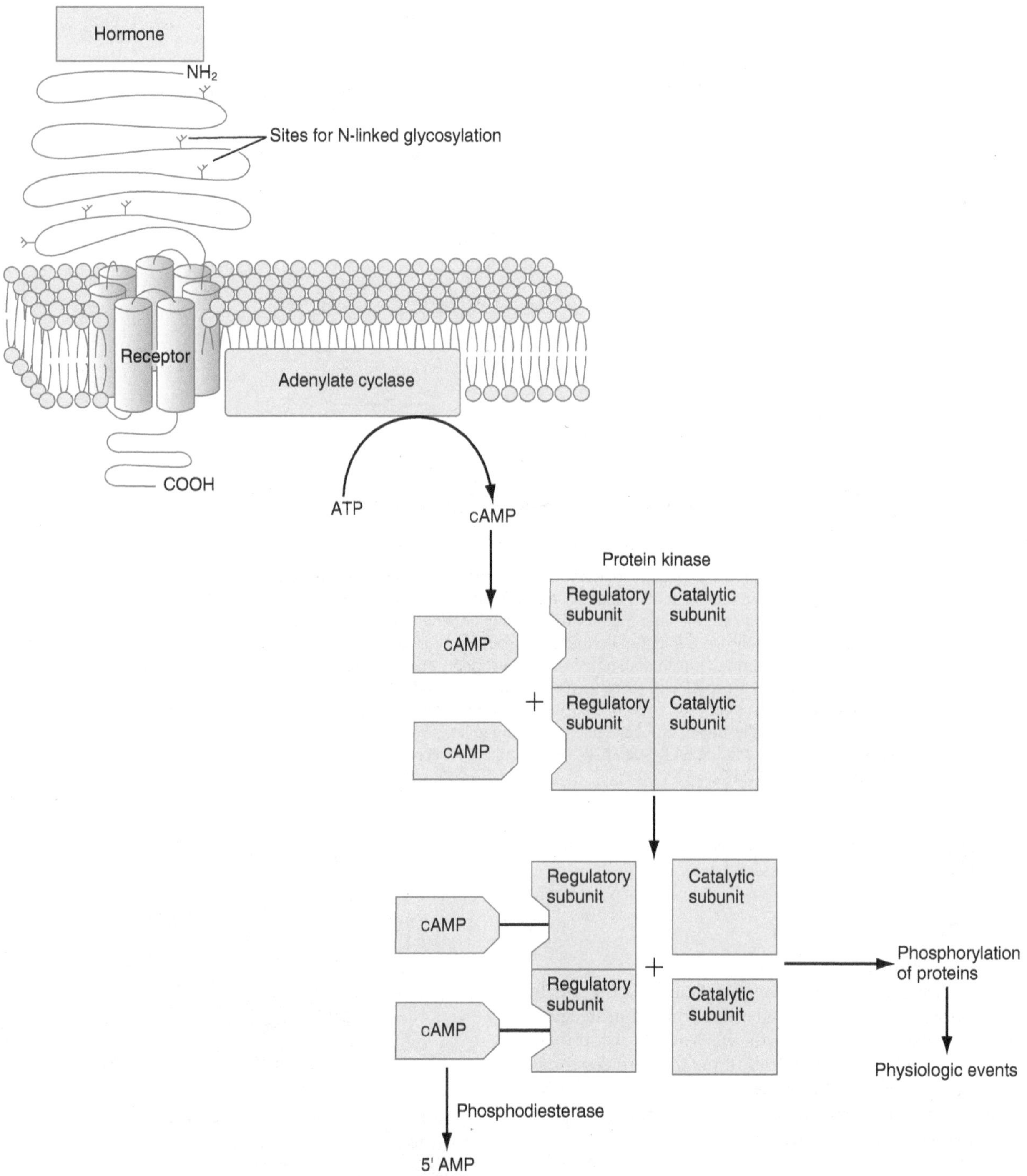


**Figure 4.9** Upon binding to their receptor, the gonadotropins activate cyclic AMP-dependent protein kinases (see text). (Modified from Speroff L, Friz M, eds. *Clinical Gynecologic Endocrinology and Infertility.* New York: Lippincott Williams & Wilkins; 2005:71-72.)

**androstenedione.** These hormones are the chief secretory products of the maturing follicle, the corpus luteum, and the ovarian stroma. The ovary also secretes, in varying amounts, estrone (a less potent estrogen), pregnenolone, 17-hydroxyprogesterone, testosterone, and dehydroepiandrosterone (DHEA). Because of the lack of the appropriate enzymes, the ovary does not synthesize mineralo- or glucocorticoids.

Steroids are lipids that have a basic chemical structure or nucleus (Fig. 4.10). The nucleus consists of three six-carbon rings (A, B, and C) joined to a five-carbon atom (D) ring. The carbon atoms are numbered as shown in Figure 4.10. Functional groups above the plane of the molecule are preceded by the β symbol and shown in the structural formula by a solid line, whereas those below the plane are indicated by an α symbol and a dotted

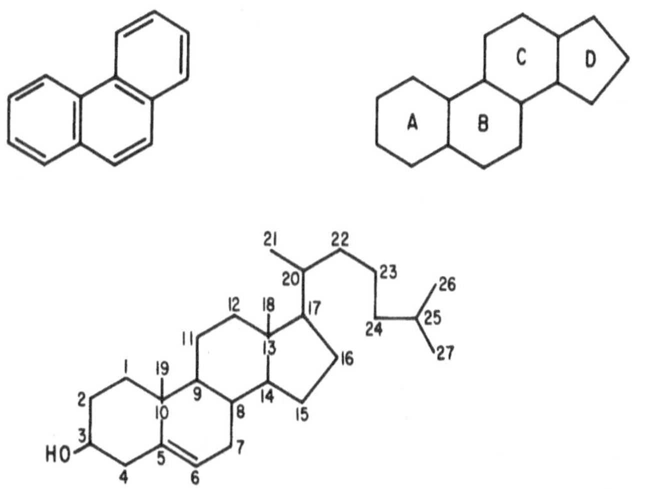


**Figure 4.10** Phenanthrene *(top left).* Cyclopentanoperhydrophenanthrene nucleus *(top right),* which incorporates the three six-carbon rings of the phenanthrene ring system *(A, B,* and *C)* and a five-carbon ring *(D),* which resembles cyclopentane. Cholesterol *(bottom)* is the common biosynthetic precursor of steroid hormones. Numbers 1 to 27 indicate the conventional numbering system of the carbon atoms in steroids. (From Stanczyk FZ. Steroid hormones. In: Lobo RA, Mishell DR, Paulson RJ, Shoupe D, eds. *Mishell's Textbook of Infertility, Contraception and Reproductive Endocrinology.* 4th ed. Malden, MA: Blackwell Science; 1997.)

line. All steroids, whether secreted by the ovary, testis, or adrenal, are derived from **acetate** (a two-carbon compound), which, in a series of complex reactions, is transformed into **cholesterol** (a 27-carbon steroid) (Fig. 4.11.)

The sex steroids (as well as the corticosteroids) are then derived from a stepwise transformation of the cholesterol molecule into steroids with 21 carbon atoms (the corticosteroids, pregnenolone, 17-hydroxy pregnenolone, progesterone, and 17-hydroxyprogesterone), 19 carbon atoms (androgens such as DHEA, androstenedione, and testosterone), and 18 carbon atoms (estrogens such as estradiol and estrone). In the first step, cholesterol is transferred from the outer mitochondrial membrane to the inner membrane, where cytochrome P450 enzyme is located. The latter will split off the cholesterol side chain, which is the first enzymatic step in steroid biosynthesis. Being lipophilic, cholesterol is unable to cross the aqueous phase between these two membranes on its own. It is now believed that steroidogenic acute regular protein (StAR) assists in that role. The next steps in steroid biosynthesis require participation of a variety of enzymes, most of which are part of the cytochrome P450 superfamily of heme-based enzymes. First is the transformation of cholesterol into pregnenolone by hydroxylation of C-20 and C-22 and cleavage between these two atoms, reducing the C-27 cholesterol to the C-21 compound pregnenolone. At this point, ovarian steroid biosynthesis proceeds along two major pathways, controlled by specific enzymes at each step: (1) the *$\Delta^5$ pathway* through 17-hydroxypregnenolone and DHEA to $\Delta^5$ androstenediol and (2) the *$\Delta^4$ pathway* via progesterone and 17-hydroxyprogesterone to the androgens, androstenedione and testosterone.

### *Aromatase Enzyme*

Androgens are converted to the estrogens estrone or estradiol by the enzyme **aromatase,** through the loss of the C-19 methyl group and the transformation of the A-ring to an aromatic state (hence the enzyme's name) through oxidation and subsequent elimination of a methyl group. The aromatic (or phenolic) ring is characteristic of the estrogens (Fig. 4.12).

Aromatase is a complex enzyme comprising two proteins. The first, P450arom (also a member of the cytochrome P450 superfamily of genes), catalyzes the series of reactions required for the formation of the phenolic A ring. The second is NADPH-cytochrome P450 reductase, a ubiquitous protein required for transferring reducing equivalents from NADPH to any microsomal form of cytochrome P450 with which it comes into contact. (All microsomal P450 enzymes require this reductase for catalysis. Disruption of this reductase has lethal consequences, as shown in knockout mice.)

The aromatase enzyme is found in many tissues besides the gonads, such as the endometrium, brain, placenta, bone, skin, and others. It is also particularly relevant to note that in humans, in contrast to other species, estrogens are also synthesized in adipose tissue, which in the postmenopausal woman becomes the major site of estrogen biosynthesis. The tissue-specific expression of the *CYP19* aromatase gene is regulated by the use of different promoters. For instance, expression in the ovary uses a promoter element proximal to the start of translation, whereas expression in adipose tissue uses distal elements. Overall, the $C_{18}$ estrogen produced in different tissue sites of biosynthesis is rather specific and dependent on the nature of the $C_{19}$ steroid presented to the aromatase enzyme: in the ovary, the main androgen source is ovarian testosterone and thus the main estrogen product from the ovary is estradiol, whereas in adipose tissue the main androgen source is circulating androstenedione (produced by the adrenals) and hence the principal estrogen produced is estrone. (The greater the amount of fat present, the greater the amount of androstenedione that is converted to estrone via aromatase.)

Mutation of *CYP19* leads to the **aromatase deficiency syndrome,** which is inherited in an autosomal recessive way (Morishima, 1995). In these female patients, accumulation of androgens during pregnancy may lead to virilization at birth. Individuals of both sexes have abnormal pubertal maturation and are tall because of the lack of estrogen to affect epiphyseal closure. Female patients have primary amenorrhea. Aromatase inhibition evidently leads to profound hypoestrogenism. Aromatase inhibitors have become useful in the management of patients with estrogen receptor positive tumors—for example, in breast cancer.

Interconversion between androstenedione and testosterone and estrone and estradiol can occur outside the ovaries. Oxidation of the latter to the former reduces biologic potency because both androstenedione and estrone have weaker biologic activity. Estrone is also converted to estrone sulfate, which has a longer half-life and is the largest component of the pool of circulating estrogens. Estrone sulfate is not biologically active; however, sulfatases in various tissues (such as breast and endometrium) can readily convert it to estrone, which in turn can be converted to the more biologically active estradiol. Steroids are in general insoluble in water but dissolve readily in organic solvents. In contrast, steroids that have a sulfate or glucuronide group attached (conjugated steroids)—such as, for example, estrone sulfate, dehydroepiandrosterone sulfate (DHEAS), or pregnanediol glucuronide—are water soluble.

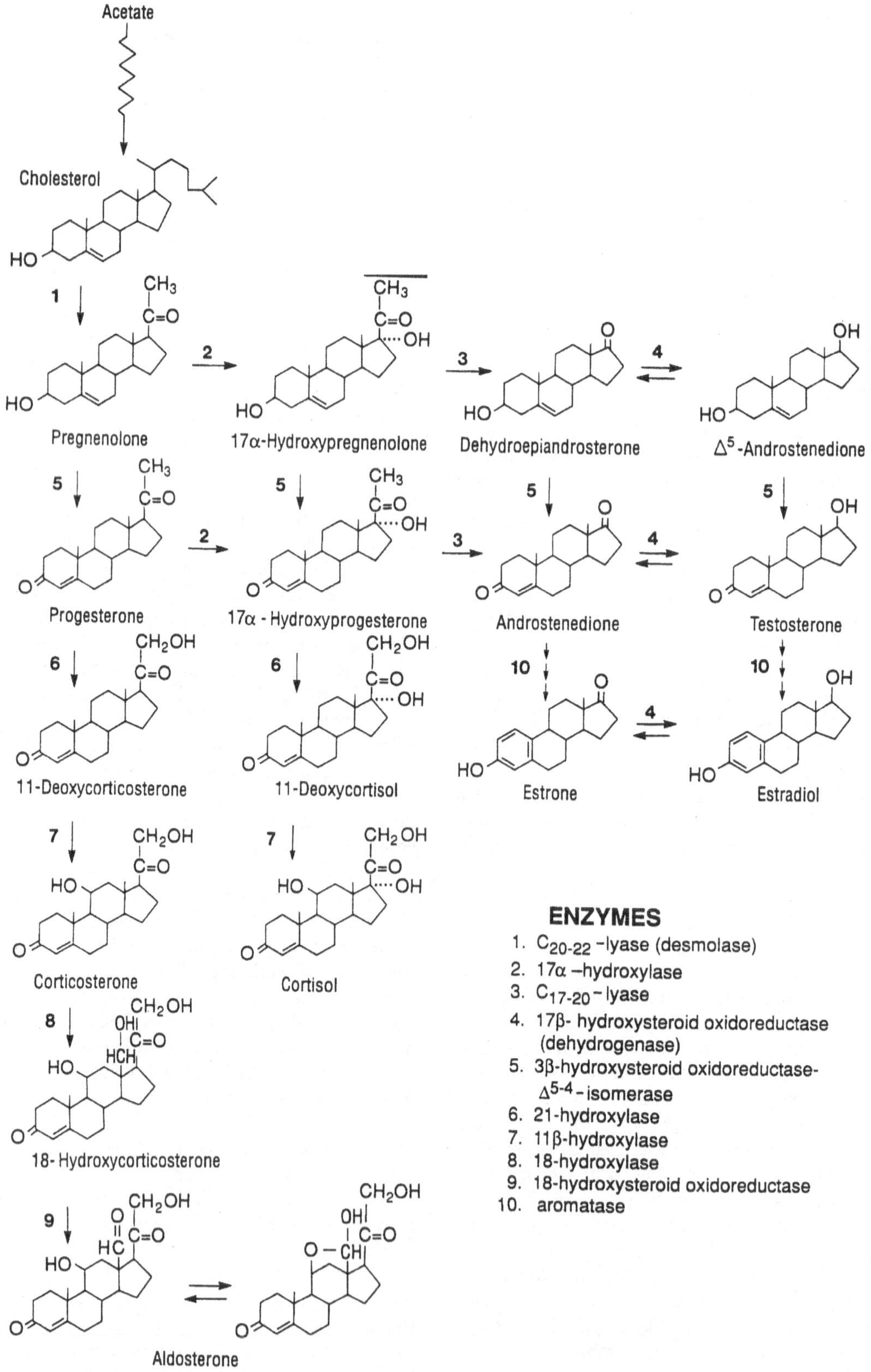


**Figure 4.11** Biosynthesis of androgens, estrogens, and corticosteroids. (From Stanczyk FZ. Steroid hormones. In: Lobo RA, Mishell DR, Paulson RJ, Shoupe D, eds. *Mishell's Textbook of Infertility, Contraception and Reproductive Endocrinology.* 4th ed. Malden, MA: Blackwell Science; 1997.)

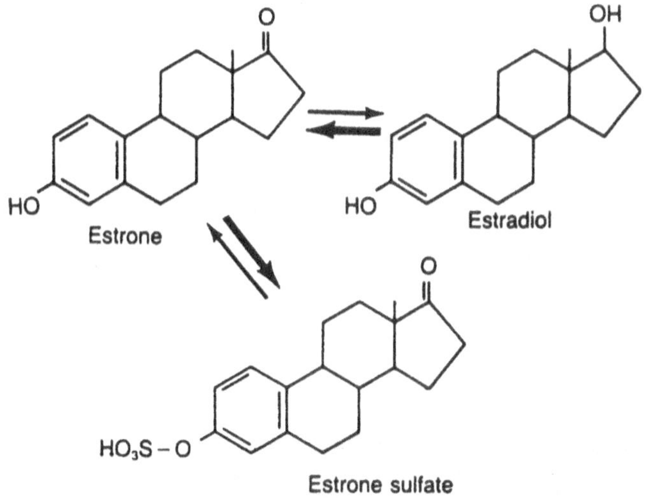


**Figure 4.12** Interconversion of the three main circulating estrogens. (From Stanczyk FZ. Steroid hormones. In: Lobo RA, Mishell DR, Paulson RJ, Shoupe D, eds. *Mishell's Textbook of Infertility, Contraception and Reproductive Endocrinology.* 4th ed. Malden, MA: Blackwell Science; 1997.)

### *Ovarian Steroids: Blood Transport and Metabolism*

After release into the circulation, sex steroids bind to a steroid-specific transport protein, **sex hormone–binding globulin (SHBG)** (a β-globulin synthesized by the liver), to the non–steroid-specific albumin, or circulate in an unbound or "free" form. (There is a separate steroid-specific protein, corticosteroid-binding protein [CBG; transcortin], which binds primarily adrenal steroids, and to a lesser degree progesterone.) Both SHBG and CBG have a high affinity (by definition) but low capacity for steroids. Albumin, in contrast, has a high capacity but binds with low affinity; thus steroids can readily dissociate from its binding and enter target cells.

The free and loosely albumin-bound steroids are believed to be the most biologically important fractions because the steroid is free to diffuse or be actively transported through the capillary wall and bind to its receptor. (There is also evidence, however, that uptake of protein-bound hormone may also play a role.) SHBG binds primarily dihydrotestosterone, testosterone, and estradiol, in order of decreasing affinity. Thus in premenopausal women, 65% of testosterone is bound to SHBG, 30% to albumin, and 5% is free, whereas 60% of estradiol is bound to SHBG, 38% to albumin, and 2% to 3% is free. The metabolic clearance rate of sex steroids is inversely related to their affinity to SHBG. It is thus important to remember that the level of SHBG, and therefore the level of free active hormone, may be influenced by various clinical conditions. For instance, circulating levels of SHBG are increased by estrogens (oral contraceptives, pregnancy) and by thyroid hormone (hyperthyroidism) and are lowered by androgens and in hypothyroidism.

The major sites of steroid metabolism are the liver and kidney. Steroids are mainly oxidized by cytochrome P450 oxidase enzymes, through reactions that introduce oxygen into the steroid ring, allowing a breakdown by other enzymes to form bile acids as final products. These bile acids can then be eliminated through secretion from the liver. In another process, which involves conjugation, the steroids are transformed from lipophilic compounds, which are only sparingly soluble in water, into metabolites that are readily water soluble and can be eliminated in urine. Examples are estradiol-17 glucuronide, estrone sulfate, and pregnanediol-3-glucuronide (the major urinary metabolite of progesterone).

### *Prostaglandins*

Prostaglandins (a subclass of eicosanoids and prostanoids) are in general mediators of inflammatory and anaphylactic reactions. Their most abundant precursor is arachidonic acid, itself formed from linoleic acid supplied in the diet. Their biosynthesis can be inhibited by several groups of compounds, including the nonsteroidal anti-inflammatory drugs (NSAIDs) type 1 (aspirin and indomethacin), which inhibit endoperoxide formation (the immediate precursor of eicosanoids), and type 2 (phenylbutazone), which inhibits the action of endoperoxidase isomerase and reductase. Corticosteroids also can inhibit prostaglandins synthesis.

In contrast to steroid hormones, which are stored and act at targets distant from their source, prostaglandins are produced intracellularly shortly before they are released and generally act locally. Specific prostanoids can have variable effects on different tissues, as well as variable effects on the same organ, even when released at the same concentration, hence the difficulty of studying their actions. One important effect is their ability to modulate the responses of endogenous stimulators and inhibitors, such as ovarian stimulation by LH, which is modulated by prostaglandin F2α (PGF2α), which in turn regulates ovarian receptor availability.

Prostaglandins play an important role in ovarian physiology. They help control early follicular growth by increasing blood supply to certain follicles and inducing FSH receptors in granulosa cells of preovulatory follicles. Both PGF2α and PGE2 are concentrated in follicular fluid of preovulatory follicles and may assist in the process of follicular rupture by facilitating proteolytic enzyme activity in the follicular walls. Many prostanoids are produced in the endometrium. Concentrations of PGE2 and PGF2α increase progressively from the proliferative to the secretory phase of the cycle, with highest levels at menstruation. These prostaglandins may help regulate myometrial contractility and may also play a role in regulating the process of menstruation.

## COMMUNICATION WITHIN THE HYPOTHALAMIC-PITUITARY-OVARIAN ENDOCRINE AXIS

### *STEROID RECEPTORS*

Gonadal steroids are integrated into every aspect of reproduction, and disruption of their signaling pathways, which obviously require initial binding to their receptors, leads to reduced fecundity and aberrations in multiple organ system. For the sex steroid feedback loops (discussed later) to be active, there must be steroid receptors in the appropriate regions of the hypothalamus and pituitary gland to respond to the ovarian signals.

As opposed to peptide or protein hormone receptors that reside on the cell membrane (discussed earlier), steroid receptors reside in the nucleus or in the cytoplasm, in between which they may shuttle in the absence of hormone (Fig. 4.13). The

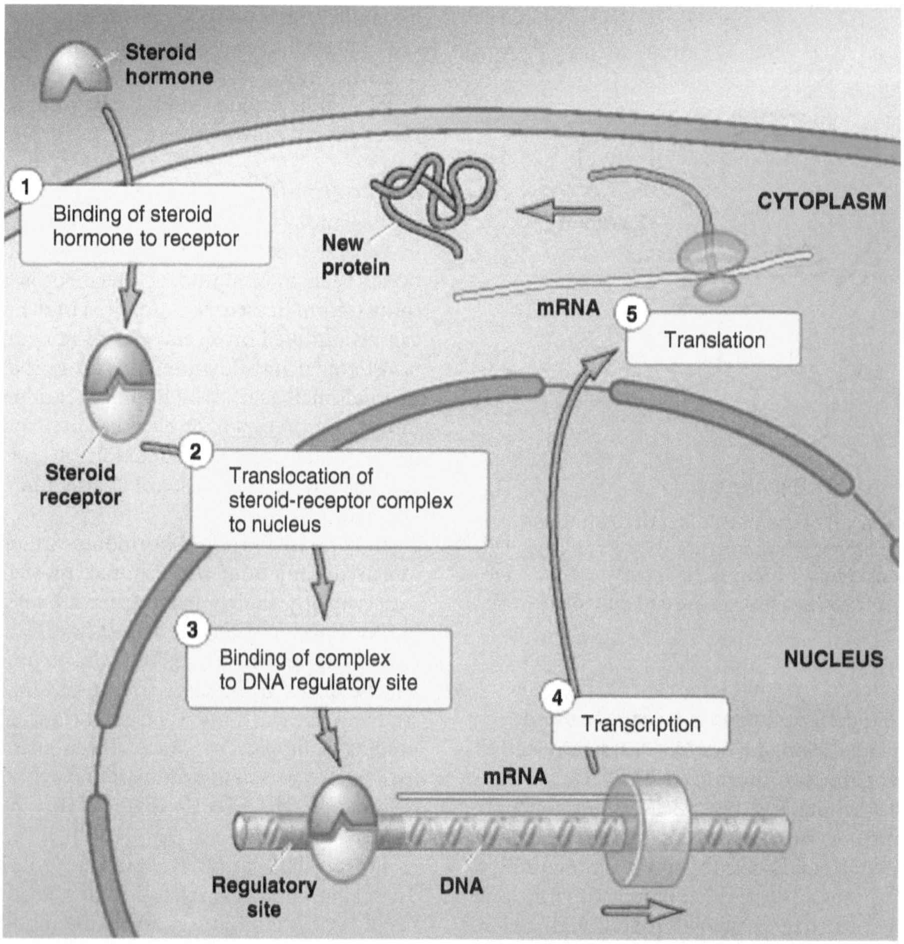


**Figure 4.13** The steroid receptor activation process. As opposed to protein hormones receptors, which reside on the cell membrane, steroid receptors reside in the nucleus or in the cytoplasm. See the text for details.

cytoplasmic receptor is sequestered (hence in an "inactive" state) within a multiprotein inhibitory complex that includes heat shock proteins. Hormone binding leads to dissociation from the heat shock proteins. The lipophilic steroids freely diffuse across the nuclear membrane to bind to their cognate receptor. This binding leads to conformational changes that transform the receptor into an "activated" state, which allows it to bind to a **hormone responsive element (HRE)**, the specific DNA-binding site to which steroid receptors bind conferring hormone sensitivity within target gene promoters. Nuclear receptors can inhibit or enhance transcription by recruiting an array of co-activator or co-repressor proteins to the transcription complex (Fig. 4.14) (Ellmann, 2009). mRNA is then generated from a segment of nuclear DNA in the process of transcription. Transcription is the most important process regulated by steroid hormones. All genes share a common basic design composed of a structural region in which the DNA encodes the specific amino acids of the protein and a regulatory region that interacts with various proteins to control the rate of transcription. Co-activators and co-repressors modify the chromatin state and recruit/activate or hinder the basal transcriptional machinery. Members of the sarcoma (SRC) family of co-activators, including SRC-1, SRC-2, and SRC-3, and the nuclear receptor co-repressor (NCoR1), interact with both the estrogen and progesterone receptors (see Fig. 4.14) (Ellmann, 2009; Horwitz, 1996). The mRNA migrates into the cytoplasm, where it translates information to ribosomes to synthesize the required new protein.

Several alternative receptor mechanisms besides the classic one outlined previously appear to exist. Some are plasma membrane steroid signaling events that are mediated through various kinases and second messengers including cAMP. These are independent of nuclear interactions and do not involve direct steroid activation of gene transcription (nongenomic). As opposed to the longer time required by the genomic pathway (hours to days), these alternate mechanisms may be responsible for some of the rapid effects of steroids—for instance, as activated by the negative steroid feedback loop (discussed later), which occurs within minutes.

Members of the steroid receptor superfamily share amino acid homology and a common structure. They contain key structural elements that enable them to bind to their respective ligands with high affinity and specificity and to recognize and bind to discrete response elements within the DNA sequence of target genes with high affinity and specificity. For instance, estrogen receptors will bind natural and synthetic estrogens, but not androgens or progestins. The affinity of a receptor for a steroid also correlates with

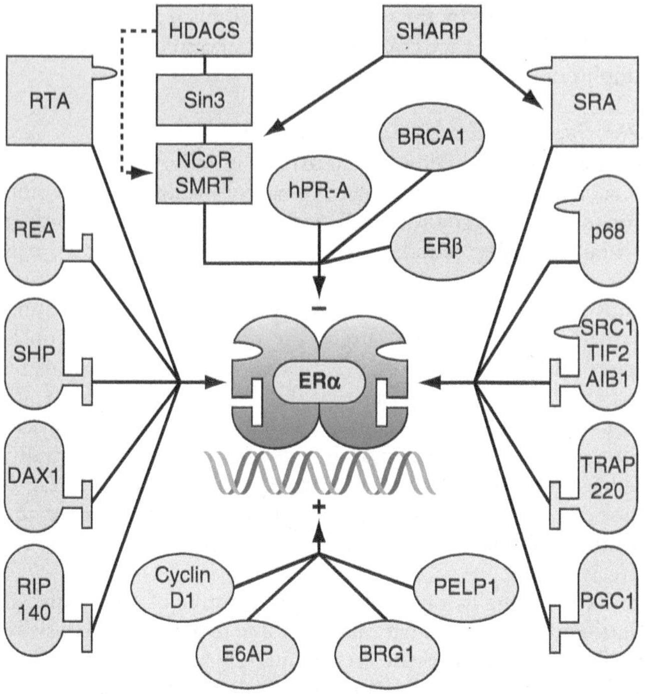


**Figure 4.14** A connections map for the human estrogen receptor (ER). The ER interacts with a large number of proteins that can either positively or negatively regulate target gene transcription. ERα cofactors interact with different target proteins linking the receptor to other signal transduction pathways. Some of the key connections that positively (+) or negatively (−) regulate ERα transcriptional activity are shown. (From McDonnell DP, Norris JD. Connections and regulation of the human estrogen receptor. *Science.* 2002; 296:1642-1644.)

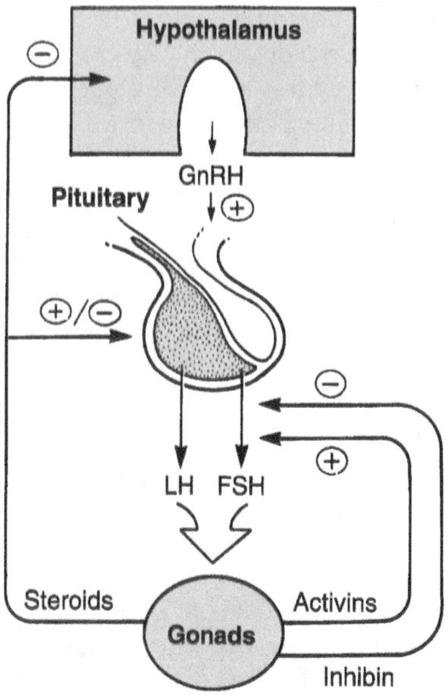


**Figure 4.15** The rapidly acting negative feedback loop of steroids on GnRH and both gonadotropins release is supplemented by a slower-acting negative feedback loop by the inhibins. (From Hylka VW, di Zerega GS. Reproductive hormones and their mechanisms of action. In: Mishell DR Jr, Davajan V, Lobo RA, eds. *Infertility, Contraception and Reproductive Endocrinology.* 3rd ed. Cambridge, MA: Blackwell Scientific; 1991.)

steroid potency; for example, the estrogen receptor has a greater affinity for estradiol than for estrone and estriol, which are much less potent than estradiol. Overall, the magnitude of the signal to the cell and of the cell response to the steroid depends on the concentration of the hormone and of the receptors, as well as on the affinity of the receptor to the hormone.

In the human, there are actually two estrogen receptors, ER-α and ER-β, which are distinct receptor forms encoded by separate genes. There are also two forms of the progesterone receptor, but these are isoforms (differing only by minor structural differences), which are encoded by the same gene.

## OVARIAN-HYPOTHALAMIC-PITUITARY FEEDBACK LOOPS

FSH and LH act on the ovaries to induce morphologic changes and ovarian steroid secretion. Morphologic processes include folliculogenesis (i.e., the cyclic recruitment of a pool of follicles to produce a mature follicle ready for ovulation) and the formation of a corpus luteum. These processes occur in sequence, conferring a monthly rhythm to the reproductive cycle. Granulosa and theca cells within the follicle and luteal cells respond to LH by synthesizing and releasing ovarian steroids, mainly estradiol-17β and progesterone. The type and amount of hormone released depend on the status of the follicle and the corpus luteum (see Menstrual Cycle, presented later).

Feedback communication between the ovaries and the hypothalamic-pituitary unit is an essential component to the physiology of the reproductive cycle. It is important for the brain and pituitary gland to modulate their secretion in response to the minute-to-minute activity status of the ovary. Through their receptors, both in various areas of the hypothalamus and in the anterior pituitary gland, the two ovarian steroids, estradiol and progesterone, play a major role in these feedback communications. More recent evidence shows that several nonsteroidal compounds are also involved in these feedbacks.

### *Negative Steroid Feedback Loop*

As in other endocrine systems, the major ovarian to brain/pituitary feedback loop is inhibitory (the **negative feedback loop**), whereby the steroid secreted by the target organ (the ovary) regulates the hypothalamic-hypophyseal unit to adjust GnRH and gonadotropin secretion appropriately (Fig. 4.15).

**Estradiol-17β** is a potent physiologic inhibitor of GnRH and of gonadotropin secretion. The threshold for the negative feedback action of estradiol is such that even small increases in the levels of the hormone induce a decrease in gonadotropins. Levels of LH and FSH during the follicular phase vary in accord with the changes in estradiol concentrations that accompany maturation of the follicle. Thus as circulating estradiol levels increase during the follicular phase, gonadotropin concentrations decrease. In postmenopausal women or women who have undergone ovariectomy or have aromatase enzyme deficiency, all of whom lack estradiol secretion, sustained increases in LH and FSH release occur because of the absence of an active negative feedback loop. In these conditions, administration of physiologic doses of estradiol results in a rapid and sustained decrease in LH and FSH to levels equivalent to those seen during the menstrual cycle. The estradiol negative feedback loop acts to decrease LH secretion rapidly, mainly by controlling the *amplitude* of each LH pulse. Most evidence suggests that this action is secondary to inhibitory effects on the GnRH pulse, most probably relayed by estrogen-receptive kisspeptin and possibly GABA neurons. Effects on the pituitary gonadotrope, whereby estradiol decreases the gonadotropin response to GnRH, may also take place.

**Progesterone**, at high concentrations such as those observed during the luteal phase of the cycle, also exerts an inhibitory effect on gonadotropin secretion. In contrast to estradiol, progesterone affects mainly the GnRH pulse generator by slowing the frequency of pulses. This effect is responsible for the significant decrease in LH pulse frequency observed during the luteal phase of the cycle, when high levels of progesterone are present, and which becomes more pronounced as the luteal phase progresses (discussed later).

There is good evidence that the slowing action of progesterone on GnRH-LH pulse frequency is mediated by central β-endorphin. Indeed, brain levels of this opioid peptide, as measured in hypophyseal portal blood in the nonhuman primate, are elevated during the luteal phase (Fig. 4.16, *A*). Furthermore, naloxone administration (an opiate antagonist) in women during the luteal phase results in a significant acceleration in pulse frequency (see Fig. 4.16, *B*).

In view of these estradiol and progesterone inhibitory feedback loops, it is not surprising that the characteristics of pulsatile LH secretion vary greatly with the stage of the menstrual cycle. During the estrogenic stage or follicular phase, pulses of high frequency but of low amplitude are seen, whereas during the progesterone stage or luteal phase, there is a progressive reduction in the frequency of the LH pulse, with pulse intervals reaching 200 minutes or more by the end of the luteal phase. This decreased pulse frequency is accompanied by a significant increase in pulse amplitude.

### *Positive Estradiol Feedback Loop*

At higher physiologic concentrations, estradiol can also exert a separate stimulatory effect (**positive feedback loop**) on gonadotropin secretion. This positive feedback is dependent on rapidly rising estradiol levels, in combination with a small but significant progesterone rise, both produced by the mature dominant follicle and responsible for the generation of the preovulatory LH and FSH surge. The positive feedback loop is observed in many species: it serves as the critical signal to the hypothalamic-pituitary axis that the dominant follicle is ready to ovulate. In most species, a GnRH surge precedes the LH surge, suggesting that the positive feedback loop acts centrally. However, there is also ample evidence that high levels of estradiol can increase GnRH pituitary receptors and augment the pituitary response to GnRH, suggesting effects at the pituitary site as well.

Experimentally, late follicular phase estradiol levels infused during the early follicular phase are able to activate the positive feedback loop and release an LH surge, however inappropriate and untimely, because no mature follicle is present at the time (Fig. 4.17).

### *Ovarian Peptides Feedback Loops*

In addition to the negative steroid feedback loop, there is also evidence that nonsteroid ovarian factors exert negative feedback effects on the anterior pituitary. Such are the **inhibins**, which are a family of glycoproteins that consist of a dimer with two dissimilar α and β subunits. The two subunits are coded by different

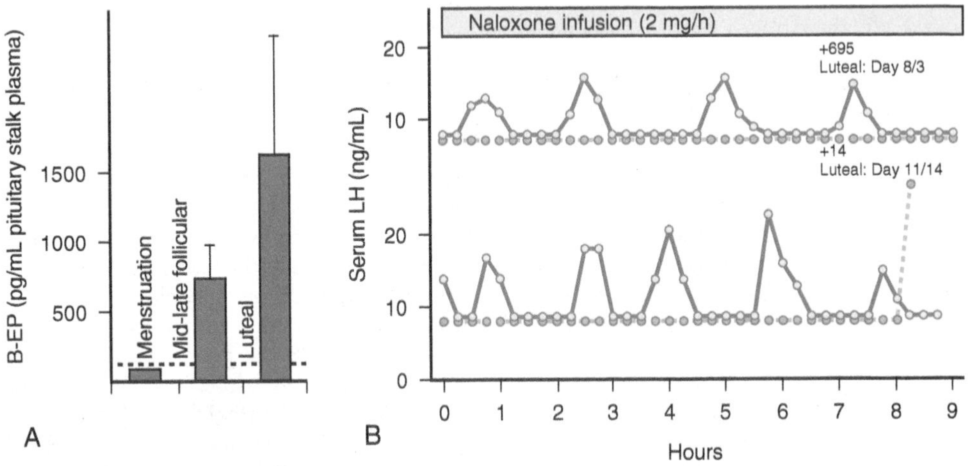


**Figure 4.16** The endogenous opiates and the menstrual cycle. **A,** Changes in hypothalamic β-endorphin activity (as determined by its secretion into the pituitary stalk portal vasculature) during the menstrual cycle in the nonhuman primate. In the presence of low ovarian steroids, such as at menstruation, endorphin levels are lowest. They are highest in the presence of progesterone during the luteal phase. **B,** Role of β-endorphin in modulating the negative feedback action of progesterone during the luteal phase; note the dramatic increase in LH pulse frequency after endogenous opiate antagonism by naloxone *(dark circles)* compared with controls receiving saline *(light circles)*. (**A,** From Van Vugt DA, Lam NY, Ferin M. Reduced frequency of pulsatile luteinizing hormone secretion in the luteal phase of the rhesus monkey: Involvement of endogenous opiates. *Endocrinology.* 1984;115:1095. **B,** From Ferin M, Van Vugt D, Wardlaw S. The hypothalamic control of the menstrual cycle and the role of endogenous opioid peptides. *Rec Prog Horm Res.* 1984;40:441.)

genes. Two forms of the β subunit have been identified, and thus inhibin can exist as α-βA (**inhibin A**) and as α-βB (**inhibin B**) (Fig. 4.18), both of which are detected in serum in women during the reproductive years. The ovaries are the only source of circulating dimeric inhibins.

The inhibins are characterized by their preferential inhibition of FSH over LH through their own negative feedback loop (see Fig. 4.15). This negative feedback loop, however, functions at a significantly slower rate (hours) than that of the steroid negative feedback loop (which is activated within minutes) and is directed mainly at the pituitary gland. It is believed that the decline in FSH after its peak in the early follicular phase of the normal cycle results from a negative feedback action of inhibin B at the pituitary level. At menopause or in premature ovarian failure, data show a decreased secretion of inhibin with reproductive aging, suggesting that inhibin B negative feedback may be an important factor controlling the early monotropic increase in FSH with aging (reflecting the decreasing number of small antral follicles recruited in each cycle and the consequent insufficient inhibin B production).

The circulating patterns of inhibin A and B during the menstrual cycle are different: plasma concentrations of inhibin B rise rapidly on the day after the intercycle FSH rise (discussed later), remain elevated for a few days, then fall progressively during the remainder of the follicular phase. After a short-lived peak following the ovulatory gonadotropin surge, inhibin B falls to a low concentration during the luteal phase. In contrast, inhibin A concentrations rise only in the later part of the follicular phase and are maximal during the midluteal phase (Fig. 4.19) These different patterns of circulating inhibin B and inhibin A during the human menstrual cycle suggest different physiologic roles (discussed later).

Other dimers of the β subunit have also been described, such as **activin** A (A-β/A-β), which in contrast to the inhibins stimulate FSH release from the pituitary (see Fig. 4.18). This effect is probably not significant because of the irreversible binding of activin to follistatin, which neutralizes activin's bioactivity.

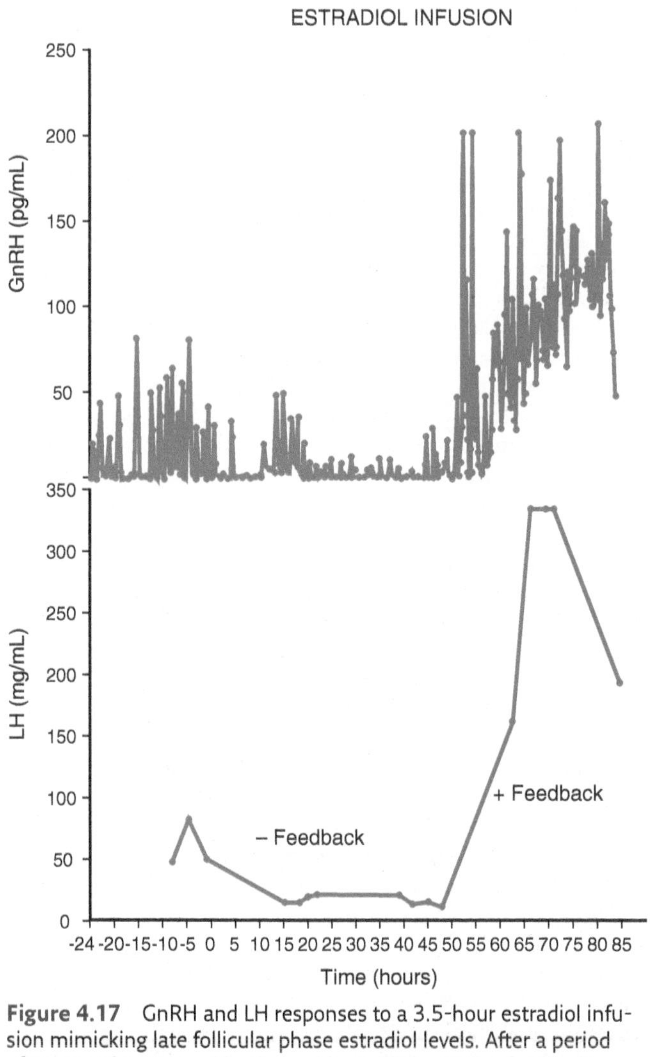


**Figure 4.17** GnRH and LH responses to a 3.5-hour estradiol infusion mimicking late follicular phase estradiol levels. After a period of suppression (caused by the rapid estradiol negative feedback), note the large increase in both GnRH and LH (caused by the positive estradiol feedback). (From Xia L, van Vugt D, Alston EJ, Luckhaus J, Ferin M. A surge of gonadotropin-releasing hormone accompanies the estradiol-induced gonadotropin surge in the rhesus monkey. *Endocrinology.* 1992;131:2812-2820.)

## MENSTRUAL CYCLE

The menstrual or ovulatory cycle involves a remarkable coordination of morphologic changes and hormonal secretion occurring not only at several levels of the hypothalamic-pituitary-ovarian axis but also in organs outside of this main axis, such as the uterus and the cervix, and expressed in an orderly sequence of events. The initial stimulus from the brain under the form of GnRH pulses is crucial to proper gonadotropin responses, which in turn instigate folliculogenesis, ovulation, and the formation of the corpus luteum. Essential to the coordination of these events is the communication between the ovaries and the hypothalamic-pituitary unit through the hormonal feedbacks, which provide continuous information of the ovarian status to the brain, which in turn responds with the proper pattern of GnRH pulses and of gonadotropin release. Humans are spontaneous ovulators (as opposed to light or seasonally related) in that the gonadotropin surge, the initiator of ovulation, is triggered by the endogenous changes in estradiol that accompany the maturation of the follicle.

This sequence of events is such that the reproductive process in the human occurs in a cyclic process at about monthly intervals. The primate menstrual cycle is divided into two phases: the follicular phase followed by the luteal phase. These are separated by the ovulatory period. The mean duration of the menstrual cycle is 28 ± 7 days. The length of the follicular phase is more variable, whereas the life span of the corpus luteum is about 14 days. In many women, the length of the follicular phase usually decreases from about 14 days to about 10 days in women over 40 years old. However, menstrual cycle length also varies in an individual woman: it is most variable in the 2 years following menarche and preceding menopause, times of life during which anovulatory cycles are most frequent. The mean age of menarche (the first menstruation) occurs around age 12, whereas menopause (the end of the reproductive phase) usually occurs between ages 45 and 55. Endocrine changes during the menstrual cycle are illustrated in Figure 4.19.

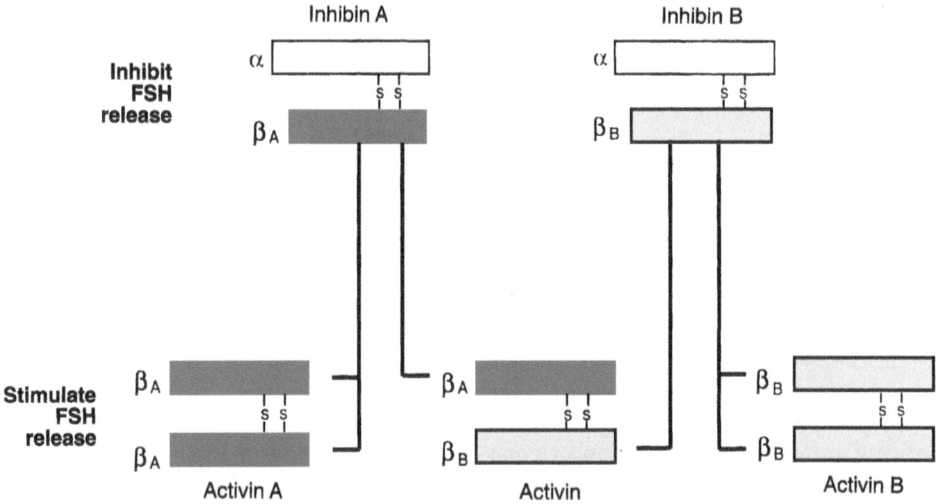


**Figure 4.18** Chemical relationships of inhibins and activins. *S*, Disulfide bond. (From Hylka VW, Di Zerega GS: Reproductive hormones and their mechanisms of action. In: Mishell DR, Davajan V, Lobo RA, eds. *Infertility, Contraception and Reproductive Endocrinology.* 3rd ed. Cambridge, MA: Blackwell Scientific; 1991.)

## FOLLICULAR PHASE

The follicular phase can be subdivided into three periods; these denote the successive recruitment of a cohort of antral follicles, the selection of a dominant follicle, and the growth of the selected dominant follicle.

### Recruitment of a Cohort of Antral Follicles

When cohorts of growing follicles reach the early antral stage (Fig. 4.20; see also Fig. 4.7), continuing growth requires a proper gonadotropin stimulatory action. **FSH** provides the critical signal for the recruitment of a **cohort** of preantral follicles. This FSH signal (cyclic recruitment) is the major survival factor that rescues the follicles from their programmed death (atresia) and allows them to start growing, increasing in size and beginning to synthesize steroids. In fact, the start of each follicular phase is characterized by a small but significant increase in the FSH:LH ratio (see Fig. 4.19), resulting in the recruitment of a cohort consisting of about three to seven secondary preantral follicles. (Only preantral follicles are able to respond to the FSH signal; follicles at an earlier stage of development lack an independent vascular system so that the signal does not reach them.)

**Ovarian reserve** is a term used to denote the number of antral follicles in the ovaries and therefore to determine the capacity of the ovary to provide oocytes that are capable of being fertilized. The determination of the ovarian reserve is an important tool in the treatment of infertility. Mainly, it can be assessed by the following means: (1) by a measurement of **FSH** on day 2 to 3 of the cycle: higher FSH levels denote ovarian aging (resulting from a decreased activity of the estradiol negative feedback loop), hence fewer recruitable follicles; (2) by a sonographic **antral follicle count**; (3) by the measurement of **inhibin B** on day 2 to 3 of the cycle, the recruitment of the follicle cohort being reflected by an increase in this hormone produced and secreted by these recruited follicles, thus inhibin B levels provide an early indicator of the number of recruited follicles and of their secretory activity (see Fig. 4.20); and (4) by the measurement of **anti-müllerian hormone (AMH)** (also named müllerian inhibiting substance [MIS]). AMH belongs to the transforming growth factor-β superfamily. It is a secretory product of granulosa cells in preantral and in small antral follicles. Together with other factors, AMH appears to inhibit the initiation of premature follicle growth. AMH levels decline with age, in parallel with the reduced follicle pool. Data have indicated that in the treatment of infertility, the measurement of AMH in conjunction with sonography offers a more useful assessment of ovarian reserve and a better correlation with the number of oocytes retrieved than that provided by FSH measurement. Unlike FSH, AMH may be measured at any time of the menstrual cycle, with minimal variation. AMH is increasingly used in clinical practice to identify women with premature ovarian insufficiency or polycystic ovary syndrome; very high levels of AMH may reflect polycystic ovary syndrome (La Marca, 2009). Studies show significantly lower age-specific AMH levels in women currently using oral contraceptives with an increase in AMH levels after discontinuation of oral contraceptives (Dolleman, 2013; van den Berg, 2010). It remains to be determined whether AMH measured during oral contraceptive use is an accurate reflection of individual ovarian reserve.

### Selection of a Dominant Follicle

Although several primary preantral follicles are recruited at the start of each cycle as part of a cohort, in the primate usually only one (the **dominant follicle**) is selected to complete growth to maturity (see Fig. 4.20), while the other follicles in the cohort become atretic. Although the process of selection is not well understood, it most probably reflects the competitive advantage of the dominant follicle, characterized by a well-vascularized theca layer, allowing a better access of the gonadotropins to their target receptors. This results in a greater local estradiol secretion, which in turn increases the density of gonadotropin receptors and promotes cell multiplication.

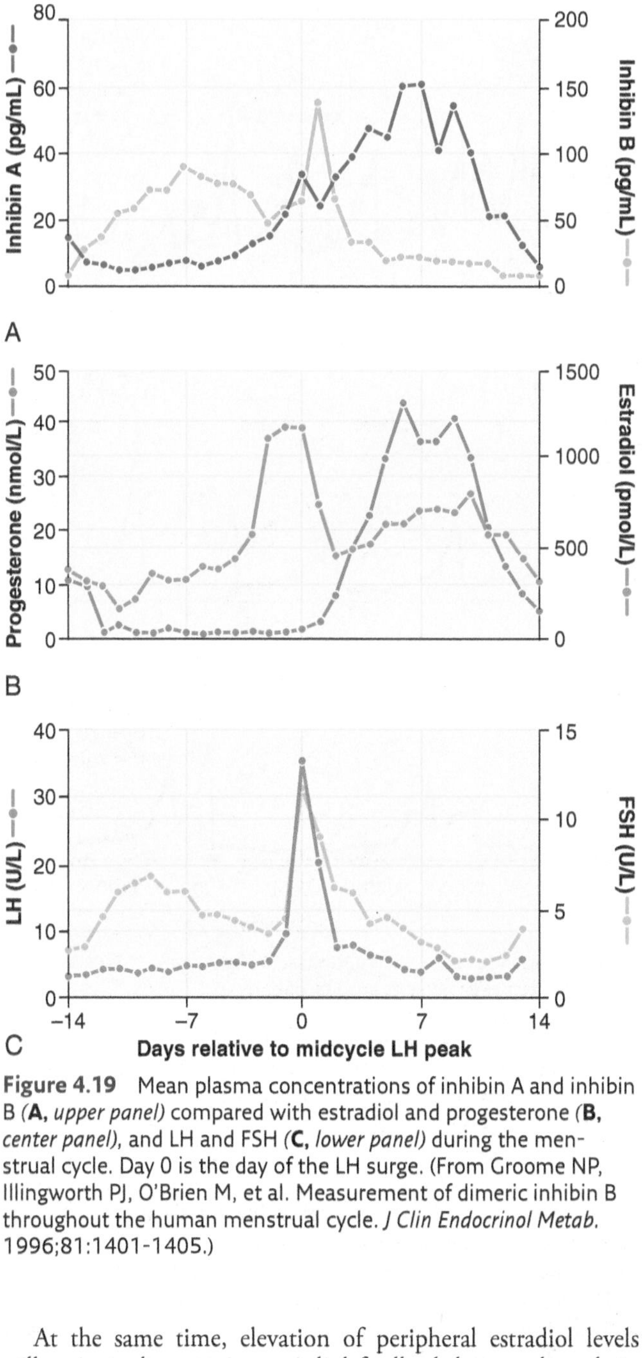


**Figure 4.19** Mean plasma concentrations of inhibin A and inhibin B (**A,** *upper panel*) compared with estradiol and progesterone (**B,** *center panel*), and LH and FSH (**C,** *lower panel*) during the menstrual cycle. Day 0 is the day of the LH surge. (From Groome NP, Illingworth PJ, O'Brien M, et al. Measurement of dimeric inhibin B throughout the human menstrual cycle. *J Clin Endocrinol Metab.* 1996;81:1401-1405.)

At the same time, elevation of peripheral estradiol levels will activate the negative estradiol feedback loop and result in a decrease in circulating FSH to a concentration insufficient to sustain growth in the other follicles of the cohort. Experimentally in the nonhuman primate, this process can be overridden by injecting antibodies to estradiol; this prevents the estradiol negative feedback loop from decreasing FSH secretion and results in the maturation of several follicles at the same time. In addition to estradiol, granulosa cells of the recruited follicles also secrete inhibin B (discussed earlier), the action of which selectively suppresses FSH secretion, further decreasing the stimulus to maturation. The dominant follicle, however, continues to grow because of its greater density of FSH receptors and greater vascularization of its theca cell layer, allowing more FSH to reach its receptors.

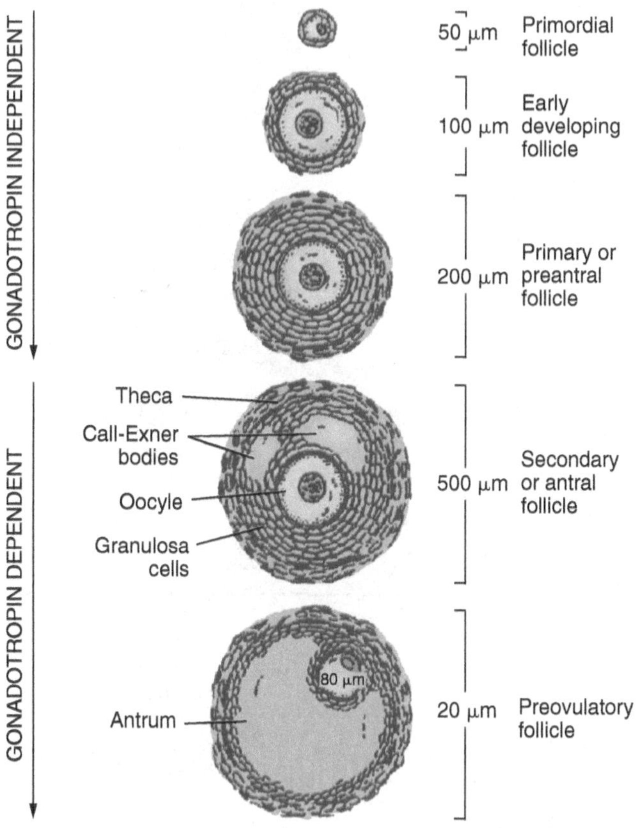


**Figure 4.20** Follicle development. Note that progress beyond the primary or preantral follicle stage depends on FSH stimulation. (From Paulson RJ. Oocytes: from development to fertilization. In: Mishell DR, Davajan V, Lobo RA, eds. *Infertility, Contraception and Reproductive Endocrinology.* 3rd ed. Cambridge, MA: Blackwell Scientific; 1991.)

The process of selection is completed by day 5 of the follicular phase. At this point, if the dominant follicle is experimentally destroyed, no surrogate follicle is available to replace it during that cycle.

### *Growth of the Dominant Follicle: The Maturing Secondary or Antral Follicle*

GnRH pulse frequency at this time of the follicular phase is at its maximum, at about 1 GnRH pulse/90 minutes (Fig. 4.21, *A*). This is the optimal pulse frequency to activate the proper gonadotropin response to increase steroid biosynthesis and the production of estradiol within the ovary. The main role of the gonadotropins and of locally produced estradiol is to continue to stimulate growth of the dominant follicle during the remainder of the follicular phase.

Production of estradiol requires successive events within different locations in the growing follicle (Fig. 4.22). **FSH receptors** are located within the avascular **granulosa** cell layer of the antral follicle. Stimulation by FSH of its receptors activates production of the enzyme **aromatase** (responsible for the biosynthesis of estrogens) within these cells. An important change in the structure of maturing follicles is the acquisition of the **theca** cell layer, which surrounds the granulosa layer and rapidly differentiates into the theca interna and the theca externa. The theca layer rapidly becomes well vascularized

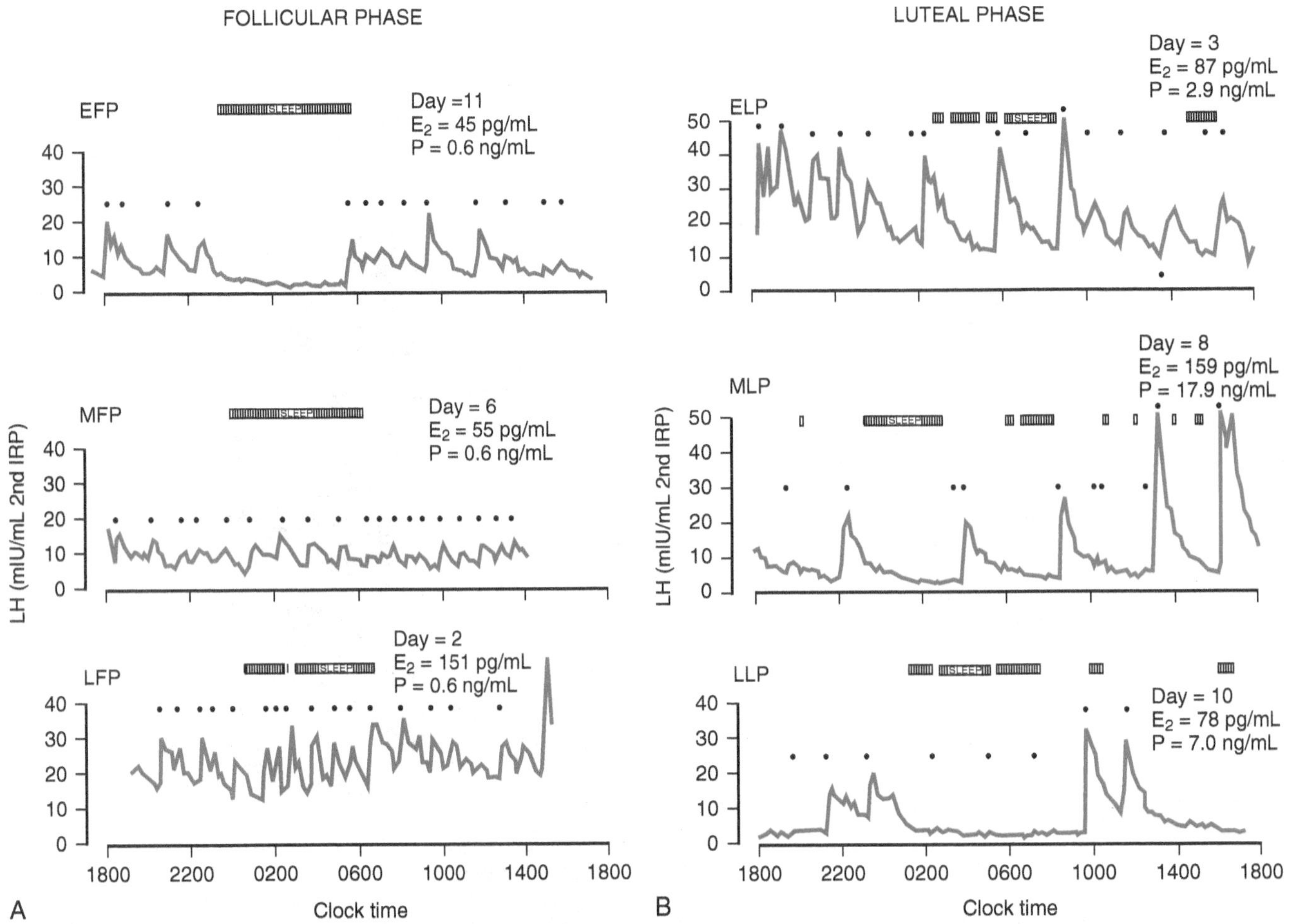


**Figure 4.21** Contrasting patterns of pulsatile LH secretion throughout the follicular phase (**A,** *left panels)* and luteal phase (**B,** *right panels)* of the menstrual cycle. Representative examples of early *(EFP)*, mid *(MFP)*, and late *(LFP)* follicular phases are shown. LH pulses are indicated by bullets. $E_2$, estradiol; *P*, progesterone. (Note that in about 20% of volunteers, there is a suppression of pulsatility during deep sleep in EFP. This does not appear to interfere with the normal cycle.) (From Filicori M, Santoro N, Merriam GR, et al. Characterization of the physiological pattern of episodic gonadotropin secretion throughout the menstrual cycle. *J Clin Endicrinol Metab.* 1986;62:1136.)

(in contrast to the granulosa layer, which remains avascular) through an active angiogenesis process, characterized by the presence of several vascular growth-promoting proteins such as vascular endothelial growth factor (VEGF), which stimulates growth of new blood vessels. This allows access of blood, and the hormones and nutrients it carries, to reach the follicle and to diffuse through to the granulosa layer. Circulating FSH now stimulates **LH receptor** synthesis within stromal cells of the **theca interna**. LH, in turn, promotes steroid biosynthesis by theca cells and the production of **androgens**. These androgens, following diffusion into the granulosa layer where the enzyme aromatase is located, are then biotransformed into **estradiol**. This leads to an overall increase in estradiol production, increased intraovarian estradiol levels, and increased estradiol secretion into the peripheral circulation, which parallels follicular parameter (Fig. 4.23).

Thus the growing dominant follicle generates its own estradiol microenvironment. Estradiol, being a mitogenic hormone, in turn directly promotes its exponential growth. (Testosterone, on the other hand, increases follicular atresia in the absence of adequate aromatase activity, which converts it to estradiol.) Indirectly, estradiol also promotes follicular growth through the activation of several regulatory protein and peptide hormones, such as inhibins, activin, folliculostatins, insulin-like growth factors (IGFs), and others. For instance, various IGFs have been shown to stimulate granulosa cell proliferation and aromatase activity. Most actions of these factors remain, however, to be elucidated in the primate. By the time the follicle reaches the preovulatory stage, the number of granulosa cells has increased from about 50 at the primordial stage to $5 \times 10^7$. This is accompanied by an exponential increase in peripheral estradiol levels (see Fig. 4.22).

As the dominant follicle grows, an **antrum** (cavity) forms into which follicular fluid accumulates. This fluid contains several steroids, peptide and protein hormones, and nutrients. The growth pattern of the dominant follicle can be documented by ultrasonography, which is well correlated with the endocrine pattern: indeed, increases in both follicle diameter

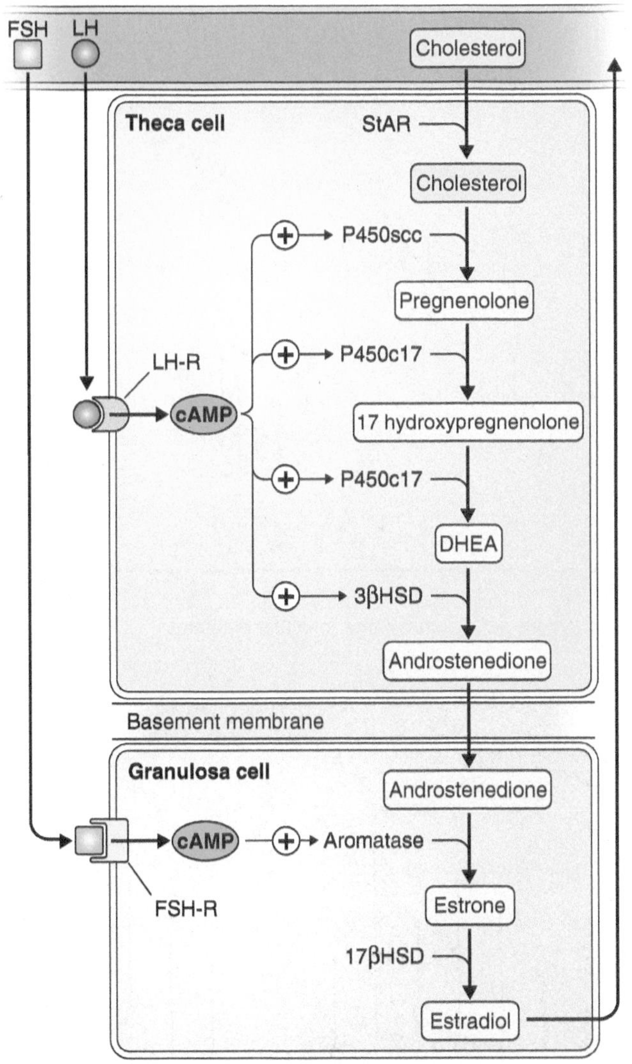


**Figure 4.22** Production of estradiol within the growing dominant follicle requires successive events within different locations (see text). FSH receptors are located within the avascular granulosa cell layer, whereas synthesis of LH receptors, stimulated by FSH, occurs within stromal cells of the theca interna. The enzyme aromatase (responsible for the biosynthesis of estrogens) stimulated by FSH originates within the granulosa cells. LH, in turn, promotes steroid biosynthesis by theca cells and the production of androgens. These androgens, following diffusion into the granulosa layer where the enzyme aromatase is located, are then biotransformed into estradiol.

and volume parallel the increase in estradiol levels in blood. At maturation, the dominant follicle reaches a mean diameter range of 18 to 25 mm.

Within the dominant follicle, the oocyte also develops and becomes surrounded by the **zona pellucida**. This is a mucopolysaccharide coat containing specific protein sites that later will allow only spermatozoa to penetrate and fertilize the ovum. Underneath the zona pellucida is the **vitelline membrane** that surrounds the ooplasm. At the end of the follicular phase, the antral follicle contains oocytes that are fully grown but are unable to undergo normal activation if retrieved and fertilized in vitro. Activation will have to await the ovulatory LH surge.

## *OVULATORY GONADOTROPIN SURGE AND OVULATION*

Maturation of the dominant follicle is marked by high blood levels of estradiol. When a threshold is reached, estradiol activates the positive feedback loop, thereby signaling to the hypothalamus and anterior pituitary gland that the follicle is ready for ovulation and that a large gonadotropin surge is to be released (see Fig. 4.17). (A small but significant increase in progesterone is also secreted by the follicle before the LH surge; because administration of a progesterone receptor antagonist delays the timing of the surge, it is thought that these low levels of progesterone help to synchronize the surge.)

In the nonhuman primate, the gonadotropin surge has been shown to be preceded by a surge of GnRH, as measured centrally, suggesting a major hypothalamic site for the positive feedback loop. For reasons unknown, this **GnRH surge** significantly outlasts the LH surge. Because GnRH cannot be measured in the human in peripheral blood, the relative importance of the sites of action of estradiol during the spontaneous surge remains to be established. (Studies in GnRH-deficient women receiving exogenous GnRH replacement in an unchanging 60-minute pulse frequency provide evidence for the relevance of pituitary sensitization to GnRH in the presence of high estradiol, as abrupt LH increases can be observed under this experimental protocol.)

During the ovulatory surge, LH levels increase 10-fold over a period of 2 to 3 days, whereas FSH levels increase about 4-fold. This gonadotropin surge is an absolute requirement for the final maturation of the oocyte and the initiation of the follicular rupture.

The LH surge initiates germinal vesicle (or nucleus) disruption, and the fully grown oocyte resumes meiosis (**meiotic maturation**). Thus it progresses from the diplotene stage of the first meiosis (which was initiated during fetal life; discussed earlier) to metaphase II of the second meiotic division. As the oocyte enters metaphase II, the first polar body appears. (Three haploid polar bodies are produced during the two-step meiosis process, at ovulation and fertilization.) To conserve nutrients, most of the cytoplasm is concentrated into the oocyte or egg. The polar bodies generated from the meiotic events contain relatively little cytoplasm, and the oocyte eventually discards them. At ovulation, meiosis is arrested again (the **second meiotic arrest**). The second meiotic division will only be completed at the time of fertilization. The oocyte's ability to be fertilized coincides with the completion of meiotic maturation and the associated increased secretion of specific proteins such as the $IP_3$ receptor, glutathione and calmodulin-dependent protein kinase II, and others.

**Ovulation** (follicle rupture) occurs about 32 hours after the initial rise of the LH surge and about 16 hours after its peak (Table 4.1). Ultrasonographic pictures of ovaries with antral follicles, a preovulatory follicle and a hemorrhagic corpus luteum are shown in Figure 4.24. The LH surge induces a cascade of molecular events and changes in the mature follicle that are associated with ovulation. Studies of these have been complex, with the result that the precise mechanisms underlying ovulation remain to be completely understood. Currently, it is postulated that the LH surge induces an acute inflammatory-like reaction; inflammatory cytokines, such as interleukins, and countless genes are also upregulated. There is

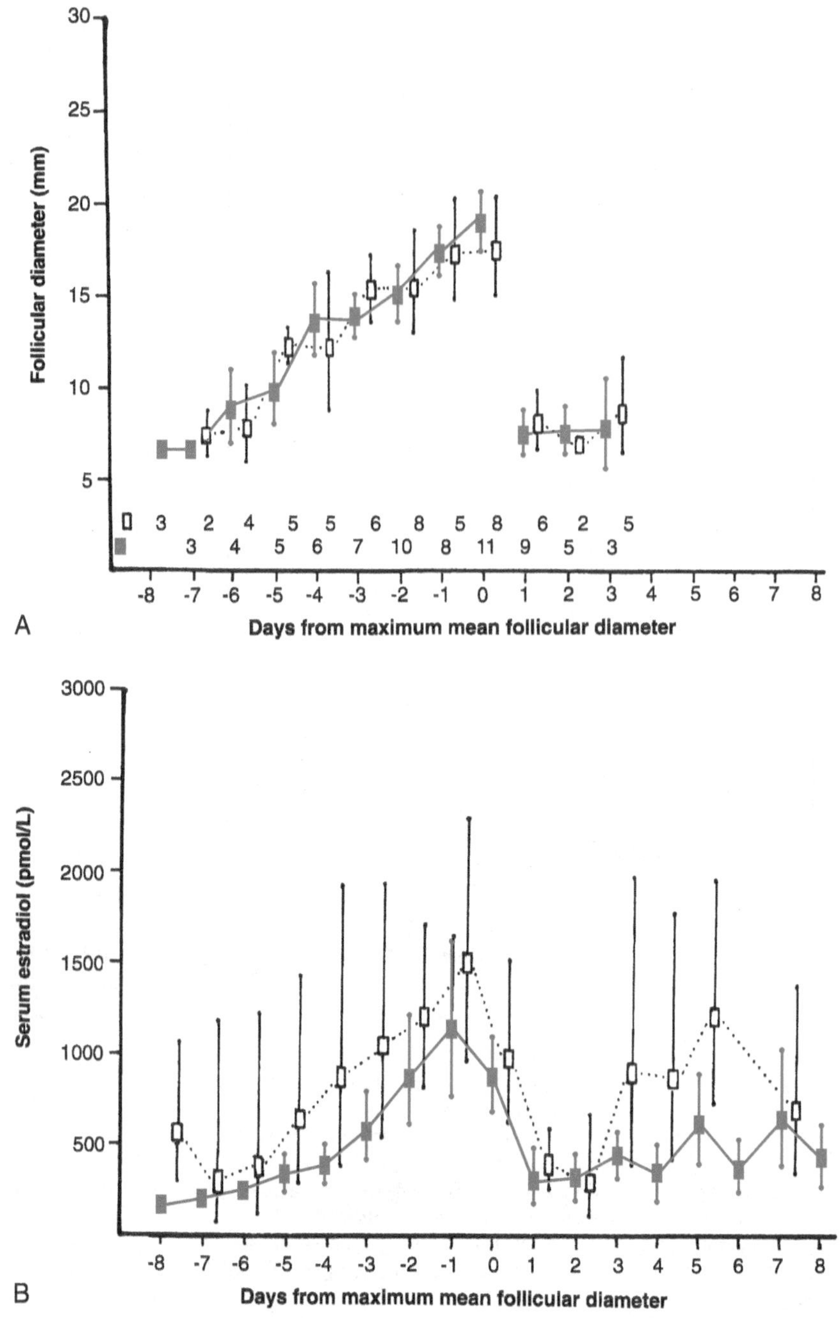


**Figure 4.23** Correlation of follicular growth, as indicated by follicular diameter (**A**), with serum estradiol levels (**B**), in spontaneous *(black bars)* and in induced conception *(blue bars)* cycles. (Modified from Eissa MK, Obhrai Ms, Docker MF, et al. Follicular growth and endocrine profiles in spontaneous and induced cycles. *Fert Ster.* 1986;45:191.)

**Table 4.1** Range of Observed Times from Defined Hormonal Events and Time of Ovulation

| | Time of Ovulation (hr) from Rise to Peak | | | |
|---|---|---|---|---|
| | First Significant Rise | | Peak | |
| *Hormone* | *Median* | *Range* | *Median* | *Range* |
| 17β-Estradiol | 82.5 | 48-168 | 24.0 | 0-48 |
| LH | 32.0 | 24-56 | 16.5 | 0-48 |
| FSH | 21.1 | 8-24 | 15.3 | 8-40 |
| Progesterone | 7.8 | 0-32 | — | — |

From World Health Organization. Temporal relationships between ovulation and defined changes in the concentration of plasma estradiol-17 beta, luteinizing hormone, follicle-stimulating hormone, and progesterone. I. Probit analysis. World Health Organization, Task Force of Methods for the Determination of the Fertile Period, Special Programme of Research, Development and Research Training in Human Reproduction. *Am J Obstet Gynecol.* 1980;138:383-390.

an increase in cyclooxygenase, which catalyzes the conversion of arachidonic acid into several prostanoids, which include the **prostaglandins** that are produced intracellularly. Prostaglandins then act locally—for instance, to induce the hyperemia and edema seen in the first hours of the process of ovulation and that result from increased blood flow and vascular permeability. Intense protease activity is generated in the follicle. The resultant **proteolytic cascade**, which among others involves collagenases and plasminogen activator (which converts plasminogen into the proteolytic enzyme plasmin), leads to the degradation of the follicular layers and wall, which plays an essential role in follicle rupture. Plasmin helps in detaching the cumulus cell-enclosed oocyte from the granulosa cells, which initiates the process of extrusion of the oocyte and cumulus when the follicle ruptures. (It is worthwhile to point out that

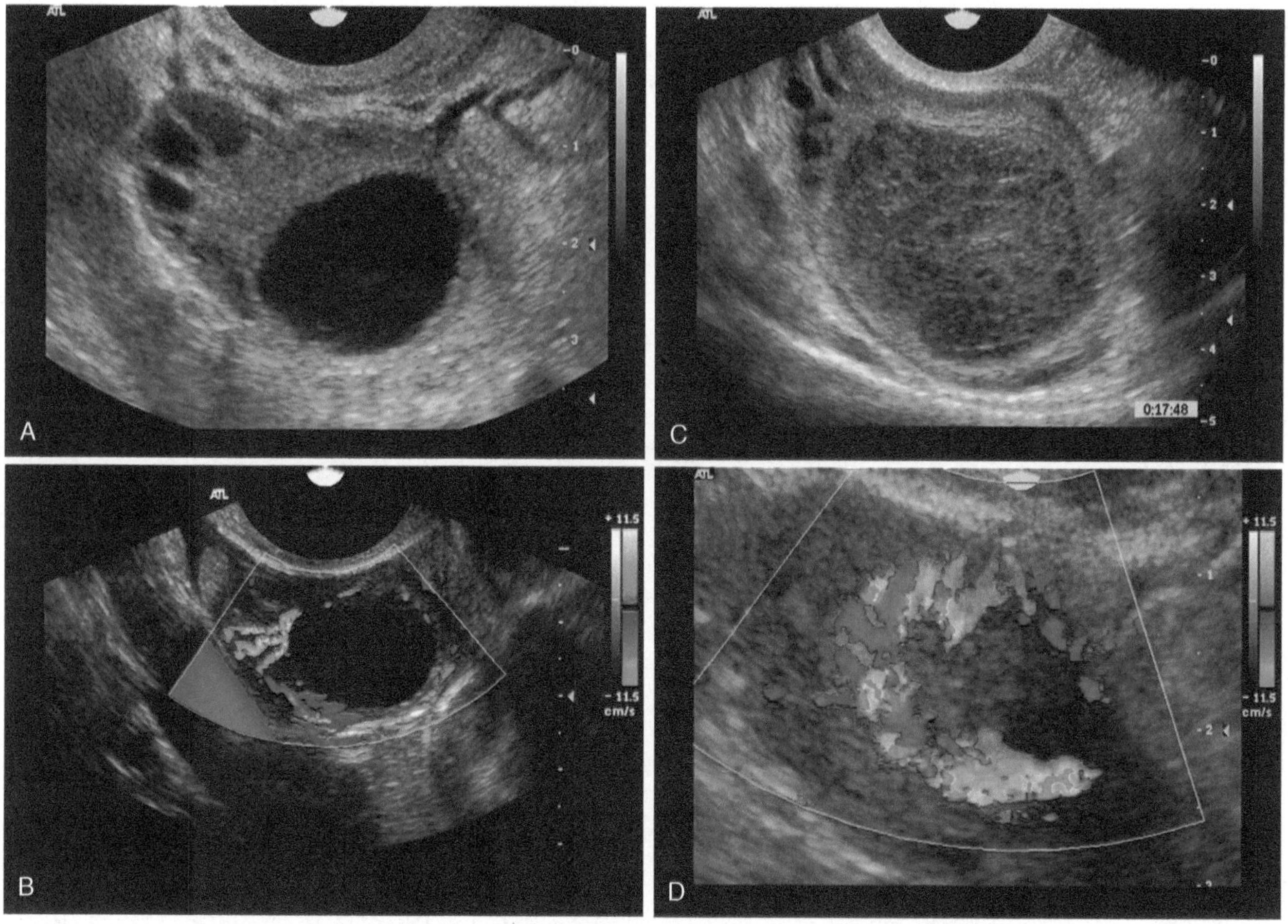


**Figure 4.24** Ovary and corpus luteum during a natural menstrual cycle. **A,** On day 12 after menstruation, a dominant follicle is visualized in the central portion of the image and several subordinate follicles from the wave (2 to 5 mm) are observed in the left lateral aspect of the ovary. **B,** Color flow Doppler image demonstrating perifollicular vascularity around a preovulatory follicle. **C,** A blood-filled corpus luteum, called a *corpus hemorrhagicum*, demonstrating thick walls of peripheral luteal tissue and a central hemorrhagic clot with an interspersed fibrin network. **D,** Color flow Doppler image of a recently ovulated follicle/new luteal glands on the day of ovulation. (From Chizen D, Pierson R. Transvaginal ultrasonography and female infertility. *Glob Libr Women's Med [ISSN: 1756-2228]*. 2010.)

the LH surge paradoxically stimulates the expression of both proteolytic enzymes and their inhibitors. This allows for a tight regulation of proteolytic activity during both the follicle rupture process and the formation of the corpus luteum out of the remaining follicle.)

## LUTEAL PHASE

After the oocyte is extruded from the mature dominant follicle, the amount of follicular fluid is markedly reduced, the follicular wall becomes convoluted, and the follicular diameter and volume greatly decrease. As a result, a new ovarian structure evolves from the ovulated follicle, the **corpus luteum**.

The corpus luteum is the result of two important events initiated at ovulation. First, granulosa and theca cells hypertrophy, take up increasing amounts of lipids, and acquire organelles associated with steroidogenesis. Simultaneously, tissue-specific gene transcription results in the activation of new key steroidogenic enzymes; the hallmark of the human corpus luteum is its secretion primarily of **progesterone**. Although there is a significant drop in estradiol and androgen secretion at ovulation, 17-hydroxylase and aromatase are present in the corpus luteum, so it also secretes 17-hydroxyprogesterone and estradiol. Significant amounts of inhibin A are also produced. Second, the basal lamina, which separated the granulosa and theca cell layers, is disrupted, and capillaries from the theca interna now invade the granulosa layer (which up to now had been avascular) to form an extensive capillary network. The result is that each steroidogenic cell within the corpus luteum is in close proximity to blood vessels.

Like the dominant follicle, growth and development of the corpus luteum occur rapidly. Vascular growth plays a central role in this process. Angiogenic factors, such as vascular endothelial growth factor (VEGF), are present in high quantity in the forming and developing corpus luteum. In nonhuman primates, experimental treatment that interferes with normal VEGF activity in the early and midluteal phase of the cycle suppresses vascular development and hence luteal growth; luteal function is compromised, as indicated by a marked fall in plasma progesterone levels.

### *Endocrine Factors and the Corpus Luteum*

Normal function of the corpus luteum depends primarily on LH stimulation throughout the luteal phase. This has been demonstrated in hypophysectomized women, in whom ovulation was induced by LH treatment. In these patients, continuing injections of small amounts of LH were essential to maintain the secretory viability of the corpus luteum. Other studies have shown that GnRH antagonist treatment (by interrupting LH secretion) readily disrupts luteal cell morphology and suppresses plasma progesterone levels.

Progesterone dominance in the luteal phase results in a significant activation of the **progesterone negative feedback loop** on the GnRH pulse generator, which acts to decrease GnRH pulse frequency. Thus during the luteal phase, there is progressive slowing down of LH pulse frequency, from 1 pulse/90 minutes at the beginning of the luteal phase to 1 pulse/3 hours or even less toward the later luteal phase (see Fig. 4.21, *right panel*). This negative progesterone feedback effect is not directly exerted on the GnRH pulse generator as it is mediated by central **β-endorphin** (an endogenous opioid peptide). β-endorphin neurons are preferentially concentrated in the arcuate nucleus, in close proximity to GnRH neurons. Studies in the nonhuman primate have shown that β-endorphin release from the hypothalamus is significantly increased in the presence of progesterone, such as in the luteal phase, and lowest in its absence, such as after ovariectomy or at menstruation. Experimental administration of a competitive β-endorphin antagonist, such as naloxone, is particularly effective in accelerating LH pulse frequency when given in the luteal phase (see Fig. 4.16, *right panel*).

Progesterone dominance during the luteal phase also affects the hypothalamic thermoregulatory center, such that a small increase in **basal body temperature** (BBT) reflects increased progesterone secretion during the luteal phase. Thus the typical BBT curve of the ovulatory menstrual cycle is biphasic (i.e., elevated during the duration of the luteal phase). (This small temperature rise does not, however, reflect the quantity of progesterone increase in that it occurs when progesterone reaches the low threshold level of 2 to 3 ng/mL.)

### *Corpus Luteum Regression (Luteolysis)*

In primates, the life span of the corpus luteum is limited to a period of about 14 days. Histologically and biochemically, the corpus luteum reaches maturity 8 to 9 days after ovulation, after which time luteal cells start to degenerate and its secretory capability begins to decline. Thus after a progressive increase in progesterone, estradiol, and inhibin A levels in the first half of the luteal phase, the period after the midluteal peak is paralleled by a decline in these hormones. (Only rapidly rising concentrations of **chorionic gonadotropin** [hCG] [secreted by the syncytiotrophoblast] following conception can rescue the corpus luteum and maintain the production of progesterone.)

Structural luteolysis is a complex process responsible for the elimination of the corpus luteum, and little progress has been made in defining the factors responsible for luteolysis in the primate. Steroidogenic luteal cells undergo characteristic degenerative changes, with intense cytoplasmic vacuolization and invasion by macrophages. It has been postulated that regression of the corpus luteum may be related to an alteration in age-dependent luteal cell responsiveness to LH and is dictated by various luteotropic and luteolytic agents, the existence and dynamics of which remain to be investigated in the human. (Although uterine prostaglandin $F_{2\alpha}$ seems to be an important luteolytic signal in nonprimate species, the primate uterus is not the source of luteolytic agents because hysterectomy does not result in a prolonged luteal phase in the human.) Degradation of the luteal cells terminates in a perimenstrual apoptotic wave, and menstruation follows ovulation by 13 to 15 days, unless conception has occurred ("the missed menses").

## *LUTEAL-FOLLICULAR TRANSITION*

The end of the luteal phase is characterized by a dramatic decrease in progesterone, estradiol, and inhibin A. This is accompanied by a characteristic divergence in the FSH:LH ratio, now favoring a specific rise in FSH (see Fig. 4.19). The increase in the FSH:LH ratio heralds a new menstrual cycle and the recruitment of a new cohort of follicles.

The increase in the FSH:LH ratio most probably reflects the following interacting phenomena: (1) a rise in FSH may be the result of the rapid decline in estradiol accompanying the demise of the corpus luteum because FSH seems to be slightly more sensitive to the estradiol negative feedback loop than LH; (2) the end of the luteal phase is also characterized by a decline in inhibin A, a hormone that specifically suppresses FSH; and (3) the rise in FSH also reflects the differential effects of GnRH pulse frequency on the synthesis of LH and FSH: the lower GnRH pulse frequency throughout the luteal phase favors FSH β-subunit synthesis over that of the LH β-subunit (discussed earlier), and thus a larger pituitary pool of FSH is available for release at the end of the luteal phase. The naturally occurring slowing of GnRH pulse frequency during the luteal phase is very relevant to a timely passage to a new cycle: indeed, imposed changes in the normal pulse frequency of this hypophysiotropic signal during the luteal phase results in significant disturbances in cyclicity.

The decrease in progesterone levels at the end of the cycle results in decreased activity in central β-endorphin, and consequently there is a resultant increase in GnRH pulse frequency. The return to a 1/pulse/90-minute frequency is essential to create the optimal conditions for the new menstrual cycle.

## MENSTRUAL CYCLE AND THE ENDOMETRIUM

Integration and synchronization between cyclic changes within the hypothalamic-pituitary-ovarian axis and the endometrium is an essential prerequisite for viable reproduction. The primary goal is to ensure an appropriate environment for the implantation of the developing conceptus.

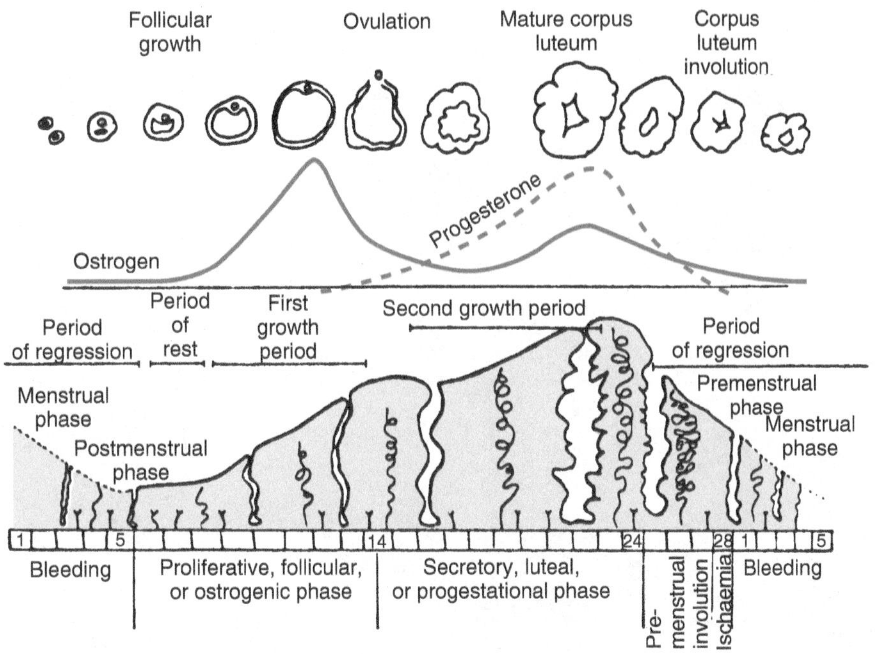


**Figure 4.25** Diagram of changes in normal human ovarian and endometrial cycles. (From Shaw ST, Roche PC. Menstruation. In: Finn CA, ed. *Oxford Review of Reproductive Endocrinology*. vol 2. London: Oxford University Press; 1980.)

Human endometrium (the glandular part of the uterus) is made up of two major layers: (1) the stratum basale, which lies on top of the myometrium (the muscle part of the uterus), consists of primordial glands and densely cellular stroma, which change little during the menstrual cycle and do not desquamate at menstruation; and (2) the stratum functionale, which lies between the basale and the lumen of the uterus, is composed of two layers. The superficial layer (stratum compactum) consists of the neck of the glands and densely populated stromal cells. The lower layer (stratum spongiosum) consists primarily of glands with less populated stroma and large amounts of interstitial tissue. Differences in structure in the two layers reflect different biologic functions: whereas the upper layer serves as the site of blastocyst implantation and provides the metabolic environment for it, the lower layer maintains the integrity of the mucosa. Changes in hormones during the menstrual cycle affect mainly the stratum functionale. A diagrammatic representation of endometrial changes during the menstrual cycle is presented in Figure 4.25.

## ENDOMETRIUM IN THE PROLIFERATIVE (FOLLICULAR) PHASE

Immediately after menstruation, the endometrium is only 1 to 2 mm thick and consists mainly of the stratum basale and a few glands. As estradiol levels increase with the growth and maturation of the dominant follicle, the number of estradiol receptors in the endometrium increases and the stratum functionale proliferates greatly by multiplication of both glandular and stromal cells. Synthesis of DNA is increased, and mitoses are numerous. Toward the late follicular phase, the straight glands become progressively more voluminous and tortuous. At the time of onset of the LH surge and before ovulation, subnuclear vacuoles appear at the base of the cells lining the glands. This is the first indication of an effect by progesterone, reflecting the small but significant increase in progesterone seen at that time. Sonography during the follicular phase shows that endometrial thickness, including both anterior and posterior layers, increases from a mean of about 4 mm in the early follicular phase to about 12 mm at the time of ovulation. Examples of structural changes of the endometrium during the menstrual cycle are shown in Figure 4.26.

## ENDOMETRIUM IN THE SECRETORY (LUTEAL) PHASE

After ovulation, the proliferative endometrium undergoes a rapid **secretory** differentiation: well-developed subnuclear glycogen-rich vacuoles appear in every cell of a given gland. This correlates with a total lack of mitoses in all glands. Both effects can be attributed to rising levels of postovulatory progesterone. Progesterone antagonizes the mitotic action of estradiol by decreasing estrogen receptors and by increasing the progesterone-specific enzyme 17 β-hydroxydehydrogenase, which converts estradiol into the much less active estrone.

As progesterone levels increase during the first part of the luteal phase, the glycogen-containing vacuoles ascend progressively toward the gland lumen. Soon thereafter, the contents of the glands are released into the endometrial lumen. The peak of intraglandular content and its release into the lumen coincides well with the arrival of the free-floating blastocyst, which reaches the uterine cavity by about 3.5 days after fertilization. This release of glycogen-rich nutrients is crucial in that it provides energy to the energy-starved free-floating blastocyst.

Appropriately timed exposure to estrogen and progesterone alters gene transcription in the endometrium resulting

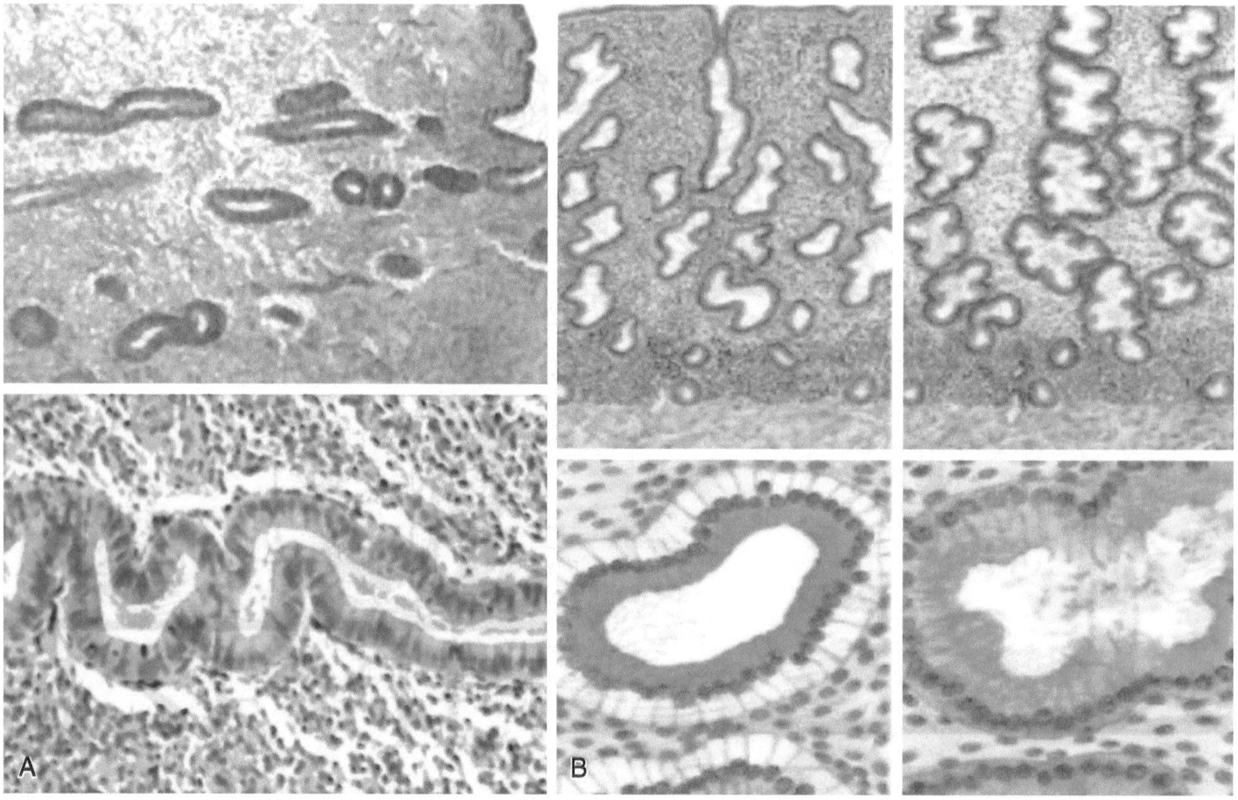


**Figure 4.26** Histology of proliferative (**A**) and secretory (**B**) endometrial tissue.

in a "receptive endometrium" that is prepared to engage in a molecular dialog with the blastocyst. The window of implantation (WOI) is typically defined as days 20 to 24 of a 28-day menstrual cycle, with implantation occurring about 1 week after fertilization. Multiple signaling pathways are activated in the endometrium to ensure successful embryo implantation (Fig. 4.27) (Cha, 2012). Several proteins, including glycodelin, insulin-like growth factor binding protein 1 (IGFBP-1), homeobox A10, and leukemia inhibitory factor, are produced by secretory phase endometrium and may play integral roles in endometrial function.[15] Glycodelin is also known as *PP14* or *progestagen-associated endometrial protein.* Although it has also been referred to as *pregnancy-associated endometrial alpha-2-globulin,* it is actually not a placental protein but rather a major secretory product of the glandular endometrial epithelium during the secretory phase. Circulating levels of glycodelin correlate well with serum progesterone levels. Glycodelin is a glycoprotein of which there are three distinct forms, with identical protein backbones but different glycosylation profiles. These glycoproteins appear to have essential roles in producing a uterine environment suitable for pregnancy and in the timing and occurrence of the appropriate sequence of events in the fertilization process.

After the first week of the luteal phase, changes in the stroma rather than in the glands become more important and relevant. The stroma becomes more edematous as a result of increased capillary permeability. Endothelial proliferation results in the coiling of capillaries and vessels, particularly in the upper functionale level producing vascular clusters. (These changes have been postulated to be mediated by prostaglandin F2α [PGF2α] and prostaglandin E [PGE2], the production of which is stimulated by estradiol and progesterone.) These changes are essential in the steps that will lead to the predecidual transformation of stromal cells.

**Predecidual stromal cells** are precursor forms of gestational decidual cells. (These cells are not involved in the implantation process because they develop after implantation.) In the nongestational endometrium, predecidual cells are engaged in phagocytosis and digestion of extracellular collagen matrix. These cellular activities may contribute to the breakdown of the endometrium at menstruation. (Predecidual cells also have metabolic functions related to pregnancy; for example, they secrete prolactin, which is related to osmoregulation of amniotic fluid. These cells also play a supportive role to the endometrial mucosa and appear to control the invasive nature of the normal trophoblast: in their absence, the trophoblast may invade the myometrium leading to placenta accreta.) Decidualization succeeds predecidualization if pregnancy occurs.

Clinically, the measurement of hormonal levels in parallel with the use of quantitative morphometric endometrial measurements produce a significant correlation with chronologic dating of the length of the luteal phase. Clinical dating of the endometrium, however, is somewhat subjective and is rarely carried out today. Sonography shows that endometrial thickness remains at the same level reached at ovulation (8 to 14 mm) throughout the luteal phase.

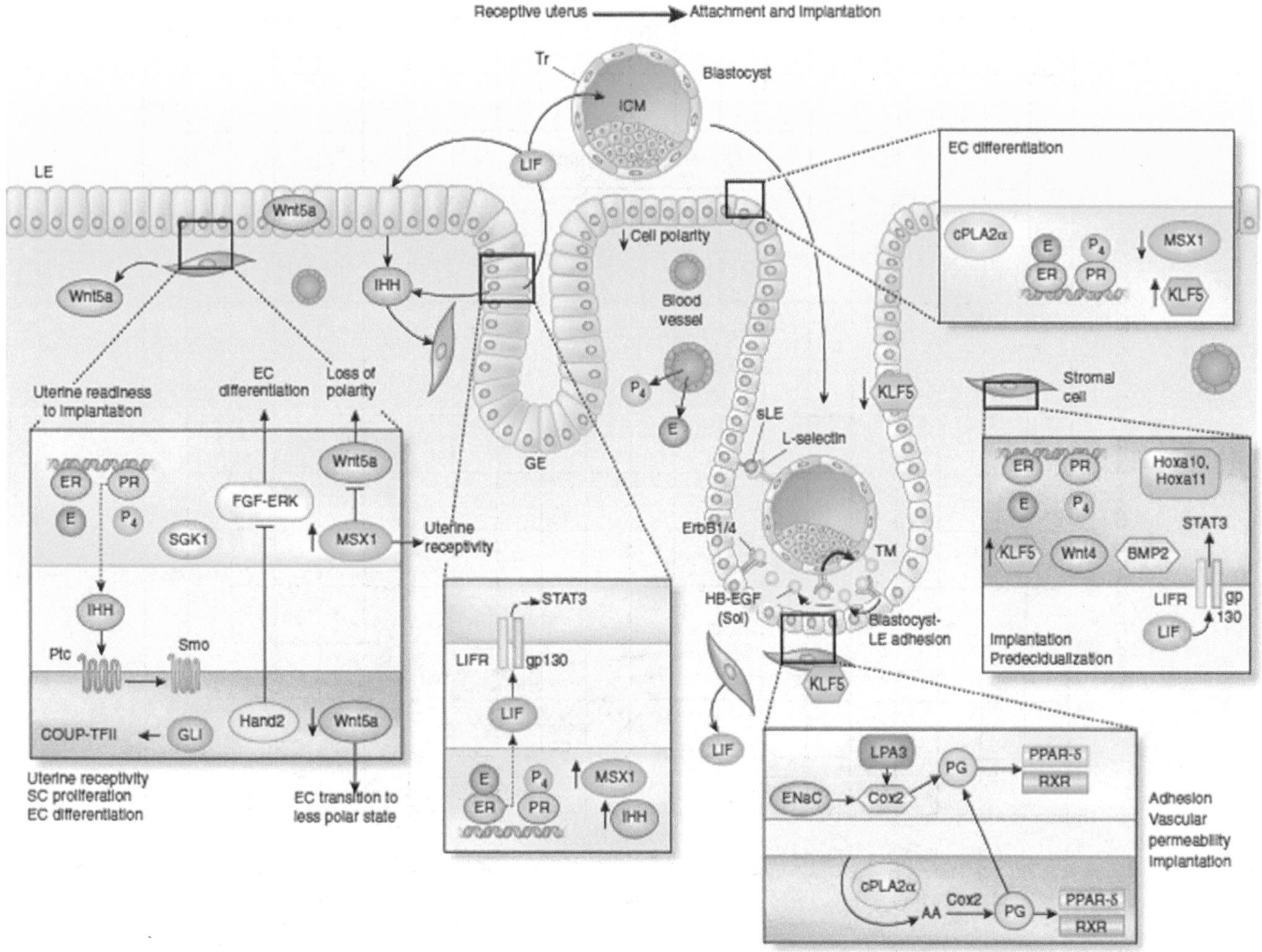


**Figure 4.27** Signaling network for uterine receptivity and implantation. This is a hybrid cartoon based on mouse and human studies, portraying compartment- and cell-type-specific expression of molecules and their potential functions necessary for uterine receptivity, implantation, and decidualization. (From Cha J, Sun X, Dey SK. Mechanisms of implantation: strategies for successful pregnancy. *Nat Med.* 2012;18:1754-1767.)

## *MENSTRUATION*

If implantation of the blastocyst does not occur in the late luteal phase and hCG is not produced to maintain the corpus luteum, the endometrial glands begin to collapse and fragment. Subsequently, polymorphonuclear leukocytes and monocytes infiltrate the glands and stroma, autolysis of the stratum functionale occurs, and desquamation begins.

Current data support the contention that cyclic elimination of the endometrium functional layer through menstrual bleeding results from intense tissue breakdown by proteolytic enzymes, mainly members of the matrix **metalloproteinase** family (**MMPs**), and that these enzymes are stimulated by the products of an inflammatory process. A number of MMPs, capable of degrading both interstitial matrix and basement membrane components, have been localized to perimenstrual endometrium, and the focal nature of their production suggests local regulation. There are probably important relationships between cells of the immune system (such as mast cells, eosinophils, neutrophils, and macrophages) and the local production and activation of MMPs.

The degrading actions by MMPs lead to the loss of integrity of blood vessels, the destruction of endometrial interstitial matrix, and the resultant bleeding characteristic of menstruation. Regular menstruation usually lasts for 3 to 5 days, but anywhere from 2 to 7 days is considered normal. Menstrual intervals vary depending of age and time of initiation of the premenopause period (Fig. 4.28). The average blood loss is 35 mL with 10 to 80 mL considered within the normal range. A similar volume of nonhematogenous fluid is also shed during menstruation. Many women also notice shedding of the endometrial lining that appears as tissue mixed with the blood. (Sometimes, this may be erroneously thought to indicate an early term miscarriage of an embryo.) The enzyme plasmin tends to inhibit the blood from clotting. Because of the blood loss, premenopausal women have higher dietary requirements for iron to prevent iron deficiency.

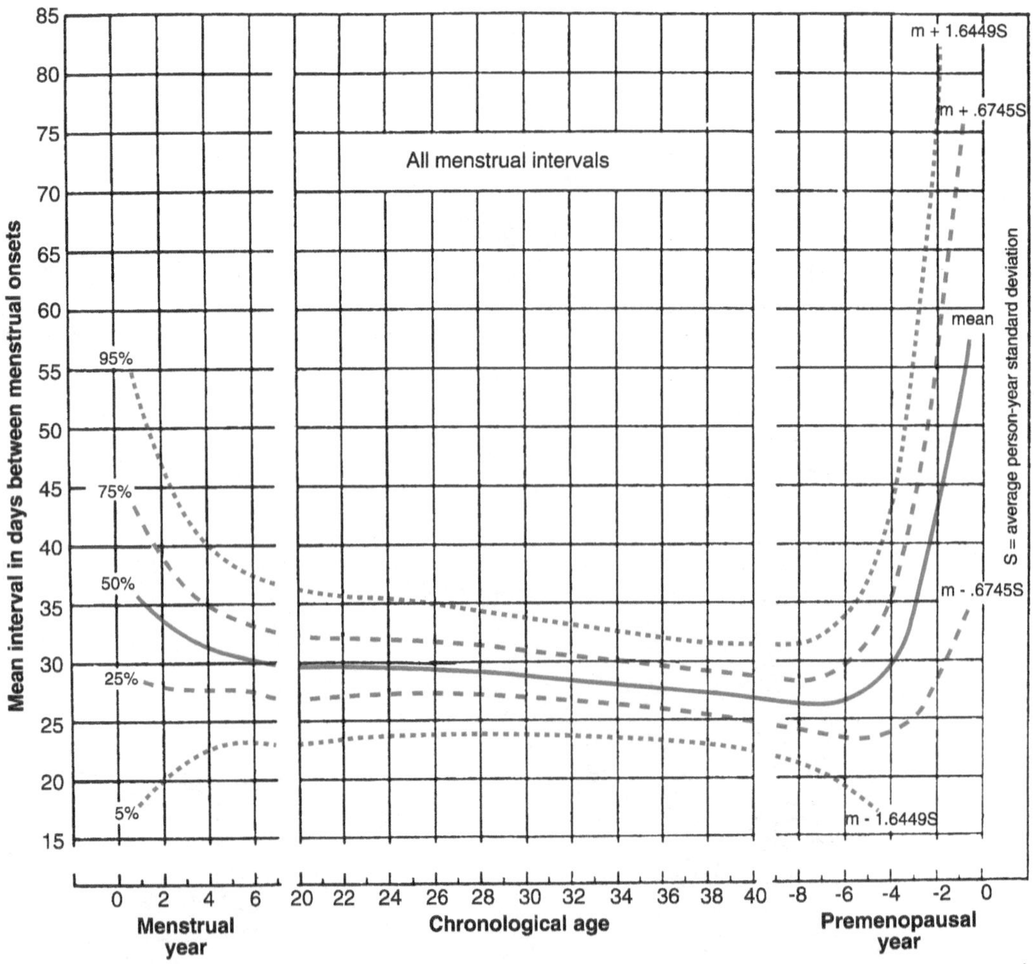


**Figure 4.28** Normal curve contours for the distribution of menstrual intervals in three zones of menstrual life. (From Treloar AE, Boynton RE, Brown BW. Variation of the human menstrual cycle through reproductive life. *Int J Fert.* 1967;12:77.)

## MENSTRUAL CYCLE AND THE CERVICAL GLANDS

The cervix plays a substantial role in fertility. Changes in the production and property of mucus secreted by the cervical glands are closely correlated to changes in estradiol and progesterone during the menstrual cycle. Enhanced production of cervical mucus and the presence of crypts within the endocervix facilitate the transport and storage of spermatozoa around midcycle. Cervical mucus is produced in copious amounts in response to high estradiol levels at the end of the follicular phase: it has a clear, water-like appearance, which is acellular, takes the aspect of a "fern" when it dries as viewed under the microscope, and is "stringy," referred to as "spinnbarkeit" (i.e., cervical mucus that can stretch on a slide at least 6 cm). So characteristic are these findings that the appearance of this type of mucus signifies the "fertile period" in women practicing natural family planning methods. In contrast, one of the actions of progesterone (as seen after ovulation during the luteal phase or as used in the "minipill") is to thicken the cervical mucus, thereby making it less conducive for sperm transport, thus providing a contraceptive effect.

From a fertility testing perspective, postcoital tests examining spermatozoa within the cervical canal at midcycle to rule out a cervical factor are seldom used in today's practice. The subjective nature of this testing makes it not highly predictive of the ability to conceive.

## HORMONE ASSAY TECHNIQUES

### IMMUNOASSAYS

No other method has had such an impact on the measurement of hormones as immunoassay methods. These techniques provide ways of measuring very small amounts of hormone in small quantities of serum or plasma rapidly and relatively specifically. The use of these techniques, pioneered by Yalow and Berson, has indeed increased the knowledge of reproductive endocrinology exponentially since the 1960s. Immunoassays and their variants have rapidly replaced previously used cumbersome bioassays. They are comparatively much faster and much easier to perform, have a much enhanced sensitivity, and usually require far less than 1 mL of serum or plasma. It should be kept in mind, however, that these techniques measure the immunologic property of a hormone, not its biologic activity (as tested by bioassays). These two effects may differ in magnitude under certain physiologic or pathologic conditions.

The basic principle of an immunoassay involves the competition between an unlabeled antigen (the hormone in the blood sample) and a labeled antigen, both of which are present in excess, for binding sites on a limited amount of antibody. The following is a brief description of the several steps required in the creation of such an assay. Even though the availability of commercial assays for a large number of hormones has greatly facilitated the measurement of hormones, proper interpretation of the generated data requires a general knowledge of these steps.

### *Preparation of Antibodies*

The first step in setting up an immunoassay is the production or availability of an antibody to the analyte (here, the hormone) to be measured. Antibodies used in immunoassays are either polyclonal or monoclonal. **Polyclonal antibodies** are usually produced following the injection of the hormone in larger animals such as sheep or rabbits. For many **protein hormones**, this means injecting the purified hormone, which the host will recognize as foreign. In the natural immune reaction that follows, the host will produce polyclonal antibodies against the hormone. In contrast to protein hormones, **steroid hormones** are too small to produce an immune reaction on their own (haptens) and are not recognized as foreign because they are the same in most species. To become antigenic, they must be attached to a carrier protein (usually bovine serum albumin). This conjugated compound is now perceived as a foreign body to the host animal and large enough to induce antibody formation.

Even with the injection of a purified antigen, polyclonal antibodies may "cross-react" with other closely related hormones and thus in some assays may lack specificity to the concerned hormone. To increase assay specificity, one may now choose to produce **monoclonal antibodies**, which provide unique specificity by recognizing only one epitope (antigenic determinant). These antibodies are produced by first injecting the antigen into a mouse to induce an immunogenic reaction in its spleen. The spleen cells are then screened to identify and separate those clones capable of secreting a single antibody type. These cells are then fused with a myeloma cell from the same species to form a hybrid cell (hybridoma), which can then be maintained in culture. Because of its immortality, the hybridoma continues to produce homogenous antibodies as long as the culture is maintained.

### *Choice of Assay Markers*

The second step in preparation for an immunoassay is the availability of a **labeled analyte** (hormone) in the competitive immunoassay or a **labeled second antibody** to the analyte in a reagent excess immunoassay. The choice of labels to be attached to the analyte or antibody is multiple.

In the initially developed radioimmunoassays, these labels were radioactive, such as iodine $I^{125}$. Although these assays were initially the norm, they mostly have been replaced by new types of immunoassays, which do not require the use of radioactive elements and thus avoid the attendant problems related to their use and to radioactivity disposal.

Major advances in the identification of nonradioactive labels and of new measurement equipment to detect and quantitate these have occurred. Presently, most current assays use nonradioactive labels. Enzyme immunoassays (enzyme-linked immunosorbent assays, or ELISA; immunometric assays) use enzymes as labels, such as horseradish peroxidase or alkaline phosphatase. Chemiluminescent immunoassays (CIA) use luminol. Fluorimetric immunoassays (FIA) use fluorescent compounds (such as fluorescein) as labels.

### *Separation of Bound and Unbound Antigen*

The third step requires a method to separate antibody-bound antigen from unbound antigen in order to determine how much antigen is bound to the antibody. In commercial assays, antibodies can be attached to solid surfaces such as to plastic tubes, beads or plates, or cellulose particles. Separation can then be ensured by washing off the unbound antigen.

Separation can also be performed by the use of a second antibody-label conjugate, which is directed against an antigenic site different from that recognized by the first antibody (see sandwich assays, discussed later).

### *Immunoassay Reaction*

In step 1, a specific antibody (ab) to the hormone (which served as the antigen, ag) binds in the patient's blood sample to the antigen during a fixed period of incubation. A set amount of labeled form of the hormone ($ag^x$) is added to compete with the unlabeled hormone to bind to the antibody, resulting in the following reaction:

$$ab + ag + ag^x \leftrightharpoons ab.ag + ab.ag^x$$

In this competitive reaction, the amount of labeled antigen bound to the antibody will be inversely proportional to the amount of antigen (hormone) present in the blood sample. For measurement, the bound antigen is then separated from the free antigen by washing or other approaches.

Immunometric assays (also referred to as "sandwich assays") use a labeled second antibody, which is usually attached to a solid phase, such as the assay tube or assay plate, in the following reactions. The second antibody is directed against an antigenic site different from that recognized by the first antibody:

$$Ab1 + ag \leftrightharpoons ab1.ag$$

$$Ab1.ag + ab^x2 \leftrightharpoons ab1.ag.ab^x2$$

Because the sandwich assay depends on occupancy of the binding sites rather than competition for these sites, an excess of reagents is used.

### *Standard Curve*

To allow for the actual measurement of the hormone levels in the blood sample, a standard curve must accompany each assay. A standard preparation of the hormone to be measured is used at various increasing or decreasing concentrations, and each concentration is then processed as for the measurement of the sample with unknown concentrations. A standard curve is then constructed by plotting the measured end points. The result for each unknown sample is then located on the ordinate of the standard curve. By drawing a perpendicular line to the abscissa, the amount of hormone present in the unknown sample can be determined. Currently, these determinations are rapidly computed.

Standard curves require varying amounts of pure preparations of hormone. This is no problem for steroid hormones, which are available in chemically pure preparations. Thus the amount added to construct the standard curve to determine the amount in the patient's sample can be expressed in terms of absolute mass or weight, such as nanograms (ng; $10^{-9}$gram) or picograms (pg; $10^{-12}$ gram). Sometimes, the results may be expressed in nanomoles (nmol). For most steroids, 1 ng/mL is equivalent to about 3 nmol/L.

Because proteins have higher molecular weights and are more complex, it is not always possible to obtain these in their pure form. In these cases, the results are usually expressed in terms of the amounts of a standard reference preparation used for the standard curve. Standard preparations are obtained by extracting the hormone from large collections of blood, urine, or tissues (such as the pituitary gland for FSH and LH). These protein standards are then most often an international reference preparation with the results expressed as international units. However, because of the use of different standard preparations, data obtained from different laboratories or assays may not agree. Thus clinicians should be aware of the normal levels reported by each laboratory reporting to them. Further complicating interpretation is the observation that protein hormones may also circulate in several forms varying slightly by amino acid or carbohydrate content.

## ASSAY EVALUATION

When evaluating the value, accuracy, and relevance of an assay, four items must be examined:

1. **Sensitivity** measures the least hormone that can be measured with accuracy. This will set the lower limit of the assay.
2. **Specificity** is the ability of the assay to measure only the specific hormone of interest. Frequently with polyclonal antibodies, results may be altered by the presence of other cross-reacting substances also recognized by the antibody, although usually at lower levels of detection. This is important to know because cross-reaction may influence the precise measurement of the hormone of interest. In such instance, a preassay separation of the cross-reacting hormones may be necessary.
3. **Accuracy** is the ability to measure the exact amount of the hormone present in the sample. Controls containing varying low and high amounts of the hormone must be always assayed alongside the patient's samples in each assay.
4. **Precision** is the ability of the assay to consistently reproduce the same results. Precision is determined by two measurements. The first, the **intraassay coefficient of variation (intraassay CV)** measures the within assay variation. It is calculated by determining the results obtained from measuring a known sample in a number of replicates (usually 10) in the same assay. The second measurement is the **interassay coefficient of variation (interassay CV)**, which is calculated by measuring known samples in multiple assays.

### *MASS SPECTROMETRY ASSAYS*

There has been an increase in the use of mass spectrometry (MS) assays in both clinical and research laboratories. A particular strength of MS assays is the ability to measure large numbers of structurally similar compounds. MS assays have high specificity, sensitivity, and throughput.[16] MS is the most powerful assay method for defining defects in steroid hormone metabolism. In larger reference laboratories, these assays have replaced the conventional radioimmunoassays, which are cumbersome and time-consuming, and direct immunoassays, which lack specificity or sensitivity. The MS technology has been implemented successfully for routine analysis of steroid hormones in major clinical diagnostic laboratories. Although the high cost of MS instrumentation, related operating costs, and the requirement for technical expertise have prohibited smaller laboratories from using this instrumentation for routine testing of steroid hormones, this situation is changing and MS assays are becoming much more widely used.

## *KEY POINTS*

- GnRH analogues are synthesized by substitution of amino acids in the parent molecule at the 6 and 10 positions. The various agonists have greater potencies and longer half-lives than the parent GnRH.
- LH and FSH have the same α subunit of thyroid-stimulating hormone (TSH) and human chorionic gonadotropin (HCG). The β subunits of all these hormones have different amino acids and carbohydrates, which provide specific biologic activity.
- LH acts on the theca cells to produce androgens, which are then transported to the granulosa cells, where they are aromatized to estrogens.
- Pregnenolone, 17-hydroxypregnenolone, progesterone, 17-hydroxyprogesterone, and corticosteroids have 21 carbon atoms; androgens (testosterone and androstenedione) have 19 carbon atoms; estrogens have 18 carbon atoms and a phenolic ring A.
- Kisspeptin (KISS1) plays a key role in the regulation of GnRH release.
- Because the ovaries lack 21-hydroxylase, 11-β-hydroxylase, and 18-hydroxylase reductase activity, they are unable to synthesize mineralocorticoids or glucocorticoids.
- Sex hormone–binding globulin (SHBG) primarily binds dihydrotestosterone, testosterone, and estradiol. About 65% of circulating testosterone is bound to SHBG and 30% to albumin. Approximately 2% remains unbound or free.
- Estrogen stimulates the synthesis of both estrogen and progesterone receptors in target tissues, and progestins inhibit the synthesis of both estrogen and progesterone receptors.
- With ultrasound it has been found that there is a steady increase in follicular diameter and volume that parallels the rise in estradiol. The dominant follicle has a maximal mean diameter of about 19.5 mm, with a range of 18 to 25 m just before ovulation. The mean maximal follicular volume is 3.8 mL, with a range of 3.1 to 8.2 mL.
- Ovulation occurs about 24 hours after the estradiol peak, as well as 32 hours after the initial rise in LH, and about 12 to 16 hours after the peak of LH levels in serum.

## KEY POINTS—cont'd

- Progesterone levels in serum are less than 1 ng/mL before ovulation and reach midluteal levels of 10 to 20 ng/mL.
- After menstruation, regeneration of the endometrium comes from cells in the spongiosum that were previously a portion of the secretory endometrium and not from the stratum basale as previously believed.
- Enzyme-linked immunosorbent assay (ELISA), or "sandwich," techniques have been developed to measure protein hormones (e.g., LH, FSH, HCG) with the use of monoclonal antibodies against the α and β subunits. The end point is a color reaction and can be read in a spectrophotometer.
- There are four characteristics of hormone assays that establish their reliability: sensitivity, specificity, accuracy, and precision.

## KEY REFERENCES

Ahima RS, Flier JS. Leptin. *Annu Rev Physiol.* 2000;62:413.

Bernard V, Young J, Chanson P, Binart N. New insights in prolactin: pathological implications. *Nat Rev Endocrinol.* 2015;11:265.

Cha J, Sun X, Dey SK. Mechanisms of implantation: strategies for successful pregnancy. *Nat Med.* 2012;18:1754.

Dolleman M, Verschuren WM, Eijkemans MJ, et al. Reproductive and lifestyle determinants of anti-Mullerian hormone in a large population-based study. *J Clin Endocrinol Metab.* 2013;98:2106.

Douglas NC, Thornton MH 2nd, Nurudeen SK, et al. Differential expression of serum glycodelin and insulin-like growth factor binding protein 1 in early pregnancy. *Reprod Sci.* 2013;20:1376.

Ellmann S, Sticht H, Thiel F, et al. Estrogen and progesterone receptors: from molecular structures to clinical targets. *Cell Mol Life Sci.* 2009;66:2405.

Hanna CB, Hennebold JD. Ovarian germline stem cells: an unlimited source of oocytes? *Fertil Steril.* 2014;101:20.

Horwitz KB, Jackson TA, Bain DL, et al. Nuclear receptor coactivators and corepressors. *Mol Endocrinol.* 1996;10:167.

Jayasena CN, Abbara A, Comninos AN, et al. Kisspeptin-54 triggers egg maturation in women undergoing in vitro fertilization. *J Clin Invest.* 2014;124:3667.

La Marca A, Broekmans FJ, Volpe A, et al. Anti-Mullerian hormone (AMH): what do we still need to know? *Hum Reprod.* 2009;24:2264.

Morishima A, Grumbach MM, Simpson ER, et al. Aromatase deficiency in male and female siblings caused by a novel mutation and the physiological role of estrogens. *J Clin Endocrinol Metab.* 1995;80:3689.

Skorupskaite K, George JT, Anderson RA. The kisspeptin-GnRH pathway in human reproductive health and disease. *Hum Reprod Update.* 2014;20:485.

Smith JT, Acohido BV, Clifton DK, et al. KiSS-1 neurones are direct targets for leptin in the ob/ob mouse. *J Neuroendocrinol.* 2006;18:298.

Tsai PS, Gill JC. Mechanisms of disease: Insights into X-linked and autosomal-dominant Kallmann syndrome. *Nat Clin Pract Endocrinol Metab.* 2006;2:160.

van den Berg MH, van Dulmen-den Broeder E, Overbeek A, et al. Comparison of ovarian function markers in users of hormonal contraceptives during the hormone-free interval and subsequent natural early follicular phases. *Hum Reprod.* 2010;25:1520.

Xu X, Veenstra TD, Fox SD, et al. Measuring fifteen endogenous estrogens simultaneously in human urine by high-performance liquid chromatography-mass spectrometry. *Anal Chem.* 2005;77:6646.

Suggested Readings can be found on ExpertConsult.com.

# 5
# Evidence-Based Medicine and Clinical Epidemiology

*Jonathan R. Foote, Laura J. Havrilesky*

Hippocrates, whom most consider to be the "father of western medicine," introduced the notion that an individual's disease originated from natural causes that could be observed and described within the environment. Medicine has come a long way since the era of Hippocrates, but his idea of diseases having natural causes was the first consideration that the practice of medicine and the treatment of diseases should be based on evidence. The idea of evidence-based medicine is no longer just an idea; it is the foundation of western medicine. Since the 1960s, there has been an explosion of research and knowledge in the basic and clinical sciences. The main goal of this research is to gain knowledge of disease processes, identify cause and effect of disease states, and develop and assess treatments, interventions, and their efficacy. The leap from the lab to clinical practice has presented a unique challenge to researchers and clinicians. Published results do not necessarily translate into meaningful clinical utility, namely related to constraints inherent in research study design. This chapter discusses traditional clinical study designs and explores modern research constructs, comparative effectiveness research (CER), and health services research (HSR).

## INTRODUCTION TO EVIDENCE-BASED MEDICINE

Evidence-based medicine aims to guide clinical decision making using our full body of knowledge from well-designed and conducted research. Research evidence rarely applies directly to a particular individual or clinical problem. Clinical decisions must be formulated within a specific context of patient care, integrated with clinical expertise, and coincide with the values and wishes of a particular patient. Clinical decision making must incorporate the most recent and valid information regarding disease prevention, diagnosis, prognosis, and treatment.

The basis for clinical evidence-based studies and the practice of evidence-based medicine starts with epidemiologic studies. The World Health Organization (WHO) defines epidemiology as "the study of distribution and determinants of health-related states or events (including disease), and the application of this study to the control of disease and other health problems" (www.who.int). More simply stated, epidemiology studies the cause and effect of a particular disease within a defined population. The basic purpose of an epidemiologic study is to estimate the relationship between an exposure and an outcome in order to assess an association or causality.

One of the most influential studies in gynecology, the Women's Health Initiative, began after epidemiologic data exhibited an association between the use of hormone replacement therapy (HRT) and the prevention of coronary heart disease and osteoporosis. The collection of this observational data led to one of the largest randomized controlled trials and U.S. prevention studies with more than 160,000 postmenopausal women enrolled. Interestingly, this trial did not demonstrate a cardioprotective effect of HRT, but rather showed an increased risk of coronary heart disease. It also demonstrated an increased risk of venous thromboembolism, stroke, and breast cancer, which were unexpected results (Rossouw, 2002). This study presents a good example of the limitations of observational epidemiologic study design. It also demonstrates the importance of developing well-designed experimental clinical trials to test, when plausible, prior observations and associations.

Epidemiologic studies can be classified as either observational or experimental. The three most common types of observational epidemiologic studies include cohort, case-control, and cross-sectional studies. Case series can also be included among these, although their data are of lower quality. The gold standard of experimental study is the randomized control trial (RCT), largely due to its ability to control for confounding variables through the process of eligibility criteria and randomization. Although the RCT is the gold standard, it often does not directly represent the therapeutic population seen in the real world. Since the early 2000s, comparative effectiveness research (CER) has created a niche to help bridge the gap between research and clinical practice. CER is geared toward assisting "consumers, clinicians, purchasers, and policy makers to make informed decisions that will improve health care at both the individual and population levels" (Iglehart, 2009). Another field of research emerging in modern medicine is health services research (HSR), which examines how patients get access to care, the cost and quality of that care, and ultimately the result of delivery of care. A particular area of interest developing within HSR is health economic analysis. There are several forms of economic analysis with the most common being cost-effectiveness analysis (CEA), which is used to compare the relative cost and effectiveness of alternative strategies, usually using a standard willingness-to-pay threshold. In the sections that follow, we will review both traditional clinical study design and emerging clinical research methods.

## TRADITIONAL CLINICAL STUDY DESIGN

Traditional clinical study designs are not created equal when it comes to their quality of evidence. Table 5.1 demonstrates a grading system assessing clinical study design and evidence quality. Blinded, randomized controlled trials offer the highest quality of evidence. Some authorities advocate that systematic reviews and meta-analyses of these types of trials produce an equal quality of evidence, although the validity of such studies relies on the quality and validity of the chosen articles (Grondin, 2011). The next level of evidence comes from cohort studies and case-control studies. The lowest quality of study design can be found in case series, case reports, and expert opinion. Table 5.2 compares the advantages, limitations, and statistical considerations of each study design. Whether experimental or observational, these clinical studies are invaluable to modern medicine and impact our day-to-day care of patients. This section will discuss each clinical study design.

**Table 5.1** Levels of Evidence in Clinical Study Design

| Level | Evidence |
|---|---|
| 1a | Systematic review (with homogeneity) of randomized controlled trials |
| 1b | Individual randomized controlled trials |
| 2a | Systematic review (with homogeneity) of cohort studies |
| 2b | Individual cohort study |
| 2c | "Outcomes research" and ecological studies |
| 3a | Systematic review of case-control studies |
| 3b | Individual case-control study |
| 4 | Case series |
| 5 | Expert opinion without explicit critical appraisal, or based on physiology, bench research, or "first principles" |

Modified from Oxford Centre for Evidence Based Medicine: Levels of Evidence, 2009, www.cebm.net.

## OBSERVATIONAL STUDIES

The term *observational study* describes a wide range of study designs. Observational studies can be classified as analytic or descriptive. Analytic studies contain a control group for comparison, which includes nonrandomized prospective and retrospective cohort studies, case-control studies, and cross-sectional studies. Descriptive studies lack a control or comparison group and consist of case reports and case series. Observational studies play an important role in evidence-based medicine and provide an important source of information when randomized controlled trials cannot be performed. The descriptive aspect of all observational studies is an invaluable attribute in clinical research, providing statistics about incidence, prevalence, and mortality rates of diseases in particular populations. Observational studies provide clinicians with the context of a disease within a population. However, observational studies cannot determine causality, regardless of how logical or plausible an association may seem. They are unfit to test hypotheses or answer etiologic questions, but they play a major role in generating new hypotheses to be tested by a more formal, experimental study design.

### Case Reports and Case Series

The basic element or unit of observational studies, as described by Grimes and Schulz, is the case report (Grimes, 2002). Case reports and case series are the least methodologically robust. This is not to say that case reports are not valuable. Case reports often describe rare or new entities in medicine and offer an opportunity to describe characteristics about a disease and allow for the postulation of hypotheses of pathophysiology. It was through case reports of unusual infections and disturbed immunity that AIDS was first described (CDC, 1981). Case reports can describe infrequent adverse events associated with medications or drugs. They can also report on the plausibility and early use of novel treatment methods or surgery. The biggest limitation of this study design is the lack of a comparison group, which does not allow for any clinical conclusions to be drawn. The scientific audience is led to use historical controls or other less robust objective considerations in order to interpret the meaning of noted observations. Case reports, or case series, should be considered no more than "the first step toward more sophisticated research" (Gehlback, 2002).

**Table 5.2** Comparison of Traditional Clinical Study Designs

| Study Design | Advantages | Limitations | Statistical Analysis |
|---|---|---|---|
| Randomized controlled trials | Gold standard; prospective; multiple study groups; randomization; can determine causality or a treatment advantage; time-consuming; expensive; internal validity | Selection bias; confounding factors; performance bias; detection bias (RCT can control for confounding factors and biases with double-blinding and randomization); limited external validity | Relative risk (RR); absolute or attributable risk (AR); confidence interval (CI); number needed to treat (NNT) |
| Cohort studies | Prospective; can assess many outcomes over time | Take many years to complete; expensive; selection bias; confounding factors; patients can be lost to follow-up; changing exposure profile | Incidence; relative risk (RR); absolute or attributable risk (AR) |
| Case-control studies | Efficient; inexpensive; can study multiple exposures; can study rare disease | Retrospective; recall bias; sampling bias; confounding factors; good external validity | Odds ratio (OR) |
| Cross-sectional studies | Can determine the frequency of disease or outcomes; highlights possible associations; efficient | Capture one moment in time; cannot determine incidence or causality; sampling bias; participation bias; recall bias | Prevalence |
| Case series | Descriptive of rare or new entities; hypothesis generating | Lack of comparison group; no clinical conclusions | No statistical analysis |

### *Cross-Sectional Studies*

Cross-sectional studies examine the relationship between exposure and the outcomes of interest in a defined population at a single point in time. In other words, cross-sectional studies are prevalence studies. *Prevalence* is defined as the number of cases in a population at a given point in time. It is a ratio, or proportion, of affected individuals in relation to a pooled population. Cross-sectional studies cannot determine incidence, or the number of new cases in a population over a period of time. They are snapshots of a disease and a population. With reference to only a designated moment in time, these studies are not able to provide causal evidence. Case reports and cross-sectional studies can highlight possible associations that deserve additional evaluation, but they cannot determine causality.

One advantage of cross-sectional studies is efficiency. Because the study population is examined at one moment in time, conclusions can be generated at the same time as data collection. There is no waiting for outcomes or observations. However, cross-sectional studies also have their disadvantages. They capture only a moment in time and thus cannot determine the incidence of disease nor a true association or causality. It is the age-old question, "Which came first, the chicken or the egg?" Population selection, participation bias, and recall bias are all possible limitations. If a tertiary care center or major referral center is conducting a research study and the study population is taken from patients who present to these facilities, they are unlikely to accurately represent the general population, or even a more specific population of patients with a particular disease undergoing therapy within the community. In 1990, Gayle and colleagues published data regarding the prevalence of HIV among university students, examining more than 17,000 specimens from 19 universities (Gayle, 1990). Thirty students, or 0.2%, had detectable HIV antibodies, which was higher than prior studies within the public. The media sensationalized these data, reporting that more than 25,000 college students across the nation may be infected with HIV. However, patient selection in this study was poor, as specimens collected for examination were not random but rather represented those students who presented to student health whose condition warranted a blood sample. Researchers must be careful that patients selected for cross-sectional studies are to be representative of the study population desired. Participation bias arises when selected subjects do not participate, such as in survey studies. If 100,000 surveys are sent out, but only 10,000 are filled out, participation bias becomes an issue. The minority of patients who respond may not be representative of the desired study population. Recall bias becomes an issue when self-reporting, as in survey studies, is a part of study design. Patients often report inaccurate information regarding certain exposures or events. However, well-conducted cross-sectional studies have their place in evidence-based medicine. They are simply prevalence studies and allow us to determine frequencies of disease or outcomes within particular populations or groups.

### *Case-Control Studies*

The purpose of a case-control study is to determine if an exposure is associated with an outcome (i.e., a disease of interest). Study participants are selected on the basis of already having the outcome of interest (the case group) or of not having that outcome (the control group). Case-control studies are always retrospective as they start with an outcome then trace back to evaluate exposures or habits. Figure 5.1 illustrates the differences in methodologies between case-control studies as compared with cohort studies. Participants in the case group must be carefully defined and should include all cases of new-onset disease drawn from an identifiable population. Controls should be sampled from that same population. The purpose of the control group is to allow for comparison in frequencies of exposures of a case group with the outcome of interest versus the control group without that outcome. In 1971, Herbst and associates published a case-control study of 8 cases and 32 matched controls identifying a strong association between vaginal adenocarcinoma and in utero exposure to diethylstilbestrol (DES) (Herbst, 1971). Although further cohort studies were required to confirm causality, this case-control study allowed for identification of a suspected culprit (exposure) for the development of vaginal adenocarcinoma in young women (outcome of interest).

Case-control studies offer the advantages of being relatively inexpensive, simple to conduct, and efficient. They are retrospective and thus do not require a prolonged period of data collection. They are able to study multiple exposures as they relate to a particular outcome of interest, and they offer the ability to study rare diseases. The quality of the results from these studies is dependent on uniform, meticulous selection of cases, control groups, and data collection among the groups. There are also disadvantages to case-control studies. Recall bias is a particular issue, as cases and controls are likely to recount historical exposures differently. Patients or families coping with an illness may recall in great detail all events they believe might be associated with the illness, whereas healthy controls may not remember similar exposures. Recall bias may also occur when information on the case group is obtained by chart review, whereas information on the control group is obtained either by interview or mail survey. It may ultimately be impossible to eliminate recall bias. Sample selection, or sampling bias, is also an issue, and it arises if the cases selected do not appropriately represent a particular disease or outcome. This is similar to sample selection issues in cross-sectional studies. Sampling bias can also occur within the control group if a representation of the desired general population either underestimates or overestimates exposures. Matching, or selecting control group participants similar in characteristics to the case group, helps to decrease bias in the selection of controls. Matching also helps to decrease possible confounding. Confounding occurs when factors relate both to the measured outcome and measured exposures. "Confounding is the epidemiologist's eternal triangle.... Are we seeing cause and effect, or is a confounding factor exerting its unappreciated influence?" (Gehlback, 2002). Controlling sample selection and

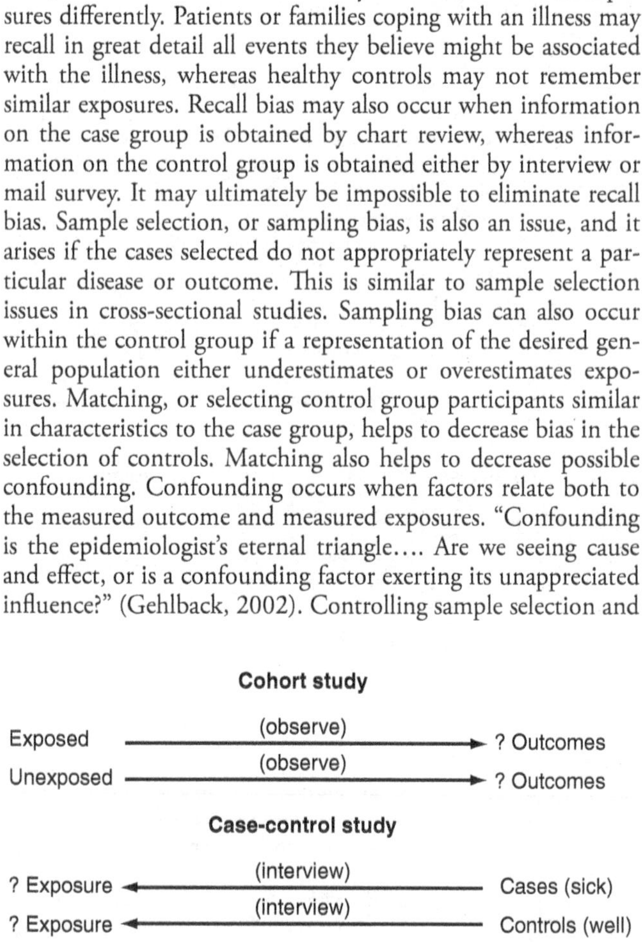


**Figure 5.1** Schematic diagram of clinical study design comparing cohort studies and case-control studies.

confounding factors allows for external validity, or the generalizability of the study to the desired population. Often statistical techniques, such as multivariate analysis and logistic regression, are used to help eliminate confounders.

Because case-control studies are by design retrospective, they are limited in their statistical analysis. They cannot provide data on incidence, relative risks, or attributable risks between an exposure and a measured outcome. Case-control studies report an odds ratio, which is the odds that an individual affected by the specific disease being studied has been exposed to a particular risk factor (case group) divided by the odds that the control group has been exposed. It is loosely considered a reasonable estimate of relative risk, but it is not a true calculation of relative risk.

### *Cohort Studies*

A cohort study selects a group of individuals at risk for an outcome of interest and divides them into subgroups based on the presence or absence of one or more exposures to be studied. Subgroups are then followed prospectively, watching for the development of the outcome of interest. Cohort studies are unique in that the study participants select their exposure, rather than having the investigator select an exposure. In experimental research, the investigator selects, either knowingly or unknowingly, the exposure. An excellent example is the Nurses' Health Study (NHS). The NHS was started in 1976 to survey more than 120,000 female nurses regarding medical history, hormonal use, and many other points of interest. The investigators have updated the study every 2 years by mailing out questionnaires to the original enrolled patients. In 2001, Grodstein and coworkers published data regarding the use of postmenopausal hormone therapy and the secondary prevention of coronary events (Grodstein, 2001). The results demonstrated a short-term increased risk of coronary events in patients with a history of coronary disease, whereas the study showed a decreased risk in long-term hormonal use.

A strength of cohort studies is the possibility of assessing many different outcomes over time and also being able to calculate incidence rates, relative risks, and attributable risks. Incidence is defined as the number of new outcomes of interest in a given population over a set period of time. In cohort studies, incidence can be calculated for the population as a whole, but it is most often calculated for populations with and without an identifiable risk factor. Relative risk (RR), or risk ratio, can be calculated from these incidence rates. RR should be thought of as a simple ratio. It is a ratio of the probability of an outcome (disease) occurring within an exposed population as compared with a nonexposed population. It is calculated as the ratio of the incidence in a population exposed to the risk factor over the incidence in the unexposed population. Attributable risk, or absolute risk, represents the absolute additional risk in the exposed population over what may be considered the baseline occurrence in the population. It is determined by calculating the difference between the incidence in the exposed population and that in the unexposed population.

Cohort studies also have their disadvantages. They are often time consuming, take many years to complete, and often become costly. The NHS is a clear example of the time and money it takes to complete a prospective cohort study. As with all analytic-observational studies, subject selection is important to control for selection bias and confounding factors. Matching of patients in control and study groups will help limit these issues. To the extent that information is collected about known or suspected confounding factors, it is also possible to control for their effect in the statistical analysis. Adjustment techniques can work only for confounding variables that an investigator knows about and measures. Participants may also be lost to follow-up given these studies take years to complete. Investigators must be diligent in keeping accurate follow-up records of each subject. In the same manner, researchers should be aware that patient habits may change over time, and thus their exposure risks may change.

## *EXPERIMENTAL STUDIES: RANDOMIZED CONTROLLED TRIALS*

Randomized controlled trials (RCTs) are considered the gold standard of clinical study design. Within the constructs of epidemiologic studies, RCT is another type of analytic study. In cohort studies, the patient controls the exposure to a factor of interest, whereas in RCTs, the clinical investigator controls exposure to the factor of interest. RCTs are designed to establish evidence of causal associations. They are characterized by the prospective assignment of study participants to a study group (who receive the factor of interest, typically a new treatment) or a placebo, no treatment, or standard care group. Although there are often only two study arms or groups within an RCT, investigators frequently develop designs involving multiple study groups. These groups are followed over time to evaluate for differences in outcomes. Outcomes of interest may include prevention or cure of a disease, reduction in severity of a condition, or differences in costs, quality of life, or side effects between treatments. An example is the Women's Health Initiative already mentioned, which examined the use of hormone replacement therapy (HRT) and the prevention of coronary heart disease, osteoporosis, and the like. The trial did not demonstrate a cardioprotective effect of HRT, but rather showed an increased risk of coronary heart disease. Although it did demonstrate protection against osteoporosis and colon cancer, it showed an increased risk of venous thromboembolism, stroke, and breast cancer (Rossouw, 2002).

RCTs have key design features that make them the gold standard. One of the main features is randomization, a feature that eliminates selection bias and allows for better control of known and unknown confounding factors. Confounding factors are also controlled with strict eligibility criteria, eliminating possible interference from any contributing factors. This is also referred to as *internal validity*, or the ability to control for confounding factors to demonstrate a true causal association. An additional feature of most RCTs is blinding. Performance bias is encountered when systemic differences exist in the care delivered to subjects. In other words, performance bias is when a patient receives less or more therapy based on knowing what particular group or treatment a patient is receiving on trial. Detection bias occurs when systemic differences exist in assessment of a particular outcome. It arises when patients are evaluated more intensely as a result of being in the study group of interest. The double-blinded RCT is a superior study design, as the blinding of both subjects and investigators is preferred to control for any performance or detection bias while also controlling for selection bias and confounding factors. Despite the theoretic design superiority of the RCT approach, these studies provide the best evidence only if the study has been thoughtfully designed, implemented, analyzed, and reported.

Although RCTs remain the gold standard of research design and evidence quality, they are not without their own limitations. Both ethical and practical considerations may limit the use of RCTs to answer clinical questions. It is clearly unethical to expose patients to potential disease-causing factors just to learn about their negative effects on a particular outcome of interest. Additional ethical concerns arise when designing treatment groups to be studied. A placebo control group is often most efficient to study the effect of a given treatment. However, if an effective treatment already exists, it is not ethical to use a placebo control group, causing harm to patients with the lack of a known, effective treatment. The concept of *primum non nocere*, or "first, do no harm," also applies in clinical research. If a condition is mild, the treatment period is brief, or effective treatment is not generally available, most investigators believe that a placebo control group is ethical. Most often in RCTs, study groups will be similar, or at least balanced with regard to benefits and harms. The question at hand is, what treatment is preferred? Is there an advantage of one treatment over the other? This uncertainty can be defined as therapeutic equipoise. It is a general uncertainty of the benefits and harms of competing treatments and is often the reason for conducting RCTs. It provides patients with an equal chance to undergo at least "standard of care" treatment versus a possible improved treatment plan. In this nature, RCTs allow an unbiased assessment of determining a preferred treatment. RCTs are also ideal to study outcomes over short periods of time. RCTs intended to study long-term or rare outcomes are much more difficult to carry out. They are time consuming and ultimately cost prohibitive. As already discussed, cohort studies may be more appropriate to evaluate rare outcomes. Unfortunately, for many clinical questions, the time, effort, and expense involved in carrying out an RCT become prohibitive.

A practical consideration in RCTs is that subjects and controls among groups are often special populations that may not be generalizable to the public, or even a specific subset of the public. In 1971, Cochrane noted this issue, stating "Between measurements based on RCTs and benefit...in the community there is a gulf which has been much under-estimated" (Cochrane, 1971). Although the RCT's strength of design is a strong internal validity, it often lacks strong external validity. External validity is the ability of a result to be generalizable in the real world. Often, the more complex the study protocol, the greater the difference between RCT results and general clinical outcomes. RCTs also often use surrogate markers to substitute for clinical outcomes. A surrogate marker is "an outcome measure that substitutes for a clinical event of true importance...an intermediate measure... commonly laboratory measurements or imaging studies thought to be involved in the causal pathway to a clinical event of interest" (Grimes, 2005). An ideal surrogate marker is a measurable event that is necessary along the pathway to the clinical end point. For example, Skaznik-Wikiel and colleagues demonstrated in a retrospective analysis of 124 women that normalization of cancer antigen 125 (CA-125) levels in ovarian cancer after three cycles of chemotherapy has been associated with an improved overall survival (Skaznik-Wikiel, 2011). However, this is a retrospective analysis, and there are no studies demonstrating an association between the response of CA-125 and overall survival, or any other clinical outcome. Researchers must be careful when using surrogate markers, as they may not always equate with the disease process being assessed. For example, the effects of a medication on lowering cholesterol are not necessarily the same as preventing heart attacks, which is the desired clinical end point. When interpreting randomized trials, surrogate markers must be used with caution. Grimes and Schulz have emphasized that surrogate markers should, among other characteristics, have similar confounders and influences, and they should show a near identical response to a treatment as the desired clinical end point. They cite an example of fluoride treatments, which improve a surrogate marker, bone mineral density, but increase fractures, which is the true clinical end point of interest. Occasionally, authors will use a "combined outcome," which includes a surrogate marker and a valid clinical outcome. This combined outcome should be interpreted cautiously because the relative effect of treatments on the various components is unknown.

Researchers may also report "secondary outcomes," or subgroup analyses, within an RCT. These outcomes may or may not have similar validity as the set of primary outcomes. RCTs are designed to test hypotheses on primary outcomes, controlling for confounding variables that affect the primary outcome. Often, secondary outcomes were not considered in the study design, and thus confounding factors affecting secondary outcomes were not controlled for. Many epidemiologists suggest results of secondary outcomes be interpreted with caution and as hypothesis generating, unless the original study design had internal validity regarding these subgroups. This is particularly true when secondary outcomes and subgroup analyses are incorporated into a meta-analysis, which will be addressed later.

## STATISTICAL INTERPRETATION

Epidemiologic studies use a quantitative approach to describing both exposures and outcomes. Whether an RCT, cohort study, or case-control study, all of these studies attempt to present their results as a single number, usually referred to as the *point estimate*, that quantifies the relationship between the exposure and the outcome. This number is an estimate of the truth rather than the truth itself, because each study, however large, includes only a sample of all the people who are affected by the exposure-outcome relationship. The point estimate expresses the strength of the association between the exposure and outcome. In an RCT or a cohort study, the point estimate is the relative risk (RR). Risk in the study subjects is the number of cases or outcomes that occur over time. The RR is simply the risk of disease (or other outcome) among the exposed or treated subjects divided by the risk in the unexposed subjects. As already discussed, case-control studies do not measure risk directly but rather an odds ratio (OR), which is generally considered a rough estimate of RR. The point of any study design is to show a strong association or causality.

Interpretations of RR and OR are similar. As the ratio approaches 1.0, there is little to no association. For both RRs and ORs, the further away the value is from 1.0, the stronger the relationship between the exposure and the outcome. Values less than 1.0 represent a negative association, or a decreased risk of an exposure-outcome relationship. Values greater than 1.0 represent a positive association, or a greater risk of an exposure-outcome relationship. A strong positive RR may be greater than 2.0 and a strong negative RR may be less than 0.5. Weaker associations can often be explained by confounding variables. However, enthusiastic investigators, worried patients, or sensationalistic media frequently overinterpret weak associations. One must also remember that an OR or RR is based on results of a specific study group and may not represent the general population. This possible difference is understood as a sampling error, or the possible difference in statistics of a study compared with the actual unknown statistics within a population. As a result, investigators will use a confidence interval (CI) to express the precision of a point estimate. Researchers do not rely solely on the traditional *P* value to detect whether a study's findings are due to a chance occurrence, especially when discussing ratios and risks. Confidence intervals represent with high probability (95%) the values within which the actual population point estimate would fall. A narrow CI indicates strong precision and is most often found with larger studies or studies with very little variance. A wide CI indicates poor precision and may be representative of an underpowered study or considerable variance among results. It must be stated that a CI does not address uncertainty in the results because of confounding factors or poor study quality. As well, a wide CI does not mean there is no association between the exposure and the outcome. A CI is a measure of precision. Even an imprecise point estimate remains the best explanation of the relationship until a larger or better study is performed. With regard to understanding graphic representation of confidence intervals, they are most often drawn as a straight line around a point estimate to show the width of their range. This is a poor representation of the actual true point estimate, as it is better understood as a bell-shaped curve centered on the point estimate. Figure 5.2 demonstrates examples of point estimates and their respective confidence intervals.

Calculating RR does not take into account the incidence or the importance of the problem being evaluated. A relative risk of 4 says that the outcome increases 400% in exposed individuals compared with unexposed individuals. However, the relative risk must be interpreted in the context of the frequency of the outcome. For instance, the incidence of venous thromboembolism (VTE) in young women while not using oral contraceptives is about 1 in 10,000 and the incidence while using oral contraceptives is 4 in 10,000; thus the relative risk is 4. However, the absolute risk of VTE is still low in both groups of women with a difference in risk of 3 in 10,000. This difference in risk is considered the absolute risk, or attributable risk (AR). It is very useful for putting large relative risks into a clinically useful perspective. It can also be reported as the absolute risk reduction when a benefit is identified or the absolute risk increase when a harm is identified.

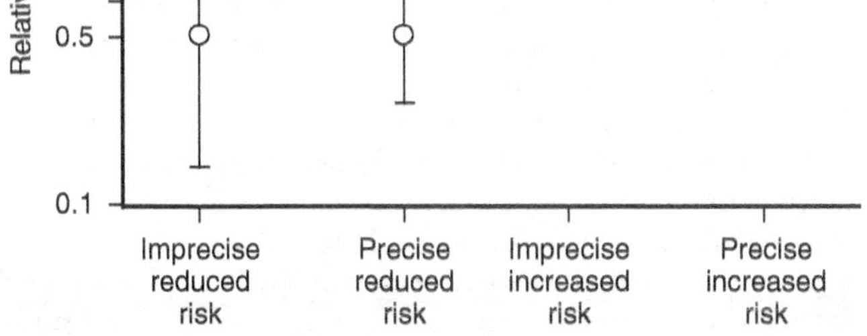

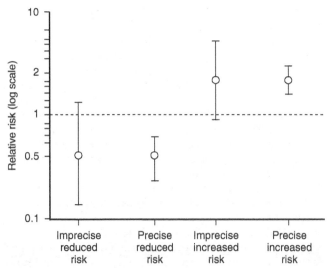


**Figure 5.2** Schematic diagram of point estimates *(open circles)* with varying confidence intervals *(lines with crossbars)*. X-axis represents interpretation of respective point estimate and confidence interval. If the confidence interval crosses 1.0, the change in risk is statistically insignificant.

An alternative calculation to AR looks at a complementary concept: how many patients need to be treated to observe one benefit or one adverse event? This concept is referred to as the *number needed to treat (NNT)*, or the number of patients who need to be treated to achieve an additional positive outcome. It is the reciprocal of the absolute risk reduction (the risk difference for good outcomes). If the effect is dangerous, the value is called the *number needed to harm (NNH)*. The number of patients who, if they received the treatment, would lead to one additional patient being harmed, compared with patients not receiving the treatment, is the reciprocal of the absolute risk increase (the risk difference for bad outcomes). Thus using the example of oral contraceptives, with an AR risk of VTE of 3 in 10,000, the number needed to harm (NNH, that is, to experience one extra VTE) is 3,333. It is simply the reciprocal of 3 in 10,000. Calculations of NNT and NNH are essential to determine the potential benefits and harm of therapies, preventive services, and screening tests. Another benefit of these calculations is that they allow us to compare benefits and harm across different treatment strategies. A caution about NNT and NNH is that the number may vary over time. The data from which an NNT is calculated are often specific and may not be generalizable to a person's lifetime or the course of a disease. NNT and NNH derived from a meta-analysis should be viewed with caution. If the studies are from varied populations or used slightly different methods, the NNT and NNH may not always apply to an individual patient or be a simple arithmetic summation.

## COMPARATIVE EFFECTIVENESS RESEARCH

Pervasive problems in the quality of delivered care, a lack of high-quality evidence to guide clinical practice and health policy, and concerns about health care spending led to a major initiative, comparative effectiveness research (CER). The Institute of Medicine has defined CER as follows:

> *The generation and synthesis of evidence that compares the benefits and harms of alternative methods to prevent, diagnose, treat, and monitor a clinical condition or to improve the delivery of care. The purpose of CER is to assist consumers, clinicians, purchasers, and policy makers to make informed decisions that will improve health care at both the individual and population levels* (IOM, 2009).

The formal process of developing a CER focus was initiated in the 2003 Medicare Modernization Act, which appropriated $50 million to conduct research to address the needs and priorities related to improve outcomes, clinical effectiveness, and appropriateness of certain services and treatments. Data from these earlier efforts were first integrated into coverage for these interventions in 2006, when the Centers for Medicare and Medicaid Services (CMS) provided support to the concept of including evidence-based decision making and research into coverage determination policies (Havrilesky, 2013a). Analysis of costs linked to health-related quality of life was later included as part of CER. In its 2007 definition of CER, the Congressional Budget Office (CBO) included costs as a factor relevant to comparison of different interventions but took a narrow view of interventions by focusing solely on treatment for individual medical conditions (CBO, 2007). CER studies often incorporate different practice settings, a wide range of subgroups, and patient-reported outcomes. Several aspects of CER are depicted in Figure 5.3 and discussed in this section.

## META-ANALYSES, SYSTEMATIC REVIEWS, AND EVIDENCE-BASED GUIDELINE DEVELOPMENT

Meta-analyses were developed in response to the problem of conflicting and inconclusive results of individual studies. Uncommon diseases or conditions are hard to study because of the small numbers of patients, which often leads to studies lacking sufficient numbers of patients and power to report significant results. In a meta-analysis, a researcher combines the results of multiple studies to enlarge the group of patients being studied. The ultimate goal of a meta-analysis is to produce a more precise result with a tighter confidence interval. However, not all meta-analyses are created equal. A meta-analysis involving well-constructed and well-performed RCTs is ideal. Meta-analyses of observational studies must be interpreted with extreme caution. Each individual study varies in population, entry criteria, case definition, and exposure definitions, which makes combining data in observational studies problematic. This is particularly true if the analysis combines data from published tables rather than combining the raw data from the original studies. Meta-analyses differ from pooled analyses in that a pooled analysis reexamines the original raw data from multiple individual studies for statistical consideration, whereas a meta-analysis does not reexamine the raw data. If the results from individual studies disagree in direction or report very different results, then the meta-analysis is

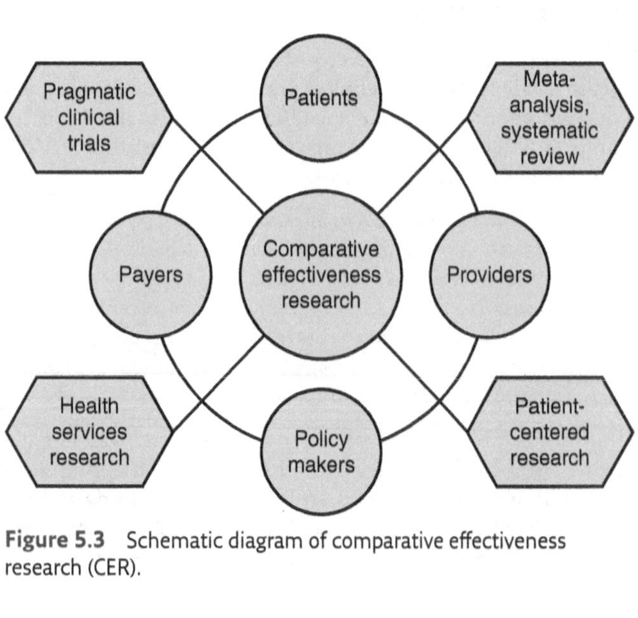


**Figure 5.3** Schematic diagram of comparative effectiveness research (CER).

not an appropriate tool to answer the question. A pooled analysis can control for heterogeneity by controlling for confounding factors in the original data. A meta-analysis can provide the same type of control by inclusion of similar, high-quality studies. One can argue that the main value of a meta-analysis is the rigorous approach to collecting and evaluating all of the relevant data on a particular clinical problem from multiple sources. A risk of meta-analysis is evaluating many published studies that are small and finding a significant effect that is not accurate. Hennekens and colleagues have suggested that when multiple studies are analyzed together to produce a new finding, the results should be interpreted with caution and viewed as hypothesis generating until a large RCT with adequate power can be performed (Hennekens, 2009). This is particularly true when the additional reported results are secondary outcomes. Neither meta-analyses nor pooled analyses are appropriate for conclusions regarding secondary outcomes, although meticulous examination of original raw data can generate associations for further study.

The clinical need for good evidence and the need for synthesis of evidence that goes beyond opinion have led to the development and use of additional approaches to reviewing evidence. Evidence-based systematic reviews include a comprehensive review and evaluation of the literature. A systematic review is a review of a clearly formulated question that uses systematic and explicit methods to identify, select, and critically appraise relevant research, and to collect and analyze data from the studies that are included in the review (Higgins, 2011). Systematic reviews are reported using a standardized format that must include a detailed description of the search strategy used to identify the relevant literature and the results of the search. Systematic reviews also carry out critical appraisal of the studies they evaluate. Critical appraisal employs a rigid standardized assessment of the relevance and quality of each study. The goal of systematic reviews is to examine the literature regarding a specific clinical question and to use an approach that will minimize bias and random error. Systematic reviews are often performed in conjunction with a meta-analysis.

In 1996, to address the suboptimal reporting of meta-analyses, an international group of researchers released the Quality of Reporting of Meta-analyses (QUOROM) statement to improve standards. In 2009, the guideline was updated to address several conceptual and practical advances in the science of systematic reviews and was renamed PRISMA (Preferred Reporting Items of Systematic reviews and Meta-Analyses). PRISMA provides a 27-item checklist that describes the content of a systematic review including the title, abstract, methods, results, discussion, and funding, as well as a flow diagram that represents the flow of information through the different phases of a systematic review. It characterizes information about the number of records identified in the literature searches, the number of studies included and excluded, and the reasons for exclusions (http://www.prisma-statement.org/statement.htm). For example, in 2013, Havrilesky and coworkers published a systemic review and meta-analysis of the use of oral contraceptive pills (OCPs) as primary prevention for ovarian cancer (Havrilesky, 2013b). This study employed methodology that followed PRISMA guidelines. In a flow diagram, the authors described literature searches, abstract screening, number of studies included and excluded, as well as explanations for exclusions. It also illustrates the advantage of systemic review and meta-analysis, which is to provide an answer to focused research questions through a rigorous and transparent form of literature review. In this case, the authors confirmed previous large studies demonstrating a duration dependent protective effect of OCP use on the incidence of ovarian cancer.

The Cochrane Collaboration is a major source of systematic reviews (www.cochrane.org). This international organization aims to help people make well-informed decisions about health care by preparing, maintaining, and promoting the accessibility of systematic reviews of the effects of health care interventions. Cochrane funding comes from proceeds from the Cochrane Library and other Cochrane products, along with donations from national and international governments, private foundations, and private funders. Of note, the organization does not accept commercialized donations to prohibit undue commercial influence.

The Agency for Healthcare Research and Quality (AHRQ) also works with a number of partners to publish systematic reviews. The AHRQ lists its mission as "producing evidence to make health care safer, higher quality, more accessible, equitable, and affordable, and to work within the U.S. Department of Health and Human Services and with other partners to make sure that the evidence is understood and used." The AHRQ also works in conjunction with the U.S. Preventive Services Task Force (USPSTF) to perform systematic reviews regarding clinical preventive services. These are published in both book form and, increasingly, electronic form. Many professional groups issue practice guidelines to help translate these often lengthy reviews into briefer, clinically useful documents, ultimately assisting clinicians in making patient care decisions. An electronic collection of such guidelines is now available at the National Guideline Clearinghouse (NGC; www.guideline.gov).

## PRAGMATIC CLINICAL TRIALS

As noted earlier, the RCT is the gold standard for evaluating the effects of treatment; however, RCTs are often not generalizable due to the tightly controlled environment in which they are carried out. In recent years, clinicians and policy makers have made a concerted effort to distinguish between the *efficacy* and the *effectiveness* of an intervention. RCTs are efficacy trials (explanatory trials) whose purpose is to determine whether an intervention produces the expected result under ideal circumstances. On the other hand, pragmatic clinical trials (PCTs) are effectiveness trials, measuring the benefit of treatment under real-world circumstances or routine clinical practice. In 1967, Schwartz defined a PCT as a trial "for which the hypothesis and study design are formulated based on information needed to make a decision" (Schwartz, 1967). PCTs address real questions of cost, risk, and benefits that arise in everyday clinical practice, providing direct, useful information to providers, patients, payers, and other decision-makers (Roland, 1998). They resemble RCTs in the use of randomization, but PCTs do not place strict constraints on the setting of the trial, target patients, or intervention delivery. Traditional RCT approaches prioritize internal validity and efficacy, testing whether the intervention has the intended effect in ideal, highly controlled settings. In contrast, PCTs prioritize external validity, or generalizability to the public. Pragmatic trials test effectiveness, or the degree of beneficial effect in everyday clinical practice.

In a document released by the AHRQ and the Patient Centered Medical Home (PCMH), there are five ways in which PCTs differ from RCTs: They (1) compare clinically relevant alternatives, (2) enroll diverse study populations, (3) recruit from a variety of practice settings, (4) measure a broad range of outcomes, and (5) adapt the intervention being tested to the local context. However, even PCTs have disadvantages. Although PCTs have excellent external validity, there is a tradeoff for internal validity. Effects of a particular treatment may be lessened or heightened, as the results were obtained in a more real-world setting. It also may be more difficult to determine what component of an intervention is responsible for a certain outcome, as the interventions can be heterogeneous. PCTs also require a great number of resources to keep meticulous records of implementation and to be sure that the study design is upheld. Regardless, the PCT is an excellent alternative to the traditional RCT in certain clinical settings. An example of the benefits of this study design is a study that examined the standard care of atrial fibrillation versus atrial fibrillation-specific management strategy (the SAFETY trial). This trial was designed as a pragmatic, randomized controlled trial. The standard group received routine primary care as well as hospital discharge follow-up. The SAFETY group included a home visit, a Holter monitory for 7 to 14 days, prolonged follow-up by a specialized cardiac nurse, and multidisciplinary support as needed. The SAFETY group was associated with more days alive out of the hospital, but no change in prolonged event-free survival (Stewart, 2015). This trial demonstrates the nature of PCTs focusing on the generalizability of an intervention to patients in the community, while holding true to RCT study design. It also demonstrates the amount of planning and support required to conduct a PCT. As the use of the PCT continues to grow, clinicians and researchers will have to learn where it will fit into our understanding of quality of evidence.

## PATIENT-CENTERED OUTCOMES RESEARCH INSTITUTE

The Patient-Centered Outcomes Research Institute (PCORI) is an independent nonprofit, nongovernmental organization established by the 2010 Patient Protection and Affordable Care Act. PCORI's purpose is to assist patients and clinicians in making informed health decisions by advancing the quality and relevance of evidence concerning a broad range of health conditions. PCORI directs research to improve prevention, diagnosis, management, and monitoring of disease in varied patient subpopulations (Patient Protection and Affordable Care Act, 2010). Patient-centered outcomes research (PCOR) differs from CER in its primary target. The institution's primary goal is to inform individual patient decision making rather than targeting a wider range of audiences such as payers and policy makers. According to a working definition approved in March 2012 by the PCORI board of governors, the purpose of PCOR is to help patients and their providers communicate and make informed health care decisions by allowing the patient's voice to be heard in assessing the value of health care options. One way that PCORI operationalizes the focus on individuals in PCOR is through examination of outcomes "that people notice and care about such as survival, function, symptoms, and health related quality of life" (D'Arcy, 2012). PCORI aims to achieve this mission by producing and promoting the use of high-integrity, evidence-based information stemming from research guided by patients, caregivers, and the broader health care community.

PCORI funds comparative clinical effectiveness research and supports work that will improve the methods used to conduct such studies.

## HEALTH SERVICES RESEARCH

The AHRQ defines health services research (HSR) as a

> *multidisciplinary field of scientific investigation that studies how social factors, financing systems, organizational structures and processes, health technologies, and personal behaviors affect access to health care, the quality and cost of health care, and ultimately, our health and well-being.*

In 1993, the National Institutes of Health (NIH) Revitalization Act created a National Information Center on Health Services Research and Health Care Technology (NICHSR), which had the following goal:

> *To make the results of health services research, including practice guidelines and technology assessments, readily available to health practitioners, health care administrators, health policy makers, payers, and the information professionals who serve these groups; to improve access to data and information needed by the creators of health services research; and to contribute to the information infrastructure needed to foster patient record systems that can produce useful health services research data as a by-product of providing health care* (http://www.nlm.nih.gov/hsrinfo).

As the cost of health care in the United States continues to increase, amounting to almost $3 trillion in 2013, HSR has the ability to make major contributions to the future of medicine. Clinical research has long shaped the practice of medicine, but HSR looks to study the infrastructure of practicing medicine. The following sections contain examples of HSR.

### DATA REGISTRY STUDIES

Large national and state registries provide the patient health care data needed for HSR. In 1971, the National Cancer Act provided funding to the National Cancer Institute (NCI) to detect, treat, and perform research on cancers in the United States. In 1973, the Surveillance, Epidemiology, and End Results (SEER) Program of NCI was established as the first national cancer registry. The SEER registry "collects and publishes cancer incidence and survival data from population-based cancer registries...on patient demographics, primary tumor site, tumor morphology and stage at diagnosis, first course of treatment, and follow-up for vital status" (http://seer.cancer.gov). The SEER database is updated annually and provided to the public. Since 1998, the Centers for Disease Control and Prevention (CDC), the American Cancer Society (ACS), the NCI, and the North American Association of Central Cancer Registries have collaborated on the Annual Report to the Nation on the Status of Cancer. Countless researchers and clinicians, along with legislators and policy makers, use SEER data. In 2015, Dinkelspiel and colleagues published SEER data on ovarian cancer from 1988 to 2012 comparing the causes of death by stage, age, and interval time after diagnosis (Dinkelspiel, 2015). SEER and CMS have also partnered to form the SEER-Medicare database. SEER continues to collect clinical and demographic information, whereas CMS provides Medicare claims for covered health care services of patients with Medicare eligibility until death. The linkage of these two data sources allows for a unique collaboration incorporating epidemiologic and health services research. Forde and associates used the SEER-Medicare database to examine the cost of treatment for elderly women with ovarian cancer in the Medicare population. Neo-adjuvant chemotherapy (NACT) and primary debulking surgery (PDS) were compared for cost and effectiveness (Forde, 2015). NACT and PDS were comparable in stage IIIC disease, whereas PDS was associated with a 12% increase in cost in stage IV disease. In both groups, NACT was associated with a decreased 5-year overall survival (OS) with hazard ratio (HR) of 1.27 and 1.19, respectively. Although cancer registries have been mentioned here, there are a number of data registries for patients. CMS and the National Institute of Diabetes and Digestive and Kidney Disease (NIDDK) have collaborated on the United States Renal Data System (USRDS) to collect and analyze data on patients with end stage renal disease (www.usrds.org).

### QUALITY IMPROVEMENT

Quality improvement (QI) is a unique format of HSR, encompassing both research and QI program development to improve the quality of health care. The Institute of Medicine (IOM) defines quality in health care as a direct correlation between the level of improved health services and the desired health outcomes of individuals and populations (www.iom.edu). QI projects can be developed and conducted within small practices, in large hospital systems, or on a much larger national and international scale. The Health Resources and Services Administration (HRSA) under the U.S. Department of Health and Human Services provides a toolkit to help QI programs develop and implement QI projects (www.hrsa.gov). There are numerous organizations and committees whose sole purpose is to examine the issue of health care quality. In 1990, the National Committee for Quality Assurance was founded as a not-for-profit organization to help build consensus around important health care quality issues. It has a simple formula: "measure, analyze, improve, repeat" (www.ncqa.org). The National Quality Forum (NQF) is a not-for-profit, nonpartisan, membership-based organization whose mission is to "lead national collaborations to improve health and healthcare quality through measurement" (qualityforum.org). Its vision is "to be the convener of key public and private sector leaders to establish national priorities and goals to achieve healthcare that is safe, effective, patient-centered, timely, efficient, and equitable." The American Medical Association (AMA) also convenes the Physician Consortium for Performance Improvement (PCPI). It is a physician-led program with a mission "to align patient-centered care, performance measurement and quality improvement" (www.ama-assn.org). The U.S. Centers of Medicare and Medicaid Services (CMS) Physician Quality Reporting System (PQRS) is a quality reporting program on the care given to Medicare beneficiaries. In 2015, the CMS will begin applying a negative payment adjustment to providers and groups who did not meet requirements of reporting data to PQRS. In 2018, PQRS will begin using these reported quality measures to make reimbursement decisions based on quality of care given to Medicare beneficiaries. The role of quality improvement is also felt heavily in surgical specialties.

CMS and other payers are increasingly refusing to pay for complications of surgery that are deemed preventable. The American College of Surgeons National Surgical Quality Improvement Program (ACS NSQIP) helps surgeons and hospitals identify preventable surgical complications. Data are collected directly from patients' charts by a surgical clinical reviewer (SCR), in contrast to collecting data from billing codes. In 2009, Hall and colleagues published data on 118 hospitals nationally participating in ACS NSQIP from 2006 to 2007 reporting that 82% of hospitals had improved risk-adjusted complication rates and 66% of hospitals had improved risk-adjusted mortality as compared to their own prior rates reported the year prior (Hall, 2009). By the end of 2007, ACS NSQIP had enrolled 183 hospitals, reporting that participating hospitals avoided on average 52.5 complications per year. ACS NSQIP helps identify and rectify preventable surgical outcomes; QI projects are a necessity for all health care providers and health care institutions.

## COST-EFFECTIVENESS ANALYSIS

The term *cost-effectiveness analysis* has become a catch phrase referring to all health economic analyses. As the cost of health care continues to rise in the United States, now expected to exceed $3 trillion in 2015, health economic analysis is more relevant than ever. There are four methods of health economic analysis, with cost-effectiveness analysis (CEA) being one of the more commonly used methods. The other three methods include cost-utility analysis (CUA), cost-minimization analysis (CMA), and cost-benefit analysis (CBA). CEA and CUA are used most often. CEA is most often used among economic analysis tools and is a comparison of relative costs and outcomes of varying treatments. It is a measure of cost per unit of effectiveness (additional survival time, number of adverse events, etc.). It determines incremental cost-effectiveness ratio (ICER), or the ratio of the difference in costs to the difference in effectiveness between two strategies. It is most often used in the allocation of resources for treatment or intervention. CUA takes into account the quality of life associated with each intervention. The number of quality-adjusted life years (QALY) is the most common metric used for comparison and represents the differences in survival and quality of life between interventions. CUA is an important effectiveness measure when morbidity and mortality are affected by an intervention. CMA assumes comparable effectiveness among intervention strategies and thus is just a comparison of the mean cost of each intervention. CBA incorporates not only the monetary expense of intervention but also the costs of the consequences of each intervention.

In CEA an intervention has traditionally been considered cost-effective if the ICER is less than $50,000 per QALY, with some leeway. It is important to understand that the term "cost-effective" does not represent that an intervention saves money but rather means that the additional cost of that intervention is worthwhile based on the improved effectiveness achieved. In 2009, Kim and coworkers published a CEA on the addition of the human papillomavirus (HPV) vaccination to routine cervical cancer screening in women older than 30 years in the United States. The estimated ICER for the addition of the vaccine ranged from $116,950 to 381,590 per QALY, which greatly exceeds the standard threshold of $50,000. It was concluded that the addition of the HPV vaccination to routine screening in women over the age of 30 years in the United States is not cost effective (Kim, 2009). These types of studies are flourishing as the cost of health care in the United States continues to rise. They are an integral part of understanding the costs and quality of health care.

## NEW HORIZONS: VALUE IN HEALTH CARE

The discussion of value in health care is currently gaining interest. Value in health care is defined as "the health outcomes achieved per dollar spent" (Porter, 2006). Outcomes are inherently linked to the medical condition of interest, whereas the dollar spent represents the total amount spent during a cycle of care, not the cost of individual service. Porter argued:

> *The proper unit for measuring value should encompass all services or activities that jointly determine success in meeting a set of patient needs. These needs are determined by the patient's medical condition, defined as an interrelated set of medical circumstances that are best addressed in an integrated way...and that value should be measured for everything included in that care* (Porter, 2010).

Large clinical societies are getting involved with defining the value of health care. The American Society of Clinical Oncology (ASCO) is developing a conceptual framework to assess the value of cancer treatment options (Schnipper, 2015). As the cost of new treatments for cancer continues to rise, the value of this care is an important question. Value in health care is in its infancy but shows promise in navigating the ever-increasing costs of health care.

## ACKNOWLEDGMENT

The authors wish to acknowledge the contributions of Dr. Vern Katz, the author of the previous edition of this chapter.

## KEY POINTS

- Evidence-based medicine seeks to improve the care of patients and the delivery of care to patients.
- Descriptive-observational studies, including cross-sectional studies and case series, help generate hypotheses and characterize the context of disease.
- Cohort studies allow us to study many outcomes over time.
- Case-control studies allow us to study rare diseases and evaluate for a wide range of exposures.
- RCTs are considered to be the gold standard of experimental clinical study design.
- PCTs are designed to study the effectiveness of an intervention in the real world.
- CER encompasses patient-centered research, PCTs, meta-analyses, systematic reviews, evidence-based guidelines, and health services research to study the benefits and harms of an intervention to improve patient care on the individual and population level.
- Estimating the value of health care involves an assessment of the quality and integration of care, as well as the overall cost to provide all services included in that care.

## KEY REFERENCES


Centers for Disease Control and Prevention (CDC). Pneumocystis pneumonia—Los Angeles. *MMWR.* 1981;30(21):250-252.

Cochrane AL. *Effectiveness and efficiency: Random reflections on health services.* London: Nuffield Provincial Hospitals Trust, 1971.

Congressional Budget Office (CBO). *Research on the Comparative Effectiveness of Medical Treatments: Issues and Options for an Expanded Federal Role.* Washington, DC: CBO; 2007.

D'Arcy LP, Rich EC. From comparative effectiveness research to patient-centered outcomes research: policy history and future directions. *Neurosurg Focus.* 2012;33(1):E7.

Dinkelspiel HE, Champer M, Hou J, et al. Long-term mortality among women with epithelial ovarian cancer. *Gynecol Oncol.* 2015;138(2):421-428.

Forde GK, Chang J, Ziogas A, et al. Costs of treatment for elderly women with advanced ovarian cancer in a Medicare population. *Gynecol Oncol.* 2015;137(3):479-484.

Gayle HD, Keeling RP, Garcia-Tunon M, et al. Prevalence of the human immunodeficiency virus among university students. *N Engl J Med.* 1990; 323(22):1538-1541.

Gehlback SH. *Interpreting the Medical Literature.* 4th edition. New York: McGraw-Hill; 2002.

Grimes DA, Schulz KF. Descriptive studies: what they can and cannot do. *Lancet.* 2002;359:145-149.

Grimes DA, Schulz KF. Surrogate end points in clinical research: hazardous to your health. *Obstet Gynecol.* 2005;105:1114-1118.

Grodstein F, Manson JE, Stampfer MJ. Postmenopausal hormone use and secondary prevention of coronary events in the Nurses Health Study. *Ann Intern Med.* 2001;135(1):1-8.

Grondin SC, Schieman C. Evidence-based medicine: levels of evidence and evaluation systems. In: *Difficult Decisions in Thoracic Surgery.* London: Springer-Verlag; 2011.

Hall BL, Hamilton BH, Richards K, et al. Does surgical quality improve in the American College of Surgeons National Surgical Quality Improvement Program: an evaluation of all participating hospitals. *Ann Surg.* 2009;250(3):363-376.

Havrilesky LH, et al. Comparative effectiveness research in gynecologic oncology. In: Barakat RR, Berchuck A, et al. eds. *Principles and Practice of Gynecologic Oncology.* 6th edition. Philadelphia: Lippincott Williams & Wilkins; 2013a:501-521.

Havrilesky LJ, Moorman PG, Lowery WJ, et al. Oral contraceptive pills as primary prevention for ovarian cancer: a systematic review and meta-analysis. *Obstet Gynecol.* 2013b;122(1):139-147.

Hennekens CH, DeMets D. The need for large-scale randomized evidence without undue emphasis on small trials, meta-analyses, or subgroup analyses. *JAMA.* 2009;302:2361-2362.

Herbst AL, Ulfelder H, Poskanzer DC. Adenocarcinoma of the vagina: association of maternal stilbestrol therapy with tumor appearance in young women. *N Engl J Med.* 1971;284(16):878-881.

Higgins JPT, Green S, eds. *Cochrane Handbook for Systematic Reviews of Interventions* Version 5.1.0 [updated March 2011]. The Cochrane Collaboration; 2011. Available at. www.cochrane-handbook.org.

Iglehart JK. Prioritzing comparative-effectiveness research—IOM recommendations. *N Engl J Med.* 2009;361(4):325-328.

Institute of Medicine (IOM). *Initial National Priorities for Comparative Effectiveness Research.* Washington, DC: The National Academies Press; 2009.

Kim JJ, Ortendahl J, Goldie SJ. Cost-effectivenes of human papillomavirus vaccination and cervical cancer screening in women older than 30 years in the United States. *Ann Intern Med.* 2009;151:538-545.

Patient Protection and Affordable Care Act, 42 U.S.C. § 18001, 2010.

Porter ME, Teisberg EO. *Redefining Health Care: Creating Value-Based Competition Based on Results.* Boston: Harvard Business School Press; 2006.

Porter ME. What is value in healthcare? *N Engl J Med.* 2010;363(26): 2477-2481.

Roland M, Torgerson DJ. What are pragmatic trials? *BMJ.* 1998; 316(7127):285.

Rossouw JE, Anderson JL, Prentice RL, et al. Risks and benefits of estrogen plus progesterone in health postmenopausal women: principle results from the women's health initiative randomized controlled trial. *JAMA.* 2002;288(3):321-333.

Schnipper LE, Davidson NE, Wollins DS, et al. American Society of Clinical Oncology Statement: A conceptual framework to assess the value of cancer treatment options. *J Clin Oncol.* 2015;33(23):2563-2577.

Schwartz D, Lellouch J. Explanatory and pragmatic attitudes in therapeutic trials. *J Chronic Dis.* 1967;20(8):637-648.

Skaznik-Wikiel ME, Sukumvanich P, Beriwal S, et al. Possible use of Ca-125 level normalization after the third chemotherapy cycle in deciding on chemotherapy regimen in patients with epithelial ovarian cancer: brief report. *Int J Gynecol Cancer.* 2011;21(6):1013-1017.

Stewart S, Ball J, Horowitz JD, et al. Standard versus atrial fibrillation-specific management strategy (SAFETY) to reduce recurrent admission and prolong survival: pragmatic, multicenter, randomized controlled trial. *Lancet.* 2015;385:775-784.


Suggested Readings can be found on ExpertConsult.com.

# 6 Medical-Legal Risk Management

*James M. Kelley III, Gretchen M. Lentz*

The word *malpractice* evokes guttural responses in physicians and health care providers. This is perhaps most true in the areas of obstetrics and gynecology, where the physical damages are often catastrophic and the economic damages reach the millions of dollars. The fear of being unjustly involved in litigation and judged by nonphysicians as liable—despite having provided reasonable and appropriate care—seems unavoidable to many conscientious health care providers. The little known reality, however, is that the growing consensus of empirical data on outcomes of malpractice actions shows that the legal system actually works for the health care provider more often than it does not. Understanding how the system works and making minor practice modifications can greatly minimize the risk of legal exposure by avoiding claims and adverse outcomes.

A medical negligence case is composed of three basic elements: a deviation from the standard of care, proximate causation, and damages. Each of these elements is required to be proved by way of "competent" expert testimony. The definition of "competent" varies state to state, but all states are uniform in requiring a physician to agree that malpractice occurred and that it directly resulted in injury. A deviation from the standard of care, though a cumbersome legal phrase, is simply a failure to act reasonably as compared with another health care provider in the same or similar clinical circumstance. A deviation from the standard of care can be an act (intraoperative bowel perforation, administration of the wrong medication, etc.) or an omission (failure to run the bowel intraoperatively if a bowel injury is possible or failure to review laboratory results in a timely manner).

Proximate causation is often a more medically complex component of a malpractice action. The law requires that the deviation from the standard of care be *a* direct, proximate cause of injury to the plaintiff. It is important to note that the deviation does not have to be *the* exclusive cause of injury, but rather need only be *a* direct proximate cause. Proximate cause, legally, merely means that with appropriate or reasonable treatment, the injury would not have occurred.

The final element of a malpractice claim is damages. Damages can be both economic and noneconomic. Economic damages include easily quantifiable losses as past and future medical bills and past and future wage losses. Noneconomic damages contemplate factors such as past and future physical pain, emotional suffering, and, in certain instances, wrongful death. To be successful, the plaintiff must prove each of these elements to a probability, through expert testimony, in order to win. A failure on any one of the elements will result in a verdict for the defendant.

As mentioned, many health care providers will be surprised to learn what the growing consensus of empirical data reflects regarding medical claims. A review of approximately 1400 closed malpractice claims from five different liability carriers showed that only 3% of claims filed had no verifiable medical injuries to justify a claim. Additionally, 37% of the 3% did not involve errors but rather would be what a physician would commonly refer to as "frivolous." Despite common perceptions about runaway juries and lottery verdicts levied against faultless physicians, the study demonstrated that 84% of the claims that did not involve errors nonetheless resulted in nonpayment. Conversely, approximately six times that rate of claims resulted in nonpayment to the plaintiff, despite the presence of medical errors and verifiable injuries (Studdert, 2006) (Box 6.1).

Although these data should be heartening for health care providers, they do little to eliminate burdens of excessive litigation costs, time away from practice and families, and the stress of participating in litigation. The goal for conscientious providers must be one focused on risk management: balancing improved patient care and minimizing medical legal risk.

A safe health care system must further incorporate efficient redundancies that promote safety without being cost prohibitive. "Errors can be prevented by designing systems that make it hard for people to do the wrong thing and easy to do the right thing" (IOM, 2000).

Realizing lawsuits will inevitably occur, what follows is a brief historical overview along with practical insights aimed at helping one enhance patient care and communication, minimize the risk of involvement in meritless litigation, and provide the best defense in the event a claim is made.

**Box 6.1 What Constitutes Medical Practice?**

To successfully maintain a medical malpractice action, a plaintiff must be able to establish three distinct elements of his or her case by way of expert testimony:

1. *Deviation from the standard of care:* The health care provider deviated from what a reasonable provider would have done in the same or similar circumstances.
2. *Causation*: The deviation was a direct cause of the injury suffered.
3. *Damages*: Economic and noneconomic damages were suffered as result of the injury.

## HISTORICAL PERSPECTIVE

*A doctor who knows nothing of the law and a lawyer who knows nothing of medicine are deficient in essential requisites of their professions.*

—David Paul Brown 1795-1872

British North America inherited its law, as its language, from England. Most European countries originally occupied by the Romans adopted a form of law based on the Roman law codes. That law is called *civil law.* England's law, on the other hand, was based mainly on Scandinavian (Danish) law with a dose of folk law of undetermined origin thrown in. It was called the *common law.* One should not be deceived by its name. It was not law designed to protect the common man. It takes its name from the fact that it was the law that was common to all of England by about the year 1240. The two forms of law differ significantly.

Civil law is a codified system of laws. That is, the laws are spelled out in a series of written statutes adopted by the jurisdiction. Civil law therefore tends to be fairly static. Common law is largely law made by judges. It may incorporate some statutory elements on specific issues, but even statutes are subject to judicial interpretation. Judges in the civil law are academics specially trained for their positions and act as prosecutor, judge, and jury. Civil law is therefore inquisitorial in nature and heavily dependent on the written word. In contrast, common law is an adversarial system in which the oral argument between the parties plays a much larger role. Judges are chosen from the practicing bar and are not usually academics. The judge is essentially a referee and instructs the jury, which makes the ultimate decision on the merits of the case. In common law, the law is made by judges who hear a disputed case on appeal. Those decisions become precedent for future cases. However, higher appellate courts or future appellate courts of the same level can overturn or overrule a prior decision if circumstances change or new information develops. Therefore change, albeit slow and irregular, is a constant element of the common law.

Under the early common law to bring a civil action a King's Writ was needed, therefore little attention was paid to compensating the individual for personal wrongs (tort law). Doctors were essentially immune from suit for malpractice. Technically some suits might have been pursued as contract suits, but written contracts were highly unusual between a physician and his patient, and without the written document such suits became almost impossible for the plaintiff to win.

In 1346 the bubonic plague arrived in Italy. It spread over Europe rapidly but did not reach England until 1348. The major effect of the epidemic occurred between 1348 and 1351, but the bubonic plague became endemic and continued more or less uninterrupted until 1381. It is estimated that between 1348 and 1351, 50% of the population died, and by 1381 two thirds of the English population was decimated by the epidemic. (Because there was no accurate census at the time, such figures are estimates based on church records, burial records, tax rolls, and contemporary accounts.)

The loss of manpower was a major blow to the English economy. Overnight, people became as important as real property (land) and personal property (including livestock) in the English economy. Therefore a physician's mistake that deprived the economy of a worker became an important enough matter to be brought before the courts. Physicians suddenly lost their immunity for practice errors. Actually it was an even worse scenario: the physician became strictly liable for an unfavorable outcome, and because there was no tort law (law compensating the individual for personal wrongs), the physician was prosecuted under the criminal law for mayhem. By 1364, it had become obvious that this was too draconian a remedy, and two property terms that had been previously used in livestock cases were introduced to permit civil malpractice cases. *Trespass* (trespass by force and arms) was charged for direct injury and *trespass on the case* for indirect injury.

These same concepts, refined over the centuries, were brought to the North American colonies and adopted almost entirely by the American court system after independence. In the early 1800s the modern concept of negligence replaced trespass and trespass on the case. In the period of rapid industrialization following the Civil War, American courts refined these claims. The four elements of a cause of action for medical negligence are as follows:

1. *Duty:* The obligation created through physician patient relationship.
2. *Breach:* A deviation from the "standard of care" for a reasonable practitioner in the same clinical circumstance.
3. *Proximate causation:* A direct and foreseeable connection between breach and injury.
4. *Damages:* Economic (medical costs, wage loss, etc.) and noneconomic (physical and emotional pain and suffering).

There is no greater asset in risk management for the clinician than a strong physician-patient relationship. Patients are typically trusting and respectful of their providers, which gives the best opportunity to avoid litigation. The typical patient will become a plaintiff when he or she loses trust in the provider or fails to get understandable answers to the complex medical issues surrounding a less than optimal outcome. "I don't know or understand either what happened or how this happened?" is the question that begins nearly all inquiries into the quality of care. This chapter provides insights that will allow the physician to supply answers to the patient, to document appropriately, and to participate more functionally in a medical-legal claim while maintaining a high level of care and professionalism.

## REPRODUCTIVE MEDICINE AND THE COURTS

No area of medicine receives more court scrutiny, legal scholarly review, or social commentary (even including presidential directives) than the fields of obstetrics and gynecology. In addition, it is common that the most expensive category of malpractice claims arise from the obstetrician/gynecologist's practice (pregnancy/birth claims, failure to diagnose breast cancer, failure to diagnose cervical cancer). Practically speaking, nearly every malpractice issue that has been litigated in American courts deserves a volume of its own to discuss and dissect adequately. Indeed, a single chapter in a general textbook of gynecology can do little but cover the generalities and touch on the more important issues the courts have addressed. Overall, applying the four elements noted previously to most claims, a malpractice case is typically a review of case facts applied to the "standard of care" and "proximate cause" through medical testimony to determine if care was simply "reasonable." It is important to note that the care does not have to be perfect nor do all decisions have to be correct. Instead, if care is attentive and the decisions rational, the provider will have a strong defense position regardless of outcome.

## PRACTICAL INSIGHT

Medical-legal risk management, at its core, centers on communication in both the written and verbal form. Awareness of the common pitfalls in the processes employed in communicating information to patients, as well as concurrent and subsequent care providers, will be invaluable if problems or litigation arise. The medical record, institutional policies and guidelines, and information communicated to patients (prospective plaintiffs) will be the only information attorneys, claim representatives, and reviewing expert physicians have available to judge the validity of a potential malpractice claim. The following discussion examines good practices to improve communications with patients (both before and after treatment), improve the accuracy of the medical records, and provide useful information about navigating the litigation process to your best outcome.

### *COMMUNICATION WITH THE PATIENT*

Physicians well understand that the relationship with a patient is in large measure a relationship of trust. More often than not, a perceived breach of that trust is the impetus for a patient to seek the advice of an outsider for explanations about unfortunate medical outcomes. It must become a routine practice for physicians to thoroughly and carefully discuss potential problems with their patients prior to treatment. Taking the time necessary to assess a patient's understanding of the procedures and possible outcomes, and answering all questions the patient may have, are critical to managing and controlling expectations. Concurrent notations in the record that you have in fact reviewed all risks and benefits of a potential treatment, thoroughly explained alternative treatments or procedures, and answered all patient questions will provide important evidence of careful and appropriate treatment, should it later become necessary (Box 6.2).

The eleven words in the sample progress note are an invaluable resource in the event of a complication or litigation. Although this is brief documentation, it does indicate the physician personally reviewed the critical elements mentioned earlier and allowed for questions. This note portrays the provider discussing the case with the patient, which will supplement the standard preprinted consent that is more "legalese" than substantive.

**Box 6.2 Practice Tip**

**Sample Progress Note**
Risks/benefits/alternatives discussed with patient. All questions answered in full.

### *POOR OUTCOME*

In the unfortunate event of a poor outcome, it is imperative for the physician to communicate more, not less, with the patient or the patient's family where appropriate. Health care providers often dramatically change—or end entirely—their relationship with patients following a maloccurrence. For example, in situations in which the patient may have ongoing care issues but is transferred to a tertiary center or a different specialist, there is often minimal or no ongoing relationship. Despite what may be the urge to distance yourself from an unpleasant or uncomfortable interaction, keep in mind that your patient and his or her family members will begin to assess whether you are forthcoming with them at this very time. If there is an attempt to avoid interaction it can, and likely will, be misperceived as an attempt to avoid explaining the cause or causes of the bad outcome. It is important that your trust relationship with the patient and the patient's family continues at this crucial time and that they feel you are willing to answer all questions.

When discussing the outcome or problem, revisit the discussion of risks and outcomes at the time of the informed consent. Reiterate the information you previously provided, and explain how this result is related to the risks previously discussed, if appropriate. Finally, it is also important that you are involved in establishing the plan for care going forward, even if it is outside of your specialty. Remaining involved preserves the physician-patient relationship. Patients are far less likely to file claims against physicians with whom they have an ongoing, trusting relationship. It is therefore important to make yourself available as long as is necessary to assure the patient and his or her family that you are answering all of their questions. Absence or avoidance will create suspicion by the patient or another family member and can ultimately lead them to seek answers to their questions from an outside source, most often an attorney.

Once again, it is imperative you write contemporaneous and accurate notes. The timing of such notes, combined with their detail and clarity, will begin to establish a good defense in the event the records are reviewed for a possible claim. It is easy to defend conscientious care, regardless of outcome, if the record supports you (Box 6.3).

### *CANCELLATIONS AND "NO SHOWS"*

Cancellations and "no shows" of patients' follow-up appointments are often ignored in the busy clinic or office. They can be, and are, frequently responsible for subsequent malpractice suits. Each cancellation or no show should be documented in the chart. The treating physician should then review the chart and, where appropriate, a letter or phone call should be made to the patient. All efforts to communicate with the patient should be documented.

### *COVERAGE ARRANGEMENTS*

As mentioned earlier, improper coverage arrangements may lead to charges of abandonment. Poor communication among coverage groups frequently leads to offended patients and can be the first step on the path to a malpractice suit.

**Box 6.3 Practice Tip**

Communication with the patient when a problem occurs is an opportunity to explain how the poor outcome happened, despite vigilance. Patients will naturally have questions, and most who contact a malpractice attorney are doing so to get answers to questions they feel were not sufficiently answered by the health care provider.

## MEDICATION ERRORS

About 1.5 million people are injured each year in the United States due to medication errors, the Institutes of Medicine of the National Academy of Sciences revealed in a 2006 review of medication management in the U.S. heath care system (IOM, 2007). The study reveals medication errors make up a large share of medical malpractice cases. The results can range from minor allergic response to death. Medications pose risk to both the institution and the provider for liability.

The reasons behind this include, but are not limited to, the frequency with which patients are being prescribed medication, the popularity of at-home prescription administration, and the many look-alike, sound-alike, drugs. The Institute of Medicine report states, "The extra medical cost of treating drug-related injuries occurring in hospitals alone conservatively amounts to $3.5 billion a year, and this estimate does not take into account lost wages and productivity or additional health care costs" (IOM, 2007).

Medication errors are always preventable, through system and personal practice modifications. Data show that 400,000 preventable drug-related injuries occur each year in hospitals (IOM, 2007). Another report states that adverse drug events cause more than 770,000 injuries and deaths each year and cost up to $5.6 million per hospital (AHRQ, 2015).

The National Coordinating Council for Medication Error and Prevention has approved the following definition of medication error:

> *Any preventable event that may cause or lead to inappropriate medication use or patient harm, while the medication is in the control of the health care professional, patient, or consumer. Such events may be related to professional practice, health care products, procedures, and systems including: prescribing; order communication; product labeling, packaging and nomenclature; compounding; dispensing; distribution; administration; education; monitoring; and use* (FDA, 2016).

### Practical Tip

The reality of practice is that many orders are verbal, telephonic, or standing. Verbal or telephonic orders should always be read back to the provider to verify drug, dosage, frequency, and method of administration. This minimizes the likelihood of a communication lapse. Furthermore, telephonic orders are frequently later signed after the medication is administered. Closely review these to be sure you are not validating the error as your own order. Litigation is often more than a year later, and memory of the details will be a challenge with a record that is inconsistent. If upon review an error is noted, correct it in the record with a single line and the corrected information at the side. Time and date your correction as well.

Be aware of your orders as well as those of other providers, anesthesia, infectious disease, and so on to be aware of interactions of medications also. Standing orders often pose a risk in this circumstance.

## COMMUNICATION THROUGH MEDICAL RECORDS

Once the litigation process has commenced, a plaintiff attorney's best friend is inaccurate or inconsistent documentation of the care provided. Inaccurate documentation can stem from a genuine standard-of-care issue; however, inaccuracies can also arise from use of inappropriate nomenclature. In either situation, the health care provider will be in the untenable position of attempting to defend a narrative note or deposition testimony that is factually inconsistent with literature, policies, or objective data in the medical record. Needless to say, in a courtroom, inconsistencies never favor the inconsistent party. Careful attention to record keeping will not only demonstrate attentive care and rationally based treatment decisions but will ultimately become a provider's best defense in a courtroom.

Within your hospital, facility, office, and charts, you must use nomenclature designed to standardize the verbiage utilized among providers. Unfortunately, despite the attempts at standardization, many health care providers have been slow to adapt. This is often based on variable levels of education by authors and is also generational. This increases not only the risk of inaccurate communication between health care providers but also the risk of a medical record replete with inconsistencies. Inconsistencies can be easily used to portray a provider as incompetent or disingenuous.

From a medicolegal risk management standpoint, it is critical to keep in mind when a plaintiff's counsel attempts to determine whether medical malpractice may have occurred, the medical record is the primary (and often the only) source of information available to evaluate the potential claim. Any narrative notes supplied will be read against subsequent health care providers' notes and the objective data such as lab results and imaging. As stated earlier, clearly noted and accurate recognition and description of reassuring and nonreassuring findings in the record will demonstrate attentive and competent care. However, inaccurate terminology, when read against the objective data, could result in the commencement of litigation.

Beyond the initial review phase of a potential claim, inconsistent and inaccurate nomenclature and record keeping will continue to present obstacles to a favorable resolution of the claim during the testimonial phase of trial. When a witness employs modified or nonstandardized nomenclature, other health care providers, including expert medical witnesses, do not necessarily understand the full extent of what is meant. This unclear communication can result in actual medical errors among providers or, at a minimum, the appearance of errors within a medical record (Box 6.4).

The example shows how the inappropriate and inconsistent nomenclature forced the physician to be critical of the nurse's actions, while the nurse attempted to separate herself from her own charting. This is not only a difficult posture to defend, but also it reflects poorly on the competency and truthfulness of the parties involved. Simply employing appropriate, consistent nomenclature would have provided an easy defense (Box 6.5).

## ALTERATION OF RECORDS

A medical malpractice case can go from defensible to indefensible immediately with an alteration of the record. An alteration is typically defined as an entry added to or redacted from the record to avoid culpability. An alteration in many states is a basis for punitive damages (noninsured). Furthermore, it may invalidate coverage under some professional policies. Most providers do not add for the purpose of deceit but to make the record more

**Box 6.4 Factual Scenario**

In a previous deposition, a physician was questioned regarding a nursing narrative note:

Q. Dr. Doe, do you expect the nurse to relay to you if there are any postoperative changes?
A. Any relevant postoperative changes should be relayed to me, particularly if there are more than one.
Q. By relevant change, do you mean if any vital signs manifest persistent change?
A. I do not understand what that means. However, if a nurse sees vitals change, I want to know about it immediately, especially if it persists.

The narrative notes within the case included the nurse describing labile blood pressures. Utilizing charting terminology such as *labile* created a scenario in which the physician had expectations of being told immediately and a medical record suggesting the call should have been made. Further testimony demonstrated that no information regarding these changes was relayed. The nurse testified as follows:

Q. Did you relay to Dr. Doe that the blood pressures were labile?
A. No.
Q. Why not?
A. Because I felt it was not necessarily significant and may be routine post-op fluctuations.
Q. So you felt it was unstable but not labile?
A. Yes.
Q. So when you chart the word *labile*, you want the jury to believe it doesn't mean labile?
A. I guess.

**Box 6.5 Practice Tip**

The consistent use of appropriate nomenclature not only minimizes risk in the defense of a medical legal action but also allows the physicians and nurses to communicate clearly by ensuring they are discussing the same findings and placing the same significance.

"complete" after an unfortunate outcome. Accordingly, it is not typical to chart after a shift has passed. In the event it is necessary, clearly note the entry as a "late entry" and date when it is entered and to when it refers. There is nothing wrong with a late entry if you accurately describe it as such. Today, technology can discern the sequence through impression as to when notes were written and if the ink is the same through infrared light. A record that can be alleged to be altered will cause a loss of credibility with any jury and may expose you to personal liability.

## COMMUNICATION CONSISTENT WITH INSTITUTIONAL POLICIES

Published institutional policies and procedures should be reviewed regularly and integrated into your daily practice. The purpose of the policies or protocols is not merely for JCAHO, or to fill shelf space, but to effectuate patient care and create a consistent safe administration of the medication and care to patients. However, each individual patient obviously deserves individual care and modifications to the policy or protocol as may be necessary. Policies and protocols relevant to the issues that are the bases of any litigation should be familiar to you *before* providing sworn testimony under oath. Because these written policies can form the basis of an accepted standard of care in your institution, any testimony or records inconsistent with these policies can be viewed by a jury as being outside the standard of care, or negligent (Box 6.6).

**Box 6.6 Factual Scenario**

Many gynecologic cases involve the failure to recognize postoperative bowel perforations or significant bleeding. Total abdominal hysterectomy usually carries with it a specific physician's postoperative orders or, more commonly, a hospital's postoperative policy or protocol. It is of critical importance that the nurse and physician both have an understanding of the specific details of the policy or protocol prior to executing care and prior to testifying regarding these issues. The following example highlights why this is important:

Q. Are you aware as to whether or not there is a postoperative policy at this facility?
A. I don't know. I guess there probably is.
Q. Do you agree that you, as a reasonable nurse, have a duty to follow the policy here at the facility?
A. I don't really know what the policy says, but I'm sure it's reasonable and yes I should probably follow it.
Q. If you failed to follow the policy, can we agree that you would have been acting unreasonably and beneath the accepted standards of care?
A. I probably should follow a policy if it exists. I guess if I didn't, I was beneath the standard of care.

The nurse went on to define terms differently from the definition contained in the policy and testified that the physician with whom she was working was aware of her actions. When the physician was questioned, he testified as follows:

Q. Do you expect the nurses to follow your specific orders and, when orders are not present specific to the chart, to follow policies or protocols that are in place for the delivery of health care to patients?
A. Absolutely.
Q. For this patient, did you write a specific postoperative order?
A. No.
Q. Your order says, "post total abdominal hysterectomy protocol"?
A. Yes.
Q. Does that mean the nurse should follow the hospital's policy or protocol?
A. Absolutely.
Q. Is a reasonable nurse allowed to deviate from that policy or protocol without calling you first?
A. No.

In the boxed example, a lack of familiarity with the standard policy within the hospital created a scenario in which the physician and nurse were uncertain as to what the hospital expected. Compounding matters, the lack of familiarity with the policy and protocol prior to deposition created a scenario in which not only did the nurse provide testimony that she deviated from the policy but also she was forced to acknowledge a total lack of familiarity with the same. In short, knowledge of and compliance with institutional policies, guidelines, and resources can demonstrate the implementation of appropriate care and documentation can be the shield of your defense; conversely, ignorance of and deviation from such policies can provide a documented deviation from the standard of care that will be the sword of the plaintiff.

### *WHEN A CLAIM IS MADE*

The institution of a claim varies from state to state and is defined differently among various insurance policies. It is imperative that you have an understanding through your institution, insurance policy, and within your state as to what constitutes knowledge or notice of a claim. When notice of a claim is received, it is imperative that you immediately notify your hospital or group administrator and your insurance company. A failure to timely notify individuals can jeopardize insurance coverage or compromise your defense, and in a worst-case scenario may potentially result in a default judgment for failure to timely respond. Although the legal system does move slowly, there are certain parameters, and timely responses are mandatory at the beginning of litigation.

Participation in a claim is aggravating, frightening, and an imposition on your professional or personal time. However, it is critical to avoid procrastination or de-prioritization of the claim regardless of the level of merit or damages perceived by you. A lawsuit is typically commenced by the filing of a legal pleading known as a "complaint." Thereafter, there will be a statutory amount of time for an "answer" to be filed on your behalf. The first portion of litigation is thereafter referred to as "discovery." This is where each side exchanges information either through documents or sworn testimony between the sides—first regarding factual information, then regarding expert opinions in the claim. A deposition is simply the opposing attorney's opportunity to ask questions under oath that are reasonably calculated to lead to relevant discoverable evidence.

Your deposition is an obligation, not an opportunity. In that regard, it is critical that you meet with your attorney in advance of your deposition so that you can be prepared for the relevant issues. A critical review of your care with your attorney is important so that you that can anticipate all areas of questioning and avoid surprise questioning under oath. The answers you give under oath are sworn testimony in the case, and often depositions circulate through the legal community even after the case closes. It is recommended that you meet at least 1 week in advance of your deposition with counsel for a preparatory session, which will allow you adequate time in the event your practice requires rescheduling that meeting, before you actually give your testimony at deposition. Additional preparation could include a mock deposition, or simulation in a question-and-answer format, with another attorney to give you a sense of the actual deposition. This can be very useful to isolate and review medically complex issues and to enhance your preparation for giving sworn testimony.

Your deposition testimony, along with that of the other factual witnesses, will supplement the medical record for the expert witnesses retained by all parties to litigation to utilize in formulating their opinions and testimony. All of which, in turn, will ultimately become the evidence jurors will use to judge which positions they find most reasonable. Accordingly, just as accurate, concise, and consistent communication in your medical record is a priority, so too should it be within your deposition.

Following discovery, cases are usually scheduled for jury trials based on individual court docket systems. You should plan on attending each day of your trial and participating in the trial all day and some evenings. Although it is no physician's desire to take time away from his or her practice to be in a courtroom, it is imperative that when you arrive, you have an accurate medical record and deposition to support the reasonableness of the decisions you made at the time that you made them (Box 6.7).

**Box 6.7 Practice Tip**

1. Secure and isolate the patient's complete medical record.
2. Make no additions, modifications, or alterations to that chart.
3. Immediately notify either your institutional administrative or insurance representative of the claim, in order to preserve malpractice coverage.
4. Participate fully—and as a priority—in the defense of the quality of your care.

### *FRAUD AND ABUSE*

In 1972, as part of the first amendments to the Medicaid and Medicare rules and regulations, Congress passed antifraud and abuse regulations. The first such laws were hardly more than a slap on the wrist. However, in 1977 Congress made those laws draconian. False statements include the following:

1. Knowingly and willfully making or causing to be made any false statement or representation of a material fact in seeking to obtain any benefit or payment
2. Fraudulently concealing or failing to disclose information affecting one's rights to a payment
3. Converting any benefit or payment rightfully belonging to another
4. Presenting or causing to be presented a claim for a physician's service knowing that the individual who furnished the service was not licensed as a physician

These also encompass false claims, bribes, kickbacks, rebates, or "any remuneration" and are felonies with a maximum penalty of 5 years in jail and a $25,000.00 fine possible for each such offense. (The law states that any provider who knowingly and willfully solicits, pays, offers, or receives any remuneration, in cash or in kind, directly or indirectly, overtly or covertly, to induce or in return for arranging for or ordering items or services that will be paid for by Medicare or Medicaid will be guilty of a felony.) These rules and regulations essentially made it impossible to practice without violating some aspect of the fraud and abuse laws. It was, however, 10 years before the laws were refined in the Medicaid-Medicare Patient Protection Act of 1987, which provided some safe harbors to free normal course-of-business procedures. Since 1987, the government has pursued fraud and abuse cases with ever-increasing vigor. In 2003, settlements in fraud and abuse cases netted the government close to $2 billion (WSJ, 2004). The real danger to the physician is not the fine that may force him or her into bankruptcy or the unusual imposition of jail time (to date, the government has seemed more interested in recovering cash and calling a halt to illegal practices than it has in jailing doctors), but the felony conviction that may result in the automatic loss of the license to practice. Thus Medicare/Medicaid fraud and abuse is a far more dangerous hazard than is malpractice.

#### *Practical Tip*

Have your patients sign in regardless of whether they have come for an office visit or just a procedure. If you are worried about privacy issues, use a privacy sign-in sheet to prevent subsequent signers from seeing previous signers. (Colwell Publishing provides several styles of such sheets, and they are likely supplied by local firms as well.)

Do not unbundle procedures that are supposed to be bundled on a physician's visit. Do not unbundle surgical procedures. Do not charge for procedures done by another licensed provider or charge for a physician's services if the physician is not physically present. Send your personnel to an accredited coding course, and make sure your coding is being done in an accurate manner. Do not be tempted to code up. Time studies and statistics are against you. Finally, beware of the "coding consultant" who promises to increase your accounts receivable.

## *LABORATORY TESTS*

In my experience, one of the most common reasons for malpractice suits is the unreported abnormal laboratory or x-ray finding. The usual story is that the pathologist or radiologist returns the report and the efficient clerk, receptionist, or nurse staples it in the medical record and then files the record. The alternative story is that the report is never sent and there is no follow-up. Of course, normal clerical errors do occur in any business; nevertheless, the physician's fiduciary duty extends to communicating the results and meanings of all abnormal tests to the patient. Therefore the failure to communicate the results of an abnormal Pap smear, glucose tolerance test, or mammogram to a patient can have disastrous legal consequences.

### *Practical Tip*

A gynecologist must have a system to track and document all laboratory and diagnostic tests and imaging studies ordered. There is no totally satisfactory way to do this. Old-fashioned "tickler" files are the least efficient, but they are better than nothing. Some office-generated computer programs have been highly successful, and some of the commercially available programs even generate an automatic notification letter. In any case, the physician must track all ordered tests and make every reasonable effort to notify the patient. The notification and follow-up must be documented. Telling the patient to call for the test results does not relieve the physician of his or her duty to notify. Finally, use the information you secure. Do not order laboratory or other diagnostic tests and then ignore or belittle those results.

## CAP STRATEGY

CAP (**c**ommunication, **a**nticipation, and **p**reparation) should be the cornerstone of simple practice philosophies that, when effectively put into practice by qualified, trained health care providers in a safe medical system, will increase patient safety and thereby "cap" exposure to liability (Fig. 6.1).

The optimal health system will assimilate CAP between and among the care providers within any given institution or health system. Applying the principles of CAP will ensure, by employing efficient written, verbal, and policy guidelines, that the right health care providers will have the correct information necessary to effectuate optimal care. There is no single greater way to reduce medical liability than to increase patient safety.

Next we will review how these simple, sound, and commonsense approaches can be incorporated to increase patient safety. Errors have and will continue to occur in any system that involves people performing duties or tasks. "The most extensive study of adverse events is the Harvard medical practice study, a study of more than 30,000 randomly selected discharges from 51 randomly selected hospitals in New York State in 1984. Adverse events, manifested by prolonged hospitalization or disability at the time of discharge, or both occurred in 3.7% of the hospitalizations. The proportion of adverse events attributed to errors (i.e., preventable adverse events) was 58% and the proportion of adverse events due to negligence was 27.6%." These data were corroborated in the 1992 studies in Colorado, Utah, and New York state (IOM, 2000). Errors can be diagnostic, treatment based, preventive, or other (Leape, 1993).

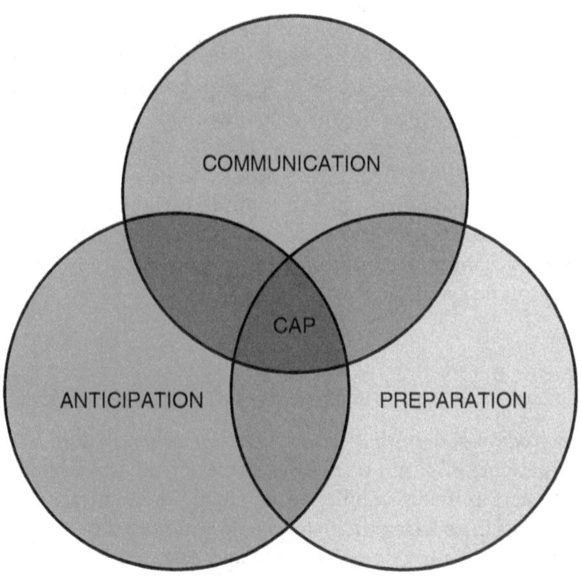


**Figure 6.1** Communication + Anticipation + Preparation = Patient safety and reduced medicolegal risk.

The American College of Obstetrics and Gynecology (ACOG) Committee Opinion 447 further placed patient safety in obstetrics and gynecology on the forefront (ACOG, 2009). The committee opinion set forth that a culture of safety should be the framework for any effort to reduce medical errors. The goal is to encourage obstetricians and gynecologists to adopt and develop safe practices that will reduce the likelihood of system failures that can cause adverse outcomes in their patient populations.

## COMMUNICATION

As explained previously, communication is the bedrock of safety and efficiency in every high-risk organization. Health care communications can be written in the medical record, published as guidelines and literature, treated as verbal communications, and accepted as cultural norms within an institution. In its analysis of sentinel events, The Joint Commission found that almost two thirds of the events involved communication failure as a root cause (TJC, 2004). Communication training is now becoming increasingly recognized as the cornerstone of any patient safety program. AHRQ developed the TeamSTEPPS trademark program to address this issue (AHRQ, 2015). Obvious times for increased risk in communication slipped through the cracks at patient handoffs, patient transfers, or shift changes. ACOG found that an increased awareness of the importance of clear communication between all members of the health care team will measurably enhance the safety of the care delivered by obstetricians and gynecologists. Training around these issues for all health care providers is highly recommended.

Communication requires, first, a basic understanding of roles and responsibilities. Team members must be clearly trained in their roles and familiar with the appropriate policies, guidelines, or procedures for delivering routine and emergent care. Through enhanced communication, and clear communication, medical errors can be avoided.

## ANTICIPATION

Anticipation is defined as an expectation or prediction. Within each patient's clinical presentation there are varying degrees of a health care provider's ability to anticipate outcomes. Anticipation assists in ensuring the right people and necessary equipment are in place to provide appropriate and safe care when needed. Anticipation requires an understanding of the patient's clinical presentation, hospital resources, and any likely encumbrance to the delivery of safe and effective care.

## PREPARATION

The Joint Commission has recommended and mandated, at various levels, simulation programs or training. Simulations are a way for institutional practices to be perfected prior to one's handling of life-threatening emergencies. The concept of a simulation, though basic and simple, requires more than just the simple actions that day. The preparation required includes appropriate staffing; reasonable, updated, and appropriately disseminated policies and guidelines that include definitions of roles and responsibilities; and planned simulations of foreseeable emergencies.

## CONCLUSION

In the broadest sense, medical malpractice is defined by whether or not conduct and decisions were reasonable. The fear of all physicians is that they will be judged ultimately by lesser-trained individuals who identify more with the patient than with the provider. The tests of reasonableness they will utilize are often as simple as asking the question, based on the care and the testimony you provided. Would the jurors be comfortable being treated by you? If the answer to that question is yes, regardless of the complications, decision making, and outcomes, then the most likely jury verdict will be in favor of the defendant physician. However, if the care appears to be inattentive or inconsistent and the records or depositions are inaccurate, the chance to explain your decision and the reasonableness you feel is behind it may be lost through no one's fault but your own.

Breakdowns in the systems of communication—with patients, care providers, or through the medical records—can create a host of problems for physicians, nurses, and health care institutions in the event of an unfavorable treatment outcome. By focusing attentively on both system-wide and individual best practices for accurate and contemporaneous communications, many problems can be avoided or quickly resolved. Awareness that your patients will have serious questions about unexpected, often life-altering, outcomes is integral to avoiding legal problems. Only when patients feel that they have not received satisfactory answers from their care providers will they seek those answers elsewhere—most likely from an attorney.

Focusing on communication, anticipation, and preparation will ensure the appropriate people are in the appropriate place with the appropriate information to deliver health care within a timely manner. The concept of capping one's liability is far too often looked at retrospectively through litigation or discussed after an error occurs. In reality, the best ways to cap liability is through enhanced communication and the development of a cohesive system of health care, which are both patient focused and health care provider friendly.

Balancing practice modifications that become oppressive or interfere with the delivery of reasonable and efficient health care can be challenging. However, ensuring adequate layers of redundancies and safeguards to make certain a single or perhaps even two human errors are protected by a well-designed cohesive system will prevent an undesirable outcome or patient harm (Fig. 6.2).

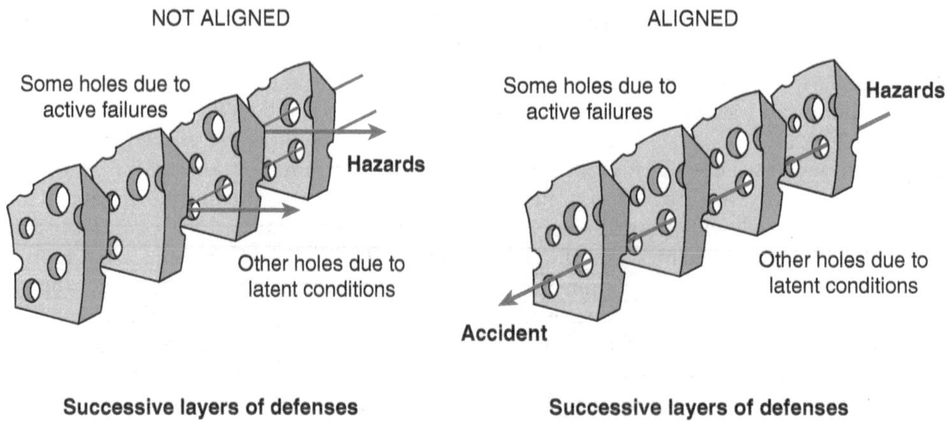


**Figure 6.2** Swiss cheese model system errors and benefits of redundancies.

## KEY REFERENCES


Agency for Healthcare Research and Quality (AHRQ). *TeamSTEPPS®: Strategies and Tools to Enhance Performance and Patient Safety.* Rockville, MD: AHRQ; 2015. Available at http://www.ahrq.gov/professionals/education/curriculum-tools/teamstepps/index.html.

American College of Obstetricians and Gynecologists. ACOG Committee Opinion No. 447: Patient safety in obstetrics and gynecology. *Obstet Gynecol.* 2009;114(6):1424-1427.

Institute of Medicine (IOM). *To Err is Human: Building a Safer Health System.* Washington, DC: The National Academies Press; 2000.

Institute of Medicine (IOM), et al. *Preventing Medication Errors: Quality Chasm Series.* Washington, DC: The National Academies Press; 2007. doi: 10317226-11623.

Leape LL, Lawthers AG, Brennan TA, et al. Preventing medical injury. *QRB Qual Rev Bull.* 1993;19(5):144-149.

Palmisano DJ. Many physicians fear making honest apology. (letter) *Wall Street Journal,* June 11, 2004:A13.

Studdert DM, Mello MM, Gawande AA, et al. Claims, errors and compensation payments in medical malpractice litigation. *N Engl J Med.* 2006;354(19):2024-2033.

The Joint Commission (TJC). *Sentinel Event Alert, Issue 30: Preventing infant death and injury during delivery;* July 21, 2004. Available at http://www.jointcommission.org/assets/1/18/SEA_30.PDF.

U.S. Food and Drug Administration (FDA). *Medication Errors;* 2016. Available at http://www.fda.gov/Drugs/DrugSafety/MedicationErrors/default.htm.


Suggested Readings can be found on ExpertConsult.com.

# 7

# History, Physical Examination, and Preventive Health Care

*Vicki Mendiratta, Gretchen M. Lentz*

The first contact a physician has with a patient is critical. It allows an initial bond of trust to be developed on which the future relationship may be built. The patient will share sensitive medical, reproductive, and psychosocial information. The physician will gain her confidence and establish rapport by the understanding and nonjudgmental manner in which he or she collects these data. Today's obstetrician/gynecologist (OB/GYN) will care for women from around the globe, with varying cultural, social, and religious beliefs and values. Women will be of differing socioeconomic status, may have physical or mental disabilities, and may identify as lesbian, bisexual, or transgender. Open communication, with an awareness of and sensitivity to the vast diversity of our patient population, will help to create a collaborative environment in which to explore health issues.

The annual well-woman visit is a crucial part of general medical care. During this visit, the health care provider can attend to current gynecologic concerns, promote disease prevention, assess risks for potential disease, and provide the indicated physical examination or tests. This annual health encounter should include healthy lifestyle counseling, as well as screening and immunizations as appropriate, based on the patient's age and risks.

The first visit generally involves taking a complete history, performing a complete physical examination, and ordering appropriate screening or laboratory tests. The physician practicing obstetrics and gynecology should not assume that others are caring for the patient's general medical needs. It may be appropriate to assume the role of her primary physician, with your care including attention to preventive health services, depending on the physician's training and skills. In other circumstances, a referral to a primary care provider may be more appropriate to better serve the patient.

This chapter focuses on the appropriate manner that an obstetrician/gynecologist should use to conduct a history and physical examination and discusses the appropriate ingredients of ongoing health maintenance.

## DIRECT OBSERVATIONS BEFORE SPEAKING TO THE PATIENT (NONVERBAL CLUES)

When meeting a patient, it is important to *look* at her even before speaking. Differing cultural backgrounds and belief systems may greatly affect the information transfer and challenge effective communication. The general demeanor of the patient should be evaluated. Many new patients are apprehensive about meeting a new physician and the pelvic examination. This apprehension may create barriers to an open and positive first encounter.

By observing nonverbal clues, such as eye contact, posture, facial expressions, or tone of voice, the physician can determine the appropriate approach for conducting the interview. The act of greeting the woman by name, making eye contact, and shaking hands is a formal but friendly start to the visit.

Four qualities have been recognized as potentially important in caring communication skills: comfort, acceptance, responsiveness, and empathy. Despite the busy demands of clinical practice, effective communication skills enhance patient satisfaction and patient safety and decrease the likelihood of medical liability litigation. Box 7.1 lists some components of effective physician communication.

## ESSENCE OF THE GYNECOLOGIC HISTORY

### *CHIEF COMPLAINT*

The patient should be encouraged to tell the physician why she has sought help. The chief complaint is a concise statement describing the woman's problem in her words. Questions such as "What is the nature of the problem that brought you to me?" or "How may I help you?" are good ways to begin.

### *HISTORY OF THE PRESENT ILLNESS (HPI)*

The patient should be able to present the problem as she sees it, in her own words, and should be interrupted only for specific clarification of points or to offer direction if she digresses too far. During the interview the physician should face the patient with direct eye contact and acknowledge important points of the history. This approach allows the physician to be involved in the problem and demonstrates a degree of caring to the patient. Now that electronic medical records (EMRs) are almost universally utilized, the ability to sit and just listen to the patient and provide that direct eye contact can be challenging, as providers are often documenting while the patient is sharing her

**Box 7.1 Components of Effective Physician Communication**

Be culturally sensitive.
Establish rapport.
Listen and respond to the woman's concerns (empathy).
Be nonjudgmental.
Include both verbal and nonverbal communication.
Engage the woman in discussion and treatment options (partnership).
Convey comfort in discussing sensitive topics.
Abandon stereotypes.
Check for understanding of your explanations.
Show support by helping the woman to overcome barriers to care and compliance with treatment.

story. When the patient has completed the history of her current problem, pertinent open-ended questions should be asked with respect to specific points. This process allows the physician to develop a more detailed database. Directed questions may be asked where pertinent to clarify points. In general, however, the patient should be encouraged to tell her story as she sees it rather than to react with short answers to specific questions. Under the latter circumstance, the physician may get the answers he or she is looking for, but they may not be accurate answers. When the HPI is documented in the medical record, it represents a chronologic history of the current concerns.

A general outline for a gynecologic and general history is given in Box 7.2. The outline is given in a specific order for general orientation. The information, however, may be collected through any comfortable discussion with the patient that seems appropriate in the circumstances. It is important that all aspects be covered.

**Box 7.2 History Outline**

I. Observation—nonverbal clues
II. Chief complaint
III. History of gynecologic problem(s)
   A. Menstrual history—last menstrual period, previous menstrual period
   B. Pregnancy history
   C. Vaginal and pelvic infections
   D. Gynecologic surgical procedures
   E. Urologic history
   F. Pelvic pain
   G. Vaginal bleeding
   H. Sexual status
   I. Contraceptive status
IV. Significant health problems
   A. Systemic illnesses, including bleeding problems
   B. Surgical procedures
   C. Other hospitalizations
V. Medications, habits, and allergies
   A. Medications taken
   B. Medication and other allergies
   C. Smoking history
   D. Alcohol usage
   E. Illicit drug usage
VI. Family history
   A. Illnesses and causes of death of first-order relatives
   B. Congenital malformations, mental retardation, and reproductive loss
VII. Occupational and avocational history
VIII. Social history
IX. Review of systems
   A. Constitutional—such as fever, fatigue
   B. Head, eyes, ears, nose, mouth, throat
   C. Cardiovascular—such as chest pain
   D. Respiratory—such as cough or shortness of breath
   E. Gastrointestinal—such as constipation, bloating, diarrhea, abdominal pain
   F. Genitourinary—such as incontinence, urinary frequency or urgency
   G. Musculoskeletal—such as back pain
   H. Skin
   I. Neurologic
   J. Psychiatric—such as sadness, feeling down or anxious; a short depression screening inventory can be administered; a frequently utilized inventory is the Patient Health Questionnaire 9
   K. Endocrine—such as significant weight gain or loss
   L. Hematologic—easy bleeding from gums or nose
   M. Allergic/immunologic
X. Physical abuse
   A. Sexual abuse—incest, rape, sexual touching

## *PERTINENT GYNECOLOGIC HISTORY*

A pertinent gynecologic history can be divided into several parts. It begins with a menstrual history, in which the age of menarche, duration of each monthly cycle, number of days during which menses occurs, and regularity of the menstrual cycles should be noted. The dates of the last menstrual period should be obtained. In addition, the characteristics of the menstrual flow, including the color, the amount of flow, and accompanying symptoms, such as cramping, nausea, headache, or diarrhea, should be noted. In general, menstruation that occurs monthly (range 21 to 35 days), lasts 4 to 7 days, is bright red, and is often accompanied by cramping on the day preceding and the first day of the period are all characteristics of an ovulatory cycle. Menstruation that is irregular, often dark in color, painless, and frequently short or very long may indicate lack of ovulation. Often adolescents or premenopausal women have **anovulatory cycles** with resultant irregular menstruation. Any vaginal bleeding not related to menses (intermenstrual bleeding) should be noted, as well as its relationship to the menstrual cycle and to other events, such as coitus (postcoital bleeding), the use of tampons, or the use of a contraceptive device. For the postmenopausal woman, the age at last menses, history of hormone replacement therapy, and any postmenopausal bleeding should be noted.

The second pertinent point in the gynecologic history is that of previous pregnancies. The woman should be asked specifically to list all pregnancies, including chemical pregnancies, all abortions (spontaneous and induced), molar and ectopic pregnancies. For deliveries, the following information should be obtained: year of birth, gestational age at delivery, the type of delivery, infant birth weight, and any complications that may have occurred. For all other pregnancies, the circumstances under which they took place, the method by which they were concluded (dilation and curettage [D&C], methotrexate, etc.), and any complications should be obtained.

Next, a history of vaginal and pelvic infections should be obtained. The patient should be asked what types of infection she has had, what treatment she received, and what complications

**Box 7.3 United States Preventive Services Task Force Definitions of High Risk for HIV and Gonorrhea**

**Gonorrhea Risk**

History of previous gonorrhea infection
Treatment or presence of other STDs
New or multiples sexual partners
Inconsistent condom use
Sex trade work
Drug use

**HIV Risk**

Men and women having unprotected sex with multiple partners
Past or present injection drug use
Women who exchange sex for money or drugs or who have partners who do
Women whose past or present partners were/are HIV-infected, bisexual or intravenous drug users
Women being treated for STDs
Women with a history of blood transfusion between 1978 and 1985
Women receiving health care in a high prevalence or high-risk clinical setting

Modified from Campos-Outcalt D. US Preventive Services Task Force: the gold standard of evidence-based prevention. *J Fam Pract.* 2005;54:517-519.
*STDs*, Sexually transmitted diseases.

she experienced. Risk factors for human immunodeficiency virus (HIV) infection, such as intravenous drug abuse or coitus with drug abusers or bisexual men, should be sought by direct questioning and HIV screening offered where appropriate (Box 7.3). The 2013 U.S. Preventive Services Task Force (USPSTF) report states with "high certainty that the net benefit of screening for HIV infection in adolescents, adults and pregnant women is substantial" (Moyer, 2013). Part of this rationale stems from the fact that 20% to 25% of individuals living with HIV infection are unaware they are infected. All hospitalizations should be reviewed as to cause and outcome.

The physician should obtain a Pap smear screening history, including the date of the last Pap smear, the frequency of screening, and any abnormal tests and the treatment. The patient's human papilloma virus (HPV) vaccination status should be determined.

The woman's contraceptive history should be investigated, including methods used, length of time they have been used, effectiveness, and any complications that may have arisen.

All instances of gynecologic surgical procedures should be noted, including office procedures, such as endometrial biopsies; vulvar, vaginal, or cervical biopsies. For any minor or major procedures, such as laparoscopy or laparotomy, the following data should be collected: dates, types of procedures, diagnoses, and significant complications. In cases where pertinent, past records, particularly operative and pathology reports, should be sought.

A complete sexual history should be obtained (Box 7.4), and specific problems should be evaluated. The history should include whether the patient is currently sexually active or has been in the past. Patients should be asked if they have one or more current partners and if they have sex with men, women, or both. The provider should also inquire about any sexual dysfunction such as dyspareunia or anorgasmia.

Symptoms of pelvic pain or discomfort should be discussed fully. Six common questions should be asked about the pain:

**Box 7.4 Important Points of Sexual History**

1. Sexual activity (presence of)
2. Types of relationships
3. Individual(s) involved
4. Satisfaction? Orgasmic? Desire/interest?
5. Dyspareunia
6. Sexual dysfunction
   a. Patient
   b. Partner

location; timing; quality, such as throbbing, burning, colicky; radiation to other body areas; intensity on a scale of 1 to 10, with 10 being the worse pain imaginable; and duration of symptoms. Additional questions about what causes the pain to worsen or subside; the context of the pain symptoms; and associated triggers, signs, and symptoms may be helpful. The pain should be described, noting the presence or absence of a relationship to the menstrual cycle and its association with other events, such as coitus or bleeding and bladder and bowel symptoms.

## GENERAL HEALTH HISTORY

The woman should be asked to list any significant health problems that she has had during her lifetime, including all hospitalizations and operative procedures. It is reasonable for the physician to ask about specific illnesses, such as diabetes, hypertension, or heart disease, that seem likely based on what is known about the woman or about her family history. Many physicians use a history checklist of the most common conditions.

Medications taken and reasons for doing so should be noted, as should allergic responses to medications. The woman should be encouraged to bring all medications, both prescription and over-the-counter drugs, including herbal preparations, to subsequent health maintenance visits. Most women who use complementary and alternative medicines do not offer this information to physicians.

A history of smoking should be obtained in detail, including amount, length of time she has smoked, and attempts at quitting smoking. She should be questioned about the use of illicit drugs, including heroin, methamphetamines, cocaine, and prescription drug abuse with narcotics. Any affirmative answers should be followed by specific questions concerning length of use, types of drugs used, and side effects that may have been noticed. Her use of alcohol should be detailed carefully, including the number of drinks per day and any history of binge drinking or previous therapy for alcoholism.

## FAMILY HISTORY

A detailed family history of first- and second-degree relatives (parents, siblings, children, aunts, uncles, and grandparents) should be taken and a family tree constructed if relevant (Fig. 7.1). Serious illnesses or causes of death for each individual should be noted. If the woman desires fertility now or in the future, an inquiry should be made about any congenital malformations, mental retardation, or pregnancy loss in either the woman's or her spouse's family. Such information may offer clues to hereditarily determined causes of reproductive problems.

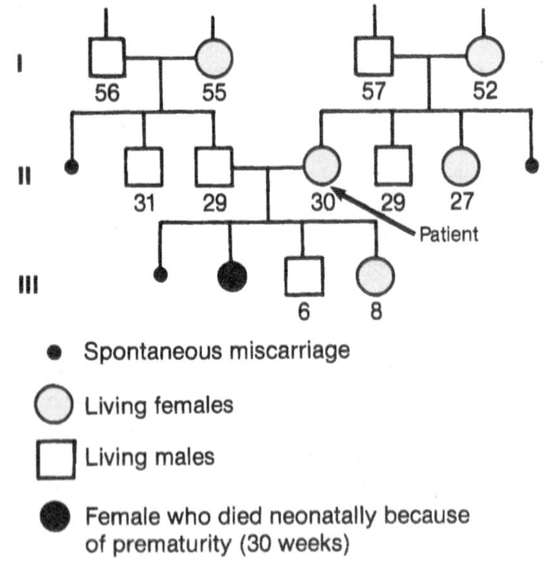


**Figure 7.1** Family tree of typical gynecologic patient.

### *Occupational and Social History*

The woman should be asked to detail her occupation. A nonjudgmental way to approach this could be to ask if she is currently working outside of the home. It is very important to determine if she is currently exercising, what type of activity she engages in, and the frequency of exercise.

Additional information that may be relevant include hobbies and other avocations that may affect health or reproductive capacity, where and with whom the woman lives, other individuals in the household, areas of the world where the woman has lived or traveled, or unusual experiences that may affect her health.

## *SAFETY ISSUES*

The patient should be questioned about safety matters. She should be asked about the use of seat belts and helmets (if she rides a bicycle, motorcycle, or horse). She should be asked whether there are firearms in her household and, if so, whether appropriate safety precautions are taken. A question about intimate partner violence is appropriate and can be asked in a nonthreatening manner, such as "Has anyone in your household threatened or physically hurt you?" Sexual violence is a widespread problem, and as more is being learned about prevention, providers should be knowledgeable about resources (Senn, 2015).

## *NUTRITIONAL AND DIETARY ASSESSMENT*

It is important to inquire about dietary choices that our patients make. Assessment of folic acid is important in reproductive-aged women. Asking about fruits and vegetables as well as calcium-containing foods should be standard. Vegetarians and vegans may need additional discussion about adequate protein and vitamin/mineral intake. A referral to a certified nutritionist may be a valuable addition to routine preventive health care.

## *REVIEW OF SYSTEMS*

A complete review of systems (ROS) should be obtained and documented. (See Box 7.2 for comprehensive ROS and some relevant examples.)

# ESSENCE OF THE ANNUAL EXAMINATION

The scope of services and examination provided by an OB/GYN in the ambulatory setting will vary from practice to practice. In 2014, the American College of Obstetricians and Gynecologists (ACOG) reaffirmed its recommendation that the annual examination include obtaining vital signs, determining body mass index (BMI), palpating the abdomen, palpating inguinal lymph nodes, and making an overall assessment of the patient's health (ACOG Committee Opinion, No. 534, 2014). The extent to which additional examination is performed is based on many factors, such as age, patient concerns, family history, and whether the patient has a primary care provider whom she also sees for routine and concern-driven care. Not all women will require a clinical breast exam or pelvic exam at each annual visit. Refer to Table 7.1 for examination and screening recommendations.

## *PHYSICAL EXAMINATION*

The patient should disrobe completely and cover herself with a hospital gown that ensures warmth and modesty. During each step of the examination she should be allowed to maintain personal control by being offered options whenever possible. These options begin with the presence or absence of a chaperone. The chaperone, a third party, usually a woman, serves a variety of purposes. She may offer warmth, compassion, and support to the patient during uncomfortable or potentially embarrassing portions of the examination. She may help the physician to carry out procedures and in some cases act as a witness to the doctor-patient interaction. Although the presence of a chaperone is not imperative in every physician-patient relationship, one should be immediately available for any encounter.

The examination should begin with a general evaluation of the patient's appearance and affect. Her weight, height, and blood pressure should be taken initially. A body mass index (BMI) should be calculated and is an important "vital sign" to track over time. Most currently used electronic medical records (EMRs) will automatically calculate BMI when height/weight data are entered. Postmenopausal women should have their height measured routinely to document evidence of osteoporosis, which causes loss of height from vertebral compression fractures. Some institutions require a pain scale reporting at each visit and consider it a fourth vital sign.

Most gynecologists will not perform a comprehensive screening head, eye, ears, neck, and throat (HEENT) examination. The American Academy of Ophthalmology (AAO) recommends that adults with no signs or risk factors for eye disease should receive a baseline comprehensive eye evaluation at age 40 and then every 2 to 4 years until age 55; every 1 to 3 years through age 64: and yearly to every other year for individuals 65 years old or older (AAO, 2015).

The thyroid gland should be palpated for irregularities or increase in size (goiter). Discrete areas of enlargement, hardness,

**Table 7.1** Examination, Screening, and Immunization Recommendations for the Annual Health Maintenance Visit

| | Age (Years) | | |
|---|---|---|---|
| | **19-39** | **40-64** | **65+** |
| Vital signs | Ht, Wt, BMI, BP | Ht, Wt, BMI, BP | Ht, Wt, BMI, BP |
| Neck | Adenopathy, thyroid | Adenopathy, thyroid | Adenopathy, thyroid |
| Clinical breast exam[§] | q 1-3 years, beginning at 20 | Yearly | Yearly |
| Abdomen | Yearly | Yearly | Yearly |
| Pelvic/speculum | 21+ periodically* | Annually/periodically* | Annually/periodically* |
| Additional exams | As indicated | As indicated | As indicated |
| Pap | 21+, q 3 years | q 5 with co-test (preferred) or q 3 Pap | Discontinue if negative adequate screening and no hx of CIN2+ |
| Chlamydia/gonorrhea | <26 and sexually active, yearly | As indicated | As indicated |
| Colon cancer screening | n/a | 50+, colonoscopy q 10 years[†] | Colonoscopy q 10 years |
| Diabetes testing | As indicated | 45+, q 3 years | q 3 years |
| Mammogram | If indicated | Annually[‡] | Annually[‡] |
| Lipids | If indicated | 45+, q 5 years | q 5 years |
| Thyroid-stimulating hormone | If indicated | 50+, q 5 years | q 5 years |
| Bone mineral density | | If indicated | q 2+ years |
| Immunizations | HPV, Tdap once, TD q 10 years; influenza yearly | Tdap once, TD q 10 years; influenza yearly; herpes zoster once (>59) | Influenza yearly; Tdap once, TD q 10 years; pneumococcus once |
| HIV | Offered routinely[#] | Offered routinely[‖] | Offered routinely[‖] |

Additional data from American the Congress of Obstetricians and Gynecologists (ACOG). Well-woman care: assessment and recommendations (http://www.acog.org/wellwoman).

*No evidence supports or refutes the annual pelvic exam, speculum, bimanual exam for low-risk, asymptomatic patients. Decisions about the examination for this group should be shared between patient and provider (ACOG Committee Opinion, #534).

†The American College of Gastroenterology recommends African Americans initiate screening at age 45 due to a higher earlier incidence of colorectal cancer. Colonoscopy is preferred but other methods include fecal occult blood testing, flexible sigmoidoscopy, double contrast barium enema, computed tomography colonography, stool DNA (interval for testing varies based on method utilized).

‡Per ACS/ACOG, however USPSTF: start age 50 and q 2 years.

§ACS and National Comprehensive Cancer Network.

‖CDC: Advisory Committee on Immunization Practices.

¶CDC recommends "routine" testing in all patients, frequency to be determined by patient and provider.

General recommendations for low-risk populations. High-risk populations may have more recommended vaccines.

High-risk groups based on lifestyle, concurrent medical conditions, and family history may have other testing or intervals for testing. Chart represents recommendations for the general populations.

*BMI*, Body mass index; *BP*, blood pressure; *HIV*, human immunodeficiency virus; *Ht*, height; *hx*, history; *q*, every; *Wt*, weight.

and tenderness should be described. The patient's neck should be palpated for evidence of adenopathy along the supraclavicular and posterior auricular chains.

In a comprehensive preventive health examination, both the chest and cardiac systems should be evaluated. Whether this is necessary in an annual well-woman visit for a healthy woman is at the discretion of the provider. A nongynecologic primary care provider or subspecialist will likely care for women with medical conditions such as hypertension or diabetes. When performing the chest exam, the chest should be inspected for symmetry of movement of the diaphragm and observed for respiratory effort. This is followed by palpation, percussion, and auscultation.

The heart should be examined by palpation for points of maximum impulse, percussed for size, and auscultated for irregularities of rate and evidence of murmurs and other adventitious sounds. The patient's heart should be auscultated in both the lying and the sitting positions. An older woman's neck should be auscultated for evidence of vascular bruits.

## BREAST EXAM

There is no evidenced-based recommendation for when to begin clinical breast exam (CBE) screening in the low-risk, asymptomatic woman. ACOG, American Cancer Society (ACS), and National Comprehensive Cancer Network (NCCN) all recommend CBE every 1 to 3 years for women ages 20 to 39 and yearly thereafter (ACOG Committee Opinion, No. 534, 2014). A careful breast examination should be carried out in a systematic fashion. To summarize a detailed clinical breast examination, refer to Box 7.5. Research has shown the following factors are associated with a high-quality breast examination: longer duration, thorough coverage of the breast, a consistent exam pattern, use of variable pressure with the finger pads, and use of the three middle fingers. ACOG, ACS, and NCCN all recommend the teaching of breast self-awareness, including teaching breast self-examination. Women are no longer instructed to examine their own breasts monthly but rather if they feel or see any concerning symptom or abnormality such as redness, pain, skin changes, or a mass.

## ABDOMINAL EXAM

The abdomen should first be inspected for symmetry, scars, masses, distension, and visible organomegaly. The hair pattern should be noted. The typical female escutcheon is that of an inverted triangle over the mons pubis. A male escutcheon involves hair growth between the area of the mons pubis and the umbilicus, also known as a *diamond pattern,* and may indicate excessive androgen activity in the patient (Fig. 7.2).

The physician should listen (auscultation) for bowel sounds. Hypoactive or absent bowel sounds may imply an ileus caused by peritoneal irritation of the bowel. Hyperactive bowel sounds may imply intrinsic irritation of the bowel or partial or complete bowel obstruction.

Next, abdominal percussion affords the ability to differentiate fluid waves and to outline solid organs and masses. Localized percussion tenderness may suggest peritoneal inflammation.

Finally, the abdomen should be palpated for organomegaly, particularly involving the liver, spleen, kidneys, and uterus, and for adnexal masses, which may be palpated abdominally, if large. Palpation affords the possibility of noting a fluid wave, which would suggest either ascites or hemoperitoneum. Palpation also yields evidence for rigidity of the abdomen, which would imply spasm in the rectus muscles secondary to intraabdominal irritation. Where the irritation is caused by intraabdominal hemorrhage or infection, this rigidity is often evidence of an acute abdomen. During the palpation of the abdomen, the physician should elicit the phenomenon of *rebound*, which also signifies intraabdominal irritation, by gently pressing the abdomen and then releasing. The release may cause pain either under the spot (direct rebound) or in a different portion of the abdomen (referred rebound). It should be noted, however, that sudden, deep pressure may cause pain even in a normal patient. Gentle pressure carried out systematically may elicit painful "trigger points." With the woman straining or simulating an abdominal sit-up, an abdominal or incisional hernia may be visualized and the fascial defect palpated.

The groin should be palpated for adenopathy and inguinal hernias.

**Box 7.5 Clinical Breast Examination Elements**

1. With patient sitting up, position her hands at her hips and ask her to gently push inward. Visualize for symmetry. Ask patient to put hands together above head and press inward. Visualize for symmetry. With arms at side, palpate axilla bilaterally, feeling for lymph nodes.
2. In the supine position, ask patient to place arms above her head. Pay attention to entire breast tissue from midsternum to the posterior axillary line and from the inframammary crease to the clavicle.
3. Inspection and palpation (a variety of palpation techniques exist):
   Skin flattening or dimpling
   Skin erythema
   Skin edema
   Nipple retraction
   Nipple eczema
   Nipple discharge
   Breast fixation
   Tissue thickening
   Palpable masses
   Tenderness

## PELVIC EXAMINATION

In 2014, ACOG continues to recommend that the pelvic exam, including an external genital evaluation, speculum exam, and bimanual exam, be performed yearly in adult women (ACOG Committee Opinion, No. 534, 2014). However, also in 2014, the American College of Physicians published their own new guidelines based on a systematic review of the literature obtained since the 1950s. The authors concluded that annual screening pelvic exams in asymptomatic, nonpregnant adult women do not offer benefit and can, in fact, cause harm. They recommended against such examinations (Qaseem, 2014). This new guideline certainly prompted much debate among physician leaders in all primary care fields. The decision to perform this exam and the frequency of the exams remain in the hands of the provider together with the patient. All symptomatic women should have a pelvic exam.

The pelvic examination is conducted with the patient lying supine on the examining table with her legs in stirrups and a sheet draped across her. The physician should be sure the patient is as relaxed as possible and should take a few minutes to describe the procedure and allow the patient to prepare herself. Suggesting that the patient allow her legs to fall wide apart and concentrate on relaxing her abdominal muscles may be helpful.

### *INSPECTION*

The vulva and introitus should be carefully inspected beginning with the mons pubis. The quality and pattern of the hair on the mons and the labia majora should be noted. During the inspection of the pubic hair, the physician should look for evidence of body lice (pediculosis). Next, the skin of the vulva/perineum is inspected for erythema, excoriation, discoloration, or loss of pigment and for the presence of vesicles, ulcerations, pustules, warty growths, or neoplastic growths. In addition, pigmented nevi or other pigmented lesions should be noted, as should varicose veins. Skin scars denoting previous episiotomy or other obstetric lacerations should be noted.

Next, the specific structures of the vulva should be systematically evaluated. The clitoris should be noted and its size and

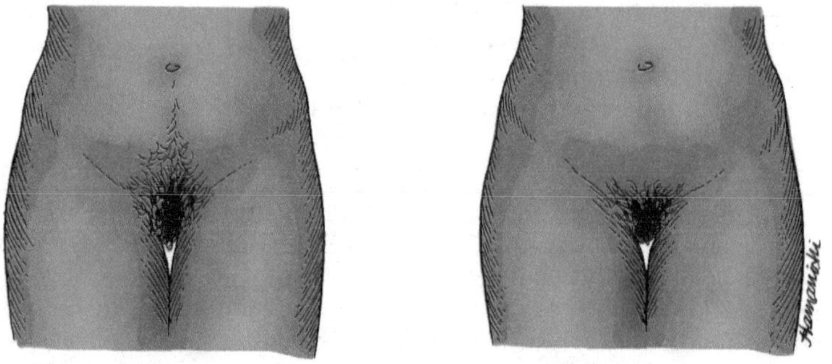

**Figure 7.2** Normal female pubic hair pattern *(right)* and hair pattern of female showing male (androgenized) pattern *(left)*.

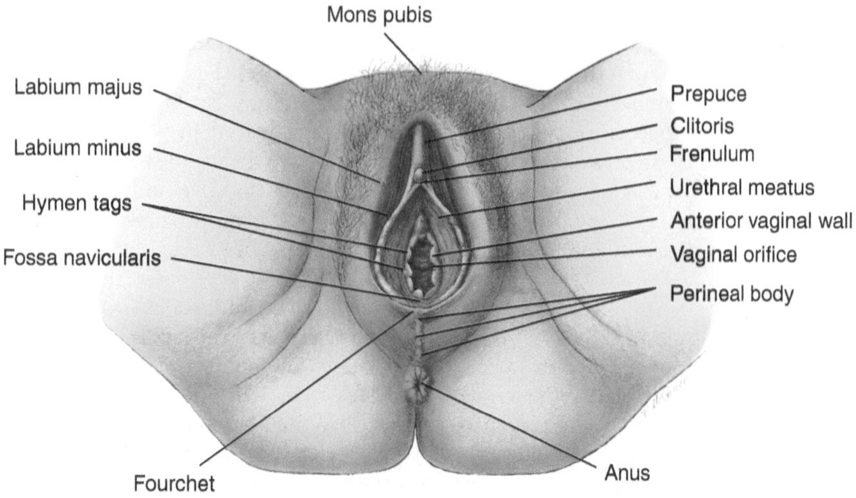


**Figure 7.3** Normal female perineum. (Modified from Krantz KE. Anatomy of the female reproductive system. In: Benson RC, ed. *Current Obstetric and Gynecologic Diagnosis and Treatment.* 5th ed. Los Altos, CA: Lange Medical; 1984.)

shape described. Normally it is 1 to 1.5 cm in length. Any irregularities or abnormalities of the labia majora or minora should be noted and carefully described. At times these areas are injured by trauma related to coitus, accidental injury, or childbearing. The patient should be questioned about evidence of trauma when appropriate.

The introitus should be observed closely. Whether the hymen is intact, imperforate, or open and whether the perineum gapes or remains closed in the usual lithotomy position should be noted.

The perineal body, the area at the posterior aspect of the labia where the muscles of the superficial perineal compartment come together, should be inspected. It represents the focal point of support for the perineum and is between the vagina and the rectum. The perianal area is then inspected for evidence of hemorrhoids, sphincter injury, warts, and other lesions (Fig. 7.3).

## PALPATION

The next step in the examination of the perineum involves palpation. The labia minora are gently separated, and the urethra is inspected and the length of the urethra is palpated and "milked" with the middle finger. In this way, irregularities and inflammation of Skene glands (periurethral glands), expressed pus or mucus, or a suburethral diverticulum can be noted. Any pus expressed from the urethra should be submitted for Gram stain and cultured, because it is occasionally found to contain gonococci. Next, the area of the posterior third of the labia majora is palpated by placing the index finger inside the introitus and the thumb on the outside of the labium. In this way, enlargements or cysts of Bartholin glands are noted. This exam should be performed on each side.

The opening of the vagina should be inspected. The presence of a cystocele or a cystourethrocele should be noted. This would be seen as a bulging of vaginal mucosa downward from the anterior wall of the vagina. The presence of this abnormality may be noted either by simply observing or by asking the patient to bear down (Fig. 7.4). Likewise, the posterior wall should be observed

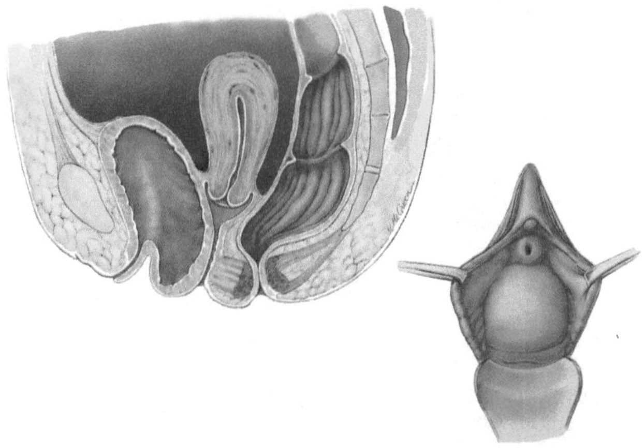

**Figure 7.4** Side and direct views of cystocele. (Modified from Symmonds RE. Anatomy of the female reproductive system. In: Benson RC, ed. *Current Obstetric and Gynecologic Diagnosis and Treatment.* 5th ed. Los Altos, CA: Lange Medical; 1984.)

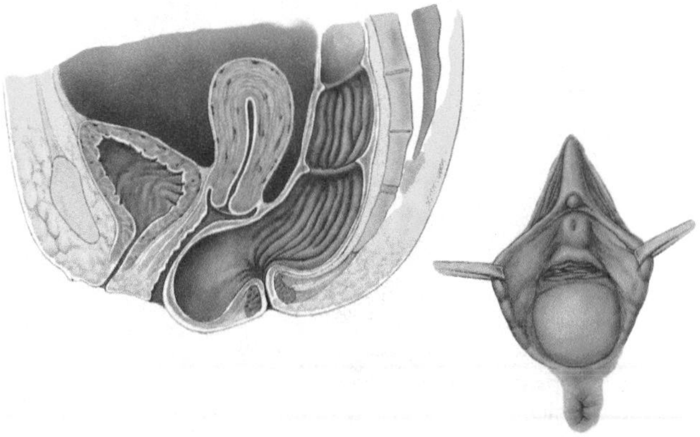

**Figure 7.5** Side and direct views of rectocele. (Modified from Symmonds RE: Relaxations of pelvic supports. In: Benson RC, ed. *Current Obstetric and Gynecologic Diagnosis and Treatment.* 5th ed. Los Altos, CA: Lange Medical; 1984.)

for a bulging upward, which would represent a rectocele (Fig. 7.5). A cystic bulge in the cul-de-sac may represent an enterocele (Fig. 7.6). Also, with the patient bearing down, the cervix may become visible, indicating prolapse of the uterus (Fig. 7.7). Each of these observations is evidence for relaxation of the pelvic supports. Accurate evaluation of pelvic organ prolapse is improved by examining the woman standing with her legs spread apart and with a Valsalva maneuver. Pelvic organ prolapse and pelvic floor dysfunction are defined and extensively discussed in Chapter 20.

## SPECULUM EXAMINATION

After palpation, the physician chooses the appropriate speculum for the patient. The most commonly utilized are the Grave and the Pederson specula. The Pederson speculum is narrower and may be more appropriate for virginal or nulligravid women, women with a history of sexual abuse, vaginal pain or dyspareunia, or postmenopausal women. Each is available in several sizes corresponding to length of the blades (small, medium, large, extra large) (Fig. 7.8).

The speculum should be warmed, either by a warming device or by being placed in warm water, and then touched to the patient's leg to determine that she feels the temperature is appropriate and comfortable. Judicious use of a water-based lubricant can facilitate a more comfortable exam for the patient. The speculum is then inserted by placing the transverse diameter of the blades in the anteroposterior position and guiding the blades through the introitus in a downward motion with the tips pointing toward the rectum. Because the anterior wall of the vagina is backed by the pubic symphysis, which is rigid, pressure upward causes the patient discomfort. This is avoided by following the described method of introducing the speculum. Also, in the resting state the vagina lies on the rectum and actually extends posteriorly from the introitus. Placing two fingers into the introitus and pressing down may facilitate the procedure.

Once the blades are inserted, the speculum should be turned so that the transverse axis of the blades is in the transverse axis of the vagina. The blades should be inserted to their full length and then opened so that the physician may inspect for the position of the cervix. If the cervix cannot be visualized with repositioning of the speculum, the physician should inspect for the position of the cervix with his or her finger and then reinsert the speculum accordingly. Once the blades are inserted and the cervix is visualized, the speculum should be opened and the introitus widened so that the cervix can be adequately inspected and any indicated specimens obtained.

The physician then inspects the vagina and cervix. The vaginal canal is inspected during the insertion of the speculum and upon its removal. The vaginal epithelium should be noted for

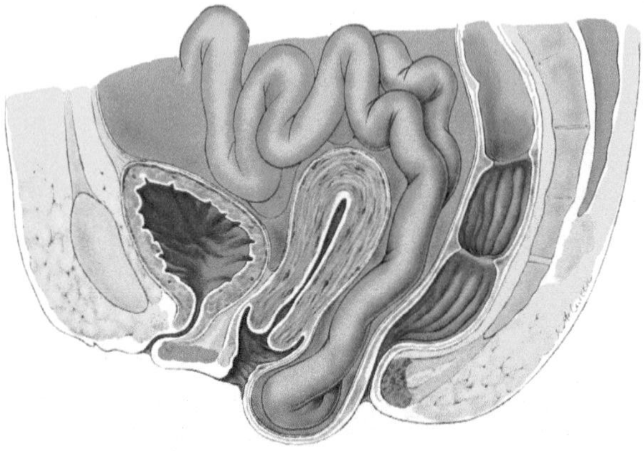

**Figure 7.6** Lateral view of enterocele. (Modified from Symmonds RE: Relaxations of pelvic supports. In: Benson RC, ed. *Current Obstetric and Gynecologic Diagnosis and Treatment.* 5th ed. Los Altos, CA: Lange Medical; 1984.)

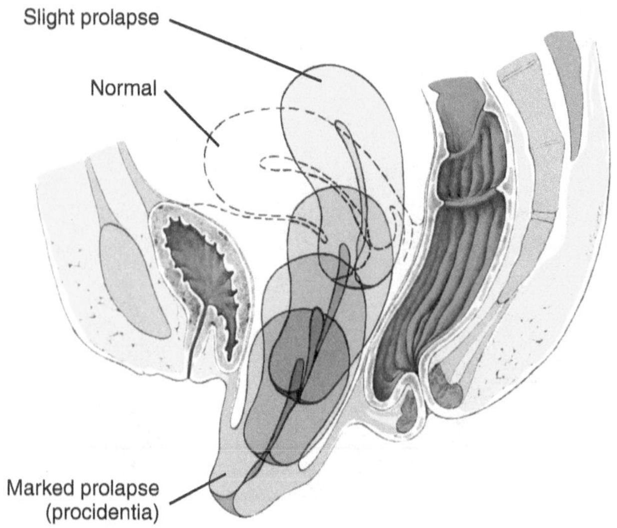


**Figure 7.7** Depiction of prolapse of uterus. (Modified from Symmonds RE: Relaxations of pelvic supports. In: Benson RC, ed. *Current Obstetric and Gynecologic Diagnosis and Treatment.* 5th ed. Los Altos, CA: Lange Medical; 1984.)

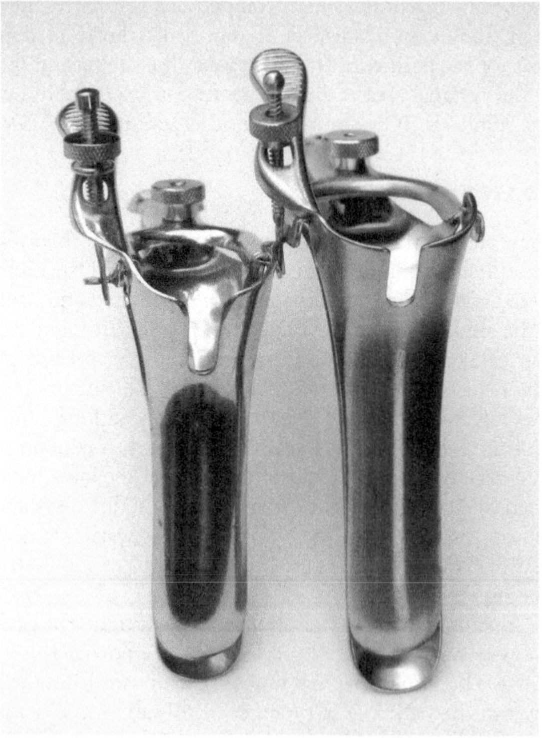

**Figure 7.8** Graves *(left)* and Pederson *(right)* specula.

evidence of erythema or lesions. Vaginal lesions, such as areas of adenosis (see Chapter 11), clear cystic structures (Gartner cysts), or inclusion cysts on the lines of scars or episiotomy incisions, should be noted.

Any concerning fluid discharge is collected for wet mount and potential culture. Saline wet mount allows for visualization of normal vaginal epithelial cells as well as any abnormal findings such as motile *trichomonads*, clue cells (vaginal epithelial cells studded with adherent coccobacilli, indicative of bacterial vaginosis), or polymorphonuclear leukocytes (indicative of inflammation).

A potassium hydroxide wet mount includes the whiff-amine test, which, if positive for a distinct fishy odor, may indicate bacterial vaginosis. In addition, inspection of the slide may reveal hyphae and budding yeast, indicative of *Candida* vaginitis.

In many instances, particularly with women younger than 26 years, it is appropriate to screen for chlamydia and gonorrhea using swabs that sample secretions from the endocervical canal or the vagina. The gold standard is **nucleic acid amplification testing (NAAT)** of the urine or vaginal/cervical discharge, rather than a culture. Yearly chlamydia testing is recommended for all sexually active women up to age 25 (ACOG, Well-Woman Care, 2014) (see Chapter 23).

Next, the cervix is inspected. It should be pink and without lesions. In a nulliparous individual, the external os should be round. When a woman is parous, the external os takes on a slitlike appearance, and if there have been cervical lacerations, healed stellate lacerations may be noted (Fig. 7.9). Normally, the transformation zone (i.e., the junction of squamous and columnar epithelium) is just barely visible inside the external os. Occasionally, glandular epithelium may be present on the **portio vaginalis**, moving the transformation zone onto the portio. This is common in teenage girls, women who have been exposed to diethylstilbestrol in utero, some women with vaginitis, or women immediately postpartum or postabortion. Generally, this is cleared by a process of **metaplasia**, in which squamous epithelium covers the columnar epithelium. This process, however, may leave small areas of irregularities and inclusion cysts, called **nabothian cysts**, which may be seen in various sizes and shapes. They are typically translucent and range from a few millimeters to up to 3 cm in size. These cysts are common benign findings and require no additional evaluation or treatment.

Cervical ectropion occurs when the endocervical epithelium is exposed to the vaginal environment and takes on a reddish appearance, similar to granulation tissue. This **ectropion** is not a pathologic condition.

Any lesions of the cervix should be noted and, where appropriate, a biopsy should be performed. In a patient with acute herpes simplex, vesicles or ulcers may be noted. In a patient infected with human papillomavirus, warts (condylomata acuminata) on the cervix may also be observed.

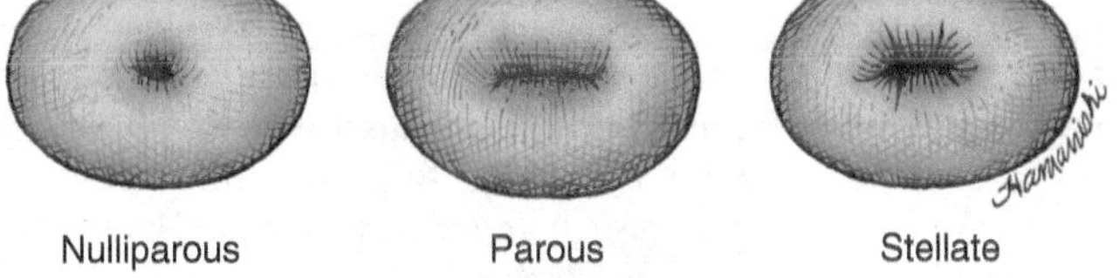


**Figure 7.9** Nulliparous, parous, and stellate lacerations of cervix.

## PAPANICOLAOU SMEAR

At this point in the examination a Pap smear is usually taken, if indicated. In 1943, Papanicolaou and Trout published their now classic monograph demonstrating the value of vaginal and cervical cytology as a screening tool for cervical neoplasm. With the use of the Pap smear in screening programs, the incidence of invasive cervical cancer has been reduced by 50%. In 2012, ACOG together with ACS and U.S. Preventive Services Task Force (USPSTF) recommended that initial screening should begin at age 21 regardless of sexual activity. For women ages 21 through 29, screening should occur every 3 years. Women ages 30 to 65 can either have co-testing (Pap plus high-risk human papillomavirus [HPV] testing) or just a routine Pap test. Repeat co-testing occurs every 5 years, whereas Pap testing alone continues on an every 3-year basis. Pap smear screening is no longer recommended in women after age 65, if she has had normal adequate testing over the past 10 years and she has not been treated for high-grade dysplasia within the past 20 years. Exceptions to the above schedule include HIV seropositive women, immunosuppressed women, and women exposed to DES in utero, all of whom should be screened annually (Saslow, 2012). It is crucial to educate women that this extended interval between Pap smears is based on long-term, excellent analysis of the existing data. The importance of this cancer screening should continue to be highlighted during annual preventive visits, as we know that 50% of cervical cancer cases develop in women who have never had a Pap test, and an additional 10% occur in women who have been underscreened (Saslow, 2012). No Pap smear screening is necessary after a complete hysterectomy done for benign conditions. However, if a supracervical hysterectomy was performed, the same screening guidelines pertain as if there had been no hysterectomy, since the cervix remains in situ.

The goal of the Pap smear is to collect cells from the transformation zone of the cervix. The presence of adequate endo- and ectocervical cells ensures that this area is captured in the specimen. After excess mucus is gently removed (routine swabbing may cause insufficient cells to be sampled), the endocervical canal is sampled with a Cytobrush, which is placed into the canal and rotated. A spatula is then used to collect ectocervical cells (Figs. 7.10 and 7.11). A single broomlike sampling device can also be used to collect both populations of cells in a single step. The collected material is placed in the liquid preservative solution. HPV testing can be concurrently ordered from the collected sample, as indicated (Video 7.1).

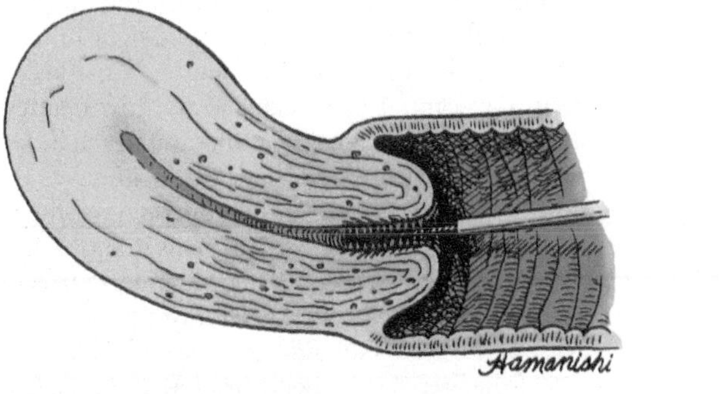


**Figure 7.10** Obtaining cells from endocervix using a Cytobrush.

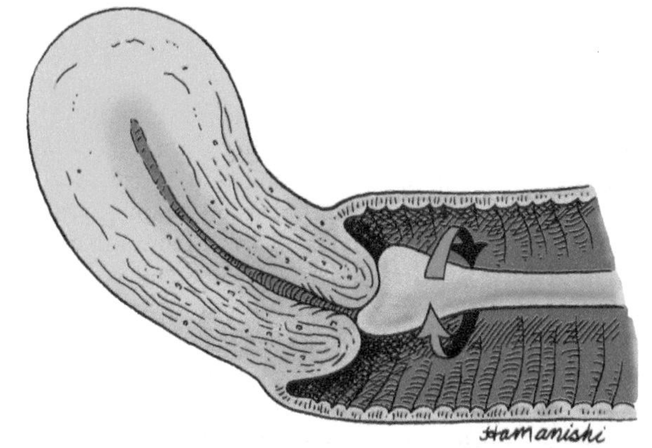


**Figure 7.11** Obtaining cells from transformation zone using Ayers spatula.

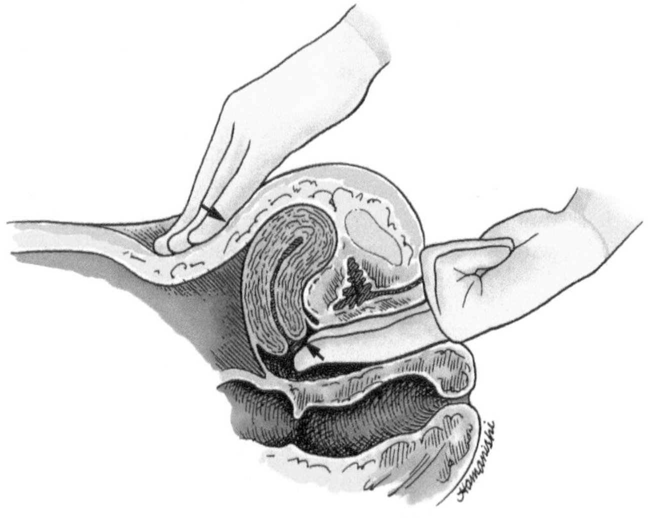


**Figure 7.12** Bimanual examination of uterus.

Chapter 28 discusses cervical dysplasia, classifications of abnormalities, surveillance, and treatment options.

### BIMANUAL EXAMINATION

The bimanual examination allows the physician to palpate the uterus and the adnexa. The lubricated index and middle fingers of the dominant hand are placed within the vagina, and the thumb is folded under so as not to cause the patient distress in the area of the mons pubis, clitoris, and pubic symphysis. The fingers are inserted deeply into the vagina so that they rest beneath the cervix in the posterior fornix. The physician should be in a comfortable position at this point, generally with the leg on the side of the vaginal examining hand on a table lift and the elbow of that arm resting on the knee. The opposite hand is placed on the patient's abdomen above the pubic symphysis. The flat of the fingers are used for palpation. The physician then elevates the uterus by pressing up on the cervix and delivering the uterus to the abdominal hand so that the uterus may be placed between the two hands, thereby identifying its position, size, shape, consistency, and mobility. In the normal and nonpregnant state, the uterus is approximately 6 cm × 4 cm and weighs approximately 60 g. It may be somewhat larger in a woman who has had children (Fig. 7.12).

Enlargement of the uterus should be described in detail. Size may be estimated in centimeters or by comparing with weeks of normal gestational age. The majority of women will have a uterus that is anteverted with the uterine fundus tipped forward. In the anteflexed uterus, the fundus points anteriorly as well. The uterus may be retroverted, in which the entire uterus tips posteriorly, and may also be retroflexed, in which the fundus points posteriorly as well. If it is positioned in a straight line with the vagina, it is said to be midposition or neutral. A markedly retroverted uterus that cannot be brought forward by manipulation is best inspected by rectovaginal examination, which is described later in the chapter. The general shape of the uterus is that of a pear, with the broadest portion at the upper pole of the fundus. Generally, the uterus is mobile, and if it fails to move, it may be fixed by adhesions. The surface should be smooth; irregularities may indicate the presence of uterine leiomyomas (fibroids).

The shape of the uterus should also be described in detail. The consistency of the uterus is generally firm but not rock hard, and this should be noted in the examination. Any undue tenderness caused by palpation or movement of the uterus should be noted, because it may imply an inflammatory process.

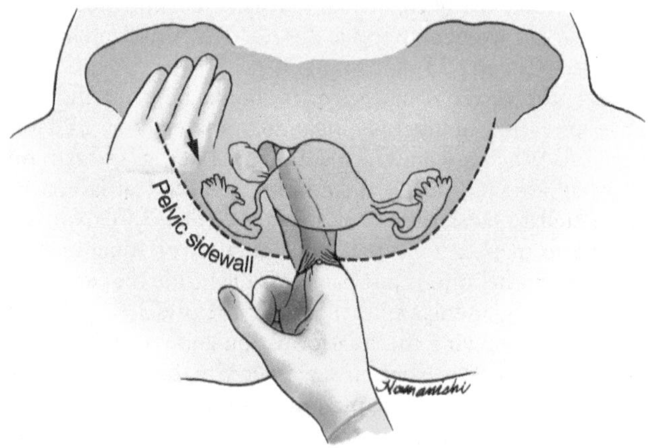


**Figure 7.13** Bimanual examination of adnexa.

Attention is then turned to examination of the adnexa. If the right hand is the pelvic hand, the first two fingers of the right hand are then moved into the right vaginal fornix as deeply as they can be inserted. The abdominal hand is placed just medial to the anterior superior iliac spine on the right, the two hands are brought as close together as possible, and with a sliding motion from the area of the anterior superior iliac spine to the introitus, the fingers are swept downward, allowing for the adnexa to be palpated between them. A normal ovary is approximately 3 × 2 cm (about the size of a walnut) and will sweep between the two fingers with ease unless it is fixed in an abnormal position by adhesions. When the adnexa are palpated, its size, mobility, and consistency should be described. When the right adnexa has been palpated, the left adnexa should be palpated in a similar fashion by turning the vaginal hand to the left vaginal fornix and repeating the exercise on the left side (Fig. 7.13). Adnexa are usually not palpable in postmenopausal women because of involution and retraction of the ovary to a position higher in the pelvis. A palpable organ in such an individual may need further investigation for ovarian pathology if enlarged, although they are mostly benign or no disease is found.

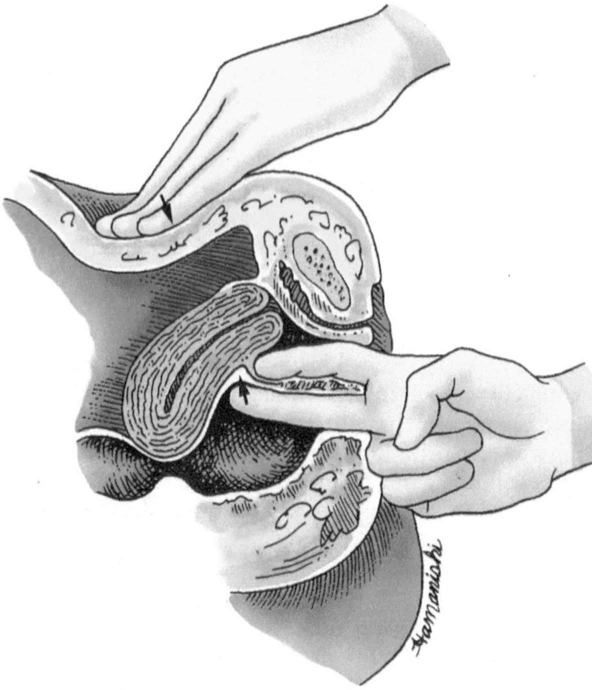

Figure 7.14 Rectovaginal examination.

## RECTOVAGINAL EXAMINATION

Historically, the rectovaginal (RV) exam has been a part of the annual examination. In fact, however, the sensitivity of the RV examination in detecting pathology is very low, limiting its capacity as a screening test. The RV exam should therefore only be performed as indicated based on patient symptoms or complaints or based on findings from the pelvic examination.

After completing the vaginal portion of the bimanual examination, the middle finger is relubricated with a water-soluble lubricant and placed into the rectum. The index finger is reinserted into the vagina. In this fashion the rectovaginal septum is palpated between the two fingers, and any thickness or mass is noted. The finger should also attempt to identify the uterosacral ligaments, which extend from the posterior wall of the cervix posteriorly and laterally toward the sacrum. Any thickening or nodularity of these structures may imply an inflammatory reaction or endometriosis. If the uterus is retroverted, that organ should be outlined for size, shape, and consistency at this point. It may be examined appropriately using the fingers inserted into the vagina and the rectum, as well as using the abdominal hand (Fig. 7.14).

## RECTAL EXAMINATION

The USPSTF and the ACS find that a digital rectal exam, by itself, is not adequate screening for colorectal cancer. Furthermore, testing a single stool specimen for fecal occult blood is also inadequate. Therefore, routine assessment of the rectum is not recommended during female pelvic exams. Colon cancer screening recommendations are described later in this chapter.

Like the RV exam, a rectal examination should only be performed based on patient symptoms, concerns, or findings on the pelvic examination. As noted earlier, simple inspection of the perianal area can reveal abnormalities such as genital warts, hemorrhoids, or skin lesions.

The rectum is then palpated in all dimensions with the rectal examining finger. It should be possible to palpate as many as 70% of distal bowel lesions with the rectal finger. The physician should also note the tone of the anal sphincter and any other anal abnormalities, such as hemorrhoids, fissures, or masses. At the end of the examination the physician should give the patient some tissue or a washcloth so that she may remove the lubricating gel from her perineum before she dresses.

It is important that each step of the examination be explained to the patient and that she is reassured about all normal findings. Wherever possible, abnormal findings should be pointed out to the patient either by allowing her to palpate the pathologic condition or by demonstrating it to her using a hand mirror. It may also be appropriate to demonstrate normal structures to the patient, such as the cervix and portions of the vagina that she may be able to see with her hand mirror. The physician should use the examination as a vehicle for teaching the patient about her body.

# ANNUAL VISIT

The annual visit is important for both health maintenance and preventive medicine reasons. Although the visit varies in emphasis depending on the patient's age, the long-term goals should be to maintain the woman in the best health and functional status possible, to promote high-quality longevity, and to aid in early detection of disease. Long-term continuity of care may improve health status. Major preventable problems must be discussed because patient behavior can make a difference. Various medical groups update recommendations for primary and preventive screening services regularly. Much of this chapter utilizes guidelines from the United States Preventive Services Task Force (USPSTF), American College of Obstetricians and Gynecologists (ACOG), Centers for Disease Control and Prevention (CDC), Morbidity and Mortality Weekly Report (MMWR), other subspecialty guidelines, and the Agency for Healthcare Research and Quality. The latter is a clearinghouse of evidence-based guidelines that allows comparison of differing recommendations, as many societies do not always agree on these guidelines. Their websites can be checked for updates.

It is important not to confuse screening with diagnosis. Screening is looking for a condition in an asymptomatic woman. Diagnostic tests are performed to clarify the etiology of a woman's complaints (symptoms) and are not screening. So when one of the organizations such as the USPSTF makes a recommendation for screening for chlamydia yearly up to age 25, it does not mean you should not test a 26-year-old woman who has symptoms of vaginal discharge or a new sexual partner. Furthermore, screening recommendations must be considered in light of local prevalence of disease and additional risk factors an individual patient might present. The USPSTF also makes recommendations that are qualified by a grade: A = strongly recommends, B = recommends, C = no recommendation for or against, D = recommends against, and I = insufficient evidence to recommend for or against.

A 2004 article published in the *Journal of the American Medical Association* estimated the root causes of American deaths and attributed 18% to tobacco, 15% to poor diet and physical inactivity, 3.5% to alcohol, 4% to microbial agents, 1% to illicit drug use, 2% to toxic agents, 1.2% to firearms, 1.8% to motor vehicles, and 1% to sexual behavior (Mokdad, 2004). Obviously, patients taking an active role in changing their behavior can alter many of these factors, and physicians have the opportunity to advise them at the annual visit. Although the gynecologist may or may not function as the sole primary care provider for women, the annual visit is an opportunity to discuss patient choices, lifestyle, and habits. It offers a perfect environment to provide education about healthy lifestyle and prevention strategies to reduce harm and improve health. In 1618, an English clergyman observed, "Prevention is so much better than healing because it saves the labor of being sick." In 1973, Belloc reported that in a study of women past the age of 45, the life expectancy was 7 years greater for those who routinely practiced six of seven important health habits as compared with those who practiced three or fewer (Box 7.6) (Belloc, 1973). These recommendations hold true today according to a 2009 report from the Agency for Healthcare Research and Quality (AHRQ). During the annual visit, physicians should therefore discuss nutrition regarding (1) proper caloric intake to maintain the patient's weight near her optimum and avoid obesity, (2) restricting saturated fat and cholesterol, and (3) understanding the need for adequate calcium and vitamin D in the diet.

At each checkup the physician should also encourage the patient to develop an exercise program appropriate for her abilities and taking into account her overall health status and recommendations from any other health care providers. Table 7.2 presents the CDC recommendations for types/duration of exercise by age group.

For patients who smoke, benefits of reduction and cessation should be addressed and resources provided. Tobacco use is a leading preventable cause of death in the United States. It is the most important modifiable risk factor associated with adverse pregnancy outcomes, and pregnancy is often a time when a woman will be motivated to quit smoking. The nonreproductive negative health effects of smoking include cancer, coronary artery disease, peripheral vascular disease, respiratory disorder, peptic ulcer disease, and osteoporosis. The five "A"s of smoking cessation are important for providers to know: ask (about use), advise (about use), assess (willingness to quit), assist (in planning and counseling), and arrange (regular contact and follow-up). Counseling strategies have been published and show that 5 to 15 minutes of motivational interviewing and problem-solving strategies will result in a 5% to 10% quit rate. More intensive options to aid in smoking cessation include pharmacotherapy with nicotine replacement, bupropion, or varenicline.

Any alcohol or drug use and potential abuse should also be discussed. Short alcohol use screening questionnaires such as CAGE are utilized in many primary and specialty care clinics.

The physician should discuss possible stressors in the patient's life, such as her relationship with her husband or partner and other family members, her satisfaction or dissatisfaction with her job, and other social problems that she may be experiencing. It is appropriate to ask questions that assess her sexual activity and gratification and questions that detect abuse or intimidation in her life. As OB/GYNs continue to care for women well past menopause, it may also appropriate to discuss the physical and emotional implications of loss and grief. Everyone suffers loss during his or her lifetime, and the older the patient the more likely that this is the case. Grief may be the result of a loss of a spouse or loved one, a pet, a job, a body part, or the ability to perform activities the patient has enjoyed (see Chapter 9).

The patient should provide updated information about all medications/supplements that she takes. This will give the physician the opportunity to review with the patient why she is taking each one and also to assess for potential adverse drug interactions. It may also be possible to tie specific drug use to an undesirable symptom the patient may be experiencing.

**Box 7.6 Good Health Habits**

- Eat moderately
- Eat a healthy diet focusing on fruits, vegetables, whole grains, and foods low in saturated fats*
- Eat breakfast
- Be tobacco free
- Exercise regularly; 30 minutes or more on most days of the week
- Use alcohol in moderation or not at all
- Sleep 7 to 8 hours per night
- Stay at a healthy weight†

*Modified from original according to AHRQ recommendations.
†Added to original according to AHRQ recommendations.

**Table 7.2** CDC Exercise Recommendations

| | Minimum Exercise | | |
|---|---|---|---|
| **Age (Years)** | **Option 1** | **Option 2** | **Option 3** |
| 18-64 | 2.5 hours moderate-intensity aerobic activity/week* and muscle-strengthening‡ activities 2+ days/week | 75 minutes vigorous-intensity aerobic activity/week† and muscle-strengthening activities 2+ days/week | Equivalent mix of moderate and vigorous aerobic activity and muscle-strengthening† activities 2+ days/week |
| 65+ | 2.5 hours moderate-intensity aerobic activity/week* and muscle-strengthening‡ activities 2+ days/week | 75 minutes vigorous-intensity aerobic activity/week† and muscle-strengthening activities 2+ days/week | Equivalent mix of moderate and vigorous aerobic activity and muscle-strengthening† activities 2+ days/week |

Data from Centers for Disease Control and Prevention (CDC). Physical activity basics. How much physical activity do adults need? 2015. Available at http://www.cdc.gov/physicalactivity/basics/adults/index.htm and Centers for Disease Control and Prevention (CDC): Physical Activity Basics. How much physical activity do older adults need? 2015. Available at http://www.cdc.gov/physicalactivity/everyone/guidelines/olderadults.html.
*Moderate-intensity aerobic activity: brisk walking, water aerobics, pushing lawn mower.
†Vigorous-intensity aerobic activity: running, swimming labs, basketball.
‡Muscle-strengthening activities: weight lifting, resistance bands, pushups, heavy gardening, yoga. Older adults need to adjust both type and intensity of exercise. Increasing overall time of aerobic exercise beyond the minimal recommendations further increases health benefits.

The annual visit is an opportunity for the physician to screen for a variety of illnesses affecting not only the reproductive organs but also all of the organ systems. The visit should include an interim health history and an age-appropriate physical examination. The weight, height, and blood pressure measurements with calculated BMI should be obtained. A neck and abdominal exam should be performed. Whether the breast, pelvic, and speculum exams are performed depends on the patient's age, concerns, and agreement between the provider and the patient (see Table 7.1).

In 2013, the American College of Obstetricians and Gynecologists published online the *Well-Woman Care: Assessments & Recommendations,* which recommended screening examinations, immunizations, and laboratory tests for the annual visit for women in different age groups (see Table 7.1). Women with concurrent medical conditions such as obesity or hypertension, women with certain lifestyle choices such as tobacco use, and women with certain family history will be directed to screening that may be sooner or more frequent than that recommended for the general population. The USPSTF and ACOG recommend referral for genetic counseling and evaluation for the breast cancer susceptibility gene *(BRCA)* for women whose family history is associated with an increased risk for deleterious mutations in the *BRCA1* or *BRCA2* genes. Ninety percent of breast cancers are sporadic, but 10% are due to inherited disorders. The prime findings in the history include multiple family members with breast or ovarian cancer, breast and ovarian cancer in a single individual, or early age of breast cancer onset. With women having a one out of eight chance of developing breast cancer in their lifetime, it makes sense to counsel even low-risk women about healthy lifestyle interventions that can lower their risk of cancer, including eating a healthy diet, exercising, and maintaining a normal body weight.

In 2009, the USPSTF published substantial changes in the mammography recommendations that have been extremely controversial. Routine screening mammography was no longer recommended in women 40 to 49 years old. Instead, the decision about when to begin regular screening should be individualized. This received a "C," which means the organization did not recommend for or against. Reasons for this change are that while breast cancer mortality does decrease with screening in this age group, it is a small net benefit. Furthermore, there were concerns about the potential harm of mammography in terms of excess radiation exposure, excess need for additional imaging and breast biopsies (false-positive tests), and patient worries and anxiety about the testing. The recommendation does leave room for an open a discussion with the individual woman. ACOG and ACS continue to recommend mammography screening yearly starting at age 40.

In 2009, screening for ages 50 to 74 was also changed from annual to biennial with a "B" recommendation by the USPSTF. In 2015, the USPSTF issued new draft guidelines regarding screening mammography (USPSTF, 2015).[8] Final updated guidelines should be available in the later half of 2015. ACOG and ACS still recommend yearly mammograms for women 50 and older. Mammograms are reported with the Breast Imaging Reporting and Data System (**BI-RADS**), which classify abnormalities identified by mammography with standardized reporting (see Chapter 15).

A variety of other screening tests are recommended during annual gynecologic visits. See Table 7.1 for ACOG recommendations. Important screening includes tests for diabetes, hyperlipidemia, thyroid disorders, osteoporosis, HIV, and colorectal cancer. The 2008 American College of Gastroenterology guidelines stated that the preferred test for colorectal cancer screening is colonoscopy every 10 years. The alternatives include fecal occult blood testing, flexible sigmoidoscopy, double contrast barium enema, CT colonography, and stool DNA (interval for testing varies based on the method utilized) (Levin, 2008). African Americans should begin routine screening at age 45. A family history of polyps does not evoke earlier onset of screening unless the polyps were advanced adenomas. If a single first-degree relative had colorectal cancer diagnosed after age 60, routine screening is recommended. Otherwise, 10 years before the age at which the family member developed colorectal cancer is the time to begin screening.

Other screening tests, such as tests for hepatitis C and tuberculosis, should certainly be considered for women in high-risk groups, with comorbid medical conditions, or with certain family histories. The USPSTF also recommends offering one-time screening for hepatitis C in adults born between 1945 and 1965.

Cancer screening besides breast, cervix, and colorectal are more symptom based. Endometrial cancer recommendations for early detection consist of advising women at menopause of their risk factors and the symptoms of endometrial cancer. Those symptoms include unexpected vaginal bleeding or spotting. Even in women known to be at increased risk of endometrial cancer, there is insufficient evidence to recommend screening (unopposed estrogen treatment, tamoxifen therapy, late menopause, nulliparity, infertility or anovulation, obesity, hypertension, and diabetes). Women at very high risk should have an annual endometrial biopsy starting at age 35 (known hereditary nonpolyposis colorectal cancer, genetic mutation carrier, or strongly suspected carrier). Regular health exams to include the thyroid, ovaries, lymph nodes, oral cavity, and skin should be offered, but no special recommendations have been made.

The best source of updated recommendations for adult immunization schedules is the CDC's MMWR website (see Table 7.1). All women should have a Tdap booster once in their adult lifetime and in each third trimester of pregnancy to facilitate some passive immunity to the fetus against *Bordetella pertussis.* Then, every 10 years, the regular TD (tetanus-diphtheria) booster is given. Influenza vaccination is recommended annually as well.

Three highly efficacious human papillomavirus (HPV) vaccines are available. In 2006, the Advisory Committee on Immunization Practices (ACIP) and then ACOG recommended vaccinating all girls and young women ages 9 to 26 with the quadrivalent vaccine Gardasil. The U.S. Food and Drug Administration (FDA) approved this in 2009. Then in 2011, ACIP recommended this vaccination for boys and young men as well. A second HPV vaccine, Cervarix, was ACIP approved in 2009. Most recently, a third HPV vaccine, the 9-valent HPV vaccine, Gardasil 9, became available. This vaccine was FDA approved in December 2014 and recommended by ACIP in February 2015. This vaccine contains virus-like particles not only for HPV types 6, 11, 16, and 18 but also for five more high-risk strains of HPV: 31, 33, 45, 52, and 58. This vaccine has been approved for females ages 9 to 26 and males ages 9 to 15. This vaccine affords more thorough coverage against the top HPV virus strains that can lead to cervical, vaginal, and vulvar cancer. Ideally, the vaccine should be administered before the onset of sexual activity to prevent cervical dysplasia and cancer and other diseases caused by low and high-risk strains of HPV. Both vaccines have excellent safety profiles and contain virus-like particles (VLPs), but no infectious virus, and are given in a three-dose series. The bivalent vaccine contains VLPs for HPV types 16 and 18, which protect against 70% of cervical cancer cases. The quadrivalent vaccine contains VLPs for HPV types 16, 18, 6, and 11. HPV types 6 and 11 cause 90% of genital warts. Because both vaccines prevent new infection against the vaccine containing VLP types but are not effective in preventing disease in individuals already exposed to these types, every effort should be made to target HPV-naive individuals. A new 9-valent vaccine will likely be available after this printing. See the discussion of intraepithelial neoplasia of the cervix in Chapter 28 for further details.

For women in high-risk groups, MMR and hepatitis B vaccine should be given if indicated. Pneumococcal vaccine should be offered to women with chronic lung, liver, or cardiovascular disease; diabetes; asplenia; cochlear implants; and immunocompromising conditions. Herpes zoster vaccine (for shingles) is recommended for women age 60 and over. For women who are 65 and older, the pneumococcal vaccine should be given once.

In addition, women in all age groups should be offered appropriate immunizations and vaccinations when they travel to other countries. The hepatitis A vaccine is available and should be offered to women of all ages. In particular, the hepatitis A vaccine should be given to women who are traveling to areas with a high or intermediate endemicity of hepatitis A, use injection drugs, have chronic liver disease, receive clotting factor concentrates, or work with primates infected with hepatitis A.

Physicians should discuss risk behavior annually with their patients. In line with injury prevention, the patient should be reminded about the use of seat belts and helmets and other safety concerns mentioned earlier in this chapter. Fall precautions can be discussed with elderly patients.

Exposure of the skin to ultraviolet radiation and proper precautions to avoid overexposure should be discussed. Regular dental checkups should be encouraged. Adequate calcium and vitamin D intake for proper bone health and age-appropriate intake recommendations should be reviewed at the annual visit (Table 7.3).

Table 7.3 Recommended Intakes of Calcium and Vitamin D

| Age (Years) | Intake Calcium (mg) | Intake Vitamin D (IU) |
|---|---|---|
| 14-18 | 1300 | 600 |
| 19-50 | 1000 | 600 |
| 5170 | 1200 | 600 |
| 71+ | 1200 | 800 |
| Pregnancy and lactation | 1000 | 600 |

From Institute of Medicine, Food and Nutrition Board. *Dietary Reference Intakes for Calcium and Vitamin D*. Washington, DC: National Academy Press; 2010. Available at http://iom.nationalacademies.org/Reports/2010/Dietary-Reference-Intakes-for-Calcium-and-Vitamin-D/DRI-Values.aspx.

Many women will ask their physician about prophylactic aspirin use. The U.S. Preventive Services Task Force (USPSTF, 2009). recommends that women with no history of heart disease or stroke aged 55 to 79 years use aspirin to prevent stroke when the benefit of aspirin use outweighs the potential harm of gastrointestinal hemorrhage or other forms of serious bleeding. The latest research suggests that most healthy women under age 65 should not take aspirin, as the risk of gastrointestinal bleeding outweighs the benefits (van Kruijsdijk, 2014). A woman's individual risk factors must be weighed.

Promoting good health is a continuing responsibility for both the physician and the patient. It represents a challenge that includes education and observation on the physician's part and motivation on the patient's part. The U.S. Department of Health and Human Services has a division devoted to women's health titled the Office on Women's Health. Its website (www.womenshealth.gov) offers accurate patient information on screening recommendations for both healthy and at-risk women. Furthermore, the website lists symptoms of serious health conditions for heart attack and stroke as well as for reproductive, breast, lung, digestive, bladder, skin, mental health, and muscle or joint problems. ACOG similarly has a comprehensive document for providing screening and prevention suggestions for women (www.acog.org/wellwoman).

## SPECIAL POPULATIONS

The 2010 United States Census data estimated there were 56 million noninstitutionalized people with a self-care disability. Women with disabilities have some unique barriers to gynecologic care. Aside from communication obstacles and nonavailability of facilities with exam tables to make routine pelvic exams easily performed, there may be ignorance or negative attitudes about a woman's life with disabilities. Women with disabilities undergo screening for cervical and breast cancer less often than recommended. Contraception, sexuality issues, childbearing plans, and abuse issues may all have to be addressed.

Data from the 2006-2008 National Survey of Family Growth revealed that 1.1% and 3.5% of women identify as lesbian or bisexual, respectively. ACOG reflects that women in this group face barriers to health care, including discriminatory attitudes and treatment, confidentiality and disclosure concerns, limited health care access, and perhaps limited understanding of their risks. Physicians should not assume all women are heterosexual, and asking about sexual activity can be done in a sensitive manner. Physicians sometimes conclude, incorrectly, that lesbian women do not need sexually transmitted infection or Pap screening because they are considered low risk. Fertility services should not be influenced by sexual orientation. ACOG has developed a committee opinion with background and recommendations (ACOG, Committee Opinion #525, 2012). Other populations that may encounter problems accessing gynecologic care include transgendered individuals and incarcerated, abused, or drug-addicted women.

## KEY POINTS

- Strive to become a culturally sensitive and aware physician with a nonjudgmental approach to women regardless of race or ethnicity, age, faith, disabilities, profession, sexual orientation, or activities.
- Menstrual history includes age of menarche, number of days of cycle, number of days of flow, presence of bleeding between menstrual periods, the date of the last menstrual period, and the date of the previous menstrual period.
- A complete gynecologic evaluation should always include a sexual history, contraceptive history, and history of physical or sexual abuse.
- The specific components of the annual exam will be based on patient age, health concern, and risk factors. Whether to perform breast or pelvic exams is a joint decision between individual providers and their patients.
- Cervical cytology screening should begin at age 21 regardless of the onset of sexual activity.
- Pap smears should be performed every 3 years until age 29, then either every 3 or 5 years, depending on the addition of HPV testing. Screening should continue until between age 65 and 70, at which time adequately screened women and those with negative screening can stop undergoing cervical cancer screening.
- Sexually active women should be evaluated at appropriate intervals for sexually transmitted diseases, with annual chlamydia screening for women age 26 and under. Counseling women on safe sex practices to avoid contracting sexually transmitted diseases is important.
- Goals of preventive medicine include maintaining good health and function and promoting high-quality longevity.
- The physician should maintain an immunization record for each patient and offer appropriate vaccinations as recommended by public health guidelines.

## KEY REFERENCES

ACOG Committee on Health Care for Underserved Women. ACOG committee opinion no. 525: health care for lesbians and bisexual women. *Obstet Gynecol.* 2012;119(5). 1977–1080.

American Academy of Ophthalmology (AAO). Policy statement: frequency of ocular examinations. San Francisco; 2015. Available at http://www.aao.org/clinical-statement/frequency-of-ocular-examinations–november-2009 Accessed July 30, 2015.

Belloc NB. Relationship of health practices and mortality. *Prev Med.* 1973;2(1):67–81.

Levin B, Lieberman DA, McFarland B, Smith RA, Brooks D, Andrews KS, et al. Screening and surveillance for the early detection of colorectal cancer and adenomatous polyps, 2008: a joint guideline from the American Cancer Society, the US Multi-Society Task Force on Colorectal Cancer, and the American College of Radiology. *CA Cancer J Clin.* 2008;58(3): 130–160.

Mokdad AH, Marks JS, Stroup DF, et al. Actual causes of death in the United States, 2000. *JAMA.* 2004;291(10):1238–1245.

Moyer VA. Screening for HIV: U.S. Preventive Services Task Force Recommendation Statement. *Ann Intern Med.* 2013;159:51–60.

Qaseem A, Humphrey LL, Harris R, Starkey M, Denberg TD. Clinical Guidelines Committee of the American College of Physicians: Screening pelvic examination in adult women: a clinical practice guideline from the American College of Physicians. *Ann Intern Med.* 2014;161(1):67–72.

Saslow D, Solomon D, Lawson HW, Killackey M, Kulasingam SL, Cain J, et al. American Cancer Society, American Society for Colposcopy and Cervical Pathology, and American Society for Clinical Pathology screening guidelines for the prevention and early detection of cervical cancer. *CA Cancer J Clin.* 2012;62(3):147–172.

US Preventive Services Task Force (USPSTF). Aspirin for the prevention of cardiovascular disease: US Preventive Services Task Force Recommendation Statement. *Ann Intern Med.* 2009;150(6):396–404.

US Preventive Services Task Force (USPSTF). *Breast cancer screening draft recommendations.* 2015. Available at http://screeningforbreastcancer.org/?ds=1&s=breast%2520cancer%2520screening. Accessed August 11, 2015.

Suggested Readings can be found on ExpertConsult.com.

# 8 Interaction of Medical Diseases and Female Physiology

*Sarah K. Dotters-Katz, Fidel A. Valea*

This chapter highlights the interactions and influences of female physiology on major medical disease processes. The chapter also reviews how medical diseases affect female physiology. Many disease processes act directly; for example, renal failure commonly induces abnormal uterine bleeding. Other diseases act indirectly through their therapies, such as cancer chemotherapy, which may lead to ovarian failure. Multiple chapters in this text discuss important aspects of female physiology. This chapter serves as an addendum to those discussions. When considering specific drug interactions and doses, the clinician is encouraged to review current pharmacologic literature.

In general, the impact of female physiology on medical disease is primarily via the effects of estrogen and to a lesser extent progesterone. Other hormones, such as prolactin, oxytocin, and gonadotropins, play minor roles. Estrogen and progesterone affect almost all major organ systems in both tonic and cyclic modes. The effects of the female hormones are mediated directly through receptors (estrogen alpha, estrogen beta, progesterone) as well as indirectly through their effects on other organ systems, such as smooth muscle relaxation and changes in prostaglandin levels. The responses induced by estrogen and progesterone may be theorized, in a teleologic sense, as promoting successful reproduction. Pathology occurs when the normal hormonal effects overlap a disease process that is already present.

Medical diseases affect female physiology at all levels of the hypothalamic-pituitary-ovarian-genital axis, from anovulation to vaginal atrophy. Medical diseases also affect female physiology in a horizontal manner, throughout every stage of a woman's life. Thus medical diseases must be seen in both a vertical and a horizontal context (i.e., a three-dimensional manner). The gynecologist acts as a consultant to other health professionals. As such, we are frequently asked to help with complications stemming from gynecologic issues. Though different clinicians direct the treatment of lupus, multiple sclerosis, or epilepsy, modulating the effects of female physiology on these disease processes is the role of the gynecologist.

## PULMONARY DISEASE

Asthma is more common in boys up until puberty. After puberty, the ratio reverses with women more prone to asthma until menopause. Asthma is one of several major diseases in which the severity of symptoms is increased around the time of menses (Box 8.1). Premenstrual asthma is well described, affecting up to 40% of reproductive-age women who have asthma, with symptoms including increasing cough, wheezing, and shortness of breath. Up to 50% of hospitalizations for asthmatic women in their 20s will occur around the time of menses. Women with premenstrual asthma have been shown to have a measurable decline in respiratory function with the end of the cycle (Dratva, 2010). Data suggest that combination oral contraceptives (OCPs) may blunt this effect and mildly decrease the severity of the asthma (Dratva, 2010). The variability of symptoms between cycles may be caused by the hormonal fluctuations from one cycle to the next.

There are several mechanisms by which hormones can affect symptoms. One theory is that the increased symptomatology is related to the estrogen and progesterone-mediated increase in both serotonin and histamine release from granulocytes and mast cells (van den Berge, 2009). Estrogen also increases eosinophilic adhesion to the bronchial lining. In addition, progesterone induces degranulation of eosinophils. Interestingly, both estrogen and progesterone also have anti-inflammatory properties, and it may be that the withdrawal of estrogen and progesterone at the end of the cycle contributes to the fluctuation in prostaglandin levels that lead to increased bronchial reactivity and premenstrual asthma.

Regarding the effects of asthma on female physiology, a few small series have noted an increased incidence of abnormal menstrual cycles in women with severe asthma (Real, 2007). Whether this is due to glucocorticoid medications or whether this is a direct effect from severe pulmonary disease on the hypothalamus is unclear. It should be noted that multiple studies have found that women with early menarche have twice the risk of asthma in early adulthood (Fida, 2012). Women who are taking inhaled glucocorticoids may be an increased for osteopenia and osteoporosis (Aljubran, 2014). Clinicians who care for women with asthma beyond their third decade should obtain vitamin D levels and council the women about adequate calcium intake. There are conflicting reports about the effect of menopause and hormone replacement therapy on asthma symptoms and severity; some have noted an improvement in symptoms, whereas others have noted a worsening (Tam, 2011; van den Berge, 2009).

**Box 8.1 Major Diseases in Which Menstrual Hormonal Changes Affect Symptoms**

Asthma
Atopic reactions
Epilepsy
Eating disorders
Irritable bowel syndrome
Menstrual migraines
Mental health disorders
Multiple sclerosis
Inflammatory bowel disease
Rheumatoid arthritis
Supraventricular tachycardia
Sickle cell disease
Type 1 diabetes

It is now common for women with cystic fibrosis (CF) to reach reproductive age. Tsang and colleagues, in a review of reproductive problems, noted that women with cystic fibrosis tend to have shorter stature, delayed puberty with delayed growth spurts, and delayed menarche (Tsang, 2010). The degree of delay is related to the severity of the disease. Additionally, due to the effects of estradiol on mucin production, periods of the menstrual cycle with high estradiol levels are associated with worse lung function (Tam, 2011). Girls with cystic fibrosis tend to be as sexually active as their peers; however, they tend to have less counseling regarding contraception than their peers. Estrogen-based contraceptives are acceptable for women with cystic fibrosis as long as they do not have pulmonary hypertension, active liver disease, or a history of thromboembolism (Tsang, 2010). Long-acting reversible contraception (LARCs), including the progesterone intrauterine devices (IUDs) or progesterone implants, are also safe, effective, and a practical option for these young women. Issues of sexuality may be problematic for young women with severe cystic fibrosis because of poor body image secondary to chronic disease, infections, and gastrointestinal disturbances from pancreatic problems, as well as sometimes enlarged rib cages from chronic hyperventilation. Thus counseling on sexuality should occur in conjunction with contraceptive counseling.

There is an emerging body of evidence suggesting that fertility is affected in women with cystic fibrosis. Cervical mucus is thicker in women with cystic fibrosis and may lead to altered fertility. Oligomenorrhea, amenorrhea, and ovulatory dysfunction are increased in women with cystic fibrosis related to the degree of severity of disease. Finally, alterations in uterine levels of bicarbonate, which affects sperm capacitation, also affect fertility in women with cystic fibrosis (Ahmad, 2013). Though a full discussion of the management of subfertility and infertility treatment options is beyond the scope of this chapter, intrauterine insemination, intracytoplasmic sperm injection, and in vitro fertilization have all been successfully performed in women with CF.

## IMMUNE AND ALLERGIC DISEASE

The profound effect that female physiology has on immunity is best exemplified by the remarkably increased survival of women compared with men from infectious causes. Estrogen and progesterone have multiple effects on the immune processes, through numerous cellular sites. This is manifest in multiple disease processes (Box 8.2). In most women the effects are mild, but in women constitutionally or genetically predisposed to atopic reaction or autoimmune disease, the effects can be significant.

**Box 8.2 Effects of Estrogen and Progesterone on Cellular Processes of the Immune System**

**B Cell**
Inhibited bone marrow B-cell lines with high concentrations of estrogen
Increased antibody production through inhibition of T-cell suppression
Enhanced interleukin-10 response

**T Cell**
Lower doses of estrogen are stimulatory, higher doses of estrogen are inhibitory, primarily through TNF
Stimulation of inhibitory T-cell pathways and T-cell cytokines
Low-level stimulation of interleukins

**Monocytes**
Increased monocyte apoptosis inhibiting differentiation
Inhibited dendritic cell differentiation (in vitro)
Inhibited migration of inflammatory cells with decreased migration at higher estrogen levels

**Mast Cells and Granulocytes**
Estrogen increases serotonin and histamine release through estrogen alpha-receptors
Progesterone promotes IgE production

**General Inflammation**
Increased presence of estrogen beta-receptors over estrogen alpha receptors with generalized inflammation
Increased sensitization of sensory neural tissue leading to increased neurogenic inflammation
Increased fibroblast activity and improved wound healing
Increased stimulation of the hypothalamus-pituitary-adrenal axis
Increased anaphylaxis* and allergic reactions

*Includes drug-induced and radiologic contrast media induced.
Data from Chen A, Rogan WJ. Isoflavones in soy infant formula: a review of evidence for endocrine and other activity in infants. *Annu Rev Nutr.* 2004;24:33-54; Lang JT, McCullough LD. Pathways to ischemic neuronal cell death: are sex differences relevant? *J Transl Med.* 2008;6:33; Straub RH. The complex role of estrogens in inflammation. *Endocr Rev.* 2007;28(5):521-574.

The overall effect may be grossly simplified in noting estrogen's effect on the B cell as an immune enhancer (Lang, 2004). In contrast, on T cells, estrogen tends to act as an inhibitor (Lang, 2004). Importantly, estrogen effects vary by the level and type of estrogen. At lower levels, as in most of the menstrual cycle, estrogen stimulates immune responses. However, at high estrogen levels such as with pregnancy, estrogen generally inhibits immune cellular responses. The effects of estrogen on inflammation have important implications for wound healing. Women heal much better than men because estrogen stimulates fibroblast activity and nerve growth. Estrogen's positive effect on reepithelialization lasts until several years after menopause (Straub, 2007). Interestingly, hormone replacement therapy improves wound healing (Perželʼová, 2016).

B-cell–dominated autoimmune diseases have a higher incidence and severity in women (Straub, 2007). Estrogen enhances the hypersensitivity responses from both B-cell activity and granulocyte action in allergic responses (Chen, 2008). Women are more prone than men to eczema, atopic irritations, hypersensitivity, and

Table 8.1 Medical Disorders with Contraindicated Contraceptive Options

| Medical Disorder | Contraindicated Contraception | Rationale/Complication |
|---|---|---|
| Systemic lupus erythematosus with antiphospholipid antibodies or thrombosis | Estrogen-containing contraception* (ECC) | Increased venous thrombosis (VTE) risk |
| Crohn disease | Any oral contraception<br>ECC† | Decreased absorption<br>Increased VTE risk |
| Severe dyslipidemia | ECC | Increased VTE risk |
| Hypertension with risk factors‡ | ECC | Increased VTE, stroke, and myocardial infarction risk |
| Renal transplant | ECC | Increased VTE risk<br>Increased metabolism |
| Thrombophilias | ECC | Increased VTE risk |
| Diabetes with risk factors§ | ECC | Increased VTE risk |
| Malabsorptive bariatric surgery | Any oral contraception | Decreased absorption |
| Migraine with aura | ECC | Increased VTE |
| Epilepsy on enzyme-inducing antiepileptic drugs | Progesterone-only oral contraception<br>Progesterone implant | Increased metabolism |

Modified from Centers for Disease Control and Prevention. U S. medical eligibility criteria for contraceptive use, 2010. *MMWR Recomm Rep*. 2010;59(RR-4):1-86.
*Includes combined oral contraception, vaginal ring, and the transdermal patch.
†In cases of extensive or active disease, prior bowel resection, very active disease, corticosteroid use, or immobilization.
‡Risk factors include: poor control, tobacco use, age >35, other chronic medical condition leading to vascular degradation, end organ damage, use of anti-hypertensives.
§Risk factors include end-organ damage, vascular disease, hyperlipidemia, poorly controlled disease.

anaphylaxis from foods, medications, radiologic contrast media, and anesthesia (Chen, 2008). Granulocytes, eosinophils, mast cells, and basophils are enhanced by estrogen (Chen, 2008). Estrogen also enhances serotonin and histamine release. In contrast, cellular-mediated immune mechanisms, primarily controlled through T cells, tend to be functionally inhibited by estrogen. At high, pregnancy levels of estrogen, there is functional inhibition of T-cell function, leading to improvement of T-cell–mediated autoimmune diseases during pregnancy such as rheumatoid arthritis or multiple sclerosis (Straub, 2007). During periods of estrogen withdrawal, late luteal phase, menstruation, postpartum, and early menopause, there are often clinical rebounds and an increase in disease flares with the release of T-cell suppression.

For the gynecologist asked to consult on women with autoimmune diseases, important strategies include ensuring that any pregnancy is planned, not only to allow time for medication optimization balancing disease stability with fetal risk but also because the best pregnancy outcomes occur when autoimmune diseases are quiescent. Thus effective contraception is essential. Estrogen-containing contraceptives (ECCs) (including the vaginal ring, the transdermal patch, and combined oral contraceptive pills) are acceptable for women with systemic lupus erythematosus (SLE), if they do not have antiphospholipid antibody syndrome or a history of thrombosis (Table 8.1) (Centers for Disease Control and Prevention [CDC], 2010). Women with SLE are also prone to menstrual irregularities, thus hormonal contraceptive may also help with cyclic regulation (Tseng, 2011). However, LARC methods are also safe, have similar benefits as far as cyclic regulation, are more effective contraceptives, and are less susceptible to user error than all ECCs, but especially OCPs. ECCs have not been shown to increase the severity of disease or the number of flares in premenopausal women with SLE (Sanchez-Guerrero, 2005).

In general, most of the autoimmune diseases are not worse around the time of menses. For the women with menstrual exacerbation, hormonal contraceptives may help to decrease periodic variability. SLE does not seem to affect menses or the timing of menopause. However, some anti-inflammatory medications,

Table 8.2 Antineoplastic and Chemotherapeutic Agents That May Produce Ovarian Failure

| Major Risk | Moderate Risk | Minimal Risk |
|---|---|---|
| Cyclophosphamide | Cisplatin | Methotrexate |
| Melphalan | Adriamycin | 5-fluorouracil |
| Busulfan | Paclitaxel* | Vincristine |
| Chlorambucil | | Bleomycin |
| Procarbazine | | Actinomycin |
| Nitrogen mustard | | |

Modified from Sonmezer M, Oktay K. Fertility preservation in young women undergoing breast cancer therapy. *Oncologist*. 2006;11(5):422-434.
*Unquantified risk at this time.

including glucocorticoids and antineoplastic agents, will affect not only the hypothalamic-pituitary-ovarian (HPO) axis but the ovarian follicles as well (Table 8.2). Women with severe end-organ disease may develop down-regulation of the HPO axis (see Chapter 26). Hormone replacement therapy (HRT) has been shown to increase the number of mild, but not severe, flares in lupus patients (Sammaritano, 2012).

Multiple sclerosis (MS), is another autoimmune condition that merits discussion. Women are more frequently affected but usually have a less severe disease course than men (Ghezzi, 2008). Evidence is mixed regarding the effects of menstruation in disease flares. However, for women with cyclic disease flares, hormonal contraceptives are safe (Ghezzi, 2008). Women with severe multiple sclerosis have an increased risk of sexual dysfunction. Though data are limited, HRT may be useful for postmenopausal women with MS.

## GASTROINTESTINAL DISEASE

Estrogen and progesterone are critical in the modulation of the gastrointestinal tract. Estrogen plays a role in the secretory and absorptive function in gut epithelium, affects the gut's microbiome composition, and has receptors on enteric neurons, which regulate neurogenic reflexes (Mulak, 2014). Progesterone is known to affect the motility of the gut, as well as the growth and metabolism of the bacteria in the gastrointestinal tract (Mulak, 2014). Thus it is no surprise that many gastrointestinal disease processes affect women differently than they affect men.

Irritable bowel syndrome (IBS) is perhaps the best example of this effect. With a female-to-male prevalence as high as 5:1, up to half of women with IBS will have exacerbations of symptoms with menses. The rapid progesterone withdrawal at the end of the luteal phase and the increase in systemic prostaglandins both lead to exacerbations of symptoms, including bloating and abdominal pain (Mulak, 2014). OCPs have been shown to decrease symptoms in women with IBS. For women in whom menstrual effects become debilitating, the use of GnRH agonists or continuous OCPs has been suggested. The incidence of IBS tends to decrease after menopause.

Celiac disease, like other autoimmune diseases, tends to preferentially affect women. Females are at twice the risk for developing celiac disease (Liu, 2014). Women with undiagnosed or poorly controlled celiac disease have more irregular menstrual cycles and secondary amenorrhea. A meta-analyses regarding fertility and celiac disease suggested that women with unexplained infertility should be tested for celiac disease, but that women with well-controlled disease do not have decreased fertility compared with women without celiac (Tersigni, 2014).

Women with Crohn disease and ulcerative colitis tend to have symptomatic exacerbations around the time of menses, specifically worsening nausea, constipation, and diarrhea. Inflammatory bowel disease (IBD) has also been shown to have a negative effect on body image and sexuality (Moleski, 2011). Dyspareunia is common, especially in those with Crohn disease. Women also cite abdominal pain, fear of incontinence, and diarrhea as reasons for decreased levels of sexual activity (Moleski, 2011). Effective contraception is important for women with IBD, as unplanned pregnancy in the setting of active disease is associated with worse maternal and fetal outcomes (Moleski, 2011). Though OCPs are not associated with disease relapse, there are some data suggesting decreased absorption in women with Crohn disease as well as in those women with increased intestinal transit secondary to previous bowel resection. For women with IBD who are at an increased risk for venous thrombosis (VTE), including those with extensive or active disease, corticosteroid use, vitamin deficiencies, or immobilization, ECCs are not recommended (CDC, 2010). LARC methods are considered safe and very effective in women with IBD, independent of disease severity, and thus often are preferred over oral contraceptive options and ECCs. It is also important to note that women with IBD are at increased risk for osteoporosis and osteopenia, and they should be screened accordingly.

Estrogen has been noted to have a protective effective on the development and progression of liver disease. Women with hepatitis C have a better response to therapy and a slower rate of disease progression than men (Rodríguez-Castro, 2014). Research also suggests estrogen plays a significant role in preventing carcinogenesis in the liver (Zhang, 2013). As such, hepatocellular carcinoma is less common in women. Some reports have also detailed the use of hormone replacement in postmenopausal women to inhibit liver fibrosis (Zhang, 2013). In contrast, autoimmune-mediated liver diseases, such as primary biliary cirrhosis and autoimmune hepatitis, are more common in women. It is also important to note that for women with cirrhosis or severe liver disease, estrogen-containing contraceptive options are contraindicated.

## VASCULAR AND HYPERTENSIVE DISEASES

In general, estrogens have a positive effect on the vascular system through improved lipid profiles. The presence of estrogen is associated with lower rates of atherogenic dyslipidemia, cardiovascular disease, and metabolic syndrome (Pellegrini, 2014). This effect is lost in postmenopausal women. However, women with dyslipidemias may have complications with estrogen because of its procoagulant effects, especially after the third or fourth decade. Women with a dyslipidemia should avoid estrogen-based contraceptives and hormone replacement therapy. However, progesterone-based contraceptives, including LARC methods, are safe and effective for these women, independent of age.

In contrast, vascular and hypertensive diseases have important effects on women. Studies indicate that women with hypertension have much higher than expected levels of sexual dysfunction with impaired genital congestion and decreased arousal (Doumas, 2006). Data regarding the effects of antihypertensive medications on sexual function are mixed. Though beta-blockers are consistently associated with worsening sexual function, multiple studies have noted that adequate blood pressure control with medication leads to an improvement in sexual function (De Franciscis, 2013; Doumas, 2006; Fogari, 2004). Women with coronary artery disease, as well as survivors of myocardial infarction, have less sexual activity and increased sexual dysfunction (Basson, 2007). Thus it is helpful for gynecologists to inquire about sexual issues in women with cardiovascular disorders.

Hormonally based contraceptives may be problematic in women who are taking antihypertensive medications or those with poorly controlled hypertension. If there is no associated thrombosis, guidelines from the American College of Obstetricians and Gynecologists (ACOG) suggest that women may use ECCs as long as their blood pressures are well controlled (ACOG, 2006; World Health Organization [WHO], 2015). A return office visit 2 or 3 months after initiation of any ECC to assess blood pressure and potential side effects is appropriate. Studies have shown a small increase in stroke and myocardial infarction in women on oral contraceptives with hypertension, but the absolute risk is quite small (ACOG, 2006; WHO, 2015). It should also be noted that women with a history of pregnancy-related hypertension who are currently normotensive are also at a slightly increased risk for myocardial infarction and VTE, though again, the absolute risk is small (ACOG, 2006; WHO, 2015). As long as a woman does not use tobacco or does not have other aspects of vascular disease besides mild hypertension, ECCs may be reasonable. However, LARC methods are preferable, especially after age 35.

Cardiac arrhythmias are also affected by gender, though the exact pathophysiologic reasons for this are unclear. Atrioventricular nodal reentrant tachycardia occurs twice as frequently in women as in men, though Wolff-Parkinson-White syndrome is more common in males (Curtis, 2012). Supraventricular tachycardias and ectopic ventricular beats occur more frequently and last longer in the luteal phase of the menstrual cycle (Curtis, 2012). The QT interval tends to be longer in women, increasing the risk for torsades de pointes. Though rates of atrial fibrillation are lower in women, women with atrial fibrillation are less likely to be anticoagulated, undergo ablative procedures, and are more likely to suffer a stroke (Curtis, 2012). Sudden cardiac death affects both genders equally.

### *Renal Disease*

Women with end-stage renal disease (ESRD) have high prolactin levels as well as gonadotropin-mediated disruption of the luteinizing hormone (LH) surge (Guglielmi, 2013). These hormonal alterations result in anovulatory cycles, amenorrhea, oligomenorrhea, menorrhagia, infertility, and decreased libido. The effects of chronic disease (see Chapter 26) on the HPO axis also contribute to an increased likelihood of anovulatory bleeding in this population. Though many women with ESRD or on dialysis have irregular menstrual cycles and problems with infertility, many are sexually active, and thus contraception should be discussed with them.

Women with end-stage renal disease have higher rates endometrial hyperplasia, likely related to anovulatory cycles. There is also an increased incidence of cervical dysplasia, thought to be due to increased susceptibility to human papillomavirus (HPV) infection. Mammography can be challenging in this population due to increased vessel calcifications. To avoid unnecessary procedures, the patient's history should be provided to the radiologist (Holley, 2007). Ca-125 is also often falsely elevated in this population and should be interpreted with caution (Holley, 2007). Women with ERSD or who have undergone renal transplant have been shown to have a higher risk of surgical complications during gynecologic procedures (Heisler, 2010).

Up to 70% of women who are on hemodialysis, with chronic renal disease, and those who have had renal transplants have some degree of sexual dysfunction, including arousal disorders, decreased libido, and decreased genital blood flow, issues with lubrication, and orgasm problems. This may be related to lower levels of circulating estrogen. These women also go through menopause at an earlier age, 47 compared with 51 in nondialyzed females, further exacerbating problems with sexual dysfunction (Guglielmi, 2013).

Peritoneal dialysis has many specific considerations in women. Fertility in this population is lower than in women receiving hemodialysis, likely related to a disruption in the ovum's path to the fallopian tube (Guglielmi, 2013). Additionally, these women may experience cyclic hemoperitoneum, usually related to retrograde menstruation (Guglielmi, 2013). The hemoperitoneum is often asymptomatic, though rarely may cause obstruction to the dialysis catheter (Guglielmi, 2013). If the hemoperitoneum is recurrent or problematic, it may be treated with tubal ligation or hormonal suppression of ovulation (Guglielmi, 2013). Finally, women who undergo peritoneal dialysis may be at increased risk for uterine prolapse possibly related to changes in intraabdominal pressure associated with the dialysis.

## HEMATOLOGIC AND THROMBOTIC DISEASES

Estrogen affects hematologic diseases primarily through its prothrombotic effects. Progesterone decreases smooth muscle venous tone, which leads to increased clotting potential. Routine screening for thrombophilias in women without a history of thrombosis, prior to the use of ECCs or hormone replacement, is not indicated. Women with a personal history of thrombosis related to estrogen should avoid estrogen-containing medications (WHO, 2015). Women with known thrombophilias are great candidates for LARC methods but can also use progesterone-based oral contraceptives. Because supplemental estrogen is contraindicated in women with thrombophilias, these women may be more prone to osteoporotic problems over time. These women should be regularly screened for a dietary history of calcium intake as well as serum levels of vitamin D, with appropriate supplementation given.

Women with sickle cell disease (SCD) tend to go through menarche at a later age but do not have an increased rate of irregular cycles (Smith-Whitley, 2014). The menstrual cycle is often associated with increased pain crises. Progesterone stabilizes red-cell membranes and significantly decreases the frequency of sickling crises, thus women with SCD may benefit from progesterone-containing contraceptives. Injectable medroxyprogesterone acetate has been used in women with frequent crises as an adjunct therapy with very good results (Smith-Whitley, 2014). The pain-mediating effects of progesterone-based IUDs and implants have not yet been well documented, though these are considered a safe contraceptive option for women with SCD. ECCs and HRT do not improve sickling but are not contraindicated (WHO, 2015).

Women who receive oral anticoagulants (OA), for either treatment or prophylaxis, experience increased vaginal bleeding, menorrhagia, and metrorrhagia (Huq, 2011). One series of women noted that after starting the OA, the duration of bleeding increased, the percentage of women reporting heavy bleeding increased to almost 75%, and the number of women seeking medical treatment nearly doubled (Sjalander, 2007). Anovulatory cycles may be particularly troublesome for these women. Progesterone-based IUD or progesterone supplementation for the 14 days at the end of the cycle may be necessary to decrease heavy bleeding. Estrogen-containing contraceptives are not recommended for women on anticoagulation (CDC, 2010). Though the copper-containing IUD does not increase the risk of thrombosis, it is also generally not recommended given its associated increased menstrual bleeding (Huq, 2011). Women on OA are also at an increased risk for ovulation bleeding and associated hemoperitoneum.

The most common inherited bleeding diathesis is von Willebrand disease. The association of von Willebrand disease and vaginal bleeding is discussed in Chapter 26. LARC methods are safe in these women. However, because estrogen increases von Willebrand factor, ECCs may be advantageous for women with excessive bleeding or ovarian cysts (Committee on Adolescent Health Care, 2013). Women with rare bleeding disorders fall into similar categories, and ECCs may be helpful for them. A consensus report discussed other therapies including endometrial ablation or hysterectomy as potential options in women with bleeding disorders who do not desire fertility (James, 2009).

## *ENDOCRINE DISEASE*

Women with type 2 diabetes or who are obese have increased rates of anovulation, infertility, and endometrial hyperplasia. ECCs are acceptable in women with isolated diabetes (type 1 or 2) without end-organ damage, as are progesterone-based contraceptives (CDC, 2010). However, because many women with diabetes have coexisting vascular disease or hyperlipidemia, it is recommended that ECCs be limited to women who are nonsmokers and younger than 35 with no other significant pathology. LARC methods are safe, effective, and recommended for women with diabetes. In addition to the contraceptive effects, LARC methods also protect the endometrium in women who are anovulatory (ACOG, 2010).

Studies of sexuality in women with diabetes have noted increased sexual dysfunction, particularly for those with type 1 diabetes and those with long-standing disease. Sexual dysfunction is due to end-organ disease, with decreased genital blood flow, decreased lubrication, and orgasmic dysfunction. Young women with type 1 diabetes are also more likely to suffer from longer menstrual cycles and heavier menses when compared with nondiabetic women (Gaete, 2010). Though these issues are worse in women with higher HbA1cs, the problems persisted in women with well-controlled disease (Gaete, 2010). It should also be noted that insulin requirements and glycemic control vary with the hormonal fluctuations of the menstrual cycle, especially in the luteal phase and around menses. Discussion of this normal variation with younger women is important.

Obese women present an interesting conundrum regarding contraceptive options. Most studies related to contraceptive efficacy exclude morbidly obese and super morbidly obese women. Thus existing data have limited generalizability to this population, though the evidence that does exist is reassuring that efficacy of many contraceptive options is maintained (Robinson, 2013). It should also be stated that given the increased risks of pregnancy in this population, some contraceptive effect is better than no contraception. The progestin-based IUD or progestin-based implant have the highest success rate, independent of weight, and should be considered a first-line treatment in the obese population (Robinson, 2013). Given the increased incidence of anovulation with obesity, the local effects of the progestin-based IUD are especially protective against endometrial hyperplasia as well. However, OCPs are also an acceptable option in the population (Robinson, 2013). There are some data suggesting decreased efficacy of transdermal contraception in obese patients; thus other methods are preferred. Obese women also describe higher rates of sexual dysfunction than normal weight-women. However, this seems to improve with weight loss and improvement in body image (Kolotkin, 2012). This is true with both natural weight loss and bariatric surgery.

Obese women undergoing bariatric surgery should also be counseled about contraception and pregnancy planning. Malabsorptive procedures, specifically the Roux-en-Y procedure, have the potential to affect absorption of all oral contraception, including emergency contraception, and thus these methods should be discouraged in women who are undergoing or have undergone this sort of operations (Robinson, 2013). The efficacy of nonoral methods is not affected by bariatric surgery; thus the LARC methods are a good option for this population. After surgery, women may transition from being anovulatory to regular ovulation with improved glucose control. It is recommended that women wait 12 to 18 months prior to attempting pregnancy after bariatric surgery, another reason that the LARC methods are a good choice for these women (Mody, 2014).

Women with congenital adrenal hyperplasia (CAH) are usually treated with glucocorticoid replacement. These women are exposed to an androgenic environment throughout their lives, thus hormonally based contraceptives, including OCPs, are a good form of contraception. Though many of these women have increased problems with hirsutism, they should not be treated with spironolactone because it may affect mineralocorticoid regulation. Infertility secondary to chronically increased progesterone and androgen levels may occur, though this condition is correctable with steroid maintenance therapy (Reichman, 2014). Women with more severe phenotypes may need mineralocorticoid as well as progesterone suppression (Reichman, 2014). Women with CAH may also have problems with dyspareunia, vaginal stenosis, and lower sexual satisfaction (Nordenstrom, 2011). Sexual counseling for these women is helpful. Of note, thyroid disease is discussed in detail in Chapter 26.

## CENTRAL NERVOUS SYSTEM DISEASE

### SEIZURE DISORDERS

Estrogen and progesterone have significant effects on a woman's susceptibility to seizures. Estrogen is a pro-convulsant, decreasing seizure threshold. Estrogen increases neuronal excitability directly on nerve cells, as well as secondarily through inhibition of the GABA system. More potent, though, are the effects of progesterone, which acts primarily via its metabolite allopregnanolone, a neurosteroid. Allopregnanolone acts rapidly and directly on the GABA receptors to enhance their activity, producing potent neural inhibition throughout the central nervous system (CNS). Withdrawal of progesterone (even in small amounts such as periovulatory) leads to a significant decline in seizure threshold and an increase in seizure frequency and severity.

More than 1 million women in the United States are affected with seizure disorders, and many have increased seizure activity related to changes in menstrual hormones. Catamenial epilepsy (from the Greek *katomenios,* meaning "monthly") has been defined as seizures that occur from 3 days prior to 4 days after the onset of menses. Pure catamenial epilepsy affects 10% of all women with epilepsy (Crawford, 2009). However, nearly 80% of women have an increase in seizure activity related to menstrual cycles (Crawford, 2009). Progesterone-based contraceptives or a small amount of progesterone add-back during menses has been used to decrease seizure frequency. Continuous OCPs with an every-3-month withdrawal may also be helpful. It is unclear if the progesterone-based IUD produces systemic progesterone levels high enough to affect the seizure threshold.

Though hormonal contraception is acceptable for women with seizure disorders, estrogen affects metabolism of some antiepileptic drugs (AEDs) (Table 8.3). Women who experience menstrual-related seizures should have serum levels of their anticonvulsant medications checked during menses. Some of these women will benefit from perimenstrual adjustments of their medications. In contrast, some antiepileptic drugs, referred to as *enzyme-inducing AEDs* (see Table 8.3), affect the metabolism of hormonal contraception. For women on this family of AEDs, progesterone-only pills have decreased efficacy and are not recommended (Crawford, 2009). Similarly, progesterone implants are contraindicated in this population (Luef, 2009). Emergency contraception can be used in women with epilepsy, but those on enzyme-inducing AEDs may need a higher dose (Crawford, 2009).

Table 8.3 Interactions of Anticonvulsants (AEDs) and Oral Contraceptives

| Enzyme-Inducing AEDs | Non-Enzyme-Inducing AEDs |
|---|---|
| Barbiturates | Gabapentin |
| Carbamazepine | Lamotrigine |
| Phenytoin | Valproic acid |
| Topiramate | Ethosuximide |
| Vigabatrin | Levetiracetam |

Modified from the American College of Obstetricians and Gynecologists (ACOG) Practice Bulletin #72, 2006, Use of Hormonal Contraception in Women with Coexisting Medical Conditions.

Almost one third of women with epilepsy exhibit some degree of sexual dysfunction, ranging from decreased interest to orgasmic dysfunction (Crawford, 2009). Thus providers caring for women with epilepsy should query patients regarding sexual function and satisfaction. Epilepsy may predispose women to earlier menopause. Seizures often increase in the perimenopausal transition, then decrease after menopause, especially in women who suffer from catamenial epilepsy (Luef, 2009). HRT is associated with an increase in seizure frequency. Finally, women with epilepsy are at increased risk for osteoporosis related to the effects of AEDs on bone metabolism (Erel, 2011). Calcium and vitamin D supplements are recommended in this population as well as monitoring of bone mineral density (Crawford, 2009).

### *MIGRAINE HEADACHES*

In general, women have three times more migraines than men. Fourteen percent of all women with migraines have pure menstrual migraines; 46% have exacerbation of severity and frequency of their migraines during menses. Approximately 17 million women are affected by this problem. A menstrual migraine is defined as a migraine headache, without aura, occurring within the last 2 days of the menstrual cycle and the first 3 days of menses and affecting two of every three cycles (Brandes, 2012). After menopause, the incidence of migraines decreases by two thirds, and women and men have equal frequencies.

The etiology of menstrual migraines is related to estrogen withdrawal. Migraines are primarily vascular headaches, and the withdrawal of the estrogen leads to a relative vascular instability (Mathew, 2013). Estrogen also affects the CNS serotonin receptors. The change in serotonin metabolism as estrogen is withdrawn affects the brain stem, which controls cerebral blood flow. Serotonin uptake is blocked by triptans, and triptans are noted to be extremely effective for both abortive treatment of menstrual migraines as well as short-term prophylaxis (prevention) (Mathew, 2013). When menstrual migraines and menstruation-related migraines are diagnosed, therapeutic choices include modifying estrogen withdrawal with therapies such as the continuous OCPs, transdermal patches, or small amounts of estrogen add-back in the appropriate time window (Brandes, 2012). Preventive therapies include tricyclic antidepressants, beta-blockers, and other medications (Brandes, 2012).

Women who have migraines with aura are more susceptible to stroke, and thus the use of estrogen-containing contraceptives in women with migraines with aura is contraindicated (WHO, 2015). However, progestin-only contraception and LARC methods are safe in this population.

**Box 8.3 Emotional Symptoms Affected by Changes in Estrogen and Progesterone**

Anger
Anxiety
Appetite change
Decreased self-esteem
Depression
Feelings of phobia
Increased sense of fatigue
Inhibited control of limbic system sensations
Irritability
Loss of pleasure
Memory problems
Mood lability
Temperature fluctuations
Vulnerability

Modified from Pinkerton JV, Guico-Pabia CJ, Taylor HS. Menstrual cycle-related exacerbation of disease. *Am J Obstet Gynecol.* 2010;202(3):221-231.

## MENTAL HEALTH ISSUES

Changes in estrogen and progesterone levels have profound effects on psychiatric and psychological symptomatology and on psychiatric diseases (Box 8.3). Estrogen and progesterone are neuromodulators, thus exacerbation of mental health conditions may occur with menstrual hormonal fluctuations. Premenstrual exacerbation has been shown to occur with anxiety disorder, panic disorder, obsessive-compulsive disorder, bipolar disease, eating disorders, and psychotic disorders (Pinkerton, 2010). Women without mental health disorders handle these fluctuations well, but women who have a predisposition to mental health disorders may be strongly affected by the hormonal fluctuations.

Premenstrual dysphoric disease (PMDD) affects up to 5% of women and is discussed in Chapter 37. Other mental health disorders are best managed by mental health providers. However, the gynecologist may help to provide hormonal stability. Continuous combined oral contraceptives can help improve depression that occurs around the time of menses (Pinkerton, 2010). Sexual dysfunction may be a symptom of depression, but it can also be a side effect of antidepressant medications, including the serotonin reuptake inhibitors (SSRIs).

New onset depression or worsening of known depression often occurs during the menopausal transition. Studies suggest this occurs in as many as half of all women (Pinkerton, 2010). Screening for depression in this age group is important given the high incidence of disease. Treatment with antidepressant medications is the first-line therapy for moderate to severe depression in the menopausal transition (Pinkerton, 2010). If there are only mild to moderate symptoms and the woman is an appropriate candidate, estrogen-containing HRT may be helpful (Pinkerton, 2010). Black cohosh and St. John's wort may also be beneficial in the treatment of perimenopausal depression, though they should be used with caution as safety data and production regulation are limited (Pinkerton, 2010).

## CANCER

The gynecologist can play a valuable role in improving quality of life for women with cancer. Sexuality in cancer patients should be addressed from the beginning of cancer therapy. Issues of depression and sexual dysfunction are enhanced by ovarian failure, loss of hair, changes in body image, and changes in relationships (Lamb, 1995). Abnormal vaginal bleeding in the first few cycles of chemotherapy is frightening, and the role of the gynecologist is important at this phase of treatment.

Chemotherapy produces toxic effects on ovarian function that are related to dose, duration, and type of chemotherapy. Agents that are particularly toxic to the ovary are listed in Table 8.2. Of these, alkylating agents are the most toxic to the ovaries, but women who receive antineoplastic agents for control of severe autoimmune disease can also develop ovarian failure. Young women treated with oophorotoxic agents often become amenorrheic, but their menses and ovarian function may return after a few or several months (Sonmezer, 2006). They generally undergo menopause earlier. For older women, their chemo-induced menopause is usually permanent. Radiation to the ovaries greater than or equal to 20 Gy may also produce ovarian failure, though oophoropexy to remove the ovaries from the field of radiation may mitigate this reaction (Mahajan, 2015).

In addition to the effects that chemotherapy has on the ovaries, the effects on the bone marrow, thrombocytopenia specifically, can lead to gynecologic issues. GnRH analogues have been shown to be effective in reducing episodes of severe vaginal bleeding associated with thrombocytopenia, without the potential risks associated with the estrogen-based options, especially venous-thromboembolism (Bates, 2011). GnRH analogues may be used as prophylaxis for menorrhagia/menstrual suppression in women with expected thrombocytopenia for more than 30 days (Bates, 2011). Acute menorrhagia in women undergoing treatment for most cancers can be treated with tranexamic acid, relying on hormonal therapies as second-line agents (Bates, 2011).

Young women wishing to preserve ovarian function and fertility need consultation prior to treatments. Mature oocytes are the most susceptible to chemotherapy, whereas immature oocytes in the prepubertal females are somewhat resistant. Thus investigators have used GnRH antagonists to suppress follicular maturity and attempt to preserve ovarian function. The results are mixed, though a Cochrane review supports their usage (Chen, 2011). Other potential options to save oocyte function and preserve fertility include in vitro fertilization with freezing of embryos, harvesting/freezing of mature oocytes after ovarian stimulation, and ovarian cryopreservation, which is still in the investigational stage. The American Society of Clinical Oncology currently recommends discussion of both embryo and oocyte cryopreservation as methods of fertility preservation (Loren, 2013). The options should be reviewed in light of the patient's needs, fertility desires, and clinical situation. Early and urgent referral to a reproductive endocrinologist with expertise in potential therapies to preserve fertility is important (McLaren, 2012).

## SUMMARY

The interaction of female physiology and medical disease is complex. The gynecologist has several roles in the treatment of these women. All providers who address women's health should regularly discuss issues of sexual function, particularly in the setting of coexisting disease. Additionally, the exacerbation of symptoms around the time of menses should be reviewed. Hormonal changes that increase the symptoms of women will change over the course of a woman's reproductive life. Disease manifestation in a woman's 20s will not be the same as symptoms in her 40s or in her 60s. There are many treatment options that can improve quality of life. Though gynecologists may not be the primary providers for nongynecologic diseases, they are best suited to act as consultants for adjunctive therapy, which may enhance the efficacy and treatment of medical disease.

## KEY POINTS

- LARC methods are safe, effective, and have minimal risk of user error, thus they have become the recommended option for most women with complicated chronic illnesses.
- The severity of asthma symptoms increases around the time of menses.
- Many women with IBS and IBD will have exacerbations of symptoms with menses.
- Women with chronic renal disease often experience menorrhagia.
- Estrogen-containing contraceptives are not recommended in women with hypertension who are over 35, use tobacco, have poorly controlled disease, or are on medications for hypertension.
- Progesterone stabilizes red cell membranes and significantly decreases the frequency of sickling crises.
- Withdrawal of progesterone (even in small amounts such as periovulatory) leads to a significant decline in the seizure threshold and an increase in seizure frequency and severity.
- Women who have migraines with aura are more susceptible to stroke, and thus the use of ECC in women with migraines with aura is contraindicated.
- Early referral of women with cancer to a reproductive endocrinologist with expertise in potential therapies to preserve fertility is important.

## KEY REFERENCES

ACOG: ACOG Practice Bulletin. No. 73. Use of hormonal contraception in women with coexisting medical conditions. *Obstet Gynecol.* 2006;107(6):1453-1472.

ACOG: ACOG Practice Bulletin No. 110. Noncontraceptive uses of hormonal contraceptives. *Obstet Gynecol.* 2010;115(1):206-218.

Ahmad A, Ahmed A, Patrizio P. Cystic fibrosis and fertility. *Curr Opin Obstet Gynecol.* 2013;25(3):167-172.

Aljubran SA, Whelan GJ, Glaum MC, et al. Osteoporosis in the at-risk asthmatic. *Allergy.* 2014;69(11):1429-1439.

Basson R, Schultz WW. Sexual sequelae of general medical disorders. *Lancet.* 2007;369(9559):409-424.

Bates JS, Buie LW, Woodis CB. Management of menorrhagia associated with chemotherapy-induced thrombocytopenia in women with hematologic malignancy. *Pharmacotherapy.* 2011;31(11):1092-1110.

Brandes JL. Migraine in women. *Continuum (Minneap Minn).* 2012;18(4):835-852.

Centers for Disease Control and Prevention (CDC). U.S. Medical Eligibility Criteria for Contraceptive Use, 2010. *MMWR Recomm Rep.* 2010;59(RR-4):1-86.

Chen H, Li J, Cui T, et al. Adjuvant gonadotropin-releasing hormone analogues for the prevention of chemotherapy induced premature ovarian failure in premenopausal women. *Cochrane Database Syst Rev.* 2011;(11):CD008018.

Chen W, Mempel M, Schober W, et al. Gender difference, sex hormones, and immediate type hypersensitivity reactions. *Allergy.* 2008;63(11):1418-1427.

Committee on Adolescent Health Care; Committee on Gynecologic Practice. Committee Opinion No.580: von Willebrand disease in women. *Obstet Gynecol.* 2013;122(6):1368-1373.

Crawford PM. Managing epilepsy in women of childbearing age. *Drug Saf.* 2009;32(4):293-307.

Curtis AB, Narasimha D. Arrhythmias in women. *Clin Cardiol.* 2012;35(3):166-171.

De Franciscis P, Mainini G, Messalli EM, et al. Arterial hypertension and female sexual dysfunction in postmenopausal women. *Clin Exp Obstet Gynecol.* 2013;40(1):58-60.

Doumas M, Tsiodras S, Tsakiris A, et al. Female sexual dysfunction in essential hypertension: a common problem being uncovered. *J Hypertens.* 2006;24(12):2387-2392.

Dratva J. Use of oestrogen only hormone replacement therapy associated with increased risk of asthma onset in postmenopausal women. *Evid Based Med.* 2010;15(6):190-191.

Erel T, Guralp O. Epilepsy and menopause. *Arch Gynecol Obstet.* 2011;284(3):749-755.

Fida NG, Williams MA, Enquobahrie DA. Association of age at menarche and menstrual characteristics with adult onset asthma among reproductive age women. *Reprod Syst Sex Disord.* 2012;1(3).

Fogari R, Preti P, Zoppi A, et al. Effect of valsartan and atenolol on sexual behavior in hypertensive postmenopausal women. *Am J Hypertens.* 2004;17(1):77-81.

Gaete X, Vivanco M, Eyzaguirre FC, et al. Menstrual cycle irregularities and their relationship with HbA1c and insulin dose in adolescents with type 1 diabetes mellitus. *Fertil Steril.* 2010;94(5):1822-1826.

Ghezzi A, Zaffaroni M. Female-specific issues in multiple sclerosis. *Expert Rev Neurother.* 2008;8(6):969-977.

Guglielmi KE. Women and ESRD: modalities, survival, unique considerations. *Adv Chronic Kidney Dis.* 2013;20(5):411-418.

Heisler CA, Casiano ER, Gebhart JB. Hysterectomy and perioperative morbidity in women who have undergone renal transplantation. *Am J Obstet Gynecol.* 2010;202(3). 314 e311-314.

Holley JL. Screening, diagnosis, and treatment of cancer in long-term dialysis patients. *Clin J Am Soc Nephrol.* 2007;2(3):604-610.

Huq FY, Tvarkova K, Arafa A, et al. Menstrual problems and contraception in women of reproductive age receiving oral anticoagulation. *Contraception.* 2011;84(2):128-132.

James AH, Kouides PA, Abdul-Kadir R, et al. Von Willebrand disease and other bleeding disorders in women: consensus on diagnosis and management from an international expert panel. *Am J Obstet Gynecol.* 2009;201(1):12 e11-18.

Kolotkin RL, Zunker C, Østbye T. Sexual functioning and obesity: a review. *Obesity (Silver Spring).* 2012;20(12):2325-2333.

Lamb MA. Effects of cancer on the sexuality and fertility of women. *Semin Oncol Nurs.* 1995;11(2):120-127.

Lang TJ. Estrogen as an immunomodulator. *Clin Immunol.* 2004;113(3):224-230.

Liu E, Lee HS, Aronsson CA, et al. Risk of pediatric celiac disease according to HLA haplotype and country. *N Engl J Med.* 2014;371(1):42-49.

Loren AW, Mangu PB, Beck LN, et al. Fertility preservation for patients with cancer: American Society of Clinical Oncology clinical practice guideline update. *J Clin Oncol.* 2013;31(19):2500-2510.

Luef G. Female issues in epilepsy: a critical review. *Epilepsy Behav.* 2009;15(1):78-82.

Mahajan N. Fertility preservation in female cancer patients: an overview. *J Hum Reprod Sci.* 2015;8(1):3-13.

Mathew PG, Dun EC, Luo JJ. A cyclic pain: the pathophysiology and treatment of menstrual migraine. *Obstet Gynecol Surv.* 2013;68(2):130-140.

McLaren JF, Bates GW. Fertility preservation in women of reproductive age with cancer. *Am J Obstet Gynecol.* 2012;207(6):455-462.

Mody SK, Han M. Obesity and contraception. *Clin Obstet Gynecol.* 2014;57(3):501-507.

Moleski SM, Choudhary C. Special considerations for women with IBD. *Gastroenterol Clin North Am.* 2011;40(2):387-398. viii-ix.

Mulak A, Tache Y, Larauche M. Sex hormones in the modulation of irritable bowel syndrome. *World J Gastroenterol.* 2014;20(10):2433-2448.

Nordenstrom A. Adult women with 21-hydroxylase deficient congenital adrenal hyperplasia, surgical and psychological aspects. *Curr Opin Pediatr.* 2011;23(4):436-442.

Pellegrini M, Pallottini V, Marin R, et al. Role of the sex hormone estrogen in the prevention of lipid disorder. *Curr Med Chem.* 2014;21(24):2734-2742.

Perželová V, Sabol F, Vasilenko T, et al. Pharmacological activation of estrogen receptors-alpha and -beta differentially modulates keratinocyte differentiation with functional impact on wound healing. *Int J Mol Med.* 2016;37(1):21-28.

Pinkerton JV, Guico-Pabia CJ, Taylor HS. Menstrual cycle-related exacerbation of disease. *Am J Obstet Gynecol.* 2010;202(3):221-231.

Real FG, Svanes C, Omenaas ER, et al. Menstrual irregularity and asthma and lung function. *J Allergy Clin Immunol.* 2007;120(3):557-564.

Reichman DE, White PC, New MI, et al. Fertility in patients with congenital adrenal hyperplasia. *Fertil Steril.* 2014;101(2):301-309.

Robinson JA, Burke AE. Obesity and hormonal contraceptive efficacy. *Womens Health (Lond Engl).* 2013;9(5):453-466.

Rodríguez-Castro KI, De Martin E, Gambato M, et al. Female gender in the setting of liver transplantation. *World J Transplant.* 2014;4(4):229-242.

Sammaritano LR. Menopause in patients with autoimmune diseases. *Autoimmun Rev.* 2012;11(6-7):A430-436.

Sanchez-Guerrero J, Uribe AG, Jimenez-Santana L, et al. A trial of contraceptive methods in women with systemic lupus erythematosus. *N Engl J Med.* 2005;353(24):2539-2549.

Sjalander A, Friberg B, Svensson P, et al. Menorrhagia and minor bleeding symptoms in women on oral anticoagulation. *J Thromb Thrombolysis.* 2007;24(1):39-41.

Smith-Whitley K. Reproductive issues in sickle cell disease. *Blood.* 2014;124(24):3538-3543.

Sonmezer M, Oktay K. Fertility preservation in young women undergoing breast cancer therapy. *Oncologist.* 2006;11(5):422-434.

Straub RH. The complex role of estrogens in inflammation. *Endocr Rev.* 2007;28(5):521-574.

Tam A, Morrish D, Wadsworth S, et al. The role of female hormones on lung function in chronic lung diseases. *BMC Womens Health.* 2011;11:24.

Tersigni C, Castellani R, de Waure C, et al. Celiac disease and reproductive disorders: meta-analysis of epidemiologic associations and potential pathogenic mechanisms. *Hum Reprod Update.* 2014;20(4):582-593.

Tsang A, Moriarty C, Towns S. Contraception, communication and counseling for sexuality and reproductive health in adolescents and young adults with CF. *Paediatr Respir Rev.* 2010;11(2):84-89.

Tseng JC, Lu LY, Hu JC, et al. The impact of systemic lupus erythematosus on women's sexual functioning. *J Sex Med.* 2011;8(12):3389-3397.

van den Berge M, Heijink HI, van Oosterhout AJ, et al. The role of female sex hormones in the development and severity of allergic and nonallergic asthma. *Clin Exp Allergy.* 2009;39(10):1477-1481.

World Health Organization (WHO). *Medical Eligibility Criteria for Contraceptive Use.* 5th ed. Geneva: WHO; 2015.

Zhang B, Wu ZY. Estrogen derivatives: novel therapeutic agents for liver cirrhosis and portal hypertension. *Eur J Gastroenterol Hepatol.* 2013;25(3):263-270.

# 9

# Emotional Aspects of Gynecology

## Depression, Anxiety, Posttraumatic Stress Disorder, Eating Disorders, Substance Use Disorders, "Difficult" Patients, Sexual Function, Rape, Intimate Partner Violence, and Grief

*Deborah S. Cowley, Gretchen M. Lentz*

Gynecologists follow women across the life cycle, from puberty through old age. The gynecologist may be a woman's primary health care provider for much of this time and thus is in an important position to help her to navigate normal developmental stages and challenges, to share in critical life events from adolescence to late life, and to provide or obtain counseling for her as she works her way through emotional adjustments and problems. Normal development includes challenges such as building an identity and self-esteem; dealing with sexuality and sexual development; forming meaningful relationships; pregnancy and motherhood; life roles and transitions; and inevitable losses, such as loss of relationships, loss of important career and life roles, loss of physical or mental abilities through illness or accident, and loss of loved ones through separation or death. In addition to these normal developmental transitions and challenges, a woman may have to deal with trauma related to difficult early childhood experiences, abuse, rape, or intimate partner violence. Psychiatric disorders such as depression, anxiety, posttraumatic stress disorder, and eating disorders are common in women, and conditions such as alcohol and drug use disorders often have a different presentation and course in women compared with men.

This chapter reviews common psychiatric disorders occurring in gynecologic patients, sexual function and disorders, and psychosocial issues and traumas that may arise during a woman's lifetime, and it offers suggestions as to how the physician can aid the patient.

## DEVELOPMENTAL ISSUES IN CHILDHOOD AND ADOLESCENCE

Self-esteem begins to develop in early childhood and is affected by the positive efforts of parents and others in the child's immediate environment. Continuous reinforcement of a child's worth as an individual, by verbal and nonverbal means, should be encouraged. Praise for the child's positive actions and setting consistent, predictable limits that are socially acceptable within the framework of the family are reasonable steps. Punishment should be limited to reinforcing the needs for the limits that have been set. Intimidation by verbal or physical means should be avoided. The physician may have the opportunity to suggest help for parents by offering reading material, discussing issues directly with them, or referring them to parenting classes. In general, positive reinforcement of the child's worth as an individual, mixed with appropriate warmth and love, tends to build self-esteem, whereas negative statements or actions tend to tear it down. A child has little basis for comparison, and if she is given negative information about herself, she will tend to believe it.

Girls and women, starting in childhood, often are highly invested in maintaining relationships, caring for others, not being "selfish" in pursuing their own goals and desires, and striving for ideal standards of appearance and behavior. These characteristics make it difficult, throughout life, to effectively and constructively express anger, be appropriately assertive, and know or pursue individual goals, and they may predispose girls and women to conditions such as depression and eating disorders, which are discussed later in the chapter. The physician can help by recognizing these characteristics and conditions early and providing support and referrals for mental health treatment as needed.

Physical, sexual, or emotional abuse in childhood and adolescence can have serious consequences for the child's development. Evidence of abuse must be addressed vigorously. The health care professional should communicate to the child or adolescent that she is a victim and is in no way responsible for what has happened. Reporting to child protective services may be legally mandated. Issues of abuse are discussed more fully later in this chapter.

## DEPRESSION

Major depression is common in women, with a lifetime prevalence of 20% to 25%. Although boys and girls are equally likely to experience depression, major depression is about twice as common in women as in men, starting in adolescence. Worldwide, depression is one of the leading causes of functional impairment and disability. The diagnosis of major depression refers to persistent sadness or lack of interest or pleasure in usual activities, lasting for at least 2 weeks, and accompanied by symptoms such as changes in eating habits, trouble sleeping, lack of energy and motivation, poor memory or concentration, and feelings of guilt, worthlessness, hopelessness, and despair. In severe cases, depression may lead to suicidal thoughts and attempts. The diagnostic criteria for major depression are listed in Box 9.1. The Patient Health Questionnaire (PHQ-9) (Table 9.1) is a useful screening tool for major depression, can be filled out quickly by the woman in the waiting room or in the office prior to a visit, and helps in identifying depression, monitoring effects of treatment, and educating the woman about her own characteristic symptoms of depression. Scores of 5, 10, 15, and 20 are cutoff scores indicating mild, moderate, moderately severe, and severe depression, respectively.

**Box 9.1 Diagnostic Criteria for Major Depressive Episode**

Five or more of the following symptoms have been present during the same 2-week period and represent a change from previous functioning; at least one of the symptoms is either (1) depressed mood or (2) loss of interest or pleasure.

1. Depressed mood most of the day, nearly every day, as indicated by either subjective report (e.g., feels sad or empty) or observation made by others (e.g., appears tearful)
2. Markedly diminished interest or pleasure in all, or almost all, activities
3. Significant weight loss (when not dieting) or weight gain, or decrease or increase in appetite
4. Insomnia or hypersomnia
5. Psychomotor agitation or retardation observable by others
6. Fatigue or loss of energy
7. Feelings of worthlessness or excessive or inappropriate guilt
8. Diminished ability to think or concentrate, or indecisiveness
9. Recurrent thoughts of death (not just fear of dying), recurrent suicidal ideation, or a suicide attempt or specific suicide plan

Symptoms cause clinically significant distress or impairment.

Modified from American Psychiatric Association. *Diagnostic and Statistical Manual of Mental Disorders*. 5th ed. (DSM-5). Washington, DC: American Psychiatric Association; 2013:160-161.

The cause of major depression is unclear. It may occur without a clear stress or precipitant, especially in women with a strong family history of depression who are genetically predisposed. A family history of depression, a prior depressive episode, and older age are all risk factors for depression. In addition, environmental stressors such as loss of relationships and loved ones, divorce, role transitions, interpersonal conflicts, medical illness, or feelings of being trapped in a stressful situation without a way to escape or cope can precipitate depression. The cause of depression in a particular person may be uniquely determined by individual factors, such as family relationships while growing up and past experiences that are highly meaningful and evoke negative feelings and memories triggered by current situations or events.

Loss of a parent during childhood is an important factor predisposing to later depression. Although there is conflicting literature—confounded by other consequences of parental loss such as financial problems, the nature of substitute caregiving, and potential family disruption—it appears that both boys and girls are at heightened risk for later depression if they lose their primary caregiver in childhood. That risk is higher if the lost caregiver is of the same gender as the child.

The increased rate of depression in women starting at menarche has also been thought to result from hormonal factors. There are clear increases in risk for depressive symptoms premenstrually, with some women only experiencing mood symptoms

**Table 9.1** Patient Health Questionnaire (PHQ-9)

Over the past 2 weeks, how often have you been bothered by any of the following problems?

| | Not at All | Several Days | More than Half the Days | Nearly Every Day |
|---|---|---|---|---|
| 1. Little interest or pleasure in doing things | 0 | 1 | 2 | 3 |
| 2. Feeling down, depressed, or hopeless | 0 | 1 | 2 | 3 |
| 3. Trouble falling or staying asleep, or sleeping too much | 0 | 1 | 2 | 3 |
| 4. Feeling tired or having little energy | 0 | 1 | 2 | 3 |
| 5. Poor appetite or overeating | 0 | 1 | 2 | 3 |
| 6. Feeling bad about yourself—or that you are a failure or have let yourself or your family down | 0 | 1 | 2 | 3 |
| 7. Trouble concentrating on things, such as reading the newspaper or watching television | 0 | 1 | 2 | 3 |
| 8. Moving or speaking so slowly that other people could have noticed, or the opposite—being so fidgety or restless that you have been moving around a lot more than usual | 0 | 1 | 2 | 3 |
| 9. Thoughts that you would be better off dead or of hurting yourself in some way | 0 | 1 | 2 | 3 |
| Total Score | ___ | +___ | +___ | +___ |

If you checked off any problems, how difficult have these problems made it for you to do your work, take care of things at home, or get along with other people?

___ Not difficult at all ___ Somewhat difficult ___ Very difficult ___ Extremely difficult

From Spitzer RL, Kroenke K, Williams JBW. For the Patient Health Questionnaire Primary Care Study Group. Validation and utility of a self-report version of PRIME-MD: the PHQ Primary Care Study. *JAMA*. 1999;282:1737-1744; Spitzer RL, Williams JBW, Kroenke K, et al. Validity and utility of the Patient Health Questionnaire in assessment of 3000 obstetrics-gynecologic patients. *Am J Obstet Gynecol*. 2000;183:759-769.

The PHQ was developed by Drs. Robert L. Spitzer, Janet B.W. Williams, Kurt Kroenke, and colleagues. PRIME-MD is a trademark of Pfizer Inc. 

at this time and others noting a worsening of underlying depression in the week or two prior to menses (for a discussion of premenstrual dysphoric disorder, see Chapter 37). The postpartum period is a high-risk time for depression and is the highest risk time in a woman's life for psychiatric hospitalization. There is also an increase in depressive symptoms at the time of menopause and the menopausal transition.

The differential diagnosis of major depression includes adjustment disorder, persistent depressive disorder (dysthymia), depression related to drugs and alcohol or secondary to a medical condition, and bipolar disorder. Adjustment disorder is a stress-related, short-term emotional or behavioral response to a stressful life circumstance. Depressive symptoms begin within 3 months of the onset of the stressor and resolve within 6 months once the stressful circumstance ends. The symptoms do not meet criteria for major depression. The physician can help a woman with an adjustment disorder by helping her to problem solve and cope with the situation she is in or by referring her for short-term therapy or counseling.

Persistent depressive disorder (previously called *dysthymic disorder*) is a chronic, low-grade depression, with symptoms present more than half the time for at least 2 years and no more than 2 months without depressive symptoms during that time. The best treatment is antidepressant medication and psychotherapy, but this condition is often harder to treat than major depression because of its chronicity. Symptoms of major depression can also be caused by alcohol or drug use, or by medical conditions, such as hypothyroidism, vitamin $B_{12}$ deficiency, anemia, or cancer (most classically pancreatic cancer). Women presenting with depression should be screened for medical disorders and asked about use of alcohol and drugs.

Probably the greatest dilemma in deciding to prescribe antidepressants is the concern that if the woman has bipolar disorder, antidepressants can cause a "switch" into a manic episode. Manic episodes are characterized by feelings of euphoria or irritability and increased energy or goal-directed activity, with symptoms such as decreased need for sleep, increased activity or agitation, talkativeness, racing thoughts, grandiose and unrealistic plans, and impulsive and risky behavior. If a woman has been hospitalized for mania or has had such symptoms for a week or more in the past, the diagnosis may be clear. However, people often do not recall their manic symptoms or have little insight into them, or they may have had briefer periods of a few days (hypomania) that still predispose them to mania with antidepressants. It is often difficult to make the diagnosis of bipolar disorder, especially just from the woman's report. Any suspicion of this condition is an indication for psychiatric consultation, because bipolar depression requires treatment with a mood stabilizer instead of, or combined with, an antidepressant.

Treatment of major depression can include antidepressant medication, psychotherapy, or both. Because both antidepressant medication and psychotherapy are effective, the initial choice of treatment can be made according to the woman's preference, although for more severe depression medication is indicated. Commonly prescribed antidepressant medications and dosages are listed in Table 9.2. A 2009 meta-analysis by Cipriani and associates suggested that the best combination of efficacy and tolerability is for sertraline or escitalopram (Cipriani, 2009). Because of their more benign side effect profiles, it is reasonable to start a selective serotonin reuptake inhibitor (SSRI) as the first antidepressant in most cases. SSRI side effects include gastrointestinal symptoms (nausea, diarrhea, vomiting), which are minimized by taking the medication with a meal. Other common side effects include initial dizziness and headaches, as well as sexual dysfunction, most commonly delayed orgasm or anorgasmia. Doses of the SSRI citalopram exceeding 40 mg daily (>20 mg /day age 60 or higher) are not recommended due to the risk of QT prolongation. SSRIs may also cause uncomfortable withdrawal symptoms if discontinued suddenly. Withdrawal symptoms can include gastrointestinal symptoms, headache, dizziness, and "electric shock" sensations. Fluoxetine, an SSRI with a long half-life, is not generally associated with withdrawal symptoms and women discontinuing other SSRIs can be switched to fluoxetine to minimize withdrawal. Fluoxetine also has the strongest

**Table 9.2** Commonly Prescribed Antidepressants

| Antidepressant | Dose Range (mg/day) | Comments |
|---|---|---|
| **Serotonin Reuptake Inhibitors (SSRIs)** | | |
| Citalopram | 20-40 | FDA warning of QT prolongation at doses >40 mg/day (>20 mg /day age 60 or higher) |
| Escitalopram | 10-20 | S-enantiomer of citalopram |
| Fluoxetine | 20-80 | Long half-life; unlikely to cause withdrawal symptoms with discontinuation or missed doses; best evidence base for use in children and adolescents |
| Paroxetine | 20-50 (25-62.5 controlled release) | High rate of withdrawal symptoms |
| Sertraline | 50-200 | |
| **Serotonin and Norepinephrine Reuptake Inhibitors (SNRIs)** | | |
| Duloxetine | 60-120 | May also be effective for neuropathic pain, urinary incontinence |
| Venlafaxine | 75-375 | Risk of elevated blood pressure |
| **Other** | | |
| Bupropion | 300-450 | Elevated risk of seizures, especially at doses above 450 mg/day; contraindicated in patients with bulimia; may be effective for comorbid attention deficit disorder; activating; does not cause sexual dysfunction or weight gain; effective for smoking cessation |
| Mirtazapine | 15-45 | Sedating; causes weight gain |
| Trazodone | 25-100 (for insomnia) | Sedating; used as adjunctive treatment for insomnia |

evidence base for treatment of major depression in children and adolescents.

Serotonin and norepinephrine reuptake inhibitors (SNRIs) include venlafaxine and duloxetine. Venlafaxine is associated with a dose-related risk for gradual onset of hypertension, and blood pressure should be monitored carefully on this medication. SNRI side effects include gastrointestinal side effects, headaches, dizziness, anorgasmia, activation, and anxiety. Bupropion appears to exert its therapeutic effect by enhancing effects of dopamine and norepinephrine. It increases energy and can cause insomnia, increased anxiety, headaches, and gastrointestinal side effects. Bupropion also lowers the seizure threshold, especially at doses above 450 mg daily, and should not be used in women with a history of a seizure disorder or bulimia. Mirtazapine is an alpha$_2$-adrenergic, 5-HT2, and 5-HT3 receptor antagonist, which also has antihistaminic effects. Its common side effects include sedation and weight gain. Trazodone is a highly sedating serotonergic antidepressant that is used primarily at low doses (25 to 100 mg at bedtime) for insomnia. Tricyclic and monoamine oxidase (MAO) inhibitor antidepressants are infrequently prescribed currently because of side effects, in addition to dietary restrictions and the risk of hypertensive crisis with MAO inhibitors. It is important to warn women that antidepressant medication can take up to 4 to 6 weeks to work, and to schedule a follow-up visit within that time to monitor treatment adherence, side effects, and therapeutic response. The Food and Drug Administration (FDA) has required black box warnings regarding increases in suicidal ideation with antidepressants, especially in adolescents and young adults. The mechanism for this is unclear but may be in part an increase in energy and motivation before improvement in mood. Women should be warned of this potential phenomenon and instructed to stop the medication and call the provider if this occurs. Overall, antidepressants reduce depression and risk for suicide, but this potentially serious side effect is another indication for close follow-up early in treatment.

Effective psychotherapies for depression include cognitive behavioral therapy (CBT) and interpersonal therapy (IPT). Cognitive behavioral therapy addresses the negative, distorted thinking that is characteristic of depression, such as the belief that things are bad now, have always been bad, and will always be bad, or thoughts of worthlessness and guilt. In addition, behavioral activation, or scheduling activities that provide a sense of accomplishment, mastery, or pleasure, is helpful in depression, and exercise has been shown to decrease depressive symptoms. Interpersonal therapy addresses the life changes and interpersonal challenges that contribute to depression, especially in women. These include grief, conflicts in interpersonal relationships including marital or intimate partner conflicts, transitions in roles within work or the family, and social isolation with a lack of supportive relationships. These therapies are usually weekly for an hour for 3 to 4 months. In cases of clear-cut couple's issues, couples therapy may be indicated, especially after the woman has recovered from depression sufficiently to participate in such therapy. Other nonmedication treatments for depression include morning light for seasonal or winter depression, and electroconvulsive treatment (ECT) or repetitive transcranial magnetic stimulation (rTMS) for depression that does not respond to medication and psychotherapy.

Both medication and psychotherapy are significantly more effective than placebo for treatment of major depression, with response rates varying between about 50% and 70%, depending on the patient population. Combined treatment with both psychotherapy and medication is more effective and is indicated for more severe depression.

The goal of treatment for depression is complete remission, or resolution of all depressive symptoms, as even mild residual symptoms increase the risk of relapse. There are several measures that can increase rates of remission (Cameron, 2014). First, close follow-up, with visits every 1 to 2 weeks at first and then every 2 to 4 weeks, will enhance adherence and response rates. One third of people prescribed an antidepressant discontinue the medication within 30 days. There is considerable stigma associated with taking psychotropic medication or having a psychiatric diagnosis, so addressing the woman's concerns that depression is a weakness or a character flaw can be helpful. Frequent visits also allow early identification of side effects that decrease adherence. Patient education about the lag in response to antidepressants and the need to take the medication every day for at least 6 to 12 months is important. Tracking symptoms with a scale such as the PHQ-9 is helpful in monitoring progress and identifying residual symptoms. If there is little response in 2 to 4 weeks, a dose increase should be considered, and only partial response at 8 weeks should prompt reassessment of the diagnosis, ensuring that the patient is taking the maximal tolerated dose of the antidepressant, and consideration of switching medications, adding an augmentation agent such as lithium, an atypical antipsychotic, or triiodothyronine (T3), or referral to a psychiatrist. Women who have had three or more episodes of major depression should be continued on maintenance antidepressant treatment.

Suicide is a feared and tragic outcome of depression and other mental health conditions. In the United States, there were 41,149 suicide deaths in 2013, 5.5 per 100,000 women and 20.2 per 100,000 men committed suicide, and suicide was the 10th leading cause of death. Rates of suicide are highest among people aged 45 to 64 years compared with other age groups and in whites, Native Americans, and Native Alaskans compared with other ethnic groups. There are 12 to 25 suicide attempts per every suicide death. Risk factors for suicide include depression or other mental health disorders, substance use disorders, a prior suicide attempt, a family history of psychiatric or substance use disorders, family violence including physical or sexual abuse, access to means such as firearms in the house, and exposure to suicidal behavior by others such as family members, peers, or celebrities. All depressed women should be asked about suicidal thoughts. This can include asking about whether the woman feels hopeless, has had thoughts that life is not worth living, or thoughts of ending her life, followed by more specific questions about whether she has made specific plans and how far she has gone to carry these out. Active suicidal thoughts and plans are a psychiatric emergency. The woman should not be left alone. The physician or staff should call 9-1-1 to have her taken to the nearest emergency room. Even in less acute cases, it is important to engage family members and other supportive people as possible, to remove firearms and other means of suicide from the home, to have someone else supervise the woman's medication, and to seek psychiatric or other mental health consultation as soon as possible.

## EATING DISORDERS

Anorexia nervosa, bulimia nervosa, and binge eating disorder are the major eating disorders and have a lifetime prevalence of 0.6%, 1%, and 3%, respectively (for a review of eating disorders, see Treasure, 2010). Eating disorders primarily affect younger people and have their peak onset between the ages of 10 and 19. In a report from the Centers for Disease Control and Prevention (2011), 61% of female high school students reported they were trying to lose weight. In the preceding 30 days, 11% had not eaten in 24 hours or more, 5% took diet pills, powders or supplements, and 4% took laxatives or induced vomiting to avoid weight gain. These disorders are more common in women than in men. Many young women with eating disorders are secretive about their disorder, do not view it as a problem, and do not seek treatment for it. Gynecologists may see such girls or women for related problems, such as amenorrhea, menstrual dysfunction, low bone density, sexual dysfunction, infertility, anxiety, depression, hyperemesis gravidarum, or other pregnancy complications. Because the woman may not volunteer information about disordered eating, it is important to have a high index of suspicion for eating disorders. A simple, five-question self-rating scale, the "SCOFF" (Box 9.2), is highly sensitive and specific in detecting eating disorders in primary care settings, and thus is a useful screening tool. The *Diagnostic and Statistical Manual*, Fifth Edition (DSM-5), diagnostic criteria for anorexia nervosa, bulimia nervosa, and binge eating disorder are listed in Box 9.3. Of note, the DSM-5 diagnosis of anorexia nervosa is also specified by current severity, with a body mass index (BMI) of 17 kg/m$^2$ being mild, 16 to 16.99 kg/m$^2$ moderate, 15 to 15.99 kg/m$^2$ severe, and less than 15 kg/m$^2$ extreme.

Anorexia nervosa is characterized by a disturbed body image; fears of becoming fat or gaining weight, even though the woman's body weight is less than expected; and amenorrhea. Weight loss is achieved by restricting food intake, over-exercising, self-induced vomiting, or use of laxatives, emetics, and diuretics. Anorexia is most common in white teenage girls in industrialized Western societies. Societal pressures and standards of attractiveness for women, which emphasize thinness, have long been considered to increase the risk for anorexia nervosa, and a preoccupation with dieting is common in girls at menarche. Increasing evidence indicates, however, that there is clearly a significant genetic contribution to anorexia nervosa and other eating disorders, with heritability estimates of 50% to 80%. Other risk factors include a history of childhood sexual abuse and psychological traits of low self-esteem, perfectionism, and obsessive thinking.

Medical signs and symptoms associated with anorexia nervosa include bradycardia, hypotension, hypothermia, leukopenia, hair loss, skin changes, and constipation. Vomiting

### Box 9.2 SCOFF Screening Questionnaire for Eating Disorders

1. Do you make yourself sick because you feel uncomfortably full? ____ Yes ____ No
2. Do you worry you have lost control over how much you eat? ____ Yes ____ No
3. Have you recently lost more than one stone (14 pounds) in a 3-month period? ____ Yes ____ No
4. Do you believe yourself to be fat when others say you are too thin? ____ Yes ____ No
5. Would you say that food dominates your life? ____ Yes ____ No

Two or more "yes" answers indicate that the patient may have an eating disorder.

Modified from Morgan JF, Reid F, Lacey JH. The SCOFF questionnaire: assessment of a new screening tool for eating disorders. *BMJ*. 1999;319:1467-1468.

### Box 9.3 Diagnostic Criteria for Eating Disorders

**Anorexia Nervosa**

A. Restriction of energy intake relative to requirements, leading to a significantly low body weight in the context of age, sex, developmental trajectory, and physical health. *Significantly low weight* is defined as a weight that is less than minimally normal or, for children and adolescents, less than that minimally expected.
B. Intense fear of gaining weight or becoming fat, or persistent behavior that interferes with weight gain, even though at a significantly low weight.
C. Disturbance in the way in which one's body weight or shape is experienced, undue influence of body weight or shape on self-evaluation, or persistent lack of recognition of the seriousness of the current low body weight.

**Coding note:** The ICD-9-CM code for anorexia nervosa is **307.1**, which is assigned regardless of the subtype. The ICD-10-CM code depends on the subtype (see below).

*Specify* whether:

**(F50.01) Restricting type:** During the last 3 months, the individual has not engaged in recurrent episodes of binge eating or purging behavior (i.e., self-induced vomiting or the misuse of laxatives, diuretics, or enemas). This subtype describes presentations in which weight loss is accomplished primarily through dieting, fasting, and/or excessive exercise.

**(F50.02) Binge-eating/purging type:** During the last 3 months, the individual has engaged in recurrent episodes of binge eating or purging behavior (i.e., self-induced vomiting or the misuse of laxatives, diuretics, or enemas).

Specify if:

**In partial remission:** After full criteria for anorexia nervosa were previously met, Criterion A (low body weight) has not been met for a sustained period, but either Criterion B (intense fear of gaining weight or becoming fat or behavior that interferes with weight gain) or Criterion C (disturbances in self-perception of weight and shape) is still met.

**In full remission:** After full criteria for anorexia nervosa were previously met, none of the criteria have been met for a sustained period of time.

*Specify* current severity:

The minimum level of severity is based, for adults, on current body mass index (BMI) (see below) or, for children and adolescents, on BMI percentile. The ranges below are derived from World Health Organization categories for thinness in adults; for children and adolescents, corresponding BMI percentiles should be used. The level of severity may be increased to reflect clinical symptoms, the degree of functional disability, and the need for supervision.

**Mild:** BMI ≥ 17 kg/m$^2$
**Moderate:** BMI 16-16.99 kg/m$^2$
**Severe:** BMI 15-15.99 kg/m$^2$
**Extreme:** BMI < 15 kg/m$^2$

*Continued*

**Box 9.3 Diagnostic Criteria for Eating Disorders-cont'd**

**Bulimia Nervosa**

A. Recurrent episodes of binge eating. An episode of binge eating is characterized by both of the following:
   1. Eating, in a discrete period of time (e.g., within any 2-hour period), an amount of food that is definitely larger than most individuals would eat in a similar period of time under similar circumstances.
   2. A sense of lack of control over eating during the episode (e.g., a feeling that one cannot stop eating or control what or how much one is eating).

B. Recurrent, inappropriate compensatory behaviors in order to prevent weight gain, such as self-induced vomiting; misuse of laxatives, diuretics, or other medications; fasting; or excessive exercise.

C. The binge eating and inappropriate compensatory behaviors both occur, on average, at least once a week for 3 months.

D. Self-evaluation is unduly influenced by body shape and weight.

E. The disturbance does not occur exclusively during episodes of anorexia nervosa.

Specify if:

**In partial remission:** After full criteria for bulimia nervosa were previously met, some, but not all, of the criteria have been met for a sustained period of time.

**In full remission:** After full criteria for bulimia nervosa were previously met, none of the criteria have been met for a sustained period of time.

*Specify* current severity:

The minimum level of severity is based on the frequency of inappropriate compensatory behaviors (see below). The level of severity may be increased to reflect other symptoms and the degree of functional disability.

**Mild:** An average of 1-3 episodes of inappropriate compensatory behaviors per week.

**Moderate:** An average of 4-7 episodes of inappropriate compensatory behaviors per week.

**Severe:** An average of 8-13 episodes of inappropriate compensatory behaviors per week.

**Extreme:** An average of 14 or more episodes of inappropriate compensatory behaviors per week.

**Binge-Eating Disorder**

A. Recurrent episodes of binge eating. An episode of binge eating is characterized by both of the following:
   1. Eating, in a discrete period of time (e.g., within any 2-hour period), an amount of food that is definitely larger than what most people would eat in a similar period of time under similar circumstances.
   2. A sense of lack of control over eating during the episode (e.g., a feeling that one cannot stop eating or control what or how much one is eating).

B. The binge-eating episodes are associated with three (or more) of the following:
   1. Eating much more rapidly than normal.
   2. Eating until feeling uncomfortably full.
   3. Eating large amounts of food when not feeling physically hungry.
   4. Eating alone because of feeling embarrassed by how much one is eating.
   5. Feeling disgusted with oneself, depressed, or very guilty afterward.

C. Marked distress regarding binge eating is present.

D. Binge eating occurs, on average, at least once a week for 3 months.

E. The binge eating is not associated with the recurrent use of inappropriate compensatory behavior as in bulimia nervosa and does not occur exclusively during the course of bulimia nervosa or anorexia nervosa.

Specify if:

**In partial remission:** After full criteria for binge-eating disorder were previously met, binge eating occurs at an average frequency of less than one episode per week for a sustained period of time.

**In full remission:** After full criteria for binge-eating disorder were previously met, none of the criteria have been met for a sustained period of time.

*Specify* current severity:

The minimum level of severity is based on the frequency of episodes of binge eating (see below). The level of severity may be increased to reflect other symptoms and the degree of functional disability.

**Mild:** 1-3 binge-eating episodes per week.

**Moderate:** 4-7 binge-eating episodes per week.

**Severe:** 8-13 binge-eating episodes per week.

**Extreme:** 14 or more binge-eating episodes per week.

From American Psychiatric Association. *Diagnostic and Statistical Manual of Mental Disorders.* 5th ed, DSM-5. Washington, DC: American Psychiatric Association; 2013, pp 338-339, 345, 350.

or laxative use may cause hypokalemia. Endocrine changes include low estrogen and testosterone levels, amenorrhea, decreased libido, hypercortisolemia, and low bone density. Prolonged QT interval is a serious sequela of anorexia nervosa and has been associated with sudden death. The mortality rate of anorexia nervosa from all causes is 5% to 6% per decade of illness.

Psychiatric symptoms associated with anorexia nervosa include depression, anxiety, social difficulties, sleep disturbance, agitation, poor emotion regulation, rigidity, obsessional thinking, and compulsive behaviors. Interestingly, these symptoms occur in individuals without anorexia nervosa during starvation and resolve with weight gain and so are most likely caused, or at least exacerbated, by the illness.

Anorexia nervosa is difficult to treat. Women do not usually seek help themselves but instead are brought to treatment by concerned family members. They fear gaining weight, do not see their illness as a problem, are frequently nonadherent to treatment, feel isolated and do not engage with treatment providers, and may have multiple relapses. About one third recover completely, but this may take a number of years. Early recognition and treatment improve outcome. Family members often become frustrated with the woman's multiple relapses, lack of insight, and apparent lack of cooperation with treatment and may need support themselves in dealing with her illness.

The best treatment for anorexia nervosa involves referral to a multidisciplinary team, with medical, nutritional, psychological, and psychiatric expertise in this area. The focus is on gradual refeeding to achieve weight gain, and outpatient treatment, with hospitalization only for acute, dangerous medical or psychiatric complications. In adolescents, family therapy or, in nonintact families, adolescent-centered individual psychotherapy is most effective (Lock, 2010). There is little evidence supporting any specific type of psychotherapy in adults, but treatment by a therapist with expertise in anorexia nervosa is more effective than support from a nonspecialist. From one randomized controlled trial (RCT), focal psychodynamic therapy seemed to help recovery at 1 year and enhanced cognitive behavioral therapy was more effective with speed of weight gain and improvement in eating disorder thinking (Zipfel, 2014). There is no clear evidence supporting treatment with psychotropic medications. An early study showing efficacy of fluoxetine to maintain weight gain has not been replicated. Preliminary trials of atypical antipsychotics, with the goal of addressing distorted thinking about weight and body shape, have shown initial promise.

Bulimia nervosa is characterized by binge eating, combined with inappropriate compensatory mechanisms to avoid weight gain, such as self-induced vomiting, misuse of laxatives or diuretics, or fasting or excessive exercise. Binge eating and compensatory behaviors occur an average of once a week for 3 months (see Box 9.3 for full diagnostic criteria). Bulimia, like anorexia, is most common in young women, has a significant genetic component, may follow teasing or criticism about the woman's weight or shape, and is thought to involve disturbances in hunger-satiety pathways, the drive system and rewarding characteristics of food, or self-regulation. Comorbidity with mood and anxiety disorders, addictions, and suicidal thoughts and behaviors is common. All-cause mortality rates, including suicide rates, are elevated, with a mortality rate of 3.9% over 8 to 25 years of follow-up.

Women with bulimia nervosa and purging may develop hypokalemia, hyponatremia, hypochloremia, a metabolic alkalosis as a result of vomiting, or a metabolic acidosis with laxative abuse. Recurrent self-induced vomiting can result in loss of dental enamel, parotid gland enlargement, or calluses and scars on the dorsal aspect of the hand. Rare but serious complications include esophageal tears, gastric rupture, rectal prolapse, and cardiac arrhythmias.

There is strong evidence for the efficacy of cognitive behavioral therapy for bulimia nervosa, although complete remission of binging and purging occurs in only 30% to 40%. Other therapies that have some evidence for efficacy are interpersonal therapy, dialectical behavior therapy focusing on emotion regulation, and family therapy in adolescents. Antidepressants are superior to placebo in treatment of bulimia, with the agent of choice being fluoxetine 60 mg daily. Of note, the antidepressant bupropion is contraindicated in women with a history of bulimia because of an elevated risk of seizures, presumably because of electrolyte abnormalities. The outcome of bulimia is full recovery in 45%, significant improvement in 27%, and a chronic, protracted course in about 23%.

In binge eating disorder, the woman binge eats (as in bulimia nervosa) an average of once a week for at least 3 months, but she does not engage in compensatory behaviors such as purging, fasting, or excessive exercise. As a result, she may also develop obesity but does not develop the medical complications associated with purging or low weight. Treatment for binge eating disorder includes nutritional consultation, diet, physical activity, education, and specific psychotherapies. There is strong evidence for the efficacy of cognitive-behavioral therapy in binge eating disorder and other psychotherapies, such as dialectical behavior therapy (DBT) and interpersonal therapy (IPT), are also effective. Medication treatments include antidepressants such as SSRIs. Weight loss agents, topiramate, and stimulants may also be effective.

## OBESITY

The prevalence of obesity has dramatically increased in the United States. The World Health Organization (WHO) definitions for body weight are shown in Table 9.3. Weight classification by body mass index (BMI) is outlined in Table 9.4. Based on this definition, more than 35% of U.S. adults are obese and 69% are overweight or obese. The prevalence of obesity is higher in middle-aged adults, minority women, and low-income women and varies by geographic regions. In particular, African American and Hispanic women are at double the risk of non-Hispanic white women. WHO describes a global epidemic of obesity, which is a major burden to worldwide chronic disease and disability. Of note, women taking psychotropic medications, especially antipsychotics, are at heightened risk for obesity and metabolic syndrome.

There is a strong relationship between mortality and increased BMI above 25 $kg/m^2$ (and below 20 $kg/m^2$) (Fig. 9.1). Even in healthy people who have never smoked, at age 50 years, there is still an elevated risk of death for persons whose BMIs are between 25 and 30 (Adams, 2006). The risk of death increased 20% to 40% in the overweight group and by two to three times among obese persons. Severe obesity is a health hazard that carries a 12-fold increase in mortality. Increased central adiposity is associated with increased risk of morbidity and mortality as well as BMI, so waist circumference can easily be measured. Using a tape measure at the level of the iliac crest, the waist circumference is taken. For women with a BMI of 25 to 34.9 $kg/m^2$, a waist circumference of over 35 inches is associated with heart disease and diabetes mellitus. Because of these risk factors, many organizations, including the American College of Obstetricians and Gynecologists, recommend screening for obesity.

Often these individuals suffer complicating factors, such as hypertension, diabetes mellitus, dyslipidemias, heart disease, stroke, arthritis, increased operative morbidity and mortality, and compromised pulmonary function (sleep apnea). Obesity has been linked to multiple obstetric and gynecologic problems, including spontaneous abortion, endometrial hyperplasia, and endometrial and breast cancer, to name a few. One meta-analysis of increased BMI and cancer risk found a strong association between a five-point BMI increase and endometrial cancer (relative risk [RR] 1.59, $P < .0001$), gallbladder cancer (RR 1.59, $P = .04$), esophageal adenocarcinoma (RR 1.51, $P < .0001$), and renal cancer (RR 1.34, $P < .0001$). A weaker positive association was found with postmenopausal breast, pancreatic, thyroid and colon cancer plus leukemia, multiple myeloma, and non-Hodgkin lymphoma. The mechanisms of cancer association with obesity may be linked to hormone systems like insulin, insulin-like growth factor, sex steroids, adipokines, and other substances.

Diet, exercise, and behavior modification provided by lay supervision is appropriate for those suffering from mild obesity; diet, exercise, and behavior modification under medical

**Table 9.3** Body Mass Index Table

| BMI | 19 | 20 | 21 | 22 | 23 | 24 | 25 | 26 | 27 | 28 | 29 | 30 | 31 | 32 | 33 | 34 | 35 |
|---|---|---|---|---|---|---|---|---|---|---|---|---|---|---|---|---|---|
| **Height (inches)** | | | | | | | | **Body Weight (lbs)** | | | | | | | | | |
| 58 | 91 | 96 | 100 | 105 | 110 | 115 | 119 | 124 | 129 | 134 | 138 | 143 | 148 | 153 | 158 | 162 | 167 |
| 59 | 94 | 99 | 104 | 109 | 114 | 119 | 124 | 128 | 133 | 138 | 143 | 148 | 153 | 158 | 163 | 168 | 173 |
| 60 | 97 | 102 | 107 | 112 | 118 | 123 | 128 | 133 | 138 | 143 | 148 | 153 | 158 | 163 | 168 | 174 | 179 |
| 61 | 100 | 106 | 111 | 116 | 122 | 127 | 132 | 137 | 143 | 148 | 153 | 158 | 164 | 169 | 174 | 180 | 185 |
| 62 | 104 | 109 | 115 | 120 | 126 | 131 | 136 | 142 | 147 | 153 | 158 | 164 | 169 | 175 | 180 | 186 | 191 |
| 63 | 107 | 113 | 118 | 124 | 130 | 135 | 141 | 146 | 152 | 158 | 163 | 169 | 175 | 180 | 186 | 191 | 197 |
| 64 | 110 | 116 | 122 | 128 | 134 | 140 | 145 | 151 | 157 | 163 | 169 | 174 | 180 | 186 | 192 | 197 | 204 |
| 65 | 114 | 120 | 126 | 132 | 138 | 144 | 150 | 156 | 162 | 168 | 174 | 180 | 186 | 192 | 198 | 204 | 210 |
| 66 | 118 | 124 | 130 | 136 | 142 | 148 | 155 | 161 | 167 | 173 | 179 | 186 | 192 | 198 | 204 | 210 | 216 |
| 67 | 121 | 127 | 134 | 140 | 146 | 153 | 159 | 166 | 172 | 178 | 185 | 191 | 198 | 204 | 211 | 217 | 223 |
| 68 | 125 | 131 | 138 | 144 | 151 | 158 | 164 | 171 | 177 | 184 | 190 | 197 | 203 | 210 | 216 | 223 | 230 |
| 69 | 128 | 135 | 142 | 149 | 155 | 162 | 169 | 176 | 182 | 189 | 196 | 203 | 209 | 216 | 223 | 230 | 236 |
| 70 | 132 | 139 | 146 | 153 | 160 | 167 | 174 | 181 | 188 | 195 | 202 | 209 | 216 | 222 | 229 | 236 | 243 |
| 71 | 136 | 143 | 150 | 157 | 165 | 172 | 179 | 186 | 193 | 200 | 208 | 215 | 222 | 229 | 236 | 243 | 250 |
| 72 | 140 | 147 | 154 | 162 | 169 | 177 | 184 | 191 | 199 | 206 | 213 | 221 | 228 | 235 | 242 | 250 | 258 |
| 73 | 144 | 151 | 159 | 166 | 174 | 182 | 189 | 197 | 204 | 212 | 219 | 227 | 235 | 242 | 250 | 257 | 265 |
| 74 | 148 | 155 | 163 | 171 | 179 | 186 | 194 | 202 | 210 | 218 | 225 | 233 | 241 | 249 | 256 | 264 | 272 |
| 75 | 152 | 160 | 168 | 176 | 184 | 192 | 200 | 208 | 216 | 224 | 232 | 240 | 248 | 256 | 264 | 272 | 279 |
| 76 | 156 | 164 | 172 | 180 | 189 | 197 | 205 | 213 | 221 | 230 | 238 | 246 | 254 | 263 | 271 | 279 | 287 |

| BMI | 36 | 37 | 38 | 39 | 40 | 41 | 42 | 43 | 44 | 45 | 46 | 47 | 48 | 49 | 50 | 51 | 52 | 53 | 54 |
|---|---|---|---|---|---|---|---|---|---|---|---|---|---|---|---|---|---|---|---|
| 58 | 172 | 177 | 181 | 186 | 191 | 196 | 201 | 205 | 210 | 215 | 220 | 224 | 229 | 234 | 239 | 244 | 248 | 253 | 258 |
| 59 | 178 | 183 | 188 | 193 | 198 | 203 | 208 | 212 | 217 | 222 | 227 | 232 | 237 | 242 | 247 | 252 | 257 | 262 | 267 |
| 60 | 184 | 189 | 194 | 199 | 204 | 209 | 215 | 220 | 225 | 230 | 235 | 240 | 245 | 250 | 255 | 261 | 266 | 271 | 276 |
| 61 | 190 | 195 | 201 | 206 | 211 | 217 | 222 | 227 | 232 | 238 | 243 | 248 | 254 | 259 | 264 | 269 | 275 | 280 | 285 |
| 62 | 196 | 202 | 207 | 213 | 218 | 224 | 229 | 235 | 240 | 246 | 251 | 256 | 262 | 267 | 273 | 278 | 284 | 289 | 295 |
| 63 | 203 | 208 | 214 | 220 | 225 | 231 | 237 | 242 | 248 | 254 | 259 | 265 | 270 | 278 | 282 | 287 | 293 | 299 | 304 |
| 64 | 209 | 215 | 221 | 227 | 232 | 238 | 244 | 250 | 256 | 262 | 267 | 273 | 279 | 285 | 291 | 296 | 302 | 308 | 314 |
| 65 | 216 | 222 | 228 | 234 | 240 | 246 | 252 | 258 | 264 | 270 | 276 | 282 | 288 | 294 | 300 | 306 | 312 | 318 | 324 |
| 66 | 223 | 229 | 235 | 241 | 247 | 253 | 260 | 266 | 272 | 278 | 284 | 291 | 297 | 303 | 309 | 315 | 322 | 328 | 334 |
| 67 | 230 | 236 | 242 | 249 | 255 | 261 | 268 | 274 | 280 | 287 | 293 | 299 | 306 | 312 | 319 | 325 | 331 | 338 | 344 |
| 68 | 236 | 243 | 249 | 256 | 262 | 269 | 276 | 282 | 289 | 295 | 302 | 308 | 315 | 322 | 328 | 335 | 341 | 348 | 354 |
| 69 | 243 | 250 | 257 | 263 | 270 | 277 | 284 | 291 | 297 | 304 | 311 | 318 | 324 | 331 | 338 | 345 | 351 | 358 | 365 |
| 70 | 250 | 257 | 264 | 271 | 278 | 285 | 292 | 299 | 306 | 313 | 320 | 327 | 334 | 341 | 348 | 355 | 362 | 369 | 376 |
| 71 | 257 | 265 | 272 | 279 | 286 | 293 | 301 | 308 | 315 | 322 | 329 | 338 | 343 | 351 | 358 | 365 | 372 | 379 | 386 |
| 72 | 265 | 272 | 279 | 287 | 294 | 302 | 309 | 316 | 324 | 331 | 338 | 346 | 353 | 361 | 368 | 375 | 383 | 390 | 397 |
| 73 | 272 | 280 | 288 | 295 | 302 | 310 | 318 | 325 | 333 | 340 | 348 | 355 | 363 | 371 | 378 | 386 | 393 | 401 | 408 |
| 74 | 280 | 287 | 293 | 303 | 311 | 319 | 326 | 334 | 342 | 350 | 358 | 365 | 373 | 381 | 389 | 396 | 404 | 412 | 420 |
| 75 | 287 | 295 | 303 | 311 | 319 | 327 | 335 | 343 | 351 | 359 | 367 | 375 | 383 | 391 | 399 | 407 | 415 | 423 | 431 |
| 76 | 295 | 304 | 312 | 320 | 328 | 336 | 344 | 353 | 361 | 369 | 377 | 385 | 394 | 402 | 410 | 418 | 426 | 435 | 443 |

Evidence Report of Clinical Guidelines on the Identification, Evaluation, and Treatment of Overweight and Obesity in Adults, 1998, http://www.ncbi.nlm.nih.gov/books/NBK2003/pdf/Bookshelf_NBK2003.pdf.

supervision is appropriate for those suffering from moderate obesity; and operative intervention is appropriate for those suffering from severe obesity if conservative measures have failed. Patients suffering from severe obesity almost always have medical complications, and these often improve with weight reduction.

Unless behavior is modified, weight loss is usually not maintained. One study of 145 patients who were approximately 60% overweight and divided them into three groups. Treatment continued for 6 months, and there was at least 1 year of follow-up in 99% of those who completed the therapy. Group 1 underwent behavior modification using Ferguson's *Learning to Eat* manual. They lost an average of 11.4 kg and regained only 1.8 kg during the follow-up year. Group 2 received medication therapy with an appetite suppressant, fenfluramine hydrochloride (Pondimin). They lost an average of 14.5 kg but regained 8.6 kg during the follow-up period.

**Table 9.4** Weight Classification by Body Mass Index (BMI)

| Weight | BMI* |
|---|---|
| Normal weight | 18.5-24.9 |
| Overweight | 25.0-29.9 |
| Obesity | >30 |
| Class I | 30.0-34.9 |
| Class II | 35.0-39.9 |
| Class III | >40 |

*BMI calculation = weight in kilograms/height in square meters.

The third group was treated with a combination of behavior modification and medication and lost an average of 15 kg but regained 9.5 kg during the follow-up period. The authors concluded that behavior modification without medication was the most appropriate therapy for moderate obesity. Setting goals is important in

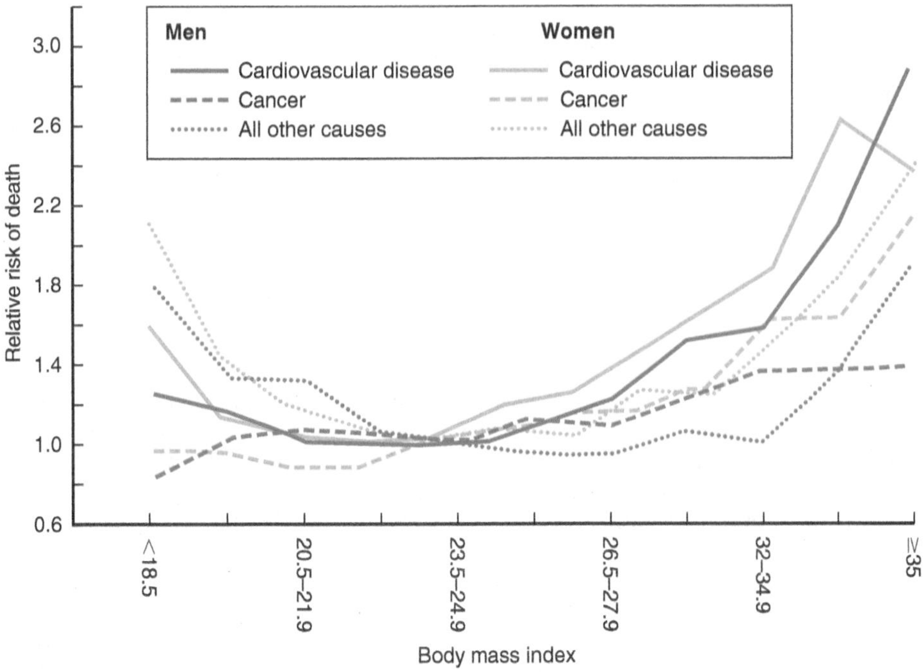


**Figure 9.1** Relation between mortality and body mass index in men and women who have never smoked. (Data from Calle EE, Thun MJ, Petrelli JM, et al. Body-Mass Index and mortality in a prospective cohort of U.S. adults. *N Eng J Med*. 1999;341:1097-1105.)

behavior therapy, and a 5% to 10% loss of total body weight is realistic over 6 months and can decrease the severity of comorbid diseases. A systematic review of 12 trials, involving 3893 participants supported these findings with intensive behavioral counseling, diet (reducing intake by ≥500 kcal/day) and exercise (≥150 minutes of walking/week) leading to clinically meaningful weight loss of 0.3 kg to 6.6 kg over 6 months (Wadden, 2014).

Many individuals embrace fad diets and look for magic cures. However, if placed on a nutritionally appropriate limited-caloric diet, they generally do well if their attitudes toward eating and response to various stimuli are modified. Lay groups, such as Weight Watchers or Take Off Pounds Sensibly (TOPS), may be successful for motivated individuals. Tracking calorie intake, utilizing a smart phone app for weight loss, avoiding food binges, avoiding eating at night, and practicing stress reduction or mindfulness-based training could benefit some women. In a meta-analysis of named diet programs, 48 randomized trials were reviewed and reported the largest weight loss was associated with the low-carbohydrate diets and low-fat diets (Johnston, 2014). The differences in weight loss between the programs were minimal. It is more important to find a healthy diet that a person can adhere to long term. One study suggested that if these structured weight loss programs could be provided free of charge to participants, both retention and average weight loss may be far better than when participants pay for these programs. Many diet programs prescribe or sell low-fat foods in an attempt to achieve a diet containing about 20% to 30% fat. Because fat represents 9 Cal/g and protein and carbohydrate represent 4 Cal/g, it is possible by changing eating habits to allow a patient a considerable quantity of food without high numbers of calories. The use of portion-controlled servings has been demonstrated to be effective for weight loss because obese persons tend to underestimate the amount of food they consume. Educating patients to change eating habits in this fashion is the key not only to losing weight but also to maintaining the weight loss. Weight loss done sensibly takes a long time. Setting a realistic goal of 5% loss of body weight over 6 months is helpful. The major problem with such individuals is maintaining weight loss, and, in fact, most do not maintain the weight loss.

Exercise is a useful addition to diet regimens. Several studies have demonstrated that although similar weight loss can be obtained by both diet alone and diet plus exercise programs, the latter will allow for a greater loss of fat stores while maintaining muscle mass. To maintain this advantage, exercise programs must be maintained. Although exercise alone is not a good method for losing weight, studies indicate exercise is very beneficial for long-term weight management and overall health. One study looked at amount of physical activity and weight gain in women and concluded that physical activity is inversely related to weight gain in women of normal weight, but not in women who are overweight (Lee, 2010). Getting more active might be manageable for some women via their work commute. A United Kingdom study found that people who commuted to work by active (bike or walk) or public transport had significantly lower BMI and percentage body fat than people who used private transportation (Flint, 2014). Presumably, utilizing public transportation required more walking each day.

The FDA has approved medications for weight loss, although there have been many concerns about safety. Generally the medication must be continued for sustained benefit or weight gain recurs. Medications are mainly recommended for BMI >30 kg/m$^2$ or BMI >27 kg/m$^2$ when comorbid conditions are present. Orlistat inhibits dietary fat absorption and is considered first-line treatment because of its better safety profile than other medications. Most subjects can expect about 3% loss of initial weight. It has side effects of fecal urgency, flatulence, and oily stools. Sibutramine inhibits reuptake of neurotransmitters and affects satiation. Adverse effects include increases in heart rate

Table 9.5 Guide to Selecting Treatment

| | Body Mass Index Category | | | | |
|---|---|---|---|---|---|
| **Treatment** | **25-26.9** | **27-29.9** | **30-34.9** | **35-39.9** | **>40** |
| Diet, physical activity, and behavior therapy | With comorbidities | With comorbidities | + | + | + |
| Pharmacotherapy | | With comorbidities | + | + | + |
| Surgery | | | | With comorbidities | With comorbidities |

From The Practical Guide: Identification, Evaluation, and Treatment of Overweight and Obesity in Adults. National Heart, Lung, and Blood Institute and North American Association for the Study of Obesity. Bethesda, MD: National Institutes of Health; 2000.
The + represents the use of indicated treatment regardless of comorbidities.

and blood pressure, so sibutramine was removed from the market. Lorcaserin is a serotonin 2c receptor agonist, which reduces appetite. It is a more selective serotonin agent so is thought to be less likely to cause cardiac valve problems. Over 1 year, about 50% of patients lost at least 3% of their body mass. Side effects include headache, dizziness, fatigue, nausea, and constipation. More patients (67% to 70%) will lose weight on phentermine plus topiramate-extended release and up to 9% weight loss for the top dose (Yanovski, 2014). Warnings include metabolic acidosis, increased heart rate, anxiety, insomnia, and increased creatinine levels. Both lorcaserin and phentermine-topiramate have warnings about memory, attention, and depression. All these medications have limited long-term safety and efficacy data. Another option is metformin for women with type 2 diabetes. A guide to selecting treatment for obesity is given in Table 9.5.

Eligible candidates for bariatric surgery include those with a BMI >40 $kg/m^2$ or a BMI >35 $kg/m^2$ if serious comorbid conditions are present, if nonsurgical weight loss measures have failed, if the woman is motivated and well-informed, and there is acceptable surgical risk. One meta-analysis found the majority of postsurgical obesity patients have resolution or improvement in comorbid conditions such as diabetes, hypertension, dyslipidemia, and obstructive sleep apnea (Puzziferri, 2014). In looking at 29 studies and 7971 patients, gastric bypass had better outcomes than gastric banding for long-term weight loss, type 2 diabetic control and remission, hypertension, and hyperlipidemia. Gastric bypass and sleeve gastrectomy reported weight loss exceeding 50% and only 31% in gastric band studies. Surgical options can provide long-term weight loss but are not without complications. Bariatric procedures used (gastric bypass, laparoscopic gastric band, vertical banded gastroplasty, and biliopancreatic diversion and switch) result in a 20% complication rate and 1% mortality. A patient with a BMI of 35 to 39 $kg/m^2$ appears to do better with surgery as well as the morbidly obese. In fact, there is even one randomized trial on laparoscopic adjustable gastric banding in adults with a BMI of 30 to 35 $kg/m^2$. The surgery was significantly more effective at reducing weight, resolving the metabolic syndrome, and improving quality of life at 2 years after the intervention.

Obesity in adolescence is a variant of the problem in the general population. The percentage of young people who are overweight has more than tripled since 1980. Seventeen percent of young people (2 to 19 years old) are obese, although this did not change between 2003-2004 and 2011-2012. Being overweight in adolescence is a more powerful predictor of morbidity from cardiovascular disease than being overweight in adulthood. Because the risk for progression with increasing morbidity and mortality is great, prompt support and behavior modification are most important. School and parental involvement are important aspects of controlling the problem. Where an obese parent is also present, best results seem to be achieved when both the parent and the child undergo therapy but in separate counseling sessions. One study of 42 obese adolescents, ages 12 through 16, divided them into three groups and used 16 weeks of treatment. When the child alone attended group therapy, there was an average 3.3-kg weight loss; when the child and mother were treated together, there was an average 5.3-kg weight loss; and when the child and mother were both treated but separately, there was an 8.4-kg weight loss. After 1 year of follow-up, the group in which the mother and child were treated separately maintained their weight loss at a mean of 7.7 kg, whereas the other two groups had regained their previous baseline levels. The Cochrane Collaboration reviewed interventions for treating obesity in children in 2009, and although 64 randomized controlled trials were found, the data quality was limited. However, combined behavior lifestyle modifications with dietary changes, physical activity, or behavioral therapy were favored over standard or self-care for meaningful weight control. In obese adolescents, pharmacologic treatment warranted consideration in addition to the combined lifestyle modifications.

The Centers for Disease Control and Prevention (CDC) mentions the following promising approaches for preventing obesity: (1) breastfeeding, which is associated with a reduced risk of overweight children; (2) regular physical activity; (3) increasing physical activity in overweight people to prevent the complications associated with obesity; and (4) decreasing children's time watching television. Beyond the individual, population-based strategies and policies are being studied.

## ANXIETY DISORDERS, OBSESSIVE-COMPULSIVE DISORDER, AND POSTTRAUMATIC STRESS DISORDER

Anxiety disorders are the most common psychiatric disorders in the general population. They usually have their onset in childhood, adolescence, or early adulthood and are more common in women than in men. Anxiety is a normal, adaptive response to danger or threat and is associated with physical symptoms (e.g., increased heart rate, sweating, shaking) and cognitive symptoms (e.g., worry, fear). Increases in anxiety are common with life stressors, including medical appointments, diagnoses, and procedures. In addition, anxiety may result from a number of drugs (e.g., caffeine, cannabis, cocaine, methamphetamine, withdrawal of alcohol or opiates), medications (e.g., theophylline, steroids),

**Box 9.4 Specifier for a Panic Attack**

**Note:** Symptoms are presented for the purpose of identifying a panic attack; however, panic attack is not a mental disorder and cannot be coded. Panic attacks can occur in the context of any anxiety disorder as well as other mental disorders (e.g., depressive disorders, posttraumatic stress disorder, substance use disorders) and some medical conditions (e.g., cardiac, respiratory, vestibular, gastrointestinal). When the presence of a panic attack is identified, it should be noted as a specifier (e.g., "posttraumatic stress disorder with panic attacks"). For panic disorder, the presence of panic attack is contained within the criteria for the disorder and panic attack is not used as a specifier.

An abrupt surge of intense fear or discomfort that reaches a peak within minutes, and during which time four (or more) of the following symptoms occur:

**Note:** The abrupt surge can occur from a calm state or an anxious state.

1. Palpitations, pounding heart, or accelerated heart rate
2. Sweating
3. Trembling or shaking
4. Sensations of shortness of breath or smothering
5. Feeling of choking
6. Chest pain or discomfort
7. Nausea or abdominal distress
8. Feeling dizzy, unsteady, lightheaded, or faint
9. Chills or heat sensations
10. Paresthesias (numbness or tingling sensations)
11. Derealization (feelings of unreality) or depersonalization (being detached from oneself)
12. Fear of losing control or "going crazy"
13. Fear of dying

**Note:** Culture-specific symptoms (e.g., tinnitus, neck soreness, headache, uncontrollable screaming or crying) may be seen. Such symptoms should not count as one of the four required symptoms.

From American Psychiatric Association. *Diagnostic and Statistical Manual of Mental Disorders*, 5th ed, DSM-5. Washington, DC: American Psychiatric Association; 2013, p.214.

or medical conditions (e.g., asthma, arrhythmias, temporal lobe epilepsy). Some people experience primary anxiety disorders, involving excessive anxiety that interferes with daily functioning, without apparent explanation or out of proportion to any stressor. Primary anxiety disorders include panic disorder, generalized anxiety disorder (GAD), social anxiety disorder, and specific phobias. Obsessive-compulsive disorder (OCD) and posttraumatic stress disorder (PTSD), although categorized separately from anxiety disorders in DSM-5, also involve significant anxiety and fear.

Panic disorder is characterized by sudden, intense attacks of fear (Katon, 2006). The symptom criteria for a panic attack are shown in Box 9.4. People with panic disorder have recurrent, unexpected panic attacks, with at least one of the attacks followed by a month or more of persistent concern about having additional attacks or worry about their consequences (e.g., losing control, having a heart attack, going crazy) or a maladaptive change in behavior because of panic attacks (e.g., avoiding certain situations for fear of having an attack). About one third of people in the general population have at least one panic attack during their lives, so that a woman presenting with a single panic attack can be reassured that this is very common. Panic attacks can be precipitated by frightening situations or heightened stress, in which case they are called *situational panic attacks*. People with only situational panic attacks are not diagnosed with panic disorder. Panic attacks without apparent precipitant are called *spontaneous*.

Panic disorder occurs in 1% to 2% of the population and is about twice as common in women than in men. Risk factors include a family history of panic disorder and significant life stress in the year before the development of symptoms. The disorder has a genetic component, with a heritability of about 30%. Complications include depression in about two thirds of people, and one third are depressed at the time of clinical presentation. Especially as panic attacks are unpredictable, they frequently lead to anticipatory anxiety (anxiety about having the next panic attack) and phobic avoidance, or avoidance of situations in which the person has had or would fear having a panic attack. These situations commonly include crowds, being in lines or in the middle of an audience, driving (especially in tunnels, over bridges, or in freeways), or other situations in which the woman would feel trapped, unable to get out, or publicly embarrassed. With time, the fear and avoidance surrounding panic attacks often become significantly more distressing and disabling than the attacks themselves and may lead to agoraphobia, or avoidance of multiple situations and activities. Panic disorder, like other anxiety disorders, is also associated with an increased rate of alcohol abuse as a form of self-medication. Finally, panic and other anxiety disorders are associated with an increased risk for suicide attempts. Thus even though a woman presents with anxiety and does not endorse depression, she should be asked about hopeless or suicidal thoughts.

The treatment of panic disorder includes reassurance, education, general measures, medication, and psychotherapy. Fortunately, treatment response rates are high, so it is possible to be optimistic that the woman has a highly treatable condition. She may fear that she is dying, has a life-threatening or serious medical illness, or that she is "going crazy," and she can be reassured that, although panic attacks are terrifying, none of these fears is true. Presenting a model of panic attacks as being the body's natural, healthy "alarm system" that is malfunctioning and being triggered for no reason is often helpful. As general measures, the woman should be counseled to avoid exacerbating factors, such as caffeine, alcohol, stimulants, or other illicit drugs and to examine possible modifiable sources of increased life stress.

Panic disorder responds well to both medication and psychotherapy (Roy-Byrne, 2006). In more severe cases or with significant comorbid phobic avoidance, a combination of both treatments is preferable. However, because both are effective, the approach to treatment can be determined by the woman's preference. The first-line medication treatment for panic disorder is serotonin reuptake inhibitor antidepressants (SSRIs). There are two important differences in prescribing these medications for panic disorder versus for depression. First, people with panic disorder are frequently very sensitive to medication side effects. Because panic attacks involve feeling out of control of physical sensations and one's own body, side effects can initially increase anxiety and panic. Thus although ultimately doses need to be similar to antidepressant doses, it is wise to start treatment at a low dose (e.g., a daily dose of 12.5 mg sertraline, 5 mg citalopram), increasing the dose rapidly after a few days if the woman has no side effects. Second, whereas antidepressants take 4 to 6 weeks or less to relieve depression, they can take up to 12 weeks to have their full effect on panic and anxiety, with some effect expected by 6 weeks. It is important to educate the woman about this delayed and gradual onset of action. Many women present in distress and ask about something that will act more rapidly. In cases of disability resulting from panic attacks (e.g., inability to function, work, or go to school), it is reasonable to prescribe a benzodiazepine along with an SSRI, with the expectation that the SSRI will be the long-term treatment and the benzodiazepine will be tapered after at most 12 weeks. A benzodiazepine such as clonazepam, which has a longer half-life, requires only twice a day dosing, and maintains more constant blood levels, is preferable to shorter-acting agents such as alprazolam. For women with a history of substance use disorders or who need to avoid the potential slowed reflexes, psychomotor impairment, and cognitive slowing associated with benzodiazepines, other alternative adjuncts to reduce anxiety and panic quickly could include hydroxyzine or gabapentin. Buspirone has not been proved effective for panic disorder. In women who do not tolerate SSRIs, most other antidepressants (e.g., venlafaxine, mirtazapine) are also effective for the long-term treatment of panic disorder, with the exception of bupropion, which increases anxiety symptoms.

Psychotherapy is a highly effective treatment for panic disorder. The best established therapy treatment is cognitive behavioral therapy (CBT), which focuses on addressing the catastrophic thoughts associated with panic attacks (e.g., "I'm dying," "I'm going to crash my car and kill myself and other people"), learning coping and anxiety reduction strategies (e.g., relaxation, paced breathing to combat hyperventilation), and gradual approach to feared situations to decrease disability. CBT for panic disorder is a weekly therapy for about 12 to 16 weeks, has significant improvement rates equal to or better than the 70% response rate with medication, yields long-term benefits after therapy is over, and increases the patient's sense of mastery and control, which is valuable in a disorder that makes people feel out of control. CBT can also help patients tolerate medication side effects and benzodiazepine withdrawal symptoms.

Overall, of the varied symptoms of panic disorder, panic attacks are the easiest to treat and quickest to resolve with both medication and therapy. Phobic avoidance and anticipatory anxiety usually linger for a longer time, because of the unpredictability of panic attacks. People with panic disorder in most cases have a relapsing and remitting condition that requires long-term medication treatment (at least a year and frequently longer) and may recur in periods of increased stress.

In contrast with the sudden attacks of fear in panic disorder, generalized anxiety disorder (GAD) is characterized by excessive anxiety and worry about a number of life situations (e.g., work, school, family members) occurring more days than not for at least 6 months. The patient experiences her worries as excessive and difficult to control and as causing significant distress or trouble functioning. In addition, she has three or more of the following symptoms associated with her anxiety and worry: restlessness, insomnia, muscle tension, fatigue, trouble concentrating, or irritability. GAD usually begins early in life, is about twice as common in women than in men, has a genetic component, and has a lifetime prevalence of 5%. This is often a chronic disorder, with other lifetime psychiatric diagnoses (depression, other anxiety disorders, substance use disorders) superimposed in up to 90% of people. The restlessness and trouble concentrating associated with GAD and anxiety in general may lead to a misdiagnosis of attention deficit disorder.

The treatment of GAD often depends on the need to treat comorbid psychiatric conditions, which may have actually led the woman to seek medical help. In general, though, GAD responds to general measures such as avoiding caffeine, alcohol, and illicit drugs; medication; and psychotherapy. Antidepressants are effective for GAD, and the first-line long-term medication treatment is an SSRI. Buspirone 30 to 60 mg daily is effective for GAD and has few side effects. Hydroxyzine and beta-blockers have been shown to be effective, as are benzodiazepines. However, given the chronic, often lifelong course of GAD, benzodiazepines are not recommended. Psychotherapy for GAD focuses on addressing and coping with worry ("What if" thoughts).

Social anxiety disorder (or social phobia) refers to anxiety in and avoidance of social situations, where the woman is or feels the center of attention and fears humiliation, embarrassment, or being judged negatively by other people (for diagnostic criteria, see Box 9.5). Symptoms of social anxiety disorder can include full-blown panic attacks, but these are provoked by social situations and are not spontaneous. In many cases, social anxiety disorder is restricted to specific situations, most often public speaking or other public performances. Some women have a more pervasive form of this disorder, in which fears and avoidance relate not just to public performance but to most social situations and interactions, such as meeting new people, parties,

**Box 9.5 Diagnostic Criteria for Social Anxiety Disorder (Social Phobia)**

A. Marked fear or anxiety about one or more social situations in which the individual is exposed to possible scrutiny by others. Examples include social interactions (e.g., having a conversation, meeting unfamiliar people), being observed (e.g., eating or drinking), and performing in front of others (e.g., giving a speech).

**Note**: In children, the anxiety must occur in peer settings and not just during interactions with adults.

B. The individual fears that he or she will act in a way or show anxiety symptoms that will be negatively evaluated (i.e., will be humiliating or embarrassing; will lead to rejection or offend others).
C. The social situations almost always provoke fear or anxiety.

**Note:** In children, the fear or anxiety may be expressed by crying, tantrums, freezing, clinging, shrinking, or failing to speak in social situations.

D. The social situations are avoided or endured with intense fear or anxiety.
E. The fear or anxiety is out of proportion to the actual threat posed by the social situation and to the sociocultural contexy.
F. The fear, anxiety, or avoidance is persistent, typically lasting for 6 months or more.
G. The fear, anxiety, or avoidance causes clinically significant distress or impairment in social, occupational, or other important areas of functioning
H. The fear, anxiety, or avoidance is not attributable to the physiological effects of a substance (e.g., a drug of abuse, a medication) or another medical condition.
I. The fear, anxiety, or avoidance is not better explained by the symptoms of another mental disorder, such as panic disorder, body dysmorphic disorder, or autism spectrum disorder.
J. If another medical condition (e.g., Parkinson's disease, obesity, disfigurement from burns or injury) is present, the fear, anxiety, or avoidance is clearly unrelated or is excessive.

Specify if:

**Performance only:** If the fear is restricted to speaking or performing in public.

From American Psychiatric Association. *Diagnostic and Statistical Manual of Mental Disorders*. 5th ed, DSM-5. Washington, DC: American Psychiatric Association; 2013, pp 202-203.

initiating and maintaining conversations, dating, group projects, speaking with authority figures, or asserting oneself.

In epidemiologic studies, the lifetime prevalence of social anxiety disorder ranges from 3% to 13%. Age of onset is usually early in life, and women are more commonly affected than men. In Asian cultures, social anxiety frequently focuses on fears of giving offense to other people—for example, through making inappropriate eye contact, body odor, flatulence, or blushing. There is evidence for a genetic or familial risk for this condition. Women with social anxiety disorder may have associated poor self-esteem, difficulty asserting themselves, depression, or alcohol abuse. Social anxiety disorder exists on a continuum with, and may be difficult to differentiate from, normal shyness, although by definition social anxiety disorder involves marked distress or impairment in functioning.

Treatment of social anxiety disorder also includes medication and psychotherapy (Stein, 2008). Serotonin reuptake inhibitors (SSRIs) are the first-line medication treatment and, as in other anxiety disorders, may take up to 12 weeks to have their full therapeutic effect. MAO inhibitors, though effective, bring with them dietary restrictions and risk of hypertensive crisis. Beta-blockers are helpful for performance anxiety but not for more generalized social anxiety disorder. Benzodiazepines are effective but should be used with caution because of the chronicity of this disorder and the comorbidity with alcohol use disorder. There is some evidence for efficacy of gabapentin. Women with social anxiety restricted to public speaking may benefit from attending Toastmasters and thus practicing public speaking in a safe setting. Cognitive behavioral therapy (CBT) for social anxiety disorder is very effective. CBT includes individual treatment focusing on distorted thoughts about social situations (e.g., thoughts that the patient will make a fool of herself, has embarrassed herself, and that this will have catastrophic consequences) and on problem solving around and role-playing feared situations. Surprisingly, group cognitive behavioral therapy is also effective for social anxiety disorder.

Specific phobias occur in up to 20% of the general population and include fears of specific animals (e.g., snakes, spiders), phenomena (e.g., lightning), or situations (e.g., heights, flying in airplanes, driving, medical or dental procedures). People usually come to medical attention for specific phobias when these interfere with daily life or with their medical treatment. For example, people may develop specific phobias related to repeated medical events like chemotherapy treatments or to necessary aspects of their daily life, such as driving or traveling by plane. The best treatment for a specific phobia is desensitization, or gradually confronting the feared situation with the aid of an anxiety reducing strategy such as relaxation or imagery. In an acute situation, a benzodiazepine may help the woman to get through the particular event, but this will not reduce her future fear of the same situation.

Obsessive-compulsive disorder (OCD) is characterized by persistent, repetitive thoughts, ideas, or images that the patient finds irrational and intrusive (obsessions), with repetitive behaviors or rituals (compulsions) designed to decrease the anxiety caused by obsessions. Common obsessions include fears of contamination, dirt, germs, and illness; doubts (e.g., about having locked the door, turned off the oven, run over someone in one's car); needing to have things in order; and sexual or religious images or preoccupations. Compulsions include repetitive and excessive washing, cleaning, checking, putting things in order, or asking for reassurance. These obsessions and compulsions are distressing, time-consuming, or interfere with functioning. The full diagnostic criteria are shown in Box 9.6. Although most

**Box 9.6 Diagnostic Criteria for Obsessive Compulsive Disorder**

A. Presence of obsessions, compulsions, or both:

Obsessions are defined by (1) or (2):

(1) Recurrent and persistent thoughts, urges, or images that are experienced, at some time during the disturbance, as intrusive and unwanted, and that in most individuals cause marked anxiety or distress.

(2) The individual attempts to ignore or suppress such thoughts, urges, or images, or to neutralize them with some other thought or action (i.e., by performing a compulsion).

Compulsions are defined by (1) and (2):

(1) Repetitive behaviors (e.g., hand washing, ordering, checking) or mental acts (e.g., praying, counting, repeating words silently) that the individual feels driven to perform in response to an obsession or according to rules that must be applied rigidly.

(2) The behaviors or mental acts are aimed at preventing or reducing anxiety or distress, or preventing some dreaded event or situation; however, these behaviors or mental acts are not connected in a realistic way with what they are designed to neutralize or prevent, or are clearly excessive.

Note: Young children may not be able to articulate the aims of these behaviors or mental acts.

B. The obsessions or compulsions are time-consuming (e.g., take more than 1 hour per day), or cause clinically significant distress or impairment in social, occupational, or other important areas of functioning.

C. The obsessive-compulsive symptoms are not attributable to the physiological effects of a substance (e.g., a drug of abuse, a medication) or another medical condition.

D. The disturbance is not better explained by the symptoms of another mental disorder (e.g., excessive worries, as in generalized anxiety disorder; preoccupation with appearance, as in body dysmorphic disorder; difficulty discarding or parting with possessions, as in hoarding disorder; hair pulling, as in trichotillomania [hair-pulling disorder]; skin picking, as in excoriation [skin-picking] disorder; stereotypies, as in stereotypic movement disorder; ritualized eating behavior, as in eating disorders; preoccupation with substances or gambling, as in substance-related and addictive disorders; preoccupation with having an illness, as in illness anxiety disorder; sexual urges or fantasies, as in paraphilic disorders; impulses, as in disruptive, impulse-control, and conduct disorders; guilty ruminations, as in major depressive disorder; thought insertion or delusional preoccupations, as in schizophrenia spectrum and other psychotic disorders; or repetitive patterns of behavior, as in autism spectrum disorder).

Specify if:

**With good or fair insight:** The individual recognizes that obsessive-compulsive disorder beliefs are definitely or probably not true or that they may or may not be true.

**With poor insight:** The individual thinks obsessive-compulsive disorder beliefs are probably true.

**With absent insight/delusional beliefs:** The individual is completely convinced that obsessive-compulsive disorder beliefs are true.

Specify if:

**Tic-related:** The individual has a current or past history of a tic disorder.

From American Psychiatric Association. *Diagnostic and Statistical Manual of Mental Disorders.* 5th ed, DSM-5. Washington, DC: American Psychiatric Association; 2013, p 237.

people with OCD realize that their obsessions and compulsions are irrational, some have poor or absent insight and think that their OCD-related beliefs may be true.

Obsessive-compulsive disorder has a lifetime prevalence of 2% to 3% and is more common in monozygotic than dizygotic twins and in first-degree relatives of affected individuals than in the general population. Rates are similar in men and women. However, males have an earlier peak age of onset than females (6 to 15 years old vs. 20 to 29 years old) and a higher comorbidity with Tourette's syndrome and tic disorders. In people with OCD, the incidence of Tourette's is 5% to 7% and of tics is 20% to 30%. Other conditions commonly associated with OCD, in both genders, include major depression, anxiety disorders, hypochondriacal concerns, and excessive use of alcohol and sedatives.

Treatment of OCD includes both medications and psychotherapy (Grant, 2014). The first-line treatment is serotonergic antidepressants, specifically SSRIs and clomipramine, which is a highly serotonergic tricyclic antidepressant. People with OCD may require higher doses of these medications than do depressed patients and take about 12 weeks for a full response. Response rates tend to be lower than in anxiety disorders and are generally 40% to 60%. It is uncommon for a patient with OCD to have complete resolution of symptoms, and this is usually a chronic, relapsing, and remitting disorder requiring ongoing treatment. The specific psychotherapy treatment most helpful in OCD is exposure and response prevention. This treatment involves gradually increasing exposure to the feared situation, without performing the compulsive ritual (e.g., exposure to dirt without the ability to wash one's hands). Patients who agree to this treatment must tolerate significant anxiety, which, however, subsides with time after each exposure and diminishes over the course of treatment.

Posttraumatic stress disorder (PTSD) refers to a characteristic set of responses to a traumatic situation that involves exposure to actual threatened death, serious injury, or sexual violence, either to oneself or experienced by witnessing the trauma occurring to others, learning that the trauma has happened to a close friend or family member, or working in a setting with repeated or extreme trauma exposure. The characteristic responses include symptoms of reexperiencing the event, avoidance of stimuli associated with the event, negative thoughts and mood associated with the trauma, and increased arousal. The full diagnostic criteria and lists of symptoms are given in Box 9.7. It is common for people to experience symptoms like this in the first month following a major trauma, in which case the diagnosis is acute stress disorder. After a month, when most people would have recovered, persistent symptoms are then diagnosed as PTSD.

PTSD has an estimated lifetime prevalence of 8% in adults in the United States. Rates of PTSD vary from one third to over half of people exposed to specific traumas, such as combat, rape, or captivity. Risk factors for development of PTSD in people exposed to a specific trauma include female sex, younger age, severity and duration of the event, lack of social support, history of prior trauma, or history of preexisting psychiatric disorders. There is also evidence that people with greater autonomic arousal (higher heart rate and blood pressure) following the trauma are at increased risk. Although PTSD would appear to be a quintessentially environmentally determined disorder, the risk of development of PTSD following trauma appears to be heritable. PTSD is associated with depression, panic attacks and anxiety, substance abuse and dependence, suicidal thoughts and attempts, and, in severe cases, psychotic symptoms such as hallucinations or paranoia.

Several types of individual and group psychotherapy are effective in the treatment of PTSD. These therapies include coping with current life problems and triggers, gradual exposure and reexperiencing of the trauma with desensitization, and examining any distorted thoughts about the trauma, such as guilt that the woman brought this upon herself or could have done more to prevent or stop it. It is important to recognize that many people are retraumatized and their symptoms worsened by retelling the story of the trauma, especially if this is not in the context of a structured, ongoing psychotherapeutic treatment.

Medications are frequently used to address symptoms of PTSD. For example, SSRIs are effective in reducing depression, anxiety, and emotional numbing. Medications such as valproate may help with impulsivity and anger. Hypnotics may be helpful for insomnia. Prazosin, an alpha-adrenergic antagonist, has been shown to be helpful in reducing trauma-related nightmares and more general PTSD symptoms. Benzodiazepines should be used with caution, given the comorbidity with substance use disorders and reports of increased impulsivity in patients with PTSD given these medications. Acute management immediately following a rape is discussed further later in the chapter.

## PSYCHOTROPIC MEDICATIONS AND ORAL CONTRACEPTIVES

The gynecologist frequently sees women who are taking psychotropic medications for one of the disorders described earlier or for other less common psychiatric disorders such as bipolar disorder or schizophrenia and may be called upon to advise them about options for birth control. There are several psychotropic medications that alter the metabolism and efficacy of oral contraceptives (OCs) or whose metabolism is in turn altered by OCs (Oesterheld, 2008).

Induction of the hepatic cytochrome P450 3A4 enzyme can increase OC metabolism and cause contraceptive failure. Psychotropic medications that induce 3A4 and that have been associated with spotting, breakthrough bleeding, or unwanted pregnancy include the mood stabilizers carbamazepine (Tegretol) and oxcarbazepine (Trileptal), topiramate (Topamax; at doses above 200 mg daily), and the wakefulness-enhancing agent modafinil (Provigil). St. John's wort, commonly used over the counter as an antidepressant, also induces 3A4 and can cause contraceptive failure. OC activity may be increased or prolonged by 3A4 inhibitors such as the antidepressants fluoxetine (Prozac) and possibly fluvoxamine (Luvox).

Oral contraceptives are themselves moderate 1A2 and 2C19 inhibitors and mild 2B6 and 3A4 inhibitors. Thus OCs can increase levels and effects of amitriptyline (Elavil), bupropion (Wellbutrin), chlordiazepoxide (Librium), chlorpromazine (Thorazine), clozapine (Clozaril), diazepam (Valium), imipramine (Tofranil), and possibly olanzapine (Zyprexa). Drugs whose clearance is increased with OCs and therefore have lower blood levels include nicotine and the mood stabilizers lamotrigine (Lamictal) and valproic acid (Depakote). Lamotrigine levels have been found to be 84% higher in the week off ethinyl

**Box 9.7 Diagnostic Criteria for Posttraumatic Stress Disorder (PTSD)**

**Note:** The following criteria apply to adults, adolescents, and children older than 6 years.

A. Exposure to actual or threatened death, serious injury, or sexual violence in one (or more) of the following ways:
  1. Directly experiencing the traumatic event(s)
  2. Witnessing, in person, the event(s) as it occurred to others
  3. Learning that the traumatic event(s) occurred to a close family member or close friend. In cases of actual or threatened death of a family member or friend, the event(s) must have been violent or accidental
  4. Experiencing repeated or extreme exposure to aversive details of the traumatic event(s) (e.g., first responders collecting human remains; police officers repeatedly exposed to details of child abuse).

  **Note:** Criterion A4 does not apply to exposure through electronic media, television, movies, or pictures, unless this exposure is work related.

B. Presence of one (or more) of the following intrusion symptoms associated with the traumatic event(s), beginning after the traumatic event(s) occurred:
  1. Recurrent, involuntary, and intrusive distressing memories of the traumatic event(s).

     **Note:** In children older than 6 years, repetitive play may occur in which themes or aspects of the traumatic event(s) are expressed.
  2. Recurrent distressing dreams in which the content and/or effect of the dream are related to the traumatic event(s).

     **Note:** In children, there may be frightening dreams without recognizable content.
  3. Dissociative reactions (e.g., flashbacks) in which the individual feels or acts as if the traumatic event(s) were recurring. (Such reactions may occur on a continuum, with the most extreme expression being a complete loss of awareness of present surroundings.)

     **Note:** In children, trauma-specific reenactment may occur in play.
  4. Intense or prolonged psychological distress at exposure to internal or external cues that symbolize or resemble an aspect of the traumatic event(s).
  5. Marked physiologic reactions to internal or external cues that symbolize or resemble an aspect of the traumatic event(s).

C. Persistent avoidance of stimuli associated with the traumatic event(s), beginning after the traumatic event(s) occurred, as evidenced by one or both of the following:
  1. Avoidance of or efforts to avoid distressing memories, thoughts, or feelings about or closely associated with the traumatic event(s).
  2. Avoidance of or efforts to avoid external reminders (people, places, conversations, activities, objects, situations) that arouse distressing memories, thoughts, or feelings about or closely associated with the traumatic event(s).

D. Negative alterations in cognitions and mood associated with the traumatic event(s), beginning or worsening after the traumatic event(s) occurred, as evidence by two (or more) of the following:
  1. Inability to remember an important aspect of the traumatic event(s) (typically due to dissociative amnesia and not to other factors such as head injury, alcohol, or drugs).
  2. Persistent and exaggerated negative beliefs or expectations about oneself, others, or the world (e.g., "I am bad," "No one can be trusted," "The world is completely dangerous," "My whole nervous system is permanently ruined").
  3. Persistent, distorted cognitions about the cause or consequences of the traumatic event(s) that lead the individual to blame himself/herself or others.
  4. Persistent negative emotional state (e.g., fear, horror, anger, guilt, or shame).
  5. Markedly diminished interest or participation in significant activities.
  6. Feelings of detachment or estrangement from others.
  7. Persistent inability to experience positive emotions (e.g., inability to experience happiness, satisfaction, or loving feelings).

E. Marked alterations in arousal and reactivity associated with the traumatic event(s), beginning or worsening after the traumatic event(s) occurred, as evidenced by two (or more) of the following:
  1. Irritable behavior and angry outbursts (with little or no provocation) typically expressed as verbal or physical aggression toward people or objects.
  2. Reckless or self-destructive behavior.
  3. Hypervigilance.
  4. Exaggerated startle response.
  5. Problems with concentration.
  6. Sleep disturbance (e.g., difficulty falling or staying asleep or restless sleep).

F. Duration of the disturbance (Criteria B, C, D, and E) is more than 1 month.

G. The disturbance causes clinically significant distress or impairment in social, occupational, or other important areas of functioning.

H. The disturbance is not attributable to the physiological effects of a substance (e.g., medication, alcohol) or another medical condition.

*Specify* whether:

**With dissociative symptoms:** The individual's symptoms meet the criteria for post-traumatic stress disorder, and in addition, in response to the stressor, the individual experiences persistent or recurrent symptoms of either of the following:
  1. **Depersonalization:** Persistent or recurrent experiences of feeling detached from, and as if one were an outside observer of, one's mental processes or body (e.g., feeling as though one were in a dream; feeling a sense of unreality of self or body or of time moving slowly).
  2. **Derealization:** Persistent or recurrent experiences of unreality of surroundings (e.g., the world around the individual is experienced as unreal, dreamlike, distant, or distorted).

**Note:** To use this subtype, the dissociative symptoms must not be attributable to the physiological effects of a substance (e.g., blackouts, behavior during alcohol intoxication) or another medical condition (e.g., complex partial seizures).

From American Psychiatric Association. *Diagnostic and Statistical Manual of Mental Disorders.* 5th ed, DSM-5. Washington, DC: American Psychiatric Association; 2013, pp 271-272.

estradiol. Given the risk of Stevens-Johnson syndrome with fluctuating levels of lamotrigine and the likelihood of worsening mood symptoms with variations in blood levels of mood stabilizers such as lamotrigine and valproic acid, it is best to advise women taking these medications to use a continuous daily OC or another form of birth control.

## SUBSTANCE USE DISORDERS

Women have lower rates of alcohol and drug use and substance use disorders than men. However, substance use disorders are common in women and the rates are increasing. In the 2013 National Survey on Drug Use and Health, rates of illicit drug use in individuals

12 years and older were 11.5% in men and 7.3% in women. Among pregnant women ages 15 to 44, the rate was 5.4%, compared with 11.4% in nonpregnant women in the same age group. Rates of past-year alcohol use disorder were 8.7% in men and 4.6% in women. In contrast to a male: female ratio for alcohol use disorders of 5:1 in the 1980s, a 2010 survey by Greenfield and colleagues showed a ratio of about 3:1. Alcohol, tobacco, and other drug uses in women are of particular concern to gynecologists, not only because of the risks to the woman but also because of the risks to her children through teratogenic risks and effects on parenting abilities (Albright, 2009).

Women consistently have been noted to have an accelerated progression of substance use disorders, with a shorter time between first use of a substance to onset of dependence and then first treatment. This phenomenon is known as *telescoping* and is best established for alcohol, cannabis, and opiates. Women generally present for treatment with a more severe form of the disorder and more social, behavioral, and medical complications than men, despite a shorter period of heavy use. They are more likely than men to suffer psychosocial consequences, such as violence and victimization, and to have psychiatric comorbidity, especially depression, anxiety, eating disorders, and posttraumatic stress disorder. About 72% of women, as opposed to 57% of men, have coexisting psychiatric disorders, and in women these other disorders are more likely to have preceded, and to exacerbate, the substance use disorder. Thus it is important to recognize and treat other mental health problems in women with alcohol and drug abuse and dependence. Heavy drinking in women increases general health risks, as it does in men, but also is associated with amenorrhea, anovulation, luteal phase dysfunction, and early menopause. The DSM-5 criteria for alcohol use disorder are shown in Box 9.8, and DSM-5 includes similar criteria for other substances.

Patients frequently do not report excessive alcohol or drug use or may not recognize their use as excessive. As in primary care and mental health settings, patients seeing gynecologists are far less likely to be recognized as having a substance use disorder based on physician assessment and documentation. There are several screening tests that can help identify these disorders (Box 9.9; Bradley, 1998). The CAGE is a brief and widely used screening test. Although it is generally helpful in detecting heavy drinking, it is less sensitive in women and minorities. The T-ACE is a variation on the CAGE, which replaces the "guilt" about drinking item with a question about tolerance. The T-ACE was developed specifically for use in pregnant women, given the high rate of guilt in women who consume any alcohol during pregnancy, and is recommended by the American College of Obstetrics and Gynecology for screening (ACOG, 2011). Another effective screening test in detecting heavy alcohol use in groups of women of mixed ethnicity is the

**Box 9.8 Diagnostic Criteria for Alcohol Use Disorder**

A problematic pattern of alcohol use leading to clinically significant impairment or distress, as manifested by at least two of the following, occurring within a 12-month period:

1. Alcohol is often taken in larger amounts or over a longer period than was intended.
2. There is a persistent desire or unsuccessful efforts to cut down or control alcohol use.
3. A great deal of time is spent in activities necessary to obtain alcohol, use alcohol, or recover from its effects.
4. Craving, or a strong desire or urge to use alcohol.
5. Recurrent alcohol use resulting in a failure to fulfill major role obligations at work, school, or home.
6. Continued alcohol use despite having persistent or recurrent social or interpersonal problems caused or exacerbated by the effects of alcohol.
7. Important social, occupational, or recreational activities are given up or reduced because of alcohol use.
8. Recurrent alcohol use in situations in which it is physically hazardous.
9. Alcohol use is continued despite knowledge of having a persistent or recurrent physical or psychological problem that is likely to have been caused or exacerbated by alcohol.
10. Tolerance, as defined by either of the following:
    a) A need for markedly increased amounts of alcohol to achieve intoxication or the desired effect
    b) A markedly diminished effect with continued use of the same amount of alcohol.
11. Withdrawal, as manifested by either of the following:
    a) The characteristic withdrawal syndrome for alcohol (refer to Criteria A and B of the criteria set for alcohol withdrawal, pp. 499-500).
    b) Alcohol (or a closely related substance, such as a benzodiazepine) is taken to relieve or avoid withdrawal symptoms.

Specify if:

**In early remission:** After full criteria for alcohol use disorder were previously met, none of the criteria for alcohol use disorder have been met for at least 3 months but for less than 12 months (with the exception that Criterion A4, "Craving, or a strong desire or urge to use alcohol," may be met).

**In sustained remission:** After full criteria for alcohol use disorder were previously met, none of the criteria for alcohol use disorder have been met at any time during a period of 12 months or longer (with the exception that Criterion A4, "Craving, or a strong desire or urge to use alcohol," may be met).

Specify if:

**In a controlled environment:** This additional specifier is used if the individual is in an environment where access to alcohol is restricted.

**Code based on current severity:** Note for the ICD-10-CM codes: If an alcohol intoxication, alcohol withdrawal, or another alcohol-induced mental disorder is also present, do not use the codes below for alcohol use disorder. Instead, the comorbid alcohol use disorder is indicated in the 4th character of the alcohol-induced disorder code (see the coding note for alcohol intoxication, alcohol withdrawal, or a specific alcohol-induced mental disorder). For example, if there is comorbid alcohol intoxication and alcohol use disorder, only the alcohol use disorder is mild, moderate, or severe: F10.129 for mild alcohol use disorder with alcohol intoxication or F10.229 for a moderate or severe alcohol use disorder with alcohol intoxication.

*Specify* current severity:

**305.00 (F10.10) Mild:** Presence of 2-3 symptoms.
**303.90 (F10.20) Moderate:** Presence of 4-5 symptoms.
**303.90 (F10.20) Severe:** Presence of 6 or more symptoms.

From American Psychiatric Association. *Diagnostic and Statistical Manual of Mental Disorders.* 5th ed, DSM-5. Washington, DC: American Psychiatric Association; 2013, pp 490-491.

TWEAK. The AUDIT is a longer, 10-item screening test that has been well validated and includes self-reports of quantity and frequency of drinking. Women who score at or above the cutoff score on any of these screening tests, or who endorse use of an illicit drug or tobacco, should be questioned further about the frequency, amount, and consequences of their use of alcohol and illicit drugs. Although women with severe alcohol use disorders may have abnormalities in laboratory tests such as hepatic enzymes (ALT, AST, GGT) or mean corpuscular volume (MCV), questionnaires provide a significantly more sensitive method of detecting problem drinking.

The gynecologist is frequently a woman's primary care provider and is in an ideal position to help the patient seek help for a substance use disorder. The patient may not realize that her use is problematic or dangerous. It can be useful to educate her about "safe" levels of alcohol use, for example. Consuming more than two drinks per day on average is considered heavy drinking for a woman and has been linked to increases in mortality, cirrhosis, and breast cancer. Women may benefit from education about adverse effects of alcohol, tobacco, and drugs to the fetus and newborn.

Once the patient has been educated, her motivation to engage in behavior change or specific substance abuse treatment can be enhanced using motivational interviewing, an efficient and highly effective brief counseling technique that aims to accomplish behavior change by helping people explore and resolve ambivalence. Advice alone is often not sufficient to bring about behavior change, and patients vary in their stage of "readiness to change" (Box 9.10). The goal of motivational interviewing is to move people through the stages of change listed in this box. Motivational interviewing was developed for substance use disorders but is also highly effective in promoting weight reduction, exercise, safe sex practices, and regular use of contraception.

Motivational interviewing emphasizes reflective listening, rather than advice giving. In the context of a trusting relationship, the physician expresses empathy and understanding of the patient's ambivalence and the obstacles to change, avoids arguments, points out discrepancies between the patient's behavior and her goals, helps problem solve ways to succeed in meeting goals, and supports the patient's own motivation and efforts to change. Training in motivational interviewing is readily available. Motivational

**Box 9.9 Substance Use Disorder Screening Tests**

**Audit**

The following questions pertain to your use of alcoholic beverages during the past year. A "drink" refers to a can or bottle of beer, a glass of wine, a wine cooler, or one cocktail or shot of hard liquor.

1. How often do you have a drink containing alcohol? (never, 0 points; monthly or less, 1 point; 2-4 times per month, 2 points; 2-3 times per week, 3 points; 4 or more times a week, 4 points)
2. How many drinks containing alcohol do you have on a typical day when you are drinking? (1-2 drinks, 0 points; 3-4 drinks, 1 point; 5-6 drinks, 2 points; 7-9 drinks, 3 points; 10 or more drinks, 4 points)
3. How often do you have 6 or more drinks on one occasion? (never, 0 points; less than once a month, 1 point; monthly, 2 points; weekly, 3 points; daily or almost daily, 4 points)
4. How often during the past year have you found that you were not able to stop drinking once you had started? (same scoring as question 3)
5. How often during the past year have you failed to do what was normally expected from you because of drinking? (same scoring as question 3)
6. How often during the past year have you needed a first drink in the morning to get yourself going after a heavy drinking session? (same scoring as question 3)
7. How often during the past year have you had a feeling of guilt or remorse after drinking? (same scoring as question 3)
8. How often during the past year have you been unable to remember what happened the night before because you were drinking? (same scoring as question 3)
9. Have you or someone else been injured as a result of your drinking? (no, 0 points; yes, but not in the past year, 2 points; yes, during the past year, 4 points)
10. Has a relative or friend, or a doctor, or other health care worker been concerned about your drinking or suggested you cut down? (same scoring as question 9)

Scoring: Add up points; score 0-40; score of 4 or above indicates possible alcohol abuse or dependence for women.

**CAGE**

C Have you ever felt you ought to cut down on your drinking?
A Have people annoyed you by criticizing your drinking?
G Have you felt bad or guilty about your drinking?
E Have you ever had a drink in the morning (eye opener) to steady your nerves or get rid of a hangover?

Scoring: 1 point for each "yes"; any yes response warrants further assessment.

**TWEAK**

T Tolerance: How many drinks can you hold (6 or more indicates tolerance) or how many drinks does it take before you begin to feel the first effects of the alcohol? (3 or more indicates tolerance)
W Worried: Have close friends or relatives worried or complained about your drinking in the past year?
E Eye opener: Do you sometimes take a drink in the morning when you first get up?
A Amnesia: Has a friend or family member ever told you about things you said or did while you were drinking that you could not remember?
K Kut down: Do you sometimes feel the need to cut down on your drinking?

Scoring: 2 points each for Tolerance or Worried; 1 point each for others; total Possible = 7 points; 2 points or more warrants further assessment in women.

**T-ACE**

T Tolerance: How many drinks does it take to make you feel high? (3 or more indicates tolerance)
A Annoyed question from CAGE
C Cut down question from CAGE
E Eye opener question from CAGE

Scoring: 2 points for tolerance, 1 point each for "yes" on other items; 1 or more points warrants further assessment in women.

Modified from Bradley KA, Boyd-Wickizer J, Powell SH, Burman ML. Alcohol screening questionnaires in women: a critical review. *JAMA.* 1998;280:166-171.

**Box 9.10 Stages of Readiness for Change**

- Precontemplation—The patient does not believe a problem exists. ("I won't get pregnant!")
- Contemplation—The patient recognizes a problem exists and is considering treatment or behavior change. ("Maybe I could get pregnant and there are things I could do to prevent this.")
- Action—The patient begins treatment or behavior change. ("I'll take that prescription for birth control pills.")
- Maintenance—The patient incorporates new behavior into daily life. ("I'm taking the pill every day.")
- Relapse—The patient returns to the undesired behavior. ("The pill makes me sick. I think I'll stop.")

From ACOG Committee Opinion. Motivational interviewing: a tool for behavior change. *Obstet Gynecol.* 2009;113:243-246.

interviewing has been shown to be a highly effective intervention, and practicing this technique adds an average of only 3 minutes to a clinic visit. Resources and videos are listed in the 2009 American College of Obstetricians and Gynecologists (ACOG) Committee Opinion regarding motivational interviewing.

Once a patient has expressed interest in cutting down use of drugs or alcohol, she may be able to do this on her own. If not, treatments include Alcoholics Anonymous, Women for Sobriety, Cocaine Anonymous, or Narcotics Anonymous; psychotherapy; or outpatient and inpatient substance abuse treatment centers. The Substance Abuse and Mental Health Services Administration (SAMHSA) provides a convenient list of drug and alcohol treatment programs by state and local area at http://www.samhsa.gov/find-help.

Specific substances of abuse are associated with particular gender differences in patterns of use and treatment success. Alcohol use in women is associated with the phenomenon of telescoping, or an accelerated course from onset of use to significant alcohol-related problems. Several biologic factors may contribute to this more rapid course, including the lower percentage of body water in women, lower levels of alcohol dehydrogenase in the gastric mucosa and thus decreased first pass metabolism, and slower rates of alcohol metabolism. Women also appear to have different motives for drinking, with a higher likelihood of drinking in response to stress, negative emotions, and underlying primary coexisting psychiatric disorders. Women are less likely to seek treatment, perhaps related to childcare responsibilities, financial resources, and greater stigma related to women's use of alcohol. Female patients may benefit from women-only treatment settings or groups addressing women's issues. Effective pharmacologic treatments for alcohol dependence in both genders include naltrexone, acamprosate, and topiramate (Jonas, 2014; Guglielmo, 2015). Alcohol use during pregnancy is associated with fetal alcohol syndrome and fetal alcohol effects, and most women avoid alcohol once they know that they are pregnant.

In 2013, 31.1% of men, 20.2% of women, and 15.4% of pregnant women in the United States reported using nicotine in the past month. Although rates are higher in men than in women, women are at increased risk for heart attacks, chronic obstructive pulmonary disease, and lung cancer secondary to nicotine (Benowitz, 2010). Nicotine also is associated with early menopause and with spontaneous abortion, low birth weight, and preterm birth with in utero exposure. Only 3% of smokers are able to quit in any given year, and women appear to have more difficulty quitting than men. Women have more success quitting in the follicular versus the luteal phase of their cycle, but they are more likely to relapse because of weight gain associated with smoking cessation and have a high rate of relapse (about 65%) even if they have quit during pregnancy. Specific smoking cessation treatments, such as the nicotine patch, bupropion, and varenicline, show equal efficacy in men and women in short-term treatment trials. Bupropion may be particularly useful in women who have comorbid depression.

Cannabis abuse is more common in men, but it has a more rapid progression in women. Cannabis is associated with impaired memory, attention, and motivation; increases risk for the onset of panic attacks; may increase vulnerability to depression and psychotic disorders; and has been associated with shorter gestation, decreased birth weight, and possible impairments in executive functioning with in utero exposure. Treatments such as cognitive behavioral therapy and therapeutic communities appear equally effective for both genders.

Women may be more vulnerable than men to the reinforcing effects of stimulants, especially during the follicular phase when estrogen levels are high. The diagnosis of attention deficit disorder is increasingly being made in women, with a corresponding increase in therapeutic use of stimulants. Illicit use of stimulants more than doubled in the general population in the decade between 1995 and 2005, and about 5% to 10% of college students are estimated to misuse stimulants. The literature regarding stimulant effects during pregnancy is conflicting, but growth restriction, decreased birth weight, decreased gestational age, and maternal hypertension have been reported.

Use of heroin and other intravenous drugs is less frequent in women than in men, and women are more likely to inject drugs if their partner uses IV drugs and introduces them to injection. In contrast, overuse of prescription narcotics is more common in women than in men. Use of opiates, including methadone, during pregnancy is associated with neonatal abstinence syndrome, respiratory depression, preterm delivery, premature rupture of membranes, fetal growth restriction, and meconium-stained amniotic fluid.

## "DIFFICULT" PATIENTS

In a study of more than 500 adult patients seen in a primary care clinic, Jackson and Kroenke (1999) found that physicians described more than 15% of their patients as "difficult." "Difficult" patients were more likely to have a depressive or anxiety disorder, poor level of functioning, unmet expectations, low levels of satisfaction, and higher use of health care services. It is always possible for a physician to have a personality clash with an individual patient, but "difficult" patients are a subset of patients who evoke negative feelings in many, if not most, physicians. These patients may be angry, argumentative, threatening, mistrustful, demanding, dissatisfied; may misuse habit-forming prescribed medications or appear "drug seeking"; may challenge the physician's approach and not comply with treatment recommendations; or may be difficult to engage in a productive treatment alliance. In a classic 1978 paper, Groves described "hateful patients" as people who "kindle aversion, fear, despair, or even downright malice in their doctors." Feeling frustration, anxiety, or dislike in seeing patients significantly reduces a physician's satisfaction with providing medical care.

"Difficult" patients have also been described as "heartsink" patients, referring to the feeling that the provider has on seeing the patient's name on his or her schedule (O'Dowd, 1988). This term emphasizes the physician's response to the patient, rather than attributing the difficulty of the interaction entirely to the patient. Indeed, there are physician characteristics that have been associated with describing patients as "difficult." A secondary analysis of the Physicians Worklife Survey divided 1391 family medicine, general internal medicine, and medical subspecialty physicians into quartiles based on the percentage of their patients they estimated as being "generally frustrating to deal with." Those in the top quartile, reporting the highest percentage of frustrating patients, were more likely to be younger (<40 years), to work more than 55 hours per week, to report higher stress, to practice in a medical subspecialty, and to have a higher number of patients with psychosocial problems or substance abuse (Krebs, 2006). Physicians have also related difficult patient encounters to patient factors but also to their own anxiety, perfectionism, need to be loved by patients, defensiveness, and being "overly nice" (Steinmetz, 2001), and physicians with high scores on psychosocial orientation to care find fewer patients to be "difficult."

A woman may not comply with treatment because of denial and fear of illness; cultural factors; having a different explanatory model of the symptoms, their cause, and their optimal treatment; or a misunderstanding of the diagnosis, treatment, or the physician's instructions and expectations. In these cases, education, reassurance where appropriate, use of a skilled interpreter, or gaining a better understanding of the woman's culture and view of her symptoms and illness may be very helpful. In some cases, a formal cultural consultation may be needed. Although such situations may be challenging, their health care providers do not generally experience these women as being "difficult" or "hateful."

Groves grouped "hateful patients" into four different categories—"dependent clingers," "entitled demanders," "manipulative help-rejecters," and "self-destructive deniers"—and described their behavior patterns and ways in which the physician can intervene to work with them more effectively. In a more recent paper, Strous and associates (2006) revisited Groves' original categories and suggested an overall framework for approaching these people based on empathy and an understanding of the physician's own responses. Empathy refers to understanding another person's feelings, motives, and point of view. It is not synonymous with sympathy, because empathy does not involve pity. Understanding what a woman is experiencing and where the woman is coming from allows the physician to more calmly take a nonblaming, problem-solving approach. In addition, the physician can use his or her own responses to understand the woman better. For example, a woman who is feeling helpless and angry may, by complaining or demanding, evoke similar responses of helplessness or anger in her health care provider, allowing the provider insight into the woman's state of mind.

Groves' first group of "hateful patients," which he called "dependent clingers," appears insatiable in their escalating demands for medical care and to represent a "bottomless pit." They require constant reassurance and inordinate amounts of time and attention, interfering with the rest of the physician's personal as well as professional life. These women may frequently and intrusively page, e-mail, call the physician at home or on the physician's cell phone, feeling unable to cope on their own. The physician cannot possibly fulfill all of the woman's demands, feels overwhelmed and angry, and tries to withdraw from caring for her. Groves suggested intervening as the woman's demands escalate and setting firm but reasonable limits (e.g., not giving out personal contact information, limiting visits or calls). The physician can empathically understand that the woman feels overwhelmed and unable to cope, but in order to preserve an effective treatment relationship the physician needs to be clear about what he or she realistically can and cannot do for the woman.

The second group, which Groves called "entitled demanders," is similarly dependent and needy but displays a sense of entitlement, aggressively makes demands of the physician (e.g., for controlled substances, expensive diagnostic tests), and may make implicit or explicit threats, such as threats of litigation. This often leads the physician to feel angry and resist complying with the demands, even if some are reasonable. Groves has recommended validating the woman's entitlement to good medical care but focusing on a shared therapeutic goal and the woman's role in working with the treatment team to accomplish that goal. Empathically recognizing the woman's fear of loss of control may allow the physician to respectfully point out destructive patterns of behavior and attempt to establish a more collaborative decision-making process.

"Manipulative help-rejecters" seek care but do not improve despite extensive workups and multiple attempts at treatment. Groves has suggested that these patients are afraid of losing the relationship with the physician if they improve. He recommended setting up a schedule of regular appointments that do not depend on having acute symptoms, much as one would do with a patient with chronic somatization and multiple physical symptoms of unclear etiology.

Finally, "self-destructive deniers" persist in self-destructive behavior such as drinking, smoking, risky sexual behavior, and use of drugs, despite obvious and significant medical problems that have resulted from this behavior. Groves conceptualized these people as having a form of chronic suicidal behavior and recommended ruling out depression, if needed with the help of a psychiatric consultation. In general, in cases in which the physician feels angry or overwhelmed and does not wish to treat the woman, consultation with colleagues, consultation with a psychiatrist, and having the woman see a psychiatrist, if she is willing to do so, can be very helpful in better understanding and managing the woman and the physician-patient relationship.

Women with the diagnosis of borderline personality disorder are often challenging for physicians to treat, given their chronic suicidal thoughts, self-harm behavior such as suicide attempts and cutting, intense and rapidly changing emotions, anger, and difficulty regulating and controlling their emotions rather than acting on them. Women with borderline personality disorder may also see one or more members of the treatment team as wonderful and other members of the team as being punitive or bad. This can lead to "splitting" within the treatment team, with team members having quite different views of and responses to the woman and resulting disagreements within the team about how to best manage the woman's care. It is important in these cases for the members of the team to have a unified approach, focusing on the best care of the woman and avoiding being overly punitive or gratifying. Psychiatric consultation can be very helpful, and there are well-validated, effective psychotherapies for people with this condition (for a review of borderline personality disorder, see Leichsenring, 2011).

Women who seek and misuse habit-forming prescription medications are another class of "difficult" patients and may evoke feelings of anger, helplessness, and confusion in providers. Such women may be quite skilled in presenting plausible reasons for their needing the medication, or they may present as "entitled demanders" and make actual or veiled threats. It is important to have clear limits regarding the circumstances under which the physician will or will not be willing to continue prescribing the medication and to convey these to the woman empathically and with the woman's best interests in mind. It may be necessary to establish a formal treatment agreement with her, spelling out how the medication will be prescribed, in what amounts, and what will happen in the case of lost prescriptions or early refill requests. In an institutional setting, such as a hospital or clinic with multiple providers, it is important to include this treatment agreement in the medical record and make sure that it is consistent with institutional policies and values. Psychiatric consultation and addressing substance abuse or dependence issues directly may be necessary.

An understanding of attachment styles can be useful in interacting with "difficult patients" as well as less extreme problems in delivering the best possible medical care. Attachment theory was first elaborated by John Bowlby, a British psychiatrist, in the 1950s, and it posits that early interactions with caregivers in the first years of life influence an individual's later interpersonal relationships. These relationships include those with health care providers. When people become ill, often they "regress," become more vulnerable and childlike, and are less able to use more effective coping strategies. The position of being ill, with associated worries about loss of control, loss of health, needing to depend on others, and uncertainty about the future, amplifies any maladaptive patterns of attachment and interpersonal interactions stemming from relationships with early caregivers.

Thompson and Ciechanowski (2003) described the application of attachment theory to primary care settings. Most people have secure attachment styles and assume both that they themselves are deserving of care and that others can be trusted. There are three insecure attachment styles that affect relationships with medical providers and the quality of medical care: dismissing, preoccupied, and fearful attachment styles.

People with a dismissing attachment style have not been able to rely on early caregivers, have had to fend for themselves, and are compulsively self-reliant. They deny their own needs, tend to minimize symptoms or disability, have difficulty seeking and complying with medical care, and avoid seeking help or support. Women with this attachment style are hard to engage in regular care, especially for chronic illnesses, and may have worse health outcomes. Patients with diabetes with a dismissing attachment style have been shown to have significantly lower levels of exercise, foot care, and adherence to oral hypoglycemic medications (Ciechanowski, 2002a). Such patients may either fall through the cracks in a busy practice or be frustrating for the physician who tries to engage them in more active treatment. Engaging such women requires respecting their need for autonomy and respect, being flexible about appointment frequency and duration, giving them control over their care where possible, and using tracking systems and appointment reminders to make sure that they are being followed appropriately.

A preoccupied attachment style is characterized by compulsive care seeking. These people have received inconsistent responses to their needs in the past and feel they must exaggerate their symptoms and distress to evoke consistent care and support. In a study of 701 female primary care patients (Ciechanowski, 2002b), those with a preoccupied attachment style reported more physical symptoms, despite comparable medical morbidity, and had the highest health care costs and utilization. Such women respond best to brief, frequent, regularly scheduled appointments and to a physician who is responsive, but calm, consistent, and unflappable.

The main feature of a fearful attachment style is mistrust of oneself and others, usually based on a history of mistreatment or abuse in the past. The woman seeks help, but she mistrusts and may reject it. She seems anxious, demanding, and highly distressed on the one hand, but she misses appointments and is nonadherent on the other. For example, in the study by Ciechanowski and coworkers (2002b) of 701 female primary care patients mentioned previously, women with a fearful attachment style reported considerable distress and symptoms but had the lowest health care costs and utilization. A major challenge in treating these women is to be patient, accept them as they are, and not withdraw from care. Thompson and Ciechanowski (2003) recommended providing care through a number of different clinic providers or a treatment team if possible, so that the woman can develop a relationship with the clinic rather than needing to trust a single person.

Understanding attachment styles and that women's interactions with the health care system reflect earlier formative relationships can be helpful in maintaining a nonpejorative stance toward the woman and in achieving the best health care outcome possible. In general, seeking an empathic understanding of the woman's point of view can allow the physician not to become caught up in the negative feelings these women can evoke. Understanding the woman's fears and wishes does not mean that the physician needs to or should do what the woman wishes. However, it may help the physician to be able to set reasonable limits and expectations and pursue an approach that is in the woman's ultimate best interests, without feeling cruel, withholding, or intimidated. All physicians find some of their patients to be "difficult." Each physician can also increase his or her ability to manage these situations and reduce personal feelings of frustration, anger, or guilt, through consultation with colleagues, participating in a Balint group to discuss the psychological aspects of patient care, collaborating with other team members in discussing and making a plan for dealing with a patient, or consulting with a mental health specialist for or about the patient.

## SEXUAL FUNCTION AND DYSFUNCTION

Sexual satisfaction is one of the more important human experiences, yet it has been estimated that as many as 51% of women experience some sexual dissatisfaction or dysfunction. But self-reported distress about a woman's sex life was much less common, estimated to be 11% (Mitchell, 2013). Although there is a strong physiologic basis for sexual function, it is impossible to separate sexual response from the many emotional, social, and other contributing factors that may influence a relationship. Cultural or religious beliefs have influence on sexual function and dysfunction. For example, many African and some Asian and Middle Eastern countries practice female circumcision to varying degrees. The more extreme genital cutting or the trauma from the experience can result in reduced sexual activity, pain, and lowered frequency of orgasm.

In 1966, Masters and Johnson published their now famous book *Human Sexual Response,* which was a discussion of observations made on the sexual cycles of 700 subjects. It is on this important work that our early understanding of the female sexual response was based. Masters and Johnson described four phases of the sexual response: excitement, plateau, orgasm, and resolution (Fig. 9.2).

The excitement phase may be initiated by a number of internal or external stimuli. Desire may be activated in the hypothalamus with dopaminergic activity. As shown in Box 9.11, physiologically this phase is associated with deep breathing, an increase in heart rate and blood pressure, a total body feeling of warmth associated often with erotic feelings, and an increase in sexual tension. There is generalized vasocongestion, which leads to breast engorgement and the development of a

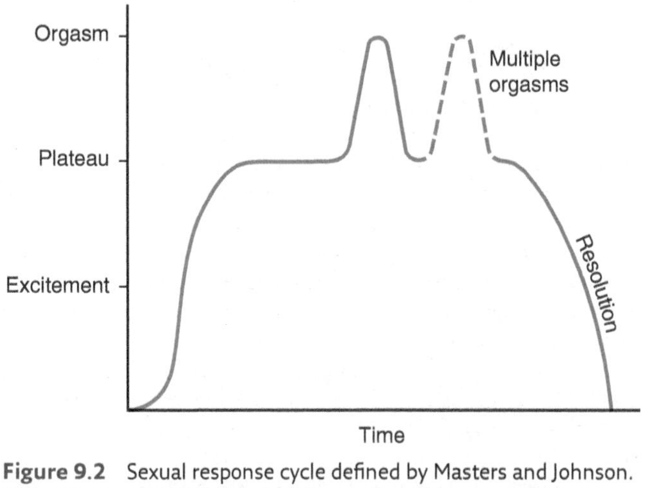


**Figure 9.2** Sexual response cycle defined by Masters and Johnson. (From Masters WH, Johnson VE. *Human Sexual Response.* Boston: Little, Brown; 1966.)

**Box 9.11 Characteristics of the Excitement Phase of the Sexual Response Cycle in the Female**

Deep breathing
Increased pulse
Increased blood pressure
Warmth and erotic feelings
Increased tension
Generalized vasocongestion
Skin flush
Breast engorgement
Nipple erection
Engorgement of labia and clitoris
Vaginal transudation
Uterine tenting

maculopapular erythematous rash on the breasts, the chest, and the epigastrium, which is called the sex flush. There is also engorgement of the labia majora (seen particularly in multiparous women) and of the labia minora. The clitoris generally swells and becomes erect because of increased genital blood flow and the neurotransmitter nitric oxide, causing it to be tightly applied to the clitoral hood. The dilation of the sinusoidal vascular spaces of the corporal tissue of the clitoris, vestibular bulbs, and spongiosal tissue lead to that engorgement. The vagina "sweats" a transudative lubricant, and the Bartholin glands may secrete small amounts of liquid. With the increasing deep breathing, the uterus may tent up into the pelvis, perhaps as a result of the Valsalva maneuver. There is also a myotonic effect, which is most notable in nipple erection. Much of the response in the excitement phase is caused by stimulation of the parasympathetic fibers of the autonomic nervous system. Dynamic genital magnetic resonance imaging (MRI) studies enable the visualization of the physiologic arousal response that provides the direct observation of the time course and magnitude of this response, along with the variability that appears to occur in women with sexual arousal disorder. In some cases, anticholinergic drugs may interfere with a full response in this stage. A diabetic woman with peripheral neuropathy may complain of poor arousal because of lack of sensation.

Next is the plateau stage, which is the culmination of the excitement phase and is associated with a marked degree of vasocongestion throughout the body. Breasts and their areolae are markedly engorged, as are the labia and the lower third of the vagina. The vasocongestion in the lower third of the vagina is such that it forms what has been called the *orgasmic platform,* causing a decrease in the diameter of the vagina by as much as 50% and thus allowing for greater friction against the penis. At this stage, the clitoris retracts tightly against the pubic symphysis, and the vagina lengthens, with dilation of the upper two thirds. Uteri in the normal anteflex position tend to tent up more. Retroverted uteri do not.

The next stage is orgasm, in which the sexual tension that has been built up in the entire body is released. Characteristics of orgasm are listed in Box 9.12. A myotonic response involves muscle systems of the entire body. There is contraction of the muscles surrounding the vagina, as well as the anal sphincter. The uterus may also contract. Muscle contraction occurs 2 to 4 seconds after the woman begins to experience the orgasm and repeats at 0.8-second intervals. The actual number and intensity of contractions vary from woman to woman. Some women observed to have orgasmic contractions are not aware that they are having an orgasm. Masters and Johnson feel that prolonged stimulation during the excitement phase, during masturbation, or in conjunction with the use of a vibrator may lead to more pronounced orgasmic activity. Whereas the excitement phase is under the influence of the parasympathetic portion of the autonomic nervous system, orgasm seems to be related to the sympathetic portion. The release of endogenous opioids, serotonin, prolactin, and oxytocin also has

**Box 9.12 Characteristics of Orgasm in the Female**

Release of tension
Generalized myotonic contractions
Contractions of perivaginal muscles and anal sphincter
Uterine contractions

been reported. Medication such as antihypertensive or antidepressant drugs, particularly SSRIs, may affect orgasmic response. A spinal cord injury may result in orgasmic disorder.

The resolution stage is last and represents a return of the woman's physiologic state to the preexcitement level. Although a refractory period is typical of the sexual response cycle in the male, no such refractory periods have been identified in women. Therefore new sexual excitement cycles may be stimulated at any time after orgasm. During the resolution phase, the woman generally experiences a feeling of personal satisfaction and well-being. Increased brain serotonergic activity has been recorded as well as decreased dopamine release.

Alternative models of the human sexual response have been proposed that differ from the linear progression of Masters and Johnson's (1966) model and also incorporate women's motivations and reasons for engaging in sex. Basson (2006) proposed that the phases overlap and may even occur in a different order. She proposed a more intimacy-based, circular model. Women in established relationships may engage in sex, not because of sexual desire but because of a desire for intimacy with their partner (Fig. 9.3).

## SEXUAL RESPONSE AND MENOPAUSE

Many factors contribute to sexual changes as a woman enters menopause. Aging in general is associated with the slowing of sexual response and decreases in the intensity of response. Specifically, arousal may be slower and orgasms may be less intense and less frequent. Aging may also lead to psychosocial changes affecting self-esteem in relation to desirability. Of course, hormonal changes are a factor. The postmenopausal woman who is not on hormone replacement therapy (HRT) may experience progressive atrophy of vaginal epithelium, a change in vaginal pH, a decrease in quantity of vaginal secretions, and a decrease in the general circulation to the vagina and uterus. Although estrogen clearly plays a role in maintaining the integrity of the vaginal mucosal epithelium and promotes lubrication, there is no direct link between estrogen levels and sexual desire or symptoms. If quality of life is poor from menopausal vasomotor symptoms and poor sleep, then estrogen can improve overall well-being without directly impacting sexual

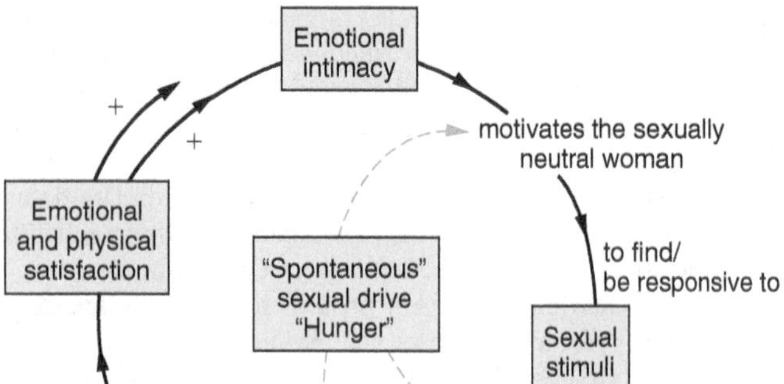

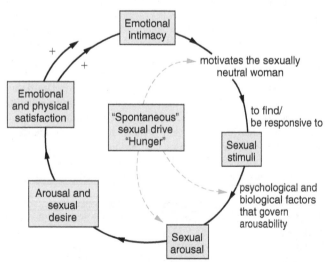


**Figure 9.3** Blended intimacy-based and sexual drive-based cycles. (From Basson R. Female sexual response: the role of drugs in the management of sexual dysfunction. *Obstet Gynecol.* 2001;98:350-353.)

desire complaints. Testosterone is the predominant androgen in women. Both the ovaries and adrenal gland produce androgens, even after the menopause and the ovarian production ceases with oophorectomy, which may lead to lower circulating levels of testosterone. Decreased testosterone levels are associated with decreased sexual desire, arousal, sensation, and orgasm, but levels of endogenous androgens do not predict sexual function.

A postmenopausal woman may experience other sexual problems relating to her partner, or if she is single, widowed, or divorced, to her lack of availability of male partners. In addition, her general health and the general health of her partner will play a role in her ability to respond sexually in a satisfactory manner. Pelvic organ prolapse and poor levator ani muscle function may contribute to poorer sexual function. Couples with marital or communication problems may find that menopause is an appropriate excuse to cease sexual activities. A concerned physician can help a couple sort out their needs and desire for sexual compatibility at this stage of life. Frequently, counseling aimed at dealing with problems of the relationship will alleviate sexual response difficulties.

Male partners of older women may suffer from medical conditions or be affected by medications, with a resultant decrease in arousal and difficulties in acquiring or maintaining an erection sufficient for intercourse. The physician should ask women about sexual function, and if male dysfunction is evident, they should make suggestions for appropriate referral to physicians or other health care workers who may deal with male sexual dysfunction.

## SEXUAL DYSFUNCTION

Female sexual dysfunction is quite common, particularly the loss of desire for sex. Higher percentages of dysfunction are seen in couples presenting for marital therapy and some women with loss of libido fear losing their partner. Both patient and physician wish for an easy solution, but the problem is often complex and not easily treated with drugs. Physicians caring for women should make a special effort to uncover sexual dysfunction or poor sexual response, as patients often do not bring up the problem unless asked. The Prevalence of Female Sexual Problems Associated with Distress and Determinants of Seeking Treatment (PRESIDE) study (Shifren, 2008) found low sexual desire accompanied by personal distress in 10% of women aged 30 to 39 years, 11% in women aged 40 to 49 years, 13% in women aged 50 to 59 years, and 10% in women aged 60 to 69 years. A 2009 report with the PRESIDE data of 31,581 respondents found the prevalence of a desire disorder was 10%, but reduced to 6.3% for those without concurrent depression. Overall, 40% of those respondents with sexual disorder of desire, arousal, or orgasm have concurrent depression.

Obviously, assembling a careful history by asking general and directed questions is appropriate when dealing with a patient in a gynecologic visit. The patient should be asked if she is sexually active; if she is active with men, women, or both; if intercourse is comfortable and enjoyable (if heterosexual); and if she experiences orgasm. Depending on the answer to these questions, more specific questioning should follow with the objective of outlining the extent of any problem and determining if there is distress related to the problem.

Sexual response problems may be the result of a previous negative sexual experience or may be secondary to emotional or physical illness. Primary medical conditions causing female sexual dysfunction can be hormonal, anatomic, vascular, or neurologic. The problem may also be related to difficulties in the current relationship or to alcohol or drug abuse. Although an occasional alcohol drink may decrease inhibitions and improve sexual response, in general, alcohol is a depressant and decreases the woman's ability to become sexually aroused and to become vaginally lubricated. Drugs with antihypertensive and anticholinergic activity, as well as those active at the α- and β-adrenergic receptors, may decrease arousal or inhibit sexual interest. Narcotics, sedatives, and antidepressant drugs, such as SSRIs, may also depress sexual responsiveness. Finally, decreased arousal or ability to remain aroused may be due to distractions in the woman's life such as concerns for children, job, or other problems that may enter her consciousness during arousal.

Hypoactive sexual desire disorder is the most common sexual dysfunction and is reported by 5% to 14% of women surveyed. This is defined as persistent or recurrent deficiency of sexual desire that causes distress. Because each individual has his or her own libidinal drive, it is not surprising that couples may have some incompatibility of needs. It is important, however, that these needs and desires be discussed openly and that reasons for lack of sexual desire that may involve experiences or problems inherent in the relationship be resolved. At times the problem may be merely a failure to set aside appropriate time and effort for intimacy. The couple should be encouraged to give sexual activity a high priority within their relationship rather than leaving it last on the list of priorities. Couples should be encouraged to use arousal and seduction techniques that are appropriate for their relationship. Satisfactory foreplay of a mutually enjoyable nature should be encouraged. Sexual arousal disorder is characterized by a persistent inability to sense genital arousal. There may be difficulty attaining adequate lubrication and swelling response of sexual excitement. The prevalence of this disorder is uncertain but possibly 5% and often coexists with decreased sexual desire, chronic medical conditions, or vaginal atrophy.

Hormonal levels are frequently obtained in evaluating desire disorders. However, there is no evidence that low testosterone levels distinguish women with sexual desire disorder from others. A report on 1021 women who had androgen levels drawn from a random recruitment in Australia found neither total nor free testosterone nor dehydroepiandrosterone sulfate (DHEAS) levels discriminated between the women with and those without low sexual function. Testosterone testing in women is not recommended because the commonly available tests are not sensitive enough to detect the low concentrations in women, and the normal range in women has not been established.

There is one FDA-approved medication for hypoactive sexual desire disorder called *flibanserin.* It is approved for premenopausal women, and daily use increased satisfying sexual events by only 1 per month. Alcohol must not be consumed. Side effects include drowsiness, hypotension, and syncope. There are no other FDA-approved medications to treat desire disorders other than estrogen for vaginal atrophy. Estrogen may improve sexual desire if hypoestrogenism is causing an overall lack of well-being from nighttime hot flashes and poor sleep or genital discomfort from atrophy. The risks of estrogen are discussed elsewhere. Androgen therapy is not at present FDA approved in women, but randomized controlled trials have noted some benefits in postmenopausal women with hypoactive sexual desire disorders and arousal disorders. Levels of endogenous androgens therapy that increase serum concentrations to the upper limit of normal have consistently been shown to improve female sexual desire and sexual activity. The transdermal testosterone patch has been evaluated with the higher dose patch (300 μg) showing increases in desire over a 6-month study in selected populations of postmenopausal women. Improvements are modest. The group that has the most response to testosterone is women who have had surgical menopause. The FDA has not approved the patch, as long-term safety and efficacy data are not available and there are particular concerns about cardiovascular risk. Testosterone use remains controversial. Phosphodiesterase inhibitors have not been found to be effective. Bupropion has shown some effectiveness, even in women without depression, but further studies are needed. Ospemifene is a selective estrogen receptor modulator that is approved for vulvovaginal atrophy and dyspareunia in postmenopausal women. This would be appropriate for women with hypoactive sexual desire disorder thought to be from pain from vaginal atrophy.

Because sex is a biopsychosocial experience, it is not surprising that no one treatment for low libido stands out. Studies narrowly focusing on orgasm, genital function, or frequency of intercourse without addressing satisfaction or quality of life may not get at the essence of the sexual experience. At present, a sound approach to female sexual dysfunction is complex and needs to assess sexual education knowledge, a women's relationship with her partner, all forms of abuse including emotional abuse or traumatic experiences, body image issues, religious or cultural ideals, depression, concerns about sexually transmitted diseases, pain, other medical problems, and everyday fatigues and stresses. Exercise to improve blood flow to the pelvis and decrease fatigue, changing SSRI medication for depression if negative sexual side effects occur, and psychotherapy/sex therapy can all be beneficial.

Sexual arousal disorders have received relatively little scientific inquiry. Masters and Johnson taught women sensate focus using masturbation training and working with the partners with apparently good results. Vaginal or systemic estrogen therapy improves arousal disorder by improving vaginal blood flow and lubrication in postmenopausal women. The FDA-approved EROS–CTD (Clitoral Therapy Device, UroMetrics, Inc., St. Paul, MN) is a cup that sits over the clitoris and a gentle vacuum is applied via a battery-powered device. The EROS-CTD has been reported to improve clitoral blood flow, engorgement, and genital sensation, which is effective in the ability to reach orgasm. Exercise may improve genital blood flow.

Sexual pain disorders include dyspareunia and vaginismus. Vaginismus is a condition in which the woman has difficulties allowing vaginal entry of a penis. It is thought to be secondary to involuntary contraction of vaginal introital and levator ani muscles. Because of this spasm, penetration is either painful or impossible. With time, there can be fear of pain and phobic avoidance. Lamont has attempted to classify the degrees of vaginismus and, in a group of 80 patients, noted that 27 (34%) had first-degree vaginismus, defined as perineal and levator spasm relieved by reassurance during pelvic examination. Another 21 (26%) had second-degree vaginismus, defined as perineal spasm maintained throughout the pelvic examination. Another 18 (22.5%) demonstrated third-degree vaginismus, defined as levator spasm and elevation of the buttocks. A total of 10 (12.5%) had fourth-degree vaginismus, defined as levator and perineal spasm with withdrawal and retreat. Four of the 80 patients refused pelvic examination. These patients frequently complain not only of pain or fear of pain with coitus or pelvic examination but also of difficulty in inserting a tampon or vaginal medication. The condition may be primary, in which case the individual has never experienced successful coitus. This problem is generally based on either early sexual abuse or aversion to sexuality in general. This leads to a form of conversion disorder or to a lack of appropriate learning about sex secondary to cultural or familial teaching that sex is evil, painful, or undesirable. Vaginismus may also occur in patients who have been sexually active when an injury or vaginal infection has led to vaginal pain with attempted coitus. This has been seen in rape victims and in women who have had painful episiotomy repairs, severe yeast vaginitis, or vulvodynia. When the underlying cause for the vaginismus is understood, the matter may be discussed frankly with the patient and her partner to effect a relearning process that is conducive to relieving the symptoms. Cognitive and behavioral therapy is encouraged, and then desensitization treatment can begin. Once desensitized to the fear and panic and by helping the woman feel in control, the actual vaginal spasm then may be relieved by teaching the patient muscle relaxation, then self-dilation techniques, using fingers or dilators, in which she and her partner can participate. This is often greatly facilitated by having the woman working with a skilled pelvic floor physical therapist. The period of therapy is usually short and the results good. There are little data from controlled trials, although one trial compared two desensitization techniques, which were both effective.

Dyspareunia is a sexual dysfunction in which genital pain occurs before, during, or after intercourse that frequently has an organic basis. The prevalence is estimated to be 8% to 22% of women. The physician should obtain a careful history of when the dyspareunia occurs (i.e., on insertion of the penis, at the midvagina during thrusting, with deep penetration of the vault, with orgasm or after intercourse), because facts obtained by this history may point to organic causes, such as poor lubrication and vaginal atrophy, a painful bladder disorder, vulvodynia, poorly healed vaginal lacerations or episiotomy, and diseases such as pelvic inflammatory disease, pelvic congestion syndrome, or endometriosis. Box 9.13 lists some causes of dyspareunia. Vulvodynia is chronic pain and burning in the vulva and affects 6 million women and the cause is largely unknown. When no organic cause can be found for the dyspareunia, techniques similar to those used in evaluating and managing vaginismus are appropriate. Pelvic floor physical therapy may be beneficial for vaginismus, vulvodynia, and dyspareunia as well as sex therapy. With all the sexual pain disorders, it is not uncommon to treat the underlying organic cause with success and find the pain continues. It is often muscle tension problems from the pain-tension-pain cycle that remain (Fig. 9.4). Specific pathologic conditions should, of course, be treated. At times, changing coital position can relieve dyspareunia. Couples should be encouraged to experiment with female-dominant and side-by-side positions to see if the pain can be prevented. An algorithm for thinking about sexual dysfunction is shown in Figure 9.5.

**Box 9.13 Causes of Dyspareunia**

- Vulvar pain caused by a specific disorder
  - Infectious
    - Vaginitis - yeast or other infectious agents
    - Desquamative inflammatory vaginitis
  - Inflammatory
    - Lichen planus
    - Lichen sclerosis
    - Dermatitis (contact or eczematous)
  - Neoplastic
  - Neurologic
    - Neuroma
    - Post herpetic
  - Trauma
    - Female genital cutting
  - Iatrogenic
    - Radiation for cancer of the vulvar, vagina or pelvis
  - Hormonal
- Vulvodynia
  - Localized
  - Provoked
- Urologic
  - Urinary tract infection (UTI)
  - Painful bladder syndrome/Interstitial cystitis
  - Urethral diverticulum
- Episiotomy
- Pelvic floor myalgia (hypertonus)
- Endometriosis
- Leiomyomata
- Pelvic inflammatory disease
- Adnexal pathology

Orgasmic dysfunction is less common at 3% to 6% of women and is often situational. It is defined as persistent or recurrent delay in or absence of orgasm. As many as 10% to 15% of women have never experienced an orgasm through any form of sexual stimulation, and another 25% to 35% will have difficulty reaching an orgasm on any particular occasion. Many women may be orgasmic secondary to masturbation or oral sex but may not be orgasmic with penile intercourse. It is important to discern by history the extent of the patient's problem and to place it into proper perspective. If the patient is anorgasmic during intercourse but has experienced orgasms, communication with her partner may aid in bringing about an orgasm during intercourse by allowing her or her partner to stimulate her clitoral area with the intensity and timing necessary to bring about an orgasm. If the woman is anorgasmic, she may be given permission to learn masturbatory techniques and sensate focus exercises to become comfortable with her own body until she has an orgasm. Then these techniques may be applied to the coital situation, thereby developing the desired response during coitus. Couples should be encouraged to communicate their sexual needs so that appropriate stimulation is offered during the arousal period and during intercourse. For situational orgasmic disorder, the focus of dialogue should be the relationship. Developing this type of dialogue is often difficult but can be aided by counseling with a sensitive physician or sex therapist.

Sexual response is a complex problem involving physiologic responses and psychosocial influences, which makes research

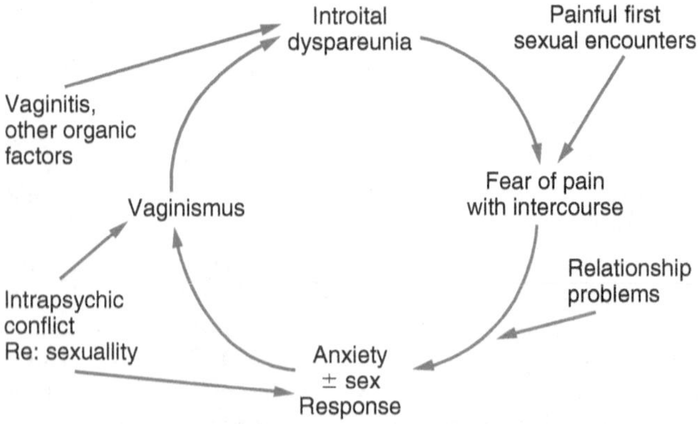


**Figure 9.4** Dyspareunia and vaginismus cycle. (From Steege JF. Dyspareunia and vaginismus. *Clin Obstet Gynecol.* 1984;27:750-759.)

studies hard to conduct. Although physicians and women may desire a pharmacologic solution, at present there is a paucity of good quality evidence. In fact, in the clinical trials of drug treatments for female sexual dysfunction, the placebo responses have been substantial. Whether attention to sexual function or changes in sexual behavior during a trial result in the marked placebo response, this definitely complicates the studies and needs to be considered in any treatment offered. Psychosexual counseling is often appropriate, as well as a comprehensive medical evaluation.

## LESBIAN, GAY, BISEXUAL, AND TRANSGENDER HEALTH CARE

Before 1990, there was little information in the literature regarding lesbian, gay, bisexual, and transgender (LGBT) health care or health issues. In 2014, the Association of American Colleges released a comprehensive curriculum to improve the health care of LGBT individuals so that medical schools can be guided in training physicians and faculty. Early uncontrolled studies were the first to suggest increased rates of depression, abuse, and substance abuse (Bradford, 1994). A systematic review and meta-analysis (King, 2008) found an increased rate of depression, anxiety disorders, and substance abuse and dependence in lesbian, gay, and bisexual individuals. The risk for suicide attempts in LGBT youth was four times as likely in comparison with heterosexual peers. Lesbian and bisexual women had a particularly high rate of alcohol and drug dependence and, again, this was more pronounced in adolescents. A number of studies have now documented that lesbian women use mental health services at high rates, with 70% to 80% having been in therapy, primarily for depression and relationship problems. The reasons for the higher rates of mental health and substance use disorders are unclear but may

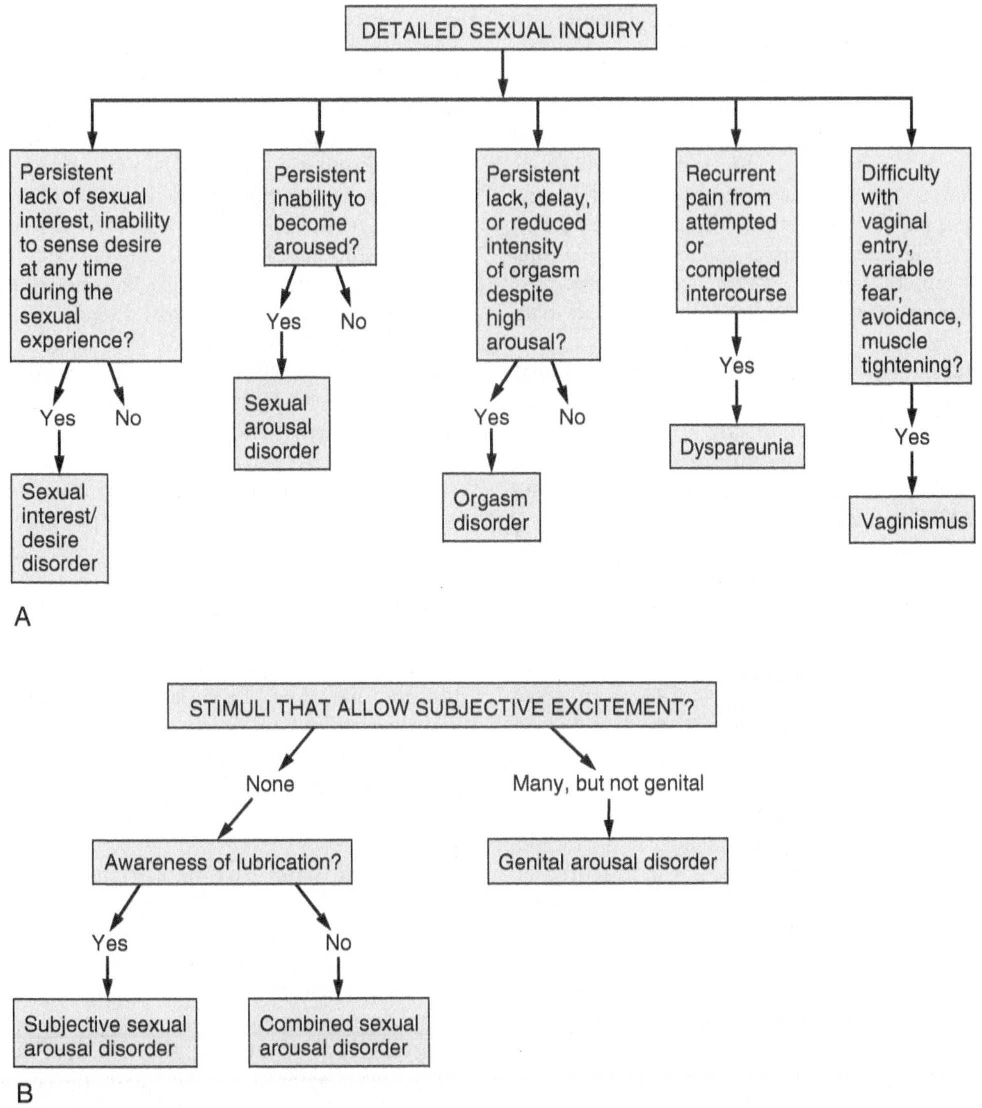


**Figure 9.5** **A,** Detailed sexual inquiry. **B,** Further assessment of arousal disorder. (From Basson R, Althof D, Davis S. Summary of the recommendations on sexual dysfunctions in women. *J Sex Med.* 2004;1:24-34.)

include a higher rate of childhood sexual abuse, being a member of a stigmatized minority group, and dealing with conflict and secrecy regarding sexual orientation.

Lesbians have a higher rate of cardiovascular risk factors, such as obesity and smoking. Smoking rates are especially high in lesbian adolescents. Lesbian and bisexual women are twice as likely to be obese as heterosexual women. That may be interrelated with studies showing LGBT youth are less likely to participate in moderate or rigorous sports activities. Since the 1990s, lesbian women have become increasingly willing to disclose their sexual orientation to health care providers and to seek routine physical examinations. Nonetheless, their rates of routine physicals and Pap smears are lower than national guidelines and lower than those of their heterosexual peers, and adolescents in particular have difficulty disclosing their sexual orientation to physicians. LGBT youth report that they think their health care provider should know their sexual orientation to provide the best possible care, but two thirds do not disclose this information. Lesbians prefer female and preferably lesbian health care providers and frequently use alternative health care providers such as nonphysicians, acupuncturists, and massage therapists. Lesbian women are 10 times less likely to be screened for cervical cancer than heterosexual women, even though their risk of developing the disease is comparable. This has been thought to be due to lack of concern and a belief that lesbian women were at low risk for cervical cancer. However, studies show human papillomavirus (HPV) screening and Pap smear frequency should be the same as the recommendations for heterosexual women. Sexually transmitted diseases also occur in lesbian women, particularly those who have had male partners.

Lesbians are increasingly having children through artificial insemination and adoption. Couples wishing to have children through donor insemination have concerns about coming out to their obstetrician, involving the nonpregnant partner, legal issues, family support, and parenting issues. Obstetrician-gynecologists need to be comfortable treating and advising LGBT women and couples, not just for pregnancy but also for general health issues, or should refer them to an appropriate provider.

## RAPE, SEXUAL ASSAULT, AND INTIMATE PARTNER VIOLENCE

### RAPE

Rape, or the sexual assault of children, women, and men, is a common act. Sexual assault encompasses many acts, including rape and unwanted genital touching. *Rape* is a legal term and refers to any penetration of a body orifice with threat of force or actual force and nonconsent. Sexual violence is defined as any sexual act performed by one person on another without that person's consent. Unfortunately, this is a common problem all over the world. A 2014 worldwide systematic review found 7.2% of women had ever experienced nonpartner sexual violence. The rates were 8% to 13% in North America with higher rates in sub-Saharan Africa and lower in Asia. Another study found 18% of women reported they had experienced attempted or completed rape. In separating out by female age groups, 11% of high school adolescents reported having been forced to have sex. The percentage increases the younger the adolescent is for involuntary first intercourse. Twenty to 25% of women in college have been victims of actual or attempted sexual assault during college. Among women 18 years of age or older, 31.5% who were raped sustained physical injury, and 36% of injured female victims received medical treatment. Of the rape victims who came to the emergency room, two thirds had general body trauma. This type of crime, however, is often underreported, and the actual incidence may be much higher. Victims are often reluctant to report sexual assault to the authorities because of embarrassment, fear of retribution, feelings of guilt, assumptions that little will be done, or simply lack of knowledge of their rights. Homeless women and women with mental illness are particularly vulnerable to sexual assaults compared with the general population.

In the past, society has held many misconceptions about the rape victim, particularly female victims. These included the notion that the individual encouraged the rape by specific behavior or dress and that no person who did not wish to be raped could be raped. Furthermore, the feeling that rape was an indication of basic promiscuity was widely held. To some extent, many of these societal misconceptions are held today.

Sexual assault happens to people of all ages and races in all socioeconomic groups. The very young, the mentally and physically handicapped, and the very old are particularly susceptible. Although men can be victims of sexual violence, most victims are female. Sexual violence can be unwanted touching and rape, but it also includes nonphysical distressing acts of sexual harassment, threats, peeping, and taking nude photos without consent. The Centers for Disease Control reported in 2006 that high school black (9.3%) and Hispanic (7.8%) students had higher rates of forced sexual intercourse than white students (6.9%). Although the perpetrator may be a stranger, he or she is often an individual well known to the victim. In fact, for first rape experience in women, 30.4% of the time the perpetrator was known to be an intimate partner, 23.7% a family member, and 20% of the time an acquaintance.

Some situations have been defined as variants of sexual assault. These include marital rape, which involves forced coitus or related acts without consent but within the marital relationship, and "date rape." In the latter situation the woman may voluntarily participate in sexual play, but coitus is performed, often forcibly, without her consent. Date rape is often not reported because the victim may believe she contributed by partially participating. This, however, can be a traumatic event and scar her self-esteem.

Almost all states have statutes that criminalize coitus with females under certain specified ages. Such an act is referred to as *statutory rape.* Consent is irrelevant because the female is defined by statute as being incapable of consenting.

During a rape, the victim loses control over his or her life for that period and frequently experiences anxiety and fear. When the attack is life threatening, shock with associated physical and psychological symptoms may occur. Burgess (1974) identified two phases of the rape-trauma syndrome. The immediate, or acute, phase lasts from hours to days and may be associated with a paralysis of the individual's usual coping mechanisms. Outwardly, the victim may demonstrate manifestations ranging from complete loss of emotional control to a well-controlled behavior pattern. The actual reaction may depend on a number of factors, including the relationship of the victim to the attacker, whether force was used, and the length of time the victim was held against his or her will. Generally, the victim appears disorganized and may complain of both physical and emotional symptoms. Physical complaints include specific injuries or general complaints of soreness, eating problems, headaches, and sleep disturbances. Behavior patterns may include fear, mood swings, irritability, guilt, anger, depression, and difficulties in concentrating. Frequently, the victim will complain of flashbacks of the attack. Medical care is often sought during the acute period, and at this point it is the physician's responsibility to assess the specific medical problems and also to offer a program of emotional support and reassurance.

The second phase of the rape-trauma syndrome involves long-term adjustment and is designated the reorganization phase. During this time, flashbacks and nightmares may continue, but phobias may also develop. These may be directed against members of the offending sex, the sex act itself, or nonrelated circumstances, such as a newly developed fear of crowds or heights. During this period the victim may institute a number of important lifestyle changes, including job, residence, friends, and significant others. If major complications such as the contraction of a sexually transmitted infections (STIs) or a pregnancy occur, resolution may be more difficult. The reorganization period may last from months to years and generally involves an attempt on the part of the victim to regain control over his or her life. During this time, medical care and counseling must be nonjudgmental, sensitive, and anticipatory. When the physician realizes that the patient is contemplating a major lifestyle change during this period, it is probably appropriate to point out to the patient why the change is being contemplated and the complicating effects it may have on the patient's overall well-being.

In some women, rape, like other trauma, can lead to ongoing, persistent posttraumatic stress disorder (PTSD, discussed earlier in this chapter), with disabling nightmares, flashbacks, hyperarousal, avoidance, depression, anxiety, and panic. Individuals with a prior history of trauma before the rape; greater severity, duration, and life-threatening nature of the assault; poor social support; and a past history of depression or anxiety are more susceptible to developing PTSD. Approximately 15% to 20% of women ages 18 to 50 have chronic pelvic pain of more than a year's duration. An estimated 40% to 50% of those women have a history of physical or sexual abuse.

### Physician's Responsibility in the Care of a Rape Victim

Although any individual may become a rape victim, this discussion will be limited to the care of a female, as is appropriate for a gynecology textbook. The physician's responsibility may be divided into three categories: medical, medicolegal, and supportive, as shown in Box 9.14.

### Medical

The physician's medical responsibilities are to treat injuries and to perform appropriate tests for, to prevent, and to treat infections and pregnancies. It is important to obtain informed consent before examining the patient and collecting specimens. In addition to addressing legal requirements, it helps the victim to regain control over her body and her life. After acute injuries have been determined and stabilized, a careful history and physical examination should be performed. It is important to have a chaperone present while taking the history, performing the examination, and collecting the specimen, to reassure the victim and to provide support. The presence of such a third party probably reduces feelings of vulnerability on the part of the victim. She should be asked to state in her own words what happened; if she knew the attacker, and if not, to describe the attacker; and to describe the specific act(s) performed. A history of previous gynecologic conditions, particularly infections and pregnancy, use of contraception, and the date of last menstrual period, should be recorded. It is necessary to determine whether the patient may have a preexisting pregnancy or be at risk for pregnancy. It is also important to ascertain whether she has had a preexisting pelvic infection.

Experience derived at the Sexual Assault Center in Seattle, Washington, demonstrated that between 12% and 40% of victims who are sexually assaulted have injuries. Most of these, however, are minor and require simple reparative therapy. Only about 1% require hospitalization and major operative repair. Lack of genital injury does not rule out assault. Nonetheless, the victim will perceive the experience as having been life threatening, as in many cases it may have been. Many injuries occur when the victim is restrained or physically coerced into the sexual act. Thus the physician should seek bruises, abrasions, or lacerations about the neck, back, buttocks, or extremities. Where a knife was used as a coercive tactic, small cuts may also be found. Erythema, lacerations, and edema of the vulva or rectum may occur because of manipulation of these areas with the hand or the penis. These are particularly common in children or virginal victims but may occur in any woman and should be looked for. Superficial or extensive lacerations of the hymen, posterior

**Box 9.14 Physician's Responsibilities in Caring for a Rape-Trauma Victim**

**Medical**
- Treat injuries
- Diagnose and treat STDs
- Prevent pregnancy

**Medicolegal**
- Document history carefully
- Examine patient thoroughly and specifically note injuries
- Collect articles of clothing
- Collect vaginal (rectal and pharyngeal) samples for sperm
- Comb pubic hair for hair samples
- Collect fingernail scrapings where appropriate
- Collect saliva for secretion substance
- Turn specimens over to forensic authorities and receive receipts for chart

**Emotional Support**
- Discuss degree of injury, probability of infection, and possibility of pregnancy
- Discuss the general course that can be predicted
- Consult with a rape-trauma counselor
- Arrange a follow-up visit for a medical and emotional evaluation in 1 to 4 weeks
- Reassure as much as possible

fourchette, or vagina may occur in virginal victims or in the elderly. Lacerations may also be noted in the area of the urethra, the rectum, and at times through the vaginal vault into the abdominal cavity. In addition, bite marks may be noted in any of these regions. Occasionally, foreign objects are inserted into the vagina, the urethra, or the rectum and may be found in situ.

Most victims are concerned about possible infections incurred as a result of the rape. To determine actual risk, it is important to know the prevalence of existing STIs in the victim population. One study (Jenny, 1990) examined 204 girls and women within 72 hours of a rape and discovered that 88 (43%) were harboring at least one STI. These included *Neisseria gonorrhoeae* in 13 of 204 (6% of all tested), cytomegalovirus in 13 of 170 (8%), *Chlamydia trachomatis* in 20 of 198 (10.1%), *Trichomonas vaginalis* in 30 of 204 (14.7%), herpes simplex virus in 4 of 170 (2.4%), *Treponema pallidum* in 2 of 199 (1%), human immunodeficiency virus (HIV)-1 in 1 of 123 (0.8%), and bacterial vaginosis in 70 of 204 (34.3%). In 109 patients (53%) who returned for follow-up (excluding those who were found to be infected on the first visit or who were treated prophylactically), there were 3 of 71 (4%) cases of gonorrhea, 1 of 65 (0.02%) of chlamydia, 10 of 81 (12%) of trichomoniasis, and 15 of 77 (19%) of bacterial vaginosis. These authors concluded that women who are raped have a higher than average prevalence of preexisting STIs but are also at a substantial risk of acquiring such diseases as a result of the assault.

A review on the risk of infection in rape victims found it was difficult to separate new from existing infection but placed the prevalence of STIs as follows: *N. gonorrhea* 0 to 26.3%, *C. trachomatis* 3.9% to 17%, *Treponema pallidum* 0 to 5.6%, *Trichomonas vaginalis* 0 to 19%, and HPV 0.6% to 2.3%. Few studies are available to predict the actual risk of acquiring an STI, but *Chlamydia trachomatis* may be the most commonly acquired infection incurred under these circumstances. Most victims fear acquiring HIV as a result of a sexual attack, but current risks are probably not high depending on the population involved and the sexual acts performed. Some studies place the risk for adult rape victims of acquiring syphilis as high as 3% to 10%. These authors did not believe the risk of acquiring STIs can be quantified, but they noted that the acquisition of viral sexually transmitted diseases (STDs), including HIV, has been reported both in adults and children. In consensual sex, the risk for HIV transmission from vaginal intercourse is 0.1% to 0.2% and for receptive anal intercourse it is 0.5% to 3%.

Commercial "evidence kits" are available. State crime lab testing may include urine or serum for "date rape" drugs when amnesia or sedation is present. A speculum exam is not always necessary, but if bleeding is reported or noted on external vulvar exam, it is appropriate. It must be remembered that infection may not be limited to the vagina but may also include the pharynx or the rectum. Specific history to raise a suspicion of this possibility should be sought. Urine or nonculture nuclear amplification tests (NAATs) for *Neisseria gonorrhoeae* and *Chlamydia trachomatis* are preferred according to the Centers for Disease Control 2015 guidelines. In addition, conventional cultures of the rectum and of the oral pharynx are indicated when the history suggests that this would be productive. A wet mount for *Trichomonas vaginalis* and bacterial vaginosis and a potassium hydroxide mount for *Candida albicans* are also useful (Box 9.15). Investigation for syphilis (rapid plasma regain [RPR]) is not routinely recommended at the Sexual Assault Center in Seattle, Washington, but may be done in follow-up.

**Box 9.15 Sexually Transmitted Diseases and Tests Available to Physicians Caring for a Rape-Trauma Victim**

**Should Perform**

NAATs for *Neisseria gonorrhoeae*
NAATs for *Chlamydia trachomatis*

**Could Perform**

Herpes simplex—culture lesion or serology
Hepatitis B—screening serology
HIV—serology
Cytomegalovirus—serology
Condyloma virus—study lesion
*Trichomonas*—saline wet mount preparation and culture or point-of-care testing
Bacterial vaginosis—pH, saline wet mount preparation
*Candida*—potassium hydroxide wet mount preparation
Syphilis—rapid plasma regain (RPR)

Data from Centers for Disease Control website, www.cdc.gov/std/treatment/2010/STD-Treatment-2010-RR5912.pdf; Harborview Sexual Assault Center.

Because the victim is also at risk for infection by the herpesvirus, hepatitis B virus, cytomegalovirus, HIV, condyloma acuminatum, and a variety of other STIs, the physician may wish to screen for those that seem appropriate at the time the victim is seen in the acute stage. Hepatitis B and HPV vaccination may be appropriate if the victim is not previously vaccinated and of appropriate age. Tetanus prophylaxis is appropriate in some cases as well. At follow-up visits the patient should again be investigated for signs and symptoms of the STIs, and appropriate repeat cultures, NAATs, and serologies should be obtained. Be aware that compliance with follow-up visits is poor. Prophylactic antibiotics are useful in acute rape management when the patient is concerned about contracting an STI or knows the assailant to be high risk. The CDC recommends the woman can be given a single dose of ceftriaxone 250 mg intramuscularly, for gonorrhea prophylaxis plus single dose azithromycin, 1 g PO for chlamydia prophylaxis plus metronidazole 2 grams orally in a single dose or tinidazole 2 grams PO in a single dose for trichomonas. If the patient is pregnant, consider giving no medications, and follow-up screening should be done in 2 weeks. If prophylaxis is desired, these antibiotics are class B drugs in pregnancy (except doxycycline which should not be given and is class D). This should prevent gonorrhea and *Chlamydia* infection but will have no effect on herpes, condylomata, or many of the other problems mentioned. Postexposure therapy with combination therapy is controversial for HIV prevention, as the benefit is unknown and extrapolated from needle-stick injuries in health care workers. It should be discussed with individuals initiating care less than 72 hours after assault and particularly if the victim has genital or rectal trauma. It is recommended if the assailant is known to be HIV or AIDS positive.

## Pregnancy

The patient's menstrual history, birth control regimen, and pregnancy status should be assessed. If the patient is at risk for pregnancy at the time of the assault, an appropriate emergency contraception or "morning after" prophylaxis can be offered as long as the pregnancy test was negative and if given within

120 hours after unprotected intercourse (1.5 mg levonorgestrel). This subject is discussed more fully in Chapter 13 . In the experience of most sexual assault centers, the chance of pregnancy occurring is quite low. Some have estimated that approximately 5% of victims having a single, unprotected coitus will become pregnant. However, if the patient has been exposed at midcycle, the risk will be higher.

### *Medicolegal*

To be meaningful, medicolegal material must be collected shortly after the assault takes place and definitely within 96 hours. The woman can be reassured that laws in all 50 states strictly limit use of past STIs or past sexual history during a trial so as not to discredit her testimony. Commercially manufactured "evidence kits" are available and may help with preserving the "chain of evidence" for a legal case. Victims should be encouraged to come immediately to a center where they can be evaluated before bathing, urinating, defecating, washing out their mouths, changing clothes, or cleaning their fingernails. The United States Department of Justice, Office of Victims of Crime, supports Sexual Assault Nurse Evaluation (SANE) programs, which have models for acute care for sexual assault. Some institutions have Sexual Assault Response Teams (SARTs), so experts are available to do the appropriate psychological, medical, and legal evaluation. You should know the resources available in your community.

In general, evidence for coitus will be present in the vagina for as long as 48 hours after the attack, but in other orifices the evidence may last only up to 6 hours. Appropriate tests should document the patient's physical and emotional condition as judged by her history and physical examination and should include data that document the use of force, evidence for sexual contact, and materials that may help identify the offender. To document that force was used, the physician should carefully describe each injury noted and illustrate with either drawings or photographs. Detail is important, because injuries suffered by sexual assault victims have common patterns. Because *rape* and *sexual assault* are legal terms, they should not be stated as diagnoses; rather the physician should report findings as "consistent with use of force." Documentation of sexual contact must begin with a history of when the patient had intercourse before the attack. If sperm or semen is found in the vagina or cervix of a victim, it must not be confused with such substances deposited during the victim's prior consenting sexual acts. Sexual contact will be verified by analysis of secretions from the vagina or rectum by identifying motile sperm. Nonmotile sperm may be present as well if the attack occurred 12 to 20 hours previously. In some instances, motile sperm will be noted for as long as 2 to 3 days in the endocervix. Vaginal wet mount is no longer recommended for identifying sperm as it lacks reproducibility. Manufactured evidence kits are available.

It is difficult to ascertain whether ejaculation occurred in the mouth, because residual seminal fluid is rapidly destroyed by bacteria and salivary enzymes, making documentation of such an event difficult after more than a few hours have passed. Seminal fluid may be found staining the skin or the clothing several hours after the attack, and this should be looked for. Because acid phosphatase is an enzyme found in high concentrations in seminal fluid, substances removed for analysis should be tested for this enzyme. Table 9.6 demonstrates the survival time of sperm in the pharynx, rectum, and cervix.

**Table 9.6** Survival Time of Sperm

| Source | Motile Sperm | Sperm | Acid Phosphatase |
|---|---|---|---|
| Vagina | Up to 8 hr | Up to 7 to 9 days | Variable (up to 48 hr) |
| Pharynx | 6 hr | Unknown | 100 IU* |
| Rectum | Undetermined | 20 to 24 hr | 100 IU* |
| Cervix | Up to 5 days | Up to 17 days | Similar to vagina |

From Anderson S. *Sexual assault—medical-legal aspects: an unpublished training packet for pediatric house staff.* Seattle, WA: Harborview Medical Center; 1980.
*Minimum detectable.

In addition to documenting that intercourse has taken place, an attempt should be made to identify the perpetrator. In this regard, all clothing intimately associated with the area of assault should be collected, labeled, and submitted to legal authorities. In addition, smears of vaginal secretions or a Pap smear should be made to permanently document the presence of sperm. Vaginal secretions needed for DNA typing should be collected by wet or dry swab and refrigerated until a pathologist can process them. In the near future tests may also be available to identify prostate-specific antigen and seminal vesicle–specific antigen in vaginal secretions. Highly sensitive DNA fingerprinting is now readily available and is admissible in many jurisdictions. Pubic hair combings should be performed in an attempt to obtain pubic hair of the assailant. Saliva should be collected from the victim to ascertain whether she secretes an antigen that could differentiate her from substances obtained from the perpetrator. Finally, fingernail scrapings should be obtained for skin or blood if the victim scratched the perpetrator. Specific blood or DNA typing may be conducted to help identify the attacker. All materials collected should be labeled and turned over to the legal authority or pathologist, depending on the system used by the medical unit. A receipt should be obtained, and this should be documented in the patient's chart.

### *Emotional Support of the Victim*

After the physical needs of the patient have been met and after the physician has carefully documented the information concerning the sexual contact, he or she should discuss with the victim the degree of injury, probability of infection or pregnancy, general course that the victim might be expected to follow with respect to these, and how follow-up to aid prevention will be carried out. The physician must allow the victim to vent anxieties and correct misconceptions. The physician should reassure her, insofar as possible, that her well-being will be restored. In doing this, the physician may call on other health personnel, such as individuals trained to help rape-trauma victims, to facilitate counseling and follow-up. The patient should not be released until specific follow-up plans are made and the patient understands what they are. A follow-up visit should be planned within 1 to 4 weeks to reevaluate the patient's medical, infectious disease, pregnancy, and psychological status. At this point, follow-up counseling should be encouraged. It is important at each visit to emphasize to the patient that she was a victim and holds no blame. At each step she must be allowed to vent her feelings and to discuss her current conceptions of the problem. It is important that the physician realize that some patients will appear to have excellent emotional control when seen immediately after a rape. This is an acute expression of the patient's defense mechanisms and should not be misinterpreted to indicate that the patient is coping with the circumstances. All the recommendations just listed should be followed *regardless* of the patient's apparent condition. Specific plans for follow-up are equally important in such an individual, because it must be anticipated that she will follow the same post-rape emotional process as anyone else. Finally, it is important to emphasize and reemphasize that at no time during the management or follow-up care of the rape victim should any comments be made by health care professionals suggesting that the patient was anything other than a victim. These women are sensitive to any accusations and insinuations and may even believe that they may have in some way been responsible for the rape. Their future well-being may be severely affected by creating such an impression.

### Female Circumcision

A form of sexual abuse only recently observed in the Western world is female circumcision or genital cutting. It is a practice growing out of cultural and traditional beliefs dating back several thousand years. The World Health Organization estimates that between 85 and 200 million women undergo these procedures each year. Although they are often performed in parts of Africa, the Middle East, and Southeast Asia, they are rarely performed in the United States or the rest of the Western world. About 168,000 women who have undergone such procedures currently live in the United States, and physicians may see the results of these procedures in patients who emigrate from countries where they are practiced.

The various forms of female genital mutilation include removal of the clitoral prepuce, excision of the clitoris, or removal of the clitoris and labia minora. Occasionally, the labia majora are also partially removed and the vagina partially sutured closed. The procedures are often performed between early childhood and age 14 and frequently without anesthesia under unsterile conditions by untrained practitioners. Therefore a variety of complications often occur, including infection, tetanus, shock, hemorrhage, and death. Long-term problems include chronic infection, scar formation, local abscesses, sterility, and incontinence. In addition, depression, anxiety, sexual dysfunction, dyspareunia, obstetric complications, and the psychosomatic conditions associated with sexual abuse may be seen. Physicians who care for women with this condition must develop an understanding of the cultural mores that lead to the performance of the procedure and the current implications on these cultural beliefs that remedial surgery may imply. Certainly the patient and her sexual partner should be involved in all decisions concerning intervention.

## ABUSE

### Intimate Partner Violence

*Domestic violence, partner abuse, intimate partner violence (IPV), the battered woman,* and *spouse abuse* are terms that refer to violence occurring between partners in an ongoing relationship even if they are not married. A battered woman is defined as any woman over the age of 16 with evidence of physical abuse on at least one occasion at the hands of an intimate male partner. The *battered wife syndrome* is defined as a symptom complex occurring as a result of violence in which a woman has at any time received deliberate, severe, or repeated (more than three times) physical abuse from her husband or significant male partner in which the minimal injury is bruising. *Intimate partner violence* (IPV) is the CDC's currently preferred term because it allows for males or females to be the victim and intimate partners can be the same or opposite sex. Actual or threatened physical, sexual, or psychological abuse by a current or former spouse (including common-law spouses), dating partner, boyfriend, or girlfriend is considered intimate partner violence. The American Medical Association has treatment guidelines and defines IPV as a "pattern of coercive behaviors that may include repeated battering and injury, psychological or emotional abuse, sexual assault, progressive societal isolation, economic deprivation, intimidation and stalking." The actual physical abuse may vary from minimal activity, such as verbal abuse or threat of violence, to throwing an object, throwing an object at someone, pushing, slapping, kicking, hitting, beating, threatening with a weapon, or using a weapon. These acts may be spontaneous or intentionally planned. Most such violence is accompanied by mental abuse and intimidation. Partner abuse is often seen in conjunction with abuse of children and elderly persons in the same household. A 2008 study by Breiding and colleagues investigated risk factors for IPV in noninstitutionalized adults and found the victims to be female, of ethnic/racial minority, to have a lower income, to be less educated, and to be older. There remain significant societal, cultural, and economic barriers for victims to seek help.

It is difficult to ascertain the specific incidence of domestic violence, but it has been estimated that 4.5 million cases of IPV occur in the United States each year, and some authors have stated that at least 50% of family relationships are violent. In a 1984 U.S. Department of Justice study, 57% of 450,000 annual acts of family violence were committed by spouses or ex-spouses, and the wife was a victim in 93% of cases. In at least one fourth of these cases the violent acts had occurred at least three times in the previous 6 months. In 1990, statistics gathered by the Federal Bureau of Investigation (FBI) reported similar findings. A 2008 phone survey of noninstitutionalized adults provided some of the best IPV prevalence data to date. Nineteen percent of women reported threatened physical violence over their lifetime, 14.5% reported attempted physical violence, and 20.2% completed physical violence. The frequency of unwanted sex for an intimate partner was 10.2%. Within the previous 12 months, 1.4% of women reported completed physical or sexual violence.

In addition, it has been estimated that between one third and one half of female homicide victims are murdered by their male partners, whereas only 12% of male homicide victims are killed by their female partners. In 1992, the American Medical Association (AMA) published guidelines for the diagnosis and treatment of domestic violence. The association noted that 47% of husbands who beat their wives do so three or more times per year, that 14% of ever-married women reported being raped by their current or former husbands, and that rape is a significant or major form of abuse in 54% of violent marriages. The AMA guidelines also summarized various studies noting that battered women may account for 22% to 35% of women seeking care for any reason in emergency departments (the majority of whom are seen by medical or nontrauma services) and 19% to 30% of injured women seen in emergency departments. This was confirmed in a 2005 study in which 17% of women seeking care in an emergency department reported current abuse. Nine percent to 14% of women seen in ambulatory care internal medicine clinics currently suffer IPV, and 26% to 28% of such women have been battered at some time. The study states that 25% of women who attempt suicide, 25% who are receiving psychiatric services, and 23% of pregnant women seeking prenatal care have been victims of domestic violence. In addition, 45% to 59% of mothers of abused children have been abused, and 58% of women older than 30 who have been raped have been abused. In a gynecologic clinic in England, John and colleagues surveyed a cohort of 825 women. Twenty-one percent reported physical abuse, and of those, 48% also had forced sexual activity. A 2005 report confirmed the prevalence rates in health care facilities with 35% of obstetrics and gynecology patients reporting IPV and 13% of women seeking care reporting current abuse. Therefore it can be seen that domestic violence and battered women are common in our society today.

The most common sites for injury are the head, neck, chest, abdomen, breast, and upper extremities. Minor injuries such as scratches, bruises, sore muscles, and welts are common. The upper extremities may be fractured as the woman attempts to defend herself. Broken teeth, burns, laceration, head injury, and strangulation are also frequently observed. In a study from Yale, 84% of the injuries were severe enough to require medical treatment, and in 81% of the cases patients stated that the assailant had beaten them with the fists. In an English study of 100 women brought to a hostel for battered women, 44% suffered from lacerations and 59% stated that they had been kicked repeatedly. All women stated that they had been hit with a clenched fist. Fractures occurred in 32, and 9 of the women had been beaten and taken to the hostel unconscious. A 2006 study also found significant injury among victims; of 519,031 cases, 41% of assaults caused observable injuries and 28% required medical treatment.

Murder and suicide are frequent components of the domestic violence problem. In a large study from Denver, Walker reported that three quarters of the battered patients felt that the batterer would kill them during the relationship, and almost half felt that they might kill the batterer. Of these victims, 11% stated that they had actually tried to kill the batterer, and 87% believed that they themselves would be the ones to die if someone were killed. This is not an exaggeration, as IPV resulted in 1544 deaths in 2004. One third of these women stated that they seriously considered committing suicide. Walker noted that victims and their attackers frequently are depressed and may move rapidly between suicidal and homicidal intent.

There is a strong relationship between spouse battering and child abuse. In Walker's study, 53% of men who abused their partners were noted also to abuse their children. Another one third had threatened to abuse their children. Interestingly, in the same relationship, 28% of the wives who themselves were abused stated that they had abused their children while living in the violent household, and an additional 6% thought that they might abuse their children at the time they were evaluated.

Physical abuse in pregnancy is common and may be referred to as *prenatal child abuse.* The incidence is somewhere between 1% and 20%, depending on the study population. In one study, 81 of 742 (10.9%) patients visiting a prenatal clinic stated that they had been victims of abuse at some time in the past, and 29 of these women stated that the abuse had continued into the pregnancy. Violence may increase postpartum. One fifth of these noted an increase in abuse during pregnancy, and one third noted a decrease. In a study of a group of Medicaid-eligible postpartum women, a constellation of factors associated with violence during pregnancy was noted. Of the patients in this study, 7% suffered battering, and significant correlates including anxiety, depression, housing problems, inadequate prenatal care, and drug and alcohol abuse were identified. The women in the study who were battered during pregnancy suffered a more severe constellation of symptoms than did those who were battered only prior to pregnancy. In the case of pregnant patients, most studies note that battering is frequently directed to the breasts and abdomen.

It is important that physicians increase their ability to recognize the signs of domestic violence and spouse abuse. A study by Hilberman and Monson (1977) demonstrated that 25% of women treated for injuries in an emergency room were victims of wife battering. The physicians who were treating these patients made the correct diagnosis originally in only 3% of cases. Viken has listed a profile of the characteristics of the abused wife. These include a history of having been beaten as a child, raised in a single parent home, married as a teenager, and pregnant before marriage. Such women frequently visit clinics and emergency rooms with a variety of somatic complaints, including headaches, insomnia, choking sensation, hyperventilation, gastrointestinal symptoms, and chest, pelvic, and back pain. Noncompliance with the advice of physicians with respect to these complaints is frequent (Box 9.16).

In visits to the physician's office or emergency room, the patient often appears shy, frightened, embarrassed, evasive, anxious, or passive and often cries. The batterer may accompany the patient on such visits and stay close at hand to monitor what she says to the physician. Thus the woman may be hesitant to provide information about how she was injured, and the explanation given may not fit the injuries observed. Alcohol or other drug abuse is common in such individuals.

**Box 9.16 Somatic Complaints in Abused Women**

Headaches
Insomnia
Choking sensation
Hyperventilation
Chest, back, or pelvic pain

**Other Signs and Symptoms**

Shyness
Fright
Embarrassment
Evasiveness
Jumpiness
Passivity
Frequent crying
Often accompanied by male partner
Drug or alcohol abuse (often overdose)
Injuries

From ACOG Technical Bulletin Number 124: *The Battered Woman.* January 1989.

Physicians should become comfortable with asking the patient whether she has been physically abused. Every pregnant woman should be screened for intimate partner violence. Introductory questions such as "Has anyone hurt you or tried to injure you?" "Has an intimate partner ever threatened you with physical violence?" and "Have you ever been physically abused either recently or in the past?" are appropriate. The physician should follow up on any positive answers in a nonjudgmental manner in an attempt to learn what is happening. Physical examinations should be complete with particular attention to bruises, lacerations, burns, improbable injury, and other signs of injury. If the patient is wearing sunglasses, she should be asked to remove them so that the physician can determine whether there are eye injuries. If the patient is pregnant, bruises seen on the breasts or abdomen should always be discussed. Physicians should carefully note evidence for abuse in the patient's record.

Battering acts tend to run in cycles consisting of three phases. The first phase is tension building, in which tension between the couple gradually escalates, manifested by discrete acts that cause family friction. Name-calling, intimidating remarks, meanness, and mild physical abuse such as pushing are common. The batterer often expresses dissatisfaction and hostility in a somewhat chronic form. The victim may attempt to placate the batterer in hopes of pleasing him or calming him. She may actually believe at this point that she has the power to avoid aggravating the situation. She may not respond to his hostile actions and may even be successful from time to time in apparently reducing tensions. This, of course, will reinforce her belief that she can control the situation. As the tension phase builds, the batterer's anger is less controlled, and the victim may withdraw, fearing that she will inadvertently set off explosive behavior. Often this withdrawal is the signal for the batterer to become more aggressive. Anything may spark the hostile act, and the acute battering then takes place. This is the cycle's second phase and is represented by an uncontrollable discharge of tension that has built up through the first phase. The attack may take the form of both verbal and physical abuse, and the victim is often left injured. In self-defense the victim may actually injure or kill the batterer. In approximately two thirds of cases reported by Walker, alcohol abuse was involved. However, the alcohol use may have been the excuse rather than the reason for the battering. After the abuse has taken place, the third phase generally follows. In this situation, the batterer apologizes, asks forgiveness, and frequently shows kindness and remorse, showering the victim with gifts and promises. This gives the victim hope that the relationship can be saved and that the violence will not recur. Batterers are often charming and manipulative, offering the victim justification for forgiveness. The cycles, however, do repeat themselves, with the first phase increasing in length and intensity, the battering becoming more severe, and the third phase tending to decrease in both duration and intensity. The batterer learns that he can control the victim without obtaining much forgiveness. The victim becomes more demoralized and loses her ability to leave the situation even if she has the means and opportunity to do so.

Batterers, too, tend to have a specific profile in most cases. They are men who refuse to take responsibility for their behavior, blaming their victims for their violent acts. They often have strong controlling personalities and do not tolerate autonomy in their partners. They have rigid expectations of marriage and sexual behavior and consider their wives or partners as chattel. They wish to be cared for in their most basic needs, frequently make unrealistic demands on their wives, and show low tolerance for stress. Depression and suicide attempts are often a part of their behavior pattern, but in general they are aggressive and assaultive in most of their behavior, generally using violence to solve their problems. On the other hand, they are often charming and manipulative, especially in their relationships outside the marriage. They often exhibit low self-esteem, feelings of inadequacy, and a sense of helplessness, all of which are generally made worse by the prospects of losing their wives. It is typical behavior for male batterers to exhibit contempt for women in their usual activities. Therapy is usually ineffective and seems to work only when the man can be made to give up violence as his primary means of solving problems.

Once the physician discovers that a woman is living in an abusive relationship, it is important to acknowledge to the patient the seriousness of the situation. To do otherwise is to give the impression that the physician approves or at least accepts the violent condition. It is important to attend to the patient's injuries and to assess the patient's emotional status from the standpoint of a psychiatric condition such as a suicidal ideation, depression, anxiety, or signs of abuse of drugs, alcohol, or other medications. The physician should also attempt to estimate the woman's ability to assess her own situation and her readiness to take appropriate action. If problems involving mental illness are present, a referral to an appropriate mental health worker who is sensitive to the issues of domestic violence should be made. Physicians should determine community resources available for handling family violence. The police department, crisis hotline, rape relief centers, domestic violence programs, and legal aid services for abused women can offer help in the acute situation. Hospital emergency rooms and shelters for battered women and children are also excellent resources. Health care workers in these organizations or private practitioners who specialize in the care of battered women, their spouses, and their children can offer counseling and follow-up care. Such individuals may be social workers, psychologists, psychiatrists, or other mental health workers trained specifically for this purpose. The physician's job is to recognize the problem and either offer counseling or get counseling for the patient so that she understands her rights and alternatives and learns to protect herself and her children from future harm. The victim of abuse likely will not wish to leave her home because of economic concerns and a fear that the batterer may continue to pursue her. Although she may have the batterer arrested and served with restraining orders, she may be convinced that she and her children cannot be protected from the batterer. She may also believe that there is a possibility of reconciliation and of change in behavior on the part of the batterer. It is therefore reasonable to discuss an exit plan with the victim to be used should the violence recur. This exit plan should include the following:

1. Have a change of clothes packed for both her and her children including toilet articles, necessary medications, and an extra set of keys to the house and car. These can be placed in a suitcase and left with a friend or family member.
2. Keep some cash, a checkbook, and a savings account book with the friend or family member.
3. Other identification papers, such as birth certificates, social security cards, voter registration cards, utility bills, and

driver's license, should be kept available, because children will need to be enrolled in school and the woman may have to seek financial assistance.
4. Have something special, such as a toy or book, for each child.
5. Have financial records available, such as mortgage papers, rent receipts, and an automobile title.
6. Determine a plan on exactly where to go regardless of the time of day or night. This may be to a friend or relative's house or to a shelter for battered women and children.
7. Ask neighbors to call police if violence begins.
8. Remove weapons.
9. Teach children to call 9-1-1.

Rehearsing an exit plan as one would conduct a fire drill makes it possible for the battered woman to respond even under the stress of the battering. Long-term aid and referral of the patient, her children, and the batterer to the appropriate resources is an important aspect of the care of such patients. The American College of Obstetricians and Gynecologists has prepared a patient education brochure that physicians can keep in their offices and give to individuals who suffer from this problem. Making the brochures available in the office waiting room may encourage women with these needs to get help.

These women often suffer from severe psychiatric problems, such as anxiety, depression, posttraumatic stress disorder (PTSD), and other pathologic conditions that may require psychotherapy. Women who are both physically and sexually assaulted have significantly higher levels of PTSD compared with women who are physically abused only. However, women who suffer any abuse, including emotional abuse without physical or sexual abuse, have a higher rate of mental health problems, including postpartum depression. Group counseling or individual counseling may also help them to rebuild their lives as single individuals or single parents. It is frequently necessary to help them develop a skill that will enable them to be employable. Counseling programs take these things into consideration. Children of victims who may be victims as well also require counseling to avoid behavior patterns that will lead to aggressive behavior in their later lives.

Intimate partner violence is a common problem that affects the family unit in particular and society in general. It can occur in all segments of society and reflects the violence that is a part of life today and the behavior of many. Physicians should learn to detect its presence in their patients and offer ways the victim can seek help. The help may include counseling for the victim, batterer, and children or constructing a plan for the woman to exit the relationship and rebuild her life in safety. There are many possible barriers for physicians screening for IPV and acting on their suspicions (Box 9.17). Ferguson's 2010 presidential address about IPV gave multiple recommendations regarding clinical practice, education and training, and research needs in this area in hopes of "ending this blight against women."

If the male batterer has not undergone anger management therapy, family counseling or intervention can be extremely dangerous, as it often raises issues that exacerbate the violence and increase the risk of serious harm to the woman and her children. Therefore this should not be advised until such time as the male batterer has addressed and eliminated his violent behavior. In general, success in such attempts with respect to the male partner is usually minimal.

Although all states have requirements for reporting child abuse, not all states require the reporting of domestic violence. However, many states have aggressive programs for intervening in domestic violence cases, and physicians should become aware of the programs in effect in their area. The patient should always be encouraged to leave a violent situation and may need community resources to help with economic and social adjustment, as well as protection for herself and her children from the violent partner. The American College of Obstetricians and Gynecologist's website has a page on resources for violence against women and lists each state's coalitions for sexual assault and domestic violence (www.acog.org/departments/dept_web.cfm?recno=17).

### *The Elderly*

The Select Committee on Aging, in investigating domestic violence against the elderly, held hearings before the Subcommittee of Human Services of the House of Representatives in 1980. The committee noted that approximately 500,000 to 2.5 million cases involving abuse of the elderly occur per year in the United States. The committee documented that abuse of the elderly may be as large a nationwide problem as child abuse. Usually, the abused person is a woman older than age 75, often with a physical impairment. She is generally white, widowed, and living with relatives. The abuser is generally an adult child living within the family but may also be a spouse. Counseling issues involve the entire family but particularly the individual causing the abuse. Physicians who care for geriatric patients should be alert for signs and symptoms of this type of domestic abuse; when it is found, community resources should be activated. All 50 states have passed legislation protecting the elderly from domestic violence and neglect. Forty-two states have mandatory reporting laws.

## GRIEF AND LOSS

The term *grief* is usually used to refer to the emotional, behavioral, and functional response to the death of a loved one. However, many people experience symptoms of grief in

**Box 9.17 Possible Barriers to Physician Screening for Intimate Partner Violence (IPV)**

Belief that "someone else will take care of it"
Forgetfulness
Not a physician's responsibility/role
IPV "should be private"
"Cannot offer much"
Lack of scientific evidence that screening improves outcomes
Cynicism: "nothing will happen"
Legal entanglement
Worry about offending/angering patients
Screening will take too much time
Insufficient training
Uncertainty about training requirements
Uncertainly about legal implications if screen is positive
Uncomfortable discussing issues of IPV
"Do not need to ask; the patient will volunteer the information"
Beliefs about victims of spouse abuse
Fear of retaliation against patient
Frustration over lack of patient disclosure
Not scientific, "sexy"

From Ferguson JE 2nd. Why doesn't SOMEBODY do something? *Am J Obstet Gynecol.* 2010;202(6):635-643.

response to losses other than death, such as losing a marriage, a job, one's health, or hope of having children, as in infertility. Gynecologists are likely to see women at times of uncomplicated grief, complicated grief, or grief-related major depression. Recognizing when a grief reaction is following an expectable course, as opposed to being complicated or involving major depression, is important in ensuring that the woman receives needed treatment.

Uncomplicated or "normal" grief has been postulated to follow defined stages, including initial numbness or shock, then sadness and depression, reorganization, and recovery. However, the literature suggests that grief experiences vary significantly among different cultures, people, and individual losses, often with intermingling of different "stages" of grief at the same time. Grief is currently thought to be a process with a wide spectrum of individual responses and a variable course, including not only painful feelings but also positive emotions and memories.

Shear (2015) has reviewed the nature of uncomplicated grief, complicated grief, and grief-related depression. Acute grief occurs early after the loss, is intensely painful, and includes sadness, longing, preoccupation with thoughts of the deceased or of the loss, disturbed sleep and appetite, trouble concentrating, and separation from and lack of interest in other people and usual activities. Bereavement may include benign hallucinations, such as hearing the voice, seeing, or sensing the presence of the deceased. Such experiences are normal and not of clinical concern. The loss of a loved one is associated with heightened risks of health problems such as myocardial infarction and Takotsubo (stress) cardiomyopathy, as well as depression, anxiety, and substance use disorders. Within a few months, acute grief gives way to integrated grief, a state in which the deceased or what has been lost is thought of often with sadness, but the woman is not preoccupied and can once more participate in pleasurable and meaningful activities and relationships. Triggers, including birthdays, anniversaries, or situations that remind her of the loss, may precipitate waves of grief, which gradually become less intense and less frequent over time. Uncomplicated grief does not require formal treatment, but instead gradually lessens with the support of family, friends, and community such as church and clergy; reassurance; information about the expected course of grief; and sometimes the help of support groups.

Complicated grief, or prolonged grief disorder, occurs in about 10% to 20% of people who lose a romantic partner and is more common than this with the death of a child. It is more likely when the death is sudden or violent (e.g., homicide or suicide). Symptoms include intense pain and longing, difficulty accepting the loss, anger, intrusive thoughts and ruminations, guilt, feelings of estrangement from other people, and suicidal thoughts. Risk factors include a history of mood and anxiety disorders, multiple losses, adverse life events, and other stressors reducing the woman's ability to cope. Complicated grief requires treatment to avoid becoming chronic and unremitting. Treatment should include psychotherapy and often also antidepressant medication.

Acute grief is commonly associated with symptoms that meet the criteria for major depression; 40% to 50% of bereaved people meet criteria at 1 month, about 20% to 25% at 2 months, and about 16% at 1 year (Zisook, 2009). There is considerable controversy about when to treat major depression occurring in the context of bereavement, especially because bereavement-related depression is similar in clinical characteristics, course, and treatment response to major depression occurring after a range of other stressors or without any identifiable trigger. Women with a past history of depression, or moderate to severe depressive symptoms as part of grief, should be treated aggressively, even in the first month or two after the loss, with antidepressant medication and psychotherapy, whereas those with milder depression can be monitored or referred for psychotherapy alone.

Obstetricians and gynecologists may need to counsel patients experiencing grief related to several areas of reproduction, including spontaneous abortion, perinatal loss, and infertility. About 15% of pregnancies end in miscarriage. Following a miscarriage, a woman may experience sadness, guilt, anger, posttraumatic stress disorder (PTSD) symptoms, and anxiety about future pregnancies. Men are also affected, although they tend to talk less about their feelings and may feel that they need to be strong to support their partner. In most cases, there is little discussion within the couple about the loss. A miscarriage most commonly represents the loss not of an established relationship but of hopes and expectations for the future, including pregnancy and motherhood. Despite this difference in the nature of the loss, the feelings of grief after miscarriage resemble those that may arise after losing a loved one, and the course of recovery is similar to that of other types of grief (Brier, 2008). Acute symptoms usually lessen significantly within about 6 months or sooner if the woman becomes pregnant again.

Several studies have examined psychological interventions after miscarriage. For example, Swanson and associates (2009) studied 341 couples, randomized to four different interventions at 1, 5, and 11 weeks after the miscarriage. Interventions were couples-focused counseling by a nurse in the couple's home for three sessions, a set of three video and workbook modules, a combination of one nurse counseling session with the three-video and workbook modules, and no intervention. All interventions used previously established models, Swanson's Caring Theory and the Meaning of Miscarriage Model, took a supportive approach, and focused on discussing the miscarriage, losses and gains resulting from the miscarriage, sharing the loss and rejoining public life, "getting through it," and trying again. The most effective intervention overall, for both depression and grief, was the three sessions of counseling by the nurse. In the absence of this resource, the obstetrician-gynecologist can help the patient and couple by normalizing feelings of depression and grief, giving the expectation that these will resolve, but also monitoring carefully for more severe or persistent symptoms of depression, PTSD, or suicidal thoughts indicating a need for referral for mental health treatment.

Perinatal loss, or stillbirth, occurs in 1% or less of pregnancies. In the weeks following a stillbirth, women commonly experience sadness, irritability, feelings of guilt, physical symptoms, depression, and anxiety, characteristic of grief; 20% continue to have symptoms a year later (Badenhorst, 2007). Women with poor social support or preexisting mental health problems are at higher risk for more intense and prolonged grief. PTSD is reported in about 20% of women during the next pregnancy, and women who hold their dead baby are at higher risk. Fathers also experience similar symptoms of grief after a stillbirth, experience anxiety and PTSD with the next pregnancy, and are also reported to have a higher risk of subsequent PTSD if they hold the dead baby. Loss of a baby may cause relationship strain or breakup, especially if the intensity or timing of grief differs significantly between the two parents. In addition, siblings may, depending on their age, be confused about what has happened, feel that they are to blame, or feel loss. Parents preoccupied by their own grief may have difficulty recognizing or helping their other children with these feelings.

Recommendations for clinicians include giving the woman and her partner clear information about what is going wrong and what is being done, involving the parents in decision making as possible, ensuring that the woman has access to postpartum medical care (e.g., suppression of lactation, contraception, help with gynecologic and sexual problems), and holding a meeting 1 to 2 months later to review what is known about the cause of the baby's death and to answer questions regarding future pregnancies. Couples are commonly advised, at the time of the loss, to create memories of the child, including holding the dead baby, giving the baby a name, taking photographs, and having a funeral. Many parents may want this and find it very important. However, especially holding the dead baby has been associated with poorer psychological outcome, increased rates of PTSD in the next pregnancy, and poor attachment to the subsequent baby. Couples may benefit from support groups, and those women or their partners who experience more severe or persistent depression, grief, anxiety, PTSD, or suicidal thoughts should be referred for mental health treatment with psychotherapy and medication, as indicated.

A special counseling challenge involves the care of a woman with an unplanned pregnancy. Such individuals often suffer conflicting feelings, which may include shame and guilt, a genuine desire to have a child, fear of social and family consequences, and fear for their own future and physical well-being. In addition, they may suffer from guilt about the termination of pregnancy if abortion is considered. Although many such women have good social support (e.g., family, significant others, friends, and religious counselors), others will rely on the physician for advice and direction. The physician should discuss all possible options with the woman, including having and raising the child, offering the child for adoption, or terminating the pregnancy. Issues involving the role of the baby's father, the effect of any decision on the future life of the woman, and the risks of procedures should be considered. The woman should be aided in reaching the most appropriate decision for her circumstances and supported in carrying out her decision. When necessary, appropriate referrals to social agencies (e.g., adoption, abortion counseling, or welfare services) should be made. The woman may experience depression, anxiety, or grief in this situation, even when making what she thinks is the best decision possible.

The inability to have a child, or infertility, affects about 1 in 10 couples and can precipitate feelings of isolation, inadequacy, poor self-esteem, guilt, anger, loss of control over one's life, depression, difficulty being around pregnant women or couples with young children, changes in one's identity and sense of meaning, and relationship strain. Infertility treatment involves significant cost, medical treatments and procedures, and psychological stress. Among women presenting for infertility treatment in one study, 40% met criteria for a psychiatric disorder, including 23% with an anxiety disorder and 17% with major depression (Burns, 2007). Failed infertility treatment engenders further stress and depression. Psychological distress has been reported to be the primary reason for dropout from infertility treatment, and pretreatment depression is predictive of dropout after one in vitro fertilization (IVF) cycle. There is some evidence that higher levels of psychological stress are associated with lower success rates of infertility treatment. Only about 50% of couples have a child as a result of infertility treatment, and those not succeeding commonly experience a grief reaction.

Many infertile women gain information and support from the Internet, although using this as one's sole source of support has been linked with higher levels of psychological distress. Women and their partners may benefit from support groups or individual or group psychotherapy. Interventions proved effective in reducing distress, and in some studies in improving conception rates, include cognitive behavioral therapy, ongoing counseling and education throughout the infertility treatment process, relaxation, stress management, coping skills, and group support. Cognitive behavioral therapy and fluoxetine have been shown to reduce both distress and depressive symptoms in mildly to moderately depressed infertile women (Faramarzi, 2013). Women with severe depression, grief, or suicidal thoughts should be referred for evaluation and antidepressant or other psychotropic medication treatment.

## DEATH AND DYING

Gynecologists, especially gynecologic-oncologists, care for women who are dying. There are several challenges for physicians caring for dying patients. First, physicians have been shown to be optimistic and inaccurate in their prognoses for terminally ill patients and to overestimate their ability to combat disease. This makes it difficult to know when to shift the conversation with a patient from a focus on cure or fighting the disease to a focus on palliative care. Making this transition may be difficult for the physician, who does not wish to give up hope prematurely. On the other hand, most patients are very concerned about issues of quality of life in confronting dying and hope for a process in which they can retain dignity, feel like themselves as much as possible, have adequate time and opportunity to put their "house in order," and have maximal possible comfort and pain relief. It is important for physicians to help women by discussing with them issues of "do not resuscitate" (DNR) orders, treatment of pain, referral to hospice, and other end-of-life issues. In fact, introducing palliative care discussions earlier in treatment appears to be helpful. For example, in a study of 151 patients with metastatic non-small-cell lung cancer, patients randomized to early palliative care integrated with oncologic care had a better quality of life and mood, less aggressive care at the end of life, and longer survival (Temel, 2011).

Psychological issues for dying patients are highly variable, depending on the person's stage of life, sense of the meaning of her life and of the illness, coping style, relationships and family support, spiritual beliefs, and economic circumstances. Feelings of grief, sadness, despair, fear, anxiety, and loneliness are present at some stage for nearly all dying patients, but some are able to achieve a high degree of equanimity and acceptance.

Developmentally, young adults with terminal illness commonly struggle with anger about the unfairness of the illness, grief and loss about life experiences they will not have, and issues related to being dependent on their parents for care. Parents of young children are concerned about the impact of their illness and death on their children, losing the opportunity to see their children grow up, and how to maintain a normal life and routine for their children and family in the face of their illness. For women in later stages of life, feelings about death depend on the degree of satisfaction and meaning that they feel with their life and what they have done, the kinds and quality of attachments they have, whether they feel robbed of retirement and later life, and whether they have lost their spouse or intimate partner already.

Block (2006) provided a comprehensive overview of psychological issues faced by dying patients and ways to explore with them issues related to the meaning of the illness, meaning of their life and achievements, spirituality, relationship issues, other life stressors, maintaining a sense of self, and fears and hopes that the patient has. Terminally ill patients benefit from the treatment of depression or anxiety states, in order to improve the quality of the remainder of their lives. Dying patients also benefit from psychological interventions, including listening, the opportunity to share feelings, and the chance to reflect on past experiences and future hopes. The gynecologist can help a dying woman by maintaining an engaged, genuine relationship with the woman as an individual throughout the dying process, helping the woman and family to anticipate and address practical issues such as enrolling in hospice and other palliative care services, and maximizing comfort and pain control.

## KEY POINTS

- Depression, anxiety disorders, obsessive-compulsive disorder, and posttraumatic stress disorder are treatable with medications or psychotherapy.
- A history of manic or hypomanic symptoms increases the risk for a "switch" into mania with antidepressant treatment.
- Close follow-up, in 1 to 2 weeks, is recommended to monitor for increases in suicidal thoughts with antidepressants, especially in adolescents and young adults.
- Active suicidal thoughts and plans are a psychiatric emergency.
- Eating disorders are life-threatening conditions that are often unrecognized.
- Girls or women presenting with amenorrhea, menstrual dysfunction, low bone density, sexual dysfunction, infertility, anxiety, depression, or hyperemesis gravidarum should be screened for eating disorders.
- Women with anxiety disorders (especially panic disorder and posttraumatic stress disorder) are at increased risk for suicide and should be asked about suicidal thoughts or plans.
- Anxiety disorders respond well to reassurance, education, and treatment with psychotherapy and medications (especially SSRI antidepressants).
- Many substance use disorders, such as alcoholism, have a more rapidly progressive course in women than in men ("telescoping").
- More than two drinks per day on average is considered heavy drinking for a woman.
- Motivational interviewing is a highly effective, brief intervention that increases women's engagement in substance abuse treatment and other behavior change.
- In cases of misuse of potentially habit-forming medications, a formal treatment agreement may be necessary.
- Understanding attachment styles can help providers to work effectively with "difficult" patients.
- Nonpharmacologic treatments for hypoactive sexual desire disorder include lifestyle changes for reducing stress and fatigue, recognizing and treating depression, increasing quality time with the partner, improving body image, and bringing novelty into the sexual repertoire.
- Lesbian and bisexual women require routine gynecologic care, have a high rate of mental health and substance use problems, and prefer female, preferably lesbian, health care providers.
- Lesbian and bisexual women have an elevated rate of mental health problems, substance use disorders, and suicide attempts, especially during adolescence.
- Intimate partner violence crosses all ethnic, racial, educational, age, and socioeconomic lines and has a large burden of social, physical, mental, and public health implications.
- The physician has a responsibility to screen and acknowledge intimate partner violence and abuse, identify the community resources for immediate referrals, assess safety, assist with reporting if necessary or desired, document appropriately using medicolegal tools, and provide ongoing clinical care.
- Gynecologists are often called on to provide or refer women for counseling related to grief; losses such as miscarriage, perinatal loss, and infertility; and end-of-life issues.
- Women suffering losses as a result of miscarriage, perinatal loss, unplanned pregnancy, or infertility benefit from support, counseling, and screening for depression and posttraumatic stress disorder.
- Complicated grief and grief accompanied by symptoms of depression benefit from antidepressant medication treatment in addition to psychotherapy.
- Women with terminal illness benefit from an engaged, genuine relationship with physicians and other health care providers, treatment of depression and anxiety states, psychological interventions and psychotherapy, and early integration of palliative care into treatment.

## KEY REFERENCES


ACOG Committee on Health Care for Underserved Women. ACOG Committee Opinion No. 423: Motivational interviewing: a tool for behavior change. *Obstet Gynecol.* 2009;113(1):243-246.

ACOG. ACOG Committee Opinion No. 496: At risk drinking and alcohol dependence: obstetric and gynecologic implications. *Obstet Gynecol.* 2011;118:383-388.

Adams KF, Schatzkin A, Harris TB, et al. Overweight, obesity, and mortality in a large prospective cohort of persons 50 to 71 years old. *N Engl J Med.* 2006;355:763-778.

Albright BB, Rayburn WF. Substance abuse among reproductive age women. *Obstet Gynecol Clin North Am.* 2009;36(4):891-906.

Badenhorst W, Hughes P. Psychological aspects of perinatal loss. *Best Pract Res Clin Obstet Gynaecol.* 2007;21(2):249-259.

Basson R. Sexual desire and arousal disorders in women. *N Engl J Med.* 2006;354:1497-1506.

Benowitz NL. Nicotine addiction. *N Engl J Med.* 2010;362:2295-2303.

Block SD. Psychological issues in end-of-life care. *J Palliat Med.* 2006;9:751-766.

Bradford J, Ryan C, Rothblum ED. National lesbian health care survey: implications for mental health care. *J Consult Clin Psychology.* 1994;62(2):228-242.

Bradley KA, Boyd-Wickizer J, Powell SH, Burman ML. Alcohol screening questionnaires in women: a critical review. *JAMA.* 1998;280(2):166-171.

Breiding MJ, Black MC, Ryan GW. Prevalence and risk factors of intimate partner violence in eighteen US states/territories. *Am J Prev Med.* 2008;34:112-118.

Brier N. Grief following miscarriage: a comprehensive review of the literature. *J Womens Health.* 2008;17:451-464.

Burgess AW, Holmstrom LL. Rape trauma syndrome. *Am J Psychiatry.* 1974;131(9):981-986.

Burns LH. Psychiatric aspects of infertility and infertility treatments. *Psychiatr Clin N Am.* 2007;30:689-716.

Cameron C, Habert J, Anand L, Furtado M. Optimizing the management of depression: primary care experience. *Psychiatry Research.* 2014;220(S1):545-557.

Centers for Disease Control and Prevention (CDC). School health guidelines to promote healthy eating and physical activity. *MMWR Recomm Rep 16.* 2011;60(RR-5):1-76.

Ciechanowski PS, Hirsch IB, Katon WJ. Interpersonal predictors of HbA1c in patients with type I diabetes. *Diabetes Care.* 2002a;25:731-736.

Ciechanowski PS, Walker EA, Katon WJ, Russo JE. Attachment theory: a model for health care utilization and somatization. *Psychosom Med.* 2002b;64:660-667.

Cipriani A, Furukawa TA, Salanti G, et al. Comparative efficacy and acceptability of 12 new-generation antidepressants: a multiple-treatments meta-analysis. *Lancet.* 2009;373:746-758.

Faramarzi M, Pasha H, Esmailzadeh S, et al. The effect of cognitive behavioral therapy and pharmacotherapy on infertility stress: a randomized controlled trial. *Int J Fertil Steril.* 2013;7(3):199-206.

Ferguson 2nd JE. Why doesn't SOMEBODY do something? *Am J Obstet Gynecol.* 2010;202(6):635-643.

Flint E, Cummins S, Sacker A. Associations between active commuting, body fat, and body mass index: population based, cross sectional study in the United Kingdom. *BMJ.* 2014;349:g4887.

Grant JE. Clinical practice: obsessive-compulsive disorder. *N Engl J Med.* 2014;371(7):646-653.

Greenfield SF, Back SE, Lawson K, et al. Substance abuse in women. *Psychiatr Clin North Am.* 2010;33:339-355.

Groves JE. Taking care of the hateful patient. *N Engl J Med.* 1978;298:883-887.

Guglielmo R, Martinotti G, Quatrale M, et al. Topiramate in alcohol use disorders: review and update. *CNS Drugs.* 2015;29(5):383-395.

Hilberman E, Monson K. Sixty battered women. *Victimology.* 1977;2:460.

Jackson JL, Kroenke K. Difficult patient encounters in the ambulatory clinic. *Arch Intern Med.* 1999;159:1069-1075.

Jenny C, Hooton TM, Bowers A, et al. Sexually transmitted diseases in victims of rape. *N Engl J Med.* 1990;322:713-716.

Johnston BD, Kanters S, Bandayrel K, et al. Comparison of weight loss among named diet programs in overweight and obese adults: a meta-analysis. *JAMA.* 2014;312(9):923-933.

Jonas DE, Amick HR, Feltner C, et al. Pharmacotherapy for adults with alcohol use disorders in outpatient settings: a systematic review and meta-analysis. *JAMA.* 2014;311(18):1889-1900.

Katon WJ. Panic disorder. *N Engl J Med.* 2006;354:2360-2367.

King M, Semlyen J, Tai SS, et al. A systematic review of mental disorder, suicide, and deliberate self-harm in lesbian, gay, and bisexual people. *BMC Psychiatry.* 2008;8:70.

Krebs EE, Garrett JM, Konrad TR. The difficult doctor? Characteristics of physicians who report frustration with patients: an analysis of survey data. *BMC Health Serv Res.* 2006;6:128.

Lee IM, Djoussé L, Sesso HD, et al. Physical activity and weight gain prevention. *JAMA.* 2010;303(12):1173-1179.

Leichsenring F, Leibing E, Kruse J, et al. Borderline personality disorder. *Lancet.* 2011;377:74-84.

Lock J, LeGrange D, Agras WS, et al. Randomized clinical trial comparing family-based treatment with adolescent-focused individual psychotherapy for adolescents with anorexia nervosa. *Arch Gen Psychiatry.* 2010;67:1025-1032.

Mitchell KR, Mercer CH, Ploubidis GB, et al. Sexual function in Britain: findings from the third National Survey of Sexual Attitudes and Lifestyles (Natsal-3). *Lancet.* 2013;382(9907):1817-1829.

O'Dowd TC. Five years of heartsink patients in general practice. *BMJ.* 1988;297:528-530.

Oesterheld JR, Cozza K, Sandson NB. Oral contraceptives. *Psychosomatics.* 2008;49:168-175.

Puzziferri N, Roshek 3rd TB, Mayo HG, et al. Long-term follow-up after bariatric surgery: a systematic review. *JAMA.* 2014;312(9):934-942.

Roy-Byrne PP, Craske MG, Stein MB. Panic disorder. *Lancet.* 2006;368:1023-1032.

Shear MK. Clinical practice: complicated grief. *N Engl J Med.* 2015;372:153-160.

Shifren JL, Monz BU, Russo PA, et al. Sexual problems and distress in United States women prevalence and correlates. *Obstet Gynecol.* 2008;112(5):970-978.

Stein MB, Stein D. Social anxiety disorder. *Lancet.* 2008;371(9618):1115-1125.

Steinmetz D, Tabenkin H. The "difficult patient" as perceived by family physicians. *Fam Pract.* 2001;18(5):495-500.

Strous RD, Ulman AM, Kotler M. The hateful patient revisited: relevance for 21st century medicine. *Eur J Intern Med.* 2006;17:387-393.

Swanson KM, Chen HT, Graham JC, et al. Resolution of miscarriage and grief in the first year after miscarriage: a randomized controlled clinical trial of couples focused interventions. *J Womens Health.* 2009;18:1245-1257.

Temel JS, Greer JA, Admane S, et al. Longitudinal perceptions of prognosis and goal of therapy in patients with metastatic non-small-cell lung cancer: results of a randomized study of early palliative care. *J Clin Oncol.* 2011;29(17):2319-2326.

Thompson D, Ciechanowski PS. Attaching a new understanding to the patient-physician relationship in family practice. *J Am Board Fam Pract.* 2003;16:219-226.

Treasure J, Claudino AM, Zucker N. Eating disorders. *Lancet.* 2010;375:583-593.

Wadden TA, Butryn ML, Hong PS, et al. Behavioral treatment of obesity in patients encountered in primary care settings: a systematic review. *JAMA.* 2014;312(17):1779-1791.

Yanovski SZ, Yanovski JA. Long-term drug treatment for obesity: a systematic and clinical review. *JAMA.* 2014;311(1):74-86.

Zipfel S, Wild B, ANTOP Study Group, et al. Focal psychodynamic therapy, cognitive behaviour therapy, and optimised treatment as usual in outpatients with anorexia nervosa (ANTOP study): randomised controlled trial. *Lancet.* 2014;383(9912):127-137.

Zisook S, Shear MK. Grief and bereavement: what psychiatrists need to know. *World Psychiatry.* 2009;8(2):67-74.


Suggested Readings can be found on ExpertConsult.com.

# 10

# Endoscopy: Hysteroscopy and Laparoscopy

## Indications, Contraindications, and Complications

*Sarah M. Carlson, Jay Goldberg, Gretchen M. Lentz*

This chapter presents an overview of frequently used endoscopic procedures in gynecology. Indications, contraindications, and complications are included for each procedure. For those unfamiliar with the procedures, the diagnostic uses are described. Therapeutic uses and pitfalls are introduced, but complex surgical procedures are better covered in focused gynecologic surgical textbooks.

Since the 1960s, there have been significant changes in the use of endoscopy in gynecologic practice. The fiberoptic bundle and more versatile light sources, as well as the incorporation of advances in technology, have dramatically increased the diagnostic and therapeutic capabilities of the hysteroscope and laparoscope.

The tremendous advances in technology have led to the emergence of more office-based procedures. Many gynecologic surgeries done by laparotomy in years past have been converted to ambulatory, outpatient procedures. Other cases traditionally completed only by laparotomy are now more likely to be performed laparoscopically with shorter hospital stays and recovery time. This chapter serves as an introductory overview of gynecologic endoscopy.

## HYSTEROSCOPY

Hysteroscopy is the direct visualization of the endometrial cavity via the cervix using an endoscope and a light source. The earliest hysteroscope was nothing more than a hollow tube with an alcohol lamp and mirror for a light source. In 1869, Pantaleoni reported the successful removal of an endometrial polyp through the scope. Modern hysteroscopes are modifications of cystoscopes with channels to introduce light via fiberoptics. Various infusion media are used for uterine cavity distention, which is necessary for inspection. Many surgical instruments and devices are available for diagnostic biopsy and pathology removal and therapeutic procedures. Office and operating room hysteroscopy requires knowledge of instrumentation, techniques, indications, contraindications, and complication management. If office hysteroscopy is used, proper office safety protocols are needed. Unfortunately, many physicians do not have the equipment and staffing available to perform hysteroscopy in the office.

Inserting a hysteroscope for diagnostic purposes only is a low-risk procedure. The key is predicting which diagnostic procedures may be challenging from severe cervical stenosis or which complex operative hysteroscopic procedures may be more safely accomplished in the operating room setting. Office hysteroscopy saves time for both the patient and physician, saves money, and is convenient. It makes sense when performing hysteroscopic procedures in the office to initially gain experience with simpler surgeries. Once expertise has been gained from sufficient operative hysteroscopic procedural volume, the more involved and challenging hysteroscopic procedures can be moved from the operating room to the office setting.

### *HYSTEROSCOPIC INDICATIONS AND CONTRAINDICATIONS*

The popularity of hysteroscopy has grown because it is a simple technique that most gynecologists are trained to perform. It is most frequently used in the evaluation of abnormal uterine bleeding for both pre- and postmenopausal women. Women with recurrent abnormal uterine bleeding, particularly postmenopausal patients with persistent bleeding following a negative endometrial biopsy, are good candidates for hysteroscopy. Endometrial biopsy and dilation and curettage (D&C) procedures frequently miss focal lesions and pedunculated structures. One study (Feldman, 1994) evaluated 286 women with perimenopausal bleeding who had had a D&C or an endometrial biopsy. Nine of 86 (10.5%) who had negative findings initially, but continued to bleed, had carcinoma or complex hyperplasia on follow-up biopsy. Hysteroscopy with directed biopsy can be useful in this setting, although controversy exists regarding the spread of endometrial cancer with hysteroscopy. Hysteroscopy can also assist in directly visualizing and removing intrauterine foreign bodies like a partially perforated or broken intrauterine device (IUD) or retrieving an IUD with missing strings. Other indications include performing hysteroscopic sterilization, evaluation of recurrent miscarriage, uterine synechiae, abnormal hysterosalpingography (HSG) or sonohysterography, and infertility. More involved operative procedures include resection of submucous myomas, lysis of synechiae, incision of uterine septa, and removal of endometrial polyps or ablation of the endometrium. Box 10.1 lists common indications.

There are few contraindications to hysteroscopy. Absolute contraindications include acute pelvic or vaginal infections including genital herpes, because of the potential for disease spread by the distention media. One exception may be for the retrieval of an IUD if the pelvic infection is related to the device. Pregnancy is a contraindication, as is recent uterine perforation. Active bleeding is a relative contraindication. If the bleeding is brisk, the hysteroscopic view might be unsatisfactory. Other relative contraindications include extensive adhesions and leiomyomata that are largely (>50%) intramyometrial rather than submucous. Cervical and uterine cancers are cited as absolute contraindications. There continues to be debate over risking endometrial cancer dissemination into the peritoneal cavity by pushing endometrial cancer cells out the fallopian tubes with the distending media. A 2010 systematic review by Polyzos and colleagues found hysteroscopy resulted in a significantly higher rate of malignant peritoneal cytology (odds ratio 1.78) when done before surgery and therefore disease upstaging, although it is unclear if the outcome is adversely affected. Gynecologists are often doing hysteroscopy to discover the etiology of abnormal bleeding, and the diagnosis of endometrial cancer is sometimes made as a result.

**Box 10.1 Possible Hysteroscopic Indications**

Abnormal uterine bleeding
- Premenopausal
- Postmenopausal

Persistent abnormal uterine bleeding after negative endometrial biopsy
Postmenopausal endometrial thickening and negative endometrial biopsy
Endometrial polyp
Submucosal myoma or possibly <50% intramural
Uterine septum
Uterine synechiae
Retained IUD
Sterilization
Endocervical lesions

## HYSTEROSCOPIC EQUIPMENT AND TECHNIQUES

Rigid hysteroscopes vary in diameter. The smaller caliber scopes, 3 to 5 mm in diameter, are used for diagnostic purposes. Several are available that have views from 0 to 70 degrees, but those with views of 12 to 30 degrees are most commonly used. Similar to a cystoscope, the outer sleeve of a rigid hysteroscope contains several channels that extend the full length of the instrument. Figure 10.1 shows the anatomy of a hysteroscope and names of the various sections. For office hysteroscopy, often a 4-mm telescope with a 7-mm outer sheath is used, so there is a channel for seven French flexible or semirigid instruments such as scissors, or biopsy or grasping forceps. The outer sheath also allows for inflow of the distending media. Although a 5-mm hysteroscope often passes without cervical dilation, a 7-mm diameter scope usually does not. Large scopes, with diameters of 8 to 10 mm, may be used for high flow of distending media and have a second channel for outflow of blood and fluid. These are used for moderate to complex procedures. Flexible minihysteroscopic instruments and microendoscopes are convenient and well tolerated in the office for diagnostic and simple operative procedures such as directed biopsies. There is generally less pain with the small flexible hysteroscopes, but the visual quality is poorer. They do allow more ease when lysing intrauterine adhesions in difficult locations (Fig. 10.2).

The cavity of the uterus is a potential space. The success of hysteroscopy depends on the media used to expand this space. Many distending media are available, including 32% dextran 70, which is highly viscous; 5% dextrose and water ($D_5W$), which has low viscosity; 1.5% glycine; Ringer's lactate; normal saline; and carbon dioxide gas. The surgeon must know which is ideal for the particular case and instrumentation and the potential risks (Table 10.1). High-molecular-weight dextran (average molecular weight, 70,000 Da in 10% glucose) is extremely viscous fluid and is biodegradable, nontoxic, nonconductive, and has good optical qualities. Most important, dextran is immiscible with blood, which helps to keep the field clear during intrauterine surgery, especially when there is active bleeding. Dextran has two drawbacks: it is antigenic, and anaphylaxis has been

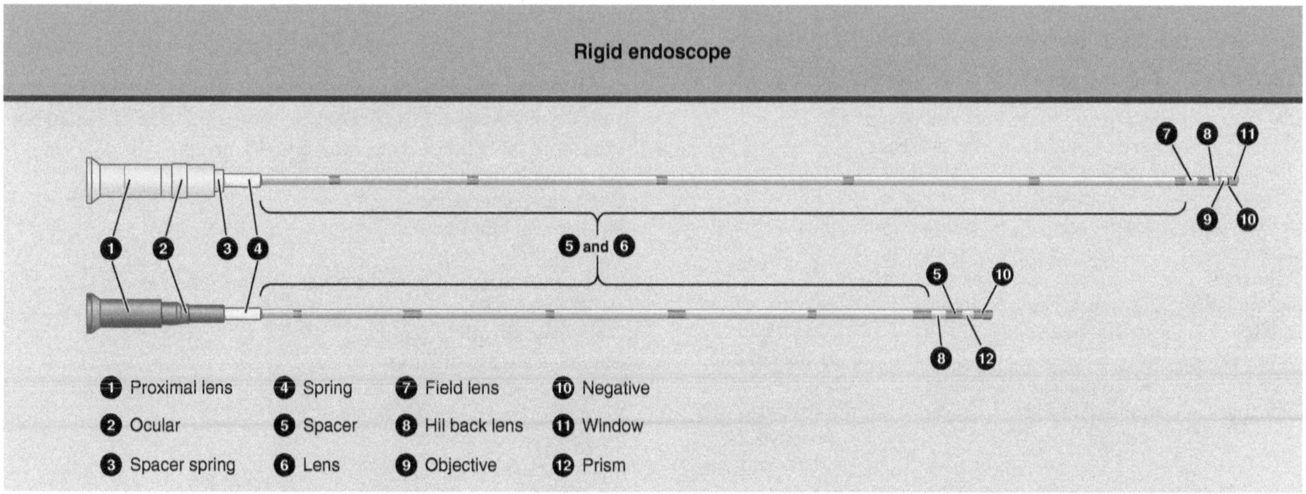


**Figure 10.1** Anatomy of a rigid endoscope. (From Beiber EJ, Sanfilippo JS, Horowitz IR. *Clinical Gynecology*. Philadelphia: Elsevier, 2006.)

reported. It also rapidly crystallizes; thus endoscopic instruments must be cleaned shortly after the procedure. It is sticky to work with and can lock the valves. Rare cases of pulmonary edema and coagulopathies from intravascular dextran have been reported. Dextran can osmotically draw fluid many times its own volume into the intravascular space if extravasation occurs. A different distention medium is recommended if one predicts that greater than 500 mL of dextran will be needed. Carbon dioxide must be infused with special equipment (not a laparoscopic insufflator) that carefully limits flow to less than 100 mL/min and maintains the pressure at approximately 60 to 70 mm Hg. Because no fluid is involved, there is no mess. If the patient has patent fallopian tubes, the $CO_2$ gas can cause diaphragmatic irritation and discomfort. The major precaution with $D_5W$ is the monitoring of total fluid intake so as not to produce water intoxication. In contrast, office hysteroscopy with the smaller flexible scopes most commonly incorporates the use of saline or lactated Ringer's solution because either is easier to use, causes less pain, and avoids the risk of electrolyte and osmolar imbalances. For operative hysteroscopy, it is necessary to carefully and frequently monitor the intake and outflow of distention media. Fluid management systems are available that calculate these values continuously. Guidelines exist for terminating a procedure when fluid deficits reach a set amount. For nonelectrolyte media, the recommended cutoff is 1000 to 1500 mL; for an electrolyte medium it is 2500 mL, but other factors should be considered such age, comorbid conditions, cardiovascular disease, and patient body mass index. For operative procedures with electrocautery, saline or isotonic solutions cannot be used because they conduct electricity (except bipolar cautery).

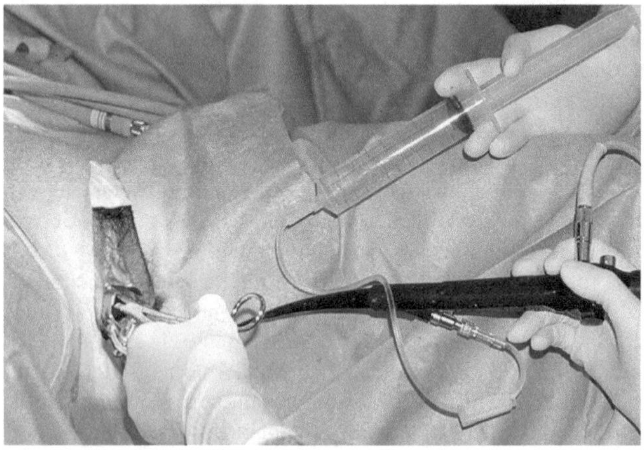

**Figure 10.2** Flexible hysteroscopy. Uterine distention is maintained with normal saline or lactated Ringer's solution injected through intravenous extension tubing. (From Goldberg JM, Falcone T. *Atlas of Endoscopic Techniques in Gynecology.* London: WB Saunders; 2000:185.)

Hysteroscopy techniques are fairly similar whether performed as an office procedure or in an operating room. A list of general equipment needed for office hysteroscopy is given in Box 10.2. A complete history and physical exam is needed; in particular, a relevant allergies and medication list must be confirmed. Appropriate tests may include a Papanicolaou smear, pregnancy test, hemoglobin or hematocrit testing, and gonorrhea or chlamydia testing. Hysteroscopy can be performed at any time during the menstrual cycle, but it is best scheduled in the early to middle proliferative phase. Endometrial pretreatment with hormonal agents may be considered prior to hysteroscopic sterilization procedures, hysteroscopic myomectomies, resectoscopic ablations, and nonresectoscopic ablations. Thinning the endometrium facilitates visualization and may aid in tissue destruction during an ablation. A bimanual examination is performed to note the size of the uterus and direction of the uterine fundus. Knowing whether the uterus is anteverted or retroverted is important to avoid uterine perforation, and a rectovaginal exam can aid in determining position. It is helpful to explain to the patient that she will experience discomfort if cervical dilation is needed and uterine cramping during the short time that the hysteroscope is inside the uterus. A single-toothed tenaculum may be used to secure the anterior cervical lip. Gentle traction on the tenaculum straightens out the uterine axis to facilitate endocervical passage of the instruments. Techniques have been described for diagnostic hysteroscopy with a small scope diameter than do not utilize a tenaculum and thus avoid causing that pain. The exocervix is then cleaned of mucus and bacteria. Many physicians will cleanse the cervical os with an iodine solution prior to introducing the scope. The most frequent problem in performing hysteroscopy is cervical stenosis or spasm. When this is encountered, the optimal method to relieve pain and overcome resistance is a

**Table 10.1** Comparison of Hysteroscopic Distention Media

| Medium | Advantage | Disadvantage | Risk |
|---|---|---|---|
| $CO_2$ | Safe<br>Ease of use<br>Rapidly absorbed | Poor visibility in the presence of bleeding | |
| Normal saline<br>Lactated Ringer's | Isotonic | Not suitable for monopolar electrosurgery | Fluid overload |
| Glycine 1.5%<br>Sorbitol<br>Mannitol 5% | Electrolyte free<br>Nonconductive | Hypotonic | Hypotonic fluid overload<br>Hyponatremia |
| Hyskon (32% dextran) | Nonconductive<br>Immiscible with blood | Difficult to deliver | Hypertonic fluid overload<br>Anaphylactic reaction |

From Beiber EJ, Sanfilippo JS, Horowitz IR. *Clinical Gynecology.* Philadelphia: Elsevier; 2006.

**Box 10.2 Equipment for Office Hysteroscopy**

- Procedure table that elevates to 46 to 48 inches
- Comfortable behind-the-knee padded stirrups
- Open-sided speculum
- Paracervical block equipment
- Tenaculum
- Hysteroscope with 4-mm diameter and fore-oblique 25- to 30-degree lens
- Diagnostic sheath of 5 mm
- Operative sheath of 7 mm
- Flexible or semirigid scissors and biopsy and grasping forceps
- Rigid scissors and biopsy and grasping forceps
- Ring forceps
- Myoma grasping forceps
- Emergency kit
- Foley catheter with 30-mL balloon

paracervical block with 1% lidocaine. Liberal use of paracervical block in difficult procedures allows the physician to be successful in obtaining endometrial biopsy tissue in more than 95% of cases, so this is likely true for hysteroscopy as well. Subsequently, the cervix can be dilated with tapered plastic or metal dilators, and the hysteroscopy can be completed. Unlike with larger rigid scopes, most patients will not require anesthesia for diagnostic procedures in the office. The infusion line should be flushed through the scope prior to insertion; otherwise bubbles will be introduced and obscure the view.

When inserting the hysteroscope, it is useful to wait a few seconds to let the distending media open the internal cervical os so that the uterine cavity can be entered more easily by following the fluid flow. Then angle of the telescope view is opposite the direction of the light post. This point must be remembered in the context of viewing an anteverted versus retroverted uterus. If the light post is pointing upward, the view is downward. If uterine cavity vision is obscured, it may be due to insufficient distention fluid, bleeding, or being up against the uterine wall or pathology. Withdraw the hysteroscope slowly while slightly increasing the distention fluid. Never advance the hysteroscope without good visualization because perforation can occur. The cavity should be inspected thoroughly and systematically. First, an overall view can be seen on entry looking for the general cavity shape, polyps, myomas, and foreign bodies. As the hysteroscope is advanced, it is rotated clockwise and counterclockwise to see the cornua and tubal ostia. On removal, endocervix is viewed. Overzealous cervical dilation can create a poor seal between the cervix and scope, allowing the fluid to run out of the cervix and poor uterine distention. Short-term complications are listed in Table 10.2.

Vaginal and oral misoprostol (prostaglandin $E_1$) given the night before the procedure, in dosages of 200 to 800 mcg can aid in the transcervical passage of the hysteroscope. This can be useful for women at risk for cervical stenosis such as those with prior cervical surgery and nulliparous women. In postmenopausal women, pretreatment with vaginal estrogen for 2 weeks before surgery may augment the cervical dilation caused by misoprostol. Women should be warned of the side effects of misoprostol, including diarrhea, cramping, uterine bleeding, and fever. Concomitant nonsteroidal anti-inflammatory drugs (NSAIDs) can reduce side effects and help with postoperative pain. Anxious patients may be pretreated with an anxiolytic such as alprazolam. For more involved procedures, intravenous analgesia and conscious sedation may be needed, and proper protocols are needed to ensure patient safety. If extensive resections are anticipated via hysteroscopy, then the procedure is better performed on an outpatient basis in the surgical suite.

For the severely stenotic cervix, having the right instruments available is critical. Lacrimal duct dilators (from ophthalmologic surgery) come in graduated sizes down to 1 mm in diameter. This can lead to cervical access when barely a dimple is seen in the external cervical os. Then, the usual tapered metal or plastic cervical dilators can facilitate complete dilation. Also, real-time ultrasonography can help the surgeon to visualize the tip of the dilator, direct the surgeon along the right track into the endometrial cavity, and prevent the surgeon from making a false cervical path or uterine perforation.

**Table 10.2** Short-Term Complications of Hysteroscopy

| Complication | Rate (%) |
|---|---|
| **Overall Complication Rate** | |
| Diagnostic hysteroscopy | 0.95 |
| Operative hysteroscopy | 2 to 3 |
| Hysteroscopic myomectomy | 1 to 5 |
| **Uterine Perforation** | |
| Operative hysteroscopy | 1 |
| Endometrial ablation—resectoscope | 2 to 2+ |
| Endometrial ablation—nonresectoscope | 1 |
| Fluid overload | 0.06 to 2 |
| Bleeding | 0.03 to 3 |
| Pelvic infection | 0.01 |
| Death—fluid overload or septicemia | 0.01 |
| Embolism; gas, air | * |
| Cervical laceration | * |
| Creation of false cervical passage | * |
| Failure to complete the procedure | * |
| Electrocautery injury | * |
| Urinary tract or bowel injury | * |
| Pulmonary and cerebral edema | * |
| Dissemination of cervical or endometrial cancer | * |

*Rare complication or exact rate of complication unknown.

## OPERATIVE HYSTEROSCOPY TECHNIQUES

The variety and extent of surgery performed transcervically with the hysteroscope has expanded significantly with technologic advances. Endoscopic procedures have progressed from snaring small polyps to hysteroscopic tubal sterilization, complex myomectomies, and ablating the entire endometrial lining. The ability to detect, biopsy, or remove focal lesions is extremely useful for abnormal bleeding workup over blind endometrial sampling. Approximately 50% of all Essure hysteroscopic tubal occlusions performed in the United States are done in an office setting, and the percentage is rising. Operative hysteroscopy may be performed with mechanical devices such as small operating scissors, electrocautery, and modified resectoscopes and lasers. Laser hysteroscopy with carbon dioxide or neodymium:yttrium-aluminum-garnet (Nd:YAG) or argon lasers requires more expensive equipment and expertise. With the development of the second-generation technology for uterine ablation and polyp and fibroid resection, the laser and resectoscope equipment is significantly less popular and less advantageous than simpler techniques.

Women with repetitive miscarriages should have a diagnostic hysteroscopic procedure, which often leads to an operative procedure. Congenital abnormalities that interfere with the success of early pregnancies, such as septa of the uterus, may be seen and removed (Fig. 10.3). Often endometrial polyps or submucous myomas are discovered and may be removed with a resectoscope wire (Fig. 10.4) or a newer morcellator type device (Fig. 10.5). The uterine synechiae of a woman with Asherman's syndrome can be cut with microscissors, reestablishing the endometrial cavity. Because adhesions interfere with the configuration of the cavity, it can be difficult for the surgeon to identify usual landmarks. Simultaneous laparoscopy guidance is often used to avoid perforation when cutting the intrauterine adhesions. Hysteroscopic metroplasty of intrauterine septa has replaced abdominal metroplasty, as it is safer and has fewer complications than laparotomy. Simultaneous laparoscopy is often used with this procedure as well to gauge the end point of cutting the septum.

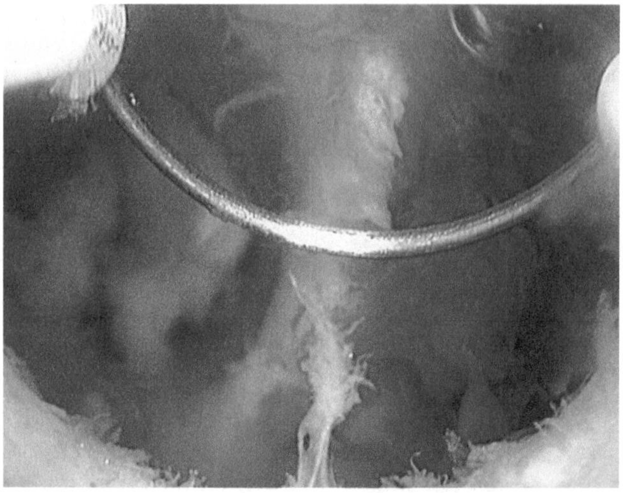

Figure 10.3 The loop is placed at the center of the apex of the septum. As the current is activated, the loop is advanced toward the fundus in small increments, always staying in the center of the septum. The septum separates, as it is divided so that no tissue must be excised. (There are small endometrial fragments in the right cornua and a small clot adherent to the left aspect of the septum.) (From Goldberg JM, Falcone T. *Atlas of Endoscopic Techniques in Gynecology.* London: WB Saunders; 2000:194.)

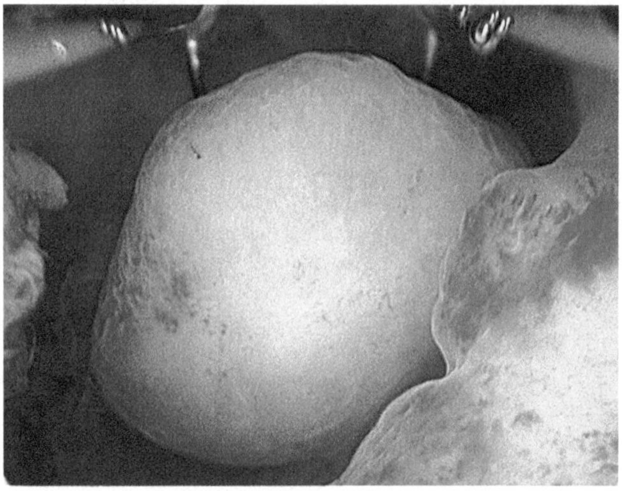

Figure 10.4 A uterine polyp with the hysteroscopic resection tool behind the polyp. (From Goldberg JM, Falcone T. *Atlas of Endoscopic Techniques in Gynecology.* London: WB Saunders; 2000:187.)

Hysteroscopy is superior to hysterosalpingogram (HSG) in discovering intrauterine disease. In comparative studies, the use of hysteroscopy revealed synechiae, polyps, or myomas in 40% of patients with normal HSGs. These abnormalities were undetected and unsuspected using radiographic techniques. The false-positive rate of HSG is 33% compared with hysteroscopy. One in three women diagnosed 5 as having an intrauterine filling defect by x-ray imaging will have a normal cavity directly visualized with the hysteroscope. Women with amenorrhea and a history of curettage who do not respond to a hormonal challenge should have an HSG or hysteroscopy. Uterine synechiae are identified by slowly injecting a water-soluble medium on HSG or by the inability to visualize the uterine cavity on hysteroscopy. If a woman has synechiae, tubal obstruction on HSG, and pelvic calcifications, a diagnosis of pelvic tuberculosis should be strongly suspected. In women with a history of recurrent abortions or infertility with a uterine abnormality seen on ultrasound, sonohysterography (SHG) is comparable to HSG and hysteroscopy in detecting uterine anomalies, especially septate and bicornuate uterus (Ludwin, 2011). SHG has the benefit of being noninvasive, cost effective, and does not expose the patient to radiation.

Submucous myomas were initially removed with a modified urologic resectoscope using a cutting 40-watt electric current and a 90-degree wire loop for shaving the myoma until it was flat with the surrounding endometrial lining. The electrocautery led to bubbles obscuring the view and the potential risk of gas or air emboli. If unsuspected perforation occurred, the risk of thermal injury was present. Greatly improved instrumentation is available with a hysteroscopic rotary or reciprocating morcellator blade for removing polyps and fibroids. It does not use electrocautery and simultaneously cuts and aspirates the pathology so that there are no bubbles and no pieces of shaved tissue floating in the cavity. Saline is used as the infusion medium as no cautery is used, which lessens the electrolyte imbalance risk. The drawback without electrocautery is that more bleeding can occur. Studies have shown successful removal of the submucous myoma at the initial hysteroscopy being 85% to 95%. The success rate of complete resection at the initial surgery is higher with myomas that are nearly completely submucous versus fibroids with a significant intramural portion. The pregnancy rate is as good as or better with hysteroscopic myomectomy than with transabdominal myomectomy.

In women with abnormal bleeding or menorrhagia who are poor surgical candidates, desire a minimally invasive procedure,

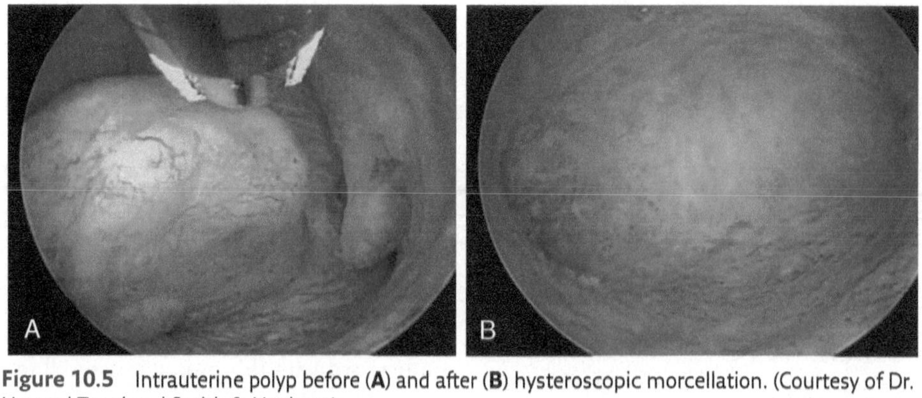


Figure 10.5 Intrauterine polyp before (**A**) and after (**B**) hysteroscopic morcellation. (Courtesy of Dr. Howard Topel and Smith & Nephew.)

or wish to preserve their uterus, the endometrial lining may be ablated or resected through the hysteroscope (Fig. 10.6). Performance of endometrial ablation or resection has decreased due to the increased usage of the levonorgestrel intrauterine device. Although endometrial ablation and levonorgestrel IUD both provide comparable reductions in menstrual blood loss, the IUD also provides contraception and protects the endometrium in women at risk for hyperplasia and carcinoma. Pregnancy following an endometrial ablation is contraindicated, but the procedure does not prevent pregnancy. Sterilization or contraception should be addressed prior to ablation. In patients with abnormal uterine bleeding following endometrial ablation, evaluation of the endometrial cavity can be hindered due to scarring. The U.S. Food and Drug Administration (FDA) has approved five global endometrial ablation devices: thermal balloon endometrial ablation (ThermaChoice, Ethicon Inc., Menlo Park, CA), radiofrequency endometrial ablation (NovaSure, Cytyc Surgical Products, Palo Alto, CA), hydrothermal endometrial ablation (HydroTermAblator, Boston Scientific, Natick, MA), cryoablation (Her Option, CryoGen Inc., San Diego, CA), and microwave endometrial ablation (Microsulis, Hampshire, England). The 2013 Cochrane database review concluded that endometrial ablation techniques offer a less invasive alternative to hysterectomies (Fergusson, 2013). All of the currently available nonresectoscopic endometrial ablation devices have limitations on acceptable endometrial cavity size and endometrial surface irregularities such as myomas. No gold standard system exists yet, as comparative studies have shown similar treatment efficacy with the available ablative systems. The second-generation devices compare favorably with the earlier used roller ball and wire loop resectoscope techniques, but they are simpler to use. Similar rates of amenorrhea and patient satisfaction have been reported, but ablation via a resectoscope is associated with longer operative times, more frequent use of general anesthesia and higher rates of irrigation fluid overload and cervical laceration compared with non-resectoscope modes.

Selective salpingography is an extension of hysteroscopy to evaluate the lumen of the fallopian tubes. The tube can be cannulized and contrast instilled for confirming proximal tubal obstruction observed on HSG.

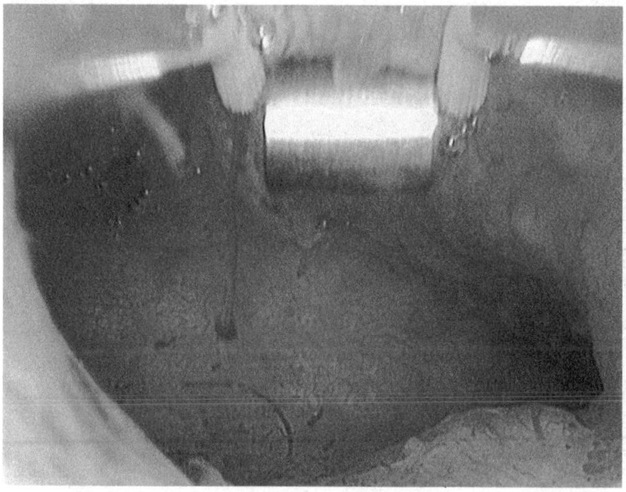

**Figure 10.6** Endometrial cavity prior to ablation with a roller ball. (From Goldberg JM, Falcone T. *Atlas of Endoscopic Techniques in Gynecology*. London: WB Saunders; 2000:197.)

Hysteroscopic sterilization may be accomplished with insertion of coils in the tubal ostia. This is desirable, as no incision is needed as for laparoscopic sterilization, and it can be performed in the office. The Essure device has been FDA approved in the United States since 2002. Under hysteroscopic viewing, the Essure coil is placed in the proximal portion of the fallopian tube. Over time, chronic inflammation around the coil leads to tubal blockage. A follow-up HSG is needed in 3 months to make sure the tubes are indeed blocked. This procedure is not reversible. Short-term efficacy studies suggest a rate equal to or greater than other tubal sterilization methods.

The risk of infection following hysteroscopy is low. Prophylactic antibiotics are not routinely administered.

## COMPLICATIONS

Complications of hysteroscopy are rare and are noted in less than 2% of the procedures. One study used a large database of 136,000 hysteroscopies and noted the significant complication rate to be 0.28% (Jansen, 2000). Complications included uterine perforation (0.12%), pelvic infection (0.01%), bleeding (0.03%), fluid overload from absorption of distending media (0.06%), and bladder or bowel injury (0.02%). Diagnostic hysteroscopy has a significantly lower complication rate than operative hysteroscopy (0.95%). The major complication of diagnostic hysteroscopy is uterine perforation, and office hysteroscopy has an incidence of 1 or 2 cases per 1000. Uterine perforation can be midline or lateral. Midline perforation rarely results in significant complications unless electrocautery or laser energy is used. Lateral perforation into the broad ligament can cause bleeding complications. Suspect uterine perforation if the operative view suddenly disappears, the fluid deficit suddenly increases, or the hysteroscope suddenly inserts farther than the fundus. Thermal injury to surrounding organs may occur with deep resections or perforations with the electrocautery instrument. If perforation is suspected during operative hysteroscopy, then an intraperitoneal evaluation may be performed either by laparoscopy or by laparotomy. Unrecognized uterine perforation might result in postoperative abdominal or pelvic pain beyond what is normally expected; abdominal distention, heavy vaginal bleeding, hypotension, nausea or vomiting or hematuria, or bowel injury, particularly thermal injuries, may present with delayed onset of symptoms and often go unrecognized.

Infection and postprocedure hemorrhage are rare. If bleeding is excessive, electrocautery coagulation at the bleeding point may be sufficient. If not, others have reported injecting dilute vasopressin at the bleeding point with caution to avoid intraarterial injection, which can result in hypertension, bradycardia, cardiovascular collapse, and even death. An inflatable 30-cc Foley balloon can be inserted via the cervix, inflated, and left for 12 to 24 hours to tamponade the uterine cavity, facilitating hemostasis. Some women develop a severe vasovagal reflex from cervical dilation and instrumentation of the uterine cavity that can result in syncope. This reflex can be diminished by giving the patient IV fluids or by performing a paracervical block. Use of the Trendelenburg position or having the patient lie supine with the legs raised can be beneficial in recovery.

Table 10.2 summarizes the complications with diagnostic and operative hysteroscopy.

The potential complications of the distending media include anaphylaxis to dextran, circulatory overload with $D_5W$, pulmonary and cerebral edema, hyponatremia, seizure, coagulopathies, and the potential of air or gas embolism with carbon dioxide. Monitoring of the patient's fluid status is important because of problems with absorption of distending media, leading to volume overload and electrolyte imbalance. Cardiac arrest has been reported with uterine insufflation with carbon dioxide when unmonitored amounts of gas were used.

Some long-term complications exist after endometrial ablation, including recurrent or persistent abnormal bleeding. In a 2013 Cochrane review comparing endometrial destruction with hysterectomy, both procedures were successful at achieving a satisfactory reduction in menstrual bleeding (Fergusson, 2013). Hysterectomy was associated with longer operative and recovery times, and patients were more likely to experience postoperative complications. Women who underwent ablation were more likely to require a future definitive surgery than those who initially had a hysterectomy. Older women have a higher success rate, because menopause occurs before the recurrent bleeding problems or obstructive symptoms occur. The inability to evaluate the endometrium if bleeding recurs and the risk of a delay in diagnosis of endometrial cancer are added concerns. Pregnancy following an endometrial ablation can occur and is often complicated by the intrauterine scarring and contracture. This can result in abnormal placentation including placenta accreta or percreta, uterine rupture, higher spontaneous abortion rates, preterm delivery, ectopic pregnancy, and fetal limb malformations. Pain from obstructed menses can occur with hematometra or postablation tubal sterilization syndrome (Sharp, 2012). Residual areas of endometrium that are not ablated or regrown can lead to trapped bleeding within the uterine cavity, leading to retrograde bleeding or cornual or uterine hematometra. (Additional risks are listed in Box 10.3.)

The American College of Obstetricians and Gynecologists (ACOG) published guidelines in 2010 that contain a section on free-standing surgical units where many operative hysteroscopy procedures are performed. Care must be taken to ensure adequate training of personnel, knowledge, uses, maintenance and cleaning of equipment, and safety protocols for sedation or anesthesia complications or surgical complications. Emergency care and hospital transfer protocols are required in writing in many states when more than minimal sedation or local anesthetic infiltration in peripheral nerves is required.

**Box 10.3 Long-Term Complications of Endometrial Ablation Devices**

Persistent bleeding
Central hematometra
Cornual hematometra
Postablation tubal sterilization syndrome (PATSS)
Retrograde bleeding
Inability to evaluate the endometrium if bleeding recurs
Delay in diagnosis of endometrial cancer
Pregnancy
Postablation cornual endosalpingoblastosis

## LAPAROSCOPY

Laparoscopy has radically changed the clinical practice of gynecology. As an often outpatient surgical technique, laparoscopy provides a window to directly visualize pelvic anatomy as well as a technique for performing many operations with less morbidity than laparotomy (Fig. 10.7).

The first human laparoscopy was first performed in 1910 in Sweden. By the mid-1970s, laparoscopy had been adopted as the method of choice for female sterilization. Once laparoscopic cholecystectomy was embraced and new instrumentation developed, the way was paved for laparoscopic hysterectomy. In 1989 the first laparoscopic hysterectomy was preformed, and by 2009, 20% of hysterectomies were laparoscopic and an additional 5% were completed using a robotic approach.

The advantages of less postoperative pain, shorter recovery time, and shorter hospital stays are obvious when laparoscopy is compared with laparotomy. This is particularly true in the obese woman who has increased risk of wound infection, thromboembolic events, and other complications from laparotomy. These events are significantly less with a laparoscopic approach. Laparoscopic visualization is excellent because the video camera and endoscope magnify the image.

### *LAPAROSCOPIC INDICATIONS AND CONTRAINDICATIONS*

The present indications for laparoscopy are almost identical to those for laparotomy, and the laparoscope is now utilized for more complicated surgery such as hysterectomy with pelvic and paraaortic lymph node dissection for endometrial cancer. The most common indication used to be female sterilization but is now diagnostic laparoscopy, and this includes the evaluation of pelvic pain. Other indications include removal of ectopic pregnancies, resection or ablation of endometriosis, ovarian cystectomy or salpingo-oophorectomy, myomectomy, hysterectomy, lysis of adhesions, removal of intraperitoneal intrauterine device, lymph node dissections, and urogynecologic procedures.

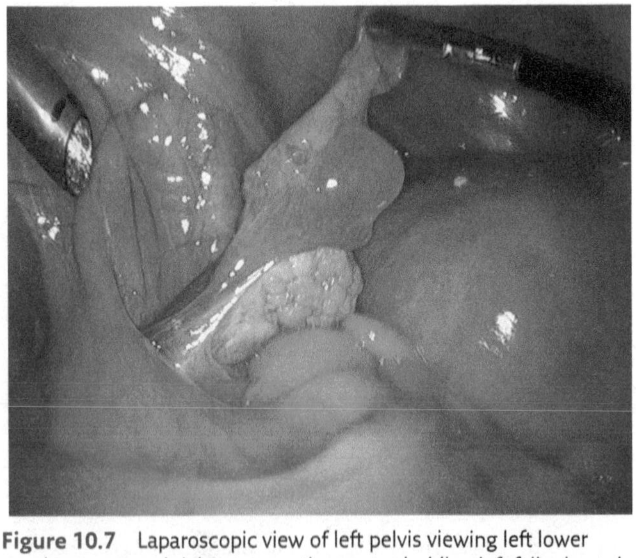

**Figure 10.7** Laparoscopic view of left pelvis viewing left lower quadrant port and right atraumatic grasper holding left fallopian tube with paratubal cyst and normal ovary. (Courtesy of Dr. Seine Chiang, University of Washington.)

Laparoscopic ovarian biopsy (for karyotyping in certain endocrine disorders) is possible. The limits and indications of surgical procedures via the laparoscope depend on the experience and judgment of the gynecologist.

Absolute contraindications to laparoscopy include intestinal obstruction, hemoperitoneum that produces hemodynamic instability, severe cardiovascular or pulmonary disease, and tuberculous peritonitis. Relative contraindications, in which each case must be individualized, include morbid obesity, large hiatal hernia, advanced malignancy, generalized peritonitis or peritonitis following previous surgery, inflammatory bowel disease, and extensive intraabdominal scarring. Even with these relative contraindications, the surgeon may attempt laparoscopy.

## *LAPAROSCOPIC EQUIPMENT AND TECHNIQUES*

Laparoscopy may be performed under local, regional, or general anesthesia. For simple procedures, many prefer local anesthesia for its safety, with the addition of conscious sedation by intravenous medication. Regional anesthesia is possible, but the Trendelenburg position needed for gravity to keep the bowels in the upper abdomen can be bothersome to the patient and restrict respiration. The risks associated with general anesthesia are one of the major hazards of laparoscopy. However, when operative laparoscopy is contemplated, general anesthesia is recommended and ensures adequate muscle relaxation, patient comfort, and the ability to manipulate intraabdominal organs. The standard diagnostic laparoscope is 10 mm in diameter, but laparoscopes come in sizes varying from 2 to 10 mm. The microlaparoscopes are used primarily for diagnostic evaluation. The 5-mm and 10-mm forms are widely utilized. Laparoscopic telescopes come in 0-degree to 30-degree lens angles, but the 0-degree type is most commonly used. Most laparoscopes are 30 cm long and provide a field of vision of 60 to 75 degrees. The inferior margin of the umbilicus is the preferred site of entry, as this is the thinnest area of the abdominal wall. Alternative sites are detailed in Figure 10.8. The choice of gas to develop the pneumoperitoneum depends on the choice of anesthesia. Nitrous oxide is preferable with local anesthesia, but carbon dioxide is the choice with general anesthesia. Nitrous oxide is nonflammable but does support combustion. Carbon dioxide quickly forms carbonic acid on the moist parietal peritoneal surface, which results in considerable discomfort to a patient without regional or general anesthesia.

A Veress needle (Fig. 10.9; radially dilating trocar with Veress-type needle) has a retractable cutting point that is used for entry into the abdominal cavity for the purpose of insufflating the abdomen with gas for laparoscopy. A trocar is a blunt, bladed, or optical device for entering the abdominal cavity for laparoscopy and is the cannula for holding the laparoscope or laparoscopic instruments (Fig. 10.10). Secondary puncture trocars vary from 5 mm (bipolar forceps, 5-mm telescope, suction/irrigation device, vessel sealing, cutting or coagulation devices), 7 or 8 mm in width (Filshie clips for sterilization), to 10 to 12 mm for pouches to remove specimens, or a morcellating device for removing fibroids or a uterus.

There are three techniques to access the abdomen. First, Veress needle insertion is used to create a pneumoperitoneum followed by trocar placement. Second, direct trocar placement in a noninsufflated abdomen has been described. Third, an open or Hasson technique can be used when adhesions are expected, particularly under the umbilicus. When using the Veress technique,

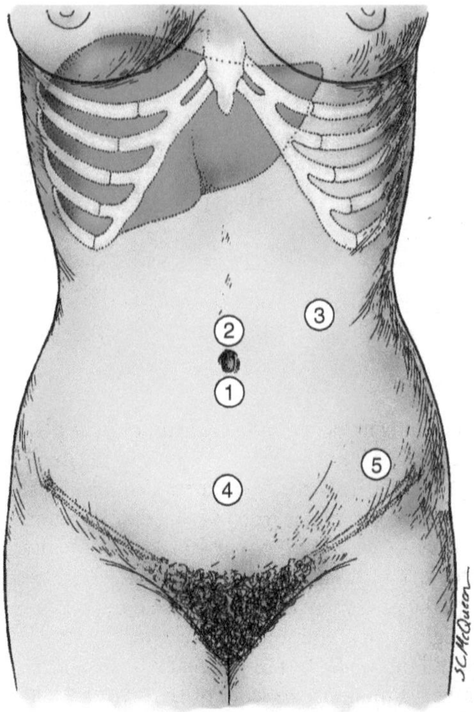


**Figure 10.8** Usual sites for insertion of insufflating needle in laparoscopy: *(1)* infraumbilical fold, *(2)* supraumbilical fold, *(3)* left costal margin, *(4)* midway between umbilicus and pubis, and *(5)* left McBurney's point. (From Corson SL. Operating room preparation and basic techniques. In: Phillips JM, ed. *Laparoscopy*. Baltimore: Williams & Wilkins; 1977. Copyright 1977 by the Williams & Wilkins Co., Baltimore.)

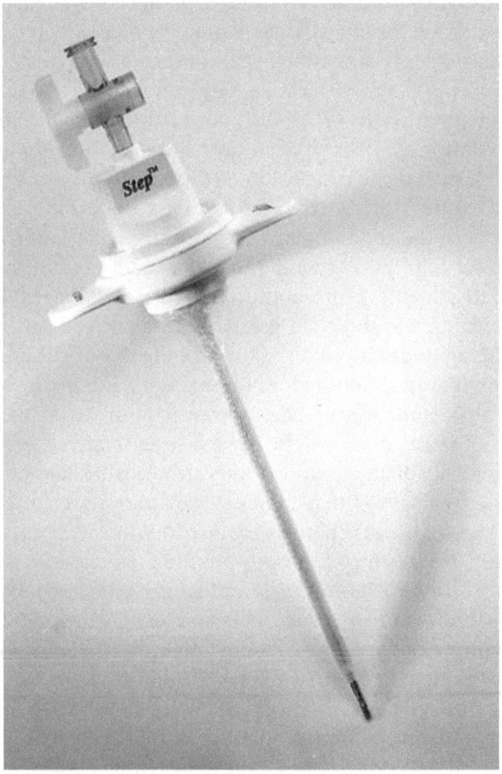


**Figure 10.9** Radially dilating trocar with Veress-type needle. (From Beiber EJ, Sanfilippo JS, Horowitz IR. *Clinical Gynecology*. Philadelphia: Elsevier; 2006.)

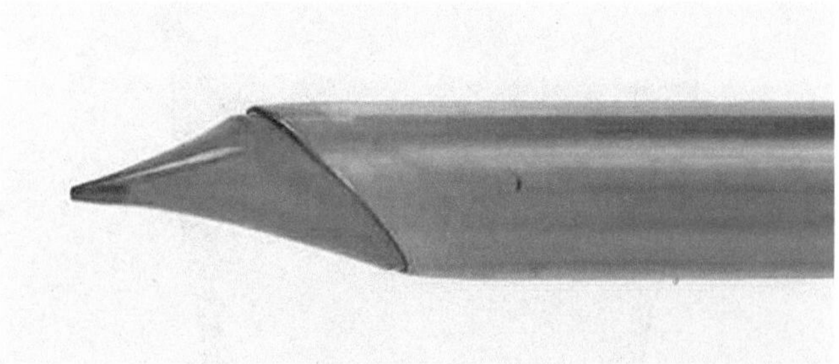

**Figure 10.10** Blunt-tip trocar for primary port. (From Beiber EJ, Sanfilippo JS, Horowitz IR. *Clinical Gynecology*. Philadelphia: Elsevier; 2006.)

a skin incision is made large enough to hold the planned trocar, which is usually 10 mm if using the umbilical site. The angle of the Veress needle insertion should vary according to the body mass index of the woman from 45 degrees in a normal weight woman to 90 degrees in an obese woman. Veress intraperitoneal pressure of ≤10 mm Hg is a reliable indicator of correct intraperitoneal needle placement, and insufflation of the carbon dioxide gas can begin. Left upper quadrant (Palmer point) laparoscopic entry should be considered in patients with suspected or known periumbilical adhesions, presence of an umbilical hernia, or after three failed insufflation attempts at the umbilicus.

Once the abdomen is insufflated to 15 mm Hg, the primary trocar can be inserted. Because it has been recognized that primary trocar placement leads to the majority of vascular and bowel injuries, many surgical products are available to potentially lessen these injuries, but none has proved safer than another. A bladed, blunt, or radial dilating trocar can be passed. A bladed cutting trocar may come with automatic blade retraction or a shield for safety. These require significantly less force to insert through the abdominal wall compared with blunt trocars. The resulting fascial defects are larger for cutting trocars than radial dilating trocars. The port may not be as fixed in this case. It is recommended that bladed port sites ≥10 mm should have fascial closure at the conclusion of the surgery to avoid postoperative hernia formation. Blunt trocars require more force for passage into the abdomen but theoretically cause fewer vascular and bowel injuries. A systematic review of 8 randomized trials with 720 patients (Antoniou, 2013) reported that abdominal wall bleeding was threefold greater with bladed trocars (9% vs. 3% with an odds ratio of 0.42), as was the risk of complications when excluding abdominal wall bleeding (0.7% vs. 0.2%). This argues that blunt trocars have a lower risk of trocar site bleeding, but a larger study will be needed to estimate visceral injury rates. Radially dilating blunt trocars are available, and one of the touted advantages is that even 10-mm port sites do not need fascial closure because hernias are rare in nonbladed port sites.

Direct trocar entry has been proposed to alleviate the difficulties with preperitoneal or intestinal gas insufflation with the Veress needle and to reduce operative time. There are studies supporting this technique. Disposable optical trocars are available to use a cannula that allows the laparoscope to visualize passing through the abdominal wall. They do not seem to reduce vascular and visceral injury, however, but do save time.

Open laparoscopy, often called the *Hasson technique*, may be used as an alternative to the Veress needle option. Instead of blind entry into the peritoneal cavity, a small incision is made in the fascia and parietal peritoneum. The cone is placed in the abdominal cavity under direct visual control. The fascia is secured to the sleeve of the cone to obtain an airtight seal. Open laparoscopy has not been proved to reduce the rate of bowel injury, but that is the theoretic benefit. Also, if the Veress needle technique fails to result in pneumoperitoneum, open laparoscopy is often an option. It is the procedure of choice if the patient has a history of multiple abdominal operations.

Once the primary trocar is in place, the telescope and camera can be attached and the pelvis visualized. Secondary trocars can be placed under direct visualization, which is why there are fewer vascular and bowel injuries with these trocars. Third and fourth puncture sites are often required for complex cases. Because each puncture site is a potential gas leak, high-flow insufflation equipment is necessary. In addition, several video monitoring screens are employed so that both the surgeon and assistant can work effectively. Unlike the short time needed for diagnostic laparoscopy, operative laparoscopy may require several hours.

Operative laparoscopy may be performed with mechanical instruments, including an extensive variety of scissors, scalpels, endoscopic syringes, myoma screws, suture devices, electrocautery instruments (both unipolar and bipolar), harmonic and vessel sealing devices for hemostasis and cutting, suction, irrigation, stapling devices, endoscopic clips, and laser instruments. During operative laparoscopy, stabilization of the pelvic organs is essential, such as traction and countertraction on the edges of an adhesion. Multiple trocar sites are needed so that the primary surgeon and assistant can use both hands. Uterine manipulators are particularly useful in laparoscopic hysterectomy. They are designed to aid in stabilizing and manipulating the uterus and identifying the cervicovaginal junction for cervix amputation.

The FDA approved robotic-assisted laparoscopy for use in gynecology in 2005. The only currently available system in the United States is the da Vinci Surgical System. The equipment is bulky and consists of a robot with three or four arms that hold the camera and surgical instruments, the camera and vision system, the console where the surgeon sits away from the patient bedside, and the wristed instruments that insert through the robotic arms and are controlled by the surgeon at the console. The camera is actually two cameras and allows for three-dimensional visualization via the computer image integrator. Other advantages include the added dexterity with the wristed instruments and ergonomic benefits for the surgeon. This can aid in surgeries that require a lot of suturing such as myomectomies or abdominal sacral colpopexy and complex gynecologic oncology or severe endometriosis procedures. Disadvantages include the high cost of the system and maintenance, lack of haptic feedback for the surgeon at the console, and increased operative time for docking the robot and the actual procedure.

## LAPAROSCOPIC PROCEDURES

Laparoscopy has made outpatient sterilization available to women throughout the world. Cumulative 10-year pregnancy rates vary between 8/1000 and 37/1000. Sterilization is accomplished with electrocautery, titanium, or spring-loaded clips. Because of the serious complications with unipolar cautery, most cautery sterilization procedures are performed with bipolar coagulation of approximately 3 cm of the isthmic portion of the fallopian tube without division. Use of a current meter is recommended

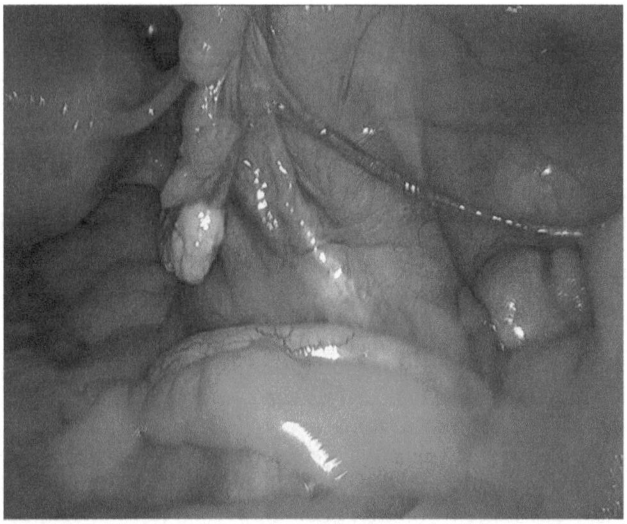

**Figure 10.11** Laparoscopic view of a woman with right lower quadrant pain and an adhesion stringing between the fallopian tube and the bowel near the cecum. Normal-appearing appendix inferiorly. (Courtesy of Dr. Seine Chiang, University of Washington.)

to indicate when complete coagulation has occurred, as visual inspection is not an accurate indication. Mechanical occlusion devices commonly used in the United States include the silicone rubber band (Falope ring), the spring-loaded clip (Hulka-Clemens clip), and the titanium clip lined with silicone rubber (Filshie clip). The ring or clip should be placed on the narrow isthmus so that the size of the appliance conforms to the diameter of the fallopian tube.

There are both diagnostic and therapeutic indications for laparoscopy in infertile women. Tubal patency and mobility can be directly observed via the laparoscope. Laparoscopy is a more sophisticated and accurate method of diagnosing tubal problems during an infertility investigation than HSG. Chromopertubation with an innocuous dye, such as indigo carmine, demonstrates tubal patency during laparoscopy. Comparative studies have documented that HSG discovers only 50% of the peritubal disease diagnosed by direct visualization via the laparoscope. Laparoscopy is able to confirm or rule out intrinsic pelvic disorders, such as endometriosis or chronic pelvic inflammatory disease with adhesions. It is possible not only to describe and stage the extent of endometriosis or pelvic adhesions but also to treat them. Adhesions can be lysed, endometrioma cysts can be removed, and areas of endometriosis can be ablated by electrocautery, laser, or completely excised, which is necessary for deep endometriotic implants (Fig. 10.11).

The management of pelvic pain has been dramatically changed by the laparoscope. The differential diagnosis of acute pain may be defined by direct visualization of the fallopian tubes, ovaries, and appendix. Laparoscopy may be used in the management of acute pelvic infection, taking direct bacterial cultures of purulent material from the tubes, draining a tubo-ovarian abscess, or removing a tubo-ovarian abscess complex with unilateral salpingo-oophorectomy. These direct transabdominal cultures have changed our opinions concerning the clinical management of polymicrobial pelvic infections. The classic violin string adhesions between the liver and the abdominal wall are sometimes noted by directing the laparoscope into the upper right quadrant in women with

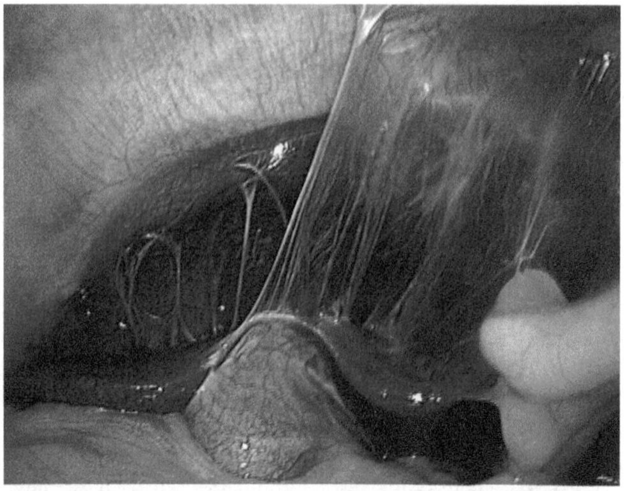

**Figure 10.12** Fitz-Hugh-Curtis syndrome in a patient with previous pelvic inflammatory disease. (From Goldberg JM, Falcone T. *Atlas of Endoscopic Techniques in Gynecology*. London: WB Saunders; 2000:71.)

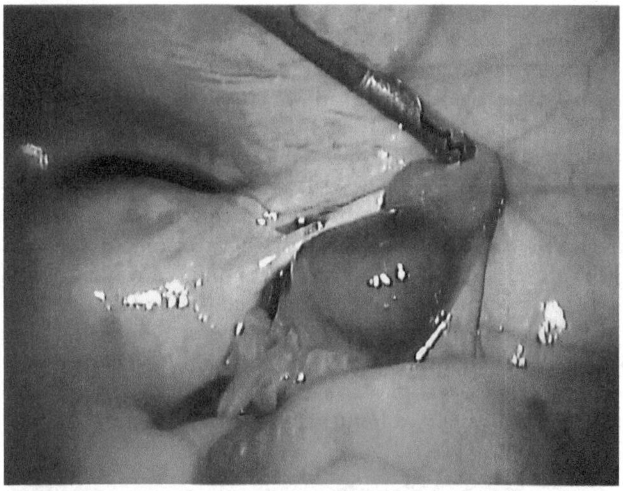

**Figure 10.13** Ectopic pregnancy in the right fallopian tube. (Courtesy of B. Beller, MD, Eugene, OR.)

prior pelvic inflammatory disease (Fig. 10.12). Sometimes the enigma of chronic pelvic pain may be solved by the findings at laparoscopy. Following the procedure, a plan for long-term management of the pain can be discussed with the patient.

Laparoscopic treatment of ectopic pregnancy most often involves salpingotomy but also may include salpingectomy (Fig. 10.13). HCG titers must be followed after conservative surgery (salpingotomy) until the titers fall to zero (usually 3 to 4 weeks) to ensure that all trophoblastic tissue has been removed. Tubal patency and subsequent pregnancy rates are comparable between laparoscopic techniques and laparotomy.

Laparoscopic hysterectomy is one area of considerable research. If vaginal hysterectomy cannot be done (which has lower complication rates, lower costs, and better outcomes), then laparoscopic hysterectomy should be considered over abdominal hysterectomy. Many considerations must go into this decision, such as the size of the uterus, adnexal disease with risk for ovarian cancer, severe endometriosis, or adhesions. The Cochrane Database of Systematic Reviews (Nieboer, 2009) considered 34 randomized trials of hysterectomy route. Laparoscopic hysterectomy compared with abdominal hysterectomy was associated with faster return to normal activity, shorter hospital stay, lower intraoperative blood loss, fewer wound infections, longer operating time, and a higher rate of bladder and ureter injuries. Figure 10.14 shows the beginning of a laparoscopic hysterectomy for uterine fibroids with creation of the bladder flap.

Laparoscopic myomectomy has been studied in two randomized controlled trials with comparison with myomectomy by minilaparotomy. This can be technically challenging laparoscopically because of the dissection and suturing required. The laparoscopic approach resulted in less blood loss, reduced length of postoperative ileus, shorter hospital stay, reduced use of pain medications, and more rapid return to normal activities, but a longer operative time. For unexplained infertility, both approaches improved reproductive outcomes similarly.

Operative laparoscopy has additionally been used for laparoscopic-assisted hysterectomy, salpingo-oophorectomy, salpingostomy and fimbrioplasty, tubal reanastomosis, appendectomy, uterosacral ligament transection, presacral neurectomy, retropubic bladder neck suspensions, and complex urogynecologic procedures. Laparoscopy may be used for major cancer staging, including paraaortic and pelvic lymphadenectomy.

Newer laparoscopic equipment using robotics has increased the ease at which minimally invasive major pelvic surgery can occur (Fig. 10.15). Cases that can be extremely challenging with traditional laparoscopy are being done with increasing frequency with robotics. Most of the published studies to date are nonrandomized and retrospective case series comparing robotic cases with historical controls. There are data showing safety and feasibility of robot-assisted surgery for numerous procedures, including tubal reanastomosis, myomectomy, hysterectomy, adnexectomy, pelvic, and paraaortic lymph node sampling and abdominal sacral colpopexy for pelvic organ prolapse. Compared with conventional laparoscopic surgery, robotic surgery achieved reduced blood loss and fewer conversions to laparotomy during the staging of endometrial cancer.

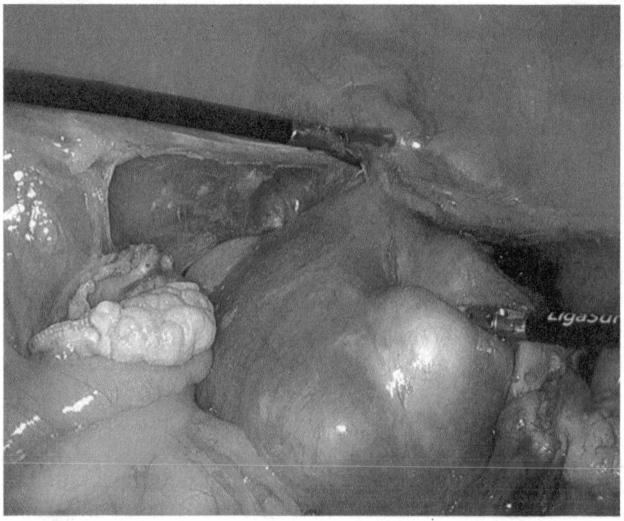

**Figure 10.14** The beginning of a laparoscopic hysterectomy for uterine fibroids showing the creation of the bladder flap with the left grasper elevating the bladder peritoneum and a bipolar/cutting device in the right hand. (Courtesy of Dr. Seine Chiang, University of Washington.)

There has been a rapid industry-driven increase in the performance of robotic-assisted hysterectomy. Although only 0.5% of all hysterectomies were performed robotically in 2007, the number increased to 9.5% in 2010 (Wright, 2013). Growth has continued to increase at an estimated 25% per year. This increased gynecologic utilization of the robot for primarily benign hysterectomies has occurred despite limited outcomes data demonstrating patient benefit compared to alternative surgical methods.

Robotic hysterectomy has been shown to have increased surgical complications, operating room time, and costs. A 2014 study by Dayaratna and Goldberg reported that mean total hospital costs for vaginal hysterectomy were \$7903, \$10,069 for laparoscopically assisted vaginal hysterectomy (LAVH), \$11,558 for laparoscopic, and \$13,429 for robotic hysterectomy ($P < .0001$). Net hospital income (insurer reimbursement – hospital cost) was \$1260 for vaginal hysterectomy. The hospital incurred losses of \$1306 for LAVH, \$4049 for laparoscopic hysterectomy, and \$4564 for robotic hysterectomy ($P = .03$).

Robotic hysterectomy has shown benefit over total abdominal hysterectomy (TAH) in regard to shorter hospitalization and a faster recovery. The same improvements over TAH, however, have been demonstrated with vaginal hysterectomy and laparoscopic hysterectomy, with more outcomes data. In appropriate candidates, the vaginal route of surgery is always preferable.

In 2013, ACOG recommended that robotic hysterectomy be limited for unusual and complex clinical conditions in which improved outcomes over standard minimally invasive approaches have been proved (Breeden, 2013).

## LAPAROSCOPIC SURGERY IN PREGNANCY

Laparoscopic surgery can sometimes be safely performed on the pregnant patient. The benefits to this approach over an open procedure are the same as in the nonpregnant patient. In addition, laparoscopic surgery may provide better visualization and less manipulation of the gravid uterus.

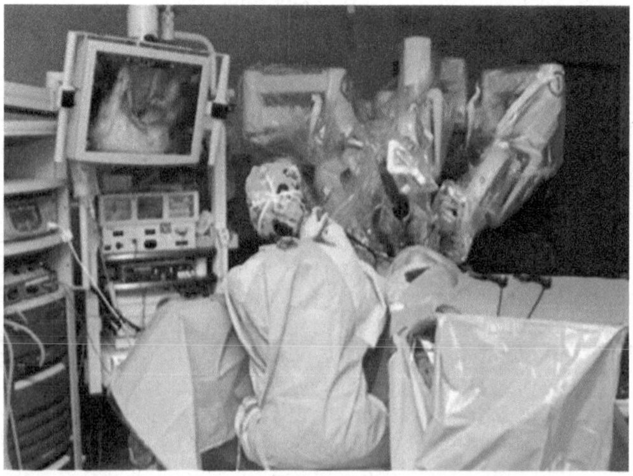

**Figure 10.15** Robotic surgery being performed. (Courtesy of Rosanne Kho, MD.)

Indications for laparoscopy in pregnancy include, but are not limited to, suspected appendicitis, ovarian torsion, and gallbladder disease. Laparoscopic surgery can be undertaken in all of pregnancy's trimesters; however, the optimal time to operate is early in the second trimester. In the third trimester, surgery may be technically difficult due to the enlarged uterus. Although currently used general anesthetic agents are not believed to have significant teratogenic effects, the data are limited.

To reduce compression of the vena cava and the subsequent effect on cardiac output and placental blood flow, pregnant patients are positioned in supine or lithotomy with a leftward tilt. Insufflation of the abdomen to pressures above 15 mm Hg may affect maternal and fetal physiology, including a reduction of maternal cardiac output, an increased risk for maternal respiratory acidosis, and a decrease in placental perfusion. Thus it is best for intraabdominal pressure to be maintained between 8 to 12 mm Hg.

In the second and third trimesters of pregnancy, initial abdominal entry has an increased risk of inadvertently injuring the enlarged uterus. To decrease this risk, an open entry technique or entry in the left-upper quadrant at the Palmer point should be considered. Subsequent trocars are inserted under direct visualization. Uterine manipulators that are placed through the cervix should not be used. Instead, a sponge stick in the vagina can be used to gently tilt the uterus.

The American College of Chest Physicians (ACCP) guidelines recommend thromboprophylaxis for all pregnant patients undergoing surgery. Mechanical compression devices are reasonable for shorter laparoscopic procedures. The addition of low-molecular-weight heparin is suggested for procedures lasting longer than 45 minutes. Early ambulation should be encouraged postoperatively. Prophylactic tocolytics are not routinely recommended. If the fetus is of a viable gestational age, fetal heart rate monitoring may be performed before and after the surgical procedure.

## LAPAROSCOPIC COMPLICATIONS

The major categories of complications with laparoscopy are laceration of blood vessels, intestinal and urinary tract injuries, including trocar and thermal injuries, incisional hernias, and cardiorespiratory problems arising from the pneumoperitoneum (Box 10.4). One complication has remained unchanged for 25 years. At least 50% of the major laparoscopic complications arise before the planned surgery starts and occur with accessing the abdomen. Most of these injuries are with the primary trocar placement at the umbilicus and involve major vascular injuries or the bowel. A Cochrane review (Ahmad, 2012) compared an open-entry technique with the Veress needle and did not find a difference in the incidence of visceral or vascular injury; however, an open-entry technique did reduce the rate of failed entry.

Several studies have evaluated the incidence of complications with operative laparoscopy. A large, multicenter French study of 29,966 laparoscopies showed a high frequency of trocar injuries with a total complication rate of 4.64 per thousand laparoscopies. Complications increase with the age of the patient and the complexity of the procedure. The overall rate of complications from large series of operative laparoscopy varies from 0.2% to 2%. Data were compiled from a series of injuries resulting from abdominal entry and laparoscopic access injuries reported to large insurance data banks (Chandler, 2001). The series included general surgery as well as gynecology from both the United States and other countries. Over a 20-year period, the data bank collected 594 reports of organ injury, 33% in gynecology patients. Importantly, 50% of bowel injuries were unrecognized for 24 hours or more. Sixty-five deaths were reported. Age older than 59 years and delayed diagnosis of injury were independently associated with mortality in this series. A systematic review of gynecology bowel injury from 90 studies found the overall incidence was 1 in 769 cases (Llarena, 2015). More complex surgeries resulted in higher injury rates. Hysterectomy led to the highest bowel injury incidence at 1 in 256. Most injuries occurred during abdominal access and insufflation using a Veress needle or trocar. A meta-analysis of 27 randomized controlled trials compared laparoscopy and laparotomy for benign gynecologic procedures. The overall risk of complication was 8.9% with laparoscopy compared with 15.2 with laparotomy (relative risk 0.6). The risk of major complications was the same at 1.4%, so the risk of minor complication was higher in the laparotomy group.

Laceration of the aorta, inferior vena cava, or iliac vessels is a surgical emergency. Because abdominal wall hematomas are usually subfascial in location, care must be taken to avoid the epigastric vessels. For safety, it has been recommended that lateral trocars be placed at least 5 cm above the symphysis and at least 8 cm from the midline (Hurd, 1994). The Veress needle or the trocar may produce intestinal injuries. Thermal injuries may be recognized at the time of surgery, but if they are not recognized intraoperatively, significant delays in recognition can lead to septicemia and death. The incidence of ureteral injuries varies from 1% to 4% with laparoscopic dissection of the cardinal ligaments.

The risk of incisional hernia is increased for port sites of 12 mm or greater and extraumbilical sites (0.17% to 0.23%). Many of these herniations occur despite fascial closure at the initial surgery. Clinical symptoms include a bulge at the incision site, which may be painful to a bowel obstruction or infarction.

Complications directly related to the pneumoperitoneum include pneumothorax, diminished venous return, gas embolism, and cardiac arrhythmias. It is important not to develop pressures greater than 20 mm Hg in establishing the pneumoperitoneum. High pressures impede venous return and limit excursion of the diaphragm. A rare but life-threatening complication of laparoscopy is gas embolism, which produces hypotension

**Box 10.4 Intraoperative and Delayed Laparoscopic Surgery Risks**

- Bleeding
  Laceration of major blood vessels; epigastric, obturator, iliac, vena cava, aorta
  Surgical site bleeding
- Trocar or Veress needle injury
- Intestinal injury; thermal or direct instrument
- Urinary tract injury; thermal or direct instrument
- Anesthetic complication
- Equipment malfunction
- Other endoscopic instrument injury
- Other thermal injury
- Subcutaneous emphysema

and the classical "mill wheel" murmur that can be heard over the entire precordium. The patient with this complication should be turned on her left side and the frothy blood aspirated by a central venous catheter directed into the right side of the heart. Other rare complications include incisional hernias at the site of the 10- to 12-mm trocar sites. This has been estimated to occur in 1 in 5000 procedures. Metastases from ovarian malignancies to the laparoscopic wound site are also a rare but real problem.

### CONTROVERSY REGARDING POWER UTERINE OR FIBROID MORCELLATION

Power or electrical morcellators are composed of a rapidly rotating cylindrical sharp blade within a tube through which strips of cut tissue are then extracted. By enabling removal of pieces of uterine or fibroid tissue through small incisions, power morcellation has allowed the performance of laparoscopic or robotic supracervical hysterectomy and myomectomy. Primarily through industry driven efforts, the number of laparoscopic and robotic hysterectomy has significantly increased. Although the goal should be converting many procedures from a laparotomy to a laparoscopic approach, many hysterectomies that should be performed vaginally have similarly moved to laparoscopic or robotic routes due to physician preference.

The reported prevalence of uterine sarcoma, a type of malignancy that includes leiomyosarcoma, in women undergoing hysterectomy or myomectomy for suspected fibroids is approximately 1 in 350. During the morcellation process, small pieces of uterine tissue may be disseminated and left within the abdomen.

On November 24, 2014, the U.S. FDA issued a communication entitled *UPDATED Laparoscopic Uterine Power Morcellation in Hysterectomy and Myomectomy: FDA Safety Communication* (FDA, 2014). Due to the risk of spreading the sarcoma tissue within the abdomen, decreasing survival, "the FDA is warning against the use of laparoscopic power morcellators in the majority of women undergoing myomectomy or hysterectomy for the treatment of fibroids." As a result of this communication, the majority of hospitals have banned the usage of power morcellation for gynecologic surgery. Many manufacturers have completely taken their power morcellators off the market. Thus laparoscopic and robotic supracervical hysterectomy and myomectomy can no longer be performed. Instead alternative routes for these procedures, such as vaginal or minilaparotomy, should be considered.

In summary, laparoscopy, more than any other advance, has changed the clinical practice of gynecology since the 1970s. Today's obstetric/gynecologic residents have a difficult time contemplating the practice of the specialty prior to the introduction of the "silver tube." Laparoscopy provides a window for the diagnosis of infertility, pelvic pain, ectopic pregnancy, abdominal and pelvic trauma, staging the extent of pelvic disease, and the visual diagnosis of abnormal anatomy. Therapeutic uses of the laparoscope vary from female sterilization to hysterectomy and node sampling. The role of robotics is still being established, but benefits exist over laparotomy in nonrandomized but controlled trials, particularly in the gynecologic oncology population.

## PATIENT SAFETY IN THE SURGICAL ENVIRONMENT

Many regulatory agencies, hospitals, medical societies and organizations, physicians, and staff have been striving for improvements in patient safety. Wrong-site surgery, wrong-patient surgery, wrong-side surgery, wrong-part surgery, and retained foreign objects have all been reported. Many factors have been associated with wrong-site surgery, including multiple surgical teams being involved in a case, multiple procedures being done during a single case, time pressures, and morbid obesity. In 2015, the Joint Commission for Hospital Accreditation published national patient safety goals for improving surgical safety. The protocol recommended a preprocedure verification process, marking the operative site and performing a "time out." A time out promotes patient safety by checking items such as confirming correct patient in two ways, correct surgical site, and procedure(s). The commission further recommends labeling all medications in syringes, cups, and basins. The World Health Organization published a suggested surgical safety checklist to further improve care. Before induction of anesthesia, the first checklist set is done and might include items for team review like patient allergies, airway risks, and estimated blood loss. Before the skin incision, another team review occurs with introductions of all personnel and roles, antibiotic prophylaxis infused if indicated, deep vein thrombosis prophylaxis given or in place if indicated, any equipment issues or concerns voiced, and essential imaging displayed. Before the conclusion of the procedure, the third part of the checklist is completed and includes the name of the procedure, the correct instrument, and sponge and needle counts; the checklist also ensures that specimens are properly labeled and key concerns for the patient recovery are discussed. Good communication between team members appears to be another important factor in patient safety.

## KEY POINTS

- The most frequent problem in performing endometrial sampling is cervical stenosis or spasm; it is also a problem for hysteroscopy, and this increases the risk of uterine perforation.
- Major indications for hysteroscopy include abnormal uterine bleeding, removal of endometrial polyps or submucous myomas, endometrial ablations, retained IUDs, desire of no incision sterilization, intrauterine adhesions diagnosis and treatment, infertility, resection of a uterine septum, and recurrent pregnancy loss.
- The endometrial lining may be ablated through the hysteroscope in women with abnormal bleeding or menorrhagia who have a normal uterine cavity and are poor surgical candidates, those who wish to retain their uterus, and those who do not desire further childbearing.
- Older resectoscopic and second-generation nonresectoscopic endometrial ablation devices appear to be equivalent with respect to successful reduction in menstrual flow and patient satisfaction at 1 year.

## KEY POINTS—cont'd

- Vaginal misoprostol administration the night before the hysteroscopic procedure can aid in cervical softening.
- A paracervical block with local anesthetic is the best method of pain control for outpatient hysteroscopy compared with topical or intracervical anesthesia.
- Complications of hysteroscopy include uterine perforation with risk of injury to the surrounding vascular and visceral structures, pelvic infection, bleeding, and absorption of the distending media.
- The primary laparoscopic trocar placement leads to the >50% of vascular and bowel injuries in gynecologic laparoscopy.
- Absolute contraindications to laparoscopy include a hemoperitoneum that has produced hemodynamic instability, bowel obstruction, advanced malignancy, large abdominal masses, severe cardiovascular disease, and tuberculous peritonitis.
- The incidence of complications with operative laparoscopy varies from 0.2% to 2%. Thermal bowel injuries often go unrecognized intraoperatively, and diagnostic delays can be life threatening.

## KEY REFERENCES


Ahmad G, O'Flynn H, Duffy JMN, Phillips K, Watson A. Laparoscopic techniques. *Cochrane Database Syst Rev.* 2012;2. CD006583.

American College of Obstetricians and Gynecologists (ACOG). Patient safety in the surgical environment. ACOG Committee Opinion No. 464. *Obstet Gynecol.* 2010;116:786-790.

Antoniou SA, Antoniou GA, Koch OO, Pointner R, Granderath FA. Blunt versus bladed trocars in laparoscopic surgery: a systematic review and meta-analysis of randomized trials. *Surg Endosc.* 2013;27(7):2312-2320.

Breeden JT. *Statement on robotic surgery by ACOG President James T.Breeden, MD*; 2013. Available at http://www.acog.org/About-ACOG/News-Room/News-Releases/2013/Statement-on-Robotic-Surgery.

Chandler JG, Corson SL, Way LW. Three spectra of laparoscopic entry access injuries. *J Am Coll Surg.* 2001;192:478.

Dayaratna S, Goldberg J, Harrington C, Leiby BE, McNeil JM. Hospital costs of total vaginal hysterectomy compared with other minimally invasive hysterectomy. *Am J Obstet Gynecol.* 2014;210(2):120.e1-120.e6.

Feldman S, Shapter A, Welch WR, et al. Two-year follow-up of 263 patients with post/perimenopausal vaginal bleeding and negative initial biopsy. *Gynecol Oncol.* 1994;55:56.

Fergusson RJ, Lethaby A, Shepperd S, Farguhar C. Endometrial resection and ablation versus hysterectomy for heavy menstrual bleeding. *Cochrane Database Syst Rev.* 2013;11. CD000329.

Hurd WW, Bude RO, DeLancey JOL, et al. The location of abdominal wall blood vessels in relationship to abdominal landmarks apparent at laparoscopy. *Am J Obstet Gynecol.* 1994;171:642-646.

Jansen FW, Vredevoogd CB, Van Ulzen K, et al. Complications of hysteroscopy: a prospective, multicenter study. *Obstet Gynecol.* 2000;96:266.

Llarena NC, Shah AB, Milad MP. Bowel injury in gynecologic laparoscopy: a systematic review. *Obstet Gynecol.* 2015;125(6):1407-1417.

Ludwin A, Ludwin I, Banas T, Knafel A, Miedzyblocki M, Basta A. Diagnostic accuracy of sonohysterography, hysterosalpingography and diagnostic hysteroscopy in diagnosis of arcuate, septate and bicornuate uterus. *J Obstet Gynaecol Res.* 2011;37(3):178-186.

Nieboer TE, Johnson N, Lethaby A, et al. Surgical approach to hysterectomy for benign gynaecological disease. *Cochrane Database Syst Rev.* 2009;(3). CD003677.

Polyzos NP, Mauri D, Tsioras S, et al. Intraperitoneal dissemination of endometrial cancer cells after hysteroscopy: a systematic review and meta-analysis. *Int J Gynecol Cancer.* 2010;20(2):261-267.

Sharp HT. Endometrial ablation: postoperative complications. *Am J Obstet Gynecol.* 2012;207(4):242-247.

US Food and Drug Administration (FDA). *UPDATED Laparoscopic Uterine Power Morcellation in Hysterectomy and Myomectomy: FDA Safety Communication*; 2014. Available at http://www.fda.gov/MedicalDevices/Safety/AlertsandNotices/ucm424443.htm?source=govdelivery&utm_medium=email&utm_source=govdelivery.

Wright JD, Herzog TJ, Tsui J, et al. Nationwide trends in the performance of inpatient hysterectomy in the United States. *Obstet Gynecol.* 2013;122:233-241.


Suggested Readings can be found on ExpertConsult.com.

# 11 Congenital Abnormalities of the Female Reproductive Tract

## Anomalies of the Vagina, Cervix, Uterus, and Adnexa

*Beth W. Rackow, Roger A. Lobo, Gretchen M. Lentz*

Congenital abnormalities of the female reproductive tract are common and can affect the external genitalia and müllerian structures. They can be caused by genetic errors or by teratogenic events during embryonic development. Minor abnormalities may be of little consequence, but major abnormalities may lead to severe impairment of menstrual and reproductive functions and can be associated with anomalies of the urinary tract. This chapter reviews a number of such abnormalities and discusses diagnosis and treatment. Anomalies can present at varying times in a female's life—at birth, before puberty, with the onset of menses, and during a pregnancy with adverse pregnancy outcomes—but many women with congenital anomalies of the reproductive tract are asymptomatic. Based on large studies, the incidence of müllerian anomalies is considered to be 1% to 3% (Nahum, 1998). Because of the profound psychological effects such abnormalities can have, the gynecologist must approach the problems of genital and müllerian anomalies with sensitivity and an understanding of the effects on the female and her family. Most tertiary centers have a diverse multidisciplinary team available for the evaluation, treatment, and support of the patient with a serious disorder of sexual development.

## AMBIGUOUS GENITALIA

After delivery of the neonate, the obstetrician is often the provider who identifies the gender of the neonate. Thereafter, a more detailed assessment of the neonate's genital anatomy is necessary. The physician should systematically observe the newborn's perineum, beginning with the mons pubis. The clitoris should be noted for any obvious enlargement, the opening of the urethra should be identified, and the labia should be gently separated to see if the introitus can be visualized. If it is possible to separate the labia, the hymen may be observed. Generally, the hymen is perforate, revealing the entrance into the vagina. At times the labia are joined by filmy adhesions; these adhesions generally separate during childhood or can be treated with the application of estrogen cream when medically indicated. Posteriorly the labia fuse in the midline at the posterior fourchette of the perineum. Posterior to the perineal body the rectum can be visualized, and it should be tested to be sure that it is perforate. Meconium staining around the rectum is evidence for perforation. If there is doubt, the rectum may be penetrated with a moistened cotton-tipped swab. Palpation of the inguinal area and labia for any masses is also important.

In newborns with ambiguous genitalia, a range of abnormalities involving the clitoris, urethra, labia, and introitus can be identified, and immediate evaluation is necessary. The current terminology for individuals with abnormal external genitalia and associated issues is *disorder of sexual development (DSD),* and these disorders can be related to in utero androgen exposure (too much or too little) that has affected development of the external genitalia. Females (individuals with XX karyotypes) with masculinized or virilized external genitalia are identified as 46,XX DSD, and males (with 46,XY karyotypes) with undervirilized external genitalia are identified as 46,XY DSD (Lee, 2006). For females, the timing of antenatal (embryonic) exposure to androgen influences the degree of masculinization (Fig. 11.1) (Grumbach, 2003). The vaginal plate separates from the urogenital sinus at about 12 weeks of fetal development. Androgen exposure before 12 weeks can result in labioscrotal fusion and retention of the urogenital sinus, which creates a single tract that the urethra and vagina empty into before reaching the perineum. Androgen exposure after 12 weeks presents primarily with clitoral hypertrophy (Low, 2003).

The finding of ambiguous genitalia occurs in a wide spectrum of possibilities, from labioscrotal fusion and an enlarged clitoris with a penile urethra to a urogenital sinus to clitoromegaly and a normal introitus. With labial fusion, the physician should palpate the groins and labial folds for evidence of gonads. Gonads palpable in the inguinal canal, labioinguinal region, or labioscrotal folds are almost always testes, and this finding is typically seen in a male with ambiguous genitalia rather than a virilized female. Conversely, an infant with ambiguous genitalia but without palpable testes in the scrotum is more likely to be a virilized female, most often the result of congenital adrenal hyperplasia. A rectal examination may allow palpation of a cervix and uterus, thus helping with gender assignment. If a bifid clitoris and labial fusion are noted, this anomaly is usually associated with extrophy of the bladder. As with any congenital anomaly, the neonate should be thoroughly evaluated for other congenital anomalies.

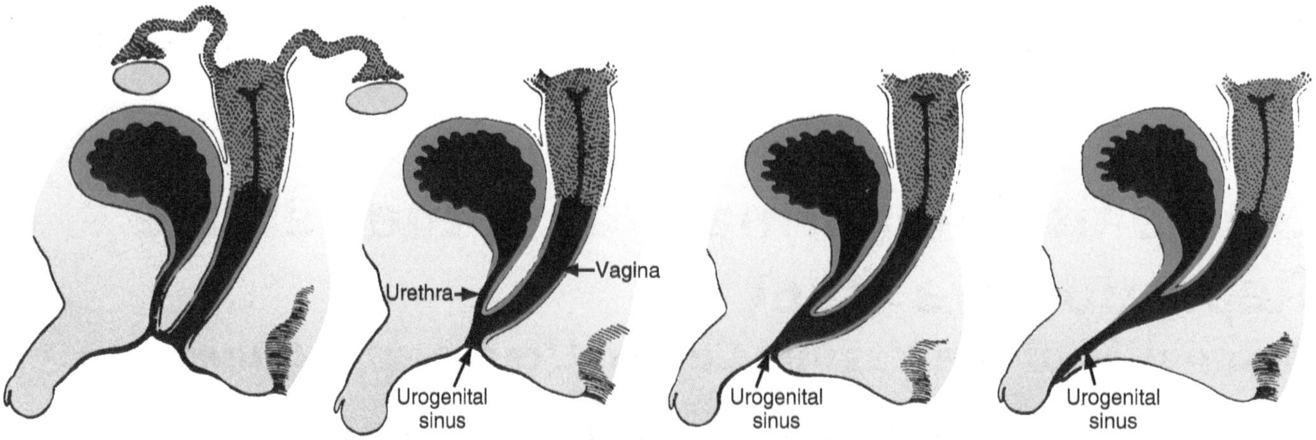


**Figure 11.1** 46,XX DSD induced by prenatal exposure to androgens. Exposure after 12th fetal week leads only to clitoral hypertrophy *(left)*. Exposure at progressively earlier stages of differentiation *(from left to right)* leads to retention of the urogenital sinus and labioscrotal fusion. If exposure occurs sufficiently early, the labia fuse to form a penile urethra. (From Grumbach MM, Hughes IA, Conte FA. Disorders of sex differentiation. In Larsen RP, Kronenberg HM, Melmed S, Polonsky KS, eds. *Williams Textbook of Endocrinology.* 10th ed. Philadelphia: WB Saunders; 2003:916.)

The initial evaluation of ambiguous genitalia involves checking a karyotype, performing a transabdominal pelvic ultrasound to assess pelvic anatomy, and obtaining blood for serum electrolytes and steroid hormone levels. In a female neonate, an ultrasound can easily identify a uterus because the estrogenized tissue is easy to visualize. If further evaluation of neonatal pelvic anatomy is necessary, cystoscopy and vaginoscopy can be performed with a pediatric cystoscope to assess the pelvic structures, including the location of the urethra and vagina and the presence of a cervix. Possible causes of 46,XX DSD include congenital adrenal hyperplasia, other genetic mutations that affect the steroid pathway, maternal ingestion of androgens, or maternal production of excess androgens (Box 11.1) (Grumbach, 2003).

It is important to systematically evaluate the newborn's genitalia to make the appropriate gender assignment, when possible. In the past, gender was assigned primarily on the principle of "phallic adequacy," with neonates with an ambiguous phallus being assigned female gender. In contrast, the current approach is to initiate a thorough evaluation of the neonate and to defer gender assignment until the clinical picture is clear. For the evaluation and management of an individual with DSD, most tertiary centers utilize a multidisciplinary team including medical genetics, pediatric urology, pediatric endocrinology, gynecology, and psychiatry (Allen, 2009).

**Box 11.1 Classification of 46,XX DSD**

**I. Androgen-Induced**

**A. Fetal Source**

1. Congenital adrenal hyperplasia
   a. Virilism only, defective adrenal 21-hydroxylation (CYP21)
   b. Virilism with salt-losing syndrome, defective adrenal 21-hydroxylation (CYP21)
   c. Virilism with hypertension, defective adrenal 11β-hydroxylation (CYP11B1)
   d. Virilism with adrenal insufficiency, deficient 3β-HSD 2 (HSD3B 2)
2. P450 aromatase (CYP19) deficiency
3. Glucocorticoid receptor gene mutation

**B. Maternal Source**

1. Iatrogenic
   a. Testosterone and related steroids
   b. Certain synthetic oral progestagens and rarely diethylstilbestrol
2. Virilizing ovarian or adrenal tumor
3. Virilizing luteoma of pregnancy
4. Congenital virilizing adrenal hyperplasia in mother*

**C. Undetermined Source**

1. Virilizing luteoma of pregnancy

**II. Non—Androgen-Induced Disturbances in Differentiation of Urogenital Structures**

From Grumbach MM, Hughes IA, Conte FA. Disorders of sex differentiation. In: Larsen RP, Kronenberg HM, Melmed S, Polonsky KS, eds. *Williams Textbook of Endocrinology.* 10th ed. Philadelphia: Saunders; 2003.

*In pregnant patient whose disease is poorly controlled or who is noncompliant, especially during the first trimester.

## PERINEAL AND HYMENAL ANOMALIES

### Clitoral Anomalies

In an adult female, the clitoris is generally 1 to 1.5 cm long and 0.5 cm wide in the nonerect state. The glans is partially covered by a hood of skin. The urethra opens near the base of the clitoris. Abnormalities of the clitoris are unusual, although it may be enlarged because of androgen stimulation. In such circumstances the shaft of the clitoris may be quite enlarged and partial development of a penile urethra may have occurred (Fig. 11.2) (Verkauf, 1970). Extreme cases of androgen stimulation are generally associated with fusion of the labia. These findings occur in infants with congenital adrenal hyperplasia and in those exposed in utero to exogenous or endogenous androgens (Fig. 11.3) (Black, 2003). Similar in appearance, males with partial androgen insensitivity syndrome have underdeveloped male external genitalia and a small phallus that appears as clitoral hypertrophy (Fig. 11.4) (Black, 2003).

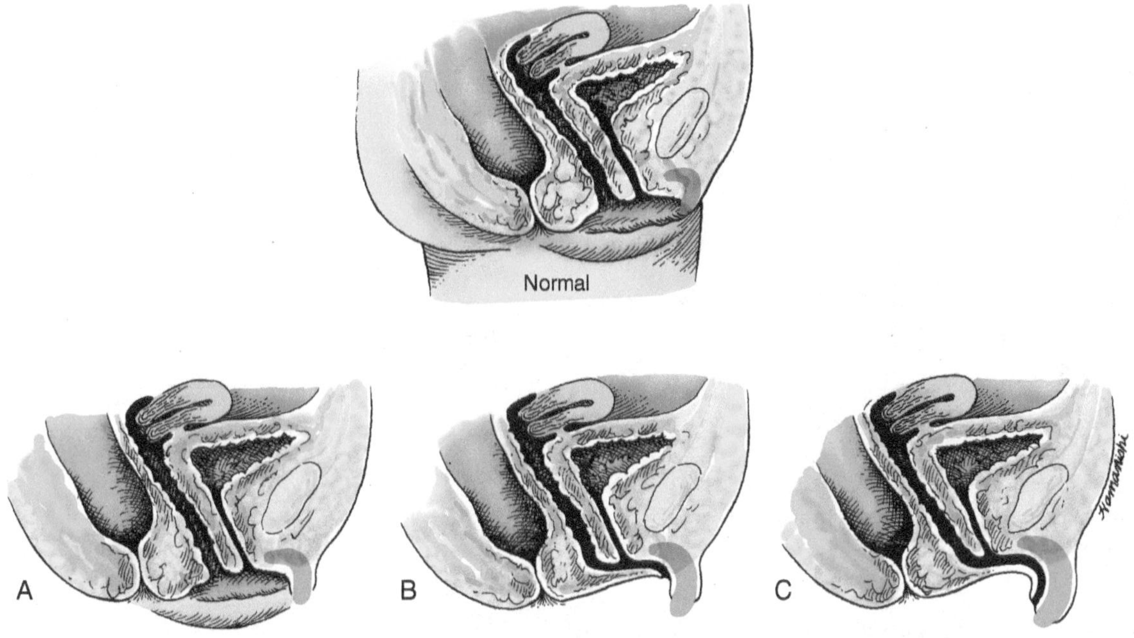


**Figure 11.2** Sagittal views of genital deformities seen in female infants who are masculinized. **A,** Minimal masculinization with slight enlargement of the clitoris. **B,** Labial fusion and more marked enlargement of the clitoris. **C,** Complete labial fusion, enlargement of the clitoris, and formation of a partial penile urethra. (Modified from Verkauf BS, Jones HW Jr. Masculinization of the female genitalia in congenital adrenal hyperplasia: relationship to the salt losing variety of the disease. *South Med J.* 1970;63:634-638.)

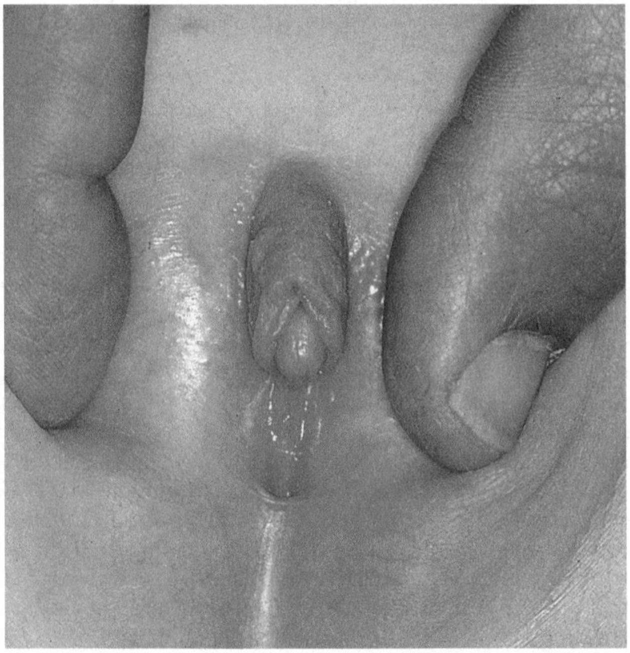

**Figure 11.3** Clitoromegaly with posterior labial fusion in a child with congenital adrenal hyperplasia. (From McKay M. Vulvar manifestations of skin disorders. In: Black M, McKay M, Braude P, et al, eds. *Obstetric and Gynecologic Dermatology.* 2nd ed. Edinburgh: Mosby; 2003:120.)

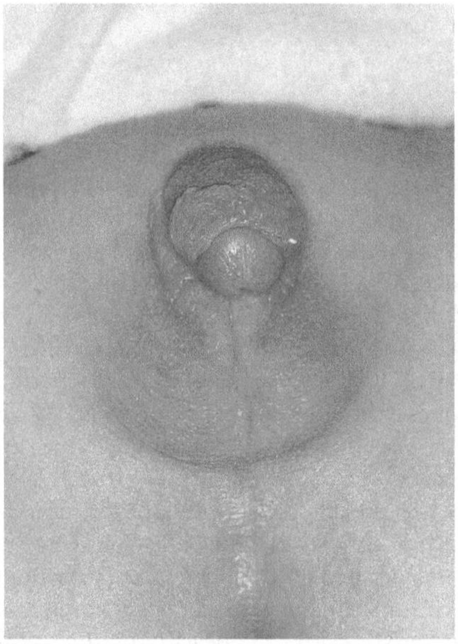

**Figure 11.4** Ambiguous genitalia in a 46,XY child with partial androgen insensitivity. (From McKay M. Vulvar manifestations of skin disorders. In: Black M, McKay M, Braude P, et al, eds. *Obstetric and Gynecologic Dermatology.* 2nd ed. Edinburgh: Mosby; 2003:121.)

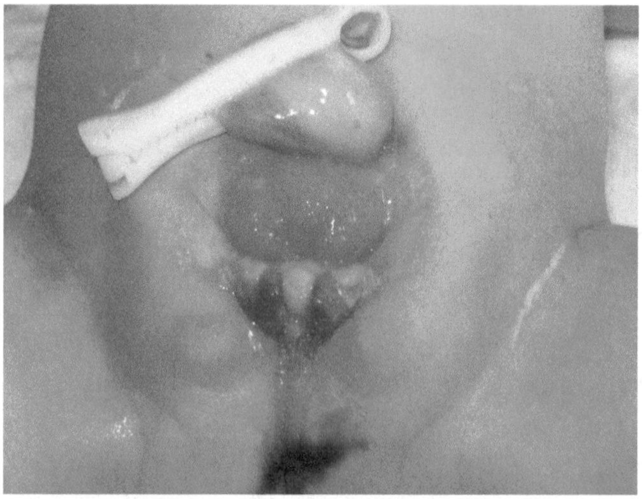

**Figure 11.5** An example of a bifid clitoris in an infant with extrophy of the bladder. (Courtesy of Richard Grady, MD.)

A bifid clitoris (Fig. 11.5) is usually seen in association with extrophy of the bladder. Extrophy of the bladder occurs rarely (1 per 30,000 births) and has a male predominance (3:1). However, when it occurs in females, it is often associated with a bifid clitoris. Approximately half of female patients with bladder extrophy may have associated reproductive tract anomalies such as vaginal anomalies and müllerian duct fusion disorders. In such cases, an anterior rotation and a shortening of the vagina with labial fusion are quite common.

### *Labial Fusion*

Labial fusion may occur without clitoromegaly. The resultant ambiguous genitalia will imply a form of DSD. 46, XX DSD or 46, XY DSD applies to individuals with a pure XX or XY karyotype but with the external genitalia of the opposite sex of the karyotype or ambiguous genitalia. The term *hermaphrodite* is no longer used and was derived from the child of the Greek gods Hermes and Aphrodite, Hermaphroditus, who was part female and part male. A true hermaphrodite is now called *ovotesticular DSD* and has both ovarian (including follicular elements) and testicular tissue, either in the same or opposite gonads. Ovotesticular DSD is extremely rare in North and South America but more common (though still very rare) in Africa.

Ovotestes are present in individuals with ovaries that usually have an SRY antigen present and testicular tissue present. The degree to which müllerian and wolffian development occurs depends on the amounts of testicular tissue present in the ovotestes and the proximity to the developing duct system. When considerable amounts of testicular tissue are present within the organ, there is a tendency for descent toward the labial/scrotal area. Thus palpation of the gonad in the inguinal canal or within the labial scrotal area is fairly common. Ovulation and menstruation may occur if the müllerian system is appropriately developed. In a similar fashion, spermatogenesis may occur as well. Where testicular tissue is present, there is an increased risk for malignant degeneration, and these gonads should be removed after puberty. Germ cell tumors, such as gonadoblastomas and dysgerminomas, have been reported in the ovarian portion of ovotestes.

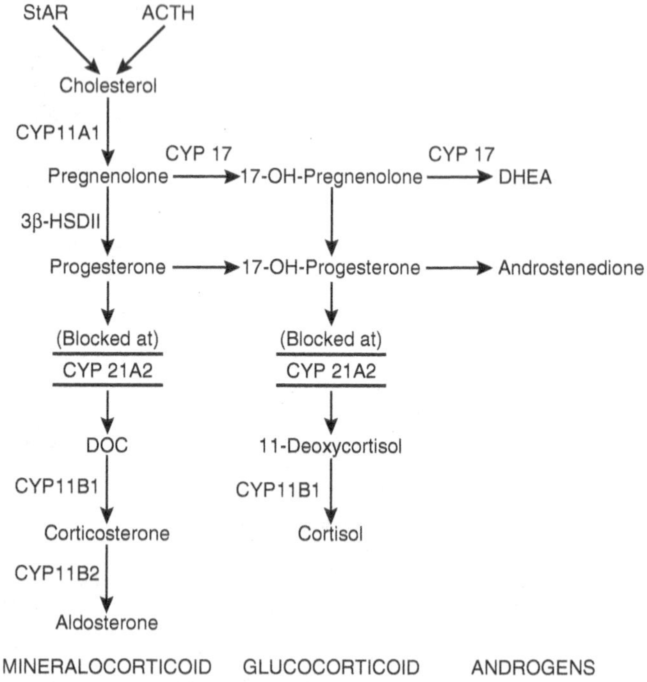


**Figure 11.6** Steroid pathway in congenital adrenal hyperplasia with absence of 21 hydroxylase. *ACTH,* Adrenocorticotropic hormone; *3β-HSDII,* 3β-hydroxysteroid dehydrogenase; *DHEA,* dehydroepiandrosterone; *DOC,* deoxycorticosterone. (From Grumbach MM, Hughes IA, Conte FA. Disorders of sex differentiation. In: Larsen RP, Kronenberg HM, Melmed S, Polonsky KS, eds. *Williams Textbook of Endocrinology.* 10th ed. Philadelphia: WB Saunders; 2003:533.)

### *Congenital Adrenal Hyperplasia*

Although labial fusion may result from exposure to exogenous androgens or be associated with defects of the anterior abdominal wall, by far the most common cause is congenital adrenal hyperplasia. The most common form of congenital adrenal hyperplasia is caused by an inborn error of metabolism involving deficiency of the 21-hydroxylase enzyme (Fig. 11.6). This condition is transmitted as an autosomal recessive gene coded on chromosome 6, and both severe and mild gene mutations have been identified. With the severe mutation, due to the absence of the 21-hydroxylase enzyme, the major biosynthetic pathway to cortisol is blocked; 17-OH-progesterone is produced instead, which is converted to the androgen androstenedione. The fetal hypothalamic-pituitary axis senses inadequate levels of cortisol and secretes excess adrenocorticotropic hormone (ACTH), which leads to increasing levels of androstenedione from the female adrenal gland and subsequent masculinization of the external genitalia. Homozygous individuals occur with an incidence as high as 1 per 490, depending on the geographic location and population studied. Screening programs have noted the incidence to be approximately 1 in 14,500 births (Pang, 1988). Depending on the population, carriers of the gene (heterozygotes) are present in a frequency ranging from 1 per 20 to 1 per 250. Two other less common enzyme defects, also transmittable as autosomal recessive traits, may produce similar abnormal findings: the 11-hydroxylase deficiency and the 3β-hydroxysteroid dehydrogenase deficiency. These two enzyme defects as well as 21-hydroxylase deficiency may cause ambiguous genitalia with masculinized females.

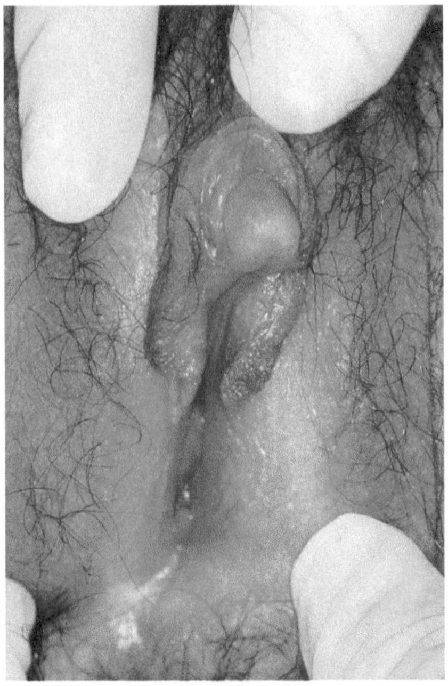

**Figure 11.7** Eleven-year-old girl with clitoromegaly and thick genital hair, who presented with facial hair and was found to have 21-hydroxylase deficiency. (From McKay M. Vulvar manifestations of skin disorders. In: Black M, McKay M, Braude P, et al, eds. *Obstetric and Gynecologic Dermatology.* 2nd ed. Edinburgh: Mosby; 2003:120.)

Congenital adrenal hyperplasia (CAH) may be demonstrated at birth by the presence of ambiguous genitalia in 46,XX individuals or present later in childhood. The majority of newborns (75%) who are homozygous for a CAH mutation are at risk for the development of a life-threatening neonatal adrenal crisis as a result of sodium loss because of lack of aldosterone production. In individuals with a milder disease presentation, delayed diagnosis may result in accelerated bone maturation due to high levels of androgens being aromatized to estradiol and thus leading to premature closure of the epiphyseal plates and short stature. The development of premature secondary sexual characteristics in males and further virilization in females may also occur (Fig. 11.7) (Black, 2003). Most states in the United States have mandatory neonatal screening for 17-OH progesterone levels to screen for CAH.

Treatment of congenital adrenal hyperplasia involves replacement of cortisol. This suppresses ACTH output and therefore decreases the stimulation of the cortisol-producing pathways of the adrenal cortex and subsequently decreases androgen production. For women known to be at risk, those diagnosed with CAH and those who have had children with CAH, antenatal therapy may be offered. After a positive pregnancy test, daily administration of dexamethasone will suppress the fetal adrenal glands until the fetal gender can be verified with prenatal diagnosis. Although this intervention remains an option, it should not be carried out routinely and is still considered experimental by the major societies (Endocrine and Pediatric Endocrine Societies). Many of the female infants exposed to high levels of androgens in utero may need corrective surgery. Children who have had initial corrective surgeries may need follow-up vaginoplasty as teenagers because of vaginal stenosis. Furthermore, because of the profound gender identity issues related to ambiguous genitalia in females with CAH, and also for women with other DSDs, ongoing psychological support and counseling are important. When available, multidisciplinary team support is recommended for the gynecologic, urologic, endocrinologic, and psychological care of these individuals.

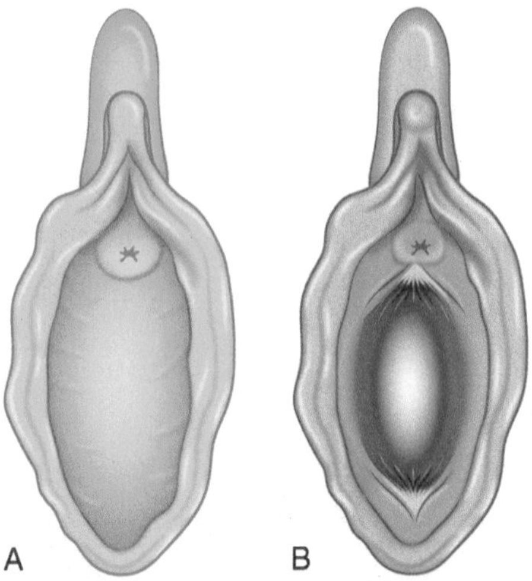


**Figure 11.8** Diagrammatic depiction of an imperforate hymen **A,** and a bulging hymen **B,** due to hematocolpos. (Modified from Dietrich JE, Miller DM, Quint EH. Obstructive reproductive track anomalies. *J Pediatr Adoles Gyn.* 2014;27[6]:396-402.)

### *Hymenal Anomalies*

The hymen represents the junction of the sinovaginal bulbs with the urogenital sinus and is composed of endoderm from the urogenital sinus epithelium. The hymen is initially a solid membrane of tissue, and the central cells of the membrane typically dissolve during late fetal development to establish a connection between the lumen of the vaginal canal and the vestibule. If this perforation does not take place, the hymen is imperforate (Dietrich, 2014) (Fig. 11.8). The incidence of an imperforate hymen is thought to be approximately 1 in 1000 live-born females (Usta, 1993). Occasionally, a hydrocolpos or mucocolpos may occur in neonates or infants when fluid or vaginal secretions build up behind an imperforate hymen. Although this fluid collection may spontaneously resolve, if it forms a mass that obstructs the urinary tract, then the hymen must be incised to release the obstructing fluid.

Menarche typically occurs within 2 to 3 years from the start of thelarche (breast development), and young women with an imperforate hymen may experience cyclic cramping but no menstrual flow. An imperforate hymen is commonly diagnosed after puberty in the setting of primary amenorrhea, hematocolpos, and possibly hematometra that can cause pelvic pain, urinary retention, and difficulty with bowel movements. In more advanced cases, due to retrograde menstruation, the menstrual blood may distend the fallopian tubes and form endometrial implants in the peritoneal cavity. Surprisingly, some females have minimal symptoms with this condition.

The diagnosis can be determined by history and physical examination; a bulging membrane with a bluish hue is appreciated at the introitus, and a vaginal mass is palpable on rectal exam. Surgical intervention is necessary to relieve the obstruction of the reproductive tract. Under anesthesia, a cruciate

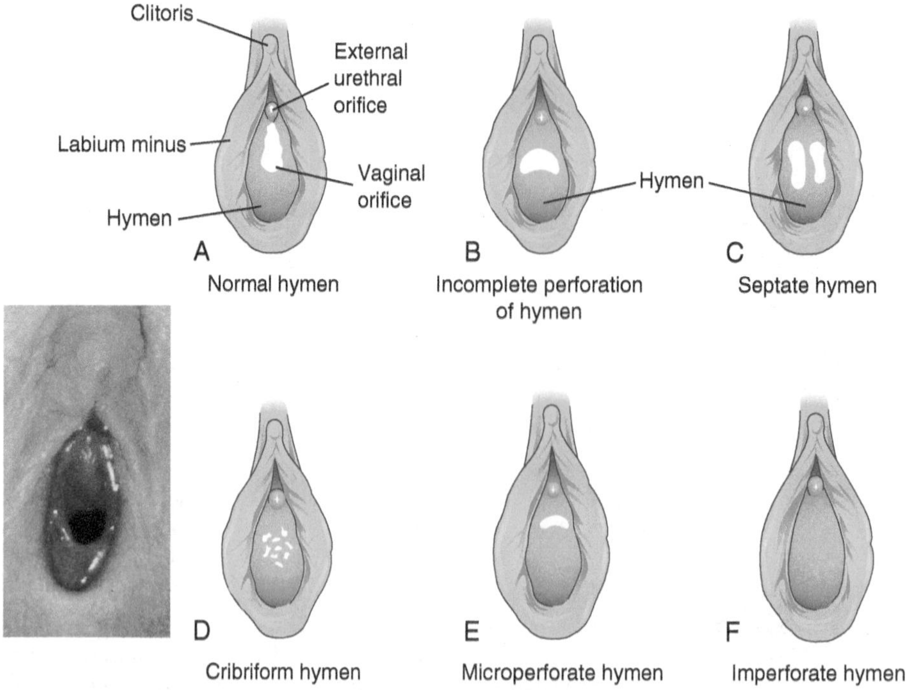


**Figure 11.9** Congenital anomalies of the hymen. Panels **A-F** show different types of hymen abnormalities. The photograph shows a normal hymen as in **A**. (From Moore KL, Persaud TVN. *The Developing Human*. 7th ed. Philadelphia: WB Saunders; 2003:322.)

incision is made into the hymen extending from 10 to 4 o'clock and 2 to 8 o'clock. Once the imperforate hymen has been carefully incised and the hematocolpos drained, the excess hymenal tissue is trimmed and hemostasis is achieved with interrupted fine absorbable sutures. The tissue often heals quickly and well, leaving a patent hymen.

Several variations exist of partial hymenal perforation: microperforate, cribriform and septate hymen, and incomplete perforate hymen (Fig. 11.9) (Moore, 2003). Females with partial hymenal perforation commonly present with difficulty inserting a tampon or difficulty with sexual activity. Occasionally, a young female is able to insert a tampon past the hymen anomaly, but once the tampon expands with blood, it cannot be removed due to the partial hymenal obstruction. Surgical correction may be necessary to remove the excess hymenal tissue and restore normal hymenal anatomy.

### Müllerian Anomalies

Müllerian anomalies, otherwise known as *congenital anomalies of the female reproductive tract,* occur due to defects in development of the müllerian ducts, which are the embryologic origin of the fallopian tubes, uterus, cervix, and a portion of the vagina. Before reviewing these disorders, it is important to understand the development of the female reproductive tract.

### Embryology

Although genetic sex is determined when sperm fertilizes the oocyte, male or female phenotype is not defined until after the sixth week of development. Between the third and fifth weeks of embryologic development, both the wolffian (mesonephric) and müllerian (paramesonephric) ducts are present. The müllerian ducts form from clefts between the mesonephros and the developing gonad. The paired wolffian ducts connect the embryologic kidney (mesonephros) to the cloaca between 5 and 10 weeks of gestation; development of the functional kidney (metanephros) is stimulated by an outgrowth of the wolffian duct, the ureteric bud. The fate of these various embryonic elements is closely entwined; an insult to or abnormal development of one embryonic element usually affects the others.

The subsequent steps of müllerian duct development are elongation, fusion, canalization, and septal resorption. The müllerian ducts elongate caudally and eventually fuse in the midline as they descend into the pelvis, reaching the urogenital sinus at an elevation known as the *müllerian tubercle.* At this point, the ducts are two solid tubes of tissue that are fused medially; this occurs by 10 weeks of gestation. Next, central absorption of the cells occurs, leading to two hollow tubes of tissue that remain fused medially. Lastly, the midline septum between the two tubes of tissue undergoes resorption, and this process commonly occurs in a caudal to cephalad direction, leading to a midline unified structure. The inferior portion of the müllerian ducts becomes the upper vagina, followed by the cervix and uterus, and the cephalad unfused portion of the ducts develops into the fallopian tubes. This process is completed by 20 weeks of embryologic development. Although this is the common theory of müllerian duct development, based on the variety of anomalies that arise from this process, many variations of this process can occur.

The vagina develops from both müllerian duct tissue and the urogenital sinus. Once the müllerian ducts reach the urogenital sinus at approximately 10 weeks of gestation, cells proliferate from the upper portion of the urogenital sinus to form solid aggregates known as the *sinovaginal bulbs.* These cell masses develop into a cord, the vaginal plate, which extends from the müllerian ducts to the urogenital sinus. This plate canalizes, starting at the hymen, which is where the sinovaginal bulb attaches to the urogenital sinus, and proceeding cranially to the developing cervix, which has by this time already canalized. The process is completed by 20 weeks of gestation.

As previously mentioned, abnormalities in any or multiple parts of müllerian and urogenital sinus development can occur and lead to a constellation of structural defects of the female reproductive tract. Anomalies in müllerian duct elongation, fusion, canalization, and septal resorption have been identified, as have anomalies in vaginal plate resorption. Common müllerian anomalies are discussed in the next few sections.

### Anomalies of Müllerian Duct Development

Müllerian anomalies are commonly classified into three categories of disordered duct development: agenesis and hypoplasia, lateral fusion defects, and vertical fusion defects. Reproductive tract abnormalities due to in utero exposure to diethylstilbestrol (DES), a synthetic estrogen that has not been used for several decades, constitute a fourth group of anomalies. Agenesis and hypoplasia can occur for a portion of or an entire müllerian duct, or for both ducts, affecting one or multiple müllerian-derived structures. Lateral fusion defects are the most common category of müllerian defects and originate due to failure of migration of one or both ducts, midline fusion of the ducts, or absorption of the midline septum between the ducts. A range of anomalies can occur, including symmetric or asymmetric and nonobstructed or obstructed müllerian structures. Vertical fusion defects occur due to disordered fusion of the müllerian ducts with the urogenital sinus or abnormal vaginal canalization, and they may present with menstrual flow obstruction. The next sections discuss specific abnormalities of müllerian duct development.

### Vaginal Agenesis

Vaginal agenesis, also known as *müllerian agenesis* or *müllerian aplasia,* occurs due to failure of müllerian duct development or marked aberrations in the typical steps of müllerian development. This condition is also known as the *Mayer-Rokitansky-Küster-Hauser (MRKH) syndrome,* named after the four physicians who discovered the syndrome (Fig. 11.10) (Baramki, 1984). This condition is characterized by congenital absence of the vagina and variable development of the uterus; 7% to 10% of women with vaginal agenesis have rudimentary uterine tissue present (Fedele, 2007). The syndrome occurs in approximately 1 in 5000 females. These individuals have normal pubertal development, normal ovarian function, and a 46,XX karyotype, and they commonly present with primary amenorrhea at 15 to 16 years of age. The cause of this disorder is currently unknown, but research into possible genetic disorders leading to MRKH is ongoing.

Complete vaginal agenesis is discovered in 75% of women with Mayer–Rokitansky–Küster–Hauser syndrome, and approximately 25% have a short vaginal pouch. Some women may have rudimentary uterine horns and can have myomas or adenomyosis in the rudimentary myometrium. If the uterine horns contain some endometrium with an epithelial lining, called *functional rudimentary horns,* menstruation into a blocked system can occur, which can lead to monthly cramping, pelvic pain, and endometriosis from retrograde menstruation. A study by Fedele and colleagues noted that 92 of 106 women with müllerian agenesis had small müllerian remnants.[13] In women with müllerian

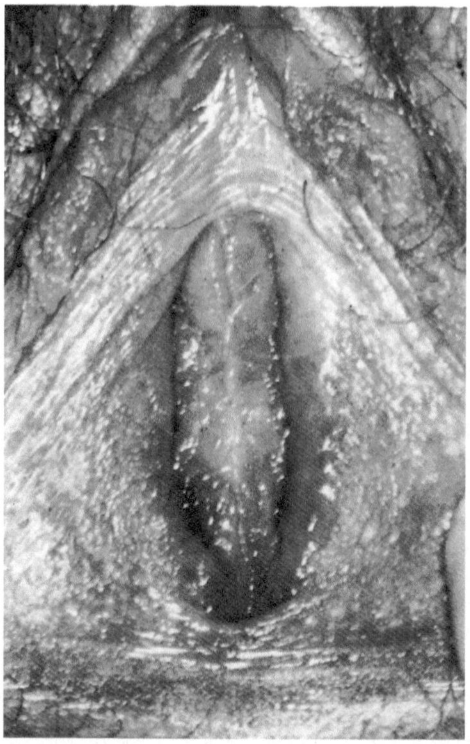

**Figure 11.10** External genitalia of a female with congenital absence of the vagina. (From Baramki TA. Treatment of congenital anomalies in girls and women. *J Reprod Med.* 1984;29[6]:376-384.)

agenesis, the ovaries are normal and the fallopian tubes are usually present.

Other congenital anomalies are associated with the diagnosis of müllerian agenesis. Due to the concomitant development of the müllerian and urinary tracts, up to 50% of women with müllerian agenesis have concurrent urinary tract anomalies. Phelan and coworkers reported that of 72 patients with vaginal agenesis, 25% had urologic abnormalities noted on intravenous pyelography (Phelan, 1953). A later study by Baramki demonstrated that 40% of 92 patients with müllerian agenesis had urologic abnormalities (Baramki, 1984). These anomalies can include renal agenesis, pelvic kidney, multicystic dysplastic kidney, and ureteral duplication. One study described a 12% incidence of skeletal anomalies, usually involving congenital fusion or absence of vertebrae in these patients. Other anomalies associated with müllerian agenesis include cardiac defects and hearing loss. Hence, women with müllerian agenesis require dedicated imaging of the urinary tract as well as other evaluation as indicated.

Females with müllerian agenesis present with normal pubertal development and primary amenorrhea. Physical examination demonstrates the absence of a vaginal opening or the presence of a short vaginal pouch, and there is an inability to palpate a uterus on rectal examination. When evaluating a female with primary amenorrhea and a distal vaginal obstruction, the differential diagnosis includes vaginal agenesis, transverse vaginal septum, imperforate hymen, and androgen insensitivity syndrome. With müllerian agenesis, measurement of reproductive hormones reveals normal levels, and the karyotype is 46,XX. Although ultrasound examination may verify the presence of normal ovaries and the absence of the uterus, magnetic resonance imaging

(MRI) offers detailed evaluation of the soft tissues of the pelvis and can confirm the diagnosis of müllerian agenesis; it can also assess if any rudimentary uterine tissue is present. Surgical evaluation by laparoscopy is not necessary unless the evaluation of pelvic pain and possible removal of functional rudimentary horns is necessary. The ovaries of these females are normal and should not be removed.

### *Androgen Insensitivity*

Although androgen insensitivity syndrome is not a müllerian anomaly, it presents in a similar manner to vaginal agenesis and therefore will be reviewed in this chapter. Androgen insensitivity occurs in individuals with a 46,XY karyotype who have certain genetic abnormalities that cause defective androgen receptors. The syndrome formerly was termed *testicular feminization syndrome.* Because the developing fetus cannot sense any testosterone, the external genitalia are feminized, and a short vaginal pouch can develop from the urogenital sinus. Due to testicular production of anti-müllerian hormone, the müllerian ducts resorb and the wolffian duct-derived tissue persists. Due to the lack of functional androgen receptors, the testes remain undescended. These individuals undergo normal pubertal development, and the testes make increasing amounts of testosterone, which is aromatized to estrogen, but without functional androgen receptors, there is no testosterone action (male muscle mass and hair production). These phenotypic females commonly present with primary amenorrhea, and they tend to be tall and have sparse to no pubic hair. After the estrogen-induced growth spurt, the undescended testes should be removed to prevent the development of a gonadoblastoma.

### *Treatment of Vaginal Agenesis*

Once the diagnosis of vaginal agenesis is determined, it is recommended that this information is shared with the female and her support system during a face-to-face conversation. This diagnosis has significant emotional, physical, sexual, and reproductive consequences for the female, and psychological counseling should be encouraged to help her cope with this diagnosis and its implications. The treatment of vaginal agenesis involves creation of a neovagina for future sexual function. Additionally, the female should be aware that achieving motherhood is possible using her own eggs and a gestational carrier, or through adoption.

There are nonsurgical and surgical methods available to achieve creation of a neovagina. The purpose of a vagina is for sexual function, although some females may wish to pursue this intervention before they are ready to become sexually active. The first-line treatment to create a neovagina is the nonsurgical option that involves the use of vaginal dilators. This is a time-consuming process that requires the daily use of dilators for 15 to 20 minutes, and it can take 3 to 6 months or longer to create a functional vagina. Each set of dilators has several sizes that increase in width and length, and the dilator is pressed at the vaginal dimple to stretch the skin. Due to discomfort, lidocaine jelly can be applied to the vagina prior to each session. Appropriate instruction should be provided prior to initiating dilation and intermittently throughout the process to make sure that proper technique is being used. Once the neovagina is created, then maintenance dilation must be performed several times per week unless the female is sexually active. These women must be counseled that they should still use condoms to protect against sexually transmitted infections.

There are multiple ways to reconstruct the vagina surgically. The goal of the operation is to develop the potential space between the bladder and the rectum and insert into this space a new tissue that will develop into a vagina. Common tissues utilized include a split-thickness skin graft, buccal mucosa, peritoneum, bowel (sigmoid or small bowel), or synthetic tissue grafts (Thomas, 2007). After the vaginal space is opened and the new tissue is inserted, the female must wear a mold for a number of months to maintain the vaginal shape as the surgical site heals. Thereafter, if she is not having intercourse regularly, she must use vaginal dilators several times per week to maintain the neovagina. Other surgical procedures to create a neovagina exist, but the discussion is beyond the scope of this chapter.

## Transverse Vaginal Septum

A transverse vaginal septum occurs due to partial canalization of the vaginal plate, leaving a band of tissue across the vagina (Fig. 11.11). This septum may be partial (perforate) or complete, and it most commonly lies at the junction between the upper third and lower two thirds of the vagina (Fig. 11.12). Transverse vaginal septae occur less frequently in the midvagina and lower vagina, and the general incidence is approximately 1 per 75,000 females. Partial transverse vaginal septa have been reported in diethylstilbestrol (DES)-exposed females. In the prepubertal state, this diagnosis is rarely made unless there is the development of a mucocolpos or mucometrium behind the septum, and an unexplained abdominal mass may form. After menarche, the presence of a complete septum leads to hematocolpos and hematometrium, similar to that seen with an imperforate hymen, except that because the obstruction is higher in the vagina and the septum is made of thicker tissue than the hymen, there is no bulging tissue at the introitus. With this anomaly, the female presents with primary amenorrhea and reports cyclic cramping and worsening pelvic pain. In contrast, the female with an incomplete (perforate) transverse septum usually menstruates

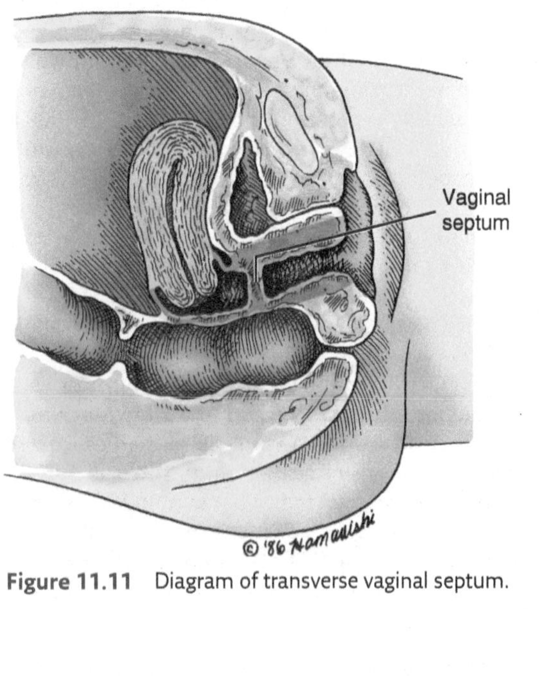


**Figure 11.11** Diagram of transverse vaginal septum.

but could develop hematocolpos over time along with foul-smelling vaginal discharge, or she could report normal menstrual function but the inability to insert a tampon or have intercourse. The transverse vaginal septum is often less than 1 cm thick; however, some septa can be more than 2 cm thick. With a thin transverse vaginal septum, the septal tissue is excised and the proximal and distal vaginal tissue are sutured together to create a normal vagina. A similar procedure is performed for a perforate transverse vaginal septum. The procedure to correct a thick vaginal septum is more difficult; once the septum is excised, a tissue graft may be needed to bridge the distance between the proximal and distal vaginal tissue edges. With all of these vaginal reconstructive procedures, the female may need to wear a stent or use dilators to prevent scarring and narrowing at the surgical site. Longitudinal septa of the vagina will be discussed with duplication of the uterus and cervix.

### *Vaginal Adenosis*

In the female who was exposed to DES in utero, the junction between the müllerian ducts and the sinovaginal bulb may not be sharply demonstrated. If müllerian elements invade the sinovaginal bulb, remnants may remain as areas of adenosis in the adult vagina. Vaginal adenosis is generally palpated submucosally, although it may be observable at the surface.

## *ABNORMALITIES OF THE CERVIX*

Cervical anomalies can occur along with uterine and vaginal anomalies or can occur in isolation. If one or both of the müllerian ducts do not fuse, do not develop, or develop incompletely, cervical duplication or agenesis can occur. Cervical duplication can result in two separate and distinct cervices or two cervices that are fused in the midline. Additionally, a septate cervix can occur when the midline septum within the cervix does not resorb. These anomalies do not typically obstruct menstrual flow. In contrast, cervical agenesis and hypoplasia occur due to incomplete or absent duct development and often present with obstructed menstrual flow with associated cyclic or chronic pain and hematometra. These rare anomalies require ultrasound or MRI to clarify the anatomic disorder. Several management options are available, including long-term menstrual suppression with hormones, cervical reconstruction, or hysterectomy. Lastly, other cervical anomalies such as hoods, collars, and adenosis are possible in women who were exposed to DES in utero.

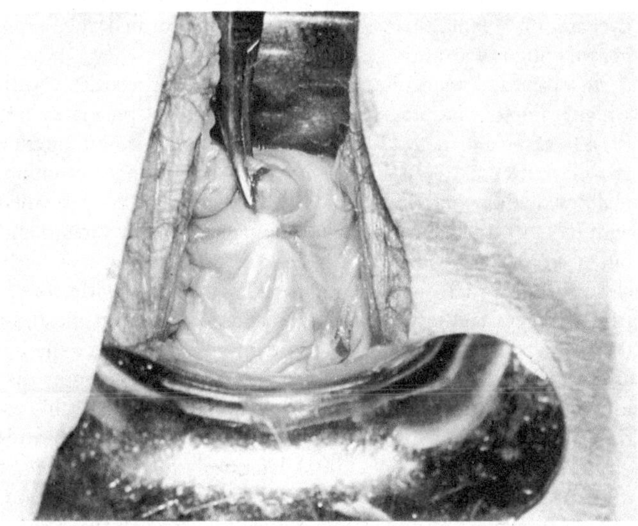

**Figure 11.12** Patient with complete transverse vaginal septum.

## *ABNORMALITIES OF THE UTERUS*

Abnormalities of the uterus are categorized as lateral fusion defects and occur due to disordered duct fusion and septal resorption. There are several classification system for müllerian anomalies; in 1988 the (American Fertility Society (Fig. 11.13) provided a straightforward classification system of uterine anomalies based on embryologic origin (American Fertility Society, 1988). A comparison of the American Fertility Society (now ASRM) system to that of the European Society of Human Reproduction and Embryology (ESHRE) found that the latter would lead to an overcalling of certain conditions that were not true anomalies (Ludwin, 2014). The hysteroscopic lysis of a uterine septum is usually straightforward and is illustrated in Video 11.1.

Hypoplasia/agenesis (category I) and unicornuate (category II) denote anomalies with developmental failure of one or both müllerian ducts; didelphys (category III) and bicornuate (category IV) describe anomalies involving a varying degree of failure of midline fusion; septate (category V) and arcuate (category VI) identify anomalies with some degree of failure of resorption of the midline septum. With this classification system, associated anomalies of the vagina, cervix, fallopian tubes, and urinary system must be documented separately. It should also be recognized that numerous anomalies exist that are exceptions to the standard theory of müllerian duct development.

Often, constellations of müllerian abnormalities occur together. A didelphys uterus is commonly seen with a duplicated vagina, and this presents similar to a longitudinal vaginal septum. In some cases, the vaginal septum obstructs one side of the duplicated system, causing a female to present with worsening pain during menstruation due to hematocolpos and hematometra on the obstructed side. A bicornuate uterus can present with a single cervix or a duplicated cervix, and a longitudinal vaginal septum can also be present. A septate uterus can present with a single, septate, or duplicated cervix and may also occur with a longitudinal vaginal septum. A unicornuate uterus may occur in isolation or be associated with a contralateral rudimentary uterine horn that may contain functional endometrial tissue. Another classification by Toaff (Toaff, 1984) depicts some of these variations (Fig. 11.14).

With uterus didelphys with an obstructed vagina and uterus or with a unicornuate uterus with a rudimentary horn, ipsilateral to the anomalous or obstructed side, urinary tract anomalies such as renal agenesis or pelvic kidney are common. Hence, in females with a müllerian anomaly, and especially in those with an obstruction of a duplicated system, imaging of the urinary tract is important to look for concomitant anomalies (Oppelt, 2007).

### *Imaging*

MRI is the gold standard for the diagnosis of these abnormalities. However, three-dimensional (3D) ultrasound (US) is also beneficial and has been considered to be equivalent in most

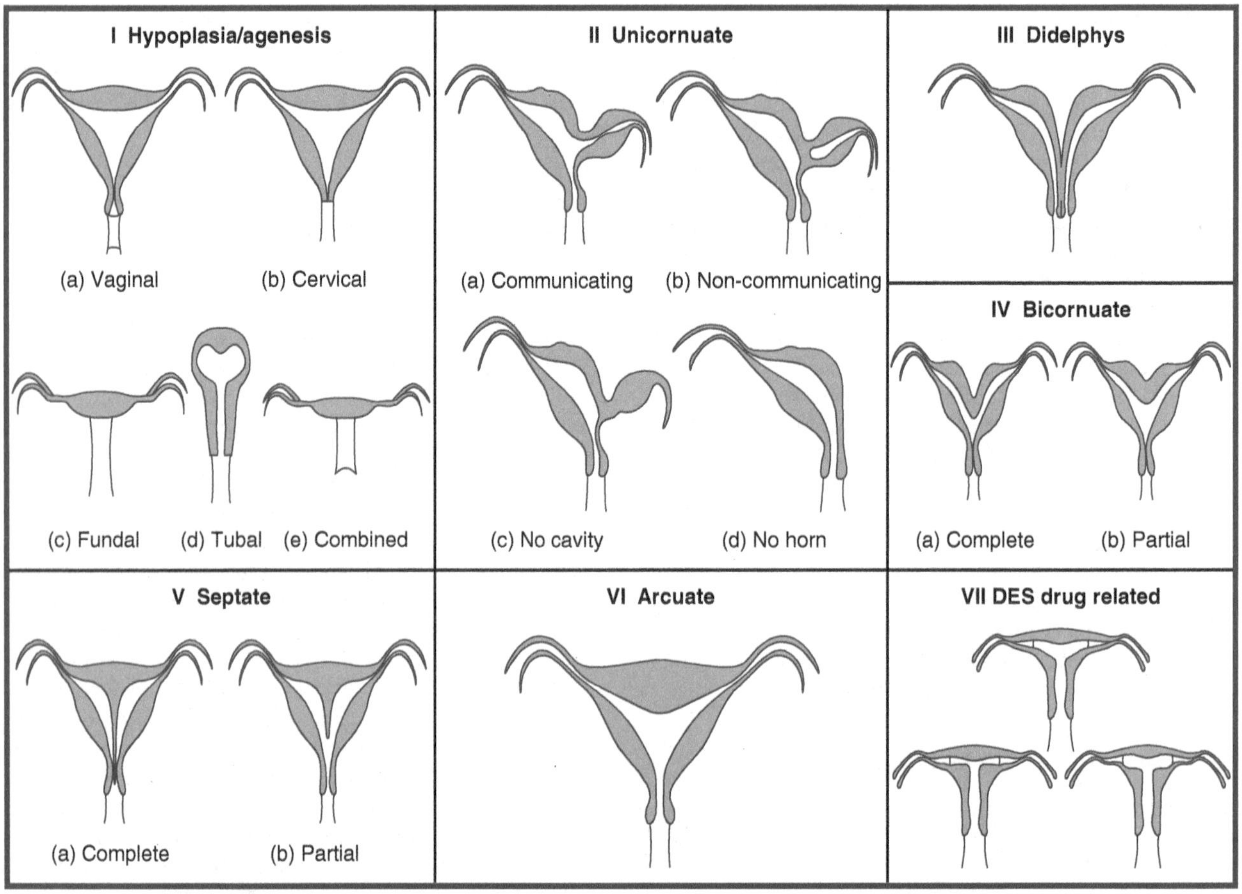


**Figure 11.13** American Fertility Society classification. (From The American Fertility Society classification of adnexal adhesions, distal tubal occlusion, tubal occlusion secondary to tubal ligation, tubal pregnancies, müllerian anomalies and intrauterine adhesions. *Fertil Steril*. 1988;49[6]:944-955.)

circumstances (Bermejo, 2010; Benacerraf, 2015). Figure 11.15 compares MRI and 3D US images of some abnormalities using the American Fertility Society classification. Imaging with a hysterosalpingogram, which can show two uterine cavities (Fig. 11.16), could be either a bicornuate uterus or a septate uterus. Conventional two-dimensional (2D) US is not able to make this distinction because it is not able to determine the external contour of the uterus, which is accomplished either by 3D US or MRI (Troiano, 2004).

### *Symptoms and Signs*

It is important to recognize several gynecologic and obstetric signs and symptoms that may indicate a uterine anomaly and to also remember that many females with congenital uterine anomalies are asymptomatic. Uterine agenesis presents with primary amenorrhea. Women with an obstructive anomaly may report cyclic or noncyclic pelvic pain and dysmenorrhea, and these symptoms can begin several months after menarche or into adulthood. Obstructive uterine anomalies are associated with hematometra, retrograde menstruation, and endometriosis. Endometriosis is a common finding in women with obstructive and nonobstructive müllerian anomalies. Abnormal bleeding can also occur with uterine anomalies and has been associated with septate uteri. Furthermore, vaginal anomalies may occur in conjunction with uterine anomalies, and abnormal bleeding may be due to a partial or microperforate vaginal obstruction or a longitudinal vaginal septum. A longitudinal vaginal septum, which is associated with septate, didelphys, and bicornuate uteri, may be a woman's first presentation with a uterine anomaly; associated symptoms include difficulty with tampon insertion, bleeding around one tampon (two are required), and dyspareunia. Hence, if a vaginal anomaly is identified, then uterine imaging is warranted.

In obstetrics, congenital uterine anomalies are associated with a higher rate of poor obstetric outcomes: recurrent pregnancy loss (RPL), first- and second-trimester pregnancy loss, intrauterine growth restriction, preterm labor and delivery, placental abruption, malpresentation, and intrauterine fetal demise. Among women with RPL, the incidence of uterine anomalies is highly variable and ranges from 6% to 38%, but based on meta-analyses it is likely closer to 12% to 16% and is as high as 25% in women with second-trimester pregnancy loss (Chan, 2011; Saravelos, 2008). In one study, the odds ratio for preterm birth less than 34 weeks with a uterine anomaly was 7.4 (Hua 2011). However, many studies identify that in women with uterine anomalies, despite the high risk of miscarriage and midtrimester pregnancy loss, the chance of a live birth is greater than 50% (Grimbizis, 2001). Uterine dysfunction is thought to occur due to diminished cavity size, impaired ability to distend, abnormal myometrial and cervical function, inadequate vascularity, or abnormal endometrial development. Due to higher rates of fetal

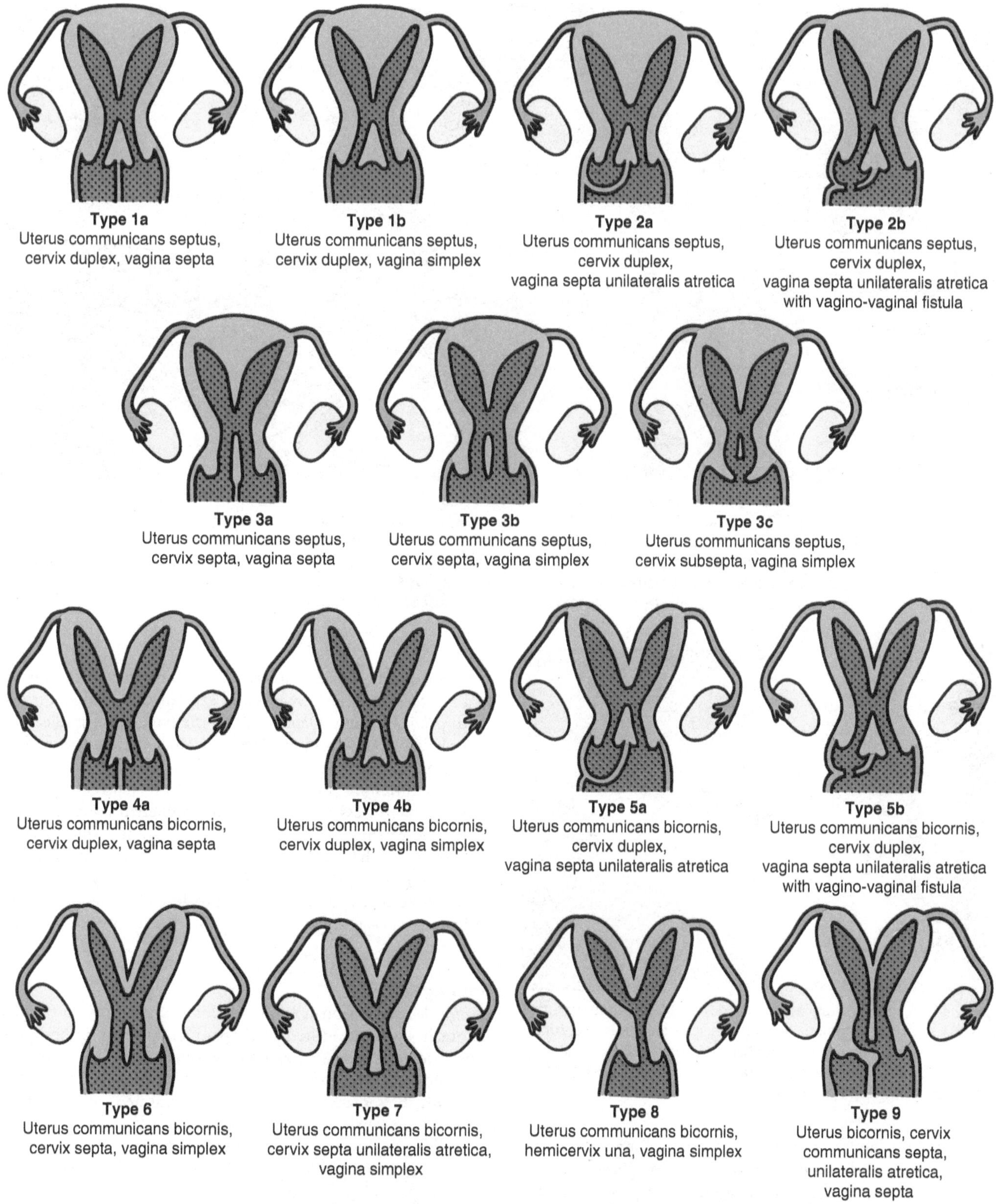


**Figure 11.14** Morphologic classification of communicating uteri. All have an isthmic communication except type 9, which has a low cervical communication. (Reprinted from Toaff ME, Lev-Toaff AS, Toaff R. Communicating uteri: review and classification with introduction of two previously unreported types. *Fertil Steril.* 1984;41[5]:661-679. Copyright 1984, with permission from The American Society for Reproductive Medicine.)

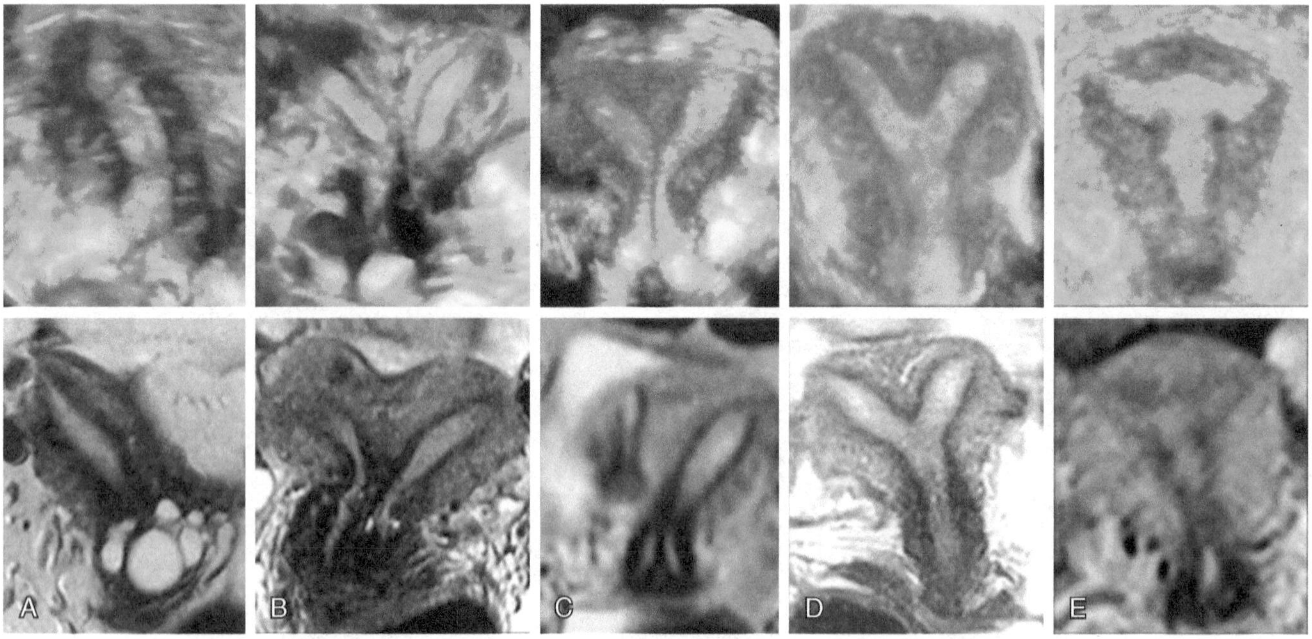


**Figure 11.15** Comparison of müllerian anomalies as viewed by 3D ultrasound and MRI. The comparisons of 3D ultrasound (top row) and MRI (bottom row) are very similar. **A,** unicornuate uterus; **B,** bicornuate bicollis uterus; **C,** complete septate uterus with two cervices; **D,** partial septate uterus; **E,** uterus with diethylstilbesterol-related malformation. (From Bermejo C, Martinez Ten P, Cantarero R, et al. Three-dimensional ultrasound in the diagnosis of müllerian duct anomalies and concordance with magnetic resonance imaging. *Ultrasound Obstet Gynecol.* 2010;35[5]:593-601.)

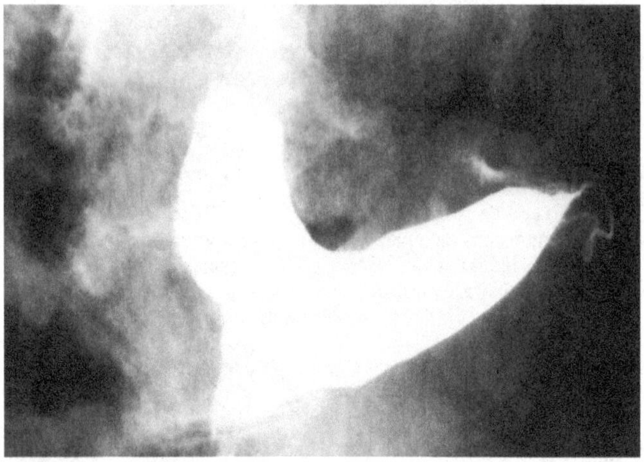

**Figure 11.16** Hysterosalpingogram (HSG) of a bicornuate uterus seen in a woman with repetitive abortions; a partial uterine septum would also look similarly on HSG. When an anomaly is appreciated on HSG, further testing is indicated to assess the myometrial contour of the uterus, which helps to make the correct diagnosis.

malpresentation, an increased rate of cesarean delivery can be seen with uterine anomalies. Additional obstetric complications, such as cervical incompetence, pregnancy-induced hypertension (due to renal anomalies), and antepartum and postpartum bleeding, are also associated with uterine anomalies. Last, pregnancy may occur in an obstructed or rudimentary uterine horn or in the fallopian tube associated with a rudimentary horn. Uterine horn pregnancies are surgical emergencies due to an 89% rate of rupture and the related morbidity and mortality (Jaysinghe, 2005).

### Diagnosis

Diagnosis of a uterine anomaly may be indicated by an individual's history, suggested by physical examination, and confirmed with pelvic imaging. Depending on the population studied and the quality of the imaging, either the arcuate uterus or the septate uterus is the most common uterine anomaly. Several imaging modalities are possible as discussed previously. In general, MRI is able to assess more complex müllerian anomalies that may involve the uterus, cervix, and vagina, and simultaneous assessment of the urinary tract is possible. It is rarely necessary to perform surgery to diagnose a uterine anomaly. It must be emphasized that with müllerian anomalies, the evaluation of the urinary tract is commonly indicated to identify any concomitant abnormalities.

### Management

Surgical intervention is indicated for women with obstructive anomalies with associated pelvic pain, endometriosis, and poor obstetric outcomes such as RPL, second-trimester loss, or preterm delivery. The goals of surgery include restoration of pelvic anatomy, preservation of fertility, and treatment of pelvic pain and endometriosis. Prior to attempting surgery for women with uterine anomalies and RPL or preterm delivery, it is important to rule out extrauterine causes of these obstetric issues. Of the uterine anomalies, the septate uterus is amenable to surgical correction (see Video 11.1). In contrast, the unicornuate uterus is never considered operable, but excision of a functional rudimentary uterine horn and the attached fallopian tube is recommended to prevent a horn or tubal gestation and to treat hematometra and pelvic pain. The bicornuate and didelphys uteri are considered operable in select circumstances; abdominal metroplasty can be performed to unify a bicornuate or didelphys uterus, but it is only performed in certain patients with poor obstetric outcomes. Furthermore, when indicated, a cervical cerclage can be utilized to attempt to improve pregnancy outcomes in women with uterine anomalies and a history of poor reproductive outcomes.

Hysteroscopic metroplasty to correct a partial or complete septate uterus can improve reproductive outcomes and is indicated in women with recurrent pregnancy loss or second-trimester pregnancy loss (Homer, 2000). During the procedure, the septum is visualized and incised with a cutting device such as scissors, an electrode, or a laser, and the cavity achieves a normal contour. After the hysteroscopic procedure, the risk of pregnancy loss or other adverse perinatal outcomes decreases dramatically; live birth rates improve from 50% to approximately 80%, and miscarriage rates decrease from 45% to approximately 15% (Grimbizis, 2001; Homer, 2000). Due to its safety, simplicity, and excellent postoperative results, the hysteroscopic approach is preferred for surgical treatment of a uterine septum, and laparoscopy can be utilized to assess the fundal contour and guide the extent of septum resection but is not mandatory. The surgical treatment of uterine septa in asymptomatic women is controversial, but some women elect to undergo surgery due to concerns regarding the obstetric risks associated with a uterine septum.

## OVARIAN ABNORMALITIES

### Accessory Ovary and Supernumerary Ovary

In 1959, Wharton defined *accessory ovary* and *supernumerary ovary*. The former term is used when excess ovarian tissue is noted near a normally placed ovary and connected to it. Supernumerary ovary occurs when a third ovary is separated from the normally situated ovaries. Printz and associates pointed out that such ovaries may be found in the omentum or retroperitoneally (Printz, 1973), and a dermoid cyst has been reported in a supernumerary ovary that occurred in the greater omentum. Wharton estimated that the occurrence of either accessory ovary or supernumerary ovary is rare, finding approximately 1 case of accessory ovary per 93,000 patients and 1 case of supernumerary ovary in 29,000 autopsies. In Wharton's review, three of four patients with supernumerary ovary and 5 of 19 patients with accessory ovary had additional congenital defects, most frequently abnormalities of the genitourinary tract (Wharton, 1959).

## KEY POINTS

- Gender identification in a newborn infant has emotional and psychological implications and should be performed as accurately as possible. However, in the setting of ambiguous genitalia, gender assignment should not be made without definitive testing and multidisciplinary participation.
- Congenital adrenal hyperplasia is an autosomal recessive condition, most commonly the result of an inborn error of metabolism involving the enzyme 21-hydroxylase. Homozygous individuals occur in 1 of every 490 to 67,000 births, averaging 1 in 14,000, and are at risk of moderate-to-severe manifestations. Heterozygotes (carriers) are present in 1 in 20 to 1 in 250 individuals and can have a more mild presentation. Differences in incidence depend on ethnic background of the population tested.
- Up to 75% of female neonates with ambiguous genitalia may develop a sodium-wasting adrenal crisis.
- The hymen develops at the junction of the sinovaginal bulb with the urogenital sinuses and is derived from endoderm, and multiple variants of hymenal anatomy exist.
- Vaginal agenesis is most often associated with Mayer-Rokitansky-Küster-Hauser syndrome or müllerian agenesis. Up to 50% of these women will have urologic abnormalities, and approximately one in eight will have skeletal abnormalities as well.
- Anomalies of the uterus and cervix demonstrate a polygenic or multifactorial pattern of inheritance and occur in approximately 2% to 3% of the female population.
- Approximately 15% of women with a history of first-trimester recurrent miscarriage and 25% of those with a second-trimester miscarriage may have a uterine anomaly.
- The uterine septum is the only uterine anomaly that can be easily corrected with a surgical procedure. In women with poor reproductive outcomes, surgery can normalize their chances of miscarriage and live birth.

## REFERENCES

Allen L. Disorder of sexual development. *Obstet Gynecol Clin North Am.* 2009;36(1):25–45.

The American Fertility Society classification of adnexal adhesions, distal tubal occlusion, tubal occlusion secondary to tubal ligation, tubal pregnancies, müllerian anomalies and intrauterine adhesions. *Fertil Steril.* 1988;49:944–955.

Baramki TA. The treatment of congenital anomalies in girls and women. *J Reprod Med.* 1984;29:376–384.

Benacerraf BR, Abuhamad AZ, Bromley B, et al. Consider ultrasound first for imaging the female pelvis. *Am J Obstet Gynecol.* 2015;212(4):450–455.

Bermejo C, Martinez Ten P, Cantarero R, Diaz D, Perez Pedregosa J, Barron E, et al. Three-dimensional ultrasound in the diagnosis of Müllerian duct anomalies and concordance with magnetic resonance imaging. *Ultrasound Obstet Gynecol.* 2010;35:593–601.

Black M, McKay M, Braude P, et al. *Obstetric and Gynecologic Dermatology.* 2nd ed. Edinburgh: Mosby; 2003:121.

Chan YY, Jayaprakasan K, Zamora J, et al. The prevalence of congenital uterine anomalies in unselected and high-risk populations: a systematic review. *Hum Reprod Update.* 2011;17:761–771.

Dietrich JE, Millar DM, Quint EH. Obstructive reproductive tract anomalies. *Pediatr Adolesc Gynecol.* 2014;27:396–402.

Fedele L, Bianchi S, Frontino G, et al. Laparoscopic findings and pelvic anatomy in Mayer-Rokitansky-Kuster-Hauser syndrome. *Obstet Gynecol.* 2007;109:1111–1115.

Grimbizis GF, Camus M, Tarlatzis BC, et al. Clinical implications of uterine malformations and hysteroscopic treatment results. *Hum Reprod Update.* 2001;7:161–174.

Grumbach MM, Hughes IA, Conte FA. Disorders of sex differentiation. In: Larsen RP, Kronenberg HM, Melmed S, Polonsky KS, eds. *Williams Textbook of Endocrinology.* 10th ed. Philadelphia: WB Saunders; 2003.

Homer HA, Li T-J, Cooke ID. The septate uterus: a review of management and reproductive outcome. *Fertil Steril.* 2000;73:1–14.
Jaysinghe Y, Rane A, Stalewski H, et al. The presentation and early diagnosis of the rudimentary uterine horn. *Obstet Gynecol.* 2005;105:1456–1467.
Lee PA, Houk CP, Ahmed SF, et al. Consensus statement on management of intersex disorders. International Consensus Conference on Intersex. *Pediatrics.* 2006;118(2):e488–500.
Low Y, Hutson JM. Murdoch Children's Research Institute Sex Study Group: Rules for clinical diagnosis in babies with ambiguous genitalia. *J Paediatr Child Health.* 2003;39:406–413.
Ludwin A, Ludwin I, Pitynski K, et al. Are the ESHRE/ESGE criteria of female genital anomalies for diagnosis of septate uterus appropriate? *Hum Reprod.* 2014;29(4):867–868.
Moore KL, Persaud TVN. *The Developing Human Clinically Oriented Embryology.* ed 7. Philadelphia: WB Saunders; 2003.
Nahum GG. Uterine anomalies—How common are they, and what is their distribution among subtypes. *J Reprod Med.* 1998;43:877–887.
Oppelt P, von Have M, Paulsen M, et al. Female genital malformations and their associated abnormalities. *Fertil Steril.* 2007;87:335–342.
Pang SY, Wallace MA, Hofman L, et al. Worldwide experience in newborn screening for classical congenital adrenal hyperplasia due to 21-hydroxylase deficiency. *Pediatrics.* 1988;81:866–874.
Phelan JT, Counseller VS, Greene LF. Deformities of the urinary tract with congenital absence of the vagina. *Surg Gynecol Obstet.* 1953;97:1.
Printz JL, Choate JW, Townes PL, et al. The embryology of supernumerary ovaries. *Obstet Gynecol.* 1973;41:246–252.
Thomas JC, Brock III JW. Vaginal substitution: attempts to create the ideal replacement. *J Urol.* 2007;178:1855–1859.
Toaff ME, Lev-Toaff AS, Toaff R. Communicating uteri: review and classification with introduction of two previously unrecorded types. *Fertil Steril.* 1984;41:661–679.
Troiano RN, McCarthy SM. Müllerian duct abnormalities: imaging and clinical issues. *Radiology.* 2004;233:19–34.
Usta IM, Awwad JT, Usta JA, et al. Imperforate hymen: report of an unusual familial occurrence. *Obstet Gynecol.* 1993;82:655–656.
Verkauf BS, Jones Jr HW. Masculinization of the female genitalia in congenital adrenal hyperplasia: relationship to the salt losing variety of the disease. *South Med J.* 1970;63:634–638.
Wharton LR. Two cases of supernumerary ovary and one of accessory ovary within an analysis of previously reported cases. *Am J Obstet Gynecol.* 1959;78:1101–1119.

Suggested Readings can be found on ExpertConsult.com.

# 12

# Pediatric and Adolescent Gynecology

## Gynecologic Examination, Infections, Trauma, Pelvic Mass, Precocious Puberty

*Eduardo Lara-Torre, Fidel A. Valea*

Gynecologic diseases are uncommon in children, especially compared with the incidence and prevalence of diseases in women of reproductive age. This chapter considers gynecologic diseases of children from infancy through adolescence. Congenital anomalies, precocious development, and amenorrhea are covered in more detail in other chapters.

The evaluation of children's gynecologic problems involves considerations of physiology, psychology, and developmental issues that are different from those of adult gynecology. The evaluation of young females is age dependent. For example, the physical presence of the mother often may facilitate examining a 4-year-old girl but may inhibit the cooperation of a 14-year-old adolescent. Thus the office visit and the gynecologic physical examination are performed differently in a prepubertal child compared with an adolescent girl or a mature reproductive-age woman.

## GYNECOLOGIC VISIT AND EXAMINATION OF A CHILD

### GENERAL APPROACH

Considerable effort should be devoted to gaining the child's confidence and establishing rapport. Young girls should feel that they are participating in their examination, not that they are being coerced or forced to have a gynecologic exam. If the interaction is poor during the first visit, the negative experience will detract from future physician-patient interactions (Lara-Torre, 2008).

The pediatric gynecologic visit may be unique to both the child and the parent. Most pediatric visits are preventive in nature. However, the pediatric gynecologic visit is usually problem oriented. This may create considerable and understandable anxiety in the child and parent. The majority of children's gynecologic problems are treated by medical, rather than surgical, means.

The most common gynecologic condition of children is vulvovaginitis. Other commonly seen diagnoses at a pediatric gynecology visit include labial adhesions, vulvar lesions, suspicion of sexual abuse, and genital trauma. Many, if not most, of these conditions will eventually require an examination to determine the etiology of the problem. An organized stepwise approach in a nonthreatening environment is more likely to result in a successful evaluation of the genitalia.

A successful gynecologic examination of a child demands that the physician adapt an exam pace that conveys both gentleness and patience with the time spent and not seem to be hurried or rushed. One excellent technique is for the physician to sit, not stand, during the initial encounter. This conveys an unhurried approach. The ambiance of the examining room may decrease the anxiety of the child if familiar and friendly objects such as children's posters are present. Interruptions should be avoided. Speculums and instruments that might frighten a child or parent should be within drawers or cabinets and out of sight during the evaluation. If a child is scheduled to be seen in the middle of a busy clinic, the staff needs to be alerted that the pace and general routine will be different during her visit.

### PERFORMANCE OF THE GYNECOLOGIC EXAM IN A CHILD

The components of a complete pediatric examination include a history; inspection with visualization of the external genitalia, non-invasive visualization of the vagina, and cervix; and, if necessary, a rectal examination (Jacobs, 2014).

Obtaining a history from a child is not an easy process. Children are not skilled historians and will often ramble, introducing many unrelated facts. Much of the history must be obtained from the parents. However, young children can help define their exact symptomatology on direct questioning. While obtaining a history, an opportunity exists to educate the child on vocabulary to describe the genital area. One way to describe genital area and breasts is to call them "private areas" and define this term as meaning areas that are covered by a bathing suit. The exam also allows a period of opportunity to counsel children, in an age-appropriate manner, about potential sexual abuse.

After the history has been obtained, the parents and the child should be reassured that the examination will not hurt. It is important to give the child a sense that she will be in control of the examination process. A helpful technique is to place the child's hand on top of the physician's hand as the abdominal examination is being performed and to give her some choices, such as having a doll or toy with her. This will give the child a sense of control as well as divert the child's attention if she is ticklish or is squirming. Emphasize that the most important part of the examination is just "looking" and there will be conversation during the entire process. To successfully examine a child, one needs the cooperation of the patient and a medical assistant.

A child's reaction will depend on her age, emotional maturity, and previous experience with health care providers. She should be allowed to visualize and handle any instruments that will be used. Many young children's primary contact with providers involves immunizations; children should be counseled and assured that this visit does not involve any "shots." It is also helpful to assure the adult that has accompanied the child that speculums are not part of the examination.

Occasionally it is best to defer the genital examination until a second visit. This is a difficult decision and is based on the extent of the child's anxiety in relation to the severity of the clinical symptoms. Physicians may elect to treat the primary symptoms of vulvovaginitis for 2 to 3 weeks, realizing that on rare occasions they could be missing something more serious. It is recommended that the examination start with the nongenital areas, such as listening to the heart and lungs; an abdominal exam and inspection of the skin should be performed. This allows one to establish a rapport and mimics the traditional visits the child has with the pediatrician. A child should never be restrained for a gynecologic examination. Often reassurance and sometimes delay until another day are the best approaches. In rare circumstances, it may be necessary to use continuous intravenous conscious sedation or general anesthesia to complete an essential examination. The most important technique to ensure cooperation is to involve the child as a partner. Children should ideally feel they are part of the exam rather than having an "exam done to them."

Draping for the gynecologic examination may produce more anxiety than it relieves and is unnecessary in the preadolescent child. A handheld mirror may help in some instances when discussing specifics of genital anatomy. It is critical to have all tools, culture tubes, and equipment within easy reach during a pediatric genital examination. Children often cannot hold still for long intervals while instruments are being located.

The first aspect of the pelvic examination is evaluation of the external genitalia (Fig. 12.1, *A* through *D*). An infant may be examined on her mother's lap. Pads should be placed in the mother's lap, as examination often is associated with urination. Young children may be examined in the frog leg position, and children as young as 2 to 3 years of age may be examined in lithotomy with use of stirrups. Lithotomy is generally used for girls 4 to 5 years of age and older.

Once the child is positioned, the vulvar area and introitus should be inspected. Many gynecologic conditions in children may be diagnosed by inspection. The introitus will gape open with gentle pressure downward and outward on the lower thigh or undeveloped thigh or labia majora area (traction) (Fig. 12.2). Asking the child to pretend to blow out candles on a birthday cake may facilitate the process. Visualization of the introitus is better achieved using the above described traction and Valsalva than separation, as it gives a deeper view of the structures and partial visualization of the vagina.

The second phase of the examination involves evaluation of the vagina. This can be accomplished without the use of any insertion of instruments. One method is to utilize the knee chest position (see Fig. 12.1, B). The child lies prone and places her buttocks in the air with legs wide apart. The vagina will then fill with air, aiding the evaluation. The child is told to have her abdomen sag into the table. An assistant pulls upward and outward on the labia majora on one side while the examiner does the same with the nondominant hand on the contralateral labia. Then an oto/ophthalmoscope is used as a magnifying instrument and light source but *is not* inserted into the vagina.

While the light from the oto/ophthalmoscope is shone into the vagina, the examiner can evaluate the vaginal walls and visualize the cervix as a transverse ridge, or flat button, that is redder than the vagina. This technique is generally successful in cooperative children unless there is a very high crescent-shaped hymen, in which case it is too difficult to shine the light into the small aperture of the vaginal introitus. A foreign object and the cervix may be visualized using this technique. Following inspection of the vagina and cervix, vaginal secretions may be obtained for microscopic examination and culture (the technique is described later).

## NORMAL FINDINGS: HYMEN AND VAGINA OF A PREPUBERTAL CHILD

The hymen of a prepubertal child exhibits a diverse range of normal variations and configurations (Fig. 12.3, *A* through *G*). Hymens are often crescent-shaped but may be annular or ring-like in configuration. They may have septums, microperforations, finger-like extensions, or be completely imperforate. There are no reported cases of congenital absence of the hymen. A mounding of hymeneal tissue is often called a *bump*. Bumps are usually a normal variant and are often attached to longitudinal ridges within the vagina. Hymens in newborns are estrogenized, resulting in a pink thick elastic redundancy. Older unestrogenized girls will have thin nonelastic hymens with significant signs of vascularity. Not every variant of hymen is normal and transections between 3 and 9 o'clock should raise a suspicion for abuse, as these are likely acquired (discussed further in Chapter 9).

The vaginal epithelium of the prepubertal child appears redder and thinner than the vagina of a woman in her reproductive years. The vagina is 4 to 6 cm long, and the secretions in a prepubertal child have a neutral or slightly alkaline pH. Recurrent vulvovaginitis, persistent bleeding, suspicion of a foreign body or neoplasm, and congenital anomalies may be indications to perform vaginoscopy and examine the inside of the vagina.

Vaginoscopy in a prepubertal child most often requires sedation with a brief inhalation or intravenous anesthetic, but it can also be performed in the office with older, cooperative children in select circumstances. The introduction of any instrument into the vagina of a young child takes skillful patience. The prepubertal vagina is narrower, thinner, and lacks the distensibility of the vagina of a woman in her reproductive years. There are many narrow-diameter endoscopes that will suffice, including the Kelly air cystoscope, contact hysteroscopes, pediatric cystoscopes, small-diameter laparoscopes, plastic vaginoscopes, and special virginal speculums designed by Huffman and Pederson. The ideal pediatric endoscope is a cystoscope or hysteroscope because the accessory channel facilitates the retrieval of foreign bodies as well as vaginal lavage. A nasal speculum or otoscope can also be used, but

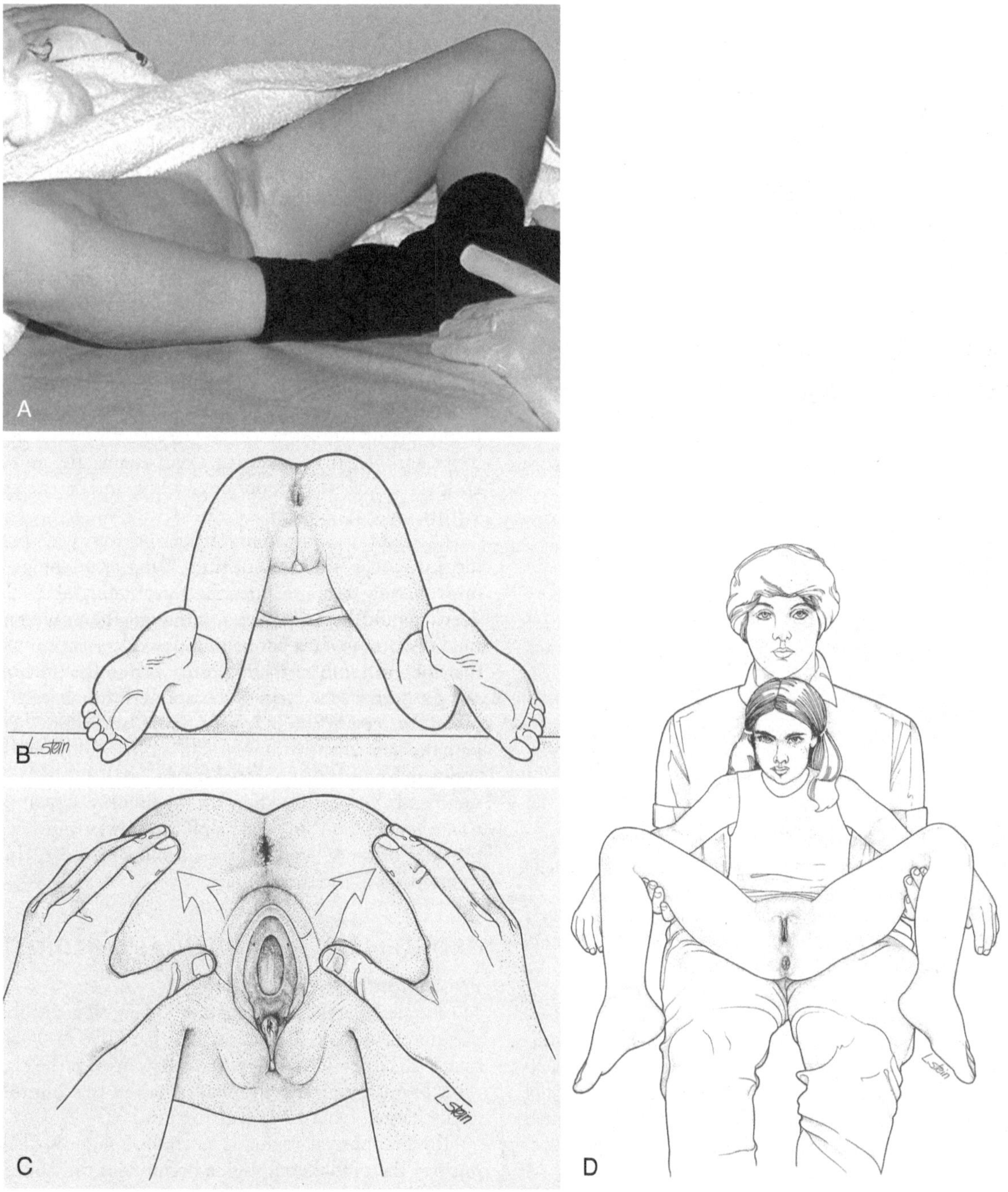


**Figure 12.1** Different exam positions for performing a gynecologic exam on a child. **A,** Frog leg position. **B,** Knee chest position. **C,** Prone position. **D,** Sitting on mom's lap. (**A,** from McCann JJ, Kerns DL. *The Anatomy of Child and Adolescent Sexual Abuse: A CD-ROM Atlas/Reference.* St. Louis: InterCorp: 1999; **B** and **C** and **D,** from Finkel MA, Giardino AP [eds.] *Medical Examination of Child Sexual Abuse: A Practical Guide*, 2nd ed. Thousand Oaks, CA: Sage, 2002, pp. 46-64.).

they are usually too short for older girls and less optimal. Local anesthesia of the vestibule may be obtained with 2% topical viscous lidocaine (Xylocaine) or longer-acting products such as lidocaine/prilocaine. **A complete vaginal evaluation should never be performed under duress or by force,** frequently the reason to use sedation when performing this examination on children.

The last step in the pelvic examination may be a rectal examination. This is often the most distressing aspect of the examination and may be omitted, depending on the child's symptoms. Common reasons to perform a rectal examination include genital tract bleeding, pelvic pain, and suspicion of a foreign body or pelvic mass. The child should be warned that the rectal examination will feel similar to the pressure of a bowel movement. The normal prepubertal uterus and ovaries are nonpalpable on rectal examination. The relative size ratio of cervix to uterus is 2 to 1 in a child, in contrast to the opposite ratio in an

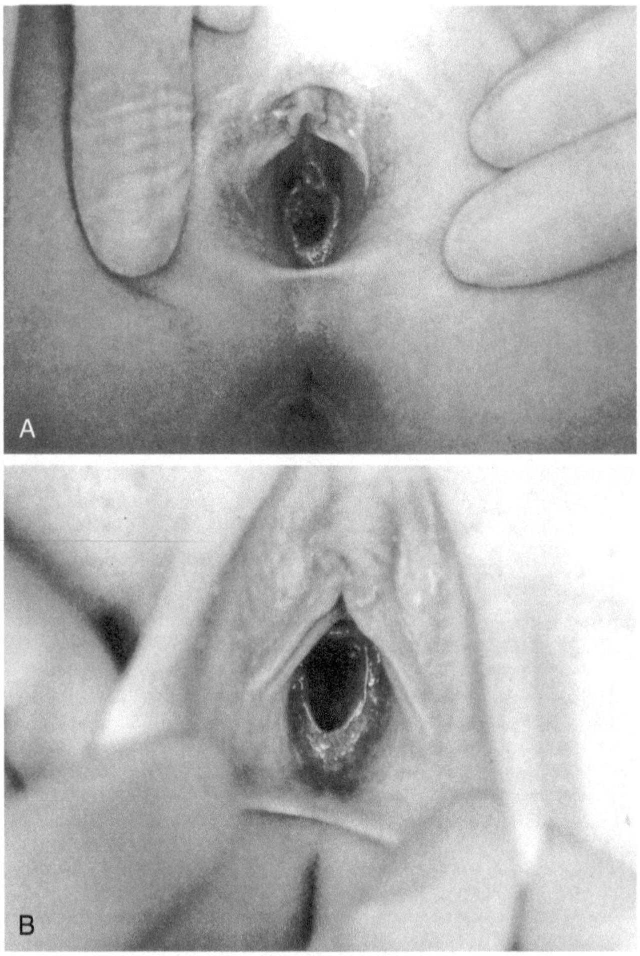

**Figure 12.2** Examination of the vulva, hymen, and anterior vagina by gentle lateral retraction (**A**) and gentle gripping of the labia and pulling anteriorly (**B**). (From Emans SJ. Office evaluation of the child and adolescent. In: Emans SJ, Laufer MR, Goldstein DP, eds. *Pediatric and Adolescent Gynecology.* 4th ed. Philadelphia: Lippincott-Raven; 1998.)

adult. Except for the cervix, any mass discovered on rectal examination in a prepubertal exam should be considered abnormal. In this age of reliable access to ultrasonography, the internal genital exam to evaluate for the uterus and ovaries can be performed with the assistance of sonography, sparing the child from a rectopelvic or pelvic examination.

## THE OFFICE VISIT AND EXAMINATION OF THE ADOLESCENT FEMALE

*Adolescence* is the period of life during which an individual matures physically and begins to transition psychologically from a child into an adult. This period of transition involves important physical and emotional changes. Before puberty, the girl's reproductive organs are in a resting, dormant state. Puberty produces dramatic alterations in the external and the internal female genitalia, as well as the adolescent's hormonal milieu. Because the pubertal changes are frequently a cause of concern for adolescent females and their parents, the gynecologist must offer the adolescent female an empathetic, kind, knowledgeable, and gentle approach. These interactions between the physician and the adolescent female will allow the physician an opportunity to gain her trust and educate the pubertal teenager about pelvic anatomy and reproduction.

The critical factors surrounding the pelvic examination of a female adolescent are different from those of examinations of children 2 to 8 years old. Many female adolescents do not want their mother, guardian, or other observers in the examining room. In many adolescent gynecology visits, a full pelvic exam is unnecessary (Lara-Torre, 2008). Frequent indications for a pelvic exam in an adolescent are listed in Box 12.1.

Each adolescent is at a different stage of development, and the approach to the exam may require variations that fit her developmental stage. A patient in early adolescence (12 to 14 years of age) may behave and need similar support as those in the prepubertal stages. They may ask for their mothers to be there, be fearful of the examination concept, and need more than one visit to achieve the goals of the visit. Those in middle or late adolescence (15 to 19 years of age) may be more acceptable to the idea of an exam and more likely to cooperate with the proper counseling and in the appropriate setting (ACOG, 2011).

Adolescents often come for examinations with preconceived ideas that it will be very painful. Slang terminology for speculums among teens includes the threatening label "the clamp." Teens should be assured that although the exam may include mild discomfort, it is not painful. Providers can counsel patients that they will inform them of each step in the process and then ask the teen if she is ready before performing each step. This places the teen in control of the tempo and allows her to anticipate the next element of the examination. Allowing them to see and touch the instruments also may assist in demystifying the exam and allow for it to flow more smoothly. Use of the "extinction phenomenon" may be helpful in this setting. The examiner provides pressure lateral to the introitus on the perineum prior to insertion of the speculum.

## PROBLEMS IN PREPUBERTAL CHILDREN

### Vulvovaginitis

*Vulvovaginitis* is the most common gynecologic problem in the prepubertal female. It is estimated that 80% to 90% of outpatient visits of children to gynecologists involve the classic symptoms of vulvovaginitis: introital irritation (discomfort/pruritus) or discharge (Table 12.1) (Farrington, 1997).

The prepubertal vagina is neutral or slightly alkaline. With puberty the prepubertal vagina becomes acidic under the influence of bacilli dependent on a glycogenated estrogen-dependent vagina. Breast budding is a reliable sign that the vaginal pH is shifting to an acidic environment.

The severity of vulvovaginitis symptoms varies widely from child to child. The pathophysiology of the majority of instances of vulvovaginitis in children involves a primary irritation of the vulva, which may be accompanied by secondary involvement of the lower one third of the vagina. Most cases involve an irritation of the vulvar epithelium by normal rectal flora or chemical irritants. This is referred to as *nonspecific vulvovaginitis.* There often are predisposing factors that lead to vulvar irritations such as the use of perfumed soaps, the pressure from tight seams of jeans or tights, and the like, which create denudation, allowing the rectal flora to easily infect the irritated epithelium. Cultures from the vagina return as normal rectal flora or *Escherichia coli.*

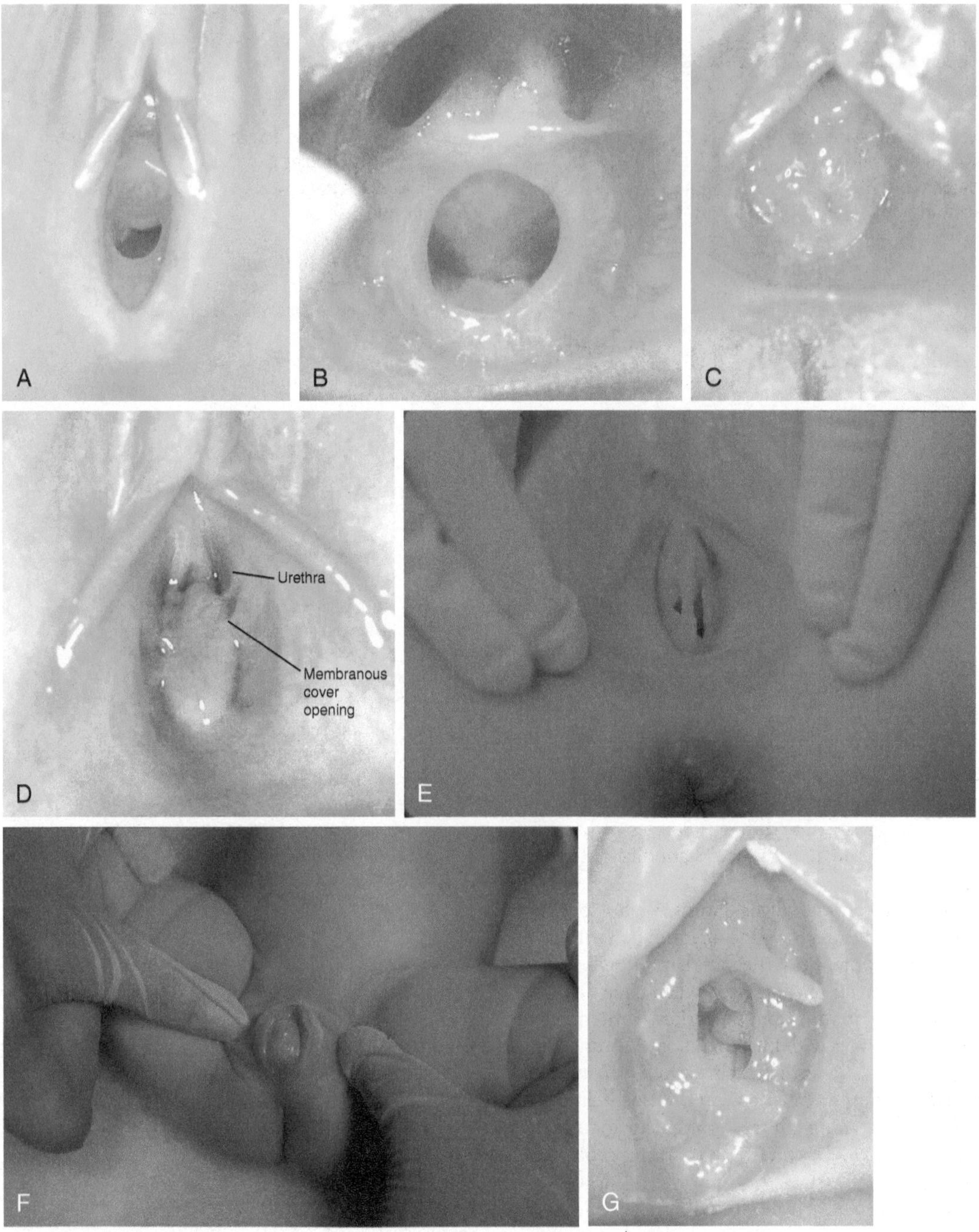


**Figure 12.3** Types of hymens. **A,** Crescentic. **B,** Annular. **C,** Redundant. **D,** Microperforate. **E,** Septated. **F,** Imperforate. **G,** Hymeneal tags. (**A** through **F**, From Perlman SE, Nakajima ST, Hertweck SP. *Clinical Protocols in Pediatric and Adolescent Gynecology.* London: Parthenon Publishing Group; 2004; **G,** From McCann JJ, Kerns DL. *The Anatomy of Child and Adolescent Sexual Abuse: A CD-ROM Atlas/Reference.* St. Louis: InterCorp; 1999.)

In a primary care setting, nonspecific vulvovaginitis accounts for the majority of vulvovaginitis cases.

There are both physiologic and behavioral reasons why a child is susceptible to vulvar infection. Physiologically, the child's vulva and vagina are exposed to bacterial contamination from the rectum more frequently than are the adult's. Because the child lacks the labial fat pads and pubic hair of the adult, when a child squats, the lower one third of the vagina is unprotected and open. There is no significant geographic barrier between the vagina and anus. The vulvar and vaginal epithelium lack the protective effects of estrogen and thus are sensitive to irritation or infection. The labia minora are thin and the vulvar skin is red because the abundant capillary network is easily visualized in the thin skin. The vaginal epithelium of a prepubertal child has a neutral or slightly alkaline pH, which provides an excellent medium for bacterial growth. The vagina of a child lacks

**Box 12.1 Common Indications for Pelvic Examination in the Adolescent**

Delayed puberty
Pelvic pain
Suspicion of intraabdominal disease
Dysfunctional uterine bleeding
Undiagnosed vaginal discharge
Inability to place tampons

Table 12.1 Clinical Features of Children Presenting with Vulvovaginitis

| Features | Number | Percentage |
|---|---|---|
| **Symptoms** | | |
| Itch | 81 | 40 |
| Soreness | 108 | 54 |
| Bleeding | 37 | 19 |
| Discharge | 104 | 52 |
| **Signs** | | |
| Genital redness | 167 | 84 |
| Visible discharge | 66 | 33 |
| Perianal soiling | 35 | 18 |
| Specific skin lesion | 28 | 14 |
| None | 5 | 2-4 |

From Pierce AM, Hart CA. Vulvovaginitis: causes and management. *Arch Dis Child.* 1992;67(4):509-512.

glycogen, lactobacilli, and a sufficient level of antibodies to help resist infection. The normal vagina of a prepubertal child is colonized by an average of nine different species of bacteria: four aerobic and facultative anaerobic species and five obligatory anaerobic species.

A major factor in childhood vulvovaginitis is poor perineal hygiene (Box 12.2). This results from the anatomic proximity of the rectum and vagina coupled with the fact that following toilet training, most youngsters are unsupervised when they defecate. Many youngsters wipe their anus from posterior to anterior and thus inoculate the vulvar skin with intestinal flora. A minor vulvar irritation may result in a scratch-itch cycle, with the possibility of secondary seeding because children wash their hands infrequently. Children's clothing is often tight fitting and nonabsorbent, which keeps the vulvar skin irritated, warm, moist, and prone to vulvovaginitis.

In some cases, nonspecific vulvovaginitis may be caused by carrying viral infections from coughing into the hands directly to the abraded vulvar epithelium. Similarly, a child with an upper respiratory tract infection may autoinoculate her vulva, especially with specific organisms (see Box 12.2). Vulvovaginitis in children may also be caused by a variety specific pathogens such as group A or group B β-hemolytic streptococci, *Haemophilus influenzae,* and *Shigella boydii; Neisseria gonorrhoeae, Trichomonas vaginalis, and Chlamydia trachomatis* may also be responsible in cases associated with abuse but are significantly less common.

Pinworms are another cause of vulvovaginitis in prepubertal children. Approximately 20% of female children infected with pinworms *(Enterobius vermicularis)* develop vulvovaginitis. The classic symptom of pinworms is nocturnal vulvar and perianal itching. At night the milk-white, pin-sized adult worms migrate from the rectum to the skin of the vulva to deposit eggs. They may be discovered by means of a flashlight or by dabbing of the vulvar skin with clear cellophane adhesive tape ideally before the child has arisen in the morning. The tape is subsequently examined under the microscope.

Despite common belief, mycotic (yeast) vaginal infections are *not* common in prepubertal children, as the alkaline pH of the vagina does not support fungal growth. Mycotic vaginal infections may be seen in immunosuppressed prepubertal girls such as HIV patients, diabetic children, or patients on chronic steroid therapy. It can also present in patients using diapers as a chronic colonization

**Box 12.2 Etiologic Factors of Premenarcheal Vulvovaginitis**

**Bacterial**

A. Nonspecific
  1. Poor perineal hygiene
  2. Intestinal parasitic invasion with pruritus
  3. Foreign bodies
  4. Urinary tract infections with irritation

B. Specific

Bacterial
1. Group A: β-hemolytic streptococci
2. *Streptococcus pneumonia*
3. *Haemophilus influenzae*/parainfluenzae
4. *Staphylococcus aureus*
5. *Neisseria meningitides*
6. *Escherichia coli*
7. *Shigella flexneri/sonnei*
8. Other enterics
9. *Neisseria gonorrhoeae*
10. *Chlamydia trachomatis*

Protozoal—*Trichomonas*

Mycotic
1. *Candida albicans*
2. Other

Helminthiasis—*Enterobius vermicularis*

Viral/Bacterial Systemic Illness
1. Chicken pox
2. Measles
3. Pityriasis rosea
4. Mononucleosis
5. Scarlet fever
6. Kawasaki disease

Other Viral Illnesses
1. Molluscum contagiosum in genital area
2. Condylomata acuminate
3. Herpes simplex type II

Physical/Chemical Agents
1. Sandbox
2. Trauma
3. Bubble bath
4. Other

Allergic/Skin Conditions
1. Seborrhea
2. Lichen sclerosus
3. Psoriasis
4. Eczema
5. Contact dermatitis

Tumors

Other
1. Prolapsed urethra
2. Ectopic ureter

From Blythe MJ, Thompson L. Premenarchal vulvovaginitis. *Indiana Med.* 1993;86(3):236-239.

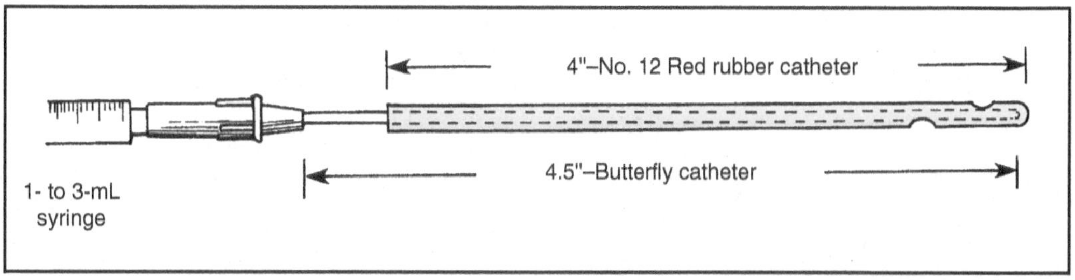


**Figure 12.4** Assembled catheter within a catheter, as used to obtain samples of vaginal secretions from prepubertal patients. (Modified from Pokorny SF, Stormer J. Atraumatic removal of secretions from the prepubertal vagina. *Am J Obstet Gynecol.* 1987;156[3]:581-582.)

(diaper rash). Other specific causes of vulvovaginitis may include systemic diseases, chicken pox, and herpes simplex infection.

There is nothing specific about the symptoms or signs of childhood vulvovaginitis. Often the first awareness comes when the mother notices staining of the child's underwear or the child complains of itching or burning. There is a wide range in the quantity of discharge, from minimal to copious. The color ranges from white or gray to yellow or green. A discharge that is both bloody and purulent is likely not from vulvovaginitis but from a foreign body (see "Vaginoscopy for Prepubertal Bleeding without Signs of Puberty," presented later in this chapter), although patients infected with some pathogens, particularly *Shigella boydii,* often present with a bloody or blood-tinged discharge. The signs of vulvovaginitis are variable and not diagnostic, but they include vulvar erythema, edema, and excoriation.

The differential diagnosis of persistent or recurrent vulvovaginitis not responsive to treatment should include considerations of a foreign body, primary vulvar skin disease (allergic or contact dermatitis), ectopic ureter, and child abuse. If the predominant symptom is pruritus, then pinworms or an irritant/nonspecific vulvitis is the most likely diagnosis.

The vulvar skin of children may also be affected by systemic skin diseases, including lichen sclerosus, seborrheic dermatitis, psoriasis, and atopic dermatitis. The classic perianal "figure-8" or "hourglass" rash is indicative of lichens scleroses with white patches and in some cases local trauma. An ectopic ureter emptying into the vagina may only intermittently release a small amount of urine; thus this rare congenital anomaly should be considered in the differential diagnosis in young children.

### Treatment of Vulvovaginitis

The foundation of treating childhood vulvovaginitis is the improvement of local perineal hygiene. Both parent and child should be instructed that the vulvar skin should be kept clean, dry, and cool, and irritants should be avoided. The child should be instructed to void with her knees spread wide apart (even while facing the toilet to improve urine draining) and taught to wipe from front to back after defecation. Loose-fitting cotton undergarments should be worn. Chemicals that may be allergens or irritants, such as bubble bath, must be discontinued. Harsh soaps and chemicals should be avoided. Instructing patients to use nonmedicated, nonscented wipes rather than toilet paper may prevent the self-inoculation of the vagina with small pieces that can initiate a chronic discharge.

Most episodes of childhood vulvovaginitis are cured solely by improved local hygiene. The majority of symptoms improve with hygienic changes and sitz baths (warm water, no soaps or chemicals). Utilizing this approach for a 2-week period should resolve most symptoms in patients with nonspecific vulvovaginitis. When this intervention fails, the suspicion for bacterial colonization is greater and a reasonable approach is the use of broad-spectrum oral antibiotics such as amoxicillin or trimethoprim sulfamethoxazole given for 10 to 14 days. Without continuation of the hygiene measures, then broad-spectrum antibiotics will only offer temporary relief, and the problem is likely to recur (Bercaw-Pratt, 2014).

If patients are going to be treated with antibiotics, one should attempt to collect a culture of the vulvovaginal discharge prior to initiation of the antibiotics. In noncooperative children, treatment should not be withheld if unable to collect a specimen and empiric treatment may be started. For attempting to collect a specimen, many techniques have been described including the use of a very slim urethral Dacron swab moistened with nonbacteriostatic saline (used for collection of male urethral cultures). Pokorny has described another method for collecting fluid from a child's vagina using a catheter within a catheter (Pokorny, 1987). This easily assembled adaptation uses a No. 12 red rubber bladder catheter for the outer catheter and the hub end of an intravenous butterfly catheter for the inner catheter (Fig. 12.4). The outer catheter serves as an insulator, and the inner catheter is used to instill a small amount of saline and aspirate into the vaginal fluid. The results of the vaginal culture may demonstrate a single organism that is a respiratory, intestinal, or sexually transmitted disease pathogen. The presence of sexually transmitted organisms in a child is usually a strong indication that sexual abuse may have taken place and appropriate referral and follow-up is necessary (see Chapter 9).

## OTHER PREPUBERTAL GYNECOLOGIC PROBLEMS

### Labial Adhesions

*Labial adhesions* literally mean the labia minora have adhered or agglutinated together at the midline. Another term sometimes used to describe this condition is *adhesive vulvitis.* Denuded epithelium of adjacent labia minora agglutinates and fuses the two labia together, creating a "flat appearance" of the vulvar surface. A telltale somewhat translucent vertical midline line is visible on physical exam at the site agglutination. This thin, narrow line in a vertical direction is pathognomonic for labial adhesions (Fig. 12.5). Labial adhesions are often partial and only involve the upper or lower aspects of the labia. Small adhesions are common

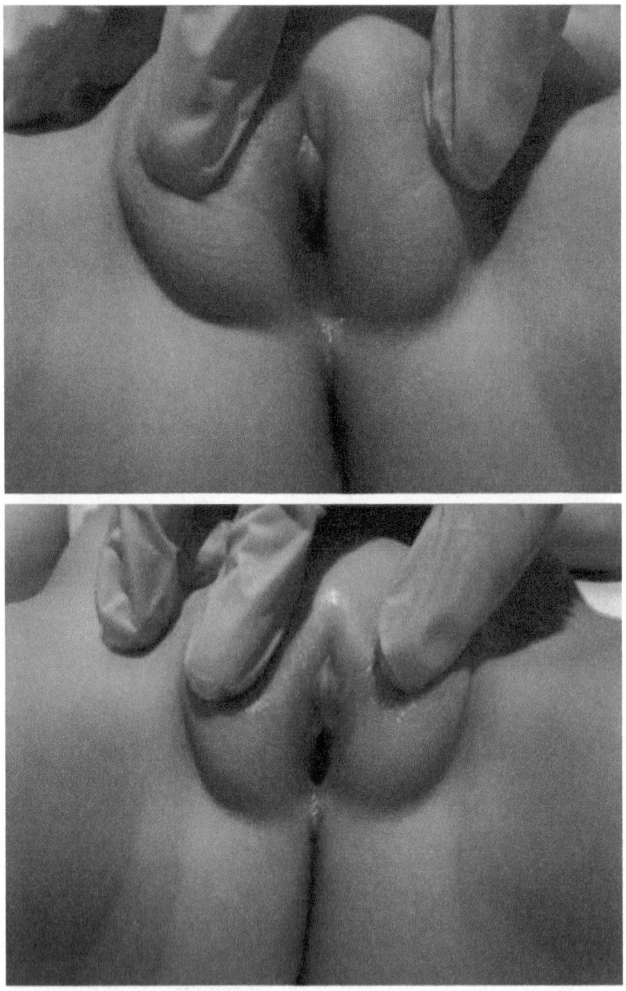

**Figure 12.5** Labial adhesions before and after treatment. (From Acker A, Jamieson MA. Use of intranasal midazolam for manual separation of labial adhesions in the office. *J Pediatr Adolesc Gynecol.* 2013;26[3]:196-198.)

in preschool children, and perhaps as many as 20% will have some degree of labial adhesions on routine examination (Bacon, 2015).

Inexperienced examiners may confuse labial adhesions for an imperforate hymen or vaginal agenesis. Although the physical exam findings are significantly different, all of these conditions may occlude the visualization of the vaginal introitus. In the patient with an imperforate hymen, the labia minora normally appear like an upside down V, and no hymeneal fringe is visible at the introitus. In vaginal agenesis, the hymeneal fringe is typically normal, but the vaginal canal ends blindly behind the hymeneal fringe.

Labial adhesions are most common in girls between 2 and 6 years of age, with up to 90% of cases occurring before age 6. Estrogen reaches a nadir during this time, predisposing the nonestrogenized labia to denudation.

There is considerable variation in the length of agglutination of the two labia minora. In the most advanced cases, there is fusion over both the urethral and the vaginal orifices. It is extremely rare for this fusion to be complete, and most children urinate through openings at the top of the adhesions, even when the urethra cannot be visualized (pinpoint opening). However, the partially fused labia may form a pouch in which urine is caught and later dribbled, presenting as incontinence. Associated urinary infections have also been reported and may be the presenting symptom leading to the diagnosis. Most patients will be asymptomatic or present with intermittent dysuria.

The recommended treatment in asymptomatic patients is observation (Bacon, 2015). Most of the time treatment requests are driven by the parental concern of a closed vagina and their interpretation that this may lead to an inability to have children in the future or engage in intercourse. Although they do not explicitly say this, upon further questioning, many parents disclose this kind of concern. With appropriate counseling and reassurance of the benign and common nature of this condition, as well as the likely resolution during puberty, most parents are reassured and follow advice. The majority of the patients will fall into this category and can be reassured and followed over time to spontaneous resolution when they produce their own endogenous estrogen. If spontaneous separation does not occur at puberty, and manual separation is required, the presence of a better estrogenized skin will decrease the chances of recurrence which in children can range from 25% to 65%.

Some children will present with symptoms and may include voiding difficulties, dysuria, frequent urinary infections, urine dribbling after voiding, recurrent vulvovaginitis, discomfort from the labia pulling at the line of adhesions, and in rare cases bleeding from the line of adhesion pulling apart.

Attempts to separate the adhesions apart in the office by pulling briskly on the labia minora should not be done. It is very painful, and the raw edges are likely to adhere again as the child will be reticent to allow application of medication after being subjected to this degree of pain. Even with local anesthesia, such as lidocaine ointments or creams, the potential pain and traumatic experience for the child should deter from this intervention, except in the well-motivated, mature child.

The most commonly utilized treatment of this condition is topical estrogen cream applied onto the labia two times per day at the site of fusion. This will usually result in spontaneous separation, usually in approximately 2 to 8 weeks. In cases when resolution takes longer than several weeks, the clinician can reexamine the patient. If increased pigmentation is noted lateral to the midline line of agglutination, the caregiver should be reinstructed to apply the cream to the line, as the lateral pigmentation indicates the estrogen is being applied lateral to the actual adhesion. The action of estrogen as well as the application over the adhesion line itself makes the treatment more effective. Care should be taken to not prolong the topical use of estrogen for more than 6 to 8 weeks. Prolonged use of topical estrogen has been associated with breast budding and in some less common cases vaginal bleeding from the peripheral effects of the absorption of estrogen. Failure of separation within the normal time frame should trigger alternate treatment.

When patients fail estrogen therapy, and symptoms persist, the use of topical corticosteroids twice a day for 6 to 8 weeks has also shown adequate results and can be consider as a first or secondary line of treatment.

Once the condition has been resolved, recurrence can often be prevented by applying a bland ointment (such as zinc oxide cream or petroleum jelly) to the raw epithelial edges for at least 1 month or even longer. As previously mentioned, recurrences are common.

McCann and colleagues reported the association between injuries of the posterior fourchette and labial adhesions in sexually abused children (McCann, 1988). Labial agglutination alone is so common that immediate suspicion of child abuse based solely on this finding in 2- to 6-year-olds is unwarranted. However, the combination of labial adhesions and scarring of the posterior fourchette, especially in children with new-onset labial adhesions after age 6, should prompt the clinician to consider sexual abuse in the differential diagnosis.

### *Physiologic Discharge of Puberty*

In the early stages of puberty, children often develop a physiologic vaginal discharge. This discharge is typically described as having a gray-white coloration, although it may appear slightly yellow but is not purulent. The physiologic discharge represents desquamation of the vaginal epithelium. The estrogenic environment allows acid-producing bacilli to become part of the normal vaginal ecosystem. The acids the bacilli produce cause a desquamation of the prepubertal vaginal epithelium. When the physiologic discharge is examined with the microscope, sheets of vaginal epithelial cells are identified.

Clinically, there is usually very little symptomatology associated with this discharge. Occasionally the thickness of the discharge causes the vulva to be "pasted" to undergarments and causes some symptoms of irritation and erythema. Usually the only treatment necessary is reassurance of both mother and child that this is a normal physiologic process that will subside with time. Symptomatic children may be treated with sitz baths and frequent changing of underwear.

### *Urethral Prolapse*

Prolapse of the urethral mucosa is not a rare event in children. The most common presentation is not urinary symptomatology but prepubertal bleeding. Often a sharp increase in abdominal pressure, such as coughing, precedes the urethral prolapse. On examination, the distal aspect of urethral mucosa may be prolapsed along the entire 360 degrees of the urethra (Fig. 12.6). This forms a red donut-like structure. The prolapse may be partial or incomplete, presenting as a ridge of erythematous tissue. It is critical to distinguish this from grapelike masses of sarcoma botryoides that originate from the vagina. Occasionally the prolapse becomes necrotic and blue-black in color.

The most common treatment is conservative and nonsurgical. Topical estrogen has been found effective in the management of this condition in many case reports and series. Although no randomized control trials exist, the short duration of treatment and shown benefits on these series supports treatment to prevent necrosis. Surgery is seldom necessary, except in rare cases where necrosis is obviously present.

### *Lichen Sclerosus*

*Lichen sclerosus* (LS), or lichen sclerosus atrophicus, is a skin dystrophy most commonly seen in postmenopausal women and prepubertal children. The cause is unclear, although there is some evidence that it may be associated with autoimmune phenomena. This has not been confirmed by prospective studies. Histologically, there is thinning of the vulvar epithelium with loss of the rete pegs. The most common symptoms are pruritus and vulvar discomfort. Other presentations may include prepubertal bleeding from trauma, constipation, and dysuria (Bercaw-Pratt, 2014).

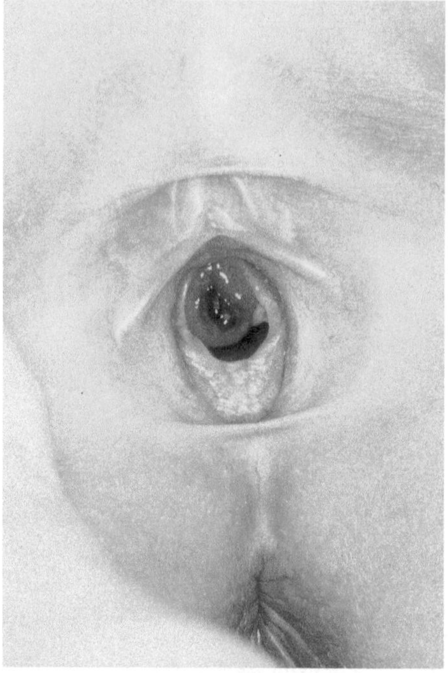

**Figure 12.6** Prepubertal urethral prolapse with high crescent-shaped hymen.

The appearance of LS varies, but lesions are always limited by the labia majora. If lesions go beyond the labia majora, the condition is unlikely to be LS. The lesion often appears in an hourglass or figure-8 formation involving the genital and perianal area (Fig. 12.7). The skin may be lichenified with a hypopigmented parchment-like appearance. Parents may note that the genital area appears whitened. Pruritus is typical presenting symptom. Secondary changes may occur subsequent to the patient excoriating the area. When this occurs, there are often signs of trauma and breaks in the integument, which in turn can become colonized with skin bacteria and create a superimposed bacterial dermatitis.

Given the abnormal appearance of LS with secondary changes, clinicians unfamiliar with this skin dystrophy often arrive at the misdiagnosis of sexual abuse. However, clinicians experienced in pediatric or postmenopausal gynecology will usually have no difficulty arriving at the correct diagnosis. Given the classic appearance in children, and the lack of association at this age with cancer, a biopsy is not necessary or indicated before treatment. In cases in which the diagnosis is unclear, or recalcitrant to therapy, a small punch biopsy may confirm the diagnosis. Performing a biopsy in prepubertal children is often difficult. Many children will not tolerate a local injection, and holding down children to perform a biopsy is clearly not acceptable. Sedation anesthesia is preferable in this situation. Rarely, children will tolerate a biopsy using local anesthesia.

The treatment of LS in children should always start with avoiding irritation or trauma to the genital epithelium. Children should be encouraged to avoid straddle activities such as bicycle or tricycle riding when symptomatic. Patients should clean the labia by soaking in sitz baths. Parents sometimes may assume lack of cleanliness is contributing to the disorder and scrub the area with soap, which may actually exacerbate the disease. Tight clothing such as jeans or tights may also abrade and irritate the vulva.

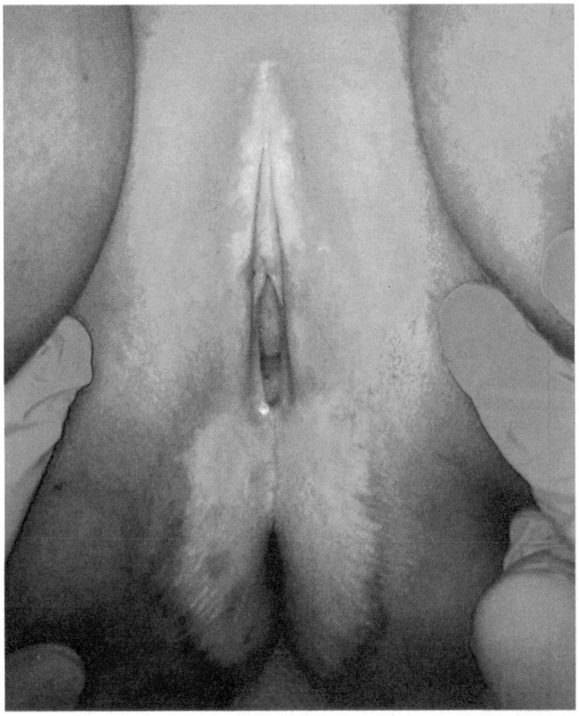

**Figure 12.7** Typical appearance of lichen sclerosus in a 9-year-old with 1-year history of vulvar pruritus. (From Bercaw-Pratt JL, Boardman LA, Simms-Cendan JS, North American Society for Pediatric and Adolescent Gynecology. Clinical recommendation: pediatric lichen sclerosus. *J Pediatr Adolesc Gynecol.* 2014;27[2]:111-116.)

The North American Society of Pediatric and Adolescent Gynecology (NASPAG) recommends the use of high-potency steroids such as clobetasol as the initial step in treatment of this condition. Tapering the steroid level should be considered as soon as a response is seen or within a 4- to 6-week interval. The tapering can be achieved by following the initial treatment with a 2- to 3-week of midpotency steroid such as betamethasone and conclude with 1% hydrocortisone for another 2 weeks (Fig. 12.8). The use of ointments is preferred over creams given there is less irritation compared with creams and the petroleum base of ointments appear to help it stay in place longer. The parents should apply the drug sparingly but consistently, avoiding application to nonaffected areas to prevent systemic effects of the drug such as adrenal suppression.

Recurrence or "flares" of the condition are common and continue for a significant period of time in most patients. Previously, many authors have asserted that LS improves with puberty. Though improvement and resolution occur sometimes, many patients will continue to have symptoms or physical findings.

## PREPUBERTAL BLEEDING WITHOUT SECONDARY SIGNS OF PUBERTY

Puberty in the female is the process of biologic change and physical development after which sexual reproduction becomes possible. This is a time of accelerated linear skeletal growth and development of secondary sexual characteristics, such as breast development and the appearance of axillary and pubic hair. The usual sequence of the physiologic events of

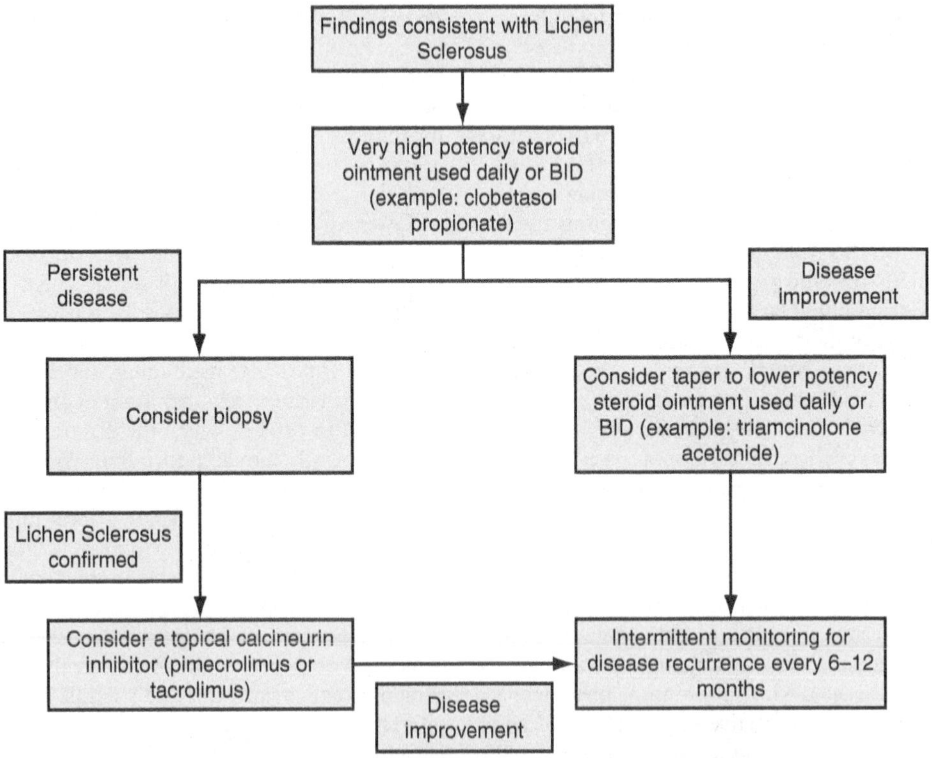


**Figure 12.8** Algorithm for treatment of lichen sclerosus in children. (From Bercaw-Pratt JL, Boardman LA, Simms-Cendan JS, North American Society for Pediatric and Adolescent Gynecology. Clinical recommendation: pediatric lichen sclerosus. *J Pediatr Adolesc Gynecol.* 2014;27[2]:111-116.)

**Box 12.3 Differential Diagnosis of Prepubertal Bleeding without Any Breast Development**

Foreign object
Genital trauma
Sexual abuse
Lichen sclerosus
Infectious vaginitis (especially from *Shigella*)
Urethral prolapse
Breakdown of labial adhesions
Friable genital warts or vulvar lesions
Vaginal tumor
Rare presentation of McCune-Albright syndrome (typically have breast development)
Isolated menarche (controversial)
Dermatologic conditions with secondary excoriation
Nongenital bleeding; mistaken as genital: rectal and urinary

puberty begins with a somatic change: an increase in growth velocity followed by either breast development (thelarche) or the appearance of pubic hair (adrenarche), followed by the period of maximal growth velocity (approximately 9 cm/year), and, last, menarche. The onset of thelarche typically precedes adrenarche in white girls. In contrast, African-American girls often have adrenarche prior to thelarche (up to 15% of girls) (Appelbaum, 2012).

A cross-sectional study of more than 1700 American girls provided contemporary data on pubertal timing (the Pediatric Research in Office Settings [PROS] study) (Herman-Giddens, 1997). In this study approximately one third of the African-American girls had thelarche or adrenarche at age 7 and almost 50% by age 8. Approximately 15% of white girls had initiated puberty by age 8 and almost 40% by age 9. Mean ages for thelarche and adrenarche were 8.9 and 8.8 for African-American girls and 10 and 10.5 years for white girls, respectively. The mean age of menarche was almost 12.2 years for the African-American girls compared with 12.8 years in the white girls. It should be noted that these ages of pubertal onset were significantly earlier, and sequences somewhat different, than previous, much older, classic descriptions of British children published by Marshall and Tanner (Marshall, 1969).

Recommendations from the PROS have included a new guideline regarding the definition of precocious development. They propose that precocious puberty should be defined as thelarche or adrenarche prior to age 6 in African-American girls or 7 in white girls. These recommendations are controversial, as some serious pathologic causes (endocrine or central nervous system [CNS]) could be overlooked if these guidelines were strictly upheld. Certainly, in girls younger than 8 with CNS or behavioral issues, a pathologic etiology of development should be entertained. A common clinical problem that is sometimes mistaken for precocious puberty is prepubertal bleeding in children without any other signs of puberty such as breast development (Box 12.3).

### *Vaginal Bleeding*

The normal sequence of puberty is that thelarche precedes menarche. In children with prepubertal bleeding without breast budding, there is almost never an endocrinologic cause, with the exception being a rare presentation of McCune-Albright syndrome (polyostotic fibrous dysplasia) or the uncommon presentation of isolated premature menarche.

The differential diagnosis of vaginal bleeding without pubertal development includes foreign body, vulvar excoriation, lichen sclerosus, shigella vaginitis, separation of labial adhesions, trauma (abuse and accidental), urethral prolapse, and friable genital warts (see Box 12.2). Rare causes include malignant tumors (sarcoma botryoides and endodermal sinus tumors of the vagina) and an unusual presentation of McCune-Albright syndrome. Lists of the differential diagnosis of prepubertal bleeding often also include accidental estrogen exposure (for example, from ingestion of a mother's birth control pills or prolonged used of estrogen topical therapy). However, in reality such exposure would rarely provide enough endometrial stimulation to produce a withdrawal bleed without breast budding. Neonates may develop a white mucoid vaginal discharge or a small amount of vaginal spotting because of the withdrawal of maternal estrogens. The discharge and vaginal spotting are self-limited.

It should be remembered that although the differential diagnosis of prepubertal bleeding includes sexual abuse, most sexually abused children do not have prepubertal bleeding. In some settings, such as emergency departments, it is more likely that prepubertal bleeding is due to sexual abuse than in primary pediatric office or a tertiary referral practice.

### *Foreign Bodies*

Symptoms secondary to a vaginal foreign body are responsible for approximately 4% of pediatric gynecologic outpatient visits. The majority of foreign bodies are found in girls between 3 and 9 years of age. The history is usually not helpful because an adult has not witnessed, nor does the child remember, putting a foreign object into the vagina. Many types of foreign bodies have been discovered; however, the most common are small wads of toilet paper. Other common foreign objects include small, hard objects such as hairpins, parts of a toy, tips of plastic markers, crayons, and sand or gravel. Some of these objects are not radiopaque. When small swabs are used to perform vaginal cultures, the examiner may note an odd sensation of touching something other than vaginal mucosa. Objects such as coins and plastic toys are often easily visible on vaginal examination, especially in the knee-chest position. Children may insert foreign bodies because the genital area is pruritic or when naturally curious children are exploring their bodies.

The classic symptom is a foul, bloody vaginal discharge. However, the discharge is often purulent and without blood. The natural history probably reflects the object initially causing irritation, creating a purulent discharge, and then as the object imbeds itself into the vaginal epithelium, bleeding and spotting may occur. There is often a lag between insertion of the object and the vaginal bleeding. Over time, the foreign body may become partially "buried" or imbedded within the vaginal wall. These imbedded objects are often difficult to remove without discomfort and may require sedation.

The presence of unexplained vaginal bleeding is an indication for a vaginoscopy. Especially in children younger than 6 years of age, without of signs of an endocrinopathy (breast budding, estrogenization of the hymen), this should be done expeditiously to rule out malignant vaginal tumors. If an object is seen on exam, the clinician may be able, in a cooperative child, to either grasp the object with a forceps or wash the object out by irrigation. The catheter technique described previously may be utilized. The use of a pediatric feeding tube with room temperature or warmed saline can also be used to "flush" the vagina. With either technique, care should be taken to minimize contact with the hymen, as it is a sensitive area at this age and the sensation can be enough for the child to stop cooperating with the procedure. In many instances this is not possible because the child cannot cooperate or because a solid object is imbedded into the vaginal wall. In these cases the object can be removed at vaginoscopy.

Children who insert foreign objects often have recurrences. This may be secondary to persistent pain or pruritus in the genital area that was not addressed at the initial encounter, and the child uses the object (solid or toilet paper) to rub or scratch the genital area. If the foreign object is toilet paper, then having the child use wipes instead of toilet paper may reduce recurrences.

#### Shigella *Vaginitis*

Approximately half of all cases of *Shigella* vaginitis present with prepubertal bleeding. There is generally no concurrent gastrointestinal symptomatology. Cultures for *Shigella* should be strongly considered in any child with no obvious cause for prepubertal bleeding. Rarely, vaginitis caused by other organisms can also present with prepubertal bleeding.

#### *Rare Causes: Vaginal Tumors and McCune-Albright Syndrome*

McCune-Albright syndrome is a rare somatic mutation that occurs during embryogenesis in neural crest cells. Because the mutation does not occur in the germline, it is not inherited. The mutation affects G protein receptors and has a variable expression, depending on how many early cells are affected (an example of mosaicism). The *GNAS1* gene is the affected area. Patients with the syndrome may manifest the classic triad of café-au-lait spots, abnormal bone lesions, and precocious puberty. Most McCune-Albright patients present with prepubertal bleeding along with thelarche. Rarely a child may present with bleeding and no breast budding. Examination of the child with prepubertal bleeding should include examination of the skin for café-au-lait spots, and the historical intake should include queries about frequent bone fractures. In cases of unexplained prepubertal bleeding, the possibility of McCune-Albright should be considered, and serial breast examinations may reveal breast budding.

#### *Sarcoma Botryoides and Endodermal Sinus Tumors of the Vagina*

Almost all cases of sarcoma botryoides of the vagina in prepubertal children occur prior to age 6 (although cases up until age 8 have been reported), and endodermal sinus tumors occur prior to age 2. Although these tumors are extremely rare causes of prepubertal bleeding, they must be considered in every young child. Both are aggressive malignancies, and prompt diagnosis is critical. In young children with no evident cause of prepubertal bleeding, a vaginoscopy should be done to rule out these malignancies.

#### *Vaginoscopy for Prepubertal Bleeding without Signs of Puberty*

Many times, no clear cause of prepubertal bleeding is defined at vaginoscopy. In these cases there likely was a small foreign object that has been expelled from the vagina or disintegrated. Even though many vaginoscopies are negative, it is especially important for clinicians to perform them promptly in young prepubertal bleeders to exclude rare but aggressive vaginal malignancies.

## ACCIDENTAL GENITAL TRAUMA

The usual cause of accidental genital trauma during childhood is a fall. Seventy-five percent of accidental trauma to the vulva and vagina involves straddle injuries. Obviously, sexual abuse is an important consideration in the differential diagnosis (Bond, 1995). Sexual abuse in a child is discussed later in this chapter.

### *VULVAR TRAUMA: LACERATIONS AND STRADDLE INJURY*

One of the most common causes of genital trauma in a child is a straddle injury. This problem occurs when a child stands, or hovers, with her legs apart over a hard object and then falls with the perineum against the object. Common straddle injuries in children occur on playground climbing structures, such as a monkey bar, or fence rails and around the edges of pools. A straddle injury generally results in unilateral and superficial injury and rarely involves the hymen. In two separate series involving more than 130 children with straddle injuries, only 3 had hymeneal transection (Dowd, 1994).

In cases of hymeneal transection with a history of straddle injury, sexual abuse should be strongly considered. In the rare cases in which the hymen is transected from accidental trauma, there is usually a history of a penetrating injury such as falling onto a stick horse or broom. If hymeneal transection has occurred, the examiner must confirm that the object has not penetrated into the vaginal wall, which could result in a dangerous hematoma, perforation into the cul-de-sac, or perforation of the abdominal cavity with potential visceral damage. A vaginoscopy or laparoscopy (or both) is generally required to rule out these possibilities. Perforations into the abdomen may not result in significant vaginal bleeding.

In children presenting with trauma and genital bleeding, the examiner must first ascertain the site, extent, and amount of bleeding. Viscous lidocaine or a longer-acting topical agent such as lidocaine/prilocaine can be applied and allowed appropriate time to provide anesthesia. Then the area can be gently washed by irrigating with sterile warmed water onto the labial area. Typical lacerations may involve denudation around the urethra or labia. The posterior fourchette is less commonly involved. In children with vulvar trauma, considerations should be given to giving a booster injection of tetanus toxoid if the last immunization was more than 5 years before the trauma.

Lacerations that are superficial (equivalent to first-degree obstetric lacerations) generally do not require repair in contrast to deeper lacerations. Often, superficial lacerations can be adequately treated by applying oxidized cellulose or similar products to stop the bleeding. Slightly deeper lacerations can be repaired with small Steri-Strips. In some deeper lacerations, one well-placed suture will stop substantial bleeding. This scenario is typical of lacerations on the inferior aspect of the labia minora. Placement of the suture may be aided by injection of lidocaine in cooperative children or by conscious sedation in the emergency department.

General anesthesia is usually required for diagnosis and treatment of extensive lacerations and deep lacerations or in children who are unable to tolerate repair in the office or emergency department. In patients in whom the extent of the laceration cannot be visualized an exam under anesthesia should be performed to prevent missing deeper lacerations than what is visualized in the emergency room. While anesthetized, the laceration should be irrigated and débrided, the vessels ligated, and the injuries repaired. Occasionally it is necessary to perform laparoscopy or an exploratory laparotomy for a suspected retroperitoneal hematoma or intraabdominal injury. Appropriate consultation with urology or pediatric surgery is recommended when the extent of the laceration is beyond the vulvar-vaginal areas.

### *Vulvar Hematomas*

If the vulva strikes a blunt object, a hematoma usually results. The lack of the mature reproductive woman's fat pad in the vulvar area predisposes a young child to bleeding from trauma. If the object is sharp, such as a fence post or skating blade, the injury may be a laceration with the potential for penetration of the perineum and injury to internal pelvic organs. Other common causes of vulvar and vaginal trauma include sexual abuse, automobile and bicycle accidents, kicks sustained in a fight, and self-inflicted wounds (Fig. 12.9).

The size of vulvar and vaginal hematomas varies widely. Initially there is bleeding into the loose connective tissue. When the pressure from the expanding hematoma exceeds the venous pressure, in most cases the hematoma will stop growing. In the majority of cases, surgical exploration should be avoided. It is rare to find a specific vessel to ligate except in cases in which the hematoma is quickly expanding over 1 to 2 minutes of observation, which likely represents a rare arterial laceration. The extent of the hematoma should be determined by both visualization and palpation. The treatment of nonexpanding vulvar hematomas is observation by serial examinations and the use of an ice pack or cool sitz bath and pain medications. Patients may have difficulty voiding secondary to urethral injury or because they are anxious to void onto abraded vulvar surfaces or secondary to urinary obstruction or a urinary injury.

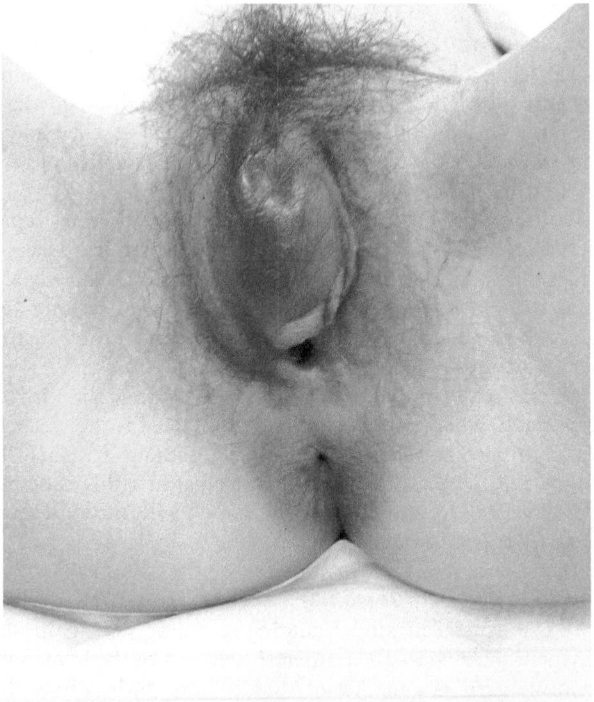

**Figure 12.9** Vulvar hematoma in an adolescent female as a result of a straddle injury. (From Mok-Lin EY, Laufer MR: Management of vulvar hematomas: use of a Word catheter. *J Pediatr Adolesc Gynecol.* 2009;22[5]:e156-e158.)

## *SEXUAL ABUSE*

Sexual abuse in reproductive women is covered in Chapter 9. This chapter contains information specifically related to sexual abuse in the prepubertal child. For a detailed and complete description of evaluation and treatment of the potentially sexually abused child, practitioners should refer to the American Academy of Pediatrics guidelines, initially published in 2009 and reaffirmed in 2013 (Kellogg, 2009), as well as the Sexually Transmitted Diseases Treatment Guidelines from the Centers for Disease Control and Prevention (CDC, 2015). These documents also contain a detailed table that describes the implications of commonly encountered sexually transmitted or sexually associated infections in the diagnosis and reporting of sexual abuse in children (Jenny, 2013).

### *Scope of the Problem*

Unfortunately, the sexual abuse of children is extremely common in the United States. Estimates indicate that approximately 20% of girls are involved in some type of sexual activity during childhood. Globally this number is even higher, with approximately one fourth of all girls victimized sexually during childhood. Although abduction cases with subsequent sexual abuse by a person unknown to the family attract national media coverage, this scenario is rare. Most perpetrators are male acquaintances known and trusted by the families. Fathers are responsible approximately 21% of the time and other male relatives 19% of the time. It is often not appreciated that mothers are involved 4% to 8% of the time. Babysitting is a common modus operandi for abusers to gain access to children.

### *History in Sexual Abuse*

There are two situations in which health care providers need to garner information regarding potential sexual abuse. One is the child or family that presents with potential sexual abuse as the chief complaint. The other situation is when the child is seen for another complaint, such as a purulent discharge, but the provider considers the possibility of sexual abuse based on historical information or physical examination.

Telephone calls regarding potential sexual abuse are a challenge for practitioners. Urgent evaluation is necessary if the abuse has occurred within 72 hours (for forensic evidence), if the child is currently in a danger of repeated abuse or self-harm, or for obvious injuries such as lacerations require treatment. If none of these criteria are encountered, the child and her family can be evaluated on a nonurgent basis. This is important, because specially trained personnel should become involved as soon as possible in these situations (pediatric forensic nurse examiners). In many settings these children can be referred to a sexual abuse team on a nonemergency basis. In settings where teams are not available, it is critical that practitioners are aware of other community resources. If at all possible, it is usually better if the child and family are interviewed separately by a qualified mental health provider (such as a social worker or psychologist) who is experienced in evaluating sexual abuse. Guidelines have been published on appropriate methods of interviewing children who may be victims of sexual abuse. Often state departments of children's services or the social work department of the community hospital can refer providers to appropriate mental health providers.

Unless there are compelling medical reasons, this interview should be performed prior to a genital examination. There are several reasons for this recommendation. First, latency age children may not be able to separate the exam from touching involved in abuse, making the history more difficult to obtain. Second, in the majority of abused children the exam is completely normal. It is important that families not rely on an exam to decide whether to seek counseling or intervention that would keep their child safe. Although providers should ask relevant questions, the more complete interview by an experienced mental health provider minimizes repetitive questioning of the child. The interview may also allow rapport to begin between the mental health professional doing the interview and the family so that the relationship can transit into therapy if indicated.

Practitioners may also consider sexual abuse based on historical complaints or physical examination findings. In this situation it is critical for the provider to query the guardian or parent in a nonthreatening manner. The approach should be "we are all on the same team and we both want to ensure the safety of your child." Queries directed to the child should be open ended and nonjudgmental. Leading questions should be avoided.

### Legal Issues in Reporting Possible Sexual Abuse

Providers must be aware of their state's laws and how to file a report alleging sexual abuse. Every state requires that suspected and known child abuse be reported. The word *suspected,* however, deserves definition. *Isolated* complaints that may be associated with sexual abuse (e.g., nightmares or genital bleeding) often do not require a report. Clinicians may suspect sexual abuse based on a variety of historical complaints and physical exam findings. Consideration to other causes of these complaints and findings is also critical. For example, in children who present with genital bleeding, the differential diagnosis may also include urethral prolapse, foreign bodies, and lichen sclerosus, vaginal tumors, or nonabusive trauma.

If a provider is unsure if a report is required, he or she should discuss the situation with local child protective services or a social worker. These professionals can help providers avoid filing vague unnecessary reports, which clog the services of overburdened state agencies. They can also aid in filing reports in borderline cases that justify exploration to obtain safety of children. In addition, discussion with agencies may help protect providers from prosecution for failure to report. It is important to document discussions in patient charts. Guidelines have been developed by the American Academy of Pediatrics regarding appropriate filing of abuse reports (Kellogg, 2009). Providers should not be hesitant to file because of fear of liability for an alleged false report. Although suits have been filed against physicians, states generally ensure immunity. It should, however, be noted that there have been successful malpractice actions against providers who have failed to diagnose or report sexual abuse.

### Physical Examination and Evaluation for Sexually Transmitted Infections

The exam of a potentially sexually abused child should include a general exam. Attention should be directed at evaluating skin for bruising, lacerations, or trauma. Parents or concerned adults should be counseled that a genital exam in children who have been abused is usually normal. Physical evidence is present in less than 5% of children. The genital exam should be carried out as described earlier in this chapter. In addition, a thorough physical exam looking for signs of physical abuse must be documented in the chart (Christian, 2000).

In situations in which abuse has occurred within 72 hours, careful collection of forensic evidence is important. Collection of all clothing and undergarments is critical. Approximately two thirds of forensic evidence is obtained from linens and clothing. Motile sperm will be present in the prepubertal vagina for approximately 8 hours, and nonmotile sperm for approximately 24 hours. Because prepubertal children do not have cervical mucous, sperm do not exist for the longer durations seen in reproductive females within the cervical canal. "Rape" kits will also often include testing for a protein specific to the prostate. Vaginal specimens may be obtained by using small swabs within the vagina, similar to the method described for obtaining vaginal cultures.

Given that only approximately 5% of abused children acquire a sexually transmitted infection (STI), providers must decide when STI testing is indicated. Both gonorrhea and chlamydia cause a vaginitis, not a cervicitis, in prepubertal children, so a vaginal culture should be done. In the United States, a vaginal *culture* for gonorrhea and chlamydia, not DNA testing, should be performed as recommended by the Centers for Disease Control and Prevention (CDC, 2015). There are several issues with the nucleic-acid amplification tests that are commonly used in reproductive females. Because nonculture methods are not labeled for use in children, positive testing may not be admissible in court. The prevalence of gonorrhea and chlamydia in children is usually lower than in appropriately screened adolescents and adults; therefore the actual positive predictive values of a positive test are lower.

Testing in prepubertal children is also influenced by typical incubation intervals of STIs. If a child was abused in an isolated incident, an STI may not be found on testing immediately after the abuse. However, a purulent discharge would prompt testing and be a red flag for possible ongoing abuse rather than an isolated incident.

When a child presents in a nonacute setting, the provider must decide whether to perform testing for STIs. It is rare for a child to have gonorrhea or chlamydia without a vaginal discharge (Bell, 1992). Standards of care regarding this issue may differ in various locations, and consultation with the local sexual assault team is warranted.

### Hymen in the Evaluation of Sexual Abuse

There is a general misunderstanding regarding the significance of hymeneal changes. The transverse diameter of the hymen was previously used as a marker of abuse. However, it is now clear that there is significant variation in children, and the state of the hymen it is not a reliable marker of abuse. Complete transections of the hymen, and clefts that extend to the junction of the hymen between 3 o'clock and 9 o'clock, are not congenital, but

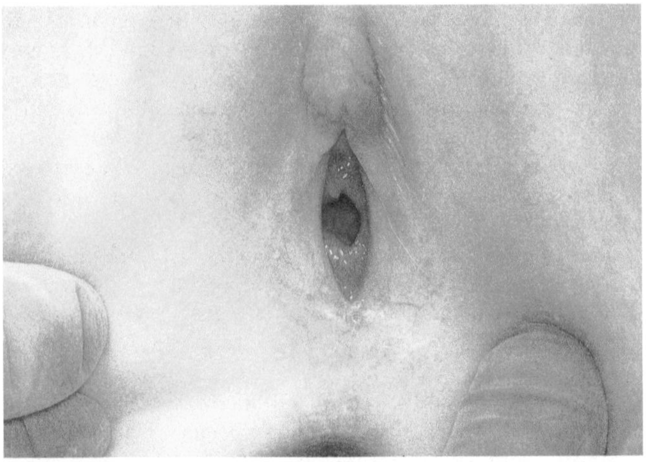

**Figure 12.10** Hymenal bump alongside of an incomplete transection of the hymen at approximately 7 to 8 o'clock.

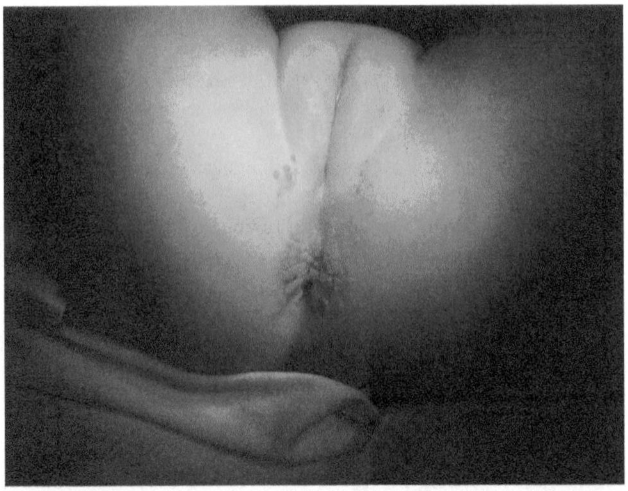

**Figure 12.11** A 3-year-old with genital warts. (From Leclair E, Black A, Fleming N. Imiquimod 5% cream treatment for rapidly progressive genital condyloma in a 3-year-old girl. *J Pediatr Adolesc Gynecol.* 2012;25[6]:e119-e121.)

if present they could be from abuse or a child inserting an object. Controversies exist as to the significance of incomplete transections (Fig. 12.10).

### *Genital Warts*

Human papillomavirus (HPV), the causative agent of genital warts, may be transmitted to children from the maternal genital tract at delivery or by sexual or nonsexual transmission after birth. The incubation interval from transmission to the presence of visible genital warts has not been defined in children; however, it appears likely that most warts appearing prior to 3 years of age are from maternal-child transmission (Fig. 12.11). If the child is 3 years of age or older, serious consideration should be given to the possibility of sexual transmission. However, genital warts "discovered" in a 4-year-old may have been present for some time prior to being noticed. This is particularly a problem in the perianal area, which may not be examined carefully even in children undergoing a cursory genital exam as part of well-child annual care (Handley, 1993).

Approximately half of lesions will regress over 5 years. Expectant management is reasonable, but parents may prefer treatment. Treatment in children is difficult. Caustic treatments such as trichloroacetic acid are painful even if children are pretreated with local anesthesia. Topical imiquimod cream is labeled for use in children 12 years and older and can cause significant vulvar irritation, but has been used successfully in younger children. If the child accidentally carries imiquimod cream to the cornea, it could cause damage to the eye. Laser and/or ultrasonic treatment is an option for significant wart tissue but must be performed under anesthesia and can be associated with significant postoperative pain.

## *THE OVARY AND ADNEXA IN PEDIATRIC AND ADOLESCENT GYNECOLOGY: CYSTS, TUMORS, AND TORSION*

Most ovarian masses in this age group are functional ovarian cysts, and if a tumor is present it most often is a benign teratoma (dermoid). However, malignancies can occur and are most often of germ cell origin, but they can also be sex-cord/stromal in origin such as a granulosa cell tumor (Amies, 2014; Lara-Torre, 2002).

Physiologic and functional cysts of the ovaries arise from gonadotropin stimulation of the follicles. They may present in the fetus, newborn, infant, at puberty, and in adolescence. The appropriate management may depend on the age and on the appearance of the cyst on ultrasound. Cysts of follicular development will be clear without significant solid components and almost always are less than 7 to 10 cm in size in reproductive adolescents. Management of adolescent functional cysts is essentially the same as the management in reproductive females. Cysts in neonates can generally be observed until resolution. Neonates and children can be observed for any signs of torsion and advised to seek immediate medical attention, unless they have exceptionally large cysts. Torsion can certainly occur and is not rare. Many neonatal cysts were initially identified on antenatal ultrasound. There are few studies, all with small numbers, regarding the natural history of antenatal or neonatal ovarian cysts. Cysts during the preschool and early grade school years are unusual, reflecting that gonadotrophins are low.

Corpus luteum cysts are often more complex than other follicular cysts. Management is similar to that in mature reproductive women, and observation is warranted unless signs of malignancy are present. Consideration should be given to dermoids and the possibility of germ cell tumors if a mass has both solid and cystic components. In rare cases of intersex, such as mixed gonadal dysgenesis, suspicion of malignancy should be high. A rare presentation of hypothyroidism is pediatric ovarian cysts.

### *Prenatal Ovarian Cysts*

Obstetric ultrasound of a female fetus frequently demonstrates a simple ovarian cyst (up to 80% of fetuses). Before a diagnosis of an ovarian cyst is made, it is critical to exclude urinary or gastrointestinal anomalies. Fetal malignancy is rare.

There is controversy regarding the management of large antenatal cysts. Antenatal aspiration for the large antenatal cyst (4 cm or more) has been proposed by some to avoid potential antenatal torsion. The obvious disadvantage is the risk of the antenatal surgery and the fact that resolution is a typical clinical course. Size and appearance enter heavily into management decisions; for example, if the cyst seems to be wandering about the abdomen on repetitive ultrasounds, it may be of greater risk of torsion. Also, large cysts (probably greater than 9 cm) may require a cesarean section.

The natural history of both antenatal and neonatal cysts is difficult to define. Data generated from a few small series may be misleading, as the outcome may be dependent on size, mobility, and how the cyst first presented. Presence of what appears to be torsion may not result in the loss of an ovary. The relative rarity of congenital absence of one ovary makes it likely that untwisting occurs. The incidence of congenital unilateral ovarian agenesis is quite rare, perhaps as rare as 1 in approximately 10,000 females. Ovarian malignancy is extremely rare in this age group and is not a consideration in the therapeutic approach. For these reasons observation is reasonable in these cases (Bryant, 2004).

### Neonatal Ovarian Cysts

Simple cystic ovarian masses in newborns and neonates are common and can be followed expectantly. Parents should be given ovarian torsion warnings, and if the infant presents with acute vomiting or abdominal pain, she should be immediately evaluated for ovarian torsion. Repeat serial ultrasonography should be performed every 4-6 weeks until the cyst resolves. Almost all will resolve if they do not undergo torsion. Malignancy is not a consideration in newborns when deciding therapy. Aspiration is an option for large cysts.

### Ovarian Cysts in Children and Adolescents

The management of cystic ovarian structures in children and adolescents should also be expectant unless they are extremely large (>10 cm), in which case the possibility of functional cysts becomes less likely. Many times, physiologic and functional cysts are discovered on an abdominal ultrasound performed for complaints such as abdominal pain. Often the presence of a cyst is incidental and unrelated to the complaint. However, in patients with pain, the possibility of ovarian torsion should be entertained. Pain from ovarian cysts generally stems from three sources: (1) expansion of the ovarian cortex (which is typical during the growth phase of follicles and lasts less than 72 hours), (2) peritoneal bleeding from rupture (particularly common in bleeding disorders and patients on anticoagulation), and (3) ovarian torsion. These causes of pain do not typically present as chronic pelvic/abdominal pain. Recurrent functional ovarian cysts may be prevented by the use of anovulatory agents, such as combined oral contraceptives in adolescents, but these agents do not assist in the resolution of cysts that are actively present.

### Ovarian Tumors in Children and Adolescents

A variety of tumors, both benign and malignant, can be seen in the childhood and adolescent years. One should always consider the possibility of a malignancy, particularly in patients with solid ovarian masses or cystic and solid components on ultrasound. A malignant diagnosis should also be considered in patients with presumed functional ovarian cysts that do not resolve during serial monitoring.

Germ cell tumors are the most common gynecologic neoplasm in this age group, and fortunately, most are benign ovarian teratomas. The most common malignant germ cell tumor is a dysgerminoma followed by endodermal sinus tumors and immature teratomas. These tumors are covered in detail in Chapter 33, but several issues are especially pertinent to children and adolescents.

Bilateral tumors are seen in 10% to 15% of dysgerminomas, but this condition is rare in all of the other germ cell tumors of the ovary except for immature teratomas. Sex cord tumors, such as granulosa and thecal cell tumors, can also be seen in this age group and often produce steroids (estrogen and testosterone respectively). Rare tumors such as gonadoblastomas, a germ cell and sex cord tumor, are seen in patients with intersex disorders such as mixed gonadal dysgenesis.

Recurrent abdominal pain is a frequent complaint of school-age children, and this common symptom is often a presenting symptom in patients with ovarian neoplasms. A young child may not be able to differentiate lower abdominal pain from pelvic pain because of the small size of the preadolescent female pelvis, making the ovaries essentially abdominal organs. One can understand why increasing abdominal girth is a frequent finding associated with ovarian enlargement.

The most common clinical manifestation of an ovarian tumor is lower abdominal pain or the presence of a mass. Some ovarian tumors in children produce only vague discomfort, such as abdominal fullness or bloating. However, adnexal masses in children are more frequently associated with acute complications—such as torsion, hemorrhage, and rupture—than are similar tumors in adults.

Ovarian tumors constitute approximately 1% of all neoplasms in premenarcheal children. Ultrasound, magnetic resonance imaging (MRI), or abdominal computed tomography (CT) may be utilized in the evaluation of a suspected pelvic mass or abdominal pain of uncertain origin in children. Abdominal ultrasonography may be used to establish that the origin of the mass is in the pelvis, whether the mass is cystic or solid, and the presence of ascites (Anthony, 2012) and should be considered as the initial imaging modality. Calcifications in an ovarian mass may appear toothlike, indicating a likely diagnosis of an ovarian teratoma.

As part of the preoperative workup, the child may be screened for elevated serum levels of tumor markers such as $\alpha$-fetoprotein, both alpha and beta human chorionic gonadotropin (HCG), inhibin (A and B), lactate dehydrogenase, estradiol, and testosterone; even tumor markers that are associated with other neoplasms can be detected in girls. HCG may be positive for either the $\alpha$ or the $\beta$ subunit, so a pregnancy test that only tests for the $\beta$ subunit is inadequate.

Ovarian tumors in preadolescent females, both benign and malignant, are usually unilateral. Thus it is imperative to be as conservative as possible in managing the opposite ovary in order to protect potential future fertility. During surgery the opposite ovary should be carefully inspected and palpated if possible. It is generally unnecessary and potentially harmful to perform a biopsy on a normal-appearing contralateral ovary in a preadolescent female. This is especially true in patients with dermoids. Careful inspection of the contralateral ovary in patients with a dysgerminoma or an immature teratoma—malignancies in which bilateral tumors are not as rare—is also appropriate, reserving biopsy only for when an abnormality is detected by clinical inspection. It was common practice to perform a "wedge biopsy" of the contralateral ovary, but that practice was not evidence based and was abandoned as it clearly increased the possibility of scarring and infertility.

Children with suspected ovarian cancer should be referred to specialists who are up to date on the most current data from research groups such as the Pediatrics Oncology Group and the Gynecologic Oncology Group, now part of NRG Oncology (Cushing, 1999). Providers should be skilled in providing their patients proper staging procedures, including lymph node assessment and evidence-based adjuvant therapy as indicated by standard national guidelines such as the guidelines of the National Comprehensive Cancer Network (NCCN) (Morgan, 2013). The role of adjuvant therapy should be individualized for each patient. The use of tumor markers to help differentiate patients with benign teratoma from malignancies is helpful in triaging appropriate referrals. However, regardless of what the makers show, referral is prudent.

Approximately 75% to 85% of ovarian neoplasms that necessitate surgery in premenarcheal females are benign, and approximately 15% to 25% are malignant neoplasms. The risk is less in young children. In a review of ovarian masses in children, Brown and coworkers reported that the risk of malignancy was only 3% up to age 8.

In summary, even though ovarian neoplasms are rare in children, this diagnosis should be considered in a young girl with abdominal pain and a palpable mass. The surgical therapy should have two goals: first, and most important, the appropriate surgical procedure including selective evaluation of lymph nodes and appropriate staging procedures; second, the preservation of future fertility, as hysterectomy is usually not necessary, even in rare cases of bilateral childhood or adolescent ovarian malignancy. The uterus should be retained to keep the patient's options for future fertility intact. Even in the absence of ovaries, fertility may be possible with artificial reproductive technology and the use of donor eggs.

### *Ovarian Torsion*

Ovarian torsion is covered in more detail in Chapter 18. Issues unique to children and adolescents are covered in this discussion. Torsion in prepubertal females may be secondary to a pelvic mass or due to mechanical factors that occur in the peripubertal interval. In early puberty, the ovaries drop from their prepubertal position at the pelvic brim into the pelvis. This drop occurs under the influence of gonadotropins that surge at puberty. Some young women may have longer supportive ligaments, predisposing them to twisting. Approximately two thirds of the time, ovarian torsion occurs on the right side, increasing the likelihood of the process being confused with appendicitis. The sigmoid colon in the left lower quadrant helps prevent the left ovary from twisting.

Although both appendicitis and torsion can present with acute pain and rebound, the gradual progression of appendicitis is quite different from the acute severe pain of torsion. Nausea and emesis often ensue immediately with torsion, owing to the severity of the pain. Appendicitis tends to present with anorexia, which gradually worsens. The young girl with an acute onset of pain and simultaneous emesis likely has ovarian torsion rather than appendicitis.

Approximately one third of ovarian torsion cases in children and adolescents are not associated with a predisposing ovarian mass such as a dermoid, large functional cyst, or malignancy. Nevertheless, even in children without an ovarian mass, after torsion the ovary will become swollen and enlarged as the lymphatic flow is blocked. In children and adolescents, the differentiation between torsion and appendicitis is a common dilemma. Radiologic evaluation to rule out appendicitis may reveal a pelvic mass. Unfortunately, the presence of vascular flow in the ovary does not rule out torsion. In fact, many cases of surgically proven torsion had normal vascular flow on ultrasound evaluation. Once a torsion is identified at the time of surgery, it is important to consider the patient's future fertility. There are numerous reports in the literature demonstrating the benefit of untwisting the gonad, regardless of its appearance, as most will regain function after the edema resolves. Risk of embolus from a thrombosed ovarian vein has not been reported in the literature. In institutions where pediatric surgeons manage these patients, consultation and co-management with gynecology will likely result in better outcomes and fewer adnexectomies.

## KEY POINTS

- It is important to give the child a sense that she will be in control of the examination process. Emphasize that the most important part of the examination is just "looking" and that there will be conversation during the entire process.
- Many gynecologic conditions in children can be diagnosed by inspection alone.
- The vaginal epithelium of the prepubertal child appears redder and thinner than the vaginal epithelium of a woman in her reproductive years.
- The prepubertal vagina is also narrower, thinner, and lacks the ability to distend like that of the vagina of a reproductively mature woman.
- The vagina of a child is 4 to 5 cm long and has a neutral pH.
- During the physical examination and rectal examination of the prepubertal child, no pelvic masses except the cervix should be palpable. The normal prepubertal uterus and ovaries are nonpalpable. The relative size ratio of cervix to uterus is 2 to 1 in a child.
- Many female adolescents do not want other observers, such as mothers, in the examining room.
- It is estimated that 80% to 90% of outpatient visits of children to gynecologists involve the classic symptoms of vulvovaginitis: introital irritation and discharge.
- Positive identification of gonorrhea, or chlamydia in a child with premenarcheal vulvovaginitis, is considered diagnostic of sexual abuse. However, many infants are infected with *Chlamydia trachomatis* during birth and remain infected for up to 2 to 3 years in the absence of specific antibiotic therapy.
- The major factor in childhood vulvovaginitis is poor perineal hygiene.
- A vaginal discharge that is both bloody and foul smelling strongly suggests the presence of a foreign body.
- In the period surrounding the time of puberty, children often develop a physiologic discharge secondary to the increase in circulating estrogen levels.

*Continued*

## KEY POINTS—cont'd

- The foundation of treating childhood vulvovaginitis is the improvement of local perineal hygiene.
- The majority of cases of persistent or recurrent nonspecific vulvovaginitis respond to improved hygiene and treatment of irritation resulting from trauma or irritating substances.
- The classic symptom of pinworms *(Enterobius vermicularis)* is nocturnal vulvar and perianal itching, the treatment for which is the antihelmintic agent, mebendazole.
- The most common vaginal foreign body in preadolescent females is a wad of toilet tissue.
- Persistent vaginal bleeding is an extremely rare symptom in a preadolescent female. However, it is important to do a thorough workup because of the serious sequelae of some of the causes of vaginal bleeding.
- Labial adhesions do not require treatment unless they are symptomatic or voiding is compromised. If necessary, small amounts of daily topical estrogen to the labia may be used for treatment.
- The usual cause of genital trauma during childhood is an accidental fall. Most such traumas involve straddle injuries.
- Accidental genital trauma often produces extreme pain and overwhelming anxiety for the child and her parents. Because of compassion and empathy, the gynecologist may underestimate the extent of the anatomic injuries.
- Small follicular cysts in preadolescent females are usually self-limiting.
- Ovarian tumors constitute approximately 1% of all neoplasms in premenarcheal children. In preadolescent females, both benign and malignant ovarian tumors are usually unilateral. Routine biopsy of the normal-appearing contralateral ovary should be avoided.
- Approximately 75% to 85% of ovarian neoplasms necessitating surgery are benign, with cystic teratomas being the most common.
- The most common malignancy in preadolescent females is a germ cell tumor.
- Even though ovarian neoplasms are rare in children, this diagnosis must be considered in a young girl with abdominal pain and a palpable mass.
- The surgical therapy of an ovarian neoplasm in a child should have two goals: the appropriate surgical removal of the neoplasm and the preservation of future fertility.
- Ovarian torsion should be managed conservatively with untwisting and preservation of the adnexa, regardless of the appearance.
- Presence or absence of Doppler flow on the ovary on ultrasound is not diagnostic of ovarian torsion, and the decision for surgical intervention should be based on the level of clinical suspicion.

## KEY REFERENCES


American College of Obstetricians and Gynecologists (ACOG). *Guidelines for Adolescent Health*. 2nd Ed. Washington, DC: ACOG; 2011.

Amies Oelschlager AE, Gow KW, Morse CB, et al. Management of large ovarian neoplasms in pediatric and adolescent females. *J Pediatr Adolesc Gynecol*. 2016;29:88–94.

Anthony EY, Caserta MP, Singh J, et al. Adnexal masses in female pediatric patients. *Am J Roentgenol*. 2012;198(5):W426–W431.

Appelbaum H, Malhotra S. A comprehensive approach to the spectrum of abnormal pubertal development. *Adolesc Med*. 2012;23(1):1–14.

Bacon JL, Romano ME, Quint EH. Clinical recommendation: pediatric labial adhesions. *J Pediatr Adolesc Gynecol*. 2015;28(5):405–409.

Bell TA, Stamm WE, Wang S, et al. Chronic Chlamydia trachomatis infections in infants. *JAMA*. 1992;267(3):400–402.

Bercaw-Pratt JL, Boardman LA, Simms-Cendan JS. North American Society for Pediatric and Adolescent Gynecology (NASPAG): Clinical recommendation: pediatric lichen sclerosus. *J Pediatr Adolesc Gynecol*. 2014;27(2):111–116.

Bond GR, Dowd MD, Landsman I, et al. Unintentional perineal injury in prepubescent girls: a multicenter, prospective report of 56 girls. *Pediatrics*. 1995;95(5):628–631.

Bryant AR, Laufer MR. Fetal ovarian cysts. *J Reprod Med*. 2004;49(5):329–337.

Centers for Disease Control and Prevention (CDC). Sexually transmitted diseases treatment guidelines, 2015. *MMWR Recomm Rep*. 2015;64(RR-12):1–140.

Christian CW, Lavelle JM, Dejong AR, et al. Forensic evidence findings in prepubertal victims of sexual assault. *Pediatrics*. 2000;106(1 Pt 1):100–104.

Cushing B, Giller R, Ablin A, et al. Surgical resection alone is effective treatment for ovarian immature teratoma in children and adolescents: a report of the Pediatric Oncology Group and the Children's Cancer Group. *Am J Obstet Gynecol*. 1999;181(2):353–358.

Dowd MD, Fitzmaurice L, Knapp J, et al. The interpretation of urogenital findings in children with straddle injuries. *J Pediatr Surg*. 1994;29(1):7–10.

Farrington PF. Pediatric vulvo-vaginitis. *Clin Obstet Gynecol*. 1997;40(1):135–140.

Handley J, Dinsmore W, Maw R, et al. Anogenital warts in prepubertal children: sexual abuse or not? *Int J STD AIDS*. 1993;4(5):271–279.

Herman-Giddens ME, Slora EJ, Wasserman RC, et al. Secondary sexual characteristics and menses in young girls seen in office practice: a study from the Pediatric Research in Office Settings network. *Pediatrics*. 1997;99(4):505–512.

Jacobs AM, Alderman E. Gynecologic examination of the pre-pubertal girl. *Pediatr Rev*. 2014;35:97–105.

Jenny C, Crawford-Jakubiak JE. Committee on Child Abuse and Neglect, American Academy of Pediatrics: The evaluation of children in the primary care setting when sexual abuse is suspected. *Pediatrics*. 2013;132(2):e558–e567.

Kellogg ND. Committee on Child Abuse and Neglect, American Academy of Pediatrics: Clinical report—the evaluation of sexual behaviors. *Pediatrics*. 2009;124(3):992–998.

Lara-Torre E. Ovarian neoplasias in children. *J Pediatr Adolesc Gynecol*. 2002;15(1):47–52.

Lara-Torre E. The physical examination in pediatric and adolescent patients. *Clinic Obstet Gynecol*. 2008;51:205–213.

Marshall WA, Tanner JM. Variations in pattern of pubertal changes in girls. *Arch Dis Child*. 1969;44(235):291–303.

McCann J, Voris J, Simon M. Labial adhesions and posterior fourchette injuries in childhood sexual abuse. *Am J Dis Child*. 1988;142(6):659–663.

Morgan Jr RJ, Alvarez RD, Armstrong DK, et al. Ovarian cancer, version 2.2013. *J Natl Compr Canc Netw*. 2013;11(10):1199–1209.

Pokorny SF, Stormer J. Atraumatic removal of secretions from the prepubertal vagina. *Am J Obstet Gynecol*. 1987;156(3):581–582.


Suggested Readings can be found on ExpertConsult.com.

# 13

# Family Planning

*Katherine Rivlin, Carolyn Westhoff*

## CONTRACEPTION OVERVIEW

Seventy percent of the 64 million U.S. women aged 15 to 44 are at risk of unintended pregnancy. In other words, these women are sexually active, capable of becoming pregnant, not currently pregnant or postpartum, and are not trying for pregnancy. Half of pregnancies in the United States are unintended, and among women who experience unintended pregnancy, more than half are not using contraception (Mosher, 2010). According to the 2011-2013 National Survey of Family Growth, 61.7% of women aged 15 to 44 in the United States, or about 90% of those at risk, are using some method of contraception (Table 13.1). The most common methods are the oral contraceptive pill (16%), female sterilization (15.5%), condoms (9.4%), long-active reversible contraception (LARC) (7.2%), or intrauterine devices (IUDs) and implants (Table 13.2) (Daniels, 2014). Thus, most women at risk of unintended pregnancy are using a method.

Because each of the currently available methods of contraception has distinct advantages and disadvantages, clinicians should be able to explain the unique features of each method. The clinician must also evaluate whether medical contraindications to a particular method exist for a woman and offer her safe and effective alternatives. The health risks associated with unintended pregnancy must always be considered in the medically challenging patient, as these risks are generally greater than those of a birth control method. In general, the best method for an individual is one that is relatively safer than pregnancy and that will be used correctly and consistently.

Table 13.1 Percentage Currently Using Any Contraceptive Method among All Women Aged 15-44, by Selected Characteristics: United States, 2011-2013

| Characteristic | Currently Using Any Method |
|---|---|
| Total | 61.7% |
| **Age in Years** | |
| 15-24 | 47.4% |
| 25-34* | 67.4% |
| 34-44* | 70.0% |
| **Hispanic Origin and Race** | |
| Hispanic | 57.3% |
| Non-Hispanic white† | 65.3% |
| Non-Hispanic black | 57.9% |
| **Education‡** | |
| Less than high school | 67.2% |
| High school or GED | 66.7% |
| Some college, no BA | 69.2% |
| BA or higher | 67.3% |

From CDC/NCHS, National Survey of Family Growth, 2011-2013. Data from Daniels K, Daugherty J, Jones J: Current contraceptive status among women aged 15-44: United States, 2011-2013. *NCHS Data Brief* (173):1-8, 2014. Available at http://www.cdc.gov/nchs/data/databriefs/db173.pdf.

*Significantly different from age group 15-24.

†Significantly different from Hispanic and non-Hispanic black women.

‡The population size referenced in this table for women aged 15-44 is 60.9 million. Analyses of education are limited to women aged 22-44 at the time of interview.

*BA*, Bachelor's degree;

*GED*, General Education Development high school equivalency diploma.

## CONTRACEPTIVE EFFECTIVENESS

All contraceptive methods have a **typical use** effectiveness (pregnancy rate given actual use, including occasional inconsistent or

Table 13.2 Percentage Distribution of Women Aged 15 to 44, by Current Contraceptive Status: United States, 2011-2013

| Characteristic | Percentage (%) |
|---|---|
| **Using Contraception** | 61.7 |
| Female sterilization | 15.5 |
| Male sterilization | 5.1 |
| Pill | 16.0 |
| Male condom | 9.4 |
| Long-acting reversible contraceptives | 7.2 |
| Depo-Provera, contraceptive ring, or patch | 4.4 |
| All other contraceptive methods | 4.1 |
| **Not Using Contraception** | 38.3 |
| Never had sexual intercourse or did not have sex in the past 3 months | 19.0 |
| Pregnant, postpartum, or seeking pregnancy | 9.5 |
| Nonuser who had sexual intercourse in the past 3 months | 6.9 |
| All other nonusers | 2.9 |

Data from Daniels K, Daugherty J, Jones J. Current contraceptive status among women aged 15-44: United States, 2011-2013. *NCHS Data Brief.* 2014;(173): 1-8. Available at http://www.cdc.gov/nchs/data/databriefs/db173.pdf.

Table 13.3 WHO Summary Table of Contraceptive Efficacy

| Method | Percentage of Women Experiencing an Unintended Pregnancy within the First Year of Use | | Percentage of Women Continuing Use at 1 Year |
|---|---|---|---|
| | Typical Use | Perfect Use | |
| No method | 85 | 85 | |
| Spermicides | 29 | 18 | 42 |
| Withdrawal | 27 | 4 | 43 |
| Fertility awareness-based methods | 25 | | |
| Standard day method | | 5 | |
| Two-days method | | 4 | |
| Ovulation method | | 3 | |
| Sponge | | | |
| Parous women | 32 | 20 | 46 |
| Nulliparous women | 16 | 9 | 57 |
| Diaphragm | 16 | 6 | 57 |
| Condom | | | |
| Female (Reality) | 21 | 5 | 49 |
| Male | 15 | 2 | 53 |
| Combined pill and progestin-only pill | 8 | 0.3 | 68 |
| Evra patch | 8 | 0.3 | 68 |
| NuvaRing | 8 | 0.3 | 68 |
| Depo-Provera | 3 | 0.3 | 56 |
| IUD | | | |
| ParaGard (copper T) | 0.8 | 0.6 | 78 |
| Mirena (LNG-IUS) | 0.2 | 0.2 | 80 |
| Implanon | 0.05 | 0.05 | 84 |
| Female sterilization | 0.5 | 0.5 | 100 |
| Male sterilization | 0.15 | 0.10 | 100 |

From Trussell J. Contraceptive efficacy. In: Hatcher RA, Trussell J, Nelson AL, et al. *Contraceptive Technology*. 20th rev. ed. New York: Ardent Media; 2012.

incorrect use) and **perfect use** effectiveness (pregnancy rate given correct and consistent use of a method with every act of intercourse). Pregnancy rates can vary widely between typical and perfect use depending on how complicated it is to use a method perfectly (Table 13.3). In general, coitus-related methods and more user-dependent methods are less effective than "forgettable methods" such as LARC. Use of two methods, or "dual method use," provides added contraceptive protection. Combining a hormonal method with a condom provides the additional health benefit of reducing sexually transmitted infection. Other multipurpose technologies are in development to concurrently prevent unintended pregnancy and reduce the risk of sexually transmitted infection, particularly HIV (Lusti-Narasimhan, 2014).

In this chapter, contraceptive methods are presented using a "tiered approach," with the most effective methods presented first followed by the less effective methods. This concept is based on the contraceptive method effectiveness communication tool offered by the World Health Organization (WHO) (Fig. 13.1).

## TIER 1 METHODS: HIGHLY EFFECTIVE (FEWER THAN 1 PREGNANCY PER 100 WOMEN IN 1 YEAR): INTRAUTERINE DEVICES (IUDs), IMPLANTS, MALE AND FEMALE STERILIZATION

### *LARC METHODS*

The top-tier contraceptive methods include all LARC methods. These methods require only one act of motivation to enable long-term use, which virtually eliminates user error once placement has occurred. LARC methods are highly effective and immediately reversible with a rapid return to fertility after removal. Very few medical contraindications to LARC exist. These methods do not require frequent visits for resupply or incur costs after placement (though upfront costs can be high). When used in the postpartum and postabortion period, LARC and permanent sterilization reduce the risk of short interval pregnancy significantly when compared to other hormonal methods (White, 2015). All of this contributes to high continuation rates and user satisfaction. As a result, the American Congress of Obstetricians and Gynecologists (ACOG) recommends that LARC methods be offered as first-line contraception to most women (ACOG, 2009).

The LARC methods currently available in the United States include a single-rod etonogestrel subdermal implant (Nexplanon), the Copper T380A intrauterine device, and several levonorgestrel intrauterine systems (LNG-IUS).

### *INTRAUTERINE DEVICES*

A safe and highly effective method of birth control with similar rates of failure for typical or perfect use, the IUD is the most commonly used reversible method of contraception worldwide. In the United States, IUD use has increased among contraceptive users from 2% in 2002 to 6.4% in 2011 to 2013 (Branum, 2015). First-year failure rates with the copper T 380A IUD and the levonorgestrel-releasing IUD are less than 1%. Pregnancy rates are somewhat related to the skill of the clinician inserting the device because correct high-fundal insertion lowers the incidence of partial or complete expulsion. Furthermore, the

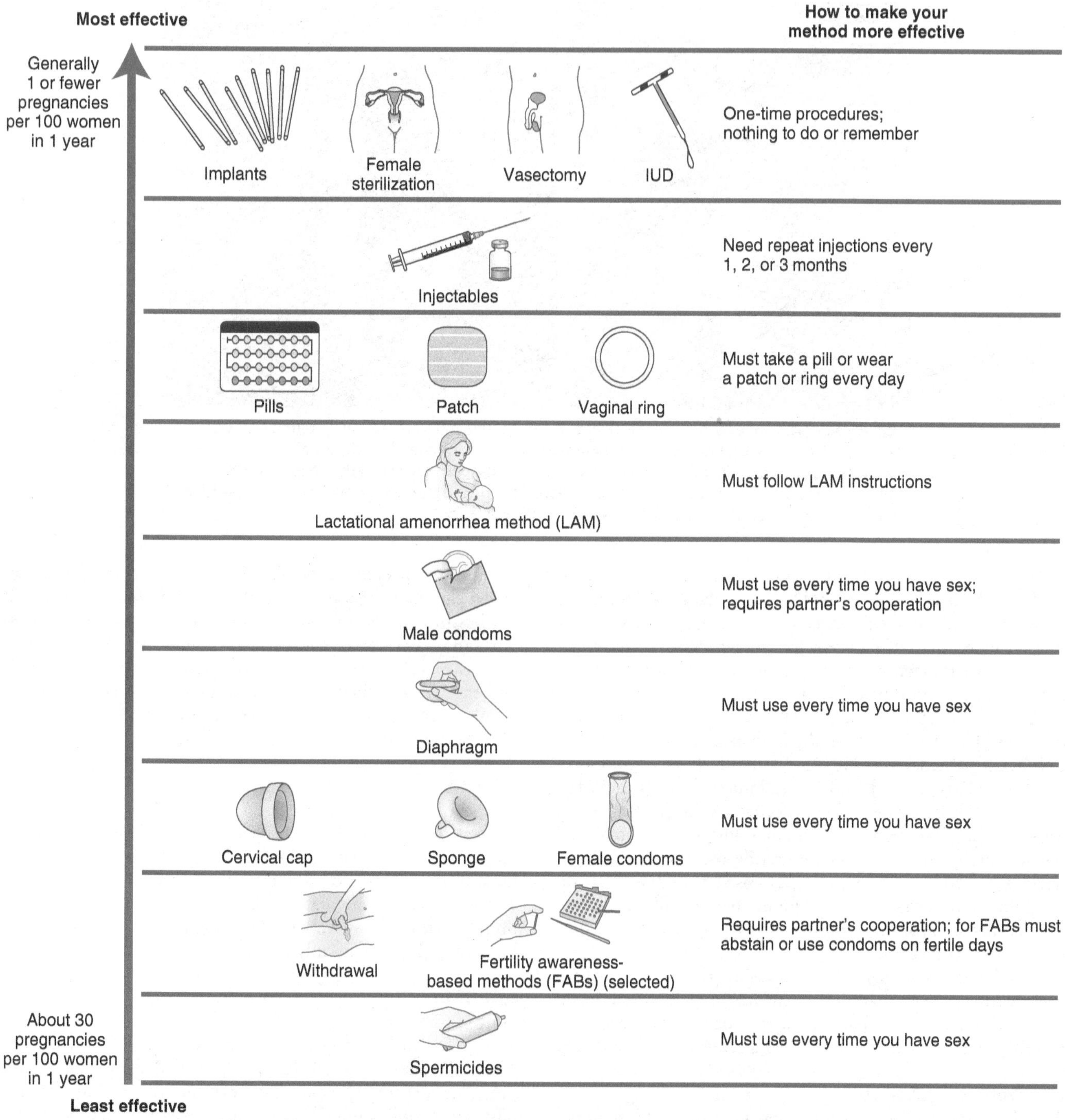


**Figure 13.1** WHO's tiered approach contraception counseling tool comparing typical effectiveness of contraceptive methods. (Redrawn from Association of Reproductive Health Professionals [ARHP]: You decide tool kit: contraceptive efficacy tools. Adapted from World Health Organization. *Comparing typical effectiveness of contraceptive methods.* [Job Aid]. Geneva, Switzerland, WHO, 2006.)

annual incidence of accidental pregnancy decreases steadily after the first year of IUD use. The cumulative pregnancy rate after 12 years of use of the copper T 380A IUD is only 1.7%, and after 5 years of use of the LNG-IUS the pregnancy rate is about 1.1%. The failure rates associated with IUDs are comparable to those achieved with surgical sterilization.

### *Types of IUDs*

The copper T 380A IUD (Paragard) (Fig. 13.2) is the only copper-bearing IUD currently marketed in the United States, although a new copper IUD (Veracept) is undergoing clinical trials. Because of the constant dissolution of copper (which on a daily basis amounts to less than that ingested in the normal

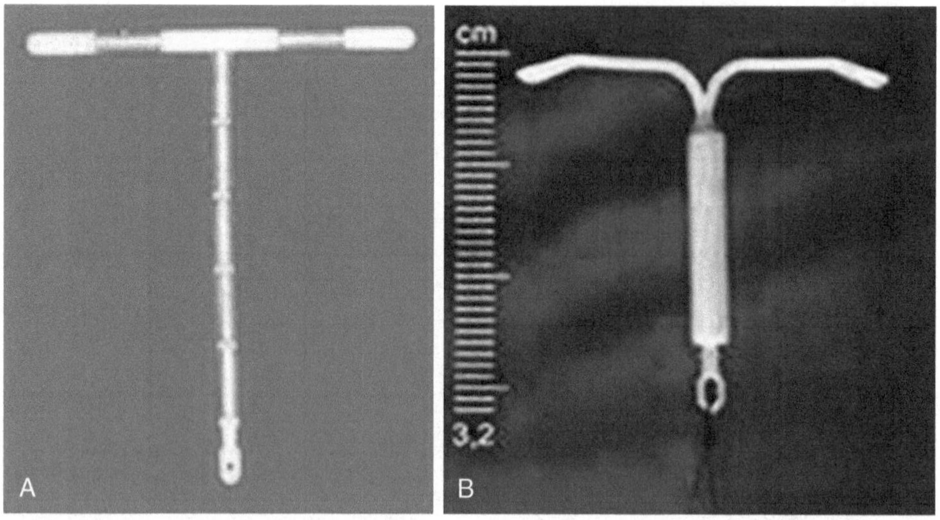


**Figure 13.2** **A,** Copper T intrauterine device. **B,** Levonorgestrel intrauterine system (LNG-IUS) *Mirena*. (**A,** From Yu J, Li H, Li J, et al. Comparative study on contraceptive efficacy and clinical performance of the copper/low-density polyethylene nanocomposite IUD and the copper T220C IUD. *Contraception*. 2008;78(4):319-323; **B,** From Searle ES. The intrauterine device and the intrauterine system. *Best Pract Res Clin Obstet Gynaecol*. 2014;28[6]:807-824.)

diet), the copper IUDs require periodic replacement. The copper T 380A is currently approved for use in the United States for 10 years and maintains its effectiveness for at least 12 years. At the scheduled time of removal, for women desiring continued contraceptive protection, the device can be removed and another inserted during the same office visit.

Adding a reservoir of a progestin to the vertical arm also increases the effectiveness of the T-shaped devices. With the LNG-IUS (Mirena) (see Fig. 13.2), about 20 μg of levonorgestrel (LNG) is released into the endometrial cavity each day. The LNG-IUS has a high level of effectiveness for at least 5 years. This IUD also reduces menstrual blood loss and has been used therapeutically to treat excessive uterine bleeding. In 2015, a new 20-μg LNG IUS device (Liletta) was approved by the Food and Drug Administration (FDA) for up to 3 years of use, though clinical trials will continue for up to 7 years, opening up the possibility for extended use.

In addition, a 13.5-μg LNG-releasing IUD device with a slightly smaller body than the Mirena has been approved for up to 3 years of use (Skyla). For the purposes of this chapter, we will be referring to the Mirena IUD when discussing the LNG-IUS.

### *Mechanisms of Action*

All IUDs induce a local inflammatory reaction of the endometrium, creating an environment that is hostile to sperm so that fertilization of the ovum does not occur. Although this sterile inflammatory reaction is the only mechanism of inert IUDs, medicated IUDs containing either copper or levonorgestrel produce additional local effects that increase their efficacy in preventing pregnancy.

#### Copper IUD

Copper markedly increases the extent of the inflammatory reaction, allowing it to accumulate throughout the uterine lumen and penetrate the cervix and probably the fallopian tubes. This affects the function and viability of gametes at many levels, preventing fertilization and lowering the chances of development of any zygote that may be formed before it reaches the uterus. In addition, copper impedes sperm transport and viability in the cervical mucus. Because of these actions of IUDs, very few, if any, sperm reach the oviducts, and the ovum usually does not become fertilized. The small numbers of fertilizations that do occur underlie the failure rate of these devices.

#### LNG-IUS

The primary effect of the progestin in the LNG-IUS is to thicken cervical mucus. This impedes sperm penetration and access to the upper genital track. Additionally, the LNG-IUS decreases tubal motility and also produces a thin, inactive endometrium. The low levels of circulating steroid sometimes inhibit ovulation. Systemic LNG levels are lower than those of the progestin implant and progestin-only pills.

### *Insertion*

#### Timing

The IUD can be safely inserted in any of the following scenarios: (1) on any day of the cycle provided the woman is not pregnant, (2) immediately postabortion, and (3) immediately postpartum following either vaginal or cesarean section delivery. Immediate postpartum insertion carries a higher risk of IUD expulsion, particularly in the case of an LNG-IUS following vaginal delivery, with expulsion rates up to 24% (Chen, 2010). In addition, the copper IUD can be used as emergency contraception for up to 5 days following unprotected intercourse. (See the Emergency Contraception, presented later in the chapter, for details.)

#### Pain

Most insertions are easy and accomplished on the first attempt. Cervical preparation with misoprostol does not increase the success of insertion and increases pain. Ibuprofen administered prior to insertion does not reduce insertion pain but may be helpful for the cramping that occurs in the hours immediately following insertion. Multiple trials show that topical anesthesia does not affect pain, although a paracervical block may decrease it. Clinicians should receive training in correct insertion technique as detailed in the product labeling (Video 13.1). If a narrow cervix prevents the passage of a uterine sound, a paracervical block should be placed and dilation performed. Difficult insertions should be referred to clinicians with expertise in family planning procedures.

### *Adverse Effects*

#### Uterine Bleeding

The majority of women discontinuing the copper IUD do so for heavy or prolonged menses or intermenstrual bleeding. The increased bleeding may be produced by an increased rate of prostaglandin release in the presence of the intrauterine foreign body. Stimulation of uterine contractions by prostaglandins may prolong menses, which is about 1 day longer in women with copper IUDs. The copper T 380A IUD is associated with as much as a 50% increase in menstrual blood loss (MBL); however, most women with a copper IUD will experience slightly increased or no change in bleeding. This heavy bleeding rarely leads to anemia.

In contrast, there is a 60% reduction of MBL during the use of the LNG-IUS. This reduction is seen as early as 3 months after insertion and persists for the duration of use of the device. After 24 months of use, 50% of users have amenorrhea and 25% have oligomenorrhea. The LNG-IUS is thus useful in the prevention and the treatment of iron deficiency anemia.

Excessive bleeding in the first few months following IUD insertion should be treated with reassurance and supplemental oral iron. The bleeding usually diminishes with time, as the uterus adjusts to the presence of the foreign body.

#### Perforation

Although rare (1 in 1000 insertions), one of the potentially serious complications associated with IUD use is perforation of the uterus, usually at the fundus. Perforation always begins at the time of insertion. IUDs correctly inserted entirely within the endometrial cavity do not migrate or wander through the uterine muscle into the peritoneal cavity. With experienced providers, the risk of perforation is less. Perforation of the uterus is best prevented by straightening the uterine axis with a tenaculum and then measuring the cavity with a uterine sound before IUD insertion.

The clinician should always suspect a perforation if the user cannot feel the threads and did not observe that the device was expelled. Sometimes the IUD is still in its correct position in the uterine cavity, but the threads have been withdrawn into the cavity as the position of the IUD has changed. To assess this situation, after pelvic examination has been performed and pregnancy excluded, a transvaginal ultrasound may be performed to locate the device. If the device is not visualized with pelvic ultrasonography, a radiograph visualizing the abdominal cavity should be performed to visualize the entire pelvis and abdomen. IUDs found to be outside the uterus usually can be removed by means of laparoscopy. In a study of 61,448 women with IUD insertions conducted with a year or more of follow-up, no IUD perforations led to serious clinical outcomes beyond the need for laparoscopic retrieval (Heinemann, 2015).

The widespread use of transvaginal ultrasound has led to the discovery that many IUDs sit in the lower uterine segment. Faúndes and colleagues found no relationship between the IUD position evaluated by ultrasound and complaints of bleeding and pain.[9] In asymptomatic individuals, the device should be left in place regardless of location within the uterine cavity. However, if the stem of the device is visible at the external cervical os, the IUD should be removed (Faúndes, 1997).

#### Complications Related to Pregnancy

A pregnancy with an IUD in place is rare. Among the few IUD users who do become pregnant, an extrauterine location is more likely than among pregnant women without an IUD. Therefore, in the case of a pregnancy, a pelvic ultrasound must be carried out to locate the pregnancy. In the event of an intrauterine pregnancy, the device should be removed regardless of whether the pregnancy is desired or undesired. As the uterus grows with the pregnancy, the threads will eventually be drawn inside the cervix and become inaccessible. If a pregnancy occurs and the IUD is not subsequently removed, the incidence of spontaneous abortion is approximately three times greater than would occur in pregnancies without an intrauterine device. Once the IUD is removed, the complication rate becomes similar to that of a pregnancy without an IUD. In the case of an undesired pregnancy, a manual vacuum aspiration can be performed with the IUD in place for removal of both the pregnancy and the device.

#### Infection in the Nonpregnant IUD User

Despite great concern among clinicians in the 1970s and 1980s that use of the IUD would markedly increase the incidence of pelvic inflammatory disease (PID), well-conducted studies provided little evidence of such an increase. A WHO combined analysis of clinical trial data including 22,908 women with IUDs showed that the PID rate was six times higher in the first 3 weeks after insertion compared with later times. Following these 3 initial weeks, the risk remained low and constant for as long as 8 years thereafter, at 0.5 cases per 1000 woman-years (Farley, 1992). The placement process, not the device itself or its thread, creates a transient risk of infection, as does any transcervical procedure.

In a meta-analysis of randomized controlled trails (RCTs), Grimes and colleagues showed that the routine use of prophylactic antibiotics preceding IUD insertion did not change outcomes, including the risk of pelvic infection (Grimes, 1999). An IUD may be placed in the absence of cervical screening for infection; however, if a provider has clinical suspicion of infectious endocervicitis, or the patient has two out of three of the following: (1) purulent vaginal discharge, (2) adnexal tenderness, or (3) cervical motion tenderness, testing for gonorrhea and chlamydia should be performed and the IUD insertion delayed.

Positive gonorrhea or chlamydia screening tests that occur with an IUD already in place (i.e., more than 3 weeks after insertion) can usually be successfully treated without removing the IUD. For a symptomatic patient continuing an IUD, an antibiotics regiment for PID approved by the Centers for Disease Control and Prevention (CDC) should be used until the woman becomes symptom free. If the infection does not improve or if there is evidence of tubo-ovarian abscess, the device should be removed after a therapeutic serum level of appropriate parenteral antibiotics has been reached, preferably after a clinical response has been observed (CDC Guidelines, 2015). An alternative method of contraception should be substituted if the IUD is removed.

*Actinomyces* organisms are often identified in routine cytology in women with IUDs in place. If the woman is asymptomatic, she may be followed without therapy at usual intervals. The IUD should not be removed from an asymptomatic colonized woman. In the rare event that a significant pelvic infection is present, the woman should be treated with long-term antibiotics (usually penicillin) and the IUD removed.

### Contraindications

It is good medical practice that IUDs not be inserted into women with any of the following six conditions: (1) pregnancy or suspicion of pregnancy, (2) acute PID, (3) postpartum endometritis or infected abortion, (4) known or suspected uterine or cervical malignancy, (5) genital bleeding of unknown origin, and (6) a previously inserted IUD that has not been removed. Few data are available to indicate whether the complications of Wilson disease or an allergy to copper are true contraindications for insertion of copper-bearing IUDs. Because of the infrequency of these conditions, it is unlikely that data will ever become available.

The high rate of complications specifically associated with the Dalkon Shield in the early 1970s reduced the confidence and enthusiasm of clinicians and women for all IUDs. It has taken 40 years, considerable research, and excellent modern medicated IUDs to reverse this trend, and IUDs are once again a mainstream method. The method was initially conservatively marketed to only parous women. However, both copper and levonorgestrel IUDs can and should be offered to young or nulliparous women.

### Overall Safety

Several long-term studies have indicated that the IUD is not associated with an increased incidence of endometrial or cervical carcinoma; rather, IUD use is associated with a reduction in risk of developing these neoplasms. Data are promising for the use of the LNG-IUS as a fertility-sparing treatment of early stage endometrial cancer (Laurelli, 2011). To date, few studies have evaluated whether hormonal IUD use changes the risk of breast cancer; however, it is an active research question.

The IUD is a particularly useful method of contraception for women who have completed their families and have contraindications to sterilization. Women in the United States who use an IUD have a higher level of satisfaction with their method of contraception than women using any of the other methods of reversible contraception.

### Subdermal Implants

Subdermal implants are among the most effective methods of contraception available, with an effectiveness equal or superior to that of sterilization and IUDs. Subdermal implants consist of one or more thin rods containing a progestin hormone. Insertion is performed in the outpatient setting, and the entire procedure takes less than 5 minutes. After skin infiltration with local anesthesia, the implant is inserted superficially into the subcutaneous tissue of the upper arm using a trocar. The insertion site is closed with adhesive, without the need for suture (Fig. 13.3). When the implant is inserted in any area of subcutaneous tissue, the steroid diffuses into the circulation at a relatively constant rate. The implant must be removed at the end of its duration of use through a small 2-mm incision, which also can be performed in the outpatient setting under local anesthesia, and closed with adhesive. Superficial insertion enhances the ease of removal; deeply implanted implants are more difficult to remove. The implant can be inserted on any day during a woman's cycle provided she is not pregnant.

The most commonly used implant in the United States is the Nexplanon, which contains 68 mg of etonogestrel (ENG). This implant is approved for use up to 3 years, is extremely effective, and is easy to insert and remove. Preliminary studies also indicate continued effectiveness for a longer duration (McNicholas, 2015). Ovulation inhibition is the main mechanism of action of this implant and thickening of the cervical mucus also occurs. Ovulation is completely inhibited for at least 30 months after insertion, and no pregnancies were reported in clinical trials of nearly 2000 women with 7500 cycles of use. Following removal of the implant, serum etonogestrel levels decline rapidly and are undetectable within 1 week after removal. Ovulation resumes rapidly, and 90% of women ovulate within 1 month after removal.

The Nexplanon implant does not result in a decrease of bone mineral density, even in women with amenorrhea. In clinical trials, continuation rates are high, with 50% to 80% of women continuing use until 2 years. Bleeding irregularities are the most common reason for discontinuation, accounting for about 60% of early removals. As with other progestin-only methods, nearly all women experience changes in their regular bleeding pattern. Amenorrhea is common, occurring in about 20% of women, and 27% have infrequent bleeding. About 12% of women have prolonged bleeding, and 6% have frequent bleeding. Unlike depo-medroxyprogesterone acetate (DMPA) or the LNG-IUS, the bleeding patterns of individual women will be unpredictable.

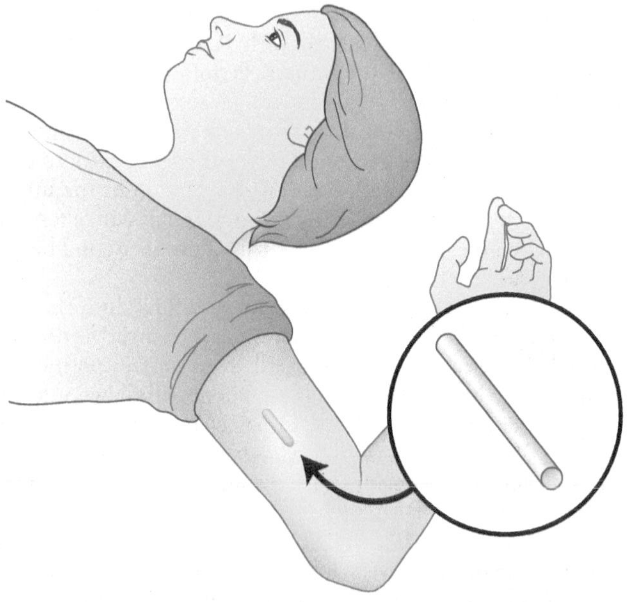

**Figure 13.3** Insertion of a contraceptive implant. (Modified and used with permission of Mayo Foundation for Medical Education and Research. All rights reserved.)

Three other implants are used worldwide but are not currently available in the United States. Jadelle is a two-rod system containing 75 mg levonorgestrel approved for up to 5 years of use. Sino-implant is also a two-rod system containing 75 mg levonorgestrel. Norplant, once widely used, is a six-rod system containing 216 mg levonorgestrel approved for 7 years of use. Insertion and particularly removal of six rods can pose challenges to providers, and the Norplant has been largely supplanted by other implants.

## PERMANENT CONTRACEPTION: STERILIZATION

Male and female sterilization are safe and highly effective methods of contraception. In contrast to the other methods of contraception, which are reversible or temporary, sterilization should be considered permanent. If women who have tubal sterilization wish to conceive, in vitro fertilization is now being performed more frequently than tubal reconstructive surgery.

Voluntary sterilization is legal in all 50 states, and the decision to be sterilized should be made solely by the individual in consultation with a provider. When a woman younger than age 30 requests sterilization, there is up to a 20% risk of regret following sterilization (Hillis, 1999).

### Male Sterilization

Male sterilization, or vasectomy, is a safe and highly effective outpatient procedure that takes about 20 minutes and requires only local anesthesia. More than 300,000 vasectomies are performed annually in the United States. The vas deferens is isolated and cut. The ends of the vas are closed, either by ligation or by fulguration, and then replaced in the scrotal sac. This occlusion of the vas prohibits sperm from passing into the ejaculate. The ejaculate is therefore sperm free, but otherwise unchanged.

Vasectomy offers several important advantages over tubal sterilization of women. The procedure is low cost (it is the most cost-effective of all contraceptive methods) and can be performed in the office with only local anesthesia. It does not involve entry into the peritoneal cavity, and efficacy is easily verified. About 13 to 20 ejaculations must occur after the operation before the ejaculate will be sterile. The absence of sperm is confirmed with a semen sample. Until that time, another method of birth control must be used. Although in the United States reversal requests range from 5% to 7% among men who have had a vasectomy, vas reanastomosis is a difficult and meticulous procedure that has a success rate of approximately 50% (ASRM, 2004).

### Female Sterilization

Approaches to female sterilization in the United States include interval sterilization using laparoscopy or hysteroscopy and postpartum sterilization at the time of cesarean section or with an infraumbilical minilaparotomy incision after vaginal delivery. Sterilization for women blocks fertilization by cutting or occluding the fallopian tubes and preventing the union of the sperm and egg. U.S. women have undergone more than 600,000 sterilization procedures annually. About half of these are performed in the postpartum period. This is the most prevalent method of contraception used by U.S. women over the age of 30 (Chan, 2010).

Female sterilization is highly effective, in the same tier of contraception effectiveness as LARC methods. The Collaborative Review of Sterilization (CREST) was a large prospective multicenter observational study of more than 10,000 women who underwent transabdominal sterilization and that included 14 years of follow-up. The CREST study found a 5-year cumulative failure probability of 13 per 1000 procedures, with failures sometimes occurring years after the sterilization procedure. Risk factors for failure included age and method of sterilization; the younger the woman, the higher the risk of failure. Postpartum partial salpingectomy carried the lowest 10-year cumulative risk of failure (7.5 per 1000 procedures), and Hulka clips (which are no longer available) carried the highest risk (36.5 per 1000 procedures) (Peterson, 1996).

The CREST study occurred prior to the introduction of Filshie clips and transcervical sterilization techniques. Some data show a 10-year cumulative failure rate of 2 to 3 per 1000 procedures for the Filshie clip (Shaw, 1999). Data are less clear for transcervical sterilization as most studies excluded women who do not return for confirmatory testing or for whom the procedure is not successfully completed at the time of insertion. Using a model to predict pregnancy probability that includes all women seeking transcervical sterilization, Gariepy and colleagues calculated a failure rate of 57 in 1000 in the first year after the initial attempt of hysteroscopic sterilization (Gariepy, 2014).

#### Transabdominal Approach

Tubal occlusion can occur at the time of cesarean section, immediately postpartum through an infraumbilical minilaparotomy while the uterus is still enlarged, or, as commonly used outside of the United States, during an interval minilaparotomy. In these cases, ligation and resection of a portion of both fallopian tubes using a technique such as the modified Pomeroy method is common (Fig. 13.4). These methods typically

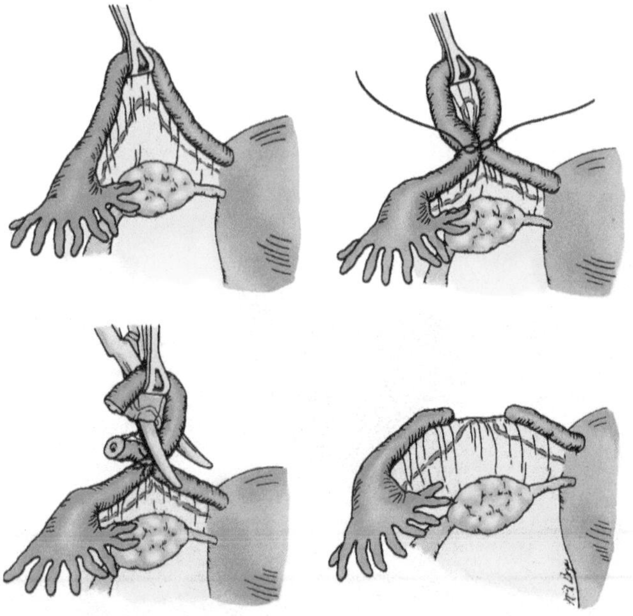

**Figure 13.4** Modified Pomeroy technique of female sterilization. (From Sciarra JJ. Surgical procedures for tubal sterilization. In: Sciarra JJ, Zatuchni GI, Daly MJ. *Gynecology and Obstetrics*. vol 6. Philadelphia: Harper & Row; 1984.)

involve general or regional anesthesia, though local anesthesia is possible.

### Laparoscopic Approach

General anesthesia is usually used for laparoscopic sterilization. Although unipolar electrosurgical techniques were popular in the early days of laparoscopic sterilization, this method was abandoned due to an increased risk of surgical complications. The most common techniques used today include bipolar cautery, the Filshie clip, and the Silastic band (Falope ring). Neither material is reactive, and the titanium does not create artifact or otherwise interfere with magnetic resonance imaging (MRI) scans.

### Transcervical Approach

Sterilization using the Essure device involves the introduction of a microinsert device transcervically through a hysteroscope (Fig. 13.5). The device is placed in the proximal portion of the fallopian tube. Over time, the device causes tissue ingrowth and permanent tubal occlusion. As with vasectomy, another method of birth control must be used to prevent pregnancy until occlusion in confirmed. A hysterosalpingogram is performed 3 months after insertion to document tubal occlusion (Fig. 13.6). Testing is under way using modified inserts that may prove to be effective much sooner. Anesthesia options include local anesthesia, intravenous sedation or general anesthesia. In a meta-analysis of 20 RCTs, the use of local anesthesia at the time of laparoscopic tubal ligation reduced postoperative pain for up to 8 hours after surgery (Harrison, 2014).

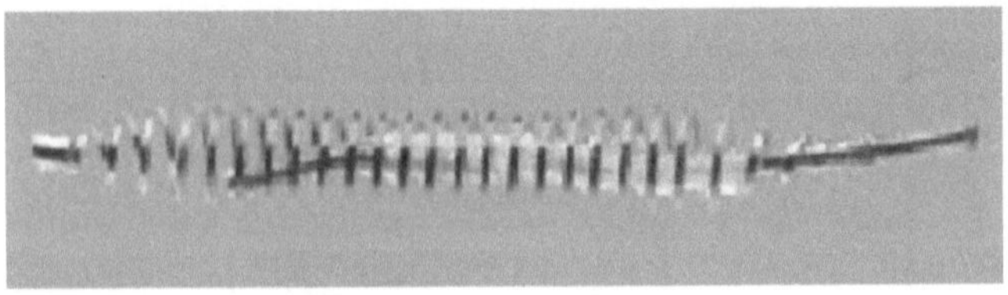

**Figure 13.5** Microinsert for transcervical sterilization in women.

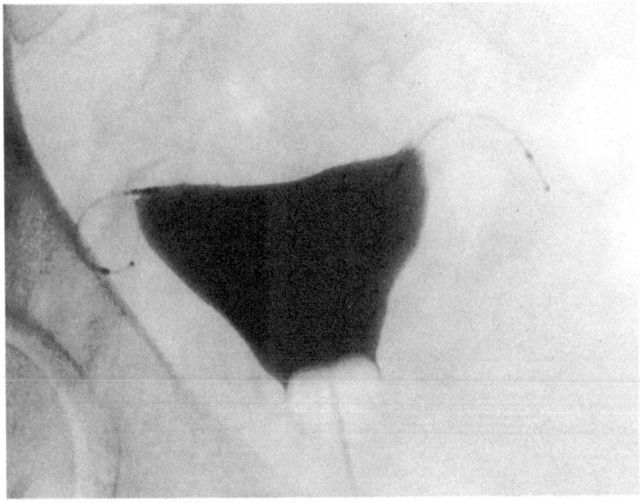

**Figure 13.6** HSG after successful Essure. (From Ogburn T, Espey E: Transcervical sterilization: past, present, and future. *Obstet Gynecol Clin North Am* 34(1):57-72, 2007.)

### Cancer Prevention

Multiple studies indicate a reduced risk of ovarian cancer following tubal ligation. Current investigations are under way to assess an improvement in risk reduction when using bilateral salpingectomy rather than simple tubal ligation (McAlpine, 2014).

## TIER 2 METHODS: VERY EFFECTIVE (6 TO 12 PREGNANCIES PER 100 WOMEN IN 1 YEAR): INJECTABLES, PILLS, PATCH, RING

### *INJECTABLE SUSPENSIONS*

Depo-Provera, or depo-medroxyprogesterone acetate (DMPA), given in a dose of 150 mg intramuscularly (IM) or 104 mg subcutaneously (SC) every 3 months, is the only injectable contraceptive available in the United States. Worldwide, other short-term injectables composed of progestin alone or a combination of progestins and estrogens are also available but will not be discussed in this chapter.

#### *Depot Formulation of MPA*

Medroxyprogesterone acetate (MPA) is a 17-acetoxy-6-methyl derivative of progesterone that has increased progestogenic potency and is longer acting (Fig. 13.7). DMPA, the long-acting injectable formulation of MPA, consists of a crystalline suspension of MPA. DMPA is an extremely effective contraceptive and involves three mechanisms of action: (1) inhibition of ovulation by suppressing levels of FSH and LH and eliminating the LH surge; (2) thickening of cervical mucus inhibiting sperm from reaching the oviduct; and (3) altering the endometrium, which causes atrophy. When used correctly and consistently, the chance of pregnancy is 0.2%. Typical failure rates are around 6%. These effectiveness rates apply to women of all body weights.

The contraceptive dosage with the IM formulation is 150 mg DMPA, given by injection deep into the gluteal or deltoid muscle, after which the progestin releases slowly into the systemic circulation. The SC formulation contains 104 mg of DMPA in 0.65 mL of diluent and is injected into the subcutaneous tissue of the anterior thigh or abdominal wall. For both formulations, the total volume injected is 1 mL.

MPA can be detected in the systemic circulation within 30 minutes after its IM injection. Although serum MPA levels vary among individuals, levels rise steadily to effective contraceptive

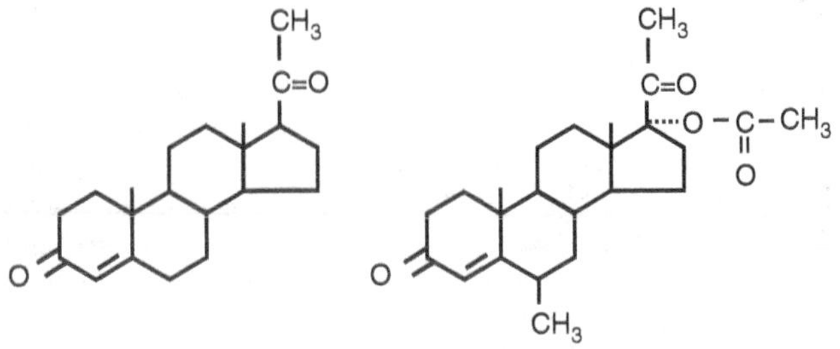


**Figure 13.7** Comparative structures of progesterone and MPA.

blood levels (>0.2 ng/mL) within 24 hours after both IM and SC injections. One RCT showed that self-administration of subcutaneous DMPA is not only feasible for women, but that continuation rates and DMPA levels were similar in women randomized to self versus clinical administration (Beasley, 2014).

### *Return of Fertility*

Because of the lag time in clearing DMPA from the circulation after both IM-DMPA and SC-DMPA, resumption of ovulation is delayed on average for 6 months and as long as 1 year after a single injection. The median delay to conception is 9 to 10 months after the last injection, with a wide range in resumption of ovulation, from 15 to 49 weeks from the last injection (Paulen, 2009).

Women who wish to become pregnant after discontinuing DMPA should know that they might experience a delay in the resumption of fertility until the drug has cleared from their circulation. After this initial delay, fecundity is similar to that found after discontinuing a barrier contraceptive (Fig. 13.8). Thus use of DMPA delays but does not prevent return of fertility.

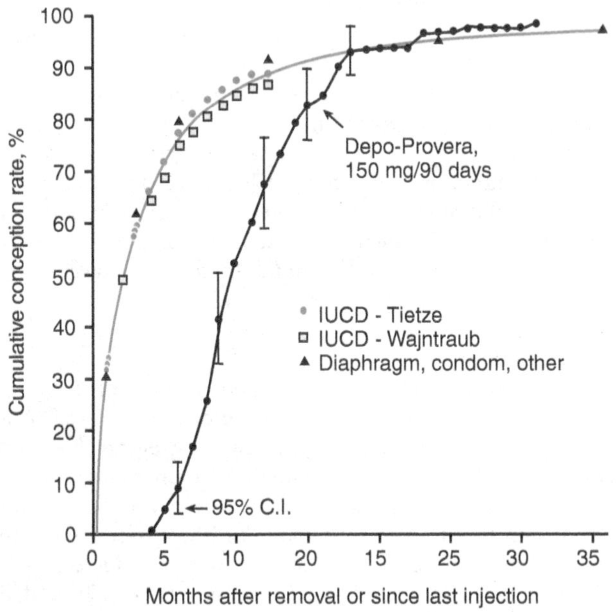


**Figure 13.8** Cumulative conception rates of women who discontinued a contraceptive method to become pregnant. *IUCD,* Intrauterine contraceptive device. (From Schwallie PC, Assenzo JR. The effect of depo-medroxyprogesterone acetate on pituitary and ovarian function, and the return of fertility following its discontinuation: a review. *Contraception.* 1974;10[2]:181-202.)

### *Clinical Side Effects*

#### Bleeding Patterns

The major side effect of DMPA is a change of the menstrual cycle. In the first 3 months after the first injection, about 30% of women experience amenorrhea and another 30% to 40% have irregular bleeding and spotting occurring more than 11 days per month. Usually light, the bleeding does not cause anemia. As the duration of therapy increases, the incidence of frequent bleeding steadily declines and the incidence of amenorrhea increases. At the end of 1 year, about 55% of women experience amenorrhea. After 2 years, about 70% of women experience amenorrhea (Fig. 13.9). Women who use this method should receive counseling that with time irregular bleeding will diminish and amenorrhea will most likely occur.

After discontinuation of DMPA, about half of women resume a regular cyclic menstrual pattern within 6 months and about three fourths have regular menses within 1 year.

#### Weight Changes

About one fourth of women using DMPA gain weight, usually in the first 6 months of use. Several longitudinal studies indicate that DMPA users gain between 1.5 and 4 kg in their first year of use and continue to gain weight thereafter. While we do not have a clear understanding of how this weight gain differs from women not on DMPA, some suggest that the injection should

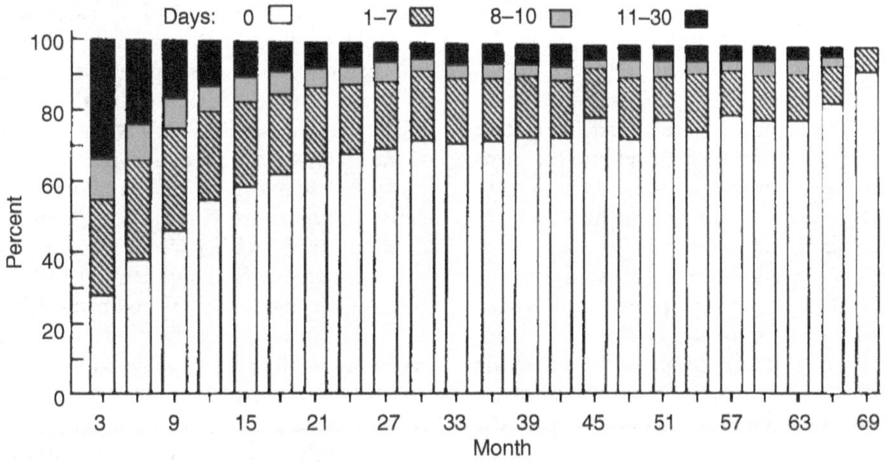


**Figure 13.9** Percentage of patients with bleeding or spotting on days 0, 1-7, 8-10, or 11-30 per 30-day cycle while receiving injectable DMPA, 150 mg, every 3 months. (From Schwallie PC, Assenzo JR. Contraceptive use: efficacy study utilizing medroxyprogesterone acetate administered as an intramuscular injection once every 90 days. *Fertil Steril.* 1973;24:331-339, from The American Society for Reproductive Medicine.)

be used with caution in patients who are already overweight or obese (Le, 2009).

#### Mood Changes

The product labeling lists depression and mood changes as side effects of DMPA. Several studies, however, indicate that the incidence of depression and mood change in women using this method of contraception is less than 5%, and thus no greater than the overall incidence of depression. No clinical trials have been performed to assess whether a causal relation between DMPA and the development of depression exists.

#### Headache

The development of headaches is the most frequent medical event reported by DMPA users and a common reason for discontinuation of its use. No comparative studies indicate that DMPA increases the incidence or severity of tension or migraine headaches and the presence of migraine headaches does not contraindicate DMPA use.

#### Bone Loss

Because DMPA suppresses production of estradiol, bone remodeling is increased and may resemble menopause. Observational studies consistently indicate that DMPA is associated with a degree of decreased bone mineral density (BMD). Longer-term studies, however, indicate that bone loss is reversible after stopping DMPA use. Measurement of bone mineral density during DMPA use is unnecessary because bone density increases after stopping DMPA and bisphosphonate therapy should not be used in DMPA users with low BMD.

#### Noncontraceptive Health Benefits

DMPA reduces the risk of developing iron deficiency anemia and PID. The reduction in risk of endometrial cancer in women on DMPA is long lasting and substantial. DMPA also reduces the incidence of primary dysmenorrhea, symptoms of endometriosis, ovulation pain, and functional ovarian cysts because it inhibits ovulation. Many believe that DMPA also reduces seizure frequency in women with epilepsy. In some studies, DMPA seems to have beneficial effects on sickle cell pain crises.

### *Clinical Recommendations*

DMPA can be started at any time during the menstrual cycle as long as the woman and her provider are reasonably certain that she is not pregnant. If given later than 7 days into the menstrual cycle, backup contraception should be used for 7 days. Women should be informed prior to receiving the first injection of the occurrence of irregular bleeding and the development of amenorrhea with DMPA with reassurance that these are normal changes. Pretreatment counseling may improve continuation rates. In addition, women need to know that the action may last as long as 1 year following the last injection if they decide to discontinue use of DMPA. If pregnancy occurs in a woman receiving DMPA, the hormone does not adversely impact the pregnancy.

## *ORAL CONTRACEPTIVES*

Because of their effectiveness and ease of administration, oral contraceptives (OCs) became the most widely used method of reversible contraception among both married and unmarried women within a few years of their introduction to the United States in 1960. The high doses of steroids in the original pill formulations caused minor side effects such as nausea, breast tenderness, and weight gain that frequently led to discontinuation of use. Since that time, other formulations have been developed and marketed with steadily decreasing dosages of both the estrogen and progestin components. Reduction in ethinyl estradiol (EE) dose has coincided with a lower incidence of severe adverse cardiovascular effects and minor adverse symptoms without increasing the failure rate. All the formulations marketed after 1975 contain less than 50 μg of EE and 3 mg or less of one of several progestins.

The most widely used methods combine EE with one of several synthetic progestins. The major effect of the progestin component is to inhibit ovulation, but progestins also contribute other contraceptive actions such as thickening of the cervical mucus and thinning of the endometrium. The major effects of the estrogen are to maintain the endometrium and thus prevent unscheduled bleeding as well as to inhibit follicular development through a synergistic effect with the progestin.

### *Pharmacology*

Synthetic steroids have greater oral potency per unit of weight than do natural steroids. The modifications in chemical structure of different synthetic progestins and estrogens affect their biologic activity. One cannot define the pharmacologic activity of the progestin or estrogen in a particular contraceptive steroid formulation based only on the amount of steroid present. The biologic activity of each steroid also has to be considered.

The three major types of OC formulations include daily progestin-only pills (POPs), also known as minipills (see Progestin-Only Pills, presented later in the chapter), fixed-dose (monophasic) combination pills, and multiphasic combination pills. The combination formulations are the most widely used. Monophasic products contain tablets with the same dose combination of an estrogen and progestin each day. In multiphasic formulations, pills containing several different dose combinations come in the same pack. A different tablet color corresponds to each dose. Depending on the number of different dose combinations, these formulations are further classified as biphasic, triphasic, or four phasic.

In the United States, most oral contraceptive regimens are packaged in a 28-day (4-week) cycle. Many combination OC formulations provide active pills continuously for 21 days (3 weeks) followed by a 7-day hormone-free interval (HFI). Most products are packaged with inactive spacer (placebo) pills during the HFI to improve compliance. Some formulations provide an iron supplement in the spacer pills. Uterine bleeding occurs secondary to hormone withdrawal during the HFI, typically 1 to 3 days after taking the last active pill. This withdrawal bleeding usually lasts 3 to 4 days and is generally lighter than during menses in an ovulatory cycle. Some formulations provide active tablets for 24 days, reducing the HFI to only 4 days, and these may be more effective than 21-day active pill formulations. Other formulations provide a small amount of EE (alone without progestin) during all parts of the 7-day HFI to reduce symptoms associated with estrogen withdrawal and the resurgence of follicle-stimulating hormone (FSH).

Newer dosing strategies include extended and continuous cycles. Extended cycle regimens contain 84 days of active pills followed by a 7-day HFI (or 7 days of EE only) that results in withdrawal bleeding only four times a year. A continuous daily LNG 90-µg /EE 20-µg regimen with 28 active pills in a treatment pack was introduced in 2007 to completely eliminate scheduled withdrawal bleeds. Some providers recommend extended use of generic, less expensive monophasic 20-µg EE OCs, instructing patients to discard the placebo pills and begin a new cycle pack after 21 days.

Randomized studies comparing cyclic and continuous dosing regimens have documented a decrease in the total scheduled bleeding days but an increase in irregular bleeding and spotting with extended or continuous use of hormonal contraceptives. Bleeding patterns typically improve over time in most users of cyclic or continuous OCs, with rates of unscheduled bleeding highest in early cycles of use. Women who experience prolonged breakthrough bleeding while taking combined OCs continuously might benefit from discontinuing the active pills for 3 days and then restarting. Greater gaps could result in ovulation and unintended pregnancy.

OCs have a 1% failure rate with perfect use and an 8% failure rate with typical use. Accidental pregnancies occurring during OC use probably do not occur because of missing just one to two pills, but rather because initiation of the new cycle of medication is delayed for a few days or because a greater number of tablets are missed. It is particularly important that the pill-free interval is not extended more than 7 days. Women should be advised that the most important pill to remember to take is the first one of each cycle. In practice, clinicians should ensure that all patients are able to easily access refills of oral contraceptives. When a woman misses two or more pills in a pack, she should take emergency contraception and use backup contraception.

### *Physiology*

#### Mechanism of Action

Combination oral contraceptives suppress gonadotropins. The estrogen component prevents a rise in follicle-stimulating hormone (FSH) and enhances the effect of the progestin component, which inhibits ovulation and, specifically, the luteinizing hormone (LH) surge. These dual actions lead to inhibition of follicle development and ovulation. The lowest amount of a progestin needed to suppress LH is the **ovulation inhibition dose**. Changes in the cervical mucus (which prevent sperm transport into the uterus), the fallopian tube (which interfere with gamete transport), and the endometrium (which reduce the likelihood of implantation) represent secondary contraceptive effects of the progestin component. Contraceptive steroids prevent ovulation mainly by interfering with release of gonadotropin-releasing hormone (GnRH) from the hypothalamus. Most studies also support that contraceptive steroids directly suppress the pituitary in addition.

With all OCs, neither gonadotropin production nor ovarian steroidogenesis is completely abolished. Levels of endogenous $E_2$ in the peripheral blood during ingestion of combination OCs are similar to those found in the early follicular phase of a physiologic cycle.

In a cohort study of U.S. women, 24-day oral contraceptive regimens containing a progestin with a long half-life had higher contraceptive effectiveness compared to 21-day regimens (Dinger, 2011). No other difference in clinical effectiveness has been demonstrated among the various combination formulations currently available in the United States.

The balance between estrogen and progestin influences the bleeding profile of a combination OC. Estrogen induces endometrial proliferation. Progestins oppose the mitotic action of estrogen, leading to a stable decidualized endometrium. Even though women taking combined OCs are exposed to both hormones at the same time rather than sequentially, they typically undergo some endometrial proliferation. The bleeding that users of combined OCs experience during the hormone-free interval is called **withdrawal bleeding**, as it occurs upon cessation of the progestin component of the pill. Bleeding that occurs during the time that active pills are ingested is called **breakthrough bleeding**.

Unscheduled (breakthrough) bleeding and absence of withdrawal bleeding (amenorrhea) occur as a result of insufficient estrogen to support the endometrium. If the user considers this problematic, increasing the amount of estrogen in the pill formulation or changing progestins often provides a solution. Otherwise absence of withdrawal bleeding is not a reason to change pills if the patient is satisfied.

#### Metabolic Effects

The synthetic steroids in OC formulations have many metabolic effects in addition to their contraceptive actions. These metabolic effects can lead to side effects and rare potentially life-threatening complications. The magnitude of these effects may be related to the dosage and potency of the steroids in the formulations. Fortunately, the more common adverse effects are relatively mild. The most frequent symptoms produced by the estrogen component include nausea (12%), breast tenderness (9%), and headache (18%). However, in placebo-controlled trials, there is no difference in the incidence of these complaints between OC users and placebo users (Redmond 1999). Reduction in EE dose to below 50 µg has greatly reduced the incidence of all of these estrogenic side effects.

OCs decrease androgen levels, which tends to reduce acne. The net effect of an OC on acne relates to three qualities: the androgenicity of the progestin component, the extent that endogenous androgens circulate freely or are bound to plasma proteins, and the activity of 5 α-reductase, the enzyme that converts testosterone to dihydrotestosterone. For most low-dose OCs, the net effect favors a reduction of acne. In two multicenter, double-blind, placebo-controlled studies, evaluating the effectiveness of triphasic norgestimate/ethinyl estradiol (Ortho Tri-Cyclen) for the treatment of acne, the OC group had a greater reduction of acne with no difference in adverse events between both groups (Redmond, 1999), a result confirmed in studies of several other OCs (O'Connell, 2008, Gallo, 2014).

Weight gain represents a common complaint of women using hormonal contraception. However, a 2013 study assessed weight gain following OC initiation in obese and normal weight women, weighing participants prior to and after 3 months of OCP use. Neither group experienced a substantial change in weight (Mayeda, 2014, Gallo, 2014).

### *Progestin-Only Pills (POPs)*

The minipill formulations consist of tablets containing a low dose of progestin and no estrogen. They are taken every day without a steroid-free interval. Because doses of a progestin are below the **ovulation inhibition dose** in the minipills that contain norethindrone or norgestrel, the other progestogenic effects become the primary mechanism of action. Clinicians should counsel their patients using the minipill that preparations should be consistently taken at the same time of day to ensure that blood levels do not fall below the effective contraceptive level. Newer POPs contain progestins that inhibit ovulation more effectively.

With minipill use, many women may still ovulate; therefore, estradiol and progesterone produced by the ovary will affect endometrial bleeding patterns. Women may experience irregular bleeding, spotting, or amenorrhea, depending on an individual woman's response.

### Coagulation Parameters

Epidemiologic studies consistently demonstrate that the risk of both venous and arterial thrombosis increases among users of combined OCs compared with nonpregnant nonusers. However, although combined oral contraceptives increase the risk of VTE, they offer significant protection against pregnancy, a condition associated with a substantially higher risk of thrombosis roughly twofold higher than that observed with OCs.

The increased risk is related to the estrogen component of the pill and is dose dependent (Gerstmann, 1991). A woman's baseline risk of venous thromboembolism (VTE) increases by three times if she ingests estrogen-containing oral contraception. If a woman already has an increased baseline risk, such as having a personal history of idiopathic VTE, she should not take an estrogen-containing contraceptive. Screening for coagulation deficiencies should only be performed before starting OC use if the woman has a family history of thrombotic events. Although progestins alone do not affect coagulation parameters, whether recent progestins increase the coagulation risk of OC use remains controversial. It has been suggested that OCs with the newer progestins increase the risk over that of the older, early generation products.

Obesity is a modest risk factor for VTE (Fig. 13.10), and extreme obesity (e.g., a body mass index [BMI] >40) should be considered a relative contraindication to use of a combined hormonal method. Use of OCs by women older than age 35 who also smoke is contraindicated due to the risk of myocardial infarction.

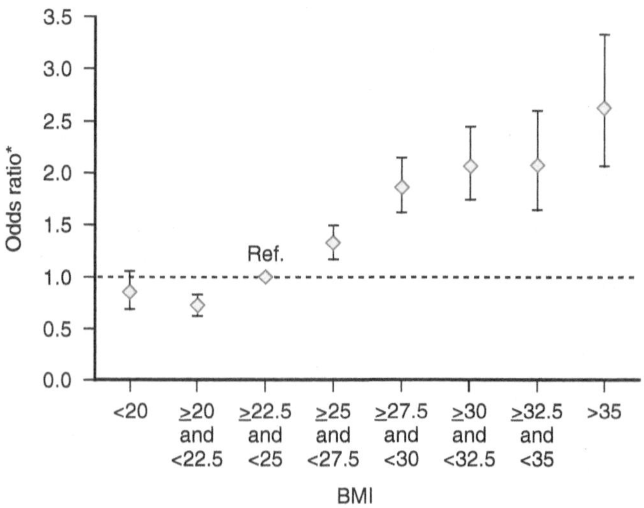


| | | | | | | | | |
|---|---|---|---|---|---|---|---|---|
| $n_p$ | 160 | 416 | 817 | 925 | 704 | 402 | 190 | 220 |
| $n_c$ | 256 | 865 | 1236 | 1102 | 626 | 311 | 154 | 133 |

*Adjusted for age and sex.

**Figure 13.10** Relative risk (with 95% confidence intervals) of deep vein thrombosis by categories of body mass (BMI). Adjusted for age and sex. (From Pomp ER, le Cessie S, Rosendaal FR, Doggen CJ. Risk of venous thrombosis: obesity and its joint effect with oral contraceptive use and prothrombotic mutations. *Br J Haematol.* 2007;139: 289-296.)

### *Return to Fertility*

After discontinuation of low-dose OCs, the suppressive effect on the hypothalamic-pituitary-ovarian axis disappears quickly. After the initial recovery, completely normal endocrine function occurs. There is little, if any, effect of duration of OC use on the length of delay of subsequent conception. There is no risk of congenital malformations or other adverse outcomes in pregnancies among women who conceive while taking OCs or shortly thereafter.

### *Neoplastic Risks and Benefits*

#### Breast Cancer

Although OC use increases the risk of breast cancer by 25%, this risk disappears after cessation of use. The absolute risk of breast cancer is low given the young age of most OC users. Some evidence indicates that those breast cancers diagnosed during OC use are more likely to be localized. The risk of developing breast cancer with OC use is not changed even in women with a high risk of developing breast cancer, including women with an immediate family history of breast cancer and those with *BRCA-1* and *BRCA-2* mutations (Milne, 2005).

#### Cervical Cancer

The epidemiologic data regarding the risk of invasive cervical cancer as well as cervical intraepithelial neoplasia and OC use are conflicting. Confounding factors could account for contrasting results in different studies. Studies indicate that the risk of cervical cancer, both invasive and in situ, for OC users compared with nonusers increases with increasing duration of OC use. These risks persist after adjusting for HPV infection, squamous cell or adenocarcinoma, number of sexual partners, cervical cytology screening, smoking, and use of barrier contraceptive (Smith, 2003, Appleby, 2007). However, some studies suggest that there may be an increased relationship between OC use and adenocarcinoma of the cervix compared with squamous cell.

There is no evidence that OC use alters the incidence or rate of the progression of cervical dysplasia to invasive cancer. Women with treated cervical dysplasia can use OCs, as can those with newly diagnosed dysplasia awaiting evaluation.

#### Endometrial Cancer

Studies have consistently demonstrated a strong protective effect between OCs and endometrial cancer. Compared with nonusers, women who use OCs for at least 1 year have an age-adjusted relative risk of 0.5 for development of endometrial cancer between ages 40 and 55. This protective effect is related to duration of use, increasing from a 20% reduction in risk with 1 year of use to a 40% reduction with 2 years of use to about a 60% reduction with 4 years of use. This protective effect persists for at least 15 years after stopping use of OCs.

Ovarian Cancer

Numerous epidemiologic studies have consistently demonstrated that OCs reduce the risk of developing ovarian cancer. The risk of ovarian cancer decreases by about 20% for every 5 years of use. For woman using OCs for 15 years or more, the risk is almost halved. One year of use may obtain a protective effect (Grimbizis, 2010). OCs reduce the risk of the four main histologic types of epithelial ovarian cancer: serous, mucinous, endometrioid, and clear-cell, and the risk of both invasive ovarian cancers and tumors of low malignant potential (borderline tumors). The protective effect continues for at least 30 years after the use of OCs ends. OC use also reduces the risk of ovarian cancer in women with *BRCA-1* and *BRCA-2* mutations and in those with a family history of ovarian cancer to the same extent as in women without these risk factors.

Liver Adenoma and Cancer

The development of a benign hepatocellular adenoma is an extremely rare occurrence. An increased risk of this tumor was reported in early OC studies of prolonged use of high-dose formulations but seems to be far lower for women taking lower OC doses. Women with active liver disease should not use hormonal contraception, as the liver is a major site for the metabolism of synthetic steroids.

Colorectal Cancer

A meta-analysis of published studies of the relationship between OCs and colorectal cancer showed that OC ever-use was associated with a 15% to 20% reduction in the risk of colorectal cancer in the eight case-control studies and four cohort studies analyzed. Thus OC use decreases the risk of developing both colon and rectal cancer (Fernandez, 2001).

### *Noncontraceptive Health Benefits*

In addition to the long-term reduction in risk of ovarian and endometrial cancer, some of the immediate benefits of OC use include improvement of menorrhagia and dysmenorrhea and decreased acne (Maguire, 2011). As a result of the antiestrogenic action of the progestins in OCs, there is less proliferation of the endometrial glands. These changes reduce the amount of blood loss at the time of endometrial shedding. This decreased blood loss makes the development of iron deficiency anemia less likely for OC users than for nonusers. OC users are significantly less likely to have menorrhagia, irregular menstruation, or intermenstrual bleeding. As OCs inhibit ovulation, they can reduce such ovulatory disorders as dysmenorrhea and premenstrual syndrome.

### *Contraindications to Oral Contraceptive Use*

The World Health Organization has published detailed guidelines listing the medical eligibility criteria for the use of contraceptive methods. These guidelines are regularly updated, and the revised fifth edition can be downloaded from the WHO website (www.who.int/reproductivehealth) (WHO, 2010).

The Centers for Disease Control and Prevention (CDC) Guidelines, specific to practice in the United States and also regularly updated, were published in 2010 and are available at the CDC website (www.cdc.gov/reproductivehealth) (CDC, 2010).

OCs can be prescribed for the majority of women of reproductive age, because these women are young and generally healthy. There are, however, certain absolute contraindications, including a history of vascular disease (thromboembolism, thrombophlebitis, atherosclerosis, and stroke) and systemic disease that may affect the vascular system (e.g., active lupus erythematosus with vascular involvement or diabetes with retinopathy or nephropathy). Cigarette smoking by OC users older than age 35 and uncontrolled hypertension are also contraindications. As breast or endometrial cancer may involve hormone-sensitive tumors, avoiding OC use is prudent. Other contraindications include undiagnosed uterine bleeding and elevated triglyceride levels.

Pregnancy is an obvious contraindication. As mentioned, OCs are not teratogenic nor will they negatively affect pregnancies occurring during or after use. Women with active liver disease should not take OCs. Women who have recovered from liver disease, such as viral hepatitis, and whose liver function tests have returned to normal can safely take OCs.

Relative contraindications to OC use include heavy cigarette smoking younger than age 35, migraine headaches, and undiagnosed causes of amenorrhea or genital bleeding. The risk of stroke, albeit low, is significantly increased in women with migraine headaches with aura who use OCs. Women who have migraine headache with aura or peripheral neurologic symptoms should not use oral contraceptives. If headache occurs only during the hormone-free interval, continuous dosing might help to control the symptoms. Women with migraine headaches without aura under 35 years of age can use OCs.

OC use may mask the symptoms produced by a prolactin-secreting adenoma. Therefore women with either galactorrhea or amenorrhea should not receive OCs until a diagnosis is established. If galactorrhea develops during OC use, OCs should be discontinued, and after 2 weeks a serum prolactin level should be measured. If elevated, further diagnostic evaluations are indicated.

Women with diabetes without cardiovascular progression can take low-dose OC formulations, because these agents do not affect glucose tolerance or accelerate diabetes mellitus.

### *Beginning Oral Contraceptives*

Adolescents

A pubertal girl who has demonstrated maturity of the hypothalamic-pituitary-ovarian axis with presumably ovulatory menstrual cycles can begin OCs without concern that their use will alter future reproductive endocrinologic function. It is also not necessary to be concerned about accelerating epiphyseal closure in the postmenarchal female. Endogenous estrogens have already initiated the process a few years before menarche, and use of contraceptive steroids will not hasten this process.

After Pregnancy

For women who deliver after 28 weeks and are not nursing, the combination pills should be initiated no sooner than 6 weeks after delivery as the increased risk of postpartum thromboembolism may be further enhanced by the hypercoagulable effects of combination OCs. Progestin-only methods can be initiated immediately.

Estrogen inhibits the action of prolactin in breast tissue receptors; therefore, the use of combination OCs (those containing both estrogen and progestin) diminishes the amount of milk produced by OC users who breast-feed their babies. The diminution of milk production is directly related to the amount of estrogen in the contraceptive formulation, and no significant health risks are associated with hormones in breast milk for the nursing infant. The major concern is that combined OCs will lower the success of initiation of lactation. Women at high risk for unintended pregnancy following delivery should consider the relative advantages of a combination pill over other methods, as well as the effect of the contraceptive on nursing success. A number of authorities, including the CDC, are not enthusiastic about the use of combined OCs until breast-feeding has been established, with many preferring to wait until 6 months have passed.

Progestins do not diminish the amount of breast milk, and progestin-only OCs are highly effective in this group of women, though not recommended by some prior to 6 weeks postpartum with breast-feeding.

### Cycling Women

Woman may find it convenient to start a pill pack on a particular day of the week. Sunday starts have been a popular recommendation; however, delaying the start of a pill pack can lead to unintended pregnancies. Starting a pill pack on the same day as a clinic visit instead of waiting until after menses allows for a quicker onset of contraception with no adverse effects on bleeding patterns and is highly acceptable to many women.[39]

### *Type of Formulation*

Estrogen dose, side effect profile, and cost should guide decisions regarding the type of formulation to prescribe. Doses with 35 μg or more of estrogen are rarely used because of the cardiovascular risks and estrogenic side effects. The U.S. Food and Drug Administration (FDA) has stated that the product prescribed should be one that contains the least amount of estrogen and progestin that is compatible with a low failure rate and the needs of the individual woman.

The progestin-only contraceptive formulations have a lower incidence of risks than do the combination formulations. Because the factors that predispose to thromboembolism are caused by the estrogen component, the incidence of thromboembolism in women taking the minipill is not increased compared to nonusers.

It is unfortunate that the infrequent adverse effects of OCs have received widespread publicity, but the more common noncontraceptive health benefits have attracted little attention.

## CONTRACEPTIVE PATCH

The contraceptive skin patch Ortho Evra (Fig. 13.11) contains 75 μg ethinyl estradiol and 6 mg norelgestromin. A generic patch is now available, and new combination patches are in development. One patch is applied to the skin each week for 3 consecutive weeks and no patch for the following week of a 4-week cycle to allow withdrawal bleeding. The patch may be applied to one of four anatomic sites: buttocks, upper outer arm, lower abdomen, or upper torso excluding the breasts. Following skin application, both steroids appear in the circulation rapidly and reach a plateau within 48 hours. Like OCs, the primary mechanism of action is the inhibition of gonadotropin release and prevention of ovulation. Contraceptive effectiveness and metabolic and clinical effects, including irregular bleeding, are similar to combination oral contraceptives. Results from clinical trials suggest that patch efficacy may be slightly lower in women with body weight more than 90 kg. In a pooled analysis of three multicenter trials, 7 out of 15 pregnancies occurred in women >80 kg. Five of the 15 pregnancies were in women >90 kg. For this reason, the Ortho Evra label indicates a possible decrease in effectiveness among overweight or obese women (Zieman, 2002). However, even in the heaviest women the patch was 90% effective. Newer patch results do not support a possible decrease in effectiveness.

## CONTRACEPTIVE VAGINAL RING

Steroids pass easily through the vaginal epithelium directly into the circulation. A flexible ring-shaped device containing 2.7 mg of ethinyl estradiol and 11.7 mg of etonogestrel (Fig. 13.12), the contraceptive ring (NuvaRing) is placed in the vagina for 21 days and then removed for up to 7 days to allow withdrawal bleeding. After this ring-free interval the woman inserts a new ring regardless of whether withdrawal bleeding has occurred. Because the steroids act systemically, the ring comes in only one size and does not have to be fitted or placed in a certain location. Like oral contraceptives, the main mechanism of action is inhibition of gonadotropins and prevention of ovulation. Because each ring delivers sufficient steroids to inhibit ovulation for 6 weeks, contraceptive action can be assumed

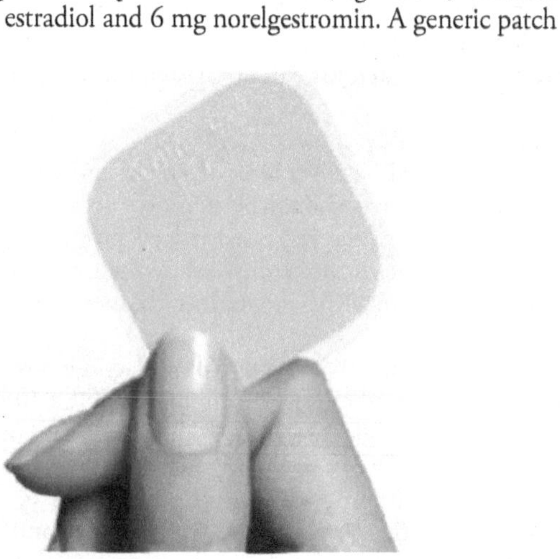

**Figure 13.11** The contraceptive skin patch releasing ethinyl estradiol and norelgestromin.

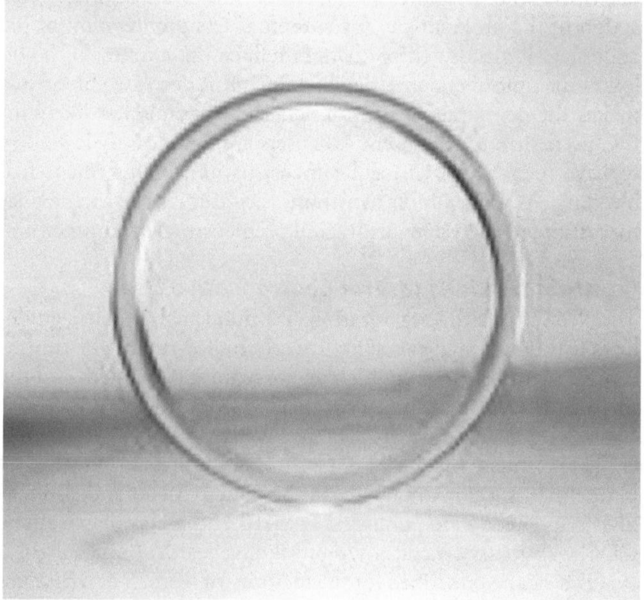

**Figure 13.12** The contraceptive vaginal ring releasing ethinyl estradiol and etonogestrel.

even if the ring is left in place beyond 21 days. Continuous use has been studied, and results are similar to those observed with continuous OCs.

Despite the low dose of ethinyl estradiol, bleeding control is good, with irregular bleeding occurring less than with OCs. Contraceptive effectiveness as well as metabolic and clinical effects are similar to that for combination oral contraceptives. Ring expulsion is uncommon, and both partners typically report high acceptability with use.

Phase III clinical trials showed no difference in efficacy for women in the heaviest weight category (>166 lb75 kg) (Westhoff, 2005), but few overweight or obese women had been enrolled. A pharmacokinetic study showed therapeutic progestogen and ethinyl estradiol levels in both normal-weight and obese women. Observed progestogen levels in obese vaginal ring users were high enough to inhibit ovulation and there was no increase in follicular activity (Dragoman, 2013).

## TIER 3 METHODS: EFFECTIVE (18 OR MORE PREGNANCIES PER 100 WOMEN IN 1 YEAR): BARRIER METHODS, LACTATIONAL AMENORRHEA, PERIODIC ABSTINENCE, COITUS-RELATED METHODS

### *BARRIER METHODS*

#### *Diaphragm and Cervical Cap*

When Margaret Sanger introduced the vaginal diaphragm to the United States in 1916, it became the most widely used female-controlled reversible contraceptive method for 4 decades prior to the introduction of oral contraceptive. The diaphragm is a thin, dome-shaped membrane of latex rubber or silicone with a flexible spring modeled into the rim. The spring allows the device to be collapsed for insertion and then allows for expansion within the vagina to seat the rim against the vaginal wall, creating a mechanical barrier between the vagina and the cervix. Traditionally, a diaphragm has been fitted by a health care provider to find the largest size that does not cause discomfort or undue pressure on the vaginal mucosa; however, no data have assessed whether a "good fit" correlates with improved effectiveness. The FDA has approved Caya, a single-size diaphragm that does not require fitting by a practitioner, intended for use over the counter (Fig. 13.13).

A cervical cap is a cup-shaped silicone or rubber device that fits around the cervix. It should be fitted to the cervix by a clinician. The only cap currently on the U.S. market is the FemCap. This product, made of soft, durable, hypoallergenic, silicone rubber, is designed to contact the vaginal walls as the dome of the device sits over the cervix (Fig. 13.14). Prescriptions of the diaphragm and cervical cap have become much less frequent.

The diaphragm and cervical cap should be used with a spermicide and be left in place for at least 8 hours after the last coital act. If repeated intercourse takes place, additional spermicide should be used vaginally. Failure rate during the first year of use for the diaphragm ranges from 13% to 17% among all users and may be as low as 4% to 8% with perfect use. The cervical cap failure rate is comparable to the diaphragm. The diaphragm and cervical cap may also reduce the risk of cervical dysplasia and cancer.

#### *Male and Female Condom*

The latex and polyurethane male condoms are the only method with FDA-approved labeling that supports use of the product to prevent both pregnancy and the transmission of sexually transmitted infections (STIs). Condoms should be encouraged as STI protection along with another more effective method for pregnancy prevention. Clinicians should review proper condom use with both men and women. The condom should be applied to the erect penis before any contract with the vagina or vulva. The tip should extend beyond the end of the penis by about half an inch to collect the ejaculate. After ejaculation, the penis must be removed from the vagina while still somewhat erect, and the base of the condom grasped to ensure the condom is removed without spillage of the ejaculate. Water-based lubrication may reduce condom breakage.

When used by strongly motivated couples, the male condom is effective. The typical use failure rate is around 15% (Hatcher, 2011).

The female condom consists of a soft, loose-fitting polyurethane sheath with two flexible rings. One ring lies at the

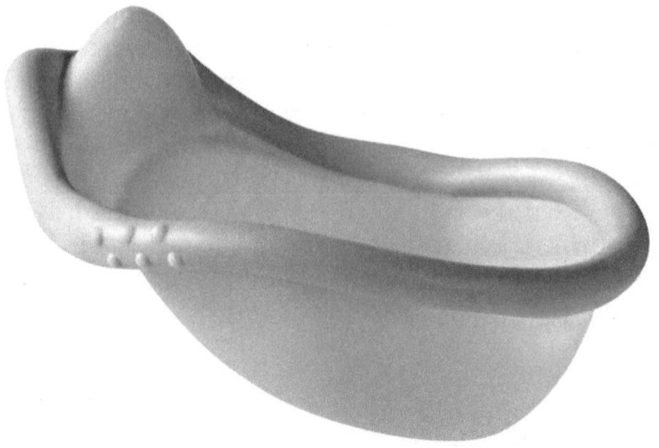

**Figure 13.13** The Caya diaphragm. (Courtesy of Kessel Medintim GmbH, www.medintim.de.)

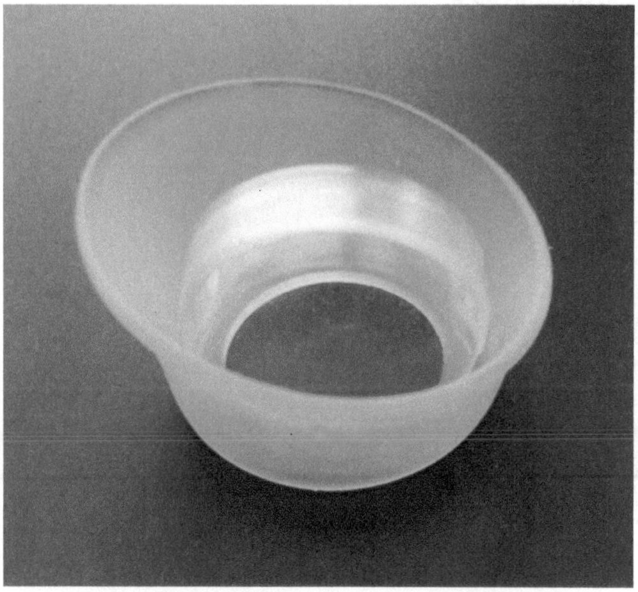

**Figure 13.14** The female barrier method FemCap.

closed end of the sheath and serves as an insertion mechanism and internal anchor for the condom inside the vagina. The outer ring forms the external edge of the device and remains outside the vagina after insertion, thus providing protection to the introitus and the base of the penis during intercourse (Fig. 13.15). The female condom is prelubricated and intended for one-time use only. Like male condoms, the device is available over the counter and does not require fitting by a health professional. It also protects against sexually transmitted diseases. It can be inserted prior to the onset of sexual activity and left in place after ejaculation has occurred. The typical use failure rate at 1 year is estimated to be 21% (Hatcher, 2011). New female condoms are forthcoming.

## LACTATIONAL AMENORRHEA METHOD (LAM)

Because prolactin inhibits gonadotropin pulsatility, nursing women typically remain amenorrheic for a variable length of time after giving birth. Higher frequency and longer duration of nursing contribute to menstrual suppression and night nursing is highly correlated with anovulation and amenorrhea.

The criteria for successful use of LAM are continuous amenorrhea and exclusive breast-feeding (no supplements) for up to 6 months after delivery. Night nursing is highly protective. When used correctly, the failure rate in the first 6 months postpartum is less than 2%.

Effective use of LAM improves with education regarding the efficacy of the method. Because breast-feeding may end sooner than anticipated, a provider should discuss in advance a reliable ongoing contraceptive plan for prompt initiation if the conditions required for success with LAM are no longer in place.

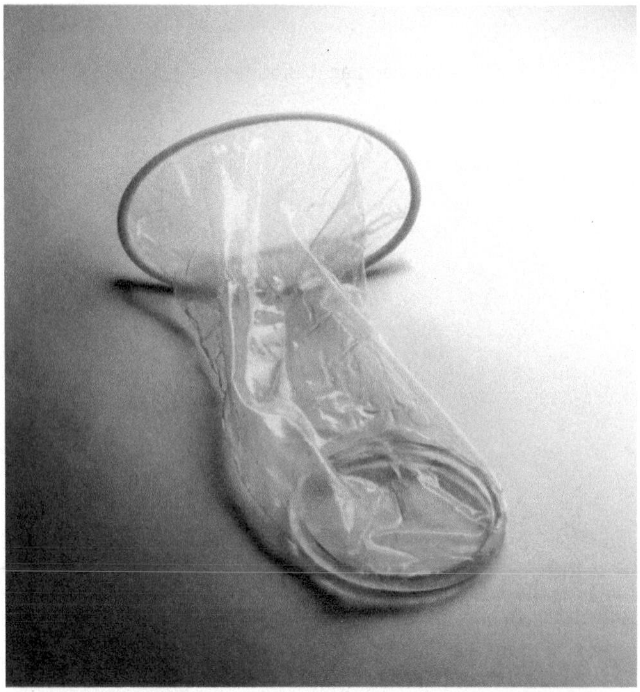

**Figure 13.15** A female condom. (From Beksinska M, Smit J, Joanis C et al. Female condom technology: new products and regulatory issues. *Contraception*. 2011;83[4]:316-321.)

## PERIODIC ABSTINENCE

Many motivated couples use abstinence from sexual intercourse or a barrier method during the days of the menstrual cycle when the ovum can be fertilized, or during the 5 days preceding ovulation or the day of ovulation. Because precisely identifying the timing of ovulation is difficult, several techniques of periodic abstinence have been utilized.

The oldest of these is the calendar rhythm method. With this method, the period of abstinence is determined by calculating the length of the individual woman's previous menstrual cycle and makes three assumptions: (1) the human ovum can be fertilized for only about 24 hours after ovulation, (2) sperm can fertilize for 3 to 5 days after coitus, and (3) ovulation usually occurs 12 to 16 days before the onset of menses. The woman therefore establishes her fertile period by subtracting 18 days from the length of her previous shortest cycle and 11 days from her previous longest cycle and abstains from coitus during this time.

Other periodic abstinence methods rely on cyclic physiologic changes. Increasing levels of progesterone occurring after ovulation cause a detectible rise in daily basal body temperature. The woman must abstain from intercourse from the cessation of menses until the third consecutive day of elevated basal temperature, or when she is postovulatory. The cervical mucus method requires that the woman recognize and interpret the presence and consistency of cervical mucus. Increasing estradiol levels increase the production of cervical mucus. Intercourse can occur after menses ends until the first day that copious, slippery mucus is observed to be present and again 4 days after the last day when the characteristic mucus was present.

The calendar, temperature, and cervical mucus methods can be used separately or in combination with one another, or the symptothermal method. Overall typical failure rates are around 24%. Women with irregular cycles should not use periodic abstinence methods, over the age of 35, or immediately following a pregnancy. Women using these methods should also have control over when intercourse occurs.

## COITUS-RELATED METHODS

### Spermicides

Spermicides consist of an active agent and a carrier. The carriers include gels, foams, creams, tablets, films, and suppositories. The active agent is a surfactant that immobilizes or kills sperm on contact by destroying the sperm cell membrane. Spermicides must be placed into the vagina before each coital act, often in combination with a barrier contraceptive to increase effectiveness. The contraceptive sponge, a cylindric piece of soft polyurethane impregnated with 1 mg of nonoxynol-9 spermicide, must be inserted into the vagina before intercourse and is effective for 24 hours. The failure rate ranges from 15% to 25%.

### Coitus Interruptus (Withdrawal)

Removal of the penis from the vagina prior to ejaculation to prevent pregnancy is an ancient male-controlled method of contraception without contraindications, devices, or cost. Withdrawal can fail because of the small numbers of sperm present in some preejaculate, the fluid produced by the penis during sexual excitement and before climax. More commonly, the method fails if withdrawal is not performed in a timely fashion. Correct and consistent use with every act of intercourse should be stressed, not only during suspected fertile times. A major drawback of the method is the lack of any protection against sexually transmitted infections. Failure rates range from 4% with perfect use to 22% with typical use.

## EMERGENCY CONTRACEPTION

Emergency contraception (EC) allows women to prevent pregnancy after an act of unprotected intercourse. Commonly misdescribed as the morning-after pill, EC can actually be used up to 120 hours after intercourse, depending on the method. Effectiveness of EC is greater the closer it is taken to the time of intercourse. Developed in the 1970s, the Yuzpe method uses various forms and doses of combined OCs that prevent pregnancy after intercourse by inhibiting ovulation. The Yuzpe method involves one dose of one to six OC tablets, depending on the brand, with a second dose 12 hours later (Table 13.4). This method reduces the pregnancy risk by about 75%. Since the 1990s, this method is used infrequently in the United States as new methods seem to have greater effectiveness.

**Table 13.4** Pills That Can Be Used for Emergency Contraception in the United States*

| Brand | Company | Pills per Dose† | Ethinyl Estradiol per Dose (μg) | Levonorgestrel per Dose (mg)‡ |
|---|---|---|---|---|
| **Antiprogestin Pills: Take One Pill** | | | | |
| Ella§ | Actavis | 1 white pill | 0 | 0 |
| **Progestin-Only Pills: Take One Dose†** | | | | |
| Plan B One-Step | Teva | 1 white pill | 0 | 1.5 |
| Generic one-dose pills (including My Way, Next Choice One Dose, Take Action, and AfterPill) | Various | 1 pill | 0 | 1.5 |
| **Combined Progestin and Estrogen Pills: Take Two Doses 12 Hours Apart** | | | | |
| Altavera | Sandoz | 4 peach pills | 120 | 0.60 |
| Amethia | Actavis | 4 white pills | 120 | 0.60 |
| Amethia Lo | Actavis | 5 white pills | 100 | 0.50 |
| Amethyst | Actavis | 6 white pills | 120 | 0.54 |
| Aviane | Teva | 5 orange pills | 100 | 0.50 |
| Camrese | Teva | 4 light blue-green pills | 120 | 0.60 |
| CamreseLo | Teva | 5 orange pills | 120 | 0.50 |
| Cryselle | Teva | 4 white pills | 120 | 0.60 |
| Enpresse | Teva | 4 orange pills | 120 | 0.50 |
| Introvale | Sandoz | 4 peach pills | 120 | 0.60 |
| Jolessa | Teva | 4 pink pills | 120 | 0.60 |
| Lessina | Teva | 5 pink pills | 100 | 0.50 |
| Levora | Actavis | 4 white pills | 120 | 0.60 |
| Lo/Ovral | Akrimax | 4 white pills | 120 | 0.60 |
| LoSeasonique | Teva | 5 orange pills | 100 | 0.50 |
| Low-Ogestrel | Actavis | 4 white pills | 120 | 0.60 |
| Lutera | Actavis | 5 white pills | 100 | 0.50 |
| Lybrel | Wyeth | 6 yellow pills | 120 | 0.54 |
| Nordette | Teva | 4 light-orange pills | 120 | 0.60 |
| Ogestrel | Actavis | 2 white pills | 100 | 0.50 |
| Portia | Teva | 4 pink pills | 120 | 0.60 |
| Quasense | Actavis | 4 white pills | 120 | 0.60 |
| Seasonale | Teva | 4 pink pills | 120 | 0.60 |
| Seasonique | Teva | 4 light-blue-green pills | 120 | 0.60 |
| Sronyx | Actavis | 5 white pills | 100 | 0.50 |
| Trivora | Actavis | 4 pink pills | 120 | 0.50 |

From Trussell J, Raymond EG, Cleland K. Emergency contraception: a last chance to prevent unintended pregnancy. 2015. Available at http://ec.princeton.edu/questions/ec-review.pdf.

*Ella, Plan B One–Step, Next Choice One Dose, My Way and Levonorgestrel Tablets are the only dedicated products specifically marketed for emergency contraception. The oral contraceptive pills listed above have been declared safe and effective for use as emergency contraceptive pills (ECPs) by the United States Food and Drug Administration. Plan B One-Step is available without age restrictions to women and men; Next Choice One Dose, My Way, and Levonorgestrel Tablets are available over the counter to women and men aged 17 and older. Ella is prescription–only regardless of age. Outside the United States, more than 100 emergency contraceptive products are specifically packaged, labeled, and marketed. Levonorgestrel-only ECPs are available either over the counter or from a pharmacist without having to see a clinician in 60 countries. For a worldwide directory of pills that can be used for emergency contraception, see http://ec.princeton.edu/worldwide/default.asp#country.

†The labels for Plan B One–Step, Next Choice One Dose, and My Way say to take the pill within 72 hours after unprotected intercourse. Research has shown that they are effective when used within 96 hours after unprotected sex. The label for Levonorgestrel Tablets says to take one pill within 72 hours after unprotected intercourse and another pill 12 hours later. Research has shown that that both pills can be taken at the same time with no decrease in efficacy or increase in side effects and that they are effective when used within 96 hours after unprotected sex.

‡The progestin in Cryselle, Lo/Ovral, Low–Ogestrel, and Ogestrel is norgestrel, which contains two isomers, only one of which (levonorgestrel) is bioactive; the amount of norgestrel in each tablet is twice the amount of levonorgestrel.

§Ella contains 30 mg ulipristal acetate.

Currently, most dedicated EC medications contain the progestin levonorgestrel. The most well known and most commonly used progestin EC is Plan B One Step (with generic forms Take Action, Next Choice One Dose, and My Way also available), a 1.5-mg levonorgestrel single dose pill or two 0.75-mg pills given 12 hours apart, both to be given within 72 hours from the time of unprotected sex. This method of EC is currently available over the counter. Plan B works by delaying or inhibiting ovulation. Because this effect is preovulatory, it is efficacious when taken during the periovulatory phase of the menstrual cycle. Effectiveness depends on the time in the cycle that it is taken. When comparing methods directly, the risk of pregnancy among women receiving the levonorgestrel only method is about half of that for women using the Yuzpe method (Raymond, 2004).

A newer type of EC is a 30-mg single dose of the selective progesterone receptor modulator ulipristal acetate (Ella). Ovulation is delayed for 5 days in women who take ulipristal acetate. Women can take it closer to the time of ovulation than other methods and still successfully delay ovulation, even after the LH surge has occurred. Thus, Ella has been approved for use up to 120 hours from the time of unprotected intercourse, and it is 42% more effective at preventing pregnancy than the levonorgestrel-only method (Glasier, 2010).

The copper IUD is the most effective form of EC. Insertion up to 5 days after unprotected intercourse is 99% effective at preventing pregnancy. When appropriate, another benefit is the fulfillment of a woman's long-term contraceptive needs. Studies evaluating Mirena placement for use as EC are under way, but currently there is insufficient evidence to recommend its use for this purpose.

Current controversies include initiation of long-term contraception at the time of EC use and EC's effectiveness in heavier women. Some data indicate that EC may be less effective when used in conjunction with long-term hormonal contraceptive methods and that it may be less effective in heavier women (Glasier, 2011). These questions are active areas of research interest. Importantly for both questions, the copper IUD is highly effective as long-term contraception even when used as EC, and its effectiveness does not depend on weight.

## INDUCED ABORTION

Induced abortion is one of the most common gynecologic operations performed in the United States and in many other countries. As determined by the landmark *Roe v. Wade* Supreme Court decision, the state may not interfere with the practice of abortion in the first trimester. In the second trimester, individual states may regulate abortion services in the interest of preserving the health of the woman.

From a public health perspective, safe and legal abortion services are a cornerstone of maternal health care. Worldwide, illegal abortion is one of the leading causes of maternal death. Despite impressive gains in contraceptive safety and use, unintended pregnancy remains a major health and social problem in the United States (see Contraception Overview, presented earlier in the chapter). Although we can and should work to reduce the number of unintended pregnancies, contraceptive failures inevitably occur, and access to safe and legal abortion services remains a keystone of reproductive health. Some abortions are performed for pregnancies that are initially intended, but abortion becomes the only recourse for maternal indications or abnormal fetal screens.

In the United States, half of pregnancies are unintended, and about 4 in 10 of these end in elective abortion (Finer, 2014). U.S. abortion rates have declined gradually since 1980 but are higher than in Western European countries. In 2011, 1.06 million abortions occurred, a 13% decline since 2008 (Fig. 13.16). By the age of 45, at least half of U.S. women will experience an unintended pregnancy, and 1 in 10 women will have an abortion by age 20, 1 in 4 by age 30, and 3 in 10 by age 45 (Jones, 2011).

Ninety percent of abortions are performed within the first 12 weeks of pregnancy, and the distribution of abortions within the first 12 weeks is becoming earlier. In September 2000, the U.S. Food and Drug Administration approved the abortion drug mifepristone to be marketed in the United States as an alternative to surgical abortion. By 2011, medication abortion accounted for 23% of all nonhospital abortions and for 36% of abortions prior to 9 weeks' gestation (Jones, 2014).

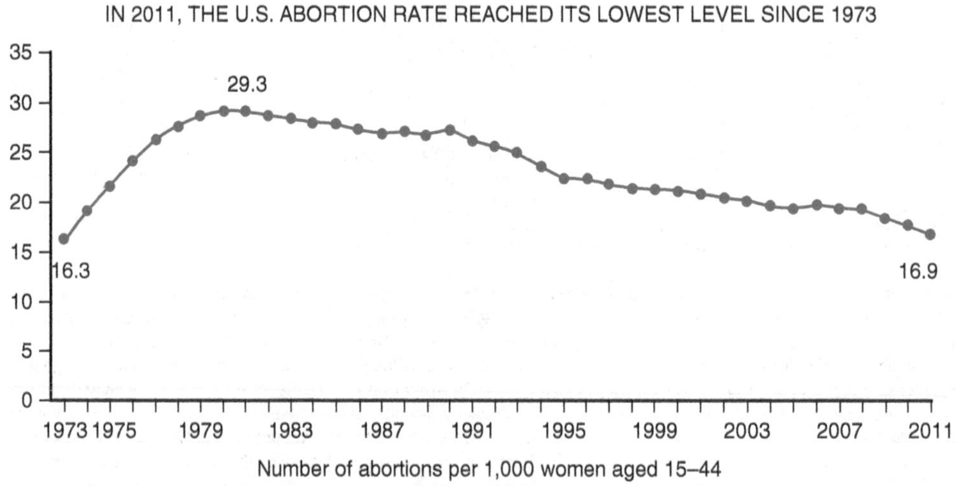


**Figure 13.16** Trends in abortion. (From Guttmacher Institute, Induced abortion in the United States, Fact Sheet, New York: Guttmacher Institute, 2014, http://www.guttmacher.org/pubs/fb_induced_abortion.html)

## METHODS OF ABORTION

### Curettage Methods

Curettage by vacuum aspiration is the predominant method of performing abortion in the first trimester. Early pregnancy aspiration can be performed with a small, flexible, plastic cannula connected to an aspiration syringe. This technique, called **manual vacuum aspiration** (MVA), can be performed up to a gestational age of 10 weeks and sometimes later. Dilation of the cervix is often required as well as some type of anesthesia, either local or with IV sedation. After 10 weeks, the uterus may be more efficiently evacuated with an electric vacuum aspiration system (EVA). In earlier gestations, randomized trials have shown similar efficacy and patient satisfaction with MVA and EVA.

Following any vacuum aspiration, good practice is to examine the tissue to determine that the gestational sac, placenta, and any fetal parts have been removed. MVA produces less disruption of small gestational sacs and may facilitate their identification. If products of conception can't be visualized, a sonogram can identify retained tissue. In the case of very early pregnancy, it can be difficult to identify a gestational sac. Serial hCG evaluation or repeat ultrasound in 1 week can ensure that pregnancy termination has occurred. If inspection reveals no gestational sac, retained products or uterine perforation should also be ruled out. The MVA technique is also a low-cost and highly efficient technique to manage miscarriage in an office setting, including incomplete or missed abortion.

Dilation and evacuation (D&E) is the surgical technique used to perform abortion beyond the first trimester. Among mid-trimester abortions performed in the United States, more than 90% are D&Es. Because a greater amount of cervical dilation is usually needed, cervical preparation with osmotic dilators may be necessary for several hours or sometimes an additional day before the procedure. The most commonly used dilators are small tents of dried and sterilized seaweed, ***Laminaria japonica***. By gently opening the cervix over several hours, the osmotic dilators substantially reduce the risk of uterine trauma, such as perforation and cervical injury. *Laminaria* can be used in concert with a single dose of mifepristone to reduce the number of *laminaria* placed without affecting dilation (Shaw, 2015). Another strategy for cervical preparation is the administration of misoprostol, a prostaglandin and $E_1$ analogue, in a dosage of 400 μg given vaginally, or buccally a few hours before vacuum aspiration or D&E. Misoprostol softens the cervix and can reduce the amount of dilation needed.

### Medical Abortion

#### First-Trimester Medication Abortion

Mifepristone, or Mifeprex, once known as RU-486, has weak progestational activity but a marked affinity for progesterone receptors in the endometrium. A competitive inhibitor of the progesterone receptor, it prevents progesterone from binding to its receptors. When mifepristone is combined with a prostaglandin up to 72 hours later, more than 95% of early pregnancies terminate. When used alone, it is only effective for two out of three pregnancies. The favorable properties of misoprostol (low cost, orally active, highly effective) have led to its widespread adoption as the preferred prostaglandin for medical abortion at all gestational ages. The FDA approved a regimen of 600 mg mifepristone followed 48 hours later by 400 μg oral misoprostol for elective termination of pregnancies of 49 days or less gestational age based on a the large multicenter trial of Spitz and associates which showed a 92% efficacy (Spitz, 1998).

Subsequent studies have evaluated lower loses of mifepristone, alternative routes of ingesting misoprostol, and alternative intervals between mifepristone and misoprostol. At this point in time, the Society of Family Planning has recommended a regimen of 200 mg of mifepristone taken by mouth, followed by 800 mg of misoprostol taken intravaginally or buccally 24 to 72 hours later at home and cite this as effective for up to 63 days gestational age (SFP, 2014). This "evidence-based" protocol reduces the cost of medical abortion, as only one 200-mg tablet of mifepristone is used and one office visit is avoided. Additional studies indicated that mifepristone remains effective to at least 70 days gestation (Winikoff, 2012).

Typical duration of bleeding after a medication abortion is 7 to 14 days. On rare occasions, prolonged bleeding can lead to the need for emergency curettage or even blood transfusion.

#### Second-Trimester Abortion

Nonsurgical midtrimester abortion through induction of uterine contractions is most commonly performed with the administration of prostaglandins vaginally, usually at a dose of 400 mg intravaginally every 6 hours. This regimen appears to be safe in women with a prior cesarean delivery, as uterine rupture is uncommon. Some advantages of a medical induction of labor over D&E include the avoidance of surgery and the chance to view or hold the fetus if desired. If no provider is available skilled in D&E, labor induction may be the only option available to a woman. Disadvantages include a longer inpatient hospitalization with a higher risk of retained products of conception and with a 30% chance of requiring further intervention for retained products, such as a D&C.

#### Ancillary Techniques

In the United States, many protocols for both medical and surgical abortion make use of ultrasound to verify gestational age and to confirm that the pregnancy is intrauterine and not ectopic. If a gestational sac is not identified, a serum quantitative β-hCG is helpful in correlation with ultrasound findings. In the first trimester, sonography is useful to determine gestational age when a substantial discrepancy occurs between the menstrual history and clinical examination; when uterine abnormalities, such as leiomyomata, are present; or when the presence of an ectopic gestation is suspected. Sonography can help to avoid inaccurate estimation of gestational age before initiating second-trimester abortions. Performing ultrasonography during a D&E may facilitate the procedure.

### Complications

Elective abortion in the United States is a very safe operation. Complications are rare, and the overall mortality is less than 1 per 100,000 procedures. Two important determinants of complications are the gestational age and method of abortion chosen. Beyond 10 weeks, abortion complication rates increase progressively with gestational age. The earlier the abortion is performed, the safer the procedure is. Therefore, access to abortion is vital to maternal safety. Legislation that delays care such as mandated waiting periods only increase the risk of complications. Induced abortion is substantially safer than the continuation of pregnancy to term. Suction curettage is the safest surgical method of abortion, followed by D&E, induction of labor, and major operations such as hysterotomy or hysterectomy.

The most common complication of surgical abortion is infection (about 1% of cases). The routine use of perioperative antibiotic prophylaxis reduces this risk. Rare complications (<1/1000 cases) include hemorrhage, the consequences of uterine perforation, and anesthetic hazards.

## KEY POINTS

- Half of all pregnancies in the United States are unintended, and among women who experience unintended pregnancy, more than half are not using contraception.
- By the age of 45, at least half of U.S. women will experience an unintended pregnancy, and one in three will have had an abortion.
- Failure rates in the first year of contraceptive use are highest for coitus-related methods (e.g., withdrawal, periodic abstinence, condoms, barrier methods) followed by combined contraceptives (pill, patch, ring) and the progestin injection. The IUD, implants, and sterilization have typical use failure rates of less than 1%, similar to that of sterilization.
- The copper IUD can increase bleeding with menses, whereas the LNG-IUS is likely to decrease bleeding with menses or lead to amenorrhea. The primary mechanism of action for the LNG-IUS is thickening of the cervical mucus.
- The contraceptive implant has an effectiveness that is equal to or superior to that of sterilization and IUDs. It inhibits ovulation and may cause irregular bleeding patterns.
- The DMPA injection completely inhibits ovulation and is likely to cause amenorrhea. Return to fertility after cessation of use can be delayed, and some DMPA users may experience weight gain.
- Combined hormonal contraceptives increase a woman's risk of VTE by about threefold to about 1/1000 per year. Women with multiple risk factors for VTE or cardiovascular disease (e.g., obesity, age >35, smoking, a personal or family history of clotting disorder) should use effective birth control methods without estrogen.
- The most effective method of emergency contraception is the copper IUD, followed by a single dose of oral ulipristal acetate (Ella). Plan B, or an oral dose of levonorgestrel, is somewhat less effective.
- First- and second-trimester medical and surgical abortion is safe and effective. Overall, abortions have a lower complication risk than carrying a pregnancy to term. Access to legal and safe abortion is a cornerstone of maternal health.

## REFERENCES


American College of Obstetricians and Gynecologists (ACOG). Committee on Gynecologic Practice; Long-Acting Reversible Contraception Working Group: ACOG Committee Opinion no. 450: increasing use of contraceptive implants and intrauterine devices to reduce unintended pregnancy. *Obstet Gynecol.* 2009;114:1434–1438.

Appleby P, Beral V, Berrington de González A, Colin D, Franceschi S, Goodhill A, et al. Cervical cancer and hormonal contraceptives: collaborative reanalysis of individual data for 16,573 women withcervical cancer and 35,509 women without cervical cancer from 24 epidemiological studies. *Lancet.* 2007;370(9599):1609–1621.

Beasley A, White K, Cremers S, Westhoff C. Randomized clinical trial of self versus clinical administration of subcutaneous depot medroxyprogesterone acetate. *Contraception.* 2014;89(5):352–356.

Branum A, Jones J. Trends in long-acting reversible contraception use among U.S. women aged 15–44. *NCHS Data Brief.* 2015;(188):1–8.

Centers for Disease Control and Prevention (CDC). *United States medical eligibility criteria (US MEC) for contraceptive use*, 2010. Available at http://www.cdc.gov/reproductivehealth/unintendedpregnancy/usmec.htm. Accessed July 31, 2015.

Chan L, Westhoff C. Tubal sterilization trends in the United States. *Fertil Steril.* 2010;94(1):1–6.

Chen B, Reeves M, Hayes J, Hohmann H, Perriera L, Creinin M. Postplacental or delayed insertion of the levonorgestrel intrauterine device after vaginal delivery: a randomized controlled trial. *Obstet Gynecol.* 2010;116(5):1079–1087.

Daniels K, Daugherty J, Jones J. Current contraceptive status among women aged 15-44: United States, 2011-2013. *NCHS Data Brief.* 2014;(173):1–8.

Dinger J, Minh T, Buttmann N, Bardenheuer K. Effectiveness of oral contraceptive pills in a large U.S. cohort comparing progestogen and regimen. *Obstet Gynecol.* 2011;117(1):33–40.

Dragoman M, Petrie K, Torgal A, Thomas T, Cremers S, Westhoff C. Contraceptive vaginal ring effectiveness is maintained during 6 weeks of use: a prospective study of normal BMI and obese women. *Contraception.* 2013;87(4):432–436.

Farley T, Rosenberg M, Rowe P. Intrauterine devices and pelvic inflammatory disease: an international perspective. *Lancet.* 1992;339:785.

Faúndes D, Bahamondes L, Faúndes A, Petta C, Díaz J, Marchi N. No relationship between IUD position evaluated by ultrasound and complaints of bleeding and pain. *Contraception.* 1997;56(1):43–47.

Fernandez E, La Vecchia C, Balducci A, Chatenoud L, Franceschi S, Negri E. Oral contraceptives and colorectal cancer risk: a meta-analysis. *Br J Cancer.* 2001;84(5):722.

Finer LB, Zolna MR. Shifts in intended and unintended pregnancies in the United States, 2001–2008. *Am J Public Health.* 2014;104(Suppl 1):S43–S48.

Gallo M, Lopez L, Grimes D, Carayon F, Schulz K, Helmerhorst F. Combination contraceptives: effects on weight. *Cochrane Database Syst Rev.* 2014;1. CD003987.

Gariepy A, Creinin M, Smith K, Xu X. Probability of pregnancy after sterilization: a comparison of hysteroscopic versus laparoscopic sterilization. *Contraception.* 2014;90(2):174–181.

Gerstman BB, Piper JM, Tomita DK, Ferguson WJ, Stadel BV, Lundin FE. Oral contraceptive estrogen dose and the risk of deep venous thromboembolic disease. *Am J Epidemiol.* 1991;133(1):32–37.

Glasier A, Cameron S, Blithe D, Scherrer B, Mathe H, Levy D, et al. Can we identify women at risk of pregnancy despite using emergency contraception? Data from randomized trials of ulipristal acetate and levonorgestrel. *Contraception.* 2011;84(4):363–367.

Glasier A, Cameron S, Fine P, Logan S, Casale W, Van Horn J, et al. Ulipristal acetate versus levonorgestrel for emergency contraception: a randomised non-inferiority trial and meta-analysis. *Lancet.* 2010;375(9714):555–562.

Grimbizis G, Tarlatzis B. The use of hormonal contraception and its protective role against endometrial and ovarian cancer. *Best Pract Res Clin Obstet Gynaecol.* 2010;24(1):29–38.

Grimes D, Schulz K. Prophylactic antibiotics for intrauterine device insertion: a metaanalysis of the randomized controlled trials. *Contraception.* 1999;60(2):57–63.

Harrison M, DiNapoli M, Westhoff C. Reducing postoperative pain after tubal ligation with rings or clips: a systematic review and meta-analysis. *Obstet Gynecol.* 2014;124(1):68–75.

Hatcher R, Trussell J, Nelson AL, Cates Jr W, et al., eds. *Contraceptive technology.* 20th revised edition. New York: Ardent Media; 2011.

Heinemann K, Reed S, Moehner S, Minh T. Risk of uterine perforation with levonorgestrel-releasing and copper intrauterine devices in the European Active Surveillance Study on Intrauterine Devices. *Contraception.* 2015;91(4):274–279.

Hillis S, Marchbanks P, Tylor L, Peterson H. Poststerilization regret: findings from the United States Collaborative Review of Sterilization. *Obstet Gynecol.* 1999;93(6):889–895.

Jones R, Jerman J. Abortion incidence and service availability in the United States.

Shaw R, Settatree R, Templeton A, Filshie G, Argent V. *Male and Female Sterilization. Evidence Based Guidelines* No. 4 In. London: Royal College of Obstetricians and Gynaecologists; 1999.

Shaw K, Shaw J, Hugin M, Velasquez G, Hopkins F, Blumenthal P. Adjunct mifepristone for cervical preparation prior to dilation and evacuation: a randomized trial. *Contraception.* 2015;91(4):313–319.

Smith JS, Green J, Berrington de Gonzalez A, Appleby P, Peto J, Plummer M, et al. Cervical cancer and use of hormonal contraceptives: a systematic review. *Lancet.* 2003;361(9364):1159–1167.

Society of Family Planning (SFP). Medical management of first-trimester abortion. *Contraception.* 2014;89(3):148–161.

Spitz IM, Bardin CW, Benton L, Robbins A. Early pregnancy termination with mifepristone and misoprostol in the United States. *N Engl J Med.* 1998;338(18):1241–1247.

Westhoff C. Higher body weight does not affect NuvaRing's efficacy. *Obstet Gynecol.* 2005;105(4):56S.

Westhoff C, Heartwell S, Edwards S, Zieman M, Cushman L, Robilotto C, et al. Initiation of oral contraceptives using a quick start compared with a conventional start: a randomized controlled trial. *Obstet Gynecol.* 2007;109(6):1270–1276.

White K, Teal S, Potter J. Contraception after delivery and short interpregnancy intervals among women in the United States. *Obstet Gynecol.* 2015;125(6):1471–1477.

Winikoff B, Dzuba I, Chong E, Goldberg A, Lichtenberg E, Ball C, et al. Extending outpatient medical abortion services through 70 days of gestational age. *Obstet Gynecol.* 2012;120(5):1070–1076.

World Health Organization (WHO). *Medical eligibility criteria for contraceptive use.* 4th ed. Geneva, Switzerland: WHO, 2010; 2009. Available at. http://whqlibdoc.who.int/publications/2010/9789241563888_eng.pdf?ua=1. Accessed July 31, 2015.

Zieman M, Guillebaud J, Weisberg E, Shangold GA, Fisher AC, Creasy GW. Contraceptive efficacy and cycle control with the Ortho Evra/Evra transdermal system: the analysis of pooled data. *Fertil Steril.* 2002;77(2 Suppl 2):S13–S18.

Suggested Readings can be found on ExpertConsult.com.

# 14

# Menopause and Care of the Mature Woman

## Endocrinology, Consequences of Estrogen Deficiency, Effects of Hormone Therapy, and Other Treatment Options

*Roger A. Lobo*

**Menopause** is defined by the last menstrual period. Because cessation of menses is variable and many of the symptoms thought to be related to menopause may occur prior to cessation of menses, there is seldom a precise timing of this event. Other terms used are *perimenopause,* which refers to a variable time beginning a few years before and continuing after the event of menopause, and **climacteric**, which merely refers to the time after the cessation of reproductive function. Although the terms *menopausal* and *postmenopausal* are used interchangeably, the former term is less correct because *menopausal* should only relate to the time around the cessation of menses. As life expectancy increases beyond the eighth decade worldwide, particularly in developed countries, an increasing proportion of the female population is postmenopausal. With the average age of menopause being at 51 years, more than a third of a woman's life is now spent after menopause. Here, symptoms and signs of estrogen deficiency merge with issues encountered with natural aging. As the world population increases and a larger proportion of this population is made up of individuals older than 50, medical care specifically directed at postmenopausal women becomes an important aspect of modem medicine. In the United States, the number of women entering menopause is expected to double in the 30 years between 1990 and 2020, and the total number of postmenopausal women is expected to be in range of 60 million (Table 14.1).

Age of menopause, which is a genetically programmed event, is subject to some variability. The age of menopause in Western countries (between 51 and 52 years) is thought to correlate with general health status; socioeconomic status is associated with an earlier age of menopause. Higher parity, on the other hand, has been found to be associated with a later menopause. Smoking has consistently been found to be associated with menopause onset taking place 1 to 2 years earlier. Hysterectomy has also been cited as resulting in an earlier menopause (Siddle, 1987), presumably because of a diminution in the blood supply to the ovary; however, the data have not been consistent. Although body mass has been thought to be related to age of menopause (greater body mass index [BMI] with later menopause), the data have not been consistent. However, physical or athletic activity has not been found to influence the age of menopause. There also appear to be ethnic differences in the onset of menopause. In the United States, black and Hispanic women have been found to have menopause approximately 2 years earlier than white women. Although parity is generally greater around the world than in the United States, the age of menopause appears to be somewhat earlier outside the United States. Malay women have menopause at approximately age 45, Thai women at age 49.5, and Filipina women between ages 47 and 48; menopause has also been reported to occur in the mid to late 40s among Indian women. Countries at higher altitude (Himalayas or Andes) have been shown to have menopause 1 to 1.5 years earlier. Because the average age of menopause in the United States is 51 to 53 years, menopause prior to age 40 is considered premature. Conversely, by age 58, 97% of women will have gone through menopause. The primary determinate of age of menopause is genetic. Based on family studies, de Bruin and colleagues[2] showed that heritability for age of menopause averaged 0.87, suggesting that genetics explains up to 87% of the variance in menopausal age. Although other estimates have not been this high, genetic programming remains extremely important.

Other than specific gene mutations that have been shown to cause **premature ovarian failure or insufficiency** (explained later in this chapter), no specific genes have been implicated to account for this genetic influence. However, several genes are likely to be involved in determining the age of menopause, and these involve immune function and DNA repair (Stolk, 2012) and may also include genes coding telomerase activity, which affects aging in general.

**Table 14.1** U.S. Population Entering the Postmenopausal Years, Ages 55 through 64

| Year | Population |
|---|---|
| 1990 | 10.8 million |
| 2000 | 12.1 million |
| 2010 | 17.1 million |
| 2020 | 19.3 million |

Modified from U.S. Bureau of the Census. *Current Population Reports: Projections of the Population of the United States 1977 to 2050.* Washington, DC: U.S. Government Printing Office; 1993.

## PREMATURE OVARIAN FAILURE AND INSUFFICIENCY

Premature ovarian failure (POF) or premature ovarian insufficiency (POI), which is the more recently used term, is defined as hypergonadotropic ovarian failure occurring prior to age 40. POI occurs in 5% to 10% of women who are evaluated for amenorrhea, thus the incidence varies according to the prevalence of amenorrhea in various populations. Estimates of the overall prevalence of POI in the general population range between 0.3% and 0.9% of women. Throughout life, there is an ongoing rate of atresia of oocytes. Because this process is accelerated with various forms of gonadal dysgenesis because of defective X chromosomes, one possible cause of POI is an increased rate of atresia that has yet to be explained. A decreased germ cell endowment or an increased rate of germ cell destruction can also explain POI. Nevertheless, about 1000 (of the original 2 million), primarily follicles, may remain. Although most of these oocytes are likely to be functionally deficient, occasionally spontaneous pregnancies occur in young women in the first few years after the diagnosis of POI. There are several possible etiologies of POI (Box 14.1).

Defects in the X chromosome may result in various types of gonadal dysgenesis with varied times of expression of ovarian failure. Even patients with classical gonadal dysgenesis (e.g., 45,XO) may undergo a normal puberty, and occasionally a pregnancy may ensue as a result of genetic mosaicism. Very small defects in the X chromosome may be sufficient to cause POI. Familial forms of POI may be related to either autosomal-dominant or sex-linked modes of inheritance. Mutations in the gene encoding the follicle-stimulating hormone (FSH) receptor (e.g., mutation in exon 7 in the gene on chromosome 2p) have been described, but these are extremely rare outside of the Finnish population, in which these mutations were originally described. An expansion of a trinucleotide repeat sequence in the first exon on the FMR1 gene (Xq 27.3) leads to fragile X syndrome, a major cause of developmental disabilities in males.

The permutation in fragile X syndrome has been shown to be associated with POI. Type 1 blepharophimosis/ptosis/epicanthus inversus (BPES) syndrome, an autosomal dominant disorder caused by mutations in the forkhead transcription factor FOXL2, includes POI. Triple X syndrome has also been associated with POI. It has been suggested that functional mutations of antimüllerian hormone (AMH) may also be associated with POI (Alvaro, 2015).

Dystrophic myotonia has also been linked to POI, although the mechanism underlying this relationship is unclear. Under the category of enzymatic defects, galactosemia is a major cause of POI that is related to the toxic buildup of galactose in women who are unable to metabolize the sugar. Even in women with fairly well-controlled galactose-free diets, POI tends to occur. Another enzymatic defect linked to POI is 17α-hydroxylase deficiency. This rare condition manifests differently from the other causes discussed here because the defect in the production of sex steroids leads to sexual infantilism and hypertension.

The degree to which autoimmunity may be responsible for POI is unclear but has been suggested to be associated in 17.5% of cases. Virtually all autoimmune disorders have been found to be associated with POI, including autoimmune polyendocrinopathies such as autoimmune polyendocrinopathy/candidiasis/ectodermal dystrophy (APECED), which is caused by mutations in the autoimmune (AIRE) gene on band 21 q22. The presence of the thymus gland appears to be required for normal ovarian function as POI has been associated with hypoplasia of the thymus. In patients who have undergone ovarian biopsy as part of their evaluation, lymphocytic infiltration surrounding follicles has been described, as well as resumption of menses after immunosuppression. Immunoassays utilizing antibodies directed at ovarian antigens have been developed and have demonstrated positive findings in some patients with POI, although the relevance of these findings remains unsettled. Ovarian autoantibodies could also conceivably be a secondary phenomenon to a primary cell-mediated form of immunity. Specific enzymes such as 3β-hydroxysteroid dehydrogenase (3βHSD) may also be the target of ovarian autoimmunity. Approximately 2% to 4% of women with autoimmunity for POI will have antiadrenal antibodies as well (Chen, 1996). This can be screened for by an assay for 21-hydroxlase antibodies. Adrenal function can practically be assessed by measuring dehydroepiandrosterone sulfate (DHEA-S) levels as well, which are higher in younger women than in menopausal women, unless the adrenal gland is affected. It may also be helpful to assess ovarian volume and follicular presence by vaginal ultrasound in these women as well. The ovaries in younger women with POI are more normal in size and have follicles present as compared with the smaller atrophic ovary in menopause.

From a practical standpoint, screening for the common autoimmune disorders is appropriate in women found to have POI. More from a theoretic standpoint, however, are abnormalities in the structure of gonadotropins, in their receptors, or in receptor binding, which could be associated with POI; these measurements are difficult. Although abnormal urinary forms of gonadotropins have been reported in women with POI, these data have not been replicated. Abnormalities of FSH receptor binding, as mediated by a serum inhibitor, have been described. A genetic defect that may lead to alterations in FSH receptor structure was mentioned previously.

Under the category of ovarian insults, POI may be induced by ionizing radiation, chemotherapy, or overly aggressive ovarian surgery. Although not well documented, viral infections have been suggested to play a role, particularly mumps. A dose of 400 to 500 rads is known to cause ovarian failure 50% of the time, and older women are more vulnerable to experiencing permanent failure. A dose of approximately 800 rads is associated with failure in all women. Ovarian failure (transient or permanent) may be induced by chemotherapeutic agents, although younger women receiving this insult have a better prognosis. Alkalizing agents, particularly cyclophosphamide, appear to be most toxic. By exclusion, the majority of women are considered to have idiopathic

**Box 14.1 Possible Causes of Premature Ovarian Failure**

Genetic
Enzymatic
Immune
Gonadotropin defects
Ovarian insults
Idiopathic

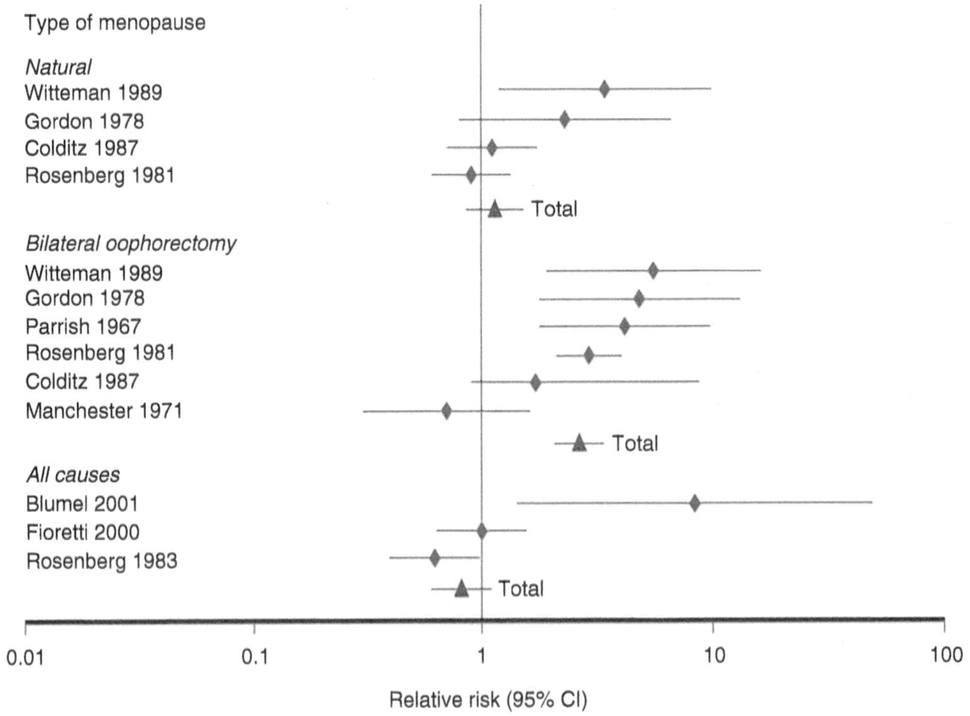


**Figure 14.1** Effect of type of "early" menopause on cardiovascular disease. Data taken from a meta-analysis. (From Atsma F, Bartelink ML, Grobbee DE, et al. Postmenopausal status and early menopause as independent risk factors for cardiovascular disease: a meta-analysis. *Menopause.* 2006;13[2]:265-279.)

POI because no demonstrable cause can be pinpointed. Among these women, small mutations in genes lying on the X chromosome or yet to be identified autosomal genes may be the cause.

## MANAGEMENT OF PREMATURE OVARIAN INSUFFICIENCY

Evaluation of POI in women younger than 30 should include screening for autoimmune disorders and a karyotype; detailed recommendations for screening of such women are available (Rebar, 2000). In addition, vaginal ultrasound may be useful for assessing the size of the ovaries and the degree of follicular development, which, if present, may signify an immunologic defect. Cases of POI caused by immunologic defects must be screened carefully for thyroid, adrenal, and other autoimmune disorders.

Treatment of all cases usually consists of estrogen replacement. Although in menopausal therapy clinicians have steered away from the term *replacement* therapy, in this specific instance of POI, estrogen treatment is truly *replacement* therapy. If fertility is a concern, the most efficacious treatment is oocyte donation. Various attempts at ovarian stimulation are usually unsuccessful; sporadic pregnancies that may occur (~5%) are just as likely to occur spontaneously as with any intervention, and often while on physiologic E2 replacement. In this setting it has been our preference not to use oral contraceptive pills for replacement in women wishing to conceive. In a long-term follow-up of a large number of women diagnosed with POI, within a year, there was spontaneous ovarian function observed in 24% of the women and over time the rate of spontaneous pregnancies was 4.4% (Bidet, 2011).

Why estrogen replacement in these young women with POI is extremely important and is not analogous to hormone therapy (HT) after menopause, is that these young women are at substantial long-term risk for osteoporosis and cardiovascular disease (CVD). Coronary heart disease and death are specifically increased in approximately 70% of women with POI; but not stroke, according to one study (Roeters van Lennep, 2014). A more extreme example of this phenomenon is with premature oophorectomy, with which the risk of CVD is many-fold increased (Fig. 14.1) (Atsma, 2006). Women with POI should be offered estrogen replacement, with some form of progestogen in women with a uterus, at least up to the natural age of menopause.

# MENOPAUSAL TRANSITION (PERIMENOPAUSE)

A workshop was convened in 2001 to build consensus on describing various stages of the menopausal transition. A more recent follow-up conference, the Study of Reproductive Aging Workshop (STRAW+10), had more streamlined bleeding criteria for the various stages and expanded the stages including the use of biochemical markers such as inhibin B and AMH in addition to FSH (Harlow, 2012) (Fig. 14.2). This scheme is important from a descriptive standpoint for the physiology behind the normal menopausal transition and is useful for characterization of women in various stages in research studies.

The ovary changes markedly from birth to the onset of menopause (Fig. 14.3). The greatest number of primordial follicles is

Menarche (at stage −5) · FMP (0) (between stages −1 and +1a)

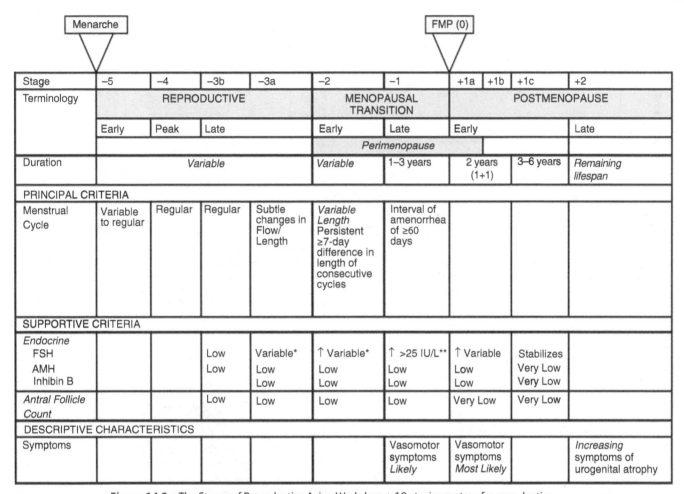

| Stage | −5 | −4 | −3b | −3a | −2 | −1 | +1a | +1b | +1c | +2 |
|---|---|---|---|---|---|---|---|---|---|---|
| Terminology | REPRODUCTIVE | | | | MENOPAUSAL TRANSITION | | POSTMENOPAUSE | | | |
| | Early | Peak | Late | | Early | Late | Early | | | Late |
| | | | | | *Perimenopause* | | | | | |
| Duration | *Variable* | | | | *Variable* | 1–3 years | 2 years (1+1) | | 3–6 years | *Remaining lifespan* |
| **PRINCIPAL CRITERIA** | | | | | | | | | | |
| Menstrual Cycle | Variable to regular | Regular | Regular | Subtle changes in Flow/ Length | *Variable Length* Persistent ≥7-day difference in length of consecutive cycles | Interval of amenorrhea of ≥60 days | | | | |
| **SUPPORTIVE CRITERIA** | | | | | | | | | | |
| *Endocrine* | | | | | | | | | | |
| FSH | | | Low | Variable* | ↑ Variable* | ↑ >25 IU/L** | ↑ Variable | | Stabilizes | |
| AMH | | | Low | Low | Low | Low | Low | | Very Low | |
| Inhibin B | | | | Low | Low | Low | Low | | Very Low | |
| *Antral Follicle Count* | | | Low | Low | Low | Low | Very Low | | Very Low | |
| **DESCRIPTIVE CHARACTERISTICS** | | | | | | | | | | |
| Symptoms | | | | | | Vasomotor symptoms *Likely* | Vasomotor symptoms *Most Likely* | | | *Increasing* symptoms of urogenital atrophy |

**Figure 14.2** The Stages of Reproductive Aging Workshop + 10 staging system for reproductive aging in women. (From Harlow SD, Gass M, Hall JE, et al. Executive summary of the stages of reproductive aging workshop + 10: addressing the unfinished agenda of staging reproductive aging. *J Clin Endocrinol Metab.* 2012;97[4]:1159-1168.)

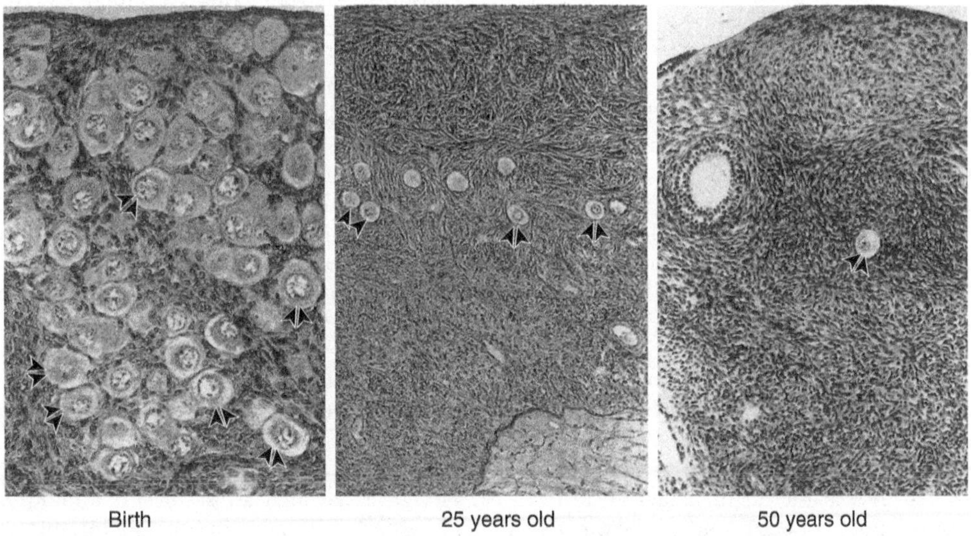


**Figure 14.3** Photomicrographs of the cortex of human ovaries from birth to 50 years of age. Small nongrowing primordial follicles *(arrowheads)* have a single layer of squamous granulosa cells. (Modified from Erickson GF. An analysis of follicle development and ovum maturation. *Semin Reprod Endocrinol.* 1986;3:233.)

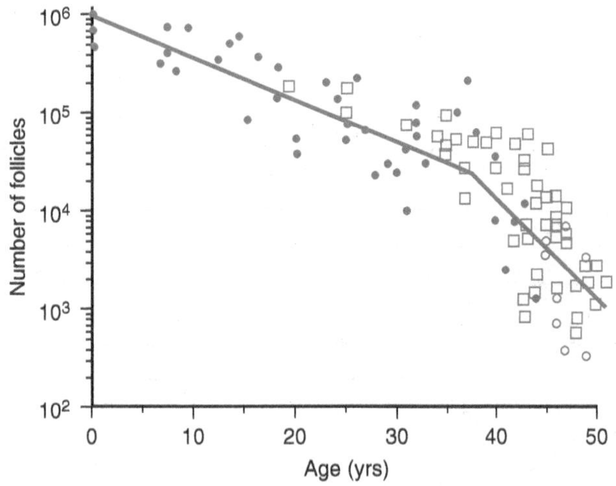


**Figure 14.4** The age-related decrease in the total number of primordial follicles (PFs) within both human ovaries from birth to menopause. As a result of recruitment (initiation of PF growth), the number of PFs decreases progressively from about 1 million at birth to 25,000 at 37 years. At 37 years, the rate of recruitment increases sharply, and the number of PFs declines to 1000 at menopause (about 51 years of age). (Modified from Faddy MJ, Gosden RJ, Gougeon A, et al. Accelerated disappearance of ovarian follicles in mid-life: Implications for forecasting menopause. *Hum Reprod.* 1992;7:1342.)

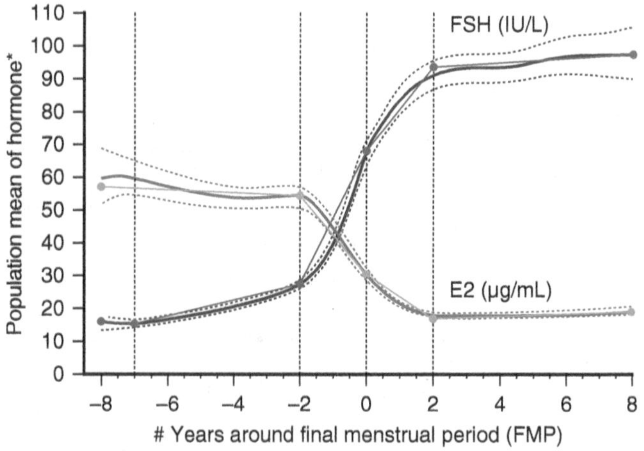


**Figure 14.5** Adjusted population means (95% CI) for segmented mean profiles for follicle-stimulating hormone and estradiol across the final menstrual period in the Study of Women's Health Across the Nation (N = 1215). (From Randolph JF Jr, Zheng H, Sowers MR, et al. Change in follicle-stimulating hormone and estradiol across the menopausal transition: effect of age at the final menstrual period. *J Clin Endocrinol Metab.* 2011;96[3]: 746-754.)

present in utero at 20 weeks' gestation and undergoes a regular rate of atresia until around the age of 37. After this time, the decline in primordial follicles appears to become more rapid between age 38 and menopause (Fig. 14.4), when no more than 1000 follicles remain. These remaining follicles are primarily atretic in nature.

These changes are reflected in circulating levels of AMH, which decline rapidly with ovarian aging (see Chapter 42). When levels of serum AMH become undetectable, menopause is likely to occur in 4 to 5 years.

## TYPES OF OVARIAN CHANGES DURING PERIMENOPAUSE

Although perimenopausal changes are generally thought to be endocrine in nature and result in menstrual changes, a marked diminution of reproductive capacity precedes this period by several years. This decline may be referred to as *gametogenic ovarian failure* and is reflected by decreased antimüllerian hormone (AMH), inhibin B levels, and antral follicle counts, and a rising FSH (Chapter 42). The concept of dissociation in ovarian function is appropriate. These changes may occur with normal menstrual function and no obvious endocrine deficiency; however, they may occur in some women as early as age 35 (10 or more years before endocrine deficiency ensues). Although subtle changes in endocrine and menstrual function can occur for up to 3 years before menopause, it has been shown that the major reduction in ovarian estrogen production does not occur until approximately a year before menopause (Fig. 14.5) (Randolph, 2011). There is also a slow decline in androgen status (i.e., androstenedione and testosterone), which cannot be adequately detected at the time of perimenopause. The decline in androgen is largely a phenomenon of aging. Products of the granulosa cell are most important for the feedback control of FSH. As the functional capacity of the follicular units decreases, the secretion of substances that suppress FSH also decreases. A marker of this is inhibin B, in which levels are lower in the early follicular phase in women in their late 30s (Fig. 14.6). Inhibin B is seldom measured clinically; rather AMH (which also reflects granulosa cell function) is most frequently assessed as noted previously. Indeed, FSH levels are higher throughout the cycle in older ovulatory women than in younger women (Fig. 14.7). The functional capacity of the ovary is also diminished as women enter into perimenopause. With gonadotropin stimulation, although estradiol ($E_2$) levels are not very different between younger and older women, total inhibin production by granulosa cells is decreased in women older than 35. From a clinical perspective, subtle increases in FSH on day 3 of the cycle, or increases in the clomiphene challenge test, correlate with decreased ovarian responses to stimulation and decreased fecundability. Müllerian inhibiting substance (MIS) or AMH serves as the most practical marker of reproductive aging. Levels decrease throughout life, being undetectable at menopause, and show less variability during the menstrual cycle compared with other markers such as FSH. However, values are lower by up to 20% in women on oral contraceptives, and this should be taken into account when assessing levels in younger women. When values reach an undetectable range (<0.05 ng/mL), menopause has been found to occur within 5 years as stated previously (Fig. 14.8).

Although there is a general decline in oocyte number with age, an accelerated atresia occurs around age 37 or 38 (see Fig. 14.4). Although the reason for this acceleration is not clear, one possible theory relates to activin secretion. Because granulosa cell-derived activin is important for stimulating FSH receptor expression, the rise in FSH levels could result in more activin production, which in turn enhances FSH action.

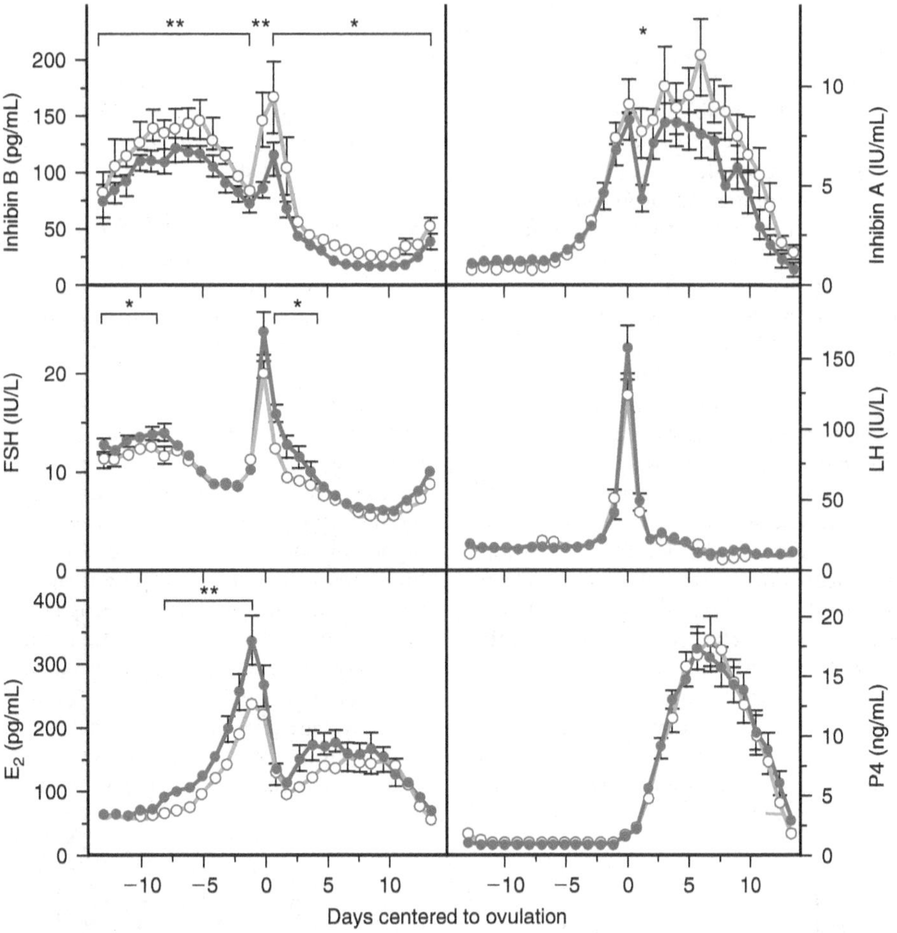


**Figure 14.6** An inhibin B, follicle-stimulating hormone (FSH), estradiol ($E_2$), inhibin A, and progesterone ($P_4$) levels in cycling women 20 to 34 years old (^) and 35 to 46 years old (•). Hormone levels are depicted as centered to the day of ovulation (*, $P < .04$; **, $P < .02$) when comparing the two age groups. (From Welt CK, McNicholl DJ, Taylor AE, et al. Female reproductive aging is marked by decreased secretion of dimeric inhibin. *J Clin Endocrinol Metab.* 1999;84[1]:105.)

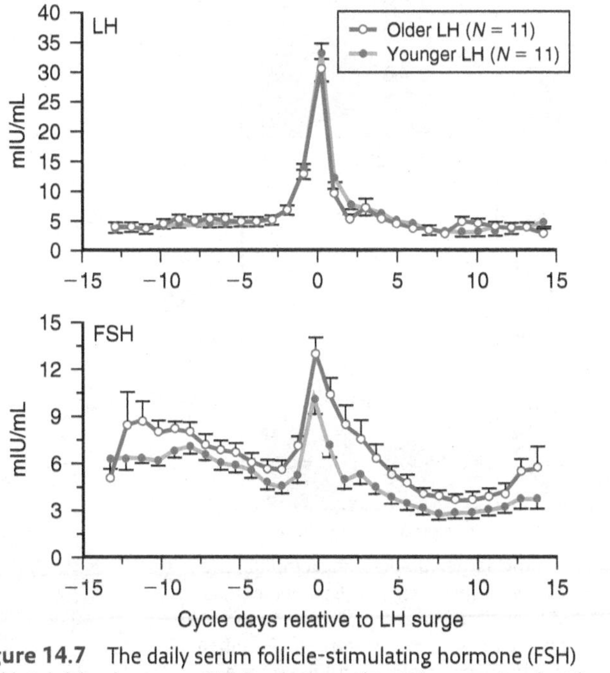


**Figure 14.7** The daily serum follicle-stimulating hormone (FSH) and luteinizing hormone (LH) levels throughout the menstrual cycle of 11 women in each group (mean ± SE). The gonadotropin secretion pattern in normal women of advanced reproductive age in relation to the monotropic FSH rise. (Modified from Klein NA, Battaglia DE, Clifton DK, et al. The gonadotropin secretion pattern in normal women of advanced reproductive age in relation to the monotropic FSH rise. *J Soc Gynecol Investig.* 1996;3:27.)

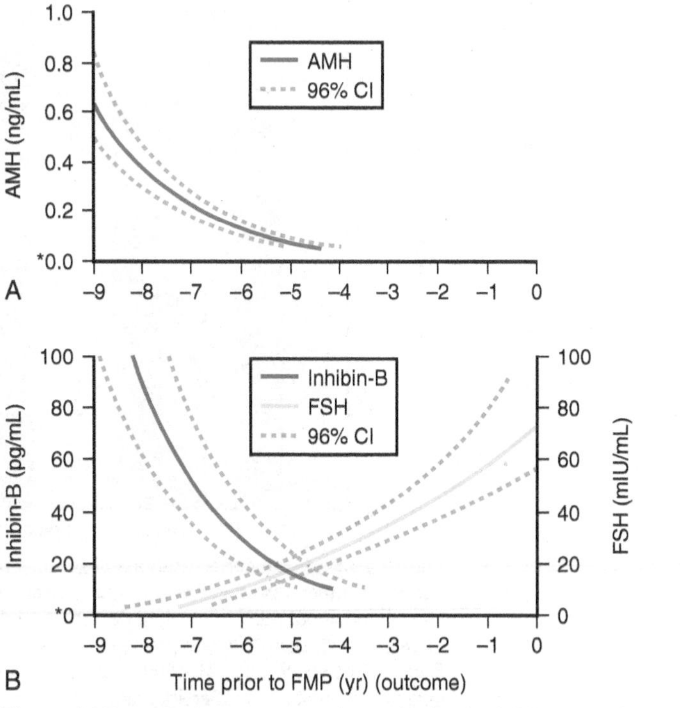


**Figure 14.8** AMH decreases to undetectable levels (0.05 ng/mL) 5 years before the final menstrual period, **A**; and inhibin B (10 pg/mL) does so 4 years before the last menstrual period, **B**. (From Sowers MR. Eyvazzadeth AD, McConnell D, et al. Antimüllerian hormone and inhibin in the definition of ovarian aging and the menopause transition. *J Clin Endocrinol Metab.* 2008;93[9]:L34768-L34783, 2008.)

A profile of elevated activin with lower inhibin B has been found in older women (Fig. 14.9). This autocrine action of activin, involving enhanced FSH action, might be expected to lead to accelerated growth and differentiation of granulosa cells. Furthermore, activin has been shown to increase the size of the pool of preantral follicles in the rat. At the same time, these follicles become more atretic. Clinical treatment of perimenopausal women should address three general areas of concern: (1) irregular bleeding, (2) symptoms of early menopause, such as **hot flushes**, and (3) the inability to conceive. Treatment of irregular bleeding is complicated by the fluctuating hormonal status. Estrogen levels may be higher than normal in the early follicular phase and progesterone secretion may be normal, or slightly decreased, although not all cycles are ovulatory. For these reasons, short-term use of an oral contraceptive (usually 20 μg ethinyl estradiol) may be an option for otherwise healthy women who do not smoke to help them cope with irregular bleeding. Early symptoms of menopause, particularly vasomotor changes, may occur as the result of fluctuating hormonal levels. In this setting, an oral contraceptive again may be an option if symptoms warrant therapy. Alternatively, lower doses of estrogen used alone may be another option. Reproductive concerns often require more aggressive treatment because of decreased cycle fecundity. Once day 3 FSH levels increase (>15 mIU/mL) and AMH levels decrease (≤0.4 ng/mL), the prognosis for pregnancy is markedly reduced.

### *Hormonal Changes with Established Menopause*

Figure 14.10 depicts the typical hormonal levels of postmenopausal women compared with those of ovulatory women in the early follicular phase. The most significant findings are the marked reductions in $E_2$ and estrone ($E_1$). Serum $E_2$ is reduced to a greater extent than $E_1$. Serum $E_1$, on the other hand, is produced primarily by peripheral aromatization from androgens, which decline principally as a function of age. Levels of $E_2$ average 15 pg/mL and range from 10 to 25 pg/mL but are closer to 10 pg/mL or less in women who have undergone oophorectomy. Serum $E_1$ values average 30 pg/mL but may be higher in obese women because aromatization increases as a function of the mass of adipose tissue. Estrone sulfate ($E_1$ S) is an estrogen conjugate that serves as a stable circulating reservoir of estrogen, and levels of $E_1$ S are the highest among estrogens in postmenopausal women. In premenopausal women, values are usually above 1000 pg/mL; in postmenopausal women, levels average 350 pg/mL. Apart from elevations in FSH and luteinizing hormone (LH), other pituitary hormones are not affected. The rise in FSH, beginning in stage −2 as early as age

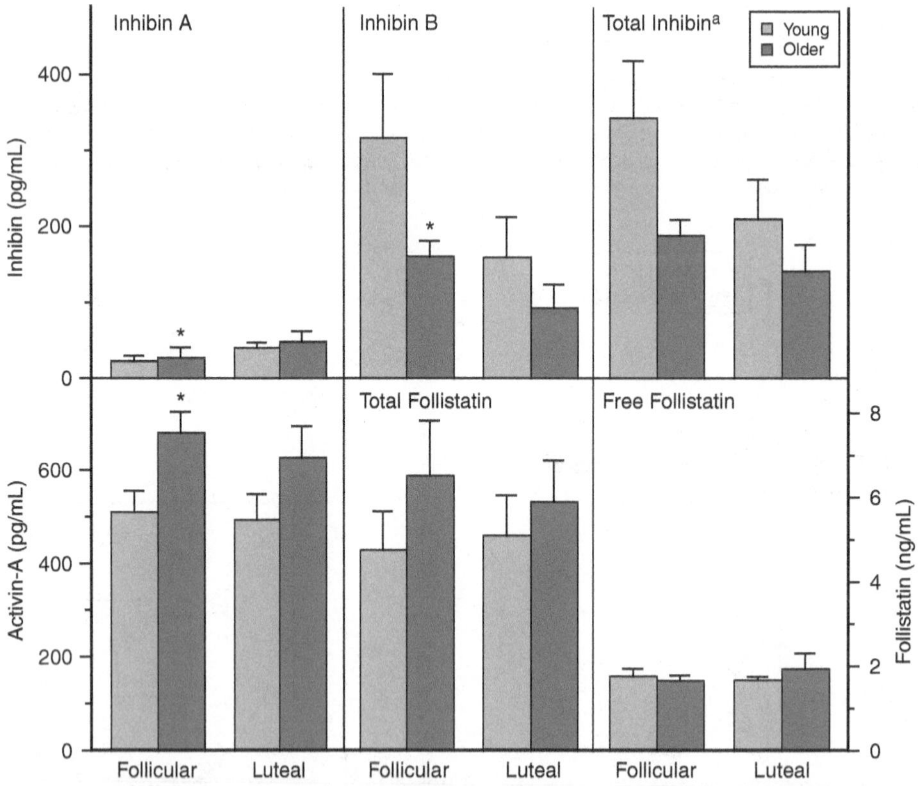


**Figure 14.9** Mean concentrations of gonadal proteins from the same subjects. Total inhibin is a derived number from the sum of inhibin A and inhibin B. *Group differences; $P < .05$. Net increase in stimulatory input resulting from a decrease in inhibin B and an increase in activin A may contribute in part to the rise in follicular phase follicle-stimulating hormone of aging cyclic women. (Modified from Reame NE, Wyman TL, Phillips DJ, et al. Net increase in stimulatory input resulting from a decrease in inhibin B and an increase in activin A may contribute in part to the rise in follicular phase follicle-stimulating hormone of aging cyclic women. *J Clin Endocrinol Metab.* 1998;83:3302.)

38 (see Fig. 14.2), fluctuates considerably until approximately 4 years after menopause (stage + 1c), when values are consistently greater than 20 mIU/mL. Specifically, growth hormone (GH), thyroid-stimulating hormone (TSH), and adrenocorticotropic hormone (ACTH) levels are normal. Serum prolactin levels may be slightly decreased because prolactin levels are influenced by estrogen status. Both the postmenopausal ovary and the adrenal gland continue to produce androgen. The ovary continues to produce androstenedione and testosterone but not $E_2$, and this production has been shown to be at least partially dependent on LH. Androstenedione and testosterone levels are lower in women who have experienced bilateral oophorectomy, with values averaging 0.8 ng/mL and 0.1 ng/mL, respectively. The adrenal gland also continues to produce androstenedione, dehydroepiandrosterone (DHEA), and dehydroepiandrosterone sulfate (DHEA-S); primarily as a function of aging, these values decrease somewhat (adrenopause), although cortisol secretion remains unaffected. Most "ovarian" testosterone production may actually arise from the adrenal by way of precursors (Couzinet, 2001). Most likely, the adrenal supplies precursor substrate (DHEA and androstenedione) for ovarian testosterone production. Although DHEA-S levels decrease with age (approximately 2% per year), data have suggested that levels transiently rise in perimenopause before the continuous decline thereafter (Fig. 14.11). This interesting finding from the Study of Women Across the Nation (SWAN) also suggested that DHEA-S levels are highest in Chinese women and lowest in African-American women.

Testosterone levels also decline as a function of age, which is best demonstrated by the reduction in 24-hour means levels (Fig. 14.12). Because of the role of the adrenal in determining levels of testosterone after menopause, adrenalectomy or dexamethasone treatment results in undetectable levels of serum testosterone. Compared with total testosterone, the measurement of bioavailable, or "free," testosterone is more useful in postmenopausal women. After menopause, sex hormone-binding globulin (SHBG) levels decrease, resulting in relatively higher levels of bioavailable testosterone or a higher free androgen index (Fig. 14.13). In women receiving oral estrogen, bioavailable testosterone levels are extremely low because SHBG levels are increased. How this relates to the decision to consider androgen therapy in postmenopausal women will be discussed later in this chapter.

Elevated gonadotropin (FSH/LH) levels arise from reduced secretion of $E_2$ and inhibin as described earlier. Although some aging effects of the brain are likely to exist, there is abundant human evidence for menopause in women to be an ovarian-induced event.

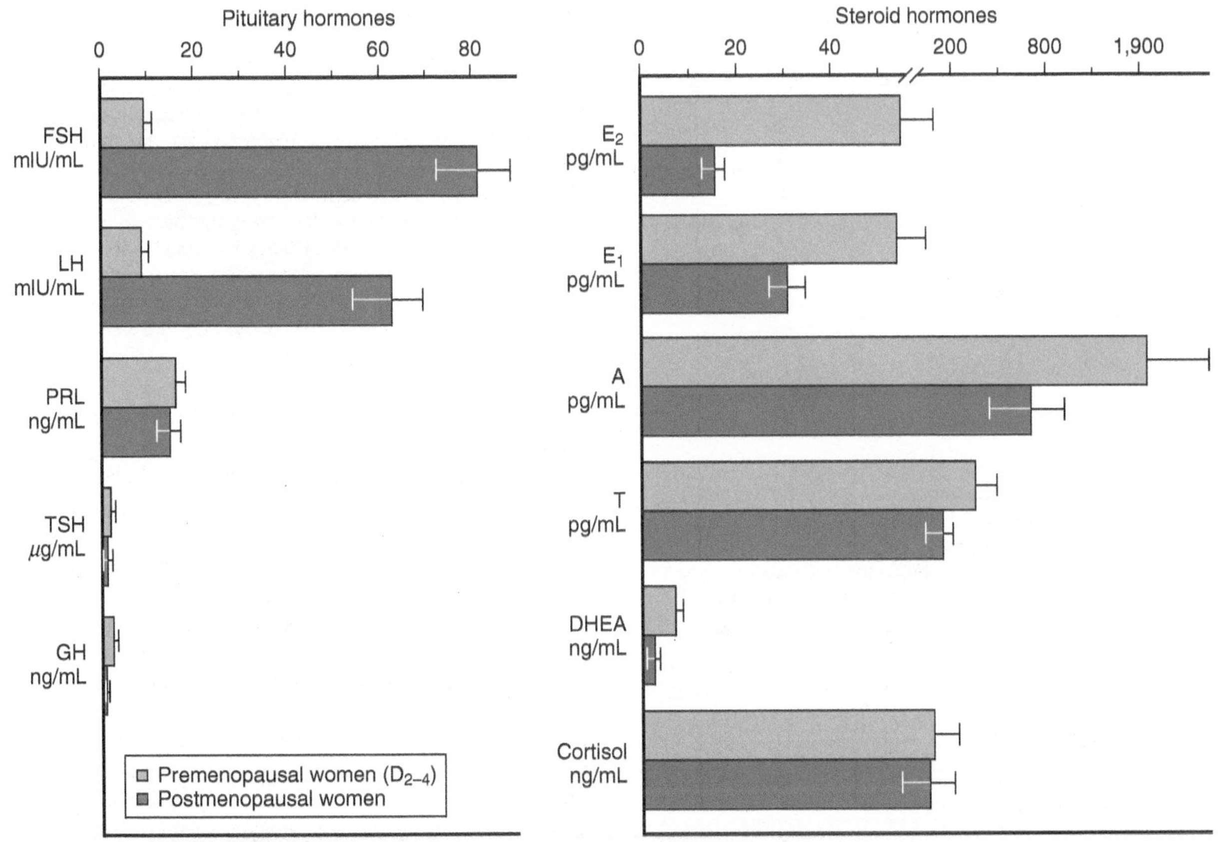


**Figure 14.10** Circulating levels of pituitary and steroid hormones in postmenopausal women compared with levels in premenopausal women studied during the first week (days 2 to 4 [$D_{2-4}$] of the menstrual cycle. *A*, Androstenedione; *DHEA*, dehydroepiandrosterone; *$E_1$*, estrogen; *$E_2$*, estradiol; *FSH*, follicle-stimulating hormone; *GH*, growth hormone; *LH*, luteinizing hormone; *PRL*, prolactin; *T*, testosterone; *TSH*, thyroid-stimulating hormone. (Modified from Yen SSC. The biology of menopause. *J Reprod Med*. 1977;18:287.)

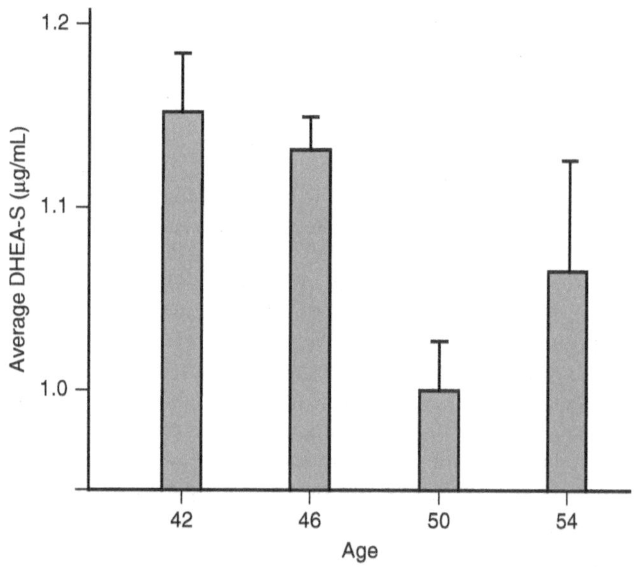


**Figure 14.11** Mean (±SE) circulating dehydroepiandrosterone sulfate (DHEA-S) at each year of age of the entire study population before and after adjustment for age, current smoking, menopausal status, log body mass index (BMI), ethnicity, site, and the interaction between ethnicity and log BMI. (Modified from Lasley BL, Santoro N, Randolf JF, et al. The relationship of circulating dehydroepiandrosterone, testosterone, and estradiol to stages of the menopausal transition and ethnicity. *J Clin Endocrinol Metab.* 2002;87: 3760-3767.)

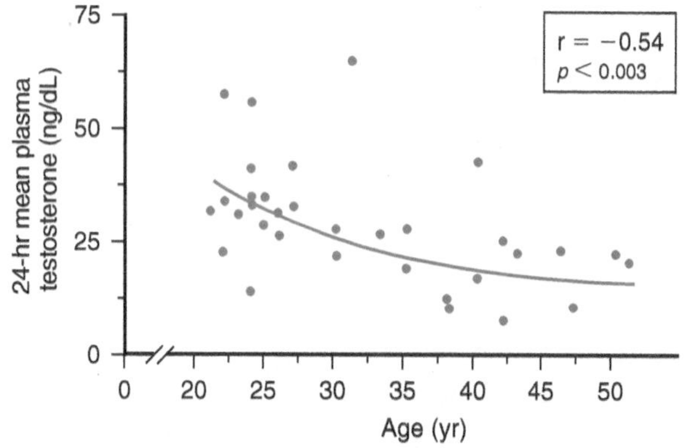


**Figure 14.12** The 24-hour mean plasma total testosterone (T) level compared with age in normal women. The regression equation was T (nmol/L) = 37.8 × age (years) − 1.12(*r* = −0.54; *P* < .003). (Modified from Zumoff B, Strain GW, Miller LK, et al. Twenty-four hour mean plasma testosterone concentration declines with age in normal premenopausal women. *J Clin Endocrinol Metab.* 1995;80:1429.)

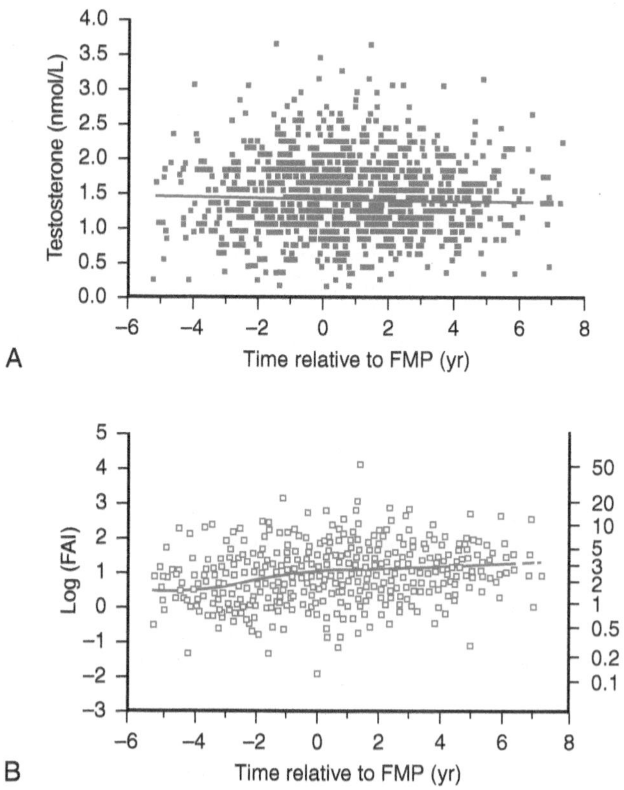


**Figure 14.13** **A,** Linear regression model: observed testosterone (T) and fitted levels of mean T across the menopausal transition. **B,** Double logistic model: observed free androgen index (FAI) and fitted levels of mean FAI across the menopausal transition. The left and right axes show FAI levels on the log and antilog scales, respectively. The horizontal axis represents time (years) with respect to first menstrual period (FMP); negative (positive) numbers indicate time before (after) FMP. (From Burger HG, Dudley EC, Cui J, et al. A prospective longitudinal study of serum testosterone, dehydroepiandrosterone sulfate, and sex hormone-binding globulin levels through the menopause transition. *J Clin Endocrinol Metab.* 2000;85:2832.)

## EFFECTS OF MENOPAUSE ON VARIOUS ORGAN SYSTEMS

### CENTRAL NERVOUS SYSTEM

The brain is an active site for estrogen action as well as estrogen formation. Estrogen activity in the brain is mediated via estrogen receptor (ER) α and ER β. Whether or not a novel membrane receptor (non-ER α/ER β) exists is still being debated. However, both genomic and nongenomic mechanisms of estrogen action clearly exist in the brain. Figure 14.14 illustrates the predominance of ER β in the cortex (frontal and parietal) and the cerebellum, based on work in the rat. Although 17β $E_2$ is a specific ligand for both receptors, certain synthetic estrogens (e.g., diethylstilbestrol) have greater affinity for ER α, whereas phytoestrogens have a greater affinity for ER β.

There are multiple actions of estrogen on the brain as reviewed by Henderson (Box 14.2), thus some important functions linked to estrogen contribute to well-being in general and, more specifically, to cognition and mood. The hallmark feature of declining estrogen status in the brain is the hot flush, which is more generically referred to as a *vasomotor episode.* The hot flash usually refers to the acute sensation of heat, and the flush or vasomotor episode includes changes in the early perception of this event and other skin changes (including diaphoresis).

Hot flushes usually occur for 2 years after the onset of estrogen deficiency but can persist for 10 or more years. Prospective data suggest that the average time for persistence of bothersome hot flushes is 7.4 years, (Avis, 2014) and up to 42% of women aged 60 to 65 years have bothersome symptoms. In 10% to 15% of women, these symptoms are severe and disabling. In the United States the incidence of these episodes varies in different ethnic groups.

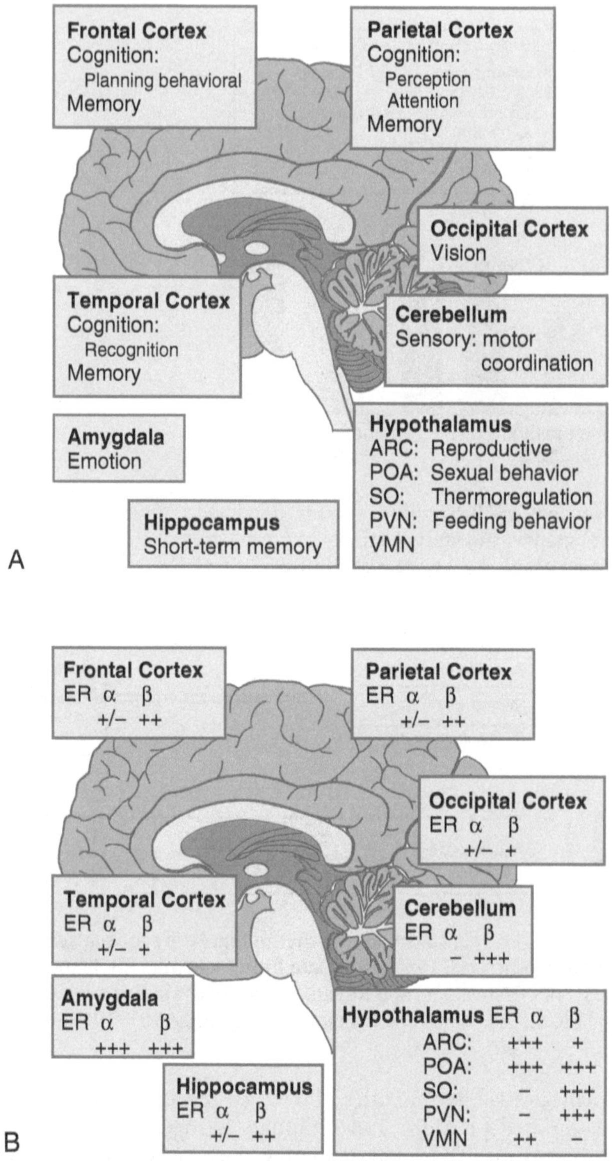


**Figure 14.14** **A,** Each region of the brain has an important role in specific brain functions. Optimal brain activity is maintained by means of the integration of different areas by neural tracts. *ARC,* Arcuate nucleus; *POA,* preoptic area; *PVN,* paraventricular nucleus; *SO,* supraoptic nucleus; *VMN,* ventromedial nucleus. **B,** Distribution of estrogen receptors ER α and ER β mRNA in the rat brain. (**B,** Adapted from Cela V, Naftolin F. Clinical effects of sex steroids on the brain. From Lobo RA [ed]. *The Treatment of the Post-menopausal Woman: Basic and Clinical Aspects.* 2nd ed. Philadelphia: Lippincott Williams & Wilkins; 1999:247-262.)

Symptoms are greatest in Hispanic and black women, intermediate in white women, and lowest among Asian women (Fig. 14.15). The severity and persistence of hot flushes for 10 or more years may cause a series of "irregular" symptoms, such as irritability, which may affect quality of life (Oldervave, 1993) (Fig. 14.16). The fall in estrogen levels precipitate the vasomotor symptoms. It has been found that some women who experience hot flushes have a thermoregulatory disruption with a much narrower temperature range between sweating and shivering. Freedman has shown that the difference in temperature at which shivering occurs, and when sweating occurs, termed the *thermoneutral zone,* is wide in asymptomatic women (Freedman, 2007). This zone is substantially more narrowed in symptomatic women, explaining their vulnerability to vasomotor symptoms (Fig. 14.17).

**Box 14.2 Effects of Estrogen on Brain Function**

**Organizational Actions**
Effects on neuronal number, morphology, and connections occurring during critical stages of development

**Neurotrophic Actions**
Neuronal differentiation
Neurite extension
Synapse formation
Interactions with neurotrophins

**Neuroprotective Actions**
Protection against apoptosis
Antioxidant properties
Anti-inflammatory properties
Augmentation of cerebral blood flow
Enhancement of glucose transport into the brain
Blunting of corticosteroid response to behavioral stress
Interactions with neurotrophins

**Effects on Neurotransmitters**
Acetylcholine
Noradrenaline
Serotonin
Dopamine
Glutamate
Gamma aminobutyric acid
Neuropeptides

**Effects on Glial Cells**

**Effects on Proteins Involved in Alzheimer Disease**
Amyloid precursor protein
Tau protein
Apolipoprotein E

Modified from Henderson VW. Estrogen, cognition, and a woman's risk of Alzheimer's disease. *Am J Med.* 1997;103(Suppl 3A):11.

Although the proximate cause of the flush remains elusive, the episodes result from a hypothalamic response (probably mediated by catecholamines) to the change in estrogen status. The flush has been well characterized physiologically. It results in heat dissipation as witnessed by an increase in peripheral temperature (fingers, toes); a decrease in skin resistance, associated with diaphoresis; and a reduction in core body temperature (Fig. 14.18). There are hormonal correlates of flush activity, such as an increase in serum LH and in plasma levels of pro-opiomelanocortin peptides (ACTH, β-endorphin) at the time of the flush, but these occurrences are thought to be epiphenomena that result as a consequence of the flush and are not related to its cause. One of the primary complaints of women with hot flushes is sleep disruption. They may awaken several times during the night and require a change of bedding and clothes because of diaphoresis. Nocturnal sleep disruption in postmenopausal women with hot flushes has been well documented by electroencephalographic (EEG) recordings. Sleep efficiency is lower, and the latency to rapid eye movement (REM) sleep is longer in women with hot flushes compared with asymptomatic women. This disturbed sleep often

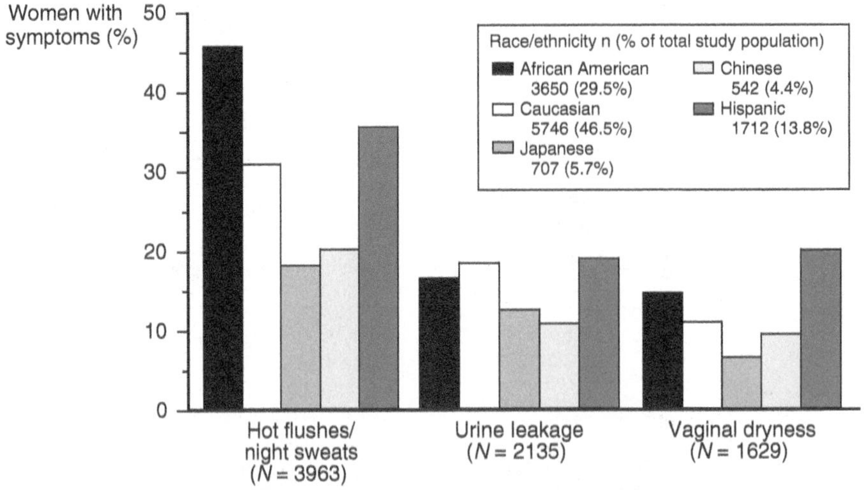


**Figure 14.15** A Study of Women's Health Across the Nation (SWAN). Symptom severity. (Modified from Gold EB, Sternfeld B, Kelsey JL, et al. Relation of demographic and lifestyle factors to symptoms in a multi-racial/ethnic population of women 40 to 55 years of age. *Am J Epidemiol.* 2000;152:463.)

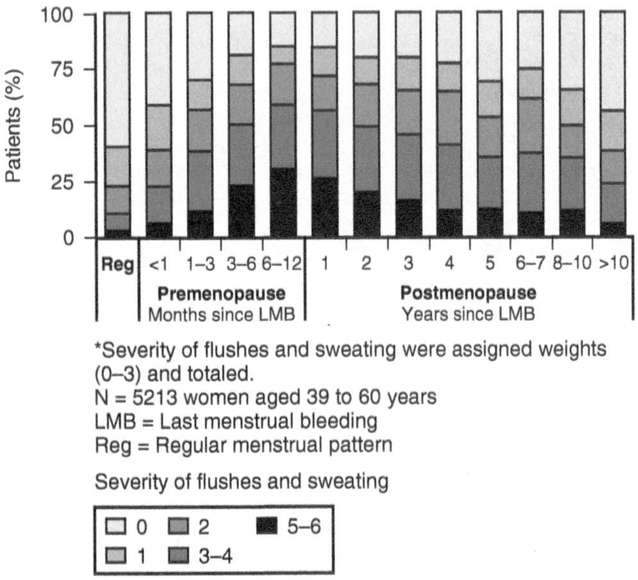


**Figure 14.16** Impact of menopause on well-being. (Modified from Oldenhave A, Jaszmann LJ, Haspels AA, et al. Impact of climacteric on well-being: a study based on 5213 women 39 to 60 years old. *Am J Obstet Gynecol.* 1993;168:772.)

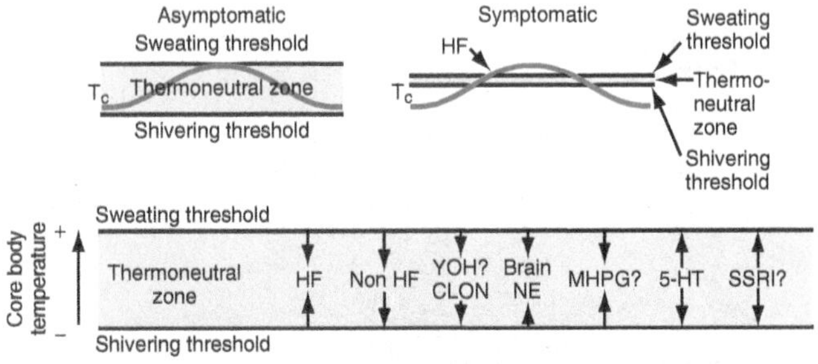


**Figure 14.17** Narrowing of the thermoregulatory zone in symptomatic women. *HF,* Hot flush. (Data from Freedman RR: Menopausal hot flashes. In: Lobo RA, ed. *Treatment of the Postmenopausal Woman.* 4th ed. New York: Academic Press; 2007:187-198.)

leads to fatigue and irritability during the day. The frequency of awakenings and hot flushes is reduced appreciably with estrogen treatment (Fig. 14.19). Sleep may be disrupted even if the woman is not conscious of being awakened from sleep. In this setting, EEG monitoring has indicated sleep disruption in concert with physiologic measures of vasomotor episodes.

In postmenopausal women, estrogen has been found to improve depressed mood regardless of whether or not this is a specific complaint (critics of some of this work point out that mood is affected by the symptomatology and by sleep deprivation). Blinded studies carried out in asymptomatic women have also shown benefit. In an estrogen-deficient state such as occurs after menopause, a higher incidence of depression (clinical or subclinical) is often manifest. However, menopause per se does not cause depression, and although estrogen does generally improve depressive mood, it should not be used for psychiatric disorders. Nevertheless, very high pharmacologic doses of estrogen have been used to treat certain types of psychiatric depression in the past. Progestogens as a class generally attenuate the beneficial effects of estrogen on mood, although this effect is highly variable.

Cognitive decline in postmenopausal women is related to aging as well as to estrogen deficiency. The literature is somewhat mixed about whether there are benefits of estrogen in terms of cognition. In more recent studies, verbal memory appears to be enhanced with estrogen and has been found to correlate with acute changes in brain imaging, signifying brain activation. Dementia increases as women age, and the most common form of dementia is Alzheimer disease (AD). Box 14.2 lists several neurotropic and neuroprotective factors related to how estrogen deficiency may be expected to result in the loss of protection against the development of AD. In addition, estrogen has a positive role in enhancing neurotransmitter function, which is deficient in women with AD. This function of estrogen has particular importance and relevance for the cholinergic system that is affected in AD. Estrogen use after menopause appears to

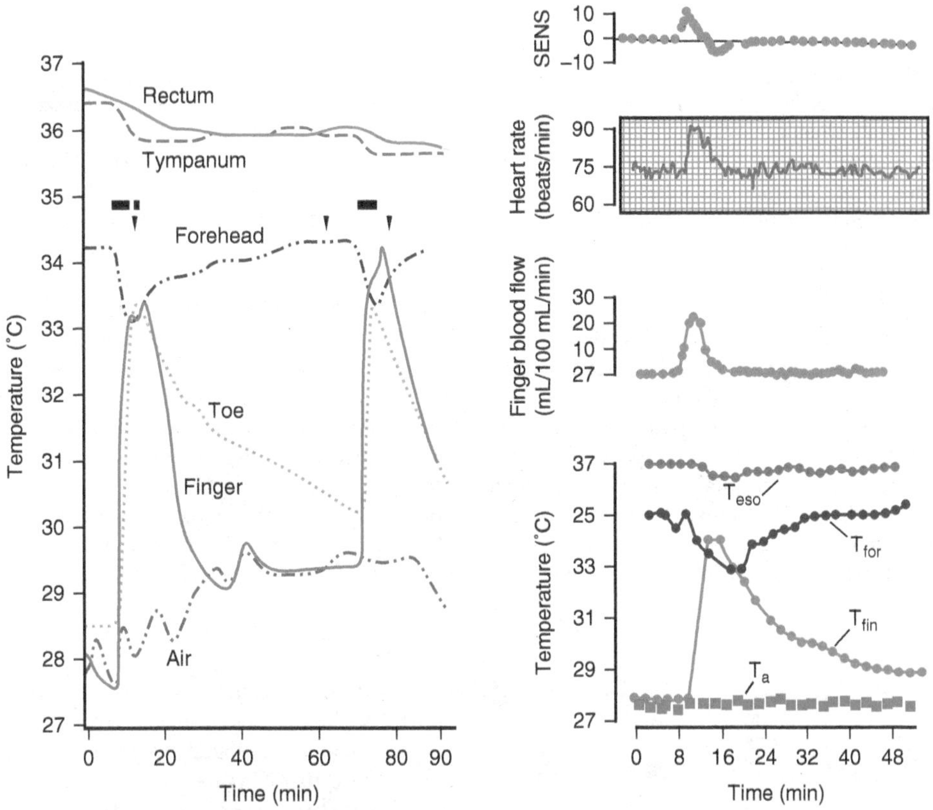


**Figure 14.18** Temperature responses to two spontaneous flashes and evoked flash. *Down arrow* indicates finger stab for blood sample. *Black bars* indicate time of flush. (Data from Molnar GW: Body temperature during menopausal hot flushes. *J Appl Physiol.* 1975;38[3]:499-303.)

decrease the likelihood of developing or delaying the onset of AD according to several observational studies and meta-analyses. However, once a woman is affected by AD, estrogen is unlikely to provide any benefit. Data from the Women's Health Initiative (WHI), however, suggested a lack of benefit of estrogen or estrogen/progestogen, or even a worsening of cognition in women initiating hormonal therapy after age 65. This suggests that timing of initiation of hormone therapy is critical, and this has also been supported by basic science studies. Here the early exposure to estrogen decreased the possibility of brain damage from free radicals and also promoted maintenance of neuronal and synaptic activity. However, prospective trials in younger women still have not been able to confirm the older observational data, suggesting a cognitive benefit of estrogen. Therefore, this area remains somewhat inconclusive. In summary, while early treatment with estrogen in younger women at the onset of menopause *may* be beneficial for cognition as it is with certain types of mood (although not proved yet), later treatment (e.g., after age 65) has no benefit and may even be detrimental, depending on the regimen of hormones used.

## COLLAGEN AND OTHER TISSUES

Estrogen has a positive effect on collagen, which is an important component of bone and skin and serves as a major support tissue for the structures of the pelvis and urinary system. Both estrogen and androgen receptors have been identified in skin fibroblasts. Nearly 30% of skin collagen is lost within the first 5 years after menopause, and collagen decreases approximately 2% per year for the first 10 years after menopause. This statistic, which is similar to that of bone loss after menopause, strongly suggests a link between skin thickness, bone loss, and the risk of **osteoporosis**. Although the literature is not entirely consistent, estrogen therapy generally improves collagen content after menopause and improves skin thickness substantially after about 2 years of treatment (Dunn, 1997). There is a possible bimodal effect with high doses of estrogen causing a reduction in skin thickness. The supportive effect of estrogen on collagen has important implications for bone homeostasis and for the pelvis after menopause. Here, reductions in collagen support and atrophy of the vaginal and urethral mucosa have been implicated in a variety of symptoms, including prolapse and urinary symptoms (Falconer, 1996). Vaginal estrogen has also been shown to reduce recurrent urinary tract infections. Symptoms of urinary incontinence and irritative bladder symptoms occur in 20% to 40% of perimenopausal and postmenopausal women. Uterine prolapse and other gynecologic symptoms related to poor collagen support, as well as urinary complaints, may improve with estrogen therapy. Although estrogen generally improves symptoms, urodynamic changes have not been shown to be altered. Estrogen has also been shown to decrease the incidence of recurrence of urinary tract infections. Restoration of bladder control in older women with estrogen has been shown to decrease the need for admission to nursing homes in Sweden. Estrogen may also have an important role in normal wound healing. In this setting, estrogen enhances the effects of growth factors such as transforming growth factor-β (TGF-β) (Ashcroft, 1997).

Although still not completely settled, it appears that oral estrogen does not improve stress urinary incontinence in postmenopausal women and may even cause such symptoms in previously asymptomatic older women. Estrogen may, however, improve urge and other irritative urinary symptoms.

### VULVOVAGINAL ATROPHY

Vulvovaginal complaints are often associated with estrogen deficiency. During perimenopause, symptoms of dryness and atrophic changes occur in 21% and 15% of women, respectively. However, these findings increase with time, and by 4 years these incidences are 47% and 55%, respectively. With this change, an increase in sexual complaints also occurs, with an incidence of dyspareunia of 41% in sexually active 60-year-old women. Estrogen deficiency results in a thin, paler vaginal mucosa. The moisture content is low, the pH increases (usually greater than 5), and the mucosa may exhibit inflammation and small petechiae.

With estrogen treatment, particularly when used locally, vaginal cytology changes have been documented, transforming from a cellular pattern of predominantly parabasal cells to one with an increased number of superficial cells. Along with this change, the vaginal pH decreases, vaginal blood flow increases, and the electropotential difference across the vaginal mucosa increases to that found in premenopausal women. Vaginal DHEA (0.25% to 1.0%) has been used with some suggested efficacy; the mechanism is presumed to be the local conversion of DHEA into estrogen, with possibly some other modulating effects as well (Labrie, 2011).

Ospenifene 60 mg, a selective estrogen receptor agonist (SERM), has been approved as an oral treatment for vulvovaginal atrophy. This SERM has particular properties of acting as an agonist in the vagina and as an antagonist in other tissues such as the breast. Information on these and other treatment options, including the use of lubricants and moisturizers, has been provided by the North American Menopause Society (Position Statement, 2013).

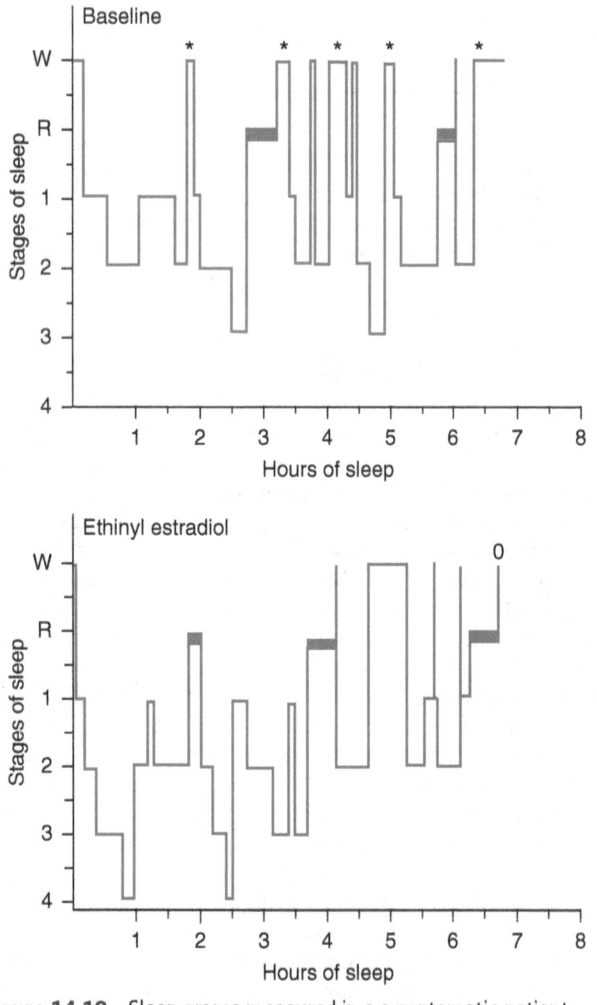


**Figure 14.19** Sleep grams measured in a symptomatic patient before and after a 30-day administration of ethinyl estradiol, 50 μg, four times daily. (Modified from Erlik Y, Tataryn IV, Meldrum DR, et al. Association of waking episodes with menopausal hot flushes. *JAMA.* 1981;245:1741.)

### BONE HEALTH

Estrogen deficiency has been well established as a cause of bone loss. This loss can be noted for the first time when menstrual cycles become irregular in perimenopause from 1.5 years before menopause to 1.5 years after menopause, spine bone mineral density has been shown to decrease by 2.5% per year, compared with a premenopausal loss rate of 0.13% per year. Loss of **trabecular bone** (spine) is greater with estrogen deficiency than is loss of **cortical bone.**

Postmenopausal bone loss leading to osteoporosis is a substantial health care problem. In Caucasian women, 35% of all postmenopausal women have been estimated to have osteoporosis based on bone mineral density. Furthermore, the lifetime fracture risk for these women is 40%. The morbidity and economic burden of osteoporosis is well documented. Interestingly, some data suggest that up to 19% of Caucasian men also have osteoporosis. Bone mass is substantially affected by sex steroids through classic mechanisms to be described later in this chapter. Attainment of peak bone mass in the late second decade (Fig. 14.20) is key to ensuring that the subsequent loss of bone mass with aging and estrogen deficiency does not lead to early osteoporosis. $E_2$ together with GH

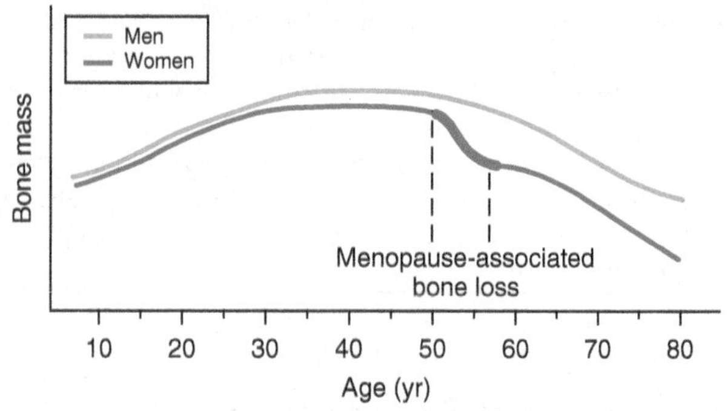


**Figure 14.20** Bone mass by age and sex. (Modified from Finkelstein JS: Osteoporosis. In: Goldman L, Bennet JC, eds. *Cecil Textbook of Medicine.* 21st ed. Philadelphia: Saunders;1999:1366-1373; Riggs BL, Melton LJ III. Involutional osteoporosis. *N Engl J Med.* 1986;314:1676.)

and insulin-like growth factor-1 act to double bone mass at the time of puberty, beginning the process of attaining peak bone mass. Postpubertal estrogen deficiency (amenorrhea from various causes) substantially jeopardizes peak bone mass. Adequate nutrition and calcium intake are also key determinants. Although estrogen is of predominant importance for bone mass in both women and men, testosterone is important in stimulating periosteal apposition; as a result, cortical bone in men is larger and thicker.

However, even in men estrogen appears to be important for bone health in that in male individuals with aromatase deficiency (inability to convert androgen to estrogen) osteoporosis ensues (Carani, 1997).

Estrogen receptors are present in osteoblasts, osteoclasts, and osteocytes. Both ER α and ER β are present in cortical bone, whereas ER β predominates in cancellous or trabecular bone (Bord, 2001). However, the more important actions of estradiol are believed to be mediated via ER α. Estrogens suppress bone turnover and maintain a certain rate of bone formation. Bone is remodeled in functional units, called *bone multicenter units* (BMUs), where resorption and formation should be in balance. Multiple sites of bone go through this turnover process over time. Estrogen decreases osteoclasts by increasing apoptosis thus reducing their life span. The effect on the osteoblast is less consistent, but $E_2$ antagonizes glucocorticoid-induced osteoblast apoptosis. Estrogen deficiency increases the activities of remodeling units, prolongs resorption, and shortens the phase of bone formation. It also increases osteoclast recruitment in BMUs, thus resorption outstrips formation. The molecular mechanisms of estrogen action on bone involve the inhibition of production of proinflammatory cytokines, which increase with a decrease in estrogen at menopause, leading to increased bone resorption (Pacifici, 1996). These cytokines include interleukin-1, interleukin-6, tumor necrosis factor-α, colony-stimulating factor-1, macrophage colony-stimulating factor, and prostaglandin $E_2$, all which may contribute to increased resorption. Estradiol also upregulates TGF-β in bone, which inhibits bone resorption. Receptor activation of nuclear factor kappa (NFκB) ligand (RANKL) is responsible for osteoclast differentiation and action. A scheme for how all these factors interact has been proposed (Fig. 14.21) (Riggs, 2000). In women, Riggs has suggested that bone loss occurs in two phases. With estrogen levels declining at the onset of menopause, an accelerated phase of bone loss occurs, which is predominantly of cancellous bone. Here 20% to 30% of cancellous bone and 5% to 10% of cortical bone can be lost in a span of 4 to 8 years. Thereafter, a slower phase of loss (1% to 2% per year) ensues, during which more cortical bone is lost. This phase is thought to be induced primarily by secondary hyperparathyroidism. The first phase is also accentuated by the decreased influence of stretching or mechanical factors, which generally promotes bone homeostasis, as a result of estrogen deficiency. Genetic influences on bone mass are more important for the attainment of peak bone mass (heritable component, 50% to 70%) than for bone loss. Polymorphisms of the vitamin D receptor gene, TGF-β gene, and the Spl-binding site in the collagen type 1 Al gene have all been implicated as being important for bone mass (Nguyen, 2000).

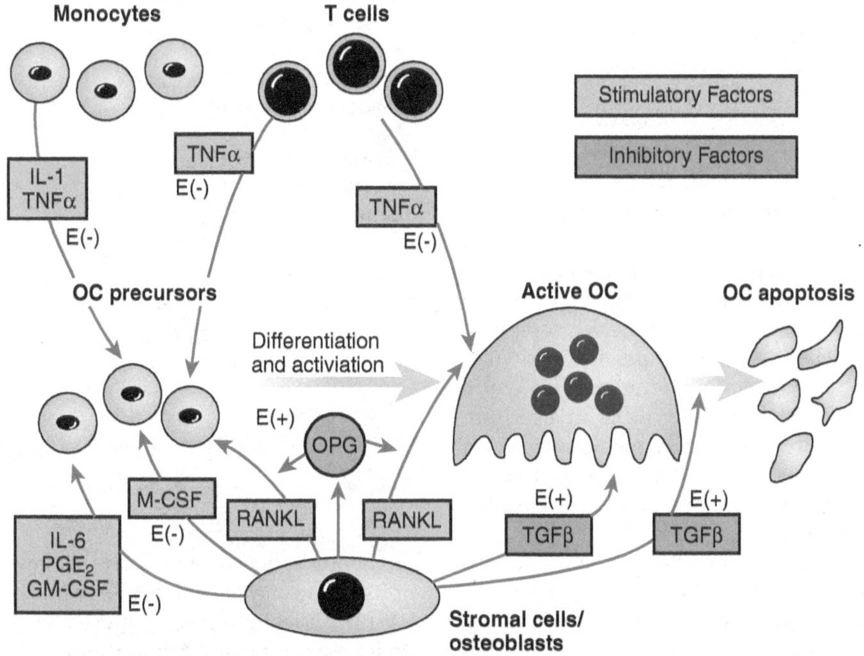


**Figure 14.21** Model for mediation of effects of estrogen *(E)* on osteoclast formation and function by cytokines in bone marrow microenvironment. Stimulatory factors are shown in orange and inhibitory factors are shown in blue. Positive (+) or negative (−) effects of E on these regulatory factors are shown in red. The model assumes that regulation is accomplished by multiple cytokines working together in concert. *GM-CSF,* Granulocyte macrophage/colony-stimulating factor; *IL,* interleukin; *M-CSF,* macrophage/colony-stimulating factor; *OC,* osteoclast; *OPG,* osteoprotegerin; *$PGE_2$,* prostaglandin $E_2$; *RANKL,* receptor activation of B ligand; *TGF-β,* transforming growth factor β. (Modified from Riggs BL. The mechanisms of estrogen regulation of bone resorption. *J Clin Invest.* 2000;106:1203.)

Table 14.2 Techniques for the Detection of Bone Mass

| | | Precision in | Examination and Analysis | Estimated |
|---|---|---|---|---|
| | **Effective** | | | |
| **Technique** | **Anatomic Site of Interest** | **Vivo (%)** | **Time (min)** | **Dose** |
| Equivalent (uSv) | | | | |
| Conventional radiographs | Spine, hip<br>2000 | NA | <5 | 2000 |
| Radiogrammetry | Hand | 1-3 | 5-10 | <1 |
| Radiographic absorptiometry | Hand | 1-2 | 5-10 | <1 |
| Single x-ray absorptiometry | Forearm, heel | 1-2 | 5-10 | <1 |
| Dual x-ray absorptiometry | Spine, hip, forearm, total body | 1-3 | 5-20 | 1-10 |
| Quantitative computed tomography | Spine, forearm, hip | 2-4 | 10-15 | 50-100 |
| Quantitative ultrasound | Heel, hand, lower leg | 1-3 | 5-10 | None |

Modified from van Kuijk C, Genant HK. Detection of osteopenia. In: Lobo RA, ed. *Treatment of the Postmenopausal Woman: Basic and Clinical Aspects*. 2nd ed. Philadelphia: Lippincott Williams & Wilkins; 1999:287-292.
*NA*, Not applicable.

Bone mass can be detected by a variety of radiographic methods (Table 14.2). Dual-energy x-ray absorptiometry (DEXA) scans have become the standard of care for detection of **osteopenia** and osteoporosis. By convention, the **T score** is used to reflect the number of standard deviations of bone loss from the peak bone mass of a young adult. Osteopenia is defined by a T score of −1 to −2.5 standard deviations; osteoporosis is defined as greater than 2.5 standard deviations.

Various biochemical assays are also available to assess bone resorption and formation in both blood and urine (Table 14.3). At present, serum markers appear to be most useful for assessing changes, with antiresorptive therapy having less variability compared with the urinary assessments. Although these biochemical measurements cannot reliably predict bone mass, they may be useful as markers of the effectiveness of treatment. For example, an increased resorption marker may decrease within months into the normal range with an antiresorptive therapy, whereas it takes 1 to 2 years to see a change in BMD with DEXA.

Fracture risk is not only determined by bone mass but by many factors, the most important of which is bone strength. This in turn is determined by bone mass as well as bone turnover for which biochemical assessments may be helpful. A research method employs a high-resolution quantitative computed tomography of bone, which is intended to provide a "virtual" bone biopsy. This may be available in the future. The World Health Organization (WHO) has made available an algorithm to predict the 10-year fracture risk of men and women living around the world. This model, called *FRAX*, can be accessed at www.shef.ac.uk/FRAX and is calculated based on individual patient history data and the results from DEXA.

Table 14.3 Bone Turnover Markers

| Marker | Specimen |
|---|---|
| **Bone Resorption Markers** | |
| Cross-linked N-telopeptide of type I collagen (NTX) | Urine, serum |
| Cross-linked C-telopeptide of type I collagen (CTX) | Urine (αα and ββ forms)<br>Serum (ββ form) |
| MMP-generated telopeptide of type I collagen (ICTP or CTX-MMP) | Serum |
| Deoxypyridinoline, free and peptide bound (fDPD, DPD) | Urine, serum |
| Pyridinoline, free and peptide bound (fPYD, PYD) | Urine serum |
| Hydroxyproline (OHP) | Urine |
| Glycosyl hydroxylysine (GylHyl) | Urine, serum |
| Helical peptide (HelP) | Urine |
| Tartrate resistant acid phosphatase 5b isoform specific for osteoclasts (TRACP 5b) | Serum, plasma |
| Cathepsin K (Cath K) | Urine, serum |
| Osteocalcin fragments (uOC) | Urine |
| **Bone Formation Markers** | |
| Osteocalcin (OC) | Serum |
| Procollagen type I C-terminal propeptide (PICP) | Serum |
| Procollagen type I N-terminal propeptide (PINP) | Serum |
| Bone-specific alkaline phosphatase (bone ALP) | Serum |

Many agents are now available for preventing osteoporosis. It is important to make a distinction about using various agents for the *prevention* of osteoporosis (e.g., in a woman who has risk factors and is osteopenic: T score above −2.5) as opposed to using drugs to *treat* established osteoporosis (T scores greater than −2.5.)

The use of estrogen will depend on whether there are other indications for estrogen treatment and whether there are any possible contraindications. Estrogen has been shown to reduce the risk of osteoporosis as well as to reduce osteoporotic fractures. A dose equivalent of 0.625 mg of conjugated equine estrogens (CEEs) was once thought to be necessary for the prevention of osteoporosis, but we now know that lower doses (0.3 mg of CEE or its equivalent) in combination with progestogens, or even with adequate calcium alone, can prevent bone loss, although there are no long-term fracture data with lower-dose therapy (Fig. 14.22). Whether the addition of progestogens by stimulating bone formation increases bone mass beyond that produced by estrogen alone is unclear. The androgenic activity of certain progestogens such as norethindrone acetate (NET) also has been suggested to play a role, by stimulating bone formation. Figures 14.23 and 14.24 provide data on changes in bone mineral density (BMD) at the spine and hip using various agents.

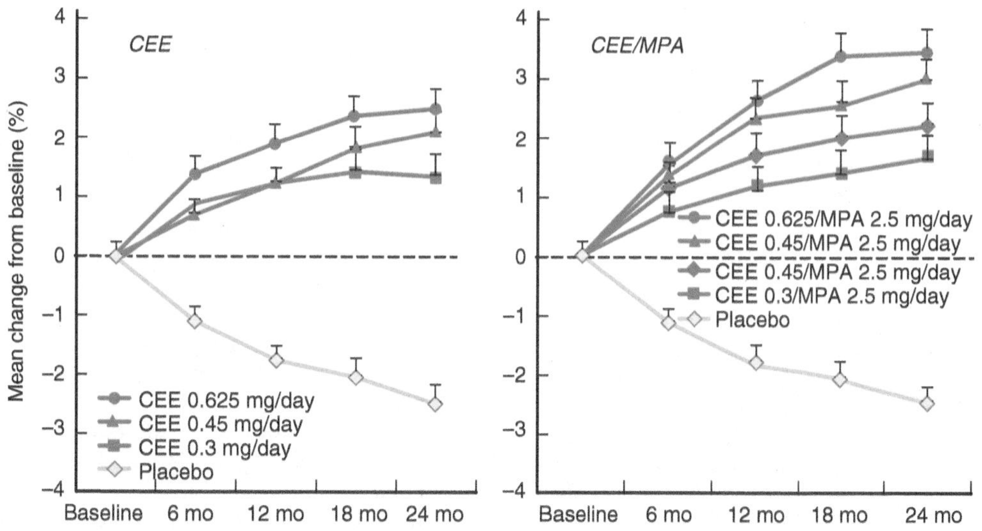


**Figure 14.22** Changes in spine bone mineral density (BMD) with hormone therapy (HT). Intent-to-treat population only. The Women's HOPE Study. *CEE*, Conjugated equine estrogens; *HOPE*, Heart, Osteoporosis, Progestin, Estrogen; *MPA*, medroxyprogesterone. (From Lindsay R, Gallagher JC, Kleerekoper M, et al. Effect of lower doses of conjugated equine estrogens with and without medroxyprogesterone acetate on bone in early postmenopausal women. *JAMA*. 2002;287:2668.)

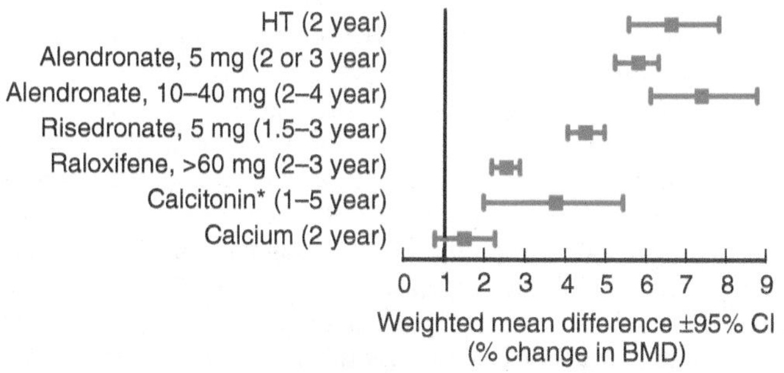


*Doses ranged from 250 to 2800 IU per week; predominantly nasal delivery.

**Figure 14.23** Meta-analysis of osteoporosis therapies: spine bone mineral density (BMD). *CI*, Confidence interval; *HT*, hormone therapy. (From Cranney A, Guyatt G, Griffith L, et al. Meta-analyses of therapies for postmenopausal osteoporosis. IX: summary of meta-analyses of therapies for postmenopausal osteoporosis. *Endocr Rev.* 2002;23:570; data from Cranney A, Tugwell P, Wells G, et al. Meta-analyses of therapies for postmenopausal osteoporosis. I. Systematic reviews of randomized trials in osteoporosis: introduction and methodology. *Endocrine Rev.* 2002;23:496.)

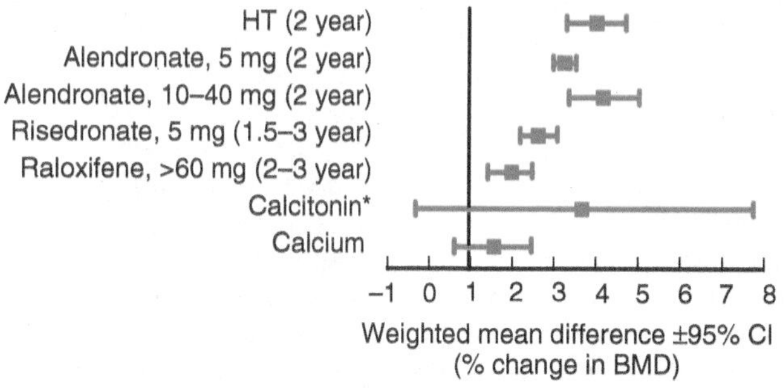


**Figure 14.24** Meta-analysis of osteoporosis therapies: total hip bone mineral density (BMD). *CI*, Confidence interval. (From Cranney A, Guyatt G, Griffith L, et al. Meta-analyses of therapies for postmenopausal osteoporosis. IX: summary of meta-analyses of therapies for postmenopausal osteoporosis. *Endocr Rev.* 2002;23:570; data from Cranney A, Tugwell P, Wells G, et al. Meta-analyses of therapies for postmenopausal osteoporosis. I. Systematic reviews of randomized trials in osteoporosis: introduction and methodology. *Endocrine Rev.* 2002;23:496.)

**Selective estrogen receptor modulators (SERMs)** such as **raloxifene**, droloxifene, and tamoxifen have all been shown to decrease bone resorption. Raloxifene has been shown to decrease vertebral fractures in a large prospective trial (Ettinger, 1999). All of these agents are used for *prevention.* In younger women, one complicating factor is that agents such as raloxifene may induce hot flushes; however, they do afford some protection for breast cancer risk, as they act as estrogen antagonists at the level of the breast. SERMs such as raloxifene act as a low-dose estrogen and can prevent vertebral fractures but not hip fractures (Fig. 14.25).

**Tibolone** (structurally related to 19-not progestins) has also been shown to be an effective treatment for the prevention of osteoporosis. Tibolone (not marketed in the United States) has SERM-like properties, but it is not specifically a SERM because it has mixed estrogenic, antiestrogenic, androgenic, and progestogenic properties, due to its metabolites. The drug does not seem to cause uterine or breast cell proliferation and also is beneficial for vasomotor symptoms. It prevents osteoporosis and has been shown to be beneficial in treatment of osteoporosis as well at a dose of 2.5 mg daily.

**Bisphosphonates** have been shown to have a significant effect on the *prevention and treatment* of osteoporosis, using similar doses for both indications. With this class of agents (etidronate, alendronate, risedronate, ibandronate, and zoledronic acid), incorporation of the bisphosphonate with hydroxyapatite in bone increases bone mass. The skeletal half-life of bisphosphonates in bone can be as long as 10 years, and their effects on the

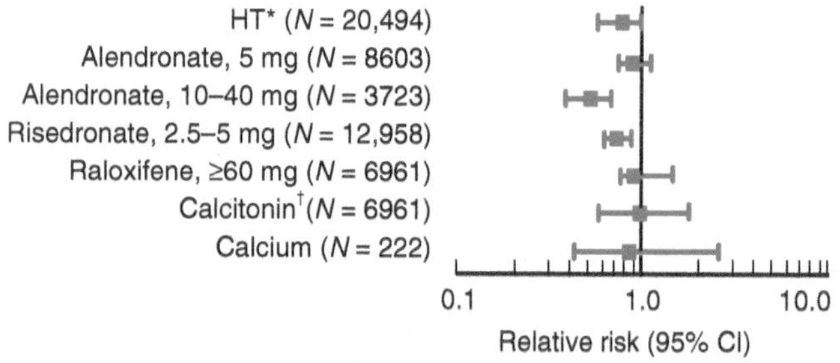


*Includes the Women's Health Initiative (WHI) trial.
†Estimate from the Prevent Recurrence of Osteoporotic Fractures (PROOF) trial.

**Figure 14.25** Meta-analysis of osteoporosis therapies: nonvertebral fractures. *CI*, Confidence interval; *HT*, hormone therapy. (From Cranney A, Guyatt G, Griffith L, et al. Meta-analyses of therapies for postmenopausal osteoporosis. IX: summary of meta-analyses of therapies for postmenopausal osteoporosis. *Endocr Rev.* 2002;23:570; data from Cranney A, Tugwell P, Wells G, et al. Meta-analyses of therapies for postmenopausal osteoporosis. I. Systematic reviews of randomized trials in osteoporosis: introduction and methodology. *Endocrine Rev.* 2002;23:496; Rosen C. Presentation for ASBMR at NIH Scientific Workshop: Menopausal hormone therapy, October 23-24, 2002.)

skeleton are sustained for a few years after discontinuation, which does not occur with other agents. These agents reduce both spine and hip fractures (see Fig. 14.25). Most data have been derived with alendronate, which, at a dosage of 5 mg daily (35 mg weekly), prevents bone loss; at 10 mg daily (70 mg weekly), alendronate is an effective treatment for osteoporosis, with evidence available that this treatment reduces vertebral and hip fractures (Cummings, 1998). Similar data are available for risedronate (35 mg weekly). Ibandronate has been approved as a once-a-month treatment (150 mg), and some data to date support the reduction in vertebral fractures. It can also be injected (3 mg) every 3 months. Zoledronic acid 5 mg is available as an intravenous infusion (over 15 minutes) once a year for the treatment of osteoporosis and every 2 years for prevention. This class of medications has the property of causing esophageal irritation, and care must be taken in administering the oral doses in an upright position with a full glass of water.

Some concern has been raised about bisphosphonates and osteonecrosis of the jaw, fractures of long bones such as the femur with long-term use, and atrial fibrillation. Jaw problems only occur with high doses when poor dentition is present. Femur fractures with long-term use are extremely rare and atrial fibrillation, although statistically increased with bisphosphonate use, is also rare. Nevertheless, we do not have long-term data (>10 years), and these drugs should not be used for more than 10 years and not with another antiresorptive agent. Its use in younger postmenopausal women (<60 years) should be limited unless there is significant osteoporosis present.

RANKL secreted by osteoblasts causes bone resorption (see Fig. 14.21). Denosumab is a monoclonal antibody that binds up RANKL, thus preventing bone resorption. It is an effective treatment for osteoporosis, and although it can also be used for prevention, it is largely viewed as a secondary agent, particularly for women intolerant to other treatments. Denosumab 60 mg is administered subcutaneously every 6 months, and it is effective both at the vertebrae and at the hip, (Cummings, 2009), with an efficacy that is similar to or greater than that of the bisphosphonates. Unlike the bisphosphonates, however, the effects wear off immediately after discontinuation of treatment. Although denosumab does not carry the small risks of jaw osteonecrosis and long bone fractures, as an immune therapy, long-term effects of immune modulation are not known.

Calcitonin (50 IU subcutaneous injections daily, or 200 IU intranasally) has been shown to inhibit bone resorption. Vertebral fractures have been shown to decrease with calcitonin therapy. Long-term effects, however, have not been established, and this is not a first-line therapy today.

Fluoride has been used for women with osteoporosis because it increases bone density. Currently, a lower dose (50 μg daily) of slow-release sodium fluoride does not seem to cause adverse effects (gastritis) and has efficacy in preventing vertebral fractures.

Intermittent parathyroid hormone (PTH) is an effective agent to increase bone mass in women with significant osteoporosis. In a randomized trial lasting 3 years, average bone density increased in the hip and spine with fewer fractures observed. This therapy, now available in the United States, is a second-tier therapy reserved for severe cases of osteoporosis. Teriparatide at 20 μg needs to be injected subcutaneously on a daily basis for no longer than 18 months (Murad, 2012).

Adjunctive measures for prevention of osteoporosis are calcium, vitamin D, and exercise. Calcium with vitamin D treatment has been shown to increase bone only in older individuals. It will not prevent bone loss in younger women at the onset of menopause. These modalities alone are not thought to be effective for the treatment of osteoporosis. A woman's total intake of elemental calcium should be 1500 mg daily if no agents are being used to inhibit resorption, and 400 to 800 IU of vitamin D should also be ingested. Caution should be exercised in prescribing excessive calcium, particularly in older individuals, as this has been linked to coronary events. Exercise has been shown to be beneficial for building muscle and bone mass and for reducing falls.

There has been the realization that many women in the United States are vitamin D deficient, particularly those in the northern parts of the country, because of less sunlight exposure. Vitamin D may also be important as an antimitotic agent that may prevent certain types of cancer. Although there is some controversy about what a normal vitamin D level should be, a blood level of 25 OH vitamin D <30 ng/mL usually warrants supplemental treatment with 25 hydroxy vitamin D.

Although it is clear that women with established osteoporosis (fractures or a T score of −2.5 or greater) should receive an antiresorptive agent (usually a bisphosphonate), there is more controversy with initiating preventive strategies with T scores in the osteopenia range (−1.0 to −2.5). Many women, however, may sustain fractures in this range of T scores. Age and risk factors (thinness, immobilization, nutritional deficiencies, family history, etc.) largely help determine the need to treat those with osteopenia. In this setting, depending on the age of the woman, her family history, and whether she has vasomotor symptoms, she may be offered hormone therapy, a SERM, or a bisphosphonate. The FRAX algorithm may also be useful as a guide to therapy.

## DEGENERATIVE ARTHRITIS

Degeneration of intervertebral discs is a process that occurs rapidly after menopause. This is consistent with changes in collagen as noted previously. There is evidence that this is benefited by estrogen after menopause.

Osteoarthritis is a source of significant distress. There is a powerful effect of estrogen in inhibiting damage to chondrocytes (Tanko, 2007). In WHI, estrogen alone (but not combination hormone therapy) significantly decreased osteoarthritis. However, much more work is needed in this area.

## CARDIOVASCULAR EFFECTS

Women have a very low incidence of cardiovascular disease (CVD) prior to menopause, but after menopause, the risk increases significantly. Data from the Framingham study have shown that the incidence is three times lower in women before menopause than in men (3.1 per 1000 per year in women ages 45 to 49). The incidence is approximately equal in men and women ages 75 to 79 (53 and 50.4 per 1000 per year, respectively). This trend also pertains to gender differences in mortality resulting from cardiovascular disease. Coronary artery disease is the leading cause of death in women, and the lifetime risk of death is 31% in postmenopausal women versus a 3% risk of dying of breast cancer.

Although CVD becomes more prevalent only in the later years following a natural menopause, premature cessation of ovarian function (before the average age of menopause) constitutes a significant risk. Premature menopause, occurring before age 35, has been shown to increase the risk of myocardial infarction two- to threefold, and oophorectomy before age 35 increases the risk sevenfold (Lobo, 2007).

When the possible reasons for the increase in CVD are examined, the most prevalent finding is an accelerated rise in total cholesterol in postmenopausal women. The changes of weight, blood pressure, and blood glucose with aging, although important, are not thought to be as important as the rate of rise in total cholesterol, which is substantially different in women after menopause versus men. This increase in total cholesterol is explained by increases in levels of low-density lipoprotein cholesterol (LDL-C). The oxidation of LDL-C is also enhanced, as are levels of very low density lipoproteins and lipoprotein (a). High-density lipoprotein cholesterol (HDL-C) levels trend downward with time, but these changes are small and inconsistent relative to the increases in LDL-C.

Coagulation balance is not substantially altered as a counterbalance of changes occurs. Some procoagulation factors increase (factor VII, fibrinogen), but so do counterbalancing factors such as antithrombin III, plasminogen, protein C, and protein S. Blood flow in all vascular beds decreases after menopause; prostacyclin production decreases, endothelin levels increase, and vasomotor responses to acetylcholine are constrictive, reflecting reduced nitric oxide synthetase activity. Most of these latter changes are due primarily to the fairly rapid reduction in estrogen levels in that with estrogen, all these parameters (generally) improve, and coronary arterial responses to acetylcholine are dilatory with a commensurate increase in blood flow.

Circulating plasma nitrites and nitrates have also been shown to increase with estrogen, and angiotensin-converting enzyme levels tend to decrease. Estrogen and progesterone receptors have been found in vascular tissues, including coronary arteries (predominantly ER β). In addition, some membrane effects are mediated by estrogen, which may or may not relate to either ER α or ER β.

Overall, the direct vascular effects of estrogen are viewed to be as important, or more important, than the changes in lipid and lipoproteins after menopause. Although replacing estrogen has been thought to be beneficial for the mechanisms previously cited, these beneficial arterial effects may only be seen in younger (stage + 1(a-c) postmenopausal women (Fig. 14.26). (Mendelsohn, 2005) Women with significant atherosclerosis or risk factors such as those studied in secondary prevention trials, who have established atherosclerosis and prior coronary disease, do not respond well to this treatment because of coronary plaque burden (see Fig. 14.26), which prevents estrogen action. Some of this lack of effect may be accounted for by increased methylation of the promoter region of ER α, which occurs with atherosclerosis and aging. Another mechanism is the significant conversion of cholesterol to 27-0H cholesterol, which also impedes estrogen's production of nitric oxide (Fig. 14.27).

In normal, nonobese postmenopausal women, carbohydrate tolerance also decreases as a result of an increase in insulin resistance. This, too, may be partially reversed by estrogen, although the data are mixed, and high doses of estrogen with or without progestogen cause a deterioration in insulin sensitivity. Biophysical and neurohormonal responses to stress (stress reactivity) are exaggerated in postmenopausal women compared with premenopausal women, and this heightened reactivity is blunted by estrogen. Whether these changes influence cardiovascular risk with estrogen deficiency is not known, but clearly estrogen treatment returns many parameters into the range of premenopausal women in early postmenopausal women. Several trials including data from both hormonal trials of the WHI have shown a reduction in the development of diabetes with hormone therapy (Bonds, 2006; Lobo, 2014).

These consistently strong basic science and clinical data for the protective effects of estrogen on the cardiovascular system together with strong epidemiologic evidence for a protective effect of estrogen (Fig. 14.28) led to the belief that estrogen should be prescribed to prevent CVD in women. Clinical trial data, however, have refuted this notion in women with established disease, as noted previously. Results from several randomized trials in women have failed to show a protective effect in women with established coronary disease. Furthermore, a trend toward increased cardiovascular events (early harm) has been observed in this setting in some women within the first 1 to 2 years. The Women's Health Initiative (WHI) trial, which compared CEE/medroxyprogesterone acetate (MPA) with placebo, came to similar conclusions. Though considered to be a primary prevention trial, it studied subjects in a large range of ages (mean age 63). These women did not have vasomotor symptoms and had more risk factors than the healthy women studied in observational cohorts as shown in Figure 14.28.

The protective effect of estrogen demonstrated in the observational trials such as the Nurse's Health Study (NHS) (see Fig. 14.28) occurred predominantly in young, healthy,

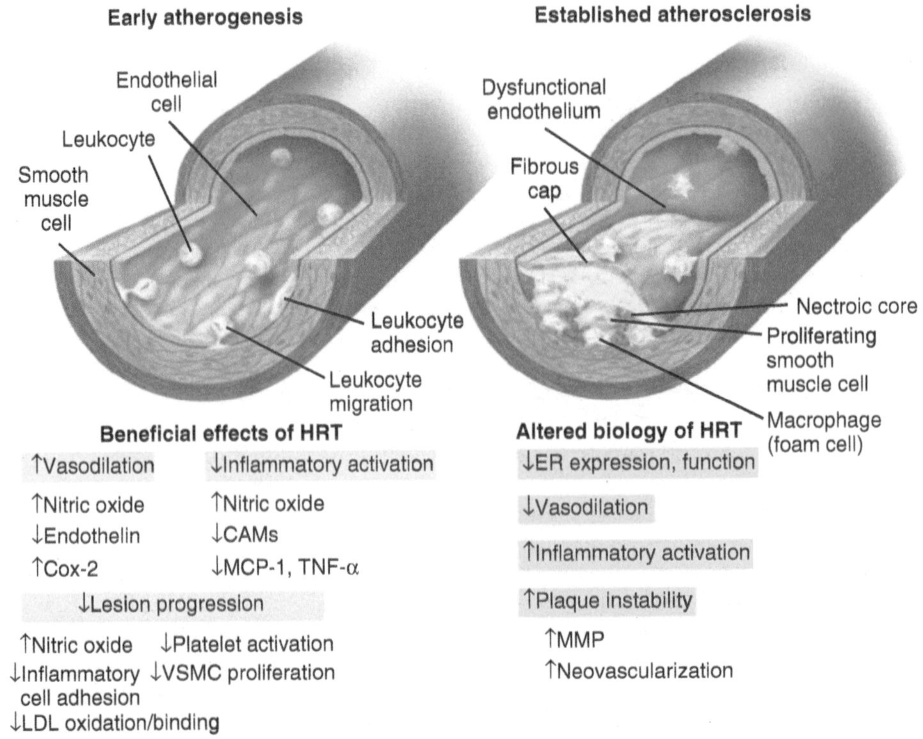


**Figure 14.26** Mechanisms of benefit of hormonal therapy with estrogen in early menopause (relatively clean coronary vessels) and the lack of effect in older women and those with significant atherosclerotic plaque burden. (From Mendelsohn ME, Karas RH. Molecular and cellular basis of cardiovascular gender differences. *Science* 2005;308[5728]:1583-1587.)

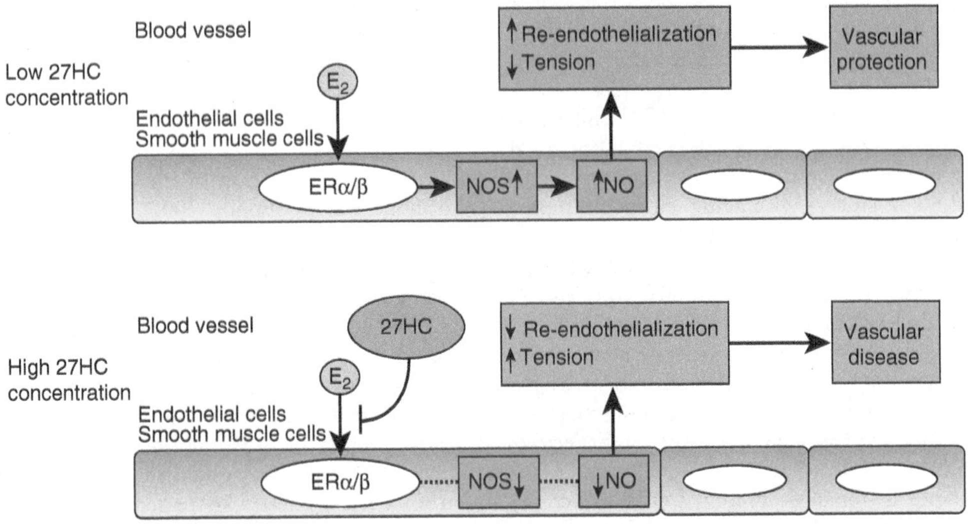


**Figure 14.27** Hypothesis of how elevated (27-hyroxycholesterol, 27HC) can influence the effect of estradiol ($E_2$). *ER*, Estrogen receptor, *NO*, nitric oxide, *NOS*, nitric oxide synthetase. (From Umetani M, Domoto H, Gormley AK, et al. 27-Hydroxycholesterol is an endogenous SERM that inhibits the cardiovascular effects of estrogen. *Nat Med.* 2007;13[10]:1185-1192.)

symptomatic women. Table 14.4 compares the demographics of the participants of WHI and the NHS. Trials carried out in the monkey model have shown a 50% to 70% protective effect against coronary atherosclerosis when estrogen is begun at the time of oophorectomy, with or without an atherogenic diet; delaying the initiation of hormonal therapy for even 2 years (in the monkey) prevents this protective effect (Fig. 14.29). This has been called the "timing" hypothesis, in which early intervention shows benefit and late intervention with hormonal therapy is possibly harmful for the cardiovascular (CV) system. Nevertheless the 13-year follow-up data from both hormonal trials of WHI do not show overall CV harm (there were no statistical changes in

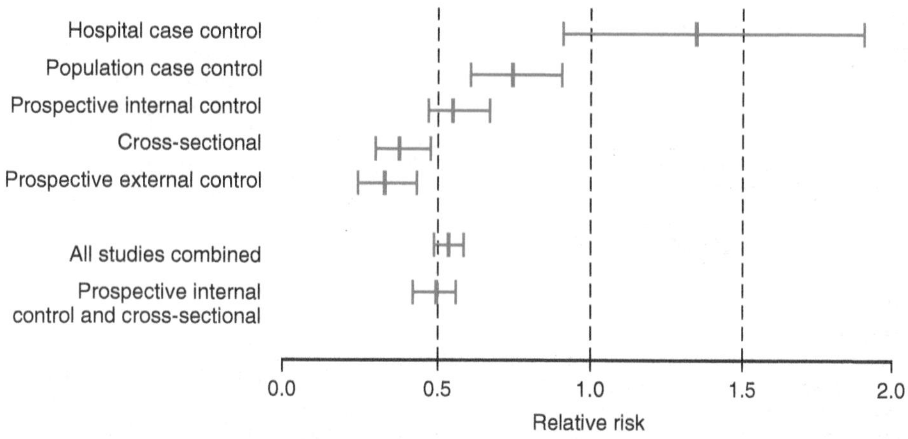


**Figure 14.28** Estrogen replacement therapy and coronary heart disease. Relationship between relative risk and study type. (Modified from Stampfer MJ, Colditz GA. Estrogen replacement therapy and coronary heart disease: a quantitative assessment of the epidemiologic evidence. *Prev Med.* 1991;20:47.)

**Table 14.4** Demographics of Women in WHI and NHS

| | WHI | NHS |
|---|---|---|
| Mean age or age range at enrollment (years) | 63 | 30-55 |
| Smokers (past and current) | 49.9% | 55% |
| Body mass index (BMI: mean) | 28.5 kg/m$^2$ | 25.1 kg/m$^2$ |
| Aspirin users | 19.1% | 43.9% |
| Menopausal symptoms | Rare | Common |

*NHS*, National health service; *WHI*, women's health initiative.

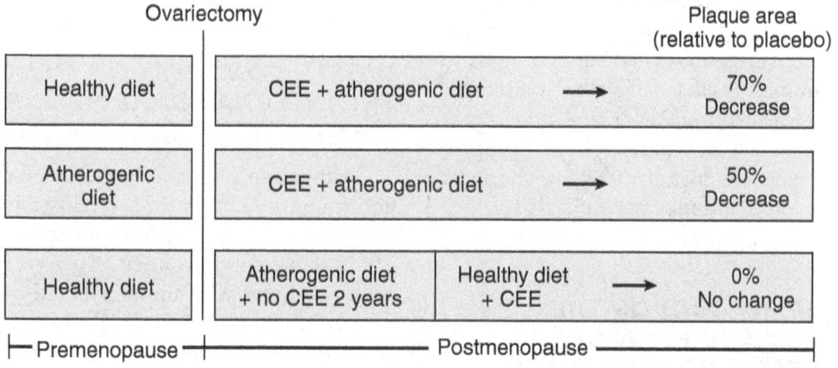


**Figure 14.29** Importance of timing of intervention on the effect of estrogens on atherogenesis in nonhuman primates. *CEE*, Conjugated equine estrogen. (Modified from Clarkson TB, Anthony MS, Jerome CP. Lack of effect of raloxifene on coronary artery atherosclerosis of postmenopausal monkeys. *J Clin Endocrinol Metab.* 1998;83:721; data from Adams MR, Register TC, Golden DL, et al. Medroxyprogesterone acetate antagonizes inhibitory effects of conjugated equine estrogens on coronary artery atherosclerosis. *Arterioscler Thromb Vasc Biol.* 1997;17:217; data from Clarkson TB, Anthony MS, Morgan TM. Inhibition of postmenopausal atherosclerosis progression: a comparison of the effects of conjugated equine estrogens and soy phytoestrogens. *J Clin Endocrinol Metab.* 2001;86:41; Williams JK, Anthony MS, Honore EK, et al. Regression of atherosclerosis in female monkeys. *Arterioscler Thromb Vasc Biol.* 1995;15:827.)

any age group when the combined data were analyzed); and benefit was demonstrated in younger women using estrogen alone (Manson, 2013). This will be reviewed in more detail later.

The perception of coronary harm and other risks in older women receiving combined CEE/MPA in WHI led to widespread confusion and concern about HT in general and led to most women stopping HT and not starting it even when there were significant symptoms. As will be discussed later, more recent data now have confirmed that HT is safe for young, healthy women, and it is particularly indicated in women with symptoms. It appears we have come full circle as many of the original concepts of cardioprotection and reduction in all-cause

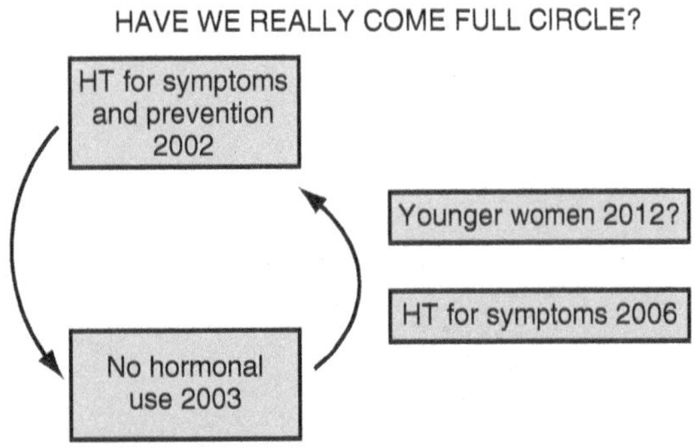


**Figure 14.30** Depiction of use of hormone therapy (HT) over time, including the current status, which is still in flux. (From Lobo RA. Where are we 10 years after the Women's Health Initiative? *J Clin Endocrinol Metab.* 2013;98[5]:1771-1780.)

mortality with estrogen have been once again confirmed from the randomized trials, when one examines the effects in younger women, close to menopause (Lobo, 2013) (Fig. 14.30). However, what we have learned from WHI is that while younger women benefit, older women do not (the timing hypothesis) and may endure harm as several secondary prevention trials (in women with established coronary disease) have shown. No clear explanation exists for what may cause the observed "early harm," but these effects were not observed in those women receiving statins concurrently. This finding suggests that HT (in the doses used) may lead to plaque destabilization and thrombosis in some women with established (although possibly silent) coronary disease. The molecular mechanisms for this effect may be due to estrogen upregulating matrix metalloproteinase-9 and inhibiting its natural inhibitor within the mural area of the plaque; the resultant disruption of the gelatinous covering then leads to thrombosis. The anti-inflammatory effects of statins inhibit this process. Additional lessons learned from WHI and more recent data are findings that **estrogen** is what is protective, and **progestogens**, depending on the type and dose, are likely to attenuate or eliminate any protective effect and may be implicated as well in the risk of breast cancer.

## WHAT ARE THE CURRENT DATA ON THE EFFECTS OF ESTROGEN AND ESTROGEN/PROGESTOGEN ON THE CARDIOVASCULAR SYSTEM?

Data from WHI first reported that the younger women, ages 50 to 59, receiving CEE alone had a significantly reduced coronary score. In 2007, WHI reported that women ages 50 to 59 receiving CEE and CEE/MPA (combined analysis) had a significant 30% reduction in all-cause mortality (Rossouw, 2007). Subsequently pooled analyses of prospective studies, including data from WHI, showed a statistical benefit in the reduction of coronary disease with estrogen in women less than 10 years from menopause or <60 years of age. A Bayesian meta-analysis (looking at retrospective and prospective studies) showed consistent data for a reduction in all cause mortality of about 30% in younger women receiving hormonal treatment (Salpeter, 2009) (Fig. 14.31).

As discussed previously, the 13-year follow-up data from WHI including the intervention and follow-up phases of the trial showed a significant benefit in younger women receiving CEE alone (Manson, 2013) (Fig. 14.32). The data with CEE/MPA were in the same direction for mortality but were less robust.

Several prospective trials in younger women deserve some discussion. The Kronos Estrogen Early Prevention Study (KEEPS) studied women within 3 years of menopause and compared the effects of CEE 0.45 mg or transdermal $E_2$ 0.05 mg, with micronized progesterone 200 mg for 12 days a month, compared with placebo, for 4 years. Carotid intima-media thickness (which reflects atherosclerosis progression) and coronary calcium were assessed as end points. The data were not able to show a benefit of estrogen compared with placebo, although estrogen provided the well-known benefits in terms of menopausal symptom relief (see Fig. 14.32). (Harman, 2014) There were very small changes in each group, and it has been suggested that the size of the trial (720 women) and the short 4 years of intervention was insufficient to show significant changes in a healthy population of women. A prospective trial in Denmark of 1000 recently postmenopausal women who received estradiol alone or estradiol and norethindrone (in women with a uterus) or no treatment for up to 10 years, with follow-up for up to 16 years, showed significant coronary benefit (Schierbeck, 2012). Cardiovascular death, myocardial infarction, and hospitalizations for congestive heart failure were significantly reduced in users of HT (Fig. 14.33). ELITE tested the "timing" hypothesis by treating women who were within 6 years of menopause and another group of women who were more than 10 years after menopause. Oral $E_2$ 1 mg or placebo was used in both groups, with vaginal progesterone for endometrial protection. The primary end point was carotid intima-media thickness, which showed a significant reduction in recently menopausal women but not in the older women, which confirmed the hypothesis (Hodis, 2014).

## WORLD CONGRESS ON MENOPAUSE OF THE INTERNATIONAL MENOPAUSE SOCIETY, MAY 1-4, 2014, CANCUN, MEXICO

A Cochrane analysis reviewed CV and overall mortality with HT and found no change in mortality when all ages and both primary and secondary prevention trials were combined (Boardman, 2015). However, in women <10 years from menopause the data were consistent with findings noted previously, with significant protective effects of 30% in all-cause mortality and 40% to 50% protection from CV mortality. It was noted, however, that there was a significant increase in venous thromboembolism (VTE), which is well known to occur with oral therapy (as also occurs with oral contraceptives) but does not affect mortality. Stroke was not affected in this younger population. The complications of VTE and potentially of ischemic stroke will be discussed later.

The two risk areas for CVD, even in younger women, at least potentially, are VTE and ischemic stroke. It is now accepted that there is a two- to threefold increase in venous thrombosis risk with oral hormonal therapy. However, the prevalence of this risk is low, particularly in young, healthy women. This two- to threefold risk is similar to that with the use of oral contraceptives. For pulmonary embolism risk, in women ages 50 to 60 years, the background risk is approximately 10 to 20 events/100,000 woman-years. Thus, with HT, the twofold increase may result in 40 events/100,000 woman-years, which is less than the rate in normal pregnancy (approximately 60/100,000 women). This risk is related to

**Study year**

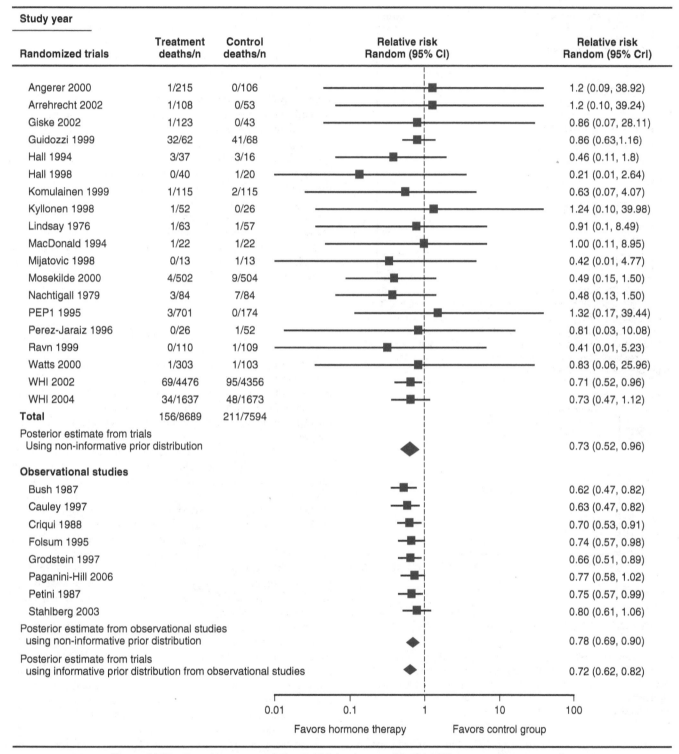

| Randomized trials | Treatment deaths/n | Control deaths/n | Relative risk Random (95% CrI) |
|---|---|---|---|
| Angerer 2000 | 1/215 | 0/106 | 1.2 (0.09, 38.92) |
| Arrehrecht 2002 | 1/108 | 0/53 | 1.2 (0.10, 39.24) |
| Giske 2002 | 1/123 | 0/43 | 0.86 (0.07, 28.11) |
| Guidozzi 1999 | 32/62 | 41/68 | 0.86 (0.63,1.16) |
| Hall 1994 | 3/37 | 3/16 | 0.46 (0.11, 1.8) |
| Hall 1998 | 0/40 | 1/20 | 0.21 (0.01, 2.64) |
| Komulainen 1999 | 1/115 | 2/115 | 0.63 (0.07, 4.07) |
| Kyllonen 1998 | 1/52 | 0/26 | 1.24 (0.10, 39.98) |
| Lindsay 1976 | 1/63 | 1/57 | 0.91 (0.1, 8.49) |
| MacDonald 1994 | 1/22 | 1/22 | 1.00 (0.11, 8.95) |
| Mijatovic 1998 | 0/13 | 1/13 | 0.42 (0.01, 4.77) |
| Mosekilde 2000 | 4/502 | 9/504 | 0.49 (0.15, 1.50) |
| Nachtigall 1979 | 3/84 | 7/84 | 0.48 (0.13, 1.50) |
| PEP1 1995 | 3/701 | 0/174 | 1.32 (0.17, 39.44) |
| Perez-Jaraiz 1996 | 0/26 | 1/52 | 0.81 (0.03, 10.08) |
| Ravn 1999 | 0/110 | 1/109 | 0.41 (0.01, 5.23) |
| Watts 2000 | 1/303 | 1/103 | 0.83 (0.06, 25.96) |
| WHI 2002 | 69/4476 | 95/4356 | 0.71 (0.52, 0.96) |
| WHI 2004 | 34/1637 | 48/1673 | 0.73 (0.47, 1.12) |
| **Total** | 156/8689 | 211/7594 | |
| Posterior estimate from trials Using non-informative prior distribution | | | 0.73 (0.52, 0.96) |
| **Observational studies** | | | |
| Bush 1987 | | | 0.62 (0.47, 0.82) |
| Cauley 1997 | | | 0.63 (0.47, 0.82) |
| Criqui 1988 | | | 0.70 (0.53, 0.91) |
| Folsum 1995 | | | 0.74 (0.57, 0.98) |
| Grodstein 1997 | | | 0.66 (0.51, 0.89) |
| Paganini-Hill 2006 | | | 0.77 (0.58, 1.02) |
| Petini 1987 | | | 0.75 (0.57, 0.99) |
| Stahlberg 2003 | | | 0.80 (0.61, 1.06) |
| Posterior estimate from observational studies using non-informative prior distribution | | | 0.78 (0.69, 0.90) |
| Posterior estimate from trials using informative prior distribution from observational studies | | | 0.72 (0.62, 0.82) |

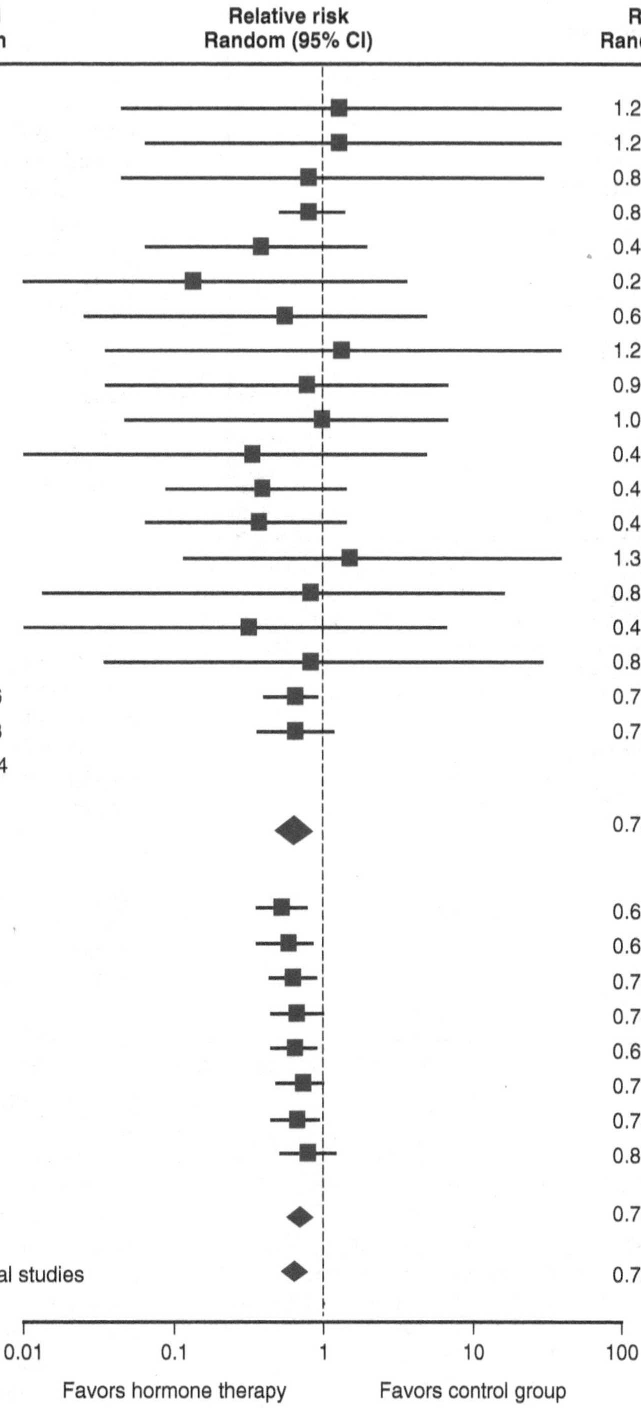


**Figure 14.31** Bayesian meta-analysis of reduction in mortality with HT in younger women. (Modified from Salpeter SR, Cheng J, Thabane L, et al. Bayesian meta-analysis of hormone therapy and mortality in younger postmenopausal women. *Am J Med.* 2009;122[11]:1016-1022.)

age, weight, dose, and route of administration of estrogen. It has also been suggested that some progestogens increase this risk further, although this has not been established. Most events (deep vein thrombosis or pulmonary emboli) occur early (within the first year) and decrease thereafter, suggesting an aberrant thrombophilic interaction with oral estrogen. The risk has been found not to be increased with transdermal estrogen (Canonico, 2008) (Fig. 14.34), which warrants consideration of the use of transdermal therapy in more high-risk women (e.g., obesity, hypertension).

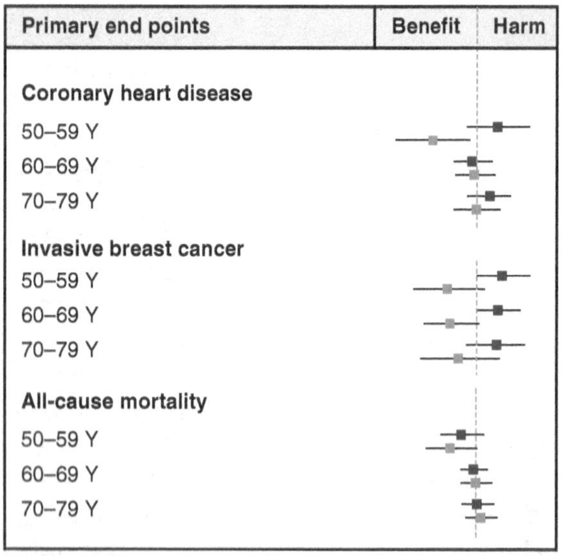


**Figure 14.32** Cumulative 13-year follow-up data, intervention and follow-up phases with CEE and CEE/MPA arms of the WHI in different age groups *(CEE, light blue; CEE/MPA, dark blue)*. (Modified from Manson JE, Chlebowski RT, Stefanick ML, et al: Menopausal hormone therapy and health outcomes during the intervention and extended poststopping phases of the Women's Health Initiative randomized trials. *JAMA* 310[13]:1353-1368, 2013.)

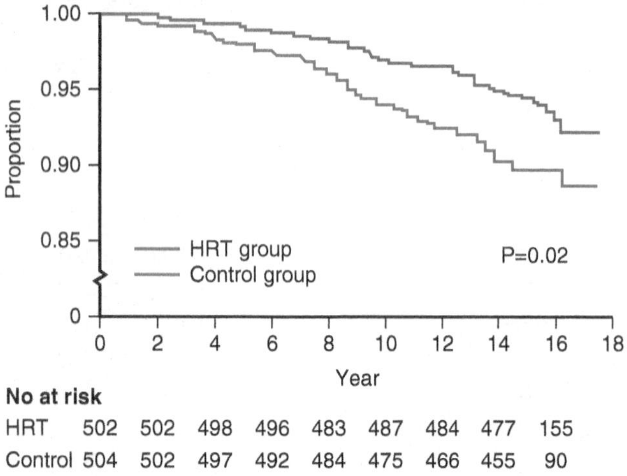


**Figure 14.33** Sixteen-year follow-up of women randomized to hormone therapy (HT) showing a reduction in death, heart failure, and myocardial infarction (MI). (Modified from Schierbeck IL, Renmark L, Tofteng CL, et al. Effect of hormone replacement therapy on cardiovascular events in recently postmenopausal women: randomized trial. *BMJ*. 2012;345:e6409.)

Stroke (ischemic, not hemorrhagic) was found to be increased in the WHI trials (both HT and Estrogen Therapy [ET]). There was an approximately 30% increase over the 5 to 6 years of the trial, but this outcome was confined primarily to older women in the trial. These data are similar to data from the NHS trial where even younger women had a very small but statistically increased risk of ischemic stroke with standard doses of oral estrogen. The increase in younger women is extremely small and may not be statistically significant. In the 13-year follow-up data from WHI (Manson, 2013) and in the Cochrane review, (Boardman, 2015), stroke was not significantly increased in the younger age groups. Thus, although a rare event, ischemic stroke risk may be increased in women taking standard doses of oral estrogen (women using CEE at 0.625 mg or more) but not with lower doses (e.g., CEE 0.3 mg). Similarly, transdermal therapy has not been associated with an increased risk. These and other data point to a thrombotic risk with oral estrogen (in susceptible women). The mechanism of ischemic stroke risk in younger women is not likely to be due to atherosclerosis as it is in coronary disease in older women but is due to acute thrombosis (Lobo, 2011) (Fig. 14.35). The thrombosis risk in younger women, much like the risk of venous thrombosis, is likely due to an aberrant interaction of estrogen with thrombotic factors, at times due to an underlying thrombophilia.

In summary, there should be no concern regarding increased cardiovascular risk for young, healthy women at the onset of menopause who are contemplating HT for treatment of symptoms. In this setting there is no evidence of increased risk, and, indeed, these women may be found to benefit from a cardiovascular standpoint.

## CANCER RISKS IN POSTMENOPAUSAL WOMEN

Just as CVD is a concern for women after menopause, the risk of cancer also increases with time after menopause, but this is a function of aging and not as a consequence of menopause per se. *Prevention* requires healthy lifestyle measures and screening for early detection, which will be emphasized again later in the chapter.

Although breast cancer is generally believed to be the leading cause of death in postmenopausal women, in fact it is lung cancer. Indeed, mortality from breast cancer tends to decrease after menopause, on an age-specific basis, but cardiovascular mortality increases, and these lines transect around the time of menopause (Fig. 14.36). The gynecologist should be well versed in the epidemiology and preventive strategies for breast, lung, cervical, endometrial, ovarian, and colorectal cancer. Further discussions of these cancers may be found in Part IV (Gynecologic Oncology) of this text. What follows is the potential effects of ET and HT on endometrial, breast, ovarian, and colorectal cancer.

**Endometrial cancer** is a common cancer in postmenopausal women and is increased in women using **unopposed estrogen therapy**. Although a woman's risk for endometrial cancer with unopposed estrogen use is two to eightfold higher than that for the general population, precursor lesions (primarily endometrial hyperplasia) signal the presence of an abnormality in most patients, and the cancer is usually well differentiated and hormonally responsive, as are hyperplasias.

One study showed that the risk of endometrial hyperplasia was 20% after 1 year of using 0.625 mg of oral CEE. In another study, the 3-year postmenopausal Estrogen/Progestin Interventions Trial, this risk of hyperplasia was approximately 40% at the end of 3 years. No cancers were reported in either of these two studies, and the addition of a progestogen essentially eliminated the hyperplasia risk. Use of CEE alone at 0.3 mg/day for 2 to 3 years results in a hyperplasia risk of 5% to 10%. With the same dose of esterified estrogens (which is less potent), no hyperplasia was found after 2 years.

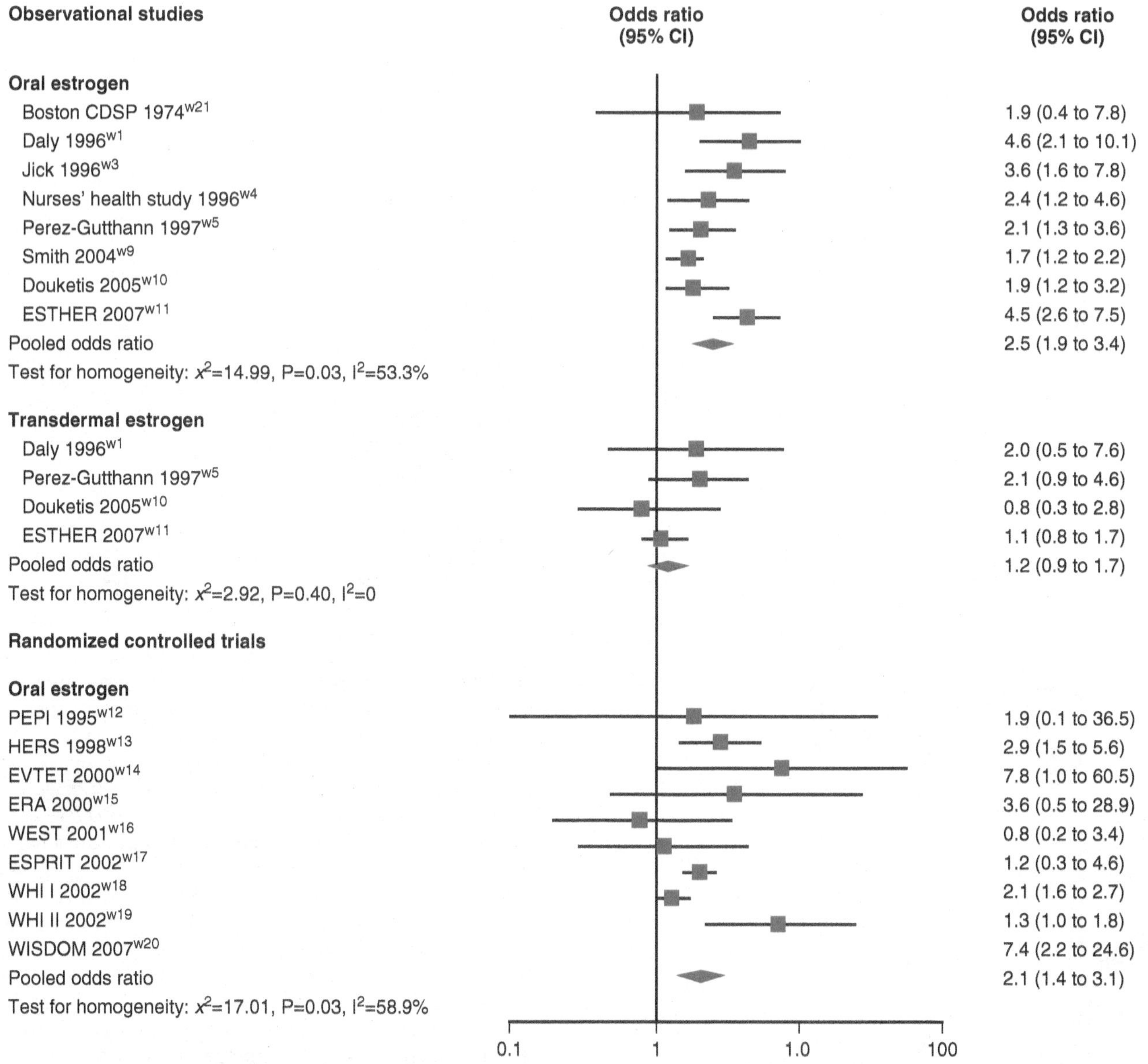


**Figure 14.34** Meta-analysis of various studies showing no increased risk of thrombosis with transdermal therapy. (Modified from Canonico M, Plu-Bureau G, Lowe GD, et al. Hormone replacement therapy and risk of venous thromboembolism in postmenopausal women: systematic review and meta-analysis. *BMJ*. 2008;336[7655]:1227-1231.)

The risk for endometrial cancer in women taking estrogen and progestogen is similar to that of women in the general population because combination therapy merely eliminates the excess risk attributed to estrogen; a few studies, however, have suggested a lower risk of endometrial cancer with **continuous combined hormone treatment**. It is important to remember that some endometrial cancers occurring in postmenopausal women are not hormonally related; thus some women may develop a serous type of cancer (poorly differentiated) while on HT, making continuous surveillance important. It could be argued that these serous cancers, which are usually receptor negative, may have arisen independently of HT use.

Although the risk for endometrial cancer is increased substantially in estrogen users, the risk of death from this type of endometrial cancer does not increase proportionately. Endometrial cancers associated with estrogen use are thought to be less aggressive than spontaneously occurring cancers, in part because tumors in women taking estrogen are more likely to be discovered and treated at an earlier stage, thus improving survival rates.

## RISK OF BREAST CANCER WITH ESTROGEN USE

Several studies and meta-analyses have shown a borderline or small statistical increase in the risk of breast cancer (relative risk [RR] 1.2 to 1.4) after approximately 5 years of estrogen use. This risk is related to the dose of estrogen, as well as duration of use. Data have pointed to the addition of progestogen as a major contributor to this increased risk of breast

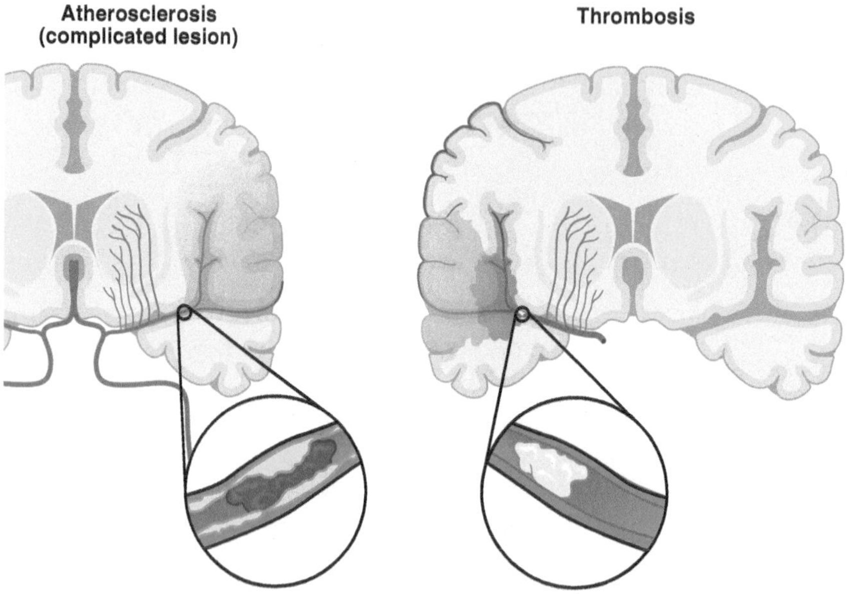


**Figure 14.35** Mechanisms of ischemic stroke risk with estrogen in older women due to atherosclerosis with complicated lesions *(left)* and due to thrombosis in younger women *(right).*

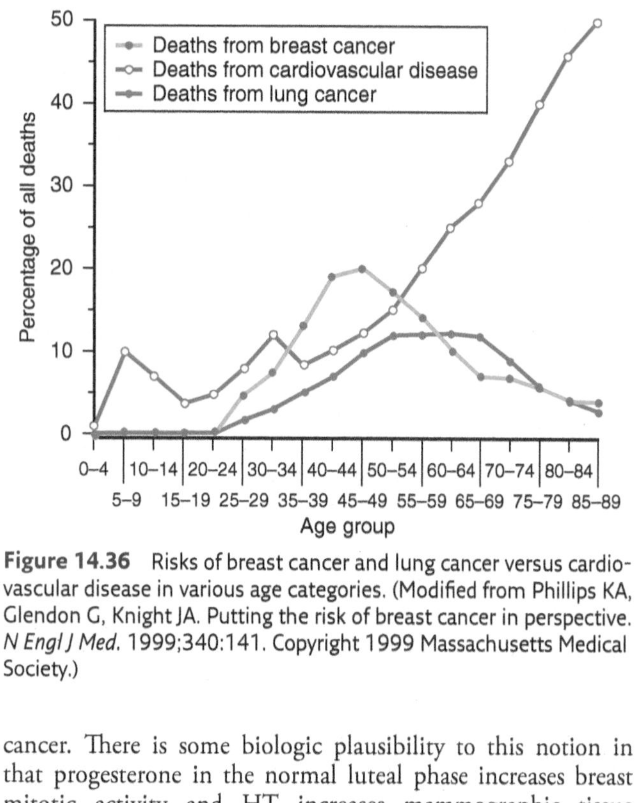


**Figure 14.36** Risks of breast cancer and lung cancer versus cardiovascular disease in various age categories. (Modified from Phillips KA, Glendon G, Knight JA. Putting the risk of breast cancer in perspective. *N Engl J Med.* 1999;340:141. Copyright 1999 Massachusetts Medical Society.)

cancer. There is some biologic plausibility to this notion in that progesterone in the normal luteal phase increases breast mitotic activity and HT increases mammographic tissue density relative to ET alone. Several small case-control studies found no increase with ET alone, but the same studies showed a statistically significant increase with progestogen use (in the range of 1.3 or 1.4 RR). In the WHI trial, the increase in breast cancer risk was of borderline significance with CEE/MPA (hazard ratio [HR] 1.24, 1.01 to 1.54). A reanalysis by Anderson and coworkers found that when correcting for variables known to affect breast cancer risk, the average risk was no longer statistically significant: 1.20 (0.94 to 1.53) (Anderson, 2006). It is important to note that the total duration of therapy is very important for the risk with estrogen/progestogen therapy. In WHI the significant increase over 5 years was only found in prior users of HT, suggesting a longer cumulative effect. *There was no statistical increase over 5 years with CEE/MPA in women in WHI who had not used HT in the past* (Anderson, 2006). A large collaborative case-control study also has shown that continuous combined estrogen-progestogen therapy is associated with increased breast cancer risk over time.

The effect of estrogen/progestogen therapy and breast cancer risk is thought to be one of promotion, rather than carcinogenesis per se. Occult breast tumors are extremely common in breast tissue and take up to 10 years of slow growth to be clinically detectable. It has been suggested that certain doses of estrogen, and particularly with estrogen/progestogen therapy, stimulate the growth of these occult receptor positive tumors, which shortens the time to clinical detection, thus allowing them to be recognized as a consequence of HT. Modeling of growth kinetics by Santen and applying these numbers to findings in WHI lend credence to this notion (Santen, 2012).

In the estrogen-only arm of WHI, after 6½ years there was a *decrease* in breast cancer risk of borderline significance HR = 0.77 (0.59 to 1.01). In a more complete analysis of these findings, Stefanick and associates found the risk to be significantly decreased for ductal cancer (0.71 [0.52 to 0.99]), and in a sensitivity analysis among adherent women, the decrease was statistically significant (0.67 [0.47 to 0.9]) (Stefanick, 2006) (Fig. 14.37). Thus, although it is unclear why there should be a decrease in breast cancer risk, we may conclude that standard dose ET (0.625 mg CEE) is not associated with a risk of breast cancer except for very long-term users. In an analysis from the NHS, Chen and colleagues found that this risk only increases significantly after 20 years (Table 14.5). This risk is predominantly seen in lean women because overweight/obese women already have an increased risk of breast cancer, which is not further increased. A theory proposed by Jordan has suggested that the decrease in risk is confined to women who did not receive hormones immediately after menopause, but some time later. The theory suggests that this lag allowed the occult breast cancers to undergo apoptosis when later exposed to estrogen, thus decreasing the risk of breast cancer (Jordan, 2015).

Putting these risks into perspective is important for patient counseling. The background risk for breast cancer in a woman between the ages of 50 and 60 is 2.8/100 women. According to data from the WHI, the overall risk for women taking CEE/MPA for 5 years was approximately a relative risk of 1.24. Note that this applies to women who had also used hormones in the past, as noted earlier. This 24% increase translates into an overall risk of 3.47/100 women, less than 1% above the background risk. This risk is expected to be even lower with different regimens including lower dose therapy, and potentially with different progestogens, such as natural progesterone, which has been shown in observational studies not to increase the risk. A relative risk of 1.24 for breast cancer is less than that for obesity alone (3.3) or for being a flight attendant (1.87) because of the increase in cosmic radiation. Furthermore, for estrogen alone, there is probably no increased risk at moderate to low doses for up to 20 years of exposure, as noted by Chen and colleagues. The risk of breast cancer is much higher with certain endogenous risk factors such as obesity and increased breast density than it is with any type of HT (Fig. 14.38).

With some exceptions in the literature, most reports have shown that the mortality rate in users of ET/HT is improved compared with those women not receiving hormones who are diagnosed with breast cancer. Figure 14.39 depicts the 10-year follow-up data from WHI with women receiving CEE alone; both breast cancer mortality and total mortality were reduced in users of estrogen (Anderson, 2012). It should be appreciated that women receiving HT are likely to have (and should have) closer surveillance (exams and mammography); accordingly, most tumors, if they occur, will be detected are at an early stage.

Family history and genetic mutations (*BRCA* 1 and 2, etc.) substantially increase the risk of a woman developing breast cancer. However, the literature suggests that the use of HT does not increase this risk further. Nevertheless, for many women it is unacceptable to consider a potentially promotional effect of using HT, and they may opt for risk reduction strategies such as the use of tamoxifen or other SERMs.

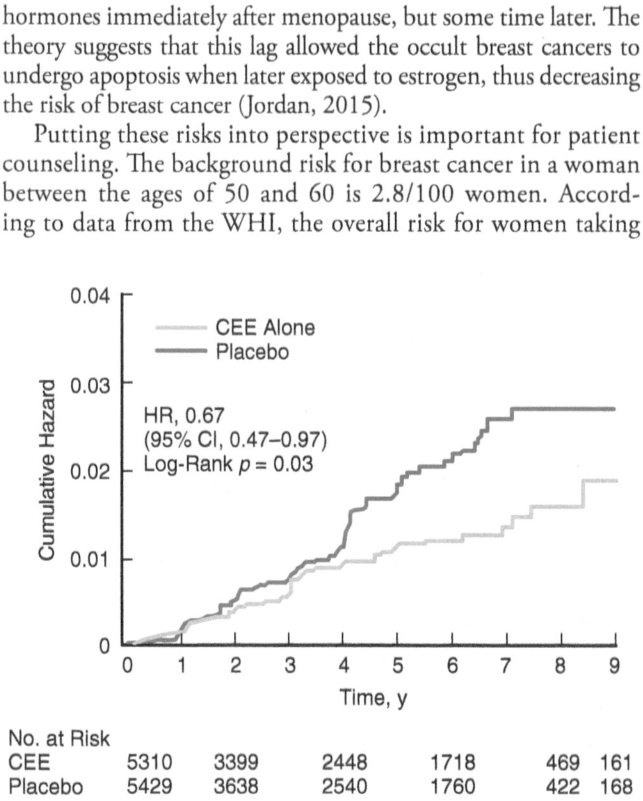


**Figure 14.37** Cumulative hazard for invasive breast cancer: sensitivity analysis. *CEE*, Conjugated equine estrogen; *CI*, confidence interval; *HR*, hazard ratio. (From Stefanick ML, Anderson GL, Margolis KL, et al. Effects of conjugated equine estrogens on breast cancer and mammography screening in postmenopausal women with hysterectomy. *JAMA*. 2006;295:1647.)

**Table 14.5** Risk of Invasive Breast Cancer by Duration of ET Use among All Postmenopausal Women Who Had Undergone Hysterectomy and Those with ER+/PR + Cancer Only*

| ET Use and Duration (Years) | All Postmenopausal Women Who Had Undergone Hysterectomy | | | | ER+/PR + Cancers Only | | | |
|---|---|---|---|---|---|---|---|---|
| | All | | Screened Cohort† | | All | | Screened Cohort† | |
| | *Cases* | *Risk* | *Cases* | *Risk* | *Cases* | *Risk* | *Cases* | *Risk* |
| Never | 226 | 1.00 | 104 | 1.00 | 87 | 1.00 | 48 | 1.00 |
| Current | | | | | | | | |
| <5 | 99 | 0.96 (0.75-1.22) | 59 | 1.06 (0.76-1.47) | 38 | 1.00 (0.67-1.49) | 26 | 1.04 (0.64-1.70) |
| 5-9.9 | 145 | 0.90 (0.73-1.12) | 95 | 0.91 (0.68-1.21) | 70 | 1.19 (0.86-1.66) | 50 | 1.08 (0.72-1.62) |
| 10-14.9 | 190 | 1.06 (0.87-1.30) | 141 | 1.11 (0.85-1.44) | 85 | 1.27 (0.93-1.73) | 77 | 1.29 (0.89-1.86) |
| 15-19.9 | 129 | 1.18 (0.95-1.48) | 95 | 1.19 (0.89-1.58) | 61 | 1.48 (1.05-2.07) | 58 | 1.50 (1.02-2.21) |
| ≥ 20 | 145 | 1.42 (1.13-1.77) | 127 | 1.58 (1.20-2.07) | 69 | 1.73 (1.24-2.43) | 74 | 1.83 (1.25-2.68) |
| *p* for trend for current use | | <0.001 | | <0.001 | | <0.001 | | <0.001 |

From Chen WY, Manson JE, Hankinson SE, et al. Unopposed estrogen therapy and the risk of invasive breast cancer. *Arch Intern Med*. 2006;166:1027.

*All cases are reported as number of cases; risks are reported as multivariate relative risk (95% CI), controlled for age (continuous), age at menopause (continuous), age at menarche (continuous), BMI (quintiles), history of benign breast disease (yes or no), family history of breast cancer in first-degree relative (yes or no), average daily alcohol consumption (0, 0.5-5, 5-10, 10-20, or ≥20 g/day), parity/age at first birth (nulliparous; 1-2 children and age at first birth ≤22 years; 1-2 children and age at first birth 23-25 years; 1-2 children and age at first birth 25 years; ≥3 children and age at first birth ≤22 years; ≥3 children and age at first birth 23-25 years; ≥3 children and age at 1st birth >25 years).

†Screened cohort defined as those women starting in 1988 who reported either a screening mammogram or clinical breast examination in the previous 2 years. All cases before 1988 are excluded.

*BMI*, Body mass index; *CI*, confidence interval; *ER+/PR+*, positive for both estrogen and progesterone receptors; *ET*, unopposed estrogen therapy.

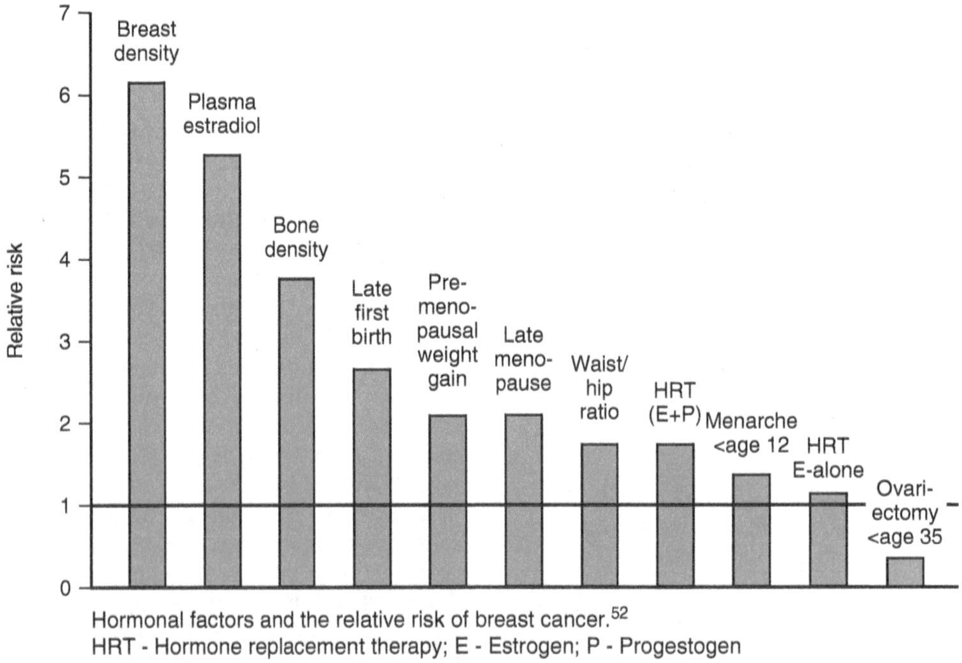


**Figure 14.38** Risks of breast cancer with various exposures and endogenous traits, particularly increased breast density. (Modified from Gompel A, Santen RJ: Hormone therapy and breast cancer risk 10 years after the WHI. *Climacteric.* 2012;15[3]:241-249.)

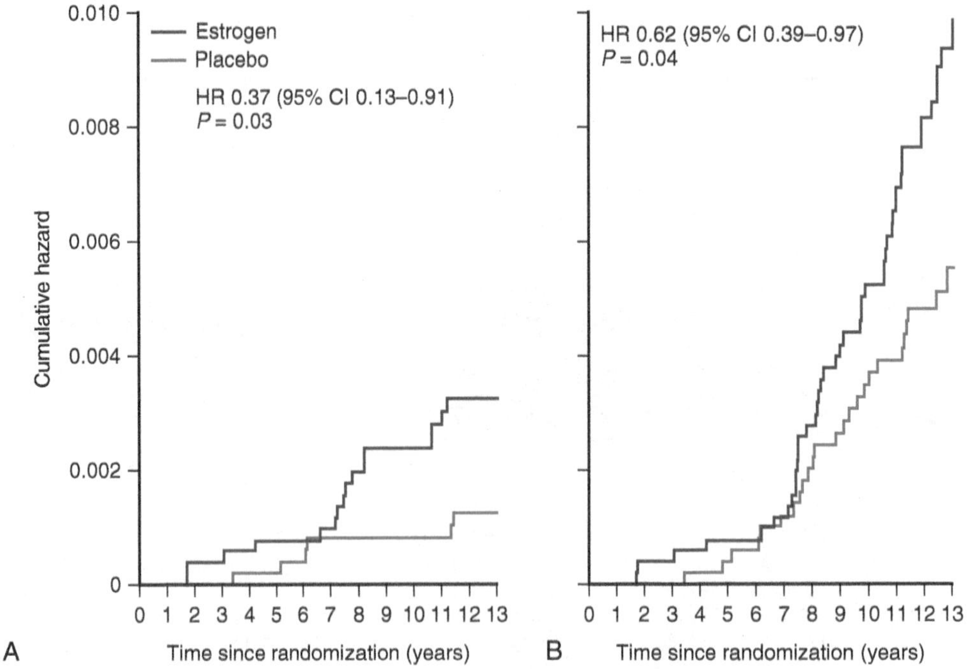


**Figure 14.39** In women with breast cancer, women taking $E_2$ had significantly reduced mortality; breast cancer (**A**) and total (**B**). (Modified from Anderson GL, Chlebowski RT, Aragaki AK, et al. Conjugated equine oestrogen and breast cancer incidence and mortality in postmenopausal women with hysterectomy: extended follow-up of the Women's Health Initiative randomized placebo-controlled trial. *Lancet Oncol.* 2012;13[5]:476-486.)

If there is a concern regarding hormones and breast cancer, it is with larger doses, a longer duration, and specifically the use of a progestogen. Accordingly, for longer-term therapy, if warranted (>5 years) lower doses of estrogen should be used, and progestogen exposure should be minimized.

### OVARIAN CANCER

Several studies have suggested an increased risk of ovarian cancer with long-duration use of ET/HT. However, the data are inconsistent, and the purported risk is less than a twofold relative risk. Prospective randomized trials such as WHI have found no statistical increase in risk. The most recent meta-analysis suggested a modest risk of 30% to 40% (Collaborative Group, 2015). In this analysis it is unclear if adequate attention was paid to confounders, and there was no association with length of exposure regarding risk, which does not make sense physiologically. Further, estrogen and estrogen/progestogens both carried some risk, whereas use of oral contraceptives are known to decrease ovarian cancer risk. According to this meta-analysis, the risk was calculated to be approximately 1 extra case of ovarian cancer per 1000 women over 5 years, which suggests if this association is real, it is extremely rare.

### COLORECTAL CANCER

The third most frequent cancer in women, colorectal cancer, is often preventable by the detection and treatment of polyps. Women older than 50 should have a colorectal evaluation by some means (detection of occult blood, sigmoidoscopy, or a colonoscopy). Data have been fairly consistent for a reduction in risk with the use of HT/ET. Several meta-analyses have shown an approximate 33% decrease in risk, as did the observational data from the NHS and the prospective randomized trial data of the CEE/MPA arm of WHI. It is unclear why in the ET arm of WHI, a decrease was not observed. No definitive mechanism for this protective effect has been found, although several theories have been advanced (changes in the composition of bile acids, anti-inflammatory effects, etc.).

### OTHER CANCERS

There has been more attention paid to lung cancer recently, in part because it is the leading cause of cancer mortality in women. The data on HT, however, has not been consistent and is without convincing evidence of any risk of lung cancer with HT use.

## CONCEPT OF DISEASE PREVENTION AFTER MENOPAUSE

*Since all major diseases such as CVD, obesity, and metabolic diseases, particularly diabetes, cancer, cognitive decline and Alzheimer's increase after menopause, menopause itself heralds an important opportunity to screen for, and prevent many of these problems (Lobo, Prevention of disease after menopause, 2014).*

Details of this approach may be found in the review cited, but in essence stresses the introduction of screening procedures for these disorders and then beginning prevention strategies such as prescribing diet and exercise regimens and the consideration of hormone therapy. Primary strategies for the prevention of CVD in men, such as statins and aspirin, have not been shown to be of benefit in women (Hodis, 2013). Thus, apart from lifestyle measures, there are no good prevention strategies for women, with the possible exception of HT. As discussed previously, in a young healthy population of women close to menopause, estrogen-based therapy has been shown to significantly decrease coronary disease and mortality, with minimal to rare risks of adverse outcomes. As Figure 14.30 shows, the use of HT was considered for prevention until the time of the various secondary prevention trials (such as the Heart and Estrogen/Progestin Replacement Study [HERS]) and then WHI, and this concept is now being reconsidered but remains controversial. Table 14.6 lists a compilation of several studies and meta-analyses that are remarkably consistent in showing a reduction in mortality in younger women receiving estrogen after menopause, which strengthens the argument of using estrogen for prevention.

Using a conservative approach fostered by the early reports of "early harm" in older women taking standard doses of CEE/MPA in secondary prevention trials or the older women in WHI, it has been suggested that women have a cardiovascular risk assessment prior to initiating HT. The American Heart Association (www.heart.org) offers an easy-to-use, rapid risk assessment calculator, which defines women at low risk if they have a <7.5% chance of sustaining a myocardial infarction in 10 years. Although some investigators have questioned the validity of this approach, risk assessment is not an unreasonable course in general, along the lines of stressing the need for *prevention* after menopause. Because most of the CV-related risks of HT relate to oral therapy, "higher" risk women may benefit more by being placed on transdermal estrogen.

In summary, apart from the need to screen carefully for all diseases at the onset of menopause, and stressing healthy lifestyle measures, the decision to initiate HT should be straightforward in symptomatic women who will benefit more in terms of absolute

**Table 14.6** Consistency in the Reduction in All-Cause Mortality in Younger Women Receiving Estrogen at the Onset of Menopause

| Study | Point Estimate (Relative Risk) |
|---|---|
| Observational meta-analysis | 0.78 (0.69-0.90)* |
| Randomized trials meta-analysis | 0.73 (0.52-0.96)* |
| Bayesian | 0.72 (0.62-0.82)* |
| WHI combined groups | 0.70 (0.62-0.82)† |
| WHI 13-year cumulative CEE | 0.78 (0.59-1.03)‡ |
| WHI 13-year cumulative CEE/MPA | 0.88 (0.70-1.1)‡ |
| Cochrane meta-analysis | 0.70 (0.52-0.95)§ |
| Finnish registry data (pre-WHI) | 0.57 (0.48-0.66)‖ |
| Finnish registry data (post-WHI) | 0.46 (0.32-0.64)‖ |

*Salpeter SR, Cheng J, Thabane L, et al. Bayesian meta-analysis of hormone therapy and mortality in younger postmenopausal women. *Am J Med.* 2009; 122(11):1016-1022.
†Rossouw JE, Prentice RL, Manson JE, et al. Postmenopausal hormone therapy and cardiovascular disease by age and years since menopause. *JAMA.* 2007;297(13):1465-1477.
‡Manson JE, Chlebowski RT, Stefanick ML, et al. Menopausal hormone therapy and health outcomes during the intervention and extended poststopping phases of the Women's Health Initiative randomized trials. *JAMA.* 2013;310:1353-1368.
§Boardman HMP, Hartley L, Main C, et al. Hormone therapy for preventing cardiovascular disease in post-menopausal women (review). *Cochrane Database Syst Rev.* 3:CD002229, 2015.
‖Tuomikoski P, Lyytinen H, Korhonen P, et al. Coronary heart disease mortality and hormone therapy before and after the Women's Health Initiative. *Obstet Gynecol.* 2014;124: 947-953. (Coronary mortality including all women but with similar point estimates as in women <60 years.)

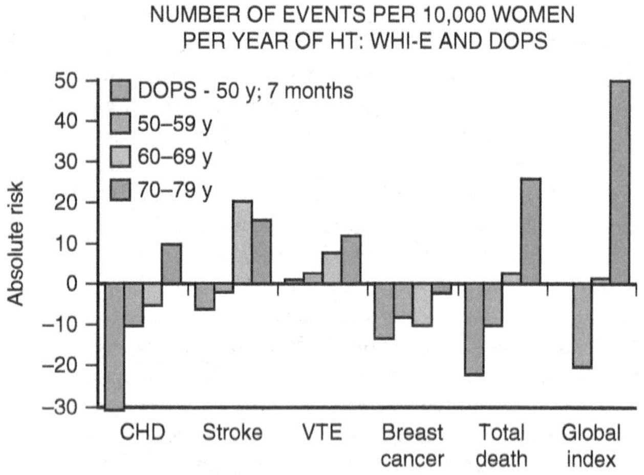


**Figure 14.40** Absolute risks in younger women receiving estrogen based on studies from the WHI (Manson, 2013), and DOPS (Schierbeck, 2012). (Courtesy of Howard Hodis, 2015.)

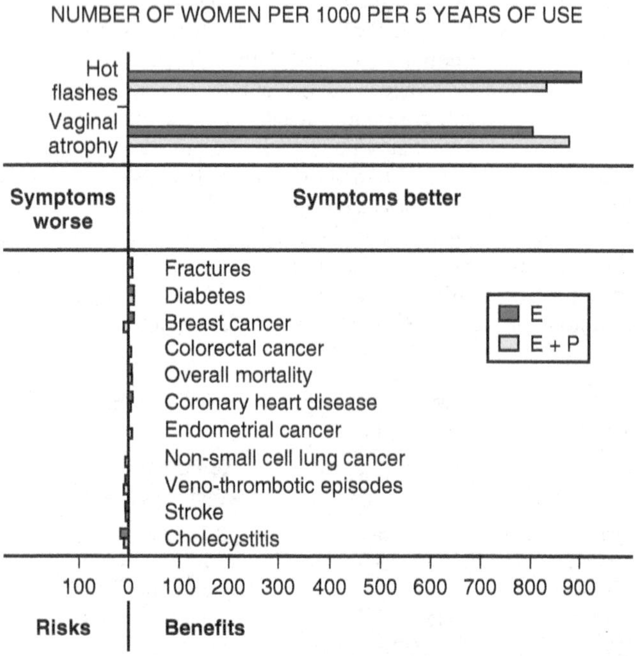


**Figure 14.41** Putting risks and benefits in perspective for the 50- to 59-year-old. (Modified from Santen R. Endocrine Society position paper. *J Clin Endocrinol Metab.* 2010;95[7 Suppl 1]:s1-s66.)

numbers of women affected by treatment (see Figure 14.41). Figure 14.40, generated from newer data and data from WHI in the 50- to 59-year-old age group, shows the absolute benefits and risks associated with the use of estrogen, strongly emphasizing benefits. However, when these absolute numbers are compared with the benefit of the reduction in hot flushes in women receiving estrogen, the latter appears to be the predominant effect (Fig. 14.41). The decision to use HT at the onset of menopause probably applies for women who are at greater risk for osteoporosis as well, based on family history and their physical characteristics. Otherwise, it is not unreasonable to consider HT in otherwise healthy women with adequate counseling and discussion of the risks and benefits. This should be an individual decision. For some women, the fear of breast cancer, particularly in those with some family history of the disease, will overshadow any potential benefits, and this view has to be respected. Women who decide to initiate HT should be made aware that this need not be a long commitment, and therapy should be reassessed annually based on needs and symptoms.

Finally, the data to date regarding protection are strongest for the use of estrogen; certain progestogens may eliminate or attenuate the benefit, and some progestogens increase the promotional risk of breast cancer. Philosophically, therefore, HT should be about using the lowest amount of a progestogen necessary to prevent endometrial disease.

## HORMONE REGIMENS

The various hormonal preparations available for treatment are listed in Box 14.3. A more complete list may be found in the Consumer section of the North American Menopause Society website at www.menopause.org. Also included are the SERMs raloxifene, bazedoxifene, and other compounds like bisphosphonates, tibolone, and human parathyroid hormone. For the clinician and patient, as noted earlier, the decision to start estrogen therapy need not involve a long-term commitment. For short-term treatment of symptoms, estrogen should be used at the lowest dose that can control hot flushes or can be administered via the vaginal route for symptoms of dryness or dyspareunia. There are no definitive data on what doses are necessary for CV protection, but whereas low doses of estrogen may be sufficient to prevent bone loss (discussed earlier) the doses necessary to afford CV protection may have to be a bit higher, although there are no data to this point in women. Therefore, lower doses are still recommended, which are sufficient for symptom control.

Oral estrogen results in higher levels of estrone ($E_1$) than estradiol ($E_2$); this is true for oral micronized $E_2$ as well as $E_1$ products. CEE is a mixture of at least 10 conjugated estrogens derived from equine pregnant urine. Estrone sulfate is the major component, but the biologic activities of equilin, 17α-dihydroequilin, and several other B-ring unsaturated estrogens, including δ5 dehydroestrone, have been documented. Table 14.7 compares the standard doses of the most frequently prescribed oral estrogens and the levels of $E_1$ and $E_2$ achieved. Much of the following clinical information may be found in systematic reviews.

Synthetic estrogens, given orally, are more potent than natural $E_2$. Ethinyl estradiol is used in oral contraceptives, with a dose of 5 μg being equivalent to the standard ET doses used (0.625 mg CEE or 1 mg micronized $E_2$). Standard ET doses are five or six times less than the amount of estrogen used in oral contraceptives. Although there are incomplete data available to compare the equivalencies of CEE and micronized estradiol (because of different end organ effects and the mixture of estrogens in CEE, which are difficult to measure), 0.625 mg CEE is probably equivalent to 1.5 mg of micronized $E_2$. Oral estrogens have a potent hepatic "first-pass" effect that results in the loss of approximately 30% of their activity with a single passage after oral administration. However, this results in stimulation of hepatic proteins and enzymes. Some of these changes are not particularly beneficial (e.g., an increase in procoagulation factors and an increase in C-reactive protein), whereas other changes are beneficial (an increase in HDL-C and a decrease in fibrinogen and plasminogen activator inhibitor-1).

$E_2$ can be administered in patches, gels, lotions, sprays, and subcutaneously. These routes of administration are not subject to

**Box 14.3 Hormonal and Osteoporosis Treatments: Available and Approved for Use in Postmenopausal Women**

**Estrogens**

**Oral**

CEE, 0.3, 0.45, 0.625, 0.9, 1.25, and 2.5 mg
Piperazine estrone sulfate, equivalent of 0.625, 1.25, and 2.5 mg
Esterified, 0.3, 0.625, 0.9, 1.25, and 2.5 mg
Micronized estradiol, 0.5, 1, and 2 mg

**Transdermal**

Estradiol patches, 0.014, 0.025, 0.0375, 0.05, 0.75, and 0.10 mg/d
Estradiol gels, 0.25 to 1.5 mg/day various brands
Estradiol spray, 1.53 mg/day

**Vaginal**

Cream, CEE (0.0625%), estradiol (0.01%)
Estradiol ring, 2 mg; vaginal tablets, 10 μg
Estradiol acetate ring for vasomotor symptoms: 50-100 μg/day for 3 months

**Parenteral**

Intramuscular injections should be avoided

**Progestins**

**Oral**

Medroxyprogesterone acetate, 2.5, 5, and 10 mg
Norethindrone acetate, 5 mg
Micronized progesterone, 100 and 200 mg

**Vaginal**

Micronized progesterone, 100 mg
Progesterone gel, 4% and 8%

**Combinations**

**Oral**

CEE + MPA (0.625 mg) + MPA (2.5 or 5 mg)
CEE + MPA (0.3 mg + MPA, 1.5 mg)
Micronized estradiol (1 mg) + norethindrone, acetate (0.5 mg)
Micronized estradiol (1 mg) + 0.5 mg drospirenone
Ethinyl estradiol 5 μg, norethindrone, 1 mg
CEE+ Bazedoxifene (SERM), 0.45 + 20 mg/day

**Transdermal**

Patch, 0.05 mg estradiol with 140 μg or 250 μg norethindrone acetate
Patch, 0.045 mg estradiol with levonorgestrel 0.05 mg

**Androgens**

**Oral**

Esterified estrogen and methyl testosterone (0.625/1.25 mg and 1.25/2.5 mg)

**Transdermal**

Patch, 150 μg/300 μg approved outside of US

**Other Nonhormonal Products**

Ospemifene (SERM), 60 mg/day for vulvovaginal atrophy
Paroxetine (SSRI), 7.5 mg/day for vasomotor symptoms

**Medications for Osteoporosis**

**Bisphosphonates**

Alendronate, 5 and 10 mg daily; 35 and 70 mg weekly
Risedronate, 5 mg; 35 mg weekly
Ibandronate, 150 mg monthly and 3l mg IV every 3 months
Zoledronic acid 5 mg once/yr
Etidronate, 200 mg (intermittent)

**Selective Estrogen Receptor Modulators (SERMs)**

Raloxifene, 60 mg

**Others for Osteoporosis**

Tibolone, 2.5 mg (not approved in the United States)
Denosumab, 60 mg subcutaneously every 6 months
Human parathyroid hormone 1-34; 20 μg subcutaneously daily

*CEE*, Conjugated equine estrogens; *MPA*, medroxyprogesterone acetate.

major hepatic effects as with oral therapy. Accordingly, there is no increase in C-reaction protein and minimal if any change in coagulation factors, but there is also only a minimal increase in HDL-C. Doses of patches are available from 0.014 mg to 0.1 mg, available for administration once or twice weekly. The ultralow-dose patch of 0.014 mg/day has been marketed for osteoporosis prevention in older women and not for treating hot flushes. Matrix patches are preferable to the older alcohol-based preparations because there is less skin reaction and estrogen delivery is more reliable. Whereas levels of $E_2$ with oral therapy may vary widely among women and within the day (peaks and valleys), levels with transdermal therapy are more constant within each woman, yet values achieved may vary from woman to woman based on absorption and metabolic characteristics. With the 0.05-mg patch, $E_2$ levels should be in the 40- to 50-pg/mL range, but an occasional woman can have values as high as 200 pg/mL or levels that are <20 pg/mL. Note also that many commercial assays for $E_2$ are not reliable and do not accurately reflect estradiol status; this is particularly the case after oral estrogen therapy, because of the increase in estrogen conjugates, which interfere with many commercial assays.

In women with vulvovaginal or urinary complaints, vaginal therapy is most appropriate. Creams of $E_2$ or CEE are available, as well as tablets and an estrogen ring. With creams, systemic absorption occurs but with levels that are one fourth of that achieved after similar doses administered orally. Absorption decreases as the mucosa becomes more estrogenized. For CEE, only 0.5 g (0.3 mg) or less is necessary; for micronized $E_2$, doses as low as 0.25 mg are sufficient. Other products (tablets and rings) are available that have been designed to limit systemic absorption. A Silastic ring is available that delivers $E_2$ to the vagina for 3 months with only minimal systemic absorption.

Estrogen may be administered continuously (daily) or for 21 to 26 days each month. If the woman has a uterus, a progestogen should be added to the regimen (see Table 14.7). For women who are totally intolerant of progestogens (regardless of the dose and route of administration) and take unopposed estrogen, even at lower doses, periodic endometrial sampling is necessary. In this setting, endometrial thickness by ultrasound may be a guide.

**Table 14.7** Mean Serum Estradiol ($E_2$) and Estrone ($E_1$)

| | Level (pg/mL) | Level (pg/mL) |
|---|---|---|
| Estrogen dose (mg) | $E_2$ | $E_1$ |
| CEE (0.3)* | 18 | 76 |
| CEE (0.625) | 39 | 153 |
| CEE (1.25) | 60 | 220 |
| Micronized $E_2$ (1) | 35 | 190 |
| Micronized $E_2$ (2) | 63 | 300 |
| $E_1$ sulfate (0.625) | 34 | 125 |
| $E_1$ sulfate (1.25) | 42 | 220 |

*Conjugated equine estrogen (CEE) contains biologically active estrogens other than $E_2$ and $E_1$.

## DEALING WITH SIDE EFFECTS

Apart from the thrombotic risks of larger doses of oral estrogen (discussed previously) there may be an "idiosyncratic" blood pressure response to oral estrogen. This has been described primarily with the use of CEE and occurs about 5% of the time. Estrogen typically causes no change in blood pressure and often can lower blood pressure, even in hypertensive women. A hypertensive response is often dealt with by changing the dose, preparation, or route of administration. The important clinical point is that blood pressure should be checked after initiation of therapy.

Other "somatic" effects of estrogen include potential breast tenderness, fluid retention, and bloating (more common with progestogens). All these symptoms are easily dealt with by changing the dose, preparation, and potentially by changing the route of administration as well. There should be a great deal of flexibility in the prescribing of estrogen, because there is no ideal product for all women.

## USE OF A PROGESTOGEN

There are many ways to administer progestogens. The most commonly used oral progestins are MPA in doses of 2.5 and 5 to 10 mg, NET in doses of 0.3 to 1 mg, and micronized progesterone in doses of 100 to 300 mg. Equivalent doses to prevent hyperplasia when administered for at least 10 days in a woman receiving ET (equivalent to 0.625 mg CEE) are as follows: MPA, 5 mg; NET, 0.35 mg; and micronized progesterone, 200 mg. Larger doses of estrogen may require larger doses and particularly more prolonged regimens. In the sequential administration of progestogens, the number of days (length of exposure) is more important than the dose. Thus, if a woman is receiving oral ET continuously, a regimen of at least 10 to 12 days exposure is preferable to a 7-day regimen.

When progestogens are administered sequentially (10 to 14 days each month), withdrawal bleeding occurs in about 80% of women. Continuous administration of both estrogen and progestogen (continuous combined therapy) was developed to achieve amenorrhea. In the first 3 to 6 months, breakthrough bleeding and spotting are common. In some women on this regimen, amenorrhea is never completely achieved. The most common combinations in the United States are single tablets containing 0.45 or 0.625 mg CEE with 1.5 and 2.5 mg of MPA, respectively, and 5 μg of $E_2$ with 1 mg NET and 1 mg micronized $E_2$ with 0.5 mg NET. A patch with $E_2$ and NET or $E_2$ and levonorgestrel is also available.

Progesterone administered vaginally (in low doses) avoids systemic effects and results in high concentrations of progesterone in the uterus. This can be accomplished with capsules, suppositories, or a 4% gel. Intrauterine delivery of progestogens is ideal for targeting the uterus and minimizing systemic effects. However, the only marketed product, the Mirena intrauterine system, delivers too high a dose of levonorgestrel (52 mg in the system) for lower doses of estrogen therapy; a 13.5 mg system (Skylar) has been made available. Progestogens, particularly when taken orally, may lead to problems of continuance or compliance because of adverse effects, including mood alterations and bleeding. This requires flexibility in prescribing habits. Most short-term clinical trials have demonstrated an attenuating effect of progestogens on cardiovascular end points that are improved with estrogen; these effects include lipoprotein changes (an attenuation of the rise in HDL-C) and arterial and metabolic effects, and potentially a further increase in thrombotic risk. The cardiovascular effects in WHI with CEE alone and CEE with MPA, which showed a more favorable effect without MPA, also suggest some detrimental effects of added progestogen. However, two different populations of women were studied in the two WHI trials, which limits any direct comparison. The most inert progestogens, such as micronized progesterone, or vaginal delivery of progesterone should have the fewest attenuating effects. As noted earlier, it is most likely that progestogen exposure is what increases the risk of breast cancer with HT. Natural micronized progesterone was found not to increase the risk of breast cancer in several French observational studies (Fournier, 2008). Progestogens should not be used in women who have had a hysterectomy.

## ANDROGEN THERAPY

In a subtle way, some women are relatively androgen deficient. Clinicians have proposed adding androgen to ET or HT for complaints or problems relating to libido and energy, which are not relieved by adequate estrogen. Although well-controlled trials using parenteral testosterone have shown benefit in younger oophorectomized women, there have been few data showing a benefit to using more physiologic therapy. Recently, however, data using a testosterone patch or pellet (with near physiologic levels) have shown improvement in several scales of well-being and sexual function (Simon, 2005). An oral preparation (esterified estrogens 0.625 mg with 1.25 mg of methyl testosterone) was shown to improve sexual motivation and enjoyment in women with hypoactive sexual desire who were unresponsive to estrogen alone. The latter findings correlated with an increase in circulating unbound testosterone levels. As newer forms and doses of androgen become available, perhaps more women may benefit from this approach. At present, androgen therapy should be individualized and considered for those women who have symptoms that are not adequately relieved with traditional hormonal therapies. It is important to note that there are no approved products for androgen therapy in the United States.

At lower doses, androgenizing side effects are infrequent. At present, small doses of methyltestosterone (1.25 and 2.5 mg) added to esterified estrogens are available in tablets, which only have the indication of relief of vasomotor symptoms. As testosterone patches are only available for men, as are gels and creams, considerable dose titration must be considered in administering testosterone to women. The low-dose testosterone patch that showed benefit for hypoactive sexual desire in hysterectomized women receiving estrogen has been approved for use in Europe but not in the United States. The U.S. Food and Drug Administration (FDA) has been concerned about long-term cardiovascular and cancer effects, although there are no data in either direction. Administration of dehydroepiandrosterone at 25 to 50 mg/day may also be an option for raising endogenous testosterone, but data have not shown it to be beneficial for symptoms such as hypoactive sexual desire.

An Endocrine Society practice guideline, supported by other major societies as well, advised against making a diagnosis of androgen insufficiency in women and suggested against its routine use in women after menopause. However, the society did suggest limited efficacy of testosterone therapy for women with hypoactive sexual desire disorder (Wierman, 2014).

Another SERM-like compound that is used worldwide but is not approved in the United States is tibolone. This progestogen-like compound exhibits estrogenic, antiestrogenic, and androgenic effects by virtue of its structure and metabolites. At 2.5 mg, tibolone suppresses hot flushes, prevents osteoporosis, and has a positive effect on mood and sexual function. There is also limited (or no) uterine stimulation. However, there is suppression of HDL-C, but at the same time a decrease in triglycerides. In the monkey, there is no deleterious effect of tibolone on coronary arteries.

### "BIOIDENTICAL" THERAPY

It has become popular to have compounding pharmacies dispense a mixture of "bioidentical" hormones in a cream or suspension for topical administration. These preparations usually contain one or more estrogens, progesterone, testosterone, and often other precursors such as pregnenolone. As an unregulated industry, without approval by the FDA, there is inadequate quality control for these products, with batch-to-batch variation and the inclusion of some steroid hormones that may not be necessary. Claims that these compounded products are safer than pharmaceutical grade hormones is completely unsubstantiated. Also "titrating" preparations to salivary hormone levels is not accurate and has never been validated. Indeed micronized estradiol, orally or estradiol as a transdermal product, and micronized progesterone, are bioidentical products approved by the FDA, and should be first-line therapy. Several major societies have come out with strong statements against the use of compounded bioidentical preparations, and there is a combined statement from the American Society for Reproductive Medicine (ASRM) and the American College of Obstetricians and Gynecologists (ACOG) (Practice Committee, 2012).

### TSEC CONCEPT

The Tissue Selective Estrogen Complex (TSEC) concept is a newer therapy for menopause. It pairs together an estrogen and a SERM, which when complexed together have specific and different tissue properties than either one would exert independently. A specific SERM, bazedoxifene (BZA)—which has agonistic effects (acting like an estrogen) on bone, antagonistic effects on the uterus and breast, and minimal effects on the CNS—when paired with CEE maintains the effects of CEE on reducing hot flushes, yet prevents endometrial hyperplasia. Accordingly, a progestogen is not needed, and this continuous regimen results in a low rate of vaginal bleeding. It is beneficial for osteoporosis protection and at least theoretically should be safer for the breast as well (Kagan, 2012). It is available as a combination product of CEE 0.45 mg and 20 mg of BZA.

## ALTERNATIVE THERAPIES FOR MENOPAUSE

There are several nonhormonal alternatives for symptoms of menopause, which are listed in Box 14.4, although none of these is as effective as estrogen. Nevertheless, for women who cannot or choose not to take a hormonal preparation, some of these are viable substitutes. Because there is a fairly significant placebo effect in the reduction in hot flushes (up to 40% reduction), at least in the short term, randomized trials against placebo are necessary to establish efficacy.

Not listed here, because this list includes non-hormonal preparations, other than estrogen or estrogen/progestogen regimens, there is an established efficacy of using progestogens alone. MPA 10 to 20 mg, and NET 5 to 10 mg (as well as other progestogen regimens) used alone, have shown some benefit in women with hot flushes, but this is less beneficial than the use of estrogen, and has more side effects, particularly with more long-term therapy (>3 months). Also if a woman cannot or will not take estrogen, it is unlikely that she would take a progestogen alone. Therefore this is often an impractical choice for dealing with symptoms.

### ANTIDEPRESSANTS (SSRIs/SNRIs) (SELECTIVE SEROTONIN REUPTAKE INHIBITORS [SSRIs]/ SEROTONIN NOREPINEPHRINE REUPTAKE INHIBITORS (SNRIs)

Several well-controlled clinical studies have shown the efficacy for several drugs in this class for hot flushes, which were initially used in women with breast cancer. These include fluoxetine (20 mg), venlafaxine (75 mg), paroxetine (12.5, 25 mg), and escitalopram (10, 20 mg) (Nelson, 2006). Apart from some side effects, such as nausea, dry mouth, and sexual dysfunction, all these agents are superior to placebo in reducing hot flushes. However, only one product, paroxetine, is approved currently by the FDA, at a lower dose of 7.5 mg. This has a moderate effect, and in breast cancer patients it may interfere with tamoxifen therapy.

### GABAPENTIN

Gabapentin has been shown to be superior to placebo in doses ranging from 300 to 900 mg. Side effects include somnolence, dizziness, fatigue, and ataxia, which are dose related. If doses are titrated up to 2400 mg (a very large dose), the efficacy has been shown to be similar to that of CEE at 0.625 mg (Reddy, 2006).

### ANTIHYPERTENSIVES

Clonidine has been the most studied, but methyldopa also has efficacy over placebo in reducing hot flushes. Typically a 0.1-mg patch is used daily. There is an obvious hypotensive response, and the efficacy is not very large, precluding its routine use unless the patient is also hypertensive.

### PHYTOESTROGENS

It has been suggested that 30% to 60% of women with symptoms at menopause seek "natural" therapies, and the majority are botanicals such as phytoestrogens. The Dietary Supplement Health and Education Act of 1994 classifies most botanical medicines as food supplements and removes them from regulatory oversight and scrutiny by the FDA. Adulteration, contamination, and poor quality control in their harvesting, manufacture, and formulation yield products of questionable efficacy and safety.

The FDA has determined that more than 25% of Chinese patent medicines are adulterated with hidden pharmaceutical drugs. These kinds of deficiencies make it difficult for consumers and practitioners to employ botanicals with confidence and

**Box 14.4 Nonhormonal Therapies for Vasomotor Symptoms**

Antidepressants (SSRIs/SNRIs)
Gabapentin
Clonidine
Isoflavones, red clover, black cohosh
Cognitive behavior therapy
Acupuncture
Stellate ganglion block

security. Furthermore, clinical trial data obtained using one brand of herbal product cannot necessarily be extrapolated to other brands using the same plant.

Phytoestrogens are a class of plant-derived estrogen-like compounds conjugated to glycoside moieties. Phytoestrogens are not biologically active in their native forms unless taken orally. After oral ingestion, colonic bacteria cleave the glycosides, producing active compounds that are subject to the enterohepatic circulation. These compounds can produce estrogen-agonistic effects in some tissues, whereas in other tissues they produce antagonistic effects.

Few randomized trials have examined the efficacy of phytoestrogens. For large daily doses (60 mg isoflavone), there appears to be some limited efficacy in relieving hot flushes, although the literature on this issue is mixed. In placebo-controlled trials, red clover and black cohosh have been found to have similar effects as placebo (Fig. 14.42) (Geller, 2009).

With doses of 30 to 40 mg of soy isoflavone, cholesterol levels may be reduced, but this is not a consistent finding. Phytoestrogens do not appear to have much of an effect on bone loss or on vaginal atrophy.

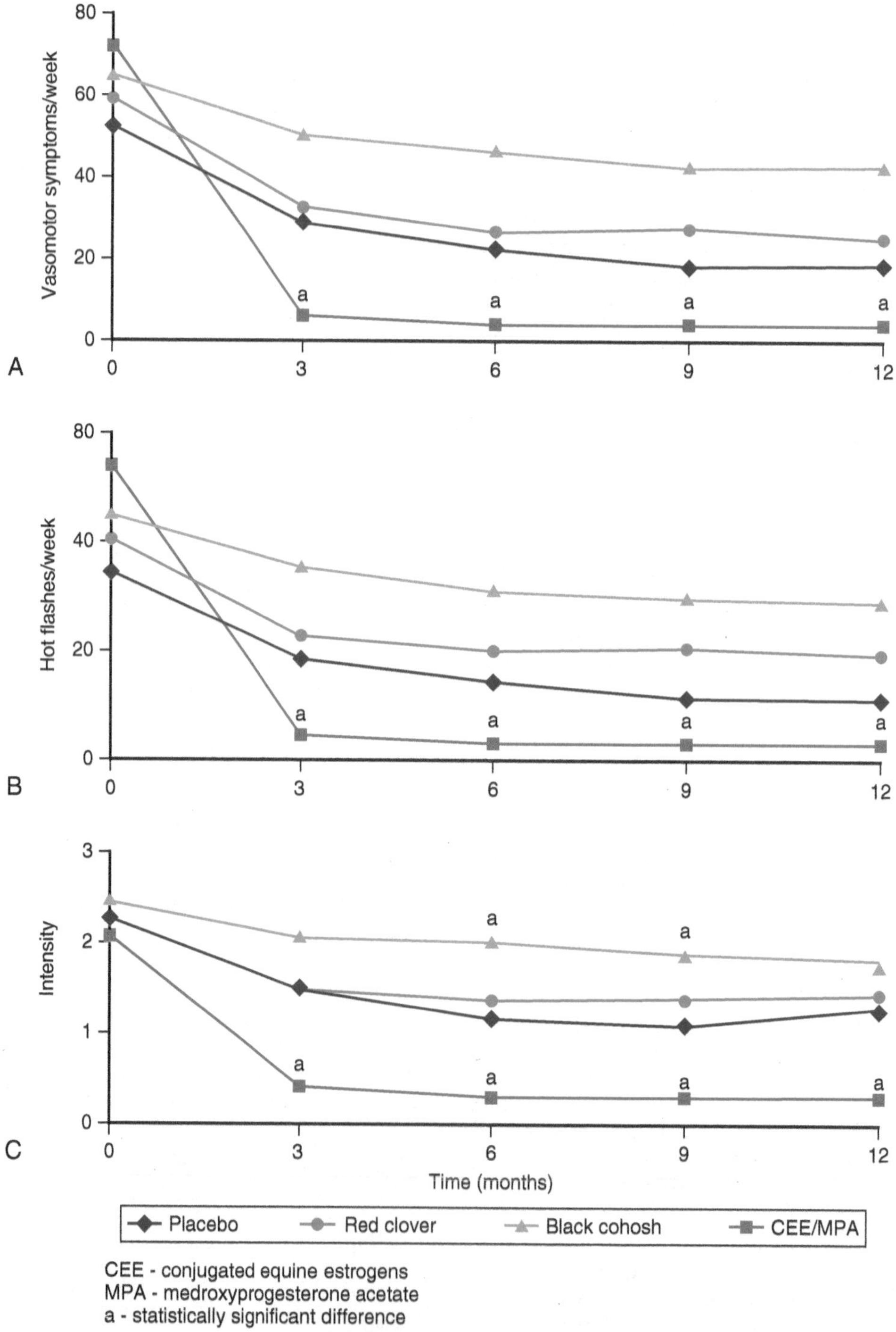


**Figure 14.42** **A** depicts the number of vasomotor symptoms per week; **B** depicts the number of hot flashes per week; and **C** depicts the intensity of the hot flashes. Black cohosh and red clover are not different from placebo. (Modified from Geller SE, Shulman LP, van Breemen RB, et al. Safety and efficacy of black cohosh and red clover for the management of vasomotor symptoms: a randomized controlled trial. *Menopause.* 2009;16[6]:1156-1166.)

### COGNITIVE BEHAVIOR THERAPY

It has been shown that "talk therapy," which teaches coping skills that may change one's cognitive appraisal of the symptoms, may be beneficial (Norton, 2013). It is not clear if this treatment will be sustained over time.

### ACUPUNCTURE

Acupuncture has been used in several trials to assess the treatment of hot flushes and other menopausal symptoms. A meta-analysis confirmed that acupuncture may be effective in alleviating the frequency and severity of hot flushes (Chiu, 2015).

### STELLATE GANGLION BLOCKADE

While somewhat invasive, needle injection of the stellate ganglion has been shown to be effective in some women, such as those being treated for breast cancer. In one study, image-guided stellate ganglion blockade with 5 mL of 0.5% bupivacaine was shown to be beneficial, compared with sham injection with saline for vasomotor symptoms (Walega, 2014).

## KEY POINTS

- The average age of menopause in the United States is 51.3 years, and it is younger in certain ethnic groups.
- Age at menopause is genetically predetermined and is not related to the number of ovulations, race, socioeconomic conditions, education, height, weight, age at menarche, or age at last pregnancy.
- Stages of menopause have been established, and the earliest clinical sign is menstrual alterations.
- The initial endocrinologic change signaling the onset of menopause is decreased AMH and ovarian inhibin-B production accompanied by an increase in FSH.
- Estradiol does not begin to significantly diminish until approximately 1 year before menopause. The rise in FSH occurs before this and stabilizes about 2 years after menopause.
- Because most diseases in women occur after menopause, the onset of menopause heralds an important opportunity to institute prevention strategies for prolonging and improving the quality of life for women.
- Bothersome vasomotor symptoms or hot flushes may persist for 10 or more years, with the mean duration of 4.5 years.
- Estrogen is the best therapy for the hot flush; other effective therapies are progestogens, selective serotonin reuptake inhibitors (SSRIs), gabapentin, clonidine, some phytoestrogens, acupuncture, and stellate ganglion blockade.
- About 1% to 1.5% of bone mass is lost each year after menopause in nonobese white and Asian women. Fractures begin to occur about age 60 to 65 in trabecular bone, such as the vertebral spine, and by age 60, 25% of these women develop spinal compression fractures. Hip fractures begin to increase after age 70.
- Dual-energy x-ray absorptiometry (DEXA) is the most accurate method to measure bone density. The bone mineral density is usually expressed as T scores and Z scores. Bone density does not completely reflect bone strength, which is what determines risk of fracture.
- In addition to estrogen (with and without progestogen), alendronate, risedronate, ibandronate, zoledronic acid, raloxifene, calcitonin, denosumab, and teriparatide will reduce postmenopausal bone loss, and some agents will stimulate bone formation as well.
- The primary indication for estrogen therapy is symptoms of menopause (hot flushes as well as quality-of-life issues); bone health may also be an indication in some women.
- In younger postmenopausal women who are receiving hormonal therapy for symptoms, the benefits outweigh risks with standard doses; lowering doses further decreases risks.
- There is no risk of coronary disease and possibly some benefit with early treatment; there are small risks of venous thrombosis and possibly of ischemic stroke, which can be minimized or eliminated with lower doses or transdermal therapy.
- There are consistent data for a reduction in all-cause mortality of 20% to 30% in younger women who initiate estrogen therapy at the onset of menopause. These data are mostly with the use of estrogen. Estrogen/progestogen therapy shows the same trend, but the data are less robust.
- These findings suggest a potential role of estrogen as a prevention therapy after menopause, although the primary indication is for symptom control and osteoporosis prevention.
- Breast cancer risk is related to dose, duration of use, and progestogen exposure. Estrogen alone and possibly the use of natural progestogen do not substantially increase the risk.
- There is no proved cognitive benefit (although this has been shown in observational studies), but there is also no evidence for harm if initiated in symptomatic women at the onset of menopause.

## KEY REFERENCES

Alvaro M, Imbert R, Demeestere I, et al. AMH mutations with reduced in vitro bioactivity are related to premature ovarian insufficiency. *Hum Reprod (Epub ahead of print)*. 2015.

Anderson GL, Chlebowski RT, Rossouw JE. Prior hormone therapy and breast cancer risk in the women's health initiative randomized trial of estrogen and progestin. *Maturities*. 2006;55:107–115.

Ashcroft GS, Dodsworth J, van Boxtel E, et al. Estrogen accelerates cutaneous wound healing associated with an increase in TGF-beta 1 levels. *Nat Med.* 1997;3:1209–1215.

Atsma F, Bartelink ML, Grobbee DE, et al. Postmenopausal status and early menopause as independent risk factors for cardiovascular disease: a meta-analysis. *Menopause*. 2006;13(2):265–279 (review).

Bidet M, Bachelot A, Bissauge E, et al. Resumption of ovarian function and pregnancies in 358 patients with premature ovarian failure. *JCEM*. 2011;96:38964–38972.

Boardman HMP, Hartley L, Main C, et al. Hormone therapy for preventing cardiovascular disease in post-menopausal women (review). *Cochrane Database Syst Rev.* 2015;3:CD002229.

Bonds DE, Lasser N, Qi L, et al. The effect of conjugated equine oestrogen on diabetes incidence: the Women's Health Initiative randomized trial. *Diabetologia.* 2006;49(3):459–468.

Bord S, Horner A, Beavan S, et al. Estrogen receptors a and b are differentially expressed in developing human bone. *Endocrinol.* 2001;86:2309–2314.

Canonico M, Plu-Bureau G, Lowe GD, et al. Hormone replacement therapy and risk of venous thromboembolism in postmenopausal women: systematic review and meta-analysis. *BMJ.* 2008;336(7655):1227–1231.

Carani C, Quin K, Simoni M, et al. Effect of testosterone and estradiol in a man with aromatase deficiency. *N Engl J Med.* 1997;337:91–95.

Chen S, Sawicka J, Betterle C, et al. Autoantibodies to steroidogenic enzymes in autoimmune polyglandular syndrome, Addison's disease, and premature ovarian failure. *J Clin Endocrinol Metab.* 1996;81(5):1871–1876.

Deutsch S, Ossowski R, Benjamin I. Comparison between degree of systemic absorption of vaginally and orally administered estrogens at different dose levels in postmenopausal women. *Am J Obstet Gynecol.* 1981;139:967.

Diokno AC, Brock BM, Brown MB, Herzog AR. Prevalence of urinary incontinence and other urological symptoms in the noninstitutionalized elderly. *J Urol.* 1986;136:1022–1025.

Ditkoff EC, Crary WG, Cristo M, Lobo RA. Estrogen improves psychological function in asymptomatic postmenopausal women. *Obstet Gynecol.* 1991;78:991–995.

dos Reis CM, de Melo NR, Meirelles ES, et al. Body composition, visceral fat distribution and fat oxidation in postmenopausal women using oral or transdermal oestrogen. *Maturitas.* 2003;46:59–68.

Dowsett M, Cantwel B, Lal A, et al. Suppression of postmenopausal ovarian steroidogenesis with the luteinizing hormone-releasing hormone agonist goserelin. *J Clin Endocrinol Metab.* 1988;66:672–677.

Dunn LB, Damesyn M, Moore AA, et al. Does estrogen prevent skin aging? Results from the First National Health and Nutrition Examination Survey (NHANESI). *Arch Dermatol.* 1997;133:339–342.

Eastell R, Hannon RA. Biochemical markers of bone turnover. In: Lobo RA, ed. *Treatment of the Postmenopausal Woman Basic and Clinical Aspects.* ed 3. St. Louis: Elsevier Academic Press; 2007:337–350.

Elia G, Bergman A. Estrogen effects on the urethra: beneficial effects in women with genuine stress incontinence. *Obstet Gynecol Surv.* 1993;48: 509–517.

Erdman JW. Jr.: Soy protein and cardiovascular disease: a statement for healthcare professionals from the Nutrition Committee of the AHA. *Circulation.* 2000;102:2555–2559.

Ericksen EF, Colvard DS, Berg NJ, et al. Evidence of estrogen receptors in normal human osteoblast-like cells. *Science.* 1988;241:84–86.

Erickson GF, Kokka S, Rivier C. Activin causes premature superovulation. *Endocrinology.* 1995;136:4804–4813.

Erickson GF. An analysis of follicle development and ovum maturation. *Semin Reprod Endocrinol.* 1986;4:233–254.

Erlik Y, Tataryn IV, Meldrum DR, et al. Association of waking episodes with menopausal hot flushes. *JAMA.* 1981;245:1741–1744.

Ettinger B, Black DM, Mitlak BH, et al. Reduction of vertebral fracture risk in postmenopausal women with osteoporosis treated with raloxifene: results from a 3-year randomized clinical trial. Multiple outcomes of raloxifene evaluation (MORE) investigators. *JAMA.* 1999;282:637–645.

Ettinger B, Friedman GD, Bush T, Quesenberry Jr CP. Reduced mortality associated with long-term postmenopausal estrogen therapy. *Obstet Gynecol.* 1996;87:6–12.

Faddy MJ, Gosden RG, Gougeon A, et al. Accelerated disappearance of ovarian follicles in mid-life: implications for forecasting menopause. *Hum Reprod.* 1992;7:1342–1346.

Falconer C, Ekman Orderberg G, Ulmasten U, et al. Changes in para-urethral connective tissue at menopause are counteracted by estrogen. *Maturitas.* 1996;24:197–204.

Fantl JA, Bump RC, Robinson D, et al. Efficacy of estrogen supplementation in the treatment of urinary incontinence: The Continence Pro-gram for Women Research Group,. *Obstet Gynecol.* 1996;88:745–749.

Fedor-Freybergh P. The influence of oestrogens on the well being and mental performance in climacteric and postmenopausal women,. *Acta Obstet Gynecol Scand Suppl.* 1977;64:1–99.

Feldman BM, Voda AM, Gronseth E. The prevalence of hot flash and associated variables among perimenopausal women. *Res Nurs Health.* 1985;8:261–268.

Fournier A, Berrino F, Clavel-Chapelon F. Unequal risks for breast cancer associated with different hormone replacement therapies: results from the E3N cohort study. *Breast Cancer Res Treat.* 2008;107(1):103–111.

Freedman RR. Menopausal hot flashes. In: Lobo RA, ed. *Treatment of the Postmenopausal Woman.* ed 3. New York: Academic Press; 2007:187–198.

Frost HM. On rho, a marrow mediator, and estrogen: their roles in bone strength and "mass" in human females, osteopenias, and osteoporosis—insights from a new paradigm. *J Bone Miner Metab.* 1998;16:113–123.

Frost HM. Perspective on the estrogen-bone relationship and post-menopausal bone loss. *J Bone Miner Res.* 1999;14:1473–1477.

Frost HM. The role of changes in mechanical usage set points in the pathogenesis of osteoporosis,. *J Bone Miner Res.* 1992;7:253–261.

Ganger KF, Vyas S, Whitehead M, et al. Pulsatility index in internal carotid artery in relation to transdermal oestradiol and time since menopause. *Lancet.* 1991;338:839–842.

Geller SE, Shulman LP, van Breemen RB, et al. Safety and efficacy of black cohosh and red clover for the management of vasomotor symptoms: a randomized controlled trial. *Menopause.* 2009;16(6):1156–1166.

Genazzani AR, Petraglia F, Facchinetti F, et al. Increase of proopi-omelanocortin-related peptides during subjective menopausal flushes. *Am J Obstet Gynecol.* 1984;149:775–779.

Geusens P, Dequeker J, Gielen J, Schot LPC. Non-linear increase in vertebral density induced by a synthetic steroid (Org OD14) in women with established osteoporosis. *Maturitas.* 1991;13:155–162.

Ghigo. *Endocrinal Metab.* 1996;81:1871–1876.

Chen WY, Manson JE, Hankinson SE, et al. Unopposed estrogen therapy and the risk of invasive breast cancer. *Arch Intern Med.* 2006;166:1027–1032.

Chen Z, Bassford T, Green SB, et al. Postmenopausal hormone therapy and body composition—a substudy of the estrogen plus progestin trial of the Women's Health Initiative. *Am J Clin Nutr.* 2005;82:651–656.

Chompootweep S, Tankeyoon M, Yamarat K, et al. The menstrual age and climacteric complaints in Thai women in Bangkok. *Maturitas.* 1993;17:63–71.

Chu MC, Cosper P, Orio F, et al. Insulin resistance in postmenopausal women with metabolic syndrome and the measurements of adiponectin, leptin, resistin, and ghrelin. *Am J Obstet Gynecol.* 2006;194(1):100–104.

Civitelli R, Pilgram TK, Dotson M. Alveolar and postcranial bone density in postmenopausal women receiving hormone/estrogen replacement therapy. *Arch Intern Med.* 2002;162:1409–1415.

Clarke SC, Kelleher J, Lloyd-Jones H, et al. A study of hormone replacement therapy in postmenopausal women with ischaemic heart disease: the Papworth HRT atherosclerosis study. *BJOG.* 2002;109:1056–1062.

Clarkson TB, Anthony MS, Jerome CP. Lack of effect of raloxifene on coronary artery atherosclerosis of postmenopausal monkeys. *J Clin Endocrinol Metab.* 1998;83:721–726.

Clarkson TB, Anthony MS, Morgan TM. Inhibition of postmenopausal atherosclerosis progression: a comparison of the effects of conjugated equine estrogens and soy phytoestrogens. *J Clin Endocrinol Metab.* 2001;86:41–47.

Clarkson TB, Anthony MS, Wagner JD. A comparison of tibolone and conjugated equine estrogens effects on coronary artery atherosclerosis and bone density of postmenopausal monkeys. *J Clin Endocrinol Metab.* 2001;86:5396–5404.

Clarkson TB. The new conundrum: do estrogens have any cardiovascular benefits? *Int J Fertil.* 2002;47:61–68.

Collins JA, Allen I, Donner A, Adams O. Oestrogen use and survival in endometrial cancer. *Lancet.* 1980;2:961–963.

Collins JA, Blake JM, Crosignani PG. Breast cancer risk with post- menopausal hormonal treatment. *Hum Reprod Update.* 2005;11(6):545–560.

Collins P, Rosano GMC, Sarrel PM, et al. Estradiol-17b attenuates acetylcholine-induced coronary arterial constriction in women but not men with coronary heart disease. *Circulation.* 1995;92:24–30.

Compagne NA, Bulfone A, Rubenstein JLR, Mellon SH. Steroidogenic enzyme p450c17 is expressed in the embryonic central nervous system. *Endocrinology.* 1995;136:5212.

Conway GS, Hettiarachchi S, Murray A, Jacobs PA. Fragile X permutations in familial premature ovarian failure. *Lancet.* 1995;346:309–310.

Cooper AR, Baker VL, Sterling EW, et al. The time is now for a new approach to primary ovarian insufficiency,. *Fertil Steril.* 2011;95(6):1890–1897.

Cooper C, Campion G, Melton LJ. Hip fractures in the elderly: a world-wide projection. *Obsteoporosis Int.* 1992;2:285–289.

Cooper GS, Sandler DP. Age at natural menopause and mortality. *Ann Epidemiol.* 1998;8:229–235.

Corpas E, Harman SM, Pineyro MA. Growth hormone (GH)-releasing hormone (I–29) twice daily reverses the decreased GH and insulin-like growth factor-I levels in old men. *J Clin Endocrinol Metab.* 1992;75:530.

Coulam CB, Kempers RD, Randall RV. Premature ovarian failure: evidence for the autoimmune mechanism. *Fertil Steril.* 1981;36:238–240.

Coulam CB, Stringfellow SS, Hoefnagel D. Evidence for a genetic factor in the etiology of premature ovarian failure. *Fertil Steril.* 1983;40:693–695.

Coulam CB, Adamson SC, Annegers JF. Incidence of premature ovarian failure. *Obstet Gynecol.* 1986;67:604–606.

Couzinet B, Meduri G, Lecce MG, et al. The postmenopausal ovary is not a major androgen-producing gland,. *J Clin Endocrinol Met.* 2001;86:5060–5066.

Coyle JT, Price DL, DeLong MR. Alzheimer's disease: a disorder of cortical cholinergic innervation. *Science.* 1983;219(4589):1184–1190.

Cummings SR, Black DM, Thompson DE, et al. Effect of alendronate on risk of fracture in women with low bone density but without vertebral fractures: results from the fracture intervention trial. *JAMA.* 1998;280:2077–2082.

Cummings SR, Black DM, Thompson DE, et al. Effect of alendronate on risk of fracture in women with low bone density but without vertebral fracture and coronary heart disease among white postmenopausal women. *Arch Intern Med.* 1989;14:2445–2448.

Damewood MD, Grochow LB. Prospects for fertility after chemotherapy or radiation for neoplastic disease. *Fertil Steril.* 1986;45:443–459.

Dawson-Hughes B, Harris SS, Krall EA, Dalla GE. Effect of calcium and vitamin D supplementation on bone density in men and women 65 years of age or older. *N Engl J Med.* 1997;337:670–676.

Dawson-Hughes B, Looker AC, Tosteson AN, et al. The potential impact of new National Osteoporosis Foundation guidance on treatment patterns,. *Osteoporosis International.* 2010;21(1):41–52.

Dawson-Hughes B, Stern D, Goldman J, Reichlin S. Regulation of growth hormone and somatomedin-C secretion in postmenopausal women: effect of physiologic estrogen replacement. *J Clin Endocrinol Metab.* 1986;63:424.

de Moraes M, Jones GS. Premature ovarian failure. *Fertil Steril.* 1967;18:440.

De Baere E, Dixon MJ, Small KW, et al. Spectrum of FOXL2 gene mutations in blepharophimosis-ptosis-epicanthus inversus (BPES) families demonstrates a genotype-phenotype correlation. *Hum Mol Genet.* 2001;15:1591–1600.

de Boer H, Blok G-J, Vand der Veen EA. Clinical aspects of growth hormone deficiency in adults. *Endocr Rev.* 1995;16:63.

de Bruin JP, Bovenhuis H, van Noord PA, et al. The role of genetic factors in age at natural menopause. *Hum Reprod.* 2001;16:2014–2018.

Dennerstein L, Dudley EC, Hopper JL, et al. A prospective population-based study of menopausal symptoms,. *Obstet Gynecol.* 2000;96:351–358.

Iranmanesh A, Lizzaralde G, Veldhuis JD. Age and relative adiposity are specific negative determinants of the frequency and amplitude of growth hormone (GH) secretory bursts and the half-life of endogenous GH in healthy men. *J Clin Endocrinol Metab.* 1991;73:1081.

Jacobs DM, Tang MX, Stern Y, et al. Cognitive function in non-demented older women who took estrogen after menopause. *Neurology.* 1998;50:368–373.

Jacobs PA. Fragile X syndrome. *J Med Genet.* 1991;28:809–810.

Jones KP, Walker LC, Anderson D. Depletion of ovarian follicles. *Biol Reprod.* 2007;77:247–251.

Jurimae J, Jurimae T. Plasma adiponectin concentration in healthy pre- and postmenopausal women: relationship with body composition, bone mineral, and metabolic variables. *Am J Physiol Endocrinol Metab.* 2007;293(1):E42–E47.

Kagan R. The tissue selective estrogen complex: a novel approach to the treatment of menopausal symptoms. *J Womens Health (Larchmt).* 2012;21(9):975–981.

Kannel WB, Hjortland MC, McNamara PM, Gordon T. Menopause and the risk of cardiovascular disease. The Framingham study. *Ann Intern Med.* 1976;85:447–452.

Karimm R, Dell RM, Greene DF, et al. Hip fracture in postmenopausal women after cessation of hormone therapy: results from a prospective study in a large health management organization. *Menopause.* 2011;18(11):1172–1177.

Kasperk CH, Wergedak JE, Farley JR, et al. Androgens directly stimulate proliferation of bone cells in vitro. *Endocrinology.* 1989;124:1576–1578.

Kaufman FR, Kogut MD, Donnell GN, et al. Hypergonadotropic hypogonadism in female patients with galactosemia. *N Engl J Med.* 1981;304:994–998.

Kawas C, Resnick S, Morrison A, et al. A prospective study of estrogen replacement therapy and the risk of developing Alzheimer's disease: The Baltimore Longitudinal study of aging. *Neurology.* 1997;48:1517–1521.

Khorram O, Laughlin GA, Yen SSC. Endocrine and metabolic effects of long term administration of [Nle 27] growth hormone releasing hormone-(I-29)-NH2 in age-advanced men and women. *J Clin Endocrinol Metab.* 1997;82:1472.

Khosla S, Riggs BL, Atkinson EJ, et al. Effects of sex and age on bone microstructure at the ultradistal radius: a population-based noninvasive in vivo assessment. *J Bone Miner Res.* 2006;21:124–131.

Kinch RAH, Plunkett ER, Smout MS, Carr DH. Primary ovarian failure: a clinicopathological and cytogenetic study. *Am J Obstet Gynecol.* 1965;91:630–644.

King RJ, Whitehead JH. Assessment of the potency of orally administered progestins in women. *Fertil Steril.* 2012;46:1062–1066.

Kingsberg S, Shifren J, Wekselman E. Evaluation of the clinical relevance of benefits associated with transdermal testosterone treatment in postmenopausal women with hypoactive sexual desire disorder. *J Sex Med.* 2007;4(4 Pt.1):1001–1008.

Klaiber EL, Broverman DM, Vogel W, et al. Individual differences in changes in mood and platelet monoamine oxidase (MAO) activity during hormonal replacement therapy in menopausal women. *Psychoneuroendocrinology.* 1996;21:575–592.

Klaiber EL, Broverman DM, Vogel W, Kobayashi Y. Estrogen therapy for severe persistent depressions in women. *Arch Gen Psychiatry.* 1979;36:550–554.

Klein NA, Illingworth PJ, Groome NP, et al. Decreased inhibin B secretion is associated with the menotropic FSH rise in older, ovulatory women: a study of serum and follicular fluid levels of dimeric inhibin A and B in spontaneous menstrual cycles. *J Clin Endocrinol Metab.* 1996;81:2742–2745.

Klein NA, Battaglia DE, Clifton DK, et al. The gonadotropin secretion pattern in normal women of advanced reproductive age in relation to the monotropic FSH rise. *J Soc Gynecol Investig.* 1996;3:27–32.

Komm BS, Terpening CM, Benz DJ, et al. Estrogen binding receptor mRNA, and biologic response in osteoblast-like osteosarcoma cells. *Science.* 1988;241:81–84.

Krall EA, Dawson-Hughes B, Hannan MT, et al. Postmenopausal estrogen replacement and tooth retention. *Am J Med.* 1997;102:536–542.

Krauss CM, Turksoy RN, Atkins L, et al. Familial premature ovarian failure due to an interstitial deletion of the long arm of the X chromosome. *N Engl J Med.* 1987;317:125–131.

Kronenberg F. Hot flashes: epidemiology and physiology. *Ann NY Acad Sci.* 1990;592:52–86.

LaBarbera AR, Miller MM, Ober C, Rebar RW. Autoimmune etiology in premature ovarian failure. *Am J Reprod Immunol Microbiol.* 1988;16:115–122.

Labrie F, Archer DF, Bouchard C, et al. Intravaginal dehydroepiandrosterone (prasterone), a highly efficient treatment of dyspareunia. *Climacteric.* 2011;14(2):282–288.

Lacey JV, Mink PJ, Lubin JH, et al. Menopausal hormone replacement therapy and risk of ovarian cancer. *JAMA.* 2002;288:368–369.

LaCroix AZ, Chlebowski RT, Manson JE, et al. Health outcomes after stopping conjugated equine estrogens among postmenopausal women with prior hysterectomy: a randomized controlled trial. *JAMA.* 2011;305(13):1305–1314.

Laflamme N, Nappi R, Drolet G, et al. Expression and neuropeptidergic characterization of estrogen receptor (ER alpha and beta) throughout the rat brain: anatomical evidence of district role of each subtype. *J Neurobiol.* 1998;36:357–378


Suggested Readings can be found on ExpertConsult.com.

# 15

# Breast Diseases

## Detection, Management, and Surveillance of Breast Disease

*Samith Sandadi, David T. Rock, James W. Orr, Jr., Fidel A. Valea*

The gynecologist's role in managing breast problems is broad and extensive, as he or she will frequently serve as a woman's primary health care advocate. Historically, gynecologists have assumed a leadership role in women's breast cancer care, having been directly involved in the organization of the American Cancer Society (formerly known as the American Society for the Control of Cancer) in 1913 and taking a major role in the initial organization of the American Society of Breast Disease in 1976. A comprehensive plan for the diagnosis and management of breast disease is a critical component of high-quality women's health care because of the prevalence and immense psychological impact of breast disease. In the United States, 7.8% of office visits by women (>51 million/year) are for breast disease. Additionally, breast cancer is the second most common cause of cancer-related death in women, and it is the leading cause of premature mortality from cancer in women as measured by total years of life lost in the United States.

Despite the high incidence and prevalence of breast disease, and the enormous personal, psychosocial, and psychosexual aspects attached to conditions of the breast, there is surprisingly little didactic and clinical teaching time devoted to the evaluation and management of breast disease during medical school and postgraduate training. Regardless, the role of the gynecologist in the management of breast disease has been addressed in a number of published clinical opinions and practice bulletins from the American College of Obstetrics and Gynecology. The role of the gynecologist includes but is not limited to the following:

- Identifying risk factors during the medical and family history
- Performing clinical breast examinations
- Offering instructions for breast self-evaluation
- Evaluating all palpable breast masses
- Encouraging women to have a routine screening mammography
- Performing diagnostic procedures or referral to those who specialize in breast disease when clinically indicated

Guidelines have questioned the benefit of breast self-examination, despite the fact that many women identify their own breast cancer. Thus the term *breast self-awareness* has been coined to imply the potential benefit of women being aware of their breasts and looking for changes, without mention of frequency or proper technique. Additionally, these guidelines indicate that there is insufficient current evidence to assess the additional benefit of clinical breast examination (CBE) beyond screening mammography in women aged 40 years or older (Siu, 2016).

Cultural and societal norms place great importance on breasts. A change or abnormality frequently ignites a fear of breast cancer and strong psychological concerns. The goal of this chapter is to present a clinically oriented approach that allows the practitioner to better understand breast anatomy, the important diagnostic and clinical aspects of benign breast disease, and the epidemiology, detection, and management of breast cancer.

## ANATOMY/EMBRYOLOGY

Breast development begins in utero during the sixth gestational week from the integument along the epithelial mammary ridges. Ducts and acini are derived from ectoderm, whereas supporting tissue arises from mesenchyme. Ductal tissue and secretory lobule development occurs under the influence of the hormonal changes that occur during puberty (see Chapter 38). Actual milk production is initiated by hormonal changes that occur during and after pregnancy.

The breasts are large, modified apocrine/sweat glands located in the superficial fascia anterior to the deep pectoralis major fascia of the chest wall. Posteriorly, the retro mammary space, a loose connective tissue plane, allows free movement over the chest wall (i.e., the breast is not firmly attached to the deep fascia). The breast tissue is suspended from the clavicle and deep clavipectoral fascia by the suspensory ligaments of Cooper that weave through the breast tissue and attach to the dermis of the skin (Fig. 15.1). These fibrous septa maintain the natural shape of the breast. Clinically, malignant involvement of these ligaments often produces skin retraction, suggesting the presence of advanced breast carcinoma.

Breast size and shape depend on genetic, racial, and dietary factors as well as age, parity, and menopausal status. On average, during the reproductive ages the adult breast weighs approximately 250 grams. Typically, a superolateral projection

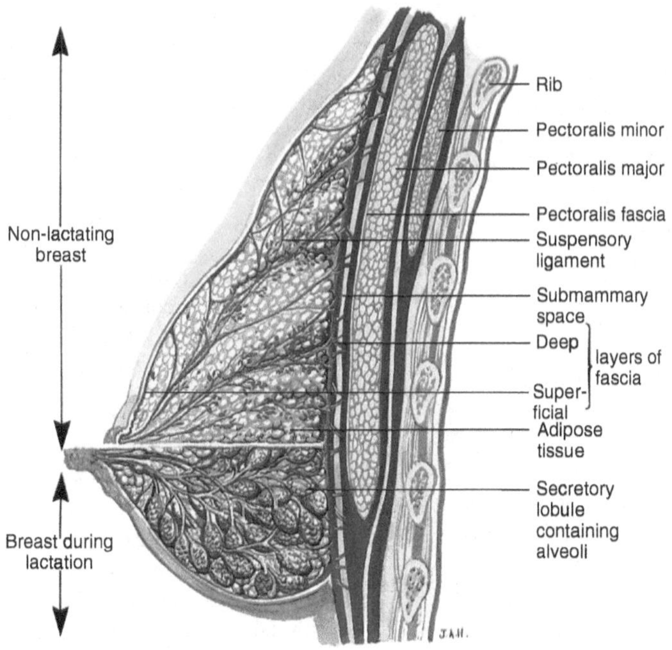


**Figure 15.1** Lactating breast. (From Shah P, ed. Breast. In: Standring S, ed. *Gray's Anatomy*. London: Churchill Livingstone; 2005: 969.)

of glandular tissue (axillary tail of Spence) pierces the deep fascia and extends toward the axilla. Glandular tissue composes approximately 20% of the mature breast with the remainder being adipose and connective tissue. Adipose tissue volume is the major determinant of breast size. Breast density refers to the proportion of fibrous/glandular tissue to adipose tissue. The periphery of the breast is predominantly adipose, and the central area contains a higher proportion of glandular tissue (Fig. 15.2). Typically, glandular tissue regresses and is replaced by adipose tissue after menopause.

A breast is composed of 12 to 20 varying-sized, triangular-shaped lobes distributed radially from the nipple. Each lobe contains its own duct system draining the 10 to 100 lobules with alveoli (acini). These functional lobules have epithelial (ductal) and stromal components and are affected by hormonal changes (estrogen, progesterone, and prolactin) resulting in development, maturation, and differentiation (Fig. 15.3). The organization of the ductal system is stimulated at puberty. Secretory cells drain into alveoli, which drain into "terminal" ducts that then coalesce into larger collecting ducts, and join with ducts from other lobules to end in lactiferous ducts, terminating at the excretory ducts of the nipple.

5 to 20 areolar (Montgomery) glands produce an oily secretion designed to keep the nipple supple and protected, particularly important during breast-feeding. They also produce a volatile compound that has been implicated in stimulating the infants' appetite through olfactory pathways (Doucet, 2009). The glands are located in the areola and even on the nipple. They are generally sensitive. Blockages or irritation result in significant problems.

The principal blood supply of the breast is derived from the perforating branches of the internal mammary arteries that originate from the internal thoracic artery. Additional sources include the lateral thoracic and thoracoacromial arteries, which originate from the axillary artery, and the posterior third, fourth, and fifth intercostal arteries, which are branches of the thoracic aorta. The inferior and central portion of the breast is the least vascular area.

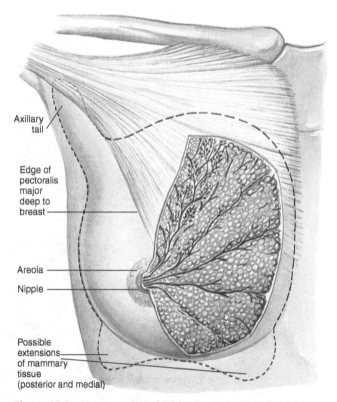


**Figure 15.2** The structures of the breast. (From Shah P, ed. Breast. In: Standring S, ed. *Gray's Anatomy*. London: Churchill Livingstone; 2005:969.)

The lymphatics of the breast converge in the subareolar plexus of Sappy. Approximately 75% of the lymphatics, particularly from the outer quadrants, drain to the 30 to 60 ipsilateral

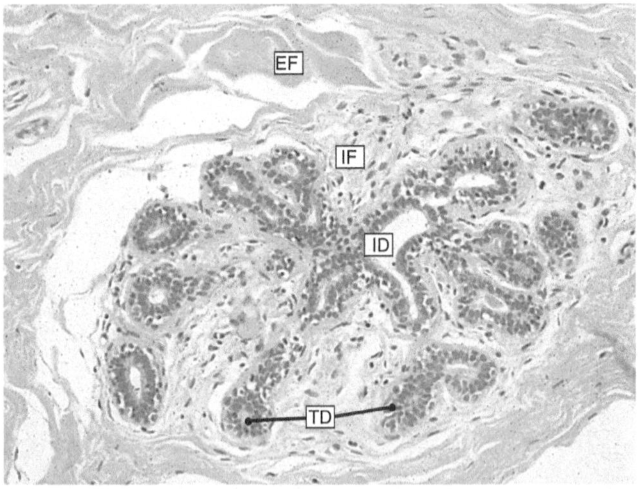


**Figure 15.3** Histologic photograph of a mammary lobule. Note the ductal tissue surrounded by fibrous tissue. Terminal ductules *(TD)* surround the central ductule *(ID)*. *EF*, extralobular fibrocollagenous tissue. (From Stevens A, Lowe J. *Human Histology*. 3rd ed. Philadelphia: Mosby; 2005:390.)

axillary regional nodes. The axillary nodes are classified by three anatomic levels defined by their relationship to the pectoralis minor muscle. Level I nodes are located lateral to the lateral border of the pectoralis minor muscle. Level II nodes are located posterior to the pectoralis minor muscle. Level III nodes include the infraclavicular nodes medial to the pectoralis minor muscle. The remaining lymphatics drain to the internal mammary or parasternal nodes, which have direct drainage to the mediastinum, the medial quadrants of the opposite breast, or the inferior phrenic nodes. The latter is important as it provides a route for metastatic disease to the liver, ovaries, and peritoneum (Fig. 15.4). Lymphatic fluid usually flows toward the most adjacent group of nodes, forming the foundation for utilizing sentinel node mapping to evaluate for nodal spread in breast cancer. In most instances, breast cancer spreads in an orderly fashion within the axillary lymph node basin based on the anatomic relationship between the primary tumor and its associated regional (sentinel) nodes. However, lymphatic metastases from one specific area of the breast may be found in any or all of the groups of regional nodes.

Breast ductal epithelium is extremely sensitive to cyclic hormonal changes. Parenchymal proliferation of the ducts is seen during the follicular phase, and there is dilation of the ductal

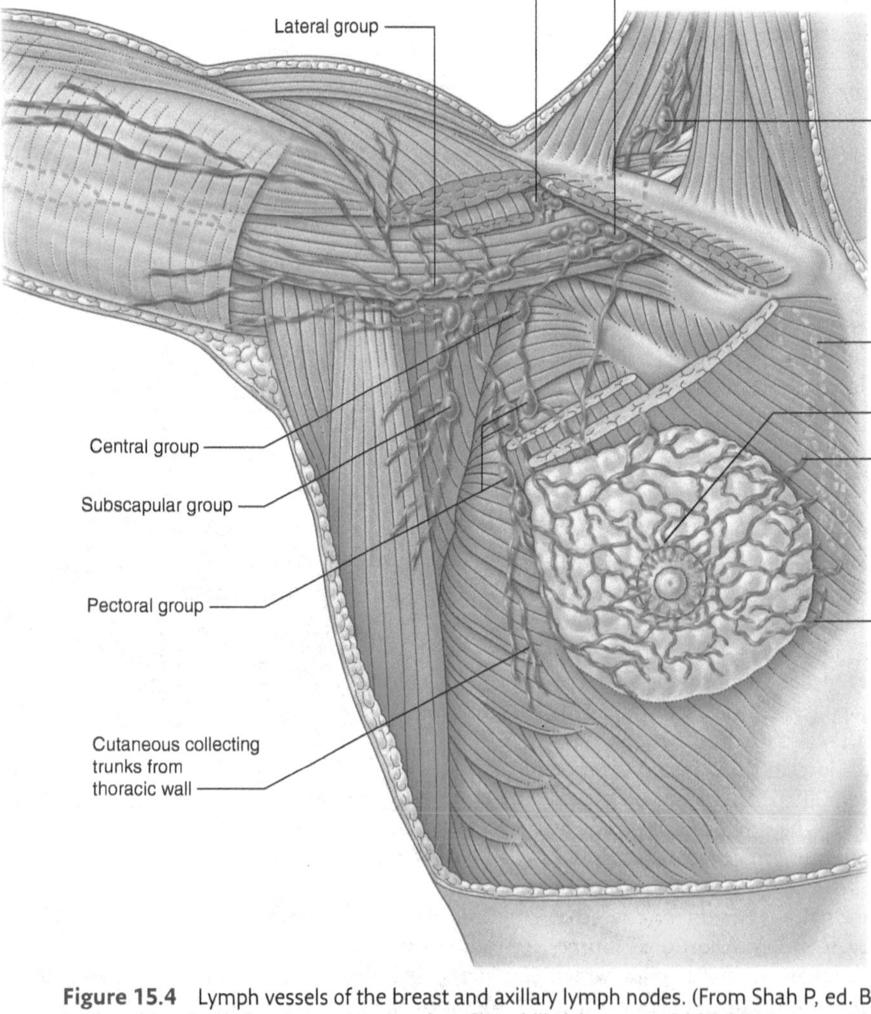


**Figure 15.4** Lymph vessels of the breast and axillary lymph nodes. (From Shah P, ed. Breast. In: Standring S, ed. *Gray's Anatomy*. London: Churchill Livingstone; 2005:971.)

system and differentiation of the alveolar cells into secretory cells during the luteal phase. Alveolar elements respond to both estrogen and progesterone. The stroma and myoepithelial cells also respond to estrogen and progesterone. Women often experience cyclic breast fullness and tenderness likely related to the 25 to 30 mL average fluctuation in volume of the premenstrual breasts. Additionally, premenstrual breast symptoms are produced by an increase in blood flow, leading to vascular engorgement, and water retention. A parallel enlargement of the ductal lumen and an increase in ductal and acinar cellular secretory activity also occur. Menstruation brings a regression of cellular activity in the alveoli and the ducts become smaller. These changes are clinically reflected by the cyclic changes noted on breast examination.

The breast undergoes normal maturational changes throughout a woman's lifetime. In addition to the pubertal and pregnancy-induced changes in the lactiferous duct lobule, the fibrous and adipose components evolve as well. The normal maturation involves a gradual increase in fibrous tissue around the lobules. With time the glandular elements are completely replaced by fibrous tissue. Women in their 20s and 30s have a gradual increase in nodularity as the lobular tissue increases with repetitive cyclic hormonal stimulation. After pregnancy and lactation, breasts may decrease in size and shape, compared with the prepregnancy state. Thus breast examination often yields different findings in the 20-year-old, the 40-year-old, as well as during and after menopause. These changes underscore the value of breast self-awareness, as each woman personally knows the changes in her body at different times in her cycle and life (Fig. 15.5).

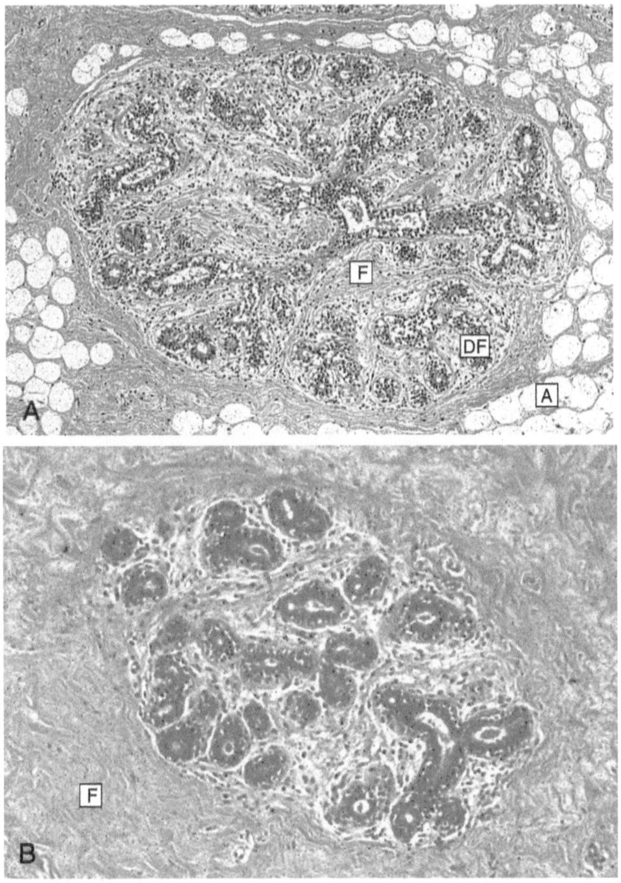


**Figure 15.5** **A,** Micrograph showing normal breast tissue from a 23-year-old woman. At the center is a breast lobule in which the system of terminal ducts and ductules is embedded in loose intralobular fibrocollagenous stroma *(F)*. There is a narrow surrounding zone of dense extralobular fibrocollagenous support tissue *(DF)*, outside of which is the soft adipose tissue *(A)* that forms the bulk of the breast. **B,** Micrograph showing normal breast tissue from a 43-year-old woman. As women age, the amount of fibrocollagenous tissue *(F)* in the breast increases, replacing some of the adipose tissue. The mammary lobules become enclosed in dense collagen. (From Stevens A, Lowe J. *Human Histology.* 3rd ed. Philadelphia: Mosby; 2005:393.)

## CONGENITAL DEVELOPMENTAL BREAST ABNORMALITIES

### *NIPPLE*

Accessory nipples can occur along the breast or milk lines that run from the axilla to the groin. Polythelia (supernumerary or accessory nipples) occurs in 1% (European descent) to 6% (Asian descent) of women. They typically present in the inframammary region (90%), may be unilateral or bilateral, and occur in equal frequency in men and women. The condition is both sporadic and familial. Sporadic cases may be associated with urologic anomalies and cardiovascular problems (hypertension and conductive or rhythm disturbances). Development may be partial or complete. When present, they have the same risk for disease as normal nipples. Treatment is generally reserved to manage irritation or to improve cosmesis.

Congenital nipple inversion occurs in 2% of women, typically in those with a family history of the same condition. The etiology is related to shortening and tethering of breast ducts and to the development of fibrous bands during intrauterine life. Nipple inversion may increase mechanical problems with breastfeeding. Surgical correction often leads to loss of sensation and inability to breast-feed.

Athelia, complete unilateral or bilateral absence of nipple and areola, can be familial (autosomal dominant) and is seen in association with amastia (absent nipple, areola, and breast tissue) or other rare syndromes (e.g., Poland syndrome). Associated ectodermal abnormalities (such as absence of the pectoral muscles) should be excluded. Treatment includes nipple and areola reconstruction commonly using tissue flaps and tattooing.

### *BREAST TISSUE*

Amastia, complete absence of both breast tissue and the nipple-areola complex, occurs with regression or failure to develop the mammary ridge. It is often associated with other ectodermal defects, including cleft palate.

Polymastia, accessory breast tissue or supernumerary breasts, occurs in approximately 1% to 2% of the general population with a female preponderance. Accessory breast tissue most commonly presents in the axilla, and multiple site occurrence is not uncommon (~33%). Initial diagnosis is common at puberty or during pregnancy when the accessory breast tissue development parallels that of normal breast tissue. Supernumerary breast tissue, be it rudimentary or fully developed, is customarily

Table 15.1 ANDI Classification of Benign Breast Disorders

| | Normal | Disorder | Disease |
|---|---|---|---|
| Early Reproductive Years (age 15-25) | Lobular development<br>Stromal development<br>Nipple eversion | Fibroadenoma<br>Adolescent hypertrophy<br>Nipple inversion | Giant fibroadenoma<br>Gigantomastia<br>Subareolar abscess |
| Later Reproductive Years (age 25-40) | Cyclical changes of menstruation<br>Epithelial hyperplasia of pregnancy | Cyclical mastalgia<br>Nodularity<br>Bloody nipple discharge | Incapacitating mastalgia |
| Involution (age 35-55) | Lobular involution<br>Duct involution<br>Dilation<br>Sclerosis<br>Epithelial turnover | Macrocysts<br>Sclerosing lesions<br>Duct ectasia<br>Nipple retraction<br>Epithelial hyperplasia | Periductal mastitis<br>Epithelial hyperplasia with atypia |

asymptomatic; however, it can cause discomfort and may be considered cosmetically unacceptable. Importantly, supernumerary breast tissue is subject to normal changes and the entire disease spectrum seen in the normal breast. Conservative management is encouraged, as surgery can be associated with unattractive scars, restriction of movement, pain, and other complications. Liposuction may useful to decrease the fatty element of accessory breasts.

Asymmetric breast development, common in adolescence and maturity, represents a benign, normal variation unless an associated palpable abnormality is present. In the extreme, a breast can be hypoplastic or absent (aplasia), and this can occur in isolation or in association with a defect in (one or both) pectoral muscles. Significant asymmetry can be deeply disturbing and affect a teenager's self-image. Full breast development usually occurs by 18 to 21 years of age and if deemed necessary, consideration of any corrective surgery, such as augmentation or reduction, should be timed appropriately.

Breast hypertrophy may be asymmetric and is separated into pubertal (virginal hypertrophy), gestational (gravid macromastia), or adult types. Medical treatment is typically not successful and reduction mammoplasty is not indicated until a significant volume of breast tissue requires removal to relieve associated symptoms such as headache, neck or back pain, upper extremity paresthesias, brassiere strap grooving, or intertrigo. Surgical outcome can be maximized when the procedure is planned after allowing for a stable breast size for 6 to 12 months.

Tubular breasts or tuberous breasts, unilateral or bilateral, are a congenital abnormality of the breasts that occurs in both sexes. During puberty breast development is stymied and the breasts fail to develop normally and fully. The transverse breast diameter is narrowed and the base constricted related to glandular hypoplasia with a deficiency in the circumferential skin envelope of the breast base. The breast appears to herniate into an oversized and protuberant areola. The exact cause of this condition is as yet unclear; however, a genetic link in a disorder of collagen deposition is suspected. Corrective procedures can be divided into operations that involve augmentation, mastopexy, combined augmentation/mastopexy, and tissue expansion followed by augmentation (Winocour, 2013).

## BENIGN BREAST DISORDERS

The majority (~90%) of breast complaints and abnormalities are associated with benign breast disorders (BBDs), a heterogeneous group of lesions or abnormalities that may present with a wide range of symptoms. They may be incidental or detected clinically or radiographically. The spectrum of BBD includes developmental abnormalities, inflammatory lesions, epithelial and stromal proliferations, and neoplasms. Benign breast diseases are often misdiagnosed and misunderstood because of their variety in presentation and anxiety about the possibility of malignancy. In fact, women with a new breast problem or complaint commonly assume the worst. Understanding the etiology and management of BBD is essential to proper clinical management and to psychologically allay patient and family fears. Unfortunately, when compared with malignancy, clinical expertise in diagnosis and management of BBD is deficient.

Numerous terminologies have been used to describe BBD. Most emphasize clinical signs, symptoms, or histologic findings. BBDs can be classified as follows:

1. Aberrations of normal development and involution (ANDI)
2. Pathologic classification
3. Clinical classification
4. Classification based on the risk for malignancy

The ANDI classification incorporates symptoms, signs, histology, physiology, pathogenesis, and degree of the breast abnormality, classified in relation to the normal processes of reproductive life and involution through a spectrum of breast conditions that range from "normal" to "disorder" to "disease" (Hughes, 1991). Thus ANDI classification suggests that BBDs are a result of minor aberrations in the normal development process, hormonal response, and involution of the breast (Table 15.1).

Additionally, BBDs can be subdivided pathologically by their potential future cancer risk:

- Nonproliferative disorders: no increased risk
- Proliferative disorders without atypia: mild to moderate increase in risk
- Atypical hyperplasia: substantial increase in risk (relative risk 5×)

Finally, a clinical classification is frequently used in which abnormalities can be subgrouped as follows:

- Physiologic swelling and tenderness
- Nodularity
- Breast pain (not usually associated with malignancy)

- Palpable breast lumps
- Nipple discharge including galactorrhea
- Breast infection and inflammation—typically associated with lactation

Most common benign breast disorders involve pain, discharge, or a mass. Infection or mastitis is less common. These symptoms and subsequent physical findings often result in denial, anxiety, and fear as patients worry that the symptoms represent cancer. The increase in size, density, and nodularity during the second half of the menstrual cycle is often associated with increased sensitivity or breast pain. Importantly, breast pain associated with cancer is generally a late symptom and is a lone presenting symptom in less than 6% of women. Nipple discharge is also a less frequent sign of cancer. The correlation of a mass with malignancy is dependent on the patient's age. The incidence of BBD begins to rise during the second decade of life and peaks in the fourth and fifth decades, as opposed to malignant diseases, whose incidence continues to increase after menopause.

Many breast symptoms stem from fibrocystic changes, previously termed *fibrocystic disease,* which are a common and natural maturation of breast tissue over time. The functional unit of the breast (the lobule), the alterations associated with the interaction among hormones, and the epithelial and stromal components of the lobule are responsible for many cases of BBDs. Initial or immature lobules, primarily developing in the early reproductive years (15 to 25 years of age), are typically replaced during pregnancy and subsequently by mature lobules. Lobular changes manifest most commonly during the menstrual cycle. Late cycle peak mitosis, followed by apoptosis, provides a milieu for stromal or ductal tissues to transform from a normal to abnormal state. Over time, these deviations produce marked differences in the structure and appearance of the breast tissue, which are histologically described as *fibrosis* or *adenosis,* frequently observed in women with no clinical complaint or finding.

Involutional breast changes, clinically apparent prior to 35 years of age, affect stromal and epithelial components of the lobules. Early stromal involution can result in the formation of microcysts from the remaining epithelial acini. Microcyst formation is common and is frequently present in healthy breasts. Ductule obstruction facilitates progression of microcysts to macrocysts. Loose, hormonally receptive connective tissue in the stroma is replaced by denser connective tissue, and epithelial involution results in gradual disappearance of the ductal elements. Epithelial involution is dependent on the continuing presence of surrounding specialized stroma. Thus cyclical and involutional changes are concurrently present for >30 years, and the involution changes will be extensive, sparing few ductal and lobular structures by menopause.

## FIBROADENOMAS

Fibroadenomas, composed of fibrous and epithelial elements, are the most common benign breast neoplasms (15% to 20%) and are often noticed accidentally while bathing. They occur most frequently in adolescents and women in their 20s (15 to 25 years of age) and are related to an aberration in normal lobular development. They demonstrate hormonal dependence, lactate during pregnancy, and involute to be replaced by hyaline connective tissue during perimenopause. Clinically they usually present as solitary slow growing, painless, freely mobile, firm, solid breast masses. The average size is 2.5 cm, and they usually remain fairly constant in size. Giant fibroadenoma, >5 cm, are rare. Hyperplastic lobules histologically resembling fibroadenomas are present in virtually all breasts. All the cellular elements of fibroadenomas are normal on conventional and electron microscopy, and the epithelium and myoepithelium maintain a normal relationship.

On clinical examination it may be difficult to distinguish a fibroadenoma from a cyst. In fact, diagnosis based solely on CBE is correct 66% of the time. Importantly, complex cysts and any cysts with solid areas should be biopsied or excised. Ultrasound is the initial, noninvasive study to differentiate a solid versus a cystic mass, as mammography is rarely indicated in a woman younger than 35 with fibroadenomas. Core needle biopsy is indicated if, and when, the cause of a palpable mass cannot be established. Surgical evaluation is appropriate for any mass (at any age) that exhibits a rapid size increase. Fibroadenomas can be followed clinically. Surgical excision of fibroadenomas should be considered if they are symptomatic or to relieve anxiety related to the palpable mass. They have a "rubbery" consistency, are usually well circumscribed, and easily delineated from surrounding breast tissue in approximately 95% of cases (Fig. 15.6). Nonoperative management can be considered for small, asymptomatic fibroadenomas, discovered in women younger than 35 if clinical exam, imaging evaluation (either mammogram or ultrasound), and biopsy (usually core needle) are 100% concordant. Approximately 35% of fibroadenomas will disappear, and approximately 10% become smaller when followed for many years. Conservative management requires continued surveillance at 6-month intervals for at least 2 years. Despite the option of conservative management, many women prefer to have the fibroadenoma excised. Excision should be performed through a cosmetically placed inframammary, axillary, or circumareolar incision. The long-term risk of invasive breast cancer in women with fibroadenomas is approximately twice that for women without fibroadenomas, as fibroadenomas are a proliferative disorder. Women with fibroadenomas should be made aware of this risk and encouraged to maintain annual mammographic screening. The postoperative risk of recurrent fibroadenoma is ~20%. Studies support the successful use of ultrasound-guided high-intensity focused ultrasound or cryoablation as an alternative treatment to surgery (Kovatcheva, 2015).

Phyllodes tumors, previously termed *Cystosarcoma phyllodes,* represent the opposite end of the spectrum of fibroepithelial tumors. Phyllodes tumors are rare, representing only 2.5% of fibroepithelial tumors and less than 1% of breast malignancies. The typical age of onset is 15 to 20 years later than fibroadenomas (fourth and fifth decades of life). They are almost exclusively seen in females and may be benign, borderline, or malignant. Differentiating benign from malignant phyllodes can be difficult and involves assessment of the size, histologic stroma/epithelium ratio, border of the lesion, stromal cellularity, number of stromal mitoses, and presence or absence of necrosis. All three generally present as a breast mass, often grow rapidly, and are typically larger at diagnosis than a fibroadenoma or ductal carcinoma. Histologically, stromal elements dominate and will invade the ducts in a leafy projection, hence the name *phyllodes,* or "leaf" (Fig. 15.7). Even the most experienced pathologists may have difficulty distinguishing between fibroadenoma, benign phyllodes tumors, and malignant

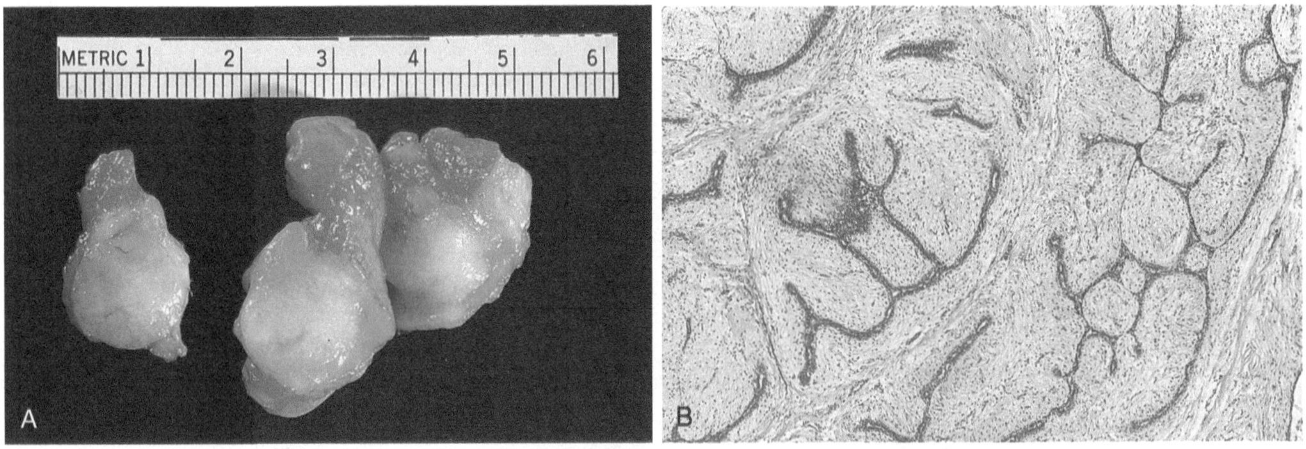


**Figure 15.6** **A,** Fibroadenoma with characteristic tan, well-circumscribed nodule. **B,** Histologic section of fibroadenoma with epithelial cells surrounded by loose mesenchymal fibrous tissue. (From Voet RL. *Color Atlas of Obstetric and Gynecologic Pathology*. St Louis: Mosby-Wolfe; 1997:204.)

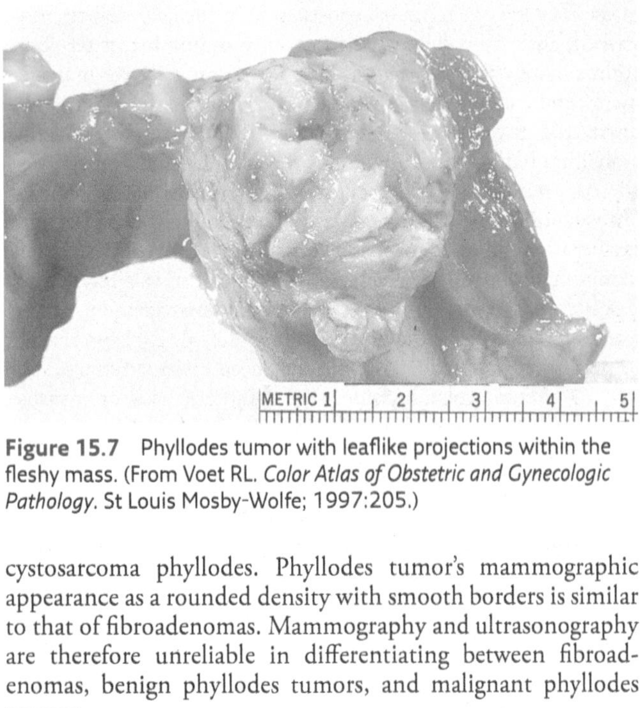


**Figure 15.7** Phyllodes tumor with leaflike projections within the fleshy mass. (From Voet RL. *Color Atlas of Obstetric and Gynecologic Pathology*. St Louis Mosby-Wolfe; 1997:205.)

cystosarcoma phyllodes. Phyllodes tumor's mammographic appearance as a rounded density with smooth borders is similar to that of fibroadenomas. Mammography and ultrasonography are therefore unreliable in differentiating between fibroadenomas, benign phyllodes tumors, and malignant phyllodes tumors.

Phyllodes tumors can be locally aggressive and require wide local excision with 1-cm margins. Unlike fibroadenomas, phyllodes tumors should not be shelled out, as it will result in an unacceptably high recurrence rate. Unfortunately, the pathologic appearance of a phyllodes tumor does not always predict the neoplasm's clinical behavior; however, risk of local recurrence of the tumor is associated with microscopic margin involvement. Malignant tumors metastasize hematogenously, and the risk of metastases is 25%; however, local recurrence is common (>20%), even with benign and borderline tumors.

## FIBROCYSTIC CHANGE

*Fibrocystic change,* previously termed *fibrocystic disease,* is the most common of all benign breast conditions. Clinicians use the nonspecific term *fibrocystic change* to describe the clinical, mammographic, and histologic findings associated with multiple irregularities in contour and texture typically associated with cyclical breast pain. Fibrocystic change presents as a spectrum of changes throughout a woman's reproductive age with significant patient variation. Fibrocystic change has an extensive list of synonyms and terminology that includes more than 35 different names and terms. The 10th revision of the *International Statistical Classification of Diseases and Related Health Problems* (ICD-10) terms this as diffuse cystic mastopathy.

The true frequency of fibrocystic change is unknown; however, autopsy evidence of histologic fibrocystic change is noted in 53% of normal breasts. Clinical evidence of fibrocystic change is evident in nearly one in two premenopausal women during breast examination; however, depending on the definition, some authors have noted that as many as 90% of women demonstrate some aspect of fibrocystic change. Although no consistent abnormality of circulating hormone levels has been proved, fibrocystic changes represent an exaggeration of normal physiologic response of breast tissue to the cyclic levels or ovarian hormones. These changes, unusual in adolescence, are most common in women of reproductive age (20 to 50 years) and unusual after menopause unless associated with exogenous hormone replacement.

Cyclic bilateral breast pain is the classic symptom of fibrocystic breast change. Clinical signs include increased breast engorgement and density, excessive breast nodularity, fluctuation in the size of cystic areas, increased tenderness, and infrequently spontaneous nipple discharge. Signs and symptoms are typically more prevalent during the premenstrual state.

Associated mastalgia is bilateral, often difficult to localize, and most frequent in the upper, outer breast quadrants. Pain may radiate to the shoulders and upper arms. Severe localized pain occurs when a simple cyst rapidly expands. The pathophysiology that produces these symptoms and signs includes cyst formation, epithelial and fibrous proliferation, and varying degrees of fluid retention. The differential diagnosis of breast pain includes referred pain from a dorsal radiculitis or inflammation of the costochondral junction (Tietze syndrome). The latter two conditions have symptoms that are not cyclic and unrelated to the menstrual cycle.

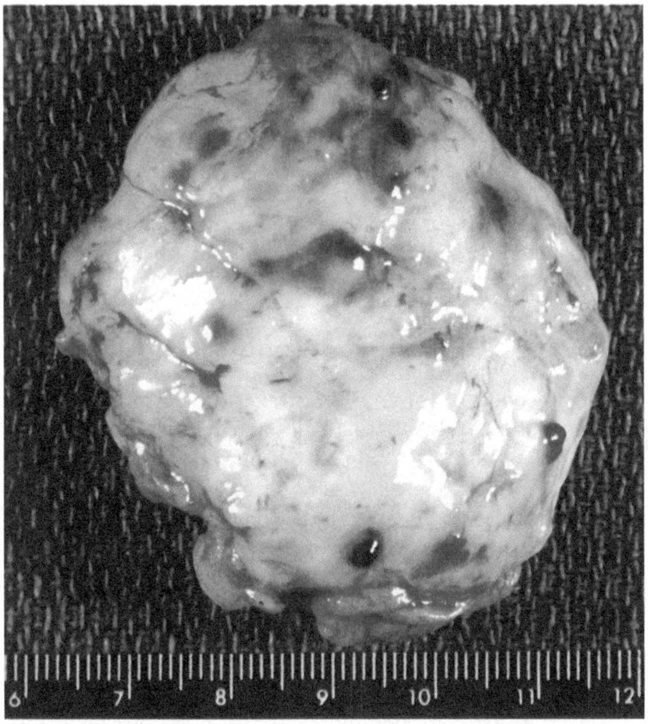


**Figure 15.8** Breast biopsy from a 38-year-old woman demonstrating the characteristic gross appearance of fibrocystic changes. Note the multiple cysts interspersed between the dense fibrous connective tissue. (Courtesy of Fidel A. Valea, MD.)

The physical findings of excessive nodularity due to fibrocystic changes have been described as similar to palpating the surface of multiple peas. There may be multiple areas of seemingly ill-defined thickening or areas of palpable lumpiness that seem more two-dimensional than the three-dimensional mass usually associated with a carcinoma (Fig. 15.8). Larger cysts may be ballotable, analogous to a water-filled balloon.

There are three general clinical stages of fibrocystic change, with each stage having characteristic histologic findings. Clinically these stages are variable and overlap, but they are described to assist in the understanding of the natural history. The first stage, mazoplasia (mastoplasia), is associated with intense stromal proliferation and occurs in the early reproductive years (20s). Breast pain is noted primarily in the upper, outer breast quadrants with most tenderness in the axillary tail.

The second clinical stage, adenosis, is characterized by marked proliferation and hyperplasia of ducts, ductules, and alveolar cells and typically occurs in women in their 30s. Premenstrual breast pain and tenderness is less severe. Multiple small breast nodules varying from 2 to 10 mm in diameter are present.

The cystic phase is the last stage and typically occurs another decade later in women in their 40s. Typically there is no breast pain unless a cyst increases rapidly in size with associated sudden pain, point tenderness, and a lump. Cysts are tender to palpation and vary from microscopic to 5 cm in diameter. Although breast cysts may occur at any age, they are generally simple and may be managed with aspiration alone. Complex cysts have internal septations, debris, or solid components and may require core needle biopsy if stability cannot be documented. The fluid aspirated from a large cyst is typically straw colored, dark brown, or green, depending on the chronicity of the cyst.

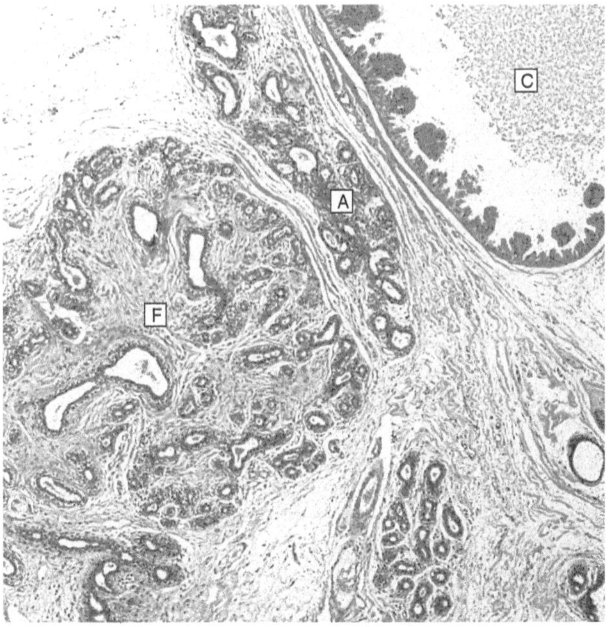


**Figure 15.9** Fibrocystic changes from histologic section. Note: Fibrosis *(F)*, adenomatous changes with increased ductal tissue *(A)*, and cysts *(C)*. (From Stevens A, Lowe J. *Human Histology*. 3rd ed. Philadelphia: Mosby; 2005:392.)

Women with a clinical diagnosis of fibrocystic change have a wide variety of histopathologic findings. The histology of fibrocystic change is characterized by proliferation and hyperplasia of the lobular, ductal, and acinar epithelium (Fig. 15.9). Usually, the proliferation of fibrous tissue occurs and accompanies epithelial hyperplasia. Many histologic variants of fibrocystic change have been described, including cysts (from microscopic to large, blue, domed cysts), adenosis (florid and sclerosing), fibrosis (periductal and stromal), duct ectasia, apocrine metaplasia, intraductal epithelial hyperplasia, and papillomatosis. Ductal epithelial hyperplasia with atypia and apocrine metaplasia with atypia are the most prominent histologic findings directly associated with the subsequent development of breast carcinoma. If either of these two conditions is discovered on breast biopsy, the chance of future breast carcinoma is increased fivefold.

Clinical management of fibrocystic change is age dependent and includes appropriate use of breast imaging. First and foremost, malignancy should be excluded, particularly in the presence of a mass or with a concerning or uncertain examination. Thereafter, successful symptom control may involve a number of medical options. Initial therapy for fibrocystic change involves mechanical support utilizing a firm support or sports bra. Dietary changes reducing methylxanthines or caffeine exposure have been helpful in relieving symptoms for some women. Although confirmatory medical studies evaluating the benefit of these dietary changes are lacking, there seems to be little harm to trying this inexpensive option for 3 to 6 months. The only dietary substance that seems, at this time, to correlate with fibrocystic symptoms is dietary fat, particularly saturated fat. Studies have demonstrated a dose-related effect between increased saturated fat and fibrocystic breast symptoms. Incorporating a low-fat, nutrient-dense diet makes sense, and limiting intake of saturated fat intake should be considered as a simple therapeutic tool for the management of women with symptomatic, refractory fibrocystic changes. Additionally, some advocate limiting or eliminating alcohol consumption to lessen estrogen levels. Diuretics are sometimes prescribed during the premenstrual phase and may lessen symptoms of breast discomfort/engorgement.

Oral contraceptives or supplemental progestins administered during the secretory phase of the cycle have also been used to treat fibrocystic changes. Oral contraceptives are reported to decrease the incidence of fibrocystic changes by 30% (Schindler, 2013). Unfortunately, 40% of women will have recurrent symptoms after discontinuation.

Danazol, dosed at 100, 200, and 400 mg daily for 4 to 6 months, suppresses gonadotropins and effectively relieves symptoms and decreases breast nodularity in ~90% of patients. Unfortunately, virilizing side effects such as hirsutism, acne, and voice changes frequently limit its use. Danazol therapy for 6 months or more should be tapered to eliminate side effects. The beneficial effects of danazol persist for several months after discontinuation.

Oral tamoxifen, 20 mg daily, is superior to placebo in randomized, double-blind trials, and pain relief is reported to be sustained in 72% of women for >1 year after discontinuation. Tamoxifen administration restricted to the luteal phase of the menstrual cycle abolishes pain in 85% of women; however, adverse side effects are frequent (21%). Following treatment, 25% of women suffer recurrent pain within 1 year. Tamoxifen 10 mg daily can be prescribed during the luteal phase of the menstrual cycle and results in similar improvements in symptoms, but with a marked reduction in adverse effects.

The selective estrogen receptor modulator (SERM) Ormeloxifene (30 mg twice weekly), a weak estrogen receptor (ER) agonist and a strong ER antagonist, demonstrated significant efficacy in the management of breast pain and fibrocystic nodularity. On rare occasions, gonadotropin-releasing hormone (GnRH) agonists may benefit women with severe fibrocystic change.

## MASTALGIA (BREAST PAIN)

Over two thirds of women will experience breast pain at some time during their reproductive years, most commonly in the perimenopausal years. Approximately 90% of conditions that cause breast pain are benign. Breast pain is typically divided into cyclic pain, related to the menstrual cycle, and noncyclic pain. Cyclic pain is diffuse and bilateral and most commonly associated with fibrocystic changes. Noncyclic breast pain is commonly localized and related to a cyst. Noncyclic breast pain should be evaluated, particularly in older women, as there is a small association with malignancy. Mammography and additional imaging can be valuable. The differential diagnosis includes a cyst, chest-wall pain, radicular pain, costochondritis, mastitis, pregnancy-related pain, prolactinomas, and medication exposure (Box 15.1). Laboratory evaluation should include an HCG and prolactin in premenopausal women. Breast cysts occur in as many as 7% of women during their lifetime and may be therapeutically aspirated if they are simple. A negative postaspiration breast examination is reassuring. Recurring simple cysts can be followed with ultrasound, typically withholding repeat aspiration for symptomatic cysts. For a more complex cyst, a more detailed workup is usually necessary. Complex cysts should have a tissue diagnosis with core needle biopsy if they are symptomatic or show progressive changes on serial sonography. Pain as a presenting symptom of malignancy is uncommon and is extremely rare in the absence of mass or skin changes. Breast pain treatment is directed at the cause; however, nonsteroidal anti-inflammatories are often useful when pain is idiopathic.

## MASTITIS AND INFLAMMATORY DISEASE

Breast infection is often subdivided into lactational, nonlactational, and postsurgical. Although decreasing in overall incidence, mastitis, infection of the ductal systems or smaller sebaceous glands, is most commonly related to *Staphylococcus aureus*. Empiric treatment with an agent that covers gram-positive organisms is appropriate. If there is poor response to the initial course of antibiotics, then cultures for methicillin-resistant *Staphylococcus aureus* (MRSA) should be performed and an agent such as a doxycycline or sulfamethoxazole/trimethoprim is indicated. These two agents are contraindicated if a woman is pregnant or lactating.

Lactational mastitis commonly occurs in the first pregnancy during the first 6 weeks of breast-feeding. Curiously, mastitis in pregnancy usually responds to first-line antibiotics such as a cephalosporin, even in the presence of MRSA; however, infection may progress to a breast abscess in 5% to 11% of patients. Continued breast-feeding or manual pumping of the affected breast is recommended to decrease engorgement.

Nonpuerperal mastitis is often associated with breast cysts and cyst rupture. Ultrasonography assists in excluding an abscess. Obviously, one should always consider and exclude the presence of malignant breast disease, particularly inflammatory cancer. Additional testing for diabetes and HIV may be indicated, particularly if yeast is the offending organism. Syphilis, tuberculosis, atypical bacterial, and fungal infections

**Box 15.1 Medications Associated with Mastalgia**

Antihypertensives
Atenolol and other beta-blockers
Hydrochlorothiazide
Methyldopa
Minoxidil
Spironolactone
Antidepressants and antipsychotic agents
Amitriptyline and other tricyclic antidepressants
Chlorpromazine/promethazine
Fluoxetine
Haloperidol
Hormonal agents
Estrogens
Progestins
Androgens
Ginseng
Clomiphene citrate
Digoxin
Chlorpropamide

may rarely cause nonpuerperal mastitis. In patients with recurrent mastitis, consider choosing an antibiotic to cover MRSA, such as clindamycin, trimethoprim-sulfamethoxazole, doxycycline, or vancomycin. Nipple piercing, particularly in smokers, is associated with mastitis and a 20-fold increase in subareolar abscess formation. As with any infection, the clinician should strongly consider removal of the foreign body. The American College of Obstetricians and Gynecologists recommends counseling women who are planning to get piercings to have a prepiercing hepatitis-B vaccine and tetanus vaccinations.

Idiopathic granulomatous mastitis (IGM), also called *idiopathic granulomatous lobular mastitis (IGLM)*, is a rare cause of breast inflammation, which may affect any age group. This disease may present with a mass, abscess, inflammation, or granuloma formation. The granulomas are often found within the lobules and on biopsy are noted to be sterile. Mammography may be equivocal or may be suspicious for malignancy. Steroid treatment has been reported to be effective in small series with equivocal results. The disease is usually self-limited, resolving within months. Skin scarring and residual small abscesses may remain, frequently necessitating surgical treatment. Chronic inflammatory diseases, such as lupus, sarcoid, and Wegner granulomatosis, are rare causes of noninfectious mastitis, and evaluation for these diseases should be performed if antibiotics are not effective. Importantly, any breast inflammation not responsive to adequate antibiotic treatment warrants a tissue diagnosis. Core needle biopsy is frequently performed when there is a lack of response to antibiotics. The diagnosis is frequently made when the biopsy demonstrates sterile granulomas after excluding other causes of granulomatous mastitis such as tuberculosis.

## NIPPLE DISCHARGE

Nipple discharge is responsible for 7% of physician visits involving breast complaints. The majority have a benign etiology; however, 55% present with a coexisting mass of which 19% are malignant. An underlying malignancy is more likely when the discharge is spontaneous (vs. induced with nipple pressure), arises from a single duct, is blood stained, and is unilateral and persistent (occurring more than twice weekly). Age is important, as an underlying malignancy is present in 3% of women under 40, 10% of women between 40 and 60, and 32% of women over 60 when nipple discharge is the *only* presenting symptom.

Intraductal papilloma and fibrocystic changes are the two most common causes of spontaneous nonmilky discharge. Galactorrhea is likely when breast discharge is bilateral, copious, pale milky in color, and occurs from multiple ducts. Importantly, numerous medications and conditions can affect the hypothalamic-pituitary axis and lead to prolactin secretion and galactorrhea. As many as 65% of premenopausal women may have a normal benign physiologic discharge with gentle squeezing of the nipple. Evaluation includes physical examination, mammography, and sonography. History may not differentiate spontaneous discharge from elicited discharge as a woman may continually attempt to express the discharge, which causes more fluid to leak.

Evaluation and diagnosis includes clinically separating the discharge into those that are spontaneous and those that only are expressed by pinching or squeezing the nipple. Nipple discharges range in color from milky to green, brown, purple, and bloody. Hemoccult testing for detection of blood in the discharge is neither sensitive nor specific. Malignancy should be excluded in any woman with a bloody discharge or any discharge associated with a mass or if the discharge originates from only one or two adjacent ducts.

Assessment of *pathologic* nipple discharge involves a careful breast examination to identify the presence or absence of a breast mass. Firm areola pressure can assist in identifying the site of any dilated duct (pressure over a dilated duct will produce the discharge); this finding helps to define where an incision should be made for any subsequent surgery. The nipple is squeezed with firm, gentle digital pressure and if fluid is expressed, the site and character of the discharge are recorded. Although bloodstained breast discharge is more likely to be associated with malignancy, fewer than 20% of patients who have a bloodstained discharge, or who have a discharge containing moderate or large amounts of blood, will have an underlying malignancy. Importantly, the absence of blood in nipple discharge does not exclude an underlying malignancy. Nipple discharge cytology can be helpful but has a poor sensitivity (<50%).

Management of a suspicious discharge begins with a physical examination and mammography, ultrasound, or magnetic resonance imaging (MRI). Any mass associated with discharge requires appropriate biopsy. A number of techniques have been evaluated to determine etiology and avoid unnecessary extirpative surgery. Ductoscopy (using a microendoscope passed into the offending duct) allows direct visualization. Ductal lavage involves duct canalization, and collection of fluid for cytologic evaluation. This technique increases cell yield by 100 times that of simple discharge cytology but can be uncomfortable for the patient. Ductography (imaging of the ductal system by infecting contrast into the symptomatic duct), also called a *galactogram*, has 60% sensitivity for detecting malignancy. This study can identify intraductal filling defects or cutoff lesions, which have a high positive predictive value for the presence of either a papilloma or a carcinoma. The procedure can be technically challenging and cause significant patient discomfort. Surgical excision of the duct and its associated lobular unit is both diagnostic and therapeutic. With the patient anesthetized, a 4-0 lacrimal probe is passed through the duct. A periareolar flap is then created, and the retroareolar duct with the probe can be identified and excised individually.

## INTRADUCTAL PAPILLOMA

Intraductal papillomas are broad-based or pedunculated polypoid epithelial lesions that may obstruct and distend the involved duct, most commonly diagnosed in perimenopausal women. Classically, their clinical presentation includes an intermittent but spontaneous discharge from one nipple involving one or two ducts. The associated discharge can be watery, serous, or bloody, and of variable volume. Approximately 75% of intraductal papillomas are located beneath the areola, are small and soft, and are often difficult to palpate, typically measuring 1 to 3 mm in diameter. During examination of the breast it is important to circumferentially put radial pressure on different areas of the areola. This technique helps to identify whether the discharge emanates from a single duct or multiple openings. When the discharge comes from a single duct, the differential diagnosis includes both intraductal papilloma and carcinoma.

Treatment of intraductal papilloma involves excisional biopsy of the involved duct and a small amount of surrounding tissue. Although these tumors tend to regress in postmenopausal women, excision should be considered to rule out malignancy. Careful surveillance at 3- to 4-month intervals is necessary if the papilloma is not surgically excised. Women with a solitary papilloma have a twofold increase in subsequent development of breast carcinoma.

### FAT NECROSIS

Fat necrosis, a benign nonsuppurative inflammatory process of adipose tissue, is a condition with a wide variety of presentations on mammography, ultrasound, and MRI. The incidence of fat necrosis of the breast is estimated to be 0.6% in the breast, representing 2.75% of all breast lesions. Fat necrosis is found to be 0.8% of breast tumors and 1% in breast reduction mammoplasty cases. The average age of patients is 50 years. Fat necrosis is most commonly the result of trauma to the breast, although it can be associated with radiotherapy, anticoagulation (warfarin), or breast procedures including breast aspiration or biopsy, lumpectomy, reduction mammoplasty, implant removal, breast reconstruction, and infection. Other rare causes for fat necrosis include polyarteritis nodosa, Weber-Christian disease, and granulomatous angiopanniculitis.

Patients commonly present with a firm, tender, indurated, ill-defined mass that may have coexisting ecchymosis, erythema, inflammation, pain, skin retraction or thickening, nipple retraction, and occasionally lymphadenopathy. As many as 70% present as an occult lesion without a history of trauma. The area of fat necrosis may liquefy and become cystic forming an oil cyst with a characteristic calcified rim. Mammography may demonstrate coarse calcifications, focal asymmetries, or microcalcifications. Treatment of fat necrosis is excisional biopsy. There is no relationship between fat necrosis and subsequent breast carcinoma.

## BREAST CARCINOMA

Globally, breast carcinoma is the most common malignancy of women, and in the United States it is the second most common cause of all cancer deaths in women. Approximately 12.3% of women (one in eight women) will develop carcinoma of the breast at some point during their lifetime. In 2014, approximately 234,190 women in the United States were diagnosed with invasive breast cancer, with 40,730 women dying from the disease (Siegel, 2015). The importance of early detection and diagnosis of breast carcinoma cannot be overemphasized. An increase in public awareness combined with improvements in mammography and newer imaging techniques have facilitated earlier detection of breast carcinoma. Earlier detection, combined with improvements with therapy, has resulted in improved survival rates. With the advent of chemoprevention in the high-risk woman, there is an opportunity to alter the natural course of the disease.

Breast carcinoma generally presents in one of two ways, either with clinical symptoms or found on screening evaluation. In the United States, most breast cancer is diagnosed as a result of an abnormal screening test. Screening includes breast self-examination, examination by a health provider (referred to as *clinical breast examination*), and imaging. The ideal time to initiate screening, along with determination of intervals, is individualized for each woman based on her risk factors. A thorough understanding of the epidemiology of breast cancer is warranted when calculating the risk of developing breast cancer. There are several models that help assess a patient's risk. If no risk factors are noted, she is said to be at average or normal risk, corresponding to the 12% (or one in eight) risk for a woman of developing breast malignancy during her lifetime. Because a woman's risk may change as her family history evolves and new findings occur on imaging, risk assessment should be ongoing.

## EPIDEMIOLOGY AND RISKS FOR BREAST CANCER

Breast cancer continues to be the most commonly diagnosed cancer in women worldwide. It is caused by a progressive accumulation of mutations in the cell's DNA. Epidemiologic studies help identify factors that through either exposure or inheritance place a woman at risk for a greater chance of cellular change. Approximately 50% of newly diagnosed breast cancers are attributable to known risk, whereas 10% are associated with simply a positive family history. The degree of risk is important to know in order to advise women and establish plans for screening or interventions.

Most epidemiologic literature when reporting breast cancer risks describes the risk from any given factor as a relative risk. Relative risk is the risk compared with subjects in an exposed group to subjects in a comparison or nonexposed group. In contrast, clinical and genetic studies usually report results as a woman's lifetime risk: the risk of developing or dying from a disease over the course of one's lifetime. The distinction can be confusing for patients and families. For example, the *BRCA* mutation causes a 10 times increase in relative risk and up to an 85% lifetime risk. Clinicians must be aware of the difference when reviewing the literature and subsequently when counseling patients and their families.

The risk factors for breast cancer may be divided into several categories (Table 15.2): demographic, estrogen exposure, lifestyle, personal breast characteristics, familial and inherited genetic mutations, and radiation exposure. Risk is generally grouped as minor and major. Minor risk factors increase a woman's lifetime risk from 12% to approximately 15%. Importantly, epidemiologic studies have also noted factors that decrease a woman's risk (Table 15.3).

## DEMOGRAPHIC ASSOCIATIONS

Age continues to remain the strongest risk factor for developing breast cancer. The risk of breast carcinoma increases directly with the patient's age (Box 15.2). Data from the Surveillance, Epidemiology, and End Results (SEER) database report the probability of a woman developing breast cancer from birth to age 39 as 0.49% (1 in 203 women) compared with 6.58% (1 in 15 women) at age 70 or older (Siegel, 2012).

**Table 15.2** Risk Factors for Breast Cancer

| Risk Factor | Qualification |
|---|---|
| Demographic—minor (less than 5 × RR) | |
| Age | Rare under age 30, common in sixth and eighth decades |
| Geographic | Common in Western countries |
| Estrogen exposures—minor | |
| Age at menarche | Younger than 12 years old |
| Age at first birth | Older than 30 years old |
| Late menopause | |
| Hormone replacement therapy | |
| Lifestyle—minor | |
| Alcohol use | Dose related (two or more drinks daily) |
| Sedentary lifestyle | |
| Obesity | |
| Postmenopausal weight gain | |
| Low vitamin D | |
| Abnormal day/night work patterns (airline attendants and variable shifts) | |
| Breast characteristics-minor | |
| Benign breast disease | Very low increased risk |
| Hyperplasia without atypia on biopsy | |
| Breast characteristics—major (increasing a woman's risk >5 × RR) | Major factors usually push a woman into the high-risk category |
| Dense breasts | Density proportional to increase in risk<br>Increased fibroglandular elements |
| Hyperplasia with atypia | |
| Previous breast cancer | |
| Familial factors—minor | |
| Multiple relatives, not first-degree, with breast cancer | |
| One first-degree relative with breast cancer | First degree—mother or sister |
| Family history—major | |
| Two or more first-degree relatives | Increased risk if the cancers are premenopausal |
| Inherited breast cancer syndrome such as *BRCA* | Very high risk |
| Radiation—minor | |
| Exposure to chest CT | |
| Radiation—major | |
| Mantle radiation for treatment of malignancy | Very high risk, which increases with age |

*CT*, Computed tomography; *RR*, relative risk.

The incidence of breast cancer varies based on geographic region. The highest rates are found in North America, Australia/New Zealand, and Western and Northern Europe. Women in Eastern Europe, South Africa, Japan, and the Caribbean form a middle group in terms of incidence. The lowest incidences are found in Asia and sub-Saharan Africa.

In the United States, white women have the highest rate of breast cancer; however, black women have a higher breast cancer mortality. Data from 2005 to 2009 report the rate of newly diagnosed breast cancer was 122 per 100,000 white women and

**Table 15.3** Factors Associated with a Decreased Risk for Breast Cancer

| Demographic | Qualification |
|---|---|
| Born and living outside Western countries | |
| Estrogen exposures | |
| Late menarche | After age 14 |
| Oophorectomy | Prior to age 35 without supplemental estrogen |
| Lactation | Proportional to total cumulative months breast-feeding |
| Age of first birth | Prior to age 20 |
| Parity | 5 or greater |
| Induced abortion | Trend (5 < *P* < .1) |
| Lifestyle | |
| Postmenopausal body mass | Minimal postmenopausal weight gain |
| Physical activity | |
| Dietary | |
| Vitamin D | Low levels associated with risk |
| Intake of vitamin D | Associated with decreased risk |
| Olive oil and omega 3 fatty acids | |
| Low-fat diet | Results suggestive but not yet conclusive |
| Medications | |
| Aspirin | Associated with decreased incidence, recurrence, and mortality |

**Box 15.2 A Woman's Risk of Having Developed Breast Cancer**

| Age | Risk |
|---|---|
| 25 | 1 in 19,608 |
| 30 | 1 in 2525 |
| 35 | 1 in 622 |
| 40 | 1 in 217 |
| 45 | 1 in 93 |
| 50 | 1 in 50 |
| 55 | 1 in 33 |
| 60 | 1 in 24 |
| 65 | 1 in 17 |
| 70 | 1 in 14 |
| 75 | 1 in 11 |
| 80 | 1 in 10 |
| 85 | 1 in 9 |
| Ever | 1 in 8 |

Data from National Cancer Institute. Painter K. Factoring in cost of mammograms. *USA Today.* December 5, 1996, p 11D.

117 per 100,000 black women. Black women more commonly presented with regional or advanced disease (45% vs. 35%) and had a 41% higher breast cancer specific mortality rate (32 vs. 22 deaths per 100,000 women) (Centers for Disease Control and Prevention [CDC], 2012). This difference may be due to several factors that include both socioeconomic aspects as well the histologic variety of tumors.

## ESTROGEN-RELATED EXPOSURE RISKS

Breast cancer risk is increased with high endogenous estrogen levels in both premenopausal and postmenopausal women. This effect is especially noted in hormone receptor–positive breast cancer. Various studies have shown that both prolonged exposure to and higher concentrations of estrogen are associated with a higher risk of breast cancer. Breast cancer is rare in the prepubertal female. Women who have breast cancer and undergo oophorectomy have a lower recurrence rate. Interestingly, the rate of recurrence in oophorectomized women is decreased, even in women with hormone-receptor-negative cancers.

Reproductive factors must also be considered in determining the risk of developing breast cancer. Nulliparous compared with parous women are at an increased risk of breast cancer, but the protective effect of pregnancy is not noted until 10 years following delivery. It is unclear whether an association exists between either multiparity or nulliparity and breast cancer. The age at which a woman delivers her first child is an important risk factor. Age at first pregnancy was analyzed in the Nurses' Health Study. When compared with nulliparous women at or near menopause, women who delivered their first child at age 20, 25, or 35 years had a cumulative incidence of breast cancer (up to age 70) of 20% lower, 10% lower, and 5% higher, respectively (Colditz, 2000). Early age at menarche is associated with a higher risk of breast cancer. Women with menarche at or after age 15 years of age compared with menarche before the age of 13 years were less likely to develop estrogen receptor–positive breast cancer. Additionally, a 16% decreased risk of estrogen receptor/negative breast cancer was noted in women with menarche at or after age 15 years.

Breast-feeding decreases the risk of breast cancer. A pooled analysis of data from 47 studies involving 50,302 women with breast cancer and 96,973 women without the disease found a direct correlation between the length of time of lactation and decreasing risk for breast malignancy (Collaborative Group on Hormonal Factors in Breast Cancer, 2002). Women who breastfed longer were more protected against breast cancer. The relative risk of breast cancer decreased by 4.3% per 12 months of breast-feeding. This decrease did not vary significantly by parity, ethnicity, age of menarche and menopause, and geographic factors. Newcomb and colleagues reported that after adjusting for parity, age at first delivery, and other confounding factors, lactation was associated with a slight reduction in the risk of breast cancer among premenopausal women compared with those who had never lactated (relative risk [RR] 0.78, confidence interval [CI] 0.6 to 0.91) (Newcomb, 1994). Overall, breastfeeding decreases the risk of breast cancer in a dose-response relationship.

Hormone replacement, specifically the use of combined estrogen and progesterone, is an established risk factor for breast cancer. Data from the Women's Health Initiative (WHI) showed that compared with the placebo group, combined hormone replacement increases the risk of breast cancer by 24%. Estrogen-only use in women with a history of a hysterectomy did not increase the risk of breast cancer (Chlebowski, 2003). The decision to use hormone replacement therapy in patients with and without other risk factors should be individualized and the risks and benefits discussed so that the woman may make an informed decision. Unlike hormonal replacement, oral contraceptives and other forms of estrogen-related contraception do not increase the risk of breast cancer. Multiple studies have noted that the oral contraceptives used since the 1980s do not pose an increased risk compared with the extremely high levels of estrogen used in oral contraceptives in the 1960s and 1970s. There is no association between abortion and breast cancer incidence.

## LIFESTYLE AND DIETARY RISK FACTORS

The relationship between dietary habits and the risk of breast cancer is not clear. A direct association between dietary fat and the risk of breast cancer has not been clearly established. Various studies have failed to show a significant association between the highest and the lowest category of consumed dietary fat and an increased risk of breast cancer. In the WHI study of postmenopausal women, the dietary arm of the study evaluated 48,835 healthy postmenopausal women who tried to reduce fat intake (Prentice, 2006). There was a minimal effect on decreasing malignancy in the breast, (RR, 0.91; CI, 0.83-1.01) after a mean follow-up of 8.1 years. Although no direct association between dietary fat intake and breast cancer risk has been established, there may be a modest effect when comparing extremes of fat intake. In the AARP Diet and Health Study, women in the highest quintile of fat intake had rates of invasive breast cancer 11% to 22% higher than those of women in the lowest quintile (Thiébaut, 2007). Although obesity is associated with a general increase in morbidity and mortality, the risk of breast cancer related to body mass index (BMI) is linked to the menopausal status of women. Obese women are at a higher risk for developing breast cancer during their postmenopausal years, with increased amounts of peripheral conversion of androstenedione to estrone. In premenopausal women, an increased BMI is associated with a lower risk of breast cancer.

Studies also have found a significant association with decreased levels of vitamin D and decreased calcium and increased risks of breast cancer and increased morbidity once breast cancer is diagnosed. Increase in plasma 25-hydroxyvitamin D (25[OH]D) levels between 27 and 35 ng/mL, were associated with a decrease in breast cancer risk in postmenopausal women (Bauer, 2013). No association between 25(OH)D levels and breast cancer risk is noted in premenopausal women. Antioxidant supplementation (vitamin A, E, or C, or beta carotene) has not been shown to be protective for breast cancer. Data regarding the effect of nonsteroidal anti-inflammatory drugs (NSAIDs) on breast cancer risk is varied. Several small studies and a nested study from the WHI noted aspirin to decrease risk for breast cancer, breast cancer recurrence, and breast cancer mortality; however, data from the Nurses' Health Study showed no association between use of aspirin, NSAIDs, or acetaminophen and the incidence of breast cancer (Zhang, 2012).

Alcohol consumption has been associated with increased risk for multiple cancers including breast cancer. Older studies reported a 40% to 50% increase in the relative risk of developing breast cancer related to alcohol consumption. The alcohol effect was primarily in estrogen receptor–positive tumors. Breast cancer risk is higher in women consuming both low and high levels of alcohol compared with no consumption. Longnecker showed that the risk of breast cancer was strongly related to the amount of alcohol consumed and that even light drinking was associated with a 10% increase in relative risk (Longnecker, 1994). A 2013 meta-analysis of 110 epidemiologic studies reported a 5% (RR 1.05%) increase in female breast cancer with light alcohol intake (Bagnardi, 2013).

Phytoestrogens are naturally occurring plant substances with a chemical structure similar to 17-beta estradiol. They consist mainly of isoflavones (found in high concentrations in soybeans and other legumes) and lignans (found in a variety of fruits, vegetables, and cereal products). There is low-quality evidence that soy-rich diets in Western women prevent breast cancer. A 2008 meta-analysis of eight studies evaluated the impact of soy food intake and breast cancer risk (Wu, 2008). A higher intake of isoflavones (≥20 mg per day) was associated with a 29% reduction in breast cancer risk in Asian women but no association with soy intake was noted among Western women. Of note, the highest level of soy intake in Western women was only about 0.8 mg daily, which may not have been an adequate amount to detect an effect.

Various miscellaneous environmental exposures have been studied for possible associations with the development of breast cancer. Megdal and associates found in a 2005 meta-analysis of 13 studies that altered day/night exposure, shift work, and increased light exposures to show an increased risk of breast cancer, RR 1.48 (CI: 1.36-1.61). Suppression of nocturnal melatonin production by the pineal gland secondary to nocturnal light exposure may contribute to the increased risk of developing breast cancer. Magnetic radiation, power lines, computer terminals, and electric blanket exposure do not increase the risk of breast cancer. Breast implants have not been shown to increase the risk for breast cancer.

## BREAST HISTORY AND BREAST CHARACTERISTICS

Women with a personal history of breast cancer or ductal carcinoma in situ are at an increased risk of developing invasive breast cancer in the contralateral breast. Analysis of SEER data showed the incidence of invasive contralateral breast cancer in women with a history of primary breast cancer was 4% during a 7.5-year follow-up period (Nichols, 2011). The risk of a contralateral breast cancer depends on the age at the time of the index breast cancer diagnosis in conjunction with the hormone receptor status of the primary tumor. The presence of ductal carcinoma in situ did not modify the rate of contralateral breast cancer.

Boyd and coworkers reported that women with dense breasts, as defined by more fibrous tissue, have a relative risk of 4.7 (CI: 2-6.2) for breast cancer (Fig. 15.10) (Boyd, 2007). This finding has been verified in other studies, and the increased risk is not due to a more difficult or later diagnosis but to the biologic characteristics of the breast itself. Women with dense breasts noted on mammograms (dense tissue involving at least 75% of the breast) have a risk of breast cancer four to five times greater compared with women with less dense tissue. Both usual and atypical hyperplasia increases the risk of breast cancer. There is a mild increase in risk when biopsies have shown hyperplasia; however, hyperplasia with atypia increases the risk by four to six orders of magnitude. The cumulative incidence of breast cancer among women with atypical hyperplasia approaches 30% at 25 years of follow-up.

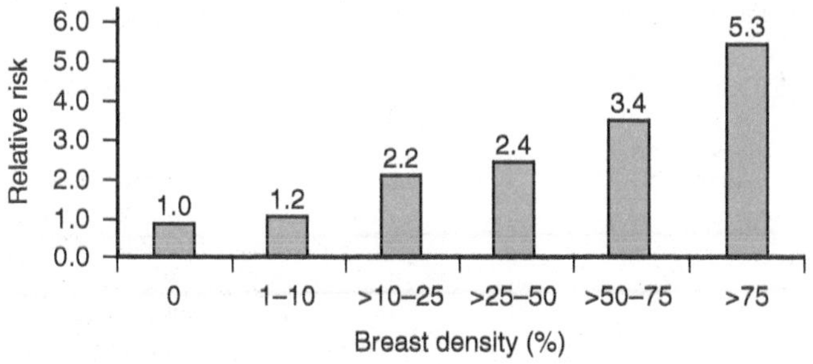


**Figure 15.10** Risks of breast cancer with increasing breast density. (Modified from Santen RJ, Mansel R. Benign breast disorders. *N Engl J Med.* 2005;353[3]:275-285.)

## INHERITED AND FAMILIAL RISKS

Most cases of breast cancer are sporadic in nature and not an inherited cancer. About 5% to 10% of all breast cancers are caused by an inherited gene mutation. There are at least four specific breast cancer syndromes, each associated with a specific mutation. Each of these syndromes is autosomal dominant and involves mutations in the proteins that repair DNA. The most common are the mutations in the breast cancer susceptibility gene 1 *(BRCA1)* and breast cancer susceptibility gene 2 *(BRCA2)*. Less common are Li-Fraumeni syndrome, associated with the *p53* gene, and Cowden syndrome, associated with the *PTEN* gene (Table 15.4).

Women with genetic syndromes tend to develop breast cancer at earlier ages and tend to have more aggressive tumors with a higher prevalence of bilateral disease. Hereditary breast and ovarian cancer (HBOC) syndrome is the most common cause of hereditary breast and ovarian cancers. This syndrome is associated with *BRCA1* and *BRCA2* mutations and is responsible for approximately 5% of breast cancer cases in the United States. Though the incidence of *BRCA* mutation is 1:250 in the United States, due to the founder effect the prevalence of *BRCA1* and *2* mutations is variable among ethnic groups and geographic area. It is highest among Ashkenazi Jews, in which approximately 2% of the population carries a deleterious *BRCA1* or *2*.

The *BRCA* genes code for very large tumor suppressor proteins. Germ line mutations in *BRCA* genes result in mutation carriers losing one of their wild-type alleles. These mutation carriers have only one functional allele of these genes in their cells. Tumors in carriers tend to demonstrate loss of the other wild-type allele through other somatic mutations or loss of heterozygosity. This genomic instability of women with *BRCA* mutations

**Table 15.4** Major Inherited Gene Mutation Syndromes Associated with Breast Cancer

| Syndrome | Gene | Incidence | Lifetime Breast Cancer Risk | Associated Cancer Risks |
|---|---|---|---|---|
| *BRCA 1* | *BRCA 1* | 1/500 to 1/1000 | 85% | Ovary and pancreas |
| *BRCA 2* | *BRCA 2* | Unclear | 85% | Ovary and pancreas |
| Cowden | *PTEN* | 1/100,000 to 1/200,000 | 50% | Thyroid and endometrium |
| Li-Fraumeni | *TP53* | 1/20,000 | 90% | Sarcoma, brain, and leukemia |

Other syndromes, including Peutz-Jeghers syndrome, ataxia telangiectasia, *CHEK2* gene mutation, and Fanconi syndrome, have much smaller lifetime risks with poorer penetrance.

causes them to be more susceptible to further mutations of DNA, which subsequently leads to malignant transformation of breast and ovarian epithelial cells.

*BRCA1* has 1863 amino acids, with several different functions, and was mapped at 17q21. In combination with several other genes including *BARD1*, *BRCA2*, *CHK1*, and *RAD51*, *BRAC* is involved in repair of double-strand DNA breaks and control of cell cycle checkpoints. Women with a *BRCA1* mutation have a risk of breast cancer of approximately 55% to 70% to age 70 and an average lifetime risk of ovarian cancer approaching 40%. The *BRCA2* gene was mapped to chromosome 13q12 and the DNA sequence determined by Schutte and coworkers in 1995. Women with a *BRCA2* gene mutation have a 45% to 70% risk of breast cancer to age 70 and a 15% to 20% lifetime risk of ovarian cancer. The risk of a contralateral breast cancer in women with a deleterious *BRCA1* or *BRCA2* mutation has been estimated to range from 10% to 65%. The contralateral breast cancer risk also depends upon age of first breast cancer presentation with the risk being higher when the age diagnosis is less than 40 compared with older than 50 years of age. *BRCA2* mutations are also associated with male breast cancers, conferring a 5% to 10% risk for a man who has inherited the mutation. Because male breast cancer is so rare, any male with breast cancer should be tested for a *BRCA* mutation.

Data also suggest a potential role of *BRCA1* and *BRCA2* mutations in sporadic breast and ovarian cancers, in particular triple-negative (i.e., breast cancers that lack expression of the estrogen receptor, progesterone receptor, and human epidermal growth factor receptor 2 [HER2]) breast cancers, some of which exhibit hypermethylation of *BRCA1*, *BRCA2*, or other downstream genes, leading to abnormal gene expression. The genomic instability of *BRCA1*- and *BRCA2*-deficient cells in hereditary and triple-negative breast cancer provides an opportunity for therapeutic development, especially drugs that target DNA repair pathways. This includes platinum-type drugs that generate double-stranded DNA breaks or poly (adenosine diphosphate-ribose) polymerase (PARP) inhibitors, which are involved in the repair of DNA single-strand breaks.

Women with a family history of breast cancer have an increased risk of developing breast cancer. Approximately 15% of breast cancers are related to familial risk. Women in such families have a combination of low penetrance polygenic inheritance contributing to their personal risk. The risk for breast cancer is significantly affected by the number of female first-degree relatives with and without cancer. The risk increases for a woman the more relatives she has with breast cancer. Additionally, the age at diagnosis of the affected first-degree relative is another factor that influences the risk for breast cancer. The risk is threefold higher if the first-degree relative was diagnosed before age 30. Models that will predict a woman's breast cancer risk are discussed later.

## RADIATION EXPOSURE

Exposure to therapeutic ionizing radiation is a recognized risk factor for the development of breast cancer. The risk of developing breast carcinoma is consistent with a linear dose-response relationship. This was first recognized in Japanese women who survived the atomic bombs, with exposed teenagers developing breast carcinoma in high incidence in their 30s. Other historical examples of ionizing radiation-induced breast cancer include women with a history of radiation treatments for postpartum mastitis, irradiation of the thymus in infancy, or multiple fluoroscopic examinations during treatment for tuberculosis. Currently, women at highest risk from radiation exposure are those who were treated with radiation for childhood malignancies, in particular Hodgkin lymphoma. Those with prepubertal exposure represent the most vulnerable age group; however, increased risk is evident in women exposed as late as 45 years of age. It is important to differentiate therapeutic ionizing radiation from radiation exposure from diagnostic imaging. One 64-slice chest computed tomography (CT) adds to a woman's lifetime risk of breast cancer by less than 1%.

## RISK ASSESSMENT AND PREVENTION

Stratification of a woman's risk of developing breast cancer is paramount. This should be an ongoing and dynamic process, as her risk increases with age and with changes in both personal and family history. The chance of developing a malignancy can be calculated based on her risk profile. This profile will influence the recommendations for both her screening as well as for preventive measures such as chemoprevention.

The risk factors that influence a woman's chances of developing a malignancy are multifactorial. With the exception of certain genetic mutations, a single risk factor is not sufficient by itself to stratify a woman into a risk group. Consequently, individualized counseling is the most effective approach to evaluating risk. Risk factors can be stratified into (1) major factors that increase relative risk greater than two times normal and (2) minor factors (see Table 15.2). A women's personal risk of developing breast cancer is divided into three levels: average, moderate, and high. Additionally, within the latter group a very high-risk group is identified for purposes of prophylactic options (Table 15.5). Women of average risk have a personal risk of about 12% of developing breast cancer, the risk of the general population. In the moderate risk group, women have personal risks from 12% to 15% of developing breast malignancy during their lifetime and have one or more minor risk factors. Women

**Table 15.5** Risk Levels for the Development of Breast Cancer

| Level | Lifetime Risk for Breast Cancer | Recommendations for Screening |
|---|---|---|
| Average | 12% | Yearly exams and mammograms beginning at age 40 |
| Moderate | 12% to 15% | Yearly exams and mammography beginning at age 40 |
| High | 15% to 20% | Yearly exams and mammography beginning at age 40; offer chemoprevention |
| Very high risk | >20% | Exams every 6 months; mammography alternating with MRI should be started on an individualized basis depending on the risk factor (e.g., for women with mantle radiation, imaging should begin at age 30 or 8 years after radiation is finished); offer chemoprevention |

in the moderate risk category do not need any changes from those of the general population in screening recommendations. Women at high risk include those who have greater than a 15% personal risk of developing breast cancer, usually from a major risk factor. In the very high-risk category, women have a personal risk over 25% and include women with a *BRCA* mutation or those who have had mantle radiation. They are often referred to breast specialists for ongoing evaluation.

Several models have been empirically developed to estimate a woman's risk of breast cancer. The most widely available and accepted tool is the Breast Cancer Risk Assessment Tool (BCRAT) developed by Dr. Mitchell Gail and is commonly known as the *Gail model*. The original model was based on data acquired from the Breast Cancer Detection and Demonstration Project to calculate the risk of a women developing breast cancer over the next 5 years till the age of 90. The model was developed in white women, taking into account age, race, age of menarche, number of births, number of first-degree relatives with breast cancer, and number of breast biopsies that have shown atypia. This model has been updated to estimate the risk for African-American women using data from the Contraceptive and Reproductive Experiences Study and for Asian-American and Pacific Islander women using data from the Asian American Breast Cancer Study (Gail, 2007; Matsuno, 2011). The BCRAT was designed for women who have never had a diagnosis of breast cancer, ductal carcinoma in situ (DCIS), or lobular carcinoma in situ (LCIS) and who do not have a strong family history suggesting an inherited gene mutation. It is not applicable to women with more than two first-degree relatives with breast cancer and does not consider more distant relatives, the age at which relatives developed breast cancer, or a family history of ovarian cancer. It is not useful for women with a strong family history of breast cancer on the paternal side. Most important, it does not estimate the risk of carrying a deleterious *BRCA1* or *BRCA2* gene.

The Clauss model, developed by Elizabeth Clauss in 1994, uses data from the Cancer and Steroid Hormone Study. This model uses first- and second-degree relatives, both maternal and paternal, to calculate risk but does not use risk factors beyond family history and also is not as robust in nonwhites. The Clauss model provides the lifetime risks for a woman over any given decade of her life.

Computerized risk prediction models have been developed to not only assess the risk of breast cancer but also the risk of carrying a deleterious *BRCA1* or *BRCA2* genes and include the BRCAPRO model (incorporates six predictive models for inherited or familial breast cancer), the International Breast Cancer Intervention Study or Tyrer-Cuzick model (incorporates both genetic and nongenetic risk factors to determine the risk of developing breast cancer and estimates of *BRCA1/2* mutation probabilities), and the BOADICEA model (developed to determine breast and ovarian cancer susceptibility because of genetic mutations).

An important role of the clinician in evaluating a woman's breast cancer risk is to determine which women should be evaluated for the inherited cancer syndromes (Box 15.3). There are several risk factors that raise suspicion for an inherited mutation. If a woman has a 5% to 10% probability of having a *BRCA* mutation, then she should be referred to a genetic counselor for a comprehensive assessment and workup of the family history. Reasons for referral to a genetic counselor for hereditary cancer risk evaluation include patients with a female breast cancer diagnosed at a young age (<50 years), a triple-negative receptor tumor, two or more synchronous primary breast cancers, male breast cancer, or invasive ovarian/fallopian tube/primary peritoneal cancer. Additional criteria include women with first-degree (sister, mother, or daughter) relatives with a history of breast cancer, a confirmed mutation in another family member, and women of Ashkenazi Jewish heritage, especially those with a family history of ovarian or breast cancer. Pre- and postgenetic counseling is essential and includes discussing the issues and implications of the results, legal and insurance aspects, noninformative results, and choices for chemoprevention or surgical prophylaxis. Women with negative or noninformative *BRCA* results may still need high-risk screening, as their risks may be greater than that of the general population.

The benefits of screening have been emphasized by major health societies and professional organizations (Table 15.6). The U.S. Preventive Services Task Force (USPSTF) recommendations updated the screening guidelines for breast cancer in 2015. The task force's recommendations were designed for women age 40 and older who do not show any signs or symptoms of breast cancer, who have no personal history of breast cancer, and who do not have a known genetic mutation or a history of chest radiation at a young age. The updated recommendations are as follows: (1) routine screening of average-risk women should begin at age 50, (2) routine screening should end at age 74, (3) women should get screening mammograms every 2 years, and (4) recommend against teaching breast self-examination. These recommendations were based on evidence that shows the value of mammography increases with age, with women ages 50 to 74 benefiting the most. In this age group screening is most beneficial and has the least amount of harm when performed every 2 years.

The American College of Obstetricians and Gynecologists (ACOG) recommends annual mammography screening for healthy women beginning at age 40. ACOG recommendations include screening mammography every 1 to 2 years for women aged 40 to 49 years and screening mammography every year for women aged 50 years or older (ACOG, 2011).

The American Cancer Society (ACS) screening guidelines for women with an average risk of breast cancer were revised in 2015. The updated recommendations are as follows: (1) regular screening mammography starting at age 45 years, (2) annual screening

**Box 15.3 Indications for Referral for Genetic Counseling for *BRCA* Gene Testing**

- Personal history of both breast and ovarian cancer
- Personal history of ovarian cancer or premenopausal breast cancer and Ashkenazi Jewish ancestry
- First-degree male relative with breast cancer
- Personal history of premenopausal breast cancer, particularly if it is triple negative
- Personal history of breast cancer and two first-degree relatives with breast cancer, any ages
- Personal history of high grace serous ovarian cancer (also primary peritoneal or fallopian tube cancers)

Modified from American College of Obstetricians and Gynecologists, et al. ACOG Practice Bulletin No. 103: hereditary breast and ovarian cancer syndrome. *Obstet Gynecol*. 2009;113:957-966.

Table 15.6 Professional Society Recommendations for Screening Mammography

| Organization | Age to Initiate Mammography | Age to Conclude Mammography | Interval between Screenings |
|---|---|---|---|
| American Academy of Family Physicians | Routinely at ≥50 y<br>Screening before age 50 should be individualized | Screening recommended to age 74 y<br>Evidence insufficient for age ≥75 y | Not stated for age 40-49 y<br>2 y for age 50-74 y |
| American Cancer Society | Routinely at ≥45 y<br>Offered for age 40-44 y | While in good health and is expected to live 10 more years or longer | 1 y for age 45-54 y<br>2 y for age ≥55 y |
| American College of Obstetricians and Gynecologists | 40 y | None stated | 1 y for all ages |
| American College of Physicians | Routinely at ≥50 y<br>40 y based on benefits, harms, preferences, and risk profile | Unclear | 2 y for all ages |
| American College of Radiology | 40 y | None stated | 1 y for all ages |
| National Comprehensive Cancer Network | 40 y | None stated | 1 y for all ages |
| U.S. Preventive Services Task Force, 2015 | Routinely at ≥50 y<br>Screening before age 50 should be individualized | Screening recommended to age 74 y<br>Evidence insufficient for age ≥75 y | 2 y for age 50-74 y |

Table 15.7 Breast Cancer Chemoprevention

| Results | Tamoxifen vs. Placebo* | Raloxifene vs. Placebo* | Raloxifene vs. Tamoxifen* |
|---|---|---|---|
| **Benefits** | | | |
| Invasive breast cancer | 0.70 (0.59-0.82) | 0.44 (0.27-0.71) | 1.02 (0.82-1.28) |
| Estrogen receptor-positive invasive breast cancer | 0.58 (0.42-0.79) | 0.33 (0.18-0.61) | 0.93 (0.72-1.24) |
| Estrogen receptor-negative invasive breast cancer | 1.19 (0.92-1.55) | 1.25 (0.67-2.31) | 1.15 (0.75-1.77) |
| Noninvasive breast cancer | 0.85 (0.54-1.35) | 1.47 (0.75-2.91) | 1.40 (0.98-2.00) |
| All-cause mortality | 1.07 (0.90-1.27) | 0.91 (0.81-1.02) | 0.94 (0.71-1.26) |
| Vertebral fracture | 0.75 (0.48-1.15) | 0.61 (0.54-0.69) | 0.98 (0.65-1.46) |
| Nonvertebral fracture | 0.66 (0.45-0.98) | 0.97 (0.87-1.09) | Insufficient data |
| **Harms** | | | |
| Thromboembolic events | 1.93 (1.41-2.64) | 1.60 (1.15-2.23) | 0.70 (0.54-0.91) |
| Coronary events | 1.00 (0.79-1.27) | 0.95 (0.84-1.06) | 1.10 (0.85-1.43) |
| Stroke | 1.36 (0.89-2.08) | 0.96 (0.67-1.38) | 0.96 (0.64-1.43) |
| Endometrial cancer | 2.13 (1.36-3.32) | 1.14 (0.65-1.98) | 0.62 (0.35-1.08) |
| Cataracts | 1.25 (0.93-1.67) | 0.93 (0.84-1.04) | 0.79 (0.68-0.92) |

Modified from Nattinger AB. In the clinic. Breast cancer screening and prevention. *Ann Intern Med.* 2010;152(7):ITC41, 2010.
*All values are risk ratio (95% CI). Four trials compared tamoxifen with placebo, two trials compared raloxifene with placebo, and one trial compared raloxifene with tamoxifen.

should be offered to women aged 45 to 54 years, (3) women 55 years and older undergo biennial screening or have the opportunity to continue screening annually, (4) women between the ages of 40 and 44 years should have the opportunity to begin annual screening, and (5) screening mammography should be continued as long as a woman's overall health is good and she has a life expectancy of 10 years or longer (Oeffinger, 2015).

No data exist regarding the ideal age at which to begin clinical breast examinations (CBEs). In the asymptomatic, low-risk patient it is unclear at what age to begin CBEs. The occurrence of breast cancer is rare before age 20 years and uncommon before age 30 years. ACOG and the National Comprehensive Cancer Network recommend that CBE be performed annually in women aged 40 years and older and every 1 to 3 years in women aged 20 to 39 years. Per the USPSTF guidelines, insufficient evidence exists to assess the additional benefits and harms of CBE beyond screening mammography in women 40 years or older. The ACS does not recommend CBE for breast cancer screening among average-risk women at any age.

## CHEMOPROPHYLAXIS AND CHEMOTHERAPEUTIC RISK REDUCTION

Breast cancer risk reduction should be considered throughout a woman's life. For women who are high risk, endocrine therapy should be discussed to reduce the risk of invasive or in situ breast cancers. The American Society of Clinical Oncology (ASCO) and the USPSTF both provide recommendations regarding the use of endocrine therapy. Selection criteria in identifying women who would benefit from endocrine therapy include age >60 years, age over 35 years with a history of lobular carcinoma in situ, ductal carcinoma in situ or atypical proliferative lesion of the breast (atypical ductal or lobular hyperplasia), women 35 to 59 years with a Gail model risk of breast cancer ≥1.66% over 5 years, and women with known *BRCA1* or *BRCA2* mutations who do not undergo prophylactic mastectomy.

Tamoxifen and raloxifene, both selective estrogen receptor modulators, are proved options that can decrease the risk of breast cancer in high-risk women (Table 15.7). Tamoxifen blocks the effects of endogenous estrogens in both the normal breast and the one with breast cancer. In the National Surgical Adjuvant Breast and Bowel Project (NSABP) B-14 trial, tamoxifen users had a significant decrease in the incidence of contralateral breast cancers compared with placebo. As a result, the Breast Cancer Prevention Trial (BCPT) was designed to assess whether tamoxifen would decrease the incidence of breast cancer in a high-risk population as determined by the Gail model for breast cancer risk assessment (Fisher, 1998). The trial enrolled 13,388 women in a double-blinded, randomized, placebo-controlled trial to evaluate the effects of tamoxifen on risk reduction. The trial was closed prematurely because of a large discordance between the two groups. Tamoxifen significantly reduced the incidence of breast cancer in this population of patients by 49% compared with controls ($P < .00001$). It did not reduce the incidence of estrogen receptor-negative cancers. A 2013 meta-analysis by the USPSTF analyzed data from four trials comparing tamoxifen to placebo (Nelson, 2013). The results showed a reduction in the risk of invasive breast cancer (RR 0.70, 95% CI: 0.59-0.82), primarily noted in estrogen receptor–positive breast cancer. A significant reduction in the incidence of nonvertebral fractures (RR 0.66, 95% CI: 0.45-0.98) was also seen (RR 0.66, 95% CI: 0.45-0.98). Additionally, the long-term follow-up results from the International Breast Cancer Intervention Study I (IBIS-1) showed a long-term reduction in the risk of hormone receptor-positive breast cancer (Cuzick, 2015). In this study of more than 7000 women, tamoxifen compared with placebo reduced the risk of invasive breast cancer between years 0 and 10 (hazard ratio [HR] 0.72, 95% CI: 0.59-0.88) and after 10 years (HR 0.69, 95% CI: 0.53-0.91). This risk reduction was observed in hormone receptor-positive breast cancer (HR 0.66, 95% CI: 0.54-0.81). Although treatment with tamoxifen compared with placebo is associated with an increased incidence in thromboembolic events and an increased incidence of endometrial cancer, the overall incidence of adverse events is small.

Raloxifene was approved by the Food and Drug Administration (FDA) for breast cancer risk reduction following the results of the Study of Tamoxifen and Raloxifene (STAR) trial (Vogel, 2006). A reduced incidence of thromboembolic events and endometrial cancer was noted in the raloxifene group compared with tamoxifen. In an 81-month median follow-up analysis, long-term raloxifene retained 76% of the effectiveness of tamoxifen in preventing invasive disease and grew closer over time to tamoxifen in preventing noninvasive disease. Less toxicity in regard to the development of endometrial cancer, uterine hyperplasia, and thromboembolic events was observed in the raloxifene group.

Aromatase inhibitors (AIs) are a reasonable alternative to SERMs for postmenopausal women. In the International Breast Cancer Intervention Study (IBIS-II), postmenopausal women at high risk of breast cancer were randomized to treatment with anastrozole or placebo for 5 years (Cuzick, 2014). After a median follow-up of 5 years, a 50% reduction in the number of invasive breast cancer was noted with anastrozole compared with the placebo group (HR 0.47, 95% CI: 0.32-0.68) along with a similar decrease in the incidence of ductal carcinoma in situ (DCIS). However, musculoskeletal side effects, vaginal dryness, and vasomotor symptoms were significantly greater in the anastrozole group.

Women with *BRCA1* mutations have significantly less benefit from tamoxifen. This is because almost all *BRCA1*-associated tumors are hormone receptor negative, unlike *BRCA2* carriers who should be offered chemoprevention. Though these medications are effective, many women do not want to take them because of the side effects related to premature or perimenopausal symptoms. These women should be offered additional medications to control the side effects.

Surgical prophylaxis is another option for the woman who wants to reduce risk. In a retrospective cohort of 639 patients, Hartmann was able to demonstrate a 90% breast cancer risk reduction for the patient with a high risk of breast cancer after prophylactic bilateral mastectomy. In a follow-up study, Hartmann was able to demonstrate a similar risk reduction in a population of women with *BRCA* gene mutations (Hartmann, 2001). Although prophylactic bilateral mastectomy provides the greatest risk reduction, it is usually reserved for the very high-risk patient because of the associated physiologic and complicated psychological consequences. Although most women who have undergone prophylactic bilateral mastectomy do not regret having undergone the procedure, approximately 5% to 20% report dissatisfaction.

## DETECTION AND DIAGNOSIS

In the United States and countries with established screening programs, most breast cancers are diagnosed as a result of an abnormal mammogram. However, a significant number are also noted during patient or clinician breast examination, and up to 15% of women are diagnosed with breast cancer not detected on mammography. Breast cancer is usually asymptomatic prior to the development of locally advanced disease. Approximately 10% of women with early breast carcinoma experience breast pain that is associated; however, focal mastalgia is usually associated with a benign condition. The classic sign of a breast carcinoma is a solitary, solid, immovable, dominant breast mass with irregular borders. About 75% of breast cancers present as a palpable breast mass. Axillary adenopathy is a potential sign of more advanced locoregional disease. Nipple discharge is an even less common symptom of breast cancer. Findings suggestive of inflammatory breast cancer include erythema, skin thickening, or skin edema causing the appearance of an orange peel (peau d'orange). With increased screening, many cancers and in situ lesions are found prior to any symptoms.

Screening utilizes tests in asymptomatic women at periodic intervals to discover breast malignancies. There is more scientific evidence regarding screening for breast cancer than for any other cancer. The kinetics of growth in breast carcinoma is the basis for the recommendations for screening and detection. The average breast mass doubles in volume every 100 days, and the diameter doubles every 300 days. A breast carcinoma grows for 6 to 8 years before reaching a diameter of 1 cm, after which it doubles in less than another year. The mean diameter of a breast mass discovered by women who perform BSE at monthly intervals is 2 cm.

The three screening modalities are breast self-examination, clinical breast examination, and imaging with mammography. BSE has the major advantages of no cost to the patient and convenience. However, studies have failed to show a beneficial effect of regular BSE in rates of breast cancer diagnosis, mortality, or tumor stage or size. BSE is associated with higher rates of breast biopsy for benign disease. Clinical breast examination (CBE) and mammography are complementary procedures and therefore the effectiveness of CBE in screening by itself is difficult to assess. As part of the screening process, the sensitivity of CBE was estimated to be 54% and specificity 94% (Barton, 1999). Various imaging modalities are available for identifying lesions that are suspicious for breast cancer. Mammography continues to be the primary choice in screening for breast cancer. It is important to note that a negative mammogram does not rule out breast carcinoma. Ultrasound is used as an adjunct to mammography for diagnostic follow-up of an abnormality seen on screening mammography. Additional imaging techniques include MRI and tomosynthesis. Current data do not support the use of MRI in screening women at average risk for breast cancer. Its use is limited to screening in high-risk patients. Newer tests, such as tomography, are under evaluation.

In summary, present protocols for screening of breast carcinoma are not ideal and continue to evolve. Nevertheless, screening tests result in a reduction in the mortality rate from breast cancer of approximately 25% to 30%.

## SELF-EXAMINATION OF THE BREASTS

Few randomized trials regarding breast self-examination exist. A 2003 Cochrane systematic review included two large population studies from China and Russia. Twice as many biopsies with benign results were performed in the screening group compared with the control group (RR, 1.89; 95% CI: 1.79-2.00) (Gemignani, 2011). Several other studies did not show an advantage of breast self-examination in the rates of breast cancer diagnosis, breast cancer death, or tumor stage or size. Although this procedure has long been advocated, breast self-examination in itself does not decrease breast cancer mortality. However, research has shown that routine breast self-examination does play a role in detecting breast cancer compared with finding a breast lump by chance or simply knowing what is normal for each woman. For this reason, some societies continue to recommend self-breast examination. ACOG recommends breast self-awareness, which for some patients includes performing a BSE and reporting changes to their physician. The ACS recommends educating women about the benefits and limitations of BSE and to report any changes. BSE is an option for women starting in their 20s. The USPSTF, however, recommends against teaching breast self-examination.

Women who choose to perform a BSE should do so when their breasts are least likely to be tender or swollen. In premenopausal women, a few days immediately after a menstrual period are the best time to detect changes in normal lumps or texture of the breasts. Postmenopausal women or women who have had a hysterectomy should be instructed to perform BSE on the same calendar days each month. Breast changes that women should be aware of include development of a lump or mass, swelling of the breast, nipple abnormalities or discharge, and skin irritation or dimpling. The examination is best done in both supine and upright positions using the finger pads of the three middle fingers. Three different levels of pressure (light, medium, and firm) are used to examine the breast. Women should be consistent in their technique used. One of the easier techniques to follow is to palpate the breasts in a clockwise fashion beginning at the nipple and gradually circumscribing larger circles; however, some advocated the vertical pattern (up and down pattern) as the most effective pattern for examining the entire breast without missing any breast tissue.

## CLINICAL BREAST EXAMINATION

Several studies have investigated the use of physical exam in addition to mammography; however, for ethical reasons no randomized trial comparing physical exam without mammography has been conducted. In meta-analysis investigating the effectiveness of CBE, Barton and colleagues included all controlled trials and case-control studies in which CBE was at least part of the screening process (Barton, 1999). CBE alone detected between 3% and 45% of breast cancers that were missed during mammography screening. The authors estimated CBE sensitivity at 54% and specificity at 94%. Factors associated with greater accuracy included longer duration of exam and a higher number of specific techniques used during the exam.

Considerable variability exists among physicians ability to detect breast lumps. Fletcher and coworkers tested the physical examination techniques of 80 different physicians using simulated breasts (Fletcher, 1985). Detection rates ranged from 17% to 83%. The ability to detect the mass was directly related to the size of the mass; 87% of 1-cm, 33% of 0.5-cm, and 14% of 0.3-cm masses were discovered. Physicians with higher discovery rates spent more time performing the examination.

Differing guidelines exist in the medical literature regarding the use of CBE in breast cancer screening protocols. However, it must be noted that no group recommends clinical breast examination alone. The ACS does not recommend clinical breast examination for breast cancer screening at any age among average-risk women. ACOG recommends clinical breast examination for everyone every 3 years from age 20 to 39, and annually thereafter. The USPSTF recommendations state that current evidence is insufficient to assess the additional benefits and harms of CBE beyond screening mammography in women 40 years or older.

Several palpation techniques exist for the clinical breast examination, and limited comparative data on the efficacy of these techniques are available. A complete breast examination involves inspecting and palpating the breasts with the patient in the sitting as well as the supine position. Initially in the sitting position with the patient arms at her sides, the clinician observes the contour, symmetry, and vascular pattern of the breasts and the skin for irritation, retraction, or edema. The patient is next asked to raise her arms over her head and any tethering of breast tissue to the chest wall should be noted. Examination of the axilla and supraclavicular nodes is best performed with the patient sitting upright. The breast examination is then performed in the supine position with both the woman's arms at her side and raised above her head. The examination includes palpation of all quadrants of the breast, axilla, supraclavicular areas, and adjacent chest wall. Palpation should use the pads of the first three fingers placed together, exerting firm but gentle pressure. It is important to examine both nipples for retraction or skin irritation. The areola should be compressed to identify any discharge. The normal

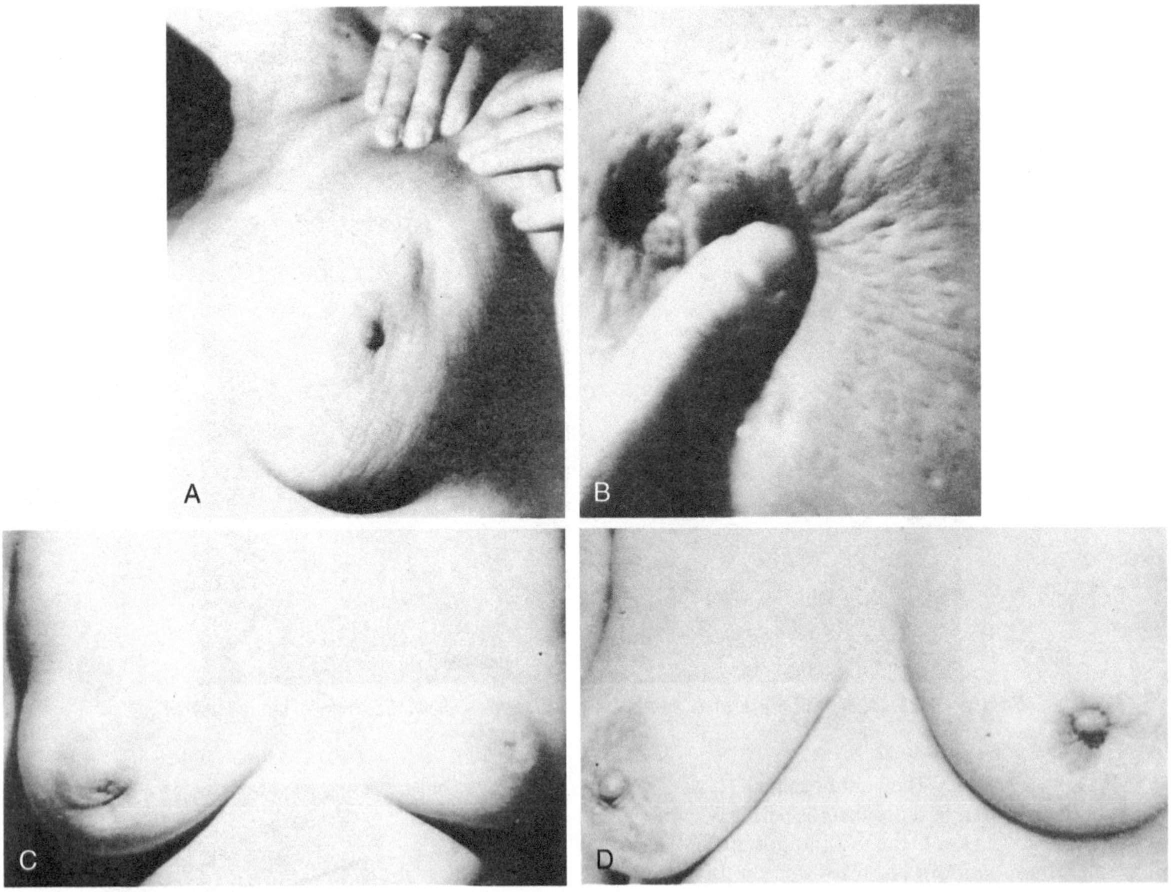

**Figure 15.11** Signs of breast carcinoma. **A,** Retraction found during physical examination. **B,** Peau d'orange from underlying carcinoma. **C,** Retraction of right nipple. **D,** Retraction of left nipple from carcinoma. (From Degrell I. *Atlas of Diseases of the Mammary Gland.* Basel, Switzerland: S Karger; 1976:20.)

breast has a small depression directly below the nipple. The skin of the breast is again carefully inspected for unusual vascular patterns, edema, erythema, or retraction (Fig. 15.11).

## MAMMOGRAPHY

The goal of screening mammography is the detection of cancer before it is clinically palpable and less likely to have progressed to the regional nodes or distant metastases. Mammography may identify cancer up to 4 years before it comes clinically evident. The 5-year survival rate for women whose breast cancer is believed to be localized to the breast with negative axillary nodes is approximately 99% versus 84% with regionalized diseased (when axillary nodes are involved). In contrast to screening mammography, diagnostic mammography is performed when women have complaints such as breast pain, a palpable lump (or mass), nipple discharge, abnormality on a screening study, or to follow women who have been treated for breast cancer.

Screening mammography is the primary imaging technique for breast cancer detection and the only breast imaging method found to reduce breast cancer related mortality. Mammography uses x-ray photons and can identify fine calcifications or small asymmetric densities associated with breast neoplasms months to years before the carcinoma enlarges to a size that may be palpated on physical examination. Nine randomized controlled trials using mammography with or without a clinical breast examination have been conducted. Systematic reviews of the trials differentiating mammogram screening with no screening indicate a protective effect among women ages 40 to 69. A 2012 meta-analysis of randomized trials showed a 20% relative risk reduction for breast cancer mortality in women who underwent screening compared with controls (Independent UK Panel on Breast Cancer Screening, 2012). However, critics suggest that breast cancer screening now may be less effective as the majority of these trials were initiated before 1990 and do not reflect modern therapy or modern imaging.

In the detection of breast cancer, the sensitivity of mammography ranges from 80% to 90% and decreases in women with dense breasts. Density is not a function of the size or firmness of the breast but refers to the ratio of glandular tissue to fatty elements. It is also a significant risk factor for the development of breast cancer. In cases where a woman is noted by plain-film mammography to have dense breasts, she should be referred for digital mammography preferably with tomosynthesis, or if she has dense breasts and she is in a known high-risk group, greater than 20% risk of the development of breast cancer, she should be offered an MRI.

Mammographic views can be generalized into two groups: standard views and supplementary views. The mediolateral

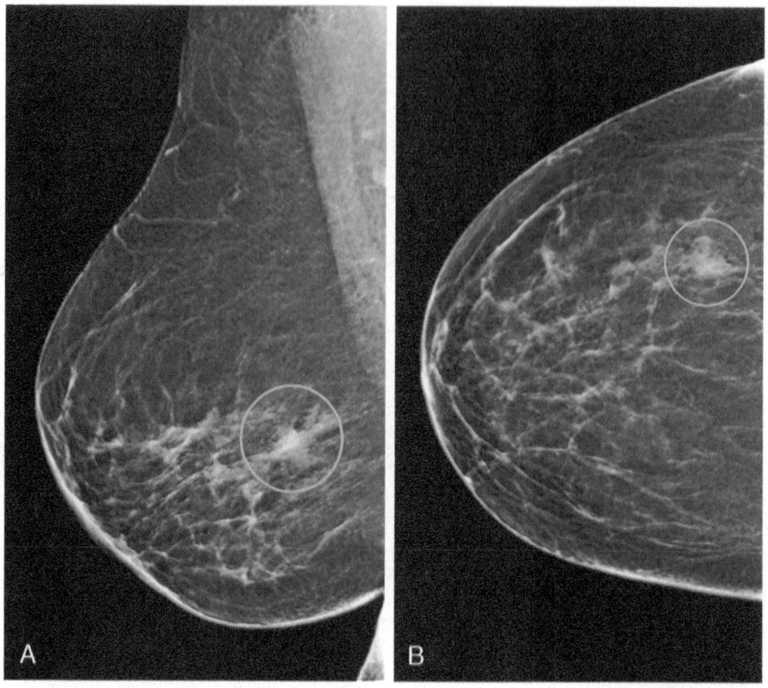


**Figure 15.12** **A,** Right breast, MLO view. **B,** Right breast, CC view. (Courtesy of Laura Isley, MD.)

oblique (MLO) view and the craniocaudal (CC) view (Fig. 15.12) are the two standard projections performed on routine screening. The MLO view is the most important projection as it depicts the greatest amount of breast tissue and is the only view that includes all of the upper outer quadrant and axillary tail. The amount of visible pectoral muscle in the MLO view determines the amount of breast tissue included in the image. This is an important factor in reducing the number of false negatives and increasing the sensitivity of mammography. Additionally, it is important to visualize the upper outer quadrant in the MLO view as most breast pathology develops in this area. An optimal CC view depicts the external lateral portion of the breast, the retromammary fat tissue (Chassaignac's bag), the pectoral muscle on the posterior edge, and the nipple.

Abnormalities noted on mammography include calcifications, masses, asymmetry, and architectural distortion. The most specific mammographic feature of malignancy is a focal mass with spiculated margins (Fig. 15.13). The positive predictive value of a mass with a spiculated margin is 81% and with irregular shape it is 73%. Clustered microcalcifications (Fig. 15.14) are noted in approximately 60% of cancers detected mammographically. Microcalcifications range from 0.1 to 1 mm in diameter, and the presence of five or more calcifications within a volume of 1 $cm^3$ is termed a *cluster*. Subsequent breast biopsies will find 25% of clusters associated with cancer and 75% with benign disease. Clustered microcalcifications can be associated with intraductal calcifications in areas of necrotic tumor or calcifications within mucin-secreting tumors. Linear branching microcalcifications have a higher predictive value for malignancy than do granular microcalcifications, particularly for high grade DCIS. Breast cancers, including DCIS, are more often diagnosed with the granular type of calcifications.

Mammographic findings are summarized employing the American College of Radiology Breast Imaging Reporting and Data System (BI-RADS) (Fig. 15.15). This reporting system was devised to standardize mammographic terminology, reduce confusing interpretations, and facilitate the monitoring of outcomes. There are six assessment categories, each associated with a specific risk of cancer. Category 0 is an incomplete assessment and therefore requires additional evaluation, which may include further imaging. Categories 1 and 2 are nonmalignant. Category 3 represents a lesion that is felt to be benign but requires interval follow-up imaging to confirm

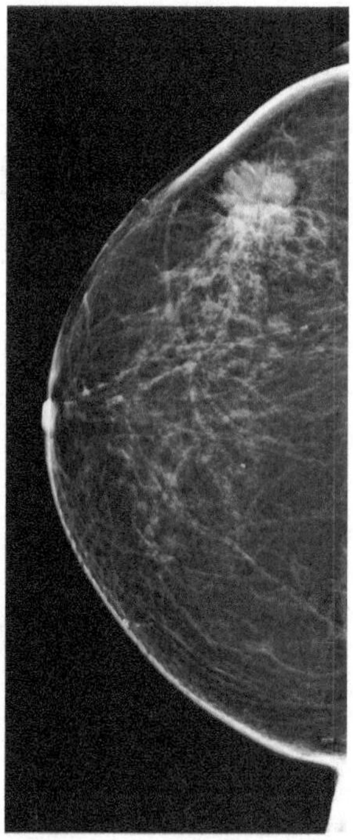

**Figure 15.13** Spiculated breast mass. (Courtesy of Laura Isley, MD.)

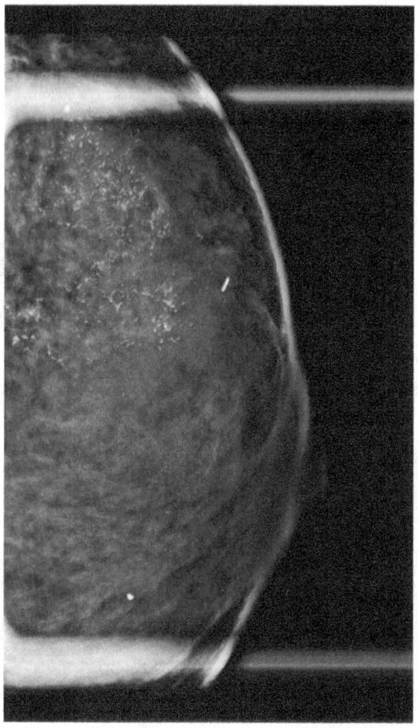

Figure 15.14 Breast microcalcifications. (Courtesy of Laura Isley, MD.)

| BI-RAD class | Description | Probability of malignancy (%) | Follow-up |
|---|---|---|---|
| 0 | Needs additional evaluation | 1 | Diagnostic mammogram, ultrasound |
| 1 | Normal mammogram | 0 | Yearly screening |
| 2 | Benign lesion | 0 | Yearly screening |
| 3 | Probably benign lesion | <2 | Short-interval follow-up |
| 4 | Suspicious for malignancy | 20 | Biopsy |
| 5 | Highly suspicious malignancy | 90 | Biopsy |

BI-RAD, Breast Imaging Reporting and Data Systems.

Figure 15.15 BI-RAD classification of mammographic lesions. (From Pazdur R, Coia LR, Hoskins WJ, Wagman LD, eds. *Cancer Management: A Multidisciplinary Approach.* 4th ed. Melville, NY: Cligott Publishing Group; 2006:143.)

stability. Categories 4 and 5 are lesions felt to be suspicious enough to warrant biopsy. Category 6 represents malignancy that has been proved. The BI-RADS final assessment is provided to standardize the reporting of mammographic findings and provide recommendations for further management.

## DIGITAL MAMMOGRAPHY

Digital mammography is the technique by which the radiographic image is obtained with digital detectors and recorded electronically in a digital format. The image is further processed and displayed as a gray-scale image that can be displayed in multiple formats. Digital mammography has several advantages compared with conventional film screen mammography.

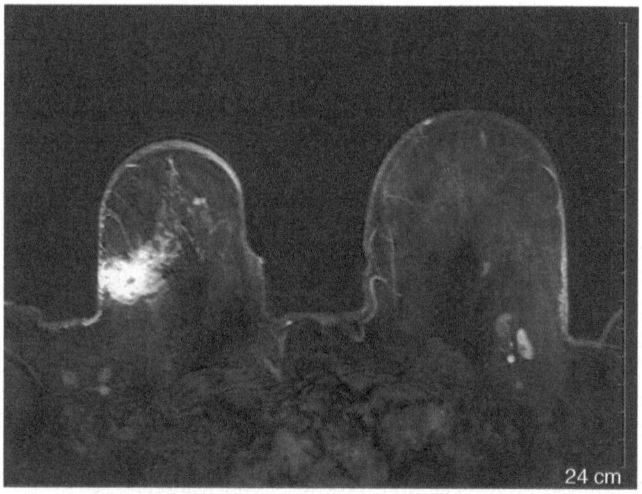


Figure 15.16 Breast MRI showing mass. (Courtesy of Laura Isley, MD.)

Image acquisition, display, and storage are much faster. Image manipulation through adjustments in contrast, brightness, and magnification of selected regions enables radiologists to obtain superior views. This technology makes it possible to subtract various layers of computerized imagery in order to examine suspicious areas and improve the ability to detect and diagnose breast carcinoma. Greater contrast resolution allows better screening of women with dense breasts and breast implants. With the ability to manipulate and postprocess the images, subtle abnormalities are increasingly detected. Images can be stored easily for future reference and can be sent electronically to be read at multiple viewing stations, thereby allowing double reading when necessary. The main disadvantages of digital mammography include the cost of the equipment and the reduced spatial resolution compared with film.

Digital mammography has been compared with film screen mammography in various studies with little difference reported in cancer detection rates. In the Digital Mammographic Imaging Screening Trial (DMIST), 49,528 asymptomatic women underwent both film and digital mammography (Pisano, 2008). Although there was no significant difference in overall diagnostic accuracy, digital mammography was more accurate for premenopausal and perimenopausal women. Furthermore, it was superior for women with dense breasts. Approximately 25,000 women aged 45 to 69 years were randomized to either digital or film screen mammography in the Oslo II Study (Skaane, 2007). The breast cancer detection rate at 2 years was significantly higher in the full field digital mammography group compared with film screen mammography (0.59% and 0.38%, respectively). In the United States, the majority of imaging centers utilize digital mammography. It may provide a small screening advantage in women younger than 50 years old. However, it must be noted that film mammography is an acceptable screening method for all women.

## MAGNETIC RESONANCE IMAGING

Magnetic resonance imaging (MRI) is another imaging modality utilized to detect breast cancer. MRI does not use ionizing radiation. Malignant tumors with increased tumor angiogenesis are differentiated from benign tumors based on the rapid uptake and release of contrast (Fig. 15.16). Lesions are classified as mass or nonmass. The reported sensitivity of MRI ranges from 71% to 100%. The lower specificity, less than 65%, is secondary to the overlap in the enhancement pattern of benign and malignant lesions. Although the specificity of MRI is lower than that for mammography, the sensitivity is higher and it is especially useful in women with dense fibroglandular breasts and implants.

Current screening recommendations are that women with a 20% or higher lifetime risk of breast cancer should be scheduled for annual MRI screening. In women of average risk, breast MRI has poor specificity. Additional potential uses or indications for MRI are to improve imaging of structures close to the chest wall, to improve imaging of women with breast implants, to detect occult primary tumors, and to evaluate for silicone implant integrity. MRI is useful in the documentation of response to neoadjuvant chemotherapy and diagnosis of recurrence and for screening of high-risk patients. MRI may be useful in the identification of multifocal, multicentric, or contralateral disease.

Several limitations of breast MRI exist. MRI cannot identify microcalcifications, and there is loss of image quality with respiratory movements. Breast MRI with gadolinium is not performed during pregnancy. MRI is contraindicated in patients with a history of gadolinium allergy, diminished renal function, cardiac pacemakers, defibrillators or other implanted devices whose operation may be disturbed by the MRI magnet.

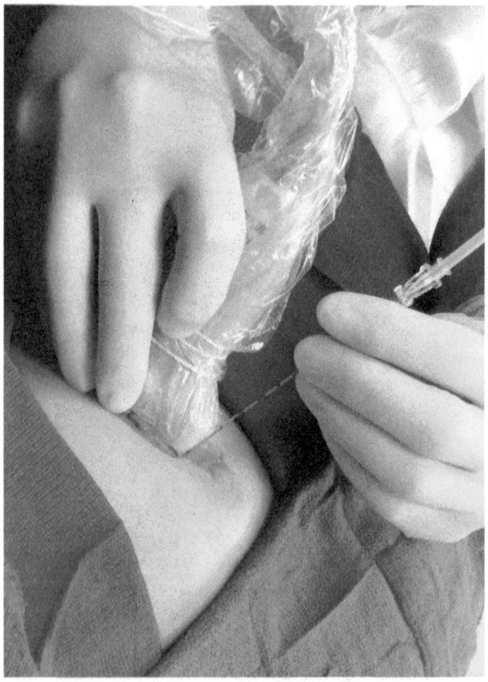

**Figure 15.17** Intraoperative ultrasound-guided wire bracketing of a nonpalpable breast lesion for excision. (Photo courtesy of David T. Rock, MD.)

### ULTRASOUND

Ultrasound has an established role in conjunction with mammography for evaluating abnormalities and is frequently used in the diagnostic follow-up of an abnormal screening mammogram. It should not be used by itself as a screening tool in average risk women. No randomized trials exist comparing combination ultrasound and mammography versus mammography alone for screening in average-risk women. However, women with dense breasts may benefit from the addition of ultrasound to screening mammography. Ultrasound screening increased the detection of otherwise occult cancers by 37% in a study involving 3626 women age 42 to 67, with dense breasts and no visible abnormalities on mammography. In women with dense breasts as their only risk factor, the American College of Radiology recognizes that ultrasound as an addition to screening mammography may be useful for incremental cancer detection.

Ultrasonography of the breast is a highly operator- and reader-dependent test with a great deal of variation among different centers. Ultrasound utilizes sound waves to image tissues and is particularly effective in differentiating cystic from solid masses. The accuracy rate of ultrasound to diagnose a cystic mass is 96% to 100%, which exceeds the combined accuracy of mammography and physical examination. It can be used in examining the axilla and determining lymph node status.

Ultrasound is frequently used to guide needle aspiration, or direct core needle biopsy. It has also been used to localize tumors intraoperatively without a guide wire with excellent success rates (Fig. 15.17). In pregnant women or women younger than 30 years old with focal breast symptoms or findings, ultrasound is the first line of imaging. Although MRI is superior at detecting silicone implant ruptures, ultrasound is usually more readily available and can be used in cases where MRI is contraindicated. In summary, ultrasound should not be used as a sole imaging technique for breast disease. Because of its lack of sensitivity and specificity for early breast carcinoma, it should not be used in an attempt to detect subclinical disease in the general population at this time.

### COMPUTED TOMOGRAPHY

CT is not routinely used for breast cancer screening or diagnosis. Due to higher radiation doses and longer study times, CT has limited value when compared with mammography. The thickness of cross-sectional slices with CT misses the majority of areas of microcalcification. It is useful for contrast-enhancing lesions, for lesions close to the chest wall, and for studying the most medial and lateral aspects of the breast. It is sometimes used for preoperative wire location of a mass that is difficult to localize by mammography. However, the increased expense and radiation exposure virtually eliminate CT scans from screening programs.

### TOMOSYNTHESIS

Breast tomosynthesis, commonly referred to as *three-dimensional (3D) mammography*, is a modification of digital mammography. The 3D image is created by taking multiple low-dose images per view along an arc over the breast. The compressed breast remains stationary while the x-ray tube rotates approximately 1 degree for each image in a 15- to 50-degree arc. The 11 to 49 acquired images are projected as cross-sectional "slices" of the breast, with each slice typically 1-mm thick. Thin slice reconstruction with tomosynthesis allows true lesions to be distinguished from spurious lesions caused by overlapping structures identified on routine mammography. Breast tomosynthesis has been approved in the United States for breast cancer screening, when used in combination with mammography. Friedewald and colleagues compared screening by digital mammography with digital mammography plus tomosynthesis (Friedwald, 2014). In this large retrospective study with data collected from 13 sites, the addition of tomosynthesis to digital mammography resulted in an overall decrease in recall rate of −16 per 1000 screens (95% CI, −18 to−14; $P < .001$) and more invasive cancers detected (4.2 cancers vs. 5.4 cancers per 1000 studies, $P < .001$). The detection rate for ductal carcinoma in situ was similar in both groups.

Disadvantages of tomosynthesis include increased radiation exposure and reading time. The radiation exposure is approximately double the usual radiation dose associated with mammography and can be even greater in patients with dense or thick breasts. Facilities with newer techniques that have a lower radiation dose are expensive and not widely available.

## BREAST TISSUE SAMPLING

The evaluation of a breast mass includes a clinical examination, imaging, and tissue sampling. This triple test has been advocated as a reliable alternative to excisional biopsy. If the physical exam, imaging findings, and cytologic evaluation of the mass all confirm the same benign process, the mass can be followed. However, if any of these assessments indicate cancer, a biopsy should be performed. The false-negative rate of triple test diagnosis approaches that of surgical biopsy, and the false-positive rate is comparable with that for frozen section.

Common indications for tissue biopsy include bloody discharge from the nipple, a persistent three-dimensional mass, or suspicious mammography. Additionally, nipple retraction or elevation and skin changes, such as erythema, induration, or edema, are also indications for breast biopsy. Imaging should precede biopsy, as the inflammation and bleeding that can occur secondary to the biopsy may significantly impair needed visualization of the breast with imaging. The choice of initial biopsy methods is dependent on the lesion characteristics, including whether it is palpable, and location. The least invasive technique that is likely to produce a diagnostic specimen should be used.

## FINE-NEEDLE ASPIRATION

Fine-needle aspiration (FNA) is the least invasive first-line sampling technique followed by core needle biopsy. FNA is a simple, office-based procedure. It is appropriate for new, well-circumscribed, usually tender masses that are thought to be simple (not complex) cysts. It is also valuable in the evaluation of ipsilateral axillary lymph nodes. If the lesion is not palpable, ultrasound guidance may be used to localize the lesion.

The skin over the breast is the most sensitive area, but the breast tissue itself has few pain fibers. Some providers choose to inject a small amount of local anesthetic (1 mL of 1% lidocaine). Care must be taken to avoid the development of a hematoma, which may obscure the mass and decrease the accuracy of the FNA. A small (18- to 21-gauge) needle is used when performing an FNA. The breast mass is secured with one hand, and the other hand introduces the needle attached to a 10- or 20-mL syringe into the mass. If the mass is found to be a cyst, the procedure can be converted into a cyst aspiration. The color of the fluid obtained via aspiration varies from clear to grossly bloody. Samples should be sent to a cytopathologist for evaluation. However, if the aspirated fluid is clear, it is not necessary to submit it for cytologic evaluation, and the patient is to be reevaluated in 1 to 2 months. If the cyst recurs, imaging should be performed to confirm their benign nature and reaspiration performed under ultrasound guidance. Less than 20% of cysts recur after a single aspiration, and fewer than 10% recur after two aspirations. A biopsy should be performed on cysts that recur within 2 weeks or that necessitate more than one repeat aspiration. In cases of a solid mass, a fixed specimen is obtained and submitted for cytopathologic evaluation. Several passes are made through the mass with continuous suction from the syringe. Moving the needle within a single tract will give a satisfactory cellular yield in the majority of cases.

Complications of needle aspiration are rare and include hematoma formation and infection. The theoretic risk of spreading cancer along the needle track has not been substantiated. Finally, it is difficult to determine the difference between carcinoma in situ and invasive cancer from the cytologic specimen obtained from FNA.

## CORE NEEDLE BIOPSY AND EXCISIONAL BIOPSY

Core needle biopsy retrieves more tissue than FNA, permitting the differentiation between invasive versus in situ cancer. A more definitive histologic assessment including tumor grade angiolymphatic invasion and hormone receptor status can be made. In addition, core needle biopsy usually provides adequate tissue for genomic analysis or cancer profiling. Vacuum-assisted directional biopsy can be used to acquire a greater volume of tissue. Excisional biopsy should be reserved for certain situations when a diagnosis is not established using the diagnostic triad.

Core needle biopsy is usually performed using a larger needle (9 to 14 gauge) than FNA. Following administration of local anesthetic, a small skin incision is made and the core biopsy needle is inserted. Three to five cores of solid tissue are collected for pathologic evaluation. A biopsy clip must be placed at the time of the biopsy for future localization of the lesion. Core needle biopsy may be performed with ultrasound, mammographic, or MRI guidance. Mammographic or stereotactic guidance is primarily used for biopsy of calcifications. The breast is imaged at 30-degree angles with 2D mammography, and the lesion is localized using computer-assisted positioning and targeting devices.

Nonpalpable breast lesions discovered by breast imaging techniques, including screening mammography, require preoperative localization by the radiologist. Under mammographic, ultrasound or MRI guidance, a wire is placed percutaneously so that the tip of the wire is fixed in the lesion. Image-guided techniques play a vital role in preoperative staging of breast cancer patients and in the planning of definitive surgery.

## CLASSIFICATION

Carcinomas make up the majority of breast malignancies and originate in the epithelium of the collecting ducts (ductal) or the terminal lobular ducts (lobular). Sarcomas are rare, constituting less than 1% of primary breast cancers, and arise

Table 15.8 Simplified Classification of Breast Carcinoma Based on Histology

| Type of Carcinoma | Percentage of All Cases Diagnosed |
|---|---|
| Ductal carcinoma | |
| In situ | 5 |
| Infiltrating | 70 |
| Infiltrating with uniform histologic appearance | 10 |
| Medullary, colloid, comedo, tubular, papillary | |
| Lobular carcinoma | |
| In situ | 3 |
| Infiltrating | 9 |
| Inflammatory carcinoma | 2 |
| Paget disease | 1 |

from stromal or connective tissue. Tumor grade is based on tubule formation, nuclear pleomorphism, and mitotic counts using the Nottingham score to determine low, intermediate, or high grade. Higher grade is associated with a poorer long-term prognosis.

Initially, breast carcinoma may be divided into invasive and in situ lesions (Table 15.8). Invasive ductal carcinoma accounts for the majority, approximately 80%, of invasive carcinomas. Invasive lobular carcinomas constitute approximately 10% to 15% of cases. Other subtypes include mucinous, tubular, medullary, micropapillary, and papillary. Both in situ and invasive carcinomas are often found in the same quadrant of the breast. Additionally, multifocal carcinomas are not uncommon, and bilateral breast carcinomas occur in 1% to 2% of newly diagnosed cases.

## DUCTAL CARCINOMA IN SITU

Ductal carcinoma in situ (DCIS) is a noninvasive lesion in which the cellular abnormalities are limited by the basement membrane of the breast ducts. The risk of DCIS increases with age and accounts for approximately 20% of newly diagnosed breast cancers. It is most commonly discovered in perimenopausal and postmenopausal women. Mammography has significantly increased the detection of this lesion. DCIS, evidenced by clustered microcalcifications, is not usually detectable by palpation. Diagnosis is confirmed with a core needle biopsy, usually using stereotactic guidance.

The histologic diagnosis of ductal carcinoma in situ includes a heterogeneous group of tumors with varying malignant potential. Classification is based on architectural pattern (comedo, micropapillary, cribriform, or solid), tumor grade (high, intermediate, or low), and evidence of necrosis. Identification of microinvasion, a minute focus of stromal invasion, is crucial as treatment recommendations may change.

The goal of treatment is to prevent the development of invasive cancer. Treatment approaches include surgery, radiation therapy, and adjuvant endocrine therapy. Mastectomy is curative for over 98% of DCIS patients. Breast-conserving surgery (lumpectomy, partial mastectomy) followed by radiation therapy has shown equivalent survival when compared with mastectomy. Chemoprevention with either a SERM or aromatase inhibitor is recommended for women with estrogen receptor–positive DCIS who have undergone breast conservation therapy to reduce the risk of developing additional invasive or noninvasive breast cancers.

## LOBULAR CARCINOMA IN SITU

Lobular carcinoma in situ (LCIS) is a noninvasive lesion arising from the lobules and terminal ducts of the breast. Historically, LCIS is found with an invasive carcinoma in approximately 5% of malignant breast specimens. Although it does not have the same malignant potential as DCIS, women with LCIS are at an increased risk of developing breast cancer. Eighty to ninety percent of cases occur in premenopausal women.

LCIS has a greater tendency to be bilateral and multifocal. The latent period for development of malignancy is longer than with DCIS. Approximately one fifth of women diagnosed with LCIS develop invasive breast carcinoma over a 20- to 25-year follow-up period. National Comprehensive Cancer Network guidelines recommend reexcision in cases where LCIS is diagnosed by core needle biopsy to rule out an invasive component. LCIS is not managed as a precursor lesion. In cases in which LCIS is diagnosed on an excisional biopsy, obtaining histologically negative margins is not mandatory as LCIS is frequently multicentric. Breast cancer chemoprevention with a SERM or an aromatase inhibitor may be indicated for women diagnosed with LCIS.

## INFILTRATING OR INVASIVE DUCTAL CARCINOMA

Infiltrating or invasive ductal carcinoma is the most common breast malignancy, comprising approximately 70% to 80% of breast malignancies. Histologically, nonuniform malignant epithelial cells of varying sizes and shapes infiltrate the surrounding tissue (Fig. 15.18). Cytologic features range from bland to highly malignant, and tumors are graded based on architectural and cytologic characteristics. Typically, infiltrating ductal carcinomas are firm and gray-white. The degree of fibrous response due to the invading malignant cells is responsible for the firm palpable mass, radiologic density, and texture during biopsy.

## INFILTRATING LOBULAR CARCINOMA

Infiltrating lobular carcinomas constitute approximately 10% to 15% of invasive lesions and are the second most common type of invasive breast cancer. These lesions are characterized by the uniformity of the small, round neoplastic cells that infiltrate the stroma and adipose tissue in a single-file fashion (Fig. 15.19). This neoplasia tends to have a multicentric origin in the same breast and tends to involve both breasts more often than infiltrating ductal carcinoma. Infiltrating lobular carcinomas are more frequently ER positive. Unlike infiltrating ductal carcinomas, the excised breast tissue frequently has a normal consistency and no mass lesion is grossly evident. Histologic subdivisions of infiltrating lobular carcinoma include small cell, round cell, and signet cell carcinomas.

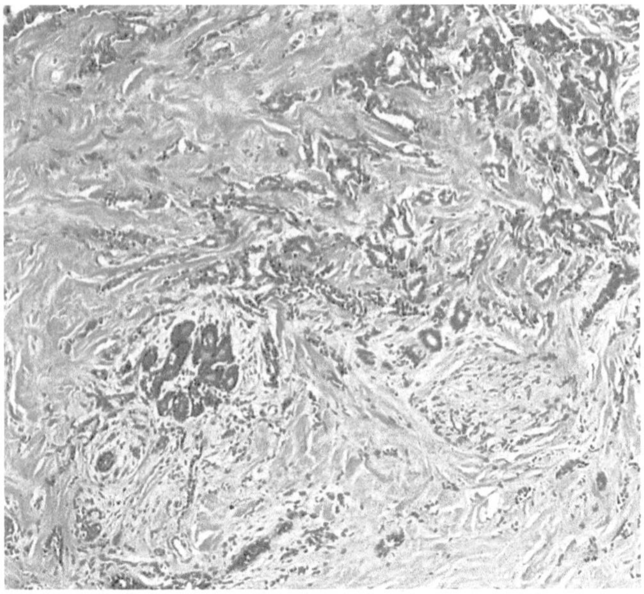

**Figure 15.18** Invasive ductal carcinoma of the breast. Malignant cells are invading the fibrous tissue. (From Stevens A, Lowe J. *Human Histology.* 3rd ed. Philadelphia: Mosby; 2005:392.)

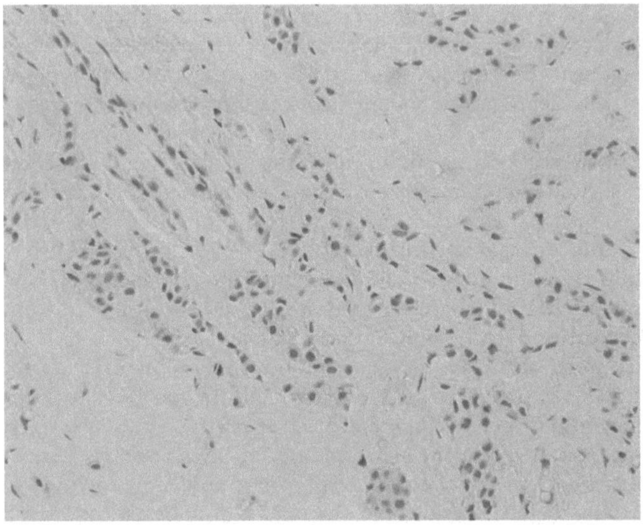

**Figure 15.19** Infiltrating lobular carcinoma of the breast. Neoplastic cells infiltrating the stroma and adipose tissue in a single-file fashion. (Courtesy of Panagiotis J. Tsakalakis, MD.)

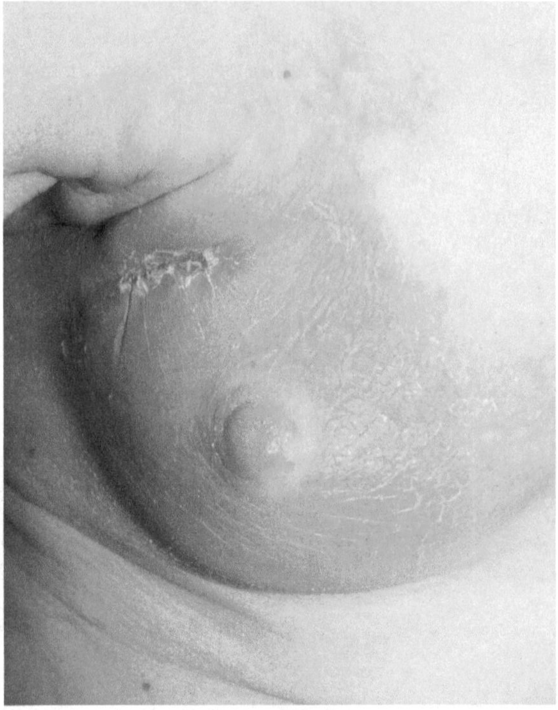

**Figure 15.20** Inflammatory breast carcinoma—cellulitic appearing plaque. (From Marks J, Miller J. *Lookingbill and Marks' Principles of Dermatology.* 4th ed. Philadelphia: Saunders; 2006.)

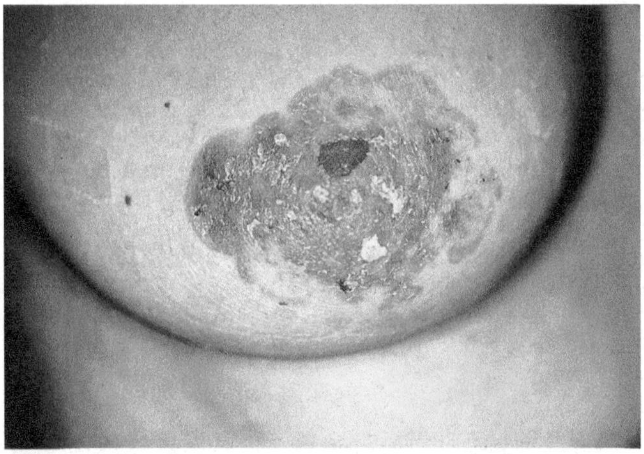

**Figure 15.21** Paget disease of the breast. Note the erythematous plaques around the nipple. (From Callen JP. Dermatologic signs of systemic disease. In: Bolognia JL, Jorizzo JL, Rapini RP, eds. *Dermatology.* Edinburgh: Mosby; 2003:714.)

## INFLAMMATORY BREAST CANCER

Inflammatory breast cancer is rare and accounts for approximately 1% to 5% of breast cancers. This type is recognized clinically as a rapidly growing malignant carcinoma with highly angiogenic and angioinvasive characteristics. Due to its aggressive features, most inflammatory breast cancers are diagnosed as either stage III or IV. Most are invasive ductal carcinomas. Infiltration of malignant cells into the dermal lymphatics of the skin produces a clinical picture that appears like a skin infection (Fig. 15.20). The breast is firm, warm, and enlarged with thickened, erythematous, peau d'orange skin changes. Histologically, dermal lymphatic invasion by malignant cells is noted.

## PAGET DISEASE

Paget disease of the breast is rare, constituting 1% to 3% of new breast carcinomas (Fig. 15.21). This lesion has an innocent appearance and looks like eczema or dermatitis of the nipple. The clinical picture of a scaly, raw, or ulcerated lesion of the nipple and areola is a result of an infiltrating ductal carcinoma that invades the epidermis. In approximately 85% of the patients, an underlying breast cancer is present with Paget disease of the breast. Punch biopsy or a full thickness wedge of the nipple is used for diagnosis. Intraepithelial adenocarcinoma cells (Paget cells) are noted on histology, presenting either singly or in small groups within the epidermis of the nipple.

## GENOMIC PROFILING

Historically, the treatment of breast cancer was based on tumor histology, axillary node status, tumor size, receptor patterns, and grade of differentiation. In addition to simplified histologic classification, a classification based on gene expression or profiling, including the presence of hormone receptors, has evolved. Identification of tumor receptor status is critical as endocrine therapy is utilized both for adjuvant therapy and in the management of advanced disease. The genomic analysis of tumors has led to the molecular subtyping of breast cancers. In the early 2000s, Perou and coworkers classified breast tumors into four different molecular subtypes: luminal, basal, HER2, and normal (Perou, 2000). Subsequently, the luminal group was further differentiated into luminal-A and luminal-B subgroups. Basal-like tumors include triple-negative tumors, tumors that are estrogen, progesterone, and HER2 negative by immunohistochemistry. A more aggressive subtype of triple-negative tumors, claudin-low tumors, has also been described. These divisions are detailed in Table 15.9.

The lactiferous ducts have two layers: the inner layer closest to the lumen and the outer layer next to the basement membrane with more myoepithelial elements. Cancers that appear to have expression of genes similar to luminal cells are usually hormonally estrogen sensitive. Luminal-A tumors make up approximately 40% of all breast cancers. These tumors are generally of the best prognosis, low grade, estrogen and progesterone receptor positive, and HER2 (Neu) negative. These are more commonly found in older women.

Luminal-B tumors account for approximately 20% of all breast cancers and have a more aggressive behavior compared with the luminal-A subtype. These tumors have overexpression of HER2 (Neu) and have a higher expression of the proliferation-related genes. Often they are estrogen and progesterone as well as *p53* gene mutation positive (these are acquired *p53* mutations as opposed to inherited mutations).

The third subtype, HER2 enriched, constitutes 10% to 15% of breast cancers. It is characterized by a high expression of both HER2 and proliferation gene clusters. These tumors are usually estrogen and progesterone negative, high grade, have a high rate of *p53* mutations, and have a poor prognosis.

The basal subtype makes up 15% to 20% of breast cancers. It is similar to basal-type duct cells in terms of expression of more myoepithelial gene profiling. These triple-negative tumors are usually high grade and exhibit a low expression of the luminal and *HER2* gene clusters. *BRCA1* tumors are up to 95% basal type.

A fifth type of breast cancer, claudin-low tumors, constitutes approximately 10% of breast cancers. Claudin-low tumors are also triple-receptor negative (estrogen, progesterone, and HER2 [Neu]). They have a high proliferation capability and are more aggressive than other subtypes.

**Table 15.9** Classification of Breast Carcinoma Based on Gene Profiling and Hormone Receptor

| Expression Type | Grade | Characteristic Behavior | Hormone Receptor Status* |
|---|---|---|---|
| Luminal A | Usually low grade | Good prognosis | E and P + |
| Luminal B | All grades | Mixed prognosis | E and P +, Her 2 (Neu) + |
| Her 2 (Neu) | Higher grades | Poor prognosis | E and P -, Her 2 (Neu) + |
| Basal | Usually grade 3 | Poor prognosis | Triple negative |
| Normal breast† | Usually low grade | Good prognosis | Triple negative |

**E*, Estrogen receptor; *P*, progesterone receptor.
†Normal breast does not express gene profiling of basal elements, myoepithelial gene expression.

### *MANAGEMENT*

A multidisciplinary team approach is necessary in the treatment of breast cancer. Local disease is treated with surgery, radiation therapy, or both. Systemic treatment includes chemotherapy, endocrine therapy, biologic therapy, or a combination of these regimens. Determination of local or systemic treatment is based on several prognostic and predictive factors including tumor histology, tumor hormone receptor status (estrogen/progesterone), tumor HER2 status, multigene testing, axillary lymph node status, evaluation of metastatic disease, patient age, comorbidities, and menopausal status.

The primary algorithm of treatment is primarily determined by the tumor stage. The tumor-node-metastasis TNM system is a widely recognized staging system based on both clinical and pathologic criteria (Table 15.10). The goal of treatment for stage 0, pure noninvasive carcinomas (LCIS, DCIS), is preventing the development of invasive disease or diagnosing the development of an invasive component when still confined to the breast. In cases of invasive disease, treatment is based on the stage-appropriate guideline for invasive carcinoma. The major objectives of treating breast carcinoma are control of local disease, treatment or prevention of distant metastasis, and improved quality of life for women treated for the disease. With multiple therapeutic options in both local and systemic therapy for breast carcinoma, women have an active role in deciding their own treatment regimen. There are several methods for controlling local disease. Breast conservation with lumpectomy or quadrantectomy is a frequent choice for the control of local disease. Sentinel node biopsy has become standard practice in the treatment of early stage breast cancer. Chemotherapy is used not only for patients with proved metastatic disease but also for women at high risk for developing distant or recurrent disease. Emphasis on conservative surgery plus radiation therapy to control multifocal cancer in the same breast and on reconstructive surgery after mastectomy has improved the quality of life for women with breast carcinoma.

**Table 15.10** TNM Staging of Breast Cancer

| | | | |
|---|---|---|---|
| **Primary Tumor (T)** | | | |
| TX | Primary tumor cannot be assessed | | |
| T0 | No evidence of primary tumor | | |
| Tis* | Carcinoma in situ; intraductal carcinoma, lobular carcinoma in situ, or Paget disease of the nipple with no tumor | | |
| T1 | Tumor is ≤2 cm in greater dimension | | |
| T1a | Tumor is ≤0.5 cm in greatest dimension | | |
| T1b | Tumor is >0.5 cm but not more than 1 cm in greatest dimension | | |
| T1c | Tumor is more than 1 cm but not more than 2 cm in greatest dimension | | |
| T2 | Tumor is >2 cm but not more than 5 cm in greatest dimension | | |
| T3 | Tumor is >5 cm in greatest dimension | | |
| T4 | Tumor of any size with direct extension to chest wall or skin | | |
| T4a | Extension to chest wall | | |
| T4b | Edema (including peau d'orange) or ulceration of the skin of the breast or satellite skin nodules confined to the same breast | | |
| T4c | Both T4a and T4b above | | |
| T4d | Inflammatory carcinoma | | |
| **Regional Lymph Node Involvement (N) (Clinical)** | | | |
| NX | Regional lymph nodes cannot be assessed (e.g., previously removed) | | |
| N0 | No regional lymph node metastasis | | |
| N1 | Metastasis to movable ipsilateral axillary lymph node(s) | | |
| N2 | Metastasis to ipsilateral axillary lymph node(s) fixed to one another or the other structures | | |
| N3 | Metastasis to ipsilateral mammary lymph node(s) | | |
| **Distant Metastasis (M)** | | | |
| MX | Presence of distant metastasis cannot be assessed | | |
| M0 | No distant metastasis | | |
| M1 | Distant metastasis (includes metastasis to ipsilateral supraclavicular lymph node[s]) | | |
| **Stage Grouping** | | | |
| Stage 0 | Tis | N0 | M0 |
| Stage I | T1 | N0 | M0 |
| Stage IIa | T0 | N1 | M0 |
| | T1 | N1* | M0 |
| | T2 | N0 | M0 |
| Stage IIb | T2 | N1 | M0 |
| | T3 | N0 | M0 |
| Stage IIIa | T0 | N2 | M0 |
| | T1 | N2 | M0 |
| | T2 | N2 | M0 |
| | T3 | N1, N2 | M0 |
| Stage IIIb | T4 | Any N | M0 |
| | Any T | N3 | M0 |
| Stage IV | Any T | Any N | M1 |

From Eberlein TJ. Current management of carcinoma of the breast. *Ann Surg.* 1994;220(2):121-136.

Paget disease associated with a tumor is classified according to the size of the tumor. Chest wall includes ribs, intercostal muscles, and serratus anterior muscle but not pectoral muscle.

*The prognosis of patients with pN1a is similar to that of patients with pN0.

### *Surgical Therapy*

The decision concerning appropriate therapy and extent of the surgical operation to treat breast carcinoma should be made by the patient in consultation with the surgeon, radiation oncologist, and medical oncologist who will treat her. The size of the tumor, the initial extent of disease, the virulence of the neoplasm, and the presence of estrogen, progesterone, or HER2 receptors are key medical factors in the decision. The initial size of the breast carcinoma is the single best predictor of the likelihood of positive axillary nodes. The presence and number of axillary node metastasis are the best predictors of survival. Traditionally, the evaluation for localized invasive disease includes bilateral diagnostic mammography, possible subsequent ultrasonography, tumor hormone receptor status, HER2 receptor status, and pathology review. MRI for the evaluation and determination of the extent of disease has been controversial. Supporters cite high sensitivity in evaluating the extent of disease, especially for invasive cancer and in dense breasts as well as the identification of second cancers. Arguments against MRI use include a high percentage of false-positive findings resulting in additional diagnostic workup or more extensive surgery than necessary.

Locoregional treatment of clinical stage I, IIA, IIB, or T3N1MO (a subset of stage IIIA) invasive breast cancer includes lumpectomy (or total mastectomy ± reconstruction) with surgical axillary staging. Intensive discussions concerning breast reconstruction or external prostheses are important to help the patient contemplate the effects of surgery on body image. Morris and coworkers have studied the psychological and social adjustments to mastectomy in 160 women, who were followed at intervals of 3, 12, and 24 months after surgery (Morris, 1977). One in four women was still having problems with depression and associated marital and sexual problems 2 years after the initial therapy. Until the 1980s, radical mastectomy was the standard operation for carcinoma of the breast. Radical mastectomy was designed to control local disease by an extensive en bloc removal of the breast and underlying pectoralis major and pectoralis minor muscles and complete axillary dissection. It is a cosmetically disfiguring operation, leaving a major deformity of the chest wall. With an increased understanding that cancer of the breast is often a systemic disease and prognosis is similar with conservative surgery, the therapeutic emphasis has changed to less radical surgery and increased use of radiotherapy and chemotherapy (Table 15.11). Often patients are not cured even with extensive local therapy. Thus protocols were established for more conservative approaches to treat local disease. The modified radical mastectomy removes

**Table 15.11** Ten-Year Disease-Free Survival Rates of Women with Breast Cancer

| | Conservation Surgery and Radiation | Radical or Modified Radical Mastectomy Alone |
|---|---|---|
| Minimal breast cancer | 92% | 95% |
| Stage I | 78% | 80% |
| Stage II | 73% | 65% |

From Montague ED. Conservation surgery and radiation therapy in the treatment of operable breast cancer. *Cancer.* 1984;53(3 Suppl):700-704.

the breast and only the fascia over the pectoralis major muscle. The pectoralis minor muscle may be removed to facilitate the axillary dissection. Simple mastectomy includes removal of the breast without underlying muscle tissue. A nipple-areolar sparing mastectomy can be considered in select patients undergoing a therapeutic mastectomy followed by immediate reconstruction. Candidates include women with small to moderate breast size with minimal ptosis and tumors smaller than 2 cm with a tumor-to-nipple areolar complex distance larger than 2 cm. Contraindications to this procedure include inflammatory breast cancer, clinical involvement of the nipple areolar complex, nipple retraction, Paget disease, or bloody nipple discharge. For patients having a mastectomy for prophylactic indications, a skin-sparing or nipple-sparing mastectomy is an option with good cosmetic results.

Breast-conserving therapy (lumpectomy, axillary sentinel lymph node biopsy followed by whole breast irradiation) has been shown to be equivalent to mastectomy and axillary lymph node dissection in the primary treatment of women with stages I and II breast cancer. Resection of a wider area of the breast than lumpectomy is referred to as a quadrantectomy. In cases of positive margins, surgical reexcision is recommended. Mastectomy may be necessary in cases of positive margins after further surgical reexcision. Contraindications to lumpectomy include the need for radiation therapy during pregnancy, extensive disease not amenable to resection by a local excision with a single incision resulting in satisfactory cosmetic outcome, and diffuse suspicious or malignant appearing microcalcifications. Relative contraindications include tumor size greater than 5 cm, history of previous radiation therapy to the breast or chest wall, and active connective tissue disease such as scleroderma and lupus that is adversely affected by radiation therapy.

Surgical axillary staging is recommended for stages I, IIA, IIB, and IIIA breast cancer. Sentinel lymph node mapping and resection is recommended in the surgical staging of the clinically negative axilla for stages I, IIA, IIB, and IIIA breast cancer. Sentinel node biopsy has decreased the need for complete axillary lymphadenectomy. Compared with standard axillary lymphadenectomy, sentinel lymph node (SLN) biopsy results in less arm/shoulder pain, lymphedema, and sensory loss. By injecting with radioactive colloid tracers and dyes, the surgeon can identify the first set of regional lymph nodes that receive lymphatic drainage from the tumor. These are termed *sentinel lymph nodes*. Subsequently, these nodes can be removed and the axillary dissection can be deleted if they are negative. In a large multi-institutional trial, Krag and colleagues were able to identify the sentinel nodes in 93% of the cases. The accuracy of sentinel node mapping in this series for predicting the status of axillary nodes was 97%. The positive predictive value was 100%, and the negative predictive value was 96% (Krag, 1998). In the American College of Surgeons Oncology Group (ACOSOG) Z0011 study, women 18 years or age or older with T1/T2 tumors, fewer than three positive SLNs, and who were undergoing breast-conserving surgery followed by whole breast radiation were randomized to SLN resection alone versus axillary lymph node (ALN) dissection. No difference was noted in local recurrence, disease-free survival, or overall survival. Locoregional recurrences at a follow-up of 6.3 years occurred in 4.1% of the ALN group and 2.8% of the SLN group ($P$ = .11). Median overall survival was 92% in both groups. No further axillary surgery is recommended in patients with a T1 or T2 tumor with less than three positive SLNs who did not receive neoadjuvant therapy and were treated with lumpectomy and whole breast radiation (Giuliano, 2010). Level I or II axillary dissection is recommended in patients with either clinically positive nodes at the time of diagnosis confirmed by FNA or core biopsy or in cases where sentinel nodes are not identified.

Breast reconstruction must be considered for any woman undergoing mastectomy for breast cancer. Although reconstruction is an optional procedure that does not influence the probability of disease recurrence or death, it is associated with an improvement in the patient's quality of life. Consultation with a reconstructive plastic surgeon should be offered. Various factors influence the type of reconstruction including patient preference, smoking history, body habitus, comorbidities, and radiation therapy plans. Obesity and smoking increase the risk of wound healing complications and flap failure.

Postmastectomy reconstruction with implants can be performed by either immediate placement of a permanent subpectoral implant or by placement of a subpectoral tissue expander implant. The pectoral muscle is stretched with gradual expansion of the expander implant by the addition of saline. Implants may contain silicone gel, saline, or a combination of both. Reconstruction techniques with autologous tissue include abdominal flaps: a transverse rectus abdominis (TRAM) flap and the deep inferior epigastric perforator (DIEP) flap, a gluteus maximus myocutaneous flap, and a latissimus dorsi flap reconstruction. There is also another option that is only offered in a few centers that does not use skin or muscle from the abdominal wall or buttocks but instead uses skin, fat, and muscle from the upper inner thigh called the *transverse upper gracilis (TUG) flap* (ACS, 2015) (Fig. 15.22). In patients undergoing postmastectomy radiation, placement of a tissue expander at the initial procedure followed by implant placement after completion of radiation therapy is preferred. If autologous tissue is used, reconstruction should be delayed until at least 6 months following completion of radiation therapy.

### Radiation Therapy

The majority of women treated with breast-conserving surgery are candidates for breast radiation therapy. After breast-conserving surgery, external beam whole breast irradiation is usually administered. In the 2011 meta-analysis by the Early Breast Cancer Trialists' Collaborative Group (EBCTCG) of 10,801 women in 17 trials, whole breast irradiation resulted in a significant reduction in the 10-year risk of any first recurrence compared with breast-conserving surgery alone (19.3 vs. 35%, RR 0.52, 95% CI: 0.48-0.56). Additionally, a significant reduction in the 15-year risk of breast cancer death (21.4% vs. 25.2%, RR 0.82, 95% CI: 0.75-0.90) was noted in the whole breast irradiation group (EBCTCG 2011a). Radiation therapy boost to the tumor bed is offered to women at higher risk of recurrence (positive lymph nodes, lymphovascular invasion, young age, or high-grade disease after lumpectomy). In women 70 years or older with node negative, stage 1 ER-positive breast cancer, postoperative radiation therapy may be omitted if they receive postoperative endocrine therapy, as the risk of an in breast recurrence is low.

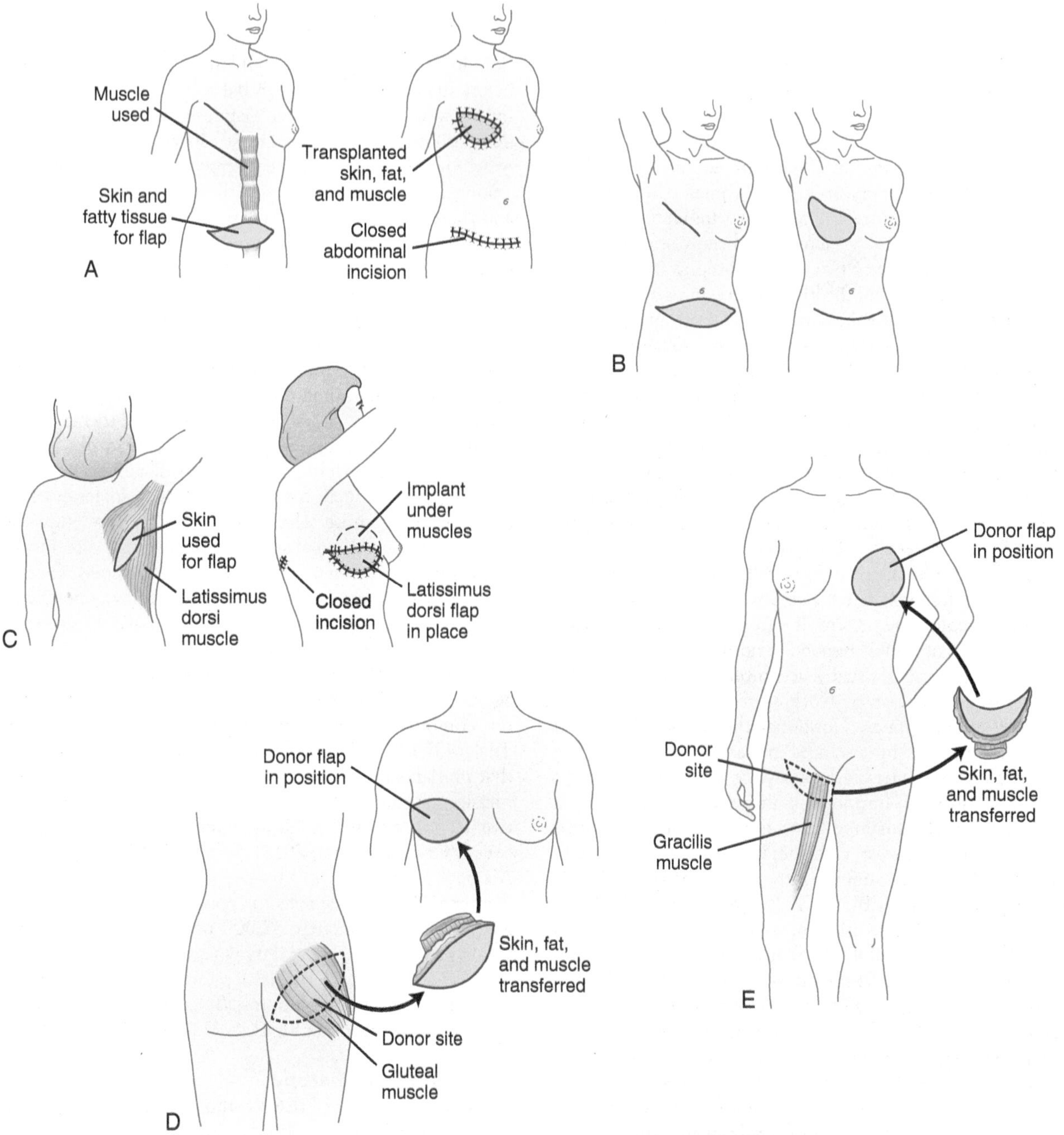


**Figure 15.22** **A,** Pedicle TRAM flap incisions through which the flap of muscle, fat, and skin are tunneled under the skin to fill the defect in the breast. **B,** Incisions used for the DIEP flap. **C,** Latissimus dorsi flap. **D,** Gluteal-free flap. **E,** Transverse upper gracilis (TUG) flap. (Modified from American Cancer Society. Breast reconstruction after mastectomy, 2015.)

Women with positive axillary lymph nodes after mastectomy and axillary lymphadenectomy are also candidates for breast radiation therapy. Randomized trials have shown both a disease-free and overall survival advantage of chest wall and regional node irradiation in these women. National Comprehensive Cancer Network (NCCN) guidelines recommend irradiation after mastectomy in women with four or more positive axillary lymph nodes and strong consideration of radiation in women with one to three positive axillary lymph nodes (NCCN, 2016). Chest wall irradiation is also recommended in women with negative nodes but with primary tumor greater than 5 cm or positive surgical margins.

### *Medical Therapy*

Along with earlier detection, advancements in systemic adjuvant therapy have resulted in a decrease in the breast cancer mortality rate. Clinicopathologic factors including stage, tumor grade, and vascular space invasion are used to calculate the risk of disease recurrence. The two major factors in predicting the likelihood of systemic disease in breast carcinoma are the diameter of the primary tumor and the number of positive axillary nodes. Women whose initial tumor is less than 1 cm in diameter and who have negative axillary nodes have excellent chances for disease-free survival. The 10-year relapse rate is less than 10%.

### Hormonal Therapy

The presence and concentration of receptors should be obtained at the initial diagnostic biopsy or surgery. Women with hormone receptor–positive breast cancer are candidates for endocrine therapy. Receptor status may change after radiotherapy or chemotherapy. Estrogen receptors are of two types, ER-alpha and ER-beta. Most laboratories test only for the ER-alpha receptors, and its biology is better understood. ER-beta receptors' role in malignancy is still under investigation. As tumors mutate and metastasize, the expression of estrogen receptors decreases. Hormonal therapies become less effective in controlling disease. Progesterone receptor positivity is a sign of better differentiation and a greater response to hormonal therapy. Progesterone receptors are often lost as tumors metastasize, as well. In general, luminal type A receptor-positive tumors are usually better differentiated and exhibit a less aggressive clinical behavior, including a lower risk of recurrence and lower capacity to proliferate. When estrogen receptors are positive, approximately 60% of breast cancers will respond to hormonal therapy; an 80% response rate is noted when both estrogen and progesterone receptors are present. If estrogen receptors are negative, less than 10% of tumors respond to hormonal manipulation.

Hormonal therapy is usually accomplished by drugs that change endocrine function by blocking receptor sites or blocking synthesis of hormones. Hormonal therapy is effective in producing a response in advanced metastatic carcinoma for approximately 1 year. Metastatic disease in soft tissue and bone is the most sensitive to hormonal manipulation. Tamoxifen, a selective estrogen receptor modulator, is a frequently prescribed hormonal agent for breast carcinoma. The 2011 EBCTCG meta-analysis compared tamoxifen treatment for 5 years with no endocrine treatment (EBCTCG, 2011b). Analysis showed a significant reduction in the risk of breast cancer recurrence at 15 years (RR 0.61, 95% CI: 0.57-0.65) and a significant reduction in the risk of breast cancer mortality at 15 years (RR 0.70, 95% CI: 0.64-0.75). Treatment with tamoxifen was associated with an increased risk of thromboembolic disease, strokes, intrauterine polyps, as well as endometrial hyperplasia and carcinoma. The overall incidence of uterine cancer was low and confined to women over 55 years. Most tamoxifen-related endometrial cancers were stage I, grade 1, and were successfully treated with surgery alone.

Tamoxifen has the greatest effect in postmenopausal women. As one would expect, tamoxifen is of greater benefit in women with tumors that have estrogen receptors than in tumors that are negative for estrogen receptors. There is no significant improvement in survival rates in patients with estrogen receptor-negative tumors. However, even in receptor-negative patients, 5 years of tamoxifen use will decrease the risk of a second primary or contralateral breast cancer by as much as 45%. Trials of tamoxifen in the adjuvant treatment setting for breast cancer showed that 10 years of tamoxifen improved outcomes when compared with 5 years. In the worldwide Adjuvant Tamoxifen: Longer Against Shorter (ATLAS) trial, approximately 13,000 women were randomized to continue tamoxifen to 10 years or stop at 5 years (Davies, 2013). Among women with ER-positive disease, continuation of tamoxifen reduced the risk of breast cancer recurrence, reduced breast cancer mortality, and reduced overall mortality. The reductions in adverse breast cancer outcomes appeared to be less extreme before than after year 10 with halve breast cancer mortality during the second decade after diagnosis. Extended tamoxifen use demonstrated no effect on breast cancer outcome in the cohort of women with ER-negative disease, and an intermediate effect among women with unknown ER status. Based on these results and those of other major trials, the American Society of Clinical Oncology updated the practice guidelines on the optimal duration of treatment of adjuvant endocrine therapy, particularly adjuvant tamoxifen (Burstein, 2014). Pre- or perimenopausal women who have received 5 years of adjuvant tamoxifen should be offered tamoxifen for a duration of 10 years. Postmenopausal women who have received 5 years of adjuvant tamoxifen should be offered the choice of continuing tamoxifen or changing to an aromatase inhibitor for 10 years total adjuvant endocrine therapy.

Aromatase inhibitors (AIs) (anastrozole, letrozole, and exemestane) block the peripheral conversion of adrenal androgens to estrone. They are ineffective in women with intact ovarian function, including those who experienced chemotherapy-induced amenorrhea, as AIs may cause an inadvertent rise in gonadotropins from the ovary, limiting their effectiveness. Cessation of ovarian function can be definitively attained by oophorectomy or pelvic radiation. Ovarian suppression can also be accomplished with pharmacologic interventions that inhibit ovarian production of estrogen, such as the gonadotropin-releasing hormone (GnRH) agonists. In premenopausal women with ER-positive breast cancer, combined results of the Suppression of Ovarian Function Trial (SOFT) and Tamoxifen and Exemestane Trial (TEXT) show that ovarian suppression plus an AI compared with ovarian suppression plus tamoxifen in premenopausal women with ER-positive breast cancer will result in better disease-free survival but not overall survival (Pagani, 2014). When compared with tamoxifen, AIs have been shown to improve outcomes for postmenopausal women with hormone receptor-positive breast cancer. In a meta-analysis of approximately 32,000 postmenopausal women with ER-positive breast cancer, AIs when compared with tamoxifen were noted to reduce recurrence rates by approximately 30%, have a higher risk of osteoporosis/fractures, and have a lower risk of endometrial cancer (EBCTCG, 2015).

### HER2-Directed Therapy

The determination of HER2 tumor status is recommended for newly diagnosed invasive breast cancers as well as for recurrences of breast cancer. The *HER2/neu* gene is an epithelial growth factor determinant (human epidermal receptor), and amplification or overexpression HER2 oncogene is found in 18% to 20% of women with breast cancer. When overexpressed on tumor cells, the *HER2/neu* gene is a poor prognostic sign and a marker for aggressive disease. Breast tumors are classified as HER2 positive if the tumor has either an immunohistochemical (IHC) stain of 3+ (defined as uniform membrane staining for HER2 in 10% or more of tumor cells), a HER2/chromosome enumeration probe 17 (CEP17) fluorescent in situ hybridization (FISH) amplification ratio $\geq 2$ or a HER2/CEP17 ratio $<2$ with an average HER2 copy number $>6$ signals/cell.

HER2-targeted therapy is recommended in patients with *HER2/neu*-positive tumors. Trastuzumab is a humanized monoclonal antibody, which is directed against the extracellular domain of the *HER2/neu* receptor. Several trials have shown significant improvement in outcome and were stopped early because of the improved outcomes compared with placebo. The drug affects multiple steps in the cell cycle and importantly sensitizes cells to other chemotherapy agents. It also increases antibody-dependent, cell-mediated cytotoxicity. Trastuzumab given for 1 year in conjunction with chemotherapy in patients with HER2-positive tumors improved disease-free and overall survival (Moja, 2012). Treatment with trastuzumab is associated with a higher risk of cardiotoxicity including congestive heart failure and a decrease in left ventricular ejection fraction. Caution must be used when patients are also receiving anthracycline-based chemotherapy, and patients should undergo routine cardiac monitoring. Pertuzumab, a monoclonal antibody that binds to HER2 and prevents dimerization of HER2 with other HER receptors, may be used in conjunction with chemotherapy and trastuzumab regimens to overcome trastuzumab resistance due to HER2:HER3 heterodimer formation. The addition of pertuzumab does not appear to increase toxicity.

### *Chemotherapy*

Chemotherapy is utilized in the treatment of breast cancer in both the adjuvant and neoadjuvant settings. Chemotherapy is recommended for the treatment of most triple-negative breast cancers, HER2-positive breast cancers, and high-risk luminal tumors. The benefit of chemotherapy is more pronounced in ER-negative tumors.

The decision to use adjuvant chemotherapy is based on several variables including the surrogate intrinsic phenotype determined by ER/PR, HER2, and Ki-67 assessment with the selective help of first-generation genomic testing. The two most commonly used molecular prognostic profiles are the Oncotype DX test and the Mammaprint assay. The Oncotype DX Breast Cancer Assay measures the expression of 16 cancer genes and 5 reference genes to produce a recurrence score (RS) from 0 to 100. It is utilized to estimate both the risk of recurrence of early-stage breast cancer and the benefit from adjuvant chemotherapy. Currently, this assay is indicated in women with node negative or 1 to 3 positive nodes and ER-positive breast cancer. The MammaPrint test analyzes 70 genes (Amsterdam 70 gene prognostic profile) and calculates either a high-risk or low-risk recurrence score for early stage breast cancer. This clinically validated prognostic profile can be used in breast cancers that are either hormone-receptor-positive or negative, node negative or one to three positive nodes, and in patients with HER2-positive disease.

Combination therapy of cytotoxic drugs is vastly superior to single-agent regimens. Anthracycline-containing combinations are more effective than regimens that do not contain anthracyclines. Paclitaxel therapy has excellent activity in breast cancer. The addition of four to five cycles of paclitaxel to four to six cycles of the Adriamycin and cyclophosphamide regimen improved disease-free and overall survival rates in patients with node-positive breast cancer. Overall, chemotherapy regimens based on anthracyclines and taxanes reduce breast cancer mortality by about one third.

In the neoadjuvant setting, chemotherapy has the potential to change unresectable tumors to resectable ones and decrease the extent of surgery necessary to achieve adequate resection. Neoadjuvant chemotherapy may be considered for patients who desire breast-conserving surgery but initially are not candidates due to tumor size. Neoadjuvant therapy is commonly used in patients with inflammatory breast cancer and may confer a survival benefit in this population of patients. The chemotherapy regimens used in the neoadjuvant setting are the same as those used in the adjuvant setting. Endocrine and HER2 targeted therapy may also be used in the preoperative setting. HER2-positive breast cancer and triple-negative breast cancer are the most chemosensitive and are excellent subtypes for neoadjuvant chemotherapy. These patients have the highest pathologic complete response rate. In HER2-positive breast cancer, neoadjuvant therapy should include trastuzumab and pertuzumab with a taxane.

## BREAST CANCER DURING PREGNANCY

Breast cancer is not frequently diagnosed during pregnancy. Less than 5% of breast cancers diagnosed before the age of 50 are during pregnancy or in the postpartum period. However, most breast cancers diagnosed during pregnancy are poorly differentiated, ER/PR negative, ALN positive, and have a large primary tumor size. Diagnosis of cancer during pregnancy is frequently delayed by 2 months or longer. Similar to nonpregnant women, in pregnant or postpartum women a breast mass is usually the presenting sign. A mass that persists for more than 2 weeks should be evaluated. Mammography is not contraindicated in pregnancy, although abdominal shielding is recommended. Breast ultrasonography can also be used to better define a mass and guide biopsy. A clinically suspicious mass should be biopsied either by FNA or core needle biopsy. Staging studies should be tailored in an effort to minimize fetal exposure to radiation.

Treatment options during pregnancy are not very different from the nonpregnant state and include mastectomy, breast-conserving therapy, and systemic therapy, but not radiation therapy. Although radical mastectomy is the most common surgery, breast-conserving therapy is an option if radiation therapy can be delayed to the postpartum period. According to the NCCN guidelines, SLN biopsy may be safely performed during pregnancy with a radiolabeled sulfur colloid. The use of blue dye is contraindicated in pregnancy. Systemic chemotherapy should be avoided in the first trimester and not be given after week 35 of pregnancy or within 3 weeks of delivery to avoid transient neonatal myelosuppression and other complications. The risk of fetal malformation during the second and third trimester is approximately 1.3%. Most data regarding chemotherapy in pregnancy are with anthracycline and alkylating chemotherapy. Fewer data exist regarding taxanes. NCCN guidelines recommend weekly administration of paclitaxel after the first trimester if indicated. Trastuzumab is not recommended for use during pregnancy and should be delayed to the postpartum period. Endocrine therapy is also contraindicated during pregnancy.

Various studies have no shown no significant difference in outcomes between women diagnosed with breast cancer during pregnancy and nonpregnant women. In a meta-analysis of 30 studies including 37,100 controls and 3628 cases of pregnancy associated breast cancer, a higher risk of death was noted in women diagnosed in the postpartum period (HR 184, 95% CI: 1.28-2.65) rather than during pregnancy (HR 1.29, 95% CI: 0.72-2.24) (Azim, 2012). Termination of pregnancy does not appear to improve survival.

## SURVEILLANCE

There are approximately 14.5 million cancer survivors in the United States as of 2014. The number of cancer survivors has increased in part due to aging and growth of the population as well as advancements in early detection and treatment. Breast cancer accounts for 41% of female cancer survivors, and close surveillance after treatment is paramount. Although most breast cancer recurrences occur in the first 5 years following treatment, recurrence may be diagnosed decades after treatment. Ongoing age-appropriate screening and preventive care for other conditions not related to breast cancer should continue as recommended for the general populations.

The NCCN guidelines are not stratified according to stage at time of diagnosis or treatment. Interval history and physical examination are recommended every 4 to 6 months for 5 years and annually thereafter, with mammography every 12 months. Women on tamoxifen are recommended to have an annual gynecologic examination every 12 months if the uterus is present. Regular bone mineral density determination is recommended for women on an aromatase inhibitor. Adherence to adjuvant endocrine therapy and maintaining an ideal body weight are also recommended. Other routine laboratory tests and imaging are not recommended for routine surveillance. The use of estrogen, progesterone, or SERMs in the treatment of osteoporosis or osteopenia is discouraged, although it may be considered in select cases. In general, bisphosphonates are preferred for bone mineral density health. Similar to the NCCN guidelines, ASCO recommendations for the follow-up and management of breast cancer include regular history, physical examination, and mammography. The ASCO guidelines recommend history and physical examination every 3 to 6 months for the first 3 years, every 6 to 12 months for years 4 and 5, and annually thereafter. Additional testing is recommended only if symptoms arise. For women who have undergone breast-conserving surgery, a posttreatment mammogram should be obtained 12 months after the initial mammogram and at least 6 months after completion of radiation therapy. Thereafter, annual mammography is recommended. Women should have regular gynecologic follow-up, and those who received tamoxifen should report any vaginal bleeding as they are at an increased risk of developing endometrial cancer.

Treatment of breast cancer with chemotherapy or hormonal therapy may cause menopausal symptoms. Women often report that sexual activity is less enjoyable and more painful. Women who have undergone mastectomy report problems with body image and interest in sex. Depression is associated with sexual dysfunction in breast cancer survivors. Physicians must regularly inquire about sexual functioning, and women with complaints of dyspareunia or other sexual disorders should be offered a referral to a sexual health expert. Women who report dyspareunia or difficulty reaching orgasm may benefit from vaginal dilators, vaginal lubricants and moisturizers, or counseling. The risks and benefits of local or vaginal estrogen therapy should be discussed and individualized based on patient symptoms and tumor characteristics. The use of vaginal estrogens in this setting is to improve the patient's quality of life and should not be underestimated.

## KEY POINTS

- The breast consists of approximately 20% glandular tissue and 80% fat and connective tissue; increasing proportions of fibroglandular to fatty tissues are the mark of denser breasts. Breast density is associated with increased risks of malignancy.
- Lymph drainage of the breast usually flows toward the most adjacent group of nodes. This concept represents the basis for sentinel node mapping in breast cancer. In most instances, breast cancer spreads in an orderly fashion within the axillary lymph node basin based on the anatomic relationship between the primary tumor and its associated regional (sentinel) nodes.
- The breast undergoes normal maturational changes throughout a woman's lifetime. The normal maturation involves a gradual increase in fibrous tissue around the lobules; with time the glandular elements are completely replaced by fibrous tissue.
- The incidence of benign breast disorders begins to rise during the second decade of life and peaks in the fourth and fifth decades. In malignant diseases, the incidence continues to increase after menopause.
- Fibroadenomas are the most common benign breast neoplasm and are most frequently present in adolescents and women in their 20s.
- Approximately 35% of fibroadenomas will disappear, and 10% will become smaller after many years.
- Over two thirds of women will experience breast pain at some time during their reproductive years, most commonly in the perimenopausal years. Approximately 90% of conditions that cause breast pain are benign.
- Cyclic bilateral breast pain is the classic symptom of fibrocystic breast change. The signs of fibrocystic changes include increased engorgement and density of the breasts, excessive nodularity, rapid change and fluctuation in the size of cystic areas, increased tenderness, and occasionally spontaneous nipple discharge.
- The majority of nipple discharge complaints have a benign etiology; however, 55% present with a coexisting mass of which 19% are malignant. An underlying malignancy is more likely when the discharge is spontaneous (vs. induced with nipple pressure), arises from a single duct, is blood stained, and is unilateral and persistent (occurring more than twice weekly).
- Intraductal papilloma and fibrocystic changes are the two most common causes of spontaneous nonmilky nipple discharge.
- Lactational mastitis commonly occurs in the first pregnancy during the first 6 weeks of breast-feeding. Continued breast-feeding or manual pumping of the affected breast is recommended to decrease engorgement.

## KEY POINTS—cont'd

- One out of eight women (12.5%) in the United States will develop carcinoma of the breast over the course of her lifetime.
- Approximately 50% of newly diagnosed breast cancers are attributable to known risk, whereas 10% are associated with a positive family history.
- Approximately 5% to 10% of breast cancers have a familial or genetic link. Genetic predisposition to develop breast carcinoma has been recognized in some families. In these families, breast cancer tends to occur at a younger age, and there is a higher prevalence of bilateral disease.
- Mutations in the *BRCA* family of genes have been identified that confer a lifetime risk of breast cancer that approaches 85%. *BRCA1* and *BRCA2* genes are involved in the majority of inheritable cases of breast cancer. These genes function as tumor suppressor genes, and several mutations have been described on each of these genes.
- Once a woman has developed carcinoma of one breast, her risk is approximately 1% per year of developing cancer in the other breast.
- Both tamoxifen and raloxifene significantly decrease the relative risk of developing breast carcinoma. AIs are a reasonable alternative to SERMs for postmenopausal women.
- Screening mammography is the primary imaging technique for breast cancer detection. The sensitivity of mammography ranges from 80% to 90% and decreases in women with dense breasts.
- The incidence of carcinoma in biopsies corresponds directly with the patient's age. Approximately 20% of breast biopsies in women age 50 are positive, and this figure increases to 33% in women age 70 or older.
- Breast cancer is usually asymptomatic before the development of advanced disease. Breast pain is experienced by only 10% of women with early breast carcinoma. The classic sign of a breast carcinoma is a solitary, solid, three-dimensional, dominant breast mass. The borders of the mass are usually indistinct.
- Microscopic metastatic disease occurs early via both hematogenous and lymphatic routes. For example, 30% to 40% of women without gross adenopathy in the axilla will have positive nodes discovered during histologic examination. With the additional assessment tools of immunohistochemical staining for the presence of cytokeratin and serial sectioning of axillary nodes, 10% to 30% of patients considered to have negative nodes by standard histologic analysis are found to be node positive.
- The initial size of the breast carcinoma is the single best predictor of the likelihood of positive axillary nodes. The presence and number of axillary node metastasis are the best predictors of survival.
- Carcinomas make up the majority of breast malignancies and originate in the epithelium of the collecting ducts (ductal) or the terminal lobular ducts (lobular). Invasive ductal carcinoma is the most common, constituting approximately 70% to 80% of malignancies.
- A multidisciplinary team approach is necessary in the treatment of breast cancer. Determination of local or systemic treatment is based on several prognostic and predictive factors including tumor histology, tumor hormone receptor status (estrogen/progesterone), tumor HER2 status, multigene testing, axillary lymph node status, evaluation of metastatic disease, patient age, comorbidities, and menopausal status.
- The primary therapy for the majority of women with stages I and II breast cancer is conservative surgery, which preserves the breast, followed by radiation therapy.
- Gynecologists should actively address the psychosexual problems that breast cancer causes in women, early in the evaluation of the disease and for several years.

## KEY REFERENCES


*American Cancer Society (ACS): Breast reconstruction after mastectomy.* 2015. Available at. http://www.cancer.org/acs/groups/cid/documents/webcontent/002992-pdf.pdf.

American College of Obstetricians-Gynecologists (ACOG). Practice bulletin no. 122: Breast cancer screening. *Obstet Gynecol.* 2011;118(2 Pt 1):372-382.

Azim Jr HA, Santoro L, Russell-Edu W, et al. Prognosis of pregnancy-associated breast cancer: a meta-analysis of 30 studies. *Cancer Treat Rev.* 2012;38(7):834-842.

Bagnardi V, Rota M, Botteri E, et al. Light alcohol drinking and cancer: a meta-analysis. *Ann Oncol.* 2013;24(2):301-308.

Barton MB, Harris R, Fletcher SW. The rational clinical examination. Does this patient have breast cancer? The screening clinical breast examination: should it be done? How? *JAMA.* 1999;282(13):1270-1280.

Bauer SR, Hankinson SE, Bertone-Johnson ER, et al. Plasma vitamin D levels, menopause, and risk of breast cancer: dose-response meta-analysis of prospective studies. *Medicine (Baltimore).* 2013;92(3):123-131.

Boyd NF, Guo H, Martin LJ, et al. Mammographic density and the risk and detection of breast cancer. *N Engl J Med.* 2007;356(3):227-236.

Burstein HJ, Temin S, Anderson H, et al. Adjuvant endocrine therapy for women with hormone receptor-positive breast cancer: American society of clinical oncology clinical practice guideline focused update. *J Clin Oncol.* 2014;32(21):2255-2269.

Centers for Disease Control and Prevention (CDC). Vital signs: racial disparities in breast cancer severity–United States, 2005-2009. *MMWR Morb Mortal Wkly Rep.* 2012;61(45):922-926.

Chlebowski RT, Hendrix SL, Langer RD, et al. Influence of estrogen plus progestin on breast cancer and mammography in healthy postmenopausal women: the Women's Health Initiative Randomized Trial. *JAMA.* 2003;289(24):3243-3253.

Colditz GA, Rosner B. Cumulative risk of breast cancer to age 70 years according to risk factor status: data from the Nurses' Health Study. *Am J Epidemiol.* 2000;152(10):950-964.

Collaborative Group on Hormonal Factors in Breast Cancer. Breast cancer and breastfeeding: collaborative reanalysis of individual data from 47 epidemiological studies in 30 countries, including 50302 women with breast cancer and 96973 women without the disease. *Lancet.* 2002;360(9328):187-195.

Cuzick J, Sestak I, Cawthorn S, et al. Tamoxifen for prevention of breast cancer: extended long-term follow-up of the IBIS-I breast cancer prevention trial. *Lancet Oncol.* 2015;16(1):67-75.

Cuzick J, Sestak I, Forbes JF, et al. Anastrozole for prevention of breast cancer in high-risk postmenopausal women (IBIS-II): an international, double-blind, randomised placebo-controlled trial. *Lancet.* 2014;383(9922):1041-1048.

Davies C, Pan H, Godwin J, et al. Long-term effects of continuing adjuvant tamoxifen to 10 years versus stopping at 5 years after diagnosis of oestrogen receptor-positive breast cancer: ATLAS, a randomised trial. *Lancet.* 2013;381(9869):805-816.

Doucet S, Soussignan R, Sagot P, et al. The secretion of areolar (Montgomery's) glands from lactating women elicits selective, unconditional responses in neonates. *PLoS One.* 2009;4(10):e7579.
Early Breast Cancer Trialists' Collaborative Group (EBCTCG), Darby S, McGale P, et al. Effect of radiotherapy after breast-conserving surgery on 10-year recurrence and 15-year breast cancer death: meta-analysis of individual patient data for 10,801 women in 17 randomised trials. *Lancet.* 2011a;378(9804):1707-1716.
Early Breast Cancer Trialists' Collaborative Group (EBCTCG), Davies C, Godwin J, et al. Relevance of breast cancer hormone receptors and other factors to the efficacy of adjuvant tamoxifen: patient-level meta-analysis of randomised trials. *Lancet.* 2011b;378(9793):771-784.
Early Breast Cancer Trialists' Collaborative Group (EBCTCG), Dowsett M, Forbes JF, et al. Aromatase inhibitors versus tamoxifen in early breast cancer: patient-level meta-analysis of the randomised trials. *Lancet.* 2015;386(10001):1341-1352.
Fisher B, Costantino JP, Wickerham DL, et al. Tamoxifen for prevention of breast cancer: report of the National Surgical Adjuvant Breast and Bowel Project P-1 Study. *J Natl Cancer Inst.* 1998;90(18):1371-1388.
Fletcher SW, O'Malley MS, Bunce LA. Physicians' abilities to detect lumps in silicone breast models. *JAMA.* 1985;253(15):2224-2228.
Friedewald SM, Rafferty EA, Rose SL, et al. Breast cancer screening using tomosynthesis in combination with digital mammography. *JAMA.* 2014;311(24):2499-2507.
Gail MH, Costantino JP, Pee D, et al. Projecting individualized absolute invasive breast cancer risk in African American women. *J Natl Cancer Inst.* 2007;99(23):1782-1792.
Gemignani ML. Breast cancer screening: why, when, and how many? *Clin Obstet Gynecol.* 2011;54(1):125-132.
Giuliano AE, McCall L, Beitsch P, et al. Locoregional recurrence after sentinel lymph node dissection with or without axillary dissection in patients with sentinel lymph node metastases: the American College of Surgeons Oncology Group Z0011 randomized trial. *Ann Surg.* 2010;252(3):426-432. discussion 432-433.
Hartmann LC, Sellers TA, Schaid DJ, et al. Efficacy of bilateral prophylactic mastectomy in BRCA1 and BRCA2 gene mutation carriers. *J Natl Cancer Inst.* 2001;93(21):1633-1637.
Hughes LE. Classification of benign breast disorders. The ANDI classification based on physiological processes within the normal breast. *Br Med Bull.* 1991;47(2):251-257.
Independent UK Panel on Breast Cancer Screening. The benefits and harms of breast cancer screening: an independent review. *Lancet.* 2012;380(9855):1778-1786.
Kovatcheva R, Guglielmina JN, Abehsera M, et al. Ultrasound-guided high-intensity focused ultrasound treatment of breast fibroadenoma-a multicenter experience. *J Ther Ultrasound.* 2015;3(1):1.
Krag D, Weaver D, Ashikaga T, et al. The sentinel node in breast cancer—a multicenter validation study. *N Engl J Med.* 1998;339(14):941-946.
Longnecker MP. Alcoholic beverage consumption in relation to risk of breast cancer: meta-analysis and review. *Cancer Causes Control.* 1994;5(1):73-82.
Matsuno RK, et al. Projecting individualized absolute invasive breast cancer risk in Asian and Pacific Islander American women. *J Natl Cancer Inst.* 2011;103(12):951-961.
Moja L, Tagliabue L, Balduzzi S, et al. Trastuzumab containing regimens for early breast cancer. *Cochrane Database Syst Rev.* 2012;4:CD006243.
Morris T, Greer HS, White P. Psychological and social adjustment to mastectomy: a two-year follow-up study. *Cancer.* 1977;40(5):2381-2387.
National Comprehensive Cancer Network (NCCN). *Breast cancer, version 1*; 2016. Available at http://www.nccn.org/professionals/physician_gls/pdf/breast.pdf.
Nelson HD, Smith ME, Griffin JC, et al. Use of medications to reduce risk for primary breast cancer: a systematic review for the U.S. Preventive Services Task Force. *Ann Intern Med.* 2013;158(8):604-614.
Newcomb PA, Storer BE, Longnecker MP, et al. Lactation and a reduced risk of premenopausal breast cancer. *N Engl J Med.* 1994;330(2):81-87.
Nichols HB, Berrington de González A, Lacey Jr JV, et al. Declining incidence of contralateral breast cancer in the United States from 1975 to 2006. *J Clin Oncol.* 2011;29(12):1564-1569.
Oeffinger KC, Fontham ET, Etzioni R, et al. Breast cancer screening for women at average risk: 2015 guideline update from the American Cancer Society. *JAMA.* 2015;314(15):1599-1614.
Pagani O, Regan MM, Walley BA, et al. Adjuvant exemestane with ovarian suppression in premenopausal breast cancer. *N Engl J Med.* 2014;371(2):107-118.
Perou CM, Sørlie T, Eisen MB, et al. Molecular portraits of human breast tumours. *Nature.* 2000;406(6797):747-752.
Pisano ED, Hendrick RE, Yaffe MJ, et al. Diagnostic accuracy of digital versus film mammography: exploratory analysis of selected population subgroups in DMIST. *Radiology.* 2008;246(2):376-383.
Prentice RL, Caan B, Chlebowski RT, et al. Low-fat dietary pattern and risk of invasive breast cancer: the Women's Health Initiative Randomized Controlled Dietary Modification Trial. *JAMA.* 2006;295(6):629-642.
Schindler AE. Non-contraceptive benefits of oral hormonal contraceptives. *Int J Endocrinol Metab.* 2013;11(1):41-47.
Siegel RL, Miller KD, Jemal A. Cancer statistics, 2015. *CA Cancer J Clin.* 2015;65(1):5-29.
Siegel R, Naishadham D, Jemal A. Cancer statistics, 2012. *CA Cancer J Clin.* 2012;62(1):10-29.
Siu AL. U.S. Preventive Services Task Force: Screening for breast cancer: U.S. Preventive Services Task Force Recommendation Statement. *Ann Intern Med.* 2016. http://dx.doi.org/10.7326/M15-2886. [Epub ahead of print].
Skaane P, Hofvind S, Skjennald A. Randomized trial of screen-film versus full-field digital mammography with soft-copy reading in population-based screening program: follow-up and final results of Oslo II study. *Radiology.* 2007;244(3):708-717.
Thiébaut AC, Kipnis V, Chang SC, et al. Dietary fat and postmenopausal invasive breast cancer in the National Institutes of Health-AARP Diet and Health Study cohort. *J Natl Cancer Inst.* 2007;99(6):451-462.
Vogel VG, Costantino JP, Wickerham DL, et al. Effects of tamoxifen vs raloxifene on the risk of developing invasive breast cancer and other disease outcomes: the NSABP Study of Tamoxifen and Raloxifene (STAR) P-2 trial. *JAMA.* 2006;295(23):2727-2741.
Winocour S, Lemaine V. Hypoplastic breast anomalies in the female adolescent breast. *Semin Plast Surg.* 2013;27(1):42-48.
Wu AH, Yu MC, Tseng CC, et al. Epidemiology of soy exposures and breast cancer risk. *Br J Cancer.* 2008;98(1):9-14.
Zhang X, Smith-Warner SA, Collins LC, et al. Use of aspirin, other nonsteroidal anti-inflammatory drugs, and acetaminophen and postmenopausal breast cancer incidence. *J Clin Oncol.* 2012;30(28):3468-3477.

Suggested Readings can be found on ExpertConsult.com

# 16

# Spontaneous Abortion and Recurrent Pregnancy Loss

## Etiology, Diagnosis, Treatment

*Sanaz Keyhan, Lisa Muasher, Suheil J. Muasher*

Pregnancy loss is a devastating event for patients and their caregivers. It often poses a medical puzzle and can be accompanied by strong emotions. Unfortunately, it is common, affecting about 15% of clinically recognized pregnancies and up to 50%, or more, of all conceptions (Kutteh, 2007). *Spontaneous abortion (SAB), miscarriage,* and *pregnancy loss* are used throughout the literature to describe the involuntary loss of a pregnancy before 20 weeks of gestation, as dated by the last menstrual period, or the loss of a fetus weighing 500 g or less. Because the term *abortion* may carry negative connotations, especially among patients, *miscarriage* is frequently substituted. Miscarriage within the first $12^{6/7}$ weeks of gestation is termed *early pregnancy loss* and denotes a nonviable intrauterine pregnancy in which the gestational sac itself is empty or contains a fetus with no cardiac activity (ACOG, 2015). After 20 weeks of gestation, pregnancy loss is called *preterm birth* or *stillbirth*, as the point of fetal viability continues to fluctuate (Kutteh, 2007).

Recurrent pregnancy loss has traditionally been defined as three or more consecutive, clinically recognized losses (Rai, 2006). More recent definitions have recommended including two or more clinically recognized losses (ASRM, 2012). The term *habitual abortion* has now been almost completely replaced by *recurrent pregnancy loss.* In addition, recurrent loss may be further stratified into primary, secondary, and tertiary. These terms denote whether the patient has ever had a viable infant or if her losses have been interspersed with deliveries of viable infants. Multiple studies have shown the risk of miscarriage approaches 45% with three previous consecutive losses. A thorough evaluation will reveal a cause of recurrent loss in over half of couples who seek treatment. The prognosis is good for these patients, with over 80% of women younger than 30 years and 60% to 70% of women ages 31 to 40 achieving a successful pregnancy within 5 years of their first visit to a physician (Lund, 2012).

This chapter discusses the epidemiology of pregnancy loss and reviews the etiology, diagnosis, and management of loss. For the purposes of this chapter, the terms *recurrent pregnancy loss* and *recurrent miscarriage* will be used interchangeably, although some groups have argued that these two adverse pregnancy outcomes have different definitions. Loss at less than 10 weeks is usually due to a chromosomal abnormality, as opposed to loss at 18 to 20 weeks' gestation, which is more often due to structural problems of the uterus or cervix (Stephenson, 2002). Some women may have more than one cause for miscarriage. Similarly, not all women with a known abnormality will suffer a loss. Because miscarriage should be viewed as a syndrome, as well as a continuum, recurrent pregnancy loss is discussed throughout the chapter.

## EPIDEMIOLOGY

Miscarriage is more common in women younger than 18 years and older than 35 years and rises both with increasing parity and number of prior losses (Fig. 16.1). Loss rates of 9% to 17% for women ages 20 to 34, 20% for women ages 35 to 40, and 40% for women over age 40 have been observed in longitudinal studies. The loss rate is believed to approach 80% in women age 45 and older (ASRM, 2012). Likewise, women with two prior losses, and no live births, have been shown to experience a loss rate of 25%, which increases to 45% with three losses (Table 16.1). The spontaneous abortion risk also increases with older paternal age, reaching 19.5% for men between ages 40 to 44 (Kleinhaus, 2006). Evaluation of the medical literature should take into account that the majority of patients will eventually have a successful pregnancy even without intervention. Remembering that 90% of pregnancy losses are not recurrent, watchful waiting may prove the best, albeit emotionally hardest, thing to do.

Nearly 80% of all clinical abortions occur in the first trimester, and the incidence declines with advancing gestational age. The loss rate remains stable through 12 weeks and decreases in the following weeks (Fig. 16.2). When a gestational sac is visualized by ultrasound, the loss rate is 11.5% but falls to 6% to 8% if embryonic cardiac activity is observed at 6 weeks and falls to 2% to 3% if cardiac activity is persistent at 8 to 12 weeks. Compared with their younger counterparts, however, women older than age 34 experience a loss rate twice as high, even after visualization of a fetal heartbeat (Achiron, 1991). Studies show

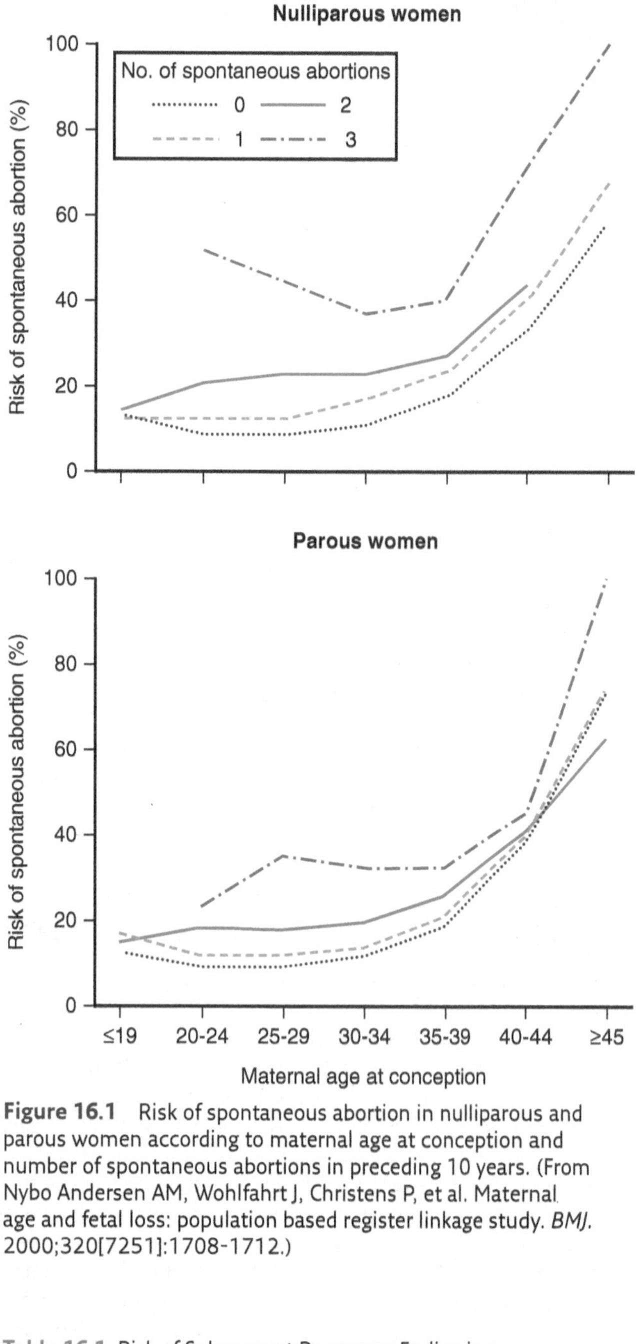


**Figure 16.1** Risk of spontaneous abortion in nulliparous and parous women according to maternal age at conception and number of spontaneous abortions in preceding 10 years. (From Nybo Andersen AM, Wohlfahrt J, Christens P, et al. Maternal age and fetal loss: population based register linkage study. *BMJ*. 2000;320[7251]:1708-1712.)

Table 16.1 Risk of Subsequent Pregnancy Ending in a Spontaneous Abortion*

| Number of Previous Abortions | Number of Pregnancies Studied | Abortion Risk (%) |
|---|---|---|
| 0 | 18,164 | 10.7 (10.3-11.2) |
| 1 | 21,054 | 15.9 (15.4-16.4) |
| 2 | 2,231 | 25.1 (23.4-27.0) |
| 3 | 353 | 45.0 (39.8-50.4) |
| 4 | 94 | 54.3 (43.7-64.4) |
| Overall | 19,737 | 11.3 (10.9-11.8) |

From Knudsen UB, Hansen V, Juul S, et al. Prognosis of a new pregnancy following previous spontaneous abortions. *Eur J Obstet Gynecol Reprod Biol*. 1991;39:31.

*The table is calculated from a 6.6% sample of the study pregnancies. Figures in parentheses: 95% confidence limits; $\chi^2$ (trend) = 728; $df$ = 1: $P < .001$.

that the majority of losses before 10 weeks are attributable to chromosomal abnormalities. Women with bleeding in the first trimester and confirmed presence of fetal cardiac activity have a 15% risk of suffering a miscarriage (Hasan, 2009).

## ETIOLOGY

Causes of pregnancy loss can be described as either maternal or fetal. Maternal factors include medical conditions, structural issues involving the uterus and cervix, and environmental exposures. Fetal reasons for loss include chromosomal abnormalities and derangement of organ development, which may or may not have a chromosomal component.

### *CHROMOSOMAL*

Chromosomal origins of pregnancy loss include embryonic errors as a result of known parental abnormalities and de novo embryonic errors in the setting of parents with normal karyotypes. Several terms are used interchangeably in the literature, often leading to flawed interpretation because the definitions vary subtly. *Congenital* means present at birth but does not infer whether a condition is inherited. *Inherited* means passed on from the parents. In other words, one or both parents have a genetic change that can be passed to their offspring. *Genetic* denotes changes in the genes or chromosomes that can be sporadic, a new mutation, or inherited. *Chromosomal* problems are all genetic, but few are inherited. Inherited chromosomal abnormalities are those resulting from familial translocations. Additional sources of chromosomal anomalies include microdeletions and microduplications. These changes are in between single gene defects and full chromosomal abnormalities and represent small portions of the DNA involving only a few genes. They may be inherited or sporadic.

Studies confirm that 50% to 60% of miscarriages are due to chromosomal anomalies and up to 85% of pregnancies shown to be nonviable by ultrasound will demonstrate aneuploidy on pathologic review following surgical evacuation. Most of the abnormal karyotypes are numeric irregularities resulting from errors during gametogenesis (chromosomal nondisjunction during meiosis), fertilization (triploidy as a result of digyny or diandry), or the first division of the fertilized ovum (tetraploidy or mosaicism). About 56% of these abnormalities are trisomic, 20% are polyploid, 18% will be chromosome X monosomies, and 4% will represent unbalanced translocations (Jacobs, 1987).

Fetal aneuploidy is the most common cause of miscarriage, with autosomal trisomies accounting for the majority of losses. Aneuploidy is usually caused by errors in the first meiotic division of the oocyte, although some trisomies are due to errors in paternal meiotic division. Trisomy 16 is the most frequently observed abnormality in abortuses, followed by trisomy 22. The most common single chromosome abnormality is monosomy 45,X; however, nearly 1 in 300 of these gestations will survive to viability (Hassold, 2007) (Table 16.2). It is important to remember that the rate of chromosomally abnormal abortuses seen in couples with recurrent pregnancy loss does not differ from their maternal and gestational age cohorts in the population at large. In women younger than age 36, recurrent loss is usually due to causes other than chromosomal abnormalities (Stephenson, 2002).

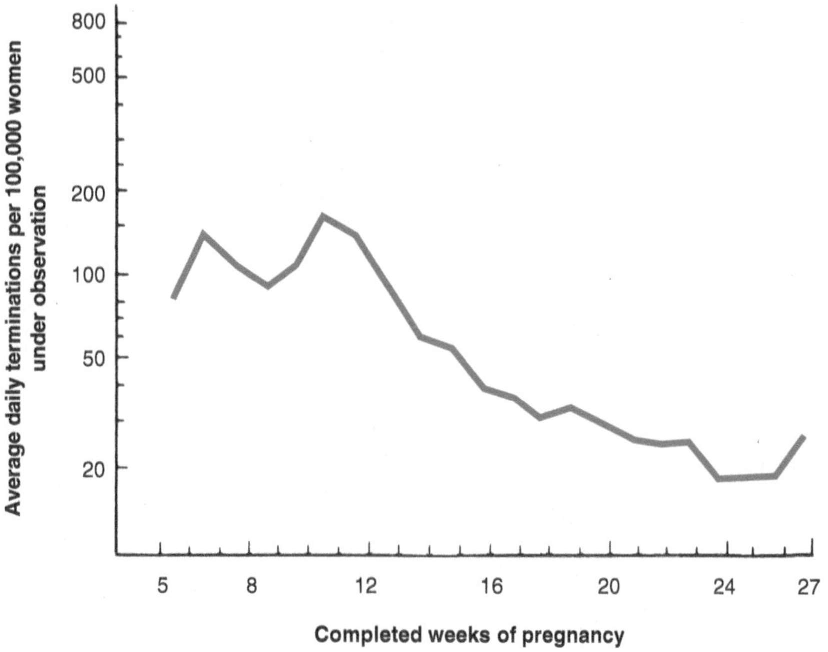


**Figure 16.2** Spontaneous abortion by week of pregnancy. (From Harlap S, Shiono PH, Ramcharan S. A life table of spontaneous abortions and the effects of age, parity, and other variables. In: Porter IH, Hook EB, eds. *Human Embryonic and Fetal Death.* New York: Academic Press; 1980.)

Although more than 98% of miscarriages due to aneuploidy occur spontaneously, some are caused by translocations in one or both parents (ASRM, 2012). In 3% to 6% of recurrent pregnancy loss, one parent, usually the woman, will carry a chromosomal abnormality (Hassold, 2007). About 50% of these will be balanced translocations, 25% are Robertsonian translocations, and another 12% are female sex chromosome mosaicism. The remainder are either inversions or other types of sporadic abnormality. Translocations are more likely to interfere with spermatogenesis than oogenesis, thus culminating in more females than males with chromosomal abnormalities attempting to conceive (Goldstein, 1994). A loss rate of 80% would be predicted if a translocation is diagnosed in one parent, but this is not actually observed as the percentage of viable, unaffected infants born depends on the type of translocation (Philipp, 2003). Large studies have shown spontaneous live birth rates of up to 71% in carriers of a structural rearrangement (Stephenson, 2006).

Loss of a chromosomally normal conceptus usually occurs at a later gestational age than one involving an embryo with chromosomal abnormalities. Although the peak incidence of euploid abortion occurs around 12 to 13 weeks' gestation, it is helpful to remember that the time of diagnosis or expulsion of products of conception does not necessarily coincide with embryonic or fetal death. Accurate timing of embryonic or fetal death is important when evaluating patients for a cause of pregnancy loss (Goldstein, 1994).

There are multiple causes for loss of chromosomally abnormal conceptions. About 2% of live-born infants will have a single gene mutation or polygenic abnormality, making these gene irregularities more common than chromosomal abnormalities, which affect 0.5% of live births. These defects may induce loss by interfering with fetal metabolism or embryonic structural differentiation (Philipp, 2003). Another theory postulates a gene that blocks normal meiotic division, as evidenced by studies of recurrent loss among women with an abnormal inactivation of one of their X chromosomes.

## UTERINE ANOMALIES

Uterine abnormalities, either congenital or acquired, may not provide the optimal environment for nourishment and survival of the embryo and thus may cause the loss of a genetically normal embryo. Congenital uterine abnormalities can be divided into those brought about by abnormal uterine fusion, those produced by maternal diethylstilbestrol (DES) ingestion, and those caused by abnormal cervical function. The last condition, the incompetent cervix, can also be acquired after mechanical cervical dilation. Uterine polyps or submucous myomas may be considered acquired.

### ANOMALIES OF UTERINE DEVELOPMENT

Congenital abnormalities of the female reproductive tract are discussed in detail in Chapter 11. The discussion in this section is limited to their importance in women with spontaneous and recurrent miscarriages.

Uterine anomalies can be observed in 4.3% (range, 2.7% to 16.7%) of the general population and in 12.6% (range, 1.8% to 37.6%) of patients with recurrent pregnancy loss. The prevalence of uterine malformations in women with recurrent pregnancy loss has varied widely due to the differences in diagnostic criteria and the imaging techniques used. The septate uterus is the most common uterine anomaly in the general population as well as in women with recurrent pregnancy loss. Women with uterine anomalies have higher rates of first- and second-trimester miscarriages compared to women with a normal uterus. Uterine

Table 16.2 Frequency of Cytogenetic Diagnoses in 420 Miscarriages from 285 Couples with Recurrent Miscarriage

| Diagnosis | Number of Miscarriages | Frequency (%) |
|---|---|---|
| Euploid, female* | 120 | 29 |
| Euploid, male† | 105 | 25 |
| Trisomy 1 | 0 | 0 |
| Trisomy 2 | 4 | 0.95 |
| Trisomy 3 | 0 | 0 |
| Trisomy 4 | 1 | 0.24 |
| Trisomy 5 | 1 | 0.24 |
| Trisomy 6 | 3 | 0.7 |
| Trisomy 7 | 3 | 0.7 |
| Trisomy 8 | 4 | 0.95 |
| Trisomy 9 | 4 | 0.95 |
| Trisomy 10 | 1 | 0.24 |
| Trisomy 11 | 1 | 0.24 |
| Trisomy 12 | 1 | 0.24 |
| Trisomy 13 | 11 | 2.6 |
| Trisomy 14 | 11 | 2.6 |
| Trisomy 15 | 22 | 5.2 |
| Trisomy 16 | 19 | 4.5 |
| Trisomy 17 | 2 | 0.48 |
| Trisomy 18 | 4 | 0.95 |
| Trisomy 19 | 0 | 0 |
| Trisomy 20 | 2 | 0.48 |
| Trisomy 21 | 11 | 2.6 |
| Trisomy 22 | 16 | 3.8 |
| Double trisomy | 9 | 2.1 |
| Sex trisomy (47,XXY) | 1 | 0.24 |
| Monosomy X (45,X) | 18 | 4.3 |
| Monosomy X and trisomy 21 | 1 | 0.24 |
| Triploidy | 27 | 6.4 |
| Tetraploidy | 10 | 2.4 |
| Unbalanced translocations | 8 | 1.9 |
| Total | 420 | 100 |

From Stephenson MD, Awartani KA, Robinson WP. Cytogenetic analysis of miscarriages from couples with recurrent miscarriage: a case control study. *Hum Reprod.* 2002;17:446-451.

*Consisting of 118 cases of 46,XX and two cases of balanced translocations.

†Consisting of 105 cases of 46,XY.

septa tend to be associated with the poorest reproductive outcome. A review by Grimbizis and colleagues found a high rate of miscarriage in women with septate (n = 499, 44.3% loss), unicornuate (n = 260, 36.5% loss), bicornuate (n = 627, 36% loss), didelphys (n = 152, 32.3% loss), and arcuate (n = 241, 25.7% loss) uteri (Grimbizis, 2001).

Several imaging modalities may be used to evaluate the uterus, including hysterosalpingogram, transvaginal ultrasonography, and sonohysterography. Magnetic resonance imaging (MRI) and three-dimensional transvaginal ultrasonography may help to better characterize the anomaly.

Hysteroscopic septoplasty is the treatment of choice for women with a septate uterus and a history of pregnancy loss, with laparotomy reserved for exceptional and complicated anomalies.

March and Israel initially reported that it was possible to incise the septum, even those thicker than 1 cm, of all of the 82 women with recurrent abortion studied, using the hysteroscope. After this treatment, the abortion rate declined from 95% to 13% (March, 1987). A large review of studies found that correction of uterine septa improved reproductive performance with live birth rate of 83.2% in 366 pregnancies. The benefits of hysteroscopic septoplasty have not yet been assessed by a randomized trial. A transfundal metroplasty technique originally described by Strassmann may be the appropriate surgical procedure for unification in women with a bicornuate uterus who have a history of recurrent pregnancy loss or previable birth. When necessary, cervical cerclage may also be used. Cervical cerclage may improve pregnancy outcomes in women with bicornuate uteri and in women with a unicornuate uterus or uterus didelphys who have a history of late-trimester pregnancy loss. Bider and coworkers reported that when cervical cerclage was used to treat women with a bicornuate uterus and recurrent pregnancy loss, the incidence of viable pregnancies markedly increased. In one series of 41 women with bicornuate uteri and recurrent abortion, 85% had a successful pregnancy outcome after cervical cerclage and the other 18 women had a term delivery following hysteroscopy (Bider, 1992). Sonographic measurements of cervical length help distinguish which patients may benefit from cerclage.

## UTERINE ANOMALIES AFTER DIETHYLSTILBESTROL

DES was prescribed to women throughout the 1950s and early to mid-1960s. Because it was withdrawn from the U.S. market in 1971, it is not a current cause of miscarriage, except in women at the end of their childbearing years. Diethylstilbestrol can lead to uterine malformations, including hypoplastic cavity, T-shaped uterus, constriction bands, a wide lower segment, and irregular borders. Studies have shown that nearly 70% of women who were exposed to DES in utero had uterine abnormalities detected on hysterosalpingography, most commonly hypoplastic T-shaped cavity (31%). Comparative studies have shown that women exposed to DES during their fetal life have a significantly greater incidence of spontaneous abortion than do controls. One study noted that the endometrial cavity of women exposed to DES in utero had a significantly smaller surface area than normal, which could perhaps contribute to the increased spontaneous abortion rate in women who had been exposed to DES in utero. No therapy, including cerclage, has been shown to significantly lower the abortion rate in women exposed to DES who have abnormalities of the uterine cavity and recurrent abortion unless they also have cervical incompetence. Because the length of gestation tends to increase with subsequent pregnancies among women who had fetal DES exposure, most of these women ultimately had a viable pregnancy.

## CERVICAL INCOMPETENCE (CERVICAL INSUFFICIENCY)

Cervical incompetence is characterized by an asymptomatic dilation of the internal cervical os, leading to dilation of the cervical canal during the second trimester of pregnancy. The consequent lack of support of the fetal membranes leads to their prolapse and rupture, which is usually followed by expulsion of the fetus and placenta. The incidence of this problem was previously estimated to vary from 1 in 57 to 1 in 1730 pregnancies. The huge range of incidence speaks to the difficulty in diagnosis. It is believed that most cases occur as a result of surgical trauma to the cervix from conization, loop electrosurgical excision procedures, mechanical dilation of the cervix during pregnancy termination, or obstetric lacerations. Cervical incompetence has also been associated with the presence of uterine anomalies, congenital defects in the cervical tissue, and fetal DES exposure. Cervical incompetence rarely causes recurrent miscarriage, as it is treated after the first occurrence of loss. There is no absolute test for the definitive diagnosis of cervical incompetence. The diagnosis is usually made by obtaining a history of second-trimester pregnancy loss without contractions or labor and in the absence of other clear etiology (e.g., bleeding, infection, ruptured membranes). Many times the patient will have mild contractions shortly before expelling the pregnancy or before an examination that finds the cervical dilatation to be advanced. Commonly, the cervix is noted to be unexpectedly dilated at the time of a mid-trimester ultrasound. Ultrasound diagnosis of cervical shortening has been shown to be a marker of preterm birth rather than cervical insufficiency. Nevertheless, cerclage may be beneficial in women with a short cervix.

History-indicated cerclages are typically placed at approximately 13 to 14 weeks. Multiple studies have shown that women at risk of cervical insufficiency can be monitored with serial transvaginal ultrasound examinations from 16 weeks to the end of 24 weeks' gestation. Ultrasound monitoring may avoid the placement of a history-indicated cerclage in more than one half of patients (Fig. 16.3). Although women with a singleton pregnancy who have a history of a prior spontaneous preterm birth at less than 34 weeks' gestation and a cervical length less than 25 mm before 24 weeks' gestation do not meet the diagnostic criteria for cervical insufficiency, studies have suggested that cerclage placement may be effective in this setting. Normal cervical length is approximately 3.5 cm or greater (Fig. 16.4, *A* and *B*). Women who are found to have cervical dilation either from digital or speculum exam at less than 24 weeks of gestation are candidates for examination-indicated cerclage, known as *emergency or rescue cerclage.* The benefit of a rescue cerclage in these women has only been demonstrated from one small randomized trial and retrospective studies.

Cerclage placement consists of a concentric nonabsorbable suture as close to the level of the internal os as possible. If strict criteria are used to diagnose cervical incompetence, fetal survival rates after cerclage have been reported to increase from 20% to 80%. However, if the criteria for diagnosis are less certain, in several randomized clinical trials, there is only a slight increase in the incidence of term deliveries after cerclage is performed. It is recommended that the suture be placed electively between 12 to 14 weeks' gestation after major embryogenesis has been completed and the incidence of spontaneous abortion caused by genetic abnormalities has markedly lessened. An ultrasound examination should be performed before the cerclage is placed to document that a normal gestation is present. Occasionally, if there is a markedly shortened cervix or placement of a cerclage has failed to maintain the pregnancy, a transabdominal cerclage may be performed. If the suture is placed externally, it is usually removed at 36 to 37 weeks' gestation, and vaginal delivery is permitted to occur. If the suture is buried as in the Shirodkar procedure, then elective cesarean delivery at or beyond 39 weeks of gestation may be considered.

## ACQUIRED UTERINE DEFECTS

### Leiomyomas

Leiomyomas are common benign uterine tumors that are present in about one third of women of reproductive age. Uterine leiomyomas may be associated with repetitive miscarriage, but there is a lack of substantial evidence and the majority of studies linking leiomyomas andspontaneous miscarriage have involved women undergoing in vitro fertilization (IVF). Leiomyomas that distort the uterine cavity, including submucosal or intramural with an intracavitary component, may result in decreased pregnancy and implantation rates as well increased risk of miscarriage. A systematic review of 11 controlled studies found the spontaneous miscarriage rate to be higher in women with submucosal and intramural fibroids (in descending order) undergoing IVF compared with women with no fibroids (Klatsky, 2008). Although a causal relationship is difficult to establish, studies have shown a significant reduction in miscarriage rates following an abdominal myomectomy. In a major review published in 1981, Buttram and Reiter reported that when abdominal myomectomy was performed in a total of 1941 women, the rate of spontaneous abortion was reduced from 41% to 19% (Buttram, 1981). A more recent, smaller study by Marchionni and colleagues showed that miscarriage rates decreased from 69% to 25% postmyomectomy (Marchionni, 2004). These data indicate that fibroids are associated with miscarriage, particularly those that distort the uterine cavity, and that a myomectomy may confer reproductive benefits. The role of intramural fibroids remains controversial. Subserosal fibroids, with greater than 50% of their mass outside the myometrium are unlikely to cause adverse pregnancy outcomes. Recurrent miscarriage is a more acceptable indication for myomectomy than a single loss. Uterine polyps are a rare cause of miscarriage based on observational studies and are found and treated hysteroscopically. The presentation is similar to that of submucous myomas. Intermenstrual spotting in this setting is an indication for hysteroscopy.

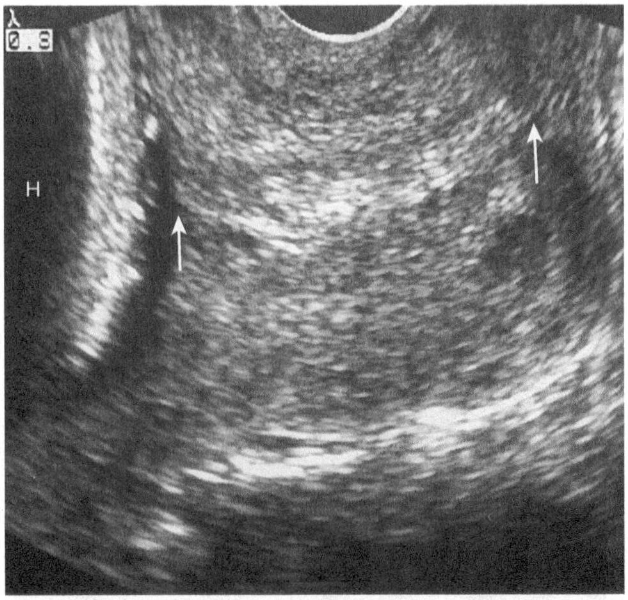


**Figure 16.3** Transvaginal ultrasound of a normal-appearing cervix. *Large arrow* to small area denotes canal from external os to internal os, respectively. *H*, Fetal head. (From Fong KW, Farine D. Cervical incompetence and preterm labor. In: Rumack CM, Wilson SR, Charboneau JW, eds. *Diagnostic Ultrasound.* 2nd ed. St. Louis: Mosby; 1998.)

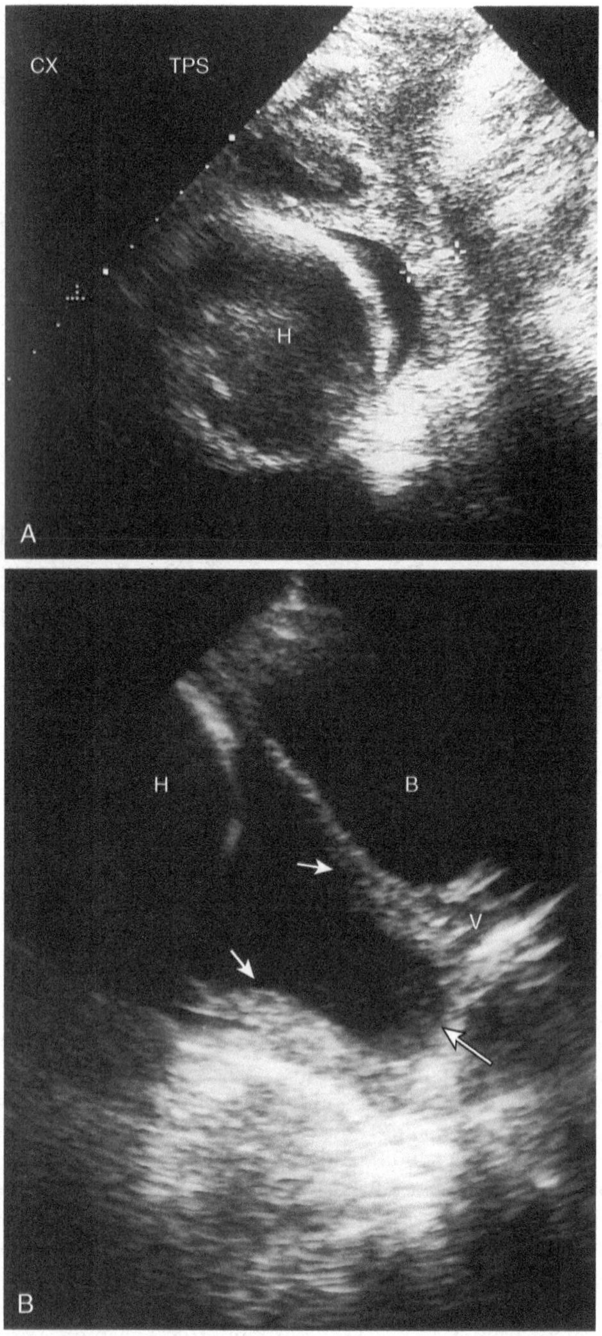


**Figure 16.4** **A,** Cervical shortening, the cervix was measured as 15 mm. Cursors are on the cervix. **B,** Advanced funneling or herniation of the membranes into the canal. This view was seen on transabdominal scan (*small arrows*, internal os; *large arrow*, external os). *B*, Maternal bladder; *CX*, cervix; *H*, fetal head; *TPS*, transperineal scan; *V*, vagina. (From Fong KW, Farine D. Cervical incompetence and preterm labor. In: Rumack CM, Wilson SR, Charboneau JW, eds. *Diagnostic Ultrasound*. 2nd ed. St. Louis: Mosby; 1998.)

### *Intrauterine Adhesions (Asherman Syndrome)*

Asherman syndrome is characterized by adhesions in the uterine cavity that can cause partial or complete obliteration of the endometrium, leading to menstrual abnormalities and amenorrhea, as well as pregnancy loss. Miscarriage is thought to be the result of insufficient endometrium to support adequate fetal growth when intrauterine adhesions (IUAs) are present. In the majority cases, adhesions result from uterine curettage for pregnancy complications such as missed or incomplete abortion as well as postpartum complications such as postpartum hemorrhage or retained placental remnants (Table 16.3). Women who undergo curettage after a pregnancy loss at a later gestational age are at higher risk compared with early pregnancy. The number of intrauterine surgical procedures seems to also increase the risk of IUA formation. In a meta-analysis of 10 prospective studies, the risk of IUA development was 2.1-fold higher for two or more curettage procedures compared with one curettage procedure (Hooker, 2014). Adhesions can also form in a nongravid uterus as a result of procedures that cause endometrial injury such as a myomectomy or curettage. In a study by Taskin and coworkers, hysteroscopic resection of multiple submucosal leiomyomas was shown to have the highest risk of IUA compared to other hysteroscopic procedures (Taskin, 2000).

**Table 16.3** Definite Causes of Intrauterine Adhesion in 1856 Cases

| | Number of Cases | Percentage |
|---|---|---|
| **Trauma Associated with Pregnancy** | | |
| Curettage after abortion | 1237 | 66.7 |
| Spontaneous | 544 | |
| Induced | 557 | |
| Unknown | 136 | |
| Postpartum curettage | 400 | 21.5 |
| Cesarean section | 38 | 2.0 |
| Evacuation of hydatidiform mole | 11 | 0.6 |
| **Trauma without Pregnancy** | | |
| Myomectomy | 24 | 1.3 |
| Diagnostic curettage | 22 | 1.2 |
| Cervical manipulation (biopsy, polypectomy, etc.) | 10 | 0.5 |
| Curettage because of menometrorrhagia | 8 | 0.4 |
| Insertion of IUD | 3 | |
| Insertion of radium | 1 | 0.3 |
| **Without Known Trauma** | | |
| Postpartum; after abortion; others | 28 | 1.5 |
| Genital tuberculosis | 74 | 4.0 |
| Total | 1856 | 100.00 |

From Schenker JG, Margalioth EJ. Intrauterine adhesions: an updated appraisal. *Fertil Steril*. 1982;37:593.
*IUA*, Intrauterine adhesion; *IUD*, intrauterine device.

The diagnosis of IUA is usually made by the finding of filling defects seen at the time of hysterosalpingogram (HSG) or by sonohysterography (Fig. 16.5). On HSG, the defects are typically irregular, with sharp contours and homogeneous opacity that persist in a series of films (Fig. 16.6). The diagnosis is best confirmed and treated by hysteroscopy.

The recommended treatment for IUA is hysteroscopic lysis of the adhesions. After adhesion lysis, a mechanical barrier such as balloon catheter or intrauterine device (IUD) is usually placed in the cavity. The balloon catheter is typically removed after 10 days and prophylactic antibiotics with doxycycline can be given while the balloon catheter is in place. High-dose estrogen is often administered postoperatively to promote reepithelialization and reduce risk of recurrent adhesions. A common regimen involves 2.5 to 5 mg of conjugated equine estrogen or 4 mg of estradiol

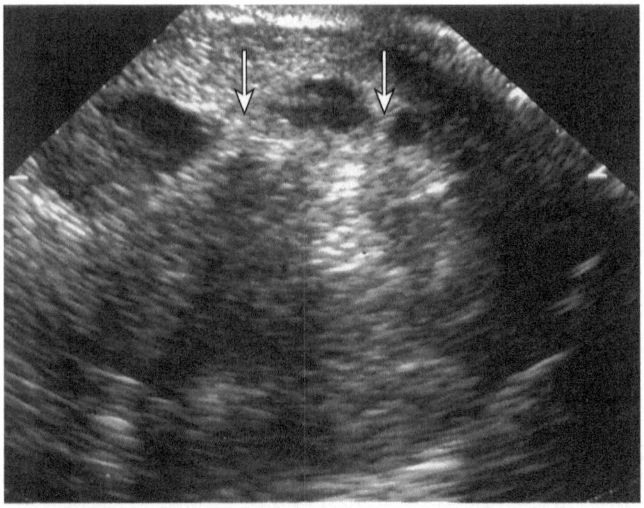

**Figure 16.5** Sonohysterography of intrauterine adhesions (*arrows*). (From Goldberg JM, Falcone T. *Atlas of Endoscopic Techniques in Gynecology*. London: WB Saunders; 2000:27.)

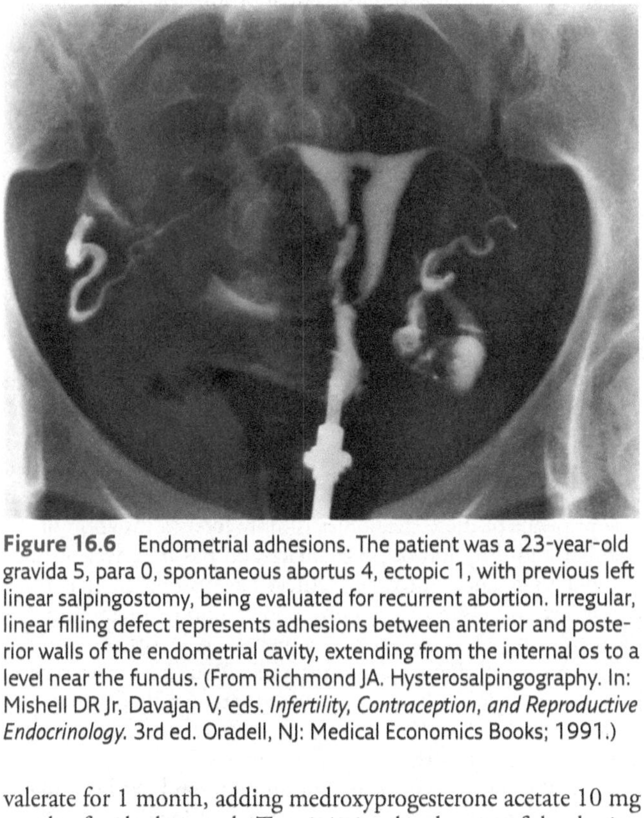

**Figure 16.6** Endometrial adhesions. The patient was a 23-year-old gravida 5, para 0, spontaneous abortus 4, ectopic 1, with previous left linear salpingostomy, being evaluated for recurrent abortion. Irregular, linear filling defect represents adhesions between anterior and posterior walls of the endometrial cavity, extending from the internal os to a level near the fundus. (From Richmond JA. Hysterosalpingography. In: Mishell DR Jr, Davajan V, eds. *Infertility, Contraception, and Reproductive Endocrinology*. 3rd ed. Oradell, NJ: Medical Economics Books; 1991.)

valerate for 1 month, adding medroxyprogesterone acetate 10 mg per day for the last week. To minimize the chances of developing IUA, curettage of the pregnant or recently pregnant uterus should be gentle and superficial and not extend deep into the muscle.

## ENDOCRINE CAUSES

### PROGESTERONE DEFICIENCY

Maintenance of the endometrium for the first 7 weeks of gestation depends on progesterone produced by the corpus luteum. After this time the corpus luteum regresses, and progesterone synthesized by the trophoblast maintains the decidual tissue. Luteal progesterone synthesis depends on human chorionic gonadotropin (HCG) produced by the trophoblast. When progesterone secretion from the corpus luteum is lower than normal or the endometrium has an inadequate response to normal circulating levels of progesterone, endometrial development may be inadequate to support the implanted blastocyst and may lead to spontaneous abortion.

The diagnosis of luteal insufficiency had historically been made by performing a histologic examination of the endometrium and finding a discrepancy of 3 days or more between the expected and actual endometrial dating pattern in at least two menstrual cycles. Investigators using this method of diagnosis have reported luteal deficiency to occur in as many as one third of women with recurrent pregnancy loss, whereas others have reported it to be an uncommon cause of miscarriage. This discrepancy may have occurred because the precision of endometrial dating by histologic examination varies among different observers, and different criteria are used for determining the day of ovulation. In fact, studies have found that diagnosing by endometrial biopsy is of limited accuracy and value because of significant inter- and intraobserver variability. Similarly, measurement of progesterone levels in the luteal phase is not considered a reliable diagnostic test due to the pulsatile release of luteinizing hormone. Moreover, there is no standard progesterone value that defines normal luteal function, as the corpus luteum function varies from cycle to cycle in normal fertile women.

Currently, most investigators believe that luteal insufficiency is rarely, if ever, the cause of recurrent spontaneous abortion. Goldstein and coworkers performed a meta-analysis of randomized control trials of the use of progestational agents given to women in early pregnancy who had a history of two or more miscarriages without a specific diagnosis of luteal deficiency. There was no significant reduction in the rate of pregnancy loss with the use of progestational agents (Goldstein, 1989). The Cochrane Collaboration Data Review evaluating 15 trials in 2013 found insufficient evidence to support the use of progesterone to prevent miscarriage, but the researchers did find a statistically significant reduced risk of pregnancy loss in women who had had three or more consecutive miscarriages (Haas, 2013). Progesterone is available as either vaginal suppositories or intramuscular progesterone beginning 3 days after ovulation and continuing throughout the first trimester.

There is no benefit to be derived by initiating progesterone therapy or administering exogenous HCG if the woman develops symptoms of threatened abortion. Low progesterone levels at this gestational age are a result, not the cause, of the abortion. When patients inquire about the use of progesterone as a rescue measure, they can be assured that if progesterone deficiency is the cause of a pregnancy loss, the pregnancy is expelled early in gestation, usually before the sixth week.

### THYROID DISEASE

Untreated overt hypothyroidism as well as subclinical hypothyroidism are also associated with miscarriage. The 2012 American Society for Reproductive Medicine (ASRM) guidelines for the treatment of recurrent pregnancy loss states that although thyroid-stimulating hormone (TSH) values of 4 to 5 mIU/L were once considered normal, the new consensus is that TSH levels above 2.5 mIU/L are outside the normal range. In fact, the Endocrine Society recommends that patients with recurrent pregnancy loss be treated to keep a TSH level of between 1 and 2.5 mIU/L. Studies regarding treating euthyroid patients with positive thyroid antibodies have been conflicting. A large prospective study of 984 euthyroid pregnant women with positive antithyroid antibodies had a significantly decreased risk of pregnancy loss if treated with levothyroxine (Negro, 2006). However, both ASRM and the Endocrine Society do not recommend routine screening for antithyroid antibodies in women with recurrent pregnancy loss.

### HYPERPROLACTINEMIA

Hyperprolactinemia has been associated with a greater risk of miscarriage. Elevated levels of prolactin can alter the hypothalamic-pituitary-ovarian axis, resulting in impaired folliculogenesis and oocyte maturation or a short luteal phase. A randomized trial found that normalization of prolactin levels with bromocriptine before pregnancy in women with a history of two or more pregnancy losses improved pregnancy outcomes. Treatment led to a live birth rate of 85.7% in the treated group compared with 52.4% in the untreated group (Hirahara, 1998).

### DIABETES MELLITUS, INSULIN RESISTANCE, AND POLYCYSTIC OVARY SYNDROME

Uncontrolled and poorly controlled diabetes mellitus is an accepted cause of miscarriage. The increased miscarriage rate is due in part to structural anomalies in the fetus. Among women with diabetes and good control of blood glucose, diabetes is an unlikely cause of miscarriage. However, diabetes without good metabolic control is associated with an increased risk of early pregnancy loss, with a direct correlation between the level of hemoglobin A1C and the rate of abortion.

Studies regarding the relationships among polycystic ovary syndrome (PCOS), elevated luteinizing hormone (LH) levels, and spontaneous abortion have been conflicting. Clifford and colleagues conducted a randomized controlled trial, which indicated that LH suppression with a GnRH analogue is not beneficial for improving live birth rates in PCOS women with recurrent abortion (Clifford, 1996). More recent evidence has supported the association among PCOS, insulin resistance, and spontaneous abortion. Insulin resistance is common in women with recurrent miscarriage and has been associated with increased risk of pregnancy loss. Proposed mechanisms include not only the inherent metabolic problems associated with higher glucose levels and decreased insulin activity such as increased inflammatory mediators but also increased levels of plasminogen activator inhibitor 1. This protein functions as a strong procoagulant and thrombophilic agent, which may result in thrombotic induction of placental insufficiency. Observational studies suggest that metformin reduces miscarriage risk in women with PCOS. In addition, metformin has been shown to be effective in insulin-resistant PCOS women with recurrent miscarriages. However, a Cochrane review in 2012 concluded that metformin treatment has no effect on the risk of miscarriage in the entire PCOS population (Tang, 2012). Currently, treatment with metformin for prevention of miscarriage is not routinely recommended for patients with PCOS.

## IMMUNOLOGIC FACTORS

### ALLOIMMUNE DISORDERS

The physiologic mechanism by which the partially foreign fetal tissue is protected from the mother's immunologic system is poorly understood. It is thought that in normal pregnancy, the maternal immune system recognizes the paternally derived antigens on embryonic tissues and produces several alloantibodies that protect the trophoblast from cytotoxic maternal immune response. Since the 1960s, investigators have postulated that miscarriage, and recurrent miscarriage in particular, may be associated with abnormalities in this maternal alloimmune response. Numerous studies have found differences in the immune mechanisms of couples with recurrent loss. However, to date, immunologic treatments have not been shown to be effective.

It has been suggested that if there is sharing of major histocompatibility locus antigens (HLA) between the male and the female in the couple with recurrent abortion, then maternal recognition of paternally derived fetal antigens is less likely to occur. Therefore the production of essential natural blocking antibodies would be hampered and abortion would be more likely to occur. Numerous studies have investigated the degree of HLA sharing at several loci in groups of couples with recurrent abortion in whom no cause for the problem could be detected. In their own study of women with three successive spontaneous abortions, Bellingard and colleagues found that there is no higher level of HLA sharing in couples with recurrent abortion than in a control group of parous women without spontaneous abortion. They also did not find a particular HLA specificity that was associated with recurrent abortion (Bellingard, 1995).

The formation of antipaternal lymphocytic antibodies is another mechanism that has been suggested as a cause of recurrent pregnancy loss. However, these antibodies have been recognized in normal pregnancies and in fact are more prevalent in fertile couples than in those with recurrent pregnancy loss. The presence of these antibodies is more likely a function of the number and duration of pregnancies and has no effect on subsequent pregnancy outcome. Others have proposed that there is a maternal failure to recognize and respond to fetal antigens by producing blocking factors, which then leaves the embryo at risk for a cell-mediated immune rejection. However, studies have shown that blocking antibodies are frequently detectable in women with recurrent pregnancy loss and are, in fact, not always present in women with normal pregnancies.

Several other aspects of the immune system have been investigated as potential causes of recurrent loss. One line of research involves the presence of natural killer cells in the early pregnancy decidua compared with the peripheral maternal circulation. Normally, there are few B lymphocytes and neutrophils but a large proportion of natural killer cells in the decidua, which are thought to contribute to control of trophoblast invasion. These proportions of uterine versus peripheral natural killer cells have been found to be different in patients with unexplained recurrent loss than in controls. However, a systematic review of 12 studies concluded that neither peripheral natural killer cell nor the peripheral killer cell number or activity predict recurrent miscarriage. Therefore the value of testing women with recurrent pregnancy loss for the levels of natural killer cells in the peripheral blood or in the uterus is questionable. The researchers recognized that there was significant heterogeneity between studies in terms of inclusion criteria, methodology of natural killer cells analysis, and outcome measurements (Tang, 2011).

Natural killer cells in the uterine decidua play a role in the cytokine response at the maternal-fetal interface. The cytokine response relevant to pregnancy is characterized as either T-helper1 (Th1) type or T-helper2 (Th2) type. Th1 responses are considered cytotoxic and associated with the release of interleukin 2, interferon, and tumor necrosis factor α, whereas Th2 responses exert a beneficial effect by inhibiting strong cellular responses and are associated with the release of interleukins 4, 6, and 10. Most women with normal pregnancies exhibit a predominant Th2 immune response. Studies have shown, however, that women with recurrent pregnancy loss have a greater Th1 response, which may be harmful to an implanting embryo. These findings support the theory that cytokine dysregulation of the immune mechanisms operating at the maternal-fetal interface may contribute to recurrent miscarriage. However, it remains unclear whether the Th1 response is the cause of pregnancy loss. The mechanism by which these factors act is not well known.

Immunotherapies developed for women with unexplained recurrent miscarriages have not been shown to be effective. A Cochrane review of 20 randomized trials concluded that immunotherapies including paternal cell immunization, third-party donor leukocytes, trophoblast membranes, and intravenous immunoglobulin do not improve the live birth rate compared with placebo treatment (Wong, 2014).

Abnormal immune responses may eventually prove for some patients to be a cause of recurrent loss, but which patients and which therapies are as of now unknown. Therefore testing for Th1 and Th2 profiles, parental HLA profiles, natural killer cells, and antiparental cytotoxic antibodies is not clinically justified.

## AUTOIMMUNE DISORDERS

Antiphospholipid syndrome (APS) is an autoimmune disorder that is associated with recurrent pregnancy loss. This disorder is characterized by the production of moderate to high levels of antiphospholipid antibodies (aPLs) as well as certain clinical features (Box 16.1). Approximately 5% to 20% of all recurrent pregnancy loss patients will test positive for aPLs, and it has been shown in a large meta-analysis that the incidence of APS is between 15% and 20% in women with recurrent pregnancy loss.

The authors of the international consensus statement recommend certain clinical criteria that should prompt testing for aPLs (Miyakis, 2006). These clinical criteria include thromboembolic events (arterial or venous) and pregnancy loss. Most pregnancy losses in women with recurrent pregnancy loss occur before 10 weeks' gestation; however, a greater proportion of losses related to aPLs occur in the fetal period greater than 10 weeks' gestation. One of the obstetric indications for aPLs testing therefore includes a single unexplained loss of a morphologically normal fetus at or beyond 10 weeks' gestation. If a pregnancy loss is diagnosed after 10 weeks' gestation but an ultrasound demonstrates that the pregnancy stopped developing before 10 weeks, testing for aPLs is not warranted. Another indication for testing is three or more unexplained consecutive losses before the 10th week of gestation excluding maternal anatomic or hormonal abnormalities and paternal and maternal chromosomal causes. Preterm severe preeclampsia and early onset placental insufficiency (intrauterine growth restriction) have been associated with APS and are therefore another indication to test for aPLs. However, there is insufficient evidence to demonstrate that screening and treatment of women with these pregnancy morbidities improves subsequent pregnancy outcomes.

The antibodies that are most commonly tested include lupus anticoagulant (LAC), anticardiolipin antibody (ACA), and anti-β2-glycoprotein 1. LAC is paradoxically named because it was first described in women with lupus, and in vitro, due to its binding with phospholipids, it will inhibit coagulation and increase the clotting time. In vivo, LAC is a strong procoagulant. To test for LAC, pathologists use specifically prepared assays, such as the kaolin clotting time or the dilute Russell viper venom test. If blood does not clot, normal serum is added to assess if the result of the clotting is due to a deficiency of clotting factors. If the blood still fails to clot with normal serum being added, then LAC is suspected. Up to 2% of normal women will have low levels of the LAC. Of note, the Venereal Disease Research Laboratory (VDRL) test for syphilis uses a phospholipid assay, and therefore the presence of LAC may induce a false-positive VDRL. Anticardiolipin antibodies are usually measured using enzyme-linked immunosorbent assays (ELISA). Both immunoglobin G and M isotypes should be measured and must be in the 99th percentile to be considered positive. Between 3% and 5% of the population will have

**Box 16.1 International Consensus Definition for the Diagnosis of Antiphospholipid Syndrome**

Diagnosis requires one of the following clinical criteria and one of the laboratory criteria:

**Clinical Criteria**

1. Vascular thrombosis
2. Pregnancy morbidity
   (a) One or more unexplained deaths of a morphologically normal fetus at or beyond the 10th week of gestation, or
   (b) One or more premature births of a morphologically normal neonate before the 34th week of gestation because of eclampsia, severe preeclampsia, or features consistent with placental insufficiency, or
   (c) Three or more unexplained consecutive spontaneous losses before the 10th week of pregnancy

**Laboratory Criteria**

1. Lupus anticoagulant present on two or more occasions at least 12 weeks apart
2. Anticardiolipin antibody of IgG or IgM isotype in medium to high titer (i.e., greater than 40 GPL or MPL, or greater than the 99th percentile) on two or more occasions, at least 12 weeks apart
3. Anti-β2-glycoprotein 1 antibody of IgG or IgM isotype in 99th percentile titer on two or more occasions, at least 12 weeks apart

Data from Committee on Practice Bulletins—Obstetrics, American College of Obstetricians and Gynecologists. Practice Bulletin No. 132: antiphospholipid syndrome. *Obstet Gynecol.* 2012;120(6):1514-1521.
*IgG*, Immunoglobulin G; *IgM*, immunoglobulin M; *GPL*, IgG phospholipid units; *MPL*, IgM phospholipid units.

low levels of immunoglobulin for ACA that is of unknown significance. Similarly, anti-β2-glycoprotein 1 is detected using ELISA and a high titer is considered sufficient to establish the diagnosis of APS. Assays for antiphospholipids other than LAC, ACA, and anti-β2-glycoprotein 1 have not been standardized and routine screening is not warranted.

Phospholipids are ubiquitous molecules that occur throughout the body and are found in almost all vasculature, particularly the placental vasculature. These antibodies react with proteins on the endothelium and induce platelet activation and thrombosis. The reaction induced by the antibody antigen complexes will induce both arterial and venous thrombosis. However, the primary mechanism by which these antibodies mediate pregnancy loss is not through thrombosis in the placental circulation, but by inducing deleterious effects on the developing trophoblast. These effects include inhibition of villous cytotrophoblast differentiation and extravillous cytotrophoblast invasion into the decidua, induction of syncytiotrophoblast apoptosis, and activation of maternal inflammatory pathways at the maternal-fetal interface (ACOG, 2012).

The treatment of antiphospholipid syndrome is both 81 mg of aspirin daily and prophylactic unfractionated heparin (usually 5000 to 10,000 units by subcutaneous injection twice a day) initiated with a positive pregnancy test. This therapy has shown to increase the live birth rate and decrease pregnancy loss. A Cochrane review in 2005 found that the combination of low-dose aspirin and unfractionated heparin reduced the pregnancy loss rate by 54% compared with aspirin alone in the treatment of APS in women with recurrent pregnancy loss (Empson, 2005). Although low-molecular-weight heparin (LMWH) has a number of advantages over unfractionated heparin, it has not shown comparable efficacy in reducing pregnancy loss in patients with APS. Similarly, other therapies including prednisone and intravenous immunoglobulin have not been proven to show any benefit and their use is not recommended. Multiple large randomized trials have evaluated the use of heparin or aspirin in women with unexplained recurrent pregnancy loss not meeting the diagnosis of APS and have not shown a benefit. Heparin and aspirin should therefore be used in women who have met the strict criteria for the diagnosis of APS.

### *Celiac Disease*

Celiac disease (sprue) is a systemic autoimmune disease caused by an allergy to gluten and is associated with miscarriage. Though its most pronounced symptoms are related to intestinal malabsorption, most patients will have minimal gastrointestinal manifestations. A strong association has been documented with adverse pregnancy outcomes, including recurrent miscarriage, intrauterine growth restriction, stillbirth, and the antibodies of celiac disease. Antigliadin antibodies appear to be toxic to trophoblasts, and suppression of the antibodies through dietary control has decreased the incidence of miscarriage. In the setting of an evaluation for miscarriage, any woman with a personal or family history of celiac disease or gluten intolerance should be tested for antigliadin and antiendomysial antibodies. The prevalence of celiac disease in first-degree relatives of patients with sprue is 10%. A study by Tursi and coworkers of women with recurrent miscarriage and celiac disease noted a decreased miscarriage rate when women were placed on gluten-free diets (Tursi, 2008).

## INHERITED THROMBOPHILIAS

An essential and vital component of a successful gestation is the healthy growth and development of the placental vasculature. The uteroplacental interface receives nearly 20% of maternal cardiac output. A self-protective physiologic adaptation is the increased thrombogenic characteristics of this interface to prevent hemorrhage during implantation, placentation, and the third stage of labor. If the mother has an inherent thrombotic tendency such as a thrombophilia, this thrombogenic microenvironment in the placenta can intensify, leading to multiple small infarctions at the uteroplacental interface. The potential for thrombosis of the microvasculature of the placenta has been used to explain the association between thrombophilia and recurrent pregnancy loss as well as adverse pregnancy outcomes such as preeclampsia, fetal growth restriction, and placenta abruption. Although there is a strong association between inherited thrombophilias and venous thromboembolism, there is still controversy whether the same is true for thrombophilias and adverse pregnancy outcomes including recurrent pregnancy loss (ACOG, 2013).

The incidence of thrombophilias, both acquired and inherited, is fairly large (>10% of the Caucasian population); thus it is difficult to equate the presence of a thrombophilia as a definitive cause of a specific adverse pregnancy event. As discussed earlier, miscarriages are frequently multifactorial, particularly recurrent loss. Thrombophilias have been associated with both early and late pregnancy loss (Box 16.2). However, the association appears to be stronger for second-trimester and later losses than for early miscarriages. In a case control trial of 3496 primarily Caucasian women with unexplained pregnancy loss and matched controls, an association was seen between factor V Leiden and prothrombin gene mutation and pregnancy loss after 10 weeks. There was no association found less than 10 weeks of gestation (Lissalde-Lavigne, 2005). This finding is logical given that placental development has not taken place very early in pregnancy. Consequently, thrombosis of placental vasculature in women with thrombophilias is less likely to explain early pregnancy loss, again highlighting that thrombophilia cannot be the only pathophysiologic mechanism playing a part. There may be individual predilections and comorbidities in addition to the thrombophilias that lead to recurrent pregnancy loss in certain women. As of yet, most of these cofactors have not been identified.

**Box 16.2 Thrombophilias Associated with Miscarriage**

Antiphospholipid antibodies—anticardiolipin, lupus anticoagulant, and anti-beta-2 glycoprotein
Antithrombin III deficiency
Elevated factor VIII levels
Factor V Leiden mutation
MTHFR mutations*
Plasminogen activator inhibitor-1 deficiency
Protein C deficiency
Protein S deficiency
Prothrombin G20210A mutation
Thrombocytosis (thrombocythemia—platelet counts >750,000)

*Methylenetetrahydrofolate reductase mutations. (Mild hyperhomocysteinemia is technically not a thrombophilia, though it may be associated with thrombosis. Many laboratories include testing for the mutations in thrombophilia panels.)

Although retrospective studies and meta-analyses of the thrombophilias indicate that there is an association between thrombophilias and miscarriage, prospective studies have shown no association. The Eunice Kennedy Shriver National Institute of Child Health and Human Development's Maternal-Fetal Medicine Units Network prospectively studied 134 pregnant women who here heterozygous for factor V Leiden and found no increase in the incidence of fetal loss (Dizon-Townson, 2005). A secondary analysis was conducted for maternal carriers of the prothrombin G20210A mutation and again no increased risk was noted (Silver, 2010).

The essential point to be made with couples is that it is almost impossible to know that a thrombophilia caused their miscarriage. Causation and association are not the same. Furthermore, there is insufficient evidence that antepartum prophylaxis with unfractionated heparin or LMWH prevents recurrence of miscarriage in these patients.

Factor V Leiden is the most common inherited thrombophilia in whites. The prevalence of this mutation in European populations is approximately 5%; however, it is rare in Asians and Africans. The Leiden mutation is a substitution of glutamine for arginine at position 506 on the factor V protein. This mutation in factor V leads to a defect in binding with the activated protein C (APC) complex. Consequently, factor Va is resistant to degradation by APC, which results in less down-regulation of thrombin. Women who are heterozygous for factor V Leiden account for approximately 40% of cases of venous thromboembolism (VTE) during pregnancy. Patients who are homozygous for factor V Leiden account for only 2% of VTE cases during pregnancy but have 80 times higher lifetime risk of thrombosis. The second most common thrombophilia is the G20210A mutation in prothrombin. The prothrombin mutation is a point mutation that is found in approximately 3% of the European population. It causes an excess concentration of prothrombin in the circulation and accounts for 17% of thromboembolism cases in pregnancy. Less common thrombophilias include deficiencies in protein C, protein S deficiency, and antithrombin III deficiency. All three of these proteins contribute to the thrombolytic pathway, and the homozygous states are not compatible with life. Protein C and antithrombin-3 levels may be assessed in pregnancy. However, protein S is an acute-phase reactant, decreasing with pregnancy, trauma, or surgery. Levels are significantly decreased by estrogen in general, and thus they should be measured at least 6 to 8 weeks after a pregnancy. Elevated factor VIII, greater than 180% of normal, and plasminogen activator inhibitor deficiency (PAI-1) have also been described as causes of thrombophilia, but they appear to have little independent risk of venous thromboembolism. Mild hyperhomocysteinemia is sometimes considered a thrombophilia. Homocysteine is an essential amino acid, which in excess may lead to damage to the vascular endothelium. One enzyme system that metabolizes homocysteine is methylenetetrahydrofolate reductase (MTHFR). Mutations in this enzyme are the most common cause of hyperhomocysteinemia and occur in 10% to 15% of the white and Asian populations. Hyperhomocysteinemia was thought to be a risk factor of VTE, but data suggest that it is a weak risk factor. There is insufficient evidence to screen for MTHFR polymorphisms or to measure fasting homocysteine levels as part of the evaluation of thrombophilias as a cause for venous thromboembolism.

Screening for inherited thrombophilias, specifically factor V Leiden and prothrombin gene mutations as well protein C, protein S, and antithrombin deficiencies, may be considered when a patient has a personal history of a VTE in the setting of a non-recurrent risk factor or has a first-degree relative with a history of a high-risk thrombophilia. Treatment of the inherited thrombophilias involves subcutaneous heparin. Either unfractionated heparin or LMWH regimens may be used. Testing for inherited thrombophilias in women with recurrent pregnancy loss or placental abruption is not recommended given insufficient evidence of an association and of treatment benefit with heparin.

## INFECTIONS

Numerous infectious agents such as *Ureaplasma urealyticum, Mycoplasma hominis, Chlamydia trachomatis, Listeria monocytogenes, Toxoplasma gondii*, rubella, cytomegalovirus, and herpes virus have all been identified in cultures from women who have had spontaneous pregnancy losses. There are fewer data regarding the relationship between these infectious agents and recurrent loss.

Although *Listeria monocytogenes* produces abortion in several animal species as well as humans in the second trimester, there is no convincing evidence that it is an abortifacient in women in the first trimester or in recurrent miscarriages. *Chlamydia trachomatis* is a common sexually transmitted pathogen, but there is no evidence that it causes miscarriage in asymptomatic women. Primary infections have been associated with pregnancy loss but not recurrent loss.

Several authors have suggested that T strain mycoplasma, both *Ureaplasma urealyticum* and *Mycoplasma hominis,* can cause miscarriage. Data indicating that *U. urealyticum* is a cause of miscarriage are stronger than for *M. hominis*. Penta and colleagues found that *U. urealyticum* and *M. hominis* were the most common bacterial species found in cultures from women who have had spontaneous pregnancy losses (Penta, 2003). Stray-Pedersen and Stray-Pedersen reported that eradication of *U. urealyticum* in the endometrium by tetracycline treatment for 10 days resulted in a significantly lower subsequent miscarriage rate (19%) (Stray-Pedersen, 1984). However, there are no randomized placebo-controlled clinical trials to prove that these organisms cause miscarriage and that treatment is effective.

The parasite *Toxoplasma gondii* may infect the embryo and lead to miscarriage. However, it is difficult to document the presence of this organism before a miscarriage occurs because there is a lack of correlation between serologic immunoassays for this organism and its detection in the endometrium by immunofluorescence.

The data for bacterial vaginosis as a cause of early miscarriage due to endometritis have been inconsistent; however, overgrowth of these bacteria has been repeatedly reported as a risk factor for late miscarriage and preterm birth.

Many viral agents may cause miscarriage if acquired as primary infections. Viral infections have been associated with both first- and second-trimester loss in cohort and case-control studies using histology and polymerase chain reaction (PCR). Parvovirus B-19 may be embryotoxic in the first trimester but is not a cause of recurrent loss. Similarly, infection from varicella, cytomegalovirus, and rubella may cause miscarriage but are not a cause of recurrent loss. Primary infection with herpes simplex virus in the genital tract has been reported to cause miscarriage. Kaproanos and coworkers were able to detect HSV by sensitive and accurate nested PCR in 41 of 95 cases (43.2%) of early pregnancy loss and in 6 of 36 cases (16.7%) of elective pregnancy termination (Kapranos, 2009). There does not appear to be an association between HSV-2 infection in pregnancy and fetal death after 16 weeks.

Given the lack of prospective studies linking any infectious agent to recurrent pregnancy loss, routinely screening for these organisms or using antibiotics empirically is not indicated.

## ENVIRONMENTAL FACTORS

### *SMOKING*

There are numerous studies evaluating smoking and miscarriage, and they all suggest an increased risk of miscarriage in a dose-dependent manner. In a large retrospective study of 47,146 women, an increased risk of pregnancy loss was seen in women who smoked as few as 10 cigarettes per day (Armstrong, 1992). A meta-analysis of 112 articles confirmed that any active smoking during pregnancy increased the risk of miscarriage and the risk of miscarriage was increased with the amount smoked (1% increase in relative risk per cigarette smoked per day) (Pineles, 2014). Cigarette smoke contains several toxic agents such as nicotine, carbon monoxide, and mutagens, which may be harmful to the developing embryo. Nicotine also has a vasoconstrictive effect that can reduce the blood flow to the placenta. Interestingly, most women who smoke do not miscarry, supporting the multifactorial nature of miscarriage. Paternal smoking also increases the risk of miscarriage. When both parents smoke, some studies have found a four times increased rate of miscarriage compared with nonsmoking controls.

### *ALCOHOL*

Kline and associates also reported that drinking alcohol, acting independently from smoking, was a risk factor for miscarriage (Table 16.4). Women who drank alcohol at least 2 days a week had an approximate twofold greater risk of having a miscarriage than women who did not drink during pregnancy (Kline, 1980). More recent studies have confirmed these findings. After studying 24,679 singleton pregnancies, Kesmodel and colleagues found more than a threefold increased risk of first-trimester spontaneous abortion for women who drank on average more than five drinks per week (Kesmodel, 2002).

### *COFFEE AND CAFFEINE*

Some epidemiologic data have suggested that moderate to heavy caffeine ingestion may be an independent risk factor for miscarriage. Studies suggest a threshold effect with more than 300 mg/day of caffeine (equivalent to three cups of coffee) is associated with a modest increase in risk for spontaneous miscarriage. A prospective study has shown that preconceptional caffeine consumption, however, is not associated with spontaneous miscarriage. Although it is not clear whether the relationship between caffeine and miscarriage is causal, women who become pregnant are recommended to limit their caffeine intake (Cnattingius, 2000).

### *IRRADIATION AND MAGNETIC FIELDS*

Animal studies have shown that ionizing radiation can produce congenital malformations, growth retardation, and embryonic and fetal death. These effects are dose related, and there is a threshold dose below which an adverse effect does not occur. Although there is evidence in the human that high-energy radiation exposure is associated with teratogenic effects and intrauterine growth restriction, there is no conclusive evidence that similar exposure increases the risk of spontaneous abortion. Because these studies will never be done, it is presumed that a threshold effect extends from teratogenicity to miscarriage.

Extrapolation from animal data indicates that the embryo is most sensitive to the lethal effect of irradiation during the day of implantation and a few days later (Table 16.5). The sensitivity decreases during the period of early embryogenesis, after which the minimum lethal dose (MLD) remains constant to term gestation. Animal and human data have shown that there is no increased risk of abortion with irradiation exposures of less than 5 rads. Diagnostic procedures, which are several-fold less than 5 rads, are therefore unlikely to cause a miscarriage even if they are administered during the time of implantation.

Exposure to magnetic fields induced by electric currents has not been associated with a significantly higher rate of miscarriage.

**Table 16.4** Frequency (%) of Alcohol Consumption among Women Experiencing Spontaneous Abortions (Cases) and Women Delivering at 28 Weeks' Gestation or Later (Controls)

| | Percentage Distribution | | | |
|---|---|---|---|---|
| **Frequency of Alcohol Consumption during Pregnancy** | **Cases** | **Controls** | **Adjusted Odds Ratio** | **95% Confidence Interval** |
| Never | 42.6 | 43.7 | 1.00 | 0.59-0.99 |
| Twice a month and less | 28.9 | 38.0 | 0.77 | 0.71-1.52 |
| Less than twice a month 10.8 } 17.9 | 10.4 } 7.9 | 1.04 } 2.36 | 1.30-2.95 | |
| 2-6 days a week 13.3 | 6.5 | 1.96 | | |
| Daily | 4.5 | 1.4 | 3.00 | 1.39-6.49 |
| Total | 648 | | | 645 |

From Kline J, Stein Z, Susser M, et al. Environmental influences on early reproductive loss in a current New York City study. In: Porter IH, Hook EB, eds. *Human Embryonic and Fetal Death*. New York: Academic Press; 1980.

Video display terminals, electric blankets, and power lines are not harmful to a pregnancy.

## ENVIRONMENTAL TOXINS

The information that exists concerning the effect of environmental toxins on human pregnancy and miscarriage is based on case reports and small case-control studies. Recommendations have been developed from data based on effects that cause fetal anomalies. These recommendations are to avoid contact.

Some, but not all, studies have shown an increased risk of pregnancy loss among women occupationally exposed to anesthetic gases, but most of these studies are retrospective questionnaires. A well-done case-control study indicated that the incidence of miscarriage in women exposed to anesthetic gases was not significantly increased. A more recent meta-analysis found that nurses exposed to anesthetic gases may be at an increased risk of spontaneous abortion; however, the strength of association was weaker in the well-designed studies. The current practice is to adequately scavenge gases in hospitals and physician's and dental offices. Similarly, women exposed to chemotherapeutic agents, such as nurses and pharmacy technicians, may have an increased risk of miscarriage (Connor, 2014).

High-quality evidence regarding a possible association between other environmental toxins and miscarriage is even less available. Heavy metals, lead, cadmium, mercury, and arsenic are embryotoxic. Of these, lead is the most common exposure and most well documented as a cause of miscarriage. If elevated lead levels are found in a patient, then chelation treatment is indicated prior to pregnancy and can be used in pregnancy as well. Organic solvents, particularly those used in the computer industry, and organic pesticides are worrisome and may induce miscarriage.

## OBESITY

Obesity, defined as body mass index (BMI) greater than or equal to 30 kg/m$^2$, has been shown to increase the risk of miscarriage. Obesity has not only been shown to increase the risk of first-trimester miscarriage but has also been shown to increase recurrence risk in patients with recurrent pregnancy loss. An observational cohort study of 372 women with recurrent early pregnancy loss found that obese women have an increased frequency of euploid miscarriages, which is a known risk factor for subsequent miscarriages (Boots, 2014). The pathophysiology of the association between obesity and miscarriage is unclear. A proposed mechanism includes leptin resistance and its detrimental effect on endometrial receptivity.

**Table 16.5** Estimation of Abortigenic Hazards of X-Irradiation to Human Embryo from Animal Experiments

| Stage of Human Gestation (Days) | Lethal Dose/50 (Rads) | MLD (Rads) |
|---|---|---|
| 1 | 70-100 | 10 |
| 14 | 140 | 25 |
| 18 | 150 | 25 |
| 28 | 220 | 50 |
| 50 | 260 | 50 |
| Late fetus to term | 300-400 | 50 |

From Brent RL. Radiation-induced embryonic and fetal loss from conception to birth. In: Porter IH, Hook EB, eds. *Human Embryonic and Fetal Death*. New York: Academic Press; 1980.

*MLD*, Minimum lethal dose.

## EXERCISE, STRESS, AND DEPRESSION

Severe stress is a well-documented cause of pregnancy loss in the animal model, and anecdotally stress has been associated with pregnancy loss in humans. Older literature, from 75 to 150 years ago, proposed that emotional stress led to adverse pregnancy outcomes. Severe stress may lead to a higher incidence of late pregnancy outcomes by affecting uteroplacental function in some cases but has not been associated with early pregnancy loss. Women who receive counseling for depression associated with recurrent loss seem to have a higher successful pregnancy rate. The interaction among stress, depression, and pregnancy outcome is complex. Currently, the relationship with pregnancy loss is equivocal at best. Many studies have repeatedly shown that employment, work, and exercise are not associated with miscarriage.

Although the Danish National Birth Cohort study, which included 92,671 pregnancies, found that moderate to intense exercise including "high-impact" exercise in the first trimester may increase pregnancy loss, the study's design was problematic and affected by recall bias (Madsen, 2007).

# DIAGNOSIS

Miscarriage is ultimately diagnosed through confirmation of a nonviable gestation. Originally, the types of abortion were described by the appearance of the patient upon presentation to the physician. They include (1) *threatened abortion*—vaginal bleeding in the setting of a viable intrauterine pregnancy and closed cervical os, (2) *missed abortion*—a nonviable intrauterine gestation less than 20 weeks with a closed cervical os, (3) *incomplete abortion*—an intrauterine gestation at less than 20 weeks with an open cervical os and partial passage of products of conception, (4) *inevitable abortion*—an open cervical os with no passage of products of conception in the setting of either a viable or nonviable intrauterine pregnancy, and (5) *complete spontaneous abortion*—passage of all products of conception in the setting of an intrauterine pregnancy. These definitions have been rendered somewhat less helpful with the widespread use of transvaginal ultrasound in the diagnosis of early pregnancy.

The level of B-hCG in a normally developing pregnancy should rise in a predictable fashion. A minimal increase of 24% in 24 hours and 53% in 48 hours was observed for viable pregnancies in a large longitudinal study. Levels may peak around 100,000 IU at 10 weeks with the steepest rate of increase observed in the first 6 weeks, followed by a slower rise and eventual fall after the peak. A "discriminatory zone" of B-hCG level has been used to predict when an intrauterine gestational sac should be visible on imaging. A B-hCG of 1500 IU has traditionally been accepted as the level at which transvaginal ultrasound should reveal an intrauterine gestational sac in a viable pregnancy. However, discussion in the literature has called this data point into question (Barnhart, 2012).

The first sonographic finding of a pregnancy is the gestational sac (Table 16.6). This is a sonographic term, not a true anatomic delineation (Goldstein, 1994). The sac is an echolucent area in the uterus surrounded by echodense-reactive endometrium (decidualized endometrium; Fig. 16.7). Intrauterine lucencies may be first visualized as early as 3 weeks after the last menstrual period, 1 week after conception, and may represent purely fluid in the secretory phase. In the interior of the sac is the developing fluid-filled chorionic sac. With visualization of the chorionic sac with secondary echoes, a true gestational sac may be defined. If the fluid is endometrial secretions, it is considered a pseudogestational sac. The first fetal structure that may be visualized on ultrasound is the yolk sac. A distorted or large yolk sac, greater than 7 mm, has been associated with pregnancy loss.

The embryonic disc is notable as a thickening on the yolk sac as early as a few days after the yolk sac appears. An embryonic disc should be visualized by approximately 5 to 6 weeks' gestational age. If the mean gestational sac diameter is more than 25 mm and no embryo is visible, an anembryonic gestation is present. The earliest cardiac activity was noted to have occurred 5 weeks after the last menstrual period in a 28-day cycle. Initially, the fetal heart rate should be in the 80 to 110 beats per minute (beats/min) range and will then often increase into the 180 to 220 bpm range for the first few months of pregnancy, but by 12 weeks it should return to 110 to 160 bpm.

Table 16.6 Ultrasound Findings in Early Pregnancy

| Ultrasound Findings | Gestational Age from LMP (days) | Approximate HCG (IU) | Approximate Risk of Miscarriage* |
|---|---|---|---|
| Gestational sac | 23-29 | 1500 | <12% |
| Yolk sac | 32-45 | 5000 | <9%† |
| Embryonic disc | 35-45 | | <8% |
| Fetal cardiac activity | >42 with CRL × 5 mm | 13,000-15,000 | <8% |
| Embryo 2 cm with heart rate | 56 | | <2% |

*If no vaginal bleeding.
†If the gestational sac is 10 mm.
*CRL*, Crown-rump length; *HCG*, human chorionic gonadotropin; *LMP*, last menstrual period.

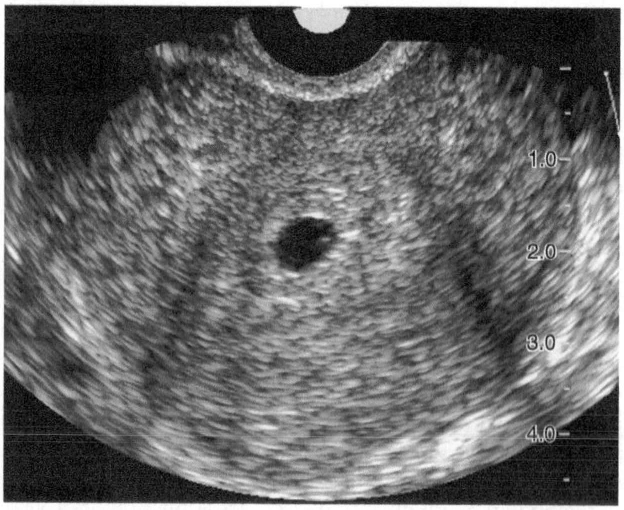


**Figure 16.7** Endovaginal ultrasound 6 days after a gestational sac, with mildly increased decidual reaction surrounding the echolucent sac. *UT*, Uterus. (From Lyons EA, Levi CS, Dashefsky SM. The first trimester. In: Rumack CM, Wilson SR, Charboneau JW [eds]: *Diagnostic Ultrasound*. 2nd ed. St. Louis: Mosby; 1998.)

Diagnosis of pregnancy loss should be made by thorough medical history and physical examination combined with ultrasound and B-hCG values. Care should be taken in basing the diagnosis on a single B-hCG level or ultrasound, as a point-in-time measurement is often unreliable. Trending of values and examination findings are usually required for accuracy. Early studies of transvaginal ultrasound for determination of fetal viability used a crown-rump length (CRL) of 5 mm without cardiac activity or an empty intrauterine gestational sac with a mean sac diameter (MSD) of 16 mm to diagnose a miscarriage. However, more recent data have prompted the Society of Radiologists in Ultrasound Multispecialty Panel on Early First Trimester Diagnosis of Miscarriage and Exclusion of a Viable Intrauterine Pregnancy to recommend more conservative guidelines These new criteria require a CRL of 7 mm or more with no heartbeat or an MSD of 25 mm or more with no embryo to diagnose an early pregnancy loss. The aim of these new criteria is to facilitate achievement of 100% specificity with a 0 false-positive rate in the diagnosis of a nonviable pregnancy. Included in these guidelines are findings suggestive, but not diagnostic, of pregnancy loss (Doubilet, 2013).

## THREATENED ABORTION

Bleeding may occur in 30% to 40% of pregnancies during the first 20 weeks, and about 50% of these will ultimately end in miscarriage (Hasan, 2009). Women who do not suffer a loss are slightly more apt to deliver preterm or encounter fetal anomalies. Ultrasound is the most useful diagnostic tool in patients with bleeding, and a subchorionic hematoma, seen as a lucency behind the brighter placental disk, will be observed in 20% of these women. About two thirds of women with bleeding will have a live fetus on ultrasound examination, and nearly 85% of these women will go on to deliver a live-born infant.

## MISSED ABORTION

The advent of early, widespread use of transvaginal ultrasound has largely made the term *missed abortion* irrelevant. Rarely will a patient have delayed diagnosis of either a fetal demise or anembryonic gestation. Retention of a dead fetus in the uterus beyond 5 weeks following the demise can be associated with consumptive coagulability and hypofibrinogenemia. The condition is usually self-limited and resolves in a few weeks without intervention. The incidence is higher with both the length of gestation and duration of fetal death, occurring uncommonly before 16 to 18 weeks.

## SEPTIC ABORTION

Infection may occur in 1% to 2% of all miscarriages, with an increased incidence following induced abortions using nonsterile equipment. A high suspicion of septic abortion should accompany symptoms of bleeding or spotting and clinical signs of infection during the first 20 weeks of pregnancy. Septic abortions may be threatened, inevitable, missed, or incomplete.

Infection can spread from the endometrium through the myometrium and eventually affect the parametrium and peritoneum. Elevated temperature, leukocytosis, lower abdominal pain, cervical motion tenderness, and a purulent vaginal discharge are all signs of septic abortion. The cause is most frequently polymicrobial, with *E. coli* and other aerobic gram-negative rods involved. Group B B-hemolytic streptococci, anaerobic streptococci, *Bacteroides*, and *Clostridium perfringens* may also be implicated. Shock can occur from the release of endotoxins.

## TREATMENT

### THREATENED ABORTION

There is no evidence to support limitation of physical activity or any medical intervention to improve the prognosis of a threatened abortion. Avoidance of excessive physical activity/exercise and coitus may serve as comfort measures. Likewise, administration of natural progesterone, synthetic progestins, or hCG should be avoided, as this may increase the probability of a missed abortion by falsely elevating monitoring levels of progesterone or B-hCG. If the patient is Rh negative, Rh immune globulin should be administered.

### DIAGNOSED ABORTION

Once a nonviable pregnancy has been diagnosed, a thorough discussion with the patient and her partner or support person should ensue. Her feelings surrounding the pregnancy, as well as cultural preferences and past experience, may influence her decision regarding intervention.

Provided there is no evidence of infection, expectant management, medical therapy, or surgical evacuation of the uterus are all viable alternatives. Multiple studies confirm that no option is superior. Whereas uterine perforation may occur with surgical intervention, heavy bleeding is more common with expectant management (ACOG, 2015).

About 50% to 70% of women will opt for expectant management. Up to 95% will successfully expel an incomplete abortion without intervention (Sotiriadis, 2005). Within 2 weeks, 25% to 85% of women with a missed abortion will spontaneously resolve the pregnancy, 37% doing so within 7 days (Luise, 2002). As there is no agreed-upon value, ultrasound should not be used to measure endometrial thickness for confirmation of completion of a miscarriage but rather solely to document the absence, thus presumed passage, of a previously seen gestational sac. Should expectant management be undertaken, the patient should have a short interval follow-up within 1 to 2 weeks.

Medical management most often employs misoprostol, a prostaglandin E1 analogue, as a means to expedite expulsion of products of conception. The majority of women, 80% to 90%, will completely expel a first-trimester loss after one or two doses. Older gestations are more apt to fail medical management. Misoprostol is administered either orally or vaginally, with the vaginal route preferred to maintain steady serum levels and to avoid gastrointestinal side effects. Candidates for medical management include women without evidence of infection, hemorrhage, anemia or a bleeding disorder. Results of a large randomized controlled trial showed success rates of 71% after a single dose and 84% after a second dose of 800 micrograms misoprostol per vagina (Zhang, 2005). Based on robust evidence, 800 micrograms of vaginal misoprostol is recommended with a repeat dose as needed in patients undergoing medical management of an early pregnancy loss. The addition of mifepristone (a progesterone receptor antagonist) to misoprostol has not been shown to be more effective than misoprostol alone (ACOG, 2015). A Cochrane review in 2013 concluded that misoprostol does not lead to higher rates of complete expulsion of products of conception than expectant management over a 7- to 10-day interval in patients with incomplete pregnancy loss (Neilson, 2013). Therefore misoprostol may not be more effective than expectant management in these women.

Surgical evacuation of the uterus should be considered in patients with hemorrhage, sepsis, or who are hemodynamically unstable. Surgical treatment may also be preferable to women who desire an immediate end point. Suction curettage has been shown superior to sharp curettage, which adds little once complete suction evacuation of the uterus has been performed. One advantage of suction evacuation is the ability to perform the procedure in an outpatient office setting using local anesthesia.

### SEPTIC ABORTION

Septic abortion carries a fatality rate of 0.4 to 0.6 per 100,000 spontaneous abortions. Women presenting with septic abortion should receive a complete blood count, urinalysis, blood chemistry, and electrolyte panel. Cervicouterine cultures should be taken, and a Gram stain may provide rapid analysis. Blood cultures, chest x-ray, and panels for coagulation and disseminated intravascular coagulation (DIC) should be obtained in women who are acutely ill. Evacuation of the uterus should occur within 2 hours of the initiation of broad-spectrum, intravenous antibiotics. Hysterectomy may be warranted for patients with severe sepsis or those whose uterus cannot be evacuated through the cervix.

## FOLLOW-UP CARE

An essential aspect of the care of women with spontaneous miscarriage is the follow-up visit. At this time, the patient should be asked open-ended questions about her experience and thoughts. Multiple studies have noted patient's anger and difficulty with the health care system during the time of a miscarriage. Dealing with those frustrations will improve interactions in the future and may also decrease the risk of depression after the loss. Grieving and depression are significant issues after miscarriage. Open-ended questions are the best way to assess a patient's mood and status. Many women experience guilt after miscarriage, believing that the loss was something that they caused by some action that they performed. In fact, one study found that 80% of women had some guilt associated with a particular act or habit that is perceived as causing the miscarriage. These issues should be addressed. Some women develop physical symptomatology with grieving that may mimic symptoms of depression, such as fatigue, anorexia, sleeplessness, and sometimes somatic symptoms such as headache and back pain.

As many as 30% of women will suffer from depression after miscarriage. If symptoms of depression are apparent, then counseling and therapy with antidepressants should be pursued. A patient should be advised that if such symptoms develop, she and her family should return. Studies have also shown that couples experiencing miscarriage are at an increased risk for breaking up compared to couples with live births.

Five percent to 20% of women may develop transient symptoms of thyroid disease after a pregnancy loss. These women have a risk of thyroid disease over the next 5 years. The symptoms should be treated with thyroid replacement for low thyroid and antithyroid medications for hyperthyroid symptoms. Treatment is usually continued for 6 to 9 months, at which point the patient is reevaluated. A free thyroxine level should be obtained.

Also, at the follow-up visit an assessment is given as to potential causes of miscarriage and possible explanations. Any testing can be ordered after two or more miscarriages. The workup that is initiated for a cause of recurrent pregnancy loss is discussed next.

Future pregnancy planning is also discussed at this visit. There is no compelling evidence showing that delaying conception after an early pregnancy loss will decrease subsequent miscarriage risk. If another pregnancy is not desired, hormonal-based contraception may be initiated immediately after completion of early pregnancy loss, if appropriate.

## RECURRENT MISCARRIAGE

Historically, recurrent miscarriage has been defined as three or more consecutive spontaneous losses. ASRM defines recurrent pregnancy loss as two or more failed clinical pregnancies, documented by ultrasonography or histopathologic examination. These criteria should be used to determine whether an evaluation for recurrent pregnancy loss is appropriate. For epidemiologic studies, however, ASRM recommends that three or more losses should be used. There are no consistent or generally accepted terms and definitions of pregnancy loss prior to viability at this time. The heterogeneity in the definition of recurrent pregnancy loss makes it difficult to compare scientific data from different research groups.

The calculated probability that a woman will have two consecutive spontaneous abortions is fewer than 5%, whereas only 1% of women will experience three or more. Approximately 50% of the time, a risk factor for the recurrent losses can be determined. Often this is a factor associated with miscarriages. The remaining couples are said to have "unexplained" recurrent miscarriage.

As discussed earlier, miscarriage risk does increase with the number of previous pregnancy losses (see Table 16.1) as well as with age. Some studies have shown that past obstetrical history of a successful pregnancy does lower the risk for another spontaneous miscarriage, whereas others have not. The frequency of chromosomally normal miscarriages is higher in women under the age of 35 with recurrent miscarriage than in those with a single spontaneous abortion. In fact, the likelihood of a normal embryonic karyotype also increases with the number of previous miscarriages and after a previous abortion with a normal karyotype. After stratifying for maternal age, the distribution of chromosomal abnormalities seen in couples with recurrent miscarriage is not different than the normal populations (Stephenson, 2002). Women with recurrent miscarriages also have a tendency to abort later in gestation, indicating that maternal or environmental factors are a more likely cause of repeated pregnancy loss.

It is recommended that diagnostic evaluation be initiated after a woman has had two failed clinical pregnancies, as one early miscarriage is relatively common. Not uncommonly a history may elicit a particular line of investigation that should be initiated even after one loss. If a pregnancy loss occurs in the second trimester, the cause is more likely to recur. Thus a diagnostic evaluation should be considered after a woman has had only one second-trimester loss.

The evaluation for women with recurrent miscarriage starts with a history and physical examination with pertinent questions regarding cervical incompetence, abnormal exposures, gastrointestinal diseases, previous gynecologic surgery, any pathologic tests that were performed on previous miscarriages, family history of miscarriages or birth defects, family history of unusual thrombosis, and open-ended questions that explore the patient's ideas about causation. Laboratory evaluation should be pointed toward clues from the history. Any history suggestive of thyroid disease may prompt studies for a TSH and antithyroid antibodies. Other studies should include prolactin, hemoglobin A1C, and antiphospholipid antibodies. An evaluation of the uterine cavity is an important part of the workup and may include a hysterosalpingogram, saline sonohysterogram, three-dimensional ultrasound, hysteroscopy, or MRI. Sonohysterography is a sensitive, specific, and accurate screening method for assessing abnormalities in the uterine cavity of women with recurrent miscarriage. A karyotype of the husband and wife should also be performed to determine if any balanced structural chromosomal abnormalities exist. More controversial screening includes the following: PCOS and insulin resistance, luteal phase progesterone, sperm DNA, alloimmune disorders such as HLA typing, and infectious agents with endocervical cultures.

If any of these tests reveals an abnormality, it may be corrected with appropriate surgical or medical therapy. If a chromosomal abnormality is found, genetic counseling is indicated. When one of the partners carries a structural genetic abnormality, several options are available to detect genetic abnormality in the offspring including IVF with preimplantation genetic diagnosis (PGD), chorionic villus sampling, or amniocentesis. IVF/PGD allows for the diagnosis of specific translocations and transfer of only unaffected embryos. Two systematic reviews have evaluated the success rates with IVF/PGS compared with natural conception and observation. These reviews reported that the live birth rates with IVF/PGD were approximately 31% to 35% per cycle and cumulative live birth rates were 55% to 74% for natural conception (ASRM, 2012). Scriven and associates performed a large intent-to-treat study evaluating 59 couples with reciprocal translocations who were undergoing PGD using the fluorescence in situ hybridization (FISH) technique. These authors found that couples would need to undergo up to three IVF cycles to achieve a 50% chance of successful live birth (Scriven, 2013). The techniques for PGS/PGD have improved since these studies were published, and therefore the live birth rates with this technology may be higher now. Given the current published evidence, however, routine preimplantation genetic testing is not recommended for couples with recurrent pregnancy loss and a structural genetic abnormality.

Approximately half of women with recurrent miscarriage will not have an identifiable factor to explain their losses. Many clinicians will offer progesterone supplementation in early pregnancy to women with unexplained recurrent miscarriages. Administration of exogenous progesterone is not recommended in women with sporadic miscarriages but may be of some benefit in women with three or more consecutive miscarriages. Regardless of any treatment, however, the majority of these women will have a successful pregnancy next time with no intervention. In fact, approximately 75% of these women will ultimately achieve a successful pregnancy. Many studies have also demonstrated that these women benefit from extensive counseling and emotional support throughout early gestation. Stray-Pedersen and Stray-Pedersen reported that when a group of women with a history of unexplained recurrent abortion were given extensive antenatal counseling and psychological support, the live birth rate was 86% (Stray-Pedersen, 1984). Clifford and associates reported that women with unexplained recurrent miscarriage given supportive care early in pregnancy had a 74% viable birth rate without other therapy. When only routine antenatal care was given to a similar group of women, the live birth rate in these three reports was between 33% and 51%, significantly less (Clifford, 1997). Thus tender loving care (TLC) defined as psychological support with routine medical and ultrasonographic examinations during early pregnancy appears to be very beneficial for improving the prognosis of couples with recurrent abortion whose cause remains undetermined.

If a woman does abort, she should be offered cytogenetic evaluation of the conceptus. Although some view karyotyping as unnecessary and expensive, other experts have reasoned that women who abort aneuploid fetuses should be spared unnecessary and costly evaluation given that the event was likely random and the greater likelihood of success with a subsequent pregnancy. However, there are drawbacks to this approach. A normal 46,XX karyotype can actually be maternal cell contamination of the tissue specimen, particularly when care is not taken to isolate only chorionic villi for cell culture. Additionally, a full evaluation of causes of recurrent pregnancy loss may be overlooked if cytogenetic assessment reveals an aneuploid abortus (ASRM, 2012).

Some authors have proposed preimplantation genetic screening (PGS) for patients with unexplained recurrent pregnancy loss to test for numerical (aneuploidy) abnormalities in order to reduce the risk of miscarriage in these patients. Investigators have argued that the percentage of aneuploidy losses in women with unexplained pregnancy loss may be underestimated given that conventional karyotyping using tissue culture is not definitive and studies on products of conception are not often performed in very early losses. Data derived from several studies have also shown a high rate of aneuploidy in patients with recurrent pregnancy loss, particularly in those over the age of 35. Garrisi and associates published a controlled clinical trial comparing the rate of miscarriage after IVF/PGS in patients with idiopathic pregnancy loss to their own expected loss rate. For patients 35 years or older, the expected loss rate was 34%, but the observed loss rate was 13.6% after IVF/PGS. These authors concluded that PGS improves pregnancy outcome in women with idiopathic recurrent pregnancy loss, particularly those older than 35 years and with two or more previous losses (Garrisi, 2009). Other studies have shown a decrease in miscarriage rate but no clear benefit of PGS in terms of live birth rate compared to natural conception in this patient population. The medical risks and financial burden of IVF/PGS must also be justified before recommending routine use of this intervention. As the technology improves, wider application of IVF with PGS is likely.

However, the possibility of having an explanation is a tool in dealing with the grief of repetitive losses. Couples with unexplained recurrent miscarriage are at even greater risk of anxiety than couples with one loss. It is that anxiety that often pushes them toward "any possible cure." The clinician is all too commonly requested to "try anything." Thus some couples are offered treatment without evidence of a diagnosis or that the treatment provides a higher chance of live birth beyond no intervention. Large studies and a *Cochrane Review* have shown that heparin, heparin and aspirin, intravenous immunoglobulin, and aspirin alone are not, and do not, increase the likelihood of a viable pregnancy. Moreover, further compelling studies are needed for interventions such as IVF with PGS. The "give it everything we've got" approach is not helpful and is potentially dangerous. The skill and art of the practitioner must be used to teach and guide families through this difficult time period with gentleness and good medicine based on the best evidence available.

## KEY POINTS

- About 15% to 20% of all human pregnancies end in a clinically recognized miscarriage, with 80% occurring in the first trimester; the incidence decreases with increasing gestational age.
- If embryonic cardiac activity is seen sonographically at 6 weeks' gestation, then the subsequent abortion rate is about 6% to 8%. If the embryo is viable at 8 weeks, then the subsequent abortion rate is 2% to 3%.
- For a woman with a reproductive history of three pregnancy losses with no live births, her chance of having a miscarriage in a subsequent pregnancy is about 45%; if she has had at least one live birth and three spontaneous abortions, the chance that her next pregnancy will result in a miscarriage is only about 30%.
- The major cause of early pregnancy loss is chromosomal. About 56% of these abnormalities are trisomic, 20% are polyploid, 18% will be chromosome X monosomies, and 4% will represent unbalanced translocations.
- Uterine anomalies can be observed in approximately 12.6% of women with recurrent pregnancy loss. Women with uterine septa have the highest risk of miscarriage.
- Women at risk of cervical insufficiency should be monitored with serial ultrasound examinations from 16 weeks to the end of 24 weeks. If strict criteria are used to diagnose cervical incompetence, fetal survival rates after cerclage have been reported to increase from 20% to 80%.

*Continued*

## KEY POINTS—cont'd

- Untreated overt hypothyroidism and subclinical hypothyroidism as well as hyperprolactinemia and uncontrolled diabetes are all potential causes of miscarriage
- The incidence of antiphospholipid syndrome is between 15% and 20% in women with recurrent pregnancy loss. The treatment is both 81 mg of aspirin daily and prophylactic heparin initiated with a positive pregnancy test.
- The prevalence of major chromosomal abnormalities present in either partner of a couple with two or more pregnancy losses is about 3%, five to six times higher than in the general population. Abnormalities occur in the female parent about twice as frequently as in the male, with balanced reciprocal translocations occurring in half of these individuals.
- Studies that have followed women who had medical, surgical, and expectant management of miscarriage have noted no difference in subsequent pregnancy rates.
- Trending B-hCG levels and serial ultrasound examinations should be used to confirm a failed pregnancy. Care should be taken to avoid a single data point to diagnose an early pregnancy loss.
- Approximately 50% of women with recurrent pregnancy loss will not have an identifiable factor to explain their loss. The majority of these women will ultimately achieve a successful pregnancy without any intervention.

## KEY REFERENCES


Achiron R, Tadmor O, Mashiach S. Heart rate as a predictor of first-trimester spontaneous abortion after ultrasound-proven viability. *Obstet Gynecol.* 1991; 78(3 Pt 1):330-334.

American College of Obstetricians and Gynecologists Women's Health Care Physicians. ACOG Practice Bulletin No. 132: Antiphospholipid syndrome. *Obstet Gynecol.* 2012;120(6):1514-1521.

American College of Obstetricians and Gynecologists Women's Health Care Physicians. ACOG Practice Bulletin No. 138: Inherited thrombophilias in pregnancy. *Obstet Gynecol.* 2013;122(3):706-717.

American College of Obstetricians and Gynecologists Women's Health Care Physicians. ACOG Practice Bulletin No. 150: early pregnancy loss. *Obstet Gynecol.* 2015;125(5):1258-1267.

Armstrong BG, McDonald AD, Sloan M. Cigarette, alcohol, and coffee consumption and spontaneous abortion. *Am J Public Health.* 1992;82(1): 85-87.

Barnhart KT. Early pregnancy failure: beware of the pitfalls of modern management. *Fertil Steril.* 2012;98(5):1061-1065.

Bellingard V, Hedon B, Eliaou JF, Seignalet J, Clot J, Viala JL. Immunogenetic study of couples with recurrent spontaneous abortions. *Eur J Obstet Gynecol Reprod Biol.* 1995;60(1):53-60.

Bider D, Kokia E, Seidman DS, Lipitz S, Mashiach S, Ben-Rafael Z. Cervical cerclage for anomalous uteri. *J Reprod Med.* 1992;37(2):138-140.

Boots CE, Bernardi LA, Stephenson MD. Frequency of euploid miscarriage is increased in obese women with recurrent early pregnancy loss. *Fertil Steril.* 2014;102(2):455-459.

Buttram VC, Reiter RC. Uterine leiomyomata: etiology, symptomatology, and management. *Fertil Steril.* 1981;36(4):433-445.

Clifford K, Rai R, Regan L. Future pregnancy outcome in unexplained recurrent first trimester miscarriage. *Hum Reprod.* 1997;12(2):387-389.

Clifford K, Rai R, Watson H, Franks S, Regan L. Does suppressing luteinising hormone secretion reduce the miscarriage rate? Results of a randomised controlled trial. *BMJ.* 1996;312(7045):1508-1511.

Cnattingius S, Signorello LB, Annerén G, et al. Caffeine intake and the risk of first-trimester spontaneous abortion. *N Engl J Med.* 2000;343(25): 1839-1845.

Connor TH, Lawson CC, Polovich M, McDiarmid MA. Reproductive health risks associated with occupational exposures to antineoplastic drugs in health care settings: a review of the evidence. *J Occup Environ Med Am Coll Occup Environ Med.* 2014;56(9):901-910.

Dizon-Townson D, Miller C, Sibai B, et al. The relationship of the factor V Leiden mutation and pregnancy outcomes for mother and fetus. *Obstet Gynecol.* 2005;106(3):517-524.

Doubilet PM, Benson CB, Bourne T, et al. Diagnostic criteria for nonviable pregnancy early in the first trimester. *N Engl J Med.* 2013;369(150):1443-1451.

Empson M, Lassere M, Craig J, Scott J. Prevention of recurrent miscarriage for women with antiphospholipid antibody or lupus anticoagulant. *Cochrane Database Syst Rev.* 2005;(2). CD002859.

Garrisi JG, Colls P, Ferry KM, Zheng X, Garrisi MG, Munné S. Effect of infertility, maternal age, and number of previous miscarriages on the outcome of preimplantation genetic diagnosis for idiopathic recurrent pregnancy loss. *Fertil Steril.* 2009;92(1):288-295.

Goldstein P, Berrier J, Rosen S, Sacks HS, Chalmers TC. A meta-analysis of randomized control trials of progestational agents in pregnancy. *Br J Obstet Gynaecol.* 1989;96(3):265-274.

Goldstein SR. Sonography in early pregnancy failure. *Clin Obstet Gynecol.* 1994;37(3):681-692.

Grimbizis GF, Camus M, Tarlatzis BC, Bontis JN, Devroey P. Clinical implications of uterine malformations and hysteroscopic treatment results. *Hum Reprod Update.* 2001;7(2):161-174.

Haas DM, Ramsey PS. Progestogen for preventing miscarriage. *Cochrane Database Syst Rev.* 2013;10. CD003511.

Hasan R, Baird DD, Herring AH, Olshan AF, Jonsson Funk ML, Hartmann KE. Association between first-trimester vaginal bleeding and miscarriage. *Obstet Gynecol.* 2009;114(4):860-867.

Hassold T, Hall H, Hunt P. The origin of human aneuploidy: where we have been, where we are going. *Hum Mol Genet.* 2007;16(Spec No. 2):R203-R208.

Hirahara F, Andoh N, Sawai K, Hirabuki T, Uemura T, Minaguchi H. Hyperprolactinemic recurrent miscarriage and results of randomized bromocriptine treatment trials. *Fertil Steril.* 1998;70(2):246-252.

Hooker AB, Lemmers M, Thurkow AL, et al. Systematic review and meta-analysis of intrauterine adhesions after miscarriage: prevalence, risk factors and long-term reproductive outcome. *Hum Reprod Update.* 2014;20(2): 262-278.

Jacobs PA, Hassold T. Chromosome abnormalities: origin and etiology in abortions and livebirths. In: Vogel F, Sperling K, eds. *Human Genetics.* Berlin: Springer-Verlag; 1987:233-244.

Kapranos NC, Kotronias DC. Detection of herpes simplex virus in first trimester pregnancy loss using molecular techniques. *Vivo Athens Greece.* 2009;23(5): 839-842.

Kesmodel U, Wisborg K, Olsen SF, Henriksen TB, Secher NJ. Moderate alcohol intake in pregnancy and the risk of spontaneous abortion. *Alcohol Alcohol.* 2002;37(1):87-92.

Klatsky PC, Tran ND, Caughey AB, Fujimoto VY. Fibroids and reproductive outcomes: a systematic literature review from conception to delivery. *Am J Obstet Gynecol.* 2008;198(4):357-366.

Kleinhaus K, Perrin M, Friedlander Y, Paltiel O, Malaspina D, Harlap S. Paternal age and spontaneous abortion. *Obstet Gynecol.* 2006;108(2):369-377.

Kline J, Shrout P, Stein Z, Susser M, Warburton D. Drinking during pregnancy and spontaneous abortion. *Lancet.* 1980;2(8187):176-180.

Kutteh WH. *Recurrent pregnancy loss, in precis, an update in obstetrics and gynecology*. Washington, DC: American College of Obstetrics and Gynecology; 2007.

Lissalde-Lavigne G, Fabbro-Peray P, Cochery-Nouvellon E, et al. Factor V Leiden and prothrombin G20210A polymorphisms as risk factors for miscarriage during a first intended pregnancy: the matched case-control "NOHA first" study. *J Thromb Haemost JTH*. 2005;3(10):2178-2184.

Luise C, Jermy K, May C, Costello G, Collins WP, Bourne TH. Outcome of expectant management of spontaneous first trimester miscarriage: observational study. *BMJ*. 2002;324(7342):873-875.

Lund M, Kamper-Jørgensen M, Nielsen HS, Lidegaard Ø, Andersen A-MN, Christiansen OB. Prognosis for live birth in women with recurrent miscarriage: what is the best measure of success? *Obstet Gynecol*. 2012;119(1):37-43.

Madsen M, Jørgensen T, Jensen ML, et al. Leisure time physical exercise during pregnancy and the risk of miscarriage: a study within the Danish National Birth Cohort. *BJOG Int J Obstet Gynaecol*. 2007;114(11):1419-1426.

March CM, Israel R. Hysteroscopic management of recurrent abortion caused by septate uterus. *Am J Obstet Gynecol*. 1987;156(4):834-842.

Marchionni M, Fambrini M, Zambelli V, Scarselli G, Susini T. Reproductive performance before and after abdominal myomectomy: a retrospective analysis. *Fertil Steril*. 2004;82(1):154-159. quiz 265.

Miyakis S, Lockshin MD, Atsumi T, et al. International consensus statement on an update of the classification criteria for definite antiphospholipid syndrome (APS). *J Thromb Haemost JTH*. 2006;4(2):295-306.

Negro R, Formoso G, Mangieri T, Pezzarossa A, Dazzi D, Hassan H. Levothyroxine treatment in euthyroid pregnant women with autoimmune thyroid disease: effects on obstetrical complications. *J Clin Endocrinol Metab*. 2006;91(7):2587-2591.

Neilson JP, Gyte GML, Hickey M, Vazquez JC, Dou L. Medical treatments for incomplete miscarriage. *Cochrane Database Syst Rev*. 2013;3:CD007223.

Penta M, Lukic A, Conte MP, et al. Infectious agents in tissues from spontaneous abortions in the first trimester of pregnancy. *New Microbiol*. 2003;26(4):329-337.

Philipp T, Philipp K, Reiner A, Beer F, Kalousek DK. Embryoscopic and cytogenetic analysis of 233 missed abortions: factors involved in the pathogenesis of developmental defects of early failed pregnancies. *Hum Reprod*. 2003;18(8):1724-1732.

Pineles BL, Park E, Samet JM. Systematic review and meta-analysis of miscarriage and maternal exposure to tobacco smoke during pregnancy. *Am J Epidemiol*. 2014;179(7):807-823.

Practice Committee of the American Society for Reproductive Medicine. Evaluation and treatment of recurrent pregnancy loss: a committee opinion. *Fertil Steril*. 2012;98(5):1103-1111.

Rai R, Regan L. Recurrent miscarriage. *Lancet*. 2006;368(9535):601-611.

Scriven PN, Flinter FA, Khalaf Y, Lashwood A, Mackie Ogilvie C. Benefits and drawbacks of preimplantation genetic diagnosis (PGD) for reciprocal translocations: lessons from a prospective cohort study. *Eur J Hum Genet EJHG*. 2013;21(10):1035-1041.

Silver RM, Zhao Y, Spong CY, et al. Prothrombin gene G20210A mutation and obstetric complications. *Obstet Gynecol*. 2010;115(1):14-20.

Sotiriadis A, Makrydimas G, Papatheodorou S, Ioannidis JPA. Expectant, medical, or surgical management of first-trimester miscarriage: a meta-analysis. *Obstet Gynecol*. 2005;105(5 Pt 1):1104-1113.

Stephenson MD, Awartani KA, Robinson WP. Cytogenetic analysis of miscarriages from couples with recurrent miscarriage: a case-control study. *Hum Reprod*. 2002;17(2):446-451.

Stephenson MD, Sierra S. Reproductive outcomes in recurrent pregnancy loss associated with a parental carrier of a structural chromosome rearrangement. *Hum Reprod*. 2006;21(4):1076-1082.

Stray-Pedersen B, Stray-Pedersen S. Etiologic factors and subsequent reproductive performance in 195 couples with a prior history of habitual abortion. *Am J Obstet Gynecol*. 1984;148(2):140-146.

Tang AW, Alfirevic Z, Quenby S. Natural killer cells and pregnancy outcomes in women with recurrent miscarriage and infertility: a systematic review. *Hum Reprod*. 2011;26(8):1971-1980.

Tang T, Lord JM, Norman RJ, Yasmin E, Balen AH. Insulin-sensitising drugs (metformin, rosiglitazone, pioglitazone, D-chiro-inositol) for women with polycystic ovary syndrome, oligo amenorrhoea and subfertility. *Cochrane Database Syst Rev*. 2012;5. CD003053.

Taskin O, Sadik S, Onoglu A, et al. Role of endometrial suppression on the frequency of intrauterine adhesions after resectoscopic surgery. *J Am Assoc Gynecol Laparosc*. 2000;7(3):351-354.

Tursi A, Giorgetti G, Brandimarte G, Elisei W. Effect of gluten-free diet on pregnancy outcome in celiac disease patients with recurrent miscarriages. *Dig Dis Sci*. 2008;53(11):2925-2928.

Wong LF, Porter TF, Scott JR. Immunotherapy for recurrent miscarriage. *Cochrane Database Syst Rev*. 2014;10. CD000112.

Zhang J, Gilles JM, Barnhart K, et al. A comparison of medical management with misoprostol and surgical management for early pregnancy failure. *N Engl J Med*. 2005;353(8):761-769.

Suggested Readings can be found on ExpertConsult.com.

# 17

# Ectopic Pregnancy

## Etiology, Pathology, Diagnosis, Management, Fertility Prognosis

*Rosanne M. Kho, Roger A. Lobo*

**Ectopic pregnancy** occurs when the fertilized ovum/developing blastocyst implants at a site outside of the endometrial cavity. It was probably first described in 963 AD by Albucasis, an Arab writer. In 1876, before the initiation of surgical therapy, the mortality rate from ectopic pregnancy was estimated to be 60%. The first successful operative treatment of ectopic pregnancy was performed in 1883 by Lawson Tait in England. In 1887, he reported that he had performed salpingectomy on four women with ectopic pregnancy and that they all survived.

## EPIDEMIOLOGY

The incidence of ectopic pregnancy has been estimated to be between 1% to 2% of all pregnancies. Although the incidence of ectopic pregnancy increased sixfold between 1970 and 1992, it has remained stable since then. In the United States in 1989, the annual ectopic pregnancy rate per 10,000 women aged 15 to 44 was 15.5, similar to that in Finland, but higher than the rate in France. The last and most recent national data reported by the Centers for Disease Control showed that the overall incidence of ectopic pregnancy had plateaued to approximately 20/1000 pregnancies in the early 1990s. The current incidence of ectopic pregnancy is difficult to estimate from available hospitalization and insurance records because the number of ectopic pregnancy cases requiring inpatient hospital treatment has decreased. The incidence varies among different countries, with rates as high as 1 in 28 and 1 in 40 pregnancies reported in Jamaica and Vietnam, respectively. The risk of ectopic pregnancy associated with assisted reproductive technology is increased compared with the general population with rates from 0.8% to 8.6%. Data from the National ART Surveillance System from 2001-2011 showed that the rate of ectopic pregnancy declined from 2% to 1.6% out of 553,577 pregnancies in the United States (Perkins, 2015).

There has been an increasing trend toward treating ectopic pregnancy conservatively (without resorting to salpingectomy) and on an ambulatory basis without overnight hospitalization. With earlier detection of ectopic pregnancy, a steadily increasing percentage of women with this problem are now being treated before tubal rupture occurs by outpatient laparoscopic procedures or by medical treatment with methotrexate. An analysis of both hospital discharge data and an ambulatory medical care survey revealed that the estimated number of hospitalizations for ectopic pregnancy in the United States declined from nearly 90,000 in 1989 to about 45,000 in 1994. However, in 1992 about half of all women with ectopic pregnancy in the United States were treated as outpatients, and the estimated number of total ectopic pregnancies in this year was 108,000, for a rate of 19.7 per 1000 reported pregnancies. Thus, in the United States in 1992, about 2 of every 100 women who were known to conceive had an ectopic gestation. The increased incidence of ectopic pregnancy is thought to be due to two factors: (1) the increased incidence of salpingitis, caused by increased infection with *Chlamydia trachomatis* or other sexually transmitted pathogens, and (2) improved diagnostic techniques, which enables the diagnosis of unruptured ectopic pregnancy with more precision and earlier in gestation, before asymptomatic resolution of the pregnancy occurs.

There is an increase in the rate of ectopic pregnancy with increasing age. However, because of the lower pregnancy rate in older women, overall only about 11% of ectopic pregnancies in the United States occur in women aged 35 to 44, whereas more than half, 58%, occur in women aged 25 to 34 years. Most ectopic pregnancies occur in multigravid women. Only 10% to 15% of ectopic pregnancies occur in nulligravid women, whereas more than half occur in women who have been pregnant three or more times. In the United States, the rates of ectopic pregnancy are similar in each section of the country, but the rates are higher for nonwhite than white women. About 3% of all reported pregnancies in nonwhite women aged 35 to 44 in the United States were ectopic.

## MORTALITY

Even with the increased use of surgery and blood transfusions and earlier diagnosis, ectopic pregnancy remains a major cause of maternal death in the United States today. From the last Centers for Disease Control and Prevention (CDC) report, 6% of pregnancy-related mortality during the period of 1991-1999 was due to ectopic pregnancies. In the United States, 876 deaths were attributed to ectopic pregnancy between 1980 and 2007. Ectopic pregnancy is the most common cause of maternal death in the first half of pregnancy. The ectopic pregnancy to mortality ratio has declined by 57% from the period 1980-1984 to 2003-2007, from 1.15 to 0.5 (Creanga, 2011). The mortality ratio was 6.8 times higher for African Americans than whites and 3.5 times higher for women older than 35 years compared with women younger than 25 years. Of the 76 deaths among women hospitalized with ectopic pregnancy between 1998 and 2007, 70% of the ectopic pregnancies were located in the fallopian tubes. Unmarried women of all races have a 1.7 times greater chance of dying of ectopic pregnancy than married women. Overall the risk of death from ectopic pregnancy is about 10 times greater than the risk of childbirth and more than 50 times greater than the risk of legal abortion.

The major cause of mortality from ectopic pregnancy is blood loss. Most cases of mortality (70%) result from gestations in the tube, and the other 30% were interstitial cornual or abdominal gestations. Because the overall incidence of ectopic pregnancy occurring in these latter locations is slightly less than 4%, interstitial and abdominal ectopic pregnancies have about a five times greater risk of being fatal. About three fourths of the women with fatal ectopic pregnancies initially developed symptoms and died in the first 12 weeks of gestation. Of the remaining one fourth who developed symptoms and died after the first trimester, 70% had interstitial or abdominal pregnancies. Patient delay in consulting a physician after development of symptoms accounted for one third of the deaths, whereas treatment delay resulting from misdiagnosis contributed to the half of the deaths.

## ETIOLOGY

### FACTORS CONTRIBUTING TO THE RISK

The major factor contributing to the risk of ectopic pregnancy is **salpingitis.** Its morphologic sequelae account for about half of the initial episodes of ectopic pregnancy. However, in about 40% of cases the cause cannot be determined and is presumed to be a physiologic disorder resulting from the delay of passage of the embryo into the uterine cavity. Ovulation from the contralateral ovary has been implicated as a cause of the delay of blastocyst transport, and it has been suggested that contralateral ovulation occurs in about one third of tubal pregnancies, although this has not been confirmed.

Another possibility in the etiology of ectopic pregnancy is a hormonal imbalance; an elevated circulating level of either estrogen or progesterone can alter normal tubal contractility. An increased rate of ectopic pregnancies has been reported in women who conceive with physiologically and pharmacologically elevated levels of progestogens. The latter condition can be produced locally with a progestogen-releasing intrauterine device (IUD), as well as systemically with progestin-only oral contraceptives. Iatrogenic, physiologically increased levels of estrogen and progesterone occur after ovulation induction and assisted reproduction techniques (ART) with either clomiphene citrate or human menopausal gonadotropins, and an increased rate of ectopic pregnancies has been reported in women conceiving after each of these treatment modalities.

Another possible cause is an abnormality of embryonic development. Although aneuploidy has been found to be prevalent in ectopic pregnancies, it may not be higher than the normal rate of aneuploidy and is unlikely to be a cause of ectopic pregnancies. Inherited genetic abnormalities are most probably not a cause of ectopic pregnancy either. Also, there is no increased incidence of ectopics among first-degree relatives.

Several epidemiologic studies indicate that cigarette smoking is associated with about a twofold increased risk of ectopic pregnancy, even when the data were controlled for the presence of other risk factors. The risk of ectopic pregnancy was directly related to the number of cigarettes smoked per day, with a fourfold increased risk noted among women who smoked 30 or more cigarettes per day. Known risk factors for ectopic pregnancy, presented as odds ratios and attributable risk, are depicted in Table 17.1 (Bouyer, 2003).

The major causes of ectopic pregnancy will be discussed in more detail next.

### TUBAL PATHOLOGY LEADING TO ECTOPIC RISK

Disruption of normal tubal anatomy from infection, surgery, congenital anomalies, or inflammatory disease such as endometriosis is a major cause of ectopic pregnancy. The agglutination of the plicae (folds) of the endosalpinx produced by salpingitis can allow passage of sperm but prevent the normal transport of the larger morula. The morula can be trapped in blind pockets formed by adhesions of the endosalpinx. In their 20-year longitudinal study, Weström and colleagues found that nearly half (45.3%) of the women with ectopic pregnancy had a clinical history or histologic findings of a prior episode of acute salpingitis (Weström, 1981). This is in agreement with the 40% incidence

**Table 17.1** Odds Ratios for Ectopic Pregnancy (Compared with Women with Recent Successful Pregnancies) and the Attributable Risks Associated with Different Risk Factors

| | Odds Ratio | Attributable Risk* |
|---|---|---|
| Probable salpingitis | 2 | |
| Confirmed salpingitis | 3.5 | |
| History of tubal surgery | 3.5 | 0.18† |
| Smoking | | 0.35 |
| Ex-smoker | 1.5 | |
| 1-9 cigarettes per day | 2 | |
| 10-19 cigarettes per day | 3 | |
| ≥20 cigarettes per day | 4 | |
| Age (years) | | 0.14 |
| 30-39 | 1.5 | |
| ≥40 | 3 | |
| Spontaneous abortion | 3 | 0.07 |
| Elective abortion | 2 | 0.03 |
| IUD history | 1.5 | 0.05 |
| Previous infertility | 2.5 | 0.18 |

From Fernandez H, Gervaise A. Ectopic pregnancies after infertility treatment: modern diagnosis and therapeutic strategy. *Hum Reprod Update.* 2004;10(6): 503-513.

Odds ratios for ectopic pregnancy (compared with deliveries) and attributable risks of the principal risk factors. *IUD*, Intrauterine device.

*From Auvergne registry data (Bouyer J, Coste J, Shojaei T, et al. Risk factors for ectopic pregnancy: a comprehensive analysis based on a large case-control, population-based study in France. *Am J Epidemiol.* 2003;157:185).

†Risk attributable to history of genital infection and tubal surgery together is 0.33.

of prior salpingitis found on histology by several groups of investigators in women with ectopic pregnancy (Fig. 17.1).

Weström and colleagues prospectively followed 900 women aged 15 to 34 years who had laparoscopically confirmed acute salpingitis and found that the subsequent ectopic pregnancy rate was 68.8 per 1000 conceptions, yielding a sixfold increase in the risk of ectopic pregnancy. The risk of ectopic after acute salpingitis increased both with the number of episodes of infection and with the increasing age of the women at the time of infection. The odds ratios for ectopic pregnancy after two and after three or more episodes of chlamydial infection were 2.1 and 4.5, respectively. Data also suggest that a history of chlamydial infection results in the production of PROKR2 protein that results in a microenvironment that predisposes to tubal implantation (Shaw, 2011).

### Endometriosis

Inflammation of the fallopian tubes due to conditions such as endometriosis is a risk factor for ectopic pregnancy. Compared with women without endometriosis, women with endometriosis had two times the risk for ectopic pregnancy (relative risk 1.9, 95% confidence interval 1.8 to 2.1) (Hjordt Hansen, 2014).

### Salpingitis Isthmica Nodosa

Salpingitis isthmica nodosa (SIN) is defined as the microscopic presence of tubal epithelium within the myosalpinx or beneath the tubal serosa (Fig. 17.2). In two histopathologic studies of tubes removed from women with ectopic pregnancy, it was found that about half contained lesions of SIN compared with 5% in a control group. With serial sectioning, it has been determined that SIN is actually a diverticulum or intrauterine extension of the tubal lumen. Associated histologic evidence of chronic salpingitis was seen in only 6% of the tubes, suggesting that SIN was not necessarily the result of infection. It has been found that the **tubal pregnancy** usually implanted in a portion of the tube distal to the SIN, indicating that mechanical entrapment of the morula is not the mechanism whereby SIN causes tubal gestation. It may be that it is SIN itself or associated tubal anomalies that may be responsible for dysfunction of the tubal transport mechanism without anatomic obstruction.

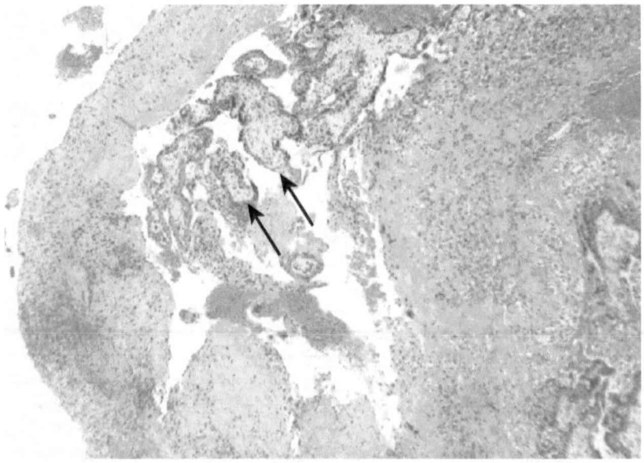

**Figure 17.1** Histology of ectopic pregnancy. Note the trophoblastic tissue *(arrows)* in the fallopian tube lumen. (Modified from www.imaging pathways.health.wa.gov.au.)

It is likely that adhesions between the tubal serosa and bowel or peritoneum may interfere with normal tubal motility and cause ectopic pregnancy because, as reported, 17% to 27% of women with ectopic pregnancy have had previous abdominal surgical procedures not involving the oviduct. On the other hand, neither endometriosis nor congenital anomalies of the tube have been associated with an increased incidence of ectopic pregnancy.

### Tubal Surgery

An operative procedure on the tube itself is a cause of ectopic pregnancy whether the tube is morphologically normal, as occurs with sterilization procedures, or abnormal, as occurs with post salpingitis reconstructive surgery. The incidence of ectopic pregnancy occurring after salpingoplasty or **salpingostomy** procedures to treat distal tubal disease ranges from 15% to 25%, probably because the damage to the endosalpinx remains. The rate of ectopic pregnancy after reversal of sterilization procedures is lower, about 4%, because the tubes have not been damaged by infection.

Women who have had a prior ectopic pregnancy, even if treated medically or by unilateral salpingectomy, are at increased risk for having a subsequent ectopic pregnancy. Of women who conceive after having one ectopic pregnancy, about 25% of subsequent pregnancies are ectopic. The rates of recurrent ectopic pregnancy after single dose methotrexate, salpingectomy and linear salpingostomy are 8%, 9.8%, and 15.4%, respectively, among women who conceive (Yao, 1997). In two large series of women with ectopic pregnancy, 7% had a history of a prior ectopic pregnancy.

### Diethylstilbestrol Exposure

Although it is less frequently encountered today, the incidence of ectopic gestation is significantly greater (four to five times) in women who have been exposed to diethylstilbestrol (DES) in utero and has been reported at the rate of 4% to 5%. This is likely due to abnormal tubal morphology and impaired function of the fimbriae. In women exposed to DES whose hysterosalpingograms demonstrated abnormalities in the uterine cavity, the ectopic pregnancy rate was as high as 13%.

## CONTRACEPTION FAILURE

For several decades, sterilization has been the most popular method of contraception used by couples in the United States.

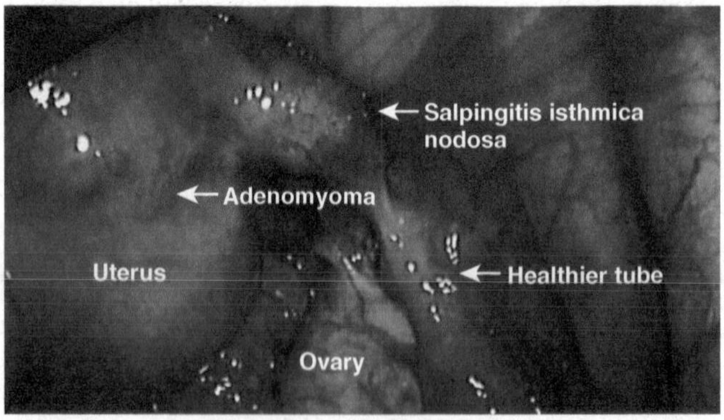


**Figure 17.2** Laparoscopic view of salpingitis isthmica nodosa in the isthmic tube and cornual regions of the uterus. Note the normal distal tube. (From www.dan martinmd.com.)

Since the development of laparoscopic surgery, female tubal sterilization is performed about twice as frequently as vasectomy. In an analysis of the long-term risk of pregnancy after tubal sterilization reported by Peterson and coworkers, it was found that within 10 years after the procedure, the cumulative life table probability of pregnancy was 1.85%. The 10-year failure rate after bipolar coagulation of the oviducts was 2.48%, which rose to 5.43% if the sterilization procedure was performed when the woman was younger than 28 years of age. These investigators reported that for all 143 pregnancies occurring after tubal sterilization, 43, or 32.9%, were ectopic pregnancies (Peterson, 1997).

Several investigators have reported that if pregnancy occurred after tubal sterilization by laparoscopic fulguration, the ectopic pregnancy rate was as high as 50%. It has been hypothesized that with the extensive tissue destruction caused by electrocoagulation, an uteroperitoneal fistula develops that allows sperm to pass into the distal segment of the oviduct and fertilize the egg (Fig. 17.3) (Corson, 1986). Such fistulas can be demonstrated radiographically in about 11% of women after laparoscopic electrocoagulation. Peterson and colleagues reported that within 10 years after the sterilization procedure, twice as many women sterilized by bipolar coagulation had ectopic pregnancies than those sterilized with metal clips or silicone bands. The overall ectopic pregnancy rate after bipolar coagulation sterilization was 1.7%.

Because about one third of pregnancies that occur after all tubal sterilizations are ectopic, women should be counseled that if they do not experience the expected menses at any time following tubal sterilization before menopause, a test to detect human chorionic gonadotropin (HCG) should be performed rapidly, and if they are pregnant, a diagnostic evaluation to exclude the presence of ectopic pregnancy is necessary. In women who have an ectopic pregnancy after sterilization with the use of electrosurgery, because the site of the fistula usually cannot be determined clinically, salpingectomies should be carried out.

Although women who become pregnant while using diaphragms or combination oral contraceptives do not have an increased chance of having an ectopic pregnancy and reliable contraception decreases the risk of all pregnancies, including ectopics, women who become pregnant while using a Copper T380 IUD or progestin-only oral contraceptives have about a 5% chance of having an ectopic pregnancy. The incidence of ectopic pregnancy in women who become pregnant with the progestogen-releasing IUDs is even higher, about 23%. The progestogen-releasing IUD inhibits tubal contractions and has a higher failure rate than the copper IUD. Women who use this method of contraception have about twice the risk of ectopic pregnancy (7.5 per 1000 woman-years) than women who use no method of contraception (3.5 per 1000 woman-years). Women using IUDs who elect to have their pregnancies terminated should have a histologic examination of the tissue removed from the uterine cavity to be certain the pregnancy was intrauterine.

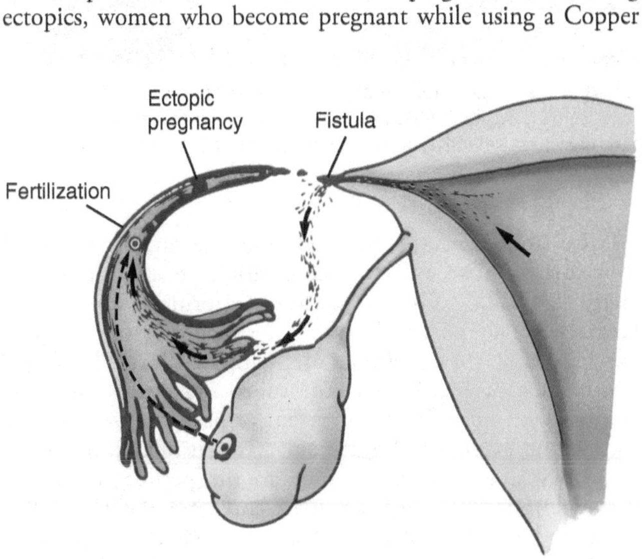


**Figure 17.3** Mechanism of ectopic pregnancy after sterilization. (From Corson SL, Batzer FR. Ectopic pregnancy: a review of the etiologic factors. *J Reprod Med.* 1986;31:78.)

## HORMONAL ALTERATIONS

As occurs with exogenous progesterone administration, if increased levels of exogenous or endogenous estrogens are present shortly after the time of ovulation, the incidence of ectopic pregnancy is increased. Several investigators have reported that the ectopic pregnancy rate is about 1.5% for conceptions that occur after ovulation has been induced with clomiphene citrate. The ectopic rate in pregnancies occurring after ovulation with human menopausal gonadotropins (HMG) has been reported to range between 3% and 4%. Fernandez and colleagues, in a case-control study, found the risk of ectopic pregnancy was increased about fourfold among ovulatory women treated with controlled ovarian hyperstimulation—clomiphene citrate, HMG, or a combination of both—for unexplained infertility (Fernandez, 1991). These reports indicate that increased levels of estrogen, as well as of progesterone, interfere with tubal motility and increase the chance of ectopic pregnancy. Ectopics occur in about 1% of pregnancies that develop after in vitro fertilization and embryo transfer. The reason for this increased incidence is likely due to one or more of several factors: increased sex steroid hormone levels, the presence of proximal tubal disease (although the ratio is similar in women with normal tubes), and flushing an embryo directly into the tube.

In vitro fertilization has been associated with an increased risk of ectopic pregnancy. Data from the National ART Surveillance system identified that 1.7% out of more than 550,000 pregnancies were ectopic between the period of 2001 and 2011. The ectopic pregnancy rate was also noted to be associated with multiple embryo transfer. The rate of ectopic pregnancy was 1.6% when one embryo was transferred compared with 1.7%, 2.2%, and 2.5% when two, three, or four or more embryos were transferred, respectively (Perkins, 2015).

## PREVIOUS ABORTION

Although some studies have suggested that a prior induced abortion increases the risk of ectopic pregnancy, there is probably no major association of increased risk.

# SITES OF ECTOPIC PREGNANCY

Most ectopic pregnancies occur in the tube. In Breen's and more recent series, (Breen, 1970; Bouyer, 2002), 97.7% of the ectopic pregnancies were tubal, 1.4% were abdominal, and less than 1% were ovarian or cervical (Fig. 17.4). The majority of tubal

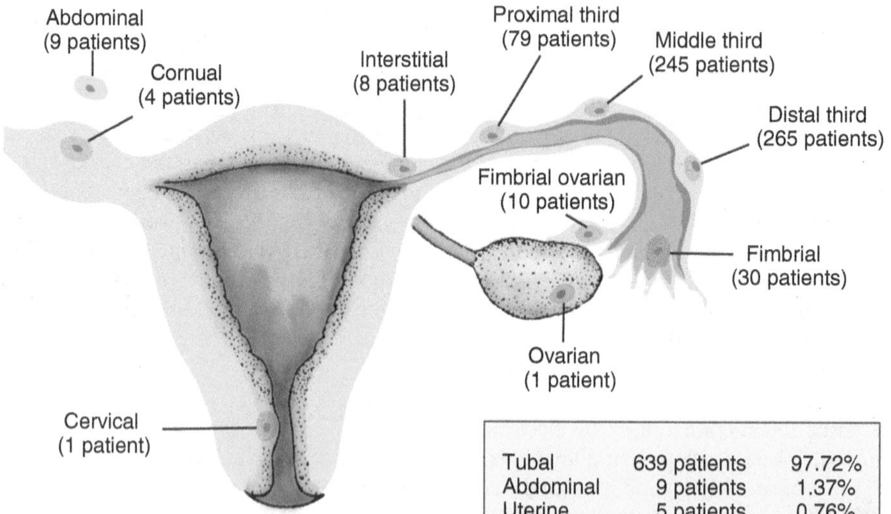


| | | |
|---|---|---|
| Tubal | 639 patients | 97.72% |
| Abdominal | 9 patients | 1.37% |
| Uterine | 5 patients | 0.76% |
| Ovarian | 1 patient | 0.15% |
| Total | 654 patients | 100.00% |

**Figure 17.4** Anatomic site of ectopic pregnancy. (From Breen JL. A 21 year survey of 654 ectopic pregnancies. *Am J Obstet Gynecol.* 1970;106:1004.)

pregnancies, 70% to 81%, were located in the ampullary portion of the tube, being about equally divided between the distal and middle third of the tube. About 12% of tubal gestations occur in the isthmus and 5% to 11% in the fimbrial region. Although Breen considered pregnancies located in the cornual area of the uterus to be uterine in origin, they are in fact pregnancies implanted in the interstitial portion of the tube. About 2% of all ectopic pregnancies are interstitial and are frequently associated with severe morbidity, because they become symptomatic later in the gestation, are difficult to diagnose, and frequently produce massive hemorrhage when they rupture (Fig. 17.5) (Bolaji, 2010). A true **cornual pregnancy** is one located in the rudimentary horn of a bicornuate uterus, and this occurrence is quite rare. In a review of 240 true cornual pregnancies reported by O'Leary and O'Leary, about 90% of them ruptured with massive hemorrhage (O'Leary, 1963).

About 1 in 200 ectopic pregnancies are true ovarian pregnancies that fulfill the four criteria originally described by Spiegelburg:

1. The tube and fimbria must be intact and separate from the ovary.
2. The gestational sac must occupy the normal position of the ovary.
3. The sac must be connected to the uterus by the ovarian ligament.
4. Ovarian tissue should be demonstrable in the walls of the sac.

Many women with ovarian pregnancies are believed to have a ruptured corpus luteum cyst, and the correct diagnosis was made during the surgical procedure only 28% of the time. The hemorrhagic mass (ovarian ectopic) should be located adjacent to the corpus luteum, never within it. **Ovarian pregnancy** is also associated with profuse hemorrhage, with 81% of reported to have a **hemoperitoneum** greater than 500 mL. Nevertheless, most can be successfully treated by ovarian resection and not oophorectomy.

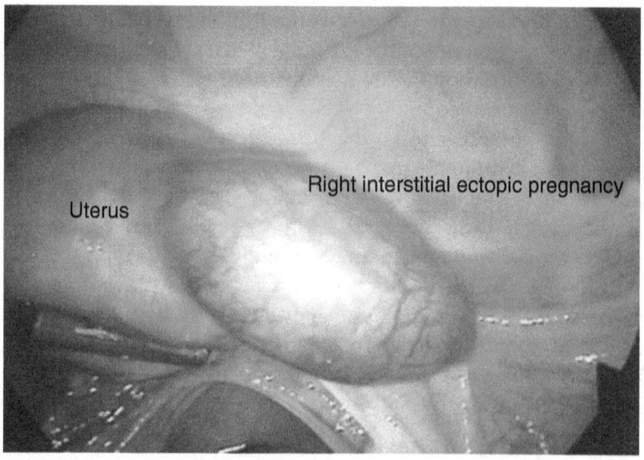


**Figure 17.5** Right interstitial pregnancy at laparoscopy. (Modified from Bolaji I, Gupta S. Medical management of interstitial pregnancy with high beta selective human chorionic gonadotropin. *Ultrasound.* 2010;18[2]:60-67.)

Most abdominal pregnancies occur secondary to **tubal abortion** with secondary implantation in the peritoneal cavity (Fig. 17.6). On rare occasions a primary **abdominal pregnancy** may occur. For the latter diagnosis to be made, the following three criteria originally set forth by Studdiford must be present: (1) the tubes and ovaries must be normal, with no evidence of recent or past injury; (2) there must be no evidence of a uteroplacental fistula; and (3) the pregnancy must be related only to the peritoneal surface and early enough in gestation to eliminate the possibility of secondary implantation after primary tubal nidation (Studdiford, 1942). An unusual type of primary abdominal pregnancy may implant in the spleen or liver and produce massive intraperitoneal hemorrhage.

The prognosis for fetal survival in abdominal pregnancy is poor, found to be 11%, and is difficult to diagnose. Once the diagnosis is established, a laparotomy with removal of the fetus should be performed immediately to prevent a possible fatal hemorrhage. An adjunctive option is to administer methotrexate. On occasion, when the placenta is tightly adherent to bowel and blood vessels, it should be left in the abdominal cavity. In such instances, the placental tissue usually resorbs. However, there may be symptoms of abdominal pain and intermittent fever for many months as well as possible partial bowel obstruction and abscess formation. Thus, it is highly desirable, if it is surgically feasible, to remove the placenta entirely. Partial removal also may result in massive hemorrhage, so the surgical approach and decision making are challenging and critical.

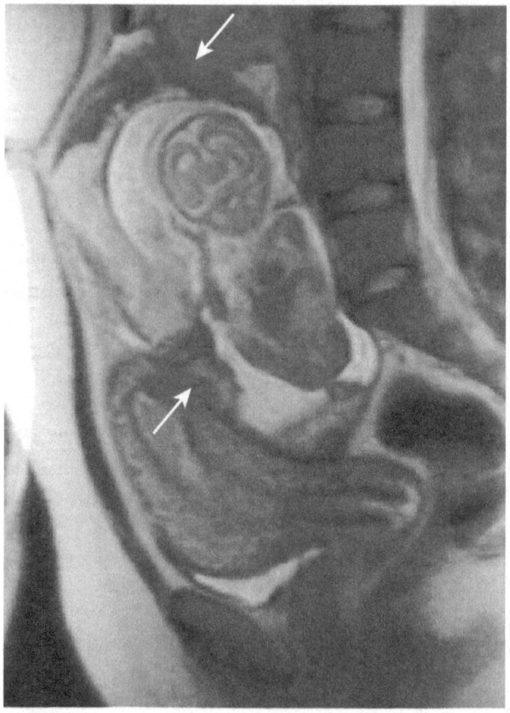

**Figure 17.6** MRI of abdominal pregnancy showing placental infarction. Note the distance of the pregnancy from the uterus. (From www.Hmer.ch/selected.)

The four pathologic criteria for the diagnosis of **cervical pregnancy** as reported by Rubin and colleagues are (1) cervical glands must be present opposite the placental attachment, (2) the attachment of the placenta to the cervix must be intimate, (3) the placenta must be below the entrance of the uterine vessels or below the peritoneal reflection of the anteroposterior surface of the uterus, and (4) fetal elements must not be present in the corpus uteri (Fig. 17.7).

The usual characteristic clinical findings of cervical pregnancy are uterine bleeding after amenorrhea without cramping pain, a softened cervix that is disproportionately enlarged, complete confinement and firm attachment of the products of conception to the endocervix, and a closed internal os.

Most cervical pregnancies are associated with previous cervical or uterine surgery such as curettage or cesarean delivery. The differential diagnosis is difficult and includes incomplete abortion, placenta previa, carcinoma of the cervix, and a degenerating leiomyoma. Although cervical ectopics previously have been associated with a high mortality because of massive hemorrhage, currently, with better methods of diagnosis and treatment, death is rare. In the past, more than half of the women with cervical pregnancy required a hysterectomy for treatment, and this was nearly always necessary if the pregnancy had advanced beyond 18 weeks. There have been several case reports in which a cervical pregnancy was successfully treated by systemic methotrexate. Other case reports have shown that after angiographic uterine artery embolization evacuation of the pregnancy can be easily

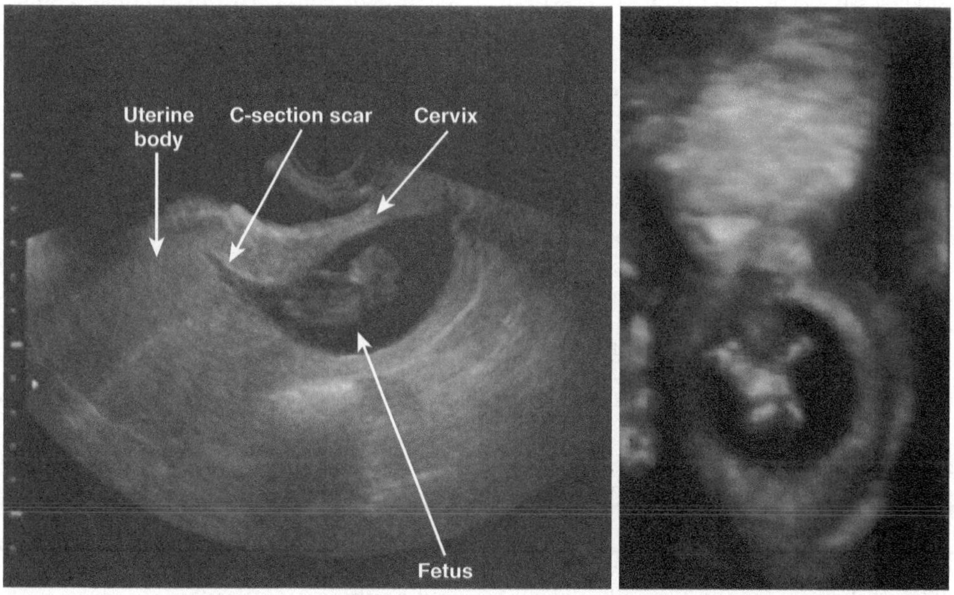


**Figure 17.7** Cervical pregnancy as viewed by 2D ultrasound *(left panel)*. Note the normal endometrium to the left of the gestational sac and the larger fetal pole. The right panel shows the same cervical ectopic on 3D ultrasound. Note the ballooned-out cervix and narrowed uterine isthmus/lower segment above it.

performed transcervically with minimal blood loss. Transvaginal ultrasound-guided injections of potassium chloride directly into the gestational sac have successfully terminated the pregnancies, as has the local injection of methotrexate, with or without uterine artery embolization.

Another uncommon form of ectopic gestation is combined intrauterine and extrauterine (heterotopic) pregnancy (94% tubal and 6% ovarian). **Heterotopic pregnancy** is traditionally considered a rare occurrence with an incidence between 1 in 16,000 or 1 in 30,000 pregnancies. With the increase of use of ovulation-inducing agents and assisted reproduction techniques (ART), the overall incidence of heterotopic pregnancy has risen to approximately 1 in 3900 pregnancies. In a series of all registered ART pregnancies in the United States from 1999 to 2002, the incidence of heterotopic pregnancy was 1.5 per 1000 ART pregnancies.[16] The incidence has been reported to be higher when tubal damage was present or four or more embryos were transferred.

A **chronic ectopic pregnancy** occurs when the intraperitoneal hemorrhage associated with tubal abortion or rupture is relatively minor and ceases spontaneously, but the ectopic gestation neither resolves completely nor implants and continues to develop as an abdominal pregnancy. The trophoblast continues to secrete HCG in small amounts, with the circulating levels less than 1000 mIU/mL in 50% of cases and less than 100 mIU/mL in 20% of cases. In one series, about 6% of all surgically treated ectopic pregnancies in one institution were classified as chronic. The most common (72%) gross pathologic finding was dense adhesions produced by the inflammatory response to the trophoblast. These adhesions attach omentum and bowel to the site of the ectopic pregnancy. In one third of the cases, a collection of clotted blood or old hematoma was present. It has been reported that because of the extensive disease, it was necessary to perform a hysterectomy in 25% of cases and an oophorectomy in 60% of women with a chronic ovarian ectopic pregnancy.

**Cesarean scar ectopic pregnancy** is a rare but potentially serious complication of early pregnancy. In this type of ectopic pregnancy, the gestational sac is located in the previous cesarean scar and is surrounded by myometrium and connective tissue. It occurs in about 1 in 2000 pregnancies and 6% of ectopic pregnancies among women with previous caesarean deliveries (Rotas, 2006). In a large series of 268 cesarean scar ectopic pregnancies, Sadeghi and colleagues reported four cases of uterine rupture including one case of fetomaternal death at 38 weeks of gestation (Sadeghi, 2010). The incidence does not appear to correlate with the number of cesarean deliveries. It is believed that the mechanism for implantation is due to the migration of the embryo through a small defect in the previous incision site or a microscopic fistula within the scar. Adenomyosis, in vitro fertilization, previous dilation and curettage, and manual removal of the placenta are also reported as risk factors.

## HISTOPATHOLOGY

When the morula implants in the tube, it does not grow mainly in the tubal lumen as has been assumed for many years. A review of the pathology of tubal gestation found that after implanting on the mucosa of the endosalpinx, the trophoblast invaded the lamina propria and then the muscularis of the tube and grew mainly between the lumen of the tube and its peritoneal covering. Growth occurred both parallel to the long axis of the tube and circumferentially around it. As the trophoblast invaded vessels, retroperitoneal tubal hemorrhage occurred that is mainly extraluminal but may extrude from the fimbriated end and create a hemoperitoneum before tubal rupture (Fig. 17.8) (Budowick, 1980).

The stretching of the peritoneum covered by this hemorrhage results in episodic pain before the final perforation into the peritoneal cavity. Rupture occurs when the serosa is maximally stretched, producing necrosis secondary to an inadequate blood supply.

Hemoperitoneum is nearly always found in advanced **ruptured ectopic pregnancy** other than that which is cervical in origin. Usually there is a combination of clotted and unclotted blood in the peritoneal cavity. The unclotted blood does not clot on removal from the peritoneal cavity because it originates from lysis of blood that has previously coagulated, similar to what occurs during menstrual bleeding. The hematocrit value of this nonclotting blood is nearly always greater than 15%, such a finding being reported in 98% of specimens obtained by **culdocentesis** in a series of ectopic pregnancies. Historically, at the time of laparotomy for a ruptured ectopic pregnancy, about half of the women have less than 500 mL of hemoperitoneum, one fourth between 500 and 1000 mL, and one fifth more than 1000 mL.

When the tube is removed and examined histologically, inflammatory cells are nearly always seen. These include plasma cells, lymphocytes, and histiocytes. The presence of chorionic villi, which are frequently degenerated or hyalinized, as well as nucleated red cells established the diagnosis of ectopic pregnancy. Decidual reaction in the tube is uncommon.

Because of limited space or inadequate nourishment, the trophoblastic tissue of most ectopic pregnancies does not grow as rapidly as that of pregnancies within the uterine cavity. As a result, HCG production does not increase as rapidly as in a normal pregnancy, and although steroid production of the corpus luteum is initiated, elevated progesterone levels cannot be maintained. Thus initially the endometrium becomes decidualized because of continued progesterone production by the corpus luteum. Sometimes the secretory cells of the endometrial glands become hypertrophied with hyperchromatism, pleomorphism,

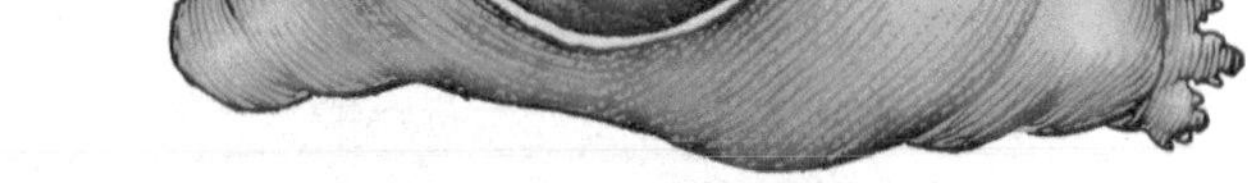

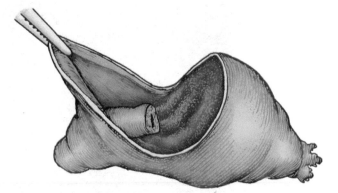

**Figure 17.8** Artist's rendition of dissected ampullary ectopic pregnancy showing space between tube and peritoneum, revealed when blood clots and placenta were removed. Toward fimbriated end, no dissection was performed and external appearance is that of a dilated tube. (From Budowick M, Johnson TRB, Genadry R, et al. The histopathology of the developing tubal ectopic pregnancy. *Fertil Steril.* 1980;34:169. Courtesy of The American Fertility Society.)

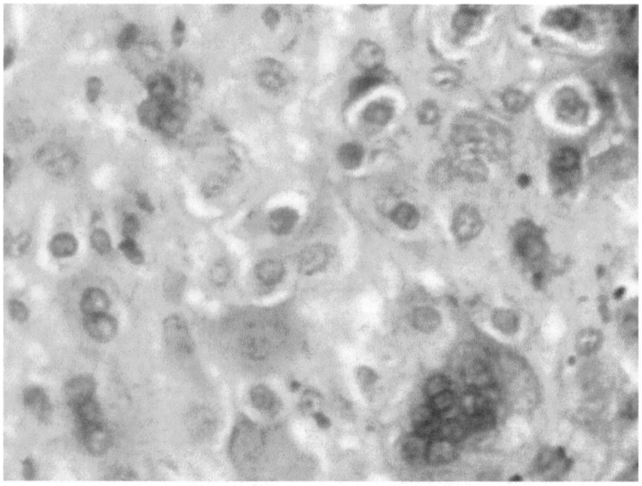

**Figure 17.9** Histology of In text, Arias-Stella reaction. Note the enlarged secretory endometrial cells, which are hypertrophied, hyperchromatic, and pleomorphic. (From www.jpathology.com.)

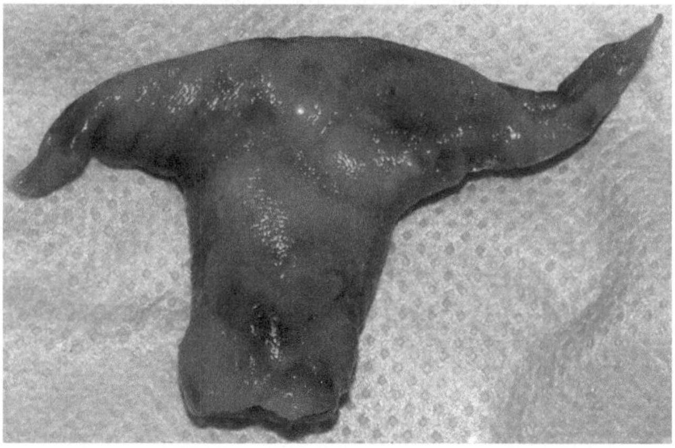

**Figure 17.10** Decidual cast. (From www.ispub.com.)

and increased mitotic activity, as originally described by Arias-Stella (Fig. 17.9). The **Arias-Stella reaction** can be confused with neoplasia, but it is not unique for ectopic pregnancy, because it can occur with an IUP as well as after ovarian stimulation with clomiphene citrate. In a histologic study of the endometrium in 84 women with ectopic pregnancies, 40% of cases had secretory endometrium, with the remainder being about equally divided among the findings of proliferative endometrium, decidual reaction, and an Arias-Stella reaction. When progesterone levels fall as a result of insufficient HCG, endometrial integrity is no longer maintained and it breaks down, producing uterine bleeding. Sometimes nearly all the decidua is passed through the cervix in an intact way, producing a **decidual cast** that may be clinically confused with a spontaneous abortion (Fig. 17.10).

## SYMPTOMS

Among women with risk factors for ectopic pregnancy, with the use of early hormonal testing and vaginal sonography, it is now frequently possible to establish the diagnosis of ectopic pregnancy before symptoms develop. However, symptoms often develop when intraperitoneal bleeding occurs from extrusion of blood through the fimbriated end of the tube in cases of tubal pregnancies or from disruption of overlying tubal, ovarian, or myometrial tissue from rupture of the gestational sac.

The most common symptoms of ectopic pregnancy are abdominal pain, absence of menses, and irregular vaginal bleeding (Table 17.2). Abdominal pain is nearly a universal symptom of intraperitoneal bleeding, but its characteristics are similar with different causes of bleeding. Before rupture occurs, the pain may be characterized as only a vague soreness or be colicky in nature. Its location may be generalized, unilateral, or bilateral. Shoulder pain occurs in about one fourth of women with ruptured ectopic pregnancy as a result of diaphragmatic irritation from the hemoperitoneum. During rupture of the tube, the pain usually becomes intense. Syncope occurs in about one third of women

**Table 17.2** Contraindications to Medical Management of Ectopic Pregnancy with Systemic Methotrexate

| Contraindication | ACOG | ASRM |
|---|---|---|
| Absolute contraindications | Breast-feeding; laboratory evidence of immunodeficiency; preexisting blood dyscrasias (bone marrow hypoplasia, leukopenia, thrombocytopenia, or clinically significant anemia); known sensitivity to methotrexate; active pulmonary disease; peptic ulcer disease; hepatic, renal, or hematologic dysfunction; alcoholism; alcoholic or other chronic liver disease | Breast-feeding: evidence of immunodeficiency; moderate-to-severe anemia, leukopenia, or thrombocytopenia; sensitivity to methotrexate; active pulmonary or peptic ulcer disease; clinically important hepatic or renal dysfunction; intrauterine pregnancy |
| Relative contraindications | Ectopic mass >3.5 cm; embryonic cardiac motion | Ectopic mass >4 cm detected by transvaginal ultrasonography; embryonic cardiac activity detected by transvaginal ultrasonography; patient declines blood transfusion; patient is not able to participate in follow-up; high initial HCG level (>5000 mIU/mL) |
| Choice of regimen based on HCG level | Multidose regimen of methotrexate may be appropriate if presenting HCG value >5000 mIU/mL | Single-dose regimen of methotrexate better in patients with a low initial HCG level |

Data from American Society for Reproductive Medicine. The Practice Committee: medical treatment of ectopic pregnancy. *Fertil Steril*. 2008;90:S206.
*ACOG*, American College of Obstetricians and Gynecologists; *ASRM*, American Society for Reproductive Medicine.

with tubal rupture. Other symptoms that occur following tubal rupture include dizziness and an urge to defecate.

The majority of women with ectopic pregnancy fail to have menses at the expected time but have one or more episodes of irregular vaginal bleeding when the decidual endometrial tissue is sloughed. The interval of amenorrhea is usually 6 weeks or more. The bleeding is usually characterized as spotting but may simulate menstrual bleeding. It is rarely as heavy as that which occurs in spontaneous abortion. About 5% to 10% of women with an advanced ectopic pregnancy will note passage of a decidual cast, as noted previously (see Fig. 17.10).

## SIGNS

The most common presenting sign in a woman with symptomatic ectopic pregnancy is abdominal tenderness, which, together with adnexal tenderness elicited at the time of the bimanual pelvic examination, is present in nearly all women with an advanced or ruptured ectopic pregnancy. It is possible to palpate an adnexal mass in half of the women, and about one third have some degree of uterine enlargement that is nearly always smaller than a normal 8-week intrauterine gestation except when an interstitial gestation is present. Tachycardia and hypotension can occur after rupture if blood loss is profuse, but temperature elevation is an uncommon finding, present in only about 5% to 10% of women with tubal rupture, and is rarely greater than 38° C.

### *DIFFERENTIAL DIAGNOSIS OF SYMPTOMATIC ECTOPIC PREGNANCY*

The diagnosis is usually obvious for women with the classic symptoms of ruptured ectopic pregnancy: a history of irregular bleeding followed by sudden onset of pain and syncope accompanied by signs of peritoneal irritation. However, before rupture the symptoms and signs are nonspecific and may also occur with other gynecologic disorders. Entities frequently confused with ectopic pregnancy include salpingitis, threatened or incomplete abortion, ruptured corpus luteum, appendicitis, dysfunctional uterine bleeding, adnexal torsion, degenerative uterine leiomyoma, and endometriosis.

In the past, studies have found that women with an ectopic pregnancy were seen multiple times before a correct diagnosis was made. Because of the possibility of a fatal outcome from undiagnosed ruptured ectopic pregnancy, it is essential that the diagnosis of ectopic pregnancy be considered in any woman of childbearing age with abdominal pain and irregular uterine bleeding even if she has had a previous tubal sterilization procedure or is using an effective method of reversible contraception.

Ectopic pregnancy should be suspected in any woman who develops the symptoms listed earlier, particularly if she has previously had a pelvic operation, especially tubal surgery, either a tubal reconstructive procedure or a sterilization procedure. Other risk factors include one or more episodes of salpingitis, a previous ectopic gestation, current use of a progesterone-releasing IUD, use of a progestin-only oral contraceptive, use of pharmacologic methods of ovulation induction, or a history of infertility. In any woman with the symptoms of ectopic gestation, the diagnosis is facilitated by a quantitative assay for HCG and pelvic ultrasonography and can be established and treated by laparoscopy or laparotomy. Culdocentesis and measurement of serum progesterone levels have also been used for diagnostic assistance. Prior to the development of pelvic vaginal ultrasound, the finding of nonclotting blood at the time of culdocentesis, especially if the hematocrit was above 15%, was of great assistance in establishing the diagnosis of ruptured ectopic pregnancy. With the use of high-resolution pelvic ultrasound, the presence of intraperitoneal fluid can be easily visualized and culdocentesis is no longer routinely done.

### *PROCEDURES USED FOR THE DIAGNOSTIC EVALUATION OF THE ASYMPTOMATIC OR MILDLY SYMPTOMATIC WOMAN WITH SUSPECTED ECTOPIC PREGNANCY*

#### *Human Chorionic Gonadotropin*

About 85% of women with ectopic pregnancy have serum HCG levels lower than those seen in normal pregnancy at a similar gestational age. However, a single quantitative HCG assay cannot be used to diagnose ectopic pregnancy because the actual dates of ovulation and conception are often not known. Even if the date of ovulation is known, 2.5% of women with normal gestations will have HCG levels lower than the normal 95% confidence limits. Furthermore, low HCG levels are also found in women with various stages of spontaneous abortion, conditions that must be considered in the differential diagnosis. Intact HCG and free β-HCG levels were measured in a large group of women in early pregnancy who presented with symptoms of ectopic pregnancy. Although mean levels of intact HCG and free β-HCG were significantly lower in the group of women with ectopic pregnancy and those who aborted than in those with viable intrauterine pregnancies, the individual HCG levels among the three conditions overlapped too much to devise a cutoff level for diagnostic purposes (Fig. 17.11) (Ledger, 1994).

Figure 17.12, as constructed by Barnhart, shows the expected changes (increases) in HCG levels in women with an intrauterine pregnancy and in spontaneous abortion. Ninety-nine percent of normal intrauterine pregnancies have an increase of at least 53% in 2 days, which is less than the rise that was previously accepted (approximately 66%). This rate of increase should be similar in single or multiple gestations (Barnhart, 2009). Note in Table 17.3 (Barnhart, 2009) the expected decline in HCG levels in women who have an abnormal pregnancy destined for a spontaneous abortion. In women with an ectopic pregnancy, the rate of rise in HCG can mimic an intrauterine pregnancy 21% of the time and can mimic a spontaneous abortion 8% of the time. Note the overlap in this increase or decrease in HCG levels as depicted in Figure 17.12.

Today, the key to the diagnosis of ectopic pregnancy is transvaginal ultrasound (TVUS). The concept of a "discriminatory zone" has been advanced and is defined as the serum HCG level above which a gestational sac should be visualized by TVUS if an intrauterine pregnancy (IUP) is present. In most institutions, a serum HCG level of 1500 to 2000 mIU/mL is used. Setting the discriminatory zone at 2000 mIU/mL instead of 1500 mIU/mL may minimize the risk of intervening when an intrauterine pregnancy is viable but may increase the risk of delaying the diagnosis of an ectopic pregnancy. When an IUP is not seen on TVUS at the set discriminatory zone, an abnormal pregnancy is diagnosed, and an ectopic pregnancy needs to be ruled out. It has been suggested further that as reliable as using the discriminatory zone is, the length of gestational sac is at least as important when accurate dating is available (as occurs with luteinizing

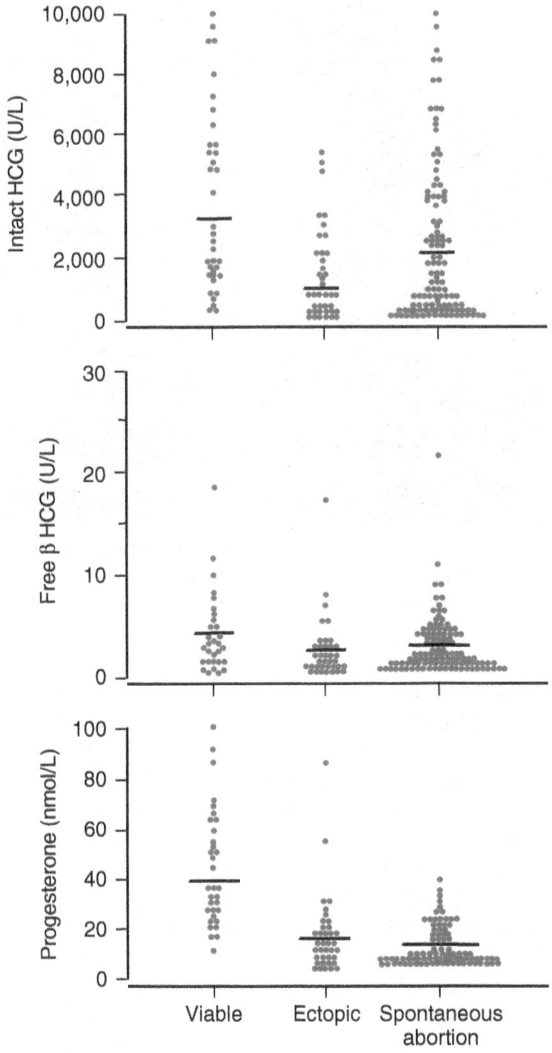


**Figure 17.11** The distribution of serum concentrations of progesterone, intact human chorionic gonadotropin (HCG), and free β-HCG in viable and ectopic pregnancies and spontaneous abortions. Means are indicated by horizontal bars (—). (From Ledger WL, Sweeting VM, Chatterjee S. Rapid diagnosis of early ectopic pregnancy in an emergency gynaecology service—are measurements of progesterone, intact and free beta human chorionic gonadotrophin helpful? *Hum Reprod.* 1994;9:157.)

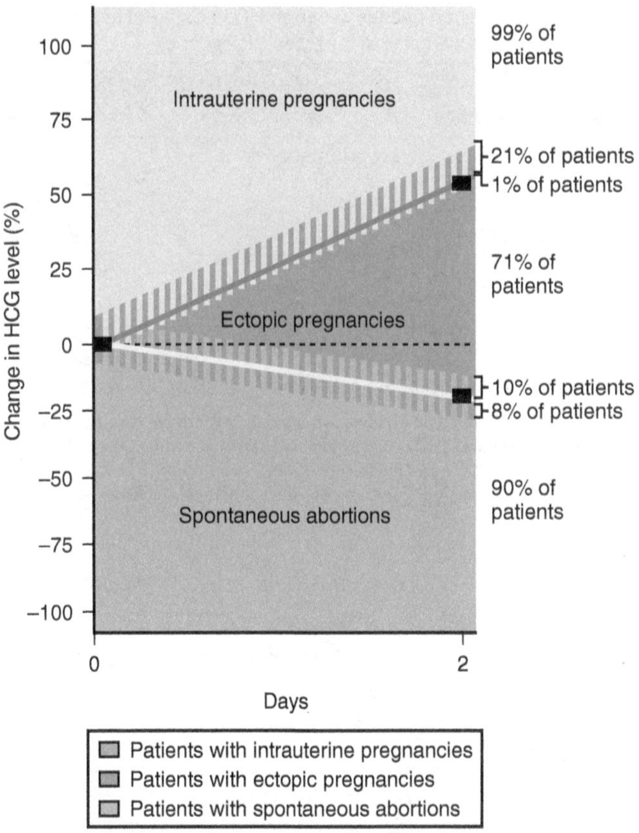


**Figure 17.12** Change in the HCG level in intrauterine pregnancy, ectopic pregnancy, and spontaneous abortion. An increase or decrease in the serial human chorionic gonadotropin (HCG) level in a woman with an ectopic pregnancy is outside the range expected for that of a woman with a growing intrauterine pregnancy or a spontaneous abortion 71% of the time. However, the increase in the HCG level in a woman with an ectopic pregnancy can mimic that of a growing intrauterine pregnancy 21% of the time, and the decrease in the HCG level can mimic that of a spontaneous abortion 8% of the time. (Modified from Barnhart K. Ectopic pregnancy. *N Engl J Med.* 2009;361[4]:384.)

hormone [LH] surge monitoring, etc.). Clearly by 5 1/2 weeks from LMP (in a woman with normal ovulatory cycle length) an intrauterine sac should be visible in a normal intrauterine pregnancy. Important ultrasound findings include visualization of a yolk sac at 5.5 weeks, a fetal pole by 6 weeks, and cardiac activity at 6.5 weeks. An abnormal pregnancy is likely if there is absence of a fetal pole with a gestational sac of 2 cm and if no cardiac activity is noted with a crown-rump length of >0.5 cm.

Thus serial measurements of HCG are of great assistance in the early diagnosis of unruptured ectopic pregnancy. However, a differentiation between ectopic pregnancies and impending spontaneous abortion cannot be made with this technique because the rate of increase of HCG in women with an ectopic pregnancy is often similar to that found in women with an impending intrauterine abortion. An algorithm for possible treatment will be presented here.

### *Progesterone*

Serum progesterone values are lower in an ectopic pregnancy, with levels in normal intrauterine pregnancies at or above 10 ng/mL. An abnormal IUP will also have low values. However, a rising progesterone level is helpful in determining that there is a normal IUP (Fig. 17.13) (McCord, 1996). The clearance of progesterone from the circulation in a failed pregnancy or ectopic is also faster than that of HCG. Therefore progesterone levels have been used as a diagnostic aide for ectopic pregnancy. Nevertheless it is not commonly used today in practice.

### *Ultrasonography*

Development of the transvaginal transducer probes with 7-MHz scanning frequency has enabled more precise imaging of the pelvic organs in early pregnancy than is possible with transabdominal ultrasonography. With these probes it is usually possible to identify an intrauterine gestational sac when the HCG level reaches 1500 mIU/mL and virtually always when the HCG level exceeds 2500 mIU/mL (First International Reference Preparation [1st IRP], now called the *Third International Standard*),

Table 17.3 Expected Change in Serum HCG Levels in First Week of Monitoring Women at Risk for Ectopic Pregnancy

| | Change in HCG (Percentage) | |
|---|---|---|
| Type of Pregnancy | After 2 Days | After 7 Days |
| **Growing Intrauterine Pregnancy** | | |
| In 50% of women | 124 | 500 |
| In 85% of women | 63 | 256 |
| In 99% of women | 53 | 133 |
| **Spontaneous Abortion*** | | |
| Initial HCG, 50 mIU/mL | -12 | -34 |
| Initial HCG, 500 mIU/mL | -21 | -60 |
| Initial HCG, 2000 mIU/mL | -31 | -79 |
| Initial HCG, 5000 mIU/mL | -35 | -84 |

From Sammel MD, Rinaudo PF, et al. Symptomatic patients with an early viable intrauterine pregnancy: HCG curves redefined. *Obstet Gynecol.* 2004;104:50-55. Data from Barnhart, *N Engl J Med.* 2009;361:4.
*This change occurred in 90% of women with spontaneous abortion. Data from Barnhart, 2009.

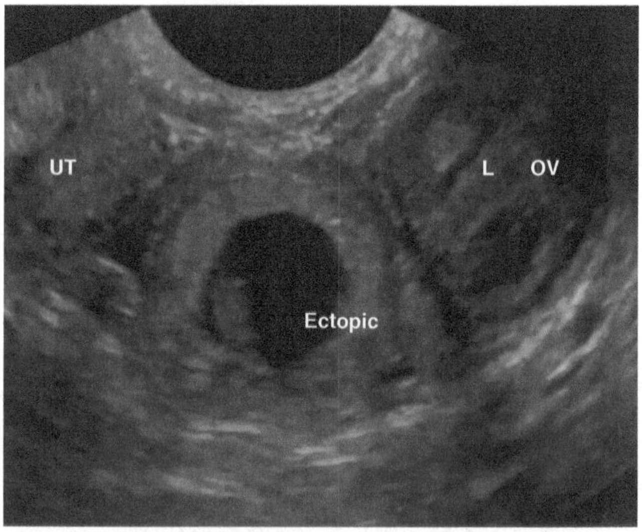


**Figure 17.14** Ultrasound showing a left tubal ectopic. Note the bagel appearance of gestational sac, which here has a fetal pole. (Modified from embryology.med.unsw.edu.au.)

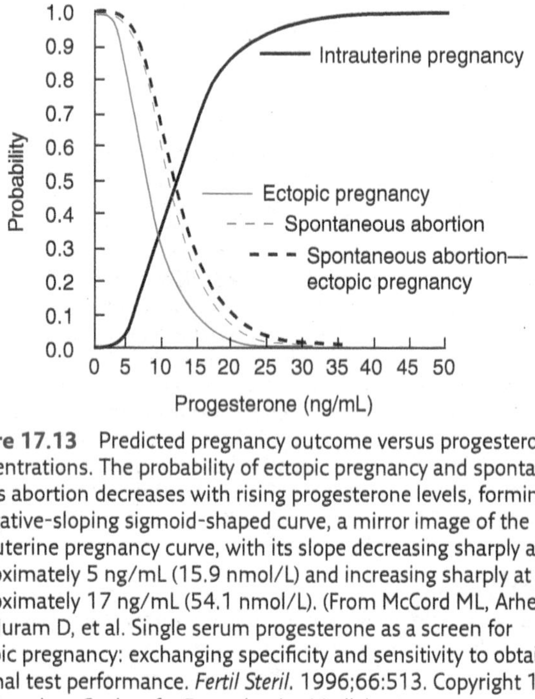


**Figure 17.13** Predicted pregnancy outcome versus progesterone concentrations. The probability of ectopic pregnancy and spontaneous abortion decreases with rising progesterone levels, forming a negative-sloping sigmoid-shaped curve, a mirror image of the intrauterine pregnancy curve, with its slope decreasing sharply at approximately 5 ng/mL (15.9 nmol/L) and increasing sharply at approximately 17 ng/mL (54.1 nmol/L). (From McCord ML, Arheart KL, Muram D, et al. Single serum progesterone as a screen for ectopic pregnancy: exchanging specificity and sensitivity to obtain optimal test performance. *Fertil Steril.* 1996;66:513. Copyright 1996, The American Society for Reproductive Medicine.)

about 5 to 6 weeks after the last menses. Kadar and colleagues reported that in both singleton and multiple gestations a gestational sac should always be seen sonographically beyond 24 days after conception, 38 days' gestational age (Kadar, 1981). Because combined extrauterine and IUP is a rare event, the finding of an intrauterine gestational sac should nearly always exclude the presence of an ectopic pregnancy. When a gestational sac is not present and the HCG level is in the discriminatory zone, a pathologic pregnancy, either an ectopic or a nonviable intrauterine gestation, is most likely present and should be suspected. Usually an adnexal mass or a gestational saclike structure can be identified in the tube when an ectopic pregnancy is present that produces levels of HCG above 2500 mIU/mL.

Thus diagnostic criteria for the ultrasonographic diagnosis of ectopic pregnancy with the use of a vaginal probe include the detection of a complex or cystic adnexal mass (often called an echogenic "bagel" sign) or visualization of an embryo fetal pole in the adnexa (Fig. 17.14). This is in the absence of an intrauterine gestational sac when the gestational age is known to be more than 38 days, or the HCG level is above a certain threshold, usually between 1500 and 2500 mIU/mL.

About two thirds of women presenting with symptoms of ectopic pregnancy have HCG levels above 2500 mIU/mL, and when this occurs, the diagnosis of ectopic pregnancy can usually be made by ultrasound. For the other one third with lower HCG levels, unless a gestational sac is evident on ultrasonography, other diagnostic techniques, such as measurement of a serum progesterone level and serial HCG determination, should be performed. Repeat ultrasonographic examinations at 3- to 5-day intervals are often helpful in establishing a correct diagnosis.

Several investigators have shown that with the use of endovaginal color Doppler flow imaging, it is possible to establish the diagnosis of ectopic pregnancy with greater sensitivity and specificity than with ordinary endovaginal sonography. With endovaginal color flow imaging of the pelvic structures in the presence of an ectopic pregnancy, about a 20% difference in the degree of tubal blood flow between the adnexa has been found compared with less than an 8% difference with intrauterine gestations. Use of endovaginal color flow compared with routine transvaginal sonography increased the sensitivity of the diagnosis of ectopic pregnancy from 71% to 95%, with a specificity of 96% to 100% in various studies (Fig. 17.15).

### *Dilation and Curettage*

When serum HCG levels are more than 1500 mIU/mL, the gestational age exceeds 38 days, or the serum progesterone level is less than 5 ng/mL and no intrauterine gestational sac is seen with vaginal ultrasonography, a curettage of the endometrial cavity (by D&C) with histologic examination of the tissue removed, by frozen section if desired, can be undertaken to determine if

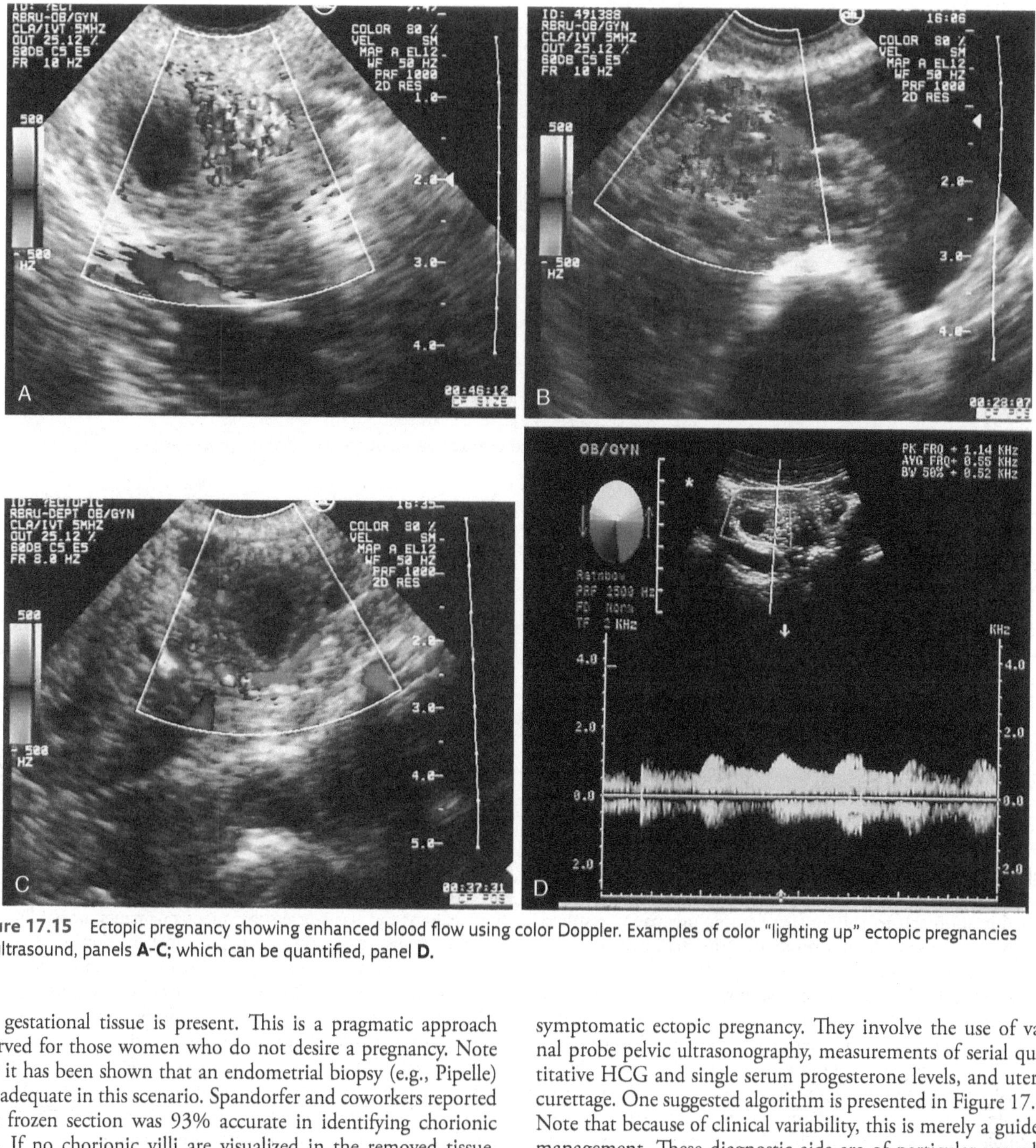


**Figure 17.15** Ectopic pregnancy showing enhanced blood flow using color Doppler. Examples of color "lighting up" ectopic pregnancies on ultrasound, panels **A-C**; which can be quantified, panel **D.**

any gestational tissue is present. This is a pragmatic approach reserved for those women who do not desire a pregnancy. Note that it has been shown that an endometrial biopsy (e.g., Pipelle) is inadequate in this scenario. Spandorfer and coworkers reported that frozen section was 93% accurate in identifying chorionic villi. If no chorionic villi are visualized in the removed tissue, serial HCGs can be followed. A presumptive diagnosis of ectopic pregnancy can be made with rising serum HCGs and treatment undertaken. An analysis by Ailawadi suggested that performing a dilatation and curettage (D&C) in this setting results in fewer complications and is at least as cost effective as the empiric use of methotrexate (Ailawadi, 2005). When chorionic villi are detected and an IUP is evacuated, the serum HCG should drop by at least 15% the day after curettage.

### *Diagnostic Evaluation of Women with Suspected Ectopic Pregnancy*

Several authors have developed flow sheets to aid the clinician in establishing the diagnosis of an asymptomatic or mildly symptomatic ectopic pregnancy. They involve the use of vaginal probe pelvic ultrasonography, measurements of serial quantitative HCG and single serum progesterone levels, and uterine curettage. One suggested algorithm is presented in Figure 17.16. Note that because of clinical variability, this is merely a guide to management. These diagnostic aids are of particular use when following an asymptomatic woman with risk factors for ectopic pregnancy, beginning shortly after conception. Performing a quantitative HCG assay twice weekly, calculating the rate of increase (measuring serum progesterone levels at 4, 5, and 6 weeks' gestational age), and performing serial ultrasonography beginning 3 weeks after ovulation will help to establish the diagnosis of ectopic pregnancy before tubal rupture. The combination of these two techniques is particularly applicable for stable women treated in institutions with adequate facilities for ultrasound and rapid serial quantitative β-HCG assays. If a woman with or without risk factors for ectopic pregnancy develops mild symptoms consistent with an ectopic gestation and is hemodynamically stable, vaginal sonography, measurement of serial

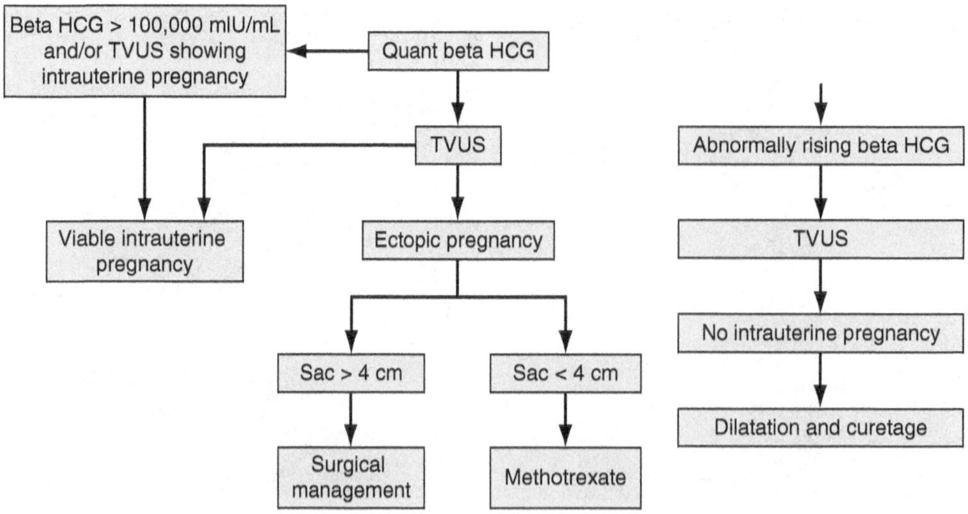


**Figure 17.16** Possible algorithm for use of methotrexate versus surgery for ectopic pregnancy.

HCG levels, and possibly serum progesterone, as well as uterine curettage if indicated, will aid in establishing the diagnosis. The use of a quantitative serum HCG assay and transvaginal sonography enables the diagnosis of ectopic gestation in hemodynamically stable women to be made with a sensitivity of 97% to 100% and a specificity of 95% to 99% (Fig. 17.17) (Gracia, 2001).

Both suggested algorithms include the use of D&C. Although, as stated previously, this approach has been deemed to be cost effective, some women, particularly those who have been attempting pregnancy, are reluctant to have this treatment. In this setting it is reasonable to continue serial HCG and ultrasound monitoring. Unless HCG falls, it will be clear that with time, treatment of a nonviable pregnancy is needed. And this could be with either a D&C or the use of methotrexate.

In an in vitro fertilization setting, if HCG criteria suggest an abnormal pregnancy of unknown location, a suction cannula can be used in an outpatient setting to aid in the diagnosis. Using this approach to rule out an ectopic pregnancy resulted in avoiding the use of methotrexate in more than two thirds of patients (Brady, 2014).

If a woman develops symptoms of a ruptured ectopic pregnancy that are of sufficient hemodynamic severity to require emergency care, a sensitive qualitative pregnancy test and vaginal sonography are usually all the diagnostic aids necessary to establish the diagnosis. If vaginal sonography is not immediately available on an emergent basis, culdocentesis may be performed. If HCG is present and peritoneal fluid is seen sonographically, it is most likely that an ectopic pregnancy is present, and laparoscopy should be performed.

## MANAGEMENT

### SURGICAL THERAPY

#### Tubal Pregnancy

Laparoscopy is the procedure of choice for ruptured ectopic pregnancy as well as for cases when medical therapy (methotrexate) is contraindicated or refused. Laparoscopy is also useful at times when an accurate diagnosis cannot be made. Older studies have suggested that there is a false-positive and false-negative rate of approximately 2% with the use of laparoscopy for ectopic pregnancies (i.e., either not being able to see the ectopic or confusing findings with hemorrhagic corpus luteal cysts, hematosalpinx, and other findings). See Video 17.1 showing laparoscopic salpingectomy for ectopic pregnancy.

Conservative treatment (i.e., preserving the tube and not performing a salpingectomy) for an unruptured ectopic pregnancy has been considered to be the method of choice for women who desire future fertility. Only recently has the first prospective randomized trial been completed, which suggested similar long-term pregnancies rates for salpingostomy versus salpingectomy and a somewhat increased rate of retained trophoblastic tissue after salpingostomy (Mol, 2014). However, in a large review by Yao and Tulandi of women with an ectopic pregnancy attempting to conceive after salpingostomy, 60% had an IUP and 15% an ectopic pregnancy. After salpingectomy, 38% had an IUP and 10% an ectopic pregnancy (Yao, 1997). The conservative surgical techniques used include salpingotomy (in which the tubal incision is closed primarily but is unnecessary and has worse subsequent pregnancy rates [discussed later]), salpingostomy (in which the tubal incision is allowed to close by secondary intention), fimbrial evacuation, and partial salpingectomy, also called *segmental resection* of the portion of the tube containing the ectopic pregnancy. Fimbrial evacuation usually traumatizes the endosalpinx and is associated with a high rate of recurrent ectopic pregnancy (24%), about twice as high as the rate after salpingectomy. In addition, this procedure may not remove the entire tubal gestation, and another procedure may be required a few days later. The best results of conservative management occur after salpingostomy (Fig. 17.18) (Leach, 1989). Tulandi and Guralnick reported that the 2-year cumulative rates of IUP after salpingotomy and salpingostomy were similar, about 45%, but the 1-year rates were twice as great when salpingostomy was performed (45% versus 21%), indicating that there is a more rapid return of normal tubal function when the incision heals by secondary intention than when it is sutured (Fig. 17.19) (Tulandi, 1991).

These techniques can be used to treat the majority of unruptured tubal pregnancies, although this long-held belief has been challenged with the randomized trial referred to earlier (Mol, 2014).

If a woman who is nulliparous has an unruptured ectopic pregnancy and strongly desires a conservative approach, salpingostomy should seriously be considered. The findings of the randomized trial

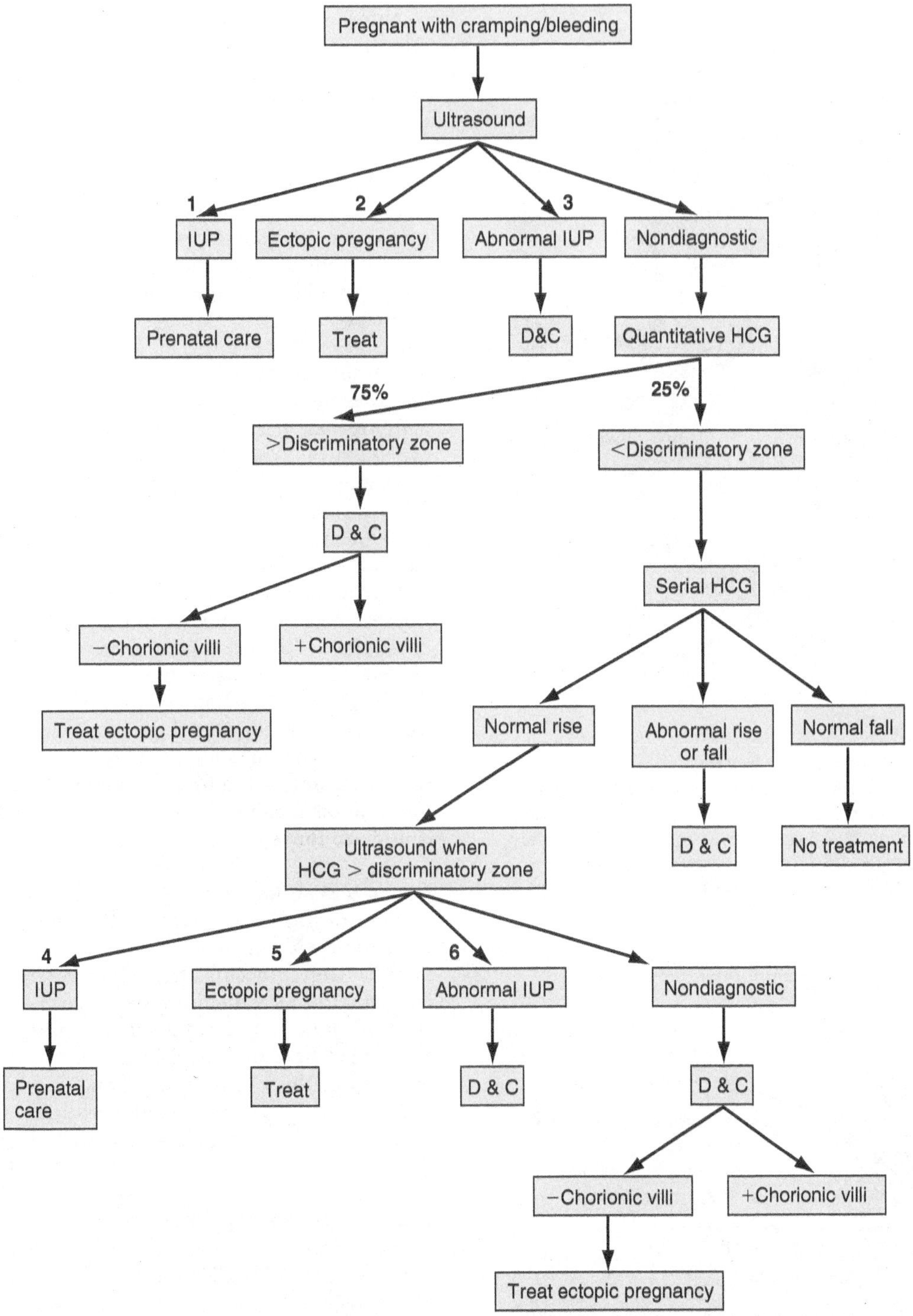


**Figure 17.17** Sample schematic of strategy 1. Numbers refer to probabilities. *D&C*, Dilatation and curettage; *IUP*, intrauterine pregnancy. (From Gracia C, Barnhart KT. Diagnosing ectopic pregnancy. *Obstet Gynecol*. 2001;97:465.)

showing equal future pregnancy rates even if salpingectomy is carried out (Mol, 2014) (Fig. 17.20) should also be weighed into the decision making.

### *Interstitial Pregnancy*

An **interstitial pregnancy** in the cornual area of the uterus can be treated laparoscopically; but it may require laparotomy with resection. A deep cornual resection is not deemed necessary and surprisingly does not decrease the risk of recurrent ectopic pregnancy. It has been proposed that a laparoscopic cornuotomy using a temporary tourniquet suture and diluted vasopressin injection can be effective for these cases (Fig. 17.21; see also Video 17.2 of laparoscopic surgery). Choi and colleagues described eight cases of patients who have undergone this technique. They described a low

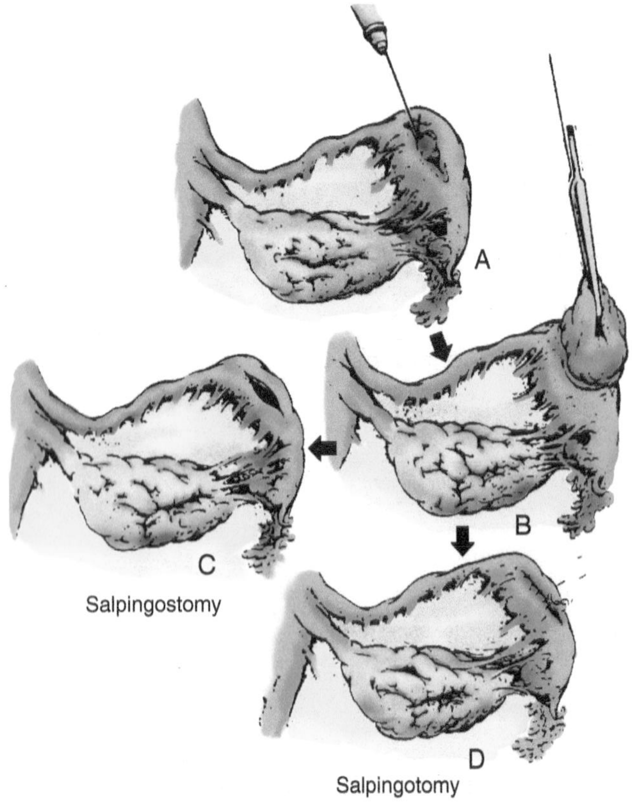


**Figure 17.18** **A,** Incision is made into the antimesenteric border of the fallopian tube. **B,** Ectopic pregnancy is gently removed from within the fallopian tube. **C,** Salpingostomy site is allowed to heal by secondary intention. **D,** Salpingotomy is completed by primary closure. (From Leach RE, Ory SJ. Modern management of ectopic pregnancy. *J Reprod Med.* 1989;34:325.)

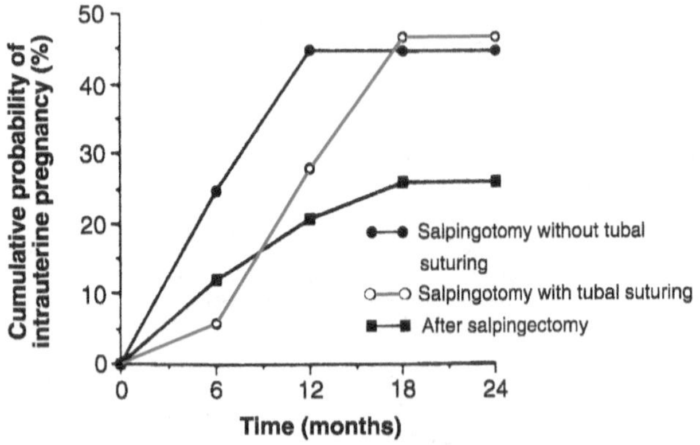


**Figure 17.19** Cumulative probability of intrauterine pregnancy after conservative surgical treatment of tubal ectopic pregnancy by salpingotomy without tubal suturing, salpingotomy with tubal suturing, and after salpingectomy. (From Tulandi T, Guralnick M. Treatment of tubal ectopic pregnancy by salpingotomy with or without tubal suturing and salpingectomy. *Fertil Steril.* 1991;55:53. Copyright 1991, The American Society for Reproductive Medicine.)

estimated blood loss (50 ± 22 mL) without major complications such as hemorrhage, and no postoperative adjuvant therapy was required. They concluded that this procedure is safe and effective in interstitial pregnancy with the advantage of preserving reproductive function compared with cornual resection (Choi, 2009).

Subsequent intrauterine pregnancies after previous cornual ectopic pregnancy should be delivered by C-section.

### *Ovarian Pregnancy*

Rare ovarian pregnancies can be treated by laparoscopic surgical excision. Many times this occurs when the expected surgery is for a ruptured tubal ectopic pregnancy or hemorrhagic corpus luteum. The surgical treatment alternatives include an ovarian wedge resection or unilateral salpingo-oophorectomy. The latter involving oophorectomy should be avoided and does not improve the subsequent pregnancy rate or lower the risk of recurrence.

### *Abdominal Pregnancy*

This is a rare situation; from an analysis of 11 abdominal pregnancy-related deaths and an estimated 5221 abdominal pregnancies in the United States, it has been estimated that there were 10.9 abdominal pregnancies per 100,000 live births and 9.2 per 1000 ectopic pregnancies; the mortality rate was 5.1 per 1000 cases. Hymel found 31 cases of late abdominal pregnancies (more than 20 weeks' gestation) from 1965 to 2012, in a literature review (Hymel, 2015). The most common sites of placental implantation were in the uterus or adnexa (47.8%), bowel (30%), and the potential spaces surrounding the uterus (8.7%). There were five cases of an intraabdominal abscess in the 14 patients in whom the placenta had been left in situ. Maternal outcomes were documented in 26 cases with seven deaths; 27 fetal outcomes were documented in 22 cases with three fetal deaths (13.6%). Treatment is always surgical and interventional radiology and endovascular surgery must be considered for assistance.

### *Cervical Pregnancy*

Surgical treatment of cervical ectopic pregnancies consists of evacuation with dilatation and curettage or vacuum aspiration. This often occurs after methotrexate treatment, which facilitates the decrease in size and vascularity of the pregnancy. What must be considered is the risk of hemorrhage. This can be avoided by a prophylactic suture ligation of the cervical branches of the uterine artery, with absorbable sutures, at 3 and 9 o'clock under transabdominal ultrasound guidance and a running-lock absorbable suture around the entire edge of the cervix.

### *Cesarean Scar Pregnancy*

Surgical treatment of cesarean scar pregnancies also consists of evacuation with dilatation and curettage or vacuum aspiration under transabdominal ultrasound guidance. To prevent hemorrhage, temporary laparoscopic bilateral artery occlusion with silicone tubing has been described (Wang, 2015). Hysteroscopy coupled with curettage followed by uterine artery embolization is also an alternative surgical approach for these cases (Qian, 2015).

## *PERSISTENT ECTOPIC PREGNANCY*

With increasing use of conservative surgical treatment instead of salpingectomy for the treatment of ectopic pregnancy, the entity of persistent ectopic pregnancy (PEP) is becoming more common. The overall mean incidence of PEP after linear salpingostomy is about 5%, being higher when the procedure is

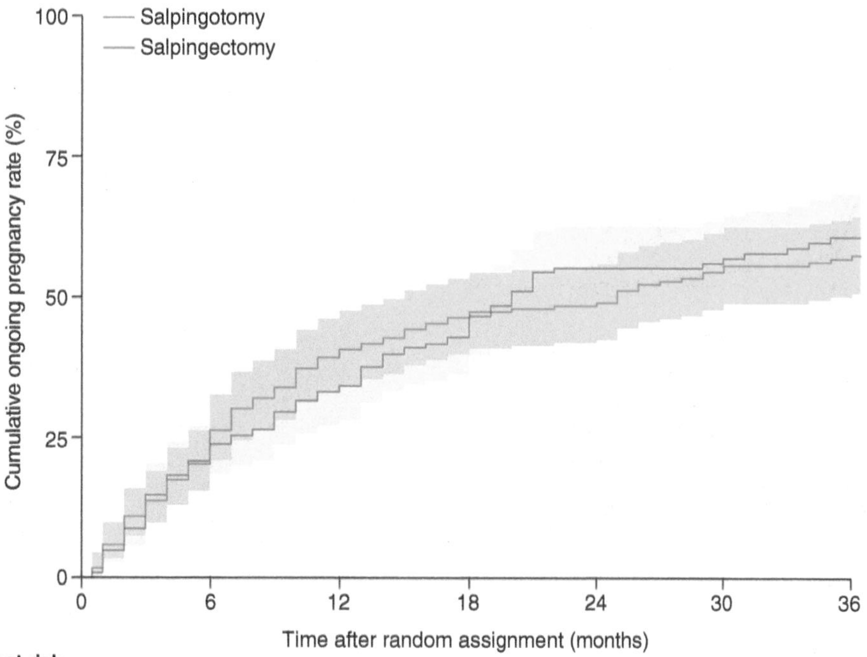


**Number at risk**

| | 0 | 6 | 12 | 18 | 24 | 30 | 36 |
|---|---|---|---|---|---|---|---|
| Salpingotomy | 215 | 158 | 128 | 92 | 65 | 48 | 40 |
| Salpingectomy | 231 | 172 | 126 | 103 | 95 | 80 | 66 |

**Figure 17.20** Kaplan-Meir curves for time to ongoing pregnancy by natural conception. Shaded areas show 95% confidence interval (CI). Median time to ongoing pregnancy by natural conception after salpingotomy was 20 months (95% CI, 17-23) and after salpingectomy was 26 months (95% CI, 15-37); cumulative rate of ongoing pregnancy by natural conception after 36 months was 60 × 7% after salpingotomy and 56 × 2% after salpingectomy. log rank $P = 0.678$; $X^2 = 0.172$ (one degree of freedom). (From Mol F, van Mello NM, Strandell A, et al. Salpingostomy versus salpingectomy in women with tubal pregnancy [ESEP study]: an open-label, multicentre, randomised controlled trial. *Lancet.* 2014;383[9927]:1483-1489.)

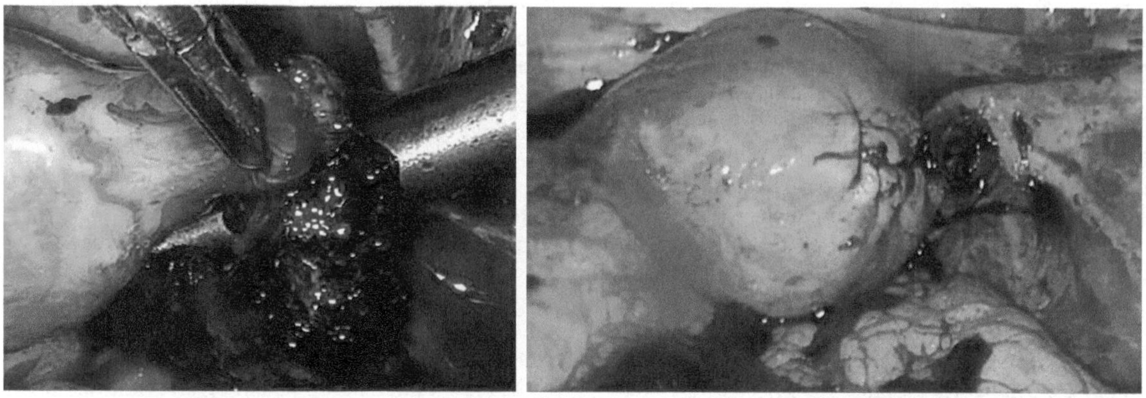

**Figure 17.21** Laparoscopic surgery for interstitial pregnancy in the cornual area of the uterus. The ectopic is evacuated after a linear incision is made and the defect is sutured as shown. (Courtesy Columbia University MIS Program.)

performed laparoscopically and lower when performed by laparotomy. After fimbrial expression or tubal abortion, the incidence of persistence ranges from 12% to 15%.

PEP is uncommon when the preoperative HCG level is below 3000 mIU/mL. When preoperative HCG levels are greater than 3000 mIU/mL, the incidence of PEP has been reported to range from about 22% to 42%. If the HCG level is above 1000 mIU/mL 7 days after surgery or is more than 15% of the original level at this time, PEP is nearly always present. If the day 7 HCG level is under 1000 mIU/mL or less than 15% of the initial value, PEP is unlikely. Vermesh and associates measured both HCG and progesterone levels preoperatively and every 3 days after conservative tubal surgery for an unruptured ectopic gestation in a group of 114 women (Vermesh 1988). Of this group, six (5.3%) had PEP, all of whom had an initial sharp drop in HCG levels to 25% of the pretreatment levels 6 days after surgery, similar to

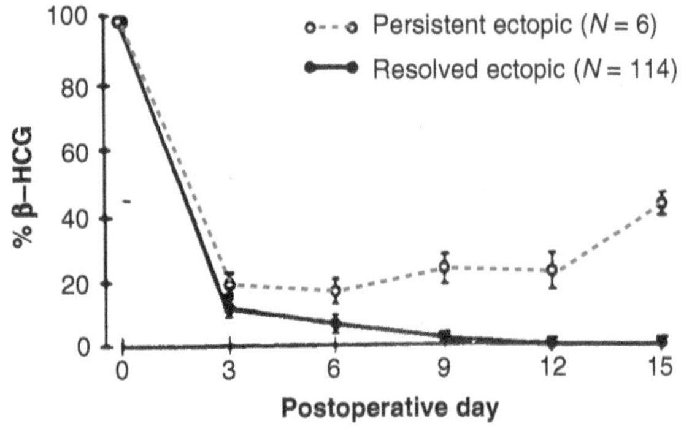


**Figure 17.22** Serum β-human chorionic gonadotropin (β-HCG) patterns in persistent and resolved ectopic gestations after conservative surgery. (From Vermesh M, Silva PD, Rosen GF, et al. Persistent tubal ectopic gestation: patterns of circulating beta-human chorionic gonadotropin and progesterone, and management options. *Fertil Steril.* 1988;50:584. Copyright 1988, The American Society for Reproductive Medicine.)

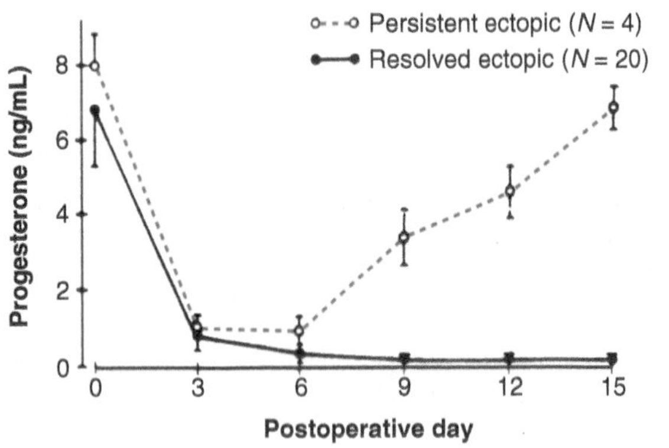


**Figure 17.23** Serum progesterone patterns in persistent and resolved ectopic gestations after conservative surgery. (From Vermesh M, Silva PD, Rosen GF, et al: Persistent tubal ectopic gestation: Patterns of circulating beta-human chorionic gonadotropin and progesterone, and management options. *Fertil Steril.* 1988;50:584. Copyright 1988, The American Society for Reproductive Medicine.)

the remainder of the group who did not have PEP. After 6 days, titers of the former group plateaued or rose slightly (Fig. 17.22).

Based on these data, PEP is presumed to be present if a day 9 serum HCG level is more than 10% of the initial level or a day 9 serum progesterone level is higher than 1.5 ng/mL (Fig. 17.23). It is now recommended that after linear salpingostomy either HCG or progesterone levels be measured initially on day 6 postoperatively and at 3-day intervals thereafter. Increasing levels of either of these hormones beyond day 6 or a day 6 level of HCG more than 1000 mIU/mL, or more than 15% of the original value are all indicators of persistent ectopic pregnancy. Because tubal rupture is likely to occur with PEP, it is best to treat the entity before this emergency situation occurs.

Methods used to treat PEP include salpingectomy, salpingostomy, methotrexate, or expectant management. Expectant management is usually reserved for the asymptomatic woman whose HCG titers plateau but do not rise. Surgical management should be utilized for women who develop symptoms of persistent lower abdominal pain. The remaining women with PEP are best treated

**Table 17.4** Multiple-Dose MTX Treatment Protocol

| Treatment Day | Laboratory Evaluation | Intervention |
|---|---|---|
| Pretreatment | HCG, CBC with differential, liver function tests, creatinine, blood type and antibody screen | Rule out spontaneous Ab<br>Rhogam if Rh negative |
| 1 | HCG | MTX 1.0 mg/kg IM |
| 2 | | LEU 0.1 mg/kg IM |
| 3 | HCG | MTX 1.0 mg/kg IM if <15% decline days 1-3<br>If >15%, stop treatment and start surveillance |
| 4 | | LEU 0.1 mg/kg IM |
| 5 | HCG | MTX 1.0 mg/kg IM if <15% decline days 3-5<br>If >15%, stop treatment and start surveillance |
| 6 | | LEU 0.1 mg/kg IM |
| 7 | HCG | MTX 1.0 mg/kg IM if <15% decline days 5-7<br>If >15%, stop treatment and start surveillance |
| 8 | | LEU 0.1 mg/kg IM |

From The Practice Committee of the American Society for Reproductive Medicine. Medical treatment of ectopic pregnancy. *Fertil Steril.* 2008;90(5 Suppl):S206-S212. Surveillance every 7 days (until HCG <35 mIU/mL). Screening laboratory studies should be repeated 1 week after the last dose of MTX.
*LEU*, leucovorin; *IM*, intramuscularly; *CBC*, Complete Blood Count; *MTX*, methotrexate; *HCG*, Human Chorionic Gonadotropin.

with methotrexate. A single dose of 50 mg/m$^2$ of methotrexate is usually sufficient to resolve PEP. Graczykowski and Mishell performed a randomized trial in which a single dose of methotrexate or placebo was given within 24 hours after salpingostomy. The use of methotrexate reduced the risk of developing PEP by nearly 90%. The prophylactic use of a single dose of methotrexate may be considered in women with larger ectopics, higher initial levels of HCG, or when the surgery had been difficult.

### *Medical Treatment*

Methotrexate (MTX) has become established as a reasonable primary treatment for ectopic pregnancy and is comparable with surgical therapy in observational studies. For medical and surgical therapy, rates of tubal pregnancy (62% to 90%) and recurrence rates (8% to 15%) are comparable.

MTX should be used in asymptomatic women who qualify for such treatment (see Fig. 17.16) and who have no contraindications (see Table 17.3) (Practice Committee ASRM, 2008). Prior to treatment, several tests should be obtained, including a complete blood count (CBC) test, liver function test, blood urea nitrogen (BUN) test, and tests of creatinine, blood type, and Rh.

There are two main protocols for MTX: multidose and single-dose regimens (Tables 17.4 and 17.5) (Practice Committee ASRM, 2008). There is also an intermediate two-dose regimen, which will be discussed later. The multidose regimen is more successful but involves more dosing and therefore potentially has more side effects. It also includes the use of leukovorin (folinic acid), an antagonist to

Table 17.5 Single-Dose MTX Treatment Protocol

| Treatment Day | Laboratory Evaluation | Intervention |
|---|---|---|
| Pretreatment | HCG, CBC with differential, liver function tests, creatinine, blood type, and antibody screen | Rule out spontaneous Ab<br>Rhogam if Rh negative |
| 1 | HCG | MTX 50 mg/m$^2$ IM |
| 4 | HCG | |
| 7 | HCG | MTX 50 mg/m$^2$ IM if β-HCG decreased <15% between day 4 and day 7 |

From The Practice Committee of the American Society for Reproductive Medicine: Medical treatment of ectopic pregnancy. *Fertil Steril* 90(5 Suppl):S206-S212, 2008.
Surveillance every 7 days (until HCG < 5 mIU/mL). ASRM Practice Committee. Treatments of ectopic pregnancy. *Fertil Steril* 2008;90(5 Suppl):S206-S212.
*HCG*, Human chorionic gonadotropin; *MTX*, methotrexate.

**Box 17.1 Treatment and Side Effects Associated with MTX**

**Treatment Effects**
Increase in abdominal girth
Increase in HCG during initial therapy
Vaginal bleeding or spotting
Abdominal pain

**Drug Side Effects**
Gastric distress, nausea, and vomiting
Stomatitis
Dizziness
Severe neutropenia (rare)
Reversible alopecia (rare)
Pneumonitis (rare)

From The Practice Committee of the American Society for Reproductive Medicine. Medical treatment of ectopic pregnancy. *Fertil Steril.* 2008;90(5 Suppl):S206-S212.

MTX, to reduce the risk of side effects. As shown in Table 17.4, the multidose regimen can be stopped if there is an appropriate decrease in HCG with treatment. The complications of MTX are listed in Box 17.1. In all regimens, the reduction in HCG is key to success, but complete resolution of HCG usually takes 2 to 3 weeks and can linger for up to 8 weeks after treatment.

Meta-analyses have confirmed the overall success of MTX to be 78% to 96%. The single-dose regimen has been reported to have a success of 88.1% (86 to 90), and the multiple-dose regimen was significantly more successful: 92 to 79 (89% to 96%). It is clear that there is a high failure rate with the single-dose regimen, and this is clearly related to the viability of the ectopic, based on its size and the level of HCG (Box 17.2). Seeing a yoke sac in the adnexa and a level of HCG >5000 mIU/mL affords a poorer prognosis of MTX single-dose therapy. Mol and associates performed a systematic review and meta-analysis comparing laparoscopic salpingostomy and methotrexate. They concluded that the clinical treatment is more cost effective with less hospitalization, faster recovery, and no significant difference in subsequent spontaneous conception rates or recurrent ectopic pregnancies (Mol, 2008).

**Box 17.2 Predictors of MTX Treatment Failure**

Adnexal fetal cardiac activity
Size and volume of the gestational mass (>4 cm)
High initial HCG concentration (>5000 mIU/mL)
Presence of free peritoneal blood
Rapidly increasing HCG concentrations (>50%/48 hours) before MTX
Continued rapid rise in HCG concentrations during MTX

From The Practice Committee of the American Society for Reproductive Medicine. Medical treatment of ectopic pregnancy. *Fertil Steril.* 2008;90(5 Suppl):S206-S212.

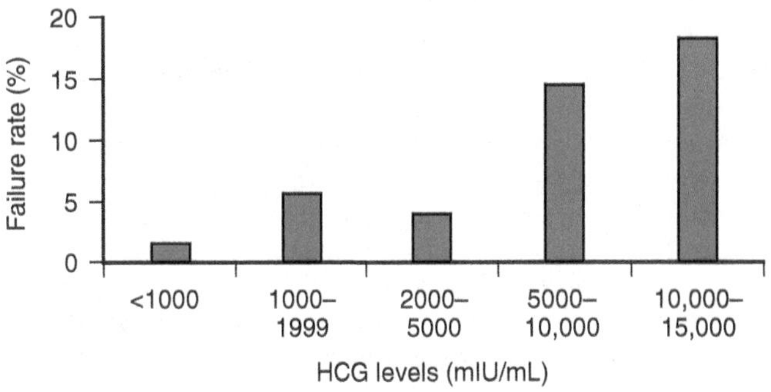


**Figure 17.24** Single-dose MTX treatment failure based on HCG level. (From The Practice Committee of the American Society for Reproductive Medicine. Medical treatment of ectopic pregnancy. *Fertil Steril.* 2008;90[5 Suppl]:S206-S212.)

Figure 17.24 provides the correlation of failure rates with high levels of HCG (Practice Committee ASRM, 2008). Box 17.2 lists the predictions of failed responses. A two-dose regimen has been proposed as well, which is intermediate between the high and multiple-dose regimens. MTX (50 mg/m$^2$) is administered on days 1 and 4 without leukovorin. This regimen may be considered for patients who have HCG levels above 5000 mIU/mL.

About 85% of patients treated with methotrexate have a transient rise in HCG level between 1 and 4 days after treatment. Between 4 and 7 days after methotrexate is administered, the HCG levels should fall at least 15%. If this amount of decrease does not occur or there is less than a 15% decrease in HCG levels in each subsequent week, an additional dose of methotrexate should be given for a maximum of three doses. If after three doses of methotrexate HCG levels do not decline by 15% weekly, a surgical procedure should be performed. Serum progesterone levels fall more rapidly than HCG levels after methotrexate, and a progesterone level of less than 1.5 ng/mL has been found to be an excellent predictor of resolution of the ectopic pregnancy. Between 3 and 7 days after initiating therapy, severe pelvic pain lasting up to 12 hours frequently occurs. This symptom, probably caused by tubal abortion, must be differentiated from the symptoms of tubal rupture. Serial monitoring of vital signs and measurement of hematocrit levels are helpful. If the woman remains hemodynamically stable and the pain disappears, a tubal abortion has probably taken place and no further therapy is necessary.

To avoid the toxicity of systemic methotrexate administration, a smaller dose of the drug has been administered directly into the tube with either laparoscopic or ultrasound visualization. In a summary of 11 series involving 295 women treated with tubal injection of methotrexate, 83% had successful resolution of the ectopic pregnancy, and subsequent tubal patency rates were 88% and fertility rates were 82%.

Because of the lower success rate and need for direct needle placement with local injection, most clinicians are now using systemic methotrexate. There have also been several reports of direct intratubal injection of other substances, including potassium chloride, hypertonic glucose, and prostaglandins, but use of these agents is generally less successful than the use of methotrexate.

Methotrexate plays an important role in the treatment of the nontubal ectopic pregnancies. It can be used be administrated intramuscularly or intraamniotically and may also be combined with other therapeutic means, such as intraamniotic administration of potassium chloride, vaginal mifepristone, or uterine artery embolization. If the treatment is considered incomplete in the patient's follow-up, additional treatments such as curettage, hysteroscopy, or even hysterectomy can be considered.

Some new drugs are being studied for the clinical management of the ectopic pregnancies, with drugs such as selective progesterone receptor modulators (i.e., mifepristone) and epidermal growth factor receptor inhibitors combined with methotrexate. Further studies are required to confirm the efficacy of these medications.

### *Expectant Management*

Although this is not a preferred plan of management, it is useful to know that certain ectopics may resolve without treatment. An overall success rate of 69% has been reported for expectant management. The lower the initial HCG level, the greater the success with spontaneous resolution.

Trio and coworkers, using multivariate analysis, reported that an initial HCG titer of less than 1000 mIU/mL and a decrease in HCG levels between the initial serum sample and one obtained a few days later were each independent predictors of successful spontaneous resolution, whereas sonographic visualization of an ectopic gestational sac was not an independent predictor of failure. In their series of 49 women managed expectantly, 88% of those with an initial HCG level of less than 1000 mIU/mL had successful resolution.

Korhonen and associates measured serial HCG levels before and during outpatient expectant management in a group of 118 women with ectopic pregnancies. This group comprised one fourth of all the women with the diagnosis of ectopic pregnancy seen at their institution during 3 years. When spontaneous resolution occurred, HCG levels declined to undetectable levels in 4 to 67 days, with a mean of 20 days. A distinct difference in the rate of decline of HCG levels in those who did and did not require surgery was not observed until 7 days after the initial examination (Fig. 17.25) (Korhonen, 1994). If HCG levels had not fallen more than two thirds of the initial level in 7 days, two thirds of this group of women needed surgical treatment for rising HCG levels, clinical symptoms, or sonographic findings of intraperitoneal bleeding. It has been reported that when serial sonography is performed, some of the tubal pregnancies can increase in size and become more vascular as they resolve. Although knowledge of these facts is important, if an unruptured ectopic pregnancy is diagnosed by β-HCG and ultrasound, it is still preferable to treat with methotrexate or perform laparoscopy, depending on the clinical situation as discussed earlier.

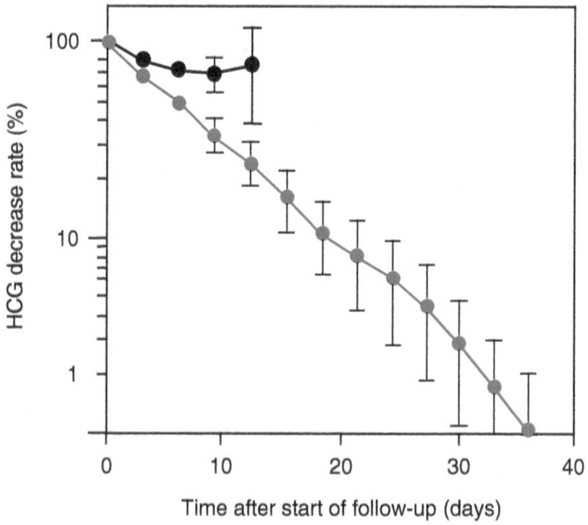


**Figure 17.25** Mean value and 95% confidence limits for ratio of serum human chorionic gonadotropin (HCG) concentrations to starting value during expectant management in patients with a spontaneous resolution *(blue circles)* and in those later treated by laparoscopy *(black circles)*. The two groups diverged at 7 days. (From Korhonen J, Stenman UH, Ylöstalo P. Serum human chorionic gonadotropin dynamics during spontaneous resolution of ectopic pregnancy. *Fertil Steril.* 1994;61:632. Copyright 1994, The American Society for Reproductive Medicine.)

## DIAGNOSIS IN WOMEN WITH A HISTORY OF INFERTILITY

In women with a history of infertility, the diagnosis of ectopic pregnancy has been subjected to a risk-scoring assessment (Fig. 17.26) (Coste, 1998). In this scenario, methotrexate therapy is preferred unless the ectopic pregnancy involves a known hydrosalpinx, in which case salpingectomy should be preferred. The Cochrane database has shown that methotrexate therapy is equivalent to laparoscopic surgery; it has also been deemed more cost effective.

## PROGNOSIS FOR SUBSEQUENT FERTILITY

If a woman wishes to conceive after having an ectopic pregnancy, three possibilities exist: she may remain infertile, she may conceive and have an intrauterine gestation (with a viable birth or spontaneous abortion), or she may conceive and have an ectopic gestation. Overall, the subsequent conception rate in women following all ectopic pregnancies is about 60%, with the other 40% remaining infertile. About one third of the pregnancies occurring after the initial ectopic pregnancy or another ectopic pregnancy, and one sixth are spontaneous abortions. Therefore only about half the pregnancies are viable, and only one third of all women with an ectopic pregnancy have a subsequent live birth. However, these overall figures are modified by several factors, particularly age, parity, history of infertility, evidence of contralateral tubal disease, whether the ectopic pregnancy is ruptured or intact, and use of an intrauterine device (IUD) at the time of the ectopic gestation. The subsequent fertility rate is significantly

**1. Calculate the score (number of points) for each risk factor:**

| Age (years) | Points | Smoking (cig/d) | Points |
|---|---|---|---|
| <35 | 0 | 0 | 0 |
| 35–39 | 3 | 1–20 | 2 |
| 40 | 6 | >20 | 4 |

| Other factors | Points YES | Points NO |
|---|---|---|
| EP history | 10 | 0 |
| Endometriosis | 9 | 0 |
| History of infection[1] | 8 | 0 |
| Clomiphene | 7 | 0 |
| Tubal surgery | 4 | 0 |

[1]Salpingitis history (confirmed or not), and/or positive serology for *Chlamydia trachomatis* (1/64)

**2. Add the points and read the absolute risk of EP according to the number of points**

| 0 | 2 | 4 | 6 | 8 | 10 | 12 | 14 | 16 | 18 | 20 | 22 | 24 | 26 | 28 | 30 | 32 | 34 | 36 | 38 | 40 | 42 | 44 | 46 | 48 |
|---|---|---|---|---|---|---|---|---|---|---|---|---|---|---|---|---|---|---|---|---|---|---|---|---|
| 1% | 2% | 2% | 3% | 5% | 7% | 11% | 15% | 21% | 28% | 37% | 47% | 57% | 66% | 74% | 81% | 87% | 91% | 93% | 96% | 97% | 98% | 99% | 99% | 99% |

For example, a woman aged 36 years, smoking 25 cigarettes/day, with an EP history and a pregnancy induced by clomiphene would have a score of 3 + 4 + 10 + 7 = 24, for an EP risk of 57%.

**Figure 17.26** Ectopic pregnancy (EP) risk scale. (From Coste J, Bouyer J, Fernandez H, Job-Spira N. Predicting the risk of extra-uterine pregnancy: construction and validation of a French risk scale. *Contacept Fertil Sex.* 1998;26:643.)

higher in parous women younger than age 30. However, if the ectopic pregnancy occurs in a woman's first pregnancy, her overall subsequent conception rate is only about 35%, being lower with a history of infertility and higher with no such history. On the other hand, women with high parity (more than three births) who develop an ectopic pregnancy have a relatively high rate, about 80%, of subsequent conception. The subsequent conception rate is lower in women who have a history of salpingitis, as well as those who have visual evidence of pathologic changes in the opposite oviduct as a result of previous salpingitis. Several studies have reported that women who were using an IUD at the time of ectopic pregnancy have normal rates of subsequent fertility and no increased risk of a subsequent ectopic pregnancy. Future fertility is significantly higher in women who have an unruptured tubal pregnancy than in those with tubal rupture, so early diagnosis is desirable. Only 65% of women with a ruptured ectopic pregnancy subsequently conceive, whereas the conception rate in women with an unruptured tubal pregnancy is approximately 82%.

In two large groups of women with unruptured ectopic pregnancy treated by conservative surgery, a high incidence of subsequent fertility (80% to 86%) and a low incidence of subsequent ectopic pregnancy (11% to 22%) have been reported. The intrauterine pregnancy (IUP) rates were 64% to 70%. In both series, the IUP rates were highest (82% to 86%) in women with no history of infertility or gross evidence of prior salpingitis. The IUP rates were significantly lower (41% to 56%) in women with infertility. It has been shown that in women with evidence of prior tubal infection or a history of infertility, subsequent IUP rates were higher when they were treated with salpingostomy (73% to 76%) than when treated with salpingectomy (43% to 44%). Most studies in the literature indicate that the overall subsequent ectopic pregnancy rate is similar among women treated by salpingostomy or salpingectomy, and the data suggest that conservative surgery is most beneficial for women with evidence of contralateral tubal damage or a history of infertility.

When comparing salpingostomy outcomes after laparoscopy or laparotomy, the women treated by laparoscopy conceived sooner than those treated by laparotomy, and there were more ectopic pregnancies in the latter group. Overall, 68% and 71% of women in the two groups, respectively, had an IUP, and 5% and 19%, respectively, had an ectopic pregnancy.

In women with an unruptured ectopic a history of infertility (particularly resulting from tubal disease), previous salpingitis, a prior ectopic pregnancy, or the presence of only one tube were each independent factors that decreased the rate of subsequent fertility and also increased the risk of subsequent ectopic pregnancy (Fig. 17.27). It has been suggested therefore that if more than one of these factors were present it would be preferable to perform a salpingectomy than to perform a salpingostomy, as 80% of the recurrent ectopic pregnancies occurred in the same tube as the initial ectopic pregnancy.

The rate of repeat ectopic pregnancies after a single ectopic pregnancy ranges from 8% to 27%, with a mean of about 20%. Because the overall pregnancy rate is in the 60% to 80% range, about one of three to four conceptions after an ectopic pregnancy is a repeat ectopic pregnancy.

Women with an ectopic pregnancy who become pregnant again should be monitored by ultrasound early in pregnancy. Only about one of three nulliparous women who have had an ectopic pregnancy ever conceives again (35%), and about one third of these conceptions are an ectopic pregnancy, for an overall rate of 13%. Risk factors for a repeat ectopic pregnancy were ectopic pregnancy as the first pregnancy, age younger than 25, evidence of tubal infection, and history of infertility (see Table 17.1). With two ectopic pregnancies, the subsequent fertility rate decreases even further. Of women who have had two consecutive ectopic pregnancies treated by

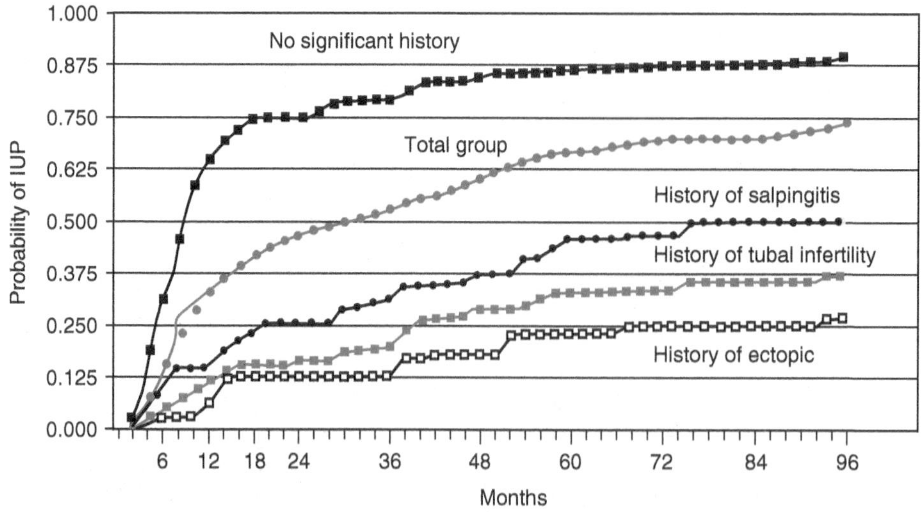


**Figure 17.27** Cumulative pregnancy rate according to the patients' history. *IUP,* Intrauterine pregnancy.

salpingostomy, about half will subsequently conceive, but the majority of these will be a repeat ectopic pregnancy. There have been several reports on salpingostomy or salpingotomy in women with an unruptured tubal pregnancy in the only remaining tube. In the great majority of the subjects, the other tube had been removed because of another ectopic gestation. Of 90 women so treated in six different centers, the conception rate was 81%, with an IUP rate of 57%. About one fourth of the women who conceived had a subsequent ectopic pregnancy, which is similar to the rate among all ectopic pregnancies. Thus conservative surgery or medical therapy may be considered when an unruptured ectopic pregnancy occurs in the only remaining tube.

More recently, Lund Karhus and colleagues performed a study of long-term reproductive outcomes in women whose first pregnancy was an ectopic. They concluded that when compared with women with a first miscarriage, women with a first ectopic pregnancy had a relative risk of a term pregnancy of 0.55, for miscarriages of 0.46, for induced abortions of 0.72, and a 4.7-fold increased risk of further ectopic pregnancy (Lund Karhus, 2013).

## KEY POINTS

- The rate of ectopic pregnancy in the United States has remained fairly constant since the early 2000s and is approximately 6.6/1000 pregnancies in women aged 15 to 24.
- The mortality rate has decreased over time and is approximately 0.5 deaths per 1000 per year.
- Risks of ectopic pregnancy include age, pelvic inflammatory disease, prior tubal surgery, smoking, and infertility.
- About 85% of women with an ectopic pregnancy have serum HCG levels lower than in normal pregnancy; the normal HCG doubling time is 1.4 to 3 days in early pregnancy. In 85% of pregnancies, there is a 66% increase every 48 hours; a rise less than 53% in 48 hours is 99% sensitive for an abnormal pregnancy.
- An intrauterine sac should be seen in a normal pregnancy when HCG levels reach 1500 to 2500 mIU/mL. The so-called discriminatory zone is a gestational age over 38 days.
- Progesterone levels below 5 ng/mL indicate an abnormal pregnancy, and levels above 25 ng/mL indicate a normal pregnancy.
- Overall, the subsequent conception rate in women with an ectopic pregnancy is about 60%. A little less than half of these pregnancies terminate in another ectopic pregnancy or spontaneous abortion; so only about one third of women with an ectopic pregnancy have a subsequent live birth.
- In women with one remaining tube, when an unruptured ectopic pregnancy is treated by salpingostomy, the conception rate is 81% with an IUP rate of 56% and a subsequent ectopic gestation rate of 24%.
- Randomized trial data suggest there is no difference in overall subsequent pregnancy outcomes between women who are treated by salpingostomy versus salpingectomy.
- The overall risk of ectopic pregnancy if a pregnancy occurs after tubal sterilization is about 30%, reaching 50% if the sterilization technique was bilateral tubal fulguration.
- The incidence of heterotopic ectopic pregnancy is about 1% of all pregnancies and is more likely to occur after ART or in vitro fertilization.
- Asymptomatic persistent ectopic pregnancy can be treated expectantly or with methotrexate (MTX). Several regimens are in use, and at least one third of women with ectopic pregnancies can be treated medically. The success of MTX depends on the size/age of the gestation and the initial HCG level. The HCG level should fall at least 15% between days 4 and 7 after the methotrexate injection and at least 15% weekly thereafter.

## KEY REFERENCES


Ailawadi M, Lorch SA, Barnhart KT. Cost-effectiveness of presumptively medical treating women at risk for ectopic pregnancy compared with first performing a dilatation and curettage. *Fertil Steril.* 2005;83(2):376.

Barnhart K. Ectopic pregnancy. *N Engl J Med.* 2009;361(4):379–387.

Bolaji I, Gupta S. Medical management of interstitial pregnancy with high beta selective human chorionic gonadotropin. *Ultrasound.* 2010;18(2):60–67.

Bouyer J, Coste J, Fernandez, et al. Sites of ectopic pregnancy: a 10 year population-based study of 1800 cases. *Hum Reprod.* 2002;17:3224.

Bouyer J, Coste J, Shojaei T, et al. Risk factors for ectopic pregnancy: A comprehensive analysis based on a large case-control, population-based study in France. *Am J Epidemiol.* 2003;157:185.

Brady P, Imudia AN, Awonuga AO, et al. Pregnancies of unknown location after in vitro fertilization: minimally invasive management with Karman cannula aspiration. *Fertil Steril.* 2014;101(2):420–426.

Breen JL. A 21-year survey of 654 ectopic pregnancies. *Am J Obstet Gynecol.* 1970;106:1004.

Budowick M, Johnson TRGB, Genadry R, et al. The histopathology of the developing tubal ectopic pregnancy. *Fertil Steril.* 1980;34:169.

Choi YS, Eun DS, Choi J, et al. Laparoscopic cornuotomy using a temporary tourniquet suture and diluted vasopressin injection in interstitial pregnancy. *Fertil Steril.* 2009;91(15):1933–1937.

Clayton HB, Schieve LA, Peterson HB, et al. A comparison of heterotopic and intrauterine-only pregnancy outcomes after assisted reproduction technologies in the United States from 1992-2002. *Fertil Steril.* 2007;87(2):303.

Corson SL, Batzer FR. Ectopic pregnancy: A review of the etiologic factors. *J Reprod Med.* 1986;31:78.

Coste J, Bouyer J, Fernandez H, et al. Predicting the risk of extra-uterine pregnancy: Construction and validation of a French risk scale. *Contracept Fertil Sex.* 1998;26:643.

Creanga AA, Shapiro-Mendoza CK, Bish CL, et al. Trends in ectopic pregnancy mortality in the United States 1980-2007. *Obstet Gynecol.* 2011;117(4):837.

Fernandez H, Coste J, Job-Spira N. Controlled ovarian hyperstimulation as a risk factor for ectopic pregnancy. *Obstet Gynecol.* 1991;78:656.

Gracia C, Barnhart KT. Diagnosing ectopic pregnancy. *Obstet Gynecol.* 2001;97:465.

Hjordt Hansen MV, Dalsgaard T, Hartwell D, et al. Reproductive prognosis in endometriosis. A national cohort study. *Acta Obstet Gynecol Scand.* 2014;93(5):483–489.

Hymel JA, Hughes DS, Gehlot A, et al. Late abdominal pregnancies(≥20 weeks gestation): A review from 1965 to 2012. *Gynecol Obstet.* 2015 (Epub ahead of print).

Kadar N, Caldwell BV, Romero R. A method of screening for ectopic pregnancy and its indications. *Obstet Gynecol.* 1981;58:162.

Korhonen J, Stenman UH, Ylostalo P. Serum human chorionic gonadotropin dynamics during spontaneous resolution of ectopic pregnancy. *Fertil Steril.* 1994;61:632.

Leach RE, Ory SJ. Modern management of ectopic pregnancy. *J Reprod Med.* 1989;34:325.

Ledger WL, Sweeting VM, Chatterjee S. Rapid diagnosis of early ectopic pregnancy in an emergency gynaecology service –are measurements of progesterone, intact and free beta human chorionic gonadotrophin helpful? *Hum Reprod.* 1994;9:157.

Lund Karhus L, Egerup P, Wessel Skovlund C, et al. Long-term reproductive outcomes in women whose first pregnancy is ectopic: a national controlled follow-up study. *Hum Reprod.* 2013;28(1):241–246.

McCord ML, Arheart KL, Muram D, et al. Single serum progesterone as a screen for ectopic pregnancy: Exchanging specificity and sensitivity to obtain optimal test performance. *Fertil Steril.* 1996;66:513.

Mol F, Mol BW, Ankum WM, et al. Current evidence on surgery, systemic methotrexate and expectant management in the treatment of tubal ectopic pregnancy: a systematic review and meta-analysis. *Hum Reprod Update.* 2008;14:309–319.

Mol F, van Mello NM, Strandell A, et al. Salpingotomy versus salpingectomy in women with tubal pregnancy (ESEP study): an open-label, multicenter, randomized controlled trial. *Lancet.* 2014;383(9927):1483–1489.

O'Leary JL, O'Leary JA. Rudimentary horn pregnancy. *Obstet Gynecol.* 1963;22:371.

Perkins KM, Boulet SL, Kissin DM, et al. Risk of ectopic pregnancy associated with assisted reproductive technology in the United States 2001-2011. *Obstet Gynecol.* 2015;125(1):70.

Peterson HB. for the US Collaborative Review of Sterilization Working Group: The risk of ectopic pregnancy after tubal sterilization. *N Engl J Med.* 1997;336:762.

Practice Committee. American Society for Reproductive Medicine: Medical treatment of ectopic pregnancy. *Fertil Steril.* 2008;90(3):S206–S212.

Qian ZD, Huang LL, Zhu XM. Curettage or operative hysteroscopy in the treatment of cesarean scar pregnancy. *Arch Gynecol Obstet.* 2015 (Epub ahead of print).

Rotas MA, Haberman S, Levgur M. Cesarean scar ectopic pregnancies: etiology, diagnosis, and management. *Obstet Gynecol.* 2006;107:1373.

Sadeghi H, Rutherford T, Rackow BW, et al: Cesarean scar ectopic pregnancy: case series and review of the literature. *Am J Perinatol* 27(2):111-20,


Suggested Readings can be found on ExpertConsult.com.

# 18

# Benign Gynecologic Lesions

## Vulva, Vagina, Cervix, Uterus, Oviduct, Ovary, Ultrasound Imaging of Pelvic Structures

*Mary Segars Dolan, Cherie Hill, Fidel A. Valea*

This chapter reviews benign gynecologic lesions; however, the symptoms and differential diagnoses of these lesions have definite similarity with those of malignant disease. As in many areas of medicine, gynecologic problems do not fall into definitive categories, and those that include malignant disease often overlap with those that include benign disease. When the diagnosis from the history, physical examination, and laboratory tests is clear, management is usually self-evident. When a specific diagnosis is unclear, tissue biopsy may be appropriate. Thus the clinical approach to patient complaints or findings must be broad and not so focused as to prematurely exclude dangerous pathologies within the differential diagnosis.

The discussions in this chapter are arranged anatomically, beginning with the vulva and subsequently covering the vagina, cervix, uterus, oviducts, and ovaries. This chapter does not attempt to be encyclopedic; rather, lesions have been selected based on their clinical importance and prevalence. Therefore extremely rare lesions have been omitted. Because several non-neoplastic abnormalities and lesions present in ways similar to those of benign tumors, this chapter also discusses entities that are not specifically abnormal growths. Clinical problems such as torsion of the ovary, lacerations of the vagina, and hematomas of the vulva are examples of common conditions included in this chapter. Gynecologic infections and associated changes are discussed in Chapter 23.

The successful clinician uses both deductive and inductive reasoning in making a diagnosis. To master both of these techniques, one must be adept at history taking and physical examination skills and be able to form a complete list of possible etiologies that may be related to the patient's complaint. An understanding of the problems discussed in this chapter will be helpful in that endeavor.

## VULVA

### *URETHRAL CARUNCLE AND URETHRAL PROLAPSE*

Urethral caruncle and urethral prolapse are conditions that primarily affect postmenopausal women and premenarchal females. They are thought to occur as a result of decreased estrogen. A urethral caruncle is a small, fleshy mass that occurs at the posterior portion of the urethral meatus of postmenopausal women (Conces, 2012). The tissue of the caruncle is soft, smooth, friable, and bright red and initially appears as an eversion of the urethra (Fig. 18.1). Urethral caruncles are generally small, single, and sessile, but they may be pedunculated and grow to be 1 to 2 cm in diameter. Urethral caruncles are believed to arise from an ectropion of the posterior urethral wall associated with retraction and atrophy of the postmenopausal vagina. The growth of the caruncle is secondary to chronic irritation or infection. Histologically, the caruncle is composed of transitional and stratified squamous epithelium with a loose connective tissue. Often the submucosal layer contains relatively large dilated veins. Caruncles are frequently subdivided by their histologic appearance into papillomatous, granulomatous, and angiomatous varieties. They are often secondarily infected, producing ulceration and bleeding. The symptoms associated with urethral caruncles are variable. Many women are asymptomatic, whereas others experience dysuria, frequency, and urgency. Sometimes the caruncle produces point tenderness after contact with undergarments or during intercourse. Ulcerative lesions usually produce spotting on contact more commonly than hematuria. The diagnosis of a urethral caruncle is established by biopsy under local anesthesia, as it can appear like a neoplasm. Initial therapy is oral or topical estrogen and avoidance of irritation. If the caruncle does not regress or is symptomatic, it may be destroyed by cryosurgery, laser therapy, fulguration, or operative excision. Following operative destruction, a Foley catheter is usually left in place for 48 to 72 hours to prevent urinary retention. Follow-up is necessary to ensure that the patient does not develop urethral stenosis. It is not uncommon for the caruncle to recur. Small, asymptomatic urethral caruncles do not need treatment.

Urethral prolapse is predominantly a disease of the premenarcheal female, although it can occur in postmenopausal women (Fig. 18.2). Patients may have dysuria; however, most are asymptomatic. The annular rosette of friable, edematous, prolapsed mucosa does not have the bright red color of a caruncle and is easily distinguished from a caruncle because it is circumferential

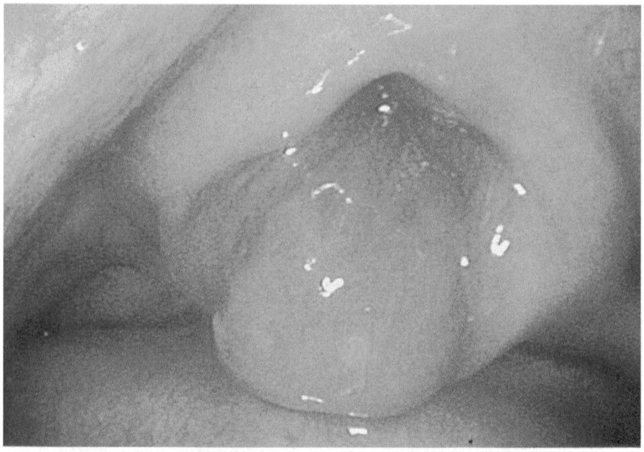

**Figure 18.1** Photo of urethral caruncle at the base of the meatus. (From Cundiff GW, Bent AE. *Endoscopic Diagnosis of the Female Lower Urinary Tract*. London: WB Saunders; 1999.)

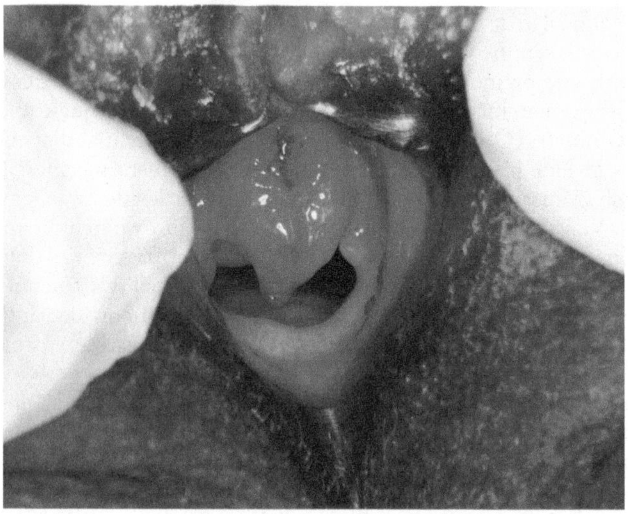

**Figure 18.2** Urethral prolapse found incidentally in a 5-year-old girl on a colposcopic examination for suspected abuse with an edematous red collar of tissue surrounding the urethral meatus. (From Hudson MJ, Swenson AD, Kaplan R, et al. Medical conditions with genital/anal findings that can be confused with sexual abuse. In: Jenny C, ed. *Child Abuse and Neglect: Diagnosis, Treatment and Evidence*. St. Louis: Elsevier; 2011.)

(Tunitsky, 2012). It may be ulcerated with necrosis or grossly edematous. Therapy of a prolapsed urethra is hot sitz baths and antibiotics to reduce inflammation and infection. Topical estrogen cream is sometimes an effective treatment. In rare cases it may be necessary to excise the redundant mucosa.

The differential diagnosis of urethral caruncles includes primary carcinoma of the urethra and prolapse of the urethral mucosa. Malignant lesions are usually hard and irregular in shape and typically are within the urethra itself (Tunitsky, 2012). Urethral carcinoma is primarily a disease of elderly women. The symptoms of a urethral carcinoma include bleeding, urinary frequency, and dysuria. The majority of urethral carcinomas are of squamous cell origin. Most of these rare carcinomas arise from the distal urethra

The differential diagnosis of a periurethral mass also includes: urethral diverticulum, leiomyoma, vaginal wall inclusion cyst,

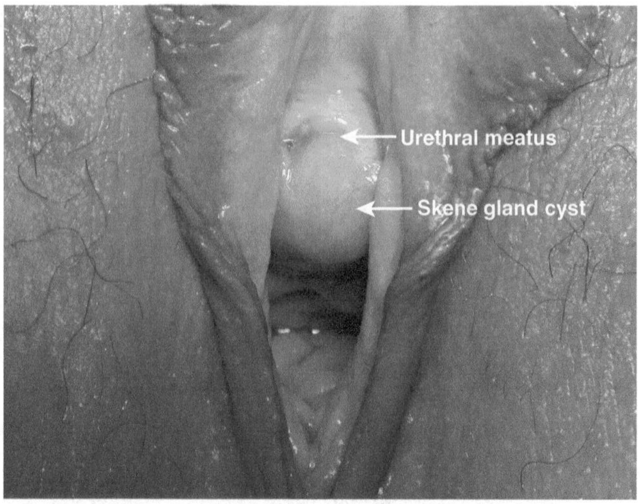


**Figure 18.3** Skene gland cyst. (From Shah SR, Nitti VW. Benign vaginal wall masses and paraurethral lesions. In: Nitti VW, ed. *Vaginal Surgery for the Urologist*. Philadelphia: Elsevier; 2012.)

Skene gland cyst or abscess, and less commonly Gartner duct cyst and ectopic ureterocele (Tunitsky, 2012). These will be discussed later in this chapter in the Vagina section.

## CYSTS

The most common large cyst of the vulva is a cystic dilation of an obstructed Bartholin duct. Bartholin glands open into the vulvar vestibule at about the 5 and 7 o'clock position, distal to the hymenal ring. Bartholin duct cysts and abscesses are fairly common, with a lifetime risk estimated to be 2% (Edwards, 2011). They occur most often during the third decade. Noninflamed cysts contain sterile, clear, mucinous fluid. They do not require treatment unless large enough to cause discomfort. Inflamed cysts may be treated with oral antibiotics or incision and drainage. A detailed review of the management of these cysts is reported by Wechter (Wechter, 2009). Lesions in the Bartholin gland can occur as carcinomas, a rare tumor that accounts for 2% to 7% of vulvar carcinomas. The median age at diagnosis is 57 years old and the incidence is highest among women in their 60s (Lee, 2015). Chapter 23 covers this topic in more detail.

Occasionally, the ducts of mucous glands of the vestibule become occluded. The resulting small cysts (usually 0.5 to 2 cm) may be clear, yellow, or blue. Similar small mucous cysts occur in the periurethral region. Wolffian duct cysts or mesonephric cysts are rare, but when they do occur, they are found near the clitoris and lateral to the hymeneal ring. These cysts have thin walls and contain clear serous fluid.

Skene duct cysts are rare, usually small, located on the anterior wall of the vagina along the distal urethra, and may present with symptoms of discomfort or be found on routine examination. These cysts arise secondary to infection and scarring of the small ducts (Fig. 18.3). The differential includes urethral diverticula. Clinically, physical compression of the cyst, unlike compression of a urethral diverticula, should not produce fluid from the urethral meatus. Imaging studies such as magnetic resonance imaging (MRI) or ultrasound may also assist in establishing the diagnosis. Asymptomatic cysts in premenopausal women may be

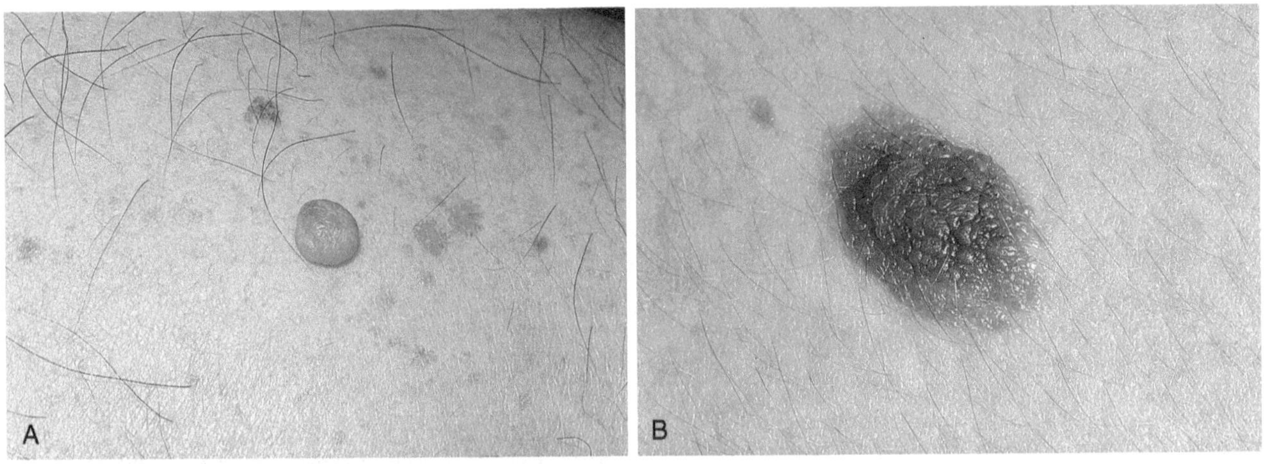


**Figure 18.4** Vulvar nevi. **A,** Dome-shaped intradermal nevus. **B,** Compound nevus with irregular pigmentation. (From Fisher BK, Margesson LJ. *Genital Skin Disorders: Diagnosis and Treatment.* St. Louis: Mosby; 1998.)

managed conservatively. Treatment is excision with careful dissection to avoid urethral injury.

The most common small vulvar cysts are epidermal cysts (epidermoid cysts). They are firm, smooth surfaced, white, yellow, slightly pink, or skin colored papules or nodules averaging 0.5 to 2 cm in size (Edwards, 2011). They are most commonly located on the hair-bearing areas. One or several lesions may be present, usually nontender and slow growing. They are firm to shotty in consistency, and their contents are usually under pressure. When noninflamed, they are asymptomatic and no treatment is necessary. If confirmation is needed, incision reveals white, caseous material, like thick cheese. Vulvar epidermal cysts do not have sebaceous cells or sebaceous material identified on microscopic examination but have keratin produced by keratinocytes in the lining of the cyst wall (Edwards, 2011). With rupture or leakage of a cyst, inflammation can occur necessitating treatment with heat applied locally and possibly incision and drainage. Cysts that become recurrently infected or produce pain should be excised when the acute inflammation has subsided. The typical epidermoid cyst develops from embryonic remnants of an anatomically malformed pilosebaceous unit.

An "inclusion cyst" may arise when bits of epithelium are implanted in the skin during surgery or trauma sufficient to break the skin surface. These may be seen at the site of an episiotomy or obstetric laceration. Large epidermal cysts may be confused with fibromas, lipomas, and hidradenomas.

## NEVUS

A nevus, commonly referred to as a *mole,* is a localized nest or cluster of melanocytes. These undifferentiated cells arise from the embryonic neural crest and are present from birth. Many nevi are not recognized until they become pigmented at the time of puberty. Approximately one of every 10 women has a pigmented vulvar lesion (Venkatesan, 2010). Vulvar nevi are one of the most common benign neoplasms in females. As with nevi in other parts of the body, they exhibit a wide range in depth of color, from blue to dark brown to black, and some may be amelanotic. The diameter of most common nevi ranges from a 3 to 10 mm. Grossly, a benign nevus may be flat, elevated, or pedunculated. The borders are sharp, the color even, and the shape is symmetrical. Dysplastic nevi are commonly 6 to 20 mm with one or more atypical features such as speckling of color, diffuse margination, additional red, white, or blue hues, and asymmetry. Other pigmented lesions in the differential diagnosis include hemangiomas, endometriosis, malignant melanoma, vulvar intraepithelial neoplasia, and seborrheic keratosis.

Vulvar nevi are generally asymptomatic. Most women do not closely inspect their vulvar skin; however, during examination, the use of a mirror held by the patient may facilitate teaching self-vulvar exam. Histologically the lesions are subdivided into three major groups: junctional (a symmetric macule), compound, and intradermal nevi (both papules) (Fig. 18.4).

Melanoma is the second most common malignancy arising in the vulva and accounts for 2% to 3% of all of the melanomas occurring in women, even though the vulva contains approximately 1% of the skin surface area of the body. The incidence of vulvar melanoma is stable or slightly decreasing. It is more common in older, white, women with a mean age at diagnosis of 68 years (Sugiyama, 2007). It is estimated that 50% of malignant melanomas arise from a preexisting nevus. Family history of melanoma is one of the strongest risk factors for the disease.

Ideally, all vulvar nevi should be excised and examined histologically. Special emphasis should be directed toward the flat junctional nevus and the dysplastic nevus, for they have the greatest potential for malignant transformation (Fig. 18.5). The lifetime risk of a woman developing melanoma from a congenital junctional nevus that measures greater than 2 cm in diameter is estimated to be approximately 10%. The lifetime risk of a melanoma forming in women with dysplastic nevi is 15 times that of the general population. Removal may be accomplished with local anesthesia or coincidentally with obstetric delivery or gynecologic surgery. Proper excisional biopsy should be three-dimensional and adequate in width and depth. Approximately 5 to 10 mm of normal skin surrounding the nevus should be included, and the biopsy should include the underlying dermis as well. Some patients are reluctant to have a "normal" appearing nevus removed. Nevi that are raised or contain hair rarely undergo malignant change. However, if they are frequently irritated or bleed spontaneously, they should be removed. Recent

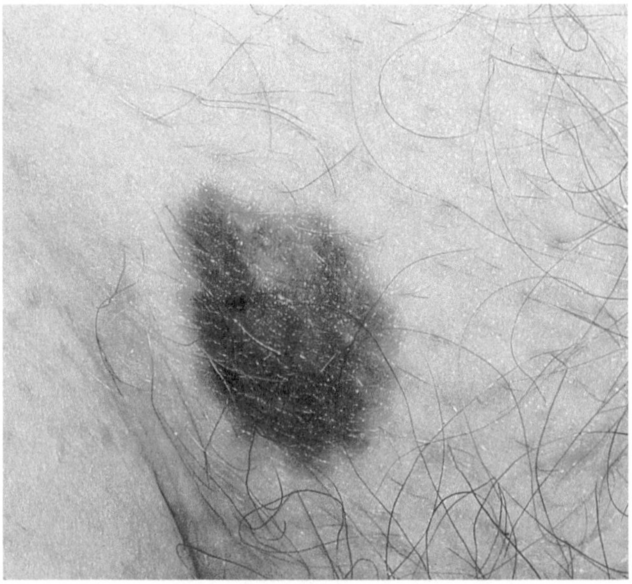

**Figure 18.5** Suprapubic dysplastic nevus with an irregular shape, reddish hue to the edges, and indistinct margins. (From Fisher BK, Margesson LJ. *Genital Skin Disorders: Diagnosis and Treatment.* St. Louis: Mosby; 1998.)

changes in growth or color, ulceration, bleeding, pain, or the development of satellite lesions mandate biopsy. The characteristic clinical features of an early malignant melanoma may be remembered by thinking ABCD: *asymmetry, border* irregularity, *color* variegation, and a *diameter* usually greater than 6 mm.

## HEMANGIOMA

Hemangiomas are rare malformations of blood vessels rather than true neoplasms. Vulvar hemangiomas frequently are discovered initially during childhood. They are usually single, 1 to 2 cm in diameter, flat, and soft, and they range in color from brown to red or purple. Histologically, the multiple channels of hemangiomas are predominantly thin-walled capillaries arranged randomly and separated by thin connective tissue septa. These tumors change in size with compression and are not encapsulated. Most hemangiomas are asymptomatic; occasionally they may become ulcerated and bleed.

There are at least five different types of vulvar hemangiomas. The strawberry and cavernous hemangiomas are congenital defects discovered in young children. The strawberry hemangioma is usually bright red to dark red, is elevated, and rarely increases in size after age 2. Approximately 60% of vulvar hemangiomas discovered during the first years of life spontaneously regress in size by the time the child goes to school. Cavernous hemangiomas are usually purple and vary in size, with the larger lesions extending deeply into the subcutaneous tissue. These hemangiomas initially appear during the first few months of life and may increase in size until age 2. Similar to strawberry hemangiomas, spontaneous resolution generally occurs before age 6. Senile or cherry angiomas are common small lesions that arise on the labia majora, usually in postmenopausal women. They are most often less than 3 mm in diameter, multiple, and red-brown to dark blue. Angiokeratomas are approximately twice the size of cherry angiomas, are purple or dark red, and occur in women between the ages of 30 and 50. They are noted for their rapid growth and tendency to bleed during strenuous exercise. In the differential diagnosis of an angiokeratoma is Kaposi sarcoma and angiosarcoma. Pyogenic granulomas are an overgrowth of inflamed granulation tissue. These lesions grow under the hormonal influence of pregnancy, with similarities to lesions in the oral cavity. Pyogenic granulomas are usually approximately 1 cm in diameter, usually a small nodule that is slightly pedunculated and appears "pinched in" at the base. They may be mistaken clinically for malignant melanomas, basal cell carcinomas, vulvar condylomas, or nevi. Treatment of pyogenic granulomas involves wide and deep excision to prevent recurrence.

The diagnosis is usually established by gross inspection of the vascular lesion. Asymptomatic hemangiomas and hemangiomas in children rarely require therapy. In adults, initial treatment of large symptomatic hemangiomas that are bleeding or infected may require subtotal resection. When the differential diagnosis is questionable, excisional biopsy should be performed. A hemangioma that is associated with troublesome bleeding may be destroyed by cryosurgery, sclerotherapy, or with the use of lasers. Cryosurgical treatment usually involves a single freeze/thaw cycle repeated three times at monthly intervals. Obviously, if the histologic diagnosis is questionable, any bleeding vulvar mass should be treated by excisional biopsy so that the definitive pathologic diagnosis can be established. Surgical removal of a large, cavernous hemangioma may be technically difficult. Lymphangiomas of the vulva do exist but are extremely rare.

Another rare malformation is the vulvar venous malformation. These lesions may become symptomatic at any age and are relatively prone to thrombosis. Venous malformations are different from vulvar varicosities, which are exacerbated with pregnancy and tend to regress postpartum. There are reports of the successful use of sclerotherapy for the treatment of the malformations.

## FIBROMA

Fibromas are the most common benign solid tumors of the vulva. They are more frequent than lipomas, the other common benign tumors of mesenchymal origin. Fibromas occur in all age groups and most commonly are found in the labia majora (Fig. 18.6). However, they actually arise from deeper connective tissue. Thus they should be considered as dermatofibromas. They grow slowly and vary from a few centimeters to one gigantic vulvar fibroma reported to weigh more than 250 pounds. Most are between 1 and 10 cm in diameter. The smaller fibromas are discovered as subcutaneous nodules. As they increase in size and weight, they become pedunculated. Smaller fibromas are firm; however, larger tumors often become cystic after undergoing myxomatous degeneration. Sometimes the vulvar skin over a fibroma is compromised by pressure and ulcerates.

Fibromas have a smooth surface and a distinct contour. On cut surface the tissue is gray-white. Fat or muscle cells microscopically may be associated with the interlacing fibroblasts. Fibromas have a low-grade potential for becoming malignant. Smaller fibromas are asymptomatic; larger ones may produce chronic pressure symptoms or acute pain when they degenerate. Treatment is operative removal if the fibromas are symptomatic or continue to grow. Occasionally they are removed for cosmetic reasons.

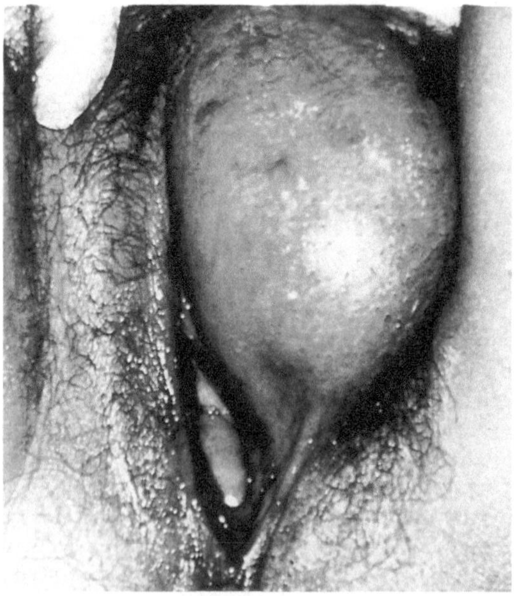

**Figure 18.6** Vulvar fibroma, the most common benign solid tumor of the vulva. (From Friedrich EG, ed. *Vulvar Disease.* 2nd ed. Philadelphia: WB Saunders; 1983.)

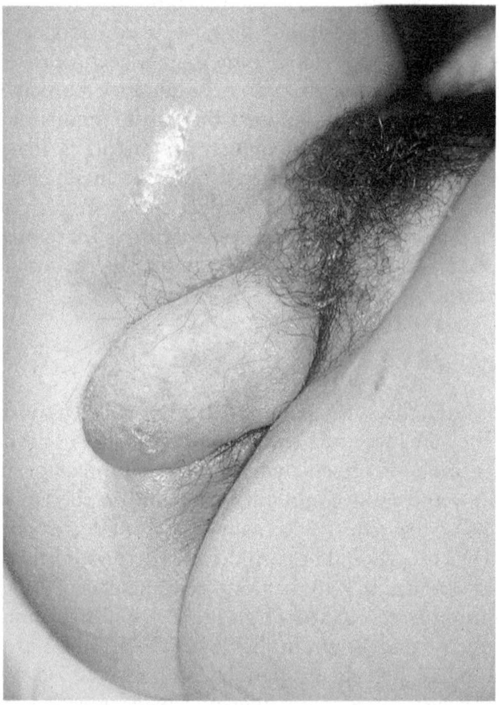

**Figure 18.7** Skin-colored pedunculated lipoma of labium major observed in a 15-year-old. (From Fisher BK, Margesson LJ. *Genital Skin Disorders: Diagnosis and Treatment.* St. Louis: Mosby; 1998.)

## LIPOMA

Lipomas are the second most frequent type of benign vulvar mesenchymal tumor. A common hamartoma of fat, lipomas of the vulva are similar to lipomas of other parts of the body. In the vulva, they are most commonly located periclitorally or within the labia majora (Edwards, 2011). When discovered they are softer and usually larger than fibromas (Fig. 18.7).

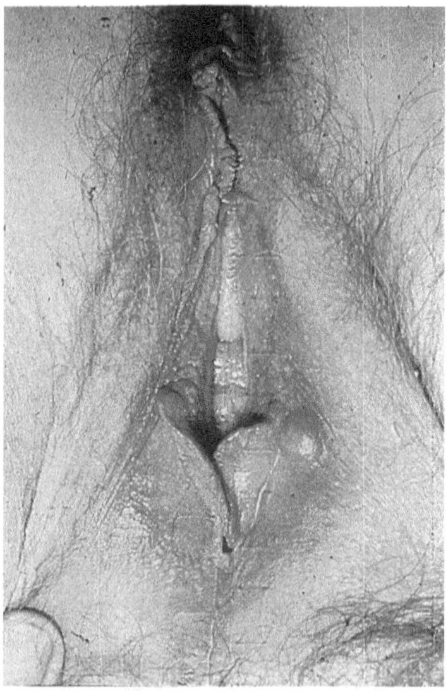

**Figure 18.8** Hidradenoma. (From Shea CH, Stevens A, Dalziel KL, et al. The vulva: cysts, neoplasms, and related lesions. In: Robboy SJ, Anderson MC, Russell P, eds. *Pathology of the Female Reproductive Tract.* Edinburgh: Churchill Livingstone; 2002.)

The majority of lipomas in the vulvar region are smaller than 3 cm. The largest vulvar lipoma reported in the literature weighed 44 pounds. They are slow growing, and their malignant potential is extremely low.

When a lipoma is cut, the substance is soft, yellow, and lobulated. Histologically, lipomas are usually more homogeneous than fibromas. Prominent areas of connective tissue occasionally are associated with the mature adipose cells of a true lipoma. Unless extremely large, lipomas do not produce symptoms. Computed tomography and MRI may be used to evaluate tumor extensions and anatomic connections with surrounding structures. MRI has been reported to facilitate the differentiation of vulvar lipomas from vulvar liposarcomas (Jayi, 2014). Excision is usually performed to establish the diagnosis, although smaller tumors may be followed conservatively.

## HIDRADENOMA (MAMMARY-LIKE GLAND ADENOMA)

The hidradenoma is a rare, small, benign vulvar tumor that is thought to be derived from mammary-like glands located in the anogenital area of women (Fig. 18.8). In a recent review of 46 cases, the tumors occurred only in postpubertal women ages 30 to 90 (Scurry, 2009). Clinically, they are small, smooth-surfaced, medium soft to firm nodules found most commonly on the labia majora or labia minora. They appear cystic and are usually asymptomatic; however, some patients report itching, bleeding, and mild pain. Hidradenomas may be cystic or solid. Approximately 50% of hidradenomas are less than 1 cm in diameter. These tumors have well-defined capsules and arise deep in the dermis. Histologically, because of its hyperplastic, adenomatous pattern, a hidradenoma may be mistaken at first glance for an adenocarcinoma. On close

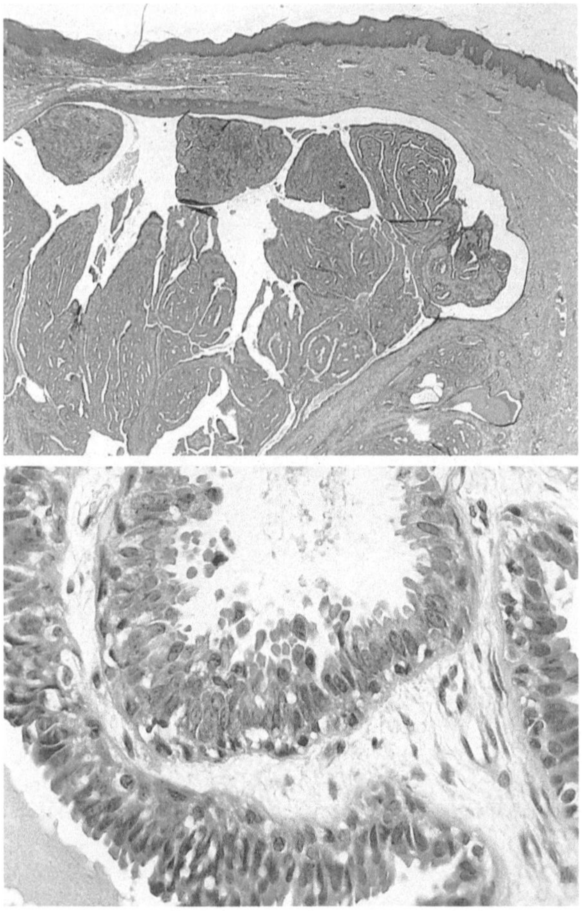

**Figure 18.9** Histology, low-, and high-power micrographs of hidradenoma. (From Clement PB, Young RH. *Atlas of Gynecologic Surgical Pathology*. Philadelphia: WB Saunders; 2000.)

inspection, however, although there is glandular hyperplasia with numerous tubular ducts, there is a paucity of mitotic figures and a lack of significant cellular and nuclear pleomorphism (Fig. 18.9). Excisional biopsy is the treatment of choice.

## SYRINGOMA

The syringoma is a benign skin adnexal neoplasm thought to be of eccrine origin. It is common on the face and eyelids but unusual on the vulva. In the vulvar area, these small, asymptomatic papules (usually less than 5 mm in diameter) are located on the labia majora. The papules are skin colored or yellow and may coalesce to form cords of firm tissue. They may be hormonally related, and pregnancy may aggravate associated pruritus. Progesterone receptor positivity has been reported (Heller, 2012). This tumor is usually treated by excisional biopsy. Cryosurgery, or laser therapy. The most common differential diagnosis is Fox-Fordyce disease, a condition of multiple retention cysts of apocrine glands accompanied by inflammation of the skin. The latter disease often produces intense pruritus, whereas syringoma is generally asymptomatic. Fox-Fordyce disease improves with pregnancy and oral contraceptive use and remits after menopause. It is treated with topical steroids, topical tretinoin cream, and oral isotretinoin.

## ENDOMETRIOSIS

Endometriosis of the vulva is uncommon. Only 1 in 500 women with endometriosis will present with vulvar lesions. The firm, small nodule or nodules may be cystic or solid and vary from a few millimeters to several centimeters in diameter. The subcutaneous lesions are blue, red, or purple, depending on their size, activity, and closeness to the surface of the skin. The gross and microscopic pathologic picture of vulvar endometriosis is similar to endometriosis of the pelvis (see Chapter 19). Vulvar adenosis may appear similar to endometriosis. The former condition occurs after laser therapy of condylomata acuminata.

Endometriosis of the vulva is usually found at the site of an old, healed obstetric laceration, episiotomy site, an area of operative removal of a Bartholin duct cyst, or along the canal of Nuck. The pathophysiology of development of vulvar endometriosis may be secondary to metaplasia, retrograde lymphatic spread, or potential implantation of endometrial tissue during operation. In one series, 15 cases of vulvar endometriosis believed to be associated with prophylactic postpartum curettage of the uterus to prevent postpartum bleeding, as there was not a single case of vulvar endometriosis in 13,800 deliveries without curettage, but 15 cases of vulvar endometriosis were associated with 2028 deliveries with prophylactic curettage. In general, symptoms do not appear for many months following implantation.

The most common symptoms of endometriosis of the vulva are pain and introital dyspareunia. The classic history is cyclic discomfort and an enlargement of the mass associated with menstrual periods. Treatment of vulvar endometriosis is by wide excision or laser vaporization depending on the size of the mass. Recurrences are common following inadequate operative removal of all the involved area and as a result, most would also recommend medical therapy with continuous oral contraceptives, progestins, or GnRH agonists.

## GRANULAR CELL MYOBLASTOMA

Granular cell myoblastoma is a rare, slow-growing, solid vulvar tumor. The tumor originates from neural sheath (Schwann) cells and is sometimes called a *schwannoma*. These tumors are found in connective tissues throughout the body, most commonly in the tongue, and occur in any age group. Approximately 7% of solitary granular cell myoblastomas are found in the subcutaneous tissue of the vulva. Twenty percent of multiple granular cell myoblastomas are located in the vulva. The tumors are usually located in the labia majora but occasionally involve the clitoris.

These tumors are subcutaneous nodules, usually 1 to 5 cm in diameter. They are benign but characteristically infiltrate the surrounding local tissue. The tumors are slow growing, but as they grow, they may cause ulcerations in the skin. The overlying skin often has hyperplastic changes that may look similar to invasive squamous cell carcinoma. Grossly, these tumors are not encapsulated. The cut surface of the tumor is yellow. Histologically, there are irregularly arranged bundles of large, round cells with indistinct borders and pink-staining cytoplasm. Initially the cell of origin was believed to be striated muscle; however, electron microscopic studies have demonstrated that this tumor is from cells of the neural sheath.

The tumor nodules are painless. Treatment involves wide excision to remove the filamentous projections into the surrounding tissue. If the initial excisional biopsy is not adequate and aggressive enough, these benign tumors tend to recur. Recurrence occurs in approximately one in five of these vulvar tumors. The appropriate therapy is a second operation with wider margins, as these tumors are not radiosensitive.

### VON RECKLINGHAUSEN DISEASE

The vulva is sometimes involved with the benign neural sheath tumors of von Recklinghausen disease (generalized neurofibromatous and café-au-lait spots). The vulvar lesions of this disease are fleshy, brownish red, polypoid tumors. Approximately 18% of women with von Recklinghausen disease have vulvar involvement. Excision is the treatment of choice for symptomatic tumors.

### OTHER ABNORMAL TISSUES PRESENTING AS VULVAR MASSES

The differential diagnosis of vulvar masses includes a large array of rare lesions and aberrant tissues, including leiomyomas, squamous papillomas, sebaceous adenomas, dermoids, accessory breast tissue and Müllerian or wolffian duct remnants, epidermal inclusion cysts, sebaceous cysts, mucous cysts, and skin diseases such as seborrheic keratosis, condylomata acuminata, and molluscum contagiosum. Some of these diseases are discussed in this chapter, others in Chapter 23.

### HEMATOMAS

Hematomas of the vulva are usually secondary to blunt trauma such as a straddle injury from a fall, an automobile accident, or a physical assault. Traumatic injuries producing vulvar hematomas have been reported secondary to a wide range of recreational activities, including bicycle, motorcycle, and go-cart riding; sledding; water skiing; cross-country skiing; and amusement park rides (Fig. 18.10). Spontaneous hematomas are rare and usually occur from rupture of a varicose vein during pregnancy or the postpartum period.

The management of nonobstetric vulvar hematomas is usually conservative unless the hematoma is greater than 10 cm in diameter or is rapidly expanding. The bleeding that produces a vulvar hematoma is usually venous in origin. Therefore it may be controlled by direct pressure. Compression and application of an ice pack to the area are appropriate therapy. If the hematoma continues to expand, operative therapy is indicated in an attempt to identify and ligate the damaged vessel. Often identification of the "key responsible vein" is a futile operative procedure. However, obvious bleeding vessels are ligated, and a pack is placed to promote hemostasis. During the operation, careful inspection and, if needed, endoscopy is performed to rule out injury to the urinary bladder and rectosigmoid.

The majority of small hematomas regress with time. However, a "chronic expanding hematoma" may become particularly problematic. The most familiar clinical example of this type of problem is the chronic subdural hematoma, but a similar situation may accompany vulvar hematomas. The underlying pathophysiology is the repetitive episodes of bleeding from capillaries in the granulation tissue of the hematoma, which result in a chronic, slowly expanding vulvar mass. Treatment of a chronic expanding hematoma is drainage and débridement.

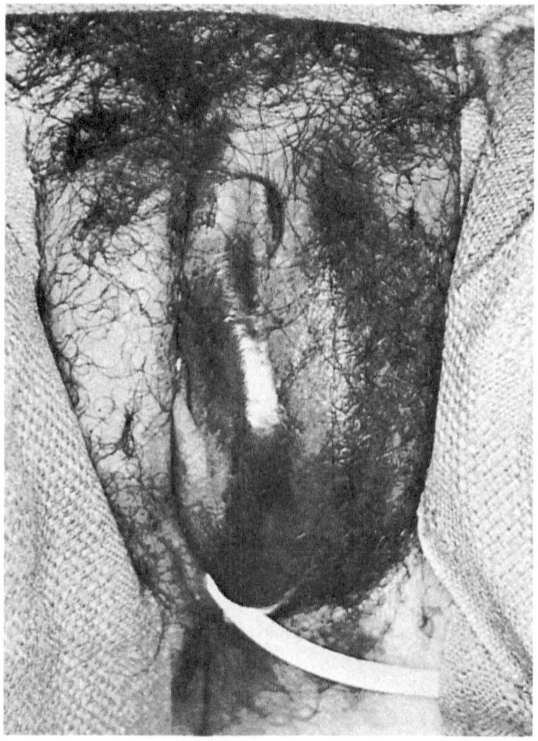

**Figure 18.10** Vulva hematoma from straddle injury that produced urethral obstruction. (From Naumann RO, Droegemueller W. Unusual etiology of vulvar hematomas. *Am J Obstet Gynecol.* 1982;142[3]: 357-358.)

## DERMATOLOGIC DISEASES

The skin of the vulva is similar to the skin over any surface of the body and is therefore susceptible to any generalized skin disease or involvement by systemic disease. The most common skin diseases involving the vulva include contact dermatitis, neurodermatitis, psoriasis, seborrheic dermatitis, cutaneous candidiasis, and lichen planus. The majority of vulvar skin problems are red, scalelike rashes, and the woman's primary complaint is of pruritus. The diagnosis and treatment of these lesions are often obscured or modified by the environment of the vulva. The combination of moisture and heat of the intertriginous areas may produce irritation; maceration; and a wet, weeping surface. Patients will commonly apply ointments and lotions, which may produce secondary irritation. Therefore it is important that the gynecologist examine the skin of the entire body, because the patient may have more classic lesions of the dermatologic disease in another location. The skin of the vulva is susceptible to acute infections produced by *Streptococcus* or *Staphylococcus,* such as folliculitis, furunculitis, impetigo, and a special chronic infection, hidradenitis suppurativa.

The nonspecific symptom complex of vulvar pruritus and burning is presented next as an introduction to the discussion of dermatologic diseases of the vulva.

## PRURITUS

Pruritus is the single most common gynecologic problem; it is a symptom of intense itching with an associated desire to scratch and rub the affected area. Not uncommonly, secondary vulvar pain develops in association or subsequent to pruritus. In some women pruritus becomes an almost unrelenting symptom, with the development of repetitive "itch-scratch" cycles. The itch-scratch cycle is a complex of itching leading to scratching, producing excoriation and then healing. The healing skin itches, leading to further scratching. Pruritus is a nonspecific symptom. The differential diagnosis includes a wide range of vulvar diseases, including skin infections, sexually transmitted diseases, specific dermatosis, vulvar dystrophies, lichen sclerosus, premalignant and malignant disease, contact dermatitis, neurodermatitis, atrophy, diabetes, drug allergies, vitamin deficiencies, pediculosis, scabies, psychological causes, and systemic diseases such as leukemia and uremia.

The management of pruritus involves establishing a diagnosis, treating the offending cause, and improving local hygiene. For successful treatment the itch-scratch cycle must be interrupted before the condition becomes chronic, resulting in lichenification of the skin, lichen simplex chronicus. Lichenification clinically is recognized by palpably thickened skin, exaggerated skin markings, and lichen-type scale. The resulting dry, scaly skin frequently cracks, forms fissures, and becomes secondarily infected, thus complicating the treatment. (See Chapter 30.)

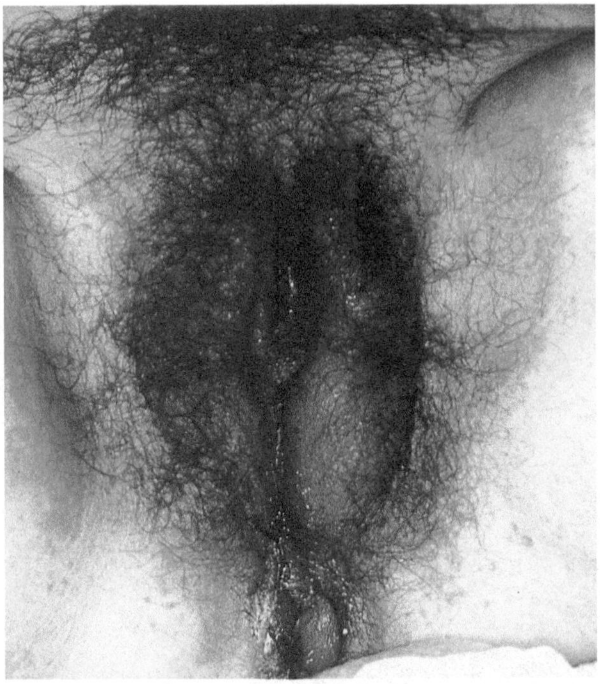

**Figure 18.11** Acute contact dermatitis to chlorhexidine. Edema and erythema are present in areas where the antiseptic chlorhexidine solution was applied. (From Stevens A, Dalziel KL. Vulvar dermatoses. In: Robboy SJ, Anderson MC, Russell P, eds. *Pathology of the Female Reproductive Tract*. Edinburgh: Churchill Livingstone; 2002.)

## CONTACT DERMATITIS

The vulvar skin, especially the intertriginous areas, is a frequent site of contact dermatitis. The vulvar skin is more reactive to exposure by irritants than other skin areas such as the extremities. Contact dermatitis is usually caused by one of two basic pathophysiologic processes: a primary irritant (nonimmunologic) or a definite allergic (immunologic) origin. In adult women, 50% of cases of chronic vulvovaginal pruritus is due to allergic and irritant contact dermatitis (Lambert, 2014). Substances that are irritants produce immediate symptoms such as a stinging and burning sensation when applied to the vulvar skin. The symptoms and signs secondary to an irritant disappear within 12 hours of discontinuing the offending substance. In contrast, allergic contact dermatitis requires 36 to 48 hours to manifest its symptoms and signs. Allergic contact dermatitis is a cell-mediated delayed-type (type IV) hypersensitivity reaction. There is development of antigen-specific T cells that may return to the skin at the next contact with the allergen. Often the signs of allergic contact dermatitis persist for several days despite removal of the allergen. Rarely, some women will be allergic to latex or semen. These reactions are type 1, IgE-mediated, immediate reactions. Angioedema and urticarial plaques and papules arise within minutes of contact. This may result in anaphylaxis. Excessive cleansing of the vulvar skin, and urinary or fecal incontinence, may precipitate an irritant dermatitis. The majority of chemicals that produce hypersensitivity of the vulvar skin are cosmetic or therapeutic agents, including vaginal contraceptives, lubricants, sprays, perfumes, douches, fabric dyes, fabric softeners, synthetic fibers, bleaches, soaps, chlorine, dyes in toilet tissues, and local anesthetic creams (Fig. 18.11). External chemicals that trigger the disease process must be avoided. Some of the most severe cases of contact dermatitis involve lesions of the vulvar skin secondary to poison ivy or poison oak. Women with a history of atopy or eczema are more prone to contact dermatitis and tend to be more sensitive to skin irritations.

Acute contact dermatitis results in a red, edematous, inflamed skin. The skin may become weeping and eczematoid. The most severe skin reactions form vesicles, and at any stage may become secondarily infected. The common symptoms of contact dermatitis include superficial vulvar tenderness, burning, and pruritus. Chronic untreated contact dermatitis can evolve into a syndrome of lichenification, with the skin developing a leathery appearance and texture, *lichen simplex chronicus* (Fig. 18.12).

The foundation of treatment of contact dermatitis is to withdraw the offending substance. Sometimes the distribution of the vulvar erythema helps to delineate the irritant. For example, localized erythema of the introitus often results from vaginal medication, whereas generalized erythema of the vulva is secondary to an allergen in clothing. It is possible to use a vulvar chemical innocuously for many months or years before the topical vulvar "allergy" develops.

Initial treatment of severe lesions is removal of all irritants or potential allergens and application of topical steroids until the skin returns to normal (Lambert, 2014). The vulvar skin should be kept clean and dry. Use of a barrier product such as zinc oxide ointment or vitamin A and D ointment may be needed to keep urine and feces away from the skin in patients with incontinence. The pain and burning can be treated with tepid water bath soaks several times a day for the first few days. Use of a lubricating agent such as petroleum jelly or Eucerin cream will reduce the pruritus by rehydrating the skin and should be applied after the

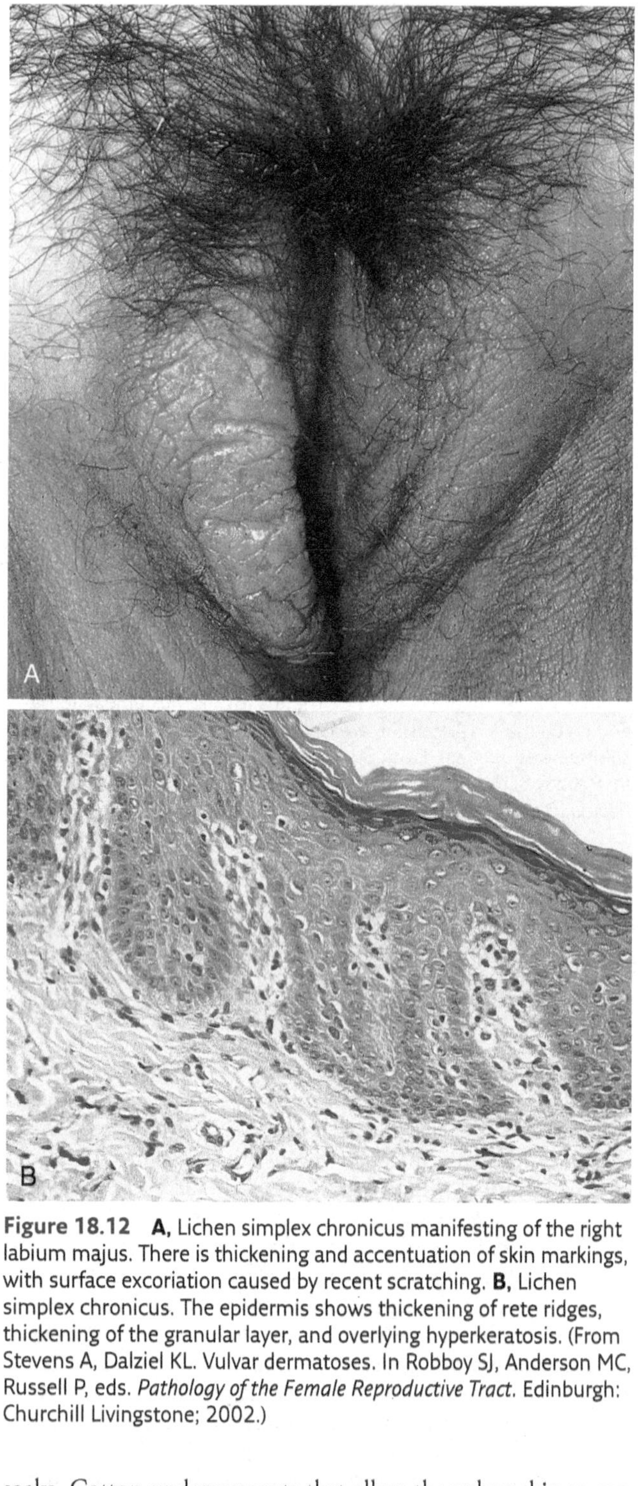

**Figure 18.12** **A,** Lichen simplex chronicus manifesting of the right labium majus. There is thickening and accentuation of skin markings, with surface excoriation caused by recent scratching. **B,** Lichen simplex chronicus. The epidermis shows thickening of rete ridges, thickening of the granular layer, and overlying hyperkeratosis. (From Stevens A, Dalziel KL. Vulvar dermatoses. In Robboy SJ, Anderson MC, Russell P, eds. *Pathology of the Female Reproductive Tract.* Edinburgh: Churchill Livingstone; 2002.)

soaks. Cotton undergarments that allow the vulvar skin to aerate should be worn, and constrictive, occlusive, or tight-fitting clothing such as pantyhose should be avoided. Use of a nonmedicated cornstarch baby powder may facilitate vulvar dryness. Hydrocortisone (0.5% to 1%) and fluorinated corticosteroids (Valisone, 0.1%, or Synalar, 0.01%) as lotions or creams may be rubbed into the skin two to three times a day for a few days to control symptoms. Synthetic systemic corticosteroids (prednisone, starting with 50 mg/day for 7 to 10 days in a decreasing dose) are sometimes necessary for treatment of poison ivy and poison oak or severe reactions. Antipruritic medications, such as antihistamines, are not of great therapeutic benefit except as soporific agents. Women often experience pruritus after steroid therapy for vulvar dermatitis. This is not necessarily a recurrence but rather represents a type of withdrawal reaction. This rebound pruritus is seen most commonly with prolonged and higher doses of steroids. After examination, the optimal treatment is a step-down to a short course of a low-potency topical steroid such as 1% hydrocortisone. Topical steroids should be continued for a month or more after clinical improvement as microscopic evidence of inflammation remains for a considerable period of time (Edwards, 2011).

## PSORIASIS

Psoriasis is a common, generalized skin disease of unknown origin. Generally, women develop psoriasis during their teenage years, with approximately 3% of adult women being affected. Approximately 20% of these have involvement of vulvar skin. The disease is chronic and relapsing, with an extremely variable and unpredictable course marked by spontaneous remissions and exacerbations. Twenty-five percent of women have a family history of the disease. Genetic susceptibility to develop psoriasis is believed to be multifactorial. Common areas of involvement are the scalp and fingernails. When psoriasis involves the vulvar skin, it produces both anxiety and embarrassment. Similar to candidiasis, psoriasis may be the first clinical manifestation of HIV infection.

Vulvar psoriasis usually affects intertriginous areas and is manifested by red to red-yellow papules. These papules tend to enlarge, becoming well-circumscribed, dull-red plaques (Fig. 18.13). Though the presence of classic silver scales and bleeding on gentle scraping of the plaques may help to establish the diagnosis, the scales are less common in the vulva than on other areas of the body.

With psoriasis on the vulvar region, the number of scales is extremely variable and frequently they are absent. Under the influence of the moisture and heat of the vulva, vulvar psoriasis may resemble candidiasis. Importantly for the diagnosis, psoriasis does not involve the vagina. Sometimes dermatologists treat refractory cases of psoriasis with oral retinoids. The margins of psoriasis are more well defined than the common skin conditions in the differential diagnosis, including candidiasis, seborrheic dermatitis, and eczema. Initial treatment for mild disease is 1% hydrocortisone cream. If the patient has pain secondary to chronic fissures, more moderate disease, a 4-week course of a fluorinated corticosteroid cream should be given. If this treatment is not successful, a dermatologist should be consulted. Several newer antipsoriatic treatments may benefit this condition, especially when it becomes moderate to severe including vitamin D analogs, topical retinoids, calcineurin inhibitors, salicylic acid, coal tar cyclosporine, and drugs that alter the immune system (biologics). Systemic steroids often produce a rebound flare-up of the disease.

## SEBORRHEIC DERMATITIS

Seborrheic dermatitis is a common chronic skin disease of unknown origin that classically affects the face, scalp, sternum, and the area behind the ears. Rarely, the mons pubis and vulvar areas may be involved. Vulvar lesions are pale to yellow-red,

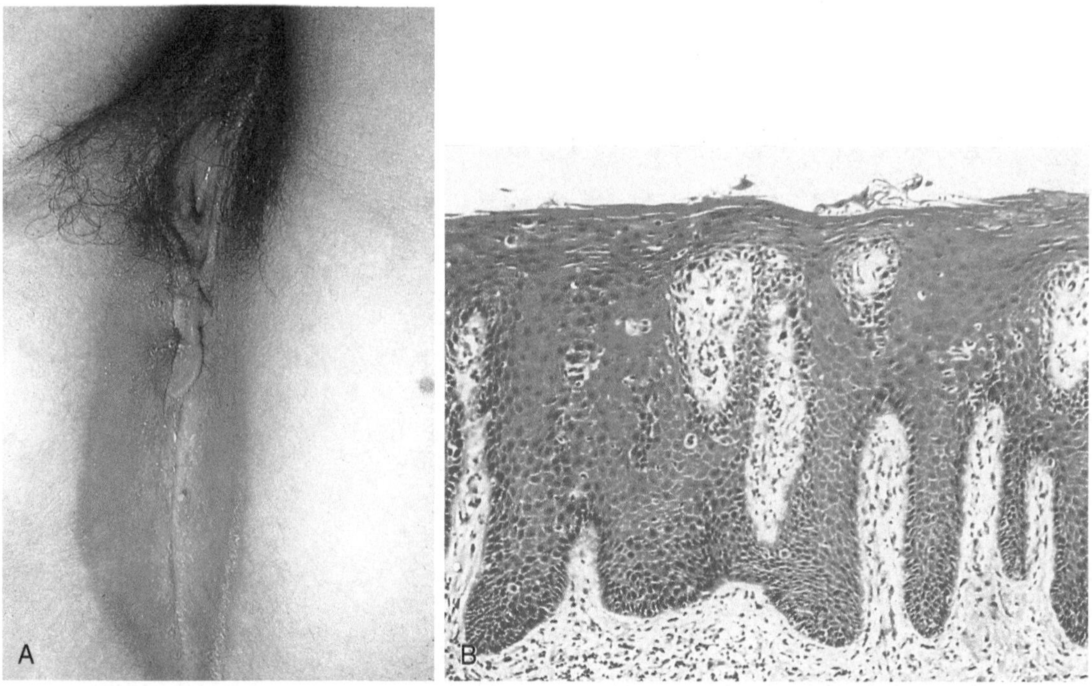


**Figure 18.13** **A,** Psoriasis of perineum and vulva. Flexural psoriasis often lacks the typical parakeratotic scale of psoriasis on other body sites. Painful erosion of the natal cleft is common. **B,** Psoriasis. There is psoriasiform hyperplasia of rete ridges with papillary dermal edema and telangiectasia. The parakeratotic scale on the skin surface is not prominent in vulvar psoriasis. (From Stevens A, Dalziel KL. Vulvar dermatoses. In: Robboy SJ, Anderson MC, Russell P, eds. *Pathology of the Female Reproductive Tract.* Edinburgh: Churchill Livingstone; 2002.)

erythematous, and edematous, and they are covered by a fine, nonadherent scale that is usually oily. Excessive sweating and emotional tension precipitate attacks. Although the cause is unknown, an abnormal reaction in the skin to a commensal yeast, *Pityrosporum ovale,* has been implicated in the pathogenesis. Treatment with topical and oral antifungal agents causes improvement; however, they are not as effective as topical steroids (Edwards, 2011). Approximately 2% to 4% of women have some form of the disease. The pruritus associated with seborrheic dermatitis varies from mild to severe. Treatment is similar to that for contact dermatitis, with hydrocortisone cream being the most effective medication. The differential diagnosis of seborrheic dermatitis includes psoriasis, cutaneous candidiasis, and contact dermatitis. Often it is difficult to differentiate between the cutaneous manifestations of psoriasis and seborrheic dermatitis. Clinically and pragmatically, the exact diagnosis is only of academic interest because the treatment is similar.

## LICHEN PLANUS

Lichen planus is an uncommon vulvovaginal dermatosis. Women complain of soreness, burning, itching, and dyspareunia. The disease presents most commonly as a hypertrophic, coalesced plaque similar to lichen sclerosis. Lichen sclerosis, though, does not involve the vagina, whereas lichen planus can. Three types of vulvar lichen planus have been described: erosive, classical, and hypertrophic. Erosive lichen planus is the most common variant occurring in 85% of the cases (Lambert, 2014). Erosive lichen planus is characterized by erosions around the introitus, clitoris, and labia majora and minora (Fig. 18.14). A lacy white edge is commonly seen. Vaginal involvement is common and patients may also present with contact bleeding, erythema, and scarring with synechiae. Many patients may also report mouth pain and have gingival lesions that appear erosive and desquamative. The classical type presents with small purple, polygonal papules, with sometimes a reticulate lace pattern. Hyperkeratotic lichen planus presents as single or multiple white-hyperkeratotic papules and plaques. Lichen planus is an inflammatory condition with unknown etiology; however, evidence suggests it to be an autoimmune disease of cellular immunity (Edwards, 2011). The autoimmune phenomenon, can be triggered by certain drugs, including beta-blockers, angiotensin-converting enzyme (ACE) inhibitors, and other medications. It may also arise spontaneously. The correct diagnosis is confirmed by a small punch biopsy of the vagina or vulva. Histologic findings (Fig. 18.15) include degeneration of the basal layers, a lymphocytic infiltrate of the dermis, as well as epidermal acanthosis.

This chronic disease tends to have spontaneous remissions and exacerbations that last for weeks to months. Treatment of local lesions is by use of a potent topical steroid ointment such as clobetasol applied twice daily. Steroid suppositories may be inserted intravaginally at night. If the patient is intensely symptomatic, oral steroids may be necessary. In postmenopausal women, topical or systemic estrogen replacement can also be crucial to avoid additional mucosal thinning. Other treatments for resistant cases include methotrexate, oral retinoids, oral griseofulvin, dapsone, azathioprine, cyclophosphamide, and topical cyclosporine. Surgery may be necessary to separate vaginal adhesions or uncover a buried clitoris. Postoperatively, the use of vaginal dilators can prevent scar reformation Women with this condition should be

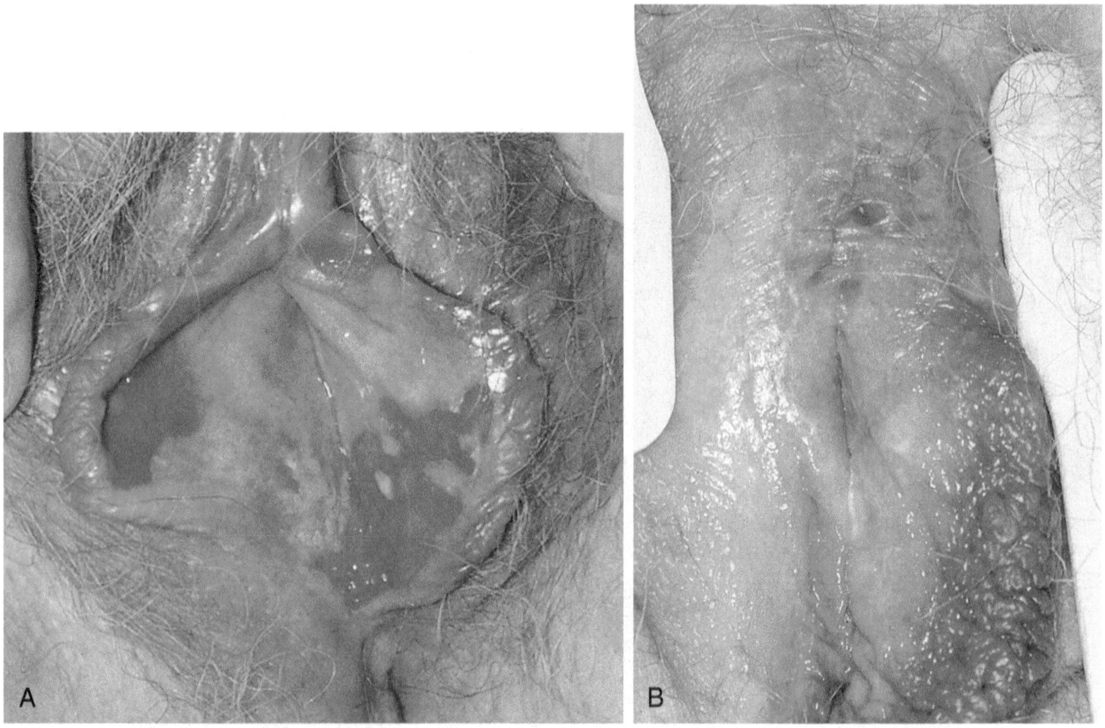


**Figure 18.14** Lichen planus. **A,** Eroded ulcers in the vulva. **B,** Lacy reticulated pattern of lichen planus with periclitoral scarring in a 71-year-old woman who has had oral lichen planus for 10 to 15 years, cutaneous lichen planus of arms and legs for 18 months, and bouts of erosive vaginal lichen planus with scarring and partial vaginal stenosis. (From Fisher BK, Margesson LJ. *Genital Skin Disorders: Diagnosis and Treatment.* St. Louis: Mosby; 1998.)

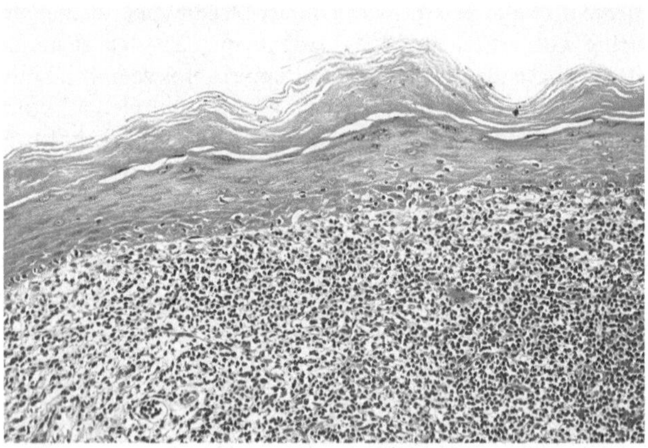

**Figure 18.15** Lichen planus, histology. Note hyperkeratosis with extensive basal layer destruction and a dense lichenoid infiltrate at the dermoepidermal junction. (From Stevens A, Dalziel KL. Vulvar dermatoses. In: Robboy SJ, Anderson MC, Russell P, eds. *Pathology of the Female Reproductive Tract.* Edinburgh: Churchill Livingstone; 2002.)

monitored at periodic intervals because of an associated increased risk of developing vulvar squamous cell carcinoma.

## BEHÇET DISEASE

Behçet disease is a rare disorder initially described as a triad of oral aphthous ulcers, genital aphthous ulcers, and uveitis. It is now known to be a multisystem disease with potential development of problems in many organ systems: skin, joints, cardiovascular, central nervous system, and gastrointestinal tract. The prevalence is high in the Mediterranean, Middle East, and Japan. Turkey has the highest prevalence with a rate of 100 to 400/100,000 individuals (Edwards, 2011). The diagnosis is made after exclusion of herpetic lesions and other ulcerative diseases. The symptoms respond to topical anesthetics. Severe disease may require antineoplastic therapy including methotrexate, steroids, or other medications.

## HIDRADENITIS SUPPURATIVA

Hidradenitis suppurativa is a chronic, unrelenting, refractory infection of skin and subcutaneous tissue that contains apocrine glands. The apocrine glands are found mainly in the axilla and the anogenital region. The disease is rare before puberty; 98% of cases are found in reproductive-age women, and most all disease regresses after menopause. As the infection progresses over time, deep scars and pits are formed (Fig. 18.16). The patient undergoes great emotional distress as this condition is both painful and is associated with a foul-smelling discharge. Current theories of the cause of this condition favor an inflammation beginning in the hair follicles (Fig. 18.17). Thus the term sometimes used synonymously is *acne inversa.* The lesions involve the mons pubis, the genitocrural folds, and the buttocks. The differential diagnosis of hidradenitis suppurativa includes simple folliculitis, Crohn disease of the vulva, pilonidal cysts, and granulomatous sexually transmitted diseases. The differentiation from Crohn disease is usually made by history with an absence of gastrointestinal (GI)

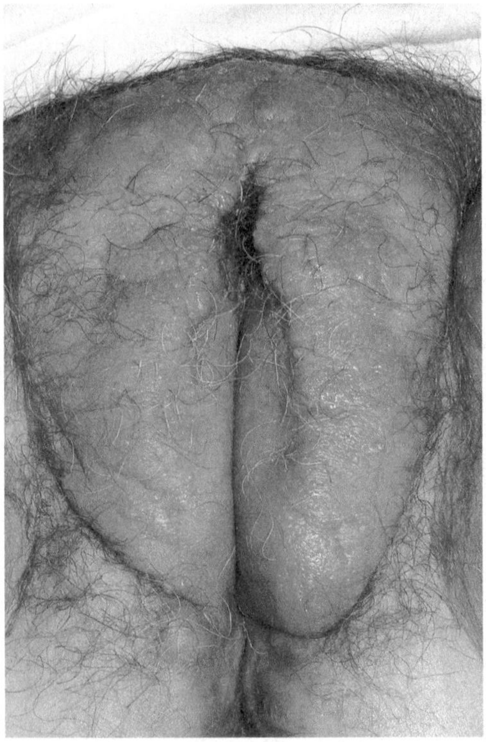

**Figure 18.16** Hidradenitis suppurativa: multiple vulvar abscesses with edema of the mons pubis and labia majora. Notice the "pitting" and "scars" from chronic infection. (From Amankwah Y, Haefner H. Vulvar edema. *Dermatol Clin.* 2010;28[4]:765-777.)

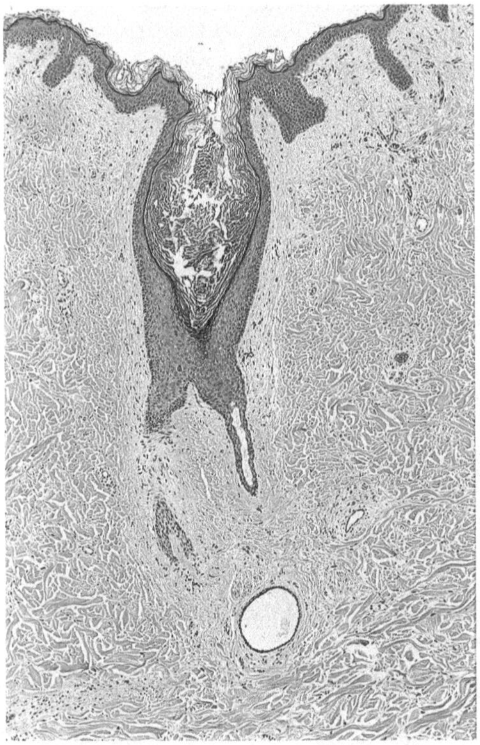

**Figure 18.17** Hydradenitis suppurativa. Biopsy with follicular plugging and connection to dilated apocrine duct. (From Kelly P. Folliculitis and the follicular occlusion tetrad. In Bolognia JL, Jorizzo JL, Rapini RP, eds. *Dermatology.* Edinburgh: Mosby; 2003.)

involvement. The early phase of the disease involves infection of the follicular epithelium, with what first appears as a boil. Erythema, involvement of multiple follicles, chronic infections that burrow and form cysts that break open and track through subcutaneous tissue, creating odiferous and painful sinuses and fistula in the vulva. The chronic scarring, fibrosis, and hyperpigmentation with foul-smelling discharge and soiling of underclothes lead to a socially debilitating condition. The diagnosis should be confirmed by biopsy.

Early on in the disease process there are small furuncles and folliculitis, for which topical and oral clindamycin is usually effective in the short term, usually requiring a 3-month course of antibiotics. Unfortunately, relapse is common; if treatment with long-term antibiotic therapy and topical steroids is unsuccessful, other medical therapies have included antiandrogens, isotretinoin, and cyclosporine. The treatment of refractory cases is aggressive, wide operative excision of the infected skin.

## EDEMA

Edema of the vulva may be a symptom of either local or generalized disease. Two of the most common causes of edema of the vulva are secondary reactions to inflammation or to lymphatic blockage. Vulvar edema is often recognized before edema in other areas of the female body is noted. The loose connective tissue of the vulva and its dependent position predispose to early development of pitting edema. Systemic causes of vulvar edema include circulatory and renal failure, ascites, and cirrhosis. Vulvar edema also may occur after intraperitoneal fluid is instilled to prevent adhesions or for dialysis. Local causes of vulvar edema include allergy, neurodermatitis, inflammation, trauma, and lymphatic obstruction caused by carcinoma or infection. Infectious diseases that are associated with vulvar edema include necrotizing fasciitis, tuberculosis, syphilis, filariasis, and lymphogranuloma venereum.

### Vulvar Pain Syndromes: Vulvar Vestibulitis, Vestibulodynia, and Dysesthetic Vulvodynia

Vulvar pain, vulvodynia, is one of the most common gynecologic problems, reported by up to 16% of women in the general population (Stockdale, 2014). Vulvodynia has been defined by the International Society for the Study of Vulvovaginal Disease as vulvar discomfort, most often described as burning pain, occurring in the absence of relevant visible findings or a specific clinically identifiable, neurologic disorder (Moyal-Barracco, 2004). It is not caused by infection, inflammation, neoplasia, or a neurologic disorder. The disease has a wide spectrum of symptomatology and response to treatment; therefore causation is most likely multifactorial. The diagnosis is made after excluding other treatable causes. A complete history identifying the onset of pain, other associated symptoms, duration of pain, medical and sexual history, treatments tried, allergies, and triggers for pain should be taken. Examination using cotton swab testing to identify areas of pain as well as pain intensity as described in The Vulvodynia Guideline (Haefner, 2005) is helpful to follow patients and response to treatment over time. Large population-based studies have noted that symptoms wax and wane, with many women having spontaneous remission. Reed and colleagues noted a 10% remission over a 2-year evaluation period. Interestingly, in the control group, approximately 2% of women developed symptoms (Reed, 2008).

The terms *vulvar pain syndrome, vulvodynia,* and *vulvar vestibulitis* are often used interchangeably. Vulvar vestibulitis is somewhat of a misnomer, because it is not inflammation. Vulvar pain syndrome is further subdivided into two categories: vestibulodynia and dysesthetic vulvodynia. The two conditions have a significant amount of overlap, although different etiologies and clinical course. In general, vestibulodynia is found in younger women, most commonly white, with onset shortly after puberty through the mid-20s. Dysesthetic vulvodynia is most common in peri- and postmenopausal women who have rarely if ever had previous vulvar pain.

The differential diagnosis of vulvar pain includes neurologic diseases, herpes simplex infection, chronic infections, abuse, pain syndromes, neoplasia, contact dermatitis, and psychogenic causes. Chronic pain is considered to be part of the vulvodynia spectrum, once the diagnoses of infection, invasive disease, and inflammation have been excluded. Severe chronic pain can be socially debilitating, and these patients have a wide spectrum of associated affective symptomatology as well. Women with vulvodynia have greater psychologic distress than women who have other vulvar problems. Importantly, these psychologic concerns must be addressed as part of the therapeutic management.

Vestibulodynia involves the symptom of allodynia, which is hyperesthesia, a pain that is related to nonpainful stimuli. The pain is not present without stimulation. The diagnostic maneuver to establish the presence of allodynia is to lightly touch the vulvar vestibule with a cotton-tipped applicator. The vulvar areas most likely to be affected are from the 4 to 8 o'clock positions along the vulvar-vaginal borders. Erythema is not always present, but when present it is confined to the vulvar vestibule (Fig. 18.18). Additionally, patients with vestibulodynia experience intolerance to pressure in the vulvar region. This pain is neurogenic in origin. The intolerance to pressure may be caused by tampon use, sexual activity, or tight clothing. The pain is described as raw and burning. It is not a spontaneous pain; it is invoked. However, it is severe in nature. Some authors have suggested that symptoms be present for at least 6 months prior to establishing the diagnosis. The symptoms may appear around the time of first intercourse, or within the next 5 to 15 years. Studies of women with vulvar vestibulodynia have found no increased incidence of sexual abuse compared with controls. However, many women are found to have erotophobia. Some even noted an increased nerve density and normal estrogen receptors compared with controls. In contrast, other investigators have noted an increase in alpha-estrogen receptors. Theories regarding the etiology cite potential immunologic, and infectious factors, though no theory has been proved to date. Oral contraceptive use in younger women and hormone replacement in older women have no association with vestibulodynia.

Vulvar dysesthesia, vulvodynia, is a non-localized pain that is constant (not provoked by touch), mimicking a neuralgia. Allodynia is rarely noted, and erythema is also much less common than in vulvar vestibulodynia. Women with vulvodynia are more often perimenopausal or postmenopausal. Dyspareunia is currently present but has usually not been present prior to the development of dysesthesia. Similar to women with vulvar vestibulodynia, there is not an increased history of sexual abuse compared with controls. Women with dysesthesia also have an increased incidence of chronic interstitial cystitis. In general, both groups of women have an increased incidence of atopy. In some, a history of inflammation from topical agents may be elicited. These agents have usually either been

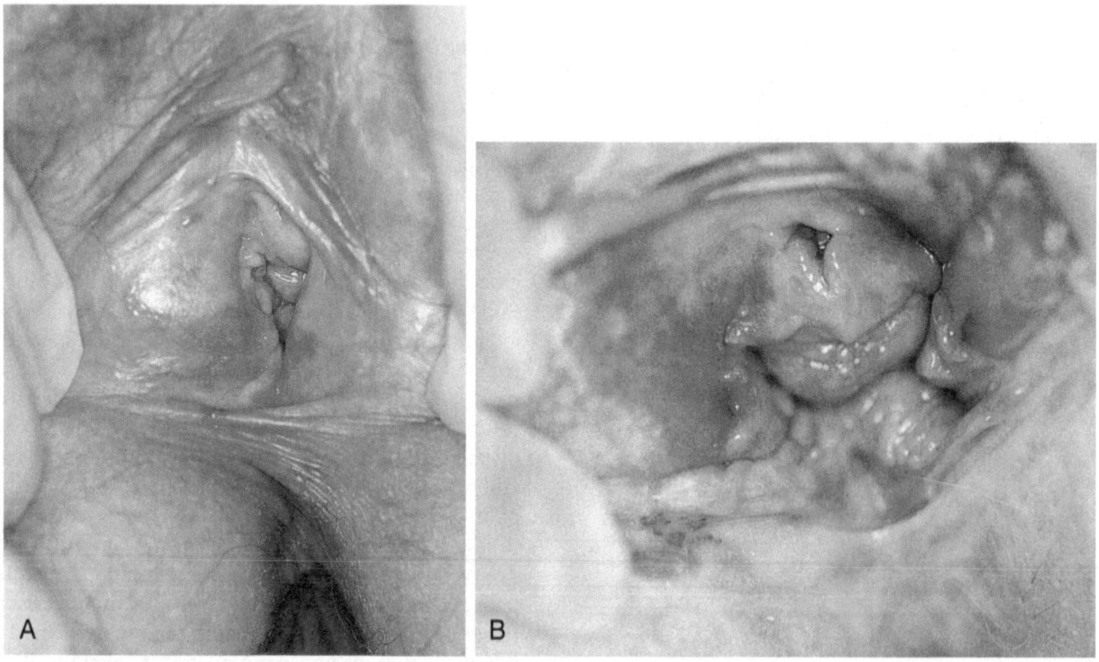


**Figure 18.18** Vulvar vestibulitis. **A,** Redness localized to the right Bartholin duct opening and, below it, vulvar vestibulitis. **B,** Discrete localized periglandular erythema in vulvar vestibulitis in a 60-year-old woman. (From Fisher BK, Margesson LJ. *Genital Skin Disorders: Diagnosis and Treatment.* St. Louis: Mosby; 1998.)

self-prescribed or prescribed by a professional to treat initially what seems to be infection. Patients are often depressed and anxious, but this is thought to be a secondary reaction to the chronic pain. An outline for evaluating these patients is presented in Box 18.1. Prior to the diagnosis, one should exclude infection from atypical Candida (which may not be obvious on inspection and should be diagnosed by culture), as well as exclusion of infection by group B streptococcus. Some would recommend that prior to extensive treatment a punch biopsy should be obtained to rule out dermatitis presenting atypically, including lichen sclerosis.

The therapeutic approach for these two conditions emphasizes a sensitivity to the debilitating social aspects of the problem. Similar to other chronic pain syndromes, tricyclic antidepressants or gabapentin have been found to be successful in several series. Doses of gabapentin range from 300 to 3600 mg, usually given with increasing doses every week. Most authors start at 300 mg daily, increase to 300 mg twice daily, then three times a day, then 600 mg three times per day to 900 three times per day and so on; the average affective dose is approximately 1800 mg a day. Approximately 66% to 75% of women have a response to treatment with gabapentin. When the medication is discontinued, it should be tapered. Biofeedback and behavior modification therapy have also produced relief. Zolnoun and coworkers reported on 61 women treated successfully for vulvar vestibulitis with 5% lidocaine ointment nightly for a period of 6 to 8 weeks (Zolnoun, 2003). In the past, women with refractory vulvar vestibulitis have been treated with surgical removal of the vulvar vestibule and reapproximation of tissue. The surgery is difficult, with a significant complication rate, but results are generally good. In one series of 126 women with vulvar vestibulitis, the complication rate was 39%; 89% of women felt that the surgery improved their condition enough to recommend it to other women. Importantly, 30% of women will have spontaneous relief of their symptoms without any treatment. Reports of multilevel nerve block given simultaneously for refractory cases have shown some response. Botulinum neurotoxin is also effective in some women, particularly for those with concurrent vaginismus and levator ani spasm. Series of treatments and combinations of treatments are often used.

For women with vestibulodynia unresponsive to other therapies, surgery is usually recommended. Vestibulectomy and modified vestibulectomy (partial or limited from 3 to 9 o'clock) have shown resolution in 60% to 90% compared with 40% to 80% for nonsurgical interventions (Stockdale, 2014). Surgery was noted to be most effective in younger women. Some advocate for partial vestibulectomy, because most pain and painful skin occurs in the lower half of the vestibule. Complications from vestibulectomy include occlusion of the Bartholin gland leading to development of cysts. This problem requires surgical "unroofing" of the duct.

**Box 18.1 Evaluation of Patients with Vulvar Pain**

- Examination of vulva for abnormal redness, erosions, crusting, ulceration, hypopigmentation
- Cotton swab test to identify areas of pain on pressure (e.g., vestibule)
- Sensory neurologic examination for allodynia and symmetric sensation
- Examination for vaginal redness, erosions, pallor, dryness
- Biopsy of specific skin findings for evaluation by dermatopathologist
- Microscopic evaluation of vaginal secretions for yeast, pH, increased white blood cells
- Culture for *Candida* (exclusive of *C. albicans*) and bacteria (especially group B *Streptococcus*)
- Evaluation for depression and impact on quality of life
- Classification of vulvar vestibulitis syndrome or dysesthetic vulvodynia

## VAGINA

### URETHRAL DIVERTICULUM

A urethral diverticulum is a permanent, epithelialized, saclike projection that arises from the posterior urethra. Most are thought to be acquired and present in women between 30 and 60 years of age (Lee, 2005). They often present as a mass of the anterior vaginal wall and represent approximately 84% of periurethral masses (Table 18.1). It is a common problem, being discovered in approximately 1% to 3% of women. Most urogynecologists have noted a decline in the prevalence of this condition since the early 1990s. The majority of cases are initially diagnosed in reproductive-age females, with the peak incidence in the fourth decade of life. The symptoms of a urethral diverticulum are nonspecific and are identical to the symptoms of a lower urinary tract infection. To diagnose this elusive condition, one should suspect urethral diverticulum in any woman with chronic or recurrent lower urinary tract symptoms. The urologic aspects of this condition are discussed in Chapter 21. Histologically the diverticulum is lined by epithelium; however, there is a lack of muscle in the saclike pocket.

Urethral diverticula may be congenital or acquired. Few urethral diverticula are present in children; therefore it is assumed that most diverticula are not congenital. The anatomy of the urethra has been described as a tree with many stunted branches that represent the periurethral ducts and glands. It is assumed that the majority of urethral diverticula result from repetitive or chronic infections of the periurethral glands. The suburethral infection may cause obstruction of the ducts and glands, with subsequent production of cystic enlargement and retention cysts. These cysts may rupture into the urethral lumen and produce a suburethral diverticulum. Persistent inflammation and stasis can lead to stone formation (10%). Malignancy has been reported in 6% to 9% of cases, mostly adenocarcinoma (Foley, 2011). Urethral diverticula are small, from 3 mm to 3 cm in diameter. The majority of urethral diverticula open

**Table 18.1** Final Diagnosis of Periurethral Mass and Frequency

| Diagnosis | *N* (%) | 95% Confidence Interval (%) |
|---|---|---|
| Urethral diverticulum | 66 (84) | 73-91 |
| Diverticulum with malignancy | 4 (6) | 2-14.8 |
| Vaginal cyst | 6 (7) | 3-15 |
| Leiomyoma | 4 (5) | 1-12 |
| Vaginal squamous cell carcinoma | 2 (2.5) | 0.03-8.8 |
| Etopic ureter | 2 (2.5) | 0.03-8.8 |
| Granuloma | 1 (1) | 0.03-6.8 |

From Blaivas JG, Flisser AJ, Bleustein CB, Panagopoulos G. Periurethral masses: diagnosis in a large series of women. *Obstet Gynecol.* 2004;103(5 Pt 1):842-847.

into the midportion of the urethra (Table 18.2). Occasionally, multiple suburethral diverticula occur in the same woman.

Classically, the symptoms associated with the urethral diverticulum are extremely chronic in nature and they have not resolved with multiple courses of oral antibiotic therapy. The most common symptoms associated with urethral diverticula are urinary urgency, frequency, and dysuria occurring about 90% of the time as the presenting symptom. Approximately 15% of women with urethral diverticula experience hematuria. Other authors have stressed the three *D*s associated with a diverticulum: *dysuria, dyspareunia,* and *dribbling* of the urine. Although for years, postvoiding dribbling has been termed a classic symptom of urethral diverticulum, it is reported by fewer than 10% of women with this condition. In Lee's series a palpable, tender mass was discovered in 56 of 108 patients (Lee, 2005). It is interesting that in most large series, approximately 20% of the women are asymptomatic. A classic sign of a suburethral diverticulum is the expression of purulent material from the urethra after compressing the suburethral area during a pelvic examination. Although the sign of producing a discharge by manual expression is specific, its sensitivity is poor.

The foundation of diagnosing urethral diverticulum is the physician's awareness of the possibility of this defect occurring in women with chronic symptoms of lower urinary tract infection. Historically, the two most common methods of diagnosing urethral diverticulum have been the voiding cystourethrography and cystourethroscopy. Approximately 70% of urethral diverticula will be filled by contrast material on a postvoiding radiograph with a lateral view. Cystourethroscopy will demonstrate the urethral opening of the urethral diverticulum in approximately 6 of 10 cases. Other diagnostic tests used to identify urethral diverticula include urethral pressure profile recordings, transvaginal ultrasound, computed tomography (CT) scans, magnetic resonance imaging (MRI), and positive-pressure urethrography. For diagnosis of urethral diverticulum, MRI sensitivity is 100% as the resolution is excellent (Tunitsky, 2012). Ultrasonography, done translabially (or introitally) may assist in the assessment of the mass being cystic or solid. Positive-pressure urethrography is done with a special double-balloon urethral catheter (Davis catheter) (Fig. 18.19). Classically, the recordings of the pressure profile of the urethra demonstrate a biphasic curve in a woman with a urethral diverticulum. If a woman has a urethral diverticulum and urinary incontinence, performing a stress urethral pressure profile will help to differentiate the etiology. The differential diagnosis includes the Gartner duct cyst, an ectopic ureter that empties into the urethra, and Skene glands cysts.

**Table 18.2** Location of the Ostium in 108 Female Patients with Diverticulum of the Urethra

| Site | Number of Patients |
|---|---|
| Distal (external) third of the urethra | 11 |
| Middle third of the urethra | 55 |
| Proximal (inner) third of the urethra (including vesical neck) | 18 |
| Multiple sites | 18 |
| Unknown | 6 |

From Lee RA. Diverticulum of the urethra: clinical presentation, diagnosis, and management. *Clin Obstet Gynecol.* 1984;27:490-498.

Several different operations can correct urethral diverticula. Excisional surgery should be scheduled when the diverticulum is not acutely infected. Operative techniques can be divided into transurethral and transvaginal approaches, with most gynecologists preferring the transvaginal approach as described by Lee (Lee, 2005). The majority of diverticula enter into the posterior aspect of the urethra. Diverticula of the distal one third may be treated by simple marsupialization. Following operations, approximately 80% of patients obtain complete relief from symptoms. Some diverticula have multiple openings into the urethra. Complete excision of this network of fistulous connections is important. The recurrence rate varies between 10% and 20%, and many failures are due to incomplete surgical resection. The most serious consequences of surgical repair of urethral diverticula are urinary incontinence and urethrovaginal fistula. Postoperative incontinence usually follows operative repairs of large diverticula that are near the bladder neck. This incontinence may be secondary to damage to the urethral sphincter. The incidence of each of these complications is approximately 1% to 2%.

## INCLUSION CYSTS

Inclusion cysts are the most common cystic structures of the vagina. In a series of 64 women with cystic masses of the vagina, 34 had inclusion cysts. The cysts are usually discovered in the posterior or lateral walls of the lower third of the vagina. Inclusion cysts vary from 1 mm to 3 cm in diameter. Similar to inclusion cysts of the vulva, inclusion cysts of the vagina are more common in parous women. Inclusion cysts usually result from birth trauma or gynecologic surgery. Often they are discovered in the site of a previous episiotomy or at the apex of the vagina following hysterectomy.

Histologically, inclusion cysts are lined by stratified squamous epithelium. These cysts contain a thick, pale yellow substance that is oily and formed by degenerating epithelial cells. Often these cysts are erroneously called sebaceous cysts in the misbelief

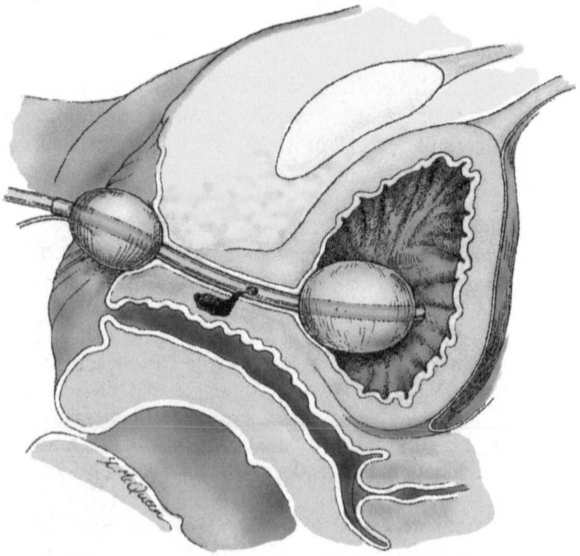

**Figure 18.19** Double-balloon catheter in use for positive-pressure urethrography.

that the central material is sebaceous. Similar to vulvar inclusion cysts, the cause is either a small tag of vaginal epithelium buried beneath the surface following a gynecologic or obstetric procedure or a misplaced island of embryonic remnant that was destined to form epithelium.

The majority of inclusion cysts are asymptomatic. If the cyst produces dyspareunia or pain, the treatment is excisional biopsy.

## DYSONTOGENETIC CYSTS

Dysontogenetic cysts of the vagina are thin-walled, soft cysts of embryonic origin. Whether the cysts arise from the mesonephros (Gartner duct cyst), the paramesonephricum (Müllerian cyst), or the urogenital sinus (vestibular cyst) is predominantly of academic rather than clinical importance. The cysts may be differentiated histologically by the epithelial lining (Fig. 18.20). Most mesonephric cysts have cuboidal, nonciliated epithelium. Most perimesonephric cysts have columnar, endocervical-like epithelium. Occasionally pressure produced by the cystic fluid produces flattening of the epithelium, which makes histologic diagnosis less reliable. Although most commonly single, dysontogenetic cysts may be multiple. The cysts are usually 1 to 5 cm in diameter and are usually discovered in the upper half of the vagina (Fig. 18.21). Sometimes multiple small cysts may present like a string of large, soft beads. A large cyst presenting at the introitus may be mistaken for a cystocele, anterior enterocele, or obstructed aberrant ureter. Approximately 1 in 200 females develop these cysts.

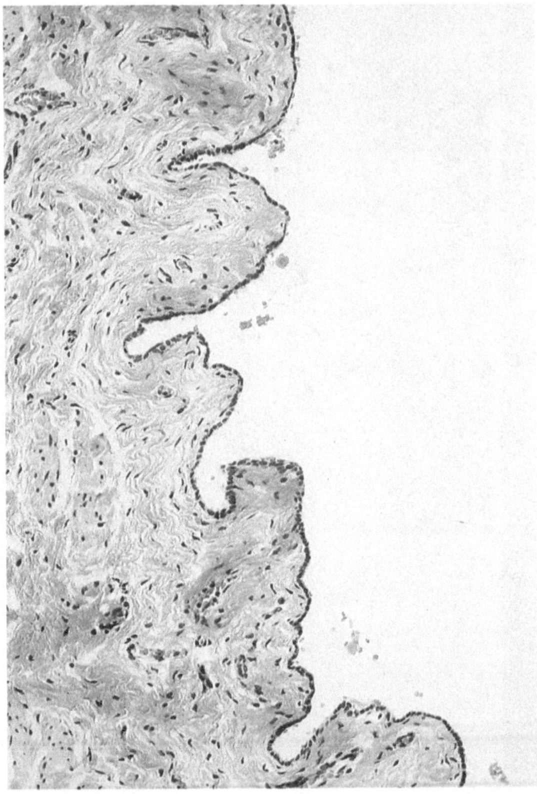

**Figure 18.20** Histology of vaginal cyst. Gartner duct cyst from the lateral vaginal wall. The cyst is lined by nonciliated cells. (From Clement PB, Young RH. *Atlas of Gynecologic Surgical Pathology.* Philadelphia: WB Saunders; 2000.)

Embryonic cysts of the vagina, especially those discovered on the anterior lateral wall, are usually Gartner duct cysts. In the embryo the distal portion of the mesonephric duct runs parallel with the vagina. It is assumed that a segment of this embryonic structure fails to regress, and the obstructed vestigial remnant becomes cystic. These cysts are most commonly found in the lower one third of the vagina.

Most of these benign cysts are asymptomatic, sausage-shaped tumors that are discovered only incidentally during pelvic examination. Small asymptomatic Gartner duct cysts may be followed conservatively. In a series of 25 women undergoing operations for symptomatic dysontogenetic cysts, a wide range of symptoms were reported, including dyspareunia, vaginal pain, urinary symptoms, and a palpable mass. Sometimes large cysts interfere with the use of tampons. MRI can be useful in delineating the course and anatomic arrangement of vaginal cysts (Wai, 2004).

Operative excision is indicated for chronic symptoms. Rarely, one of these cysts becomes infected, and if operated on during the acute phase, marsupialization of the cyst is preferred. Excision of the vaginal cyst may be a much more formidable operation than anticipated. The cystic structure may extend up into the broad ligament and anatomically be in proximity to the distal course of the ureter.

Rare tumors of the vagina include fibromas, angiomyxomas, and hemangiomas. All are usually found by the patient and require surgical excision.

## TAMPON PROBLEMS

The vaginal tampon has achieved immense popularity and ubiquitous use. It is not surprising that there are rare associated risks with tampon usage: vaginal ulcers, the "forgotten" tampon, and toxic shock syndrome. The latter, related to toxins elaborated by *Staphylococcus aureus,* is discussed in Chapter 23.

Wearing tampons for a few days has been associated with microscopic epithelial changes. The majority of women develop epithelial dehydration and epithelial layering, and some will develop microscopic ulcers. These minor changes take between 48 hours and 7 days to heal. In a study of colposcopic changes related to the tampon, Friedrich found serial changes of epithelial drying, peeling, layering, and ultimately microulceration (Friedrich, 1981). In his study, 15% of women wearing tampons only during the time of normal menstruation developed microulcerations. No clinical symptoms were associated with these microscopic changes. Theoretically, these microulcerations are a potential portal of entry for the HIV virus.

Large macroscopic ulcers of the vaginal fornix have been described in women using vaginal tampons for prolonged lengths of time for persistent vaginal discharge or spotting. The ulcers have a base of clean granulation tissue with smooth, rolled edges. One can even find tampon fibers in the biopsies of these ulcers. The pathophysiology of the ulcer is believed to be secondary to drying and pressure necrosis induced by the tampon. Obviously, many of these young women use tampons for the identical symptoms that are associated with a vaginal ulcer—that is, spotting and vaginal discharge. Often the intermenstrual spotting is believed to be breakthrough bleeding from oral contraceptives, and the possibility of a vaginal ulcer from chronic tampon usage is overlooked.

Vaginal ulcers are not uncommon secondary to several types of foreign objects, including diaphragms, pessaries, and medicated silicon rings. Management is conservative, because the ulcers heal spontaneously when the foreign object is removed. Any persistent ulcer should be biopsied to establish the cause.

A woman with a "lost" or "forgotten" tampon presents with a classic foul vaginal discharge and occasionally spotting. The tampon is usually found high in the vagina. The odor from a forgotten tampon is overwhelming. The tampon is removed using a "double glove technique" where two gloves are donned on the removal hand and, upon grasping the tampon, the outer glove is pulled over the tampon and tied as the tampon is removed. The woman should be treated with an antibiotic vaginal cream or gel (such as MetroGel or clindamycin) for the next 5 to 7 days.

## LOCAL TRAUMA

The most frequent cause of trauma to the lower genital tract of adult females is coitus. Approximately 80% of vaginal lacerations occur secondary to sexual intercourse. Other causes of vaginal trauma are straddle injuries, penetration injuries by foreign objects, sexual assault, vaginismus, and water-skiing accidents. The management of vulvar and vaginal trauma in children is discussed in Chapters 11 and 12.

The predisposing factors believed to be related to coital injury include virginity, the state of the postpartum and postmenopausal vaginal epithelium, pregnancy, intercourse after a prolonged period of abstinence, hysterectomy, and inebriation. In one series of 19 injuries from normal coitus, 12 of the women were between the ages of 16 and 25 and 5 were older than 45. The most common injury is a transverse tear of the posterior fornix. Similar linear lacerations often occur in the right or left vaginal fornices. The location of the coital injury is believed to be related to the poor support of the upper vagina, which is supported only by a thin layer of connective tissue. The most prominent symptom of a coital vaginal laceration is profuse or prolonged vaginal bleeding. Many women experienced sharp pain during intercourse, and 25% noted persistent abdominal pain. The most troublesome but extremely rare complication of vaginal laceration is vaginal evisceration. Coital injury to the vagina should be considered in any woman with profuse or prolonged abnormal vaginal bleeding. Sensitive but thorough history regarding abuse is always appropriate.

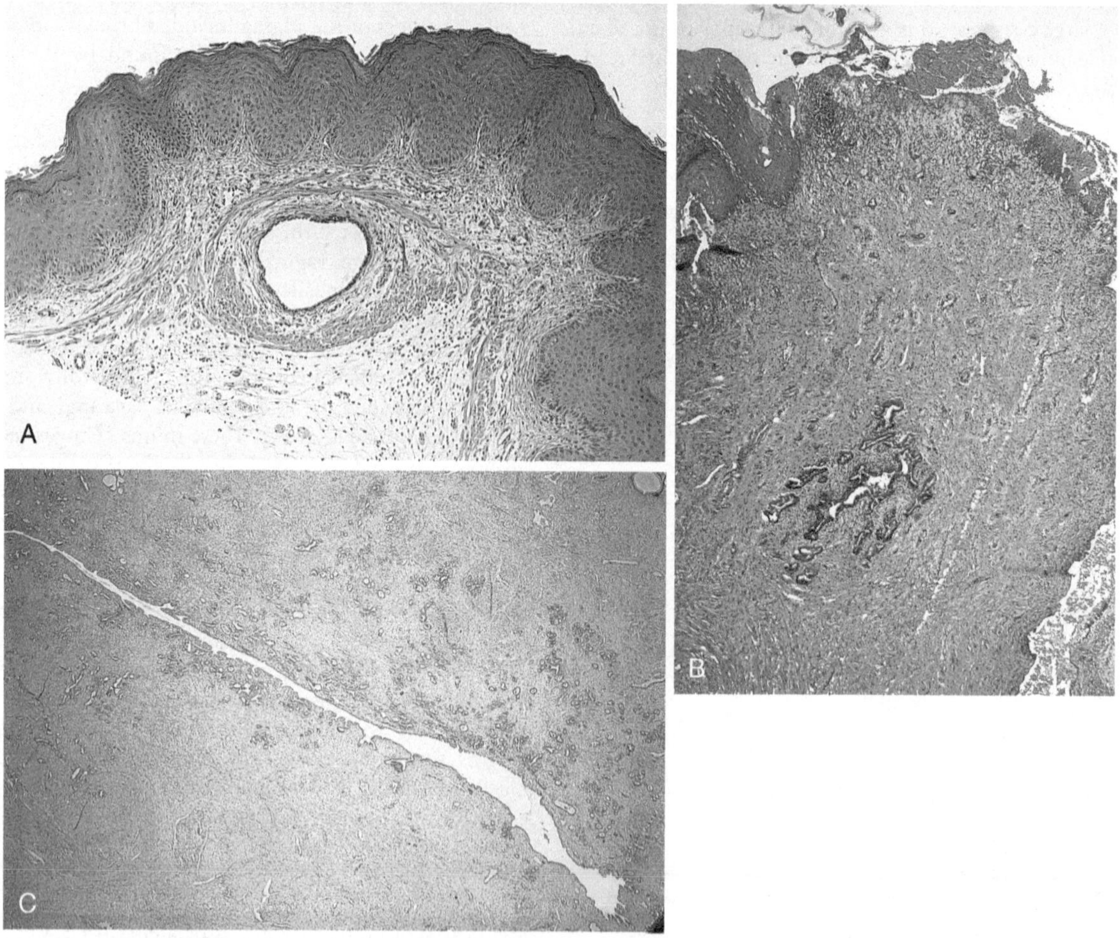


**Figure 18.21** **A,** Normal mesonephric duct. On cross section it is a single duct in the submucosa surrounded by clusters of smooth muscle bands. **B,** Mesonephric duct. The mother duct, located deep in the wall of the vagina, is surrounded by smaller arborized offshoots. **C,** Elongated mesonephric duct. (From Robboy SJ, Anderson MC, Russell P, et al. The vagina. In: Robboy SJ, Anderson MC, Russell P, eds. *Pathology of the Female Reproductive Tract.* Edinburgh: Churchill Livingstone; 2002.)

Management of coital lacerations involves prompt suturing under adequate anesthesia. Secondary injury to the urinary and gastrointestinal tracts should be ruled out.

## CERVIX

### ENDOCERVICAL AND CERVICAL POLYPS

Endocervical and cervical polyps are the most common benign neoplastic growths of the cervix, reported in 4% of gynecologic patients. Endocervical polyps are most common in multiparous women in their 40s and 50s. Cervical polyps usually present as a single polyp, but multiple polyps do occur occasionally. The majority are smooth, soft, reddish purple to cherry red, and fragile. They readily bleed when touched. Endocervical polyps may be single or multiple and are a few millimeters to 4 cm in diameter. The stalk of the polyp is of variable length and width (Fig. 18.22). Polyps may arise from either the endocervical canal (endocervical polyp) or ectocervix (cervical polyp). Endocervical polyps are more common than are cervical polyps. Often the terms *endocervical* and *cervical* polyps are used to describe the same abnormality. Polyps whose base is in the endocervix usually have a narrow, long pedicle and occur during the reproductive years, whereas polyps that arise from the ectocervix have a short, broad base and usually occur in postmenopausal women.

The hypothesis of the origin of endocervical polyps is that they are usually secondary to inflammation or abnormal focal responsiveness to hormonal stimulation. Focal hyperplasia and localized proliferation are the response of the cervix to local inflammation. The color of the polyp depends in part on its origin, with most endocervical polyps being cherry red and most cervical polyps grayish white.

The classic symptom of an endocervical polyp is intermenstrual bleeding, especially following contact such as coitus or a pelvic examination. Sometimes an associated leukorrhea emanates from the infected cervix. Many endocervical polyps are asymptomatic and recognized for the first time during a routine speculum examination. Often the polyp seen on inspection is difficult to palpate because of its soft consistency.

Histologically the surface epithelium of the polyp is columnar or squamous epithelium, depending on the site of origin and the degree of squamous metaplasia (Fig. 18.23). The stalk is composed of an edematous, inflamed, loose, and richly vascular connective tissue. Six different histologic subtypes have been described: adenomatous, cystic, fibrous, vascular, inflammatory, and fibromyomatous. Greater than 80% are of the adenomatous type. During pregnancy, focal areas of decidual changes may develop in the stroma. Often there is ulceration of the stalk's most dependent portion, which explains the symptom of contact bleeding. Malignant degeneration of an endocervical polyp is extremely rare. The reported incidence is less than 1 in 200. Considerations in the differential diagnosis include endometrial polyps, small prolapsed myomas, retained products of conception, squamous papilloma, sarcoma, and cervical malignancy. Microglandular endocervical hyperplasia sometimes presents as a 1- to 2-cm polyp. This is an exaggerated histologic response, usually to oral contraceptives.

Most endocervical polyps may be managed in the office by grasping the base of the polyp with an appropriately sized clamp. The polyp is avulsed with a twisting motion and sent to the pathology laboratory for microscopic evaluation. The polyp is usually friable. If the base is broad or bleeding ensues, the base may be treated with chemical cautery, electrocautery, or cryocautery. After the polyp is removed, the endometrium should be evaluated in women older than 40 who have presented with abnormal bleeding, to rule out coexisting pathology, as significant endometrial pathology is found in approximately 5% of asymptomatic women with endocervical polyps.

### NABOTHIAN CYSTS

Nabothian cysts are retention cysts of endocervical columnar cells occurring where a tunnel or cleft has been covered by squamous metaplasia. These cysts are so common that they are considered a normal feature of the adult cervix. Many women have

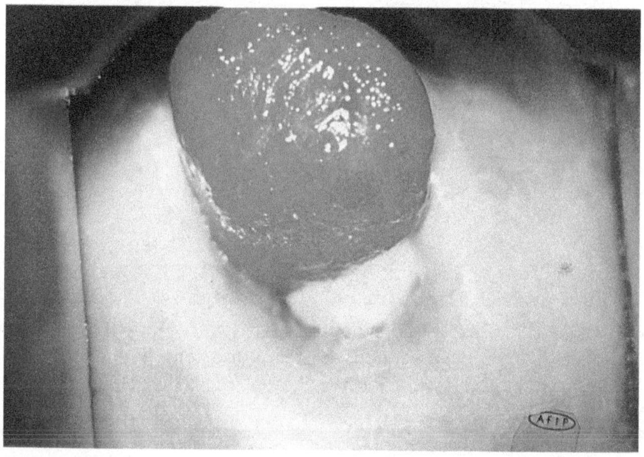


**Figure 18.22** Cervical polyp. A large polyp protrudes from the external cervical os. The surface is red and rough, covered by endocervical epithelium. (From Anderson MC, Robboy SJ, Russell P, et al. The cervix—benign and non-neoplastic conditions. In: Robboy SJ, Anderson MC, Russell P, eds. *Pathology of the Female Reproductive Tract.* Edinburgh: Churchill Livingstone; 2002.)

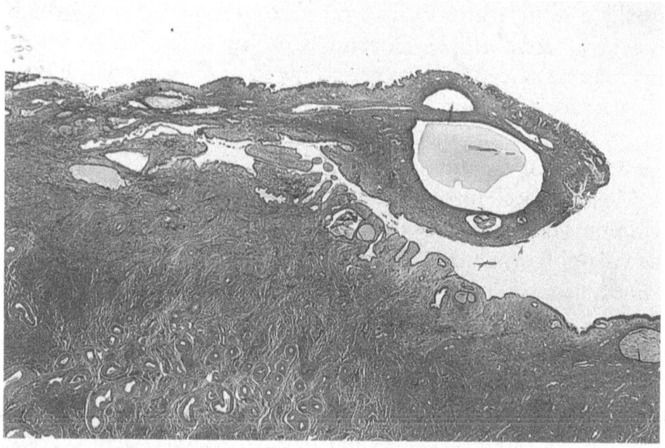

**Figure 18.23** Cervical polyp. The stroma is fibromuscular and the base contains thick-walled blood vessels. Endocervical crypts, some dilated, are present within the polyp. (From Anderson MC, Robboy SJ, Russell P, et al. The cervix—benign and non-neoplastic conditions. In: Robboy SJ, Anderson MC, Russell P, eds. *Pathology of the Female Reproductive Tract.* Edinburgh: Churchill Livingstone; 2002.)

multiple cysts. Grossly, these cysts may be translucent or opaque whitish or yellow in color. Nabothian cysts vary from microscopic to macroscopic size, with the majority between 3 mm and 3 cm in diameter. Rarely, a woman with several large nabothian cysts may develop gross enlargement of the cervix. These mucous retention cysts are produced by the spontaneous healing process of the cervix. The area of the transformation zone of the cervix is in an almost constant process of repair, and squamous metaplasia and inflammation may block the cleft of a gland orifice. The endocervical columnar cells continue to secrete, and thus a mucous retention cyst is formed. Nabothian cysts are asymptomatic, and no treatment is necessary.

## LACERATIONS

Cervical lacerations may occur during obstetric deliveries. Obstetric lacerations vary from minor superficial tears to extensive full-thickness lacerations at 3 and 9 o'clock, respectively, which may extend into the broad ligament. Lacerations may occur in nonpregnant women with mechanical dilation of the cervix. The atrophic cervix of the postmenopausal woman increases the risk of cervical laceration when the cervix is mechanically dilated for dilation and curettage or hysteroscopy.

Acute cervical lacerations bleed and should be sutured. Cervical lacerations that are not repaired may give the external os of the cervix a fish-mouthed appearance; however, they are usually asymptomatic. The use of laminaria tents to slowly soften and dilate the cervix before mechanical instrumentation of the endometrial cavity has reduced the magnitude of iatrogenic cervical lacerations. Furthermore, the practice of routine inspection of the cervix following every second- or third-trimester delivery has enabled physicians to discover and repair extensive cervical lacerations. Extensive cervical lacerations, especially those involving the endocervical stroma, may lead to incompetence of the cervix during a subsequent pregnancy.

## CERVICAL MYOMAS

Cervical myomas are smooth, firm masses that are similar to myomas of the fundus (Figs. 18.24 and 18.25). A cervical myoma is usually a solitary growth in contrast to uterine myomas, which in general, are multiple. Depending on the series, 3% to 8% of myomas are categorized as cervical myomas. Because of the relative paucity of smooth muscle fibers in the cervical stroma, the majority of myomas that appear to be cervical actually arise from the isthmus of the uterus.

Most cervical myomas are small and asymptomatic. When symptoms do occur, they are dependent on the direction in which the enlarging myoma expands. The expanding myoma produces symptoms secondary to mechanical pressure on adjacent organs. Cervical myomas may produce dysuria, urgency, urethral or ureteral obstruction, dyspareunia, or obstruction of the cervix. Occasionally a cervical myoma may become pedunculated and protrude through the external os of the cervix. These prolapsed myomas are often ulcerated and infected. A very large cervical myoma may produce distortion of the cervical canal and upper vagina. Rarely, a cervical myoma causes dystocia during childbirth.

The diagnosis of a cervical myoma is by inspection and palpation. Grossly and histologically, cervical myomas are identical to and indistinguishable from myomas of the corpus of the uterus.

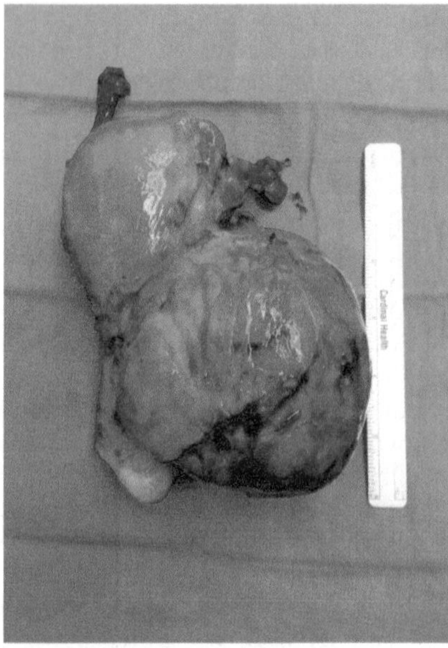

**Figure 18.24** Large fibroid originating from the lateral wall of the cervix and growing into the broad ligament. (Courtesy of Fidel A. Valea, MD.)

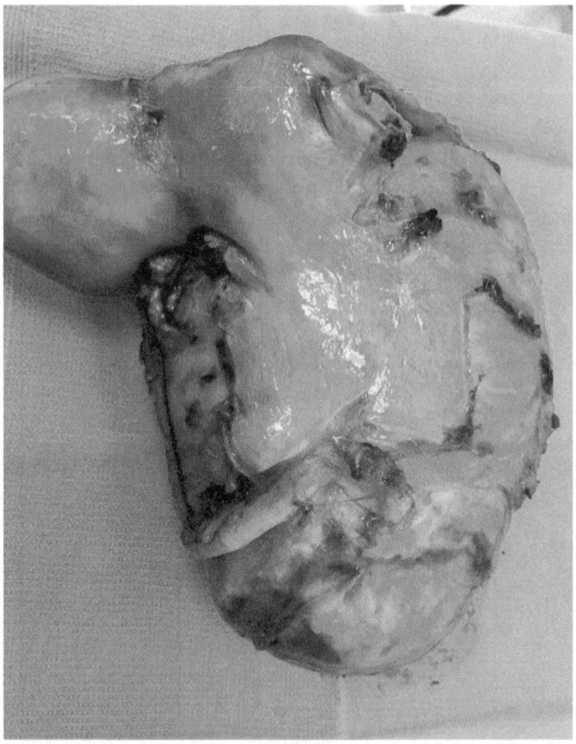

**Figure 18.25** Posterior view of the uterus with a large fibroid that is prolapsing through a very dilated cervix and completely distorts the anatomy of the lower uterine segment. (Courtesy of Fidel A. Valea, MD.)

Occasionally the histologic picture of cervical myomas will demonstrate many hyalinized, thick-walled blood vessels that are postulated to be the source of the neoplastic smooth muscle tumor. This latter subtype of cervical myoma is termed a *vascular leiomyoma.* Management is similar to that of uterine myomas in that asymptomatic, small myomas may be observed for rate of growth. The occurrence and persistence of symptoms from a cervical myoma are an indication for medical therapy with gonadotropin-releasing hormone (GnRH) agonists or myomectomy or hysterectomy, depending on the patient's age and future reproductive plans. Treatment of cervical myomas that grow laterally may become a challenge if myomectomy is the operation of choice, because of both a complex blood supply and involvement with the distal course of the ureter. Cervical myomas may be treated by radiologic catheter embolization. Prolapsed uterine myomas are discussed later in this chapter.

### CERVICAL STENOSIS

Cervical stenosis most often occurs in the region of the internal os. Cervical stenosis may be divided into congenital or acquired types. The causes of acquired cervical stenosis are operative, radiation, infection, neoplasia, or atrophic changes. Loop electrocautery excision procedure (LEEP), cone biopsy, and cautery of the cervix (either electrocautery or cryocoagulation) are the operations that most commonly associated with cervical stenosis. The volume of tissue removed and repeat excision procedures have been reported to increase the risk for cervical stenosis (Suh-Burgmann, 2000). The symptoms of cervical stenosis depend on whether the patient is premenopausal or postmenopausal and whether the obstruction is complete or partial. Common symptoms in premenopausal women include dysmenorrhea, pelvic pain, abnormal bleeding, amenorrhea, and infertility. The infertility is usually associated with endometriosis, which is commonly found in reproductive-age women with cervical stenosis. Postmenopausal women are usually asymptomatic for a long time. Slowly they develop a hematometra (blood), hydrometra (clear fluid), or pyometra (exudate).

The diagnosis is established by inability to introduce a 1- to 2-mm dilator into the uterine cavity. If the obstruction is complete, a soft, slightly tender, enlarged uterus is appreciated as a midline mass, and ultrasound examination demonstrating fluid within the uterine cavity. Management of cervical stenosis is dilation of the cervix with dilators under ultrasound guidance. If stenosis recurs, monthly laminaria tents may be used. Similarly, office follow-up and sounding of the cervix of women who have had a cone biopsy or cautery of the cervix is important to establish patency of the endocervical canal. Postmenopausal women with pyometra usually do not need antibiotics. After the acute infection has subsided, endometrial carcinoma and endocervical carcinoma should be ruled out by appropriate diagnostic biopsies. After cervical dilation, it is often useful to leave a T tube or latex nasopharyngeal airway as a stent in the cervical canal for a few days to maintain patency.

## UTERUS

### ULTRASOUND

Ultrasound, primarily endovaginal, is the most common and most efficient imaging technique for pelvic structures. For endovaginal ultrasound, transducers are configured on vaginal probes and placed in a sterile sheath, usually a glove or condom, prior to an examination. During the examination the woman is in a dorsal lithotomy position and has an empty bladder. Because the transducer is closer to the pelvic organs than when a transabdominal approach is employed, endovaginal resolution is usually superior. However, if the pelvic structures to be studied have expanded and extend into the patient's abdomen, the organs are difficult to visualize with an endovaginal probe. Most ultrasound machines are equipped with both types of transducers.

For transabdominal gynecologic examinations, a sector scanner is preferable. It provides greater resolution of the pelvis and an easier examination than the linear array. During abdominal pelvic ultrasound examination, it is helpful for the patient to have a full bladder. This serves as an acoustic window for the high-frequency sound waves. Ultrasound is more than 90% accurate in recognizing the presence of a pelvic mass, but it does not establish a tissue diagnosis.

Ultrasonography employs an acoustic pulse echo technique. The transducer of the ultrasound machine is made up of piezoelectric crystals that vibrate and emit acoustic pulses. Acoustic echoes return from the tissues being scanned and cause the crystals to vibrate again and release an electric charge. A computer within the ultrasound machine then integrates the electric charges to form the image. Present equipment provides resolution of less than 0.2 mm.

Doppler ultrasound techniques assess the frequency of returning echoes to determine the velocity of moving structures. Measurement of diastolic and systolic velocities provides indirect indices of vascular resistance. Muscular arteries have high resistance. Newly developed vessels, such as those arising in malignancies, have little vascular wall musculature and thus have low resistance. Three-dimensional ultrasound is a computer technique in which multiple two-dimensional images are compiled to render either a surface- or volume-based image that appears to occupy space, as opposed to being flat. Three-dimensional ultrasound has of yet not been shown to have a specific diagnostic advantage in gynecology compared with other modalities.

A disadvantage of ultrasound is its poor penetration of bone and air; thus the pubic symphysis and air-filled intestines and rectum often inhibit visualization. Advantages of ultrasound include the real-time nature of the image, the absence of radiation, the ability to perform the procedure in the office before, during, or immediately after a pelvic examination, and the ability to describe the findings to the patient while she is watching. One of the most reassuring aspects of sonography is the absence of adverse clinical effects from the energy levels used in diagnostic studies.

Sonographic evaluation of endometrial pathology involves measurement of the endometrial thickness or stripe. The normal endometrial thickness is 4 mm or less in a postmenopausal woman not taking hormones. The thickness varies in premenopausal women at different times of the menstrual cycle and in women taking hormone replacement (Fig. 18.26); making endometrial thickness measurements less reliable in that setting. The endometrial thickness is measured in the longitudinal plane, from outer margin to outer margin, at the widest part of the endometrium. Ultrasound is not a screening tool in asymptomatic women. However, several studies of postmenopausal women with vaginal bleeding have documented that malignancy is extremely rare in women with an endometrial thickness of 4 mm or less. Systematic reviews have noted that ultrasound may be reliably used to predict 96% to 99% of endometrial cancers in women with postmenopausal bleeding. The flip side of the coin is that 1% to 4% of malignancies will be missed using a cutoff of less than 4 mm (Tabor, 2002). In addition, papillary-serous adenocarcinomas of

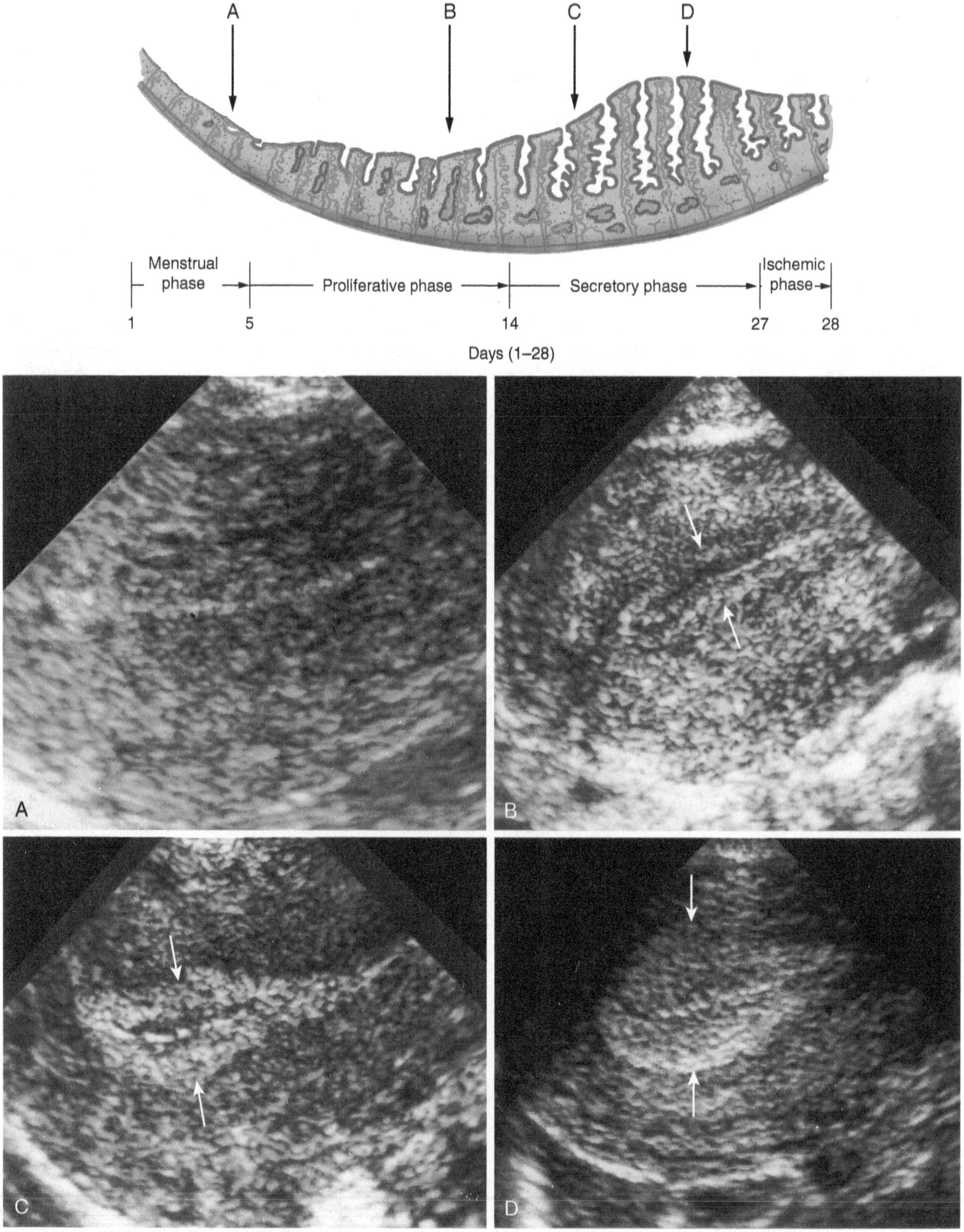


**Figure 18.26** Variation in endometrium during menstrual cycle. **A,** Early proliferative phase. **B,** Late proliferative phase. **C,** Periovulatory phase. **D,** Late secretory phase. Note increase in endometrial thickness throughout the menstrual cycle. Also note multilayered appearance in the late proliferative phase. (From Fleischer AC, Kepple DM. Benign conditions of the uterus, cervix, and endometrium. In: Nyberg DA, Hill LM, Bohm-Velez M, et al, eds. *Transvaginal Ultrasound*. St. Louis: Mosby-Year Book; 1992.)

the endometrium do not always develop the same endometrial stripe thickness as endometrioid cancer. Two caveats for using ultrasound in screening of postmenopausal bleeding are (1) ultrasound does not provide a diagnosis—a tissue specimen is necessary for a diagnosis, and (2) all women with bleeding, no matter the endometrial thickness, should have a tissue biopsy. If an endometrial biopsy obtains inadequate tissue and the endometrial thickness is 5 mm or greater, a repeat biopsy, hysteroscopically directed biopsy, or curettage should be performed.

Sonohysterography is an easily accomplished and validated technique for evaluating the endometrial cavity. The technique involves instilling saline into the uterine cavity. Sonohysterography is an alternative to office hysteroscopy. In this procedure, a thin balloon-tipped catheter or intrauterine insemination catheter is inserted through the cervical os, and 5 to 30 mL of warmed saline is slowly injected into the uterine cavity. Meta-analyses of sonohysterography have found the procedure to be successful in obtaining information in 95% of women, with minimal complications. Contraindications are active cervical or uterine infection. Some clinicians will have patients take a dose of ibuprofen prior to the procedure. Preferably, sonohysterography is performed in the proliferative phase of the cycle when the endometrial lining is at its lowest level. Sonohysterography has also been helpful in the evaluation of polyps, filling defects, submucous myomas, and uterine septae (Fig. 18.27). Importantly, sonohysterography, as with all types of ultrasound, does not make a tissue diagnosis.

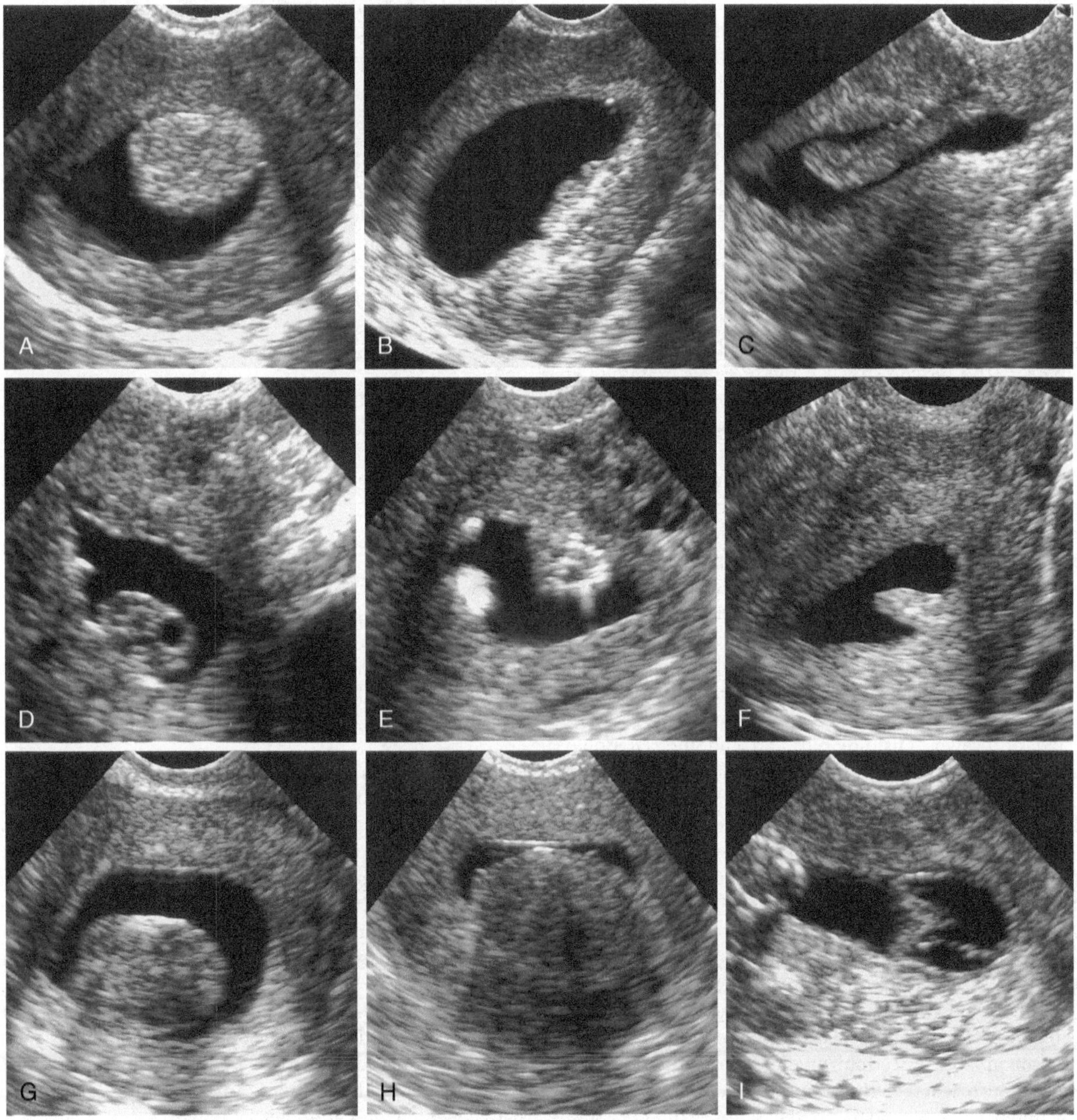


**Figure 18.27** Sonohysterograms. **A,** Well-defined, round echogenic polyp. **B,** Carpet of small polyps. **C,** Polyp on a stalk. **D,** Polyp with cystic areas. **E,** Small polyp. **F,** Small polyp. **G,** Hypoechoic submucosal fibroid. **H,** Hypoechoic attenuating submucosal fibroid. **I,** Endometrial adhesions. Note bridging bands of tissue within fluid-filled endometrial canal. (From Salem S. The uterus and adnexa. In Rumack CM, Wilson SR, Charboneau JW, eds. *Diagnostic Ultrasound,* 2nd ed. St. Louis: Mosby; 1998:538.)

Sonography is the method of choice to locate a "missing" intrauterine device (IUD). It will help in diagnosing perforation of the uterus or unrecognized expulsion of the device. Endovaginal ultrasound transducers equipped with needle guides are frequently used for oocyte aspiration as part of in vitro fertilization.

In summary, ultrasound has become an extremely valuable adjunct to the bimanual examination. In many patients, particularly obese patients, it is superior to perform bimanual examination alone. An endovaginal ultrasound of an early pregnancy has become a mainstay in the evaluation of the pregnant woman with first-trimester vaginal bleeding.

## ENDOMETRIAL POLYPS

Endometrial polyps are localized overgrowths of endometrial glands and stroma that project beyond the surface of the endometrium. They are soft, pliable, and may be single or multiple. Most polyps arise from the fundus of the uterus. *Polypoid hyperplasia* is a benign condition in which numerous small polyps are discovered throughout the endometrial cavity. Endometrial polyps vary from a few millimeters to several centimeters in diameter, and it is possible for a single large polyp to fill the endometrial cavity. Endometrial polyps may have a broad base (sessile) or be attached by a slender pedicle (pedunculated). They occur in all age groups but have a peak incidence between the ages of 40 and 49. The prevalence of endometrial polyps in reproductive-age women is 20% to 25%. Endometrial polyps are noted in approximately 10% of women when the uterus is examined at autopsy. The cause of endometrial polyps is unknown. Because polyps are often associated with endometrial hyperplasia, unopposed estrogen has been implicated as a possible etiology.

The majority of endometrial polyps are asymptomatic. Those that are symptomatic are associated with a wide range of abnormal bleeding patterns. No single abnormal bleeding pattern is diagnostic for polyps; however, menorrhagia, premenstrual and postmenstrual staining, and scanty postmenstrual spotting are the most common. Occasionally a pedunculated endometrial polyp with a long pedicle may protrude from the external cervical os. Sometimes large endometrial polyps may contribute to infertility.

Polyps are succulent and velvety, with a large central vascular core. The color is usually gray or tan but may occasionally be red or brown. Histologically, an endometrial polyp has three components: endometrial glands, endometrial stroma, and central vascular channels (Figs. 18.27 and 18.28). Epithelium must be identified on three sides, like a peninsula. Approximately two of three polyps consist of an immature endometrium that does not respond to cyclic changes in circulating progesterone. This immature endometrium differs from surrounding endometrium and often appears as a "Swiss cheese" cystic hyperplasia during all phases of the menstrual cycle (Fig. 18.29). The other one third of endometrial polyps consist of functional endometria that will undergo cyclic histologic changes. The tip of a prolapsed polyp often undergoes squamous metaplasia, infection, or ulceration. The clinician cannot distinguish whether the abnormal bleeding originates from the polyp or is secondary to the frequently coexisting endometrial hyperplasia. Approximately one in four reproductive-age women with abnormal bleeding will have endometrial polyps discovered in her uterine cavity.

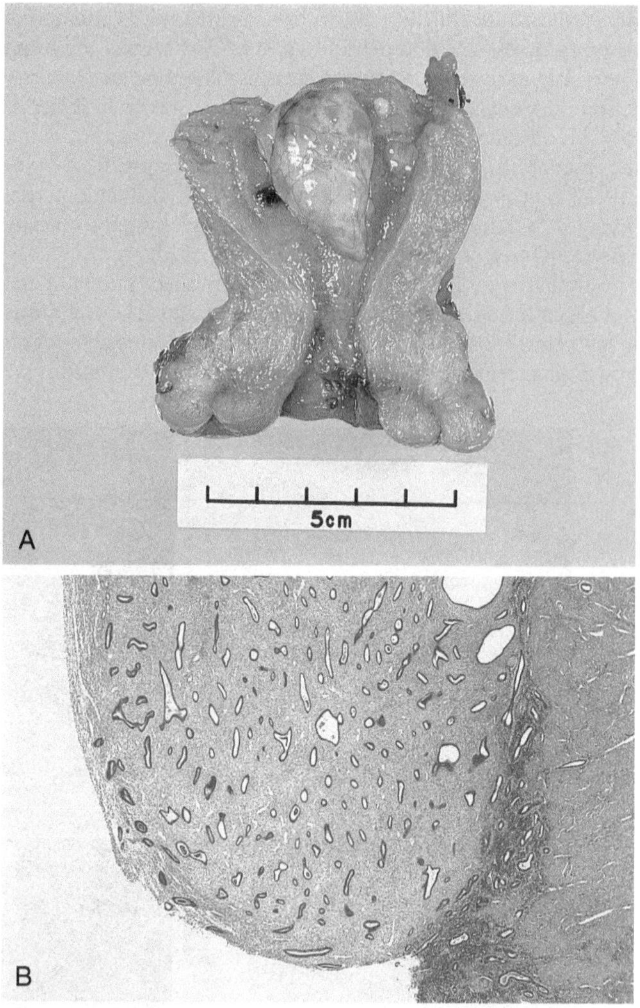


**Figure 18.28** Endometrial polyp. **A,** Note cystic glands in the polyp. **B,** The fibrous stroma of the polyp contrasts with the cellular stroma of the adjacent endometrium. (From Anderson MC, Robboy SJ, Russell P, et al. Endometritis, metaplasias, polyps, and miscellaneous changes. In: Robboy SJ, Anderson MC, Russell P, eds. *Pathology of the Female Reproductive Tract.* Edinburgh: Churchill Livingstone; 2002.)

Malignancy in an endometrial polyp is related to patient's age and is most often of a low stage and grade. In one series of 67 women from the UK with endometrial polyps, 86% were benign, 13% hyperplastic, and 3% malignant. Another series of 61 women with polyps found 88% were benign and 5% were malignant. A recent review and meta-analysis of the oncogenic potential of endometrial polyps reported among women found to have endometrial polyps; the prevalence of premalignant or malignant polyps was 5.42% in postmenopausal women compared with 1.7% in reproductive aged women. Furthermore, the prevalence of endometrial neoplasia within polyps in women with symptomatic bleeding was 4.15% compared with 2.16% for those without bleeding. Among symptomatic postmenopausal women with endometrial polyps, 4.47% had a malignant polyp compared with 1.51% in asymptomatic postmenopausal women (Lee, 2010). The question of an association with endometrial polyps and endometrial carcinoma is still debated.

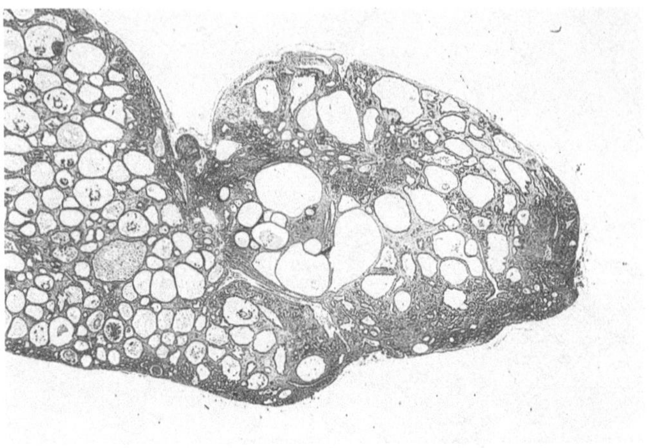

**Figure 18.29** Endometrial polyp showing multiple cystic glands with flattened epithelial lining. (From Anderson MC, Robboy SJ, Russell P, et al. Endometritis, metaplasias, polyps and miscellaneous changes. In: Robboy SJ, Anderson MC, Russell P, eds. *Pathology of the Female Reproductive Tract.* Edinburgh: Churchill Livingstone; 2002.)

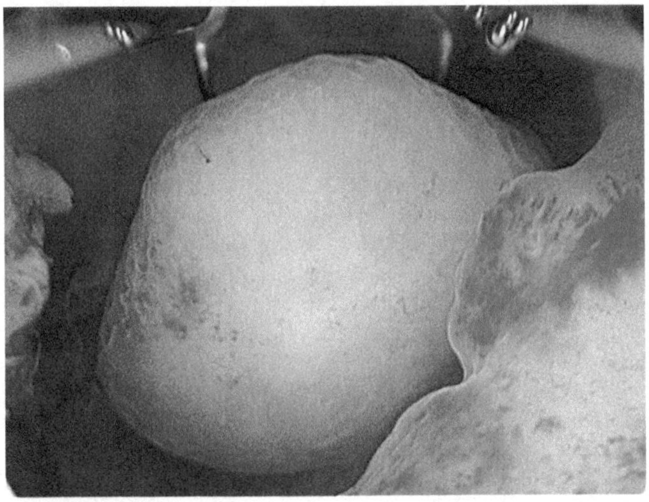

**Figure 18.30** Endocervical polyp was seen at hysteroscopy. (From Goldberg JM, Falcone T. *Atlas of Endoscopic Techniques in Gynecology.* London: WB Saunders; 2000.)

A population-based, case-control study from Sweden estimated that the increased risk of subsequent endometrial carcinoma in women with endometrial polyps is only twofold. It is interesting that benign polyps have been found in approximately 20% of uteri removed for endometrial carcinoma.

Unusual polyps have been described in association with chronic administration of the nonsteroidal antiestrogen tamoxifen. The endometrial abnormalities associated with chronic tamoxifen therapy include polyps, 20% to 35%; endometrial hyperplasia, 2% to 4%; endometrial carcinoma, 1% to 2%; and often with multiple irregular sonolucencies suggesting the presence of cysts.

Most endometrial polyps are asymptomatic, and the diagnosis is not usually established until the uterus is opened following hysterectomy for other reasons. Endometrial polyps may be discovered by vaginal ultrasound, with or without hydrosonography, hysteroscopy, or hysterosalpingography during the diagnostic workup of a woman with a refractory case of abnormal uterine bleeding or pelvic mass. Endometrial polyps are frequently confused with endocervical polyps (Fig. 18.30). A well-defined, uniformly hyperechoic mass that is less than 2 cm in diameter, identified by vaginal ultrasound within the endometrial cavity, is usually a benign endometrial polyp (see Fig. 18.27, *A-C*). Most endometrial polyps usually resolve after a few years, although new polyps can form.

The optimal management of endometrial polyps is removal by hysteroscopy with D&C. Because of the frequent association of endometrial polyps and other endometrial pathology, it is important to examine histologically both the polyp and the associated endometrial lining. Polyps, because of their mobility, often tend to elude the curette. Postcurettage hysteroscopic studies have demonstrated that routine use of a long, narrow polyp forceps at the time of curettage at best results in discovery and removal of only approximately one in four endometrial polyps. The differential diagnosis of endometrial polyps includes submucous leiomyomas, adenomyomas, retained products of conception, endometrial hyperplasia, carcinoma, and uterine sarcomas.

## HEMATOMETRA

A hematometra is a uterus distended with blood and is secondary to gynatresia, which is partial or complete obstruction of any portion of the lower genital tract. Obstruction of the isthmus of the uterus, cervix, or vagina may be congenital or acquired. The two most common congenital causes of hematometra are an imperforate hymen and a transverse vaginal septum. Among the leading causes of acquired lower tract stenosis are senile atrophy of the endocervical canal and endometrium, scarring of the isthmus by synechiae, cervical stenosis associated with surgery, radiation therapy, cryocautery or electrocautery, endometrial ablation, and malignant disease of the endocervical canal.

The symptoms of hematometra depend on the age of the patient, her menstrual history and the rapidity of the accumulation of blood in the uterine cavity, and the possibility of secondary infection producing pyometra. Thus common symptoms of hematometra include primary or secondary amenorrhea and possibly cyclic lower abdominal pain. During the early teenage years, the combination of primary amenorrhea and cyclic, episodic cramping lower abdominal pains suggests the possibility of a developing hematometra. Occasionally the obstruction is incomplete, and there is associated spotting of dark brown blood. Hematometra in postmenopausal women may be entirely asymptomatic. On pelvic examination a mildly tender, globular uterus is usually palpated. Ultrasound may be used to confirm the diagnosis.

The diagnosis of hematometra is generally suspected by the history of amenorrhea and cyclic abdominal pain. The diagnosis is usually confirmed by vaginal ultrasound or probing the cervix with a narrow metal dilator, with release of dark brownish black blood from the endocervical canal. Sometimes the blood retained inside the uterus becomes secondarily infected and has a foul odor.

Management of hematometra depends on operative relief of the lower tract obstruction. Treatment of congenital obstruction is discussed in Chapter 11. Appropriate biopsy specimens of the endocervical canal and endometrium should be obtained to rule out malignancy when the cause of hematometra is not obvious. If the uterus is significantly enlarged or if there is any suspicion that the retained fluid is infected, drainage should be accomplished first. Biopsy should be postponed for approximately 2 weeks to diminish the chances of infection or uterine perforation. Hematometra following operations or cryocautery usually resolves with cervical dilation. Rarely, a hematometra may form following a first-trimester abortion. This is treated by repeat suction aspiration of the products of conception that are blocking the internal os.

## LEIOMYOMAS

Leiomyomas, also called *myomas,* are benign tumors of muscle cell origin. These tumors are often referred to by their popular names, *fibroids* or *fibromyomas,* but such terms are semantic misnomers if one is referring to the cell of origin. Most leiomyomas contain varying amounts of fibrous tissue, which is believed to be secondary to degeneration of some of the smooth muscle cells.

Leiomyomas are the most common benign neoplasms of the uterus. The lifetime prevalence of leiomyomas is greater than 80% among African-American women and approaches 70% among white women (Baird, 2003). In general, a third of myomas will become symptomatic causing abnormal and excessive uterine bleeding, pelvic pain, pelvic pressure, bowel and bladder dysfunction, infertility, recurrent miscarriage, and abdominal protrusion. Leiomyomas are a tremendous public health burden and the most frequent indication for hysterectomy in the United States. There are significant health disparities for African-American women with fibroids (Eltoukhi, 2014). Approximately 42 per 1000 women are hospitalized annually because of fibroids, but African-American women have higher rates of hospitalization, myomectomies, and hysterectomies compared with white women (relative risk [RR] of 3.5, 6.8, and 2.4, respectively) (Wechter, 2011). In black women, vitamin D deficiency has been linked with increased fibroid risk (Baird, 2013). Why some women develop myomas while others do not is unknown. Therefore effective treatment is limited by the poor understanding of their pathogenesis.

Risk factors associated with the development of myomata include increasing age, early menarche, low parity, tamoxifen use, obesity, and in some studies a high-fat diet. Smoking has been found to be associated with a decreased incidence of myomata. African-American women have the highest incidence, whereas Hispanic and Asian women have similar rates to white women. There appears to be a familial tendency to develop myoma. Studies of twins have noted than when identical and fraternal twins are compared, a significant proportion of myoma tend to have an inherited basis. Rare genetic conditions such as hereditary leiomyomatosis and renal cell cancer (Launoned, 2001) and Alport syndrome (Uliana, 2011) feature development of myomas. The growth of myomas is dependent on gonadal steroids, and there are increased numbers of steroid receptors in myomas compared with normal myometrium. They are diagnosed only after menarche and tend to regress after menopause (Okolo, 2008). They have a limited malignant potential with less than 1% transformation into malignancy. Cytogenetically, the most fibroids are chromosomally normal and arise from a single cell (are clonal). However, the remainder share similar tumor-specific chromosomal rearrangements that are associated with tumor growth (Levy, 2012). Although fibroids are clonal in nature, heterogeneity exists and they may vary greatly in size, location, and appearance within the same uterus. There is accumulating evidence that suggests hypoxia is implicated in early cellular events that lead to the myometrial smooth muscle cell to transform into leiomyoma (Tal, 2014). Angiogenesis and vascularization are factors that control the growth of tumors. Tal and Segars reviewed the molecular regulation of the growth factors involved in angiogenesis of fibroids and described the potential implications for future therapy (Tal, 2014).

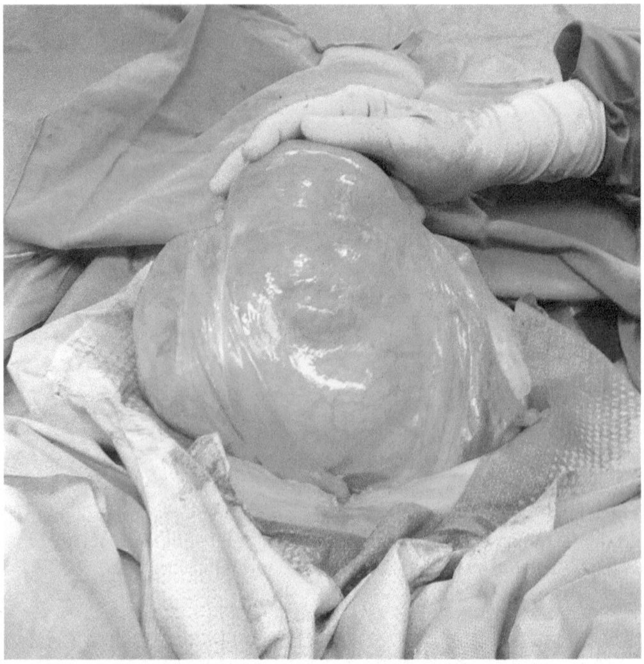

**Figure 18.31** Image of large fibroid uterus prior to hysterectomy. (Courtesy of Fidel A. Valea, MD.)

Although leiomyomas arise throughout the body in any structure containing smooth muscle, in the pelvis the majority are found in the corpus of the uterus. Occasionally, leiomyomas may be found in the fallopian tube or the round ligament, and approximately 5% of uterine myomas originate from the cervix. Rarely, myomas will arise in the retroperitoneum and produce symptoms secondary to "mass effects" on adjacent organs.

Myomas may be single but most often are multiple. They vary greatly in size from microscopic to multinodular uterine tumors that may weigh more than 50 pounds and literally fill the patient's abdomen (Fig. 18.31). Initially most myomas develop from the myometrium, beginning as intramural myomas. As they grow, they remain attached to the myometrium with a pedicle of varying width and thickness. Small myomas are round, firm, solid tumors. With continued growth, the myometrium at the edge of the tumor is compressed and forms a pseudocapsule. Although myomas do not have a true capsule, this pseudocapsule is a valuable surgical plane during a myomectomy.

Myomas are classed into subgroups by their relative anatomic relationship and position to the layers of the uterus (Fig. 18.32). The three most common types of myomas are intramural, subserous, and submucous, with special nomenclature for broad ligament and parasitic myomas (Fig. 18.33). Continued growth in one direction determines which myomas will be located just below the endometrium (submucosal) and which will be found just

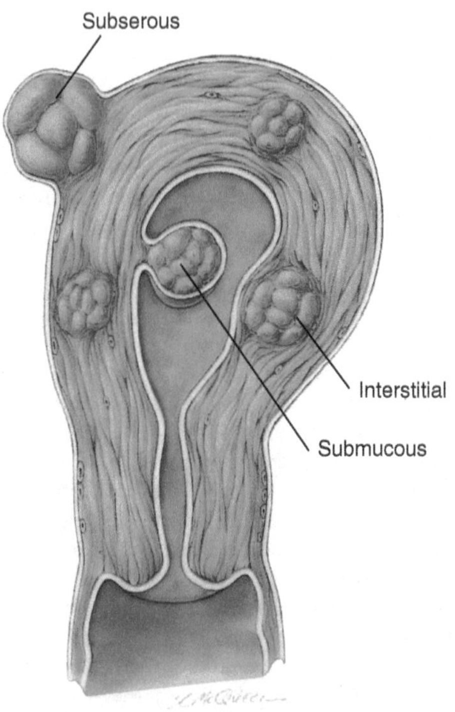


Figure 18.32 Drawing of cut surface of uterus showing characteristic whorl-like appearance and varying locations of leiomyomas. (From Novak ER, Woodruff JD, eds. *Novak's Gynecologic and Obstetric Pathology.* 6th ed. Philadelphia: WB Saunders; 1967:215.)

beneath the serosa (subserosal) (Fig. 18.34). Although only 5% to 10% of myomas become submucosal, they usually are the most troublesome clinically (Fig. 18.35). These submucosal tumors may be associated with abnormal vaginal bleeding or distortion of the uterine cavity that may produce infertility or miscarriage. Rarely, a submucosal myoma enlarges and becomes pedunculated. The uterus will try to expel it, and the prolapsed myoma may protrude through the external cervical os (see Fig. 18.25).

Subserosal myomas give the uterus its knobby contour during pelvic examination. Further growth of a subserosal myoma may lead to a pedunculated myoma wandering into the peritoneal cavity. This myoma may outgrow its uterine blood supply and obtain a secondary blood supply from another organ, such as the omentum, and become a parasitic myoma. Growth of a myoma in a lateral direction from the uterus may result in a broad ligament myoma (see Fig. 18.24). The clinical significance of broad ligament myomas is that they are difficult to differentiate on pelvic examination from a solid ovarian tumor. Large, broad ligament myomas may produce a hydroureter as they enlarge.

Though the origin of uterine leiomyomas is incompletely understood, cytogenetic studies have yielded some clues to how and why myomas develop. Each tumor develops from a single muscle cell a progenitor myocyte, thus each myoma is monoclonal. Cytogenetic analysis has demonstrated that myomas have

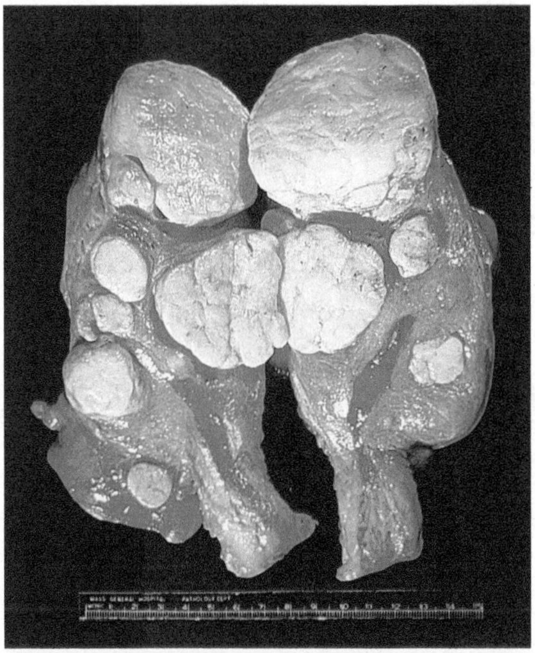

Figure 18.33 Multiple leiomyomas. These are predominantly intramural. The bulging cut surfaces are clearly shown. (From Anderson MC, Robboy SJ, Russell P. Uterine smooth muscle tumors. In: Robboy SJ, Anderson MC, Russell P, eds. *Pathology of the Female Reproductive Tract.* Edinburgh: Churchill Livingstone; 2002.)

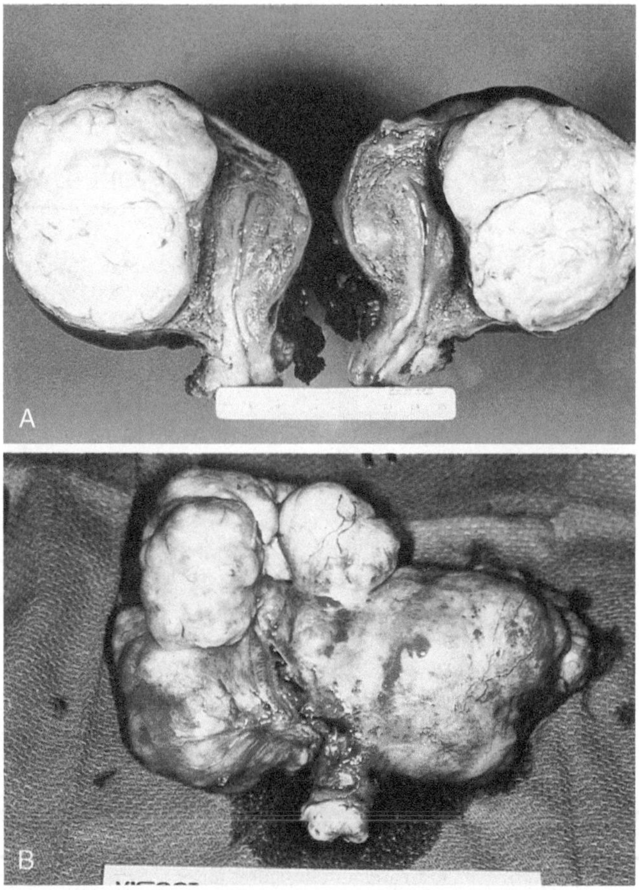


Figure 18.34 **A,** Large subserosal myoma. **B,** Hysterectomy specimen of myomatous uterus. (Courtesy of Vern L. Katz and William Droegemueller.)

multiple chromosomal abnormalities. (Each myoma would have cells with the same abnormality.) Sixty percent are normal, 46XX. The larger the myoma, the more an abnormal karyotype will be detected. Interestingly, the chromosomal anomalies of myomata have a remarkable clustering of changes. Twenty percent of abnormalities involve translocations between chromosomes 12 and 14. Seventeen percent involve a deletion of chromosome 7. Twelve percent involve a deletion of chromosome 12, and some are trisomy 12. The affected regions on chromosome 12 are also abnormal in many other types of solid tumors. The regions of chromosome 12 and 7 involve genes that may regulate growth-inducing proteins and cytokines, including transforming growth factor β (TGF-β), epidermal growth factor (EGF), insulin-like growth factors (IGF) 1 and 2, and platelet-derived growth factor (PDGF) (Fig. 18.36). Many of these cytokines have been found in significantly higher concentrations in myomas than in the surrounding myometrium. Current theory holds that the neoplastic transformation from normal myometrium to leiomyomata is the result of a somatic mutation in the single progenitor cell. The mutation then affects cytokines that affect cell growth. The growth may also be influenced by the relative levels of estrogen or progesterone. Both estrogen and progesterone receptors are found in higher concentrations in uterine myomas, as are other genomic changes that potentiate cellular proliferation. There also appear to be similarities between fibroids and keloid formation. Interestingly, Ishikawa and colleagues noted that myoma cells have an increased expression of aromatase, which further potentiates more local estrogen. Interestingly, African-American women had the highest levels of aromatase in myoma cells (Ishikawa, 2009).

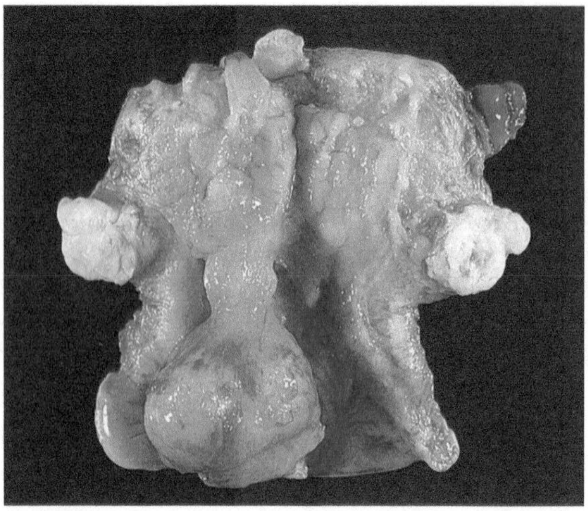

**Figure 18.35** Uterus with multiple myomata. Note the large central submucosal myoma. (From Voet RL. *Color Atlas of Obstetric and Gynecologic Pathology*. St. Louis: Mosby-Wolfe; 1997.)

Myomas are rare before menarche, and most myomas diminish in size following menopause with the reduction of a significant amount of circulating estrogen. Myomas often enlarge during pregnancy and occasionally enlarge secondary to oral contraceptive therapy. Medically induced hypoestrogenic states produce reductions in the size of myomas. Women who smoke cigarettes and are thus relatively estrogen-deficient have a lower

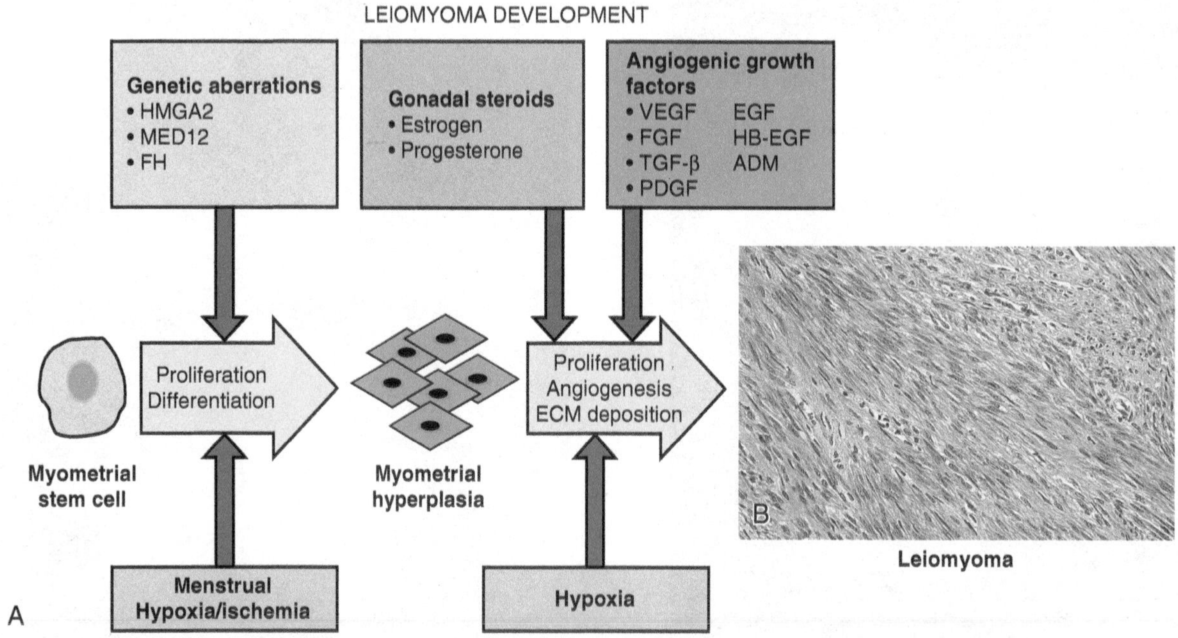


**Figure 18.36** **A,** Leiomyoma development. **B,** Leiomyoma. The smooth muscle cells are markedly elongated and have eosinophilic cytoplasm and elongated, cigar-shaped nuclei. The nuclei are uniform and mitotic figures absent or sparse. (**A,** Modified from Tal R, Segars JH. The role of angiogenic factors in fibroid pathogenesis: potential implications for future therapy. *Hum Reprod Update*. 2014; 20[2]:194-216. **B,** From Anderson MC, Robboy SJ, Russell P. Uterine smooth muscle tumors. In: Robboy SJ, Anderson MC, Russell P, eds. *Pathology of the Female Reproductive Tract*. Edinburgh: Churchill Livingstone; 2002.)

incidence of myomas. Many women, though, have small myomas that do not grow under the influence of high circulating estrogen levels. Thus the relationship between estrogen and progesterone levels and myoma growth is complex.

Grossly, a myoma has a lighter color than the normal myometrium. On a cut surface, the tumor has a glistening, pearl-white appearance, with the smooth muscle arranged in a trabeculated or whorled configuration. Histologically there is a proliferation of mature smooth muscle cells. The nonstriated muscle fibers are arranged in interlacing bundles. Between bundles of smooth muscle cells are variable amounts of fibrous connective tissue, especially toward the center of any large tumor (see Fig. 18.36). The amount of fibrous tissue is proportional to the extent of atrophy and degeneration that has occurred over time. The intracellular structure of myoma cells is different from the surrounding normal myometrium. The abnormal cells contain more collagen and what has been described as a "stiffer" cytoskeleton secondary to the intracellular pressure generated by the densely packed surrounding myoma. Less than 5% of myomas exhibit hypercellularity, and these are termed *cellular leiomyomata.* Cellular leiomyomata tend to be larger in size and solitary. There is less accompanying adenomyosis or other uterine pathology. The clinical presentation of cellular leiomyoma is more similar to that of a sarcoma (leiomyosarcoma). Other authors have noted a genomic expression that is similar, as well, to leiomyosarcomas. However, cellular leiomyomata are not precursors to sarcoma and have a benign prognosis.

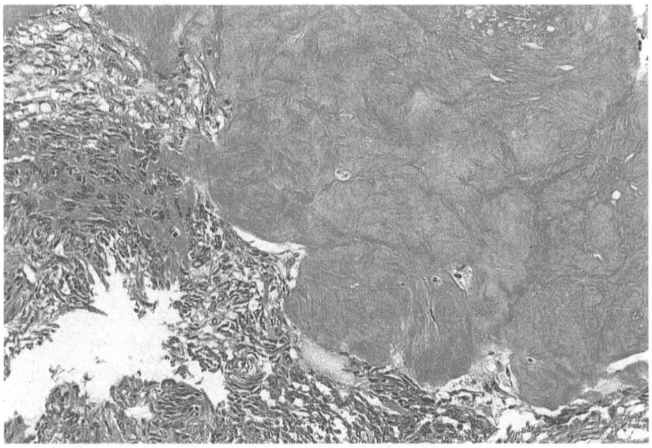

**Figure 18.37** Hyaline degeneration is a leiomyoma. There is an eosinophilic ground-glass appearance. (From Anderson MC, Robboy SJ, Russell P. Uterine smooth muscle tumors. In: Robboy SJ, Anderson MC, Russell P, eds. *Pathology of the Female Reproductive Tract.* Edinburgh: Churchill Livingstone; 2002.)

The eventual fate of some myomas is determined by their relatively poor vascular supply. This supply is found in one or two major arteries at the base or pedicle of the myoma. The arterial supply of myomas is significantly less than that of a similarly sized area of normal myometrium. Thus with continued growth, degeneration occurs because the tumor outgrows its blood supply. The severity of the discrepancy between the myoma's growth and its blood supply determines the extent of degeneration: hyaline, myxomatous, calcific, cystic, fatty, or red degeneration and necrosis. The mildest form of degeneration of a myoma is hyaline degeneration (Fig. 18.37). Grossly, in this condition the surface of the myoma is homogeneous with loss of the whorled pattern. Histologically, with hyaline degeneration, cellular detail is lost as the smooth muscle cells are replaced by fibrous connective tissue. Huang and colleagues, using transvaginal color Doppler ultrasound, documented that the intratumoral blood flow correlated with reduced tumor size and tumor volume but did not correlate with angiogenesis or cell proliferation (Huang, 1996).

The most acute form of degeneration is red, or carneous, infarction (Fig. 18.38). This acute muscular infarction causes severe pain and localized peritoneal irritation. This form of degeneration occurs during pregnancy in approximately 5% to 10% of gravid women with myomas. The condition is best treated with nonsteroidal anti-inflammatory agents for 72 hours, as long as the woman is less than 32 weeks' gestation. The ultrasound appearance of painful myomas is one of mixed echodense and echolucent areas. Serial ultrasound examinations have also

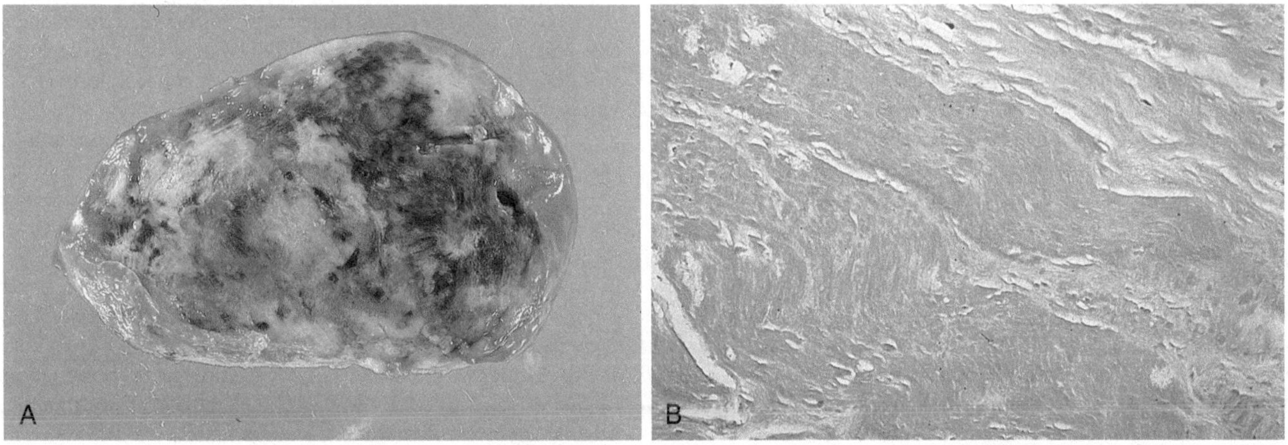


**Figure 18.38** **A,** Gross view of an infracted leiomyoma. **B,** Red degeneration; the ghosts of the muscle cells and their nuclei remain. (**A,** From Anderson MC, Robboy SJ, Russell P. Uterine smooth muscle tumors. In: Robboy SJ, Anderson MC, Russell P, eds. *Pathology of the Female Reproductive Tract.* Edinburgh: Churchill Livingstone; 2002. **B,** From Voet RL. *Color Atlas of Obstetric and Gynecologic Pathology.* St. Louis: Mosby-Wolfe; 1997.)

demonstrated that most (80%) myomas do not change size during pregnancy; if a change in size does occur, it is usually not associated with painful symptomatology. During pregnancy this complication should be treated medically, for attempts at operative removal may result in profuse blood loss. If the patient is not pregnant, acute degeneration is not a contraindication to myomectomy. The more advanced forms of degenerating myomas may become secondarily infected, especially when large necrotic areas exist. The histologic changes of degeneration are found more commonly in larger myomas. However, two thirds of all myomas show some degree of degeneration, with the three most common types being hyaline degeneration (65%), myxomatous degeneration (15%), and calcific degeneration (10%).

The literature emphasizes that the incidence of malignant degeneration is estimated to be between 0.3% and 0.7%. The term *malignant degeneration* is incorrect. It is unknown as to whether myomas degenerate into sarcomas. Given the very high prevalence of myomas, most investigators believe that sarcomas arise spontaneously in myomatous uteri. A meta-analysis of the prevalence of occult leiomyosarcoma found at surgery for presumed uterine fibroids estimated the rate of leiomyosarcoma to be 0.51 per 1000 procedures (confidence interval [CI] = 0.16 to 0.98) or approximately 1 in 2000. If only the prospective studies were included (64 studies), there was a substantially lower estimate of 0.12 leiomyosarcomas per 1000 procedures (CI = 0.01 to 0.75) or 1 in 8300 surgeries (Pritts, 2015). The possibility of a uterine tumor being a leiomyoma sarcoma is 10 times greater in a woman in her 60s than in a woman in her 40s.

The most common symptoms related to myomas are pressure from an enlarging pelvic mass, pain including dysmenorrhea, and abnormal uterine bleeding. The severity of symptoms is usually related to the number, location, and size of the myomas. However, over two thirds of women with uterine myomas are asymptomatic.

One of three women with myomas experiences pelvic pain or pressure. Acquired dysmenorrhea is one of the most frequent complaints. Various forms of vascular compromise, either acute degeneration or torsion of the pedicle, produce severe pelvic pain. Mild pelvic discomfort is described as pelvic heaviness or a dull, aching sensation that may be secondary to edematous swelling in the myoma. An enlarged myoma or myomas often produce pressure symptoms similar to those of an enlarging pregnant uterus. Sometimes a woman will notice that her abdominal girth is increasing without appreciable change in weight. Alternatively, an anterior myoma pressing on the bladder may produce urinary frequency and urgency. In general, urinary symptoms are more common than rectal symptoms. Extremely large myomas and broad ligament myomas may produce a unilateral or bilateral hydroureter.

Abnormal bleeding is experienced by 30% of women with myomas. The most common symptom is menorrhagia, but intermenstrual spotting and disruption of a normal pattern are other frequent complaints. Wegienka and colleagues evaluated the bleeding pattern of 596 women with myomas. Compared with a control group, bleeding was more frequently described as gushing. Menses were longer in duration and heavier. In this study, symptoms of bleeding were related to the size of myomas. Interestingly, the location of the myomas, submucous versus intramural, was not related to bleeding symptoms (Wegienka, 2003). The exact cause-and-effect relationship between myomas and abnormal bleeding is difficult to determine and is poorly understood. The explanation is straightforward when there are areas of ulceration over submucous myomas. However, ulceration is a rare finding. The most popular theory is that myomas result in an abnormal microvascular growth pattern and function of the vessels in the adjacent endometrium. The older theory that the amount of menorrhagia is directly related to an increase of endometrial surface area has been disproved. One of three women with abnormal bleeding and submucous myomas also has endometrial hyperplasia, which may be the cause of the symptom.

Occasionally, myomas are the only identifiable abnormality after a detailed infertility investigation. Because the data relating myomas to infertility are weak, myomectomy is indicated only in long-standing infertility and recurrent abortion after all other potential factors have been investigated and treated. Studies suggest that submucous myomas that distort the uterine cavity are the myomas that may affect reproduction. Successful full-term pregnancy rates of 40% to 50% have been reported following a myomectomy. The success of an operation is most dependent on the age of the patient, the size of the myomas, and the number of compounding factors that affect the couple's fertility. A Cochrane review of the surgical treatment of fibroids for subfertility noted "insufficient evidence from randomized controlled trials to evaluate the role of myomectomy to improve fertility" (Metwally, 2012).

Rapid growth of a uterine myoma after menopause is a disturbing symptom. This is the classic symptom of a leiomyosarcoma; however, fibroids can have growth spurts, and most guidelines (but not all) suggest rapid growth is not necessarily an indication for treatment (Stewart, 2015). Rarely, a secondary polycythemia is noted in women with uterine myomas. This syndrome is related to elevated levels of erythropoietin. The polycythemia diminishes following removal of the uterus.

Clinically, the diagnosis of uterine myomas is usually confirmed by physical examination. Upon palpation, an enlarged, firm, irregular uterus may be felt. The three conditions that commonly enter into the differential diagnosis are pregnancy, adenomyosis, and an ovarian neoplasm. The discrimination between large ovarian tumors and myomatous uteri may be difficult on physical examination, because the extension of myomas laterally may make palpation of normal ovaries impossible during the pelvic examination. The mobility of the pelvic mass and whether the mass moves independently or as part of the uterus may be helpful diagnostically. Ultrasound is diagnostic; it can easily differentiate fibroids from a pregnant uterus or adnexal mass (Stewart, 2015). Submucosal myomas may be diagnosed by vaginal ultrasound, sonohysterography, hysteroscopy, or as a filling defect on hysterosalpingography. Occasionally, an abdominopelvic radiograph will note concentric calcifications. Several reports promote CT and MRI studies of uterine myomas. However, these imaging techniques are more expensive than ultrasound. Until CT and MRI can distinguish between benign and malignant myomas, they will rarely be ordered in routine clinical management of myomas. MRI is helpful in differentiating adenomyosis or an adenomyoma from a single, solitary myoma, especially in a woman desiring preservation of her fertility. MRI with gadolinium contrast can also provide information on devascularized (degenerated) fibroids and more detail on the location of fibroids with respect to endometrial, intramural, or serosal

(Stewart, 2015). Serial ultrasound examinations have been used to evaluate progression in the size of myomas or response to therapy, although there is a strong correlation between pelvic exam and ultrasound, in determining the size of myomas.

The management of small, asymptomatic myomas is judicious observation. When the tumor is first discovered, it is appropriate to perform a pelvic examination at 6-month intervals to determine the rate of growth. The majority of women will not need surgery, especially those women in the perimenopausal period, where the condition usually improves with diminishing levels of circulating estrogens.

Cases of abnormal bleeding and leiomyomas should be investigated thoroughly for concurrent problems such as endometrial hyperplasia. If symptoms do not improve with conservative management, operative therapy may be considered. The choice between a myomectomy and hysterectomy is usually determined by the patient's age, parity, and, most important, future reproductive plans. Myomectomy is associated with longer hospital stays and more pelvic adhesions than hysterectomy. Studies suggest that myomectomy results in approximately 80% resolution of symptoms. Hysterectomy is associated with a greater than 90% patient satisfaction rate, though hysterectomy has a higher rate of urinary tract injuries, particularly abdominal hysterectomy. When myomectomies are performed to preserve fertility, care must be taken to avoid adhesions, which may compromise the goal of the operation. In the past, full-thickness myomectomies (surgeries that entered the endometrial cavity) were considered an indication for cesarean delivery prior to labor. Currently, most clinicians recommend strong consideration for cesarean section for all degrees of myomectomy other than removal of a pedunculated leiomyomata or small hysteroscopic resection.

Classic indications for a myomectomy include persistent abnormal bleeding, pain or pressure, or enlargement of an asymptomatic myoma to more than 8 cm in a woman who has not completed childbearing. The causal relationship of myomas and adverse reproductive outcomes is poorly understood. Long-standing infertility or repetitive abortion directly related to myomas is rare. Contraindications to a myomectomy include pregnancy, advanced adnexal disease, malignancy, and the situation in which enucleation of the myoma would severely reduce endometrial surface so that the uterus would not be functional. The choice between the two operations is not always an easy one.

Within 20 years of the myomectomy operation, one in four women subsequently has a hysterectomy performed, the majority for recurrent leiomyomas. Myomectomy may be performed in selected women using laparoscopic techniques. Hurst and associates have emphasized careful, multilayer closure and the use of antiadhesive barriers (Hurst, 2005). Some centers excise uterine myomas vaginally using an anterior or posterior colpotomy. They believe that vaginal myomectomy is an alternative surgical plan even in women with moderately enlarged tumors. Submucous myomas may be resected via the cervical canal using the hysteroscope. Although preliminary studies using laser surgery have been reported, most investigators advocate using an operative resectoscope. Three out of four women have long-term relief of their menorrhagia secondary to uterine myomas following hysteroscopic resection of the myomas.

The indications for hysterectomy for myomas are similar to indications for myomectomy, with a few additions. Some gynecologists selectively perform a hysterectomy for asymptomatic myomas when the uterus has reached the size of a 14- to 16-week gestation. The hypothesis is that most myomas of this size will eventually produce symptoms. However, it is impossible to predict which individual woman will develop symptoms. Rapid growth of a myoma after menopause warrants investigation and consideration for surgery. Prolapse of a myoma through the cervix is optimally treated by vaginal removal and ligation of the base of the myoma, with antibiotic coverage. Hysteroscopic resection aids the transvaginal removal of a prolapsed myoma.

There has been much controversy regarding the prevalence of undiagnosed uterine cancers among women with presumed benign fibroids at the time of hysterectomy. Morcellation is the process by which a large portion of tissue is divided into smaller pieces. The benefit of morcellation is the ability to perform a hysterectomy or myomectomy in a minimally invasive fashion, avoiding an open abdominal incision and the associated longer recovery time and higher mortality rate (Lawrence, 2014). This can be accomplished manually (i.e., with a scalpel or scissors) or via a rapidly rotating blade known as a *power morcellator*. The use of power morcellation may spread unsuspected cancer during surgery for treatment of symptomatic fibroids. There is no evidence that manual morcellation vaginally or abdominally eliminates this risk (ACOG, 2014). Wright reported that among women undergoing minimally invasive hysterectomy with morcellation, the risk of uterine cancer was 1 in 300 in women younger than 40 years of age and 1 in 1500 in women 40 to 44 years old (Wright, 2014). The Food and Drug Administration (FDA) recommends against the use of laparoscopic power morcellators in the majority of women undergoing myomectomy or hysterectomy for treatment of fibroids, thereby significantly limiting the use of morcellation to hysterectomy in premenopausal women who are not candidates for en bloc resection, and only after counseling women about the risks of power morcellation and the potential spread of cancer and offering alternatives such as morcellation in a bag that some centers are performing (USFDA, 2014). The use of an intraperitoneal bag for morcellation has been proposed to reduce tissue dissemination. Unfortunately, the current intraperitoneal bags are not designed for concurrent use with a power morcellator (ACOG, 2014).

For women undergoing minimally invasive surgery for symptomatic fibroids, preoperative considerations must be made regarding age, menopausal status, hereditary factors, uterine size, rapid uterine growth, endometrial sampling, cervical cytology, and pelvic imaging. Informed consent for these procedures should include a discussion of the risks and benefits of power morcellation. If after careful review malignancy is strongly suspected or known, then power morcellation must be avoided. After the FDA statement was released, a systematic review and meta-analysis were performed investigating survival outcomes of patients with unexpected uterine leiomyosarcoma. The pooled analysis showed a threefold increased risk of overall recurrence and fourfold increased risk of intraabdominal recurrence of leiomyosarcoma in patients undergoing uterine morcellation, whereas no increased risk of extraabdominal recurrence was demonstrated (Bogani, 2015). The data sampled were limited due to small sample size and the retrospective nature of the studies, thus more research is needed to determine the true impact of morcellation on unsuspected cancer and disease prognosis. Nonetheless, the impact of the FDA warning on clinical practice has become quickly evident. A survey of American Association of Gynecologic Laparoscopists (AAGL) and American College of Obstetricians and Gynecologists (ACOG) members showed nearly half of the respondents had increased their rate of laparotomy and nearly three quarters stopped using power morcellation during hysterectomy and myomectomy primarily due to hospital mandate, although they did not believe it resulted in improved patient outcomes (Lum, 2016).

It is possible to treat leiomyomas medically by reducing the circulating level of estrogen and progesterone. GnRH agonists, medroxyprogesterone acetate (Depo-Provera), danazol, aromatase inhibitors, and the antiprogesterone RU 486 have undergone clinical trials. Randomized controlled trials of 5 and 10 mg of mifepristone (RU486) have shown significant reduction in size, bleeding, and improvement in quality of life. Mifepristone acts through inhibition of progesterone receptors. Daily administration of 5 mg and 10 mg has shown uterine volume reductions of 48% and 52% after 1 year for both doses. Amenorrhea occurred in 65% of the women in 6 months and in 705 within a year. However, long-term use is controversial due to the potential of inducing endometrial pathology (Eisinger, 2005). The use of GnRH agonists, sometimes with add-back hormonal therapy, has also been successful in treating myomas. A Cochrane review on add-back therapy with GnRH analogues for uterine fibroids concluded there was low or moderate evidence that tibolone, raloxifene, estriol, and ipriflavone help preserve bone density and medroxyprogesterone acetate (MPA) and tibolone may reduce vasomotor symptoms. The studies included assessed only short-term (within 12 months) effectiveness and safety. Larger uterine volume was an adverse effect associated with some of the therapies (MPA, tibolone, and conjugated estrogens) (Moroni, 2015). Reductions in mean uterine volume and myoma size by 40% to 50% have been documented. However, individual responses vary greatly. With medical treatments, most of the size reductions occur within the first 3 months. After cessation of therapy, myomas gradually resume their pretreatment size. By 6 months after treatment, most myomas will have returned to their original size. During treatment, Doppler flow studies have demonstrated increased resistance in the uterine arteries and in the smaller arteries feeding the myoma. Also during treatment, the proliferative activity of the myoma and the binding of epidermal growth factor are reduced. The use of medical suppressive therapies such as GnRH agonists for women with large myomas and those with anemia may reduce blood loss at the time of hysterectomy or myomectomy. However, one study found that tourniquets at the time of myomectomy were as effective as pretreatment with GnRH agonists in decreasing blood loss.

### Therapies for Heavy Menstrual Bleeding

In women who have heavy menstrual bleeding as the primary symptom, limited data support the effectiveness of medical therapies including tranexamic acid and the levonorgestrel-releasing intrauterine device (Stewart, 2015). Tranexamic acid is an oral fibrinolytic agent that may decrease bleeding when taken only during heavy menstrual bleeding. As its mechanism of action is concerning for increased thrombotic risk, it should not be taken concomitantly with oral contraceptives. The levonorgestrel-releasing intrauterine device decreased menstrual bleeding while providing contraception; however, the rate of expulsion among women with submucosal fibroids may be as high as 12% (Stewart, 2015). Oral progestogens have not been demonstrated to reduce fibroid size or fibroid-related symptoms (Sangkomkamhang, 2013). Oral contraceptives reduce menstrual bleeding in women with fibroids according to observational data. In addition, nonsteroidal anti-inflammatory drugs decrease heavy menstrual bleeding and menstrual pain.

### Future Options for Medical Treatment

Currently, no validated medical treatment is able to eliminate fibroids; therefore surgery is the most effective treatment for symptomatic fibroids. However, there are emerging medical treatments that may be a good option for women who wish to avoid surgery, or before surgery, to reduce the invasiveness of the operation. In women with planned surgical treatment, oral ulipristal acetate controls symptoms, reduces tumor size, and improves quality of life compared with placebo and is not inferior to leuprolide acetate when used for 3 months (Perez-Lopez, 2015).

Ulipristal acetate is a selective progesterone receptor modulator that on binding to the progesterone receptor in target tissues displays antagonist and partial agonist effects (McKeage, 2011). The efficacy of ulipristal acetate has been demonstrated in three European phase III studies evaluating PGL4001 (Ulipristal Acetate) Efficacy Assessment in Reduction of Symptoms Due to Uterine Leiomyomata (PEARL I, II, and III) (Donnez 2012a, 2012b, 2014). Ulipristal acetate was approved for medical treatment for fibroids in Canada in 2013 (Singh, 2015). It is also licensed in Europe for the same indication (Trefoux, 2015). It is not FDA approved for treatment of fibroids in the United States.

Aromatase inhibitors block the synthesis of estrogen. They have been shown to reduce uterine fibroid size (up to 71% in 2 months) and ameliorate uterine fibroid symptoms, including a reduction in menstrual volume and duration of menstruation, and urinary retention (Shozu, 2003). Table 18.3 summarizes the medical options for the management of patients with uterine leiomyomas.

### Uterine Artery Embolization

Uterine myomas may also be treated with uterine artery embolization (UAE) (Fig. 18.39). Multiple embolic materials have been used including gelatin sponge (Gelfoam) silicone spheres, gelatin microspheres, metal coils, and most commonly polyvinyl alcohol (PVA) particles of various diameters. Postprocedural abdominal and pelvic pain is common for the first 24 hours and may last up to 2 weeks. Most patients remain overnight in the hospital for pain relief and observation; however, some women will go home a few hours after treatment. Large trials, including the EMMY trial (Uterine Artery Embolization for Treatment of Symptomatic Uterine Fibroid Tumors), have consistently documented shorter hospitalizations and shorter recoveries, with a similar complication rate to hysterectomy. Reviews of the large trials and reports find that the need for reoperation within the first few years after embolization is 20% to 30%, with an overall failure rate of 40%, *failure rate* being defined as a return of symptoms and decrement in quality of life measures. The 5-year failure rate from the EMMY trial as reported by van der Kooij and associates included a 28.4% subsequent hysterectomy rate (van der Kooij, 2010). Risk factors for failure with UAE included younger age at embolization, bleeding as an indication for therapy, multiple myomas, and the finding at the time of imaging of collateral ovarian vessels feeding the myoma. Thus the procedure

Table 18.3 Summary of the Medical Management Options for Patients with Uterine Leiomyomas

| Drug Class | Action | Benefits | Risks | Side Effects (%) | Authors* |
|---|---|---|---|---|---|
| COC | Inhibits ovulation; inhibits sex steroid secretion | 17% decrease in the risk of leiomyoma growth; decreases bleeding and increases hematocrit | Thromboembolic events; hepatocellular adenoma (rare) | Spotting; mastalgia; headache; gastrointestinal upset | Qin et al; Orsini et al |
| Progestogens | May inhibit ovulation and sex steroid synthesis; decidualizes endometrium, inducing a "pseudopregnancy" state | Improves bleeding in up to 70%; amenorrhea in up to 30%; may decrease uterine volume in up to 50% | Loss of bone mass (prolonged use of depot MPA) | Irregular bleeding/ spotting; ovarian follicular cysts | Venkatachalam et al; Ichigo et al |
| LNG-IUS | Endometrial atrophy | Reduces bleeding intensity in up to 99%; decreases uterine volume in about 40% | Device expulsion | Ovarian cysts; acne | Kriplani et al; Sayed et al |
| GnRH-a | Hypoestrogenism due to gonadotrophin secretion inhibition | Uterine volume decrease in up to 50%; high rates of amenorrhea | Loss of bone mass with prolonged use | Hot flashes (>90%); vaginal atrophy; headache; mood disorders | Friedman et al; Tummon et al; Dawood et al |
| SPRM | Inhibits ovulation; inhibits progesterone action on fibroid tissue | Improves bleeding in up to 98% of patients; decreases fibroid volume in up to 53% | Long term endometrial safety is unknown | Benign endometrial changes after short-term use | Donnez et al; Williams et al |

From Moroni RM, Vieira CS, Ferriani RA, et al. Pharmacological treatment of uterine fibroids. *Ann Med Health Sci Res.* 2014;4(Suppl 3):S185-S192.
*All citations are from the original source article.
*COC*, combined oral contraceptive; *GnRH-a*, gonadotropin-releasing hormone analog; *LNG-IUS*, levonorgestrel-releasing intrauterine system; *MPA*, medroxyprogesterone acetate; *SPRM*, selective progesterone receptor modulators.

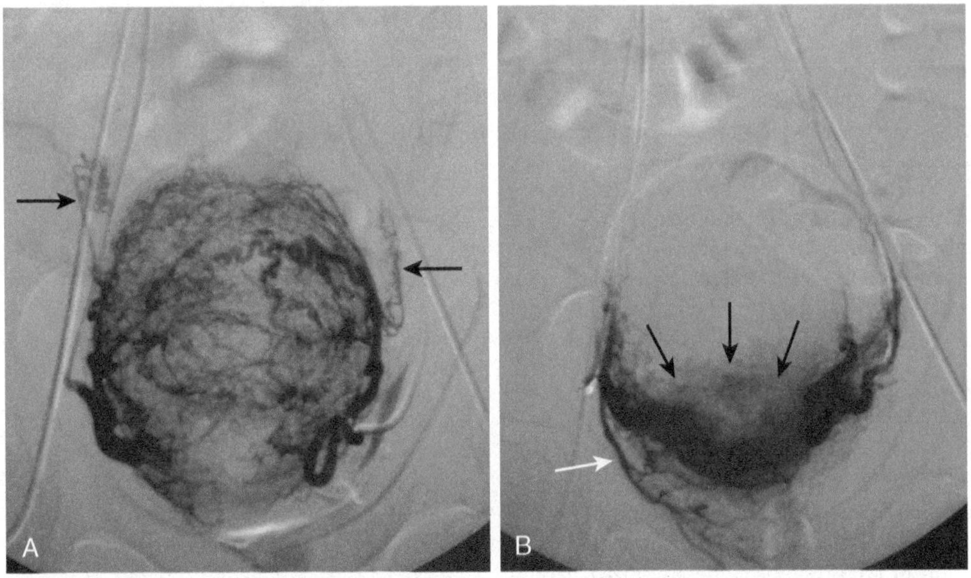


**Figure 18.39** Uterine fibroid embolization. **A,** Angiographic image of uterine leiomyoma before uterine fibroid embolization. *Arrows* point to preembolization uterine artery. **B,** Postembolization image of same devascularized myoma with normal myometrial perfusion maintained *(black arrows)*. White arrow points to patent cervicovaginal branch of uterine artery at completion of embolization. (From Spies JB, Czeyda-Pommersheim F. Uterine fibroid embolization. In Mauro MA, Murphy KPJ, Thomson KR, et al, eds. *Image-Guided Interventions.* 2nd ed. Philadelphia: Elsevier; 2014:542-546.)

itself, though a valuable alternative to hysterectomy, is not for all women, with a significant proportion of women needing follow-up procedures.

Fertility after arterial embolization is difficult to quantify. Higher than expected rates of intrauterine growth restriction, preterm delivery, and miscarriage have been reported. In general, women choosing a conservative approach to preserve fertility should have a surgical myomectomy rather than UAE.

Complications of UAE affect about 5% of patients and include postembolization fever; sepsis from infarction of the necrotic myometrium, which may occur several weeks to a few months post procedure; and ovarian failure, affecting up to 3% of cases in women younger than 45 and 15% in women older than 45. This is thought to occur from spread of emboli material into the ovarian circulation. There is, in general, a decreased ovarian reserve found in older women after embolization. Amenorrhea

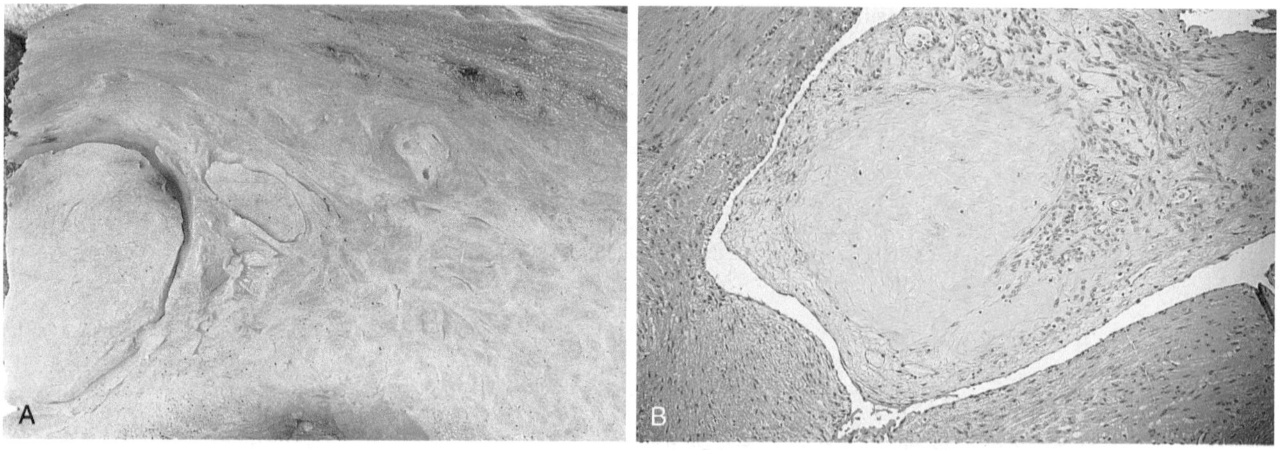


**Figure 18.40** Intravenous leiomyomatosis. **A,** Tumor masses are present within distended blood vessels. **B,** This example shows hyaline degeneration of the intravascular element. (From Anderson MC, Robboy SJ, Russell P. Uterine smooth muscle tumors. In: Robboy SJ, Anderson MC, Russell P, eds. *Pathology of the Female Reproductive Tract.* Edinburgh: Churchill Livingstone; 2002.)

may occur secondary to an endometrial hypoxic injury, as well. Rarely, necrosis of surrounding tissues may present as a complication of embolization.

Another complication of UAE is shedding of necrotic myomata or portions of myomata into the intrauterine cavity. Shedding may lead to infection or abdominal pain as the uterus tries to pass the material. This may require either a uterine curettage or hysteroscopic removal, although some authors have reported removing the necrotic material in the office. Because shedding of necrotic material is a relatively common complication, several authors have recommended that submucous myomata be removed hysteroscopically rather than attempted through UAE because these types of myomata are more prone to be shed into the uterine cavity. Intraabdominal adhesions, particularly after embolization of larger myomata, are also an uncommon but not rare complication.

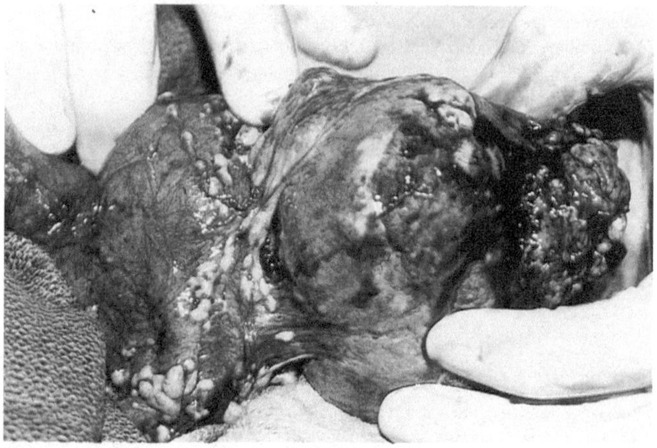

**Figure 18.41** Photograph of leiomyomatosis peritonealis disseminate. (Courtesy of William Droegemueller and Vern L. Katz.)

### *Other Minimally Invasive Interventions*

Endometrial ablation is used mainly to manage heavy uterine bleeding. It is limited to women with a normal-size uterus and uterine fibroids less than 3 cm in diameter. Compared with hysterectomy, endometrial ablation has a shorter intraoperative time, faster recovery, and fewer adverse events; however, it has inferior reduction in menstrual bleeding and lower patient satisfaction (Lethaby, 2000). Pregnancy following endometrial ablation is not recommended due to the high risk of miscarriage, ectopic pregnancy, and invasive placental disorders that may occur after this procedure.

Myolysis (the destruction of uterine fibroids or their blood supply via ultrasound, laser, cryotherapy, or other methods) has been studied as a conservative alternative for women who want to preserve their uterus but not fertility. Candidates are women with small fibroids (typically less than or equal to 5 cm) or the largest fibroid being less than 10 cm in diameter. Cheung reviewed the literature on sonographically guided high-intensity focused ultrasound for the management of fibroids, a procedure commonly used in China (Cheung, 2013). Magnetic resonance guided focused ultrasound surgery appears to be the most effective and least aggressive; however, this technique is limited by the need for costly equipment and limited data of efficacy and safety (Marret, 2012).

Two associated but rare diseases should be noted: intravenous leiomyomatosis and leiomyomatosis peritonealis disseminata. *Intravenous leiomyomatosis* is a rare condition in which benign smooth muscle fibers invade and slowly grow into the venous channels of the pelvis (Fig. 18.40). The tumor grows by direct extension and grossly appears like a "spaghetti" tumor. Only 25% of tumors extend beyond the broad ligament. However, case series and reports document tumor growth into the vena cava and right heart. The tumors may present with cardiac symptomatology and usually require surgical resection. Series from Zhang and colleagues and Worley and colleagues noted good results with single staged surgeries. Most authors recommend antiestrogen therapy with aromatase inhibitors after resection of leiomyomatosis of any degree (Worley, 2009; Zhang, 2010).

*Leiomyomatosis peritonealis disseminata* (LPD) is a benign disease with multiple small nodules over the surface of the pelvis and abdominal peritoneum. Grossly, LPD mimics disseminated carcinoma (Fig. 18.41). However, histologic examination

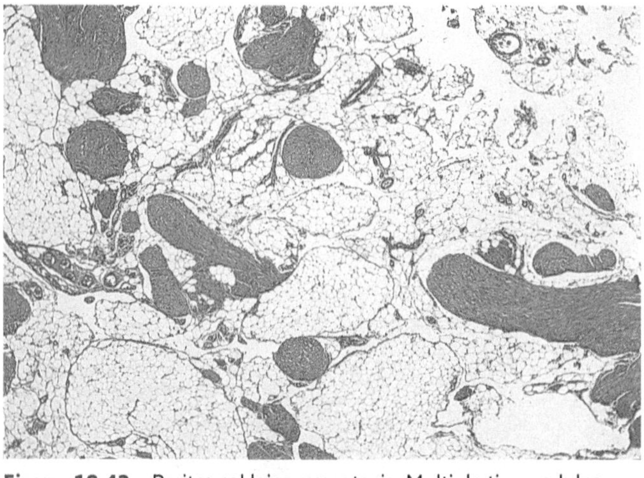

Figure 18.42 Peritoneal leiomyomatosis. Multiple tiny nodules of smooth muscle are scattered throughout the omentum. (From Anderson MC, Robboy SJ, Russell P. Uterine smooth muscle tumors. In: Robboy SJ, Anderson MC, Russell P, eds. *Pathology of the Female Reproductive Tract*. Edinburgh: Churchill Livingstone; 2002.)

demonstrates benign-appearing myomas (Fig. 18.42). This disorder is often associated with a recent pregnancy. Also, the use of power morcellation increases the risk of LPD, due to intraperitoneal spread of uterine tissue (Kumar, 2008). Therapies with progestogens, selective estrogen receptor modulators (SERMS), or aromatase inhibitors have all been used in management. A rare autosomal syndrome of uterine and cutaneous leiomyomata and renal cell carcinoma also exists. Consideration should be given to renal evaluation in families with this history and with cutaneous leiomyomas.

In summary, leiomyomas are the most common tumor in women, and certainly one of the most common problems facing the gynecologist. Symptoms will present in 30% to 50% of women with myomata. Management is individualized to fit the patient's symptoms and reproductive desires.

## ADENOMYOSIS

Adenomyosis has often been referred to as *endometriosis interna*. This term is misleading because endometriosis and adenomyosis are discovered in the same patient in less than 20% of women. More important, endometriosis and adenomyosis are clinically different diseases. The only common feature is the presence of ectopic endometrial glands and stroma. Adenomyosis is derived from aberrant glands of the basalis layer of the endometrium. Therefore these glands do not usually undergo the traditional proliferative and secretory changes that are associated with cyclic ovarian hormone production. The disease is common and may be found in up to 60% of hysterectomy specimens in women in the late reproductive years. Most studies have documented an incidence closer to 30%, with greater than 50% of these women being relatively asymptomatic. The symptoms of menorrhagia and dysmenorrhea form a spectrum and are subjective, thus delineating an incidence of associated symptomatology with adenomyosis is problematic.

Adenomyosis is usually diagnosed incidentally by the pathologist examining histologic sections of surgical specimens. The frequency of the histologic diagnosis is directly related to how

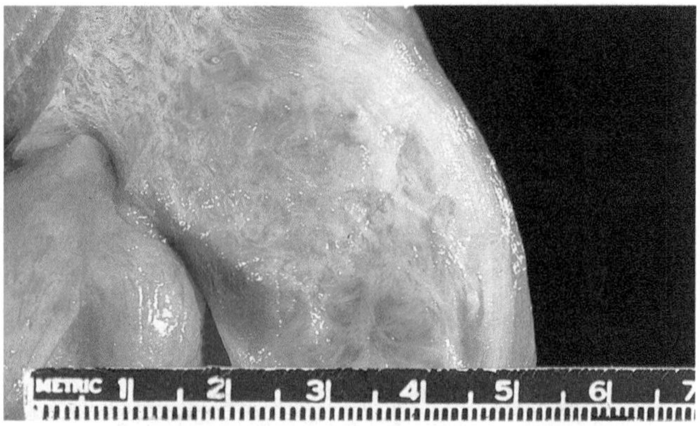


Figure 18.43 Adenomyosis. The myometrial wall is distorted and thickened by poorly circumscribed trabeculae that contain pinpoint hemorrhagic cysts. (From Anderson MC, Robboy SJ, Russell P. Uterine smooth muscle tumors. In: Robboy SJ, Anderson MC, Russell P, eds. *Pathology of the Female Reproductive Tract*. Edinburgh: Churchill Livingstone; 2002.)

meticulously the pathologist searches for the disease. Adenomyosis is also a common incidental finding during autopsy. Serial histologic slides confirm the continuity of benign growth of the basalis layer of the endometrium into the myometrium. Thus the histogenesis of adenomyosis is direct extension from the endometrial lining.

The disease is associated with increased parity, particularly uterine surgeries and traumas. The pathogenesis of adenomyosis is unknown but is theorized to be associated with disruption of the barrier between the endometrium and myometrium as one series noted a 1.7 RR (1.1 to 2.6) of a dilation and curettage with an SAB in women with adenomyosis versus control subjects. Other studies have found a higher rate of induced abortion with presumed curettage in women with adenomyosis versus controls. Panganamamula and associates noted the history of any prior uterine surgery to be a significant risk factor in a set of 412 women with adenomyosis, 1.37 RR (1.05 to 1.79) (Panganamamula, 2004). These studies and experimental work in animals strongly support the theory that trauma to the endometrial-myometrial interface is a significant factor in the etiology of this condition. However, because adenomyosis was described well before uterine curettage and may occur (though uncommonly) in nulliparous women, the full pathogenesis is yet to be determined.

### PATHOLOGY

There are two distinct pathologic presentations of adenomyosis. The most common is a diffuse involvement of both anterior and posterior walls of the uterus. The posterior wall is usually involved more than the anterior wall (Fig. 18.43). The individual areas of adenomyosis are not encapsulated. The second presentation is a focal area or adenomyoma. This results in an asymmetrical uterus, and this special area of adenomyosis may have a pseudocapsule. Diffuse adenomyosis is found in two thirds of cases.

In the more common, diffuse type of adenomyosis the uterus is uniformly enlarged, usually two to three times normal size. It is often difficult to distinguish on physical examination from uterine leiomyomas. However, the ultrasound appearance of leiomyomata helps to distinguish the two. Similarly on visual

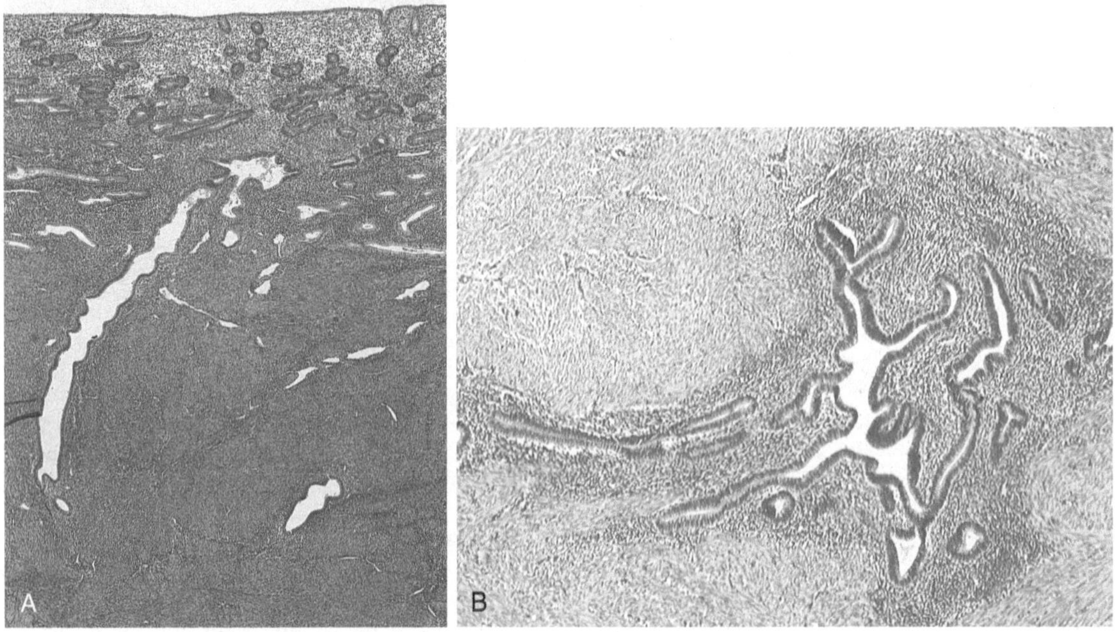


**Figure 18.44** Adenomyosis, histologic appearance. **A,** Endometrial tissue infiltrates into the myometrium. **B,** The infiltrating islands of endometrium consist of both glands and stroma. The glands are inactive and of basal pattern. (From Anderson MC, Robboy SJ, Russell P. Uterine smooth muscle tumors. In: Robboy SJ, Anderson MC, Russell P, eds. *Pathology of the Female Reproductive Tract.* Edinburgh: Churchill Livingstone; 2002.)

inspection the two entities are quite different. When a knife transects the myometrium, the cut surface protrudes convexly and has a spongy appearance. The cut surface of a uterus with adenomyosis is darker than the white surface of a myoma. Sometimes there are discrete areas of adenomyosis that are not densely encapsulated and contain small, dark cystic spaces. There is not a distinct cleavage plane around focal adenomyomas as there is with uterine myomas.

Histologic examination will note benign endometrial glands and stroma are within the myometrium. These glands rarely undergo the same cyclic changes as the normal uterine endometrium. Studies have demonstrated both estrogen and progesterone receptors in tissue samples from adenomyosis.

The standard criterion used in diagnosis of adenomyosis is the finding of endometrial glands and stroma more than one low-powered field (2.5 mm) from the basalis layer of the endometrium. The small areas of adenomyosis have the same general appearance as the basalis layers of the endometrium. Histologically the glands exhibit an inactive or proliferative pattern. Rarely, one can also see cystic hyperplasia or a pseudodecidual pattern. In general, there is a lack of inflammatory cells surrounding the fossae of adenomyosis. Although the areas do not undergo full menstrual-type changes, bleeding may occur in these ectopic areas, as evidenced by both gross and microscopic findings. It is not unusual to see histologic variability in several different areas deep in the walls of the myometrium from the same uterus. Some fossae of adenomyosis undergo decidual changes either during pregnancy or during estrogen-progestin therapy for endometriosis. The reaction of the myometrium to the ectopic endometrium is hyperplasia and hypertrophy of individual muscle fibers (Figs. 18.43 and 18.44). Surrounding most foci of glands and stroma are localized areas of hyperplasia of the smooth muscle of the uterus. This change in the myometrium produces the globular enlargement of the uterus (Fig. 18.45).

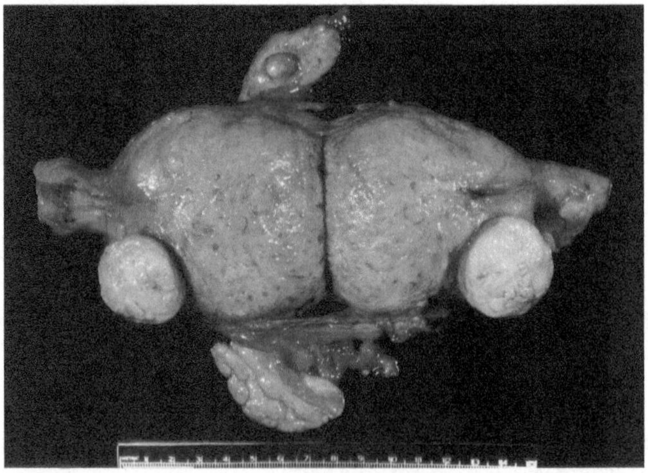

**Figure 18.45** Hysterectomy with adenomyosis. The uterine corpus is thickened and shows prominent trabeculation of the myometrium with multiple small foci of hemorrhage. (From Oliva E. Endometrial stromal tumors, mixed müllerian tumors, adenomyosis, adenomyomas and rare sarcomas. In: Mutter GL, Prat J, eds. *Robboy's Pathology of the Female Reproductive Tract.* 3rd ed. Philadelphia: Elsevier; 2014:425-458.)

### CLINICAL DIAGNOSIS

Over 50% of women with adenomyosis are asymptomatic or have minor symptoms that do not annoy them enough to seek medical care. They attribute the increase in dysmenorrhea or menstrual bleeding to the aging process and tolerate the symptoms. Symptomatic adenomyosis usually presents in women between the ages of 35 and 50. The severity of pelvic symptoms increases proportionally to the depth of penetration and the total volume of disease in the myometrium.

The classic symptoms of adenomyosis are secondary dysmenorrhea and menorrhagia. The acquired dysmenorrhea becomes increasingly more severe as the disease progresses. Occasionally the patient complains of dyspareunia, which is midline in location and deep in the pelvis. On pelvic examination the uterus is diffusely enlarged, usually two to three times normal size. It is most unusual for the uterine enlargement associated with adenomyosis to be greater than a 14-week-size gestation unless the patient also has uterine myomas. The uterus is globular and tender immediately before and during menstruation (see Fig. 18.45). LevGur and colleagues evaluated the gynecologic histories of women with diffuse adenomyosis compared with women without such a history (LevGur, 2000). In their series, the symptoms of dysmenorrhea and menorrhagia correlated with the amount of adenomyosis and the depth of myometrial invasion.

The diagnosis of adenomyosis is usually confirmed following histologic examination of the hysterectomy specimen. Frequently the clinical diagnosis is inaccurately assigned to the patient who has chronic pelvic pain. Traditionally the patient will have endometrial sampling to rule out other organic causes of abnormal bleeding. Many times adenomyosis is diagnosed retrospectively following a hysterectomy for other indications. Attempts have been made to establish the diagnosis preoperatively by transcervical needle biopsy of the myometrium. However, even with multiple needle biopsies, the sensitivity of the test is too low to be of practical clinical value. Adenomyosis may coexist with both endometrial hyperplasia and endometrial carcinoma. Approximately two of three women with adenomyosis have coexistent pelvic pathology, most commonly myomas but also endometriosis, endometrial hyperplasia, and salpingitis isthmica nodosa.

Ultrasound and MRI are both useful to help differentiate between adenomyosis and uterine myomas in a young woman desiring future childbearing. Diagnosing adenomyosis by transvaginal ultrasonography has a reported sensitivity between 53% and 89% and a specificity of 50% to 89%. In some series, MRI is more sensitive, ranging between 88% and 93%, and has a higher specificity (66% to 91%) than ultrasonography in the diagnosis of adenomyosis. Verma and associates reported the addition of sonohysterography with vaginal ultrasound, with an increase in sensitivity and specificity comparable with MRI. T2-weighted images are superior in making the diagnosis and documenting widened junctional zones (Verma, 2009). Studies indicate that three-dimensional transvaginal ultrasound is superior to two-dimensional transvaginal ultrasound and may allow for the diagnosis of early stage disease (Struble, 2016). Findings of poorly defined junctional zone markings in the endometrial-myometrial interface help confirm the diagnosis. Ascher and coworkers described high signal intensity striations emanating from the endometrium and trailing into the myometrium as helpful findings (Ascher, 2003). These bands most likely represent the glands and hypertrophied muscle of adenomyosis. MRI is clinically useful in differentiating adenomyosis from uterine leiomyoma, especially preoperatively in women who desire future fertility or who may choose uterine artery embolization for treatment of myomata. The success of uterine artery embolization for adenomyosis is unproved.

### MANAGEMENT

There is no satisfactory proved medical treatment for adenomyosis. Patients with adenomyosis have been treated with GnRH agonists, progestogens, and progesterone-containing IUDs, cyclic hormones, or prostaglandin synthetase inhibitors for their abnormal bleeding and pain. Hysterectomy is the definitive treatment if this therapy is appropriate for the woman's age, parity, and plans for future reproduction. Size of the uterus, degree of prolapse, and presence of associated pelvic pathology determine the choice of surgical approach. Women who become pregnant with adenomyosis are at increased risk of pregnancy complications such as premature labor and delivery, low birthweight, and preterm premature rupture of membranes.

## OVIDUCT

### LEIOMYOMAS

Both benign and malignant tumors of the oviduct are uncommon compared with other gynecologic neoplasms. Although these tumors are underreported, fewer than 100 women with myomas or leiomyomas of the oviduct are described in the literature. Tubal leiomyomas may be single or multiple and usually are discovered in the interstitial portion of the tubes. They usually coexist with the more common uterine leiomyomas. Myomas may originate from muscle cells in the walls of the tube or blood vessels or from smooth muscle in the broad ligament.

Leiomyomas of the tube present as smooth, firm, mobile, usually nontender masses that may be palpated during the bimanual examination. Similar to uterine myomas, they may be subserosal, interstitial, or submucosal. During laparoscopy the myomas appear as a spherical mass that protrudes from beneath the peritoneal surface. They vary from a few millimeters to 15 cm in diameter. Histologically they are identical to uterine leiomyomas.

The majority of the myomas of the oviduct are asymptomatic. Rarely, they may undergo acute degeneration or be associated with unilateral tubal obstruction or torsion. Treatment of a symptomatic tubal leiomyoma is excision.

### ADENOMATOID TUMORS

The most prevalent benign tumor of the oviduct is the *angiomyoma* or *adenomatoid tumor* (Fig. 18.46). They are small, gray-white, circumscribed nodules, 1 to 2 cm in diameter. These tumors are usually unilateral and present as small nodules just under the tubal serosa. These small nodules do not produce pelvic symptoms or signs. These benign tumors also are found below the serosa of the fundus of the uterus and the broad ligament. Microscopically, they are composed of small tubules lined by a low cuboidal or flat epithelium. Histologic studies have

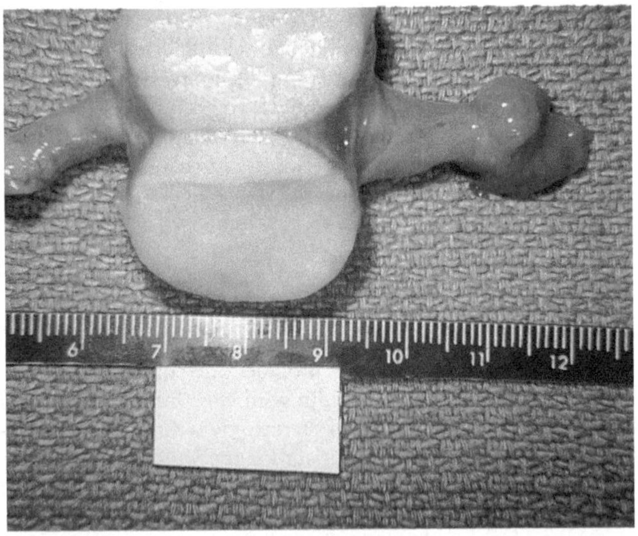

**Figure 18.46** Adenomatoid tumor. (From Anderson MC, Robboy SJ, Russell P. The fallopian tube. In: Robboy SJ, Anderson MC, Russell P, eds. *Pathology of the Female Reproductive Tract.* Edinburgh: Churchill Livingstone; 2002.)

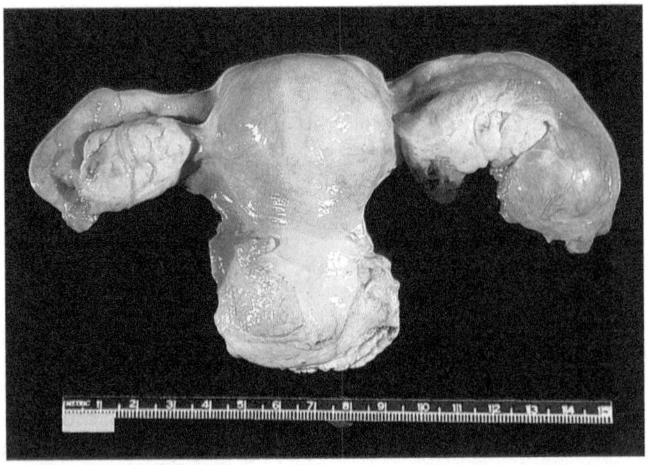

**Figure 18.48** Broad ligament cyst. This parovarian, or paratubal cyst, is thin walled and contains clear watery fluid. (From Anderson MC, Robboy SJ, Russell P. The fallopian tube. In: Robboy SJ, Anderson MC, Russell P, eds. *Pathology of the Female Reproductive Tract.* Edinburgh: Churchill Livingstone; 2002.)

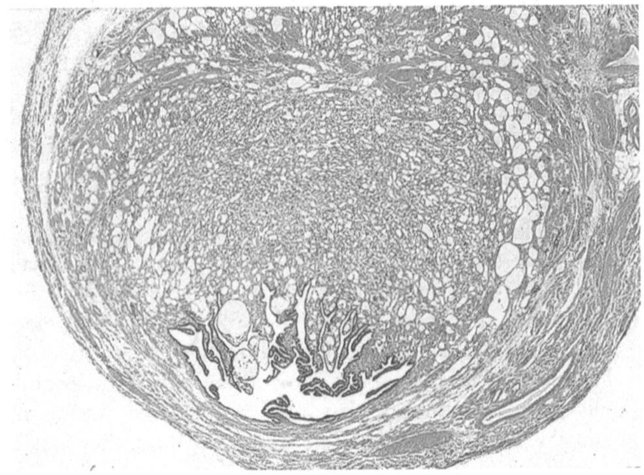

**Figure 18.47** Adenomatoid tumor arising in the fallopian tube. (From Voet RL. *Color Atlas of Obstetric and Gynecologic Pathology.* St. Louis: Mosby-Wolfe; 1997.)

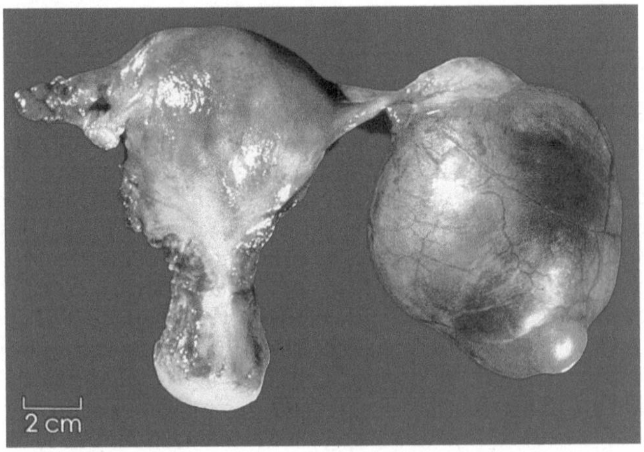


**Figure 18.49** A nonneoplastic cyst with the broad ligament abuts the normal ovary. (From Clement PB, Young RH. *Atlas of Gynecologic Surgical Pathology.* Philadelphia: Saunders; 2000.)

established that the thin-walled channels that comprise these tumors are of mesothelial origin (Fig. 18.47). These tumors do not become malignant; however, they may be mistaken for a low-grade neoplasm when initially viewed during a frozen-section evaluation.

## PARATUBAL CYSTS

Paratubal cysts are frequently incidental discoveries during gynecologic operations for other abnormalities. They are often multiple and may vary from 0.5 cm to more than 20 cm in diameter. Most cysts are small, asymptomatic, and slow growing and are discovered during the third and fourth decades of life. When paratubal cysts are *pedunculated* and near the fimbrial end of the oviduct, they are called hydatid cysts of Morgagni (Figs. 18.48 and 18.49). Cysts near the oviduct may be of mesonephric, mesothelial, or paramesonephric origin. Sometimes the histologic differentiation is difficult because of mechanically produced changes in the cells that line the cyst. These cysts are translucent and contain a clear or pale yellow fluid.

The histogenesis of the majority of paratubal cysts had been believed to be from the mesonephric duct, with the cysts arising from the main duct or accessory tubules. These latter cysts often develop between the leaves of the broad ligament in the mesosalpinx, with the ovary being separate. However, a histologic study of 79 paratubal cysts documented that 60 of the cysts were of tubal origin. Thus the majority of grossly identified "paratubal cysts" are in reality accessory lumina of the fallopian tubes. The remaining 19 cysts were of mesothelial origin. Paratubal cysts are thin walled and smooth and contain clear fluid. Often there are multiple small cysts. Occasionally there is a papillomatous proliferation on the internal wall of these cysts. Inflammatory cysts of the peritoneum may be found anywhere in the pelvis.

The majority of paratubal cysts are asymptomatic and are usually discovered incidentally during ultrasound or during gynecologic operations. When paratubal cysts are symptomatic, they generally produce a dull pain. During a pelvic examination it is difficult to distinguish a paratubal cyst from an ovarian mass. At operation the oviduct is often found stretched over a large paratubal cyst. The oviduct should not be removed in these cases because it will return to normal size after the paratubal cyst is excised. In one retrospective 10-year review of 168 women with parovarian tumors, three low-grade malignant neoplasms were found. These malignancies were in women of reproductive age who had cysts greater than 5 cm in diameter with internal papillary projections. The authors cautioned that the differentiation between benign and malignant parovarian masses cannot be made by external examination of the cyst. The practice of aspirating cysts via the laparoscope should be limited to cysts that are completely simple and associated with normal cancer antigen-125 (CA-125) levels. More recent theories of epithelial ovarian carcinogenesis suggest that serous, endometrioid, and clear cell carcinomas are derived from the fallopian tube and the endometrium rather than the ovarian surface epithelium (Erickson, 2013). The American College of Obstetricians and Gynecologists supports the view that prophylactic salpingectomy may offer clinicians the opportunity to prevent ovarian cancer in their patients, and the surgeon should discuss the potential benefits of the removal of the fallopian tubes during hysterectomy in women at population risk for ovarian cancer (ACOG, 2015).

Paratubal cysts may grow rapidly during pregnancy, and most of the cases of torsion of these cysts have been reported during pregnancy or the puerperium. Treatment is simple excision.

### TORSION

Acute torsion of the oviduct is a rare event; however, it has been reported with both normal and pathologic fallopian tubes. Pregnancy predisposes to this problem. Tubal torsion usually accompanies torsion of the ovary, as they have a common vascular pedicle. (See the discussion of ovarian torsion presented later in this chapter.) Torsion of the fallopian tube is secondary to an ovarian mass in approximately 50% to 60% of patients. The right tube is involved more frequently than is the left (Fig. 18.50). The degree of tubal torsion varies from less than one turn to four complete rotations. Torsion of the oviduct is usually seen in women of reproductive age. However, it occurs also in preadolescent children, especially when part of the tube is enclosed in the sac of a femoral or inguinal hernia.

Tubal torsion may be divided into intrinsic and extrinsic causes. Prominent intrinsic causes include congenital abnormalities, such as increased tortuosity caused by excessive length of the tube, and pathologic processes, such as hydrosalpinx, hematosalpinx, tubal neoplasms, and previous operation, especially tubal ligation. Torsion of the fallopian tube following tubal ligation is usually of the distal end. Extrinsic causes of tubal torsion are ovarian and peritubal tumors, adhesions, trauma, and pregnancy.

The most important symptom of tubal torsion is acute lower abdominal and pelvic pain. The onset of this pain is usually sudden, but it may also be gradual, and the pain is usually located in the iliac fossa, with radiation to the thigh and flank. The duration of pain is generally less than 48 hours, and it is associated with nausea and vomiting in two thirds of the cases. Usually, the pelvic pain,

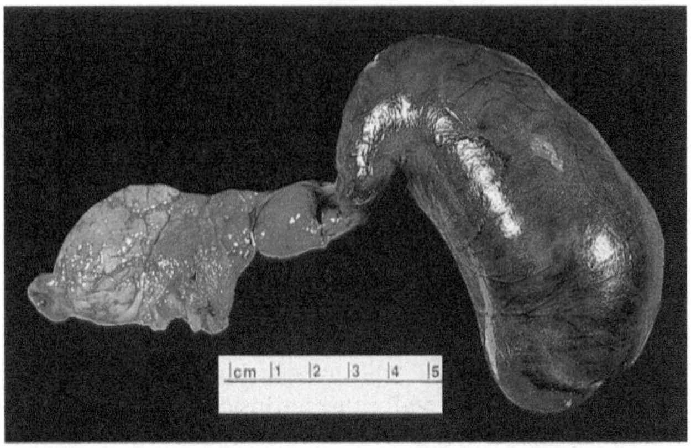


**Figure 18.50** Hematosalpinx with torsion. (From Voet RL. *Color Atlas of Obstetric and Gynecologic Pathology*. St. Louis: Mosby-Wolfe; 1997.)

secondary to hypoxia, is so intense that it is difficult to perform an adequate pelvic exam. Unless there is associated torsion of the ovary, a specific mass is usually not palpable on pelvic examination.

The preoperative diagnosis of tubal torsion is made in less than 20% of reported cases. However, the number of cases diagnosed preoperatively has increased dramatically with the use of vaginal ultrasonography. Because of the severity of the pain, a wide differential diagnosis of abdominal and pelvic pathology must be considered. The differential diagnosis includes acute appendicitis, ectopic pregnancy, pelvic inflammatory disease, and rupture or torsion of an ovarian cyst.

Exploratory operation determines the extent of hypoxia and the choice of operative techniques. With tubal torsion, usually the tubes are gangrenous and must be excised. The twisted tube is usually filled with a bloody or serous fluid. It may be possible to restore normal circulation to the tube by manually untwisting it. The tube is usually sutured into a secure position to prevent recurrence.

## OVARY

Ovarian masses are a frequent finding on pelvic examination and pelvic imaging. The task of the clinician is to determine whether the mass should be removed or may be managed expectantly. The general factors used to consider removal include the symptoms produces by the mass, the chances that the mass is malignant, and the likelihood of spontaneous resolution.

### FUNCTIONAL CYSTS

#### Follicular Cysts

Follicular cysts are by far the most frequent cystic structures in normal ovaries. They may be found as early as 20 weeks, gestation in female fetuses and throughout a woman's reproductive life. Follicular cysts are frequently multiple and may vary from a few millimeters to as large as 15 cm in diameter. A normal follicle may develop into a physiologic cyst. A minimum diameter to be considered as a cyst is generally considered to be between 2.5 and 3 cm. Follicular cysts are not neoplastic and are believed to be dependent on gonadotropins for growth. They arise from a temporary variation of a normal physiologic process. Clinically they may present with the signs and symptoms of ovarian enlargement and therefore must be differentiated from a true ovarian neoplasm. Functional cysts may be solitary or multiple. These cysts are found most commonly in young, menstruating women. Solitary cysts may occur during the fetal and neonatal periods and rarely during childhood, but there is an increase in frequency during the perimenarcheal period. Wolf and coworkers studied 149 postmenopausal women and found simple cysts ranging in size from 0.4 to 4.7 cm in 15% of them (Wolf, 1991). Large solitary follicular cysts in which the lining is luteinized are occasionally discovered during pregnancy and the puerperium. CA-125 may be used to evaluate such cysts in pregnancy. The values for CA-125 should be within the normal range past 12 weeks' gestation. Multiple follicular cysts in which the lining is luteinized are associated with either intrinsic or extrinsic elevated levels of gonadotropins. Interestingly, reproductive-age women with cystic fibrosis appear to have an increased propensity for developing individual follicular cysts.

Follicular cysts are translucent, thin-walled, and are filled with a watery, clear to straw-colored fluid. If a small opening in the capsule of the cyst suddenly develops, the cyst fluid under pressure will squirt out. These cysts are situated in the ovarian cortex, and sometimes they appear as translucent domes on the surface of the ovary. Histologically the lining of the cyst is usually composed of a closely packed layer of round, plump granulosa cells, with the spindle-shaped cells of the theca interna deeper in the stroma. In many cysts the lining of granulosa cells is difficult to distinguish, having undergone pressure atrophy. All that remains is a hyalinized connective tissue lining. The temporary disturbance in follicular function that produces the clinical picture of a follicular cyst is poorly understood. Follicular cysts may result from either the dominant mature follicle's failing to rupture (persistent follicle) or an immature follicle's failing to undergo the normal process of atresia. In the latter circumstance, the incompletely developed follicle fails to reabsorb follicular fluid. Some follicular cysts lose their ability to produce estrogen, and in others the granulosa cells remain productive, with prolonged secretion of estrogens. Occasionally, follicular cysts are better termed *follicular hematomas,* because blood from the vascular theca zone fills the cavity of the cyst.

Most follicular cysts are asymptomatic and are discovered during ultrasound imaging of the pelvis or a routine pelvic examination. Ultrasound cannot reliably differentiate a benign from a malignant process. However, several characteristics of ovarian masses correlate with malignancy, including internal papillations (echogenic structures protruding into the mass), loculations, solid lesions or cystic lesions with solid components, thick septations, and smaller cysts adjacent to or part of the wall of the larger cyst–daughter cysts (Fig. 18.51).

These cysts may rupture during examination, because of their thin walls. The patient may experience tenesmus, a transient pelvic tenderness, deep dyspareunia, or no pain whatsoever. Rarely is significant intraperitoneal bleeding associated with the rupture of a follicular cyst. However, women who are chronically anticoagulated or those with von Willebrand disease may bleed. Occasionally, menstrual irregularities and abnormal uterine bleeding may be associated with follicular cysts, which produce elevated blood estrogen levels. The syndrome associated with such follicular cysts consists of a regular cycle with a prolonged intermenstrual interval, followed by episodes of menorrhagia. Some women with larger follicular cysts notice a vague, dull sensation or heaviness in the pelvis.

The initial management of a suspected follicular cyst is conservative observation. The majority of follicular cysts disappear spontaneously by either reabsorption of the cyst fluid or silent rupture within 4 to 8 weeks of initial diagnosis. However, a persistent ovarian mass necessitates operative intervention to differentiate a physiologic cyst from a true neoplasm of the ovary. There is no way to make the differentiation on the basis of signs, symptoms, or the initial growth pattern during early development of either process. Endovaginal ultrasound examination is helpful in differentiating simple from complex cysts and is also helpful during conservative management by providing dimensions to determine if the cyst is increasing in size. When the diameter of the cyst remains stable for greater than 10 weeks or enlarges, a neoplasia should be ruled out. Oral contraceptives may be prescribed for 4 to 6 weeks for young women with adnexal masses. This therapy removes any influence that pituitary gonadotropins may have on the persistence of the ovarian cyst. It also allows for several weeks of observation. In one series, 80% of cystic masses 4 to 6 cm in size disappeared during the time the patient was taking oral contraceptives. However, randomized prospective trials found no difference in the rate of disappearance of functional ovarian cysts between the group that received oral contraceptives and the control group, perhaps because so many cysts will resolve spontaneously.

The evaluation of an asymptomatic cyst, found incidentally, is based on the principle that the cyst should be removed if there is any suspicion of malignancy. Suspicion may develop because of history, including family history, patient age, and other nongynecologic signs and symptoms. The size and physical characteristics of the cyst are as important as are other laboratory parameters. CA-125 is helpful in evaluating the adnexal mass in postmenopausal women. In premenopausal women, CA-125 is rarely helpful unless the mass is extremely suggestive of malignancy. As discussed earlier, measurement of diastolic and systolic velocities provide indirect indices of vascular resistance. Muscular arteries have high resistance. Newly developed vessels, such as those arising in malignancies, have little vascular wall musculature and thus have low resistance. When a color flow Doppler scan demonstrates vascularity, the vascular resistance can be calculated. Low resistance is associated with malignancy, and high resistance usually is associated with normal tissue or benign disease. Although color flow Doppler has been shown to be sensitive in evaluating ovarian neoplasms, it is neither sensitive nor specific enough to be used as a determining study. In most cases, simple small cysts may be observed. In general, complex cysts or persistent simple cysts larger than 10 cm should be evaluated. In women with cysts in pregnancy, if the cyst is simple with a normal CA-125, conservative management is acceptable. (CA-125 is generally not obtained in pregnant women with cysts less than 5 cm if they are simple.)

A cyst in a perimenopausal or postmenopausal woman should be removed if it is anything other than a simple cyst, if the CA-125 is abnormal (>35), or if the cyst is persistent or large (>10 cm), although observation may be reasonable in select cases. A small simple cyst in a perimenopausal or postmenopausal woman (<5 cm) with a normal CA-125 may be observed with follow-up ultrasound and CA125 testing every 6 months for 2 years. If unchanged at that point routine monitoring can be stopped. Several studies, including the large prospective series from Greenlee and colleagues, examined the issue of simple cysts in postmenopausal women with simple cysts. These studies have noted that expectant management is safe and reasonable. In the series by Greenlee, the Prostate, Lung, Colorectal, and Ovarian cancer Screening Trial, women were followed for 4 years with transvaginal ultrasound. Of 15,735 women, 2217 (14%) had at least one simple cyst. Cysts were more common in women in the 50- to 59-year-old age group and women with hysterectomies prior to age 40. Cysts were less common among smokers and older women. In all, 54% of cysts were present on scans 1 year later; 8% of women had more than one cyst. Only 0.4% of the entire population developed ovarian cancer, and half of the women who developed cancer did not have cysts. The 14% incidence of cysts in postmenopausal women is similar to rates of simple cysts in other large series. Thus women with simple cysts who are asymptomatic and with negative CA-125 may be reassured and if desired, followed expectantly (Greenlee, 2010). Management of cysts between 5 and 10 cm that are otherwise not suggestive should be individualized. Ekerhovd and coworkers reported on 927 premenopausal women and 377 postmenopausal women with ovarian cysts. Of these women, 660 had unilocular simple cysts, 3 were borderline, and 4 were malignant (total of 1%). All of the borderline and malignant tumors were found in cysts greater than 7.5 cm. In women with cysts that had echodensity and papulations (644 women), 24 (3.7%) turned out to be borderline or malignant. Cysts that were multiseptate were not included in the study. All cysts with internal structures were excised and had a much higher rate of malignancy. The authors, as well as others, have confirmed the recommendation that unilocular cysts less than 5 cm may be followed if there is no family history, a normal CA-125, or other significant findings (Ekerhovd, 2001).

In premenopausal women, operative management of nonmalignant cysts is cystectomy, not oophorectomy. Many clinicians will manage simple cysts laparoscopically. Because this procedure

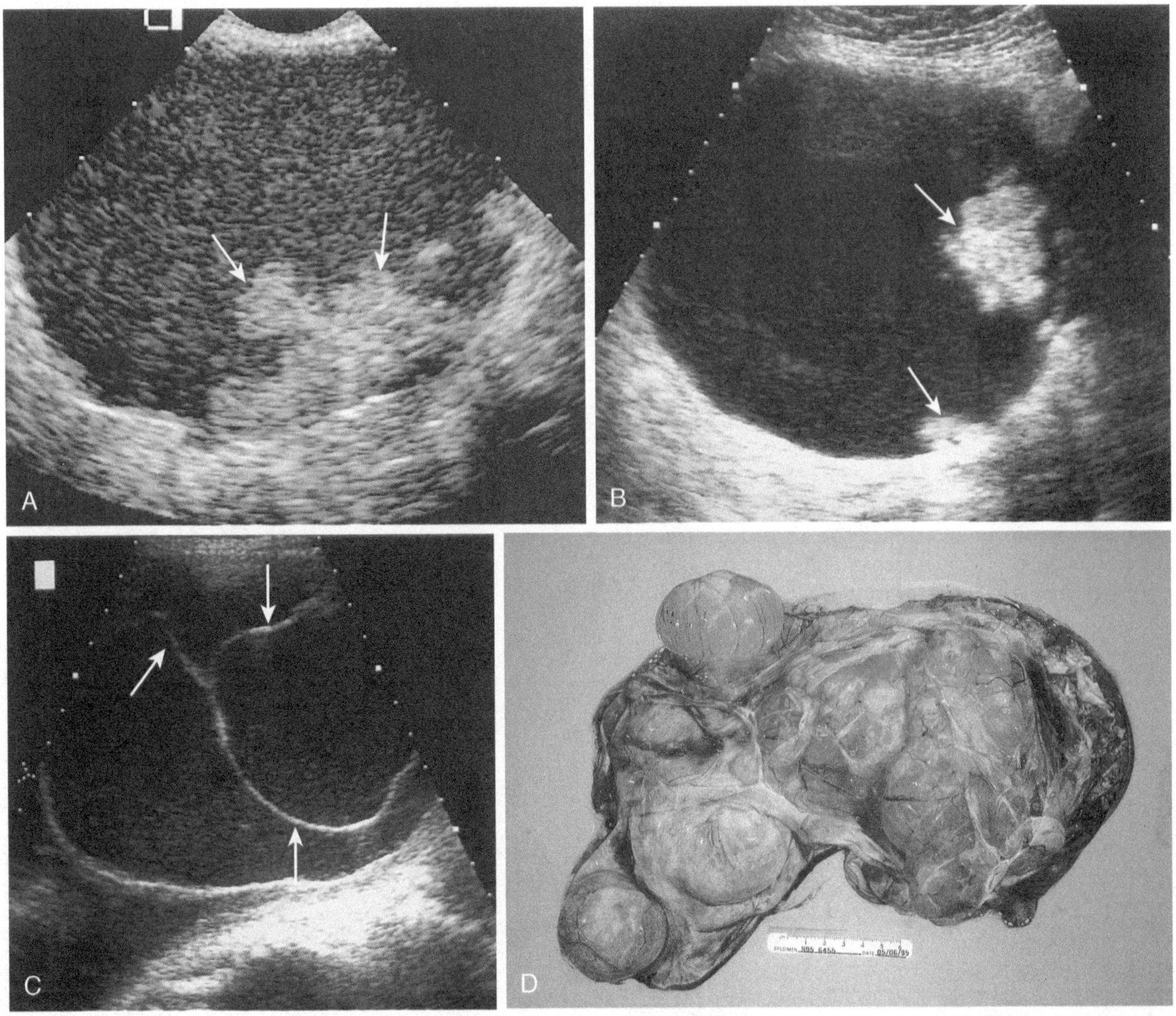


**Figure 18.51** Serous cystadenocarcinoma, varying appearances. **A,** Transvaginal scan shows large cystic mass containing multiple low-level internal echoes and solid echogenic components *(arrows)*. **B,** Transabdominal scan shows large cystic mass with irregular solid echogenic mural nodules *(arrows)* and low-level internal echoes. **C,** Mucinous cystadenoma. Transabdominal scan shows large cystic mass with multiple thin septations *(arrows)* and fine low-level internal echoes. **D,** Gross pathologic specimen shows multiple cystic loculations. (From Salem S. The uterus and adnexa. In: Rumack CM, Wilson SR, Charboneau JW, eds. *Diagnostic Ultrasound*. St. Louis: Mosby; 1998:555-556.)

has an accompanying risk of spilling malignant cells into the peritoneal cavity if the cyst is an early carcinoma, strict preoperative criteria should be fulfilled before laparoscopy is attempted. These include the woman's age; size of the mass; and ultrasound characteristics, such as nonadherent, smooth, and thin-walled cysts, without papillae or internal echoes (simple). DeWilde and associates, reporting on a series of follicular cysts averaging 6 cm in diameter, found that the recurrence rate following laparoscopic fenestration was approximately 2% (DeWilde, 1989). Higher rates of recurrence, up to 40%, have been reported for simple drainage of multiple types of benign cysts, the point being that drainage or fenestration is effective for follicular cysts and poorly effective for other cysts. When cysts are drained, it is essential to remember that cytologic examination of cyst fluid has poor predictive value and poor sensitivity in differentiating benign from malignant cysts. One report of fine-needle aspiration of ovarian cysts found sensitivity of 25%, specificity of 90%, a false-positive rate of 73%, and a false-negative rate of 12% (Higgins, 1999). If there is any suspicion of malignancy, the cyst should be removed as carefully as possible and a histopathologic evaluation obtained. The size of the cyst is not a necessary reason to avoid laparoscopy. Most simple cysts, even those larger than 10 cm, can be managed through the laparoscope.

### Corpus Luteum Cysts

Corpus luteum cysts are less common than follicular cysts, but clinically they are more important. This discussion collectively combines corpus luteum cysts and persistently functioning mature corpora lutea (Fig. 18.52). Pathologists are sometimes able to distinguish between a hemorrhagic cystic corpus luteum and a corpus luteum cyst, but at other times this difference cannot be established. All corpora lutea are cystic with gradual reabsorption of a limited amount of hemorrhage, which may form a cavity. Clinically, corpora lutea are not termed *corpus luteum cysts* unless they are a minimum of 3 cm in diameter. Corpus luteum cysts may be associated with either normal endocrine function or prolonged secretion of progesterone. The associated menstrual pattern may be normal, delayed menstruation, or amenorrhea.

Corpora lutea develop from mature graafian follicles. Intrafollicular bleeding does not occur during ovulation. However, 2 to 4 days later, during the stage of vascularization, thin-walled capillaries invade the granulosa cells from the theca interna. Spontaneous but limited bleeding fills the central cavity of the maturing corpus luteum with blood. Subsequently this blood is absorbed, forming a small cystic space. When the hemorrhage is excessive, the cystic space enlarges. If the hemorrhage into the central cavity is brisk, intracystic pressure increases and rupture of the corpus luteum is a possibility. If rupture does not occur, the size of the resulting corpus luteum cyst usually varies between 3 and 10 cm. Occasionally a cyst may be 11 to 15 cm in diameter. If a cystic central cavity persists, blood is replaced by clear fluid, and the result is a hormonally inactive corpus albicans cyst (Fig. 18.53). A corpus luteum of pregnancy is normally 3 to 5 cm in diameter with a central cystic structure, occupying at least 50% of the ovarian mass.

Most corpus luteum cysts are small, the average diameter being 4 cm. Grossly, they have a smooth surface and, depending on whether the cyst represents acute or chronic hemorrhage, are purplish red to brown. When a corpus luteum is cut, the convoluted lining is yellowish orange, and the center contains an organizing blood clot. Both the granulosa and the theca cells undergo luteinization. In chronic corpus luteum cysts, the wall becomes gray-white, and the polygonal luteinized cells usually undergo pressure atrophy. Hallatt and colleagues reviewed 173 ruptured corpora lutea with hemoperitoneum. In their institution the frequency of serious bleeding from a corpus luteum cyst compared with ectopic pregnancy was one in four (Hallatt, 1984).

Corpus luteum cysts vary from being asymptomatic masses to those causing catastrophic and massive intraperitoneal bleeding associated with rupture. Many corpus luteum cysts produce dull, unilateral, lower abdominal and pelvic pain. The enlarged ovary is moderately tender on pelvic examination. Depending on the amount of progesterone secretion associated with cysts, the menstrual bleeding may be normal or delayed several days to weeks with subsequent menorrhagia. Halban, in 1915, described

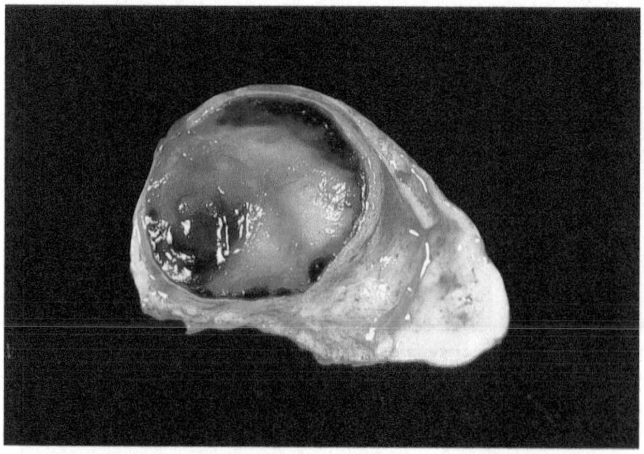

**Figure 18.52** Hemorrhagic corpus luteum with an outer yellow rim and central hemorrhage. (From Voet RL. *Color Atlas of Obstetric and Gynecologic Pathology*. St. Louis: Mosby-Wolfe; 1997.)

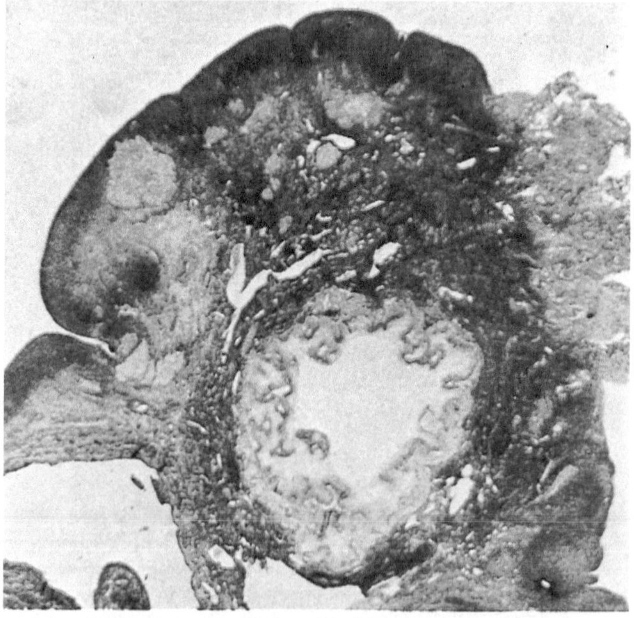

**Figure 18.53** Corpus albicans cyst. Lining of cyst is composed of hyalinized connective tissue. (From Blaustein A. Nonneoplastic cysts of the ovary. In: Blaustein A, ed. *Pathology of the Female Genital Tract*. New York: Springer-Verlag: 1977:396.)

a syndrome of a persistently functioning corpus luteum cyst that has clinical features similar to an unruptured ectopic pregnancy. Halban's classic triad was a delay in a normal period followed by spotting; unilateral pelvic pain; and a small, tender, adnexal mass. This triad of symptomatology is similar to the triad of an anomalous period or delay in a normal period, spotting, and unilateral pelvic pain that are exhibited by the classic ectopic pregnancy. The differential diagnosis between these two conditions without a sensitive pregnancy test is difficult.

Corpus luteum cysts may cause intraperitoneal bleeding. The amount of bleeding varies from slight to clinically significant hemorrhage, necessitating blood transfusion. Internal bleeding often follows coitus, exercise, trauma, or a pelvic examination. However, episodes of bleeding usually do not recur, which differs from an ectopic pregnancy. Women with a bleeding diathesis or those undergoing chronic warfarin (Coumadin) therapy are especially prone to developing ovarian hemorrhage from a corpus luteum cyst. Bleeding occurs usually between days 20 and 26 of their cycle, and these women have a 31% chance for subsequent hemorrhage from a recurrent corpus luteum cyst. Oral contraceptives are sometimes used to suppress ovulation and avoid recurrent hemorrhage.

Hallatt and colleagues reported that sudden, severe, lower abdominal pain was a prominent symptom in women with hemoperitoneum caused by a ruptured corpus luteum cyst (Table 18.4). One of three women also noted unilateral cramping and lower abdominal pain for 1 to 2 weeks before overt rupture. The right ovary was the source of hemorrhage in 66% of their series (Hallatt, 1984). Tang and coworkers have also reported a right-sided predominance in the incidence of hemorrhage from corpus luteum cysts. They postulated that the difference is related to a higher intraluminal pressure on the right side because of the differences in ovarian vein architecture (Tang, 1985). Most ruptures occur between days 20 and 26 of the cycle, although in the series of Hallatt and colleagues, 28% of the women had a delay in menses not explained by pregnancy (Table 18.5).

The differential diagnosis of a woman with acute pain and suspected ruptured corpus luteum cyst includes ectopic pregnancy, a ruptured endometrioma, and adnexal torsion. A sensitive serum or urinary assay for human chorionic gonadotropin (HCG) will help to differentiate a bleeding corpus luteum from ectopic pregnancy (see Chapter 17). Vaginal ultrasound is useful in establishing a preoperative diagnosis. Culdocentesis has been used in the past to establish the severity of the hemorrhage, but it is rarely used today. If the hematocrit of the fluid obtained from the posterior cul-de-sac is greater than 15%, operative therapy is recommended. Cystectomy is the operative treatment of choice, with preservation of the remaining portion of the ovary. In the series by DeWilde and associates reporting on persistent corpus luteum cysts treated by fenestration via the laparoscope, 6 of 44 (14%) recurred. Obviously, it was impossible for the authors to distinguish between a recurrent corpus luteum cyst and the development of a new corpus luteum (DeWilde, 1989). Unruptured corpus luteum cysts may be followed conservatively. Raziel and coworkers reported on a series of 70 women with ruptured corpora lutea. Ultrasonic evidence of large amounts of peritoneal fluid and severe pain were indications for operative intervention. In 12 of 70 patients with small amounts of intraperitoneal fluid and mild to moderate pain, observation alone was associated with resolution of symptoms (Raziel, 1993).

### *Theca Lutein Cysts*

Theca lutein cysts are by far the least common of the three types of physiologic ovarian cysts (Fig. 18.54). Unlike corpus luteum cysts, theca lutein cysts are almost always bilateral and produce moderate to massive enlargement of the ovaries. The individual cysts vary in size from 1 cm to 10 cm or more in diameter. These cysts arise from either prolonged or excessive stimulation of the ovaries by endogenous or exogenous gonadotropins or increased ovarian sensitivity to gonadotropins. The condition of ovarian enlargement secondary to the development of multiple luteinized follicular cysts is termed *hyperreactio luteinalis*. Approximately 50% of molar pregnancies and 10% of choriocarcinomas have associated bilateral theca lutein cysts (Chapter 35). In these patients the HCG from the trophoblast produces luteinization of the cells in immature, mature, and atretic follicles. The cysts are also discovered in the latter months of pregnancies, often with conditions that produce a large placenta, such as twins, diabetes, and Rh sensitization. It is not uncommon to iatrogenically produce theca lutein cysts in women receiving medications to induce ovulation. Theca lutein cysts are occasionally discovered in association with normal pregnancy, as well as in newborn infants secondary to transplacental effects of maternal gonadotropins. Rarely, these cysts are found in young girls with juvenile hypothyroidism.

**Table 18.4** Symptoms of 173 Women with Ruptured Corpus Luteum

| Location | Number | Percentage |
|---|---|---|
| Right ovary | 114 | 66 |
| Left ovary | 56 | 32 |
| Unknown | 3 | 2 |
| Abdominal pain | 173 | 100 |
| Right ovary | 21 | 72 |
| Left ovary | 8 | 28 |
| Duration | | |
| Less than 24 hours | 94 | 54 |
| 1 to 7 days | 40 | 23 |
| Over 7 days | 14 | 8 |
| Unknown | 25 | 15 |
| Nausea or vomiting or diarrhea | 60 | 35 |

From Hallatt JG, Steele CH Jr, Snyder M. Ruptured corpus luteum with hemoperitoneum: a study of 173 surgical cases. *Am J Obstet Gynecol*. 1984;149(1):5-9.

**Table 18.5** Menstrual History in 173 Women with Ruptured Corpus Luteum

| Last Menstrual Period to Operation | No. of Women |
|---|---|
| Under 14 days | 5 |
| 14 to 31 days (pregnant = 2) | 77 |
| 31 to 60 days (pregnant = 15) | 56 |
| Over 60 days (pregnant = 10) | 18 |
| No menstrual period | 14 |
| Hysterectomy | 5 |
| Amenorrhea after oral contraceptives | 5 |
| Secondary amenorrhea | 2 |
| Menarche | 1 |
| Menopause | 1 |
| History of irregular menses | 14 |
| Unknown | 3 |

From Hallatt JG, Steele CH Jr, Snyder M. Ruptured corpus luteum with hemoperitoneum: a study of 173 surgical cases. *Am J Obstet Gynecol*. 1984;149(1):5-9.

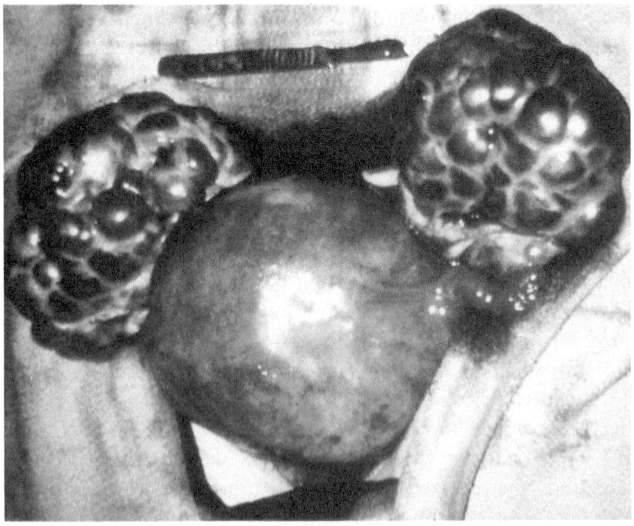

**Figure 18.54** Bilateral theca lutein cysts. (Courtesy of Daniel R. Mishell, Jr., MD.)

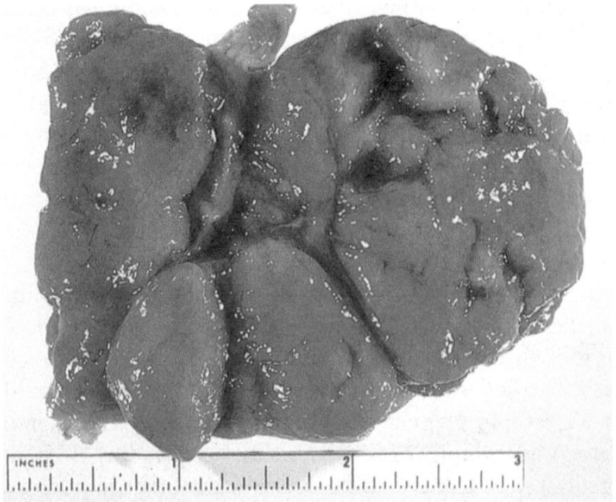

**Figure 18.55** Luteoma of pregnancy with numerous solid brown nodules. (From Voet RL. *Color Atlas of Obstetric and Gynecologic Pathology*. St. Louis: Mosby-Wolfe; 1997.)

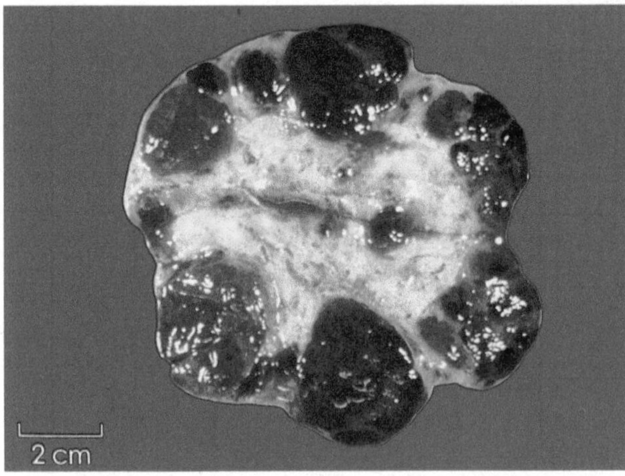


**Figure 18.56** Luteoma with multiple reddish nodules. (From Clement PB, Young RH. *Atlas of Gynecologic Surgical Pathology*. Philadelphia: WB Saunders; 2000.)

Grossly the total ovarian size may be voluminous, 20 to 30 cm in diameter, with multiple theca lutein cysts. Bilateral ovarian enlargement is produced by multiple gray to bluish-tinged cysts. The bilateral enlargement is secondary to hundreds of thin-walled locules or cysts, producing a honeycombed appearance. Grossly the external surface of the ovary appears lobulated. The small cysts contain a clear to straw-colored or hemorrhagic fluid. Histologically the lining of the cyst is composed of theca lutein cells (paralutein cells), believed to originate from ovarian connective tissue. Occasionally there is also luteinization of granulosa cells. These voluminous and congested ovaries are slow growing. The majority of women with smaller cysts are asymptomatic. Generally only the larger cysts produce vague symptoms, such as a sense of pressure in the pelvis. Ascites and increasing abdominal girth have been reported with hyperstimulation from exogenous gonadotropins. Rarely, associated adnexal torsion or bleeding may occur less than 1% of the time. Some theca lutein cysts persist for weeks after HCG levels normalize.

The presence of theca lutein cysts is established by palpation and often confirmed by ultrasound examination. Treatment is conservative because these cysts gradually regress. If these cysts are discovered incidentally at cesarean delivery, they should be handled delicately. No attempt should be made to drain or puncture the multiple cysts because of the possibility of hemorrhage. Bleeding is difficult to control in these cases because of the thin walls that constitute the cysts.

A condition related to theca lutein cysts is the luteoma of pregnancy. The condition is rare and not a true neoplasm but rather a specific, benign, hyperplastic reaction of ovarian theca lutein cells (Figs. 18.55 and 18.56). These nodules do not arise from the corpus luteum of pregnancy. Fifty percent of luteomas are multiple, and approximately 30% of those reported have bilateral nodules. In appearance they are discrete and brown to reddish brown and may be solid or cystic.

The majority of patients with luteomas are asymptomatic. The solid, fleshy, often hemorrhagic nodules are discovered incidentally at cesarean delivery or postpartum tubal ligation. Most cases have been reported in multiparous African-American women. Masculinization of the mother occurs in 30% of cases, and masculinization of the external genitalia of the female fetus may sometimes occur. These tumors regress spontaneously following completion of the pregnancy.

## BENIGN NEOPLASMS OF THE OVARY

### Benign Cystic Teratoma (Dermoid Cyst, Mature Teratoma)

Benign ovarian teratomas are usually cystic structures that on histologic examination contain elements from all three germ cell layers. The word *teratoma* was first advanced by Virchow and translated literally means "monstrous growth." Teratomas of the ovary may be benign or malignant. Although *dermoid* is a misnomer, it is the most common term used to describe the benign cystic tumor, composed of mature cells, whereas the malignant variety is composed of immature cells (immature teratoma). *Dermoid* is a descriptive term in that it emphasizes the preponderance of ectodermal tissue with some mesodermal and rare

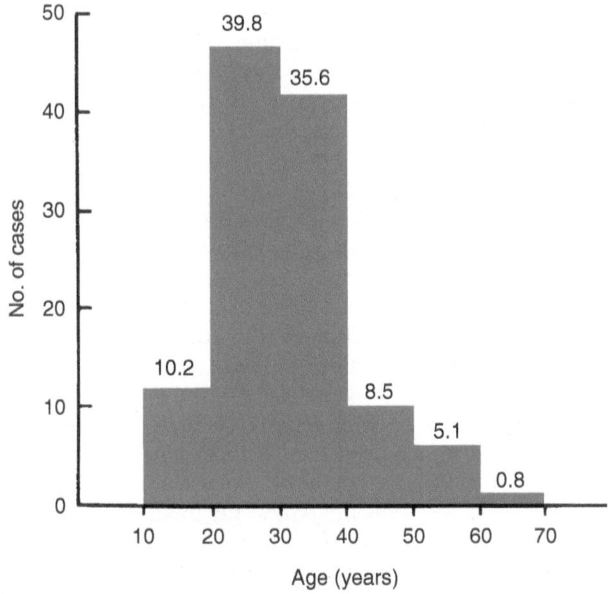


**Figure 18.57** Age distribution of cystic teratomas. (From Lakkis WG, Martin MC, Gelfand MM. Benign cystic teratoma of the ovary: a 6-year review. Originally published in *Can J Surg.* 1985;28:444.)

endodermal derivatives. Malignant teratomas that are immature are usually solid with some cystic areas and histologically contain immature or embryonic-appearing tissue. (See Chapter 33, for further discussion of malignant teratomas.) Benign teratomas may contain a malignant component, usually in women older than 40 (mean age 48). The malignant component is generally a squamous carcinoma and is found in less than 1% of cases. Non-ovarian teratomas may arise in any midline structure of the body where the germ cell has resided during embryonic life.

Benign teratomas are among the most common ovarian neoplasms. They account for more than 90% of germ cell tumors of the ovary. These slow-growing tumors occur from infancy to the postmenopausal years. Depending on the series, dermoids represent 20% to 25% of all ovarian neoplasms and approximately 33% of all benign tumors, if follicular and corpus luteum cysts are excluded. Dermoids are the most common ovarian neoplasm in prepubertal females and are also common in teenagers. More than 50% of benign teratomas are discovered in women between the ages of 25 and 50 years. In one series of 118 women with dermoids, 86% of the women were younger than 40 years of age, and 3.4% had recurrences (Fig. 18.57). With routine obstetric ultrasound, the mean age at diagnosis is expected to fall. In most large series of benign tumors in postmenopausal women, dermoids account for approximately 20% of the neoplasms.

Dermoids vary from a few millimeters to 25 cm in diameter although they have been reported to weigh as much as 7657 g in an asymptomatic woman. However, 80% are less than 10 cm. These tumors may be single or multiple, with as many as nine individual dermoids having been reported in the same ovary. Benign teratomas occur bilaterally 10% to 15% of the time. Often, dermoid cysts are pedunculated. These cysts make the ovary heavier than normal, and thus they are usually discovered either in the cul-de-sac or anterior to the broad ligament. On palpation these tumors, which have both cystic and solid components, have a doughy consistency.

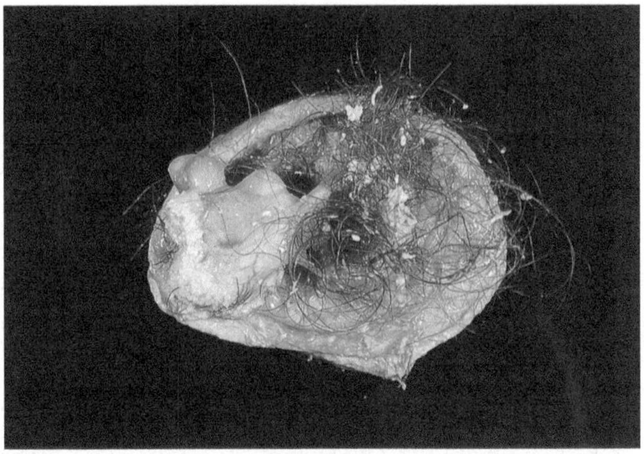

**Figure 18.58** Mature cystic teratoma (dermoid cyst) filled with hair and keratinous debris with one solid nodular area (Rokitansky protuberance). (From Voet RL. *Color Atlas of Obstetric and Gynecologic Pathology*. St. Louis: Mosby-Wolfe; 1997.)

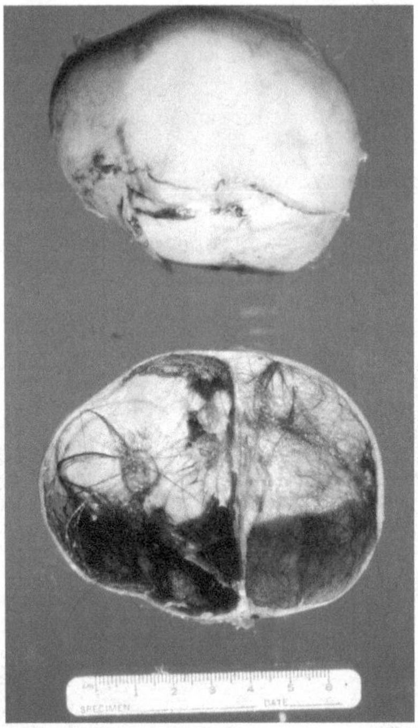

**Figure 18.59** Bilateral mature cystic teratomas in pregnancy. The cyst is bilocular. Dermal papillae are noted. Teeth are also present in the left lobule. (From Russell P, Robboy SJ, Anderson MC. Germ cell tumors of the ovaries. In: Robboy SJ, Anderson MC, Russell P, eds. *Pathology of the Female Reproductive Tract*. Edinburgh: Churchill Livingstone; 2002.)

The cysts are usually unilocular. The walls of the cyst are a smooth, shiny, opaque white color. When they are opened, thick sebaceous fluid pours from the cyst, often with tangled masses of hair and firm areas of cartilage and teeth (Figs. 18.58 and 18.59). The sebaceous material is a thick fluid at body temperature but solidifies when it cools in room air.

Benign teratomas are believed to arise from a single germ cell after the first meiotic division. Therefore they develop from totipotential stem cells, and they are neoplastic sequelae from a transformed germ cell. Dermoids have a chromosomal makeup of 46,XX and the chromosomes of dermoids were different from the chromosomes of the host, leading one to postulate that dermoids began by parthenogenesis from secondary oocytes. An alternative hypothesis was that the dermoid resulted from fusion of the second polar body with the oocyte. One thing is certain—dermoids do not arise from somatic cells nor from an oogonium before the first stage of meiosis. The first meiotic division occurs at approximately 13 weeks of gestation. Thus dermoids begin in fetal life sometime after the first trimester.

Histologically, benign teratomas are composed of mature cells, usually from all three germ layers (Fig. 18.60). A combination of skin and skin appendages, including sebaceous glands, sweat glands, hair follicles, muscle fibers, cartilage, bone, teeth, glial cells, and epithelium of the respiratory and gastrointestinal tracts, may be visualized. Teeth are predominantly premolar and molar forms. The fluid in dermoid cysts is usually sebaceous. Most solid elements arise and are contained in a protrusion or nipple (mamilla) in the cyst wall, termed the *prominence or tubercle of Rokitansky.* This prominence may be visualized by ultrasound as an echodense region, thus aiding in the sonographic diagnosis. If malignancy occurs, it is almost always found in this nest of cells. The wall of the cyst will often contain granulation tissue, giant cells, and pseudoxanthoma cells.

From 50% to 60% of dermoids are asymptomatic and are discovered during a routine pelvic examination, coincidentally visualized during pelvic imaging, or found incidentally at laparotomy. Presenting symptoms of dermoids include pain and the sensation of pelvic pressure. Specific complications of dermoid cysts include torsion, rupture, infection, hemorrhage, and malignant degeneration. Three medical diseases also may be associated with dermoid cysts: thyrotoxicosis, carcinoid syndrome, and autoimmune hemolytic anemia, the latter two being quite rare.

Adult thyroid tissue is discovered microscopically in approximately 12% of benign teratomas. Struma ovarii is a teratoma in which the thyroid tissue has overgrown other elements and is the predominant tissue (Fig. 18.61). Strumae ovarii constitute 2% to 3% of ovarian teratomas. These tumors are usually unilateral and measure less than 10 cm in diameter. Less than 5% of women with strumae ovarii develop thyrotoxicosis, which may be secondary to the production of increased thyroid hormone by either the ovarian or the thyroid gland.

Another rare finding with dermoids is the presence of a primary carcinoid tumor from the gastrointestinal or respiratory tract epithelium contained in the dermoid. One of three of these tumors is associated with the typical carcinoid syndrome even without metastatic spread. If the carcinoid is functioning, it may be diagnosed by measuring serum serotonin levels or urinary levels of 5-hydroxyindoleacetic acid. The autoimmune hemolytic anemia associated with dermoids is the rarest of the three medical complications.

Rupture or perforation of the contents of a dermoid into the peritoneal cavity or an adjacent organ is a potentially serious complication. The incidence varies between 0.7% and 4.6%. However, most series report less than 1%. Rupture is more common in pregnancy. If a rupture occurs during surgery, the abdomen should be copiously irrigated with saline, with careful removal of any particulate matter. Chemical peritonitis is reported in less than 1% of ruptured dermoids. Rupture may

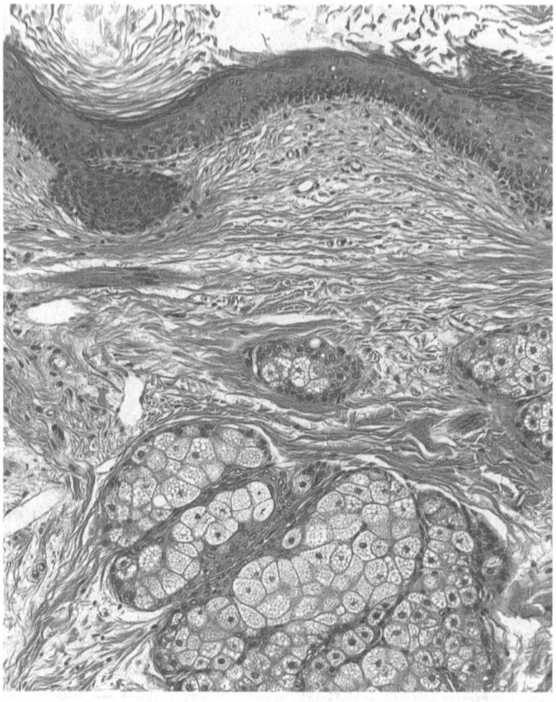

**Figure 18.60** Mature cystic teratoma. This cyst is lined by mature epidermis and is subtended by connective tissue containing exuberant dermal appendages (pilosebaceous follicles). (From Russell P, Robboy SJ, Anderson MC. Germ cell tumors of the ovaries. In: Robboy SJ, Anderson MC, Russell P, eds. *Pathology of the Female Reproductive Tract.* Edinburgh: Churchill Livingstone; 2002.)

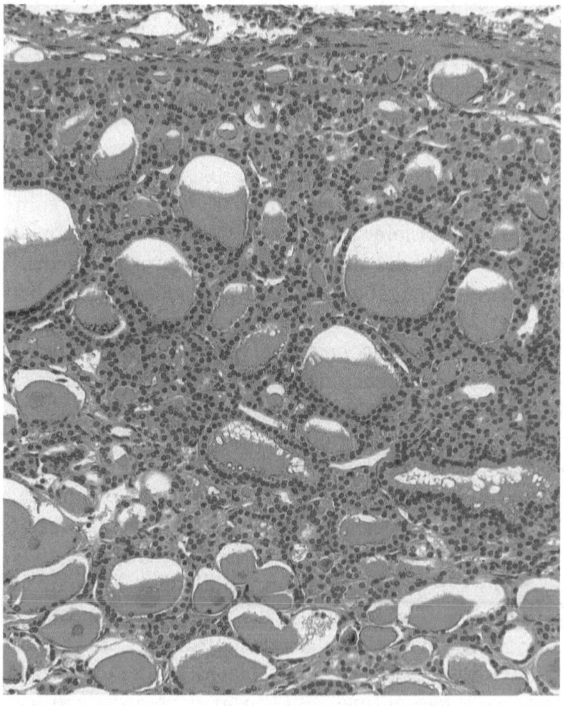

**Figure 18.61** Struma ovarii. Variably sized banal thyroid follicles. (From Russell P, Robboy SJ, Anderson MC. Germ cell tumors of the ovaries. In: Robboy SJ, Anderson MC, Russell P, eds. *Pathology of the Female Reproductive Tract.* Edinburgh: Churchill Livingstone; 2002.)

occur either catastrophically, which produces an acute abdomen, or by a slow leak of the sebaceous material. The latter is clinically more common, with the sebaceous material producing a severe chemical granulomatous peritonitis. Some warn that this possibility should be considered and a frozen section obtained so that the true diagnosis is established. Thus a young woman will not be mistakenly treated for suspected ovarian carcinoma with metastasis because of the identical gross appearance of a slow-leaking dermoid cyst. Infection, hemorrhage, and malignant degeneration are all unusual complications of dermoids, occurring in less than 1% of patients.

Torsion of a dermoid is the most frequent complication, occurring in 3.5% to 11% of cases. Because of its weight, the benign teratoma is often pedunculated, which may predispose to torsion. Torsion is more common in younger women. Small dermoid cysts, less than 6 cm in diameter, grow slowly at an approximate rate of 2 mm per year.

The diagnosis of a dermoid cyst is often established when a semisolid mass is palpated anterior to the broad ligament. Approximately 50% of dermoids have pelvic calcifications on radiographic examination. Often an ovarian teratoma is an incidental finding during radiologic investigation of the genitourinary or gastrointestinal tract. Most dermoids have a characteristic ultrasound picture. These characteristics include a dense echogenic area within a larger cystic area, a cyst filled with bands of mixed echoes, and an echoic dense cyst. Unfortunately, only one of three dermoids has this "typical picture." In one series of 45 patients with 51 biopsy-proved dermoid cysts, 24% of the dermoid cysts were predominantly solid, 20% were almost entirely cystic, and 24% were not visible. Ultrasound has a more than 95% positive predictive value and a less than 5% false-positive rate.

Operative treatment of benign cystic teratomas is cystectomy with preservation of as much normal ovarian tissue as possible. Laparoscopic cystectomy is an accepted approach. Rates of spillage are comparable with that from open laparotomy. However, adequate irrigation in such cases is essential and often more time consuming. Many authors use a 10-cm diameter cutoff as the upper limit for a laparoscopic approach.

When a teratoma is diagnosed incidentally during pregnancy, conservative management is acceptable. Though dermoids have a higher incidence of torsion and potential for rupture during pregnancy, most large series have not shown that an aggressive approach to asymptomatic teratomas less than 10 cm confers any advantage for the mother or pregnancy. Though laparoscopy is safe during pregnancy, a small periumbilical minilaparotomy may be a faster, less traumatic approach. The treatment is cystectomy, and with the recommendation for reduced intraoperative time this approach may be preferable during pregnancy.

### Endometriomas

Endometriosis of the ovary is usually associated with endometriosis in other areas of the pelvic cavity. Approximately two out of three women with endometriosis have ovarian involvement. Interestingly, only 5% of these women have enlargement of the ovaries that is detectable by pelvic examination. However, because of the prevalence of the disease, endometriosis is one of the most common causes of enlargement of the ovary. Because most authors do not classify endometriosis as a neoplastic disease, the diagnosis of endometriosis may not be given due consideration in the differential diagnosis of an adnexal mass. Ovarian endometriosis is similar to endometriosis elsewhere and is described in greater detail in Chapter 19.

The size of ovarian endometriomas varies from small, superficial, blue-black implants that are 1 to 5 mm in diameter to large, multiloculated, hemorrhagic cysts that may be 5 to 10 cm in diameter (Fig. 18.62). Clinically, large ovarian endometriomas, greater than 20 cm in diameter, are extremely rare. Areas of ovarian endometriosis that become cystic are termed *endometriomas*. Rarely, large chocolate cysts of the ovary may reach 15 to 20 cm (Fig. 18.63). Larger cysts are frequently bilateral. The surface of an ovary with endometriosis is often irregular, puckered, and scarred. Depending on their size, endometriomas replace a portion of the normal ovarian tissue.

Although most women with endometriomas are asymptomatic, the most common symptoms associated with ovarian endometriosis are pelvic pain, dyspareunia, and infertility. Approximately 10% of the operations for endometriosis are for acute symptoms, usually related to a ruptured ovarian endometrioma that was previously asymptomatic. Smaller cysts generally have thin walls, and perforation occurs commonly secondary to cyclic hemorrhage into the cystic cavity.

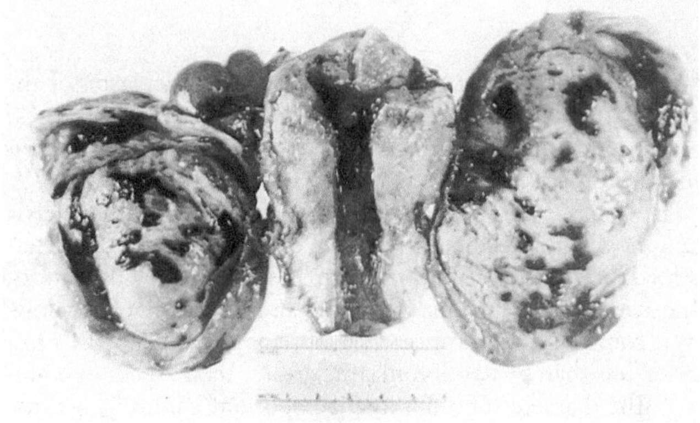

**Figure 18.62** Endometriosis of ovaries. Wall of endometriotic cyst is thickened and fibrotic. Inner surface shows areas of dark brown discoloration. (From Janovski NA, ed. *Color Atlas of Gross Gynecologic and Obstetric Pathology*. New York: McGraw-Hill; 1969:159.)

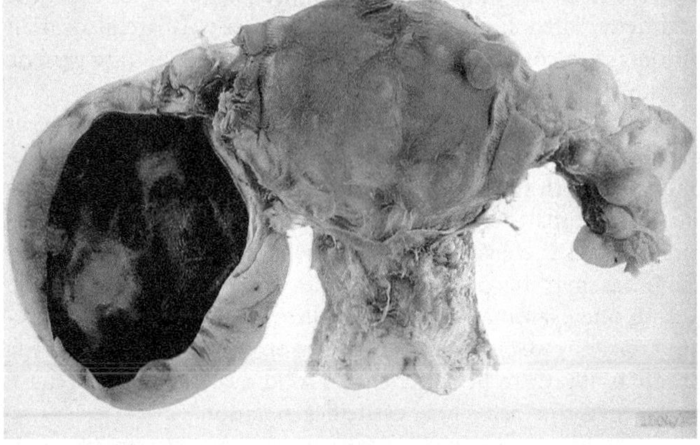

**Figure 18.63** "Chocolate cyst" of ovary. The endometrioma is large, but it has not yet completely replaced the ovary. (From Robboy SJ. Endometriosis. In: Robboy SJ, Anderson MC, Russell P, eds. *Pathology of the Female Reproductive Tract*. Edinburgh: Churchill Livingstone; 2002.)

On pelvic examination, the ovaries are often tender and immobile, secondary to associated inflammation and adhesions. Most commonly the ovaries are densely adherent to surrounding structures, including the peritoneum of the pelvic sidewall, the oviduct, the broad ligament, and sometimes the small or large bowel. Endometrial glands, endometrial stroma, and large phagocytic cells containing hemosiderin may be identified histologically (see Fig. 19-10). Pressure atrophy may lead to the loss of architecture of the endometrial glands. The ultrasound characteristics include a thick-walled cyst with a relatively homogeneous echo pattern that is somewhat echolucent. This appearance confers a greater than 95% positive predictive value in some studies.

The choice between medical and operative management depends on several factors, including the patient's age, future reproductive plans, and severity of symptoms. Medical therapy is rarely successful in treating ovarian endometriosis if the disease has produced ovarian enlargement. Often surgical therapy is complicated by formation of de novo and recurrent adhesions.

On pathologic examination, it is important to distinguish endometriosis from benign endometrial tumors, which are usually adenofibromas. The latter tumor is a true neoplasm, and there is a malignant counterpart.

### *Fibroma*

Fibromas are the most common benign, solid neoplasms of the ovary. Their malignant potential is low, less than 1%. These tumors make up approximately 5% of benign ovarian neoplasms and approximately 20% of all solid tumors of the ovary.

Fibromas vary in size from small nodules to huge pelvic tumors weighing 50 pounds. One of the predominant characteristics of fibromas is that they are extremely slow-growing tumors. The average diameter of a fibroma is approximately 6 cm; however, some tumors have reached 30 cm in diameter. In most series, less than 5% of fibromas are greater than 20 cm in diameter. The diameter of a fibroma is important clinically, because the incidence of associated ascites is directly proportional to the size of the tumor. Many ovarian fibromas are misdiagnosed and are believed to be leiomyomas prior to operation. Ninety percent of fibromas are unilateral; however, multiple fibromas are found in the same ovary in 10% to 15% of cases. The average age of a woman with an ovarian fibroma is 48. Thus this tumor often presents in postmenopausal women. The tumor arises from the undifferentiated fibrous stroma of the ovary. Bilateral ovarian fibromas are commonly found in women with the rare genetic transmitted basal cell nevus syndrome.

The pelvic symptoms that develop with growth of fibromas include pressure and abdominal enlargement, which may be secondary to both the size of the tumor and ascites. Smaller tumors are asymptomatic because these tumors do not elaborate hormones. Thus there is no change in the pattern of menstrual flow. Fibromas may be pedunculated and therefore easily palpable during one examination yet difficult to palpate during a subsequent pelvic examination. Sometimes on pelvic examination the fibromas appear to be softer than a solid ovarian tumor because of the edema or occasional cystic degeneration.

Meigs' syndrome is the association of an ovarian fibroma, ascites, and hydrothorax. Both the ascites and the hydrothorax resolve after removal of the ovarian tumor. The ascites is caused by transudation of fluid from the ovarian fibroma; the incidence of ascites is directly related to the size of the fibroma. Fifty percent of patients have ascites if the tumor is greater than 6 cm. However, true Meigs' syndrome is rare, occurring in less than 2% of ovarian fibromas. The hydrothorax develops secondary to a flow of ascitic fluid into the pleural space via the lymphatics of the diaphragm. Statistically the right pleural space is involved in 75% of reported cases, the left in 10%, and both sides in 15%. The clinical features of Meigs' syndrome are not unique to fibromas, and a similar clinical picture is found with many other ovarian tumors.

Grossly, fibromas are heavy, solid, well encapsulated, and grayish white. The cut surface usually demonstrates a homogeneous white or yellowish white solid tissue with a trabeculated or whorled appearance similar to that of myomas. The majority of fibromas are grossly edematous (Fig. 18.64). Less than 10% of fibromas have calcifications or small areas of hyaline or cystic degeneration. Histologically, fibromas are composed of connective tissue, stromal cells, and varying amounts of collagen interposed between the cells. The connective tissue cells are spindle-shaped, mature fibroblasts. They are arranged in an imperfect pattern. A few smooth muscle fibers may be occasionally identified. It is sometimes difficult to distinguish fibromas from nonneoplastic thecomas. Histologically the pathologist must differentiate fibromas from stromal hyperplasia, fibrosarcomas, and also look for epithelial elements of an associated Brenner tumor.

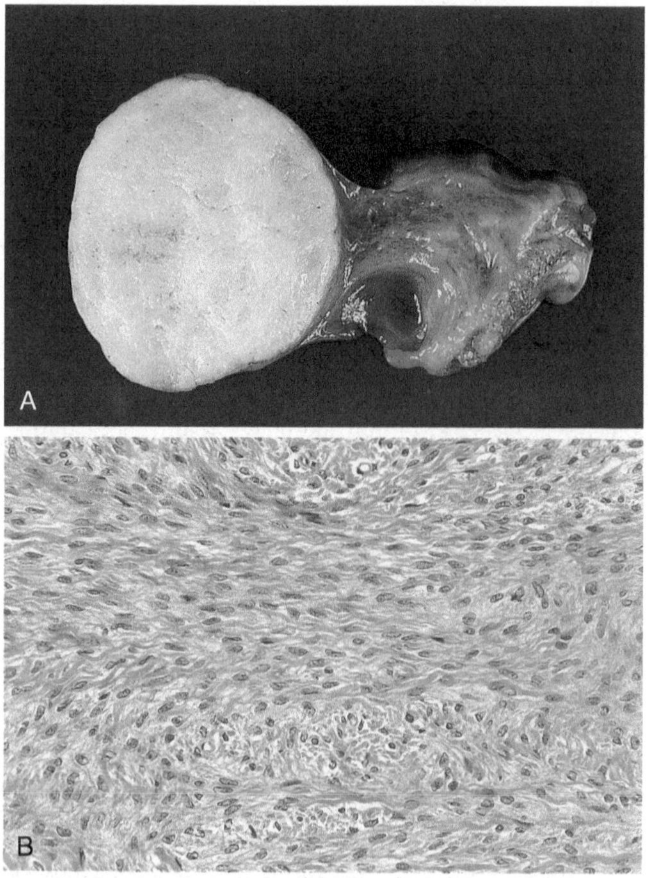


**Figure 18.64** **A,** Fibroma of the ovary with a well-circumscribed light tan mass. **B,** Histology of fibroma of the ovary, demonstrating bland fibrous differentiation. (From Voet RL. *Color Atlas of Obstetric and Gynecologic Pathology*. St. Louis: Mosby-Wolfe; 1997.)

The management of fibromas is straightforward because any woman with a solid ovarian neoplasm should have an exploratory operation soon after the tumor is discovered. Simple excision of the tumor is all that is necessary. Following excision of the tumor, there is resolution of all symptoms, including ascites. Because these tumors are frequently discovered in postmenopausal women, often a bilateral salpingo-oophorectomy and total abdominal hysterectomy are performed. Conversely, it is important to note that most women who preoperatively have the combination of a solid ovarian tumor and ascites are found to have ovarian carcinoma.

### *Transitional Cell Tumors: Brenner Tumors*

Brenner tumors are rare, small, smooth, solid, fibroepithelial ovarian tumors that are generally asymptomatic. The semantic classification of neoplasms changes, and the current preferred term for benign Brenner tumor is *transitional cell tumor*. The benign, proliferative (low malignant potential), and malignant forms together constitute approximately 2% of ovarian tumors. These tumors usually occur in women ages 40 to 60 years. Approximately 30% of transitional cell tumors are discovered as small, solid tumors in association with a concurrent serous cystic neoplasia, such as serous or mucinous cystadenomas of the ipsilateral ovary. Some are microscopic, with the entire tumor contained in a single low-powered microscopic field, and others may reach a diameter of 20 cm; the majority are less than 5 cm in diameter. The tumor is unilateral 85% to 95% of the time.

The Brenner tumor was first described in 1898. In 1932, Robert Meyer postulated that it was a distinct, independent neoplasm from granulosa cell tumors. Since that time there has been a controversy in the gynecologic pathology literature as to the histogenesis of the neoplasm. Presently, most authorities accept the theory that most of these tumors result from metaplasia of coelomic epithelium into uroepithelium. Detailed three-dimensional histologic studies have demonstrated a downward growth in a cordlike fashion of epithelium from the surface of the ovary to deeper areas in the ovarian cortex. Others have postulated that sometimes the solid nests of epithelial cells of the tumor originate from the rete ovarii or Walthard rests. Electron microscopy confirmed the histologic and ultrastructural similarity between the epithelium in Brenner tumors and transitional epithelium. These authors argue that because of the histogenesis from coelomic inclusion cysts and also the mixture of Müllerian-type epithelium in 30% of Brenner tumors, it might be appropriate to classify Brenner tumors in the epithelial group of ovarian neoplasms.

Approximately 90% of these small neoplasms are discovered incidentally during a gynecologic operation, although large tumors may produce unilateral pelvic discomfort. Postmenopausal bleeding is sometimes associated with Brenner tumors, as endometrial hyperplasia is a coexisting abnormality in 10% to 16% of cases. It is postulated that luteinization of the stroma produces estrogen with resulting hyperplasia that leads to classic findings of ovarian Brenner tumors on CT or MRI. The extensive fibrous content of these tumors results in lower signal intensity in T2-weighted images. During CT scanning, Brenner tumors characteristically demonstrate a finding of extensive amorphous calcification within the solid components of the ovarian mass.

Grossly, Brenner tumors are smooth, firm, gray-white, solid tumors that grossly resemble fibromas. Similar to fibromas, transitional cell tumors are slow growing. On sectioning, the tumor usually appears gray; however, occasionally there is a yellowish tinge with small cystic spaces (Fig. 18.65). Approximately 1% to 2% of these tumors undergo malignant change (Chapter 33). Histologically, Brenner tumors have two principal components: solid masses or nests of epithelial cells and a surrounding fibrous stroma. The epithelial cells are uniform and do not appear anaplastic (Fig. 18.66). The histology and ultrastructure

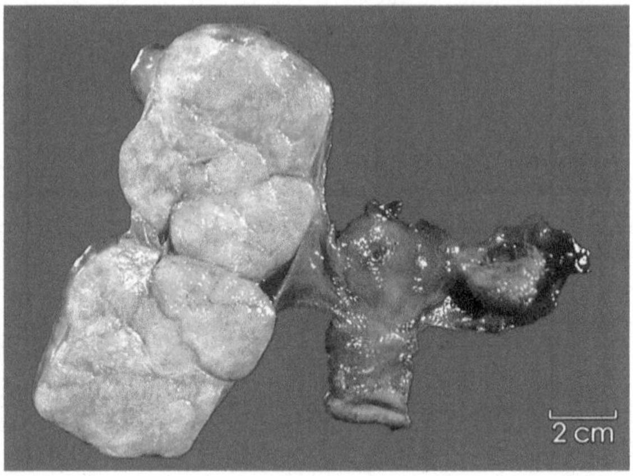


**Figure 18.65** Brenner tumor. (From Clement PB, Young RH: *Atlas of Gynecologic Surgical Pathology*. Philadelphia: WB Saunders; 2000.)

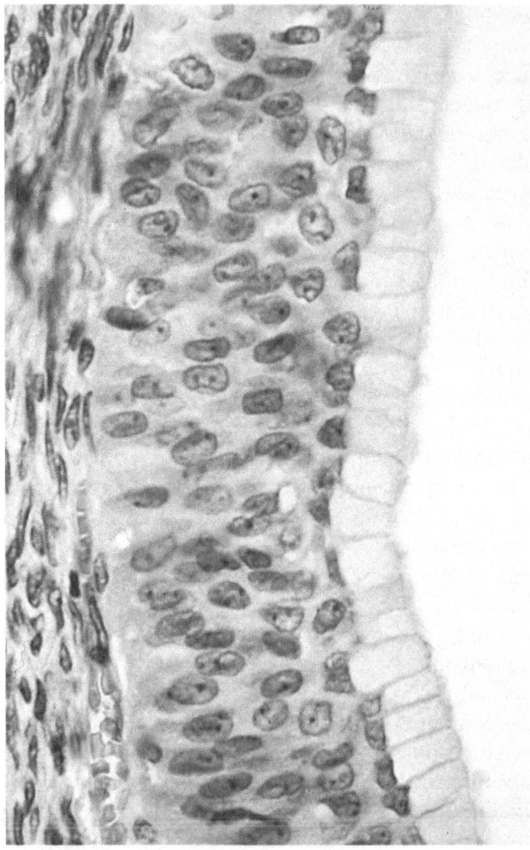

**Figure 18.66** Benign Brenner tumor. A cyst in the Brenner tumor is lined by an inner layer of endocervical-type mucinous cells and an outer layer of stratified transitional cells, a few of which have grooved nuclei. (From Clement PB, Young RH. *Atlas of Gynecologic Surgical Pathology*. Philadelphia: WB Saunders, 2000.)

of the epithelial cells of a Brenner tumor are similar to transitional epithelium of the urinary bladder. The pale epithelial cells have a coffee bean–appearing nucleus, which is also described as a longitudinal groove in the cell's nucleus.

Electron microscopy has demonstrated that the longitudinal groove during routine microscopy is produced by prominent indentation of the nuclear membrane. An additional ovarian neoplasm is frequently found associated with Brenner tumors. Balasa and colleagues, in a review of 302 tumors, reported 100 other concurrent neoplasms, with the majority being serous and mucinous cystadenomas or teratomas (Balasa, 1977).

Management of Brenner tumors is operative, with simple excision being the procedure of choice. However, as with ovarian fibromas, the patient's age is often the principal factor in deciding the extent of the operation.

### *Adenofibroma and Cystadenofibroma*

Adenofibromas and cystadenofibromas are closely related. Both of these benign firm tumors consist of fibrous and epithelial components. The epithelial element is most commonly serous but histologically may be mucinous and endometrioid or clear cell. They differ from benign epithelial cystadenomas in that there is a preponderance of connective tissue. Most pathologists emphasize that at least 25% of the tumor consists of fibrous connective tissue. Obviously, cystadenofibromas have microscopic or occasional macroscopic areas that are cystic. The varying degree of fibrous stroma and epithelial elements produces a spectrum of tumors, which have resulted in a confusing nomenclature with terms such as *papillomas, fibropapillomas,* and *fibroadenomas.*

Adenofibromas are usually small fibrous tumors that arise from the surface of the ovary. They are bilateral in 20% to 25% of women. They usually occur in postmenopausal women and are 1 to 15 cm in diameter. Grossly, they are gray or white tumors, and it is difficult to distinguish them from fibromas. Papillary adenofibromas, which project from the surface of the ovary, at first glance may appear to be external excrescences of a malignant tumor. Histologically, small precursors of adenofibromas are identified in many normal ovaries. Under the microscope, true cystic gland spaces lined by cuboidal epithelium are characteristic. However, differing from serous cystadenomas, the fibrous connective tissue surrounding the cystic spaces is abundant and is the predominant tissue of the tumor.

Smaller tumors are asymptomatic and are only discovered incidentally during abdominal or pelvic operations. Large tumors may cause pressure symptoms or, rarely, undergo adnexal torsion. A small series of the MRI features of these tumors has been reported. Similar to Brenner tumors, the fibrous component produces a very low signal intensity on T2-weighted images. This interest in imaging results from an attempt to distinguish, prior to operation, whether a predominantly solid ovarian mass is benign or malignant. Because adenofibromas are usually discovered in postmenopausal women, the treatment of choice is bilateral salpingo-oophorectomy and total abdominal hysterectomy. Because these tumors are benign and because malignant transformation is rare, simple excision of the tumor and inspection of the contralateral ovary are appropriate in younger women.

### *Torsion*

Torsion of the ovary or both the oviduct and the ovary (adnexal torsion) is uncommon but an important cause of acute lower abdominal and pelvic pain. Torsion may cause up to 3% of all acute abdomens presenting to emergency departments. Torsion of the ovary may occur separately from torsion of the fallopian tube, but most commonly the two adnexal structures are affected together.

Adnexal torsion occurs most commonly during the reproductive years, with the average patient being in her mid-20s. However, adnexal torsion is also a complication of benign ovarian tumors in the postmenopausal woman. Pregnancy appears to predispose women to adnexal torsion. Approximately one in five women are pregnant when the condition is diagnosed. Most susceptible are ovaries that are enlarged secondary to ovulation induction during early pregnancy. The most common cause of adnexal torsion is ovarian enlargement by an 8- to 12-cm benign mass of the ovary. However, smaller ovaries may also undergo torsion. Ovarian tumors are discovered in 50% to 60% of women with adnexal torsion. Torsion of a normal ovary or adnexum is also possible and occurs more frequently in children. Dermoids are the most frequently reported tumors in women with adnexal torsion. However, the relative risk of adnexal torsion is higher with parovarian cysts, solid benign tumors, and serous cysts of the ovary. The right ovary has a greater tendency to twist (3 to 2) than does the left ovary. Torsion of a malignant ovarian tumor is comparatively rare.

Patients with adnexal torsion present with acute, severe, unilateral, lower abdominal and pelvic pain. Often the patient relates the onset of the severe pain to an abrupt change of position. A unilateral, extremely tender adnexal mass is found in more than 90% of patients. Approximately two thirds of patients have associated nausea and vomiting. These associated gastrointestinal symptoms sometimes lead to a preoperative diagnosis of acute appendicitis or small intestinal obstruction. Many patients have noted intermittent previous episodes of similar pain for several days to several weeks. The hypothesis is that previous episodes of pain were secondary to partial torsion, with spontaneous reversal without significant vascular compromise. With progressive torsion, initially venous and lymphatic obstruction occurs. This produces a cyanotic, edematous ovary, which on pelvic examination presents as a unilateral, extremely tender adnexal mass. Further progression of the torsion interrupts the major arterial supply to the ovary, resulting in hypoxia, adnexal necrosis, and a concomitant low-grade fever and leukocytosis. Fever is more common in women who have developed necrosis of the adnexa. Approximately 10% of women with adnexal torsion have a repetitive episode affecting the contralateral adnexa.

Most patients with adnexal torsion present with symptoms and signs severe enough to demand operative intervention (Fig. 18.67). Some authors have reported the successful use of Doppler ultrasound to evaluate ovarian arterial blood flow to help diagnose torsion. Abnormal color Doppler flow is highly predictive of torsion of the ovary. However, approximately 60% of women with surgically confirmed adnexal torsion will have a normal Doppler flow study (Sasaki, 2014). The false-negative rate is high enough that normal Doppler studies should never trump clinical suspicion. Women with ovarian torsion may be treated via laparoscopic surgery. The most common gynecologic conditions that may be confused with

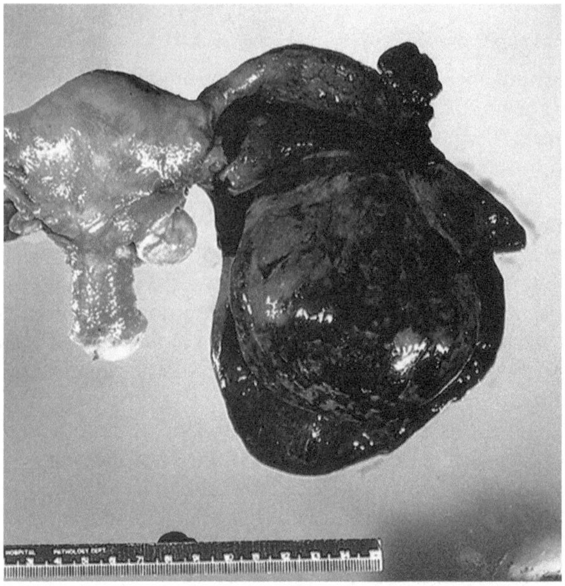

**Figure 18.67** Adnexal torsion with hemorrhagic infarction. A benign cyst was found in the ovary. (From Clement PB, Young RH: *Atlas of Gynecologic Surgical Pathology.* Philadelphia: WB Saunders; 2000.)

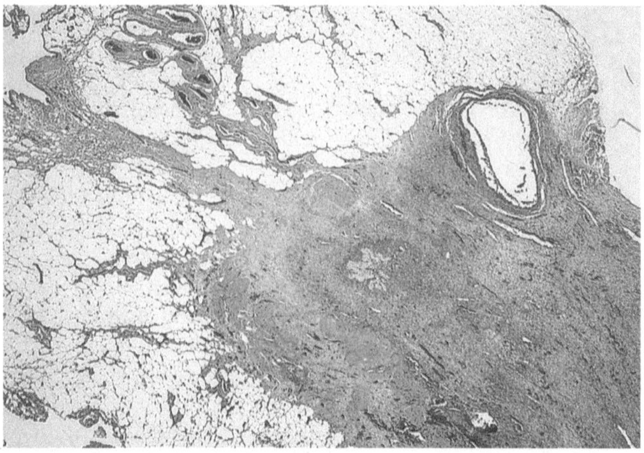

**Figure 18.68** Ovarian remnant syndrome. Ovarian tissue that was left behind at the time of oophorectomy has regrown and is functional. (From Robboy SJ, Bentley RC, Russell P, et al. The peritoneum. In: Robboy SJ, Anderson MC, Russell P, eds. *Pathology of the Female Reproductive Tract.* Edinburgh: Churchill Livingstone; 2002.)

adnexal torsion are a ruptured corpus luteum or an adnexal abscess. In series emphasizing the early diagnosis of adnexal torsion, conservative operative management has been possible in 75% of cases.

Because the majority of cases of adnexal torsion occur in young women, a conservative operation is ideal. The clinician should maintain a high index of suspicion for adnexal torsion so that early and conservative surgery is possible. With severe vascular compromise, the appropriate operation is unilateral salpingo-oophorectomy. The vascular pedicle should be clamped with care so as not to injure the ureter, which may be tented up by the torsion.

Although salpingo-oophorectomy has been the routine treatment for ovarian torsion, large series of conservative management have been reported. Conservative surgery either through the laparoscope or via laparotomy entails gentle untwisting of the pedicle, possibly cystectomy, and stabilization of the ovary with sutures. The increasing use of de-torsion may result in re-torsion. A review noted that the risk of re-torsion in pregnancy was as high as 19.5% to 37.5%; among fertile women it was 28.6%. Based on observational studies, de-torsion and fixation of the ovary is a safe procedure that reduces the risk of recurrence (Hyttel, 2015).

The risk of pulmonary embolus (PE) with adnexal torsion is small, approximately 0.2%. One series noted the risk of PE to be similar when torsion was managed by conservative surgery with untwisting or adnexal removal without untwisting.

### *Ovarian Remnant Syndrome*

Chronic pelvic pain secondary to a small area of functioning ovarian tissue following intended total removal of both ovaries is termed *ovarian remnant syndrome.* Most of the women who develop this condition had endometriosis or chronic pelvic inflammatory disease and extensive pelvic adhesions discovered during previous surgical procedures. A more recently described risk factor is laparoscopic oophorectomy.

The chronic pelvic pain is usually cyclic and exacerbated following coitus. Approximately half of women present with pain, and half with a pelvic mass. Usually the masses are small, approximately 3 cm in diameter, and most commonly located in the retroperitoneal space immediately adjacent to either ureter. Histologically, the mass contains both ovarian follicles and stroma (Fig. 18.68). If the mass cannot be palpated during pelvic examination, imaging studies such as vaginal ultrasound or MRI are often helpful. Premenopausal levels of follicle-simulating hormone or estradiol help to establish the diagnosis in a woman who has a history of a bilateral salpingo-oophorectomy. However, sometimes a small area of ovarian tissue does not produce enough circulating estrogen to suppress gonadotropins. Difficult cases have been diagnosed by challenging and stimulating the suspected ovarian remnant with either clomiphene citrate or a GnRH agonist.

Once the diagnosis is suspected, the most effective treatment is surgical removal of the ovarian remnant. The tissue should be removed by laparoscopy or laparotomy with wide excision of the mass using meticulous techniques so as to protect the integrity of the ureter. A review of 186 patients with a history of bilateral salpingo-oophorectomy who underwent removal of an ovarian remnant confirmed by pathology revealed an intraoperative complication rate of 9.6% (Magtibay, 2005). A retrospective review reported that laparoscopic and robotic surgery for the treatment of ovarian remnant syndrome had less blood loss, lower postoperative complications, and a shorter length of stay than laparotomy (Zapardiel, 2012).

## *ACKNOWLEDGMENTS*

We thank Vern Katz for his contributions to this chapter in the previous edition, as well as Martha Goetsch for her advice with portions of this chapter in the previous edition.

## KEY POINTS

- The most common large cyst of the vulva is a cystic dilation of an obstructed Bartholin duct, with a lifetime risk estimated to be 2%. These cysts occur most often during the third decade. Inflamed cysts may be treated with oral antibiotics or incision and drainage.
- The vulva contains 1% of the skin surface of the body, but 5% to 10% of all malignant melanomas in women arise from this region. Melanoma is the second most common malignancy arising in the vulva and accounts for 2% to 3% of all of the melanomas occurring in women.
- Ideally, all vulvar nevi should be excised and examined histologically. Special emphasis should be directed toward the flat junctional nevus and the dysplastic nevus, for they have the greatest potential for malignant transformation. The dysplastic nevus is characterized by being more than 5 mm in diameter, with irregular borders and patches of variegated pigment.
- The management of nonobstetric vulvar hematomas is usually conservative unless the hematoma is greater than 10 cm in diameter or rapidly increasing.
- In adult women, 50% of cases of chronic vulvovaginal pruritus are due to allergic and irritant contact dermatitis. The most common causes of vulvar contact dermatitis are cosmetic and local therapeutic agents. Initial treatment of severe lesions is removal of all irritants or potential allergens and application of topical steroids until the skin returns to normal.
- Women usually develop psoriasis during their teenage years, with approximately 3% of adult women being affected. Approximately 20% of these have involvement of the vulvar skin. The margins of psoriasis are better defined than the common skin conditions in the differential diagnosis, including candidiasis, seborrheic dermatitis, and eczema.
- Psoriasis does not involve the vagina, only the vulva.
- Lichen sclerosus does not involve the vagina, whereas lichen planus may involve the vagina.
- Vulvar pain, vulvodynia, is one of the most common gynecologic problems, reported by up to 16% of women in the general population; 30% of women will have spontaneous relief of their symptoms without any treatment.
- Classically, the symptoms associated with the urethral diverticulum are extremely chronic in nature and have not resolved with multiple courses of oral antibiotic therapy.
- Cervical stenosis may occur following loop electrocautery excision procedures (LEEPs). The volume of tissue removed and repeat excisional procedures have been reported to increase the risk for cervical stenosis.
- Endocervical polyps are smooth, soft, red, fragile masses. They are found most commonly in multiparous women in their 40s and 50s. After the endocervical polyp is removed, endometrial sampling should be performed to diagnose a coexisting endometrial hyperplasia or carcinoma.
- Endometrial polyps are noted in approximately 10% of women when the uterus is examined at autopsy. Approximately one in four women with abnormal bleeding will have an endometrial polyp.
- Leiomyomas are the most common benign neoplasms of the uterus. The lifetime prevalence of leiomyomas is greater than 80% among African-American women and approaches 70% among white women.
- Cytogenetically, leiomyomas are chromosomally normal and arise from a single cell (they are clonal). All the cells are derived from one progenitor myocyte.
- Abnormal bleeding is experienced by a third of women with myomas, the most common pattern being intermenstrual spotting. Women with myomas and abnormal bleeding should be thoroughly evaluated for concurrent causes of bleeding.
- Adenomyosis is frequently asymptomatic. If multiple serial sections of the uterus are obtained, the incidence may exceed 60% in women 40 to 50 years of age.
- Adenomyosis rarely causes uterine enlargement greater than a size that corresponds to 14 weeks' gestation unless there is concomitant uterine pathology.
- The initial management of a suspected follicular cyst is conservative observation. The majority of follicular cysts disappear spontaneously by either reabsorption of the cyst fluid or silent rupture within 4 to 8 weeks of the initial diagnosis.
- The practice of aspirating cysts laparoscopically should be limited to cysts that are completely simple and associated with normal CA-125 levels. The intraoperative spillage of malignant cystic tumors should be avoided if possible, although the true risk that spillage poses is unknown.
- The differential diagnosis of a woman with acute pain and a suspected ruptured corpus luteum cyst includes ectopic pregnancy, a ruptured endometrioma, and adnexal torsion.
- The treatment of unruptured corpus luteum cysts is conservative. However, if the cyst persists or intraperitoneal bleeding occurs, necessitating operation, the treatment is cystectomy.
- Drainage or fenestration is effective for follicular cysts and poorly effective for cystadenomas. They will tend to recur. When cysts are drained, it is essential to remember that the cytologic examination of cyst fluid has poor predictive value and poor sensitivity in differentiating benign from malignant cysts.
- Theca lutein cysts arise from either prolonged or excessive stimulation of the ovaries by endogenous or exogenous gonadotropins or increased ovarian sensitivity to gonadotropins. The condition of ovarian enlargement secondary to the development of multiple luteinized follicular cysts is termed *hyperreactio luteinalis.* Approximately 50% of molar pregnancies and 10% of choriocarcinomas have associated bilateral theca lutein cysts.
- Benign ovarian teratomas vary from a few millimeters to 25 cm, may be single or multiple, and are bilateral 10% to 15% of the time. Dermoids are believed to arise during fetal life from a single germ cell. They are 46,XX in karyotype.
- Operative treatment of benign cystic teratomas is via cystectomy with preservation of as much normal ovarian tissue as possible.

## KEY POINTS—cont'd

- Fifty percent of patients with an ovarian fibroma will have ascites if the tumor is greater than 6 cm. The incidence of associated ascites is directly proportional to the size of the tumor.
- Transitional cell tumors (Brenner tumors) are small, smooth, solid, fibroepithelial tumors of the ovary. They usually occur in women between the ages of 40 and 60 and are predominantly unilateral.
- Adnexal torsion occurs most commonly in the reproductive years, with the average age of patients being in the mid-20s. Pregnancy predisposes to adnexal torsion.
- Ovarian tumors are discovered in 50% to 60% of women with adnexal torsion.
- Abnormal color Doppler flow is highly predictive of torsion of the ovary. However, approximately 50% of women with surgically confirmed adnexal torsion will have a normal Doppler flow study.
- Conservative surgery, either through the laparoscope or via laparotomy, entails gentle untwisting of the pedicle, possibly cystectomy, and stabilization of the ovary with sutures. De-torsion and fixation of the ovary is a safe procedure that reduces the risk of recurrence.
- The risk of pulmonary embolus with adnexal torsion is approximately 0.2%. The risk is similar regardless of whether the condition is managed by conservative surgery with untwisting or adnexal removal without untwisting.

## KEY REFERENCES


American College of Obstetricians and Gynecologists (ACOG). *Power morcellation and occult malignancy in gynecologic surgery*; 2014. Available at http://www.acog.org/Resources-And-Publications/Task-Force-and-Work-Group-Reports/Power-Morcellation-and-Occult-Malignancy-in-Gynecologic-Surgery. Retrieved February 18, 2016.

American College of Obstetricians and Gynecologists (ACOG). Committee opinion no. 620: salpingectomy for ovarian cancer prevention. *Obstet Gynecol.* 2015;125(1):279-281.

Ascher SM, Jha RC, Reinhold C. Benign myometrial conditions: leiomyomas and adenomyosis. *Top Magn Reson Imaging.* 2003;14(4):281-304.

Baird DD, Dunson DB, Hill MC, et al. High cumulative incidence of uterine leiomyoma in black and white women: ultrasound evidence. *Am J Obstet Gynecol.* 2003;188(1):100-107.

Baird DD, Hill MC, Schectman JM, et al. Vitamin D and the risk of uterine fibroids. *Epidemiology.* 2013;24(3):447-453.

Balasa RW, Adcock LL, Prem KA, et al. The Brenner tumor. *Obstet Gynecol.* 1977;50:120.

Bogani G, Cliby WA, Aletti GD. Impact of morcellation on survival outcomes of patients with unexpected uterine leiomyosarcoma: a systematic review and meta-analysis. *Gynecol Oncol.* 2015;137(1):167-172.

Cheung VY. Sonographically guided high-intensity focused ultrasound for the management of uterine fibroids. *J Ultrasound Med.* 2013;32(8):1353-1358.

Conces MR, Williamson SR, Montironi R, et al. Urethral caruncle: clinicopathologic features of 41 cases. *Hum Pathol.* 2012;43(9):1400-1404.

DeWilde R, Bordt J, Hesseling M, et al. Ovarian cystostomy. *Acta Obstet Gynecol Scand.* 1989;68(4):363-364.

Donnez J, Tatarchuk TF, Bouchard P, et al. Ulipristal acetate versus placebo for fibroid treatment before surgery. *N Engl J Med.* 2012b;366(5):409-420.

Donnez J, Tomaszewski J, Vazquez F, et al. Ulipristal acetate versus leuprolide acetate for uterine fibroids. *N Engl J Med.* 2012a;366(5):421-432.

Donnez J, Vazquez F, Tomaszewski J, et al. Long-term treatment of uterine fibroids with ulipristal acetate. *Fertil Steril.* 2014;101(6):1565-1573.

Edwards L, Lynch P. Skin-colored lesions. In: Edwards L, Lynch PJ, eds. *Genital Dermatology Atlas.* 2nd edition. Philadelphia: Lippincott Williams and Wilkins; 2011:197-227.

Eisinger SH, Bonfiglio T, Fiscella K, et al. Twelve-month safety and efficacy of low-dose mifepristone for uterine myomas. *J Minim Invasive Gynecol.* 2005; 12(3):227-233.

Ekerhovd E, Wienerroith H, Staudach A, et al. Preoperative assessment of unilocular adnexal cysts by transvaginal ultrasonography: a comparison between ultrasonographic morphologic imaging and histopatholigic diagnosis. *Am J Obstet Gynecol.* 2001;184(2):48-54.

Eltoukhi HM, Modi MN, Weston M, et al. The health disparities of uterine fibroids for African American women: a public health issue. *Am J Obstet Gynecol.* 2014;210(3):194-199.

Erickson BK, Conner MG, Landen Jr CN. The role of the fallopian tube in the origin of ovarian cancer. *Am J Obstet Gynecol.* 2013;209(5):409-414.

Foley CL, Greenwell TJ, Gardiner RA. Urethral diverticula in females. *BJU Int.* 2011;108(Suppl 2):20-23.

Friedrich EG. Tampon effects on vaginal health. *Clin Obstet Gynecol.* 1981; 24(2):395-406.

Greenlee RT, Kessel B, Williams CR, et al. Prevalence, incidence, and natural history of simple ovarian cysts among women >55 years old in a large cancer screening trial. *Am J Obstet Gynecol.* 2010;202(4):373.e1-373.e9.

Haefner HK, Collins ME, Davis GD, et al. The vulvodynia guideline. *J Low Genit Tract Dis.* 2005;9(1):40-41.

Hallatt JG, Steele CH, Snyder M. Ruptured corpus luteum with hemoperitoneum: a study of 173 surgical cases. *Am J Obstet Gynecol.* 1984;149(1):5-9.

Heller DS. Benign papular lesions of the vulva. *J Low Genit Tract Dis.* 2012; 16(3):296-305.

Higgins RV, Matkins JF, Marroum MC. Comparison of fine-needle aspiration cytologic findings of ovarian cysts with ovarian histologic findings. *Am J Obstet Gynecol.* 1999;180(3 Pt 1):550-553.

Huang SC, Yu CH, Huang RT, et al. Intratumoral blood flow in uterine myoma correlated with a lower tumor size and volume, but not correlated with cell proliferation or angiogenesis. *Obstet Gynecol.* 1996;87(6):1019-1024.

Hurst BS, Matthews ML, Marshburn PB. Laparoscopic myomectomy for symptomatic uterine myomas. *Fertil Steril.* 2005;83(1):1-23.

Hyttel TE, Bak GS, Larsen SB, et al. Re-torsion of the ovaries. *Acta Obstet Gynecol Scand.* 2015;94(3):236-244.

Ishikawa H, Reierstad S, Demura M, et al. High aromatase expression in uterine leiomyoma tissues of African-American women. *J Clin Endocrinol Metab.* 2009;94(5):1752-1756.

Jayi S, Laadioui M, El Fatemi H, et al. Vulvar lipoma: a case report. *J Med Case Rep.* 2014;8:203.

Kumar S, Sharma JB, Verma D, et al. Disseminated peritoneal leiomyomatosis: an unusual complication of laparoscopic myomectomy. *Arch Gynecol Obstet.* 2008;278(1):93-95.

Lambert J. Pruritus in female patients. *Biomed Res Int.* 2014;2014:541867.

Launoned V, Vierimaa O, Kiuru M, et al. Inherited susceptibility to uterine leiomyomas and renal cell cancer. *Proc Natl Acad Sci USA.* 2001;98(6): 3387-3392.

Lawrence HC. *American College of Obstetricians and Gynecologists: ACOG Statement on power morcellation*; 2014. Available at http://www.acog.org/About-ACOG/News-Room/Statements/2014/ACOG-Statement-on-Power-Morcellation. Retrieved February 18, 2016.

Lee JW, Fynes MM. Female urethral diverticula. *Best Pract Res Clin Obstet Gynaecol.* 2005;19(6):875-893.

Lee MY, Dalpiaz A, Schwamb R, et al. Clinical pathology of bartholin's glands: a review of the literature. *Curr Urol.* 2015;8(1):22-25.

Lee SC, Kaunitz AM, Sanchez-Ramos L, et al. The oncogenic potential of endometrial polyps: a sytematic review and meta-analysis. *Obstet Gynecol.* 2010;116(5):1197-1205.

Lethaby A, Shepperd S, Cooke I, et al. Endometrial resection and ablation versus hysterectomy for heavy menstrual bleeding. *Cochrane Database Syst Rev.* 2000;(2): CD000329.

LevGur M, Abadi MA, Tucker A. Adenomyosis: symptoms, histology, and pregnancy terminations. *Obstet Gynecol.* 2000;95(5):688-691.
Levy G, Hill MJ, Beall S, et al. Leiomyoma: genetics, assisted reproduction, pregnancy and therapeutic advances. *J Assist Reprod Genet.* 2012;29(8):703-712.
Lum DA, Sokol ER, Berek JS, et al. Impact of the 2014 FDA warnings against power morcellation. *J Minim Invasive Gynecol.* 2016. [epub ahead of print].
Magtibay PM, Nyholm JL, Hernandez JL, et al. Ovarian remnant syndrome. *Am J Obstet Gynecol.* 2005;193(6):2062-2066.
Marret H, Fritel X, Ouldamer L, et al. Therapeutic management of uterine fibroid tumors: updated French guidelines. *Eur J Obstet Gynecol Reprod Biol.* 2012;165(2):156-164.
McKeage K, Croxtall JD. Ulipristal acetate: a review of its use in emergency contraception. *Drugs.* 2011;71(7):935-945.
Metwally M, Cheong YC, Horne AW. Surgical treatment of fibroids for subfertility. *Cochrane Database Syst Rev.* 2012;11:CD003857.
Moroni RM, Martins WP, Ferriani RA, et al. Add-back therapy with GnRH analogues for uterine fibroids. *Cochrane Database Syst Rev.* 2015;(3). CD010854.
Moyal-Barracco M, Lynch PJ. 2003 ISSVD terminology and classification of vulvodynia: a historical perspective. *J Reprod Med.* 2004;49(10):772-777.
Okolo S. Incidence, aetiology and epidemiology of uterine fibroids. *Best Pract Res Clin Obstet Gynaecol.* 2008;22(4):571-588.
Panganamamula UR, Harmanli OH, Isik-Akbay EF, et al. Is prior uterine surgery a risk factor for adenomyosis? *Obstet Gynecol.* 2004;104(5 Pt 1):1034-1038.
Perez-Lopez FR. Ulipristal acetate in the management of symptomatic uterine fibroids: facts and pending issues. *Climacteric.* 2015;18(2):177-181.
Pritts EA, Vanness DJ, Berek JS, et al. The prevalence of occult leiomyosarcoma at surgery for presumed uterine fibroids: a meta-analysis. *Gynecol Surg.* 2015;12(3):165-177.
Raziel A, Ron-El R, Pansky M, et al. Current management of ruptured corpus luteum. *Eur J Obstet Gynecol Reprod Biol.* 1993;50(1):77-81.
Reed BD, Haefner HK, Sen A, et al. Vulvodynia incidence and remission rates among adult women. *Am College Obstet Gynecol.* 2008;112(2 Pt 1):231-237.
Sangkomkamhang US, Lumbiganon P, Laopaiboon M, et al. Progestogens or progestogen-releasing intrauterine systems for uterine fibroids. *Cochrane Database Syst Rev.* 2013;(2). CD008994.
Sasaki KF, Miller CE. Adnexal torsion: review of the literature. *J Minim Invasive Gynecol.* 2014;21(2):196-202.
Scurry J, Van der Putte SC, Pyman J, et al. Mammary-like gland adenoma of the vulva: review of 46 cases. *Pathology.* 2009;41(4):372-378.
Shozu M, Murakami K, Segawa T, et al. Successful treatment of a symptomatic uterine leiomyoma in a perimenopausal woman with a nonsteroidal aromatase inhibitor. *Fertil Steril.* 2003;79(3):628-631.
Singh SS, Belland L. Contemporary management of uterine fibroids: focus on emerging medical treatments. *Curr Med Res Opin.* 2015;31(1):1-12.
Stewart EA. Uterine fibroids. *N Engl J Med.* 2015;372(17):1646-1655.
Stockdale CK, Lawson HW. 2013 vulvodynia guideline update. *J Low Genit Tract Dis.* 2014;18(2):93-100.
Struble J, Reid S, Bedaiwy MA. Adenomyosis: a clinical review of a challenging gynecologic condition. *J Minim Invasive Gynecol.* 2016;23(2):164-185.
Sugiyama VE, Chan JK, Shin JY, et al. Vulvar melanoma. A multivariable analysis of 644 patients. *Obstet Gynecol.* 2007;110(2 Pt 1):296-301.
Suh-Burgmann EJ, Whall-Strojwas D, Chang Y, et al. Risk factors for cervical stenosis after loop electrocautery excision procedure. *Obstet Gynecol.* 2000; 96(5):657-660.
Tabor A, Watt HC, Wald NJ. Endometrial thickness as a test for endometrial cancer in women with postmenopausal vaginal bleeding. *Obstet Gynecol.* 2002;99(4):663-670.
Tal R, Segars JH. The role of angiogenic factors in fibroid pathogenesis: potential implications for future therapy. *Hum Reprod Update.* 2014;20(2):194-216.
Tang LCH, Cho HKM, Chan SYW, et al. Dextropreponderance of corpus luteum rupture. *J Reprod Med.* 1985;30:764.
Trefoux BA, Luton D, Koskas M. Clinical utility of ulipristal acetate for the treatment of uterine fibroids: current evidence. *Int J Womens Health.* 2015; 7:321-330.
Tunitsky E, Goldman HB, Ridgeway B. Periurethral mass: a rare and puzzling entity. *Obstet Gynecol.* 2012;120(6):1459-1464.
Uliana V, Marcocci E, Mucciolo M, et al. Alport syndrome and leiomyomatosis: the first deletion extending beyond COL4A6 intron 2. *Pediatr Nephrol.* 2011; 26(5):717-724.
U.S. Food and Drug Administration (USFDA). *Laparoscopic uterine power morcellation in hysterectomy and myomectomy: FDA Safety Communication*; 2014. Available at http://www.fda.gov/MedicalDevices/Safety/AlertsandNotices/ucm424443.htm. Retrieved February 18, 2016.
Van der Kooij SM, Hehenkamp WJK, Volkers NA, et al. Uterine artery embolization vs hysterectomy in the treatment of sympotomatic uterine fibroids: 5-year outcome from the randomized EMMY trial. *Am J Obstet Gynecol.* 2010;203(2). 105.e1-13.
Venkatesan A. Pigmented lesions of the vulva. *Dermatol Clin.* 2010;28(4):795-805.
Verma SK, Lev-Toaff AS, Baltarowich OH, et al. Adenomyosis: sonohysterography with MRI correlation. *AJR Am J Roentgenol.* 2009;192(4):1112-1116.
Wai CY, Corton MM, Miller M, et al. Multiple vaginal wall cysts: diagnosis and surgical management. *Obstet Gynecol.* 2004;103(5 Pt 2):1099-1102.
Wechter ME, Steward EA, Myers ER, et al. Leiomyoma-related hospitalization and surgery: prevalence and predicted growth based on population trends. *Am J Obstet Gynecol.* 2011;205(5):492.e1-492.e5.
Wechter ME, Wu JM, Marzano D, et al. Management of Bartholin's duct cysts and abscesses: a systematic review. *Obstet Gynecol Surv.* 2009;64(6):395-404.
Wegienka G, Baird DD, Hertz-Picciotto I, et al. Self-reported heavy bleeding associated with uterine leiomyomata. *Obstet Gynecol.* 2003;101:431.
Wolf SI, Gosnik BB, Feldesman MR, et al. Prevalence of simple adnexal cysts in postmenopausal women. *Radiology.* 1991;180:65.
Worley MJ, Aelion A, Caputo TA, et al. Intravenous leiomyomatosis with intracardiac extension: a single-institution experience. *Am J Obstet Gynecol.* 2009;201(6):574.e1-574.e5.
Wright JD, Tergas AI, Burke WM, et al. Uterine pathology in women undergoing minimally invasive hysterectomy using morcellation. *JAMA.* 2014; 312(12):1253-1255.
Zapardiel I, Zanagnolo V, Kho RM, et al. Ovarian remnant syndrome: comparison of laparotomy, laparoscopy and robotic surgery. *Acta Obstet Gynecol Scand.* 2012;91(8):965-969.
Zhang C, Miao Q, Liu X, et al. Intravenous leiomyomatosis with intracardiac extension. *Ann Thorac Surg.* 2010;89(5):1641-1643.
Zolnoun DA, Hartmann KE, Steege JF. Overnight 5% lidocaine ointment for treatment of vulvar vestibulitis. *Obstet Gynecol.* 2003;102(1):84-87.

Suggested Readings can be found on ExpertConsult.com.

# 19

# Endometriosis

## Etiology, Pathology, Diagnosis, Management

*Arnold Advincula, Mireille Truong, Roger A. Lobo*

## ENDOMETRIOSIS

Endometriosis is a benign but, in many women, a progressive and aggressive disease. The wide spectrum of clinical problems that occur with endometriosis has frustrated gynecologists, fascinated pathologists, and burdened patients for years. Although endometriosis was first described in 1860, the classic studies by Sampson in the 1920s were the first to emphasize the clinical and pathologic correlations of endometriosis (Sampson, 1927). Even today, many aspects of the disease remain enigmatic.

By definition, endometriosis is the presence and growth of the glands and stroma of the lining of the uterus in an aberrant or heterotopic location. Adenomyosis is the growth of endometrial glands and stroma into the uterine myometrium to a depth of at least 2.5 mm from the basalis layer of the endometrium. Adenomyosis is sometimes termed *internal endometriosis*; however, this is a semantic misnomer because most likely they are separate diseases.

It is usually stated that the incidence of endometriosis has been increasing since the 1980s. This opinion is secondary to an enlightened awareness of mild endometriosis as diagnosed by the increasing use of laparoscopy. Since the early 2000s, diagnostic delay, the average time to the first diagnosis of the disease, has decreased dramatically. However, it has been estimated to take an average time of 11.7 years in the United States and 8 years in the United Kingdom to make the diagnosis. Evers has advanced a provocative hypothesis that endometrial implants in the peritoneal cavity are a physiologic finding secondary to retrograde menstruation, and their presence does not confirm a disease process (Evers, 1994). The overall prevalence of endometriosis in reproductive aged women has been suggested to be as high as 11% (Buck Louis, 2011). The age-specific incidence or prevalence of endometriosis is not known and has only been estimated. Many patients are diagnosed incidentally during surgery performed for a variety of other indications. Conservative estimates find that endometriosis is present in 5% to 15% of laparotomies performed on reproductive-age females. The prevalence of active endometriosis is approximately 33% in women with chronic pelvic pain. The incidence of endometriosis is 30% to 45% in women with infertility. In a compilation of eight studies encompassing 162 patients with endometriosis, the natural course of endometriosis has been reported to increase or progress 31% of the time, to remain the same 32% of the time and to regress in 38% (Taylor, 2014). The cause of endometriosis is uncertain and involves many mechanisms including retrograde menstruation, vascular dissemination, metaplasia, genetic predisposition, immunologic changes, and hormonal influences, as discussed later. In addition, there is increasing evidence that environmental factors may also play a role, including exposure to dioxin and other endocrine disruptors. Clinically, it is most difficult to predict the natural course of endometriosis in any one individual. For example, the clinician cannot know which woman with mild disease in her 20s will progress to severe disease at a later age.

The typical patient with endometriosis is in her mid-30s, is nulliparous and involuntarily infertile, and has symptoms of secondary dysmenorrhea and pelvic pain, but it must be stressed that symptoms and signs may be extremely variable. The classic symptom of endometriosis is pelvic pain. However, in clinical practice the majority of cases are not "classic." The diagnosis and treatment of infertility associated with endometriosis is discussed in Chapter 42. Aberrant endometrial tissue grows under the cyclic influence of ovarian hormones and is particularly estrogen dependent; therefore, the disease is most commonly found during the reproductive years. However, 5% of women with endometriosis are diagnosed following menopause. Postmenopausal endometriosis is usually stimulated by exogenous estrogen. Endometriosis in teenagers should be investigated for obstructive reproductive tract abnormalities that increase the amount of retrograde menstruation. Although previously thought to be rare in adolescents, in teens with pelvic pain, endometriosis has been found in approximately half the cases.

Endometriosis is a disease not only of great individual variability but also of contrasting pathophysiologic processes. It is a benign disease, yet it has the characteristics of a malignancy—that is, it is locally infiltrative, invasive, and widely disseminating. Although the physiologic levels of estrogen stimulate the growth of ectopic endometrium, the use of contraceptive steroids of various doses is usually beneficial for treatment. Another contrast often noted is the inverse relationship between the extent of pelvic endometriosis and the severity of pelvic pain. Women with extensive endometriosis may be asymptomatic, whereas other patients with minimal implants may have incapacitating chronic pelvic pain. However, as would be expected, women with deep infiltrating endometriosis, especially in retroperitoneal spaces, often experience severe episodes of pain. Pelvic lesions of endometriosis have been found to have positive immunostaining for smooth muscle as well as nerve cells (Medina, 2009).

The clinical variability in responses among women with endometriosis may relate to differences in immunologic function and variations in cytokine production.

## ETIOLOGY

There are several theories to explain the pathogenesis of endometriosis. However, no single theory adequately explains all the manifestations of the disease. Most important, there is only speculation as to why some women develop endometriosis and others do not. One popular theory is that there is a complex interplay between a dose-response curve of the amount of retrograde menstruation and an individual woman's immunologic response (these in turn may depend on ethnic and genetic variability).

### Retrograde Menstruation

The most popular theory is that endometriosis results from retrograde menstruation. Sampson suggested that pelvic endometriosis was secondary to implantation of endometrial cells shed during menstruation (Sampson, 1927). It has been suggested that the shedding of endometrial-based adult stem cells and mesenchymal cells may explain this phenomenon (Gargett, 2010). These cells attach to the pelvic peritoneum and under hormonal influence grow as homologous grafts. Indeed, reflux of menstrual blood and viable endometrial cells in the pelvis of ovulating women has been documented. Endometriosis is discovered most frequently in areas immediately adjacent to the tubal ostia or in the dependent areas of the pelvis.

Endometriosis is frequently found in women with outflow obstruction of the genital tract. The attachment of the shed endometrial cells involves the expression of adhesion molecules and their receptors. This is thought to be an extremely rapid process as demonstrated in vitro. Figures 19.1 and 19.2 depict the process of implants from retrograde menstruation and early invasion (Flores, 2007; Witz, 2001).

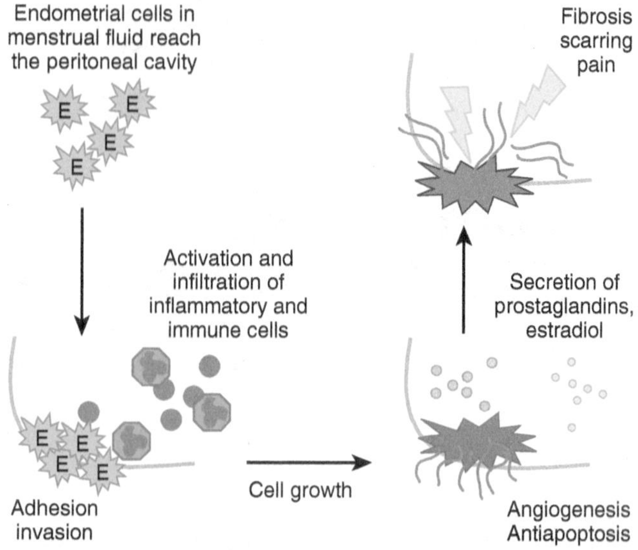


**Figure 19.1** Proposed establishment of peritoneal endometriotic implants via retrograde menstruation, attachment, proliferation, migration, neovascularization, inflammation, and fibrosis. *E*, Endometrial cell. (From Flores I, Rivera E, Ruiz LA, et al. Molecular profiling of experimental endometriosis identified gene expression patterns in common with human disease. *Fertil Steril.* 2007;87[5]:1180-1199.)

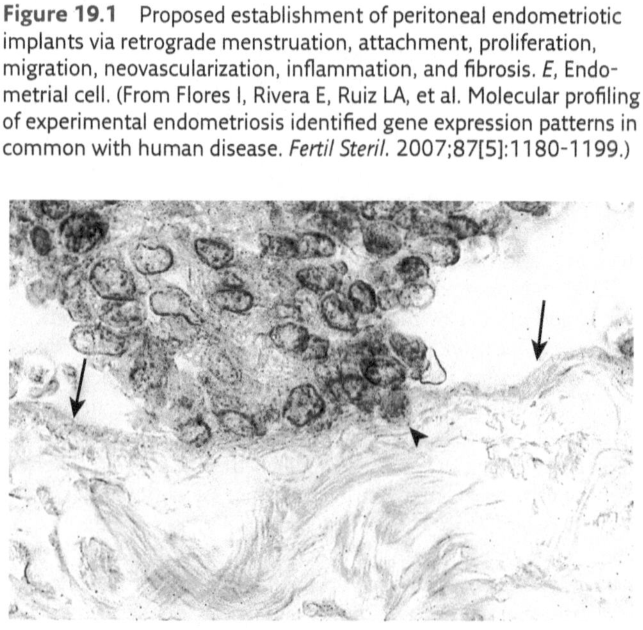

**Figure 19.2** Early Invasion of an Endometrial Implant through the Mesothelium. The mesothelium is labeled with monoclonal antibody to cytokeratin and stained with diaminobenzidine *(arrows)*. An endometrial stromal cell *(arrowhead)* passing through the mesothelium is thought to represent the initial step of invasion into the stroma of the peritoneum. Original magnification, ×31,000. Counterstained with hematoxylin. (From Witz CA, Monotoya-Rodrigueez I, Schenken RS. Whole explants of peritoneum and endometrium: a novel model of the early endometriosis lesion. *Fertil Steril.* 1999;71[1]:56-60.)

### Metaplasia

In contrast to the theory of seeding from retrograde menstruation is the theory that endometriosis arises from metaplasia of the coelomic epithelium or proliferation of embryonic rests (Meyer, 1924). The Müllerian ducts and nearby mesenchymal tissue form the majority of the female reproductive tract. The Müllerian duct is derived from the coelomic epithelium during fetal development. The metaplasia hypothesis postulates that the coelomic epithelium retains the ability for multipotential development. The decidual reaction of isolated areas of peritoneum during pregnancy is an example of this process. It is well known that the surface epithelium of the ovary can differentiate into several different histologic cell types. Endometriosis has been discovered in prepubertal girls, women with congenital absence of the uterus, and rarely in men. These examples support the coelomic metaplasia theory.

Metaplasia occurs after an "induction phenomenon" has stimulated the multipotential cell. The induction substance may be a combination of menstrual debris and the influence of estrogen and progesterone. It has been hypothesized that the histogenesis of endometriosis in peritoneal pockets of the posterior pelvis results from a congenital anomaly involving rudimentary duplication of the Müllerian system (Batt, 1989). The peritoneal pockets that they describe are found in the posterior pelvis, the posterior aspects of the broad ligament, and the cul-de-sac (Fig. 19.3). Similarly, it has been postulated that metaplasia of the coelomic epithelium that invaginates into the ovarian cortex is the pathogenesis for the development of ovarian endometriosis (Nisolle, 1997).

### Lymphatic and Vascular Metastasis

The theory of endometrium being transplanted via lymphatic channels and the vascular system (Halban, 1925) helps to explain rare and remote sites of endometriosis, such as the spinal column and nose. Endometriosis has been observed in the pelvic lymph nodes of approximately 30% of women with the disease.

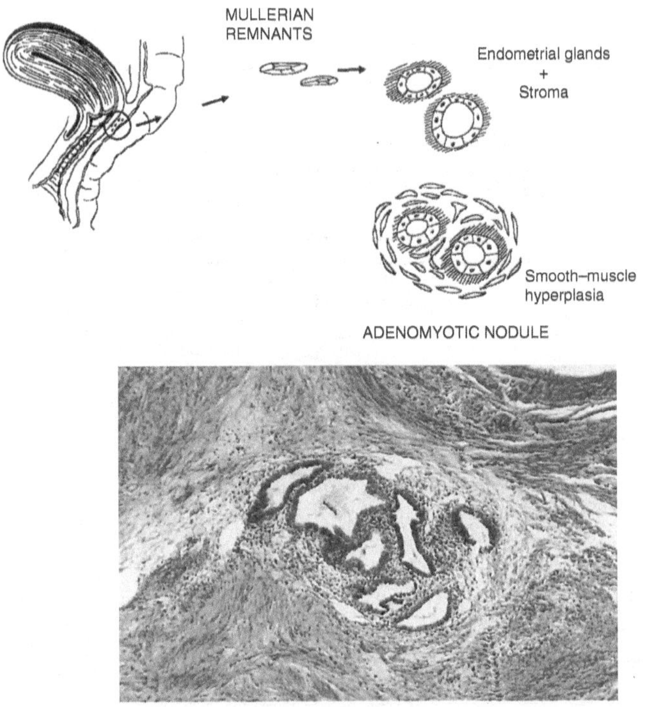


**Figure 19.3** Proposed derivation of endometriotic lesion in the rectovaginal septum. (From Strauss JF, Barbieri R. *Yen & Jaffe's Reproductive Endocrinology.* 5th ed. Philadelphia: Saunders: 2004:692-693.)

Hematogenous dissemination of endometrium is the best theory to explain endometriosis of the forearm and thigh, as well as multiple lesions in the lung.

### *Iatrogenic Dissemination*

Endometriosis of the anterior abdominal wall is sometimes discovered in women after a cesarean delivery. The hypothesis is that endometrial glands and stroma are implanted during the procedure. The aberrant tissue is found subcutaneously at the abdominal incision. Rarely, iatrogenic endometriosis may be discovered in an episiotomy scar.

### *Immunologic Changes*

One of the most perplexing, unanswered questions concerning the pathophysiology of endometriosis is that some women with retrograde menstruation develop endometriosis, but most do not. Multiple investigations have suggested that changes in the immune system, especially altered function of immune-related cells, are directly related to the pathogenesis of endometriosis. Whether endometriosis is an autoimmune disease has been intensely debated for many years. Studies have demonstrated abnormalities in cell-mediated and humoral components of the immune system in both peripheral blood and peritoneal fluid. Box 19.1 depicts various cytokines and growth factors that have been implicated in the pathogenesis of endometriosis (McLaren, 1997).

Most likely the primary immunologic change involves an alteration in the function of the peritoneal macrophages so prevalent in the peritoneal fluid of patients with endometriosis. It has been hypothesized that women who do not develop endometriosis have monocytic-type macrophages in their peritoneal fluid that have a short life span and limited function. Conversely, women who develop endometriosis have more peritoneal macrophages that are larger. These hyperactive cells secrete multiple growth factors and cytokines that enhance the development of endometriosis. The attraction of leukocytes to specific areas is controlled by chemokines, which are chemotactic cytokines (Halme, 1984) (Fig. 19.4). Changes in the expression of integrins also may be an important local factor. Following the theory of different macrophage populations in endometriosis is the finding that the destroying of normally extruded endometrial cells in endometriosis may be deficient. It has been shown that natural killer (NK) cells have decreased cytotoxicity against endometrial and hematopoietic cells in women with endometriosis. Also, peritoneal fluid of women with endometriosis has less influence of NK activity than is found in fertile women without endometriosis.

Another attractive theory is the finding of a protein similar to haptoglobin in endometriosis epithelial cells called Endo 1. This chemoattractant protein-enhanced local production of interleukin-6 (IL-6) self-perpetuates lesion/cytokine interactions. Further compounding the proliferative activity of endometriosis lesions are angiogenic factors that are increased in lesions. Here the expression of basic fibroblast factor, IL-6, IL-8, platelet-derived growth factor (PDGF), and vascular endothelial growth factor (VEGF) are all increased.

Steroid interactions also enhance the progression of disease. Estrogen production is enhanced locally, and there is evidence for upregulation of aromatase activity, increased COX-2 expression, and dysregulation of 17β-dehydrogenase activity, where there is a deficiency in 17β-dehydrogenase II activity and possibly an enhancement of type II activity favoring local estradiol production (Bulun, 2009). Figure 19.5 shows abnormalities of COX-2,

**Box 19.1 Cytokines and Growth Factors in Peritoneal Fluid**

**Concentrations Increased in Endometriosis**
Complement
Eotaxin
Glycodelin
IL-1
IL-6
IL-8
MCP-1
PDGF
RANTES
Soluble ICAM-1
TGF-β
VEGF

**Concentrations Unchanged in Endometriosis**
EGF
Basic FGF
Interferon-γ
IL-2
IL-4
IL-12

**Concentrations Decreased in Endometriosis**
IL-13

From McLaren J, Deatry G, Prentice A, et al. Decreased levels of the potent regulator of monocyte/macrophage activation, interleukin-13, in the peritoneal fluid of patients with endometriosis. *Hum Reprod.* 1997;12(6):1307-1310.
*EGF*, Epidermal growth factor; *FGF*, fibroblast growth factor; *ICAM*, intercellular adhesion molecule; *IL*, interleukin; *MCP*, membrane cofactor protein; *PDGF*, platelet-derived growth factor; *RANTES*, regulated upon activation, normal T cell expressed and secreted; *TGF*, transforming growth factor; *VEGF*, vascular endothelial growth factor. References are from the original source.

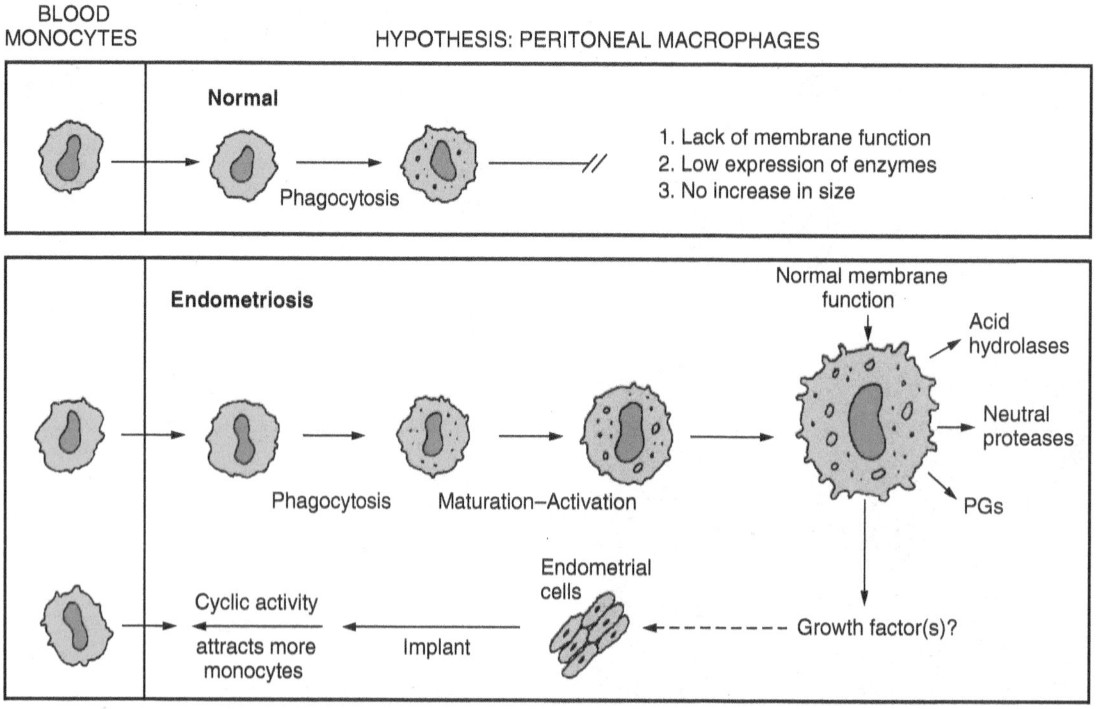


**Figure 19.4** Hypothesis regarding pathophysiologic characteristics of human peritoneal macrophages in endometriosis. *PG*, Prostaglandins. (Modified from Halme J, Becker S, Haskill S, et al. Altered maturation and function of peritoneal macrophages: possible role in pathogenesis of endometriosis. *Am J Obstet Gynecol.* 1987;156:787.)

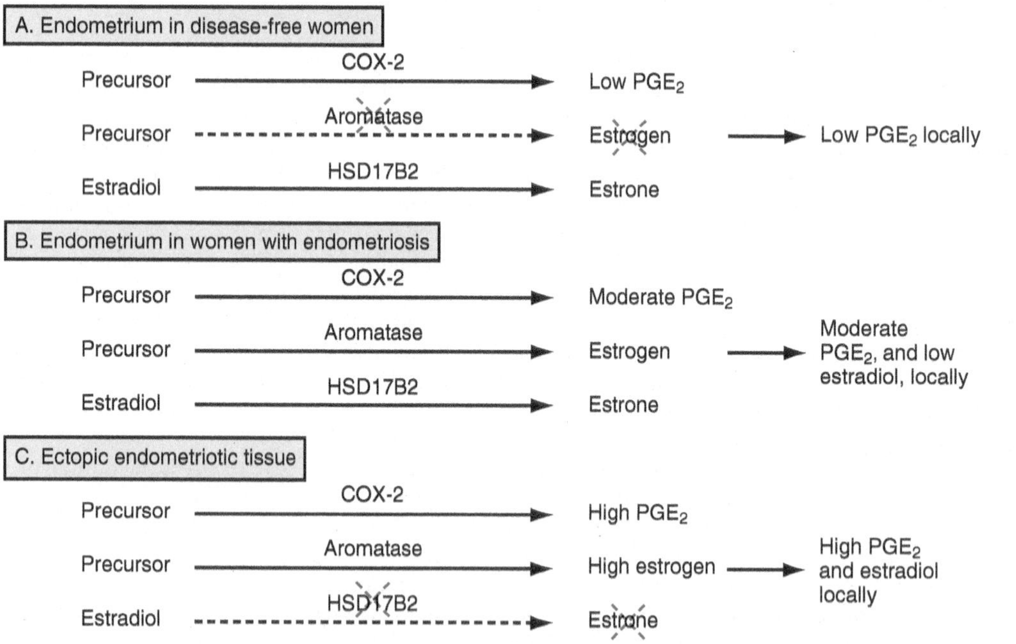


**Figure 19.5** Normal Endometrium and Endometriosis. In normal endometrial tissue *(panel A)*, activity of the enzyme cyclooxygenase-2 (CO-2), and thus production of prostaglandin $E_2$ ($PGE_2$), is low. Estrogen is not produced locally, owing to the absence of aromatase. During the luteal phase, the progesterone-dependent 17β-hydroxysteroid dehydrogenase 2(HSD17B2) enzyme catalyzes the conversion of the biologically active estradiol to estrone that is less estrogenic. In the endometrium of women with endometriosis *(panel B)*, there is a subtle increase in COX-2 activity. In ectopic endometriotic tissue *(panel C)*, full-blown molecular abnormalities include high COX-2 and aromatase levels. Increased $PGE_2$ formation in endometrial and endometriotic tissues can cause severe menstrual cramps and chronic pelvic pain. Tissue estradiol levels should be high, because estradiol is overproduced by aromatase and is not metabolized owing to deficient HSD17B2 activity. Increasing enzyme activity is denoted by the increasing thickness of arrows. (Modified from Bulun SE. Mechanisms of disease: endometriosis. *N Engl J Med.* 2009;360[3]:268-279.)

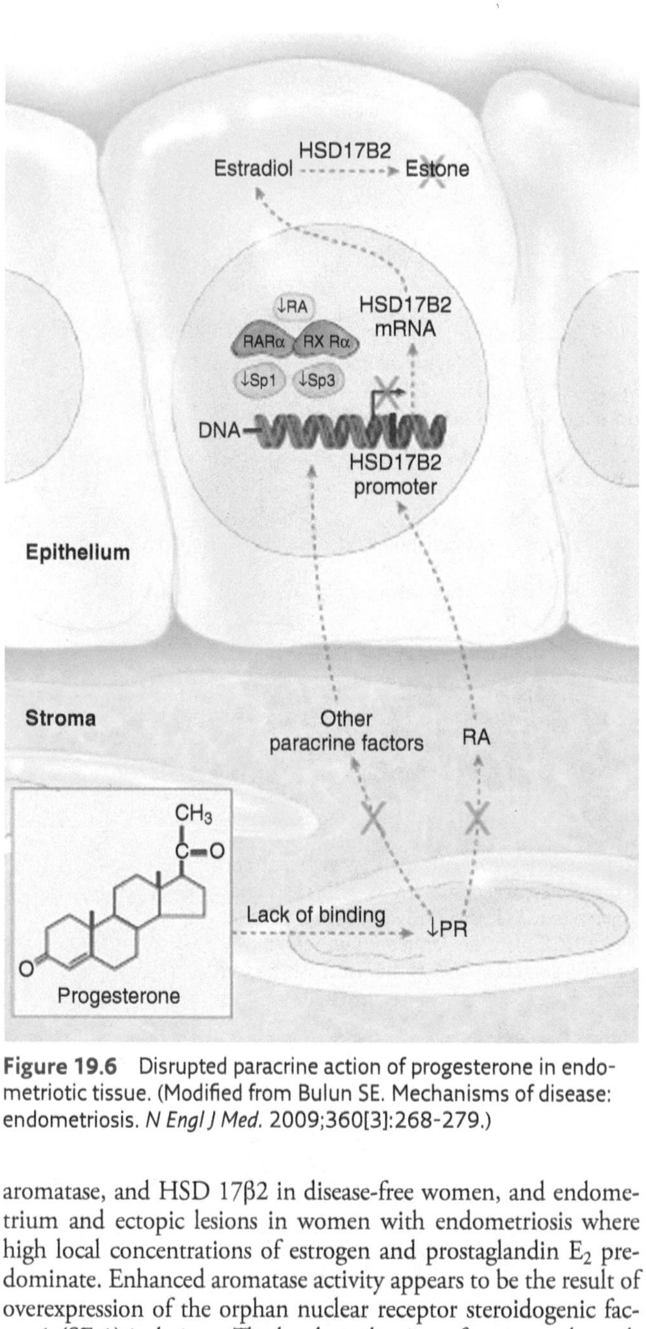


**Figure 19.6** Disrupted paracrine action of progesterone in endometriotic tissue. (Modified from Bulun SE. Mechanisms of disease: endometriosis. *N Engl J Med.* 2009;360[3]:268-279.)

aromatase, and HSD 17β2 in disease-free women, and endometrium and ectopic lesions in women with endometriosis where high local concentrations of estrogen and prostaglandin $E_2$ predominate. Enhanced aromatase activity appears to be the result of overexpression of the orphan nuclear receptor steroidogenic factor-1 (SF-1) in lesions. The local production of estrogen through aromatase activity explains why progression of lesions may occur even with ovarian suppression. Further, there is evidence for progesterone "resistance" (Bulun, 2009) (Fig. 19.6). This is occasioned by a dysregulation of the isoform B of the progesterone receptor in most endometriotic lesions where levels may be undetectable. The latter propensity may be on a genetic basis, as discussed later.

Autoimmunity may well exist in women with endometriosis, and although the findings of abnormalities of the histocompatibility locus antigen (HLA) system have not been consistent, there are reports of increased B and T cells, and serum immunoglobulin (IgG, IgA, and IgM) autoantibodies in endometriosis. A survey of the U.S. Endometriosis Association has provided suggestive evidence of the higher prevalence of other autoimmune diseases. The association of all these immune processes in the symptoms and signs of endometriosis is depicted in Figure 19.7.

### *Genetic Predisposition*

Several studies have documented a familial predisposition to endometriosis with grouping of cases of endometriosis in mothers and their daughters. An investigation by Simpson and coworkers demonstrated a sevenfold increase in the incidence of endometriosis in relatives of women with the disease compared with controls (Simpson, 1980). One of 10 women with severe endometriosis will have a sister or mother with clinical manifestations of the disease. The incidence of endometriosis in first-degree relatives, women with severe endometriosis, has been thought to be 7%. Women who have a family history of endometriosis are likely to develop the disease earlier in life and to have more advanced disease than women whose first-degree relatives are free of the disease. Studies have identified deletions of genes, most specifically increased heterogenicity of chromosome 17 and aneuploidy, in women with endometriosis compared with controls (Kosugi, 1999). Loci on 7p and 10q have also been found to increase the susceptibility for endometriosis (Painter, 2011; Treloar, 2005). The expression of this genetic liability most likely depends on an interaction with environmental and epigenetic factors, with many factors being involved. Preliminary data suggest some bilateral ovarian endometrial cysts may arise independently from different clones. Although no consistent abnormality has been found in women with endometriosis, there are several candidate genes. Box 19.2 provides a partial list of genes and gene products aberrantly expressed in endometriosis.

Several of these aberrantly expressed gene products, for example, the matrix metalloproteinases (MMPs) and integrins, have important implications for endometrial lesion attachment and for implantation defects, which may exist in infertile women with endometriosis. Reflux of MMPs into the peritoneal cavity at menstruation may contribute to peritoneal attachment in susceptible women.

Finally, Bulun and others have suggested that genetic predisposition or exposure to environmental factors (Bulun, 2009), may program fetal progenitor cells in an epigenetic way to overexpress SP1 and estrogen receptor β, which increase the risk of developing endometriosis (Bulun, 2009).

Certain ethnic groups have an increased risk of having endometriosis. This is particularly striking in Asian women, in whom a ninefold increase has been suggested (Jacoby, 2010).

### *Pathology*

The majority of endometrial implants are located in the dependent portions of the female pelvis (Fig. 19.8). The ovaries are the most common site, being involved in two of three women with endometriosis. In most of these women the involvement is bilateral. The pelvic peritoneum over the uterus; the anterior and posterior cul-de-sac; and the uterosacral, round, and broad ligaments are also common sites where endometriosis develops. Pelvic lymph nodes have been found to be involved in up to 30% of cases.

The cervix, vagina, and vulva are other possible pelvic locations. Brosens has emphasized the importance of distinguishing between superficial and deep lesions of endometriosis (Brosens, 2000). Deep lesions, penetrations of greater than 5 mm, represent a more progressive form of the disease. Distinguishing superficial implant lesions on peritoneal surfaces, including the ovary, from deep endometriotic ovarian cysts and cul-de-sac nodules is important for therapy (discussed later end parens here? in that these latter abnormalities may suggest different causes of the disease (e.g., metaplasia), which require a surgical approach.

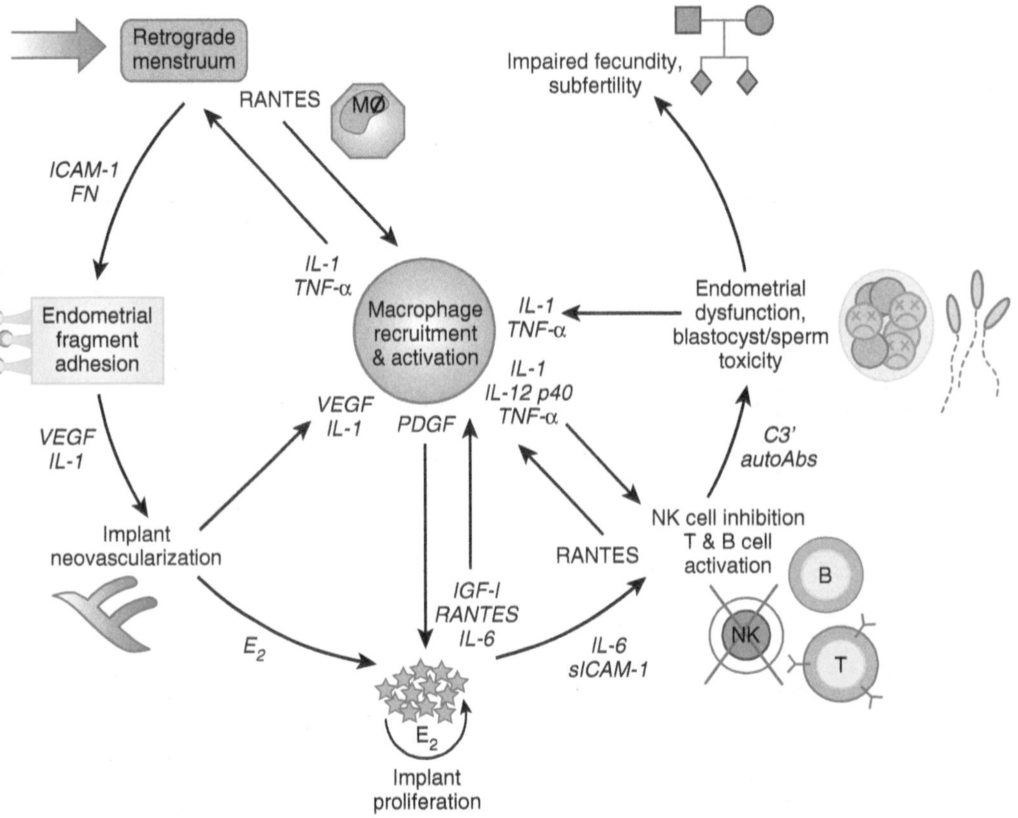


**Figure 19.7** Schematogram depicting the network of chemokines, cytokines, and growth factors in the pathophysiology of endometriosis. *autoAbs*, Autoantibodies; *C3;* complement 3; $E_2$, estradiol; *FN*, fibronectin; *sICAM*, soluble intercellular adhesion molecule; *IGF-1*, insulin-like growth factor-1; *IL*, interleukin; *MØ*, macrophage; *NK cell*, natural killer cell; *PDGF*, platelet-derived growth factor; *RANTES*, regulated on activation, normal IT cell expressed and secreted; *TNF*, tumor necrosis factor; *VEGF*, vascular endothelial growth factor.

**Box 19.2 Genes and Gene Products Aberrantly Expressed in Endometrium from Women with Endometriosis**

Aromatase
Endometrial bleeding factor
Hepatocyte growth factor
17β-hydroxysteroid dehydrogenase
*HOX* A10
*HOX* A11
Leukemia inhibitory factor
Matrix metalloproteinases 3, 7, and 11
Tissue inhibitors of metalloproteinases
Progesterone-receptor isoforms
Complement 3
Glutathione peroxidase
Catalase
Thrombospondin 1
Vascular endothelial growth factor
Integrin $\alpha_v\beta_3$
Glycodelin

Approximately 10% to 15% of women with advanced disease have lesions involving the rectosigmoid. Depending on the amount of associated scarring, endometriosis of the bowel may be difficult to differentiate grossly from a primary neoplasm of the large intestine. Endometriosis may be found in a wide variety

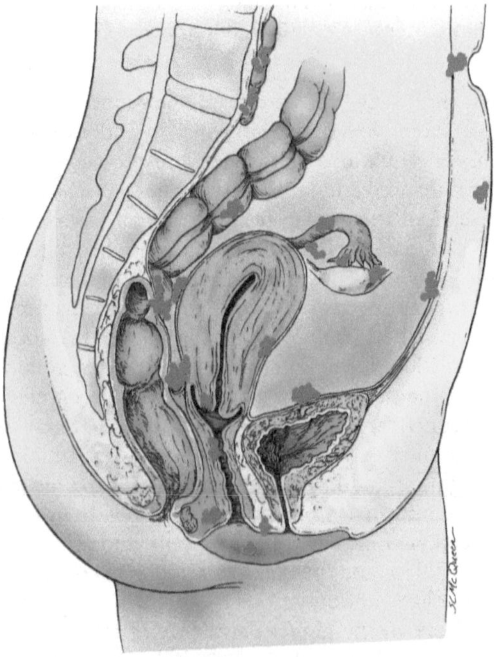

**Figure 19.8** Common pelvic sites of endometriosis.

Table 19.1 Anatomic Distribution of Endometriosis

| Common Sites | Rare Sites |
|---|---|
| Ovaries | Umbilicus |
| Pelvic peritoneum | Episiotomy scar |
| Ligaments of the uterus | Bladder |
| Sigmoid colon | Kidney |
| Appendix | Lungs |
| Pelvic lymph nodes | Arms |
| Cervix | Legs |
| Vagina | Nasal mucosa |
| Fallopian tubes | Spinal column |

Table 19.2 Preoperative Symptoms in 130 Patients Undergoing Colorectal Resection for Endometriosis

| Symptom | No. of Patients | (%) |
|---|---|---|
| Pelvic pain | 111 | (85) |
| Rectal pain | 68 | (52) |
| Cyclic rectal bleeding | 24 | (18) |
| Diarrhea | 55 | (42) |
| Constipation | 53 | (41) |
| Diarrhea and constipation | 18 | (14) |
| Dyspareunia | 83 | (64) |

From Bailey HR, Ott MT, Hartendorp P. Aggressive surgical management for advanced colorectal endometriosis. *Dis Colon Rectum*. 1994;37(8):747-753.

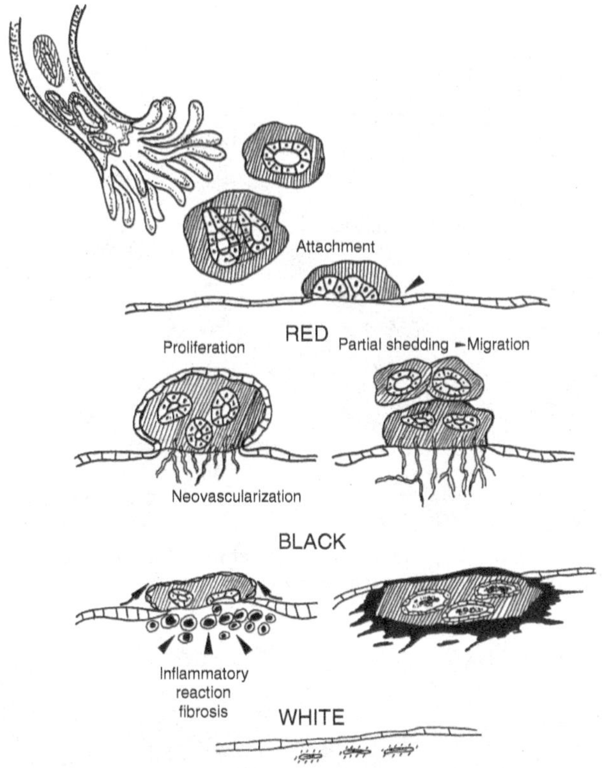


**Figure 19.9** Proposed establishment of peritoneal endometriotic implants via retrograde menstruation and the like. (From Strauss JF, Barbieri R. *Yen & Jaffe's Reproductive Endocrinology*. 5th ed. Philadelphia: Saunders; 2004:692-693.)

of sites, including the umbilicus, areas of previous surgical incisions of the anterior abdominal wall or perineum, the bladder, ureter, kidney, lung, arms, legs, and even the male urinary tract (Table 19.1).

Gross pathologic changes of endometriosis exhibit wide variability in color, shape, size, and associated inflammatory and fibrotic changes. The visual manifestations of endometriosis in the female pelvis are protean and have many appearances. Increased awareness and anticipation have focused on the subtle lesions of endometriosis. Clinicians closely inspect the pelvic peritoneum to identify abnormal areas and small, nonhemorrhagic lesions. More emphasis has been placed on biopsy confirmation of endometriosis because of increasing awareness of subtle lesions. The gross appearance of the implant depends on the site, activity, relationship to the day of the menstrual cycle, and chronicity of the area involved. The color of the lesion varies widely and may be red, brown, black, white, yellow, pink, clear, or a red vesicle. The predominant color depends on the blood supply and the amount of hemorrhage and fibrosis. The color also appears related to the size of the lesion, the degree of edema, and the amount of inspissated material (Table 19.2). Figure 19.9 depicts the spectrum of lesions with black and white lesions reflecting older lesions with inflammatory and fibrotic changes. Other peritoneal lesions that grossly appear similar to endometriosis, but on histologic examination are not, include necrotic areas of an ectopic pregnancy, fibrotic reactions to suture, hemangiomas, adrenal rest, Walthard rest, breast cancer, ovarian cancer, epithelial inclusions, residual carbon from laser surgery, peritoneal inflammation, psammoma bodies, peritoneal reactions to oil-based hysterosalpingogram dye, and splenosis.

New lesions are small, bleblike implants that are less than 1 cm in diameter. Initially these areas are raised above the surrounding tissues. Red, blood-filled lesions have been shown, by histologic and biochemical studies, to be the most active phase of the disease (see Fig. 19.9; also see Video 19.1). With time, the areas of endometriosis become larger and assume a light or dark brown color, and they may be described as "powder burn" areas or "chocolate cysts." The older lesions are white, have more intense scarring, and are usually puckered or retracted from the surrounding tissue. White or mixed colored lesions are more likely to provide histologic confirmation of endometriosis. Also, the progression from red to white lesions also seems to correlate with age.

The pattern of ovarian endometriosis is also variable. Individual areas range from 1 mm to large chocolate cysts greater than 8 cm in diameter (Fig. 19.10). The associated adhesions may be filmy or dense. Larger cysts are usually densely adherent to the surrounding pelvic sidewalls or broad ligament.

The three cardinal histologic features of endometriosis are ectopic endometrial glands, ectopic endometrial stroma, and hemorrhage into the adjacent tissue (Fig. 19.11). Previous hemorrhage can be discovered by identifying large macrophages filled with hemosiderin near the periphery of the lesion. In the majority of cases, the aberrant endometrial glands and stroma respond in cyclic fashion to estrogen and progesterone. These changes may or may not be in synchrony with the endometrial lining of the uterus. The ectopic endometrial stroma will undergo classic decidual changes similar to pregnancy when exposed to high physiologic or pharmacologic levels of progesterone.

In approximately 25% of cases of endometriosis, viable endometrial glands and stroma cannot be identified. Repetitive episodes of hemorrhage may lead to severe inflammatory changes and result in the glands and stroma undergoing necrobiosis

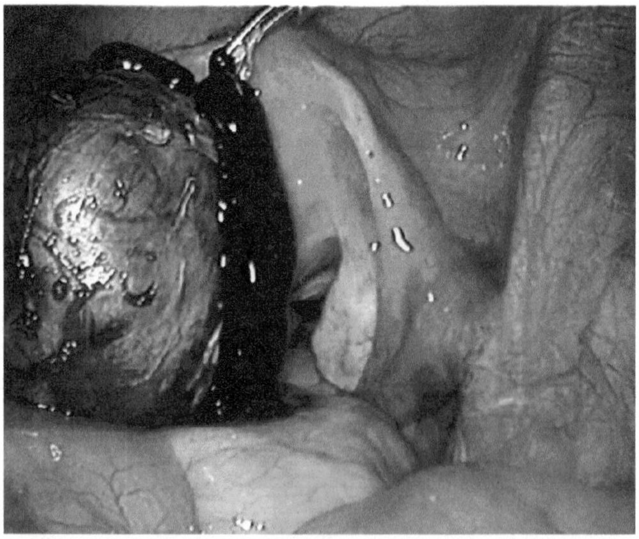

**Figure 19.10** Rupture of large endometrioma "chocolate cyst." (From www.pathologystudent.com.)

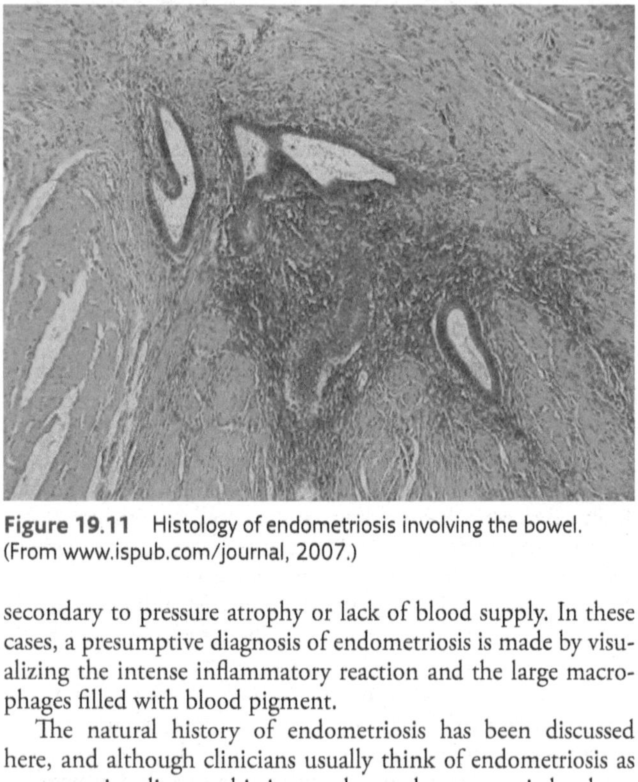

**Figure 19.11** Histology of endometriosis involving the bowel. (From www.ispub.com/journal, 2007.)

secondary to pressure atrophy or lack of blood supply. In these cases, a presumptive diagnosis of endometriosis is made by visualizing the intense inflammatory reaction and the large macrophages filled with blood pigment.

The natural history of endometriosis has been discussed here, and although clinicians usually think of endometriosis as a progressive disease, this is not always the case, as it has been shown to be progressive only about one third of the time. The pathophysiology of progression from subtle endometriosis to severe disease may be expected from the multiple mechanisms of potential disease acceleration discussed earlier, with immune function most likely involved.

## CLINICAL DIAGNOSIS

### Symptoms

It is important to reemphasize that endometriosis has many clinical presentations, with one in three women being asymptomatic. Most important, the disease has an extremely unpredictable course. The classic symptoms of endometriosis are cyclic pelvic pain and infertility. The chronic pelvic pain usually presents as secondary dysmenorrhea or dyspareunia (or both). Secondary dysmenorrhea usually begins 36 to 48 hours prior to the onset of menses. However, approximately one third of patients with endometriosis are asymptomatic, with the disease being discovered incidentally during an abdominal operation or visualized at laparoscopy for an unrelated problem. Conversely, endometriosis is discovered in approximately one of three women whose primary symptom is chronic pelvic pain.

Clinicians have appreciated the paradox that the extent of pelvic pain is often inversely related to the amount of endometriosis in the female pelvis. Women with large, fixed adnexal masses sometimes have minor symptoms, whereas other patients with only a few small foci with deep infiltration may experience moderate to severe chronic pain. The cyclic pelvic pain is related to the sequential swelling and the extravasation of blood and menstrual debris into the surrounding tissue. The chemical mediators of this intense sterile inflammation and pain are believed to be prostaglandins and cytokines. Infiltrative endometriosis, which involves extensive areas of the retroperitoneal space, often is associated with moderate to severe pelvic pain. Studies of pain mapping by laparoscopy under minimal sedation have found that pelvic pain arises from areas of normal peritoneum adjacent to areas of endometriosis.

Secondary dysmenorrhea is a common component of pain that varies from a dull ache to severe pelvic pain. It may be unilateral or bilateral and may radiate to the lower back, legs, and groin. Patients often complain of pelvic heaviness or a perception of their internal organs being swollen. Unlike primary dysmenorrhea, the pain may last for many days, including several days before and after the menstrual flow.

The dyspareunia associated with endometriosis is described as pain deep in the pelvis. The cause of this symptom seems to be immobility of the pelvic organs during coital activity or direct pressure on areas of endometriosis in the uterosacral ligaments or the cul-de-sac. Sometimes patients describe areas of point tenderness. The acute pain, experienced during deep penetration, may continue for several hours following intercourse.

Abnormal bleeding is a symptom noted by 15% to 20% of women with endometriosis. The most frequent complaints are premenstrual spotting and menorrhagia. Usually this abnormal bleeding is not associated with anovulation and may be related to abnormalities of the endometrium. On the other hand, patients with endometriosis frequently have ovulatory dysfunction. Approximately 15% of women with endometriosis have coincidental anovulation or luteal dysfunction.

An increased incidence of first-trimester abortion in women with untreated endometriosis has been reported, although this notion has been challenged and remains an unproven association. Less common, yet troublesome, are the symptoms resulting from endometriosis influencing the gastrointestinal and urinary tracts. Cyclic abdominal pain, intermittent constipation, diarrhea, dyschezia, urinary frequency, dysuria, and hematuria are all possible symptoms. Bowel obstruction and hydronephrosis may occur. One rare clinical manifestation of endometriosis is catamenial hemothorax, bloody pleural fluid occurring during menses. Massive ascites is a rare symptom of

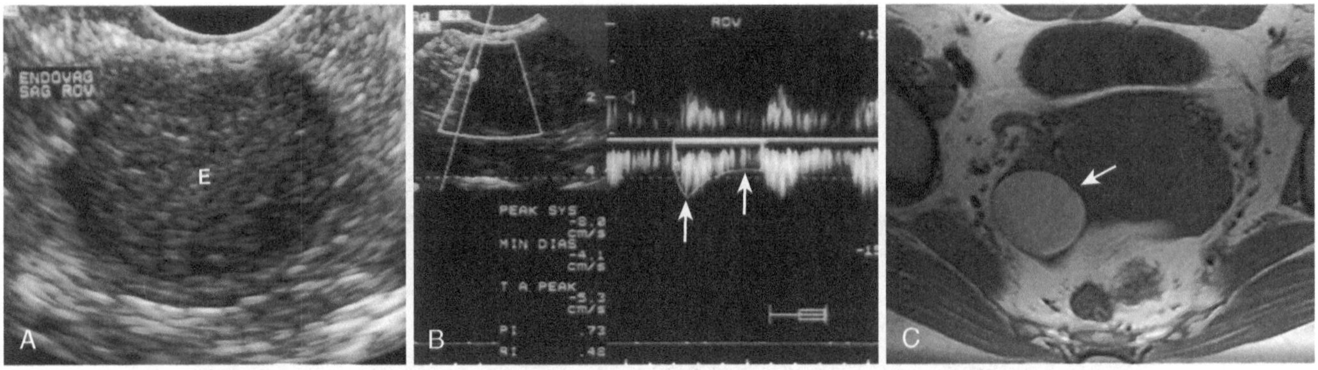


**Figure 19.12 Ultrasound of Endometriosis. A,** Endovaginal ultrasound showing an endometrioma. Note low-level echoes. **B,** Doppler showing increased flow (RI = 0.48), which suggests a malignancy. **C,** T1-weighted MRI showing an endometrioma *(arrow)* with a high-intensity similar to fat. (Modified from Web MD, img.medscape.com.)

endometriosis, but it is important because the disease process initially masquerades as ovarian carcinoma.

### *Clinical Findings (Physical Exam)*

The classic pelvic finding of endometriosis is a fixed retroverted uterus, with scarring and tenderness posterior to the uterus. The characteristic nodularity of the uterosacral ligaments and cul-de-sac may be palpated on rectovaginal examination in women with this distribution of the disease. Advanced cases have extensive scarring and narrowing of the posterior vaginal fornix. The ovaries may be enlarged and tender and are often fixed to the broad ligament or lateral pelvic sidewall. The adnexal enlargement is rarely symmetric, as one may expect in some benign pelvic conditions. Speculum examination may demonstrate small areas of endometriosis on the cervix or upper vagina. Lateral displacement or deviation of the cervix is visualized or palpated by digital exam of the vagina and cervix in approximately 15% of women with moderate or severe endometriosis. Carrying out a pelvic examination during the first or second day of menstrual flow may aid in the diagnosis as it is the time of maximum swelling and tenderness in the areas of endometriosis. The diagnosis can be confirmed in most cases by direct laparoscopic visualization of endometriosis with its associated scarring and adhesion formation. In many patients, endometriosis was discovered for the first time during an infertility investigation, although routine laparoscopy is no longer being carried out in the infertility investigation. Biopsy of selected implants confirms the diagnosis.

#### Imaging

Imaging can be a useful adjunct to the clinical presentation and physical exam for evaluation of endometriosis, especially with deep infiltrating endometriosis (DIE).

Ultrasound examination shows no specific pattern to screen for pelvic endometriosis but may be helpful in differentiating solid from cystic lesions and may help distinguish an endometrioma from other adnexal abnormalities. Because the lesions are vascular, increased Doppler flow may be demonstrated in endometriosis (Fig. 19.12). More recent studies have demonstrated a fair sensitivity from 49% to 91%, with high specificity (93% to 100%) when using transvaginal ultrasound (TVUS) to detect DIE, with the greatest sensitivity and specificity for detection of rectosigmoid lesions. Modified techniques such as rectal water contrast transvaginal ultrasound can increase the probability of detecting a DIE lesion, which is now considered to be the more sensitive technique for the diagnosis of DIE (Noventa, 2015).

Magnetic resonance imaging (MRI) provides the best overall diagnostic tool for endometriosis but is not always a practical modality for its diagnosis. With a detection ratio and specificity of around 78% for implants, MRI for endometriosis has a reported sensitivity and specificity of approximately 91% to 95%. There is a characteristic hyperintensity on T1-weighted images and a hypointensity on T2-weighted images (de Venecia, 2015).

#### Diagnostic Laparoscopy

When laparoscopy is undertaken to establish the diagnosis of endometriosis, it is important to describe systematically the extent of the pathology. The American Society for Reproductive Medicine developed a point-scoring system in 1996, designed primarily to record the extent of the disease in fertility patients (ASRM, 1997). The focus here was intended to provide characterization of disease extent for fertility and not for pain assessment. Nevertheless, there are no data supporting this correlation of scoring with pregnancy rates. More recently, a proposed scoring system by Adamson focuses on the fertility potential of patients with endometriosis, the Endometriosis Fertility Index (EFI), and it has been shown in prospective evaluation to correlate with pregnancy rates (Adamson, 2010). For example, a low score of 0.3 was shown to have a 3-year cumulative pregnancy rate of only 10% to 11%.

Figures 19.13 and 19.14 illustrate ultrasound and MRI findings in retrocervical endometriosis as well as endometriosis infiltrating the bowel.

Although a benign disease, endometriosis exhibits characteristics of both malignancy and sterile inflammation. Therefore, the common considerations in the differential diagnosis include chronic pelvic inflammatory disease, ovarian malignancy, degeneration of myomas, hemorrhage or torsion of ovarian cysts, adenomyosis, primary dysmenorrhea, and functional bowel disease.

Occasionally a large endometrioma of the ovary may rupture into the peritoneal cavity. This results in an acute surgical abdomen and brings into the differential diagnosis conditions such as ectopic pregnancy, appendicitis, diverticulitis, and a bleeding corpus luteum cyst.

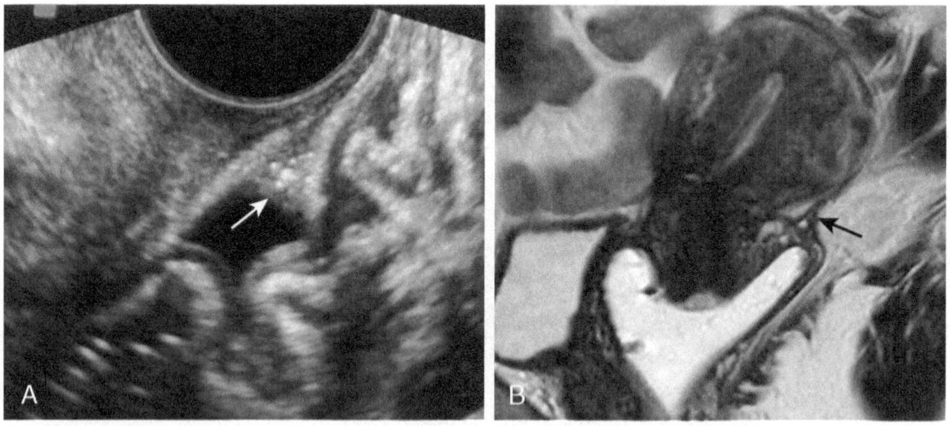


**Figure 19.13** Retrocervical endometriosis attached to posterior vaginal fornix on vaginal ultrasound (**A**) and by MRI (**B**). Arrows show the lesions in different patients. (Courtesy of Manoel Goncalves, MD, Clinica Medicina da Mulher and RDO Medicina Diagnostica, and Mauricio Abrao, MD, University of Sao Paulo, Sao Paulo, Brazil.)

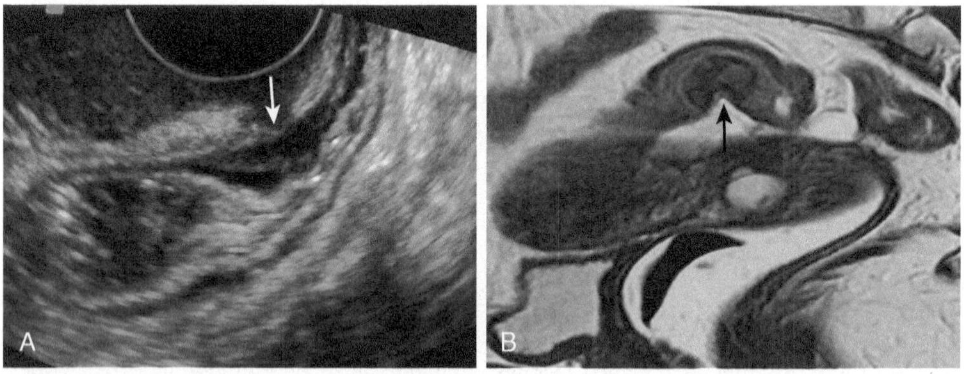


**Figure 19.14** Rectal endometriosis infiltrating part of the muscular wall of the intestine by vaginal ultrasound (**A**) and sigmoid endometriosis infiltrating part of the muscular wall of the intestine by MRI (**B**). Arrows show the lesions. (Courtesy of Manoel Goncalves, MD, Clinica Medicina da Mulher and RDO Medicine Diagnostica, and Mauricio Abrao, MD, University of Sao Paulo, Sao Paulo, Brazil.)

## MONITORING THE COURSE OF DISEASE: ARE THERE MARKERS?

Serial pelvic examinations are a poor indicator of progression of disease. Serum levels of cancer antigen-125 (CA-125) have been used as a marker for endometriosis. CA-125 levels are elevated in most patients with endometriosis and increases incrementally with advanced stages. However, assays for serum levels of CA-125 have a low specificity because they also increase with other pelvic conditions such as leiomyomas, acute pelvic inflammatory disease, and the first trimester of pregnancy. Similarly, serum CA-125 levels have a low sensitivity for the diagnosis of early or minimal endometriosis (Cheng, 2002).

Glycodelin, previously known as *placental protein 14,* has been shown to be elevated in endometriosis and is produced in endometriotic lesions. Levels also fall with removal of the disease. However, because of great variability in levels, glycodelin has not proved to be useful clinically. The most predictive markers appear to be Il-1, chemoattractant protein-1 and interferon gamma, with Il-1 being the most useful marker (Othman, 2007). There has been interest is proteomic analyses as well (Fassbender, 2012).

Although it is generally thought that endometriosis improves during pregnancy, this is not always the case, and an increase in lesions has been documented, although primarily in the first trimester. Ovarian endometriomas, which may have a different pathogenetic origin, from surface implants of endometriosis on the ovary may persist during pregnancy. Also, ovarian endometriosis rupture during pregnancy may occur.

*Endometriosis may be associated with ovarian cancer.* Not only are lesions found at the time of diagnosis of ovarian cancer, but the risk of developing ovarian cancer may increase fourfold in women with endometriosis. Loss of heterozygosity and mutations in suppressor genes, for example, *p53,* may explain this association (Dinulescu, 2005; Pearce, 2012). These findings warrant caution in the long-term follow-up of women who have extensive disease and ovarian endometriomas, particularly with large masses and those that increase in size.

The association of other cancers with endometriosis, although suggested, has not been substantiated. However, cervical endometriosis is a particular condition that can produce abnormalities in cervical cytology.

Endometriosis is dependent on ovarian hormones to stimulate growth. With natural menopause, there is a gradual relief of symptoms. Following surgical menopause, areas of endometriosis rapidly disappear. However, it is important to note that 5% of symptomatic cases of endometriosis present after menopause. The majority of cases in women in their late 50s or early 60s are related to the use of exogenous estrogen.

## TREATMENT

The two primary short-term goals in treating endometriosis are the relief of pain and promotion of fertility. The primary long-term goal in the management of endometriosis is attempting to prevent progression or recurrence of the disease process. Presently, there is a paucity of definitive, evidence-based literature to select the most appropriate method of treatment. A Cochrane review of evidence-based therapies lists a variety of agents that may be helpful but does not specify a clearly preferred agent (Hickey, 2014). This is because there have been few prospective head-to-head comparisons and because the disease is heterogeneous with vast differences in the spectrum of clinical symptoms and extent of disease from one woman to another. Therefore the treatment plan must be individualized. Choice of therapy, for women whose primary symptom is pelvic pain, depends on multiple variables, including the patient's age, her future reproductive plans, the location and extent of her disease, the severity of her symptoms, and associated pelvic pathology. Although the gold standard for making a diagnosis is laparoscopy to establish the nature and extent of endometriosis, this is not always possible, particularly in a younger population. Imaging techniques may only be helpful if a mass is identified, and the suggestion of performing an endometrial biopsy (discussed later) may be too invasive for younger nulliparous woman. If other gynecologic conditions such as chronic pelvic inflammatory disease or neoplasia have been ruled out, empiric medical therapy for 3 months is a reasonable option. Various suppressive treatments and where they act in the pathophysiology of endometriosis may be found in Figure 19.15.

Treatment of endometriosis can be medical, surgical, or a combination of both. Most of the sex steroids, alone or in combination, have been tried in clinical studies to suppress the growth of endometriosis. Optimal regression secondary to medical treatment is observed in small endometriomas that are less than 1 to 2 cm in diameter. Response in larger areas of endometriosis may be minimal with medical therapy. A poor therapeutic result may be governed by the reduction of blood supply to the mass caused by surrounding scar tissue. Some data have suggested that with certain suppressive therapies, such as the use of dienogest, there is a decrease in nerve fiber density in endometriosis lesions (Tarjanne, 2015).

Surgical therapy is divided into conservative and definitive operations. Conservative surgery involves the resection or destruction of endometrial implants, lysis of adhesions, and attempts to restore normal pelvic anatomy. Definitive surgery involves the removal of both ovaries, the uterus, and all visible ectopic foci of endometriosis. This type of surgery is analogous to cytoreductive surgery in ovarian carcinoma.

### MEDICAL THERAPY

Medical therapy is aimed at suppression of lesions and associated symptoms, particularly pain. This is best achieved by menstrual suppression, ideally without inducing hypoestrogenism. Unfortunately, once suppressive therapy is stopped, symptoms tend to recur at variable rates. The choice of medical therapy should be individualized, weighing in potential adverse effects, side effects, cost of therapy, and expected patient compliance. The clinical effectiveness, as measured by relief of symptoms and recurrence rates of current medical therapies, are largely similar. The recurrence rate following medical therapy is 5% to 15% in the first year and increases to 40% to 50% in 5 years. Obviously the chance of recurrence is directly related to the extent of initial disease. In summary, medical therapy usually suppresses symptomatology and prevents progression of endometriosis, but it does not provide a long-lasting cure of the disease. The recurrence rate in women who initially had minimal disease is approximately 35%, whereas in those women whose initial disease was severe the rate is approximately 75%. Although there are several medical therapies for endometriosis, the Food and Drug Administration (FDA) has approved only danazol and gonadotropin-releasing hormone (GnRH) agonists. Other therapies include traditional oral contraceptives (OCs), novel progestogens such as gestinone and dienogest, an oral GnRH antagonist, the levonorgestrel-releasing intrauterine system (IUS), the aromatase inhibitor letrozole, and certain selective progesterone receptor modulators.

#### *Danazol*

Although approved for use in the 1970s, clinicians rarely prescribe danazol (because of lack of familiarity, its side effect profile, and the availability of other agents) and most frequently select GnRH agonists, progestogens, or oral contraceptives. Danazol is also prescribed for women with benign cystic mastitis, menorrhagia, and hereditary angioneurotic edema. Danazol is an attenuated androgen that is active when given orally. Chemically it is a synthetic steroid that is the isoxazole derivative of ethisterone (17-α-ethinyltestosterone). Many years ago, oral androgens such as methyl testosterone were also used, as they induce endometrial atrophy. Danazol produces a hypoestrogenic and hyperandrogenic effect on steroid-sensitive end organs. The drug is mildly androgenic and anabolic leading to its side-effect profile.

Danazol induces atrophic changes in the endometrium of the uterus and similar changes in endometrial implants. It may also modulate immunologic function. Although doses of 400 to 800 mg of danazol have been prescribed, many clinicians reduce the total daily dosage of the drug to 200, and even 100, mg of danazol daily. Danazol is usually begun during menses (days 1 to 5). Because the relief of the symptoms is directly related to the incidence of amenorrhea, the lower dosages of danazol are not as effective. Side effects of the hormonal changes are encountered by 80%, and approximately 10% to 20% of women discontinue danazol because of side effects. There have been reports of deepening of the voice that did not resolve after discontinuation. Mild elevation in serum liver enzyme levels has been reported in women treated for endometriosis, and women who take danazol for longer than 6 months should have serum liver enzyme determinations. An androgenic effect on lipids occurs, with reduction in high-density lipoprotein (HDL) cholesterol and triglycerides and an increase in low-density lipoprotein (LDL) cholesterol.

The standard length of treatment with danazol is 6 to 9 months. Approximately three of four patients note significant

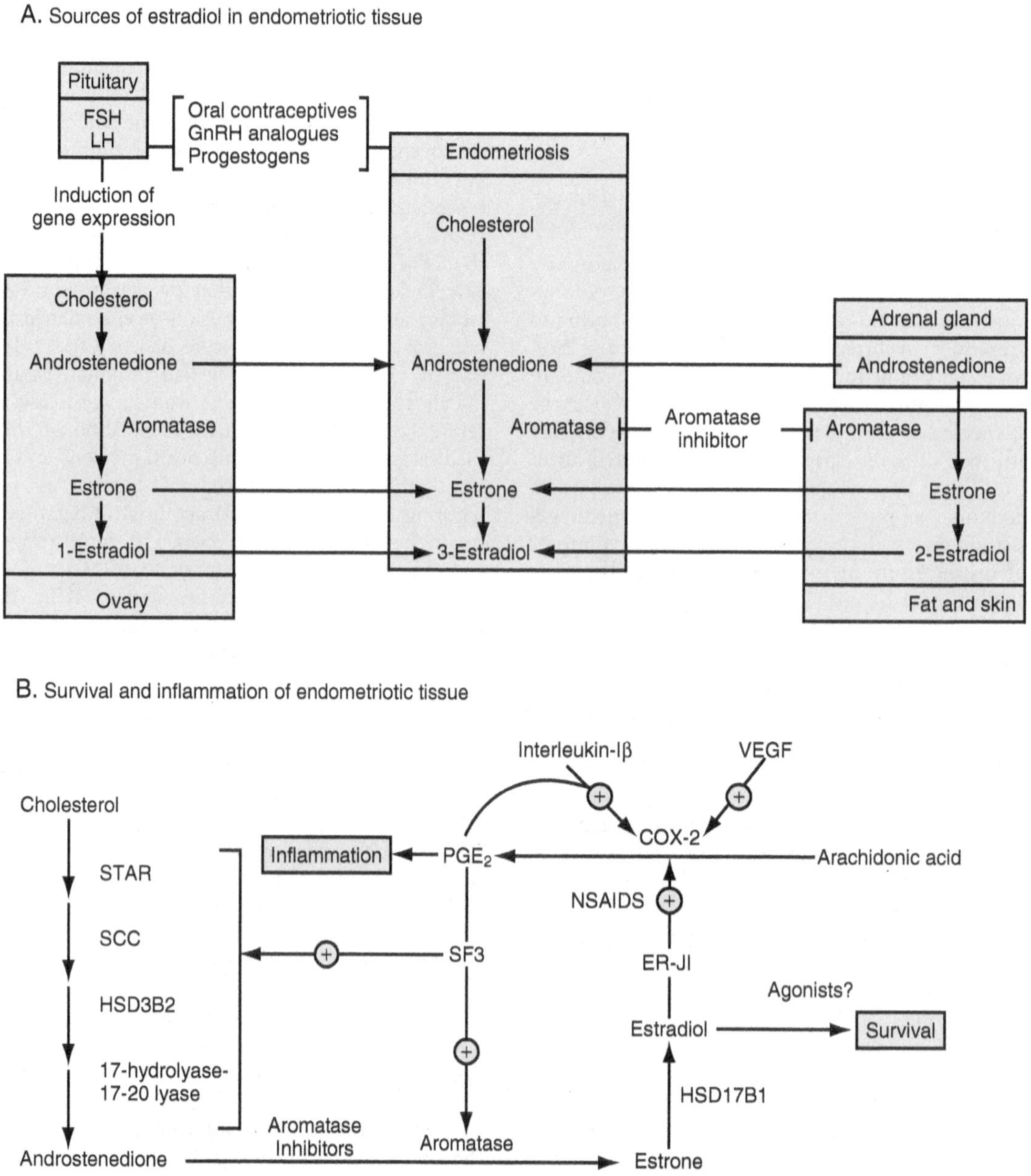


**Figure 19.15 Molecular Distinctions between Endometriotic Tissue and Endometrium.** **A,** The three sources of estradiol, biologically active estrogen, in endometriotic tissue. The first sources are follicle-stimulating hormone (FSH) and luteinizing hormone (LH), which induce the expression of ovarian steroidogenic genes, including aromatase, for biosynthesis of estradiol. Ovarian secretion of estradiol can be reduced through suppression of FSH and LH by gonadotropin-releasing hormone (GnRH) analogues, combination oral contraceptives, or progestins. The second source of estrogen is the estradiol that arises from aromatase activity in fat or skin. The third source of estradiol is local production in endometriotic tissue. Aromatase inhibition in peripheral tissue (fat and skin) and endometriotic tissue stops estradiol biosynthesis and is therapeutic in endometriosis. As shown in **B,** high levels of local estradiol and prostaglandin $E_2$ ($PGE_2$) are maintained in endometriotic tissue by autoregulatory positive-feedback mechanisms (indicated by plus signs) that involve nuclear receptors (steroidogenic factor 1 [SF1] and estrogen receptor β [ER-β]), enzymatic pathways, cytokines, and growth factors. COX-2 denotes cyclooxygenase-2, HSD17B1 17β-hydroxysteroid dehydrogenase 1, HSD3B2 3β-hydroxysteroid dehydrogenase 2, side-chain cleavage (SCC) enzyme, steroidogenic acute regulatory (STAR) protein, and vascular endothelial growth factor (VEGF). (Modified from Bulun SE. Mechanisms of disease: endometriosis. *N Engl J Med.* 2009;360[3]:268-279.)

improvement in their symptoms, and about 90% have objective improvement discovered at a second-look laparoscopy. The uncorrected fertility rate following danazol therapy is approximately 40%. Unfortunately, symptoms will recur in 15% to 30% of women within 2 years following therapy.

Several randomized, double-blind clinical studies have compared the therapeutic effectiveness of danazol with GnRH agonists. The results do not show significant differences between the efficacies of these two drugs.

## GONADOTROPIN-RELEASING HORMONE AGONISTS

Several GnRH agonists have been developed and approved for the treatment of endometriosis. Representative agonists are leuprolide acetate (Lupron, injectable), nafarelin acetate (Synarel, intranasal), and goserelin acetate (Zoladex, subcutaneous implant). The usual dose of leuprolide acetate is 3.75 mg intramuscularly once per month or an 11.25-mg depot injection every 3 months. Nafarelin acetate nasal spray is given in a dose of one spray (200 μg) in one nostril in the morning and one spray (200 μg) in the other nostril in the evening up to a maximum of 800 μg daily. Goserelin acetate is given in a dosage of 3.6 mg every 28 days in a biodegradable subcutaneous implant.

Studies have determined the dose-response curve of the GnRH agonists, establishing the optimal dose to produce sufficient down-regulation and desensitization of the pituitary to produce extremely low levels of circulating estrogen and amenorrhea. Chronic use of GnRH agonists produces a "medical oophorectomy." A dramatic reduction occurs in serum estrone, $E_2$, testosterone, and androstenedione to levels similar to the hormonal levels in oophorectomized women. There are no significant changes in total serum cholesterol, HDL, or LDL levels during therapeutic periods as long as 6 months. Endometrial samples obtained after several months of chronic agonist therapy demonstrated either atrophic or an early proliferative endometrium.

The side effects associated with GnRH agonist therapy are primarily those associated with decreased estrogen, similar to menopause. The three most common symptoms are hot flushes, vaginal dryness, and insomnia. A decrease in bone mineral content has been demonstrated in the trabecular bone of the lumbar spine by quantitative computer tomography. This decrease in bone density is not seen in the compact bone of the distal radius. There is a decrease in measured bone mass of 2% to 7% during a 6-month course of agonist therapy. However, it has been established that the decrease in bone density associated with 6 months of therapy completely recovers between 12 and 24 months.

The clinical response to agonist therapy depends on when the therapy is initiated in regard to the menstrual cycle. If agonist therapy is begun during the follicular phase, an agonist phase results in an initial rapid rise in follicle-stimulating hormone (FSH) and $E_2$ for approximately 3 weeks. FSH levels fall to basal levels by the third to fourth week of therapy. $E_2$ levels rapidly decline after 21 days of therapy. The expected surge in luteinizing hormone (LH) does not occur, and serum progesterone levels do not become elevated. Amenorrhea is induced within 6 to 8 weeks. In contrast, beginning agonist therapy during the luteal phase or if artificially manipulated by the concurrent administration of oral progestogen, serum $E_2$ levels are suppressed within 2 weeks. Amenorrhea is induced in 4 to 5 weeks. It is important to ensure that the patient is not pregnant when beginning GnRH agonist therapy during the luteal phase.

GnRH agonist therapy improves symptoms in 75% to 90% of patients with endometriosis, depending on the extent of the disease in the study group. Growth of endometriosis is arrested, diminished, or eliminated. The greatest therapeutic effects are seen when areas of endometriosis are less than 1 cm in diameter. Ovarian function usually returns to normal in 6 to 12 weeks after 6 months of GnRH agonist therapy. Large ovarian endometriomas and severe adhesive disease have not responded to hormonal therapy.

Currently, many clinicians "add back" hormone replacement therapy with dosages similar to those used in menopausal therapy in combination with chronic GnRH agonist regimens. The clinical hypothesis is that the add-back medication will reduce or eliminate the vasomotor symptoms and vaginal atrophy and also diminish or overcome the demineralization of bone. Barbieri has suggested that there is a therapeutic window that he estimates is a circulating level of approximately 30 pg/mL of $E_2$ (Barbieri, 1992). He postulated that this level of $E_2$ is enough to protect the body from substantial bone loss and is not high enough to interfere with the inhibition of growth of endometriosis (Fig. 19.16). Multiple randomized trials have demonstrated that add-back therapy does not interfere with the effectiveness of agonists to relieve the pelvic pain from endometriosis. The majority of studies have also

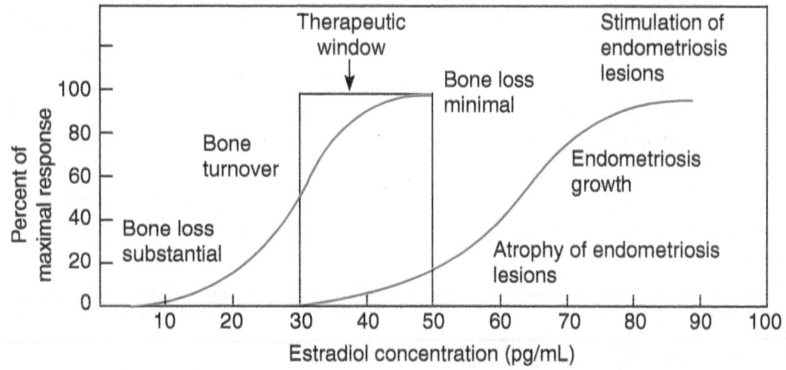


**Figure 19.16 Estradiol Therapeutic Window.** The concentration of estradiol required to cause the growth of endometriosis lesions may be greater than the concentration required to stabilize bone mineral density. (From Barbieri RL. Hormone treatment of endometriosis: the estrogen threshold hypothesis. *Am J Obstet Gynecol.* 1992;166[2]:740-745.)

demonstrated no diminished therapeutic efficacy when add-back therapy is initiated simultaneously with the GnRH agonist. Some clinicians additionally give bisphosphonates and calcium with the low-dose progestins and estrogen, but bisphosphonates are not recommended in younger women who may wish to become pregnant. Add-back regimens not only reduce or eliminate adverse clinical and metabolic side effects associated with hypoestrogenism but also facilitate safe and effective prolongation of GnRH agonist therapy for up to 12 months. Additional agents that have been used for add back therapy are tibolone and raloxifene.

GnRH antagonists have also been considered an attractive option in that they have no "flare" effect. A direct effect on lesions has also been hypothesized. Novel oral agents are also in early development. In a phase 2 randomized trial of oral elagolix (GnRH antagonist) at 150 and 250 mg versus leuprolide acetate in women with endometriosis pain, it was suggested that there was equal efficacy of elagolix with leuprolide and less bone loss with the antagonist (Ezzati, 2015).

For women not wishing to conceive, who predominantly have pain and no indication for surgery (which may include failed medical therapy), stopping and starting various treatments and interchanging them is a reasonable approach to control symptoms.

## ORAL CONTRACEPTIVES

In the late 1950s, very large doses of norethynodrel with mestranol daily were given to produce amenorrhea and a "pseudopregnancy." Most of the published studies involved the first-generation, high-estrogen–content oral contraceptives. However, more recent reports have established that the present low-estrogen monophasic combination pills, specifically the ones with a relatively high progestin potency, are equally effective when used in a continuous fashion. It has been accepted that the most economical regimen for the treatment of women with mild or moderate symptoms of endometriosis has been continuous daily oral contraceptives for 6 to 12 months. Continuous dose regimens are aimed at more complete suppression, with an advantage over cyclic use (Zorbas, 2015) and the only concern is with breakthrough bleeding, which can be dealt with in a variety of ways as with contraceptive therapy (see Chapter 13).

One potential risk of using oral contraceptives or progestogens is that there is some risk of rupture if a large endometrioma is present. Rupture of large endometriomas may result in an acute surgical abdomen during the first 6 weeks of oral contraceptive therapy. During prolonged therapy the endometrial glands atrophy and the stroma undergoes a marked decidual reaction. Some smaller endometriomas (~3 cm) can undergo necrobiosis and resorption.

The most common side effects of inducing amenorrhea with oral contraceptives include weight gain and breast tenderness. Approximately one in three women discontinues this therapy because of side effects.

The results of continuous oral contraceptive therapy include a decrease in symptomatology in approximately 80% of patients during therapy.

## NONSTEROIDAL ANTI-INFLAMMATORY DRUGS

Nonsteroidal anti-inflammatory drugs (NSAIDs) are beneficial for pain relief and as concomitant therapy may improve the bleeding control of patients on oral contraceptives. There may also be a direct therapeutic value in endometriosis. Although cyclooxygenase-2 (COX-2) inhibitors are now infrequently used because of cardiovascular concerns in older individuals, this therapy for endometriosis has a rationale in that lesions of endometriosis have been found to express high levels of COX-2 (see Fig. 19.15). In summary, anti-inflammatory agents may be beneficial for pain relief as well as potentially for the treatment of endometriosis, particularly when other suppressive therapy cannot be used.

### Other Hormonal Treatments

For women who cannot tolerate the high dosage of estrogen in an oral contraceptive or who have a contraindication to estrogen therapy, treatment with progestogens only has been successful. Medroxyprogesterone acetate (Provera) in a dosage of 20 to 30 mg orally per day or depo-medroxyprogesterone acetate (Depo-Provera) in a dosage of 150 mg intramuscularly every 3 months to a maximum of 200 mg every month will produce a prolonged amenorrhea. The medication is most appropriate for the older woman who has completed childbearing. The time of resumption of ovulation following discontinuation of injectable medroxyprogesterone is prolonged and extremely variable. Some women will not ovulate for more than a year after their last injection. Therefore this form of therapy should not be prescribed for a young woman who is contemplating pregnancy in the near future. Oral medroxyprogesterone in a dosage of 30 mg/day is an alternative mode of therapy, as is norethindrone acetate (10 to 40 mg) daily. This more androgenic progestogen, although quite effective, has a similar symptom profile to that for continuous medroxyprogesterone.

Gestrinone is a progestogen originally developed as a once-a-week oral contraceptive. This drug has undergone clinical trials for endometriosis with dosages ranging from 2.5 to 7.5 mg/week. Gestrinone acts as an agonist–antagonist of progesterone receptors and an agonist of androgen receptors and also binds weakly to estrogen receptors. At completion of therapy in a randomized trial, a tendency for prolonged pain relief was observed for gestrinone when compared with GnRH agonist, and showed similar efficacy (Gestrinone Italian Study Group, 1996).

Dienogest is a selective progestogen that causes anovulation, has an antiproliferative effect on endometrial cells, and may inhibit cytokine secretion. In clinical trials at 2 mg/day orally, it has been found to be as effective as GnRH agonists (Ferrero, 2015).

The levonorgestrel IUS has been shown to be beneficial for pain relief in women with endometriosis compared to expectant management. It is particularly suited for women who have rectocervical and cul-de-sac disease (Fedele, 2001; Petta, 2005).

**Aromatase inhibitors** (anastrozole 1 mg, and letrozole 2.5 and 5 mg) have been found to be beneficial in that not only does estrogen tend to cause proliferation of the disease but also endometriosis lesions have been found to contain the aromatase enzyme (Bulun, 2009). When given alone to premenopausal women it will cause stimulation of gonadotropins and has been used to induce ovulation; but in postmenopausal women and in the premenopausal women in combination with a progestogen or oral contraception pills there is good promise that it will be beneficial for the treatment of endometriosis (Attar, 2006).

## OTHER POSSIBLE MEDICAL THERAPIES

There are several other less well-proved therapies. These include the peroxisome proliferator-activated receptor (PPAR) ligands, which have been shown to inhibit macrophage action in animal models (Lebovic, 2007); targeting haptoglobin because of structural similarity to Endo-1; targeting MMPs; and tumor necrosis factor α and VEGF (Falconer, 2008). Newer antiprogestogens have also shown efficacy in small clinical trials, (Chabbert-Buffet, 2005); and several compounds are being studied further. ERβ agonists may also play some role in the future trials in that some of the estrogen action involved in increasing VEGF and angiogenetic factors are mediated through ERβ (see Fig. 19.15). ERβ may also modulate immune function. It should be noted that selective estrogen receptor modulators, specifically tamoxifen and raloxifene, have not been shown to be beneficial (Stratton, 2008). Another anti-inflammatory immunomodulator, pentoxifylline, has also shown promise.

Various medicinal herbs have been suggested for use based on their antiproliferative and anti-inflammatory and pain-relieving properties (Wieser, 2007). However, no rigorous clinical trial data are available at present.

## ROUTE OF ADMINISTRATION

Delivering various progestogens or danazol locally (intrauterine as with the levonorgestrel IUS or vaginally) may also enhance effectiveness. Small clinical trials have suggested the benefit of using suppositories and local agents, particularly in those women with cul-de-sac disease.

## SURGICAL THERAPY

Surgery therapy can serve as an adjunct or alternative to medical therapy and can help prevent or delay further disease progression. The main roles of surgical therapy in the management of endometriosis are to provide symptomatic relief (pain) and to improve fertility outcomes.

Surgical management includes conservative and definitive approaches that address three main categories of lesions: superficial endometriosis (see Video 19.1), endometriomas and deep infiltrating endometriosis (DIE).

Conservative surgery involves preservation of reproductive organs and restoration of normal pelvic anatomy while removing all macroscopic endometriotic lesions or endometriomas and performing lysis of adhesions. Definitive surgery involves removing the uterus and cervix along with any visible lesions while preserving or removing either one or both of the ovaries.

Minimally invasive surgical approaches such as laparoscopy and robotic surgery have largely replaced the need for laparotomy due to advantages such as improved visualization, shorter recovery period, decreased blood loss, and decreased risks of complications.

Surgical techniques for endometriosis may vary from surgeon to surgeon, but key surgical principles should be maintained. A survey of the abdomen and pelvis should always be performed while identifying key anatomic structures including the ureter (Videos 19.2 to 19.4). Restoring normal pelvic anatomy, preventing adhesions, and limiting tissue damage is essential for successful endometriosis surgery. It is often helpful to start dissections going from normal anatomy toward abnormal anatomy. Energy should be used judiciously and cautiously especially with difficult dissections with distorted anatomy and when adjacent to vital structures such as major blood vessels, the ureter, bladder, or bowel. Although both techniques of ablation and excision have shown improvement in outcomes compared to expectant management, there is still debate on which is most effective. A randomized study demonstrated no difference at 1 year, but at 5 years, excision resulted in greater reduction in pain, notably dyspareunia (Healey, 2014).

## SURGICAL MANAGEMENT FOR PAIN

In women suffering from chronic pelvic pain due to endometriosis who have failed conservative medical therapy, surgery can be an effective treatment, especially in cases of moderate or severe endometriosis in which pelvic adhesive disease is present along with the involvement of nonreproductive organs.

In a prospective randomized trial, Sutton compared the effect of laser laparoscopy over expectant management after diagnostic laparoscopy. Pain decreased by 62.5% compared with 22.6% with expectant management, and pain relief continued in 55% of women over 72 months. The placebo response was noted to be 22%. Another randomized trial demonstrated an 80% improvement in symptoms with a 30% placebo response rate from surgery. The median time to pain recurrence after surgery has been estimated to be 20 months and reported to be approximately 15% at 1 year, 36% at 5 years, and 50% by 7 years. A study by Weir and colleagues predicted that 25% of women are likely to undergo additional surgery for endometriosis within 4 years, and 10% will need a hysterectomy.

Definitive surgical treatment, involving hysterectomy, is effective for symptomatic relief with reoperation free rates of 86% (with ovarian preservation) and 91% (without ovarian preservation) at 5 years. Although removal of the ovaries may decrease the risk of disease recurrence, this should be balanced with the risks associated with removing the ovaries and therefore should be individualized based on the patient's age, clinical presentation, and goals. Approximately one out of three women will develop recurrent symptoms and subsequently have a second operation involving oophorectomy. Though debatable, postsurgical hormonal suppression with progestins or oral contraceptives may be considered in order to decrease risks of recurrence, especially if there is any residual or unresectable disease at the time of surgery.

Other surgical treatments include presacral neurectomy and photodynamic therapy. In select patients with midline pain, presacral neurectomy may be an option for short-term improvement in symptoms, but complications can include bowel and bladder dysfunction. Photodynamic therapy for endometriosis is undergoing preliminary trials. This procedure involves intravenous injection of a special dye that is concentrated in areas of endometriosis. A laser light produces a photochemical reaction to destroy the areas.

## SURGICAL MANAGEMENT FOR FERTILITY

Management of patients with endometriosis undergoing assisted reproductive treatment can be challenging. Medical therapy may sometimes be required for symptomatic control while waiting for fertility treatment; however, this is generally not recommended. There have been studies suggesting improved fertility outcomes with prolonged GnRH agonist use when administered prior to assisted reproductive treatment. Surgical management in these women can be considered, though there has been debate

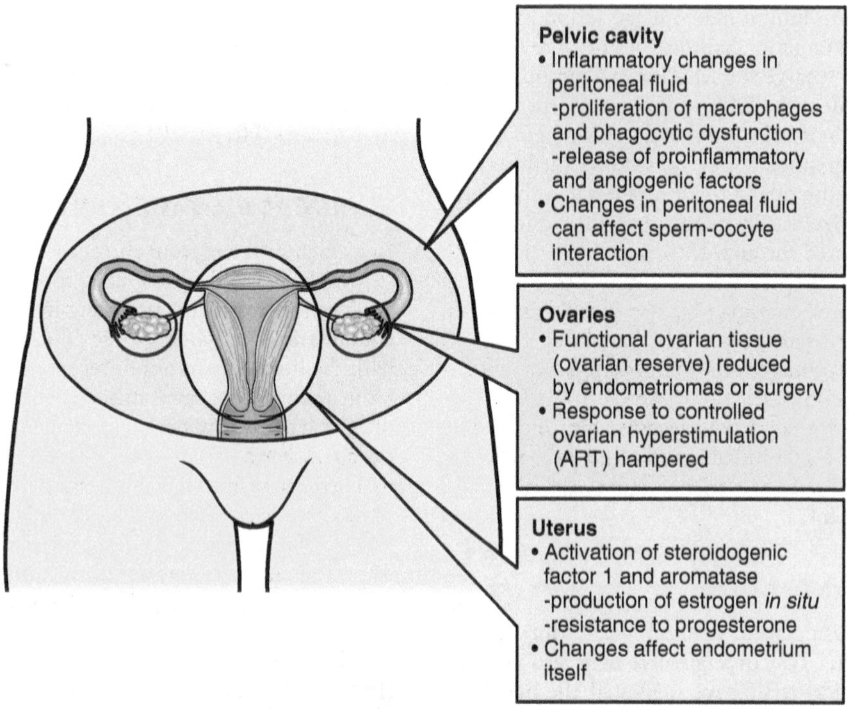
Pelvic cavity
• Inflammatory changes in peritoneal fluid
-proliferation of macrophages and phagocytic dysfunction
-release of proinflammatory and angiogenic factors
• Changes in peritoneal fluid can affect sperm-oocyte interaction
Ovaries
• Functional ovarian tissue (ovarian reserve) reduced by endometriomas or surgery
• Response to controlled ovarian hyperstimulation (ART) hampered
Uterus
• Activation of steroidogenic factor 1 and aromatase
-production of estrogen *in situ*
-resistance to progesterone
• Changes affect endometrium itself

**Figure 19.17** Mechanisms of endometriosis associated infertility. *ART,* Assisted reproductive technologies. (Modified from de Ziegler, Borghese B, Chapron C. Endometriosis and infertility: pathophysiology and management. *Lancet.* 2010;376[9742]:730-738. Data from Strauss J, Barbieri R. *Yen and Jaffe's Reproductive Endocrinology.* 7th ed. Philadelphia: Elsevier; 2014.)

about the timing and risks/benefits of surgery in the setting of in vitro fertilization (IVF).

For stage I/II endometriosis, excision or ablation of endometriosis has been shown to increase live birth and ongoing pregnancy rates and is therefore recommended when visible lesions are present. Although there is lack of randomized trials, for stage III/IV, surgical treatment has also been suggested to increase pregnancy rates (see Therapy for Subfertility later in this chapter).

### *Endometriomas*

Conservative management of endometriomas (see Video 19.2) has potential risks such as infection of the endometriomas, interfering with response to infertility treatments and oocyte retrieval, risks of complications in pregnancy, and malignancy. Endometriomas may also decrease ovarian reserve. Despite these theoretic risks, surgical removal of endometriomas is not generally recommended prior to IVF. Evidence suggests that surgery for endometriomas does not necessarily increase fertility outcome while it can further compromise ovarian reserve, increase the risk of premature ovarian failure, and induce early menopause. On the other hand, surgical treatment of endometriomas can be beneficial for certain cases such as in symptomatic patients (i.e., pelvic pain) or in those with difficult access to follicles. Surgical excision of endometriomas greater than 3 cm were previously thought to improve pregnancy rates, but studies show no difference compared to expectant management. Excision of endometriomas is preferable over ablation or drainage, as this technique has been shown to increase clinical pregnancy rates.

In patients failing to conceive spontaneously after the initial surgery, assisted reproductive therapy is recommended, as this has been shown to be more effective than repeat surgery. Although controversial, repeat surgery can be considered after failed assisted reproductive treatments, but further studies are needed to determine optimal management of such patients.

## *THERAPY FOR SUBFERTILITY*

The subfertility that occurs in women with endometriosis can be the result of multiple mechanisms (Fig. 19.17).

Medical therapy cannot be first-line treatment for endometriosis because suppression of ovulation interferes with the ability to conceive. Occasionally as an adjunct, more prolonged (than usual) GnRH agonist therapy may be used before IVF. In this section, surgical options are considered.

It is clear that for symptomatic women with ovarian endometriomas, laparoscopic surgical excision should be undertaken. However, in cases of extensive pelvic disease where in vitro fertilization/embryo transfer (IVF-ET) is a necessary approach, and when pelvic pain is not a significant issue, the removal of endometriomas is of no benefit and may be harmful in that it may compromise ovarian reserve. Some data suggest that women with endometriosis may have a lower ovarian reserve, as reflected by lower levels of anti-Müllerian hormone; surgery only decreases levels further (Roustan, 2015). The size of an endometrioma also comes into play in cases of IVF-ET; if all visible normal ovarian tissue is replaced by endometriomas (typically endometriomas around 4 cm or greater), surgical excision may be necessary. Otherwise for small lesions (~2 cm), follicle aspiration can be accomplished avoiding the endometriomas. In general, the presence of endometriomas tends to decrease the number of oocytes aspirated but may not impair oocyte or embryo quality. Again, it

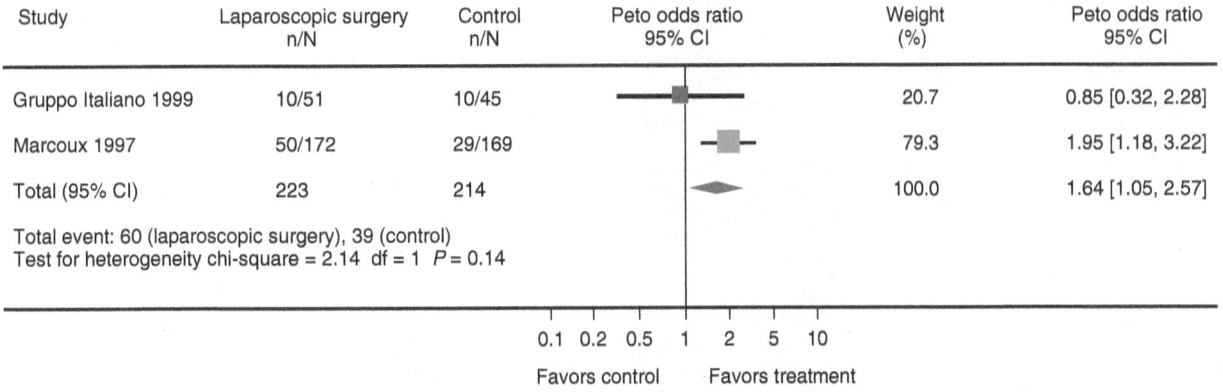

Study
Laparoscopic surgery n/N
Control n/N
Peto odds ratio 95% CI
Weight (%)
Peto odds ratio 95% CI
Gruppo Italiano 1999
10/51
10/45
20.7
0.85 [0.32, 2.28]
Marcoux 1997
50/172
29/169
79.3
1.95 [1.18, 3.22]
Total (95% CI)
223
214
100.0
1.64 [1.05, 2.57]
Total event: 60 (laparoscopic surgery), 39 (control)
Test for heterogeneity chi-square = 2.14 df = 1 P = 0.14
0.1 0.2 0.5 1 2 5 10
Favors control
Favors treatment


**Figure 19.18** Meta-analysis of the two randomized trials assessing the efficacy of laparoscopic surgery in the treatment of subfertility associated with minimal-to-mind endometriosis. Combing live birth and ongoing pregnancy data from the two studies shows an improvement with laparoscopic surgical treatment (OR 1.64, 95%; CI 1.05-2.57). *Df*, Degrees of freedom. (From Jacobson TZ, Barlow DH, Koninckx PR, et al: Laparoscopic surgery for subfertility associated with endometriosis. *Cochrane Database Syst Rev*. 2002;4:CD001398.)

is generally agreed (systemic review and meta-analysis) that surgery for endometriomas does not improve IVF rates (Hamdan, 2015); therefore the consideration for surgery should only be selected on an individual basis.

There has long been a debate as to whether treating *mild* endometriotic lesions or implants would improve fertility. Two prospective randomized trials have provided some guidance. Data from the Canadian and Italian studies, taken together, suggest that the pregnancy rates improve with implant ablation (Jacobson, 2002) (Fig. 19.18). Thus one additional pregnancy may be expected for eight surgical procedures. The way these data should be extrapolated into practice is that if a laparoscopy is being performed in a woman wishing to conceive, visible lesions should be ablated if technically possible rather than ignoring them.

Apart from the mechanical factors (endometriomas, adhesions, fibrosis) affecting pregnancy rates, in endometriosis, macrophage and cytokine abnormalities are thought to play a significant role in inhibiting fertility (see Fig. 19.17). These factors may affect oocyte quality, fertilization, and embryo quality as well as endometrial receptivity. Therefore, in addition to ablating lesions when present, several strategies have been devised to enhance fecundity. Controlled ovarian stimulation along with intrauterine insemination, an approach to enhance fecundity in women with unexplained infertility, has been found to be beneficial in women with endometriosis. Finally, if IVF-ET is undertaken (because of mechanical factors or with other failed approaches), there has been controversy as to whether pregnancy rates and live birth rates are affected by having the disease. Although an older meta-analysis suggested an approximate 20% reduction in pregnancy rates, (Barnhart, 2002) data suggest that pregnancy rates are comparable unless endometriosis is severe (Hamdan, 2015). However, at the same time, prior suppressive therapy (before initiation of an IVF cycle) has been shown to be benefit. A Cochrane systematic review of three RCTs found that prior suppression of endometriosis with a GnRH agonist for 3 to 6 months prior to IVF-ET improves outcomes with an odds ratio of 9.19 (Sallam, 2006). This reemphasizes the pathophysiologic consequences involved with having endometriosis (described earlier).

The role of surgical therapy in the management of endometriosis is very much dependent on the clinical presentation of the patient and her desire for future fertility. Although there can be a beneficial effect for fertility, a detrimental effect can also be seen. Advanced stages of disease, particularly those involving extrapelvic locations (discussed later), are often best managed in a multidisciplinary fashion.

## ENDOMETRIOSIS AT OTHER SITES

### *GASTROINTESTINAL TRACT ENDOMETRIOSIS*

The incidence of gastrointestinal tract involvement in a series of women with histologically proven endometriosis varies from 3% to 37%. Most large series document an incidence of approximately 5%. Implants that involve the gastrointestinal tract are the most common site of extrapelvic endometriosis but can be the most challenging to manage. The severity and extent of involvement of the bowel by ectopic endometrium varies from the incidental finding of a spot on the serosa of the bowel to obstruction of the rectosigmoid. In the majority of cases, endometriosis of the gastrointestinal tract involves the sigmoid colon and the anterior wall of the rectum, accounting for approximately 90% of cases (see Video 19.4).

Involvement of the appendix is the next common type of gastrointestinal (GI) tract endometriosis with an incidence reported to be between 1% and 13%. In a series of more than 100 consecutive patients with endometriosis, 13% had histologic evidence of endometriosis in the appendix, whereas only 60% of these cases are detected on gross examination. Endometriosis of the small bowel (Video 19.5) is rare, where only approximately 200 cases of endometriosis of the ileum have been reported in the literature. Of note, 48% of patients with rectosigmoid lesions will also have endometriosis of the ovaries, and 84% will have rectocervical lesions (Hemming, 2009). (Fig. 19.19; also see Video 19.3).

In most cases, the implants do not produce clinical symptoms. Classic symptoms of endometriosis of the large bowel include dysmenorrhea (cyclic pelvic cramping and lower abdominal pain) and dyschezia (rectal pain with defecation), especially during the menstrual period. Other associated symptoms include deep

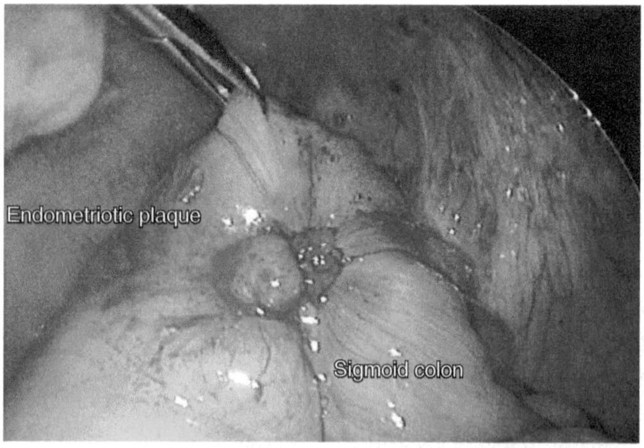


**Figure 19.19** Endometriosis involving the sigmoid colon. (From Hemmings R, Falcone T. Endometriosis. In: Falcone T, Hurd WW. *Clinical Reproductive Medicine and Surgery.* Philadelphia: Mosby; 2007.)

dyspareunia, change in bowel function, diarrhea or constipation (or both), and occasionally hematochezia. Studies have demonstrated that 25% to 35% of women with advanced endometriosis of the large bowel experience episodic rectal bleeding due to endometriosis extending into the submucosa. A distinct dysfunction of the enteric nervous system has been suggested to be the primary cause of the abnormalities of bowel function in women with endometriosis. It is difficult to differentiate the symptoms associated with endometriosis from the overlapping constellation of symptoms associated with inflammatory disease of the colon or malignancy. Hence, early diagnosis of gastrointestinal endometriosis and differentiation from other GI conditions are important. Women with a gastrointestinal malignancy usually experience intermittent rather than cyclic intestinal bleeding. Although acyclic bowel symptoms can occur with GI endometriosis, cyclic GI symptoms generally occur up to 89% cases, and therefore suspicion of GI endometriosis should be high with this type of presentation.

Physical exam can also help with diagnosis of deep infiltrating endometriosis invading the rectosigmoid such as by palpation of a pelvic mass or "rectal shelf" on rectovaginal examination. Sigmoidoscopy usually demonstrates absence of a mucosal lesion in addition to fixation and immobility of the anterior rectal wall. Donnez and coworkers speculated that endometriosis of the rectovaginal septum is a disease process more closely related to foci of adenomyosis than endometriosis (Donnez, 1997).

Endometriosis involving the GI tract is usually unresponsive to medical therapy and often requires surgical excision. Surgery should generally be performed in coordination with a multidisciplinary team. Complete excision of these lesions sometimes necessitates bowel resection. Although no consensus exists, bowel resection generally is indicated in symptomatic women when lesions are greater than 2 cm, greater than 30% of the circumference is involved, and when there is invasion into the inner muscularis layer, which may require bowel resection (see Video 19.4). When surgery is indicated, while still unclear which is better, bowel resection can be done via either segmental or discoid resection. Parameters that should be considered in surgical planning include size, number and depth of lesions, extent of bowel circumference involvement, distance to anal verge, and presence of lymph node involvement.

After surgical resection, up to 70% of patients have improvement of symptoms with a recurrence rate of 0 to 34%. Pregnancy rates have been reported to be between 24% to 66%.

## URINARY TRACT ENDOMETRIOSIS

Endometriosis in the female pelvis occasionally produces dysfunction in adjacent pelvic organs. Approximately 10% of women with endometriosis have involvement of the urinary tract, which most commonly involves endometriotic implants and associated retroperitoneal fibrosis located in the peritoneum overlying the ureter or the bladder. In most cases an incidental finding of aberrant endometrial glands and stroma is discovered on the bladder peritoneum and anterior cul-de-sac. The most serious consequence of urinary tract involvement is ureteral obstruction, which occurs in about 1% of women with moderate or severe pelvic endometriosis. The pathogenesis of endometriosis of the bladder is controversial. Interestingly, approximately 50% of women with endometriosis of the urinary tract have a history of previous pelvic surgery. The lesions may develop from implanted endometrium during cesarean delivery or may be an extension from adenomyosis of the anterior uterine wall.

Patients with endometriosis involving the urinary tract have nonspecific clinical presentations. Hematuria and flank pain are experienced by less than 25% of women. One of three women with documented complete ureteral obstruction secondary to endometriosis has no pelvic symptoms whatsoever. The clinical challenge is to diagnose minimal ureteral obstruction at an early stage, before loss of renal function. The obstruction is almost always in the distal one third of the course of the ureter. The importance of an imaging study to diagnose ureteral compromise in all women with retroperitoneal endometriosis cannot be overemphasized.

Endometriosis of the bladder is discovered most often in the region of the trigone or the anterior wall of the bladder (Video 19.6). Bladder endometriosis produces midline, lower abdominal, and suprapubic pain, dysuria, and, occasionally, cyclic hematuria. Treatment of endometriosis of the peritoneum over the bladder can be accomplished by medical or surgical means. Ureteral obstruction may be intrinsic, from active endometriosis, or extrinsic, from long-standing fibrotic reactions to retroperitoneal inflammation. Extrinsic endometriosis is three to five times more common than the intrinsic form. There are few reports of endometriosis of the ureter responding to danazol or GnRH agonists. However, long-term follow-up with serial ultrasound imaging or intravenous pyelograms must be undertaken to ensure that the disease process does not recur.

Surgical therapy is the preferred treatment for ureteral obstruction secondary to endometriosis (Video 19.7). The operations are rare and should be individualized. The most common surgical approaches include removal of the uterus and both ovaries and the relief of urinary obstruction by ureterolysis or by ureteroneocystostomy. Ureteral resection is often needed if hydronephrosis is present. If ureterolysis is performed, peristalsis in the involved segment of the ureter should be observed, along with adequate resection of the endometriosis and surrounding inflammation in the retroperitoneal space. Ureteroneocystostomy has the advantage of bypassing the urinary obstruction and making it technically easier to resect the area of endometriosis and associated retroperitoneal fibrosis.

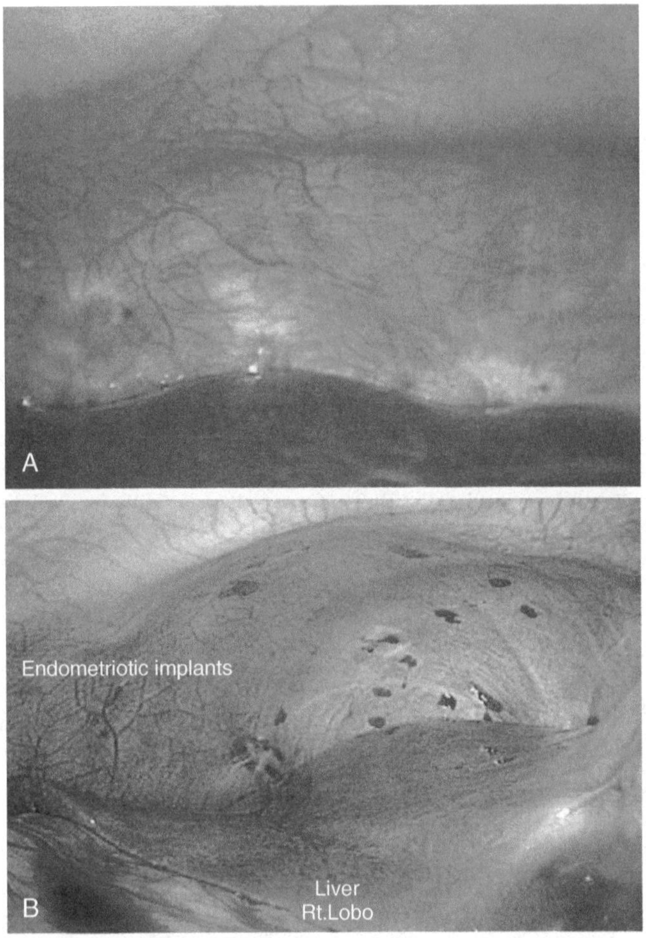


**Figure 19.20** **A,** Fibrotic-type endometriosis involving the right hemidiaphragm. The lesions are seen above the liver. Most are obscured by the liver. **B,** Hemorrhagic-type endometriosis lesions of the right hemidiaphragm. (From Hemmings RR, Falcone T. Endometriosis. In: Falcone T, Hurd WW. *Clinical Reproductive Medicine and Surgery*. Philadelphia: Mosby; 2007:741.)

## EXTRA PELVIC ENDOMETRIOSIS

Endometriosis can also involve the diaphragm (Fig. 19.20). This may be an incidental finding at laparoscopy and can be asymptomatic. However, if a patient is symptomatic, the most common presentation of diaphragmatic endometriosis is right-sided catamenial pneumothorax. Other signs and symptoms can include dyspnea, chest pain, shoulder pain, hemoptysis, and the presence of pulmonary nodules. Medical suppressive therapy is the first approach, although surgery, including pleurodesis, may be considered. These patients should be referred to thoracic surgery.

## *KEY POINTS*

- Endometriosis is a benign, usually progressive, and sometimes recurrent disease that invades locally and disseminates widely.
- Possible causal factors of endometriosis include retrograde menstruation, coelomic metaplasia, vascular metastasis, immunologic changes, iatrogenic dissemination, and a genetic predisposition.
- Endometriosis lesions produce estrogen locally and have increased secretion of prostaglandins and inflammatory cytokines, which can cause pain and contribute to infertility. There is also a relative resistance to progesterone in endometriosis lesions.
- Grossly, endometriosis appears in many forms, including red, brown, black, white, yellow, pink, or clear vesicles and lesions. Red, blood-filled lesions are in the most active phase of endometriosis.
- Approximately 10% of teenagers who develop endometriosis have associated congenital outflow obstruction.

*Continued*

## KEY POINTS—cont'd

- The two primary short-term goals in treating endometriosis are the relief of pain and the promotion of fertility. The primary long-term goal in the management of a woman with endometriosis is attempting to prevent progression or recurrence of the disease process.
- There are several established treatments for endometriosis (such as oral contraceptives and GnRH agonists and danazol) and some novel therapies undergoing trials such as the use of oral antagonists, aromatase inhibitors, progesterone receptor modulators, and cytokine inhibitors.
- The recurrence rate following medical therapy is 5% to 15% in the first year and increases to 40% to 50% in 5 years.
- The side effects associated with GnRH agonist therapy are primarily those associated with estrogen deprivation, similar to menopause. The three most common symptoms are hot flushes, vaginal dryness, and insomnia. A decrease in bone mineral content of trabecular bone has been demonstrated in the cortical bone on the lumbar spine by quantitative computed tomography.
- Many clinicians "add back" very low doses of estrogen, low doses of progestins, or both in combination with chronic GnRH agonist therapy.
- The incidence of endometriosis is 30% to 45% in women with infertility. There is probably some benefit to abrading endometriosis lesions when seen at laparoscopy. In patients with endometriosis, the success of IVF-ET decreases only in women with severe disease.
- Classic symptoms of endometriosis of the large bowel include cyclic pelvic cramping and lower abdominal pain and rectal pain with defecation, especially during the menstrual period.
- Endometriosis of the bladder is discovered most often in the region of the trigone or the anterior wall of the bladder. Bladder endometriosis produces midline, lower abdominal, and suprapubic pain, dysuria, and, occasionally, cyclic hematuria.

## KEY REFERENCES


Adamson GD, Pasta DJ. Endometriosis fertility index: the new, validated endometriosis staging system. *Fertil Steril.* 2010;94:1609–1615.

American Society for Reproductive Medicine (ASRM). Revised American Society for Reproductive Medicine classification of endometriosis: 1996. *Fertil Steril.* 1997;67:817–821.

Attar E, Bulun SE. Aromatase inhibitors: the next generation of therapeutics for endometriosis? *Fertil Steril.* 2006;85:1307–1318.

Barbieri RL. Hormone treatment of endometriosis: the estrogen threshold hypothesis. *Am J Obstet Gynecol.* 1992;166:740–745.

Barnhart K, Dunsmoor-su R, Coutifaris C. Effect of endometriosis on in vitro fertilization. *Fertil Steril.* 2002;77:1148–1155.

Batt RE, Smith RA. Embryologic theory of histogenesis of endometriosis in peritoneal pockets. *Obstet Gynecol Clin North Am.* 1989;16:15–28.

Brosens IA, Brosens JJ. Redefining endometriosis: Is deep endometriosis a progressive disease? *Hum Reprod.* 2000;15:1–3.

Buck Louis GM, Hediger ML, Peterson CM, et al. Incidence of endometriosis by study population and diagnostic method: the ENDO study. *Fertil Steril.* 2011;96:360–365.

Bulun SE. Mechanisms of disease: endometriosis. *N Engl J Med.* 2009;360(3): 268–279 (review).

Chabbert-Buffet N, Meduri G, Bouchard P, et al. Selective progesterone receptor modulators and progesterone antagonists: mechanisms of action and clinical applications. *Hum Reprod Update.* 2005;11:293–307.

Cheng YM, Wang ST, Chou CY. Serum CA-125 in preoperative patients at high risk for endometriosis. *Obstet Gynecol.* 2002;99:375–380.

de Venecia, Ascher SM. Pelvic endometriosis: a spectrum of magnetic resonance imaging findings. *Semin Ultrasound CT MR.* 2015;36(4):385–393.

Dinulescu DM, Ince TA, Quade BJ, et al. Role of K-ras and ten in the development of mouse models of endometriosis and endometrioid ovarian cancer. *Nat Med.* 2005;11:63–70.

Donnez J, Nisolle M, Gillerot S, et al. Rectovaginal septum adenomyotic nodules: a series of 500 cases. *Br J Obstet Gynaecol.* 1997;104:1014–1018.

Evers JL. Endometriosis does not exist; all women have endometriosis. *Hum Reprod.* 1994;9:2206–2209.

Ezzati M, Carr BR. Elagolix, a novel, orally bioavailable GnRH antagonist under investigation for the treatment of endometriosis-related pain. *Womens Health (Lond Engl).* 2015;11:19–28.

Falconer H, Mwenda JM, Chai DC, et al. Effects of anti-TNF-mAb treatment on pregnancy in baboons with induced endometriosis. *Fertil Steril.* 2008;89(Suppl 5):1537–1545.

Fassbender A, Waelkens E, Verbeeck N, et al. Proteomics analysis of plasma for early diagnosis of endometriosis. *Obstet Gynecol.* 2012;119:276–285.

Fedele L, Bianchi S, Zanconato G, et al. Use of a levonorgestrel-releasing intrauterine device in the treatment of rectovaginal endometriosis. *Fertil Steril.* 2001;75:485–488.

Ferrero S, Remorgida V, Venturini PL, et al. Endometriosis: the effects of dienogest. *BMJ Clin Evid.* 2015.

Flores I, Rivera E, Ruiz LA, et al. Molecular profiling of experimental endometriosis identified gene expression patterns in common with human disease. *Fertil Steril.* 2007;87:1180–1199.

Gargett CE, Masuda H. Adult stem cells in the endometrium. *Mol Hum Reprod.* 2010;16:818–834.

Gestrinone Italian Study Group. Gestrinone versus a gonadotropin-releasing hormone agonist for the treatment off pelvic pain associated with endometriosis: a multicenter, randomized, double-blind study. *Fertil Steril.* 1996;66:911–919.

Halban J. Hysteroadenosis metastica. *Zentralb Gynakol.* 1925;7:387–397.

Halme J, Hammond MG, Hulka JF, et al. Retrograde menstruation in healthy women and in patients with endometriosis. *Obstet Gynecol.* 1984;64:151–154.

Hamdan M, Omar SZ, Dunselman G, et al. Influence of endometriosis on assisted reproductive technology outcomes: a systematic review and meta-analysis. *Obstet Gynecol.* 2015;125(1):79–88.

Healey M, Cheng C, Kaur H. To excise or ablate endometriosis? A prospective randomized double-blinded trial after 5-year follow-up. *J Minim Invasive Gynecol.* 2014;21(6):999–1004.

Hickey M, Ballard K, Farquhar CM. Endometriosis. *BMJ.* 2014;348:g1752.

Jacobson TZ, Barlow DH, Koninckx PR, et al. Laparoscopic surgery for subfertility associated with endometriosis. *Cochrane Database Syst Rev.* 2002;4: CD001398.

Jacoby VL, Fujimoto VY, Giudice LC, et al. Racial and ethnic disparities in benign gynecologic conditions and associated surgeries. *Am J Obstet Gynecol.* 2010;202:514–521.

Kosugi Y, Elias S, Malinak LR, et al. Increased heterogeneity of chromosome 17aneuploidy in endometriosis. *Am J Obstet Gynecol.* 1999;180:792–797.

Lebovic DI, Mwenda JM, Chai DC, et al. PPAR-gamma receptor ligand induces regression of endometrial explants in baboons: a prospective, randomized, placebo-and drug-controlled study. *Fertil Steril.* 2007;88:1108–1119.

McLaren J, Dealtry G, Prentice A, et al. Decreased levels of the potent regulator of monocyte/macrophage activation, interleukin-13, in the peritoneal fluid of patients with endometriosis. *Hum Reprod Update.* 1997;12:1307–1310.

Medina MG, Lebovic DI. L'Endometriosis-associated nerve fibers and pain. *Acta Obstet et Gynecol.* 2009;88:968–975.

Meyer R. Zur Frage der heterotopen Epithelwucherung, insbe


Suggested Readings can be found on ExpertConsult.com.

# 20

# Anatomic Defects of the Abdominal Wall and Pelvic Floor

## Abdominal Hernias, Inguinal Hernias, and Pelvic Organ Prolapse: Diagnosis and Management

*Anna C. Kirby, Gretchen M. Lentz*

The structural supports of the abdomen and pelvis are susceptible to a number of stresses. In the female, these supports are affected by congenital anatomic weaknesses, the stresses of childbearing, injury, surgical damage, and straining. In addition, a combination of chronic stresses, such as lifting heavy objects, chronic cough, straining at stool, or activities that require frequent stretching, plus the aging process, may make older women more susceptible to such abnormalities. This chapter considers hernias of the abdominal wall and pelvic region, as well as conditions that are a result of the loss of pelvic supports.

## ABDOMINAL WALL HERNIAS

The abdominal wall is made up of the following structures beginning externally: skin; subcutaneous connective tissue; external oblique, internal oblique, and transversus abdominis muscles with their investing fascia; and parietal peritoneum. The rectus abdominis muscles run longitudinally in the midline from the xiphoid to the pubic symphysis. The investing fasciae of the external oblique, internal oblique, and transversus abdominis muscles completely encase the rectus abdominis muscles cephalad to the semilunar line. Caudally from the semilunar line the muscle is completely behind the aponeurosis of the fasciae of these muscles and lies directly on the peritoneum (Fig. 20.1). Normally the investing fasciae join in the midline after surrounding the rectus abdominis muscles.

In the male, the descent of the testes from their original retroperitoneal site to the scrotum necessitates passing through the abdominal wall to the inguinal region. At the level of the transversalis fascia where the descent begins, the internal inguinal ring is formed. The inferior epigastric artery defines the medial margin of this ring as it courses from the external iliac artery medially and superiorly into the rectus sheath. The inguinal canal runs from the internal inguinal ring obliquely downward, emerging through the external inguinal ring and opening in the external oblique aponeurosis just above the pubic spine, and then continuing into the scrotum. This allows for passage of the testes and for the presence of part of the spermatic cord.

In the female, the round ligament courses in the same direction but ends short of the labia.

An **inguinal hernia**—that is, a bulge of peritoneum through the internal inguinal ring and into the inguinal canal—is less common in the female than in the male and is frequently identified after stretching of the abdominal wall during or after pregnancy. It may be related to a congenital weakness of this area. Occasionally a femoral-type groin hernia may develop. In this case, the defect in the transversalis fascia occurs in the Hesselbach triangle, which is an area bounded laterally by the inferior epigastric artery, inferiorly by the inguinal ligament, and medially by the lateral margin of the rectus sheath (Fig. 20.2). The hernia sac passes under the inguinal ligament into the femoral triangle rather than coursing through the inguinal canal. **Femoral hernias** are more common in females than in males and have higher risk of strangulation (Fitzgibbons, 2015).

With a **reducible hernia**, the contents can be returned to the abdominal cavity. If the contents cannot be reduced, the hernia is said to be incarcerated. An **incarcerated hernia** may be acute, accompanied by pain, or long-standing and asymptomatic. If the blood supply to the incarcerated structure is compromised, the hernia is said to be *strangulated.* Because the hernia sac is primarily prolapsed peritoneum, the hernia itself is not strangulated but only its contents. On rare occasions, a portion of the wall of the hernia sac is composed of an organ such as the sigmoid colon or the cecum. In these instances, the hernia is called a **sliding hernia**.

A **ventral hernia** occurs in the abdominal wall away from the groin. Examples include **umbilical hernias**, which are caused by congenital relaxation of the umbilical ring, and **incisional hernias**, which are herniations through separation of fascial planes after operative incision. Incisional hernias generally involve the separation of the fascia of the abdominal wall with the hernia sac palpated beneath the skin and subcutaneous tissue. The sac wall is composed of peritoneum. Because the umbilicus consists of a fusion of skin, fascia, and peritoneum, an umbilical hernia generally occurs because the fascial ring is grossly separated, allowing the hernia sac to protrude. This occurs most frequently in obese women. The hernia sac itself is made up of peritoneum

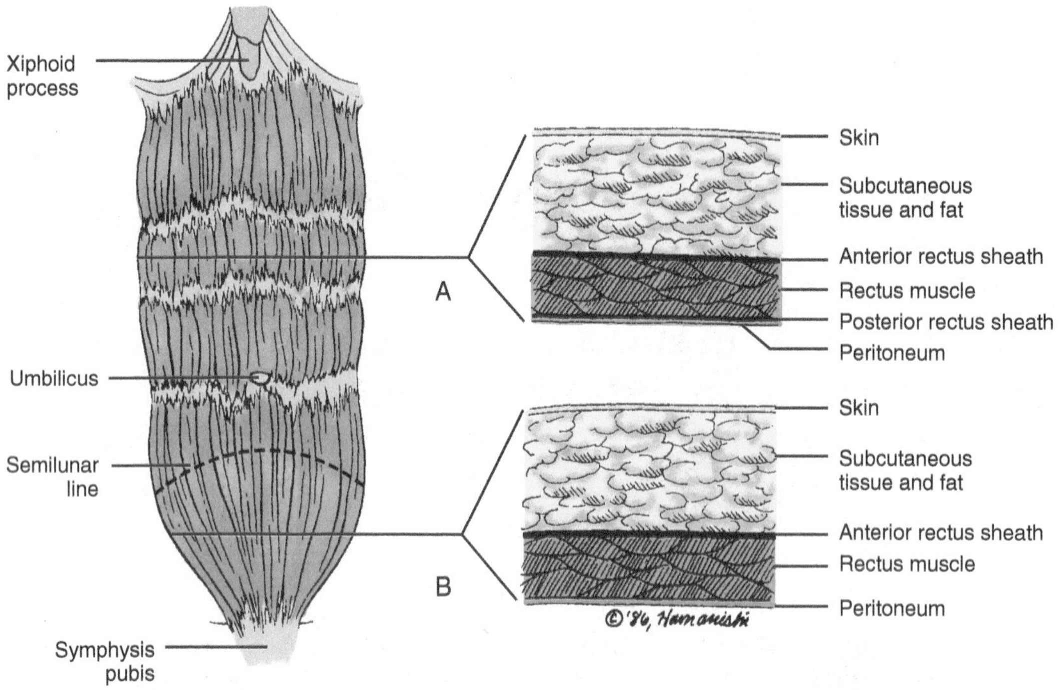


**Figure 20.1** Layers of the abdominal wall. **A,** Above semilunar line. **B,** Below semilunar line.

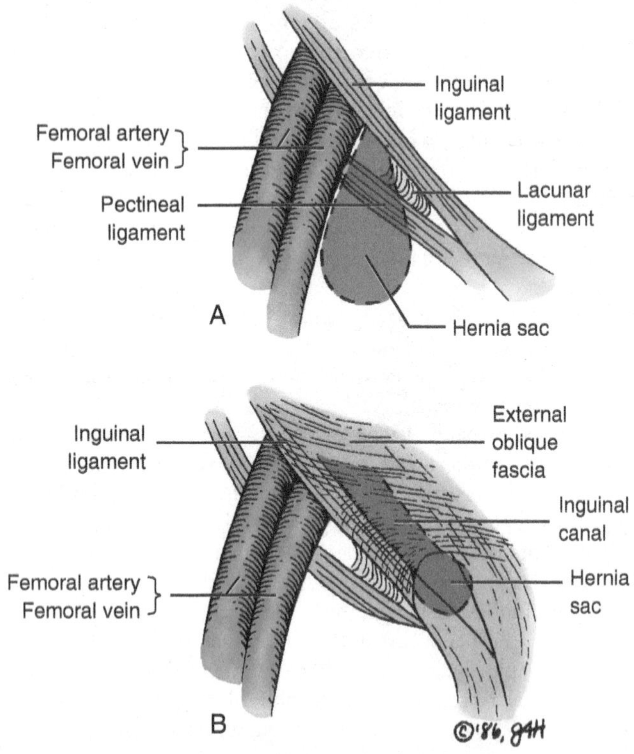


**Figure 20.2** Right femoral (**A**) and right inguinal (**B**) hernias in the female.

and subcutaneous tissue beneath the skin (Fig. 20.3). Two special ventral hernias include the epigastric hernia, which occurs in a defect of the linea alba above the umbilicus, and the rare **spigelian hernia,** which is a herniation at a point where the vertical linea semilunaris joins the lateral border of the rectus muscle.

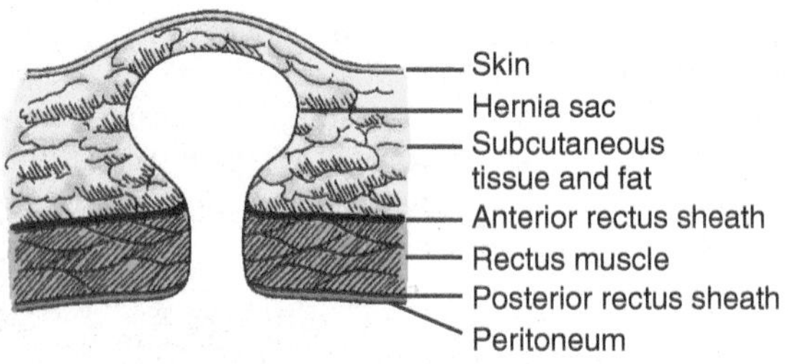


**Figure 20.3** Umbilical hernia.

Spigelian hernias are rare and result from congenital or acquired defects. These are rather rare hernias (1% to 2% of all hernias).

**Rectus diastasis** is an acquired abdominal wall defect in which the rectus muscles on either side of the midline separate. This is not a true hernia, as there is no fascial defect, but it is mentioned here for differential diagnosis purposes. Pregnancy is a common risk factor for rectus diastasis.

## *ETIOLOGY*

Hernias may be the result of a congenital malformation. The umbilical hernia is the best example. Before 10 weeks' gestation, the abdominal contents are partially herniated through the umbilicus into the extra embryonic coelomic cavity. However, after 10 weeks the viscera normally return to the abdominal cavity, and the defect in the abdominal wall closes during subsequent fetal growth. Generally at birth only the space occupied by the umbilical cord remains patent. After the cutting of the cord, the area heals so that the skin in the area of the umbilicus fuses above the closed fascial layer. Some infants at birth will show a small umbilical hernia, but in most instances the fascial defect closes during the first 3 years of life. If it does not close, an umbilical hernia will form. Black infants have umbilical hernias more often than do white infants. Occasionally, umbilical hernias occur in adults after the distention of the abdominal cavity with pregnancy or with ascites.

In rare cases the abdominal wall closure process is less complete during gestation, leading to an **omphalocele**, which is a hernia sac at the umbilicus covered only by peritoneum and including bowel and other abdominal contents. Omphaloceles are usually seen in infants with other malformations and possibly chromosome anomalies, such as trisomy 13.

Hernias that occur in adults are often associated with trauma or injury. In many instances, the hernia bulge develops slowly after years of heavy labor. It is likely that a congenital anatomic defect was always present but became exaggerated over time, leading to the development of a hernia. Zimmerman and Anson suggested that inguinal lesions resulted from inadequate muscle support at the lower area of the inguinal canal, primarily caused by a defect in the internal oblique muscle. Stretching of this area in pregnancy may initiate a hernia, but other factors, such as chronic cough caused by smoking or chronic respiratory disease, may be responsible.

Incisional hernias generally occur because of poor healing of the fascia after surgery. This may be secondary to poor nutrition, infection, obesity, or necrosis of the fascia secondary to suturing. It may also occur because absorbable suture loses its tensile strength before healing is complete or excessive wound tension. Stress and strain secondary to chronic cough or vomiting in the postoperative period may contribute to the process. Emergency surgery increases the risk of incisional hernia. Other conditions that inhibit wound healing include obesity, smoking, connective tissue disorders, and immunosuppressant medications. Incisional hernias may develop in 10% to 15% of patients after abdominal laparotomy incisions.

## SYMPTOMS, SIGNS, AND DIAGNOSIS

Bulges in the abdominal wall lead to the discovery of most ventral or groin hernias in women, either by a physician at the time of physical examination or by the patient. Occasionally, excessive straining or trauma will be implicated, and the patient may experience a feeling of tearing of tissue. Frequently the bulges are noted during an increase in intraabdominal pressure such as with coughing, pregnancy, or ascites. Most hernias are asymptomatic, but in some cases, particularly with larger ones, there may be aching or discomfort. Should intraabdominal organs move into the sac, the patient may experience some discomfort. Organs that strangulate within the sac cause acute pain and discomfort. Incarcerated organs may give nonspecific visceral pain, which is most likely the result of mesenteric stretching. An incisional hernia with incarceration may present with a bowel obstruction.

In cases in which a hernia exists but no contents are within the sac, physical examination reveals a weakening at the site of the hernia. It is often possible to feel the "ring" of the hernia as one palpates the defect through the skin and subcutaneous tissue. The patient's straining will generally accentuate the hernia, making it more palpable and visible. In the case of inguinal and femoral hernias, it may be necessary for the patient to be standing for one to palpate the hernia.

When there are intraabdominal contents within the hernia sac, the hernia is more easily palpated. The physician should then decide, based on his or her attempts to gently milk the contents from the sac back through the defect ring, whether the contents are reducible. For a hernia that does not reduce easily but in which there is no evidence of vascular compromise, it is sometimes useful to apply ice packs to the abdomen in the area of the incarcerated hernia before additional attempts are made to reduce it. In cases of **strangulated hernia**, evidence of devitalization of an organ, such as fever, leukocytosis, and evidence for an acute abdomen, may be noted.

With classic presentation of strangulated hernia on history and physical exam, surgical management should be pursued without imaging confirmation. If symptoms are present, but the exam cannot confirm a hernia, ultrasonography can be ordered. Computed tomography (CT) and magnetic resonance imaging (MRI) provide more anatomic detail and accuracy, but at increased cost and radiation exposure with CT.

## MANAGEMENT

Nonoperative management of ventral wall and incisional hernias in women is often feasible. Umbilical hernias in little girls will generally close by age 3 or 4 years and rarely become incarcerated. Unincarcerated groin hernias are often small and become uncomfortable only with an increase in intraabdominal pressure, such as occurs with pregnancy. Many authors advocate repair, however, because the small neck of these hernias may make incarceration more likely. With pregnancy, the opportunity for incarceration is reduced because the increasing size of the uterus pushes bowel contents away from the area of the herniation. Trusses and other supports are generally difficult to fit and are of little value in women.

Larger hernias, hernias that continuously contain intraabdominal contents, hernias that cause continuing discomfort, and those that have been incarcerated should be repaired. Most incisional hernias should be repaired, but asymptomatic groin hernias can be safely managed conservatively. Some general principles of operative repair can be stated. The first principle involves the anatomy of the hernia. The hernia almost always consists of a sac of peritoneum with a narrow neck and a fascial defect of some sort. In rare instances, if a peritoneal sac is broad based, it may be possible to simply reduce the sac through the fascial defect without opening it and then to repair the fascial defect. However, if a narrow-necked sac exists, it must be dissected free of the fascial defect, emptied of its contents, and then excised and sutured at the neck (base). The fascial defect is then mobilized completely to remove stress and scarring, and it is closed with permanent suture. In many cases the fascial defect may be large, and the degree of mobilization that is required may be impossible. In such instances, patching with inert material, such as polypropylene mesh, may be necessary. Mesh repairs have become the preferred technique for incisional hernias because the recurrence rate is lowered. Studies are conclusive regarding lower recurrence risk for hernia using permanent mesh. However, the infection risk is higher. Sutured repair without mesh is still acceptable for small hernias (<2 to 3 cm).

The second principle involves management of the contents of the hernia sac. Usually the hernia sac reduces with ease, but if intraabdominal contents are fixed to the sac wall by adhesions, the sac must be opened and the adhesions carefully separated. Care must be taken not to damage the organs or their blood supply. When these organs are reduced from the sac, the sac may be handled in the usual fashion. When incarceration has occurred, the organs must be inspected for viability before replacement.

### Umbilical Hernia Repair

To surgically repair an umbilical hernia, a curved incision is made at the inferior margin of the umbilicus (Fig. 20.4). The umbilicus

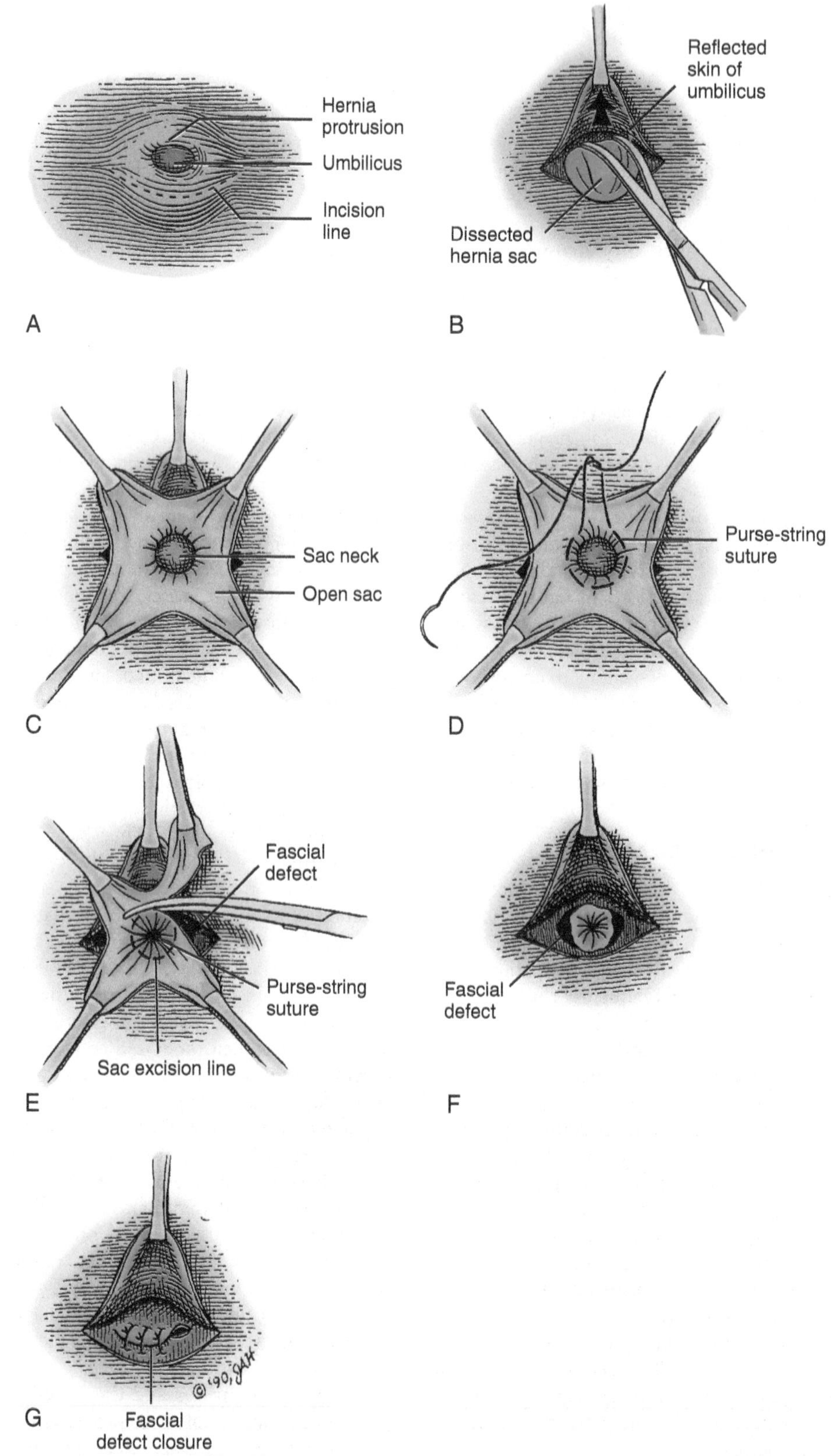


**Figure 20.4** Repair of umbilical hernia. **A,** Site of incision. **B,** Umbilicus dissected free of sac and reflected upward. **C,** Appearance of sac that is cut open. **D,** Placement of purse-string suture at neck of sac. **E,** Sac dissected free of fascial defect after suture is tied. **F,** Appearance of fascial defect after sac has been excised. **G,** Fascial defect closed; umbilicus will be tacked to it.

is dissected free of the sac and reflected upward. The sac is then dissected free of the fascial defect and either reduced or excised, depending on the circumstances. The fascial edges are freshened and either closed by direct approximation anterior to posterior using nonabsorbable sutures or mobilized and closed in a "vest over pants" manner, suturing the anterior edge to the posterior edge in an overlapping fashion. Studies have not shown that neither of these closures is superior to the other, and the approach taken generally is the one that best fits the circumstances. The umbilicus is then tacked to the fascial defect and the skin margin approximated. Large defects may require mesh placement to avoid tension on the closure (Aslani, 2010). Laparoscopic repair is also possible.

### *Incisional Hernia*

Repair of an incisional hernia can be accomplished by incising the skin through the old scar or via a parallel incision and dissecting through the subcutaneous tissue to identify both margins of the separated fascial defect. The peritoneum of the hernia sac is then isolated, dissected free of the margins, and reduced in the most appropriate fashion, with the surgeon exercising care not to damage any organs that may be fixed in the sac by adhesions. The fascial edges are then mobilized completely and closed with a mass suture technique. Outcome studies show a sutured repair is more likely to result in a recurrence than a mesh repair, although sutured repair may be adequate for small hernias (<2 or 3 cm) and when the risk of using a mesh prosthesis is unacceptable. Laparoscopic repairs are increasingly common. In a meta-analysis of five randomized controlled trials involving 611 patients, the recurrence risk and length of hospital stay were similar, but laparoscopic repairs had reduced risk of wound infection compared to open repairs (Al Chalabi, 2015).

Prevention of incisional hernias bears mention because 10% to 15% of abdominal incisions will develop a hernia. Preventing wound infection with appropriate antibiotic prophylaxis if indicated and careful surgical technique is worthwhile because the hernia rate increases to 23% with postoperative wound infection. A meta-analysis of abdominal fascial closure concluded that a continuous nonabsorbable suture closure resulted in the lowest rates of incisional hernia. Weight loss and smoking cessation should be recommended, as these are risk factors for hernia development.

## PELVIC ORGAN PROLAPSE

Pelvic organ prolapse (POP) is a condition characterized by the failure of various anatomic structures to support the pelvic viscera. It is defined as the descent of one or more of the vaginal walls or cervix: **anterior vaginal wall prolapse (cystocele, urethrocele, paravaginal defect)**, **posterior vaginal wall prolapse (rectocele or enterocele)**, **uterine/cervical prolapse**, or **vaginal vault prolapse** (after hysterectomy, often with an enterocele) (Fig. 20.5). Symptoms can include vaginal bulging, pelvic pressure, vaginal bleeding or discharge,

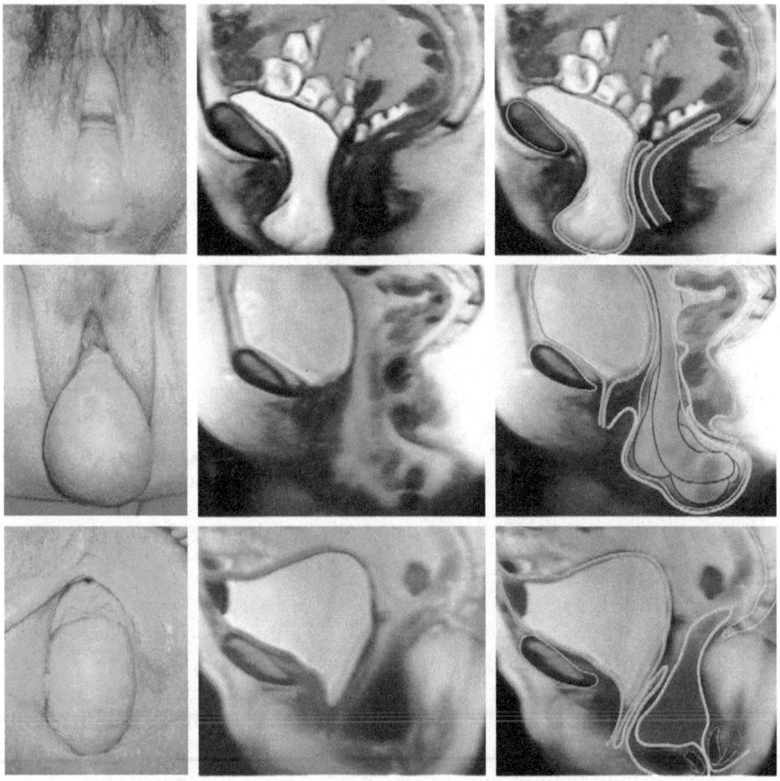

**Figure 20.5** Photographs in lithotomy position and sagittal magnetic resonance image showing vaginal wall prolapse. Prolapse might include *(top to bottom):* bladder (cystocele), small bowel (enterocele) or rectum (rectocele). Purple: bladder; orange: vagina; brown: colon, and rectum; green: peritoneum. (From Jelovsek JE, Maher C, Barber MD. Pelvic organ prolapse. *Lancet.* 2007;369:1027-1038.)

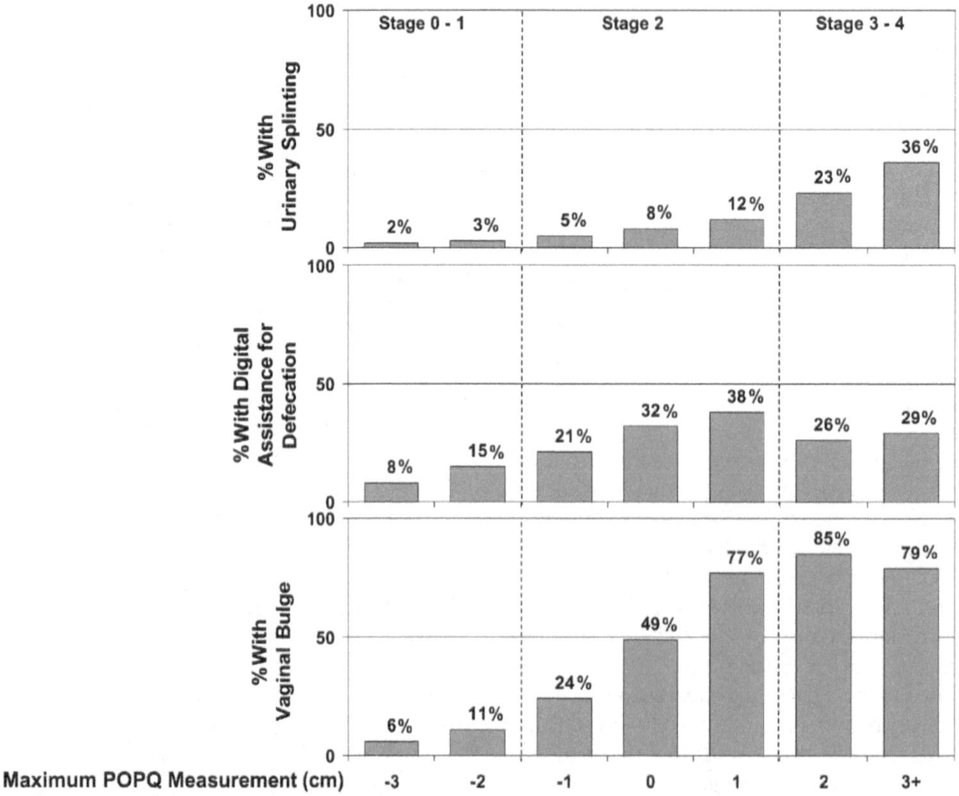


**Figure 20.6** Prevalence of prolapse symptoms per the pelvic organ prolapse quantification (POPQ) system. The percentage of patients who report urinary splinting, digital assistance, and vaginal bulge is demonstrated for each relevant POPQ measurement. (Modified from Tan JS, Lukacz ES, Menefee SA, et al. Predictive value of prolapse symptoms: a large database study. *Int Urogynecol J Pelvic Floor Dysfunct.* 2005;16:203-209.)

low backache, and the need to replace the prolapse (**splint**) in order to void or defecate (Haylen, 2010), or POP can be asymptomatic. Symptoms are more common when the prolapse extends beyond the hymen (Fig. 20.6) (Tan, 2005). POP usually involves more than one wall of the vagina.

## *RISK FACTORS*

POP is common, particularly in parous women, although many are asymptomatic. Although the prevalence of POP is 30% to 50%, the prevalence of symptomatic POP is closer to 3% (Nygaard, 2008). As demonstrated in Figure 20.7, most POP does not require treatment. A woman in the United States has a 13% lifetime risk of undergoing prolapse surgery (Wu, 2014). More than 360,000 surgical repairs are performed each year for POP in the United States (FDA, 2011). White and Latina women have four to five times higher risk of symptomatic POP compared with African-American women, and white women have the highest risk of having POP at or beyond the hymen (Whitcomb, 2009). Pelvic support structure defects have been associated with age, vaginal childbirth–related injury (neurologic or muscular or both), obesity, diabetes, connective tissue disorders, genetics/family history, and neurologic diseases (Cartwright, 2014; Memon, 2013) (Box 20.1). A single vaginal childbirth is associated with up to 10-fold higher odds of POP (Quiroz, 2010), and the risk

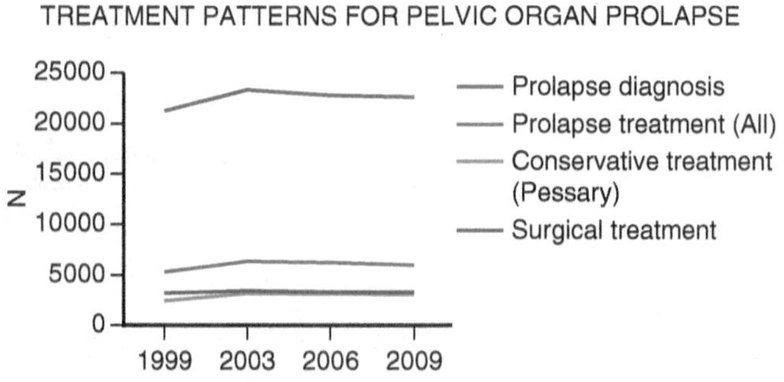


**Figure 20.7** Prolapse diagnosis and rates of different management patterns among female Medicare beneficiaries. (From Khan AA. Trends in management of pelvic organ prolapse among female Medicare beneficiaries. *Am J Obstet Gynecol.* 1015;212[4]:463.e1-463.e8.)

of surgery for POP may increase with each additional vaginal delivery (Larsson, 2009). In some cases, the injury from childbirth is subtle, but sometimes it is obvious, as shown in the images of this woman who had complete right-sided avulsion of her puborectalis (one of the levator ani muscles) after a normal vaginal delivery (Fig. 20.8).

Frequently, damage to the pelvic floor results in urinary incontinence instead of or in addition to POP. Urinary incontinence is discussed in detail in Chapter 21.

## NORMAL ANATOMY AND PATHOPHYSIOLOGY

Normal support of pelvic organs is provided by several key anatomic structures, including the pelvic floor muscles and connective tissue attachments (Fig. 20.9). Level I support of the vaginal apex and cervix is provided by the uterosacral and cardinal ligaments and associated connective tissue, level II support of the mid-vagina is provided by connective tissue attachments to the arcus tendineus fasciae pelvis on the lateral pelvic side walls, level III support of the distal (inferior) vagina is provided by the perineal membrane and muscles, (DeLancey, 1992), and all of the attachments are connected through endopelvic connective tissue.

The vagina is a hollow, fibromuscular tube composed of three layers: nonkeratinizing stratified epithelium, lamina propria (loose connective tissue), and muscularis (fibromuscular tissue with collagen and elastin). It is supported by attachments to the sacrum, coccyx, and lateral pelvic sidewalls. Anteriorly, the vagina supports the base of the bladder and urethra. The rectum is located posterior to the vagina behind the rectovaginal septum superiorly, and the perineal body is fused with the vaginal muscularis inferiorly. Although the connective tissues that lie between the vagina and surrounding organs have commonly been called *endopelvic fascia* and distinct planes can often be found during surgical dissection, DeLancey found that histologically this tissue is composed of connective tissue and muscle rather than fascia.

**Box 20.1 Risk Factors for Development of Pelvic Organ Prolapse**

Vaginal childbirth
Aging
Obesity
Diabetes
Genetic conditions/connective tissue disorders
Neurologic injury

**Possible Associations with Pelvic Organ Prolapse**

Prior pelvic surgery
Hysterectomy
Constipation
Irritable bowel syndrome
Episiotomy
Higher weight of the largest infant delivered vaginally
Chronic cough and respiratory diseases
Exercise
Heavy lifting
Lower education

The pathophysiology of POP is probably multifactorial. Bump and Norton outlined a useful concept for looking at risk factors as predisposing, inciting, promoting, or decompensating events (Fig. 20.10). Although imaging is not usually necessary in the evaluation of POP, imaging techniques including ultrasonography and MRI are increasing our understanding of support defects. Three-dimensional (3D) color thickness mapping was used to compare the levator ani of 30 women: 10 asymptomatic, 10 with urodynamic stress incontinence, and 10 with POP. Thicker, bulkier levator ani muscles were found in the asymptomatic women. Loss of levator muscle bulk was found in women with POP and stress incontinence (Fig. 20.11) (Hoyte, 2004). Theoretic explanations for these findings include muscle atrophy from denervation from childbirth injuries or muscle wasting from muscle insertion detachment also from childbirth, and possibly age and hormonal status. More women with POP had levator muscle defects and increased size of the levator hiatus on MRI compared to women with stress urinary incontinence and controls. MRI studies of POP demonstrate a more vertical vaginal axis and wider genital hiatus in women with POP compared to controls, in whom the upper two thirds portion of the vagina is nearly horizontal (Fig. 20.12).

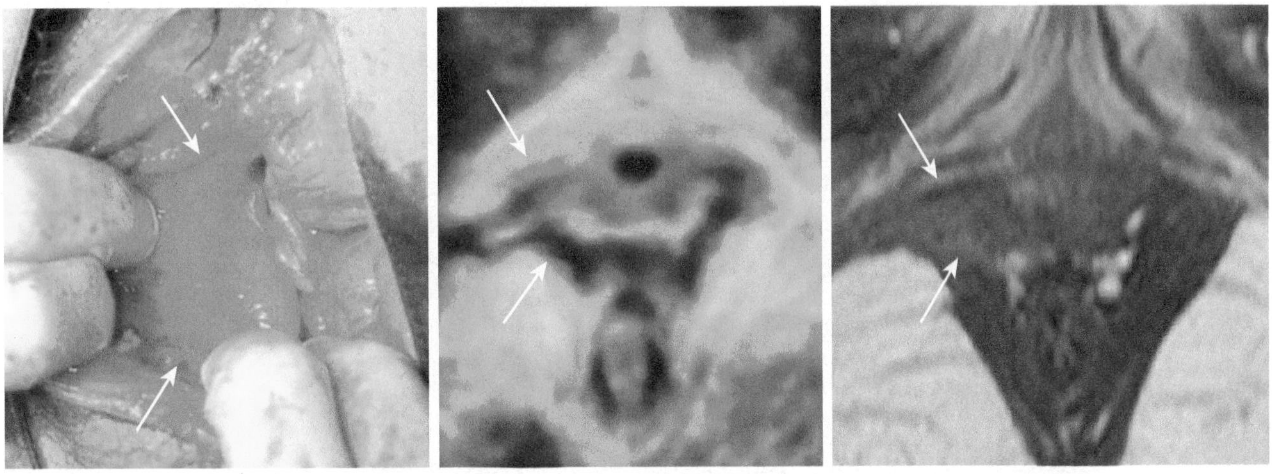

**Figure 20.8** Right-sided puborectalis avulsion after normal vaginal delivery at term. The left image shows appearances immediately postpartum, with the avulsed muscle exposed by a large vaginal tear. The middle image shows a rendered volume (axial plane, translabial three-dimensional ultrasound scan) 3 months postpartum, and the right image shows magnetic resonance imaging findings (single slice in the axial plane) at 3.5 months postpartum. *Top arrows* indicate the site of avulsion on the inferior pubic ramus, and *bottom arrows* show the retracted stump of puborectalis. (From Dietz HP, Gillespie A, Phadke P. Avulsion of the pubovisceral muscle associated with large vaginal tear after normal vaginal delivery at term: a case report. *Aust NZ J Obstet Gynaecol.* 2007;47:341-344.)

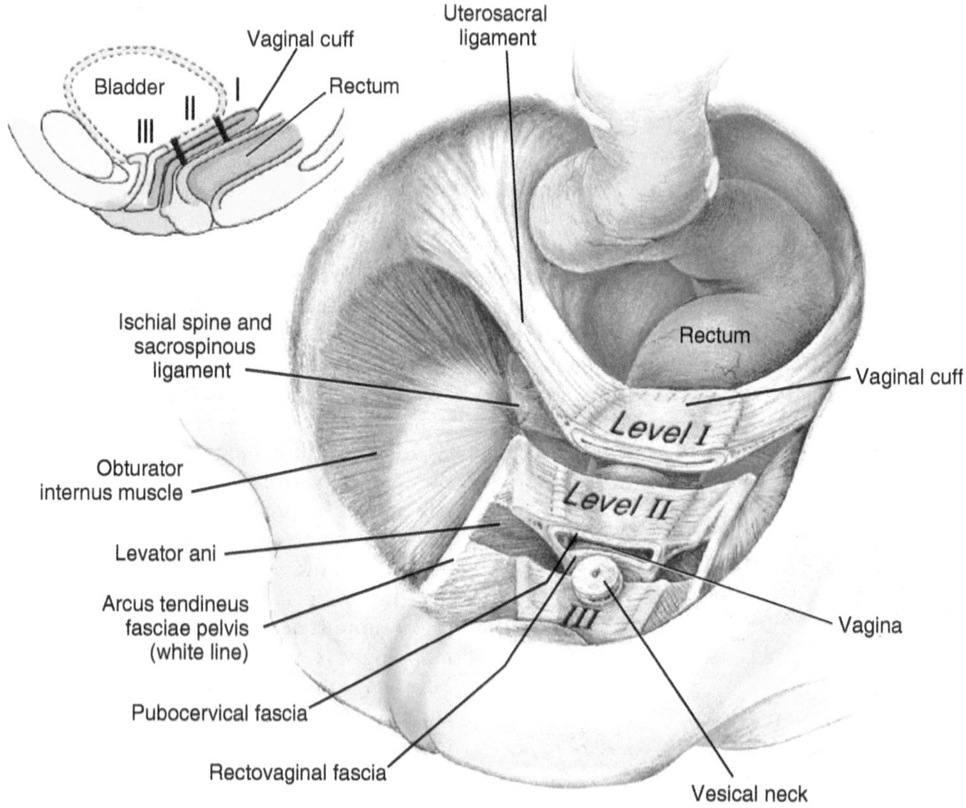


**Figure 20.9** Level I (suspension) and level II (attachment) support of the vagina. In level I the paracolpium (uterosacral ligaments) suspends the vagina from the lateral pelvic walls. Fibers of level I extend both vertically and posteriorly toward the sacrum. In level II support, the vagina is attached to the arcus tendineus fasciae pelvis and superior fascia of the levator ani by condensations of the levator fascia (e.g., endopelvic and pubocervical fascia). In level III support, the vaginal wall is attached directly to adjacent structures without intervening paracolpium (i.e., urethra anteriorly, perineal body posteriorly, and levator ani muscles laterally). (From Biggs GY, Nitti VW, Karram M. Pelvic organ prolapse. In: Nitti VW, ed. *Vaginal Surgery for the Urologist*. Philadelphia: Elsevier; 2012:17-22. Data modified from DeLancey J. Anatomic aspects of vaginal eversion after hysterectomy. *Am J Obstet Gynecol*. 1992;166[6 Pt 1]:1717-1728.)

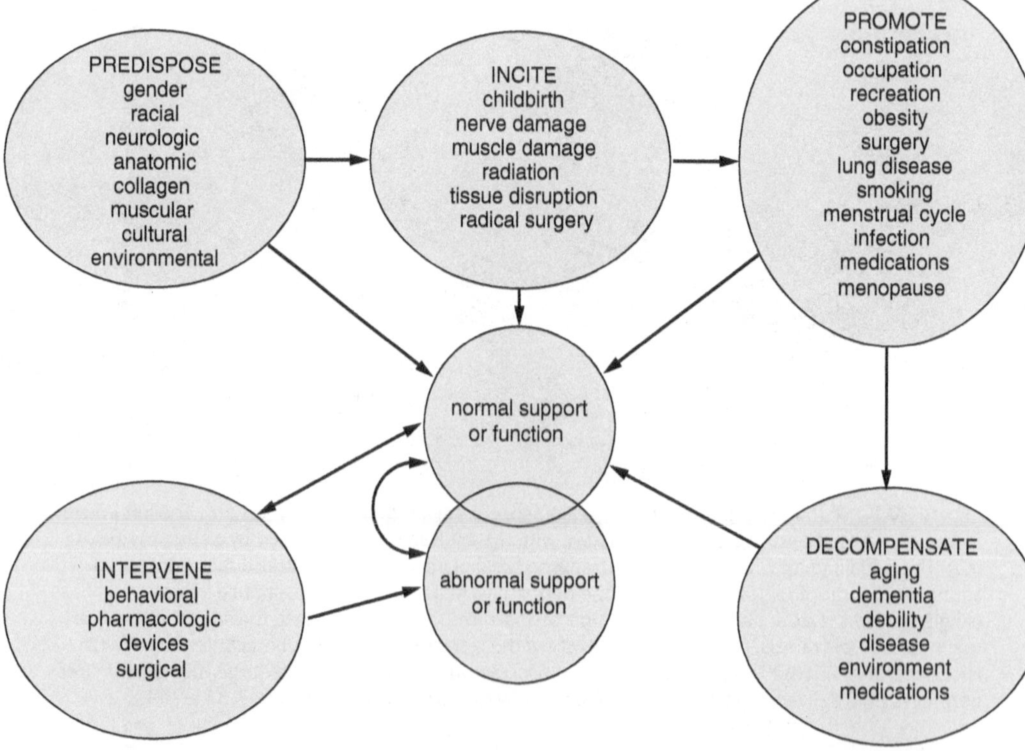


**Figure 20.10** Model for the development of pelvic floor dysfunction in women. (From Bump RC, Norton PA. Epidemiology and natural history of pelvic floor dysfunction. *Obstet Gynecol ClNA*. 1998;25[4]:723.)

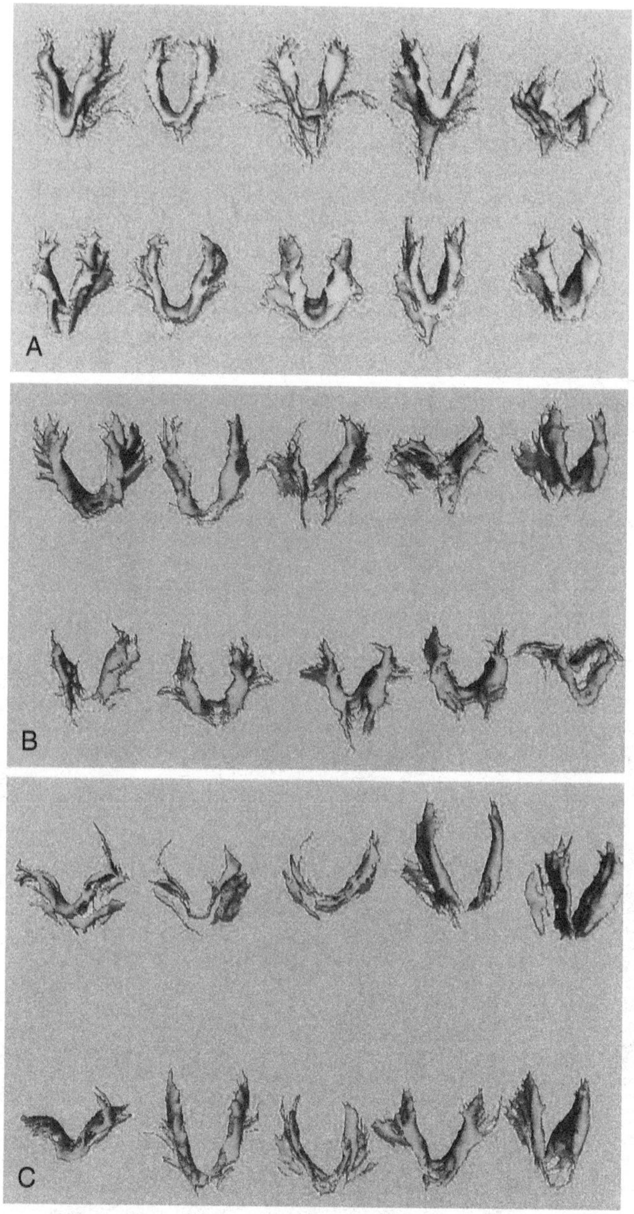

**Figure 20.11** Color images of reconstructed levator ani muscles from three subject groups: asymptomatic group (**A**), stress incontinence group (**B**), prolapse group (**C**). (From Hoyte L, Jakab M, Warfield SK. Levator ani thickness variations in symptomatic and asymptomatic women using magnetic resonance-based 3-dimensional color mapping. *Am J Obstet Gynecol.* 2004;191:856.)

## GENERAL SYMPTOM ASSESSMENT

Symptoms of POP are often not specific to the area that is prolapsing, and many women have no symptoms. The classic symptoms of prolapse include vaginal heaviness and pressure, a vaginal bulge, pelvic pain, or vaginal bleeding (from erosions of exposed vaginal epithelium). Back pain and pelvic pain are not reliably associated with prolapse. If a woman with objective prolapse does not have any bothersome symptoms or evidence of associated medical risks such as urinary retention or renal impairment from urethral or ureteral kinking, she does not need treatment. Because more than one pelvic floor disorder is often present, urinary, bowel, and sexual symptoms should be assessed in addition to prolapse symptoms in any woman with POP (Box 20.2). Urinary symptoms can include urinary incontinence, difficulty voiding, slow urinary stream, or a sensation of incomplete bladder emptying. Bowel symptoms such as constipation, straining, incomplete evacuation, fecal incontinence, or splinting (reducing the prolapse) to achieve bowel movements can be present. Sexual symptoms may include discomfort, irritation, and decreased sexual desire. She should also be asked about how these symptoms affect her quality of life, emotional health, and social interactions as well as whether or not they affect her ability to do usual daily chores, exercise, and participate in social events. Validated, self-administered questionnaires are available such as the Pelvic Organ Prolapse Quality of Life (P-QOL) scale and the Urinary Distress Inventory, which cover these categories. Understanding the woman's goals for treatment is important, because often there are multiple symptoms in each of these areas that cause varying degrees of bother and distress.

## QUANTIFICATION OF PELVIC ORGAN PROLAPSE

There are several systems for objectively measuring pelvic organ prolapse. In one system that is commonly used but imprecise, prolapse into the upper barrel of the vagina is called **first degree**, prolapse is to the introitus is **second degree**, prolapse past through the introitus is **third degree**, and complete eversion of the vagina is **fourth degree** prolapse. In the Baden-Walker system, **grade 0** is normal position, **grade 1** is descent halfway to the hymen, **grade 2** is descent to the hymen, **grade 3** is descent halfway past the hymen, and **grade 4** is maximum possible descent (Baden, 1972). Although these systems are commonly used and reasonable, they provide no information regarding which walls of the vagina are prolapsed and are rather imprecise regarding the severity of the prolapse, so in 1996 the Pelvic Organ Prolapse Quantitative (**POP-Q**) system was developed (Bump, 1996). A comparison of these measurement systems is shown in Figure 20.13.

## PELVIC ORGAN PROLAPSE QUANTITATIVE

In 1996, the International Continence Society (ICS), the American Urogynecologic Society (AUGS), and the Society of Gynecologic Surgeons (SGS) adapted a standardized terminology for the description of female pelvic organ prolapse and pelvic floor dysfunction and a standard measurement system for POP: the POP-Q (Bump, 1996). POP-Q is an objective, site-specific system for describing, quantifying, and staging pelvic support and was developed to enhance both clinical and academic communication with respect to individual patients and populations of patients. The new terminology, which refers to anterior vaginal wall, posterior vaginal wall, and vaginal vault prolapse, makes no assumptions regarding the organs behind the walls. It was designed to replace terms such as *cystocele, rectocele,* and *enterocele* with anatomic landmarks rather than organs, but the old terminology is still in wide clinical use and is often appropriate when it is known which organs are prolapsing behind the vaginal walls.

In the POP-Q system, as shown in Figure 20.14, all of the measurements are performed while the patient strains (bears down) except for total vaginal length (TVL). Point Aa is a point located in the midline of the anterior wall 3 cm proximal to the urethral meatus and is roughly the location of the urethrovesical crease (Fig. 20.15). Point Ba represents the most distal position of the anterior vaginal wall between Aa and the cervix or cuff. Point C represents either the most distal edge of the cervix or the leading edge of the vaginal cuff if a hysterectomy has been performed. Point D represents the location of the posterior fornix (pouch of Douglas) or the posterior point of attachment of the uterosacral ligaments (there is debate among the experts) in a woman with a cervix. Point Bp is a point most distal of any part of the upper posterior vaginal wall between Ap and the cervix or cuff, and point Ap is a point located in the midline of the posterior vaginal wall 3 cm proximal to the hymen. To record measurements, these points should be expressed in centimeters above or below the hymen (i.e., negative measurements are above the hymen and positive measurements are below the hymen). PB, which is the length of the perineal body between the posterior vagina and rectum, and GH, which is the genital hiatus measurement from the urethra to the posterior vagina, are measured during strain and do not have positive or negative values because they are not compared to the hymen. The most severe prolapse measurement on any of the vaginal walls can then be used to assign the **stage** of prolapse as described in Box 20.3: **stage 0**: no prolapse, **stage 1**: the most distal prolapse is more than 1 cm above (inside) the hymen, **stage 2**: prolapse between 1 cm above and 1 cm below the hymen, **stage 3**: prolapse more than 1 cm beyond the hymen but no farther than TVL - 2 cm, and **stage 4**: complete eversion/procidentia.

These organizations hope that by using this system, a clearer understanding of a patient's prolapse will be achieved and the transmittal of this information to others will be made more accurate. They also expect that this system will make it possible to standardize research information. Because the old terminology remains commonly used outside academic centers, both will be referred to in this chapter.

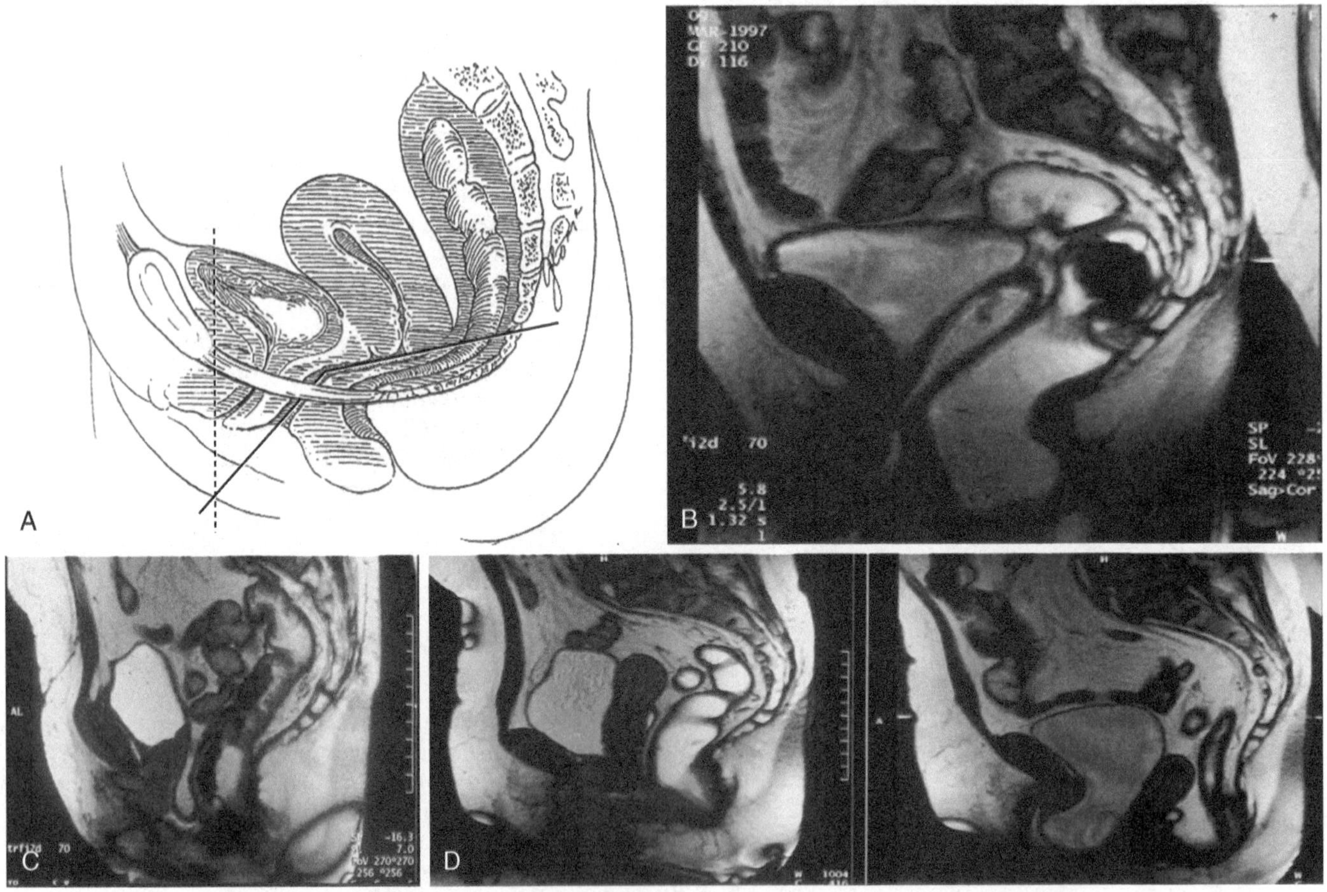


**Figure 20.12** **A** and **B,** In the nulliparous patient, the lower one third of the vagina is oriented more vertically, whereas the upper two thirds deviate horizontally, thereby maintaining the vaginal axis in an almost horizontal position. **C,** During stressful maneuvers such as coughing or straining, the levator hiatus is shortened anteriorly by contraction of the pubococcygeus muscles. **D,** In the case of genital prolapse when the levator ani support is lost, the vaginal axis becomes more vertical, the urogenital hiatus broadens, and fascial supports are strained. (From Chapple CR, Milsom I. Urinary incontinence and pelvic prolapse. In: Wein AJ, Kavoussi LR, Novick AC, et al. *Campbell-Walsh Urology.* 10th ed. Philadelphia: Elsevier; 2012:1871-1895.e7.)

## ANTERIOR VAGINAL WALL PROLAPSE (URETHROCELE AND CYSTOCELE)

Loss of anterior vaginal wall support is the most common site of primary POP. Anterior vaginal wall most commonly involves a cystocele, in which the bladder protrudes or descends with the vaginal wall relaxation, and it can less commonly include an enterocele in which the small bowel descends behind the upper vagina. Anterior compartment defects may also allow the descent of the urethra (urethrocele) and bladder neck. Normal support of the anterior vaginal wall depends on level I apical support as well as level II support from the endopelvic connective tissue and its attachments to the bony pelvis and pelvic muscles. The trapezoidal anterior vaginal wall has distal and medial attachments near the pubic symphysis, lateral attachments to the arcus tendineus fascia pelvis, and proximal and lateral attachments near the ischial spines. Anatomic studies have identified breaks in these attachments in women with POP. Lateral breaks are thought to cause paravaginal defects. Distal detachments from near the pubic symphysis may result in urethroceles or urethral hypermobility. Anterior vaginal wall prolapse can be associated with stress urinary incontinence from urethral hypermobility or urinary retention from urethral kinking that causes obstruction (Fig. 20.16).

**Box 20.2 Pelvic Organ Prolapse Symptom Categories for Clinical Evaluation**

Lower urinary tract symptoms
Urinary incontinence
Frequency, urgency, nocturia
Voiding difficulty: slow stream, incomplete emptying, obstruction
Urinary splinting

**Bowel Symptoms**
Constipation
Straining
Incomplete evacuation
Bowel splinting
Anal incontinence

**Sexual Symptoms**
Interference with sexual activity
Dyspareunia
Decreased sexual desire

**Other Symptoms**
Pelvic pressure, heaviness, pain
Presence of vaginal bulge/mass
Low back pain
Tampon not retained
Quality of life impacts

### *Symptoms and Signs*

Symptoms of POP include a sensation of fullness, pelvic pressure, vaginal bulge, and a feeling that organs are falling out. With anterior vaginal wall prolapse, the woman may also report a feeling of incomplete emptying with voiding, a slow urinary stream, or urinary urgency. The patient and the physician note a soft, bulging mass of the anterior vaginal wall. In some patients this mass must be replaced manually before the patient can void. Strain, cough, or prolonged standing often accentuates the bulge. Often POP symptoms are less bothersome in the morning and worsen later in the day after upright activities. The mass may descend to or beyond the introitus. Although urethroceles and cystoceles almost always occur in parous women, they have been noted in nulliparous women who have poor structural supports. This is particularly true in women who have congenital malformations or

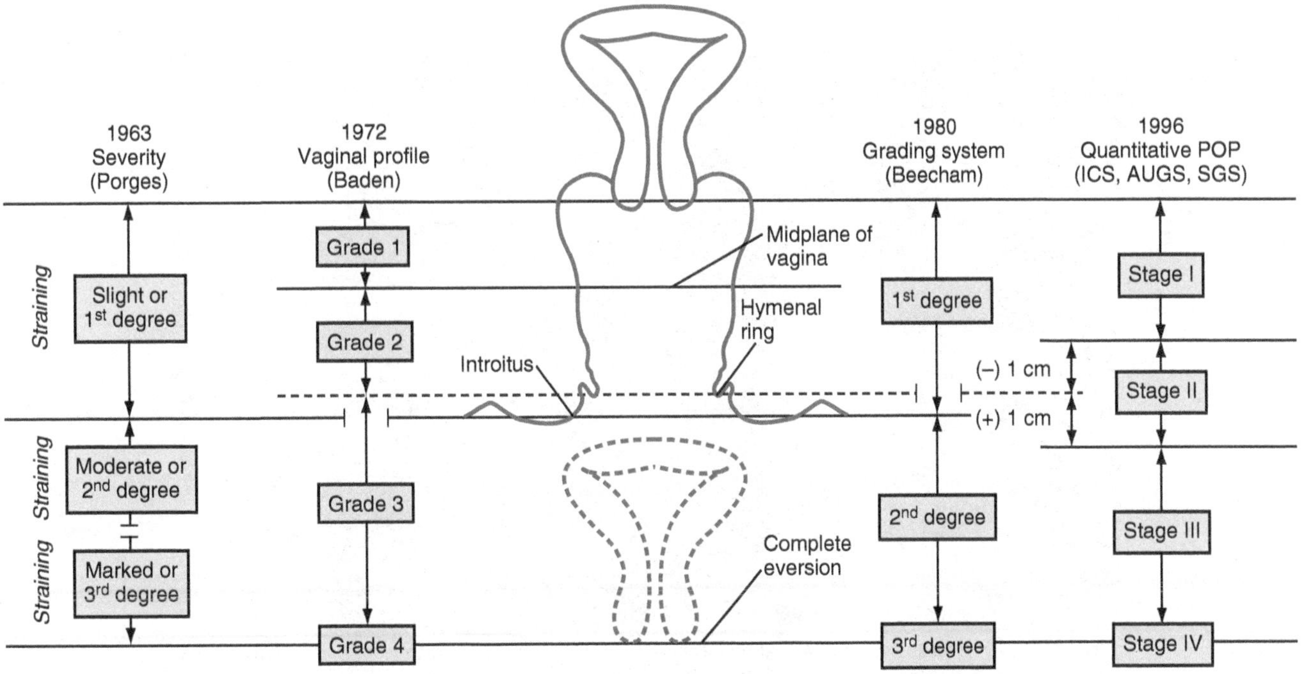


**Figure 20.13** Visual comparison of systems used to quantify pelvic organ prolapse. (From Theofrastous JP, Swift SE. The clinical evaluation of pelvic floor dysfunction. *Obstet Gynecol Clin North Am.* 1998;25[4]:783-804.)

weaknesses of the endopelvic connective tissue and musculature of the pelvic floor. Most parous women demonstrate some degree of cystocele, and when asymptomatic, they do not require therapy.

Women with prolapse often have concurrent urinary symptoms. Some women have stress incontinence caused by urethral hypermobility or weak urethral sphincter, but others are continent despite a lack of urethral support. Another group of women may have occult or latent stress incontinence (stress incontinence on prolapse reduction) because their continence depends on urethral kinking or obstruction from severe prolapse. Treating the prolapse with a pessary support or surgery could unkink the urethra and result in stress urinary incontinence.

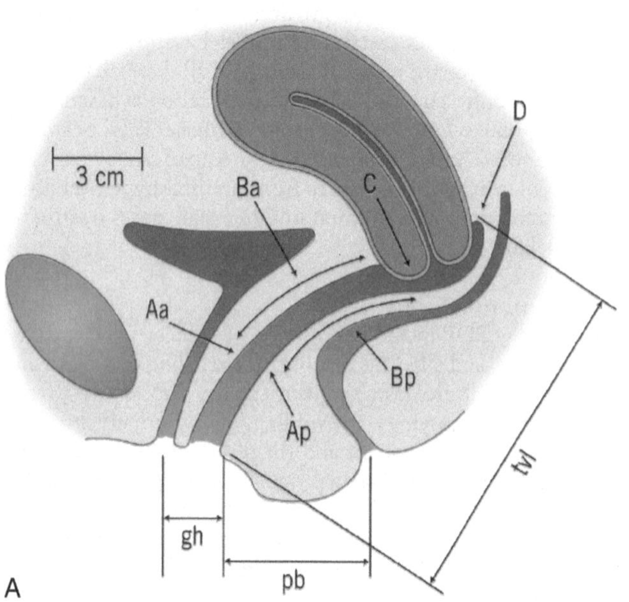


A

B

| Point | Description | Range of values |
|---|---|---|
| Aa | Anterior vaginal wall 3 cm proximal to the hymen | –3 cm to +3 cm |
| Ba | Most distal position of remaining upper anterior vaginal wall | –3 cm to +tvl |
| C | Most distal edge of cervix or vaginal cuff scar | – |
| D | Posterior fornix (N/A if post-hysterectomy) | – |
| Ap | Posterior vaginal wall 3 cm proximal to the hymen | –3 cm to +3 cm |
| Bp | Most distal position of remaining upper posterior vaginal wall | –3 cm to +tvl |
| gh (genital hiatus) | Measured from middle of external urethral meatus to posterior midline hymen | – |
| pb (perineal body) | Measured from posterior margin of gh to middle of anal opening | – |
| tvl (total vaginal length) | Depth of vagina when point D or C is reduced to normal position | – |

**Figure 20.14** **A,** Landmarks for the Pelvic Organ Prolapse Quantification System (POP-Q) system. **B,** POP-Q points of reference. (**A,** from Bump RC, Mattiasson A, Bo K, et al. The standardization of terminology of female pelvic organ prolapse and pelvic floor dysfunction. *Am J Obstet Gynecol.* 1996;175[1]:10-17. **B** from and **A** also modified from Kobashi KC. Evaluation of patients with urinary Incontinence and pelvic prolapse. In: Wein AJ, Kavoussi LR, Novick AC, et al. *Campbell-Walsh Urology.* 10th ed. Philadelphia: Elsevier; 2012:1896-1908.e30.)

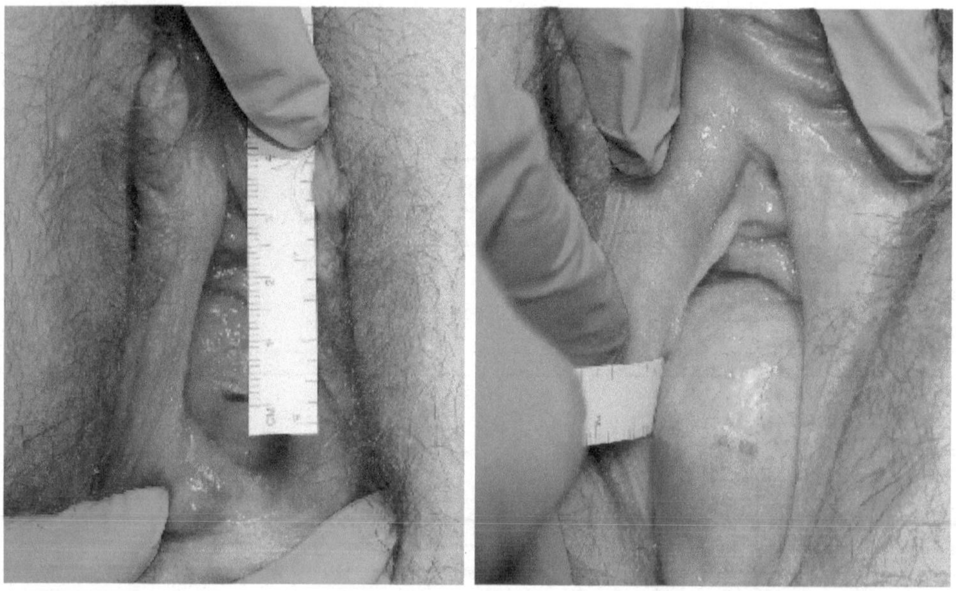

**Figure 20.15** Measuring point Aa. At rest, the Aa point is marked 3 cm proximal to the urethral meatus along the anterior vaginal wall *(left).* Then the patient is asked to strain, and the location of this point is measure in relation to the plane of the hymenal remnant *(right).* In this case, Aa is equal to +2 cm (2 cm past the hymen). In clinical practice, an imaginary mark is used. (From Reid F: Assessment of pelvic organ prolapse. *Obstet Gynaecol Reprod Med.* 2011;21[7]:190-197.)

Sexual function symptoms should be considered. Dyspareunia, vaginal dryness or irritation, and other difficulty with intercourse may occur with POP in any compartment.

### *Diagnosis*

Pelvic organ prolapse is best measured with a patient straining in the lithotomy position, although the physician should ask the patient if this reproduces her maximum bulge and, if not, repeat the examination in the standing position. Maximum prolapse is more likely to be observed with a full bladder in the standing position at the end of the day. To observe and measure anterior vaginal wall prolapse, a retractor or posterior wall blade of a Graves speculum is used to depress the posterior vaginal wall. The patient is then asked to strain, and the degree of anterior vaginal wall prolapse is noted. It is important to measure the amount of apical and posterior prolapse as well in order to not miss significant defects in the other compartments by focusing only on the most prominent prolapse. The physician should palpate the bladder neck and note whether it is well supported. Generally, if the supports of the bladder neck are adequate, the urethra is adequately supported. If a cystocele and urethrocele are present, it invariably follows that the bladder neck is not supported. Although determining the type of anterior vaginal wall prolapse—central or lateral/paravaginal—is no longer as important as once thought, a ring/sponge forceps can be used with the split speculum. If supporting the lateral anterior vaginal walls to the arcus tendineus fascia pelvis with an open ring forceps causes the cystocele to disappear with straining, a paravaginal defect is present. If apical support with the ring forceps causes the cystocele to resolve with straining, an apical or central defect is present.

It is important to perform POP-Q or at least qualitative measurements of the whole vagina, as often more than one compartment is affected. Checking the vaginal tissues for ulceration and bleeding should also be done. Pelvic floor muscle bulk, symmetry, and function should be assessed during the bimanual exam by asking the woman to tighten her muscles like she is trying to inhibit voiding or flatus.

Urethroceles should be differentiated from inflamed and enlarged Skene glands and urethral diverticula. Cystoceles must be differentiated from bladder tumors and bladder diverticula, both of which are rare but may occur. Urethroceles and cystoceles are generally soft, pliable, and nontender. Although diverticula may be reducible, a sensation of a mass is usually present. Inflamed Skene glands are generally tender. With diverticula or Skene glands, it may be possible to express pus from the urethra when they are palpated. In such cases, gonococcal, chlamydial, and other bacterial infections should be considered.

If surgical management of prolapse is being considered, the physician may want to perform a **preoperative prolapse reduction standing stress test** to evaluate for stress urinary

**Box 20.3 Staging of Pelvic Floor Prolapse Using International Continence Society Terminology**

**Stage 0**
No prolapse is demonstrated. Points Aa, Ap, Ba, and Bp are all at −3 cm, and either point C or D is between total vaginal length −2 cm.

**Stage I**
Criteria for stage 0 are not met, but the most distal portion of the prolapse is >1 cm above the level of the hymen.

**Stage II**
The most distal portion of the prolapse is ≤1 cm proximal or distal to the plane of the hymen.

**Stage III**
The most distal portion of the prolapse is >1 cm below the plane of the hymen but protrudes no farther than 2 cm less than the total vaginal length in centimeters.

**Stage IV**
Essentially complete eversion of the total length of the lower genital tract.

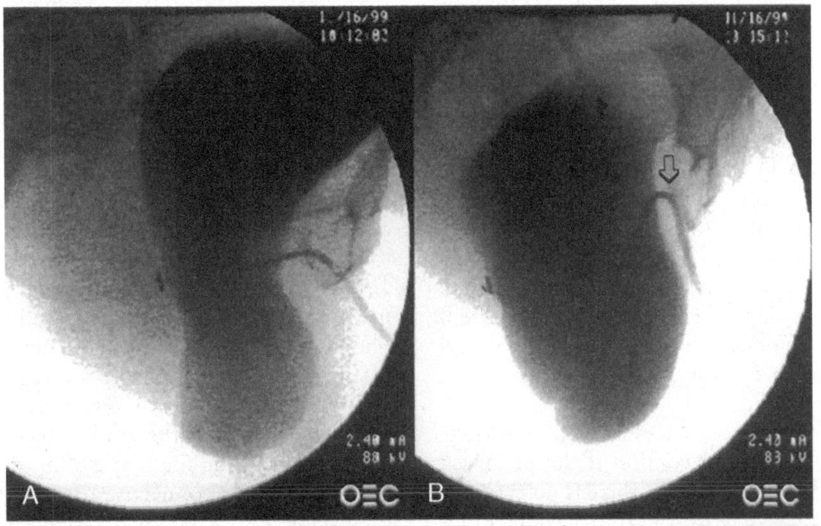


**Figure 20.16** Urethral kinking caused by large cystocele.< > Fluorourodynamic study shows a large cystocele before (**A**) and after (**B**) strain maneuver was performed. The urethra *(arrow)* clearly can be seen to "kink off" during the strain maneuver. The patient demonstrated severe stress incontinence after prolapse reduction. (From Gallentine ML, Cespedes RD. Occult stress urinary incontinence and the effect of vaginal vault prolapsed on abdominal leak point pressures. *Urology.* 2001;57[1]:40-44.)

incontinence. With a comfortably full bladder (ideally around 300 mL), usually in the standing position, the patient is asked to cough while the prolapse is replaced in its normal anatomic position. If she leaks during this test, she has latent or occult stress urinary incontinence that is likely to present after surgical repair of the prolapse. In women who underwent apical suspension for POP and were randomized to surgery with or without an anti-incontinence procedure, women with positive preoperative prolapse reduction stress tests had a 71.9% chance of urinary incontinence after surgery without a sling compared to a 29.6% chance of urinary incontinence without a sling. Women with negative preoperative prolapse reduction stress tests in this trial had a 38.1% chance of urinary incontinence without a sling and a 20.6% chance with a sling (Wei, 2012). With this information, the patient and physician can decide whether or not to do an anti-incontinence procedure at the time of prolapse repair.

### *Management*

Treatment of anterior vaginal wall prolapse may be nonoperative or operative depending on patient preferences and goals. If the patient is not bothered by the prolapse, it can be left alone and managed expectantly unless it is causing urinary retention or renal hydronephrosis. Women with mild (e.g., Stage 2) POP may elect for nonoperative management with pelvic floor physical therapy and Kegel exercises, which can decrease the risk of prolapse progression and can be effective at improving the sensation of pressure from mild POP (Kegel exercises are described in Chapter 21). Pelvic floor physical therapy can also treat associated urinary, bowel, and sexual dysfunction.

In one study, 447 women were randomized to receive individualized pelvic floor muscle training or a prolapse lifestyle advice leaflet with no muscle training (control group). At 6 and 12 months, the women assigned to pelvic floor muscle training had fewer prolapse symptoms as measured by a prolapse symptom questionnaire (POP-SS) than the control group.[19] Another randomized controlled trial investigated morphologic and functional changes after pelvic floor muscle training in 109 women with stage 1-III POP (Braekken, 2010). This supervised training led to a 44% increase in muscle strength, a 15% increase in muscle thickness, a decreased levator hiatus area, shortened muscle length, and elevation of the bladder and rectum position. It took 6 months of muscle hypertrophy training to achieve these results, so this option requires motivated patients. A follow-up study by the same group reported that 11 (19%) of women in the exercise group improved one stage on the Pelvic Organ Prolapse Quantification system compared with 4 (8%) of controls. This did correlate with reduced frequency and bother of vaginal bulging and heaviness by 74% and 67%, respectively. It is reasonable to offer pelvic floor muscle training for POP symptoms because it is without adverse effects. Women who have performed Kegel exercises on their own and have not improved may still benefit from working with a physical therapist.

In an older woman, the use of a vaginal estrogen product may improve vaginal atrophy and patient comfort if the prolapsed vaginal epithelium is irritated or ulcerated. There is no evidence that estrogen therapy will prevent or treat POP. Behavioral modification may help urinary symptoms such as urgency and will be discussed in Chapter 21.

Nonoperative support of the POP can also be achieved with a vaginal **pessary** (Fig. 20.17), or even with the intermittent use of a large tampon (pessaries are discussed in more detail under Uterine Prolapse in this chapter). If pelvic floor strengthening and pessary do not adequately control the prolapse symptoms or if a patient declines these options, then surgery can be considered. A young woman should be encouraged to avoid operative repair until she has completed her family. If pessary management is not adequate and the abnormality is so uncomfortable that repair must be performed before childbearing is complete, cesarean delivery should be considered for subsequent pregnancies.

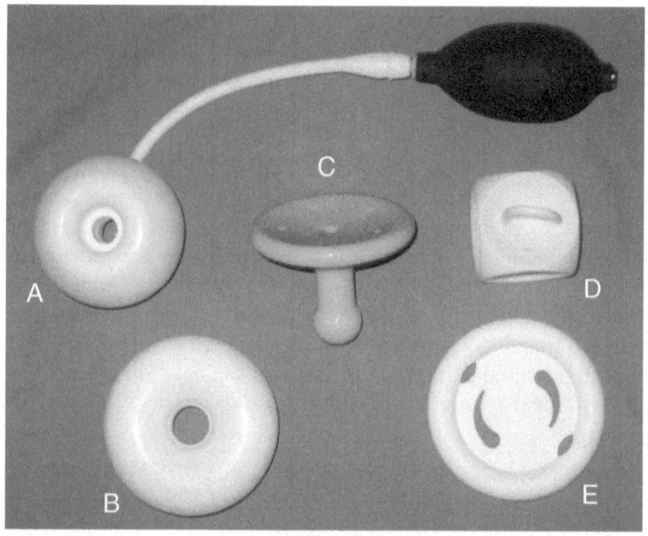

**Figure 20.17** Examples of pessaries: **A,** inflatable; **B,** donut; **C,** Gellhorn; **D,** cube; **E,** ring with support.

Operative repair of anterior vaginal wall prolapse is generally performed in conjunction with the repair of all other pelvic support defects. It is unusual for anterior supports of the vagina to relax without an accompanying relaxation of the apical compartment. Repair therefore usually consists of an anterior colporrhaphy as well as correction of uterine descensus or apical defect posthysterectomy. If noted, posterior vaginal wall prolapse may also be repaired at the same time.

Anterior wall repair (**colporrhaphy**) is performed by plicating the connective tissue of the anterior vaginal in the midline. After placement of a Foley catheter, the vaginal epithelium is incised from just distal to the anterior lip of the cervix or cuff to just proximal to the urethrovesical junction or bladder neck, which can be identified using the inflated bulb of a Foley catheter (Fig. 20.18). If the woman has undergone a hysterectomy in the past, the incision may be made approximately 1 to 1.5 cm anterior to the vaginal scar. The longitudinal incision is made by through the vaginal epithelium to but not through the underlying connective tissue. When the longitudinal incision is complete, the cut edge of the vagina is held under tension, and the fibromuscular tissue underneath (sometimes called *pubocervical fascia,* although it is technically not fascia) is separated from it using sharp and blunt dissection. This is repeated on each side. The connective tissue is imbricated in the midline by placing absorbable or delayed absorbable 0 or 2-0 sutures laterally on each side of the defect and tying them in the midline. For larger cystoceles, a two-layer plication may be needed. The excess vaginal epithelium can be trimmed and then closed over the repair using absorbable suture such as 2-0 polyglycol.

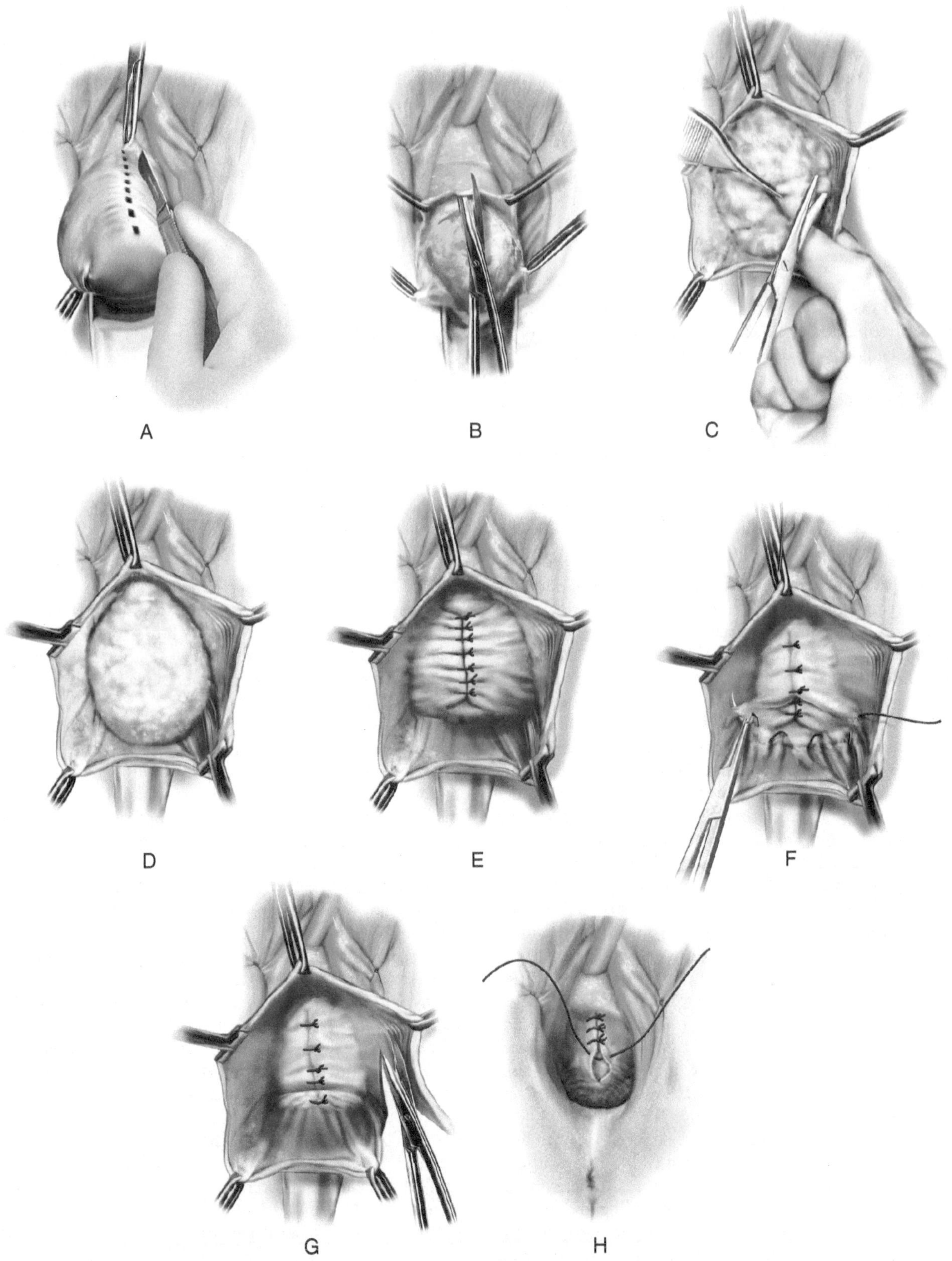


**Figure 20.18** Classic anterior colporrhaphy. **A,** The initial midline anterior vaginal wall incision is demonstrated. **B,** The midline incision is extended using scissors. **C,** Dissection of the vaginal epithelium off the underlying connective tissue and fibromuscular layer. **D,** The dissection is complete. **E,** The initial plication layer is placed. **F,** The second plication layer is placed, if needed. **G,** Trimming of excess vaginal epithelium. **H,** Closure of vaginal epithelium. (From Maher CF, Karram MM. Surgical management of anterior vaginal wall prolapse. In: Karram MM, Maher CF, eds. *Surgical Management of Pelvic Organ Prolapse*. Philadelphia: Elsevier; 2013:117-137.)

Cystoscopy should be performed to assess bladder and ureteral integrity after the procedure is completed.

Midurethral sling surgery for associated stress urinary incontinence or **stress urinary incontinence on prolapse reduction** (occult or latent stress incontinence) can then be performed through a separate incision over the midurethra. These and other anti-incontinence procedures are discussed in Chapter 21.

Alternatively, if midurethral slings are not available or depending on physician comfort, a Kelly plication can be performed to treat the urethrocele and decrease the patient's risk of stress urinary incontinence, although the success rates are lower than the success rates for other anti-incontinence surgeries, including mesh midurethral slings, Burch urethropexies, and fascial slings. In this case, the longitudinal incision can be continued under the urethra and the Kelly plication performed prior to the anterior colporrhaphy. A suture over the bladder neck (Kelly stitch) brings together the connective tissue on either side. The stitch should be placed as lateral as possible without tension, parallel to the urethra on each side, and then tied. The most appropriate tie for this closure is also 0 or 2-0 polyglycol suture.

## POSTOPERATIVE VOIDING DYSFUNCTION

Postoperatively, the bladder should be drained as long as there is a vaginal packing in place, usually for about 1 day, normally with a 16-French urethral catheter. Because there is a risk of urinary retention immediately after surgery, a voiding trial should be performed after removing any vaginal pack and prior to discharging the patient. There are two common ways to provide a **voiding trial**: back fill and auto fill. For the back fill, the bladder is retrograde filled with 300 mL of sterile saline, and then the catheter is removed. For auto fill, the catheter is removed, and the bladder is allowed to fill spontaneously. The voided volume is measured, and the residual volume is measured with a bladder ultrasound or straight catheterization in either type of voiding trial, or it can calculated after a back fill. The patient can be considered to have passed the voiding trial if she voids at least two thirds of the total bladder volume (i.e., a postvoid residual of less than 100 mL after voiding 200 mL of a 300 mL total bladder volume). Two randomized trials of the two voiding trial techniques revealed that the back fill technique was a better predictor of adequate postoperative bladder emptying than the auto fill technique, and it was also preferred by patients (Pulvino, 2010; Geller, 2011). Notably, 40% or more of patients had an unsuccessful voiding trial after prolapse or incontinence surgeries and were discharged home with a catheter. It is helpful to counsel women on this high chance of going home with a catheter, given short hospital stays after these procedures.

After an anterior repair if voiding does not occur prior to hospital discharge, the woman may be treated with a Foley catheter for continuous drainage or clean intermittent self-catheterization (CISC) for 1 to 7 days and rechecked for voiding and residual urine as an outpatient. Prophylactic antibiotics are rarely recommended; however, symptomatic lower urinary tract infections are common and should be treated as they occur.

Alternatives to voiding trials include suprapubic catheter drainage or teaching all patients how to perform CISC. With a suprapubic catheter, the drainage tube can be clamped, allowing the patient to void when she can and allowing residual urine measurements to be taken. The suprapubic technique is simple to use and seems to have a lower incidence of infection than does transurethral catheterization, but patients may complain of extravasation of urine around the site and occasionally of hematoma formation. CISC can be intimidating for patients to learn, but once learned, many patients prefer not having an indwelling catheter and can measure their own postvoid residual urine volumes. CISC is generally not necessary if short periods of catheterization are anticipated. The surgeon should decide which method is best suited to the patient's needs and develop a system that the surgeon and nursing team understand and can follow.

## POSTOPERATIVE RESTRICTIONS

Although there are no data regarding postoperative restrictions, in general patients are advised to avoid straining from constipation, heavy lifting, and strenuous activity for about 6 weeks (Nygaard, 2013). Nothing should be placed in the vagina until it heals. On the other hand, women should be able to resume other nonstrenuous normal activities as soon as they feel ready.

### *RECURRENT ANTERIOR VAGINAL WALL PROLAPSE*

Because recurrent POP is common after anterior colporrhaphy, augmentation of anterior vaginal wall prolapse repairs with graft materials has been proposed. However, although it may improve the anatomic result compared to traditional native tissue anterior colporrhaphy, it is associated with increased complications such as mesh exposure, pelvic pain, and dyspareunia. Figure 20.19 shows the excision of exposed vaginal mesh that had been placed in a prior POP surgery. In 2008, a public health notification issued by the U.S. Food and Drug Administration (FDA) summarized more than 1000 reports of surgical complications associated with mesh-augmented repairs. Subsequently in 2011, the FDA issued a Safety Communication that summarized its review of surgical mesh for transvaginal repair of POP: complications are not rare, and it is not clear that it is more effective than traditional non-mesh repair (FDA, 2011). A 2013 Cochrane Database systematic review concluded that the risk of recurrent prolapse symptoms and anterior vaginal wall prolapse on examination are decreased with the use of biologic or synthetic grafts, but disadvantages include longer operative times, greater blood loss, prolapse in other areas of the vagina, new onset stress urinary incontinence, and an 11% rate of vaginal mesh exposure (Maher, 2013). The 5-year cumulative risk for repeat surgery has been found to be higher after anterior prolapse surgeries that involved mesh than those that did not (15.2% versus 9.8%) when mesh revisions/removals were included. In this same study, the 5-year risk of recurrent surgery for POP was similar between vaginal mesh and native tissue repair groups (10.4% versus 9.3%) (Jonsson, 2013). Certainly careful patient selection, detailed patient counseling, and a skilled surgeon with proper training is needed for these procedures and to manage the complications.

Recurrent anterior vaginal wall prolapse remains a frustrating problem for gynecologic surgeons and patients. In fact, George R. White was quoted in 1909 saying, "Ahlfet states that the only problem in plastic gynecology left unsolved by the gynecologist is

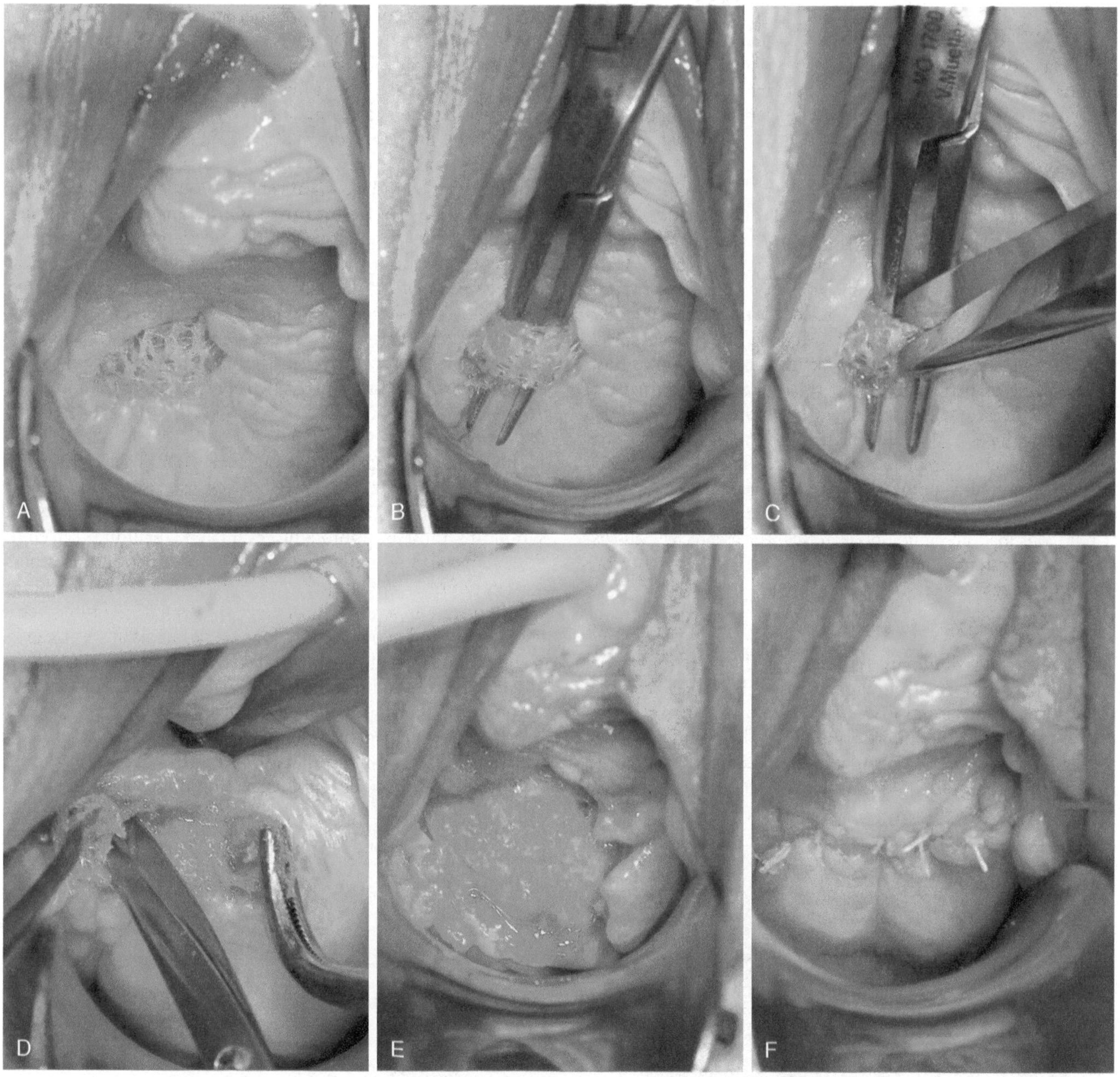


**Figure 20.19 Surgical Technique of Mesh Excision.** **A,** Anterior vaginal wall with 2- × 2-cm perigee mesh exposure. **B,** Undermining the mesh. **C,** Transecting the mesh, which has folded over on itself. **D,** Dissecting between mesh and bladder. **E,** Most of the mesh has been excised. **F,** Closure with interrupted suture. (From Margulies RU. Complications requiring reoperation following vaginal mesh kit procedures for prolapse. *Am J Obstet Gynecol.* 2008;199[6]:678.e1-678.e4.)

that of permanent cure of cystocele." It remains a problem even now, with reported failure rates of 30% to 46% after anterior colporrhaphy based on strict anatomic criteria: POP-Q stage 0 or 1, which was consistent with a 2001 National Institutes of Health (NIH) Standardization Workshop's recommendations at the time (Weber, 2001). However, it is increasingly recognized that strict anatomic "success" may not be clinically relevant for patients with POP. When this same study was reanalyzed with the more patient-centered outcomes of no POP beyond the hymen, no symptoms, and no retreatment, the success rate was 89% (Chmielewski, 2011). Because paravaginal repairs and mesh-reinforcement have not significantly decreased the rate of recurrence, and addition of mesh grafts increases the reoperation rate compared to native tissue repairs because of mesh complications as noted earlier, anterior colporrhaphy remains the procedure of choice for isolated anterior vaginal wall prolapse. Notably, the rate of recurrence has been found to significantly decrease with the addition of apical vaginal support (Eilber, 2013). In the setting of apical support defects associated with anterior vaginal wall prolapse, repairs such as uterosacral ligament suspension, sacrospinous ligament suspension, and sacral colpopexy may be indicated. These procedures are discussed later in this chapter.

## *POSTERIOR VAGINAL WALL PROLAPSE (RECTOCELE)*

The prevalence of posterior vaginal wall prolapse in community-dwelling women in the United States ranges from 18% to 40% and 9% to 76% in urogynecology clinics, depending on the definition used (Grimes, 2012).

### *Symptoms and Signs*

As with other forms of POP, the patient with a rectocele often complains of pelvic pressure, a "falling out" feeling in the vagina, a vaginal bulge, or disruption in sexual activity. Protrusion of the prolapse may worsen later in the day and be aggravated by prolonged standing or exertion. With a rectocele, the woman may also complain of constipation, difficulty with bowel movements, a feeling of incomplete emptying of the rectum, and the need to push on the vagina or perineum (splint) to have a bowel movement. Obstructed defecation symptoms may be reported by 9% to 60% of women with pelvic floor disorders, with 18% to 25% splinting, 27% straining, and 26% incompletely evacuating (Grimes, 2012). Although reported symptoms might be related to the rectocele, there are many other potential causes of evacuation problems that are not (constipation, sigmoidocele, rectal prolapse, rectal intussusception). Defecatory symptoms frequently but not always improve after rectocele repair.

### *Diagnosis*

Posterior vaginal wall prolapse is descent of the posterior vaginal wall and may include an enterocele (small bowel), a rectocele (rectum), or both. Posterior vaginal wall prolapse may be identified by retracting the anterior vaginal wall upward with one half of a Graves or Pederson speculum and asking the patient to strain (Fig. 20.20). POP-Q measurements should be performed of all compartments of the vagina. An example POP-Q for a women with isolated posterior vaginal wall prolapse is shown, although in reality POP usually involves more than one compartment, particularly after hysterectomy (Fig. 20.21). The physician should then place one finger in the rectum and one in the vagina and palpate the defect. Often the rectovaginal septum is paper thin, and the rectocele can be palpated to its upper margin. One finger in the rectum can also evaluate for the presence of a "pocket" or bulge into the vaginal canal where stool may get trapped. If an enterocele is present, it may be possible to differentiate it from the rectocele by having the patient strain. Frequently, however, the diagnosis of a small enterocele is established only at the time of operation. Evacuation symptoms suggestive of an obstructive process or seeming out of proportion to the degree of rectocele bear further investigation by an expert, possibly with anal manometry, defecography, or dynamic MRI.

### *Management*

Nonoperative management of a rectocele is similar to that mentioned for a cystocele. Pessaries, Kegel exercises, and estrogen may be useful in the appropriate situations. Gastrointestinal symptoms must be thoroughly evaluated, including screening for colorectal cancer if appropriate. If constipation and straining are issues, a dietary fiber and fluid intake review should be obtained. At least 25 g of fiber, adequate hydration, regular exercise, and allowing time for defecation after meals can be recommended to regulate bowel habits as first-line therapy. Polyethylene glycol can be used as needed if these first-line therapies do not adequately normalize stool consistency.

Operative management of posterior vaginal wall prolapse usually involves **posterior colporrhaphy** or a site-specific repair, plus or minus surgical correction of apical prolapse and

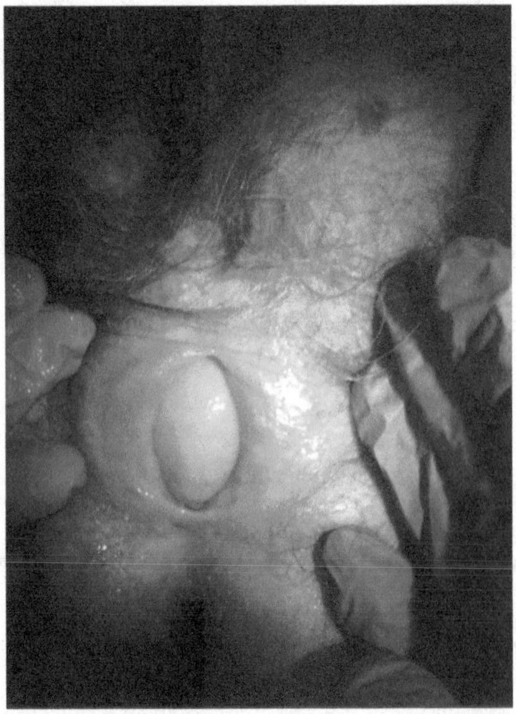

**Figure 20.20 Rectocele.** Although this may appear to be a cystocele, split speculum exam revealed a rectocele.

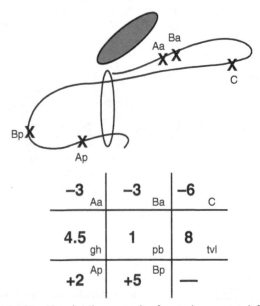

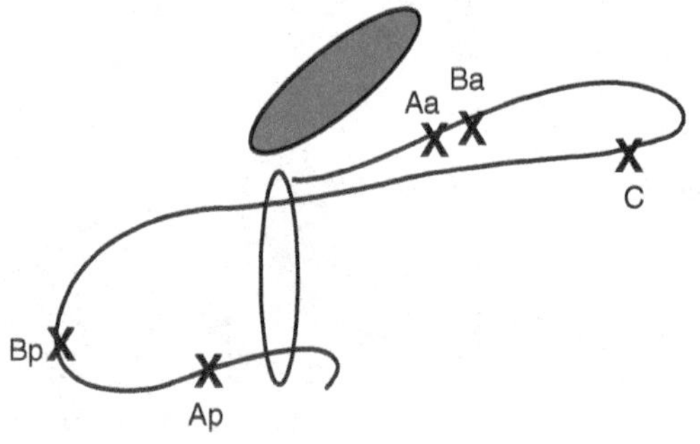


| | | |
|---|---|---|
| –3 Aa | –3 Ba | –6 C |
| 4.5 gh | 1 pb | 8 tvl |
| +2 Ap | +5 Bp | — |

**Figure 20.21** Line drawing example of posterior support defect. The anterior compartment is well supported. The leading point of the prolapse is point Bp (+5), which is 5 cm beyond the hymen. Total vaginal length is 8 cm, and point C (–6), the cuff position, has descended 2 cm. (From Bump RC, Mattiasson A, Bo K, et al. The standardization of terminology of female pelvic organ prolapse and pelvic floor dysfunction. *Am J Obstet Gynecol.* 1996;175[1]:10-17.)

anterior vaginal wall prolapse if present. Most women with posterior vaginal wall prolapse also have a gaping genital hiatus and a defect in their perineal body. Therefore, a **perineorrhaphy** to rebuild the perineal body is often performed at the same time, as shown in Figure 20.22. The surgeon should estimate at the time of starting the posterior repair what degree of perineorrhaphy he or she wishes to perform. The margins of the perineum to be narrowed are generally marked by placing Allis clamps on the hymen such that reapproximating the clamps results in a normal genital hiatus (Fig. 20.23). The tissue between these clamps is then removed with a scalpel or curved Mayo scissors. To perform a posterior colporrhaphy, the vaginal epithelium is incised in the midline to the top of the bulge or left intact depending on surgeon preference. The vaginal epithelium is separated from the underlying fibromuscular tissue laterally and proximally toward the apex of the vagina above the limit of the rectocele using sharp and blunt dissection. At this point, a site-specific repair, posterior colporrhaphy, or a combination of both can be performed to reduce the bulge. Both methods have high success rates.

To complete a posterior colporrhaphy either alone or in addition to a site-specific repair, after the vaginal wall is incised, the edges are grasped and placed under tension, and the perirectal connective tissue is separated from the vaginal epithelium by blunt and sharp (if necessary) dissection. This is carried out bilaterally until it is possible for the operator to palpate the perirectal

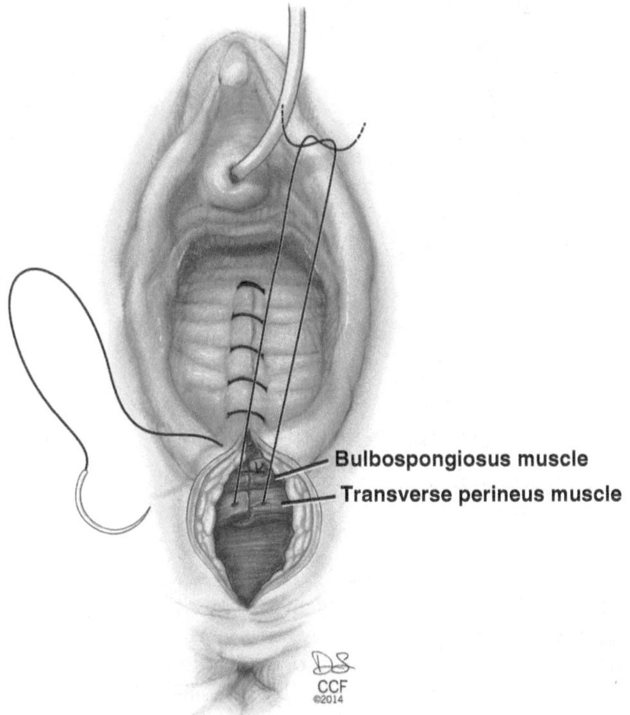


**Figure 20.22** Perineorrhaphy. Following the completion of the repair of the rectocele, the perineal body may need to be reconstructed. The bulbospongiosus and the superficial transverse peroneus muscles are plicated in the midline with absorbable sutures. (From Muir TW. Surgical treatment of rectocele and perineal defects. In Walters MD, Karram MM. *Urogynecology and Reconstructive Pelvic Surgery.* 4th ed. Philadelphia: Elsevier: 2015:342-359.)

space on each side. The operator then places a delayed absorbable suture into the perirectal fibromuscular tissue on either side and brings the tissue together in the midline. The operator may choose to place these sutures with one finger in the rectum, and if not, should at least check the rectum after the completion of the repair to ensure that no suture is placed into the rectum. When the sutures are tied, these tissues are interposed between rectum and vagina, thereby reducing the rectocele. Care must be taken to avoid creating a "shelf" in the posterior vaginal wall, which may narrow the vagina too much and lead to dyspareunia. Levator ani plication appears to increase dyspareunia, so it is not indicated in sexually active women.

To perform a site-specific posterior vaginal repair, the fibromuscularis is examined after the dissection is performed and any defects individually isolated and repaired with delayed absorbable suture.

If vaginal vault prolapse is also present, a separate repair is indicated for support of the vaginal apex, and this is discussed later. The vaginal edges are then trimmed and the vagina closed with a row of either continuous or interrupted absorbable sutures.

Attention is then turned to the perineorrhaphy when there is perineal muscle separation and a perineal body defect. It is closed in the following fashion. Absorbable sutures such as 0 Polyglycol sutures are placed in the lateral margins of the transverse incision, essentially bringing bulbocavernosal and superficial perineal muscles together from either side to the midline. The operator can be sure that the bulbocavernosal muscle insertions are included in the sutures by pulling on the suture and noting whether the tension identifies the muscle bundles. Overtightening the introitus may cause dyspareunia. The remainder of the perineal incision is then closed with a row of 2-0 polyglycol sutures to the deep tissue, and the skin of the perineum is closed with either interrupted or continuous subcuticular suture of 3-0 absorbable suture.

## RECURRENT POSTERIOR VAGINAL WALL PROLAPSE

Successful repair of posterior vaginal wall prolapse may be slightly higher for posterior colporrhaphy (96%) than site-specific repair (89%) when defined as no prolapse beyond the hymen; recurrence is uncommon. Because of low recurrence rates of posterior vaginal wall prolapse and the increased risks of augmenting posterior repairs with grafts, a Cochrane Review concluded that evidence does not support the use of any grafts at the time of posterior vaginal repair.[24] Although anatomic position is often corrected by a posterior repair, function may not be corrected. Defecatory problems may remain, so patients should be forewarned.

## ENTEROCELE

An **enterocele** is a herniation of the pouch of Douglas (cul-de-sac) between the uterosacral ligaments into the rectovaginal septum containing small bowel. It frequently occurs after an abdominal or vaginal hysterectomy and generally is the result of a weakened support for the pouch of Douglas and the loss of vaginal apical support by the uterosacral ligaments. To decrease the risk of developing an enterocele after a hysterectomy, the uterosacral and cardinal ligaments, which are the most important support

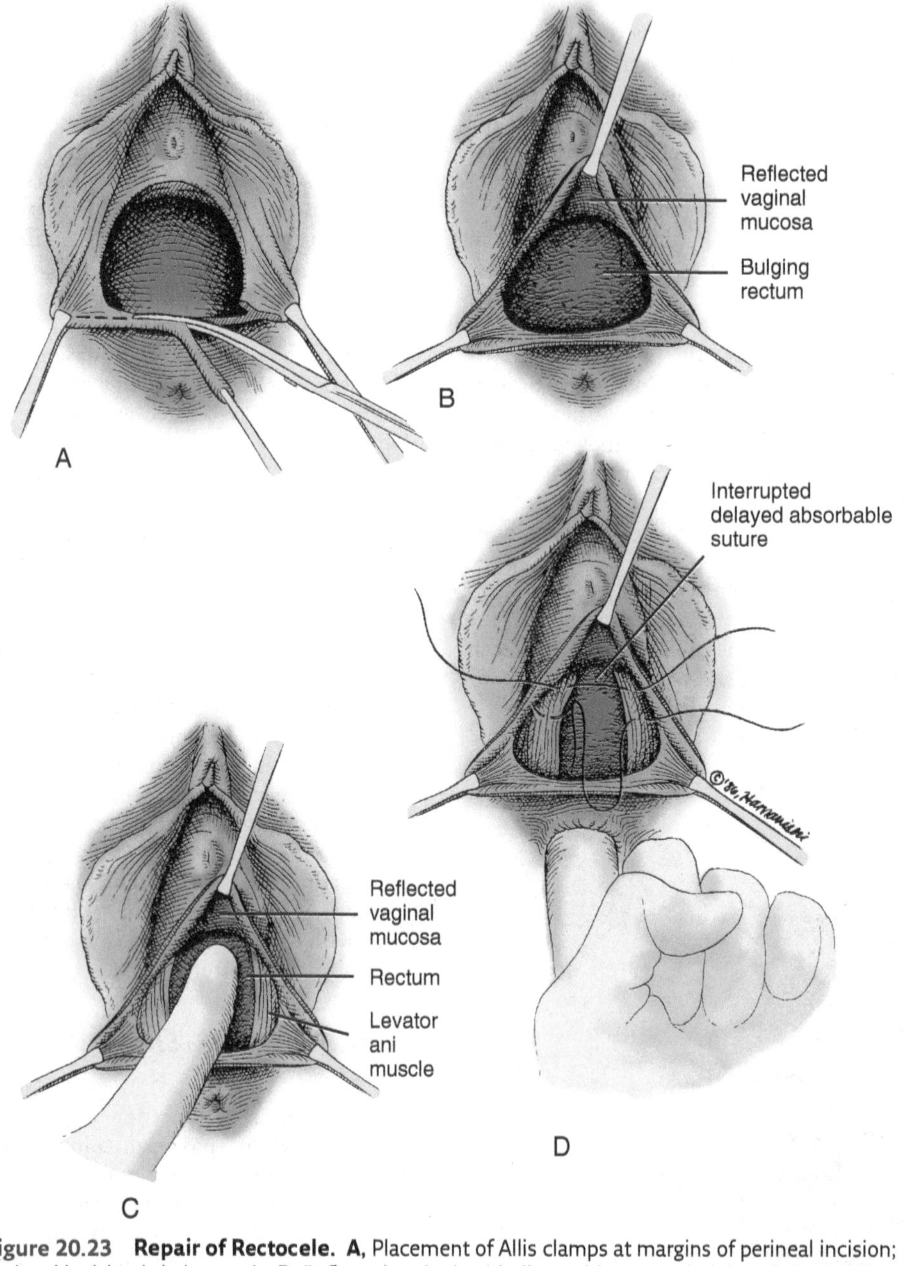


**Figure 20.23 Repair of Rectocele. A,** Placement of Allis clamps at margins of perineal incision; perineal incision is being made. **B,** Reflected vaginal epithelium with rectum bulging. **C,** Depression of rectum identifying margins of levator ani muscle. **D,** Placement of sutures in perirectal tissue and levator ani bundles.

structures for the vagina, should be incorporated into the vault repair as described later under Management.

### *Diagnosis*

An enterocele is not always easy to diagnose. It is a true hernia of the peritoneal cavity emanating from the pouch of Douglas between the uterosacral ligaments and into the rectovaginal septum (Figs. 20.24 and 20.25). It may be noticed as a separate bulge above the rectocele, and at times it may be large enough to prolapse through the vagina (Figs. 20.26 and 20.27). If such is the case, it may be possible to make the specific diagnosis of enterocele by transilluminating the bulge and seeing small bowel shadows within the sac. It may also be possible to differentiate the enterocele from a rectocele by rectovaginal examination. The contents of an enterocele are always small bowel and may also include omentum. The contents may be easily reducible or may be fixed to the peritoneum of the sac by adhesions.

### *Management*

Enteroceles may be managed expectantly if asymptomatic, or they can be treated with pessaries or surgery. They rarely occur in isolation, so surgical management usually also involves vaginal vault suspension as described later in this chapter with or without anterior and posterior repairs if indicated. When repairing an

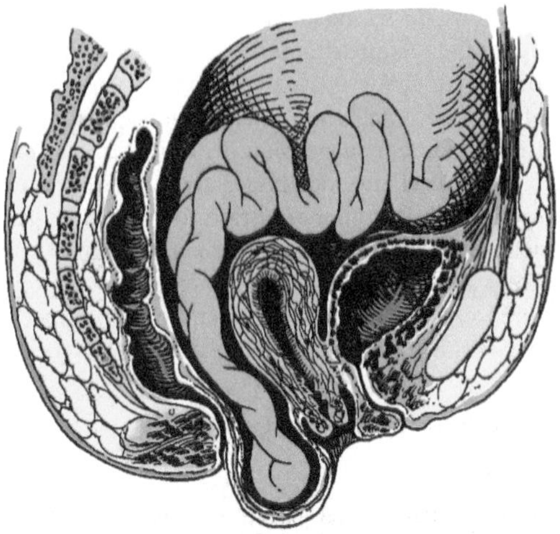

**Figure 20.24** Enterocele and uterine prolapse. (From Symmonds RE: Relaxation of pelvic supports. In Benson RC, ed. *Current Obstetric and Gynecologic Diagnosis and Treatment.* 5th ed. Los Altos, CA: Lange Medical; 1984.)

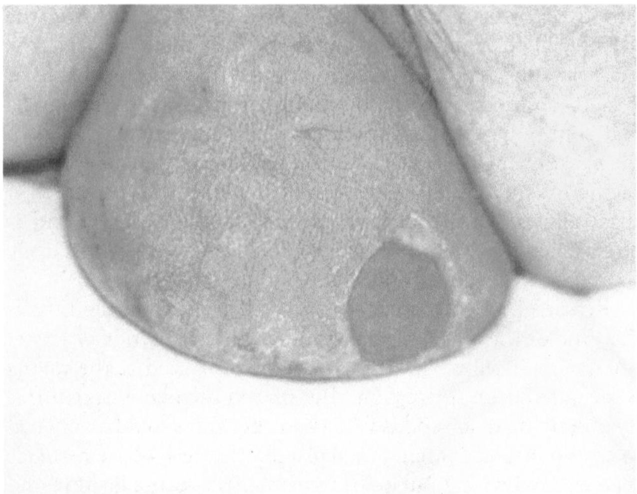

**Figure 20.26** Elderly patient with stage IV apical eversion and enterocele with vaginal ulcers.

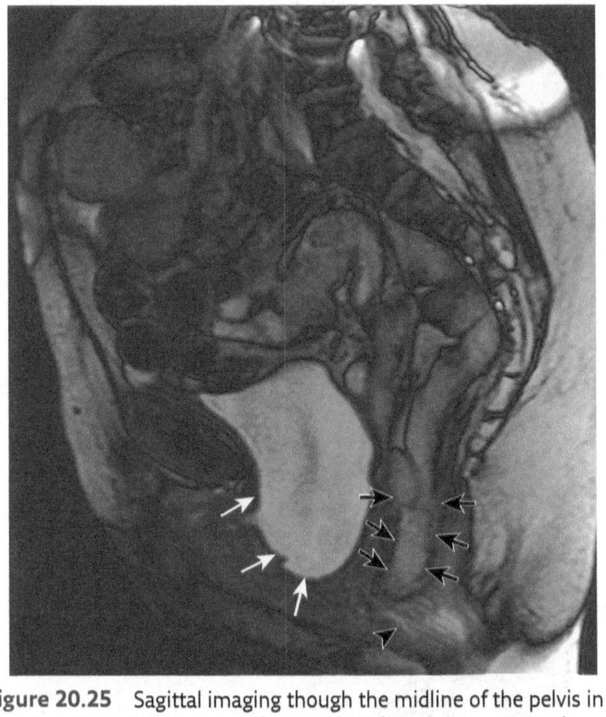

**Figure 20.25** Sagittal imaging though the midline of the pelvis in a female patient during magnetic resonance imaging proctography. A loop of small bowel has descended anterior to the rectum to form a large enterocele *(black arrows)*. Note the coexistent cystocele *(white arrows)* and small collapsed rectocele *(arrowhead)*. (From Taylor SA. Imaging pelvic floor dysfunction. *Best Pract Res Clin Gastroenterol.* 2009;23[4]:487-503.)

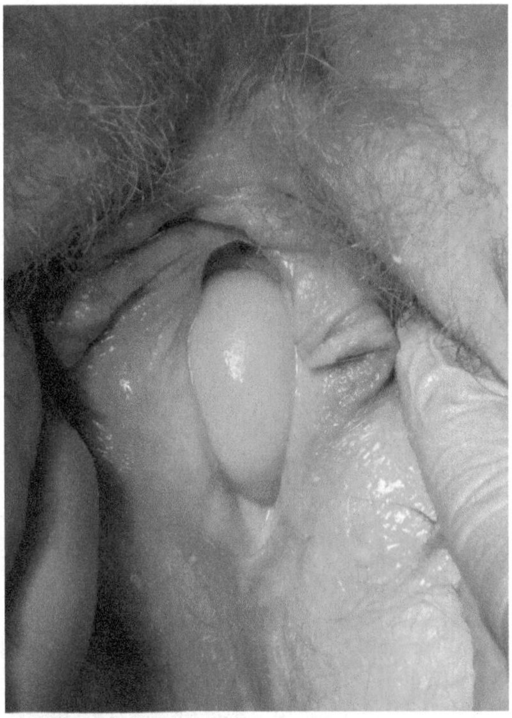

**Figure 20.27 Enterocele with Vaginal Apical Prolapse.** Split speculum exam and digital exam with palpation of bowel in the sac helped define this defect.

enterocele transabdominally, the sac should be reduced upward if possible and dissected free from the bladder and rectum. If the uterosacral ligaments are present, these may be brought together in the midline and attached to the vaginal cuff. If the uterosacral ligaments cannot be identified, as with large enteroceles after previously performed hysterectomy, concentric purse-string sutures in the connective tissue over the vagina and rectum may obliterate the cul-de-sac. Care must be taken to avoid damaging the ureters, rectum, and sigmoid colon. It is best to perform this procedure with permanent sutures. Because the enterocele has probably occurred because of weakening of the apical supports (uterosacral ligaments), an apical suspension surgery such as abdominal sacrocolpopexy is often necessary for resuspension and closure of the enterocele defect.

If uterosacral ligaments can be identified at the time of a vaginal hysterectomy, they can be used to repair and prevent enterocele formation. This can be accomplished by fixing the uterosacral ligaments to the peritoneum of the sac and the vaginal vault connective tissue using a suture of absorbable or delayed absorbable suture, beginning on one side of the vagina and continuing through the uterosacral ligament of that side, the peritoneum of the sac, and the uterosacral ligament and then vagina on the opposite side. Multiple sutures can be placed if space allows. This technique was described by McCall and is often called the *McCall stitch* or *McCall culdoplasty.* It effectively shortens the cul-de-sac and supports the enterocele neck.

Repair of an enterocele can be carried out transvaginally at the time of the apical repair with or without anterior or posterior vaginal wall repair. The sac will be visualized as the vagina is separated from the rectum. The sac can then be dissected free of underlying tissue and isolated at its neck. It should be opened to ensure that all contents are replaced. The neck of the hernia is then sutured with a purse-string permanent suture ligature and the sac excised (Fig. 20.28).

It is important to support the neck of the enterocele sac as much as possible. Approximating the anterior and posterior vaginal connective tissue is also important to close the defect. Usually with an enterocele, support of the vaginal apex such as a sacrospinous ligament suspension is needed for optimal repair.

Correctly repaired enteroceles usually will not recur. Enteroceles repaired without proper attention to ligation of the neck of the sac, closure of the anterior and posterior vaginal connective tissue of the vaginal cuff, and concurrent rectocele repair may recur. In such cases, a subsequent operation with special attention to these surgical principles is indicated.

## UTERINE PROLAPSE (DESCENSUS, PROCIDENTIA)

Prolapse of the uterus and cervix into or through the barrel of the vagina is associated with injuries of the endopelvic connective tissue and level I support structures, including the cardinal and uterosacral

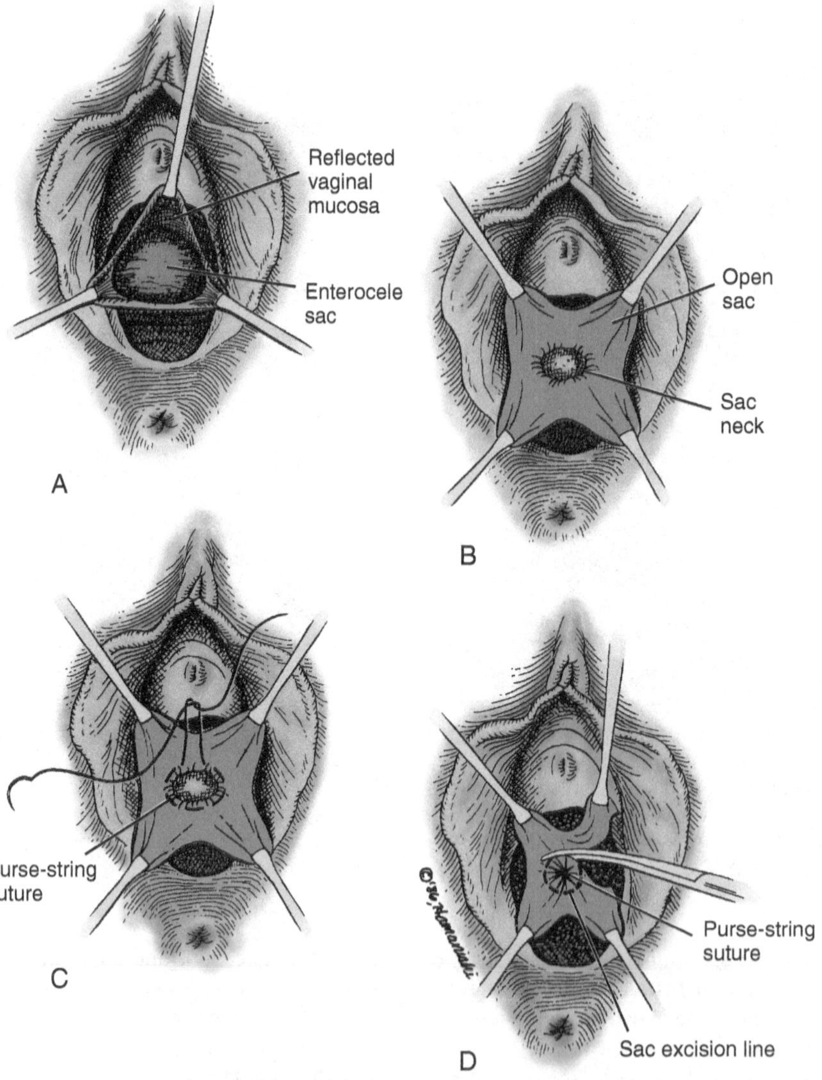


**Figure 20.28 Repair of Enterocele. A,** Appearance of enterocele sac with vaginal wall reflected. **B,** Appearance of open enterocele sac with sac neck identified. **C,** Placing of purse-string suture at the neck of the enterocele sac. **D,** Excision of enterocele sac.

ligaments, as well as injury to the neuromuscular unit with relaxation of the pelvic floor muscles, particularly the levator ani muscles (Fig. 20.29). Uterine prolapse is almost always associated with rectocele and cystocele and, at times, enterocele, supporting the concept of overall damage to the pelvic support structures.

### *Symptoms and Signs*

Again, common symptoms noted by patients with uterine prolapse are a feeling of pelvic pressure and heaviness, fullness, bulge or "falling out" in the perineal area. Because uterine prolapse is almost always associated with anterior and posterior vaginal wall prolapse, symptoms that were reported earlier for cystocele and rectocele may be present as well. In cases in which the cervix and uterus are low in the vaginal canal, the cervix may be seen protruding from the introitus, giving the patient the impression that a tumor is bulging out of her vagina. Where stage III or IV prolapse has occurred, the patient may be aware that a mass has actually prolapsed out of the introitus. In stage IV prolapse, the vagina is everted around the uterus and cervix and completely exteriorized. When this occurs, the patient is in danger of developing dryness, thickening, and chronic inflammation of the vaginal epithelium and cervix. She may also have pain and bleeding, for example, from ulcerations. There is often discharge, and secondary infection can occur. Stasis ulcers may result from edema and interference with blood supply to the vaginal wall. Evisceration of abdominal contents is a rare complication, but a surgical emergency. In almost every case of acquired prolapse, the perineal supports are poor, and the perineal body is damaged.

### *Management*

As with other forms of prolapse, mild or asymptomatic uterine prolapse does not need treatment or can be treated with pelvic floor muscle strengthening. If the prolapse is causing symptoms, infection, urinary retention, or hydronephrosis (from ureteral kinking), it can be treated with a pessary or surgery. Degrees of prolapse that place the cervix at or through the introitus probably cause greater discomfort and are usually more bothersome to the patient.

Nonoperative management of such conditions involves the use of a pessary (see Fig. 20.17). All women should be offered pessary management for prolapse. Pessary management should be particularly encouraged rather than surgery in women with medical conditions that make surgery dangerous (i.e., poor surgical candidates) and in women who have not completed childbearing. Pessaries involve replacement of the uterus to its normal position in the pelvis and then the institution of support using one of these devices. Pessaries are available in varying shapes and sizes and should be properly fitted to the patient. In general, the perineum must be capable of holding the pessary in place, or the pessary will frequently fall out. There is currently no evidence from randomized controlled trials on pessary use to direct the selection of the device or to compare pessaries with other treatments or surgery. The ring pessary is the most commonly used shape. Usually a support pessary is tried first, such as a ring or Gehrung because they are easier for the patient to use. Space-occupying pessaries such as the cube, Gellhorn, donut, and inflatoball, are a second option. Gellhorn pessaries may be more successfully fit for stage IV POP more often than rings, but it is reasonable to start with the smallest and easiest to use shapes first. A prospective trial found that 75% of 203 women fitted with a pessary successfully retained the device at 2 weeks (Fernando, 2006). Failure to retain the pessary was significantly associated with increasing parity, prior POP surgery, and past hysterectomy. Forty-eight percent of the women completed a questionnaire at 4 months. The pessary reduced symptoms of POP, including general symptoms of a vaginal bulge. It also relieved urinary symptoms such as voiding problems in 40% of women, urinary urgency in 38%, urgency urinary incontinence in 29%, bowel evacuation in 28%, fecal urgency in 23%, and urge fecal incontinence by 20%. There was no improvement in stress urinary incontinence.

Complications from vaginal pessaries are rare with proper use. This includes regular removal, cleaning, and replacement, as well as use of vaginal estrogen cream for postmenopausal women with vaginal atrophy. Complications include vaginal infections, bleeding, discomfort, vaginal erosion and ulceration, and pessary incarceration. More serious complications such as erosion into the bladder and rectum have been rarely reported, usually from neglect.

If a woman with advanced prolapse is pregnant, it is important to replace the uterus before it enlarges and becomes trapped in the lower pelvis or vagina. If this happens, edema may cause incarceration and even loss of blood supply to the uterus. In a postmenopausal woman, estrogen replacement for at least 30 days with vaginal estrogen cream may help improve the vitality of the vaginal epithelium, the cervix, and the vasculature of these organs, making fitting of a pessary or the operative procedure and the healing process more efficient.

Operative repair for prolapse of the uterus and cervix can be transabdominal or transvaginal. The surgical approach will depend on patient comorbidities, patient preferences regarding risks and durability, and surgeon expertise. Common surgical options to treat uterovaginal prolapse include vaginal hysterectomy with vault suspension to the uterosacral or sacrospinous ligaments, abdominal (open, laparoscopic, or robotic) supracervical hysterectomy with sacrocolpopexy, and colpocleisis. Other surgeries including abdominal (open laparoscopic, or robotic) uterosacral ligament suspension with or without hysterectomy, transvaginal hysteropexy with or without mesh sacrohysteropexy, and Manchester procedures can be appropriate for some patients. Sacrocolpopexy, which is described in more detail in

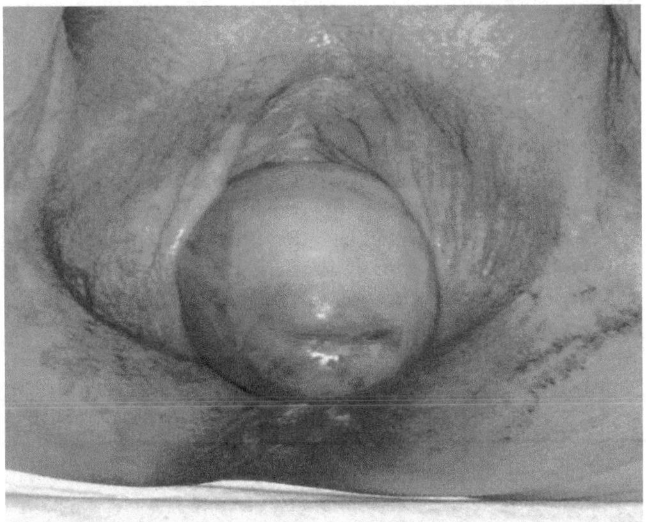

**Figure 20.29** Uterine prolapse.

the Vaginal Vault Prolapse (Apical Prolapse after Hysterectomy) section, is the most durable surgery for apical prolapse but has more surgical risks than vaginal surgeries.

Transvaginal repair usually involves a vaginal hysterectomy followed by a vaginal vault suspension to the uterosacral or sacrospinous ligaments. The uterosacral ligaments can be sutured together so that the cul-de-sac is shortened or obliterated as in a McCall culdoplasty described previously, or the vaginal vault can supported high up to the uterosacral or sacrospinous ligaments. High uterosacral ligament and sacrospinous ligament suspensions are described in the Vaginal Vault Prolapse (Apical Prolapse after Hysterectomy) section presented later in this chapter.

The American College of Obstetricians and Gynecologists' 2009 committee opinion and a Cochrane systematic review the same year suggest that vaginal hysterectomy is associated with better outcomes and fewer complications than laparoscopic or abdominal hysterectomy (ACOG, 2009). This is a general recommendation, and with POP, often there are many other considerations including concomitant procedures needed, concern about failure rates, and restoration of bowel, bladder, and sexual function. In some cases, a vaginal hysterectomy is not advisable, and the optimal route of hysterectomy depends on many factors, including the size and shape of the uterus, accessibility to the uterus, surgeon training and experience, and planned concurrent surgical procedures. In cases in which an abdominal, laparoscopically assisted vaginal, or total laparoscopic hysterectomy is preferable, an apical suspension can be performed vaginally or abdominally, and anterior and posterior colporrhaphy can be performed vaginally if needed.

In some women the cervix is hypertrophied and elongated to the area of the introitus, but the supports of the uterus itself are intact. A cystocele and rectocele may be present, and operative repair can consist of a **Manchester** (Donald or Fothergill) operation. This operation combines an anterior and posterior colporrhaphy with the amputation of the cervix and the use of the cardinal ligaments to support the anterior vaginal wall and bladder. Although it was suggested for repair in young women who wish to maintain their reproductive abilities, the loss of the cervix may interfere with fertility or lead to incompetence of the internal cervical os. The operation has value in elderly women with comorbid medical conditions who have an elongated cervix and well-supported uterus because it is technically easier and has a shorter operative time than the vaginal hysterectomy in such cases, and the entering of the peritoneal cavity is avoided.

In elderly women who are no longer sexually active, a simple and effective procedure for reducing prolapse is an obliterative procedure called a **colpocleisis**. The classic partial colpocleisis procedure was described by Le Fort in 1877 (Fig. 20.30) and involves the removal of a strip of anterior and posterior vaginal wall, with approximation of the anterior and posterior walls to each other. This procedure may be performed with or without the presence of a uterus and cervix, and when it is completed, the vaginal cavity is nearly completely closed, with small vaginal canals on either side of the opposed vaginal walls to allow drainage of any fluid from the cuff or uterus. Dissection of the vaginal wall is carried to the level of the bladder neck anteriorly and to the reflection of bladder onto the cervix at the upper margin of the vagina. Posteriorly the dissection is carried from just inside the introitus to a position just posterior to the cervix. If a hysterectomy has been previously performed, the dissection may begin approximately 1 cm on either side of the vaginal scar. Canals are left on each lateral vaginal wall to allow drainage from the cervix or apex. If the cervix and uterus are still present and intrauterine pathology occurs, bleeding through these canals can alert the physician to a potential problem. In low-risk women, no evaluation for uterine pathology is necessary prior to colpocleisis. In women with risk factors, however, a cervical or endometrial evaluation should be completed prior to colpocleisis because colpocleisis makes access to these organs difficult. If there is cervical or uterine pathology, the uterus and cervix should not be left in situ. Cystoscopy should be performed to assess bladder and ureteral integrity after the procedure is completed.

A large perineorrhaphy is usually performed in association with the colpocleisis. Together, these procedures result in a short vagina of approximately 3 cm and a small genital hiatus of about 1 to 2 cm. The patient can be reassured that her external genitalia look completely normal and that her risk of prolapse recurrence is small. Cystoscopy and rectal examination are important to ensure no bladder, rectal, or ureteral injury after prolapse surgery. An anti-incontinence operation such as a midurethral synthetic sling may be carried out if the patient has stress urinary incontinence or stress urinary incontinence on prolapse reduction, either at the time of surgery or as an interval procedure.

The **Goodall-Power modification** of the Le Fort operation (Fig. 20.31) allows for the removal of a triangular piece of vaginal wall beginning at the cervical reflection or 1 cm above the vaginal scar at the base of the triangle, with the apex of the triangle just beneath the bladder neck anteriorly and just at the introitus posteriorly. The cut edge of vaginal wall making up the base of the triangle anteriorly is sutured to the similar wall posteriorly, and the vaginal incision is then closed with a row of interrupted sutures beginning beneath the bladder neck and carried side to side to the area of the introitus. This procedure works well for relatively small prolapses, whereas the Le Fort is best for larger ones.

Prognosis for a colpocleisis procedure to reduce the prolapse and prevent recurrence is generally excellent. Case series report 91% to 100% success rates. Careful counseling must be done preoperatively to be sure the woman will never desire coital activity because occasional regret over closure of the vagina has been reported. Overall, patient satisfaction is high, and regret is low (Vij, 2014).

In a comparison of 25 elderly women (average age 82 years) in poor health with uterovaginal prolapse treated by colpocleisis with 42 younger women with similar prolapse treated with vaginal hysterectomy, anterior colporrhaphy, and posterior colporrhaphy, the average operating time for the Le Fort procedure was 75 minutes compared with 150 minutes for the vaginal hysterectomy. There was one postoperative death in the Le Fort group, but 19 of the 20 remaining Le Fort patients had excellent results for a follow-up of an average of 25 months (range of 4 to 40 months) (Denehy, 1995).

A special circumstance involves the treatment of women who wish to maintain their fertility despite the fact that they have symptomatic uterine prolapse. As noted, pessary is preferable to surgery for these women. However, there are small

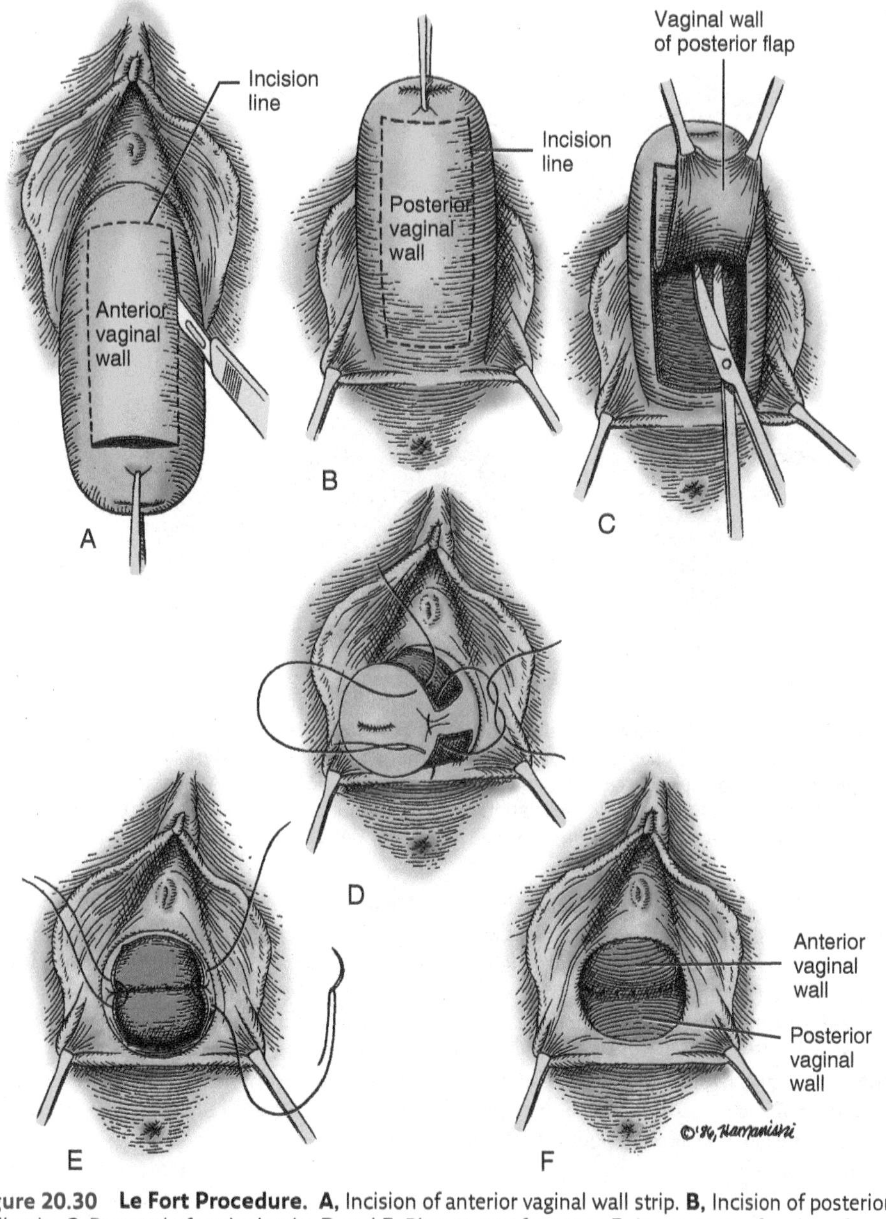


**Figure 20.30 Le Fort Procedure.** **A,** Incision of anterior vaginal wall strip. **B,** Incision of posterior wall strip. **C,** Removal of vaginal strip. **D** and **E,** Placement of sutures. **F,** Appearance of vagina after procedure is completed but before perineorrhaphy is performed.

studies suggesting surgical treatment may be an option. There was one small case series in which the authors sutured bilateral uterosacral ligaments to the sacrospinous ligaments to reduce the prolapse. Eighteen of the 19 women had good anatomic restoration, and five subsequently delivered babies (Kovac, 1993). An uncontrolled trial of laparoscopic uterosacral ligament uterine suspension versus vaginal hysterectomy and vault suspension reported excellent support as measured by POP-Q, and no laparoscopic uterine suspension patient had reoperation for recurrence (Diwan, 2006). Laparoscopic hysteropexy (sacrocervicopexy with uterine preservation) has also been described. In a case series of 40 women who desired retention of fertility, 1 year after surgery the cervix was on average 4.84 cm above the hymenal ring (Rosenblatt, 2008). With only small studies and case series, it is unclear what the role of uterine suspension should be in current practice and the longevity of such repairs. Young women with POP who desire further childbearing should be encouraged to try a pessary first.

## VAGINAL VAULT PROLAPSE (APICAL PROLAPSE AFTER HYSTERECTOMY)

Prolapse of the vaginal apex at some time remote to the performance of either abdominal or vaginal hysterectomy has been reported as occurring in 0.1% to 18.2% of patients, with 5% of women having surgery for posthysterectomy POP (Blandon, 2007). Apical prolapse may be accompanied by a cystocele, a rectocele, an enterocele, or some combination thereof. Occasionally the prolapse involves only one of those entities and not the entire vaginal apex. In a study in Munich, Richter reported that of 97 posthysterectomy prolapses,

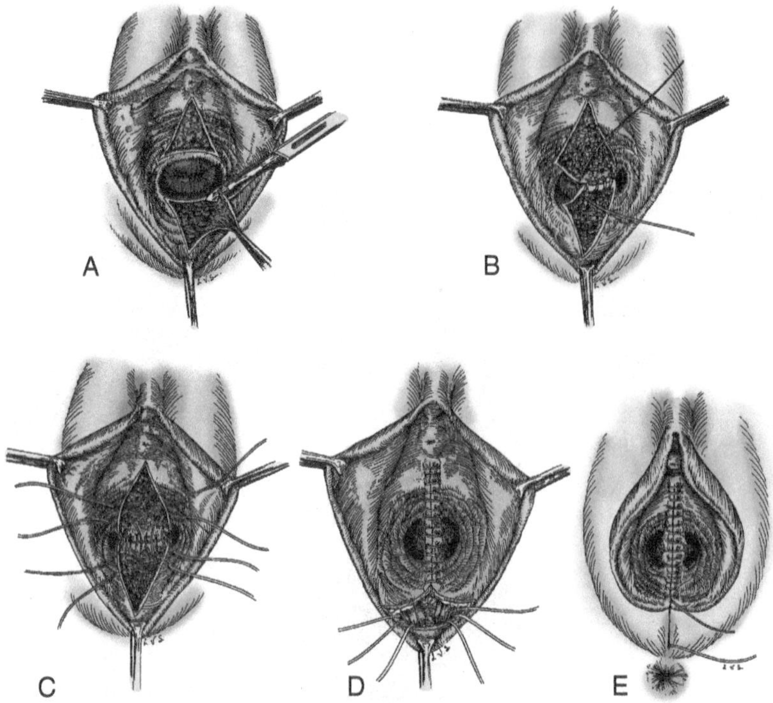


**Figure 20.31 Goodall-Power modification of Le Fort operation. A,** Representation of vaginal incision on anterior and posterior wall. **B,** Early placement of sutures. **C,** Later placement of sutures. **D,** Vaginal incision completely closed; perineorrhaphy being performed. **E,** Appearance at completion of procedure. (From Symmonds RE. Relaxation of pelvic supports. In: Benson RC, ed. *Current Obstetric and Gynecologic Diagnosis and Treatment,* 5th ed. Los Altos, CA: Lange Medical; 1984.)

6.2% were cystocele only, 5.1% rectocele only, 9.3% primarily an enterocele type, and 72.2% of mixed type (Richter, 1982). It is rare to find isolated support defects of the anterior or posterior vaginal walls or an isolated apical defect (Rooney, 2006). Vaginal vault prolapse is probably the result of continuing pelvic support defects in the connective tissues, namely, the cardinal and uterosacral ligaments attachments to the vaginal cuff. Multiple vaginal wall defects are usually found because the connective tissue defects, the pelvic floor muscles, and innervation are globally affected and usually not isolated damage to one site.

### *Symptoms and Signs*

Symptoms and signs of vaginal apex prolapse are similar to those delineated for uterine prolapse. They include pelvic heaviness, backache, a mass protruding through the introitus, vaginal bleeding or discharge, and discomfort sitting or walking. Bladder and rectal symptoms can include stress incontinence, urinary urgency, urinary frequency, incomplete bladder emptying, difficult bowel movements, and splinting to void or defecate.

### *Diagnosis*

POP-Q or other quantitative measurements should be performed, as with other forms of prolapse, to ensure that all three compartments are considered: anterior, apical, and posterior. Examination may help determine the contents of the herniation depending on where the vaginal scar is located in relation to the protruding mass and the extent to which the supports of the pelvis are lost. Rectovaginal examination is often helpful in delineating an enterocele from a rectocele.

### *Management*

As with other POP, if not bothersome and not causing excessive kinking of the urethra or ureters, vaginal vault prolapse can be managed expectantly or with pelvic floor muscle strengthening. Vaginal estrogen can be used to treat ulcerations. Pessaries should be offered and attempted if preferable to the patient; unfortunately, however, prior hysterectomy makes successful pessary fitting difficult because the pessaries are more likely to fall out.

For operative management, the first guiding principle is that the normal position of the vagina in the standing position is against the rectum and no more than 30 degrees from the horizontal (Fig. 20.32). The second principle is that pelvic relaxation is a part of the problem and dictates that an existing cystocele, rectocele, or enterocele may need to be repaired as part of the procedure, particularly if correction of the apical defect does not reduce all the prolapsed compartments. The third principle acknowledges that the perineal body is almost always severely weakened in such patients and must therefore be reconstructed as well. The choices of operative procedures are many and may be approached abdominally, vaginally, laparoscopically, robotically, or some combination thereof. Benefits of vaginal surgery are generally shorter operative times, fewer complications, and quicker return to daily activities. Benefits of abdominal (whether open, laparoscopic, or robotic-assisted laparoscopic) include improved durability but with increased operative time and risks. Randomized, controlled trials are few, but a systematic review suggests that abdominal sacrocolpopexy for apical prolapse has higher success rates than sacrospinous colpopexy with less stress

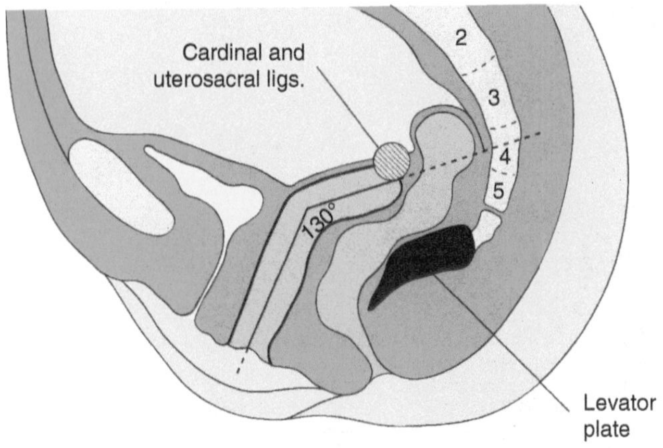


**Figure 20.32** Normal vaginal axis of nulliparous woman in the standing position. Note that the upper third of the vagina is nearly horizontal and is directed toward the S3 and S4 sacral vertebrae. (From Funt MI, Thompson JD, Birch H. Normal vaginal axis. *South Med J.* 1978;71[12]:1534.)

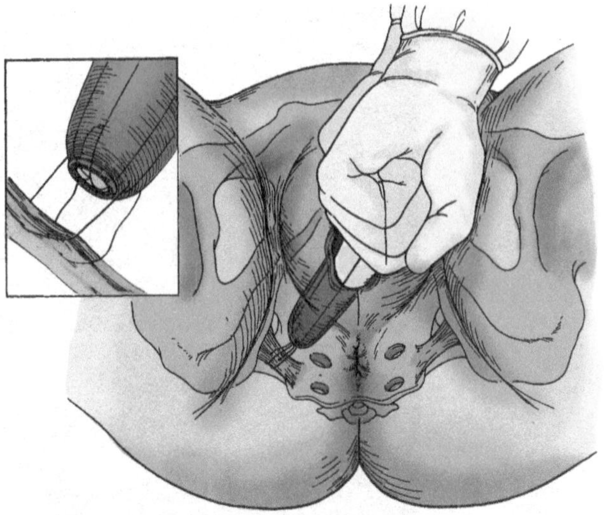

**Figure 20.33** Sutures tied to bring the vaginal apex into contact with the sacrospinous ligament. The apex should approximate the ligament such that there is no "suture bridge." (Modified from Morley GW, DeLancey JOL. Sacrospinous ligament fixation for eversion of the vagina. *Am J Obstet Gynecol.* 1988;158:872.)

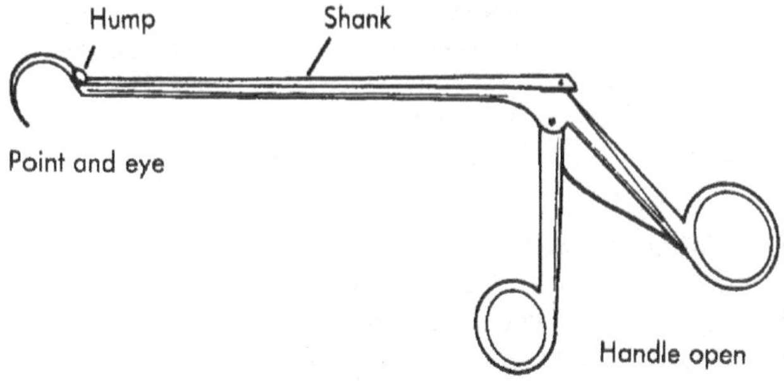


**Figure 20.34** The Miyazaki hook ligature carrier. (From Miyazaki FS. Miya hook ligature carrier for sacrospinous ligament suspension. *Obstet Gynecol.* 1987;70:286.)

incontinence and less dyspareunia. However, it has greater morbidity, including operating time, length of hospital stay, and time to return to normal activity, and it is also associated with higher cost (Barber, 2013). The material of choice for sacrocolpopexies is type 1 wide pore, monofilament polypropylene mesh.

For transvaginal procedures, goals include maintaining adequate vaginal length and supporting the vagina nearly parallel to the horizontal. A randomized controlled trial of 374 women assigned to transvaginal fixation to the uterosacral ligaments or the sacrospinous ligaments found comparably good success rates: 15% of women in the trial had prolapse beyond the hymen 2 years after surgery, and only 5% required treatment for recurrent prolapse with pessary or surgery (Barber, 2014). The overall rate of perioperative adverse events was comparable between the procedures, including less than 1% risk of urethral, major vascular, or rectal injury, and a 3% risk of blood transfusion. Vaginal granulation and suture exposures were seen in approximately 15% of patients. Neurologic pain was higher in the sacrospinous ligament group (12%) than in the uterosacral group (7%). Ureteral obstruction was only seen in the uterosacral group (3%), and all but one was recognized and successfully managed intraoperatively. Mesh augmentation for vaginal vault prolapse is an alternative with some evidence to support it in terms of anatomic outcomes; however, as noted previously, it has higher complication rates and should only be placed by surgeons with adequate training to minimize complications.

**Sacrospinous ligament suspension** is performed by dissecting the vaginal epithelium off the underlying fibromuscular tissue all the way down through the perirectal space to the right ischial spine and then clearing off the sacrospinous ligament medial to the ischial spine. The surgeon must first identify the apex of the vagina and ensure that it will reach the ligament without tension. The vaginal incision can be in the anterior, apical, or posterior vaginal wall. After the dissection is complete, sutures are placed through the sacrospinous ligament 2 fingerbreadths medial to the ischial spine while the rectum is manually deflected medially. Figure 20.33 depicts the fixation of the vaginal vault to the sacrospinous ligament and the direction of the vagina after the procedure. Care must be taken to place the sutures sufficiently medially to avoid pudendal nerve injury. This space is deep and tight, and several techniques and devices have been designed to assist with passage of the sutures through the sacrospinous ligament, including the Miyazaki hook ligature carrier (Fig. 20.34) and Deschamps ligature carrier with nerve hook, both of which require direct visualization of the ligament using Breisky-Navratil retractors. Other systems have been adopted from other fields such as the Shutt suture punch system from orthopedics (Sharp, 1993), and the Endo Stitch (Covidien) autosuturing device from laparoscopic surgery. The Capio (Boston Scientific) was specifically designed for prolapse surgery. Mesh kits for apical support procedures often have their own methods of attachment to the sacrospinous ligaments (Fig. 20.35).

Operative risks of sacrospinous colpopexy include injury to the pudendal and inferior gluteal arteries and the pudendal and sciatic nerves. Rectal injury is rare, although care must be taken when dissecting the rectal pillars to reach the ligament and to retract the bowel away when placing the sutures. The iliococcygeal ligament can be used in cases in which the vagina is not

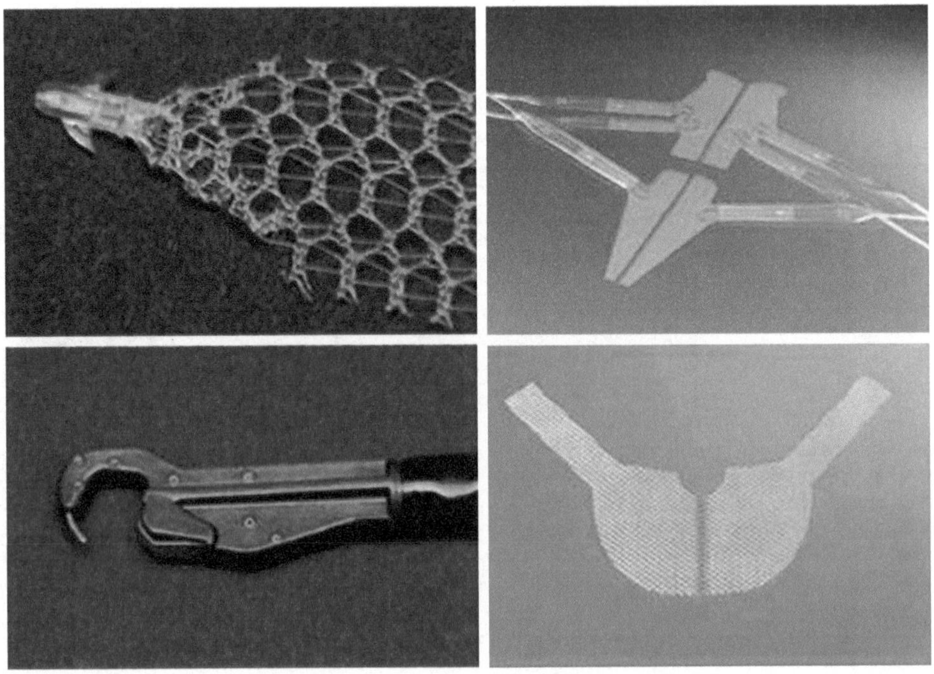

**Figure 20.35 Trocarless Mesh Delivery Systems.** *Upper left,* Elevate tined delivery system by American Medical Systems. *Lower left,* Capio needle driver for Boston Scientific products. *Upper right,* Pinnacle mesh system by Boston Scientific. *Lower right,* Uphold anterior mesh system by Boston Scientific. (From Evans J, Karram M. Repair of pelvic organ prolapse using synthetic mesh kits. In: Nitti VW, ed. *Vaginal Surgery for the Urologist.* Philadelphia: Elsevier; 2012:89-104.)

long enough to reach the sacrospinous ligament without excessive tension. It has a similar risk profile with respect to recurrent cystocele, buttock pain, and hemorrhage and only slightly inferior subjective success rates (91% compared with 94%) and patient satisfaction (71% compared with 91% on a visual analog scale 0-100) (Maher, 2001).

**Uterosacral ligament suspension** offers theoretic advantages for apical support because, unlike the sacrospinous ligaments, these units are support structures in normal anatomy and replace the vagina in its normal anatomic position. However, as noted earlier, clinical trials do not suggest any advantage over sacrospinous ligament suspension (Barber, 2014). To perform this procedure, the anterior and posterior vaginal walls are opened in the midline, and the enterocele sac is opened to enter the peritoneal cavity (Shull, 2000). It is commonly performed after vaginal hysterectomy, when the peritoneal cavity is already open, or it can be performed open or laparoscopically at the time of other abdominal or laparoscopic procedures. After packing the bowel out of the field, the uterosacral ligaments can be identified and grasped with a long Allis clamp, taking care to avoid the ureter. A series of two or three sutures are placed high in each uterosacral ligament near the level of the ischial spine and then used to resupport the vaginal apex with the anterior vaginal endopelvic connective tissue and the posterior vaginal rectovaginal septum closed together. Any enterocele defect is closed with this technique, and any residual anterior or posterior vaginal wall prolapse can be further reduced with colporrhaphy.

Cystoscopy must be performed at the end of the procedure to ensure ureteral patency by looking for brisk efflux of urine from each ureteral orifice because there is as high as 11% rate of intraoperative ureteral kinking that requires removal and replacement of the offending sutures (3% in the trial described earlier). Some surgeons prefer to perform cystoscopy midprocedure with the uterosacral sutures on tension before they are placed through the vaginal apex because they are easier to remove and replace at that time. They must repeat cystoscopy to ensure ureteral patency at the end of the procedure as well. Injury to the sacral nerves from sutures that are placed too deeply in the sidewall has also been reported and usually presents as pain.

For the abdominal surgical treatment of vaginal vault prolapse, a variety of procedures have been tried, and sacrocolpopexy appears to be the most successful. Other methods of transabdominal apical support include fixation of the vaginal vault to the anterior abdominal wall, to the lumbar spine, to the sacral promontory, to various tendinous lines in the musculature of the true pelvis (e.g., paravaginal repair to the arcus tendineus), and to the sacrospinous ligament. The anterior abdominal wall fixation increases the diameters of the pouch of Douglas and frequently adds to the risk of subsequent enterocele development, often creating a recurrence in short order. Fixation to the lumbar spine or the sacral promontory is often difficult to achieve directly and requires the interposition of a graft to perform a sacrocolpopexy. Wide-pore, monofilament polypropylene mesh is what is most commonly used today due to decrease complications compared to braided mesh with small pores and due to reduced recurrence rates compared to biologic materials such as cadaveric fascia and fascial aponeurosis from the patient (Culligan, 2005).

The technique for performing a **sacrocolpopexy** is essentially the same whether it is performed through a laparotomy, with laparoscopy, or with robotic-assisted laparoscopy. The vagina is

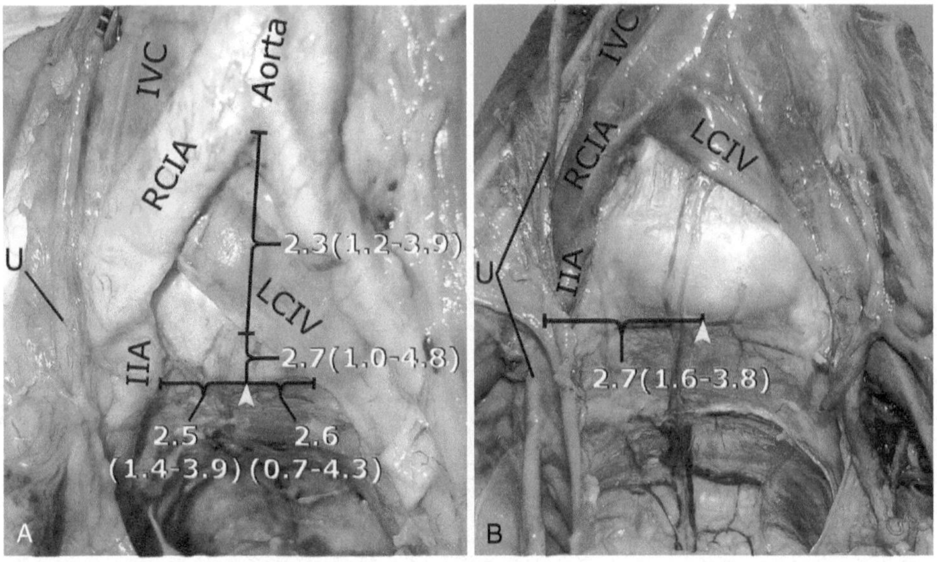


**Figure 20.36** Exposed presacral space in two unembalmed cadavers. These exposed presacral space illustrate the average distances (in centimeters) and range from midsacral promontory *(yellow arrowhead)* to (**A**) the vascular structures and to (**B**) the right ureter. Note the proximity of LCIV to the midsacral promontory in the cadaver on **A** *(left panel)*. *IIA*, Internal iliac artery; *LCIV*, the left common iliac vein; *RCIA*, right common iliac artery; *U*, ureter. (From Good MM, Abele TA, Balgobin S, et al. Vascular and ureteral anatomy relative to the midsacral promontory. *Am J Obstet Gynecol*. 2013;208[6]:486.e1-486.e7.)

dissected away from the bladder and rectum, and then the mesh graft is sutured to the anterior and posterior vaginal walls. A bridge of mesh extends to sacrum, where it is affixed to the anterior longitudinal ligament over first sacral vertebral body (S1) in a tension-free manner. Care must be taken when performing the dissection to access the anterior longitudinal ligament to avoid the middle sacral artery and the plexus of veins in its vicinity. The mesh graft should be made retroperitoneal by closing the peritoneum over it, theoretically to reduce internal hernias and adhesions that could result in small bowel obstruction, which nonetheless can occur in one in 400 of cases. After sacrocolpopexy, the pouch of Douglas may still be large enough to allow an enterocele to develop. Therefore some surgeons also perform a culdoplasty to obliterate the cul-de-sac.

Operative complications from abdominal sacrocolpopexy include cystotomy (3.1%), enterotomy (1.6%), wound problems (4.6%), ileus (3.6%), thromboembolic event (3.3%), ureteral injury (1%), hemorrhage or transfusion (4.4%), and small bowel obstruction (1% to 5%) (Nygaard, 2004). As with vaginally placed mesh, synthetic mesh for sacrocolpopexies can result in vaginal exposures or bladder or bowel erosions, although the rates of mesh complications for mesh placed abdominally is less than that for mesh placed vaginally. Some operative risks are decreased with minimally invasive techniques (laparoscopy, robot) compared to laparotomy. One of the most dreaded operative complications is presacral hemorrhage when dissecting or placing sutures over the sacrum due to the proximity of large vessels and presacral plexuses (Fig. 20.36). Care must be taken to visualize the blood vessels and be prepared in the event of hemorrhage.

As with other POP surgeries, abdominal sacrocolpopexy can unmask stress urinary incontinence. A multicenter study of 322 women with no preoperative stress incontinence symptoms were randomized to have a concomitant Burch colposuspension or not (controls). Three months after surgery, 24% of women in the Burch group and 44% of controls had stress incontinence, even though none reported stress incontinence preoperatively. Burch colposuspension significantly reduced postoperative stress incontinence when performed at the time of abdominal sacrocolpopexy, without an increase in other urinary problems (Brubaker, 2006). Now that Burch colposuspensions have largely been replaced by midurethral slings, it is less imperative to preemptively treat stress incontinence at the time of a sacrocolpopexy. Surgeons and patients have the option of concomitant anti-incontinence surgery in the form of a midurethral sling or Burch at the time of sacrocolpopexy or performing an interval midurethral sling surgery if indicated postoperatively.

In elderly women who are no longer sexually active, and particularly in those who have medical reasons to avoid a longer procedure, a Le Fort–type **colpocleisis** operation may be performed with an excellent result, low complication rate, and low recurrence rate. This procedure was discussed in detail in the uterine prolapse section of this chapter.

The question of continuing sexual activity after POP repairs is obviously an important one. With an adequate vaginal operation (with the exception of colpocleisis) or abdominal operation, intercourse is achievable in most patients who wish to maintain this activity.

## RECTAL PROLAPSE

Rectal prolapse is covered in Chapter 22.

## CONCLUSION

In all women with symptomatic pelvic organ prolapse, several areas of function must be discussed and potentially addressed, including urinary, bowel, sexual, and other pelvic complaints. Nonsurgical treatments are often effective, and women do not need any treatment if they have no symptoms or bother. Symptomatic women with mild prolapse should be offered pelvic floor physical therapy if available. Symptomatic women with any stage of prolapse should be offered a pessary fitting.

If surgical treatment is desired, there are many factors to consider, including patient characteristics and desires as well as the surgeon's skills. Recurrent pelvic organ prolapse is a substantial problem, and little is known about the prevention of pelvic organ prolapse, so much research is still needed in this field.

## KEY POINTS

- In the female, large hernias, hernias that continuously have intraabdominal contents, hernias that cause continuing discomfort, and hernias that have been incarcerated should be operatively repaired.
- Pelvic organ prolapse is defined as the descent of one or more compartments of the vagina: the anterior vaginal wall, posterior vaginal wall, uterus (cervix), or apex (vaginal vault or cuff scar after hysterectomy).
- Pelvic organ prolapse is more likely to be symptomatic when the leading edge protrudes past the hymen; it can be managed expectantly if asymptomatic.
- Renal function should be evaluated in women with advanced pelvic organ prolapse if the patient declines treatment to reduce the prolapse.
- Vaginal delivery is a major risk factor for the development of pelvic organ prolapse.
- The cardinal and uterosacral ligaments hold the uterus and upper vagina in the proper location.
- Pessaries should be offered to all women with symptomatic pelvic organ prolapse.
- Pelvic organ prolapse often includes a mixture of anterior, posterior, and apical prolapse, and each compartment should be evaluated under strain prior to determining the appropriate operative treatment.
- Surgery for pelvic organ prolapse is usually effective at decreasing a vaginal bulge, but the effects on urinary, bowel, and sexual function can vary. It is important to elicit a patient's goals before surgery.
- Vaginal vault prolapse can be repaired abdominally or vaginally. An abdominal sacral colpopexy with synthetic mesh appears to have a higher long-term success rate for the vaginal apex, but at the risk of more surgical complications.

## KEY REFERENCES


ACOG Committee Opinion No. 444: choosing the route of hysterectomy for benign disease. *Obstet Gynecol.* 2009;114(5):1156–1158.

Al Chalabi H, Larkin J, Mehigan B, McCormick P. A systematic review of laparoscopic versus open abdominal incisional hernia repair, with meta-analysis of randomized controlled trials. *Int J Surg.* 2015. [epub ahead of print].

Aslani N, Brown CJ. Does mesh offer an advantage over tissue in the open repair of umbilical hernias? A systematic review and meta-analysis. *Hernia.* 2010;14(5):455–462.

Baden WF, Walker TA. Genesis of the vaginal profile: a correlated classification of vaginal relaxation. *Clin Obstet Gynecol.* 1972;15(4):1048–1054.

Barber MD, Brubaker L, Burgio KL, et al. Comparison of 2 transvaginal surgical approaches and perioperative behavioral therapy for apical vaginal prolapse: the OPTIMAL randomized trial. *JAMA.* 2014;311(10):1023–1034.

Barber MD, Maher C. Apical prolapse. *Int Urogynecol J.* 2013;24(11):1815–1833.

Blandon RE, Bharucha AE, Melton 3rd LJ, et al. Incidence of pelvic floor repair after hysterectomy: a population-based cohort study. *Am J Obstet Gynecol.* 2007;197(6). 664 e661-e667.

Braekken IH, Majida M, Engh ME, Bo K. Morphological changes after pelvic floor muscle training measured by 3-dimensional ultrasonography: a randomized controlled trial. *Obstet Gynecol.* 2010;115(2 Pt 1):317–324.

Brubaker L, Cundiff GW, Fine P, et al. Abdominal sacrocolpopexy with Burch colposuspension to reduce urinary stress incontinence. *N Engl J Med.* 2006;354(15):1557–1566.

Bump RC, Mattiasson A, Bo K, et al. The standardization of terminology of female pelvic organ prolapse and pelvic floor dysfunction. *Am J Obstet Gynecol.* 1996;175(1):10–17.

Cartwright R, Kirby AC, Tikkinen KA, et al. Systematic review and metaanalysis of genetic association studies of urinary symptoms and prolapse in women. *Am J Obstet Gynecol.* 2014;212(2):199.e1–199.e24.

Chmielewski L, Walters MD, Weber AM, Barber MD. Reanalysis of a randomized trial of 3 techniques of anterior colporrhaphy using clinically relevant definitions of success. *Am J Obstet Gynecol.* 2011;205(1). 69 e61-68.

Culligan PJ, Blackwell L, Goldsmith LJ, et al. A randomized controlled trial comparing fascia lata and synthetic mesh for sacral colpopexy. *Obstet Gynecol.* 2005;106(1):29–37.

DeLancey JO. Anatomic aspects of vaginal eversion after hysterectomy. *Am J Obstet Gynecol.* 1992;166(6 Pt 1):1717–1724. discussion 1724-1718.

Denehy TR, Choe JY, Gregori CA, Breen JL. Modified Le Fort partial colpocleisis with Kelly urethral plication and posterior colpoperineoplasty in the medically compromised elderly: a comparison with vaginal hysterectomy, anterior colporrhaphy, and posterior colpoperineoplasty. *Am J Obstet Gynecol.* 1995;173(6):1697–1701. discussion 1701-1692.

Diwan A, Rardin CR, Strohsnitter WC, et al. Laparoscopic uterosacral ligament uterine suspension compared with vaginal hysterectomy with vaginal vault suspension for uterovaginal prolapse. *Int Urogynecol J Pelvic Floor Dysfunct.* 2006;17(1):79–83.

Eilber KS, Alperin M, Khan A, et al. Outcomes of vaginal prolapse surgery among female Medicare beneficiaries: the role of apical support. *Obstet Gynecol.* 2013;122(5):981–987.

Fernando RJ, Thakar R, Sultan AH, et al. Effect of vaginal pessaries on symptoms associated with pelvic organ prolapse. *Obstet Gynecol.* 2006;108(1):93–99.

Fitzgibbons Jr RJ, Forse RA. Clinical practice. Groin hernias in adults. *N Engl J Med.* 2015;372(8):756–763.

Food and Drug Administration (FDA). Urogynecologic surgical mesh: update on the safety and effectiveness of transvaginal placement for pelvic organ prolapse. *United States Food and Drug Administration White Paper*; July 2011:6.

Geller EJ, Hankins KJ, Parnell BA, et al. Diagnostic accuracy of retrograde and spontaneous voiding trials for postoperative voiding dysfunction: a randomized controlled trial. *Obstet Gynecol.* 2011;118(3):637–642.

Grimes CL, Lukacz ES. Posterior vaginal compartment prolapse and defecatory dysfunction: are they related? *Int Urogynecol J.* 2012;23(5):537–551.

Hagen S, Stark D, Glazener C, et al. Individualised pelvic floor muscle training in women with pelvic organ prolapse (POPPY): a multicentre randomised controlled trial. *Lancet.* 2014;383(9919):796–806.

Haylen BT, de Ridder D, Freeman RM, et al. An International Urogynecological Association (IUGA)/International Continence Society (ICS) joint report on the terminology for female pelvic floor dysfunction. *Neurourol Urodyn.* 2010;29(1):4–20.

Hoyte L, Jakab M, Warfield SK, et al. Levator ani thickness variations in symptomatic and asymptomatic women using magnetic resonance-based 3-dimensional color mapping. *Am J Obstet Gynecol.* 2004;191(3):856–861.

Jonsson Funk M, Visco AG, Weidner AC, et al. Long-term outcomes of vaginal mesh versus native tissue repair for anterior vaginal wall prolapse. *Int Urogynecol J.* 2013;24(8):1279–1285.

Kovac SR, Cruikshank SH. Successful pregnancies and vaginal deliveries after sacrospinous uterosacral fixation in five of nineteen patients. *Am J Obstet Gynecol.* 1993;168(6 Pt 1):1778–1783. discussion 1783-1776.

Larsson C, Kallen K, Andolf E. Cesarean section and risk of pelvic organ prolapse: a nested case-control study. *Am J Obstet Gynecol.* 2009;200(3). 243 e241-244.

Maher C, Feiner B, Baessler K, Schmid C. Surgical management of pelvic organ prolapse in women. *Cochrane Database Syst Rev.* 2013;4:CD004014.

Maher CF, Murray CJ, Carey MP, et al. Iliococcygeus or sacrospinous fixation for vaginal vault prolapse. *Obstet Gynecol.* 2001;98(1):40–44.

Memon HU, Handa VL. Vaginal childbirth and pelvic floor disorders. *Womens Health (Lond Engl).* 2013;9(3):265–277. quiz 276-267.

Nygaard I, Barber MD, Burgio KL, et al. Prevalence of symptomatic pelvic floor disorders in US women. *JAMA.* 2008;300(11):1311–1316.

Nygaard IE, Hamad NM, Shaw JM. Activity restrictions after gynecologic surgery: is there evidence? *Int Urogynecol J.* 2013;24(5):719–724.

Nygaard IE, McCreery R, Brubaker L, et al. Abdominal sacrocolpopexy: a comprehensive review. *Obstet Gynecol.* 2004;104(4):805–823.

Pulvino JQ, Duecy EE, Buchsbaum GM, Flynn MK. Comparison of 2 techniques to predict voiding efficiency after inpatient urogynecologic surgery. *J Urol.* 2010;184(4):1408–1412.

Quiroz LH, Munoz A, Shippey SH, et al. Vaginal parity and pelvic organ prolapse. *J Reprod Med.* 2010;55(3-4):93–98.

Richter K. Massive eversion of the vagina: pathogenesis, diagnosis, and therapy of the "true" prolapse of the vaginal stump. *Clin Obstet Gynecol.* 1982;25(4):897–912.

Rooney K, Kenton K, Mueller ER, et al. Advanced anterior vaginal wall prolapse is highly correlated with apical prolapse. *Am J Obstet Gynecol.* 2006;195(6):1837–1840.

Rosenblatt PL, Chelmow D, Ferzandi TR. Laparoscopic sacrocervicopexy for the treatment of uterine prolapse: a retrospective case series report. *J Minim Invasive Gynecol.* 2008;15(3):268–272.

Sharp TR. Sacrospinous suspension made easy. *Obstet Gynecol.* 1993;82(5):873–875.

Shull BL, Bachofen C, Coates KW, Kuehl TJ. A transvaginal approach to repair of apical and other associated sites of pelvic organ prolapse with uterosacral ligaments. *Am J Obstet Gynecol.* 2000;183(6):1365–1373. discussion 1373-1364.

Tan JS, Lukacz ES, Menefee SA, et al. Predictive value of prolapse symptoms: a large database study. *Int Urogynecol J Pelvic Floor Dysfunct.* 2005;16(3):203–209. discussion 209.

Vij M, Bombieri L, Dua A, Freeman R. Long-term follow-up after colpocleisis: regret, bowel, and bladder function. *Int Urogynecol J.* 2014;25(6):811–815.

Weber AM, Abrams P, Brubaker L, et al. The standardization of terminology for researchers in female pelvic floor disorders. *Int Urogynecol J Pelvic Floor Dysfunct.* 2001;12(3):178–186.

Wei JT, Nygaard I, Richter HE, et al. A midurethral sling to reduce incontinence after vaginal prolapse repair. *N Engl J Med.* 2012;366(25):2358–2367.

Whitcomb EL, Rortveit G, Brown JS, et al. Racial differences in pelvic organ prolapse. *Obstet Gynecol.* 2009;114(6):1271–1277.

Wu JM, Matthews CA, Conover MM, et al. Lifetime risk of stress urinary incontinence or pelvic organ prolapse surgery. *Obstet Gynecol.* 2014;123(6):1201–1206.

# 21

# Lower Urinary Tract Function and Disorders

## Physiology of Micturition, Voiding Dysfunction, Urinary Incontinence, Urinary Tract Infections, and Painful Bladder Syndrome

*Anna C. Kirby, Gretchen M. Lentz*

The gynecologist frequently consults on and treats urologic problems in the female patient. Perhaps the most commonly seen of these problems involves infection and inflammation of the lower tract. Urinary tract infections (UTIs) occur in up to 50% of women over their lifetime. Painful bladder syndrome affects fewer women, but they often have chronic pain and may make frequent visits to the gynecologist's office before a diagnosis is made. Furthermore, there is considerable overlap of symptoms with other gynecologic problems such as UTIs, overactive bladder (OAB), endometriosis, and dyspareunia, so a gynecologist should be familiar with these conditions.

Many women suffer from some degree of urinary incontinence. Various prevalence studies have reported that approximately 30% of women noted some degree of incontinence during the preceding 12 months. Ten percent of women suffer from weekly incontinence, and 5% have daily incontinence. Urinary incontinence problems increase in incidence with age and, because the number of older women in our population is increasing, this problem is growing in magnitude. A survey of pelvic floor disorders by (Nygaard, 2008) found at least one pelvic floor disorder in 24% of women. At least monthly urine leakage was reported by 7% of women ages 20 to 39, 17% ages 40 to 59, 23% ages 60 to 79, and 32% 80 years of age and older. This study may actually underpredict the prevalence of these disorders because women in the survey may have been successfully treated and not counted. Overweight and obese women were more likely to report urinary incontinence than women of normal weight.

Continence depends on a number of factors, including the neurologic control of micturition, the anatomic relationships of the urinary tract, and the specific effects of a number of systemic, infectious, and neoplastic conditions. Older women have additional challenges to the urinary system with comorbid medical conditions, ambulatory difficulties, and cognitive impairments. Not only does the prevalence of urinary incontinence increase with age, but so does the severity. Incontinence has been associated with depression, increased social isolation, falls, hip fractures, and admission to nursing homes, which has additional morbidity. Furthermore, incontinence decreases quality of life and increases costs to society. This chapter discusses the physiology of normal micturition as well as the evaluation and treatment of female lower urinary tract conditions.

## PHYSIOLOGY OF MICTURITION

A number of factors are involved in maintaining continence. The central nervous system (CNS) and peripheral ganglia coordinate function of the lower urinary system through complex neural pathways—those that maintain a urethral closure mechanism and those that affect detrusor function. It is a balance between bladder storage, which is organized primarily in the spinal cord and coordinates urethral closure and detrusor relaxation, and micturition, which is controlled by reflex mechanisms mediated by the brain. Voluntary voiding is a learned function and is not automatic, like heart rate control.

Bladder detrusor contractility is stimulated by the activity of the parasympathetic nervous system, mediated primarily through the neurotransmitter acetylcholine. This stimulates muscarinic (primarily $M_3$) receptors in the bladder wall, which then activate detrusor contraction. Sympathetic nerve $\alpha$ receptors within the bladder cause bladder relaxation when stimulated. Bladder contraction may also be affected by irritation and inflammation of the bladder wall lining, causing uninhibited contractions. Inhibitory input to the urethral smooth muscle is conveyed by nitric oxide via parasympathetic nerves. Somatic cholinergic motor nerves supply the striated muscles of the external urethral sphincter from the sacral spinal cord.

The act of voiding is under the control of four basic autonomic and somatic nervous system feedback loops. The first loop (loop I) involves a circuit from the cerebral cortex to the brain stem, which inhibits micturition by modifying sensory stimuli emanating from loop II. Loop II, which originates in the sacral micturition center (S2 through S4) and the detrusor muscle wall itself, represents sensory fibers to the brain stem, where modulation of the stimuli by loop I takes place. If cerebral inhibition is not imposed (loop I), the stimuli are returned to the sacral micturition center as a response to the bladder filling, allowing activation of loop III. Loop III involves sensory flow from the bladder wall to the sacral micturition center with returning motor fibers to the urethral sphincter striated muscle, which allows the voluntary relaxation of the urethral sphincter as the detrusor contracts. Loop IV originates in the frontal lobe of the cerebral cortex and runs to the sacral micturition center and then to the urethral striated muscle, allowing urethral voluntary muscles to relax, thus leading to the initiation of voiding. Figure 21.1 demonstrates these four loops. Table 21.1 summarizes the important aspects of each loop (Ostergard, 1979).

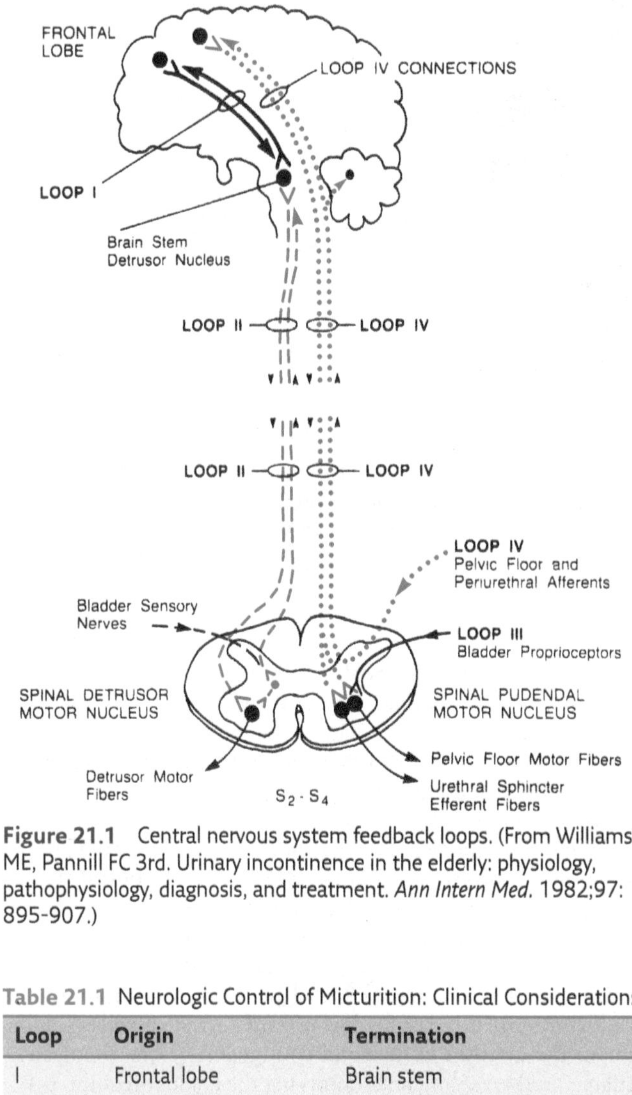


**Figure 21.1** Central nervous system feedback loops. (From Williams ME, Pannill FC 3rd. Urinary incontinence in the elderly: physiology, pathophysiology, diagnosis, and treatment. *Ann Intern Med.* 1982;97: 895-907.)

Both the parasympathetic and sympathetic nervous systems function with the CNS in these feedback loops via the pontine micturition center. The parasympathetic system is involved in the act of voiding via nuclei in S2 through S4 (micturition center) and mediates its activity through the neurotransmitter acetylcholine, directly stimulating muscarinic receptors in the bladder wall. This signal is transmitted via the pelvic nerve and causes the detrusor to contract. At the same time, the pontine micturition center (PMC) in the brain inhibits the sympathetic pathway as well as the somatic pathway to the urethra. This allows the urethra to relax so that coordinated voiding can occur. Functional brain imaging studies (e.g., positron emission tomography [PET]) during voiding show activation of the cortex, insula, and PMC. The sympathetic system, on the other hand, acts to prevent micturition. Norepinephrine is secreted via this system, stimulating both α- and β-adrenergic receptors. The bladder contains primarily β receptors, stimulation of which causes relaxation of the detrusor muscle. The urethra contains primarily α receptors. Stimulation of these α receptors causes contraction of the urethral sphincter. Thus the overall effect is to prevent micturition (Fig. 21.2). Estrogen and progesterone receptors are present in the bladder and urethra, although their role in affecting continence has not been fully elucidated. Many other neurotransmitters, neuropeptides, and receptors have been identified in the lower urinary tract, including dopamine, serotonin, nitric oxide, γ-aminobutyric acid (GABA), glutamine, neurokinin A, nerve growth factor, and adenosine triphosphate (ATP).

Because the neurogenic control of micturition is so complex and depends on the interaction of so many factors, it is understandable that a host of general systemic diseases or diseases involving the nervous system may affect bladder control. These include, but are not limited to, diabetes mellitus, vascular diseases, obesity, cognitive disorders, normal pressure hydrocephalus, demyelinating diseases (e.g., multiple sclerosis), CNS trauma, and tumors. The system can be disrupted by a stroke, which is a suprapontine lesions leading to loss of central inhibition, resulting in detrusor overactivity and reemergence of reflex micturition. A spinal cord injury above the lumbosacral level eliminates voluntary control of voiding, leading to acute urinary retention. Later, neurogenic detrusor overactivity occurs from spinal reflex pathways, which are uncoordinated, so the urethral sphincter may not relax simultaneously, leading to detrusor-sphincter dyssynergia. A lumbosacral burst fracture can result

**Table 21.1** Neurologic Control of Micturition: Clinical Considerations on Central Nervous System Reflex Loops

| Loop | Origin | Termination | Function | Associated Conditions |
|---|---|---|---|---|
| I | Frontal lobe | Brain stem | Coordinates volitional control of micturition | Parkinson disease, brain tumors, trauma, micturition |
| II | Brain stem Bladder wall | Brain stem | Detrusor muscle contraction to empty bladder | Spinal cord trauma, multiple sclerosis (MS), spinal cord tumors, neuropathy, local urinary tract disease |
| III | Sensory afferents of tumors, diabetic detrusor muscle disease | Striated muscle of urethral sphincter via pudendal motor neurons and sacral micturition center | Allows relaxation of urethral sphincter in synchrony with detrusor contraction | MS, spinal cord trauma or neuropathy, local urinary tract |
| IV | Frontal lobe | Pudendal nucleus | Volitional control of striated external urethral sphincter | Cerebral or spinal trauma or tumor, MS, cerebrovascular disease, lower urinary tract disease |

Modified from Ostergard DR. The neurological control of micturition and integral voiding reflexes. *Obstet Gynecol Surv.* 1979;34:417-423.

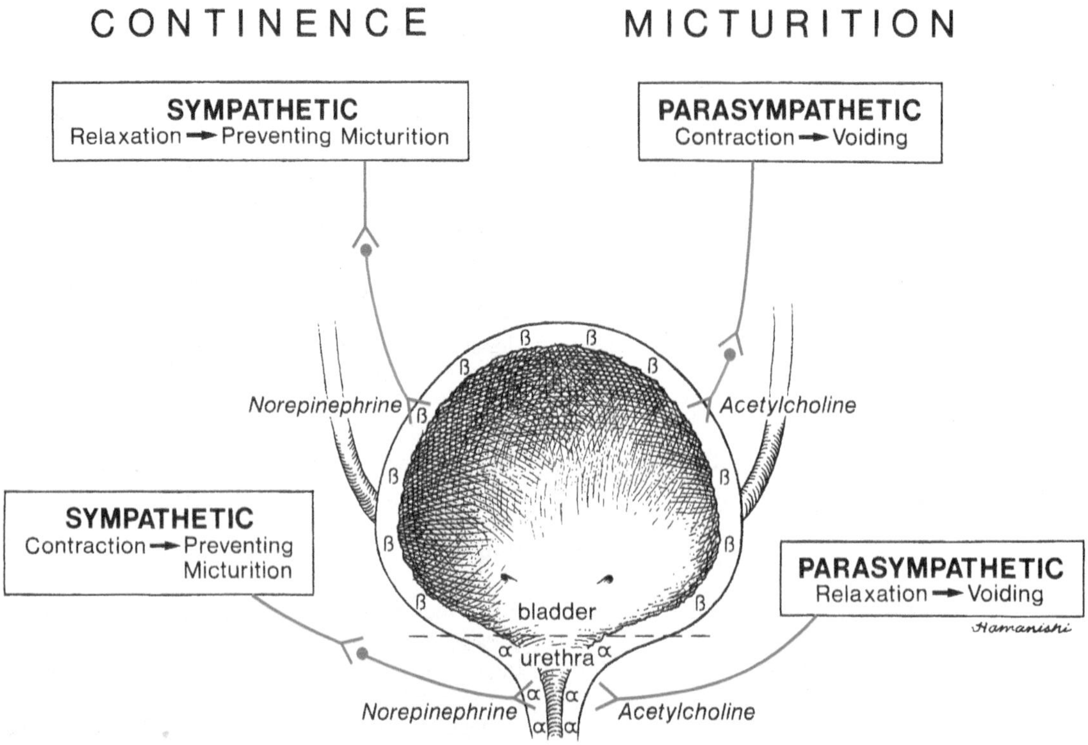


**Figure 21.2 Innervation of the Bladder and Urethra.** Parasympathetic fibers arising in S2-S4 have long preganglionic fibers and pelvic ganglia close to the bladder and urethra. These parasympathetic fibers excrete acetylcholine. Sympathetic fibers that have long postganglionic fibers discharge norepinephrine to β receptors, primarily in the bladder, and α receptors, primarily in the urethra. (Modified from Raz S. Pharmacological treatment of lower urinary tract dysfunction. *Urol Clin North Am.* 1978;5:323-324.)

Table 21.2 Drugs That Affect Continence and Micturition

| Drug | Action |
|---|---|
| **Sympathetic (Relaxes Bladder; Controls Urethral Sphincter)** | |
| Dopamine | α-Adrenergic stimulator |
| Methamphetamine | α-Adrenergic stimulator |
| Norepinephrine | α-Adrenergic stimulator |
| Phenylephrine | α-Adrenergic stimulator |
| Albuterol | β-Adrenergic stimulator |
| Isoproterenol | β-Adrenergic stimulator |
| Terbutaline | β-Adrenergic stimulator |
| **Parasympathetic (Stimulates Bladder Contraction; Relaxes Urethral Sphincter)** | |
| Pilocarpine | Stimulates acetylcholine, incontinence |
| Pyridostigmine | Stimulates acetylcholine, incontinence |
| **Sympathetic Blockers** | |
| Hydralazine | Adrenergic blocker, stress incontinence |
| Methyldopa | Adrenergic blocker, stress incontinence |
| Reserpine | Adrenergic blocker, stress incontinence |
| **Parasympathetic Blockers** | |
| Atropine | Parasympathetic inhibitor, impaired emptying |
| Papaverine | Parasympathetic inhibitor, impaired emptying |
| Scopolamine | Parasympathetic inhibitor, impaired emptying |

in detrusor overactivity with urethral sphincter hyporeflexia or sphincter hyperreflexia. A radical hysterectomy or subsacral cauda equine lesion might disrupt the local reflexes and lead to overflow incontinence because of detrusor and sphincter hyporeflexia. If the pudendal nerve is intact, the sphincter function will be normal.

In addition, medications that have an effect on the CNS or autonomic nervous system may affect bladder control. Compounds with atropine-like effects may interfere with the initiation of micturition, whereas those with cholinergic effects may cause bladder overactivity (Table 21.2).

In summary, bladder control depends on the ability of the bladder to store urine under low pressure, which involves inhibition of the detrusor muscle and contraction of the smooth and striated urethral sphincters. Emptying the bladder requires coordination with pelvic floor and urethral sphincter relaxation and detrusor contraction. Local reflexes and central inhibitory influences are involved.

## BLADDER AND URETHRAL ANATOMY AND FUNCTION

With the neurologic principles of micturition in mind, it is appropriate to assess other factors that may influence continence. The bladder and urethra are essentially a functional unit (Asmussen, 1976) with the bladder's subfunction being to store urine and the urethra's to allow it to pass. For urine to pass through the urethra, the maximum urethral pressure must be lower than the intravesical pressure. Intravesical pressure depends on the following: (1) the volume of fluid in the bladder, (2) the part of the intraabdominal pressure transmitted to the bladder, and (3) the tension in the bladder wall related to muscular and nervous system activity and elastic properties. The resting pressure in the bladder is between 20 and 30 cm $H_2O$ due to surrounding intraabdominal pressure with little or no pressure added from tension in the bladder wall in normal bladders (i.e., the detrusor pressure, which is further described in the Urodynamics section of this chapter) is 0 cm $H_2O$.

The intraurethral pressure depends on the following: (1) striated muscle fibers of the urethral wall, (2) smooth muscle fibers of the urethral wall (a circular and longitudinal layer), (3) vascular content of the urethral submucosal cavernous plexus, (4) passive elasticity of the urethral wall, and (5) the part of the intraabdominal pressure transmitted to the urethra. The urethra has primarily receptors from the sympathetic nervous system, which, when stimulated, cause contraction of the urethral sphincter. The urethral smooth and striated (skeletal) muscles add to the resting urethral tone, whereas the skeletal fibers react when intraabdominal pressure rises, such as with a cough.

Anatomically, the exact border between the bladder and urethra is difficult to determine. The functional length of the urethra, however, is that part in which the urethral pressure exceeds the bladder pressure. The urethral closure pressure (UCP) is defined as the maximum urethral pressure minus the bladder pressure (Asmussen, 1976). For continence to be present, the UCP must be higher than the bladder pressure. Urethral pressure varies with age, increasing up to the age of 20 years and then gradually decreasing until menopause. However, after menopause, the fall of this pressure is more rapid. Asmussen and Ulmsten (1976) have demonstrated that the highest pressure zone in the urethra is approximately at the midpoint of the functional urethral length. The anatomic urethral length is approximately 3 to 4 cm. This high-pressure zone is located at approximately 0.5 cm proximal to the urogenital diaphragm (Westby, 1982). Most of the functional urethral length is actually above the urogenital diaphragm (Fig. 21.3). The submucosal cavernous plexus of vessels, the bulk of the smooth and striated muscle, and the bulk of the autonomic nerve supply are most prominent in the area in which they record the maximum urethral pressure. Because the urethral pressure displays high-pressure zone oscillations that are synchronous with the heartbeat, the submucosal cavernous plexus is probably important in helping to maintain continence (Fig. 21.4). Estrogen receptors are found in the bladder and urethra. Urethral pressure can oscillate as much as 25 cm $H_2O$ in young women but seldom more than 5 cm $H_2O$ in postmenopausal women (Enhorning, 1961). The cavernous plexus is thicker walled and less elastic in older women. Thus not only is the epithelium of the bladder and bladder neck dependent on hormone stimulation, but probably so is the vascular system of these areas.

DeLancey made some interesting observations on functioning periurethral anatomy by studying serial histologic sections of intact pelvic viscera and surrounding tissue and by dissecting 22 fresh and embalmed cadavers (DeLancey, 1986). Because the length of the urethra varies among women, the topography of urethral and paraurethral structures was expressed in terms of the location along the urethra, as a percentage of the total urethra. DeLancey considered the zero location as that point at which the urethra leaves the bladder lumen and the 100th percentile as that point at which the urethra terminates on the perineum. From the standpoint of functional anatomy, there is excellent agreement among the measurements made from each of his specimens when percentiles are used; Table 21.3 depicts these anatomic relationships. It can be seen that the intramural urethra represents approximately 20% of the length of the urethra. The portion of the urethra encircled by striated urethral sphincter muscle and associated with the pubourethral ligament and vaginal levator attachment concerns the midurethra—that is, that portion from the 20th to 60th percentile along the total length. The 60th to 80th percentile of the urethral length passes through the urogenital diaphragm and is under the influence of the urethrovaginal sphincter muscles. Finally, the last 20%, or distal urethra, traverses the bulbocavernosus muscles. These urethral landmarks are depicted in Figure 21.5, which highlights the actual ranges and values. The actual anatomic relationships

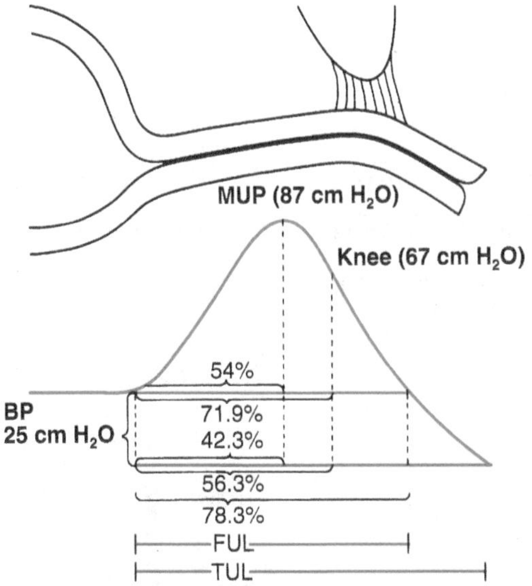


**Figure 21.3** Location of maximum urethral pressure in relation to the urogenital diaphragm (average value of 25 normal women). Knee indicates the location of the urogenital diaphragm seen on x-ray film and transformed to the pressure curve. *BP,* Blood pressure; *MUP,* maximal urethral pressure. (From Asmussen M, Ulmsten U. On the physiology of continence and pathophysiology of stress incontinence in the female. *Contrib Gynecol Obstet.* 1983;10:32-50.)

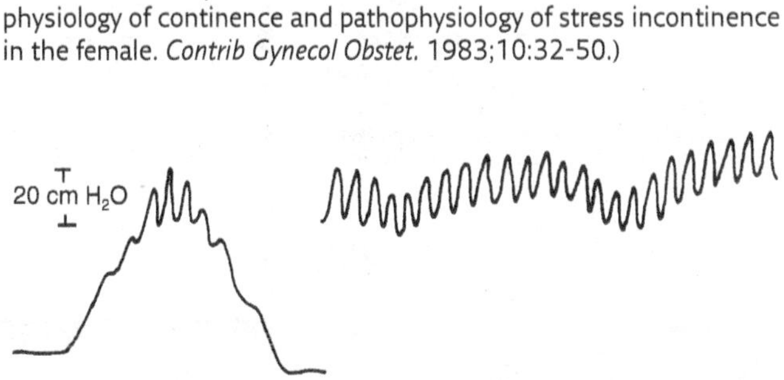


**Figure 21.4** Maximum urethral pressure shows great variation synchronously with the heartbeat. Variations of 20 cm $H_2O$ as shown in the curve are not uncommon. (From Asmussen M, Ulmsten U. On the physiology of continence and pathophysiology of stress incontinence in the female. *Contrib Gynecol Obstet.* 1983;10:32-50.)

are depicted in Figure 21.6. DeLancey's observations help correlate the anatomic relationships with the physiologic observations that others have made.

In a subsequent paper, DeLancey (1994) noted that additional anatomic factors might influence continence. Using serial histologic sections from eight female cadavers and the dissections of 34 other cadavers, he noted that the proximal urethra gets added support because the anterior vagina is attached to the muscles of the pelvic diaphragm and to the arcus tendineus fasciae pelvis. Contraction of the pelvic diaphragm thus pulls the vagina against the posterior surface of the urethra, helping to close it. At rest, the urethra is supported by its attachment to the arcus tendineus fasciae pelvis and the tone of the pelvic diaphragm muscles. Two striated muscle arches, the compressor urethrae and urethrovaginal sphincter, support the distal urethra in the region of the urogenital diaphragm. These muscles help compress the distal urethra, helping to maintain continence during a cough.

In summary, continence depends on the bladder, urethra, pelvic muscles, the surrounding connective tissue supports, and the nervous system.

Table 21.3 Topography of Urethral and Paraurethral Structures*

| Approximate Location† | Region of the Urethra | Paraurethral Structures |
|---|---|---|
| 0-20 | Intramural urethra | Urethral lumen traverses bladder wall |
| 20-60 | Midurethra | Striated urethral sphincter muscle<br>Pubourethral ligament<br>Vaginolevator attachment |
| 60-80 | Urogenital diaphragm | Compressor urethrae muscle<br>Urethrovaginal sphincter muscle |
| 80-100 | Distal urethra | Bulbocavernosus muscle |

From DeLancey JO. Correlative study of paraurethral anatomy. *Obstet Gynecol.* 1986;68:91-97.

*Smooth muscle of the urethra was not considered.

†Expressed as a percentile of total urethral length.

## DIAGNOSTIC PROCEDURES

The clinical history is useful in the diagnosis of urinary incontinence. Several validated scales are available, such as the Urogenital Distress Inventory (UDI), Incontinence Impact Questionnaire (IIQ), Bristol Female Lower Urinary Tract Questionnaire, and King's Health Questionnaire, although not one has become the preferred instrument. Useful testing can be done in the gynecologist's office without the need for sophisticated equipment. These procedures are described and their benefits noted. The description is followed by a discussion of more sophisticated diagnostic techniques requiring specialized equipment.

### URINALYSIS AND CULTURE

A simple urinalysis and urine culture may provide much information. The presence of white or red blood cells (RBCs) and bacteria in a catheterized or clean voided sample, in which the perineum around the urethra has been appropriately prepared with an antiseptic solution, may suggest a UTI, nephrolithiasis,

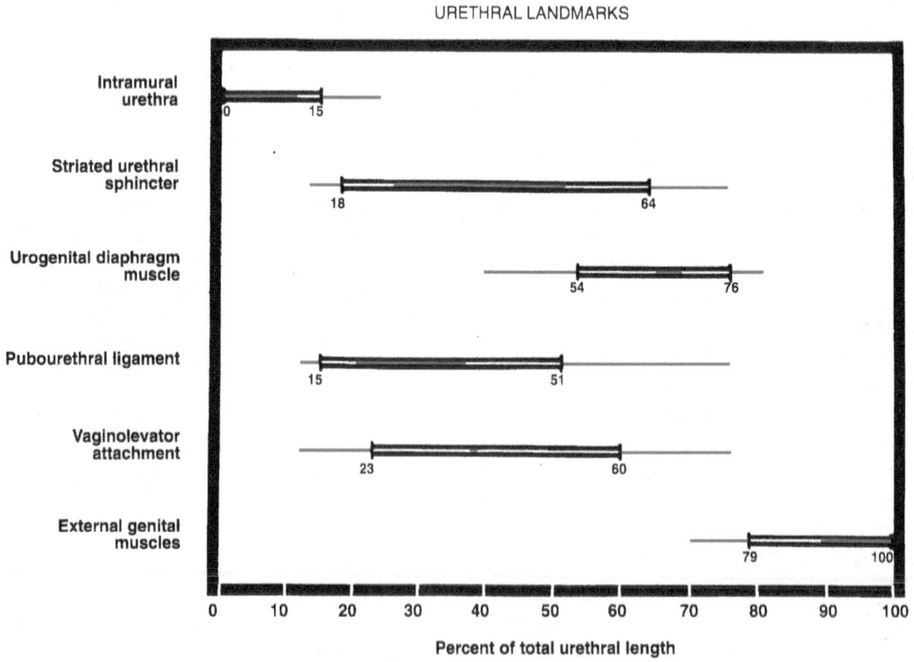


**Figure 21.5** Average spatial distribution of paraurethral structures, as well as the range of values found. Urogenital diaphragm muscles are the compressor urethrae and urethrovaginal sphincter. (From DeLancey JO. Correlative study of paraurethral anatomy. *Obstet Gynecol.* 1986;68:91-97.)

kidney disease, or even urinary tract malignancy in rare cases. UTI may be associated with urgency, frequency, dysuria, and even incontinence. In such cases, the urinalysis and urine culture may be diagnostic. Several dipstick methods are available to detect bacteriuria, pyuria, and the presence of nitrites and leukocyte esterase. The accuracy of these methods is variable, but they do have some use in screening patients who are incontinent or have symptoms suggestive of infection. In some cases, a culture should be obtained to identify the specific organism involved and verify the presence of an infection. Urinalysis is also useful to screen for microscopic hematuria (RBCs) in women with new-onset urgency and frequency because underlying urinary tract pathology may be present. A formal microscopic urinalysis should be carried out to confirm screening results because urine dipstick tests can often yield a false-positive result and actual RBCs need to be identified. A catheterized specimen should be obtained if abnormal results are questioned because of vaginal contamination. This is common in women with pelvic organ prolapse, obesity, postmenopausal bleeding, menses, or in older women with arthritis and poor hand function. Screening for asymptomatic bacteruria should only be done for pregnant women and for women planning to undergo urologic procedures.

## TEST FOR RESIDUAL URINE

This simple procedure can be extremely helpful in the evaluation of a woman with incontinence with pelvic organ prolapse, voiding symptoms such as frequency or incomplete bladder emptying, or recurrent UTIs. The woman is asked to void, and a catheter is inserted into the bladder no more than 10 to 15 minutes later.

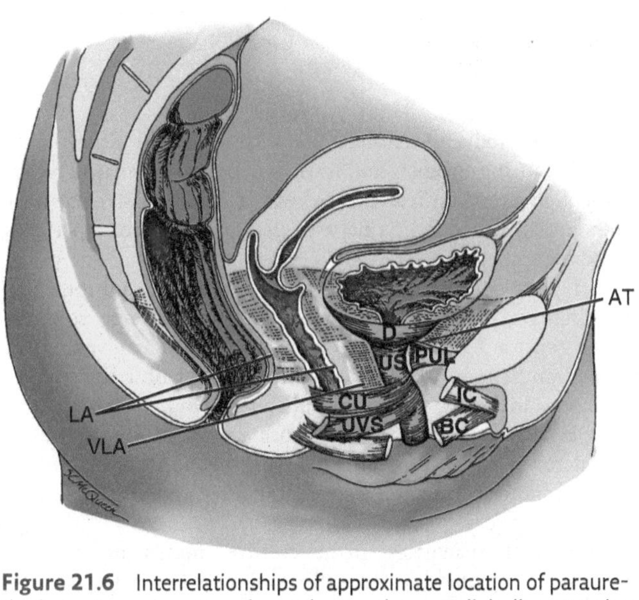


**Figure 21.6** Interrelationships of approximate location of paraurethral structures. Levator ani muscles are shown as light lines running deep to the pelvic viscera. The vaginal levator attachment is shown as a darker area. *AT,* Arcus tendineus fasciae pelvis; *BC,* bulbocavernosus muscle; *CU,* compressor urethrae; *D,* detrusor muscle; *IC,* ischiocavernosus muscle; *LA,* levator ani muscles; *PUL,* pubourethral ligament; *US,* urethral sphincter; *UVS,* urethrovaginal sphincter; *VLA,* vaginal levator attachment. (Modified from DeLancey JO. Correlative study of paraurethral anatomy. *Obstet Gynecol.* 1986;68:91-97.)

The urine remaining in the bladder is measured and may be sent for urinalysis and culture. Definitions of normal postvoid residual volumes vary, but under normal circumstances, the amount of residual urine should be less than 150 mL or less than one third of the bladder volume (e.g., 100 mL after voiding 200 mL). Large amounts of residual urine suggest urinary retention resulting from inadequate bladder emptying. A reasonably accurate measure of residual urine volume can also be obtained noninvasively by ultrasound. Bladder scan ultrasound units are available and patients prefer to avoid urethral catheterization. Postvoid residual urine volume by ultrasound may be falsely elevated in women with large uterine fibroids or a large adnexal mass. Confirmation is necessary with catheterization if this is suspected.

## BLADDER DIARY

In many cases, stress urinary incontinence can be correctly diagnosed in a primary care setting from the clinical history alone. The bladder diary appears to be a cost-effective adjunct to clinical history for diagnosing detrusor overactivity. Asking the woman to complete a bladder diary is a simple, inexpensive way to obtain information about her fluid intake, voiding habits, voided volumes, and incontinent episodes. An example diary form is shown in Figure 21.7.

## OFFICE CYSTOMETRICS

It is possible to gain a great deal of information about bladder capacity and bladder function with relatively simple tools. Once a catheter is inserted to check for residual urine, the catheter is left in place and attached to a graduated Asepto syringe without a bulb. It is possible to pour sterile saline (or sterile water) into the syringe by gravity and measure the amount of saline that first causes the woman to have the urge to void. This first urge should normally occur after 150 to 200 mL of saline has been infused. Women with normal bladder function should be able to continue to maintain continence at that level. Similarly, a strong, normally controllable urge to void usually occurs when 400 to 500 mL has been instilled. Thus a normal bladder first transmits an urge to void at 150 to 200 mL, and functional capacity is reached at 400 to 600 mL. Larger volumes can be reached without incontinence, but this is usually accomplished with a great deal of conscious effort. If, during filling, the woman reports urgency and the column of fluid in the Asepto syringe rises, leakage may be seen around the catheter and detrusor overactivity confirmed.

## COUGH STRESS TEST AND PAD WEIGHT TEST

If a bladder has been previously filled to measure capacity, it should then be emptied to approximately 250 to 300 mL of saline, or if the bladder is empty, 250 to 300 mL of saline should be instilled. The catheter is then removed and the woman is asked to cough while in the recumbent position. If urine spurts from the urethral meatus, stress incontinence may be present and a positive cough stress test (CST) is noted. After the stress test is performed in a recumbent woman, it should be repeated with the woman standing if no leakage is seen. Frequently, she will appear to be continent with stress while lying down but may demonstrate incontinence when the influence of gravity on the

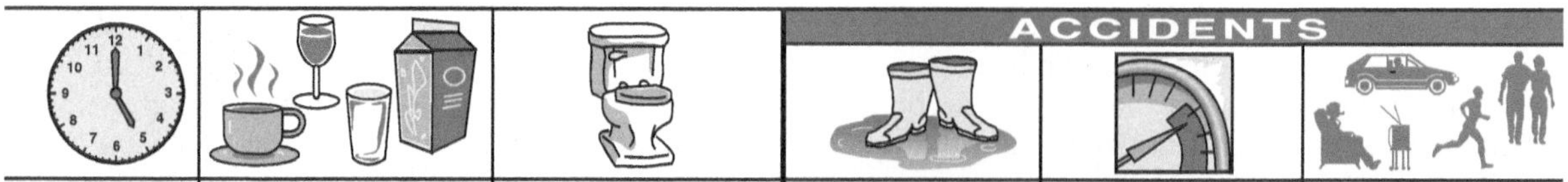
**Your Daily Bladder Diary**

This diary will help you and your health care team. Bladder diaries help show the causes of bladder control trouble. The "Example" line (below) will show you how to use the diary.

| | | | | | ACCIDENTS | | |
|---|---|---|---|---|---|---|---|
| **Time** | **Drinks** What kind? | How many? | **Urine** How many times? | How much? sm med lg | **Accidental leaks** sm med lg | **Did you feel a strong urge to go?** | **What were you doing at the time?** *Sneezing, exercising, driving, lifting, etc.* |
| Example | *coffee* | *2 cups* | *//* | ☐ ☒ ☐ | ☐ ☒ ☐ | ☒ Yes ☐ No | *Running* |
| 6–7 am | | | | ☐ ☐ ☐ | ☐ ☐ ☐ | ☐ Yes ☐ No | |
| 7–8 am | | | | ☐ ☐ ☐ | ☐ ☐ ☐ | ☐ Yes ☐ No | |
| 8–9 am | | | | ☐ ☐ ☐ | ☐ ☐ ☐ | ☐ Yes ☐ No | |
| 9–10 am | | | | ☐ ☐ ☐ | ☐ ☐ ☐ | ☐ Yes ☐ No | |
| 10–11 am | | | | ☐ ☐ ☐ | ☐ ☐ ☐ | ☐ Yes ☐ No | |
| 11–12 noon | | | | ☐ ☐ ☐ | ☐ ☐ ☐ | ☐ Yes ☐ No | |
| 12–1 pm | | | | ☐ ☐ ☐ | ☐ ☐ ☐ | ☐ Yes ☐ No | |
| 1–2 pm | | | | ☐ ☐ ☐ | ☐ ☐ ☐ | ☐ Yes ☐ No | |
| 2–3 pm | | | | ☐ ☐ ☐ | ☐ ☐ ☐ | ☐ Yes ☐ No | |
| 3–4 pm | | | | ☐ ☐ ☐ | ☐ ☐ ☐ | ☐ Yes ☐ No | |
| 4–5 pm | | | | ☐ ☐ ☐ | ☐ ☐ ☐ | ☐ Yes ☐ No | |
| 5–6 pm | | | | ☐ ☐ ☐ | ☐ ☐ ☐ | ☐ Yes ☐ No | |
| 6–7 pm | | | | ☐ ☐ ☐ | ☐ ☐ ☐ | ☐ Yes ☐ No | |

**Your name:** ______________________ **Date:** __________

**Figure 21.7** Daily bladder diary. (From Vasavada SP, Appell R, Sand PK, et al, eds. *Female Urology, Urogynecology, and Voiding Dysfunction.* New York: Marcel Dekker; 2005:127.)

pelvic organs is brought into play in the standing position. For research studies, 250 or 300 mL of saline is instilled, the woman is asked to cough 10 times, and any leakage is considered a positive CST. In clinical practice, it is also reasonable to perform the standing cough stress test if the patient has a comfortably full bladder and then calculate the volume in the bladder afterward by adding the voided volume and the postvoid residual. If around 250 mL, the volume was adequate. If the volume in the bladder was low during a negative cough stress test, it should be repeated with around 250 mL. The clinical stress test is effective in diagnosing stress incontinence.

Because urine loss with cough should be immediate if stress incontinence is the problem, it may be possible to detect evidence of detrusor overactivity by observing the time of the spurt of urine in the stress test. Typically, the detrusor reacts a few seconds after the stimulus; therefore a spurt that occurs after a delay after a cough suggests the presence of a cough-induced involuntary detrusor contraction.

If no leakage is seen and anterior vaginal wall prolapse is present, occult stress incontinence is possible. It can be challenging to determine whether a woman with anterior vaginal wall relaxation is likely to develop overt stress incontinence after a pelvic organ prolapse repair. The cough stress test is repeated with the prolapse reduced manually or with a pessary, either in the clinic or during urodynamic testing; a positive prolapse reduction cough stress test is associated with increased risk of de novo stress incontinence than a negative test, but it is not a perfectly accurate predictor.

A 1-hour pad weight test is another research tool for documenting pre- and postintervention urinary leakage volumes. Again, with a 250-mL bladder volume, a pad is given to the woman and she is asked to complete a series of activities over the hour, including walking, climbing stairs, coughing, and other events. If the pad weighs more than 2 to 3 g, the test is considered positive. Both this test and the CST are commonly used as objective measures of outcome for surgical incontinence trials.

Thus with urinalysis, urine culture, measuring postvoid residual urine, bladder diary, documented first urge to void, bladder capacity, and the cough stress test, the physician will have a great deal of information concerning the cause of the woman's urinary complaint. More sophisticated urodynamic evaluations using specific and often costly equipment should be performed by those who are trained and experienced in these tests. A short discussion of these procedures and the equipment involved follows.

## URODYNAMICS

Urodynamic investigation attempts to measure bladder and urethral function and voiding function. Cystometry, part of the urodynamic test, measures bladder pressure during the filling phase of the micturition cycle. First urge to void, normal desire to void, and bladder capacity are noted. The woman can cough or perform the Valsalva maneuver to detect stress incontinence in the absence of a detrusor contraction. Detrusor overactivity may be noted with the symptom of urgency, with or without leakage, in association with a detrusor pressure rise. Poor compliance from a nonelastic bladder is noted with a gradual pressure rise of more than 15 cm $H_2O$ from baseline rather than phasic contractions of detrusor overactivity. Pressure flow studies measure voiding in terms of detrusor and urethral function. In attempting to understand the basis of urinary stress incontinence, the practitioner must realize that what must be determined is the relationship between the simultaneous intraurethral and intravesical pressures (Fig. 21.8). For greatest accuracy, these should be measured with the woman in the sitting position as well as standing, at rest, and with straining. The ideal means of evaluating a woman for incontinence is to use a multichannel recorder that permits pressure determinations at two points within the urethra (proximal and midpoint to distal), one within the bladder, and one intraabdominally as recorded by an intrarectal sensor or by a sensor within the vagina if the vagina is in a relatively normal position (not prolapsed). Figure 21.9 shows a multichannel urodynamic study during the pressure/flow or voiding phase and highlights a woman with a voiding disorder, which was the main reason the study was ordered.

Several authors have described the concept of leak point pressure tests for evaluating urethral function in stress incontinence. Instead of measuring the intravesical pressure needed to overcome passive urethral resistance, this test measures the intravesical pressure necessary to overcome urethral resistance under stress (cough or strain). Studies have reported many variations in techniques to measure leak point pressures. The International Continence Society defines an abdominal leak point pressure (ALPP) as the lowest of the intentional or actively increased intravesical pressure that provokes urinary leakage in the absence of a detrusor contraction. This increased pressure can result from a Valsalva maneuver (VLPP) or coughing. The ALPP has been used to separate urinary stress incontinence as either related to an anatomic defect (hypermobility of the urethra) or intrinsic sphincter deficiency. However, is has become clear there is significant overlap in these conditions and using a simple cutoff of less than 60 cm $H_2O$ to define intrinsic sphincter deficiency is too simplistic. The woman's history and clinical picture must be considered carefully and not just an arbitrary cutoff point.

Maximal urethral closure pressure (MUCP) is another measure of urethral function in stress incontinence. Below 20 cm $H_2O$ is the criteria used to define intrinsic sphincter deficiency. Using the MUCP for choosing therapy in subtypes of stress incontinence or for outcome results in surgical trials has been criticized because unlike the VLPP, the test is not performed during stress. A 2010 randomized, controlled trial by Nager and colleagues studied the relationship between various measurements of urethral function and subjective scores of urinary incontinence (Nager, 2010). They found that VLPP and MUCP have moderate correlation with each other, but each had little or no correlation with the woman's subjective scores of incontinence severity or objective tests such as the supine empty bladder stress test. These data call into question the use of urodynamic measures of urethral function when they do not correlate with urinary incontinence severity. However, many stress incontinence surgical trials use the MUCP and leak point pressures to categorize incontinence and to predict risk of surgical failure, so being familiar with the tests is useful.

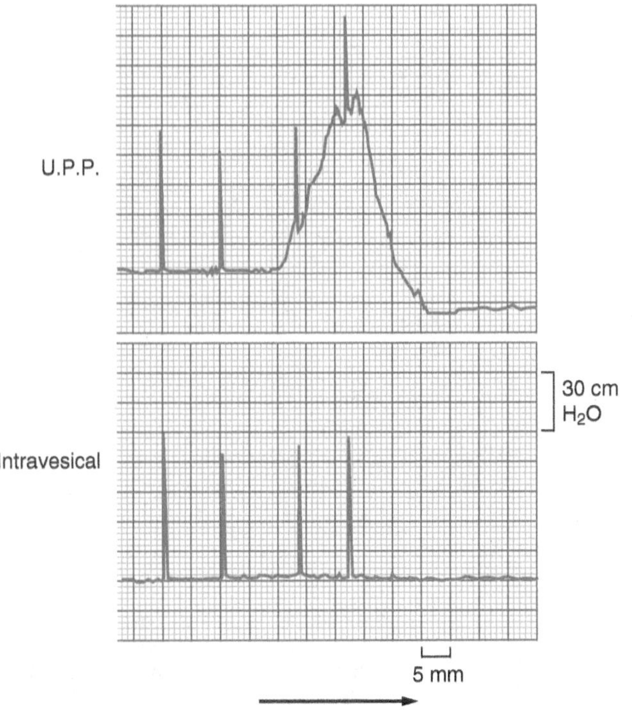


**Figure 21.8** Simultaneous recordings of urethra and intravesical pressures during coughing. Stress produces a parallel increase of bladder and urethral pressure because the intraabdominal position of the bladder and proximal two thirds of the urethra are displayed. *U.P.P.*, Urethral pressure profile. (From Raz S. Pharmacological treatment of lower urinary tract dysfunction. *Urol Clin North Am.* 1978;5:323-324.)

Other studies have called into question the usefulness of urodynamics for stress or urge incontinence symptoms in uncomplicated cases. The test correlates poorly with symptoms and often does not affect the outcome of treatment, even with stress incontinence surgery (Nager, 2008). When urodynamic testing is done, it must be correlated with the woman's symptoms and exam, as those factors may be more revealing than the test.

Multichannel devices involve more expensive equipment and require continuous maintenance. It is possible to add a video urodynamic system to the multichannel recorders, making it possible via fluoroscopy to identify reflux into the ureters in high-risk patients. The video system also makes it possible to actually observe the act of micturition, any anatomic changes, and the effect of stress. Because the data obtained by multichannel pressure recordings plus the ability to actually visualize the woman voiding offers the most accurate diagnostic information that the clinician can obtain, this technique is considered the standard against which other tests are measured.

Urodynamic testing is not necessary for beginning a conservative treatment program for stress, urge, or mixed incontinence

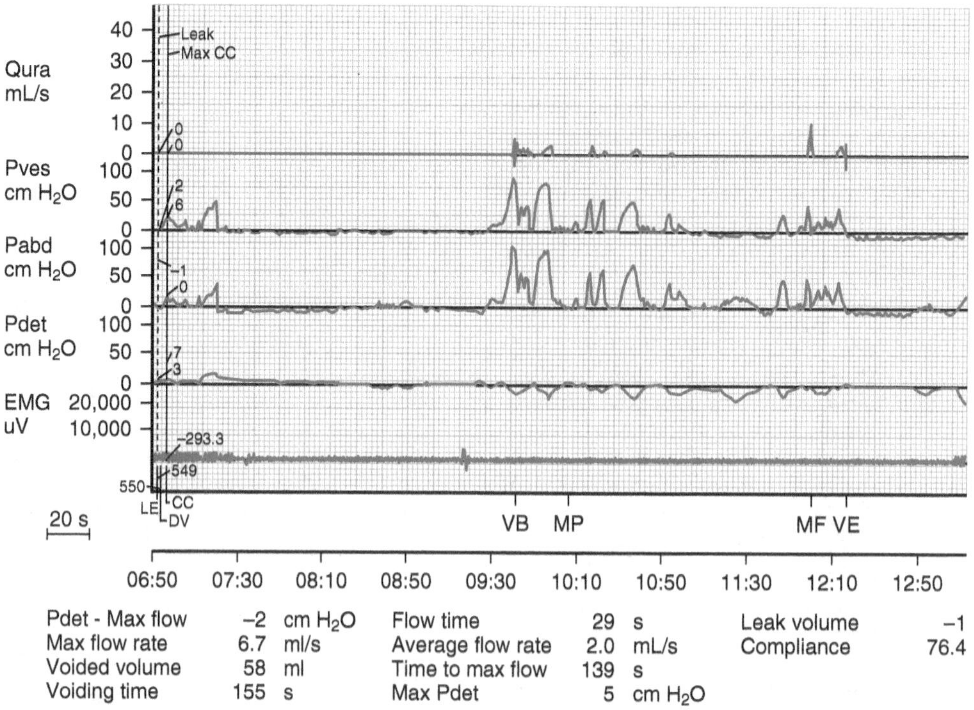


**Figure 21.9** Multichannel urodynamic study of a 44-year-old woman, G5 P1, with complaints of mixed incontinence and difficulty emptying her bladder. She had some minor neurologic symptoms suggestive of multiple sclerosis, but her evaluation had not proved a definite diagnosis. Her voiding study revealed an acontractile bladder and abdominal straining to void, with poor urine flow.

symptoms or for routine evaluation. However, if the diagnosis is unclear, the woman has failed conservative therapy, has had prior incontinence surgery, has voiding complaints, has pelvic organ prolapse beyond the hymen, or has a complicated medical history (such as neurologic disease), then urodynamic testing may provide useful information.

## CYSTOURETHROSCOPY

Cystourethroscopy, or simply cystoscopy, may be performed with a flexible or rigid telescope that allows visualization of the urethra, bladder, and ureteral orifices in an office setting (Box 21.1). Generally, saline or sterile water is used for the infusion fluid to expand the bladder. Local lidocaine jelly is inserted into the urethra for analgesia in the office. A small 17 Fr sheath is commonly used for routine inspection and a larger sheath for operative procedures. Examination of the bladder is best accomplished using a 30- or 70-degree lens, which offers the angles needed to examine the bladder in its entirety. A 0- or 12-degree lens is best for examining the urethra. The bladder may have to be flushed for optimal viewing if blood obscures the view; this can easily be done by filling, emptying, and refilling the bladder. A systematic survey should be done inspecting the bladder base and trigone, ureteral orifices, dome, and all other surfaces all the way back to the bladder neck. The bladder may be visualized and the presence of inflammation, foreign bodies, urinary tract stones, anatomic abnormalities such as a duplicated ureter (Fig. 21.10), or benign or malignant lesions noted. Urethroscopy, using the same cystoscopy equipment, is excellent for visualizing the urethra and provides information about inflammatory processes within the urethra, urethral diverticula, and other anatomic defects such as a urethral stricture or foreign body (e.g., mesh from an midurethral tape sling), and it permits some estimate of urethral tone.

**Box 21.1 Common Findings on Urethrocystoscopy**

**Normal Urothelium—Pale, Fine Blood Vessels**
- Normal—squamous metaplasia in trigone (benign overgrowth)
- Abnormal—hypervascularity
- Abnormal—cystic lesions in the trigone; could be benign cystitis (UTI)
- Abnormal—stitch or mesh from incontinence surgery
- Abnormal—bladder stone or kidney stone that has passed
- Abnormal—lesion growing from wall; biopsy, could be carcinoma
- Abnormal—grapelike clusters; biopsy, could be transitional cell carcinoma
- Abnormal—trabeculations (hypertrophied detrusor muscle), benign; seen in OAB or outlet obstruction
- Abnormal—Hunner ulcer; pathognomonic for interstitial cystitis

**Normal Urethra—Collapsed in Absence of Fluid Flow**
- Abnormal—fronds or pseudopolyps, benign response to inflammation
- Abnormal—stricture; prior surgery, especially urethral diverticulum excision

**Ureteral Orifices with Bilateral Jets of Urine Flow**
- Abnormal—sluggish flow, could mean partial obstruction
- Abnormal—no flow, could mean obstruction from current or past surgery, stone, or stricture

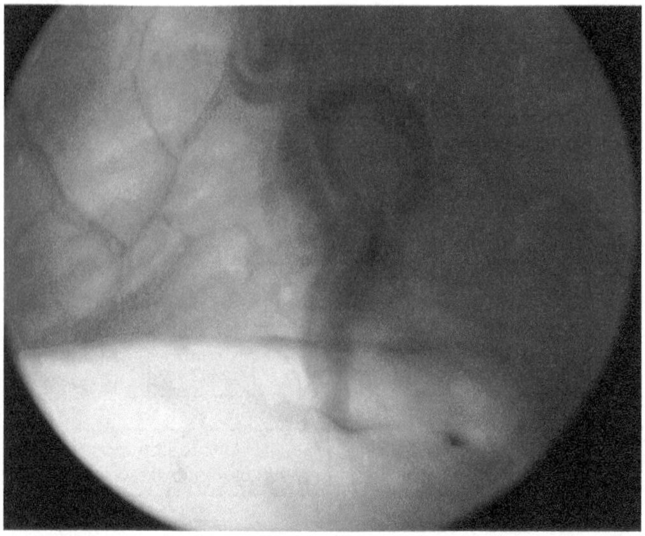

**Figure 21.10** Cystoscopy after indigo carmine was infused intravenously to confirm the duplicated ureters on the left side and that both were functioning.

## INFECTIONS OF THE LOWER URINARY TRACT

### *CYSTITIS*

A UTI (cystitis) is the most common bacterial infection seen in an outpatient setting. Infections of the urethra and bladder are almost always associated with some combination of the following: frequency, urgency, dysuria, pyuria, hematuria, acute or chronic pelvic pain, backache, and, at times, fever. As many as 50% of all women develop UTIs at some time during their life and, by age 70, as many as 10% of women will have recurrent UTIs. At times, incontinence is associated with acute and recurrent infections. Although *Escherichia coli* is the cause of most UTIs (80% to 85%), a myriad of organisms, including *Enterobacter, Klebsiella, Pseudomonas, Proteus, Streptococcus faecalis, Staphylococcus saprophyticus, Enterococcus,* and *Chlamydia,* can be found. The presence of bacteria in the urine (bacteriuria) does not necessarily prove clinical infection. Bacteriuria is fairly common in women, especially older women. For example, cumulative data from several studies have suggested that 20% of women older than 65 years will demonstrate bacteriuria, but the percentage increases from approximately 15% in the 65- to 70-year group to 20% to 50% for women older than 80 years. Bacteriuria is present in women who are on chronic catheterization and common in women in nursing homes who are chronically incontinent. Asymptomatic bacteriuria is not treated, even in older women or people with diabetes, with no change in their morbidity or mortality (Mody, 2014). Exceptions exist to this recommendation if the woman is undergoing an invasive procedure, is pregnant, has had a renal transplant, or is incontinent and her incontinence resolves with treatment. If a woman with asymptomatic bacteriuria becomes symptomatic, treatment is appropriate.

Many explanations have been offered as to why the female urinary tract is vulnerable to infection. These include the following: short female urethra, thereby allowing easier access of bacteria to the bladder; proximity of the vulva, vagina, and rectum to the opening of the urethra; effects of sexual intercourse on the entrance of bacteria into the urethra and lower urinary tract; and effect of loss of estrogen on the reproductive tract of older women. After menopause, the vaginal pH rises and may alter the vaginal flora, allowing for colonization of uropathogenic species, especially *E. coli*; it is probably appropriate to add personal immunologic and genetic variations to this list, which may make one woman more susceptible than another to certain bacteria. Genetic factors also explain why some UTIs as nonsecretors of certain blood group antigens are at increased risk.

The definition of a symptomatic UTI is a woman with dysuria, frequency, urgency, or suprapubic pain with pyuria. Uncomplicated UTIs occur in healthy women with normal urinary function. UTIs are classified as complicated when there are comorbid conditions that require longer treatment courses, such as underlying urologic abnormalities, presence of a foreign body (e.g., catheter), urinary calculi, obstruction of urine flow, diabetes mellitus, spinal cord injury, pregnancy, renal transplantation, or other illnesses. Acute uncomplicated cystitis (AUC) can often be diagnosed successfully with symptom assessment. In outpatient settings, women with at least two of three acute symptoms (dysuria, urgency, frequency) in the absence of vaginal discharge (or risk for sexually transmitted infection) have a greater than 90% probability of having AUC. Additional urine testing does not aid in the diagnostic accuracy. However, outside of those criteria, a clean-catch midstream urine sample for dipstick testing for leukocyte esterase and nitrites or a microscopic unspun urine evaluation for white blood cells (pyuria) can be helpful. Pyuria should always be seen in the urine when UTI occurs and is the most valuable test. RBCs may be present in microscopic or macroscopic numbers. Hematuria is common in acute infections, and infection is the most common cause of hematuria. Gross hematuria may occur as a result of the extravasation of blood across dilated and inflamed capillaries. If microscopic or macroscopic hematuria persists after UTI treatment, it must be evaluated. The pathogens are predictable in AUC, so culture is unnecessary and can be reserved for recurrent UTIs (≥2 in 6 months) or complicated UTIs. If a culture is done, it usually grows a single organism. The number of organisms per milliliter is not important. In cases of urethritis, the presence of as few as 100 organisms/mL may indicate an infection because of the dilution of the urine.

In 2009, the Infectious Diseases Society of America (IDSA) developed evidence-based guidelines for the treatment of acute uncomplicated cystitis (AUC). These are UTIs in nonpregnant, premenopausal women without pyelonephritis. If local *E. coli* bacterial resistance rates are less than 20%, trimethoprim-sulfamethoxazole (TMP-SMX) is recommended. Three-day therapy is adequate for AUC. The resistance of *E. coli* to TMP-SMX has increased over time. Short-course (3-day) therapy improves patient tolerability and compliance and reduces cost. This treatment strategy results in more than a 90% cure rate. Nitrofurantoin monohydrate/macrocrystals are an appropriate alternative. At least 5 days of drug treatment is recommended. Resistance rates of *E. coli* to nitrofurantoin have remained low. This should be avoided if early pyelonephritis is even suspected. The third alternative recommended is fosfomycin trometanol, 3 grams given as a single dose. This may have slightly lower efficacy than the other two options. Fluoroquinolones are not on the list, although highly efficacious, as resistance is rising, and it is recommended that these medications be reserved for

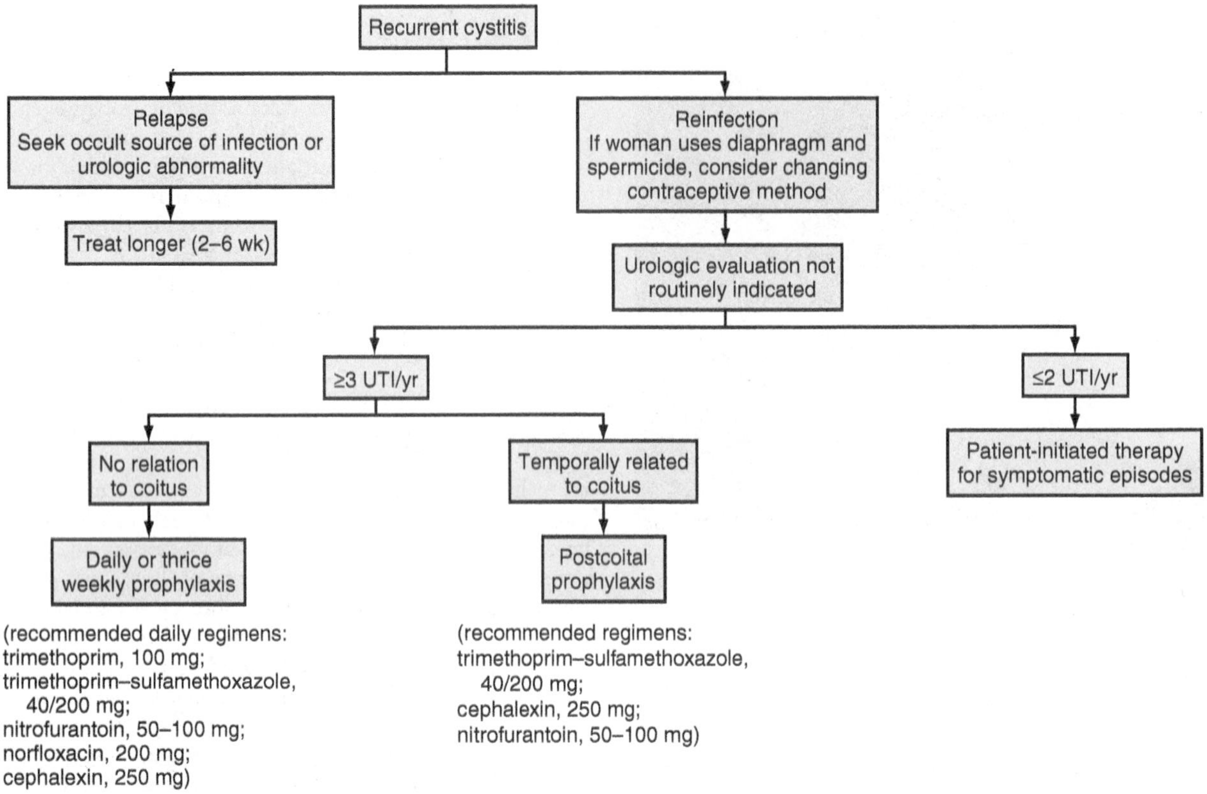


**Figure 21.11** Strategies for managing recurrent cystitis in women. (From Stamm WE, Hooton TM. Management of urinary tract infections in adults. *N Engl J Med.* 1993;329:1328-1334.)

more serious infections. With uncomplicated UTIs, progression to pyelonephritis is extremely rare. The woman should remain adequately hydrated and be encouraged to continue treatment, even though symptoms generally disappear within 48 hours. Infections frequently recur because they are not adequately eradicated. This may result from physician error (treating with too low a dose of antibiotic, the wrong antibiotic, or for too short a period of time) or patient error (not taking the medication as prescribed). For complicated UTIs, a 7- to 10-day course of a fluoroquinolone is recommended. If a culture is obtained and results are reported, the antibiotic may be changed if the organisms noted are not sensitive to the antibiotic in use.

Persistent or recurrent cystitis following the initial infection presents in approximately 20% of women (Fig. 21.11). Frequent infections with the same organism (relapse) suggest the possibility that a nidus of infection exists. Recurrent infections of different organisms (reinfection) should alert the physician to the need for a more complete evaluation. However, radiographic imaging—seeking structural abnormalities of the bladder, kidney, or ureters—is rarely useful in otherwise healthy women. More than 90% of recurrences in young women are exogenous reinfection with new isolates arising from local flora. Behavioral modification has become popular for preventing recurrent acute cystitis. Possible modifications in lifestyle include discontinuing use of a diaphragm and spermicide for contraception. Nonoxynol 9 has been associated with an increased risk of UTIs in women (Fihn, 1996).

Recurrent UTI are defined by ≥2 episodes in the past 6 months or ≥3 episodes in the past 12 months. In primary care clinics, 53% of women over 55 years of age and 36% of younger women report a recurrence within 1 year. There are several strategies for managing recurrent UTIs. One strategy is eliminating risk factors, such as use of Nonoxynol 9 or correcting vaginal atrophy. Postmenopausal women with recurrent UTIs often benefit from vaginal estrogen therapy because this restores the acidic environment of the vagina and allows normal bacteria and lactobacilli to repopulate the vagina (Raz, 1993). Many episodes of recurrent UTIs in young women occur within 24 hours of coitus. These women are excellent candidates to be treated with postcoital prophylactic antibiotics with a single dose. The antibiotics most commonly chosen for low-dose antibiotic prophylaxis include trimethoprim, TMP-SMX, nitrofurantoin, and a cephalosporin. Often women with recurrent UTIs at unpredictable times prefer self-initiated treatment with the onset of symptoms. Using the antibiotics presented here for AUC is reasonable. Continuous antibiotics are sometimes needed. Prophylaxis may be given for months without significant emergence of antibiotic-resistant bacteria. Personalized antibiotic prophylaxis remains the most effective method of managing recurrent UTIs. Non-antibiotic prevention strategies such as cranberry supplements, vitamin C, and methenamine salts lack strong evidence of benefit, but some women wish to try these options. The most evidence exists for cranberry supplements, but the correct dosage or formulation is unknown and studies are contradictory. D-Mannose also has little evidence of benefit but is being studied. Also under study are use of vaccinations, *Lactobacillus* and probiotics. Delaying treatment with antibiotics and trying ibuprofen has been studied. However, the majority of women needed antibiotics, and it just delayed the duration of symptoms (Grigoryan, 2014).

Frequent catheterizations or manipulation of the lower urinary tract will often cause UTIs. An indwelling catheter for 24 hours leads to bacteriuria in as many as 50% of patients. When left in place for 96 hours, an indwelling catheter causes bacteriuria in almost 100% of patients. There is no good evidence supporting the use of prophylactic antibiotics in patients who must continue catheter use. A woman with an indwelling catheter should be monitored for the possibility of a symptomatic UTI, be kept adequately hydrated, have a urine culture if symptoms occur, and be treated with the appropriate antibiotic. However, it is difficult to eradicate infection in the presence of an indwelling catheter. Removing the catheter or switching to clean intermittent self-catheterization would be optimal. Postoperative and debilitated patients are at greatest risk.

Although physicians commonly recommend measures to their patients for preventing UTIs, studies do not support these practices. These include wiping the rectum away from the urethra, voiding after intercourse, and drinking more fluid.

Additional circumstances that may be responsible for infections in women include the dilation of the urinary tract in pregnancy, urinary tract obstruction, urinary stones, urethral diverticulum, foreign bodies (e.g., mesh placed for a midurethral sling for incontinence), ureteral reflux, and pelvic organ prolapse. Other causes of UTIs in men and women include the need for frequent catheterization, instrumentation, and overdistention of the bladder in neurogenic conditions in which stasis becomes a problem.

### *URETHRITIS*

Patients with acute urethritis generally have the typical findings of lower tract UTIs, which include dysuria, frequency, and urgency. They often have a urethra that is tender to palpation. Under certain circumstances, it may be possible to express pus from the urethra; this is particularly common in acute infections with gonococcal or *Chlamydia* organisms. In these situations, the infection involves not only the urethra but also the periurethral glands. Herpes simplex virus has also been associated with urethritis. *Trichomonas vaginalis* has been cultured in nongonococcal urethritis but is more established as a causative agent in men.

Pus expressed from the urethra should be submitted for culture and for smear with Gram stain. Intracellular diplococci are suggestive of gonorrhea. *Neisseria gonorrhoeae* and *Chlamydia* are well known for causing urethritis, and nucleic acid amplification tests (NAATs) of the urine enable detection of both organisms. It should be kept in mind that these are reportable diseases to the state health department. Frequently, significant pyuria is noted in a first void clean-catch urine sample, particularly when taken early in the voiding. Urine obtained by the clean-catch method should also be cultured. NAATs are available at major centers for *Mycoplasma genitalium,* although not approved by the U.S. Food and Drug Administration (FDA). This organism has been implicated in recurrent urethritis in men and cervicitis and pelvic inflammatory disease in women, so is worth consideration if no other causes of dysuria are identified.

If no specific organism is identified on smear, treating as for AUC is appropriate with 3 days of TMP/SMX or nitrofurantoin for 5 days. If *Chlamydia* is found on NAAT, doxycycline, 100 mg twice daily, should be prescribed for 7 days, or azithromycin, 1 g orally, in a single dose, should be given. If gonorrhea is diagnosed, the current recommended treatment consists of dual therapy with ceftriaxone 250 mg IM (single dose), plus azithromycin 1 g (single dose). Alternative treatment is cefixime, 400 mg (single dose) with azithromycin 1 gram (single dose) (Centers for Disease Control and Prevention [CDC] 2015). Coinfections with *N. gonorrhoeae* and *C. trachomatis* are common. *Mycoplasma* and *ureaplasma* are treated with 7 days of doxycycline as for *Chlamydia,* but they have a cure rate of 31%. Azithromycin is more effective, but resistance is rising.

## PAINFUL BLADDER SYNDROME AND INTERSTITIAL CYSTITIS

Painful bladder syndrome is a more global definition adopted by the International Continence Society to deal with patients with pain syndromes of the lower urinary tract without evidence of bladder pathology or infection. By definition, painful bladder syndrome (PBS) is the complaint of suprapubic pain related to bladder filling accompanied by other symptoms, such as daytime frequency and nocturia, in the absence of proven UTIs or other pathology. Interstitial cystitis (IC) is a complex, painful bladder condition that may be the same entity as PBS or may be at the far end on the severity spectrum. There is no consensus on how to define this condition. They will be referred to together as PBS-IC or individually, according to research study definition. The cause and pathophysiology are poorly understood but are most likely multifactorial. Theories regarding cause include an altered bladder epithelial permeability, mast cell activation, and an up-regulation of sensory afferent nerves. Studies have found that C fiber bladder afferent neurons have changes in their electrical and chemical properties affecting bladder sensitivity. It is a common syndrome, seen in women more often than men, but the actual incidence is unknown, although it has been estimated to be as high as 500/100,000 women.

The most common symptoms of PBS-IC are bladder-pelvic pain, urgency, daytime frequency, and nocturia, without evidence of infection or other causes. A common feature that may distinguish PBS-IC from other conditions is increase in pain with bladder filling and relief with voiding. The so-called *urethral syndrome* is poorly characterized and has largely been abandoned. The International Continence Society standardization report in 2002 added a new genitourinary pain syndrome category and defined urethral pain syndrome as the "occurrence of recurrent episodic urethral pain usually on voiding, with daytime frequency and nocturia, in the absence of proven infection or other obvious pathology." This problem may be part of the PBS-IC group. Several symptom indices are useful for evaluating women with painful bladder complaints, although they were not developed for screening. The pain, urgency, frequency (PUF) scale (Table 21.4) and O'Leary-Sant scale are helpful in characterizing a woman's complaints, especially in light of the lack of definitive diagnostic testing. There is much overlap in PBS-IC symptomatology. It is often confused with other bladder conditions such as UTIs, overactive bladder, and urethral syndrome (an outdated term, but it may be part of the spectrum of the syndrome). The differential diagnosis also includes several gynecologic conditions such as pelvic inflammatory disease, vulvodynia, and endometriosis. Dyspareunia is also a common

Table 21.4 Pelvic Pain, Urgency, Frequency (PUF) Patient Symptom Scale

| | POINTS | | | | | |
|---|---|---|---|---|---|---|
| **Question** | **0** | **1** | **2** | **3** | **4** | **Score** |
| 1. How many times do you go to the bathroom during the day? | 3-6 | 7-10 | 11-14 | 15-19 | 20 + | |
| 2. a. How many times do you go to the bathroom at night? | 0 | 1 | 2 | 3 | 4 + | |
| b. If you get up at night to go to the bathroom, does it bother you? | Never | Occasionally | Moderate | Severe | | |
| 3. Are you currently sexually active? Yes/No | | | | | | |
| 4. a. If you are sexually active, do you now or have you ever had pain or symptoms during or after sexual intercourse? | Never | Occasionally | Usually | Always | | |
| b. If you have pain, does it make you avoid sexual intercourse? | Never | Occasionally | Usually | Always | | |
| 5. Do you have pain associated with your bladder or in your pelvis (vagina, labia, lower abdomen, urethra, perineum)? | Never | Occasionally | Usually | Always | | |
| 6. Do you still have urgency after you go to the bathroom? | Never | Occasionally | Usually | Always | | |
| 7. a. If you have pain, is it usually mild, moderate, or severe? | | Mild | Moderate | Severe | | |
| b. Does your pain bother you? | Never | Occasionally | Usually | Always | | |
| 8. a. If you have urgency, is it usually mild, moderate, or severe? | | Mild | Moderate | Severe | | |
| b. Does your urgency bother you? | Never | Occasionally | Usually | Always | | |
| Total Score: | | | | | | |

complaint in sexually active women and in women with PBS-IC. PBS-IC should be considered in the differential diagnosis of any woman with chronic pelvic pain.

A urinalysis, urine culture, and postvoid residual urine are recommended. A voiding diary will often demonstrate frequent small voids of less than 150 mL each and as many as 20 or more voids daily. Sleep can be disrupted by a frequent need to void. On examination, suprapubic and anterior vaginal wall tenderness may be found. Other assessments might include cytology (tobacco use), imaging, cystoscopy, and or laparoscopy. These are not needed to make the diagnosis. Cystoscopy may be needed to rule out other conditions. On cystoscopy, the bladder frequently appears normal during filling but, with distention under anesthesia, characteristic petechial hemorrhages resembling glomeruli usually appear. Oozing of blood is often seen. However, glomerulations may be a nonspecific finding because they can be seen in asymptomatic women. This cystoscopic finding is not diagnostic of IC, although it is used to differentiate IC from PBS in some studies. Hunner ulcers are diagnostic of IC but are infrequently seen in women with bladder pain. If a biopsy under anesthesia is taken, ulcers with granulation tissue, mucosal hemorrhage, monocytic infiltration, and mast cells in the lamina propria and detrusor muscle are often seen. Parsons has proposed that these changes are related to a defective or altered glycosaminoglycan mucus layer, which results in altered bladder permeability (Parsons, 1994). However, investigations to date have not shown whether this alteration is cause or effect. Some authors believe that these changes are the result of an autoimmune disease. The presence of immunoglobulins and complement in the bladder wall and the increase in interleukin-6 level in patients' urine may support this finding. Naturally occurring feline interstitial cystitis (FIC) shows changes in electrical currents that control neuronal excitability in sensory neurons.

To date, there is no laboratory test or urine test that is diagnostic of IC. Although urodynamic testing may reveal that these patients have early first sensation to void and low bladder capacities, there is no range in volume that is specific for IC. The potassium sensitivity test (PST) involves inserting a catheter into the bladder and instilling a saline solution, followed by a potassium chloride solution. A positive PST result is noted if increased pain occurs with the potassium solution. Current recommendations do not support using the PST for diagnosis of PBS-IC (Hanno, 2015), and it can be very painful for women.

Many treatments are available, but few have been uniformly helpful. A multipronged treatment strategy is often necessary including behavioral changes, oral medications, bladder instillations, and other surgical treatments (Hanno, 2015). Women are encouraged to see this as a chronic problem that is not malignant and to try to reduce stress, work on general management strategies, encourage family support, and avail themselves of the writings and support of the Interstitial Cystitis Association. Women should be instructed to avoid acidic, alcoholic, and carbonated beverages, spicy foods, coffee, tea, chocolate, tomatoes, vinegar, and artificial sweeteners, all of which have been associated with increased pain in patients with PBS-IC. Tobacco should also be avoided. Bladder retraining to increase the interval between voiding may help. Pelvic floor physical therapy that emphasizes relaxation techniques also can be of benefit in woman with increased pelvic floor muscle tone and tenderness.

A heparin analogue, pentosan polysulfate sodium (PPS, Elmiron), has been given orally 100 mg three times daily, with some reported improvement. PPS is the only FDA-approved oral drug for IC and may help repair the glycosaminoglycan layer of the bladder epithelium. It can take 6 months to be effective and improvements are modest; 38% of patients have a more than 50% improvement at 12 weeks. Tricyclic antidepressants may also be helpful because they can inhibit the neural activation that leads to pain. Amitriptyline is not FDA-approved for IC, but doses of 10 to 75 mg nightly have produced pain relief in two thirds of women and decreases in urgency and frequency. Unfortunately, in another trial, when reviewing all randomized subjects, amitriptyline with education and behavioral modification did not significantly improve symptoms. However, in this study, it was found that amitriptyline may benefit those who can tolerate a daily dose of 50 mg or more, although this subgroup comparison was not specified in advance. Women with PBS-IC often have trouble sleeping from the pain and nocturia and amitriptyline has anticholinergic effects to potentially reduce urgency/frequency, so taking amitriptyline at bedtime might be helpful for other reasons. The side effects of sedation, dry mouth, and constipation are often bothersome. Antihistamines such as hydroxyzine may be of benefit for patients with concurrent allergies and for decreasing mast cell degranulation, but most studies have not shown benefit. Depression treatments and antidepressants may be useful in depressed women. General chronic pain medication treatments might be of use.

Bladder instillations with various solutions have been tried. FDA-approved therapy includes dimethyl sulfoxide (DMSO) bladder instillation. DMSO is an anti-inflammatory agent that acts as a bladder anesthetic, relaxes muscles, causes mast cell inhibition, and may dissolve collagen. Many other drugs have been instilled, including heparin, lidocaine, steroids, and oxybutynin, but trials are insufficient to show a benefit. With pain flares, heparin and lidocaine may be of benefit (though not FDA approved).

Hydrodistention of the bladder under anesthesia is therapeutic in 20% to 30% of patients and is sometimes done at the initial evaluation when performing cystoscopy to rule out other pathology. However, most experts do not use hydrodistention as a diagnostic criterion any longer because the findings of glomerulations are nondiagnostic. If Hunner ulcerations are seen, they can be treated. Three to 6 months of symptom improvement occurs with distention in responders.

Hormonal suppression in premenopausal women with menstrual flares may provide benefit. There are additional fourth- and fifth-line therapies to be tried if the basic strategies have not been successful, including neuromodulation and intradetrusor Botox injections. Because PBS-IC is a complex disease, it is best treated by an experienced physician with the expertise and patience to deal with the woman and her needs over a prolonged period. Usually, multiple interventions are necessary, with a combination of behavioral changes, pelvic floor physical therapy, counseling, oral medications, and bladder instillations.

## URETHRAL DIVERTICULUM

### Causes

Urethral diverticulum is an outpouching of the urethral mucosa, usually into the vaginal tissues. Urethral diverticula occur in perhaps as many as 1% to 5% of all women at some time during their lifetime. Age distribution in published reports ranges from 19 to 76 years, but most diverticula seem to occur between the ages of 20 and 60 years. The disease occurs more frequently in black women than white women, with a ratio perhaps as high as 3:1.

A variety of causes have been suggested, including congenital, acute and chronic inflammatory, and traumatic. The congenital theory stems from the fact that rare cases have been reported in children and neonates. Most are likely acquired, however. Evidence for acute and chronic infection comes from observations noting infection and obstruction of the periurethral glands, which result in the formation of retention cysts that when repeatedly infected, may rupture into the lumen of the urethra and remain as an outpouching, giving rise to the diverticulum. Several authors have suggested that the gonococcus is the cause of this condition, but *E. coli* and other organisms have been found in such processes. Urethral trauma from multiple catheterizations or from childbirth has also been suggested as a causative factor. However, many women with diverticula have neither been catheterized nor given birth.

### Symptoms and Signs

The classic description of symptoms in a woman with urethral diverticula includes the three Ds: postvoid dribbling, dysuria, and dyspareunia. More common are complaints of postvoid dribbling and the finding of an anterior vaginal wall mass. Urinary frequency and urgency, dysuria, history of recurrent UTIs, dribbling, urethral or vaginal pain, and incontinence symptoms occur and more often will suggest other etiologies. Occasionally, hematuria occurs or stones are found in the diverticula or discharge or pus come from the urethra. Most occur in the middle or distal urethra posteriorly. There may be more than one present, and complex diverticula can even encircle the urethra or be horseshoe shaped.

### Diagnosis

Diagnosis is generally suggested by physical examination. The distal anterior vaginal wall overlying the urethra or bladder neck may be tender, or a cystic mass may be found about the distal or midurethra. Pus, blood, or cloudy urine may be expressed as the urethra and mass are massaged. A normal examination and nonclassic symptoms are often typical of how a woman presents, which is why the diagnosis is often delayed. Historically, the double-catheter balloon technique, which essentially closes the urethra at each end and forces contrast medium into the diverticulum under pressure during cystography, has been the gold standard. Now, magnetic resonance imaging (MRI) with cross-sectional imaging offers the most detailed anatomic study; it can also image diverticula that do not communicate with the urethra, as well as multiple outpouchings. Other tests are sometimes useful, such as urethroscopy, voiding cystourethrography, urodynamics (because 35% to 50% will have incontinence), and transvaginal ultrasound.

### Treatment

No treatment is indicated for asymptomatic urethral diverticula. Mild symptoms of frequency and urgency can be treated with anticholinergics and infections with antibiotics. Carcinoma has been reported in diverticula, so caution is needed if no surgical therapy is planned. A variety of procedures have been suggested for the management of urethral diverticula. Lapides has suggested a technique for transurethral marsupialization that involves the resection of the roof of the diverticulum using transurethral electrocautery (Lapides, 1978). Essentially, this technique enlarges the orifice of the diverticulum by incising its roof; however, the orifice can be challenging to identify or not found at all. Others have reported a marsupialization technique in which the diverticulum was opened and sutured to the vaginal epithelial surface. Generally, this leads to a fistula and requires secondary closure, making this technique useful in only rare circumstances and with distal diverticulum. Transvaginal diverticulectomy is the more common procedure.

Urethroscopy occasionally identifies the location of the diverticulum and careful inspection may show multiple diverticula. One study noted the diverticulum coming from the distal third of the urethra in only 10 of 85 patients, whereas 38 patients demonstrated an origin from the middle third and 13 from the proximal third, including the bladder neck (Lee, 1983). Lee noted multiple diverticula in 18 of 85 patients.

After the diverticulum is identified and evaluated, an incision is made in the anterior vaginal wall and the diverticulum is dissected free of the pubocervical connective tissue. The diverticulum's neck is noted and excised by sharp dissection, and the urethral wall is closed with a row of interrupted 4-0 polyglycol sutures. The closure line is generally in the longitudinal axis. Occasionally, however, a transverse closure is necessary because of the nature of the attachment. The pubocervical connective tissue is then reinforced with a row of 3-0 polyglycol reabsorbable interrupted sutures with attempt to avoid overlapping suture lines. Hemostasis is scrupulously secured with electrocautery, and the vaginal incision is closed with polyglycol sutures (Fig. 21.12).

Most diverticula emanate from the ventral wall of the urethra. Occasionally, however, the diverticulum is noted to be arising from the lateral wall of the urethra or even from the anterior wall. In these cases, the dissection must be carefully carried to the base of the diverticulum and the procedure carried out as stated. In all cases, a 16 French Foley or suprapubic catheter is left in place for 7 to 14 days. Postoperative voiding cystourethrogram can be performed to ensure that there are no urethrovesical fistulas before discontinuing use of the catheter.

Several nuances have been offered to make dissection and subsequent repair easier. One involves placing a ureteral catheter into the diverticulum and allowing it to coil so that the diverticulum is more easily observable during dissection. Some surgeons have attempted to dilate the neck of the diverticulum before beginning the excision and, occasionally, have even tried to pack foreign substances such as gauze through the neck to make the dissection easier. Sometimes, a Martius flap is brought into the field between the periurethral connective tissue closure and vaginal wall. This is thought to prevent fistula formation and is more commonly done with recurrent diverticulum.

### Complications

Major complications of this procedure include urethrovaginal fistula formation, development of stress urinary incontinence, recurrence of the diverticulum, missing diverticula when multiple diverticula are present, and stricture of the urethra. Reported urethrovaginal fistula rates are 5% to 8.3%. If the diverticulum recurs

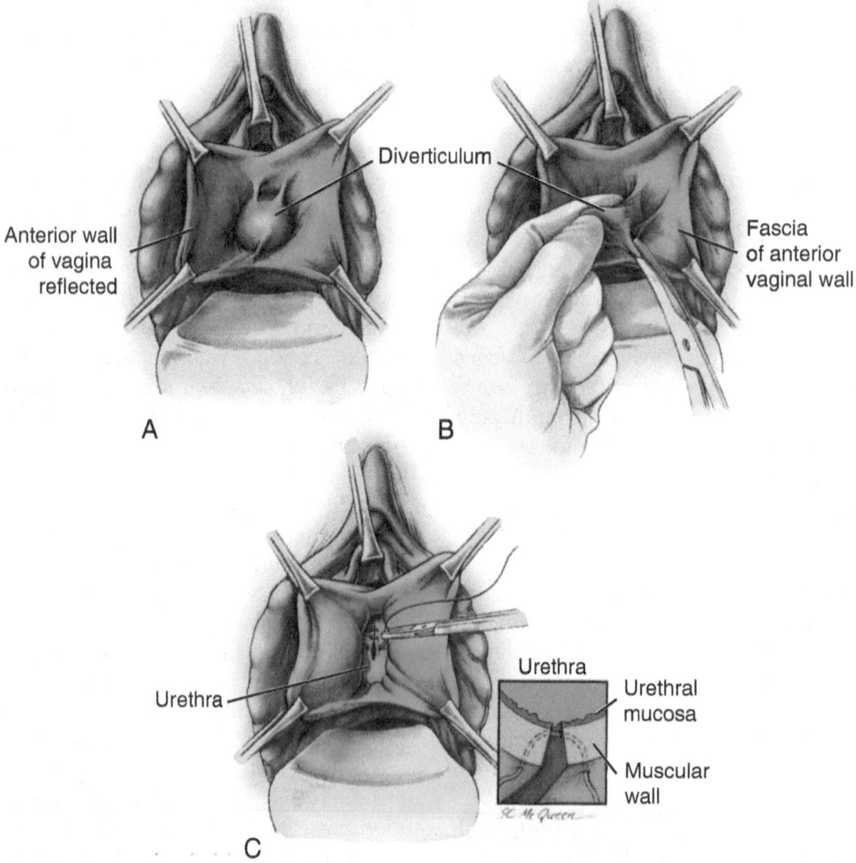


**Figure 21.12** Resection of Urethral Diverticulum. **A,** Diverticulum exposed with vaginal lining and endopelvic fascia retracted. **B,** Fingers hold diverticulum on traction, which aids in dissection and identification of ostium. **C,** After complete resection of the diverticulum, the urethra is closed with fine, interrupted extramucosal sutures. (Modified from Lee RA. Diverticulum of the female urethra: postoperative complications and results. *Obstet Gynecol.* 1983;61:52-58.)

within the first few months after operation, it may represent a second diverticulum that was overlooked or an inappropriate repair of the diagnosed diverticulum. If the diverticulum occurs after 1 year, it is probably a new lesion. Stricture of the urethra has been reported less than 5% of the time. After diverticulectomy, recurrence that requires repeat excision occurs about 10% of the time. Risk factors for recurrence included proximal diverticulum, multiple diverticula, and previous pelvic or vaginal surgery, excluding previous diverticulectomy. Some with recurrent diverticulum will have persistent pain or discomfort with urination and even with complete excision those symptoms can remain.

Stress incontinence development may be related to the dissection of the bladder neck and proximal urethra with injury to the urethral sphincter mechanism. If intrinsic sphincter deficiency results, the incontinence can be difficult to treat because of tissue compromise from repair.

## UROLITHIASIS

Urinary tract stones, renal or ureteral, may occur in patients of both genders and at any age. Approximately 5% of women will develop a symptomatic stone by the age of 70 years. These may be related to metabolic abnormalities, such as gout or errors of calcium metabolism, but usually relate to chronic infection and stasis of urine. The leading risk factor for stones is genetic. Other risk factors for calculi in women include pregnancy, during which time the urinary tract becomes dilated and stasis is more common, a history of kidney stones or family history, certain medications, excessive vitamin C intake, low calcium intake, chronic diarrhea, and dehydration.

Symptoms occur most often when a stone passes from the kidney to the ureter. Pain occurs on the side of the stone and varies from a dull ache to severe paroxysms of pain, called *renal colic.* Flank pain, lower abdominal pain, and groin pain can occur; the location can vary as the stone moves down the ureter with radiation of pain to the groin. Gross or microscopic hematuria is usually present. Noncontrast CT scanning has become the gold standard for diagnosis, particularly if the abdominal radiograph is normal. Ultrasound misses small stones but is recommended for pregnant women and is increasingly recommended for initial screening as no radiation is used.

Various treatment modalities are available, including observation with pain medications and fluids awaiting spontaneous passage, endoscopic removal, surgical removal, and destruction of the stone with laser or shockwave lithotripsy. Although not FDA-approved, alpha-blockers may aid in passage of the stone. The principal consideration, however, should be correction of the basic problem that caused the stone. Urgent intervention is necessary if the woman has fever, chills, nausea and vomiting, and pain uncontrolled by narcotics. An obstructing stone in the presence of infection can be life threatening.

## URINARY INCONTINENCE

### RISK FACTORS

Box 21.2 lists the currently known risk factors associated with incontinence, summarizing the work of several authors. Some of the factors will be highlighted in this section. The prevalence of urinary incontinence increases until approximately 50 years of age and then stabilizes before increasing again after age 65. Prevalence estimates were presented earlier in this chapter. One study compared risk factors and determinants of urodynamic stress incontinence between smokers and nonsmokers using a case-control method (Bump, 1994). In this study, 71 smokers and 118 nonsmokers were compared following a complete urogynecologic evaluation. Smokers were found to have stronger urethral sphincters and generated a greater increase in bladder pressure with coughing, but similar findings with respect to urethral mobility and pressure transmission ratios were found when compared with nonsmokers. Urodynamic stress incontinence developed in smokers despite their stronger urethral sphincter findings,

**Box 21.2 Factors Independently Associated with Urinary Incontinence in Women**

**MODIFIABLE FACTORS**

| | |
|---|---|
| **Gynecologic** | **Medications** |
| Cystocele | Diuretics |
| Uterine prolapse | Estrogen |
| Non-normal gynecologic examination | Benzodiazepines |
| Poor pelvic floor muscle contraction | Tranquilizers |
| | Antidepressants |
| | Hypnotics |
| | Laxatives |
| **Urologic and Gastrointestinal** | **Other Factors** |
| Antibiotics | Smoking |
| Recurrent urinary tract infections | High caffeine intake |
| Dysuria | Higher body mass index |
| Fecal incontinence | Functional impairment |
| Constipation | |
| Bowel problems | |
| **Comorbid Diseases** | |
| Diabetes | |
| Stroke | |
| Elevated systolic blood pressure | |
| Cognitive impairment | |
| Parkinsonism | |
| Arthritis | |
| Back problems | |
| Hearing and visual impairment | |

**NONMODIFIABLE FACTORS**

| | |
|---|---|
| **Gynecologic Factors** | **Other Factors** |
| Hysterectomy in older women | Age |
| Prolapse surgery | White race |
| | Higher education |
| | Childhood enuresis |
| | Presence of two or more comorbid diseases |
| **Pregnancy-Related Factors** | |
| Vaginal delivery | |
| Forceps delivery | |
| Cesarean section | |
| Increased parity | |
| Fetal birth weight | |

From Holroyd-Leduc JM, Straus SE. Management of urinary incontinence in women: clinical applications. *JAMA.* 2004;291(8):996-999.

probably because of more violent coughing leading to earlier development of anatomic defects.

Another area of interest involves racial and ethnic differences with respect to the presence of urinary incontinence. Black women with urinary incontinence have a different distribution of symptoms and different reasons for their incontinence than white women. Black women had a significantly lower prevalence of pure urodynamic stress incontinence than white women. The findings may possibly relate to differences in collagen and connective tissue. Several other studies have found a higher prevalence of urinary incontinence in non-Hispanic white women and Mexican-Americen woman compared with rates in Asian and black women, although at least two studies have found no difference between racial or ethnic groups.

Obesity has a strong association with incontinence and, for every five-unit increase in body mass index, the risk increases. Depression and anxiety are associated with incontinence. This has been further evaluated in overweight and obese women. These women reported a higher number of weekly incontinence episodes than women without depressive symptoms, as well as more bothersome symptoms and poorer quality of life (Melville, 2009).

Epidemiologic studies have suggested increased risk with hysterectomy but short-term clinical studies have not, so more research is needed to clarify this issue. Vaginal childbirth and higher fetal weight are risk factors in younger women, but the effect diminishes in older women, possibly because the neuromuscular decline with aging becomes a more important factor. The prevalence of incontinence is significantly higher for women in nursing homes and women with cognitive impairment and poor mobility.

## *STRESS URINARY INCONTINENCE*

Stress urinary incontinence is the involuntary loss of urine with physical exertion such as exercise, cough, or sneeze. When urine leakage is observed during a urodynamic study, with an increase in intraabdominal pressure and without a detrusor contraction, it is called *urodynamic stress incontinence* (Haylen, 2010). Stress urinary incontinence is a common condition for which nearly 14% of women in the United States will undergo surgery at some point (Wu, 2014).

Injury, particularly trauma from obstetric delivery, has been implicated in stress incontinence. The odds ratio of stress urinary incontinence in parous compared with nulliparous women is threefold (Hansen, 2012); the odds ratio after vaginal compared with cesarean delivery is twofold (Lukacz, 2006). Meyer and colleagues studied 149 patients during pregnancy and 9 weeks postpartum. They found that 36% of women who were delivered by forceps and 21% who delivered spontaneously suffered from urinary incontinence (Meyer, 1998). Bladder neck mobility was significantly increased after all vaginal births, but bladder neck position at rest was only lowered in the forceps group. Women who underwent cesarean delivery were unaffected. DeLancey and coworkers have reported MRI images showing levator ani injuries in 10% to 15% of primiparous women (DeLancey, 2003). These injuries may lead to later pelvic floor dysfunction and incontinence, although long-term follow-up studies are needed (Fig. 21.13). Considering other forms of pelvic floor trauma, Nygaard studied female American Olympic athletes and could not find a difference between the low-impact (swimmers) and high-impact (gymnasts, track and field performers) athletes with respect to the development of stress incontinence later in life (Nygaard, 1997).

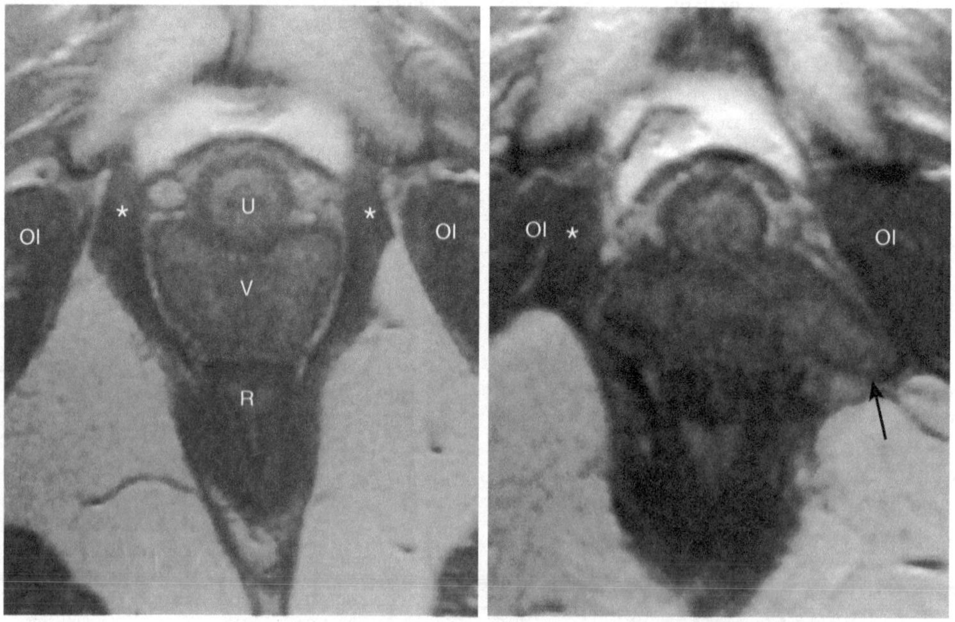


**Figure 21.13** Axial magnetic resonance imaging scan at the level of the midurethra in a normal nullipara *(left)* and a woman 9 months after vaginal birth *(right)* in whom the pubovisceral portion of the levator ani muscle has been lost. The pubovisceral muscle (*) is seen between the urethra *(U)* and obturator internus *(OI)* muscle in the normal woman but is missing in the woman on the right. *R*, Rectum; *V*, vagina. (From DeLancey JO, Ashton-Miller JA. Pathophysiology of adult urinary incontinence. *Gastroenterology*. 2004;126[Suppl 1]:S23-S32.)

### *Evaluation*

Urethral support and coaptation are both important for maintaining continence. DeLancey's hammock theory suggests that the urethra is supported by the endopelvic fascia and anterior vaginal wall (DeLancey, 1994). Because that support layer is attached to the pelvic wall via the arcus tendineus fascia pelvis and levator ani, the urethra is compressed by increases in abdominal pressure. This maintains urethral pressure above bladder pressure and prevents urinary leakage (Fig. 21.14). Urethral hypermobility, which can be measured using a "Q-tip test," corresponds to the loss of the backstop support at the bladder neck. The Q-tip test involves placing a cotton swab into the urethra to the bladder neck and observing the angle that the urethra makes with the horizontal during a strain maneuver. A large excursion from the horizontal suggests defects in the supports of the urethra but not a specific urologic diagnosis. However, this angle is useful for deciding on an appropriate anti-incontinence procedure because midurethral slings act by providing resistance to a hypermobile urethra during increases in intraabdominal pressure, whereas urethral bulking agents are not affected by urethral movement and may be more appropriate for some women with stress incontinence. These are discussed in the "Intrinsic Sphincter Deficiency" section of the chapter. A maximum Q-tip excursion angle greater than 30 degrees suggests hypermobility and is associated with higher success rates after midurethral sling surgery. Women with stress incontinence without urethral hypermobility have a 1.9-fold risk of failure after midurethral sling and may be better served by a urethral bulking agent, which improves urethral coaptation at rest and during strain (Richter, 2011). Urethral mobility can also be evaluated using the prolapse quantification system, visualization, palpation, or ultrasonography.

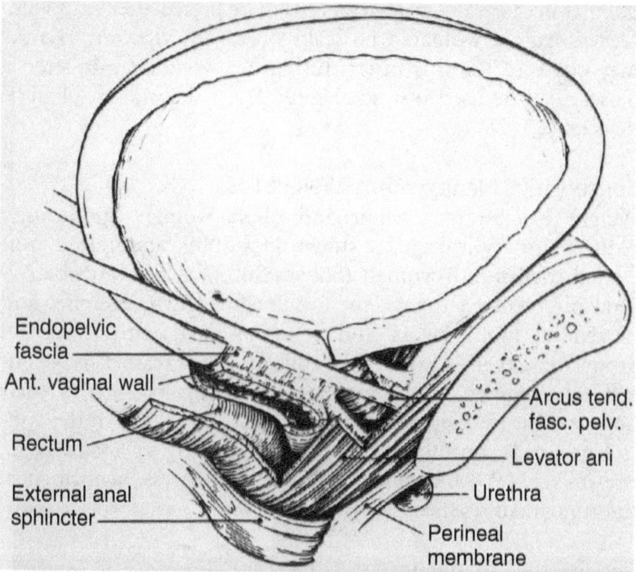


**Figure 21.14** Lateral view of the components of the urethral support system. Note how the levator ani muscles support the rectum, vagina, and urethrovesical neck. Also note how the endopelvic fascia next to the urethra attaches to the levator ani muscle; contraction of the levator muscle leads to elevation of the urethrovesical neck. (From DeLancey JO, Ashton-Miller JA. Pathophysiology of adult urinary incontinence. *Gastroenterology*. 2004;126[Suppl 1]:S23-S32.)

Urethral coaptation is affected by the urethral mucosa and vasculature, adjacent connective tissue structures, striated and smooth muscles, and involuntary and voluntary muscles that contract in response to stress. Midurethral sling and urethral bulking agents will be discussed in more detail in the Surgical Management section.

Stress incontinence may occur with injury to or degeneration of the urethral support system or urethral sphincter mechanism, and it is likely that most women with incontinence have elements of both problems. Although we try to classify women with stress incontinence as having urethral hypermobility or the more severe leakage associated with urethral musculature damage, termed *low-pressure urethra* or *intrinsic sphincter deficiency* (ISD), there is actually great overlap. The diagnosis of ISD is somewhat debatable but is given to women with low Valsalva leak point pressures or low maximum urethral closure pressures measured during urodynamics. These women may have more severe continence, and the diagnosis of ISD is also associated with higher failure rates after midurethral sling surgery as well (Nager, 2011).

Bladder neck funneling, position, and hypermobility can be evaluated by perineal ultrasound. Although the clinical uses to date are limited, it is useful in studying the pelvic structures in continent and incontinent women, and it may have clinical applications in the future. Ultrasound examination of the urethral sphincter may also be helpful in measuring length, thickness, and striated muscle volume. Athanasiou and associates, using three-dimensional ultrasound, have shown that women with stress urinary incontinence have significantly shorter, thinner, and smaller volumes of striated muscle in their urethras than continent women of comparable ages and parity (Athanasiou, 1999).

Women with anterior vaginal wall prolapse often have urethral hypermobility but may or may not have stress incontinence. If they have stress incontinence, they must have some urethral sphincter compromise along with the hypermobility. It is also possible that the prolapse kinks off the urethra, thus maintaining continence, and that reduction of the prolapse will unmask occult stress incontinence. Prolapse reduction stress testing, in which the patient is asked to cough with a comfortably full bladder while the prolapse is reduced, can help predict which women are likely to have stress incontinence after prolapse surgery. A concurrent anti-incontinence procedure can be considered in these women.

Prior to performing surgery for stress urinary incontinence, the minimum evaluation includes complete history (including urologic history, medical history, medications), urinalysis (to exclude urinary tract infection), physical examination that includes vaginal inspection and prolapse evaluation), demonstrable urinary leakage with a cough stress test, an evaluation of urethral mobility, measurement of postvoid residual volume (it should be less than 150 mL) (ACOG, 2014). This is sufficient for patients with uncomplicated stress incontinence. Multichannel urodynamic testing should be reserved for women with complicated stress incontinence, such as unclear diagnosis, large urge component, or prior anti-incontinence surgery. Inquiring about a woman's goals for treatment of stress incontinence is useful, as is identifying the most bothersome aspects of her complaints. All women should be offered conservative treatments first, and then surgery can be pursued if she fails or declines nonoperative treatments.

### *Treatment*

#### Conservative Management: Pelvic Floor Muscle Strengthening

Conservative measure should be discussed and offered to all women with stress incontinence (Box 21.3). The first-line treatment is pelvic floor muscle training directed toward the strengthening of the levator ani and pubococcygeal muscles, which affect the urethral closure mechanism. This can be affected by isometric exercises, as described by Kegel. The woman can be instructed on how to contract these muscles by being told to attempt to stop the urinary stream while she is voiding. Importantly, after she learns which muscles to contract, she should perform the exercises at other times without any relationship to voiding because contracting her pelvic floor muscles during voiding could lead to voiding dysfunction. Pelvic muscle exercise success is improved with specific training by a health professional or physical therapist. Improvement in the muscular supports may be enough to overcome the anatomic weakness that originally led to the stress incontinence.

Although these exercises have a number of modifications, one useful application is to teach the woman to contract these muscles slowly, 8 to 12 times, for a count of 6 to 8 seconds each, and to repeat this series for three sets daily. A meta-analysis of 12 randomized controlled trials found that at least 24 contractions a day for 6 weeks resulted in decreased incontinence episodes; more contractions did not result in additional improvement (Choi, 2007). Better efficacy was noted in younger women with stress incontinence than older women and women with mixed or urgency incontinence.

A Cochrane Database review of pelvic floor muscle training analyzed 21 trials involving 1281 women (Dumoulin, 2015). Women who did pelvic floor muscle training were 8 times more likely to be cured and 17 times more likely to be cured or improved compared with the control group. These exercises helped women with all types of incontinence. Again, the women with stress incontinence enjoyed more benefit. With no serious adverse effects, pelvic floor muscle training should be offered as a first-line conservative management program for women with urinary incontinence.

Many patients enjoy prolonged relief, even after stopping pelvic floor muscle exercises. Bø and Talseth studied 23 women who participated in a 6-month intensive pelvic floor muscle exercise routine and noted that 5 years later, 75% demonstrated no leakage during a stress test and 70% were satisfied with their continence (Bø, 1996). Of these patients, 70% were still exercising their pelvic muscles at least once weekly and demonstrated pelvic floor muscle strength. Nygaard noted similar findings (Nygaard, 1996). These authors noted improvement of incontinence, not only in patients with stress incontinence but also in those with urge and mixed urinary incontinence.

It is important to ensure that the woman is aware of how to perform the exercises correctly. In a study by Bump and coworkers in which 47 women were given simple verbal or written instructions, 23 (49%) had an ideal Kegel effort signified by an increase in force of the urethral closure. However, 12 subjects (25%) were performing the technique poorly and in such a way that incontinence might be promoted (Bump, 1991). The authors recommended a demonstration approach rather than a written or verbal approach.

A variation in pelvic muscle training is the use of weighted vaginal cones. This involves a set of cones of increasing weight that require pelvic muscle contraction to hold them within the vagina. Peattie and associates demonstrated an improvement in 70% of 30 premenopausal women with stress incontinence after only 1 month of exercise. A correlation was noted between decreased urine loss and the ability to retain cones of increased weight (Peattie, 1988).

Pelvic floor electrical stimulation has also been studied for improving pelvic floor muscle strength and decreasing symptoms of stress incontinence. A small, removable vaginal probe is placed in the vagina or anus and the electrical stimulation activates a pelvic muscle contraction. A randomized controlled trial by Goode and colleagues studied 200 women with stress incontinence and found that pelvic floor electrical stimulation did not increase effectiveness in a comprehensive behavioral training program (Goode, 2003).

**Box 21.3 Methods of Pelvic Muscle Strengthening**

Kegel exercises
Biofeedback
Isometric with vaginal cones (weights)
Electrical stimulation of pelvic floor

#### Conservative Management: Pessaries

An incontinence pessary is a silicone ring device with a knob placed in the vagina, with the goal of stabilizing the urethra to eliminate hypermobility and increase urethral pressure during increases in intraabdominal pressure. This is a safe and effective conservative treatment (Richter, 2010b). The FemSoft urethral insert device (Rochester Medical, Stewartville, MN) is basically a urethral plug. Although women with stress incontinence may have greatly reduced leakage when wearing the insert, it is not popular because a new device needs to be placed after each void. Occasionally a woman who leaks only with vigorous exercise may chose to use this insert during her workout, but often a pessary can be used instead. Figure 21.15 shows each of these devices.

#### Conservative Management: Weight Loss

Weight loss in overweight and obese woman significantly reduces urinary leakage, as shown in a 2009 randomized controlled trial of 338 women (Subak, 2009). A 6-month behavioral intervention for weight loss included diet, exercise, and behavioral modification and was compared with a control group that received structured education not related to weight loss. The women in the intervention group lost 8% of their body weight (7.8 kg) compared with 1.6% (1.5 kg) in the control group. Incontinence episodes declined by 47% and 28%, respectively ($P = .01$), but this was only for stress incontinence, not urge incontinence.

#### Conservative Management: Others

In postmenopausal women, estrogen therapy was thought to increase the vasculature and mucosal seal of the urethra, thereby increasing urethral closing pressure and overcoming the effects that may have led to mild degrees of stress incontinence. However, randomized studies have called into question these effects and, in fact, the opposite effect has been shown. The Heart and Estrogen/Progestin Replacement Study (HERS) found the women taking combined hormone replacement actually reported worsened incontinence (Grady, 1998). Both the Women's Health Initiative (WHI) and Nurses' Health Study also found increased risk of incontinence; the WHI found that the risk was greatest for stress incontinence. Oral estrogen is no longer advised for stress incontinence. (See Estrogen and the Lower Urinary Tract, presented later in the chapter.)

Other non–FDA-approved drugs and combinations of drugs have been studied to determine whether pharmacologic therapy can aid stress incontinent women. Imipramine, a tricyclic antidepressant, has α-adrenergic enhancement characteristics. Its action on the α receptors in the bladder neck and urethra may cause muscle contraction and could theoretically lessen stress incontinence. However, imipramine has limited benefit for treating stress incontinence, and there is weak evidence to suggest that any adrenergic drugs are better than placebo treatment.

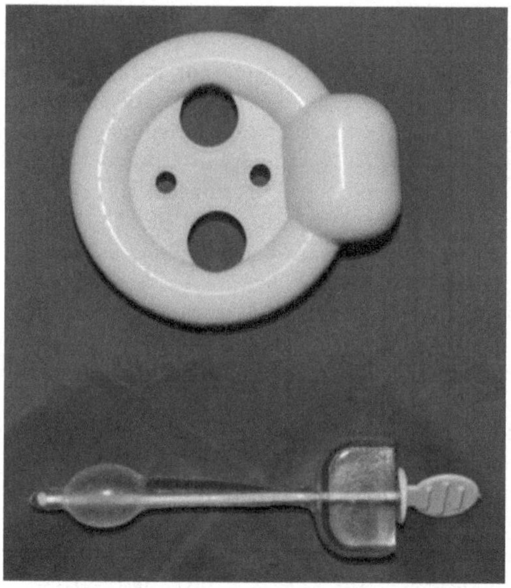

**Figure 21.15** Incontinence ring pessary and FemSoft urethral insert.

Duloxetine is not FDA approved for treating stress incontinence in the United States but has been approved in Europe. Duloxetine is a serotonin and norepinephrine reuptake inhibitor that stimulates pudendal motor neuron activity in Onuf's nucleus in the spinal cord and causes rhabdosphincter contraction in the urethra. Several large randomized trials have compared duloxetine to placebo, but reduction in incontinence is modest, and cure rates are no different than placebo. Nausea is a frequent side effect. For a woman considering treatment for depression, who also has bothersome stress incontinence, duloxetine is a reasonable medication to consider. Table 21.5 summarizes classes of other agents that may affect urinary function.

## Surgical Management

Hundreds of surgical procedures have been developed to treat stress incontinence. Today, the most commonly performed surgeries for stress incontinence are midurethral slings with synthetic mesh. These are more or as effective as other surgeries and have decreased morbidity. Before describing midurethral slings in detail, a historical review of surgeries developed to treat stress incontinence. Familiarity with these procedures is necessary because these women often present with recurrent stress incontinence. Scarring in the vagina and retropubic space can increase the risk of complications, particularly bladder injuries, from subsequent surgeries for stress incontinence.

Before the 1950s, the operative approach to treat stress incontinence primarily involved the plication of the bladder neck (Kelly plication procedure) with anterior colporrhaphy to reduce a cystocele via a vaginal approach. Published studies have demonstrated that retropubic urethropexy operations have a higher

**Table 21.5** Drugs with Possible Effects on the Lower Urinary Tract

| Class | Possible Side Effects | Drug and Usual Indication | Action |
|---|---|---|---|
| Antihypertensives | Incontinence | Reserpine, hypertension<br>Methyldopa, hypertension<br>Angiotensin-converting enzyme inhibitors<br>Alpha 1-blockers | Pharmacologic sympathectomy by depleting catecholamines<br>Side effect of cough—may worsen stress incontinence<br>Decreased urethral sphincter tone |
| Dopaminergic agonists | Bladder neck obstruction | Bromocriptine, galactorrhea<br>Levodopa, Parkinson disease | Increased urethral resistance, decreased detrusor contractions |
| Cholinergic agonists | Decreased bladder capacity and increased intravesical pressure | Digitalis, cardiotropic | Increased bladder wall tension |
| Neuroleptics | Incontinence | Major tranquilizers: prochlorperazine, promethazine, clozapine, trifluoperazine, chlorpromazine, haloperidol | Dopamine receptor blockade, with internal sphincter relaxation or decreased contractility from anticholinergic effects or mixed effects |
| β-Adrenergic agents | Urinary retention | Isoxsuprine, vasodilator<br>Terbutaline, bronchodilator | Inhibited bladder muscle contractility |
| Estrogen orally | Incontinence | | Worsens stress and mixed urinary incontinence |
| Xanthines | Incontinence | Caffeine | Increased contractility or rate of emptying<br>Decreased urethral closure pressure |
| Alcohol | Frequency, urgency | | Sedation and immobility may inhibit ability to recognize urgency |

cure rate than anterior colporrhaphies for stress incontinence when the patients are followed long term (Bergman, 1995; Harris, 1995). Anterior colporrhaphy has been largely abandoned as a surgical procedure for treating stress incontinence.

Transvaginal needle suspensions (TVNSs) were introduced in the late 1950s as a less invasive alternative to retropubic operations. Special needles were developed by Pereyra in 1959 that could be used to guide sutures from the paravaginal tissue through the space of Retzius to be suspended from the rectus fascia, just above the bladder neck. This was carried out through small suprapubic and vaginal incisions. Stamey's 1973 modification of the Pereyra procedure used a small tube of Dacron material to buttress the suture and prevent it from pulling through the rectus fascia. Many other modifications of TVNS have been described.

Several national and international organizations convened and reviewed the long-term success rates of incontinence operations when it became apparent that TVNS held up poorly after 2 to 3 years. Consensus statements suggested slings and retropubic suspensions have more durable results than TVNS or anterior repair for stress incontinence. Like anterior repairs, TVNS have rapidly declined as a primary treatment option for stress incontinence.

Before midurethral synthetic slings for woman with stress incontinence were popularized, the two most common surgeries were suprapubic urethropexies and pubovaginal bladder neck slings. The Marshall-Marchetti-Krantz suprapubic urethrovesical suspension operation was first reported in 1949 and for years was the mainstay of many surgeons attempting to alleviate stress incontinence in these patients. The space of Retzius is entered, the bladder neck is identified, generally with a 30-mL bulb Foley catheter in the bladder, and the paravaginal tissue adjacent to the bladder neck is identified and sutured to the pubic symphysis using two or three interrupted sutures on each side of the bladder neck. The surgeon must be careful not to place undue stress on the bladder neck (Fig. 21.16). A rare (1% to 2%) but painful complication of the Marshall-Marchetti-Krantz procedure is osteitis pubis. This condition is an inflammatory reaction in the periosteum of the pubic bone that is more often associated with permanent suture material.

In 1961, Burch advocated a modification of the suprapubic bladder neck suspension by suspending the vaginal wall to Cooper's ligament, now referred to as a *Burch colposuspension* or *Burch procedure* (Fig. 21.17). Polyglycol or nonabsorbable sutures are appropriate. At times, patients have difficulty voiding for prolonged periods, and the occasional woman may report that she needs to rise off the commode to a semistanding position to void.

Colombo and coworkers performed a prospective randomized clinical trial using the Burch and Marshall-Marchetti-Krantz procedures (Colombo, 1994). The follow-up was 2 to 7 years. They reported subjective and objective cure rates of 92% and 80%, respectively, for the Burch procedure and 85% and 65%, respectively, for the Marshall-Marchetti-Krantz procedure. These differences were not statistically significant. A 2005 Cochrane Database review of 39 trials of the Burch procedure noted that the success rate reported ranged from 85% to 90% at 1 year, and 70% were dry at 5 years (Lapitan, 2005). Follow-up urodynamic studies performed 10 years later in one study reported a surgical cure rate of 90.3%, but five of the seven patients who were considered failures thought that their symptoms had improved.

Pubovaginal slings are most commonly created with the patient's rectus fascia or fascia lata. Strips of fascia are then placed under the proximal urethra and attached to the abdominal wall to compress the urethra and decrease incontinence.

A 2007 multicenter randomized controlled trial compared 655 women assigned to have an autologous fascial sling or Burch procedure (Albo, 2007). At 24 months, the success rates were higher for women who had the fascial sling than the Burch procedure, 44% versus 38% ($P = .01$), using the strictest outcome criteria and 66% versus 49% ($P < .001$), respectively, if specifically considering stress incontinence outcomes. However, the fascial sling group had more complications with UTIs, voiding

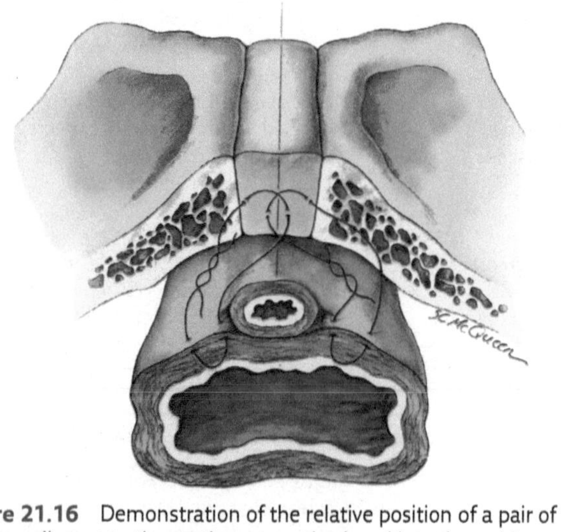

**Figure 21.16** Demonstration of the relative position of a pair of sutures adjacent to the urethra, securely placed into the pubic symphysis. (Modified from Buchsbaum HJ, Schmidt JD, eds. *Gynecologic and Obstetric Urology.* Philadelphia: WB Saunders; 1982.)

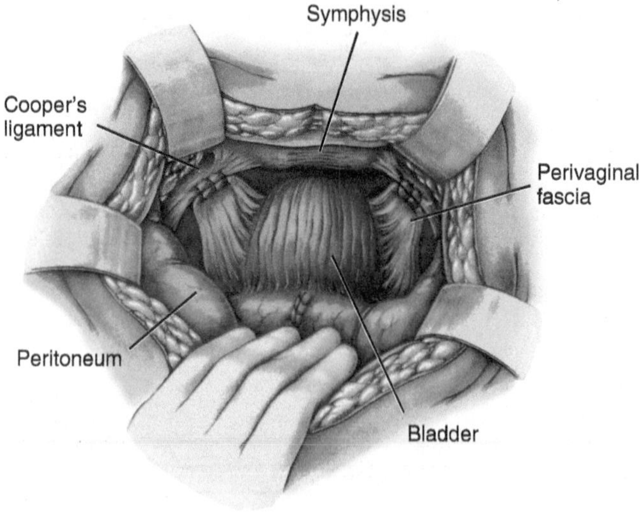


**Figure 21.17** Burch Procedure. The lateral edges of the vagina have been sutured to Cooper's ligament. (Modified from Burch JC. Urethrovaginal fixation to Cooper's ligament for correction of stress incontinence, cystocele, and prolapse. *Am J Obstet Gynecol.* 1961;81:281-290.)

difficulty, and postoperative urge incontinence. The Burch procedure can also be performed laparoscopically. Saidi and colleagues reported comparable 12-month cure rates in 70 patients undergoing laparoscopic procedures (91.4%) and 87 patients undergoing open procedures (92%) (Saidi, 1998). The laparoscopic procedures had a somewhat shorter operative time and a much shorter hospital stay. Ross followed 48 consecutive patients who underwent laparoscopic Burch procedures and found a cure rate of 93% and 89% at 1 and 2 years, respectively, using multichannel urodynamic studies (Ross, 1998).

### Surgical Management: Midurethral Slings

Tension-free midurethral slings using permanent mesh have become the most commonly used surgical procedures for stress incontinence. The first to be introduced was the retropubic tension-free vaginal tape sling (TVT). It was developed based on the theory that the tension on the pubourethral ligaments interacts with muscles of the pelvic floor and suburethral vaginal support structure. Ulmsten and coworkers published a 1996 article on 75 women treated with a midurethral sling made of permanent mesh (Fig. 21.18) (Ulmsten, 1996). The sling was placed under local anesthesia with sedation. A small vaginal incision was made under the midurethra. Small tunnels were made bilaterally to aid in passage of the trocar from the vaginal area through the retropubic space against the pubic bone, and exiting through abdominal skin punctures suprapubically. Cystoscopy was performed to evaluate for bladder perforation before the sling was brought into place. The sling was a monofilament polypropylene synthetic mesh, 1 cm wide and 40 cm long. An 84% cure rate was reported, an additional 8% were improved, and 8% failed. At 3 years after surgery, Ulmsten and colleagues reported an 86% cure rate.

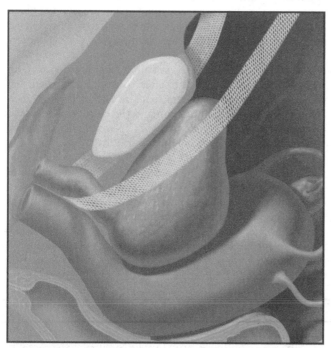

**Figure 21.18** Tension-free vaginal tape (TVT) sling with Prolene mesh placed midurethrally, without the need for fixation. (Courtesy of Gynecare, Ethicon, Somerville, NJ.)

Many other researchers worldwide have published similar success rates. Complications have included retropubic hematoma, bladder perforation, intraoperative bleeding, urinary retention, mesh exposure, and, rarely, bowel and urethral injuries. Ward, Hilton, and the UK and Ireland TVT trial group published a prospective randomized study comparing TVT with Burch colposuspension for primary urodynamic stress incontinence (Ward, 2004). With strict outcome data, the TVT procedure appears to be as effective as the Burch procedure at 2 years, with 63% and 51% cured by objective outcome data, respectively. The lower cure rates in this trial are likely because of the strict outcome criteria. Although the Burch procedure is often successful, the 2- to 3-day hospital stay, 4- to 6- week recovery, and additional risks are much less attractive than a short outpatient procedure (usually less than 30 minutes) with three small incisions and a 2-week recovery time. However, the placement of a permanent mesh has additional risks of mesh erosion and infection not seen with the Burch procedure.

Delorme introduced the transobturator tape (TOT) sling approach in 2001 with the hope of avoiding vascular, bladder, and bowel injuries (Delorme, 2001). TOT sling trocars traverse the obturator canal instead of the retropubic space and enter through small groin incisions at the level of the clitoris bilaterally. Delorme described an out-to-in passage through the obturator membrane along the inferior pubic ramus. Two years later, an in-to-out passage was described and touted to reduce urethral injury. Complications include bleeding, groin or leg pain, and urethral injuries. Objective and subjective cure rates were similar in a randomized trial comparing a TOT tape sling with a Burch colposuspension. In the largest multicenter randomized trial comparing retropubic TVT with TOT sling, 597 women were randomized, and 95% completed 12-month follow-up for treatment success analysis (Richter, 2010a). Objective treatment success required a negative cough stress test, negative pad test, and no retreatment. Objective success was 80.8% for the retropubic sling and 77.7% for a TOT sling; subjective success rates were 62.2% and 55.8%, respectively. Voiding dysfunction was significantly more common in the retropubic sling group (2.7% vs. 0%; $P = .004$). Neurologic symptoms of thigh and groin pain were higher in the TOT group (9.4% vs. 4%; $P = .01$). Because retropubic and transobturator midurethral slings have similar cure rates, the choice regarding which sling is appropriate for each patient is based on risks of complications and surgeon expertise. Either procedure can also lead to de novo development of urge incontinence, mesh erosion, mesh infection, or dyspareunia.

Single-incision mini-slings are the most recent permutation of the synthetic midurethral sling and were designed to avoid both the retropubic space and the groin by anchoring to the obturator membrane through a single vaginal incision. Meta-analyses comparing older versions of mini-slings suggested worse outcomes compared with full-length midurethral slings (Schimpf, 2014), but a more recent analysis that includes only newer mini-slings suggests comparable outcomes (Mostafa, 2014). Because they are newer to the market, there is less long-term data about them.

A 2012 review by the Society for Gynecologic Surgeons analyzed all 48 randomized controlled trials of slings with at least 12 months of follow-up (Schimpf, 2014). This group concluded that Burch and midurethral slings had similar cure rates, so the decision for one or the other should be based on minimizing risks. They recommended midurethral slings over pubovaginal slings to optimize subjective cure rates, and, similar to studies referenced earlier, found similar success rates between full-length midurethral slings.

### *POSTOPERATIVE VOIDING TRIAL*

It is usual postoperatively to check a woman for residual urine after she voids because she has a 24% chance of needing a catheter for temporary urinary retention after surgery (Richter, 2010a); after a retrograde fill of 300 mL, she should be able to void about 200 mL, and if not the catheter should be replaced for 1 to 3 days or the patient should be instructed on clean intermittent self-catheterization. The risk of continued catheterization is 6% 2 weeks after sling surgery and 2% after 6 weeks. In these circumstances, loosening or cutting the sling may be indicated. Voiding trials are discussed in more detail in Chapter 20.

### *URODYNAMICS*

As discussed in the Evaluation section of this chapter, urodynamics are no longer routinely done before stress incontinence surgery in uncomplicated cases. Studies have questioned the role of urodynamics, particularly in women with straightforward stress incontinence, no urge incontinence, no voiding complaints, and no prior incontinence surgery. One study of a carefully selected group of women at low risk of voiding problems found that preoperative urodynamic studies did not predict postoperative voiding dysfunction or the risk of surgical revision in the pubovaginal sling group (Lemack, 2008). Another study reported that the level of Valsalva leak point pressure (VLPP) and presence of detrusor overactivity did not predict the success of a Burch colposuspension or an autologous fascial sling in women with pure stress incontinence. In women with straightforward, demonstrable stress urinary incontinence randomized to undergo preoperative urodynamics or not, outcomes at 1 year were not inferior in the group that did not undergo urodynamics (Nager, 2012).

### *RISKS OF MESH*

Synthetic mesh is a permanent implant. In 2008, the U.S. Food and Drug Administration created a public health notification regarding complications from the transvaginal use of mesh for prolapse and incontinence (FDA, 2008). New data suggest that the risks from transvaginal mesh for prolapse is more of a concern than transvaginal mesh for incontinence, and so in 2011 the U.S. FDA advisory refers to prolapse only (FDA, 2011). Mesh complications from midurethral slings are uncommon but can include mesh erosions into the bladder or urethra, mesh exposures in the vagina, pain, dyspareunia, and rare complications such as severe infections. Despite the small risks associated with using a permanent implant, midurethral slings are the most studied anti-incontinence surgery in medical history and remain the most commonly performed surgeries for stress incontinence.

### *INTRINSIC SPHINCTER DEFICIENCY*

In 1981, McGuire noted the loss of intrinsic urethral tone in a number of women, particularly those with a history of pelvic trauma, radiation, underlying neurologic conditions, or scarring of the urethral sphincter. This has been termed *intrinsic sphincter deficiency* (ISD). Currently, the two types of stress incontinence, hypermobility and ISD, are thought to be interdependent and not separate entities. However, it is still useful to discuss severe stress incontinence in women with a fixed and poorly functioning urethra.

Sand and associates offered some insight into why at least some retropubic urethropexy procedures fail (Sand, 1987). In a study of 86 patients evaluated preoperatively and postoperatively with urodynamic studies, they noted that in women younger than 50 years, there was a significant risk of failure if the preoperative urethral closure pressure was less than 20 cm $H_2O$. Although low urethral closure pressure was found to be an independent risk factor in women younger than 50 years, it was not found to be the case in women older than 50. Horbach and Ostergard retrospectively evaluated 263 consecutive patients undergoing a complete urodynamic evaluation because of urinary leakage (Horbach, 1994). Intrinsic sphincter dysfunction was defined as maximum urethral closure of 20 cm $H_2O$ or less in the sitting position at maximum cystometric capacity; 132 women (50.2%) were found to have intrinsic sphincter dysfunction. Women in this group tended to be older and more likely to have undergone a hysterectomy and at least one anti-incontinence procedure compared with women with continence problems who had normal urethral pressure. By multivariate analysis, it was noted that age older than 50 years was the only independent variable that could predict the presence of intrinsic sphincter dysfunction in women with stress urinary incontinence.

At present, treatment for urinary stress incontinence caused by ISD consists of one of the following: periurethral bulking substance injections. urethral bladder neck sling procedures in select woman. midurethral synthetic sling. or use of an artificial sphincter device. A number of substances have been used for periurethral bulking injections. These include the individual's blood or fat, polytetrafluoroethylene (Teflon), bovine collagen, silicone microspheres, and pyrolytic zirconium oxide. Injection of blood or fat has provided only transient relief, and the use of Teflon has resulted in several complications, primarily caused by wandering of the Teflon to distant sites. Glutaraldehyde cross-linked (GAX) collagen has been used as a urethral bulking agent. This is a bovine dermal collagen first used by Appell and colleagues, who reported a high success rate. It has a relatively high incidence of hypersensitivity reaction and therefore women should be skin-tested before its use. Without hypersensitivity, it appears to be a relatively safe and minimally invasive means of closing the urethra. It is currently not commercially available because no companies are producing it. It seems to have a positive effect for at least 2 years, and it is possible to reinject patients. Long-term follow-up has been disappointing, with a 26% success rate at 5 years. Part of the failure may be because collagen is biodegradable and not necessarily durable. Permanent materials of silicone microimplants and pyrolytic zirconium oxide beads have been studied. Short-term success rates have ranged widely from 33% to 60% for cure or improvement. No material has proved better than another. Nonetheless, for older unfit women and women who have failed other incontinence surgeries, an injectable material for stress incontinence may be an attractive option.

Midurethral synthetic slings have been studied for ISD. The differing definitions of ISD with urethral hypermobility versus a fixed nonmobile urethra have made comparisons difficult. In published trials of a retropubic midurethral sling with hypermobility and a low maximum urethral closure pressure (MUCP), the low MUCP did not seem to affect the outcome. Reported cure rates range from 73% to 86%. One study with a 5-year follow-up found that 57% of the women were very satisfied, and another 17% had improved continence. In contrast, using a TOT approach in this circumstance resulted in more failures. In the setting of a fixed urethra, only 33% of women reported being cured of incontinence.

A variety of traditional sling procedures, including the use of fascia lata, anterior rectus fascia tissue, cadaveric fascia lata, and inert materials such as polyethylene terephthalate (Mersilene) mesh, can be used. These procedures mobilize the bladder neck, often by a vaginal or vaginal and abdominal approach, and allow the interposition of a strip of material under the proximal urethra surrounding the bladder neck, which is attached to the anterior rectus sheath. This creates support and compression to the urethra and prevents urethral movement during increased abdominal pressure. This procedure is generally effective in creating continence.

The surgeon must exercise care in determining the tension to be applied on the bladder neck when the sling is fixed. Making it too tight may interfere with voiding and may actually damage the bladder neck or lead to de novo development of urge incontinence; making it too loose will abrogate its effectiveness. Generally, with a "No." 16 or 18 Foley catheter in the urethra, it should be possible for the surgeon to judge the tension so that the sling fits comfortably against the urethra without compressing it. Concomitant cystoscopy may also be used.

Many other reports using other sling materials have shown success rates (cure or improvement) of 86% to 92%, with complications of UTIs, urinary retention, and de novo development of urgency.

An anterior rectus sheath fascial sling procedure is now generally reserved for patients with intrinsic sphincter deficiency or women whose previous anti-incontinence procedure failed and have a fixed urethra, because midurethral slings do not work as well with a fixed urethra. Fascia lata slings have been used by many surgeons and can be performed mostly vaginally in a relatively short operative time. However, the woman then has a leg incision to harvest the fascia lata, which can be painful. Autologous fascia lata is more effective than irradiated and freeze-dried donor fascia lata, with the use of the latter type leading to a concern about graft degeneration and, thus procedure failure.

The use of the artificial urinary sphincter may be a viable option for some women and will generally produce continence. Artificial urinary sphincters are generally placed by abdominal and vaginal surgical approaches. The artificial sphincter consists of a cuff surrounding the urethra. The device is controlled by a pressure balloon placed in the space of Retzius. The woman controls the device by releasing pressure via a pump in the labia when she wishes to void and reestablishing pressure when she wishes to be continent. Diokno and coworkers reported a 91% success rate in 32 patients in whom they implanted the device in 1988. Their use has been limited by side effects including erosion and mechanical problems.

## OVERACTIVE BLADDER

Overactive bladder (OAB) is defined as the symptom of urgency, with or without urge incontinence, usually with frequency and nocturia in the absence of UTI or other pathology. Urgency is the complaint of a sudden compelling desire to pass urine, which is difficult to defer. Urge incontinence is the complaint of involuntary leakage of urine accompanied by or immediately preceded by urgency. This condition is generally chronic and may wax and wane, but it is slowly progressive and associated with an urgency-frequency problem that is often accompanied by painless, involuntary urine loss. Generally, a large volume of urine is lost; leakage may occur in any position and often with a change in position. Rarely, an event usually associated with stress incontinence, such as coughing, will trigger this urge incontinence, but it is generally delayed until seconds after the stress has occurred. Large-volume urine loss is more characteristic of urge incontinence compared with stress incontinence. Stress incontinence frequently disappears when recumbent, but urge incontinence continues, often with nocturia. Table 21.6 summarizes the differences in symptoms. OAB occurs in approximately 17% of the population and the incidence increases with age. OAB patients have a lower quality of life than women with stress incontinence. Differential diagnoses include urinary tract pathology, PBS-IC, polydipsia, polyuria, nocturnal polyuria, and medical conditions that are associated with nocturia (vascular or sleep disorders).

Detrusor overactivity is a urodynamic observation; it is the result of sudden, spontaneous detrusor contraction. It has previously been termed *detrusor dyssynergia, unstable bladder*, or *detrusor instability*. The term *idiopathic detrusor overactivity* is used as a urodynamic definition when there is no defined cause of the condition. If a neurologic disorder, such as stroke, Parkinson disease, multiple sclerosis, spinal cord injury, or other CNS pathology is present, the term *neurogenic detrusor overactivity* is appropriate. In older women, urgency and incomplete bladder emptying can coexist. Dribbling often results. This condition is termed *detrusor hyperactivity with impaired contractile function* (DHIC), and these two conditions may have different causative factors.

The loss of urine in OAB is probably triggered by sudden uninhibited stimulation of receptors in the bladder wall. The problem may be caused by the breakdown of normal neurologic and inhibitory reflexes. A postal survey of 6000 women in a Washington State health maintenance organization estimated the prevalence of urinary incontinence to be 42% and major depression 3.7% (Melville, 2005). However, the depression

**Table 21.6** Typical Symptom Differences in Stress and Urge Incontinence

| Symptom | Stress Incontinence | Urge Incontinence |
|---|---|---|
| Leakage with exertion, cough, sneeze, activity | Yes | No |
| Leakage with sensation or urgency | No | Yes |
| Frequency, nocturia | No | Yes |
| Large volume urine loss | No | Yes |
| Leakage with running water, key in the door | No | Yes |
| Leakage with position change from sitting to standing | Possible | Yes |
| Leakage while recumbent | No | Possible |
| History of childhood bedwetting | No | Yes |

rate was significantly higher in women with incontinence and, in particular, women with moderate and severe incontinence (5.7% and 8.3%, respectively). It also differed by incontinence type (4.7% stress, 6.6% in urge or mixed). The study did not indicate that one condition caused the other; however, there is an increased risk of major depression in women with urinary incontinence, so it is worth screening for depression in this population. It is possible that altered neurotransmitter function, such as serotonin or norepinephrine, could alter bladder function, contributing to uninhibited detrusor contractions and urge incontinence.

Women with both stress incontinence and OAB experienced a lower cure rate after surgery than women with stress incontinence only. No relationship could be found among preoperative symptoms, age, history of previous procedures, and cystometric parameters between those who were cured and those who were not. In addition, none of these criteria could predict which woman who was detrusor-stable before surgery would develop overactivity after surgery. In some women, overactive bladder symptoms improve after stress incontinence surgery. Risks of developing OAB symptoms or having persistent OAB after surgery must be recognized and incorporated into the preoperative counseling because it may require further medical therapy.

## DIAGNOSIS

A bladder diary such as that shown in Figure 21.7 can be useful in diagnosing OAB because it can document frequency (more than eight daytime voids), nocturia (more than one nighttime void), and episodes of incontinence preceded by urgency. Additional information can be obtained about incontinence related to activity (stress incontinence), fluid intake, pad usage, and voided volumes (a measure of bladder capacity). The ideal diary duration has yet to be established, but 1 to 3 days is generally recommended. Filling cystometry, which evaluates the pressure-volume relationship of the bladder, allows the detection of spontaneous involuntary detrusor contractions in the bladder, which are noted as the bladder fills. However, even in women who clearly describe urgency urinary incontinence symptoms, the single snapshot of one urodynamic study frequently fails to detect involuntary detrusor contractions. Sensitivity is increased with standing and provocative maneuvers such as running water, but because sensitivity remains low, treatment for urgency incontinence is reasonable even if not demonstrated during urodynamic studies.

## TREATMENT: BEHAVIORAL

Behavioral therapy is first-line treatment. In women with stress and urgency urinary incontinence, it is unclear which to address first, but if the predominant symptom is urgency, this should probably be treated first. Urgency incontinence can improve, worsen (or develop de novo), or be unchanged after sling surgery, so patients who have undergone an operation for stress urinary incontinence and continue to be incontinent should be evaluated for detrusor overactivity.

Behavioral management includes fluid management, avoidance of bladder irritants, and bladder training. Because most patients with detrusor overactivity have abnormal voiding habits, bladder retraining or bladder drills are useful. This involves a programmed progressive lengthening of the period between voiding, with or without the addition of biofeedback techniques. Women need to be taught urge suppression using distraction, relaxation techniques, or pelvic floor muscle contractions. The goal is to increase the voiding interval to 2 to 3 hours with normal fluid intake. In their study, Millard and Oldenburg demonstrated improvement in 74% of women with detrusor overactivity using these techniques (Millard, 1983). Cystometric studies performed on these patients revealed a reversion to stable bladder function. However, compliance with bladder retraining by patients is often a problem. Visco and associates studied 123 women who were offered bladder retraining and found that 55% never started treatment or were noncompliant (Visco, 1999). They noted that women who were given concurrent pharmacologic therapy had a higher (87%) compliance rate. Other behavioral treatments such as scheduled voiding, fluid management, and a bedside commode may be particularly helpful for older women with OAB.

In a 2006 Cochrane Database review, it was concluded that women with incontinence who performed pelvic floor muscle training were more likely to report cure or improvement, although they averaged only approximately one less incontinence episode daily (Hay-Smith, 2006). Although women with urge incontinence may experience less benefit than women with stress incontinence, there did appear to be improvement and few adverse effects. Women also need a strategy for urge suppression to prevent leakage, and a few quick Kegel exercises followed by deep breathing and relaxation may help reduce urge. Given the noninvasive nature of muscle training, it makes sense as initial therapy for all urinary incontinence problems over a 3-month period.

## TREATMENT: MEDICAL

Anticholinergic (antimuscarinic) or beta-3 adrenergic receptor agonist drugs may be useful; Table 21.7 shows currently available drugs. These medications, in conjunction with bladder retraining, have greater efficacy than either alone. In one trial, combination therapy yielded better outcomes over time on the Urogenital Distress Inventory and Overactive Bladder Questionnaire ($P < .001$) at both time points studied for patient satisfaction and perceived improvement but not health-related quality of life (Burgio, 2000).

**Table 21.7** Medications for Overactive Bladder

| Drug | Dosage* |
|---|---|
| Oxybutynin (Ditropan IR) † | 5 mg bid, tid, qid |
| Oxybutynin (Ditropan XL)‡ | 5 to 30 mg daily |
| Tolterodine (Detrol IR) † | 1 or 2 mg bid |
| Tolterodine (Detrol LA)§ | 4 mg daily |
| Oxybutynin transdermal (Oxytrol) | 3.9-mg patch (twice weekly) |
| Darifenacin (Enablex) | 7.5 or 15 mg daily |
| Solifenacin (VESIcare) | 5 or 10 mg daily |
| Trospium (Sanctura) | 20 mg bid or 60 mg daily (ER)‡ |
| Fesoterodine (Toviaz) | 4 mg to 8 mg daily |
| Mirabegron (Myrbetriq) | 25 to 50mg daily |

**bid*, Twice per day; *tid*, three times per day; *qid*, four times per day.
†Intermediate-release (IR).
‡Extended release (XL, ER).
§Long acting (LA).

Overall, in clinical studies, antimuscarinic drugs reduce incontinence episodes by 60% to 75%, but only 20% to 40% of patients have no incontinent episodes. Although efficacy has been proven in many randomized trials, poor patient compliance is often found with these medications because of continued incontinence, expense without cure, and anticholinergic side effects. The most common side effect is dry mouth. Flexible-dosing schedules of several drugs, changing to a different drug, or using a drug patch delivery system are options for finding a tolerable drug for this chronic condition. Salvatore found that two thirds of women discontinued therapy within 4 months, likely because they do not provide long-lasting symptom relief (Salvatore, 2005). A randomized trial of adding behavioral training to medication therapy reduced incontinence frequency but did not allow the woman to stop the drug and maintain improvement. Caution must be advised in elderly patients as antimuscarinics can have more adverse effects (dizziness) and cognitive effects. One study linked higher cumulative anticholinergic use with an increased risk of dementia (Gray, 2015). Intravesical instillation of anticholinergic medication can provide an alternative delivery mechanism for women who fail or cannot tolerate oral therapy. The newer beta-3 adrenergic agonist drug Mirabegron has similar efficacy to the anticholinergics, but it works through a different mechanism to promote detrusor relaxation and facilitate urine storage. It appears to have fewer side effects than anticholinergic medications but is contraindicated in women with uncontrolled hypertension.

## TREATMENT: PROCEDURES

Women with intractable detrusor overactivity who have failed conservative and medical treatment have procedural and surgical options. Figure 21.19 shows a therapeutic pathway for OAB that demonstrates first-line through third-line options.

Pelvic floor electrical stimulation has been studied for improving a woman's ability to inhibit involuntary detrusor contractions and decreasing symptoms of urge incontinence but has mixed results. A small removable vaginal probe is placed in the vagina or anus; electrical stimulation activates a pelvic muscle contraction. This transvaginal neuromodulation appears to be of benefit compared with placebo although data is limited.

Neuromodulation is increasingly recognized as beneficial for women with refractory symptoms (failed behavioral treatments and medications over roughly 3 months). It includes direct sacral neuromodulation of S3 and peripheral neuromodulation through peripheral tibial nerve stimulation (PTNS) to the sacral nerve plexus. In practice, PTNS is done weekly for 30 minutes for 12 weeks and then every 3 to 4 weeks for maintenance therapy. There are few reported side effects except for pain during the stimulation. Many women prefer this to long-term medication use. There are many trials and a randomized trial with a sham treatment group that support efficacy (Peters, 2010). One randomized, crossover trial compared PTNS with solifenacin (Vecchioli-Scaldazza, 2013). There were fewer daily voids, nocturia episodes, and urge incontinence events in both groups, but PTNS showed greater effectiveness than solifenacin. The PTNS group also reported better quality of life and perceived effectiveness of urgency control. Much remains to be learned about patient selection criteria and long-term effects.

Another route of neuromodulation involves an implantable device, which chronically stimulates the sacral nerves and reduces symptoms. The FDA approved InterStim (Medtronic, Minneapolis, MN) for sacral neuromodulation (SNS) in 1997 for urgency, urge incontinence, and later for urinary retention (Fig. 21.20). Patients have a stimulation test with either a tined lead wire placed in the office or a potentially permanent lead wire placed in the operating room under fluoroscopy. If the results showed a ≥50% improvement in urge incontinence symptoms, the permanent stimulator is implanted. The device complication rate has decreased with improvement in the wire lead that is placed (Fig. 21.21) and other improvements in standardizing the implantation procedure, but infection, failure to improve symptoms long term, and the need for explanation problems remain. One randomized trial of SNS versus standard antimuscarinic medication in 147 subjects found that at 6 months, the success rate was 61% in the SNS group versus 42% in the medication group ($P$ = .02) (Siegel, 2015). There were significant improvements in the quality of life scores in the SNS group. Furthermore, the improved or greatly improved urinary symptom scores were 86% for SNS versus 44% in the medication group. The complication rate for the SNS device was 30.5% compared with 27.3% medication adverse event rate. Multiple long-term outcome studies have been published confirming that this is a feasible option for many women with refractory urge incontinence. Women must have good cognitive function to consider this

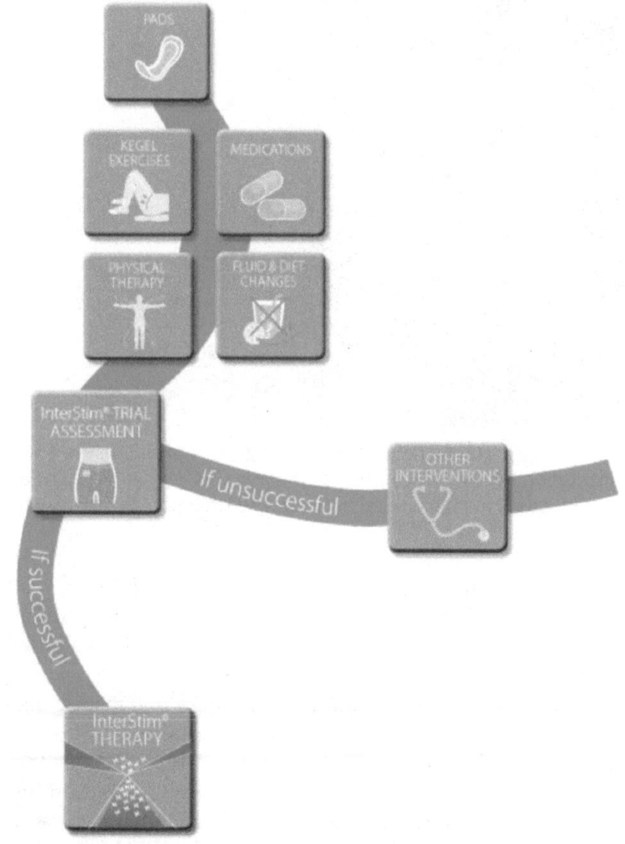


**Figure 21.19** Treatment algorithm for urge incontinence. (Courtesy of Medtronic, Minneapolis, MN.)

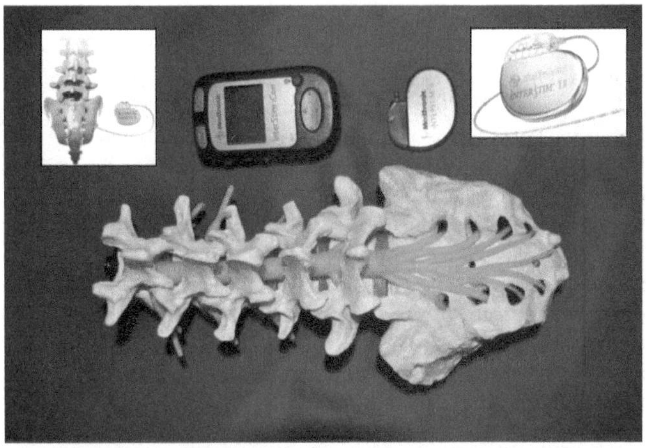

**Figure 21.20** InterStim test generator and permanent implantable generator, along with spinal cord model. (Courtesy of Medtronic, Minneapolis, MN.)

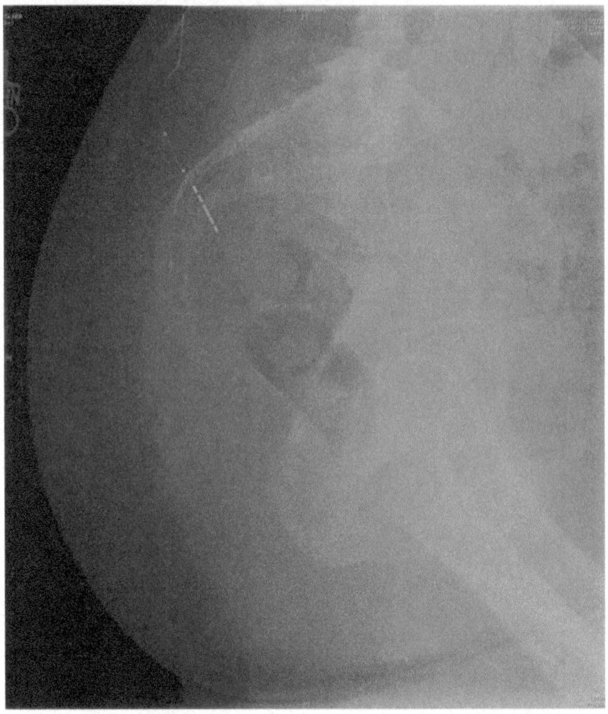

**Figure 21.21** Lateral radiograph showing the lead wire in the final implantation site at S3. (Courtesy of Dr. Jane L. Miller, Department of Urology, School of Medicine, University of Washington, Seattle, WA.)

**Table 21.8** Effective Treatment Options for Women with Urinary Incontinence by Type of Incontinence

| Treatment Option | Stress Incontinence | Urge Incontinence |
|---|---|---|
| Nonpharmacologic | Pelvic floor muscle training<br>Bladder training<br>Prompted voiding<br>Incontinence pessary | Pelvic floor muscle training<br>Bladder training<br>Prompted voiding<br>Posterior tibial nerve stimulation |
| Pharmacologic | | Anticholinergic drugs (antimuscarinic)<br>Beta agonist |
| Surgical | Midurethral synthetic sling<br>Retropubic colposuspension<br>Suburethral fascial sling | Botulinum toxin A injection<br>Sacral neuromodulation |

Modified from Holroyd-Leduc JM, Straus SE. Management of urinary incontinence in women: clinical applications. *JAMA*. 2004;291(8):996-999.

option. Reoperation is not uncommon with infection, lead movement, and battery replacement. Women cannot undergo MRI below the head, so this must be discussed and considered before ploacement.

Intradetrusor onabotulinumtoxin A blocks presynaptic acetylcholine from parasympathetic nerves, causing paralysis of the detrusor smooth muscle, although it may also affect bladder afferent or urothelial cell neurotransmitters. Onabotulinumtoxin A is injected into the bladder wall via cystoscopy either in the office or in an outpatient surgery setting. It is FDA approved, and published studies show 60% to 70% cure or improvement rates. Temporary urinary retention was reported as high as 40% with early studies using higher doses but is 5% to 10% in newer studies. Women should return for postvoid residual urine testing and be prepared to learn clean intermittent self-catheterization if needed until the drug wears off. Dose finding studies compared with placebo have found that 100 units and 150 units are superior to placebo. UTIs are more common after infection. Long-term efficacy data show that reinjection is usually necessary, but repeat injections remain as effective as initial injections. Benefit is maintained for 3 to 12 months. A randomized controlled trial directly compared onabotulinumtoxin A injection (100 units) with oral solifenacin and at 6 months; they had similar efficacy (Visco, 2012).

Table 21.8 summarizes the treatment options for the two most common types of urinary incontinence. Figure 21.22 shows an evaluation and treatment algorithm for stress, urge, and mixed incontinence.

## MIXED URINARY INCONTINENCE

As the term implies, *mixed urinary incontinence* means that a woman complains of both stress and urge incontinence. The pathophysiology and treatment of mixed incontinence have not been well studied despite the fact that it accounts for one third of incontinence complaints. Sometimes the woman can articulate which problem is worse, and treatment can begin for the more bothersome condition. Pelvic floor muscle exercises and behavioral training are appropriate first-line therapies for both types of incontinence (see the stress and urge incontinence sections presented earlier). The literature supports trying antimuscarinic drugs, which in one trial significantly reduced incontinence episodes. Of five published studies of surgical trials for mixed incontinence using slings, varied cure rates have been reported. Although the stress incontinence component of the leakage may decrease, the woman is often disappointed to still be leaking because the urge component has not improved. The risk of having

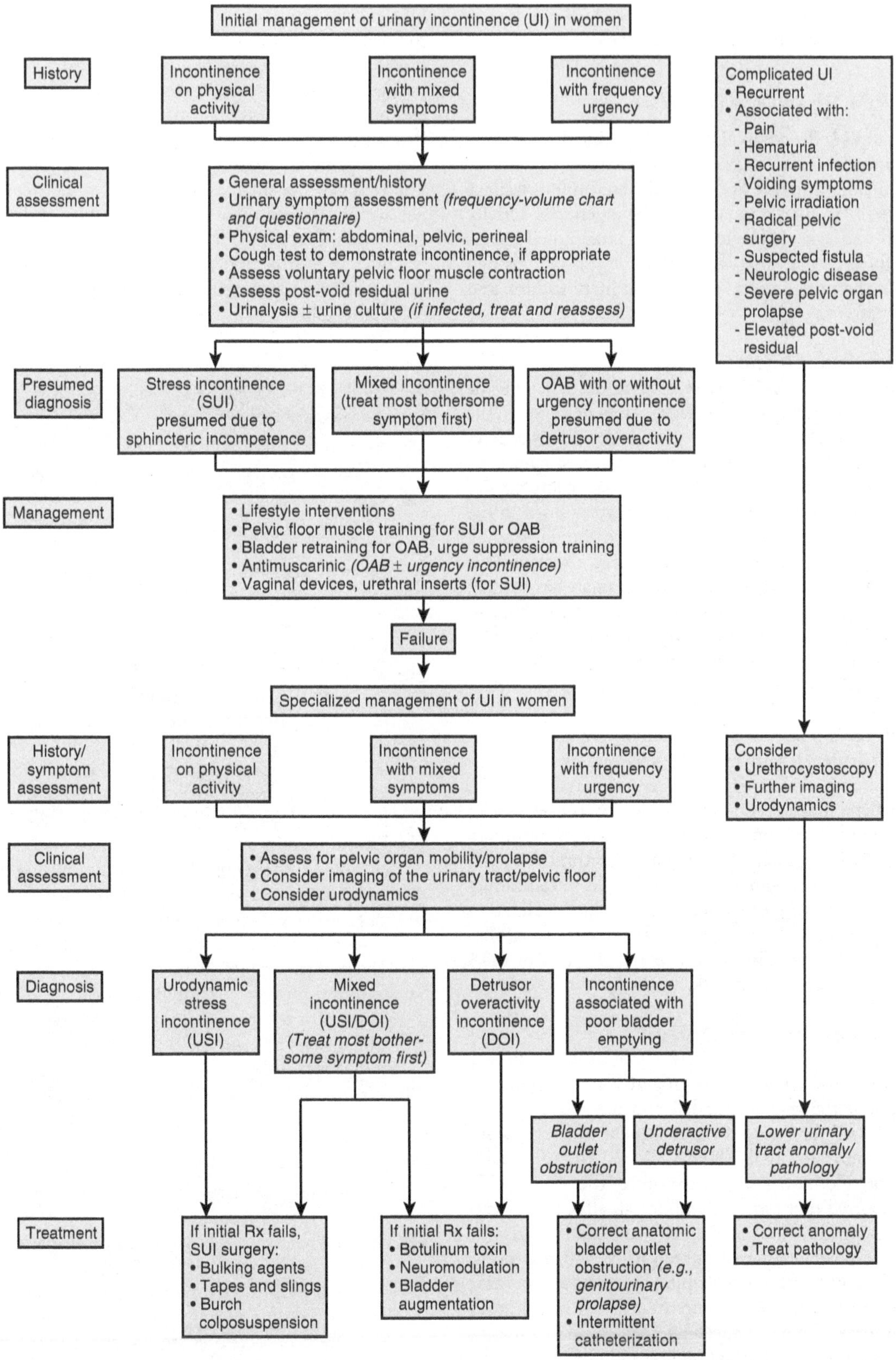


**Figure 21.22** Summary treatment algorithm for stress, urge, and mixed incontinence.

persistent detrusor overactivity after surgery must be recognized and incorporated into the preoperative counseling.

## OTHER TYPES OF INCONTINENCE

Nocturnal enuresis is the complaint of loss of urine during sleep. The term *continuous urinary incontinence* has been defined by the International Continence Society as the continuous leakage of urine where the woman does not describe urgency or activity associated with the leakage (Haylen, 2010). Extraurethral incontinence is defined as the observation of urine leakage through channels other than the urethra, including urinary fistulas, and an ectopic ureter.

### Chronic Retention of Urine

*Overflow incontinence* is the old term used to describe chronic retention of urine. It occurs when a bladder does not empty. The problem may be caused by a neurologic disorder that interferes with normal bladder reflexes, neuropathy, myogenic failure, or obstruction of the urethra. Typically, the woman complains of voiding small amounts and still feeling that there is urine in the bladder, or she may only complain of incontinence and lose small amounts of urine without any control. Typically, the bladder is not painful and may be palpable after the woman has voided. The diagnosis is made when there is persistence of a significant amount of urine left in the bladder after voiding, as confirmed with ultrasound bladder scanning or catheterization. Typically in this setting, the postvoid residual urine volume is more than 300 mL.

This condition is mostly seen in patients after incontinence surgery and in patients with multiple sclerosis, diabetic neuropathy, and trauma or tumors of the central nervous system. A complete general medical and urologic workup is necessary to clarify the patient's condition. Therapy directed at the primary cause may be beneficial, such a releasing a suburethral sling that is obstructive. Often, the woman must be trained in techniques of intermittent self-catheterization. Sacral neuromodulation is FDA approved for women with urinary retention. Alpha-blockers used for men with prostatic hypertrophy are not FDA approved for women and rarely work.

### Estrogen and the Lower Urinary Tract

Estrogen has long been known to play a role in lower urinary tract function because estrogen and progesterone receptors are found throughout the vagina, bladder, and urethra. Estrogens had been prescribed for years for the treatment of stress incontinence, until controlled trials (HERS, WHI, Nurses' Health Study) and the Hormones and Urogenital Therapy (HUT) Committee reported that estrogen was not an efficacious treatment for stress incontinence and actually increased the risk of incontinence. In postmenopausal women with vaginal atrophy, there may also be urethral mucosal epithelium atrophy because there are estrogen receptors in the urethra, which may lead to irritative symptoms. Vaginal estrogen does appear to be superior to placebo for recurrent cystitis and vaginal and urethral atrophy in the postmenopausal woman. Urethral atrophy and inflammation might contribute to irritate the bladder and lead to symptoms of urgency and frequency. A systematic review of the effects of vaginally administered estrogen has reported significant improvement in frequency, nocturia, urgency, incontinence episodes, and bladder capacity in postmenopausal women. In doses used for the treatment of genital atrophy (0.5 g of unconjugated estrogen cream three times weekly), serum levels were low and endometrial thickness unchanged. An intravaginal estrogen ring that releases very low levels of estrogen over a 3-month period is a convenient method of administration for many women. The estrogen benefit may be caused by the treatment of vaginal atrophy rather than a specific bladder and urethral effect. Possible confounding effects of progestogens and the multitudes of different estrogen preparations, oral and vaginal, hamper most studies. Progestogens have been associated with increased bladder irritability.

## KEY POINTS

- As many as 30% of all women may suffer from some degree of urinary incontinence during their lifetime.
- Continence is determined by the balance between forces that maintain urethral closure and those that affect detrusor function. Parasympathetic nervous system activity via the neurotransmitter acetylcholine stimulates receptors in the bladder wall to activate detrusor contraction. Sympathetic nervous system activation leads to bladder relaxation.
- The highest pressure zone in the urethra is approximately the midpoint in the functional urethra, which is roughly 0.5 cm proximal to the urogenital diaphragm.
- Approximately 50% of all women will develop urinary infections at some point in their lifetime and, by age 70 years, as many as 10% of women will have recurrent UTIs.
- Painful bladder syndrome–interstitial cystitis is a painful, chronic bladder condition that is not related to infection and is associated with symptoms of bladder and pelvic pain, urinary frequency, urgency, or nocturia, and often dyspareunia.
- The midurethral synthetic tape slings (retropubic and transobturator midurethral) appear to have similar efficacy for the surgical treatment of stress incontinence, with a shorter surgery and recovery time than a Burch colposuspension.
- Retropubic and transobturator midurethral slings have similar success rates for stress incontinence, although with different risk profiles. The retropubic approach has a significantly higher risk of bladder perforation, bleeding, and voiding dysfunction, and the obturator approach has a higher risk of groin and leg pain.
- Approximately 20% of women with urinary incontinence suffer from detrusor overactivity. Behavioral changes and oral medications are first-line treatments, although often they have disappointing cure rates. Neuromodulation and surgical procedures are available and effective for refractory symptoms.
- Being obese or overweight increases the risk of urinary incontinence, and weight loss can reduce stress incontinence significantly.

## KEY REFERENCES


Albo ME, Richter HE, Brubaker L, et al. Burch colposuspension versus fascial sling to reduce urinary stress incontinence. *N Engl J Med.* 2007;356(21): 2143-2155.

American College of Obstetricians and Gynecologists. ACOG committee opinion no. 603: evaluation of uncomplicated stress urinary incontinence in women before surgical treatment. *Obstet Gynecol.* 2014;123(6): 1403-1407.

Asmussen M, Ulmsten U. A new technique for measurements of the urethra pressure profile. *Acta Obstet Gynecol Scand.* 1976;55(2):167-173.

Athanasiou S, Khullar V, Boos K, Salvatore S, Cardozo L. Imaging the urethral sphincter with three-dimensional ultrasound. *Obstet Gynecol.* 1999; 94(2):295-301.

Bergman A, Elia G. Three surgical procedures for genuine stress incontinence: five-year follow-up of a prospective randomized study. *Am J Obstet Gynecol.* 1995;173(1):66-71.

Bø K, Talseth T. Long-term effect of pelvic floor muscle exercise 5 years after cessation of organized training. *Obstet Gynecol.* 1996;87(2):261-265.

Bump RC, Hurt WG, Fantl JA, Wyman JF. Assessment of Kegel pelvic muscle exercise performance after brief verbal instruction. *Am J Obstet Gynecol.* 1991;165(2):322-327. discussion 327-329.

Bump RC, McClish DM. Cigarette smoking and pure genuine stress incontinence of urine: a comparison of risk factors and determinants between smokers and nonsmokers. *Am J Obstet Gynecol.* 1994;170(2):579-582.

Burgio KL, Locher JL, Goode PS. Combined behavioral and drug therapy for urge incontinence in older women. *J Am Geriatr Soc.* 2000;48(4):370-374.

Centers for Disease Control and Prevention. Sexually Transmitted Diseases Treatment Guidelines. *MMWR Recomm Rep.* 2015;64(No. RR-3): 1-137.

Choi H, Palmer MH, Park J. Meta-analysis of pelvic floor muscle training: randomized controlled trials in incontinent women. *Nurs Res.* 2007;56(4):226-234.

Colombo M, Scalambrino S, Maggioni A, Milani R. Burch colposuspension versus modified Marshall-Marchetti-Krantz urethropexy for primary genuine stress urinary incontinence: a prospective, randomized clinical trial. *Am J Obstet Gynecol.* 1994;171(6):1573-1579.

DeLancey JO. Correlative study of paraurethral anatomy. *Obstet Gynecol.* 1986;68(1):91-97.

DeLancey JO. Structural support of the urethra as it relates to stress urinary incontinence: the hammock hypothesis. *Am J Obstet Gynecol.* 1994;170(6): 1713-1720. discussion 1720-1713.

DeLancey JO, Kearney R, Chou Q, Speights S, Binno S. The appearance of levator ani muscle abnormalities in magnetic resonance images after vaginal delivery. *Obstet Gynecol.* 2003;101(1):46-53.

Delorme E. Transobturator urethral suspension: mini-invasive procedure in the treatment of stress urinary incontinence in women. *Prog Urol.* 2001; 11(6):1306-1313.

Dumoulin C, Hay-Smith J, Habee-Seguin GM, Mercier J. Pelvic floor muscle training versus no treatment, or inactive control treatments, for urinary incontinence in women: a short version Cochrane systematic review with meta-analysis. *Neurourol Urodyn.* 2015;34(4):300-308.

Enhorning G. Simultaneous recording of intravesical and intraurethral pressure. A study on urethral closure in normal and stress incontinent women. *Acta Chir Scand Suppl.* 1961;276(Suppl):1-68.

Fihn SD, Boyko EJ, Normand EH, et al. Association between use of spermicide-coated condoms and Escherichia coli urinary tract infection in young women. *Am J Epidemiol.* 1996;144(5):512-520.

Food and Drug Administration (FDA). *FDA Public Health Notification: Serious Complications Associated with Transvaginal Placement of Surgical Mesh in Repair of Pelvic Organ Prolapse and Stress Urinary Incontinence*; 2008.

Food and Drug Administration (FDA). *FDA Safety Communication: UPDATE on Serious Complications Associated with Transvaginal Placement of Surgical Mesh for Pelvic Organ Prolapse*; 2011.

Goode PS, Burgio KL, Locher JL, et al. Effect of behavioral training with or without pelvic floor electrical stimulation on stress incontinence in women: a randomized controlled trial. *JAMA.* 2003;290(3):345-352.

Grady D, Applegate W, Bush T, Furberg C, Riggs B, Hulley SB. Heart and Estrogen/progestin Replacement Study (HERS): design, methods, and baseline characteristics. *Control Clin Trials.* 1998;19(4):314-335.

Gray SL, Anderson ML, Dublin S, et al. Cumulative use of strong anticholinergics and incident dementia: a prospective cohort study. *JAMA Intern Med.* 2015;175(3):401-407.

Grigoryan L, Trautner BW, Gupta K. Diagnosis and management of urinary tract infections in the outpatient setting: a review. *JAMA.* 2014;312(16): 1677-1684.

Hanno PM, Erickson D, Moldwin R, et al. Diagnosis and treatment of interstitial cystitis/bladder pain syndrome. AUA guideline amendment. *J Urol.* 2015;193:1545-1553.

Hansen BB, Svare J, Viktrup L, Jorgensen T, Lose G. Urinary incontinence during pregnancy and 1 year after delivery in primiparous women compared with a control group of nulliparous women. *Neurourol Urodyn.* 2012;31(4): 475-480.

Harris RL, Yancey CA, Wiser WL, Morrison JC, Meeks GR. Comparison of anterior colporrhaphy and retropubic urethropexy for patients with genuine stress urinary incontinence. *Am J Obstet Gynecol.* 1995;173(6):1671-1674. discussion 1674-1675.

Haylen BT, de Ridder D, Freeman RM, et al. An International Urogynecological Association (IUGA)/International Continence Society (ICS) joint report on the terminology for female pelvic floor dysfunction. *Neurourol Urodyn.* 2010;29(1):4-20.

Hay-Smith EJ, Dumoulin C. Pelvic floor muscle training versus no treatment, or inactive control treatments, for urinary incontinence in women. *Cochrane Database Syst Rev.* 2006;(1):CD005654.

Horbach NS, Ostergard DR. Predicting intrinsic urethral sphincter dysfunction in women with stress urinary incontinence. *Obstet Gynecol.* 1994;84(2): 188-192.

Lapides J. Transurethral treatment of urethral diverticula in women. *Trans Am Assoc Genitourin Surg.* 1978;70:135-137.

Lapitan MC, Cody DJ, Grant AM. Open retropubic colposuspension for urinary incontinence in women. *Cochrane Database Syst Rev.* 2005;3:CD002912.

Lee RA. Diverticulum of the female urethra: postoperative complications and results. *Obstet Gynecol.* 1983;61(1):52-58.

Lemack GE, Krauss S, Litman H, et al. Normal preoperative urodynamic testing does not predict voiding dysfunction after Burch colposuspension versus pubovaginal sling. *J Urol.* 2008;180(5):2076-2080.

Lukacz ES, Lawrence JM, Contreras R, Nager CW, Luber KM. Parity, mode of delivery, and pelvic floor disorders. *Obstet Gynecol.* 2006;107(6):1253-1260.

Melville JL, Delaney K, Newton K, et al. Incontinence severity and major depression in incontinent women. *Obstet Gynecol.* 2005;106:585.

Melville JL, Fan MY, Rau H, Nygaard IE, Katon WJ. Major depression and urinary incontinence in women: temporal associations in an epidemiologic sample. *Am J Obstet Gynecol.* 2009;201(5):490 e491-497.

Meyer S, Schreyer A, De Grandi P, Hohlfeld P. The effects of birth on urinary continence mechanisms and other pelvic-floor characteristics. *Obstet Gynecol.* 1998;92(4 Pt 1):613-618.

Millard RJ, Oldenburg BF. The symptomatic, urodynamic and psychodynamic results of bladder re-education programs. *J Urol.* 1983;130(4):715-719.

Mody L, Juthani-Mehta M. Urinary tract infections in older women: a clinical review. *JAMA.* 2014;311(8):844-854.

Mostafa A, Lim CP, Hopper L, Madhuvrata P, Abdel-Fattah M. Single-incision mini-slings versus standard midurethral slings in surgical management of female stress urinary incontinence: an updated systematic review and meta-analysis of effectiveness and complications. *Eur Urol.* 2014;65(2):402-427.

Nager CW, Brubaker L, Litman HJ, et al. A randomized trial of urodynamic testing before stress-incontinence surgery. *N Engl J Med.* 2012;366(21): 1987-1997.

Nager CW, FitzGerald M, Kraus SR, et al. Urodynamic measures do not predict stress continence outcomes after surgery for stress urinary incontinence in selected women. *J Urol.* 2008;179(4):1470-1474.

Nager CW, Kraus SR, Kenton K, et al. Urodynamics, the supine empty bladder stress test, and incontinence severity. *Neurourol Urodyn.* 2010;29:1306-1311.

Nager CW, Sirls L, Litman HJ, et al. Baseline urodynamic predictors of treatment failure 1 year after mid urethral sling surgery. *J Urol Aug.* 2011;186(2): 597-603.

Nygaard IE. Does prolonged high-impact activity contribute to later urinary incontinence? A retrospective cohort study of female Olympians. *Obstet Gynecol.* 1997;90(5):718-722.

Nygaard I, Barber MD, Burgio KL, et al. Prevalence of symptomatic pelvic floor disorders in US women. *JAMA.* 2008;300(11):1311-1316.

Nygaard IE, Kreder KJ, Lepic MM, Fountain KA, Rhomberg AT. Efficacy of pelvic floor muscle exercises in women with stress, urge, and mixed urinary incontinence. *Am J Obstet Gynecol.* 1996;174(1 Pt 1):120-125.

Ostergard DR. The neurological control of micturition and integral voiding reflexes. *Obstet Gynecol Surv.* 1979;34(6):417-423.

Parsons CL. The therapeutic role of sulfated polysaccharides in the urinary bladder. *Urol Clin North Am.* 1994;21(1):93-100.

Peattie AB, Plevnik S, Stanton SL. Vaginal cones: a conservative method of treating genuine stress incontinence. *Br J Obstet Gynaecol.* 1988;95(10):1049-1053.

Peters KM, Carrico DJ, Perez-Marrero RA, et al. Randomized trial of percutaneous tibial nerve stimulation versus Sham efficacy in the treatment of overactive bladder syndrome: results from the SUmiT trial. *J Urol.* 2010;183(4):1438-1443.

Raz R, Stamm WE. A controlled trial of intravaginal estriol in postmenopausal women with recurrent urinary tract infections. *N Engl J Med.* 1993;329(11):753-756.

Richter HE, Albo ME, Zyczynski HM, et al. Retropubic versus transobturator midurethral slings for stress incontinence. *N Engl J Med.* 2010a;362(22):2066-2076.

Richter HE, Burgio KL, Brubaker L, et al. Continence pessary compared with behavioral therapy or combined therapy for stress incontinence: a randomized controlled trial. *Obstet Gynecol.* 2010b;115(3):609-617.

Richter HE, Litman HJ, Lukacz ES, et al. Demographic and clinical predictors of treatment failure one year after midurethral sling surgery. *Obstet Gynecol.* 2011;117(4):913-921.

Ross JW. Multichannel urodynamic evaluation of laparoscopic Burch colposuspension for genuine stress incontinence. *Obstet Gynecol.* 1998;91(1):55-59.

Saidi MH, Gallagher MS, Skop IP, Saidi JA, Sadler RK, Diaz KC. Extraperitoneal laparoscopic colposuspension: short-term cure rate, complications, and duration of hospital stay in comparison with Burch colposuspension. *Obstet Gynecol.* 1998;92(4 Pt 1):619-621.

Salvatore S, Khullar V, Cardozo L, Milani R, Athanasiou S, Kelleher C. Long-term prospective randomized study comparing two different regimens of oxybutynin as a treatment for detrusor overactivity. *Eur J Obstet Gynecol Reprod Biol.* 2005;119(2):237-241.

Sand PK, Bowen LW, Panganiban R, Ostergard DR. The low pressure urethra as a factor in failed retropubic urethropexy. *Obstet Gynecol.* 1987;69(3 Pt 1):399-402.

Schimpf MO, Rahn DD, Wheeler TL, et al. Sling surgery for stress urinary incontinence in women: a systematic review and metaanalysis. *Am J Obstet Gynecol.* 2014;211(1). 71 e71-71 e27.

Siegel S, Noblett K, Mangel J, et al. Results of a prospective, randomized, multicenter study evaluating sacral neuromodulation with InterStim therapy compared to standard medical therapy at 6-months in subjects with mild symptoms of overactive bladder. *Neurourol Urodyn.* 2015;34(3):224-230.

Subak LL, Wing R, West DS, et al. Weight loss to treat urinary incontinence in overweight and obese women. *N Engl J Med.* 2009;360(5):481-490.

Ulmsten U, Henriksson L, Johnson P, Varhos G. An ambulatory surgical procedure under local anesthesia for treatment of female urinary incontinence. *Int Urogynecol J Pelvic Floor Dysfunct.* 1996;7(2):81-85. discussion 85-86.

Vecchioli-Scaldazza C, Morosetti C, Berouz A, et al. Solifenacin succinate versus percutaneous tibial nerve stimulation in women with overactive bladder syndrome: results of a randomized controlled crossover study. *Gynecol Obstet Invest.* 2013;75(4):230-234.

Visco AG, Brubaker L, Richter HE, et al. Anticholinergic therapy vs. onabotulintoxina for urgency urinary incontinence. *N Eng J Med.* 2012;367(19):1803-1813.

Visco AG, Weidner AC, Cundiff GW, Bump RC. Observed patient compliance with a structured outpatient bladder retraining program. *Am J Obstet Gynecol.* 1999;181(6):1392-1394.

Ward KL, Hilton P. UK, Ireland TVTTG: A prospective multicenter randomized trial of tension-free vaginal tape and colposuspension for primary urodynamic stress incontinence: two-year follow-up. *Am J Obstet Gynecol.* 2004;190(2):324-331.

Westby M, Asmussen M, Ulmsten U. Location of maximum intraurethral pressure related to urogenital diaphragm in the female subject as studied by simultaneous urethrocystometry and voiding urethrocystography. *Am J Obstet Gynecol.* 1982;144(4):408-412.

Wu JM, Matthews CA, Conover MM, Pate V, Jonsson Funk M. Lifetime risk of stress urinary incontinence or pelvic organ prolapse surgery. *Obstet Gynecol.* 2014;123(6):1201-1206.

Suggested Readings can be found on ExpertConsult.com.

# 22

# Anal Incontinence

## Diagnosis and Management

*Gretchen M. Lentz, Mukta Krane*

Anorectal disorders are common in women and anal incontinence is particularly distressing. Despite the negative impact on quality of life, women may be reluctant to discuss this with their physician because of embarrassment. As one of the most common contributing factors to anal incontinence is pregnancy and delivery, the obstetrician-gynecologist will often be the first to assess the problem. The prevalence of anal incontinence increases with age, so it is imperative that physicians are equipped to address these problems in postmenopausal women and be aware of the significant effects that these disorders can have on a woman's self-sufficiency and ability to carry out activities of daily living. Anal incontinence is a general term that refers to loss of gas or fecal material via the anus. Fecal incontinence is the inability to prevent loss of stool from the anus until desired. This chapter addresses the causes, diagnosis, and treatment of anal incontinence. *Accidental bowel leakage* is also a newer term being used.

## ANAL INCONTINENCE

Fecal incontinence (FI) is one of the most devastating of all physical disabilities but, because of the social embarrassment and psychological effects, most patients fail to report their symptoms and many physicians do not ask. Therefore the exact prevalence of this condition is unknown. Estimates range from 9% to 16% of community-dwelling women with average age of onset between 47 and 55 years. Part of this variability relates to study definition differences for fecal incontinence. Occasional fecal soiling will not be as devastating as gross fecal incontinence, but both may be reported as part of the same study definition. Approximately 10% of women will report some change in bowel habits after one vaginal delivery. Prevalence increases with age. Little is known about racial differences in fecal incontinence, but a 2010 study found a prevalence of 6.1% in noninstitutionalized African Americans aged 52 to 68 years. Over 30% of women reporting urinary incontinence also report fecal incontinence, known as *dual incontinence.* Fecal incontinence is the second leading cause of nursing home placement. Box 22.1 lists common risk factors for this condition. Late-onset fecal incontinence may have a different set of risk factors and, in one nested case-control study, bowel disturbances rather than obstetric events were more important.

Anal incontinence is the inability to defer the elimination of stool or gas until there is a socially acceptable time and place to do so. Fecal incontinence is the inability to defer the elimination of stool and can be subdivided into three groups: fecal urge incontinence, passive incontinence, and fecal seepage. Fecal urge incontinence is the loss of fecal contents despite attempts to avoid defecation. Passive incontinence refers to the involuntary discharge of feces without awareness or sensation. Fecal seepage is most often defined as the involuntary leakage of small amounts of stool. Because maintaining continence is a complex physiologic process that requires a person's ability to perceive the type of fecal bolus, store or retain when necessary, and excrete when desirable, the loss of that ability is equally complex.

In the evaluation of anal incontinence, it is important for the physician to understand the woman's symptoms, type of loss (i.e., flatus or liquid/solid stool), frequency of incontinence, effect on the quality of her life, and concurrent pelvic floor derangements. Fecal incontinence affects each woman's life in a different manner. What may be acceptable for one woman may be intolerable to another. Evaluation and treatment should be directed by the severity of the woman's symptoms and the expected goals of therapy.

### PHYSIOLOGY OF FECAL CONTINENCE

Fecal continence is significantly affected by stool consistency and volume, colonic transit time, rectal compliance, innervation of the pelvic floor and anal sphincter, and interplay among the puborectalis muscle, rectum, and anal sphincters. Loss of one or more of these functions can lead to fecal incontinence.

As a bolus of stool or gas passes from the sigmoid colon to the rectal canal, receptors in the wall of the puborectalis sense the distention of the rectum. As long as the pressure in the anal canal is maintained at a higher level than the rectal pressure, continence is maintained. Anal canal pressure depends on a competent internal anal sphincter (IAS) and external anal sphincter (EAS). The IAS is a thickened continuation of the circular muscle of the colon and provides 75% to 85% of the resting tone of the anal canal, but there is a lower rectal sphincter pressure when the anal canal is distended with stool. The IAS, under autonomic control, maintains the high-pressure zone or continence zone and, along with the EAS, keeps the anal canal closed. Disruption or dysfunction of the IAS may result in passive incontinence. The shape of the combined IAS and

EAS is almost cylindrical as it encircles the anal canal. Magnetic resonance imaging (MRI) scans from nulliparous women have shown that the EAS does not appear as a cylinder but rather has lateral winged projections. The function of this component is not known. The sphincter complex averages 18.3 mm in thickness and 2.8 cm in length in the midline anteriorly; 54% of the anterior thickness is attributable to the IAS and the remainder to the EAS. The EAS provides the voluntary squeeze pressure that prevents incontinence with increasing rectal or abdominal pressure and is related to urge incontinence. The EAS is innervated by the hemorrhoidal branch of the pudendal nerve from the S2-S4 nerve roots. Contraction of the EAS, voluntarily or through a spinal reflex, increases the anal canal pressure by 25%, but this tone cannot be maintained indefinitely because these are fatigable, fast-twitch muscles.

**Box 22.1 Risk Factors for Fecal Incontinence**

**General**
- Aging
- Obstetric anal sphincter laceration
- Operative vaginal delivery with forceps
- Neuropathy
- Bowel motility disorders
- Hemorrhoids and previous anal surgery

**Late-Onset (After Age 40)**
- Current smoking
- High body mass index
- Diarrhea
- Irritable bowel syndrome
- Cholecystectomy
- Rectocele
- Urinary incontinence
- Bariatric surgery

The third muscular component of the sphincter complex is the puborectalis muscle (Fig. 22.1). The puborectalis, part of the levator ani muscle complex, originates from the pubic bone on either side of the midline, passes beside the vagina and rectum, and fuses posteriorly behind the anorectal junction to form the U-shaped sling that cradles the rectum while sending some fibers onto the walls of the anal canal. Unlike most other striated muscles, the puborectalis, like the IAS, maintains a constant muscle tone that is directly proportional to the volume of the rectal content and pressure, and it relaxes at the time of defecation. Both the puborectalis and EAS contain a majority of type I, or slow-twitch, muscle fibers, which are ideally suited to maintaining a constant contraction or tone. Each muscle group also contains a small proportion of type II, or fast-twitch, fibers that allow for quick responses to rapid increases in intraabdominal pressure. The puborectalis is innervated by direct branches from S3 and S4 and, to a lesser degree, from the pudendal nerve. The constant contraction of the puborectalis creates a 90-degree angle between the rectum and anal canal. This angle, known as the *anorectal angle,* has been the source of much discussion and evaluation in determining its role in the maintenance of continence. Parks has postulated that this angle creates a flap valve effect that presses the anterior rectal wall down onto the upper anal canal and thereby prevents the rectal contents from entering the anal canal when intraabdominal pressure is applied. The anterior rectal wall therefore acts as a plug. However, Bartolo has found that when the anal sphincter is maximally stressed and the

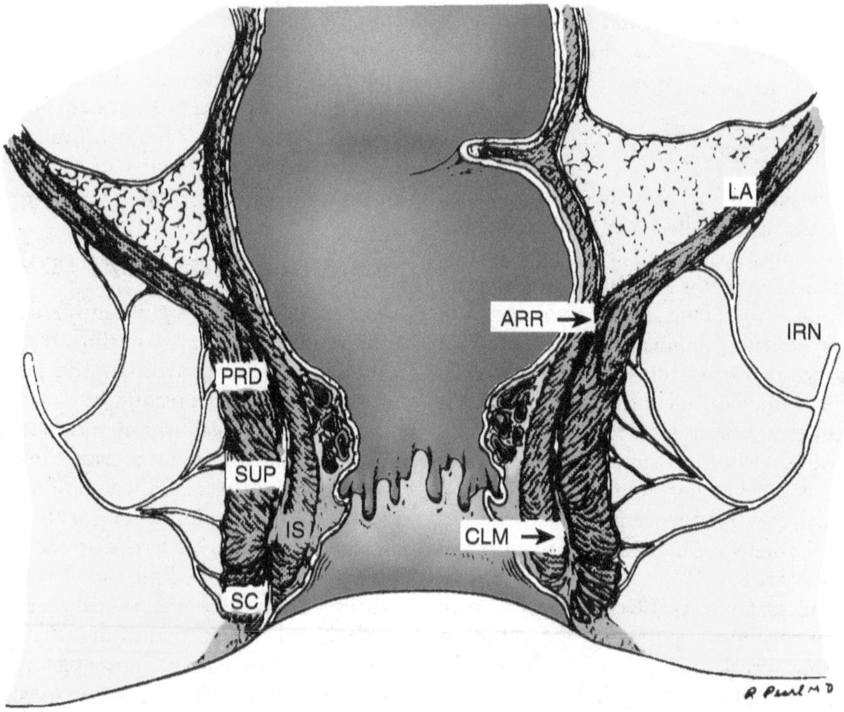


**Figure 22.1** Coronal section of the anal canal and lower rectum. *ARR,* Level of anorectal ring; *CLM,* conjoined longitudinal muscle; *IRN,* inferior rectal nerve; *LA,* levator ani muscles; *PRD,* puborectalis/deep external sphincter complex; *SC,* subcutaneous external sphincter. (From Pearl RK: In Smith L, ed. *Practical Guide to Anorectal Testing.* New York: Igaku-Shoin; 1995.)

Table 22.1 Anal Incontinence: Components of the Continence Mechanism

| Component | Function | Symptoms of Deficit |
|---|---|---|
| External anal sphincter | Provides emergency control for liquid stool and flatus | Fecal urgency; urge-related incontinence of liquid stool and flatus |
| Puborectalis | Maintains continence of solid stool | Incontinence of solid stool |
| Internal anal sphincter | Keeps anal canal closed at rest; allows sampling of stool content and enhances continence of liquid stool and flatus | Fecal soiling<br>Incontinence of liquid stool and flatus |
| Anal sensation | Allows discrimination of gas, liquid, and solid stool; provides warning of impending incontinence | Fecal soiling; fecal leakage that is promptly halted by voluntary contraction on conscious detection |
| Colonic motility | Controls stool volume, consistency, and delivery rate to the rectum | Incontinence of liquid or loose stools during prolonged or severe diarrheal states |
| Rectal reservoir | Maintains adequate reservoir under low pressure | Incontinence of solid stool associated with sudden rectal distention; fecal urgency and urge-related incontinence |

From Toglia M. Anal incontinence: an underrecognized, undertreated problem. *Female Patient.* 1996;21:27.

rectum is visualized radiographically, there is no contact between the rectal wall and anal canal (Bartolo, 1986). In addition, surgical procedures that try to recreate this angle in an attempt to restore continence have not proved effective.

When a bolus of stool or gas is sensed in the rectum, the IAS has a reflex relaxation that allows for colonic contents to be sampled by the anal canal to distinguish solid, liquid, and gas forms of fecal material. After the sampling, the IAS contracts and the fecal material is pushed back into the rectum. This reflex, known as the *rectoanal inhibitory reflex (RAIR),* is absent in patients with Hirschsprung disease. This reflex can also be inhibited by chronic dilation of the anus with fecal impaction and can lead to incontinence. If the impaction is cured, the reflex and anal tone can return to normal.

If the rectum has normal compliance and the person chooses to defer defecation, the IAS and EAS sphincters and puborectalis remain contracted until the appropriate time to eliminate. As seen in Table 22.1, loss of any of these important components can lead to incontinence of flatus, liquid, or solid stool.

**Box 22.2 Common Causes of Fecal Incontinence**

- Obstetric injury
  - Disruption of internal anal sphincter
  - Disruption of external anal sphincter
  - Pelvic floor denervation
- Trauma
  - Pelvic fracture
  - Accidental injury
  - Anal intercourse
  - Anorectal surgery
  - Rectovaginal fistula
- Diarrheal states
  - Irritable bowel syndrome
  - Infectious diarrhea
  - Inflammatory bowel disease
  - Short gut syndrome
  - Laxative abuse
  - Radiation
- Malabsorption
- Rectal neoplasia
- Rectal prolapse
- Rectocele
- Hemorrhoids
- Overflow
  - Impaction
  - Encopresis
- Neurologic disease
  - Congenital anomalies (e.g., myelomeningocele)
  - Multiple sclerosis
  - Diabetic neuropathy
  - Neoplasms or injury of brain, spinal cord, cauda equina
  - Pudendal neuropathy (e.g., from childbirth, chronic straining, perineal descent)
- Congenital anomalies of the anorectum or pelvis

## CAUSES AND PATHOPHYSIOLOGY

There are many causes of fecal incontinence (Box 22.2). One way to categorize the reasons for fecal incontinence is to separate the initial cause into those that start outside the pelvis with a normal pelvic floor from those that start with an abnormal pelvic floor. Causes that start outside the pelvis include all the pathologies that cause diarrhea or increased intestinal motility, overflow incontinence from fecal impaction, and rectal neoplasms. Known or diagnosable neurologic conditions such as multiple sclerosis, diabetic neuropathy, trauma, or neoplasms in the spinal cord or cauda equina initially begin as pathologies outside the pelvis, and the pelvic floor is presumed to be normal. As these neuropathies progress, there is damage to the pelvic floor musculature or rectal sensation, resulting in fecal incontinence.

Fecal incontinence secondary to an abnormal pelvic floor is caused by congenital anorectal malformations, surgery, obstetric injury, aging, or pelvic floor denervation without a known neurologic disease. Historically, incontinence secondary to denervation has been designated as idiopathic and represents 80% of patients with fecal incontinence. Pelvic floor denervation has been studied extensively in women with urinary and fecal incontinence, as well as pelvic organ prolapse. Denervation may be secondary to vaginal delivery, chronic straining with constipation, rectal prolapse, or descending perineal syndrome. Histologic studies of the EAS and puborectalis show fibrosis, scarring, and fiber-type grouping consistent with nerve damage and reinnervation in women with idiopathic fecal incontinence. Electromyography (EMG) studies have demonstrated reinnervation of the pelvic floor with increased fiber density and prolongation of nerve conduction on pudendal nerve terminal motor latency (PNTML) studies.

In healthy women, the most common cause of fecal incontinence is damage to the anal sphincters at the time of vaginal delivery, with or without neuronal injury. This type of incontinence is often referred to as anal incontinence. Damage can occur by mechanical disruption or separation of the IAS, EAS, or both, or by damage to the muscle innervation by stretching or crushing the pudendal and pelvic nerves. Sultan and coworkers' 1993 landmark study showed that 13% of primiparas and 23% of multiparas developed fecal incontinence or fecal urgency by 6 weeks postpartum (Sultan, 1993). By endoanal ultrasound, all but one of the women had evidence of anal sphincter disruption. The incidence of occult external anal sphincter disruption after vaginal delivery determined by endoanal ultrasound ranged from 11% to 35%. Most of the women showed pudendal nerve conduction prolongation but recovered by 6 months postpartum. Because anal sphincter injury correlated with the development of symptoms, reducing anal sphincter injury and understanding risk factors are critical to prevention. The chance of anatomic sphincter injury is increased with midline episiotomy, instrumented delivery, vaginal delivery of larger infants, and persistent occiput posterior presenting head position. Other risk factors include increasing maternal age, prolonged second stage (longer than 2 hours), epidural anesthesia, and clinically diagnosed sphincter laceration at the time of delivery. The first vaginal delivery appears to have the greatest effect on pelvic floor function and risk of EAS disruption, but subsequent deliveries can increase the risk of permanent damage, especially in women with transient symptoms of fecal incontinence after their first delivery. Not all risk factors are known, and not all women are susceptible to pelvic floor and sphincter damage with vaginal delivery.

Diabetes mellitus deserves mention because of its rising prevalence. Diabetics can develop autonomic neuropathy and can have decreased IAS resting pressure. Either of these might contribute to fecal incontinence.

## DIAGNOSIS AND ASSESSMENT

For fecal incontinence, even more than urinary incontinence, if the physician does not ask, the woman will not volunteer the information. Ideally, a question such as "How often do you leak gas, liquid, or solid stool?" should be placed on the standard office intake questionnaire. Several reports have shown that twice as many patients complain of fecal or flatal incontinence when given a written questionnaire rather than answering verbal questioning.

Because approximately 1 in 10 women will develop some fecal incontinence or fecal urgency after one vaginal delivery, it is especially important to incorporate open-ended questions concerning flatal or fecal incontinence as part of the 6-week postpartum visit. In addition, as women age, the chance of developing fecal incontinence increases, so it is also important to target older women for questioning.

### Evaluation

Assessment of the woman with fecal incontinence must include a thorough history because the origin of the problem may be the single most important criterion of therapy. Box 22.3 lists some questions to be asked when taking a history regarding fecal incontinence.

**Box 22.3 History in a Patient with Suspected Fecal Incontinence**

Onset and precipitating event(s)
Duration, severity, and timing
Stool consistency and urgency
Coexisting problems, surgery, urinary incontinence, back injury
Obstetric history—forceps, tears, presentation, repair
Drugs, caffeine, diet
Clinical subtypes—passive or urge incontinence or fecal seepage
Clinical grading of severity
History of fecal impaction

**Table 22.2** Continence Grading Scale*

| Type of Incontinence | Frequency | | | | |
|---|---|---|---|---|---|
| | Never | Rarely | Sometimes | Usually | Always |
| Solid | 0 | 1 | 2 | 3 | 4 |
| Liquid | 0 | 1 | 2 | 3 | 4 |
| Gas | 0 | 1 | 2 | 3 | 4 |
| Wears pad | 0 | 1 | 2 | 3 | 4 |
| Lifestyle alteration | 0 | 1 | 2 | 3 | 4 |

*The continence score is determined by adding points from this table, which takes into account the type and frequency of incontinence and the extent to which it alters the patient's life.

From Jorge JM, Wexner SD. Etiology and management of fecal incontinence. *Dis Colon Rectum*. 1993;36:77-97.

0= perfect, 20 = complete incontinence; never = 0 (never); rarely = < 1/month; sometimes = < 1/week, ≥ 1/month; usually = <1/day, ≥1/week; always = ≥1/day.

The history should include onset, duration, severity of the condition, effect on the woman's daily activities, pad use, frequency and consistency of bowel movements, use of laxatives, fiber intake, and dietary habits. Specific questions concerning diarrhea, amount of flatus, average number of stools per day, passage of mucus, and bloating should be asked. Physicians and patients define normal bowel function differently. Diarrhea may mean frequent bowel movements to one person but loose and watery bowel movements to another. It is best to have the woman quantitate the number of bowel movements and incontinent episodes and describe the stool consistency. A diary of bowel habits and incontinent episodes can be useful, and several standardized classification systems are available. Table 22.2 gives a frequently used scoring system developed by Jorge and Wexner (1993). The woman circles the appropriate number on each line of the scale. The numbers are then added. A perfect score, or 0, indicates no incontinence and a score of 20 indicates complete incontinence. The value of this continence grading scale is that it can be used before and after treatment to determine the efficacy of the intervention. A standardized questionnaire should be used whenever possible to direct diagnosis and treatment and assess treatment success.

The history should also identify specific complaints such as feelings of incomplete emptying, straining with bowel movements, fecal urgency, pain with defecation, and insensible loss of stool. It is important to determine whether the woman senses the need to have a bowel movement or if she is unaware

| Stool Diary | | | | | | | | |
|---|---|---|---|---|---|---|---|---|
| PLEASE RECORD YOUR STOOL HABITS FOR ONE WEEK: | | | | | | | Name: Hosp #: | |
| **Date** | **Time of bowel movement** | **Incontinence** Yes / No | **Stool seepage or straining** Yes / No | **Stool consistency** (Type 1–7) See below | **Urgency** – unable to postpone BM for more than 15 minutes Yes / No | **Use of pads** Yes / No | **Medications** | **Comments** |
| | | | | | | | | |
| | | | | | | | | |
| | | | | | | | | |
| | | | | | | | | |
| | | | | | | | | |
| | | | | | | | | |
| | | | | | | | | |
| | | | | | | | | |

Use the following descriptors for describing stool consistency:

Type 1: **Separate hard lumps.** Type 2: **Sausage-shaped but lumpy.** Type 3: **Like a sausage but with cracks on its surface.**
Type 4: **Like a sausage or snake, smooth and soft.** Type 5: **Soft blobs with clear-cut edges (passed easily).**
Type 6: **Fluffy pieces with ragged edges, a mushy stool.** Type 7: **Watery.**

**Figure 22.2** Stool diary.This is a sample stool diary for assessing patients with fecal incontinence. (From Rao SS. American College of Gastroenterology Practice Parameters Committee: diagnosis and management of fecal incontinence. American College of Gastroenterology Practice Parameters Committee. *Am J Gastroenterol.* 2004;99:1585.)

that she needs to defecate but finds stool in her undergarments. A sensory impairment or hygiene problem is implied when stool leakage occurs without warning. If the woman is aware of impending incontinence but cannot prevent the passage of stool, a motor impairment is suggested. Patients may have pseudoincontinence secondary to soiling from prolapsing hemorrhoids or rectovaginal or anovaginal fistulas. Patients should also be questioned about other pelvic floor pathologies, particularly rectal prolapse, rectovaginal fistulas, and urinary incontinence.

The review of systems should include abdominal pain or cramping, lower back or pelvic pain, any changes in pelvic or lower extremity sensation, and changes in sexual response. Changes in the neurologic function of the pelvis or lower extremities or a history of an acute onset of fecal incontinence should direct the physician to rule out a neurologic disease, such as multiple sclerosis or a neoplasm of the brain or lumbosacral spinal cord.

The past medical history should include detailed history of vaginal deliveries, including birth weights, length of second stage, episiotomies or lacerations, and use of forceps. Any breakdown or complications of episiotomy healing should be noted. The past history of abdominal and pelvic surgeries or trauma to the back or pelvis should be reviewed. Details and operative reports of any anal dilations, anal sphincterotomy, hemorrhoidectomy, rectovaginal fistula repairs, or posterior colporrhaphy should be obtained. Patients should also be questioned about previous evaluations and results of flexible sigmoidoscopy, colonoscopy, and barium enemas. Any family history of colon cancer, inflammatory bowel disease, or familial polyposis should be elicited.

Many medications also affect bowel function. The woman should not only be asked about laxatives and bowel stimulants, but a complete list of all prescription and over-the-counter medications, as well as any dietary or herbal supplements, should be reviewed. Many drugs, including anticholinergics, antidepressants, iron, narcotics, nonsteroidal anti-inflammatory drugs (NSAIDs), and pseudoephedrine, can cause chronic constipation that may contribute to overflow incontinence or pelvic floor neuropathy secondary to straining.

Women can be instructed on how to keep a daily stool diary (Fig. 22.2). This is a good baseline evaluation tool and can later be used to assess conservative treatment with dietary changes and fiber intake.

### *Physical Examination*

Undergarments or pads should be inspected for stool, mucus, blood, or pus. If material is found, the woman should be asked if this is her normal leakage. Physical examination begins with inspection of the perineum and anal region. Pruritus ani, or discoloration and irritation of the perianal skin, is commonly seen with fecal incontinence of liquid stool and chronic diarrhea. Perianal skin creases or folds should completely encircle the anus. Note the presence of protruding tissue around or from the anus and determine whether there are external hemorrhoids or mucosal or full-thickness rectal prolapse (Fig. 22.3). The dovetail sign, or loss of anterior perineal folds, indicates a defect

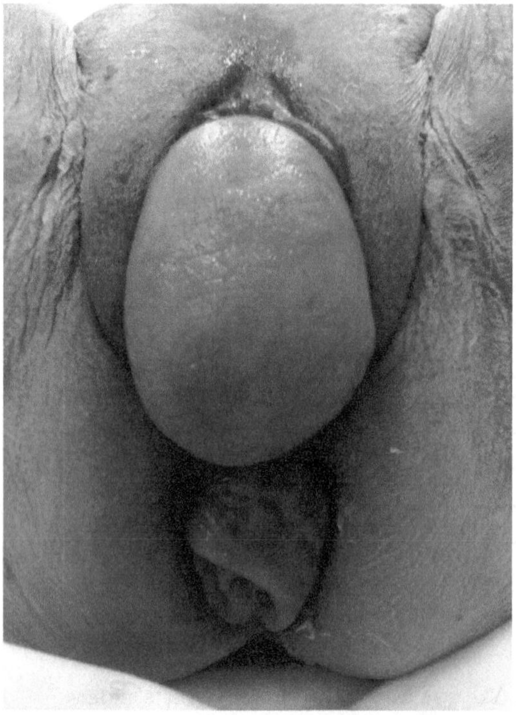

**Figure 22.3** Combined severe rectal prolapse and vaginal pelvic organ prolapse. Note the protrusion of the rectal mucosa from the anus.

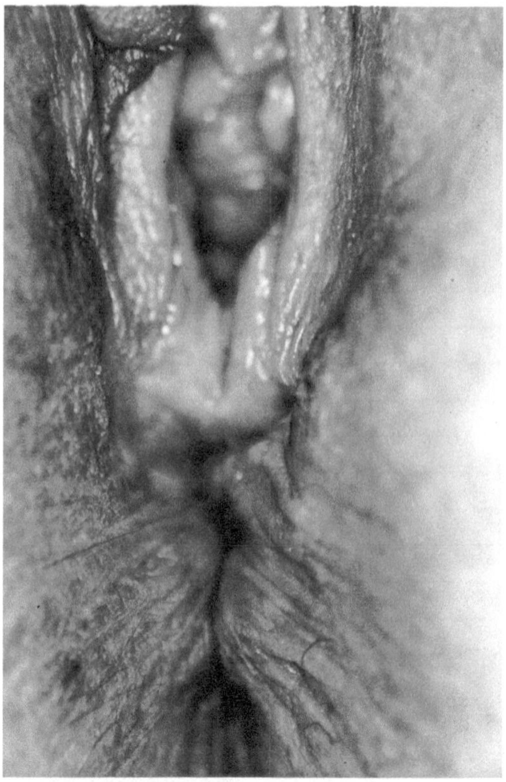

**Figure 22.4** Perineum with chronic laceration of external anal sphincter (EAS). Inspection of the perineum shows the classic dovetail sign with loss of the anal skin creases anteriorly because of a chronic third-degree laceration of the EAS. Normally, with an intact sphincter, the skin creases are arranged radially around the anus. (From Stenchever MA, Benson JT, eds. *Atlas of Clinical Gynecology.* New York: McGraw-Hill; 2000.)

in the EAS or chronic third-degree laceration (Fig. 22.4). Previous episiotomy, laceration, or surgical scars should be noted. The size of the genital hiatus and presence of genital prolapse should be assessed as an indicator of pelvic floor neuromuscular function. The innervation of the EAS can be grossly tested by eliciting the clitoral-anal or bulbocavernosus reflex. Using a cotton swab, a gentle, quick touch beside the clitoris or over the bulbocavernosus muscle should elicit a contraction of the EAS. If intact, the reflex implies that the pudendal nerve afferents and rectal or external hemorrhoidal branch of the pudendal efferent nerves are functional. Unlike men, who should always exhibit this reflex, approximately 10% of women lack this reflex naturally. However, if absent, and in the presence of fecal incontinence, further neurologic testing is indicated. Sensation in the S2-S4 dermatomes should be screened by dull and pinprick discrimination when touching the perineum. The same wooden cotton swab used to elicit bulbocavernosus reflexes can be broken and then used for pinprick (broken end) and dull (cotton end) sensation testing. Loss of sensation should direct the clinician to further neurologic or radiologic assessment of the nervous system.

Next, the woman should be asked to squeeze as if trying not to pass gas. Inspection of the perianal folds should be evaluated for a concentric contraction and some upward movement of the perineal body as she contracts the EAS and levator ani. Substitution with contraction of the buttocks, upper thighs, or abdomen should be noted. The woman should then be asked to bear down as if trying to have a bowel movement. She should be reassured that it is expected that she might pass flatus during this part of the examination. The degree of perineal descent and any prolapse of the vagina, pelvic viscera, or rectum should be noted. If there appears to be any pelvic organ prolapse, the examination should be performed with the woman in the standing position or after straining on a commode to maximize the prolapse.

Rectal examination is used to assess resting and squeeze tones of the anal canal. The resting tone of the anal canal is an indicator of IAS function. When asked to squeeze, the woman should feel a circumferential contraction and tightening. An upward movement of the rectum and posterior compartment of the pelvis should be seen as the levator ani muscles contract. Because these muscles also play an important role in anal continence, palpation of the levators for strength and symmetry should be performed by palpating the muscles on each side of the vagina at the introitus.

In addition to assessing rectal tone, the anal canal and rectum should be palpated for masses and a dilated rectum or the presence of stool in the rectal vault. A chronically distended rectum, with stool, a tumor, or an intussuscepting bowel will disrupt the normal rectoanal inhibitory reflex that allows the highly sensitive anal canal to sample the stool contents by relaxing the IAS while time-contracting the EAS to prevent incontinence. If this reflex is suppressed, the anal canal remains dilated, the EAS fatigues, and incontinence will occur.

While doing the rectal examination, the doctor asks the woman to strain to diagnose the presence of a rectocele, enterocele, rectal prolapse, or bowel intussusception. With the examiner's finger in the rectum, the integrity of the rectovaginal septum,

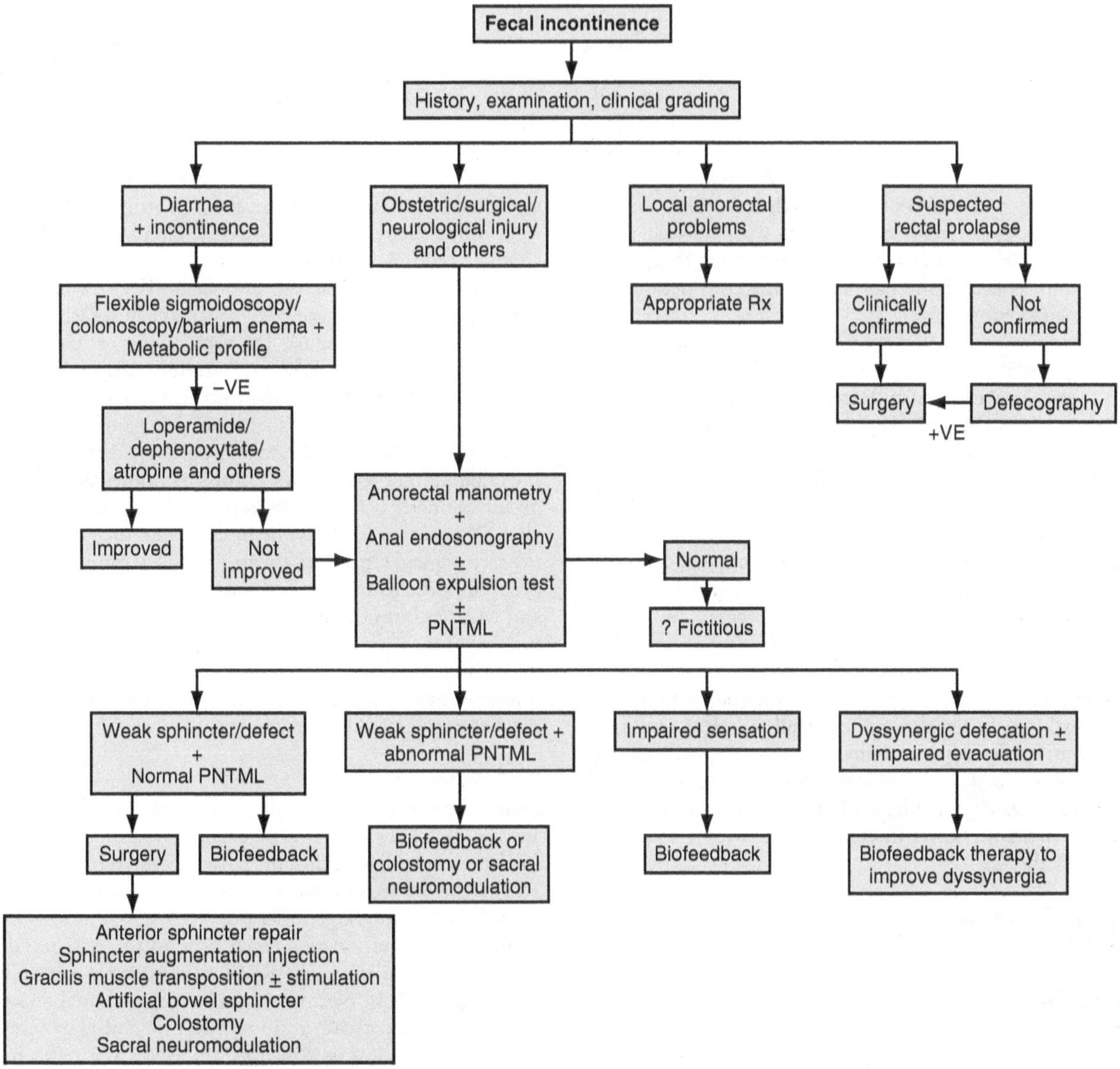


**Figure 22.5** Algorithmic approach to the evaluation and management of fecal incontinence. A detailed history differentiates incontinence of gas, liquid, or solid stool, along with frequency, onset, and effect on the patient's quality of life. The history should assess the possibility of Crohn disease, ulcerative colitis, irritable bowel syndrome, radiation to the pelvis, neurologic diseases such as multiple sclerosis, and prior anorectal surgeries. A detailed obstetric history should include type of delivery, weight of largest infant, length of second stage, episiotomy or lacerations, and use of forceps or vacuum extraction. Rectal examination should assess resting and squeeze tone, presence of a rectocele or rectal mass, and fecal impaction. Inspection of the rectum and vagina should evaluate for a rectovaginal fistula, prolapsing hemorrhoids, or rectal prolapse. Further evaluation, including radiologic and physiologic tests, have been shown in a prospective study at a tertiary colorectal referral clinic to alter the final diagnosis of the cause of fecal incontinence in 19% of cases. (From Rao SS. American College of Gastroenterology Practice Parameters Committee: diagnosis and management of fecal incontinence. American College of Gastroenterology Practice Parameters Committee. *Am J Gastroenterol.* 2004;99:1585.)

posterior vaginal wall, and perineal body can be assessed by palpating through the vagina via bimanual examination.

### *Testing*

Clinical diagnosis based on physical examination and history alone will be accurate in most patients. However, further evaluation, including radiologic and physiologic tests, have been shown in a prospective study at a tertiary colorectal referral clinic to alter the final diagnosis of the cause of fecal incontinence in 19% of cases. Which tests to consider should be based on history and physical examination, prior treatment, and proposed therapy. The algorithm outlined in Figure 22.5 recommends further evaluation based on history and the rectal tone. Normal rectal tone directs the clinician away from anal incontinence and toward a metabolic or colonic origin. Metabolic tests, including determination of thyroid-stimulating hormone and glucose levels, should be carried out. If chronic diarrhea is present with normal rectal sphincter tone, stool cultures, colonoscopy, and diarrhea evaluation are indicated. Differential diagnosis for a diarrhea workup will include lactose intolerance, celiac sprue, inflammatory bowel disease, irritable bowel syndrome, and bacterial overgrowth from diabetic gastroparesis. In cases of fecal incontinence with normal rectal sphincter tone without diarrhea, anal manometry to evaluate rectal sensation is useful and can help in the consideration of peripheral neuropathy causes.

Poor resting tone on rectal examination directs the clinician to a neuromuscular cause. A normal resting tone, but with poor squeeze, suggests an anterior sphincter defect and chronic third-degree laceration of the EAS. If poor rectal squeeze is detected, endoanal ultrasonography is the best first-line test.

Evaluation or further testing is performed not only for diagnostic purposes but also to determine which nonsurgical and surgical therapies are most likely to benefit the woman. In addition, certain tests, such as anal manometry or an anal sphincter ultrasound, can be used for baseline assessment to which post-treatment assessment or function can be compared. Whenever the woman's history does not match her physical examination findings, further testing should be considered. In addition, if the woman has had prior surgery or has other pelvic floor dysfunction, testing before treatment, especially surgical, may help direct care. It is important to remember that the woman may have more than one cause or pathology contributing to her fecal incontinence, such as pudendal neuropathy and an anal sphincter defect or irritable bowel in combination with a weakened pelvic floor (Table 22.3).

### *Diagnostic Procedures*

#### Colonoscopy

A colonoscopy is indicated for any woman with chronic diarrhea to evaluate for inflammatory bowel disease and infectious diarrhea. Endoscopic evaluation detects mucosal disease or neoplasia effectively. This is also acceptable bowel screening for any woman older than 50 years, particularly if an acute change in bowel habits is reported. In addition, any patient presenting with fecal incontinence in the setting of rectal prolapse should undergo a colonoscopy to ensure that a rectal mass is not the cause of the prolapse.

#### Endoanal Ultrasound

Endoanal ultrasound (EAUS) has significantly enhanced the ability to delineate defects of the IAS and EAS. EAUS is one of the simplest and least expensive tests for imaging sphincter defects, and a study evaluating the role of anorectal physiology testing found it to be the test that most often informed management decisions. However, EAUS is user dependent and requires significant training. It is generally performed with a 10-MHz rigid probe that creates a 360-degree circular image of the anal sphincter complex, allowing assessment of the integrity, thickness, and length of the IAS and EAS. The IAS is visible as a hypoechoic circle, and the EAS is seen as a hyperechoic or mixed echogenic circle (Fig. 22.6). The distal anal canal is characterized by the presence of the EAS but a thin or absent IAS. The IAS and EAS are both robust in the mid anal canal and the proximal anal canal is identified by visualization of the puborectalis, which forms a posterior sling. Endoanal ultrasound is most useful in the evaluation of patients for chronic third-degree lacerations or occult sphincter tears. Breaks in the EAS can be readily noted. A gloved finger should always be inserted into the vagina to oppose the rectovaginal septum to the probe to determine the size of the perineal body. Knowing the boundaries of the sphincter defect and whether both the EAS and IAS are disrupted can direct the surgeon at the time of anal sphincteroplasty. Similar information can be obtained from EMG of the EAS when used to map the sphincter defect. In general, transanal ultrasound is less painful and better tolerated by the woman.

#### Anal Manometry

Anal manometry is a commonly used test that objectively assesses rectal sensation, anal canal pressures, and the RAIR. Anal manometry is helpful for patients who have had prior surgery to the anorectal canal or radiation therapy that could have altered the rectal storage function.

Anal manometry uses a rectal balloon to assess rectal sensation, rectal compliance, the RAIR, and maximal tolerable rectal volume (Fig. 22.7). Normal values include an initial sensation of 20 mL, urge to defecate at 80 to 120 mL, and maximum tolerable capacity at 200 to 250 mL. The RAIR is a reflex response to increased pressure in the rectum from gas or stool. Normally, the IAS relaxes to allow a sampling of the rectal contents by the anal canal to determine whether the contents are gas or stool and whether it is an appropriate time to defecate or pass flatus. At the same time, the EAS squeezes to prevent incontinence.

**Table 22.3** Tests of Anorectal Function for Patients with Fecal Incontinence

| Test | Measures | Indication |
|---|---|---|
| Anal manometry | Resting anal pressures<br>Maximum squeeze pressure<br>Rectoanal inhibitory reflex<br>Rectal sensation | Low resting and squeeze pressure on rectal examination<br>Prior radiation treatment<br>Fecal urgency<br>Fecal impaction |
| Single-fiber EMG | Fiber density<br>Muscle activity | Denervation<br>Reinnervation injury<br>Map EAS defect |
| Pudendal nerve motor latency | Speed of signal along pudendal nerve | Pudendal nerve damage from childbirth or straining |
| Endoscopic ultrasound | IAS and EAS defect | Obstetric or traumatic sphincter injuries |
| Defecating proctography or MRI defecography | Movement of pelvic floor<br>Pelvic floor defects | Perineal descent<br>Posterior compartment deficits |

*EAS*, External anal sphincter; *EMG*, electromyography; *IAS*, internal anal sphincter.

In addition to rectal function, resting and squeeze pressures in the anal canal are obtained by pulling a perfusion catheter with radial ports (four or eight) through the anal canal. The IAS contributes 80% of the resting pressure. Although there are slight variations depending on the equipment and technique used, normal resting pressure is in the range of 60 to 80 mm Hg. Voluntary contraction of the EAS or squeeze pressure is assessed by the force of the squeeze, which is known as the maximum pressure, and the duration of the squeeze. Normal squeeze pressure is in the 120 to 180 mm Hg range and is sustained for 20

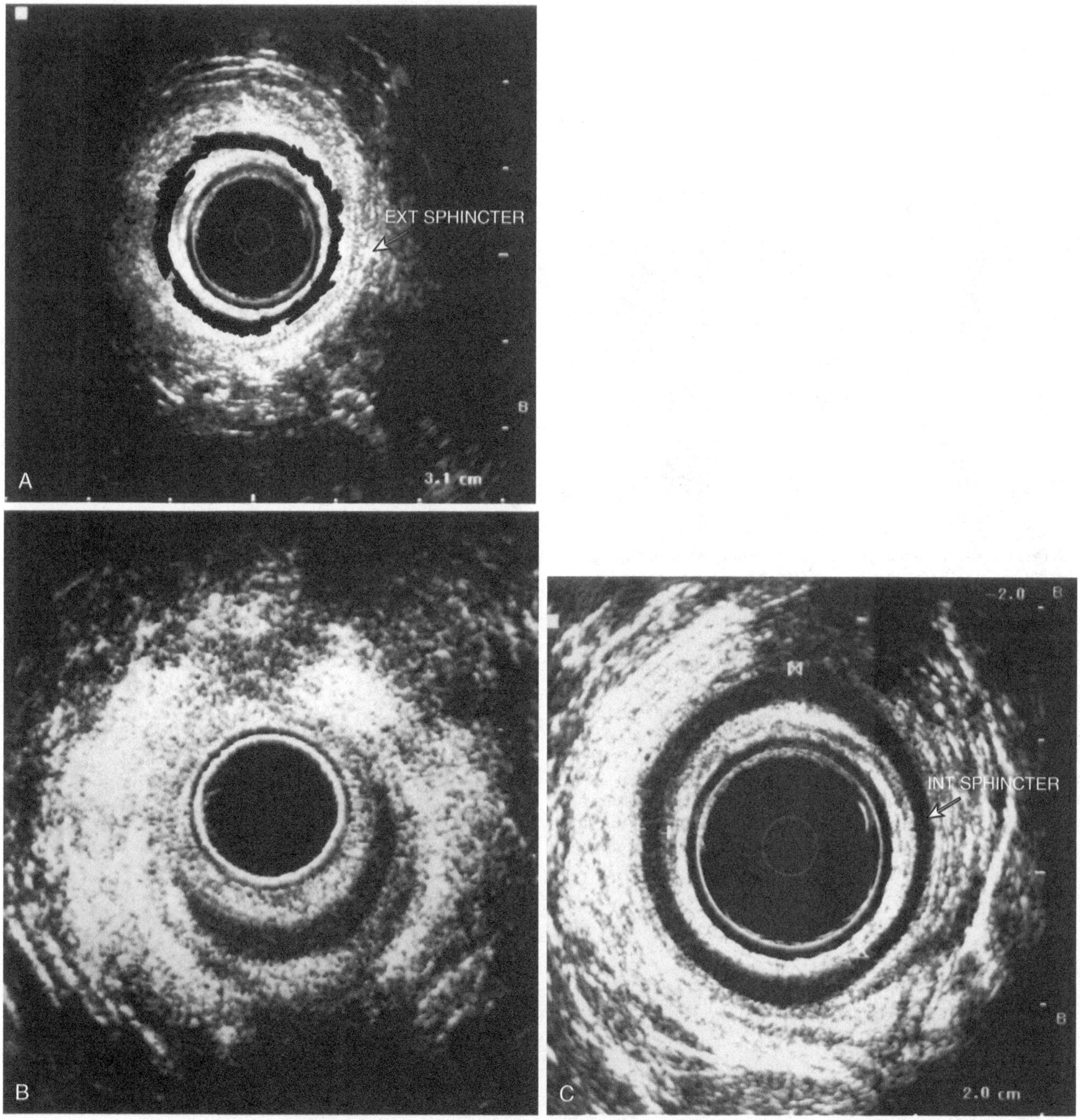


**Figure 22.6** Anal ultrasound. **A,** Anal ultrasound has significantly enhanced the ability to delineate defects of the internal and external anal sphincters. The internal anal sphincter (IAS, labeled as INT SPHINCTER) is visible as a hypoechoic circle, and the external anal sphincter (EAS, labeled as EXT SPHINCTER) is seen as a hyperechoic circle. Scarred areas have a homogeneous gray appearance. Both the IAS and EAS are intact. **B,** With the patient supine, a defect in the IAS from 3 to 9 o'clock and a defect at 12 o'clock in the EAS are shown. **C,** Again, with the vagina at the 12 o'clock position, there is an intact IAS and defect in the EAS. (From Stenchever MA, Benson JT, eds. *Atlas of Clinical Gynecology.* New York: McGraw-Hill; 2000.)

seconds (Fig. 22.8). Both resting and anal squeeze pressures are reduced in women with anorectal incontinence.

The utility of anal manometry is debated as most treatment decisions are based on symptoms rather than a manometric value. In addition, some studies have demonstrated that manometry poorly predicts response to surgical intervention and may not correlate well with incontinence scores after intervention.

### Electromyography

EMG is used for mapping the EAS defect and for determining the presence and degree of neuropathy, denervation, and reinnervation. EMG evaluates the bioelectrical action potentials generated by the depolarization of skeletal striated muscle. This evaluation consists of systematic examination of spontaneous activity, recruitment patterns, and the waveform of the motor unit action potentials (MUAPs).

Performance and interpretation of EMG of the EAS requires special training and experience. A needle electrode is inserted into the skeletal muscle of the EAS. First, spontaneous activity is heard and seen. Next, the woman voluntarily squeezes her pelvic floor and recruitment activity is recorded. Straining should decrease activity and coughing should increase recruitment. The final step in analysis is evaluation of the MUAP waveform. Following nerve damage, as seen with a vaginal delivery, reinnervation of the muscle fibers leads to a single motor unit innervating multiple muscle fibers. On single-fiber EMG, the MUAPs have larger amplitudes, longer duration, and more phases or crossings of the baseline. Because discomfort and pain can occur with needle electrodes, endoanal ultrasound has replaced EMG for assessing the anatomy of the anal sphincter.

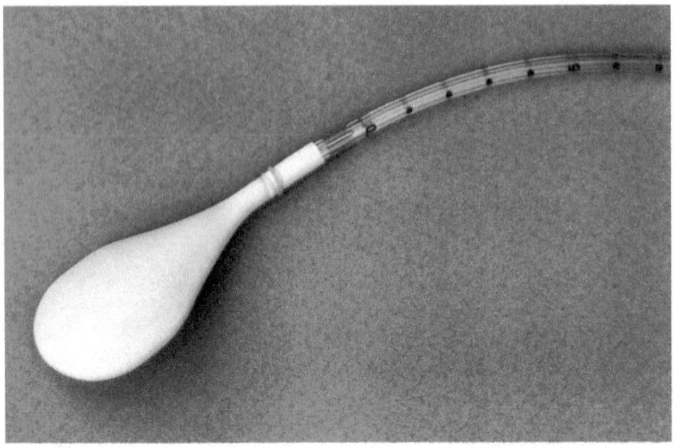

**Figure 22.7** Anal manometer, a four-channel perfusion catheter with balloon tip. There are many different types and methods for performing anal manometry. A balloon or probe is inserted into the rectum, and a pressure transducer relays information to a recorder or computer. Important manometric parameters include sphincter length, resting and squeeze pressures, rectal sensation, and presence of the anorectal inhibitory reflex (RAIR). The balloon is placed in the rectum and inflated by 10-cm$^3$ increments to determine rectal sensation and compliance. The presence of the RAIR is determined with balloon inflation and observing the IAS relax and the EAS contract to allow for the sampling of rectal contents. The four radical ports are perfused with sterile water, and resting and squeeze pressures around the anal canal are measured at 1-cm intervals along the anal canal. The catheter can be pulled at a constant rate to determine the length of the sphincter and high-pressure or continence zone.

### Pudendal Nerve Terminal Motor Latency

Nerve conduction studies measure the time from stimulation of a nerve to a response in the muscle it innervates. The PNTML is determined by using a glove-mounted electrode known as a *St. Mark's pudendal electrode,* connected to a pulsed stimulus generator; with the examiner's index finger in the vagina or anus, the pudendal nerve is stimulated at the ischial spine.

The latent period between the pudendal nerve stimulation and the electromechanical response of the muscle is measured. Normal PNTML is 2.0 ± 0.2 milliseconds. A normal PNTML is the measurement of the fastest response of the pudendal nerve and does not necessarily mean that the entire nerve is normal (Fig. 22.9). Prolonged PNTMLs have been found in patients with idiopathic fecal incontinence and in patients with rectal prolapse and may be predictive of continence following surgical repair. Gilliland's 1998 study suggested that PNTML was the most sensitive predictor of functional outcome of overlapping EAS repairs (Gilliland, 1998). However, these tests are rarely performed now because newer research shows poor correlation of prolonged pudendal terminal latencies with clinical symptoms, and PNTML does not seem to directly reflect nerve function in the way that quantitative EMG can.

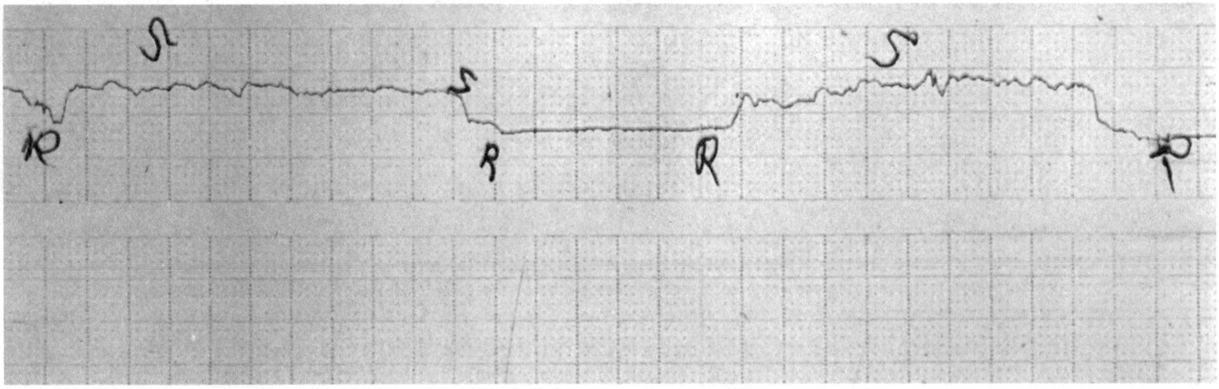


**Figure 22.8** A single-channel recording of the resting pressure of the anal canal *(R)* and the squeeze pressure *(S)*. The IAS contributes 80% of the resting pressure. Voluntary contraction or squeezing of the EAS should double the resting pressure.

### Defecography

Dynamic cystoproctography, or defecography, is an imaging technique that has been widely used in the evaluation of anorectal function and anatomy, dating back to the mid-1960s. Defecography may be used as an adjunct to physical examination in patients with chronic constipation and pelvic floor defects or hernias that may be contributing to their fecal incontinence. Rectal intussusceptions, rectal prolapse, and sigmoidocele can be seen on defecography, along with rectoceles that do not empty at the time of defecation. Stool retained in the rectocele can cause chronic distention of the rectum and loss of rectal sensation. The loss of rectal sensation leads to chronic constipation or impaction, causing further neuromuscular damage to the pelvic floor and ultimately fecal incontinence. Perineal descent and the anorectal angle can be objectively measured using defecography.

Fluoroscopic defecography usually involves the insertion of radio-opaque contrast transanally. The patient is then often placed into a seated position and asked to defecate, and real-time fluoroscopic images are obtained. Defecography is user dependent, and there may be significant interobserver differences in the interpretation of these images.

### Magnetic Resonance Imaging of the Anal Sphincters

MRI of the anal sphincters can evaluate muscular and connective tissue supports of the pelvis. Advances in MRI technologies using the endoanal coil, rapid sequencing, and cinematic display have replaced defecography for the evaluation of the pelvic floor and defecation disorders in some centers. Muscular defects, along with pelvic organ prolapse and perineal descent, can be assessed. Specialized dynamic MRI has the advantage of evaluating other pelvic anatomy, which may assist in the interpretation of the images. A common criticism of MRI defecography is that it is often performed in the supine position, which is not physiologic. Although open MRI technology addresses this issue, it is not readily available at most centers.

### Transit Study

A colonic transit study is used to evaluate colonic motility and is most often used for the evaluation of chronic constipation. For patients for whom fecal impaction or overflow incontinence is high on the differential, a transit study may be indicated. There are numerous variations of the study. The woman ingests a Sitzmark capsule containing 20 or 25 radiopaque rings. She does not take any laxatives or bowel stimulants. On days 1, 3, and 5 after taking the capsule, an abdominal flat radiographic plate is obtained. Normally, 80% of the capsules should have been passed. Diffuse or global colon dysfunction is indicated if the rings are dispersed throughout the colon or segmental abnormalities can be seen if the rings are clustered in one area or trapped in a rectocele.

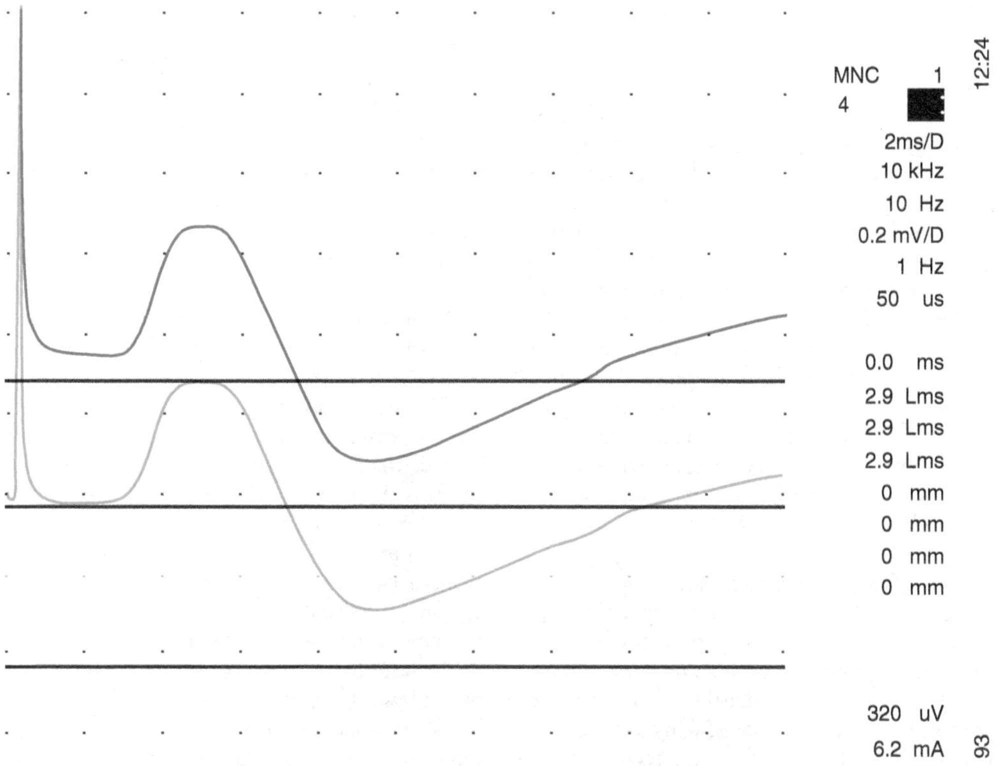


**Figure 22.9** Pudendal nerve terminal motor latencies (PNTML). Normal bilateral PNTML have been shown to be 2.0 ± 0.2 milliseconds. The latency response is measured from the onset of the stimulus to the onset of the response in the EAS. A normal PNTML is the measurement of the fastest response of the pudendal nerve and does not necessarily mean that the entire nerve is normal, and neither does an abnormal latency indicate abnormal muscle function. A damaged nerve can heal and reinnervate the muscle and, although the PNTML may be slightly prolonged, the muscle functions normally. (From Stenchever MA, Benson JT, eds. *Atlas of Clinical Gynecology*. New York: McGraw-Hill; 2000.)

Table 22.4 Treatment of Fecal Incontinence

| Management | Option |
|---|---|
| Education and lifestyle interventions | Regular bowel evacuation, optimization of stool consistency, unclear role for caffeine restriction, weight reduction, smoking cessation, gastrointestinal medication review and change, treatment of reversible causes of diarrhea |
| Diet | Dietary manipulation with soluble fiber for avoiding loose stools and for mild FI |
| Anal sphincter exercises or biofeedback training | Weak evidence suggesting efficacy for exercises, but safe, noninvasive treatment; biofeedback has insufficient evidence to recommend because of inadequate trials, but is noninvasive |
| Electrical stimulation | Insufficient evidence to recommend but small trials show some benefit |
| Medications | Loperamide, diphenoxylate plus atropine (concern of central nervous system side effects) for diarrhea; enemas, laxatives, suppositories for complete bowel emptying |
| Sacral nerve stimulation | Approved by the U.S. Food and Drug Administration in 2011, and multiple studies show benefit up to 5 years |
| Surgery | Anal sphincteroplasty indicated for postobstetric laceration or highly symptomatic women who have failed conservative measures with defined sphincter defect |

## TREATMENT

Treatment of fecal incontinence includes lifestyle changes, dietary management, biofeedback, electrical stimulation, medications, devices, sacral nerve stimulation, and surgery (Table 22.4). Obstructive devices, including transanal plugs, have been marketed but are not widely used. A vaginal pessary-like bowel control device that inflates posteriorly to obstruct the bowel is recently approved and shows some promise. Obviously, fecal incontinence should be treated based on the diagnosis as in medications or surgery for inflammatory bowel disease or surgery for a neoplasm of the cauda equina. Treatment of any underlying conditions that may be causing fecal incontinence is the first step in management. For all women with fecal incontinence, maintaining normal stool consistency and frequency is essential first-line treatment. For women with associated liquid or watery stools, dietary modifications and medications are first-line therapy.

### *Education, Diet, and Lifestyle Interventions*

Education regarding good bowel function makes sense, but little research exists to support this strategy. Having a predictable, regular bowel evacuation program and optimizing stool consistency to avoid the loose stool or frank diarrhea that taxes the system seems to improve fecal incontinence. Having a larger and formed stool, rather than liquid stool, allows for rectal distention and sensation that may provide earlier warning and better emptying.

Increasing dietary fiber with diet changes, bulking agents, or fiber supplements such as methylcellulose or psyllium helps increase stool size. Eating high-fiber cereals and drinking hot coffee or tea at breakfast are encouraged to stimulate the gastrocolic reflex and elimination before leaving home. There is reasonable evidence that adding soluble dietary fiber compared with placebo in women with loose stools reduces the rate of FI. However, women must be warned that fiber supplements can worsen diarrhea and cause bloating in some people. Increases in fiber also had benefit for women with mild FI, without loose stools. By keeping a food diary, women may identify offending foods (e.g., lactose, fructose) that aggravate their FI and learn to avoid those foods. Nicotine can hasten rectosigmoid transit time and stimulate distal colonic motility, so it may exacerbate fecal urgency. In a nursing home study, a daily exercise program with education around toileting opportunities improved FI. Brisk exercise, particularly after meals, may precipitate FI because of increased colonic activity.

### *Biofeedback*

For fecal incontinence, like urinary incontinence, biofeedback requires a motivated woman, feedback device, and planned exercise program. Although the woman may not perceive normal sensation or be able to contract her pelvic floor voluntarily, she must be neurologically intact to benefit from biofeedback. No correlation has been seen with premanometry testing as long as some neuromuscular function is present.

One trial has reported 60% to 70% of patients with fecal incontinence secondary to an abnormal pelvic floor will have a 90% reduction in incontinence with biofeedback. Further studies have shown varying success rates of 38% to 100%. A National Institutes of Health (NIH) consensus statement has concluded that biofeedback is effective in the first year postpartum for reversing some pregnancy-related fecal incontinence. The largest prospective study, by Norton and others, compared standard care with biofeedback (Norton, 2003). The improvement was 54% in the biofeedback group and 53% in the standard care group. Although this questions the effectiveness of biofeedback, it is important to consider that the standard group received nine 40- to 60-minute sessions with a nurse specialist on diet, fluid management, bowel evacuation techniques, bowel training, and use of antidiarrheal medications. Also, biofeedback helped over 50% of patients with this difficult problem. The other lesson from this trial is that more than 50% of patients improved with conservative measures.

Biofeedback of any type is based on the woman hearing, seeing, or sensing a response from a planned exercise. A measuring device, electrode or pressure transducer, is used transvaginally or transanally to record and provide feedback to the woman on how she is squeezing the pelvic floor. She then uses this feedback to increase or lengthen the pelvic floor contraction. If the woman has incontinence secondary to a sensory deficit in the rectum, rectal balloons can be used to "retrain" the woman to perceive rectal distention while squeezing her external sphincter in response to rectal distention. The woman can be taught by a physical therapist, who not only provides encouragement but also instructs on proper technique. Although initially labor-intensive, biofeedback has no side effects or morbidity and can be used in conjunction with other treatment modalities, including surgery. The American College of Gastroenterology recommends biofeedback therapy despite imperfect evidence to support its use. In addition, for patients with urinary and fecal incontinence, a single therapy may improve both conditions.

Biofeedback is often used in conjunction with pelvic floor physical therapy and in a single-center randomized control trial the addition of biofeedback to a regimen of pelvic floor exercises resulted in 44% of patients reporting complete continence at 3 months compared with 21% in patients undergoing pelvic floor exercises alone ($P = .008$).

### *Electrical Stimulation Therapy*

Functional electrical stimulation therapy has been shown to improve fecal incontinence in patients with a weakened pelvic floor who are unable to contract their EAS or puborectalis on command. Because of the expense, electrical stimulation is generally reserved for patients who are unable to respond to traditional biofeedback protocols. Both transvaginal and transrectal probes are available. Most protocols recommend high-frequency stimulation at a maximum tolerable stimulation of 50 Hz for 15 to 20 minutes twice daily. Response to therapy is usually seen in 6 weeks, with maximum improvement by 12 weeks, but reported benefits are slight. New stimulation protocols with both biofeedback and electrical stimulation in a 2010 randomized trial of 158 patients were promising at 3 months, with a 50% continence rate.

#### Devices

A vaginal bowel-control system that looks like a pessary with an inflatable posterior balloon has been tested. One multicenter study found 61 of 110 women (56%) were successfully fit with the device. The success rate at 3 months was 86%, which meant the women considered their bowel symptoms to be "much better" or "very much better" with improvement in quality of life (Richter, 2015). Pelvic cramping or discomfort occurred in 23%. This is a promising nonsurgical option and is just becoming clinically available.

#### Percutaneous Tibial Nerve Stimulation

Tibial nerve stimulation is thought to lead to changes in anorectal neuromuscular function because of shared sacral segmental innervation. Some initial trials were promising. Unfortunately, the most recent randomized controlled trial of 227 patients given percutaneous tibial nerve stimulation (PTNS) like that used for urinary urge incontinence showed no significant benefit over sham stimulation (Knowles, 2015). In the PTNS group, 38% had a greater than 50% reduction in episodes of fecal incontinence per week compared with 31% in the sham stimulation group. Although this was not statistically significant, it may have been a clinically relevant improvement to individual patients. The study was not large enough to look at subgroups, but patients with marked fecal urgency and inability to delay defecation would be a further group to study.

### *Medications*

No specific medication is approved for fecal incontinence except for antidiarrheal medications. A Cochrane review concluded that there is little evidence to guide clinicians in the selection of pharmacologic agents to treat fecal incontinence. To slow intestinal transit and allow for increased water absorption, several medications (Table 22.5) are available. Loperamide is an antidiarrheal agent that slows small and large bowel peristalsis, thereby increasing transit time through the gastrointestinal tract. Loperamide appears more effective than diphenoxylate for fecal urgency–related incontinence and also increases IAS tone and decreases sensitivity of the RAIR. In addition, loperamide is almost completely metabolized in the liver, resulting in minimal levels entering the systemic circulation. Also, unlike diphenoxylate, it does not cross the blood-brain barrier and therefore has fewer central nervous system (CNS) side effects. Amitriptyline, a tricyclic antidepressant, has also been shown in a small study of 42 patients to significantly improve symptoms of fecal incontinence, likely by increasing colonic transit time. In addition, in some patients who fail to respond to loperamide, cholestyramine has proved to be effective. Hyoscyamine is recommended for women with fecal incontinence after meals. Taking this before meals is recommended. For some patients, a daily cleansing of the rectum with an enema allows for several hours of freedom from their incontinence.

**Table 22.5** Medications for Treatment of Diarrhea

| Drug | Dosage* | Mechanism of Action |
|---|---|---|
| Loperamide | 2 mg tid or 4 mg followed by 2 mg after loose bowel movement<br>Maximum, 8 mg/day | Inhibits circular and longitudinal muscle contraction |
| Diphenoxylate with atropine | 5 mg qid initial dose | Direct action of circular smooth muscle to decrease peristalsis |
| Hyoscyamine sulfate | 0.375 mg bid timecaps | Anticholinergic |
| Cholestyramine | 4-mg pack qid or bid | Binds bile acids after cholecystectomy |

**bid*, Twice a day; *tid*, three times per day; *qid*, four times per day.

### *Surgery*

Surgical management of fecal incontinence includes sacral neuromodulation, repair of rectal prolapse, anal sphincteroplasty, radiofrequency treatment of the anal canal, injectable perianal bulking materials, anal sphincter neomuscular flaps, and implantation of artificial sphincters. Unfortunately, postanal repair or posterior levatorplasty has not been shown to be effective for the treatment of fecal incontinence in most patients and will not be discussed here. Patients with anatomic defects that may be causing or contributing to their fecal incontinence including full thickness or hemorrhoidal prolapse, fistula in ano, and rectovaginal fistula should have these repaired first as this often improves or resolves the incontinence.

#### Injectables

Perianal injection of bulking agents for fecal incontinence has been done with several materials, including silicone, collagen, and carbon-coated microbeads. The goal is for the bulking agent to augment the IAS closing the anal canal or raising pressure inside the anal canal. A double-blinded trial randomized patients who had failed conservative measures to either nonanimal stabilized hyaluronic acid (NASHA Dx) (n = 136) or sham treatment (n = 70) (Graf, 2011). Patients with persistent complaints of fecal incontinence at 1 month were offered retreatment. At 6 months, 71 patients (52%) in the treatment group compared with 22 patients (31%) in the sham group reported ≥50% improvement from baseline in the number of fecal incontinent episodes ($P = .0089$). However, whereas patients in the treatment group had a higher number of incontinence-free days, incontinence scores were not significantly different between the two groups. Danielson evaluated quality of life 2 years after injection of bulking agents for the treatment of fecal incontinence and found that patients who received two injections were more likely to achieve 50% improvement compared with those receiving one injection (Danielson, 2013). However, only patients who achieved at least a 75% improvement in symptoms reported a benefit in terms of quality of life (Danielson, 2013). A Cochrane review from 2013 concluded that although several studies demonstrated short-term benefits, the overall quality of the data is poor and long-term follow-up is still needed (Maeda, 2013). Injection of bulking agents is contraindicated in patients with full-thickness rectal prolapse, rectocele, anorectal malformations, active inflammatory bowel disease, and a history of anorectal radiation.

#### SECCA Procedure

The SECCA procedure, or radiofrequency anal sphincter remodeling, involves delivering temperature-controlled radiofrequency waves to the anal canal resulting in denatured collagen and changes to tissue compliance potentially narrowing the anal canal. A review of the literature reveals that most studies are small, single institution series with short follow-up. Data from randomized control trials are lacking, but one small trial with a 12-month follow-up showed modest improvement (Frascio, 2014). Complications, including pain, bleeding, and ulceration, are rare. The procedure is contraindication in patients previously treated with injection of a bulking agent.

#### Anterior Sphincteroplasty

Sphincteroplasty is a common surgical treatment for persistent anal incontinence after obstetric anal sphincter lacerations, but long-term results remain disappointing. The literature is conflicting regarding overlapping versus end-to-end sphincteroplasty techniques. Anterior overlapping sphincteroplasty is performed through a curvilinear incision in the perineum over the outer edge of the EAS defect. The entire sphincter complex is dissected widely to the anorectal ring. The incision should not extend beyond 180 degrees of the circumference to avoid injury to the pudendal nerves posterior laterally. Since it is important to dissect out to healthy sphincter muscle, this technique should not be used for sphincter injuries that extend greater than 180 degrees of the circumference. The scar is divided anteriorly and overlapped to create a narrowed anal opening being careful to avoid stenosis. Using 2-0 or 3-0 prolonged absorbable sutures, mattress sutures are placed through the sphincters (Fig. 22.10). The perineal body is reapproximated and the anoderm closed loosely with interrupted 3-0 chromic sutures, allowing space for drainage. Alternatively a drain may be placed in the perineal closure. It is important to avoid separating the internal and external sphincters or excising the scar. The advantage of the overlapping sphincteroplasty over the traditional end-to-end repair is decreased tension to prevent separation of the suture line once anesthesia no longer prevents sphincter contraction.

Overlapping anterior anal sphincteroplasty provides symptomatic control of incontinence in 60% to 80% of patients with anatomic EAS defects in the short term. Repair of an anal sphincter laceration includes not only repair of the EAS but also identification and repair of any IAS defects. Because the IAS maintains the resting tone of the anus, it is important to restore sphincter integrity, especially for control of flatus. Unfortunately, symptomatic relief is often not durable, and overlapping sphincteroplasty cure rates 5 to 10 years after surgery may be as low as 1% to 28% (Table 22.6). This has called into question the use of overlapping sphincteroplasty as the primary surgical treatment for fecal incontinence particularly in women who develop symptoms years after their initial sphincter injury.

A number of studies have attempted to identify factors associated with sphincteroplasty outcomes, but no single variable has proved predictive. Unilateral or bilateral pudendal nerve injury has been associated with worse outcomes in some reports, and therefore patients who have an anal sphincter defect and prolonged PNTML should be counseled that their chance of continence following surgery may be decreased (Gilliland, 1998).

When anal sphincter injury occurs during vaginal delivery, the type of repair needed has been debated. To date, according to only a few studies, there is no significant difference between end-to-end and overlapping anal sphincteroplasties. The outcome of anal sphincteroplasties after delivery is unacceptably poor, with 47% to 67% of women complaining of defecatory symptoms such as flatus incontinence, fecal urgency, and fecal incontinence. Although frank fecal incontinence is reported at a much lower rate, 2% to 9%, the other defecatory symptoms are nonetheless bothersome to women. Furthermore, endoanal ultrasound examinations after sphincteroplasty show persistent anatomic defects in 40% to 85% of repairs.

Because the outcome after anal sphincteroplasty is suboptimal, prevention emerges as an even more important consideration. Vaginal childbirth injury to the anal sphincter is such a common cause of fecal incontinence that prevention should start here. Midline episiotomy has been shown repeatedly in various studies to be strongly associated with anal sphincter damage. Avoidance of routine episiotomy and consideration of a mediolateral episiotomy when absolutely necessary could be beneficial in prevention efforts.

### *Sacral Nerve Stimulation*

In 2011, a sacral nerve stimulation device was FDA approved for treating chronic fecal incontinence. In one randomized controlled trial, 54 of 120 patients with severe fecal incontinence improved with the test stimulation and had the permanent generator placed, and 22 (47%) were continent. Observational studies have reported similar improvements. A 2010 study reported on long-term outcomes in a cohort analysis of consecutive patients. Treatment success was defined as a more than 50% reduction in episodes of fecal incontinence compared with baseline. Temporary sacral nerve stimulation was performed in 118 patients and 91 (77%) were considered suitable for permanent implantation. The median follow-up period was 22 months (range, 1 to 138 months); 70 patients were followed for 1 year, with success in 63 (90%). Of 18 patients followed for 5 years, 15 (83%) reported continued success—11 (61%) maintained full efficacy, 4 (22%) reported some loss, and 3 (17%) reported complete loss. Three patients with a 10-year follow up had no loss in efficacy. A systematic review reported that 79% of patients experienced at least 50% improvement in weekly fecal incontinence episodes in the short term and 84% in the long term (>36 months) based on a pooled analysis of all current studies in the literature (Thin, 2013). When these pooled data were analyzed on an intention-to-treat basis, 63% of patients achieved improvement of at least 50% in the short term and 35% reported 100% continence in

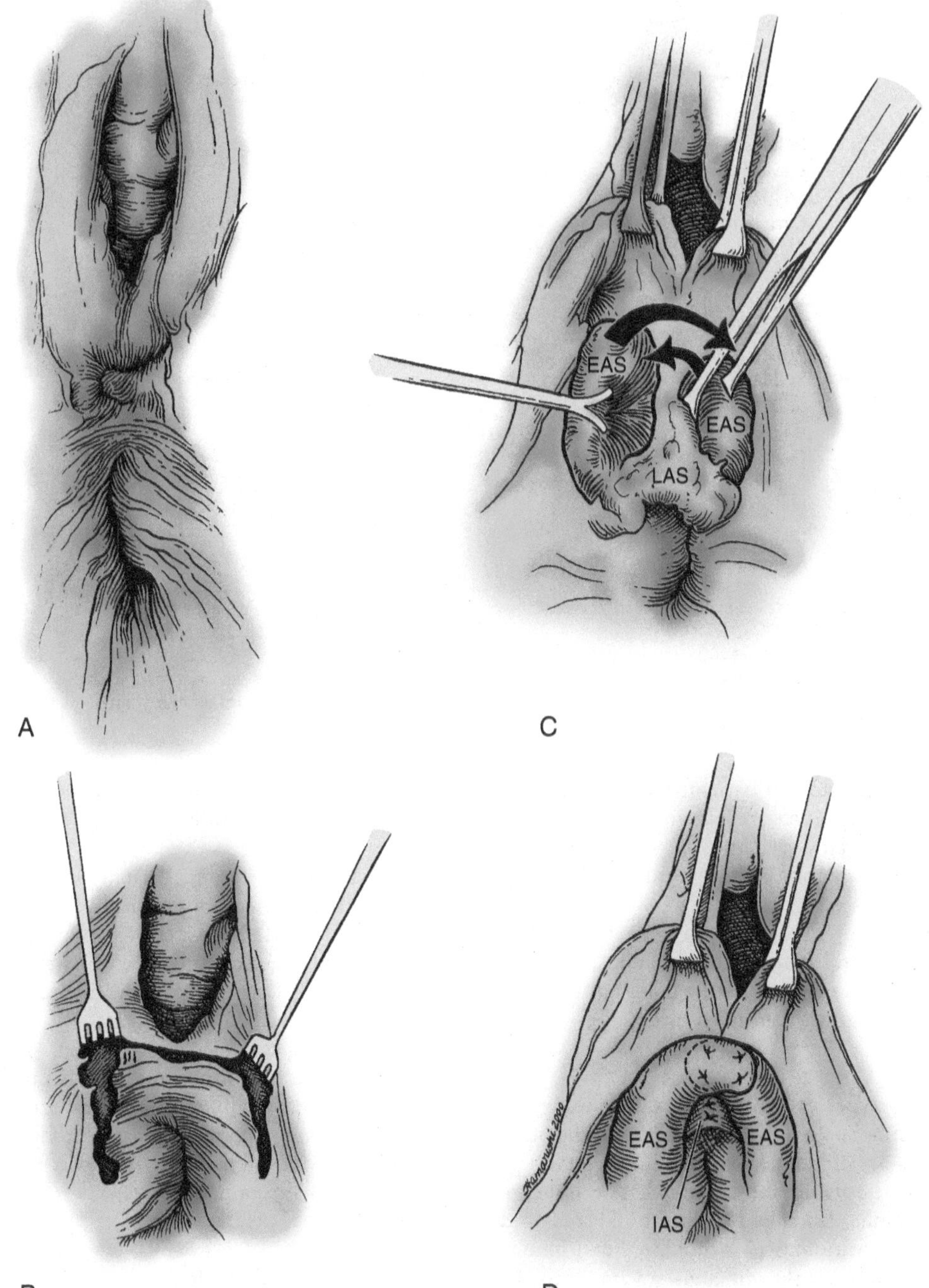


**Figure 22.10** Sphincter drawing. **A,** Dovetail sign with loss of anal skin creases anteriorly. **B,** Transperineal incision. **C,** EAS identified. **D,** Overlapping sphincteroplasty and IAS repaired.

the long term. A large, prospective, multi-institutional, nonrandomized study found that 89% of patients achieved greater than 50% improvement in fecal incontinence episodes and at 5 years 36% of patients had complete continence (Hull, 2013). The infection rate was reported at 10.8% and at 5 years 24.4% of patients had undergone at least one revision or replacement.

Sacral neuromodulation was initially viewed as a treatment for patients who had failed an anterior sphincteroplasty or did not have a sphincter defect, but it is increasing being seen as an alternative to other surgical options and according to the latest practice parameters of the American Society of Colon and Rectal Surgeons it may be considered a first-line surgical treatment of fecal incontinence (Paquette, 2015). A study that included 91 patients with no sphincter defect and 54 patients with a complete external sphincter defect confirmed with ultrasound showed that the presence of a sphincter defect did not affect the outcome of sacral neuromodulation (Johnson, 2015). Significant improvements in fecal incontinence scores have been seen in patients with up to a 120-degree sphincter defect (Tjandra, 2008). In fact, symptomatic relief may be

Table 22.6 Outcomes after Sphincteroplasty

| Study, Year* | Institution | No. of Patients | Follow-up Period (mean [range]; mo) | Outcome | |
|---|---|---|---|---|---|
| | | | | Success (%) | Improved (%) |
| Fang et al, 1984 | Minnesota | 76 | 35 (2-62) | 82 | 89 |
| Browning and Motson, 1988 | St. Marks | 83 | 39.2 (4-116) | 78 | 91 |
| Ctercteko et al, 1988 | Cleveland Clinic, Ohio | 44 | 50 | 75 | |
| Laurberg et al, 1988 | St. Marks | 19 | 18 (median, 9-36) | 47 | 79 |
| Yoshioka and Keighley, 1989 | Birmingham | 27 | 48 (median, 16-108) | | 74.1 |
| Wexner et al, 1991 | Cleveland Clinic, Florida | 16 | 10 (3-16) | 76 | 87.5 |
| Fleshman et al, 1991 | Washington University | 55 | 0 (12-24) | 72 | 87 |
| Simmang et al, 1994 | Washington University | 14 | 0 (6-12) | 71 | 93 |
| Engel et al, 1994 | St. Marks | 55 | 15 (6-36) | 60.4 | |
| Engel et al, 1994 | Amsterdam | 28 | 46 (median, 15-116) | 75 | |
| Londono-Schimmer et al, 1994 | St. Marks | 94 | 58.5 (median, 12-98) | 50 | 75 |
| Sitzler and Thompson, 1996 | St. Marks | 31 | 0 (1-36) | 74 | |
| Felt-Bersma et al, 1996 | Vrije University | 18 | 14 (3-39) | | 72 |
| Oliveira et al, 1996 | Cleveland Clinic, Florida | 55 | 29 (3-61) | 70.1 | 80 |
| Nikiteas et al, 1996 | Birmingham | 42 | 38 (median, 12-66) | 60 | |
| Gilliland et al, 1998 | Cleveland Clinic, Florida | 100 | 24 (median, 2-96) | 55 | 69 |
| Malouf et al, 2000† | St. Marks | 474 | 77 (60-96) | | 50 |
| Grey et al, 2007‡ | Manchester | 47 | >60 | | 60 |

From Gilliand R, Altomare DF, Moreira H, et al. Pudendal neuropathy is predictive of failure following anterior overlapping sphincteroplasty. *Dis Colon Rectum*. 1998;41:1516-1522.

*All references from the original source (Gilliand et al, 1998), except the last two.

†Malouf AJ, Norton CS, Engel AF, et al. Long-term results of overlapping anterior anal-sphincter repair for obstetric trauma. *Lancet*. 2000;355:260-265.

‡Grey BR, Sheldon RR, Telford KJ, Kiff ES. Anterior anal sphincter repair can be of long-term benefit: a 12-year case cohort from a single surgeon. *BMC Surg*. 2007;7:1.

achieved with neuromodulation in patients with a history of sphincter defect, previous sphincter repair, and pudendal neuropathy (Brouwer, 2010). However, there have been no randomized control trials comparing sacral neuromodulation to overlapping sphincteroplasty.

Sacral neuromodulation is a less invasive treatment than other surgical alternatives and has few complications, so it is a promising option that is gaining popularity. Long-term follow-up is required, though, to ensure continued success.

### Neosphincters

There are basically two types of neosphincters, one using the woman's own skeletal muscle, usually the gracilis, and the other using an artificial Silastic cuff connected to a fluid reservoir to occlude the anal canal. The gracilis muscle wrap has been shown to have inconsistent results. Initially described by Pickrell and colleagues in 1952, the entire muscle is mobilized and its distal portion wrapped snugly around the anus, anchored to the contralateral ischial tuberosity (Pickrell, 1952). The addition of chronic, low-frequency electrical stimulation of the nerve or muscle has been used to convert fatigue-prone type II to fatigue-resistant type I muscle fibers. Once converted, the muscle may be continuously stimulated, resulting in prolonged closure of the anal canal. A report by Baeten and colleagues for the Dynamic Graciloplasty Therapy Study Group reported on 123 adults treated at 20 institutions with dynamic graciloplasty and found that 63% of patients reported a 50% or greater improvement in incontinent events 1 year after surgery (Baeten, 2000). Another 11% noted some improvement, and 26% reported no improvement or worsened incontinence. There was one surgery-related death; 74% of patients experienced an adverse event related to the treatment, with 40% of patients requiring additional surgery. Despite these frequent complications, most patients showed a significant improvement in quality of life postsurgery.

Artificial sphincters are indicated for patients with anal incontinence caused by neuromuscular disease, congenital malformations, sphincter defects greater than 180 degrees, or patients who have failed all other treatments. A Silastic cuff is connected to a fluid reservoir that encircles the anal canal to cause closure. The cuff is deflated before defecation. Although most studies are small and retrospective, there have been a few prospective studies that have shown improvement in symptoms if the device is retained without complication (Ruiz Carmona, 2009; Wong, 2011). However, complications including infection, anorectal ulceration, device migration, pain, device erosion, and mechanical breakdown are common.

### Stoma Creation

A stoma may be offered if all other acceptable treatments have failed or the patient does not want to pursue other surgical options. Although this sounds extreme, it can greatly improve the quality of life for women with severe fecal incontinence.

## RECTOVAGINAL FISTULAS

Although not a true source of fecal incontinence by definition, rectovaginal fistulas (RVFs) are common enough complications of vaginal birth and gynecologic surgeries to be addressed under this heading. An RVF is an abnormal connection between the vagina and rectum. Whenever a woman presents with complaints of fecal or flatal incontinence, an RVF should be included in the differential diagnosis.

Table 22.7 Origin of Rectovaginal Fistula

| Category | Condition | Mechanism |
|---|---|---|
| Traumatic | | |
| Obstetric | Prolonged second stage of labor | Pressure necrosis of rectovaginal septum |
| | Midline episiotomy | Extension directed into rectum |
| | Perineal lacerations | |
| Foreign body | Vaginal pessaries | Pressure necrosis |
| | Violent coitus | Mechanical perforation |
| | Sexual abuse | Mechanical perforation |
| Iatrogenic | Hysterectomy | Injury to anterior rectal wall |
| | Stapled colorectal anastomosis | Staple line includes vagina |
| | Transanal excision of anterior rectal tumor | Deep margin of resection into vagina |
| | Enemas | Mechanical perforation |
| | Anorectal (e.g., incision and drainage of intramural abscesses) | Mechanical perforation |
| Inflammatory | Crohn disease | Transmural inflammation-perforation |
| | Pelvic radiation | Early tumor necrosis |
| | Pelvic abscess | Late transmural inflammation |
| | Perirectal abscess | Late transmural inflammation |
| Neoplastic | Rectal | Local tumor growth into neighboring structure |
| | Cervical | |
| | Uterine | |
| | Vaginal | |
| | Primary or recurrent tumors | |

From Stenchever MA, Benson JT, eds. *Atlas of Clinical Gynecology*. New York: McGraw-Hill; 2000.

The causes of RVF, as seen in Table 22.7, include traumatic, inflammatory, and neoplastic origins, but obstetric injuries are the most common cause. It is estimated that 0.1% of vaginal births will result in an RVF.

A fistula occurring caudad or adjacent to the EAS is termed an *anovaginal fistula* and is managed differently from an RVF. Fistulas that occur more than 3 cm above the anal verge are true RVFs. Most RVFs secondary to obstetric injury occur in the lower third of the vagina and may be associated with a sphincter defect in the EAS. It is important to evaluate the EAS (discussed earlier) with transanal ultrasound or EMG to map any defects prior to surgical treatment.

Fistulas secondary to surgical trauma, malignancy, or an inflammatory process may occur at any point along the vaginal wall, including the apex. If a fistula develops after a difficult surgery, such as after pelvic inflammatory disease, or radiotherapy, it is important to check for more than one fistula prior to repair. If the woman has a history of malignancy, examination with biopsy specimens should be performed to rule out cancer as the cause of the fistula.

Depending on the size and location of the fistula, the woman may be almost asymptomatic or complain of a small amount of flatus passing into her vagina with a low small fistula. With a large fistula, she may have formed stool coming through the vagina with every bowel movement, causing significant distress and hygiene problems. Rectal bleeding is more likely to be reported with a neoplastic process or post–pelvic radiation.

Evaluation of a woman includes a history and physical examination to determine cause. If there is suspicion of inflammatory bowel disease, a colonoscopy is warranted. Perineal skin and rectal examinations are important to visualize the fistula tract and determine the integrity of the anal sphincters and quality of the tissues surrounding the fistula, and to palpate for abscesses and other masses. Most obstetric-related RVFs show the fistula along the scar line. Methylene blue mixed in lubricant and placed in the rectum can help identify the fistula. If still not identified, a dilute methylene blue enema with a tampon in the vagina may help in isolating the fistula. If the vaginal orifice is found, but not the rectal opening, insertion of an angiocatheter with a squirting of hydrogen peroxide can show bubbling on the rectal side. A small lacrimal duct probe may allow passage through the vaginal tract to identify the rectal exit site.

An office anoscopy or proctoscopy may also help evaluate the surrounding tissues. In general, a mature epithelialized fistula that is not infected is not painful on digital examination. If the examination in the office is not successful in locating the fistula or is too painful for the woman, she should be taken to the operating room for examination under anesthesia. If the fistula has still not been identified, filling the vagina with water and insufflating the rectum should produce bubbling in the vagina that can be traced to the opening. A barium enema may also be helpful for identifying high fistulas. Vaginography using dilute barium solution may also help to identify a fistula.

Surgical management of an anovaginal or anoperineal fistula is accomplished by opening the fistula tract, curetting the tract, and leaving the tract open to heal secondarily. Excision of the tract and primary closure will result in recurrent fistula formation in most cases.

Many surgical procedures have been described for the treatment of RVF. Regardless of the procedure chosen, basic surgical principles must be followed. The tissue must be healthy, well vascularized, and free of infection and induration. This may require waiting for up to 3 months following the original trauma or surgery for complete healing. If there is significant fecal contamination, prior radiation, or persistent abscess, a diverting colostomy should be considered. After a colostomy, a delay of 8 to 12 weeks is generally required for the inflammation and cellulites around the fistula to heal. At the time of repair, a Martius fat pad graft can be used to increase the vascular supply to the area. Preoperatively, the woman should have a complete mechanical bowel preparation starting several days before the surgery to prevent liquid stool from contaminating the field. Some surgeons may place the woman on a liquid diet several days before surgery with no mechanical bowel preparation except enemas until clear the night before surgery. The goal is to have no liquid stool in the rectum and to have the woman's first postoperative bowel movement, several days after surgery, be soft but formed. Antibiotic bowel prophylaxis is warranted.

Other surgical principles include excision of the entire fistulous tract, wide mobilization of the rectal tissue, and broad tissue-to-tissue closure without tension. The rectal side is the high-pressure side and requires attention to repair. The vaginal side may be closed or left open to drain, if indicated, and should close spontaneously. A delayed absorbable suture, such as 3-0 Polysorb (glycolide-lactide copolymer), is used on all layers. Alternatively, a monofilament delayed absorbable suture such as Maxon (monofilament polyglyconate) or PDS (polydioxanone) may lower the risk of infection over a braided suture. Permanent sutures are not used.

Transvaginal and transrectal repairs have been described, but gynecologists generally prefer the transvaginal approach. Depending on the location and need to repair the anal sphincters, an uncomplicated fistula can be repaired as for a fourth-degree laceration as a perineoproctotomy with layered closure. After cutting from the perineal body, through the sphincters and to the fistulous tract, care must be taken to excise the tract and any surrounding scar tissue. A two-layered closure of the rectum and anal canal is then performed, as in a fourth-degree closure. Care should be given to closing the EAS.

To preserve an intact sphincter, the RVF can be cored out by placing a pediatric Foley transvaginally, filling the balloon on the rectal side, and then using the Foley for traction by pulling upward. After excision, depending on the size, a small fistula can be closed with two-layer purse-string sutures or with an interrupted two-layer closure.

Transrectal repairs, preferred by many colorectal surgeons, generally involve the development of rectal mucosal flaps, mobilized and brought down or lateral to cover the excised fistula site. In 23 patients treated at the Cleveland Clinic with rectal advancement flaps, fistulas were successfully cured in 77% of patients with obstetric or surgical injury and 60% of patients with Crohn disease.

Postoperatively, the woman's diet and medications should be managed to keep her bowel movements soft, but formed. In most cases, a clear liquid diet is continued for the first 3 days after surgery, followed by a low-residue diet. Broad-spectrum antibiotics should be continued for 2 weeks. Sitz baths, two or three times daily, followed by the use of a blow dryer or heat lamp, keep the area clean and dry.

## KEY POINTS

- Estimates of fecal incontinence range from 11% to 15% of community-dwelling women older than 64 years.
- Over 30% of women reporting urinary incontinence also report fecal incontinence, known as *dual incontinence.*
- The IAS, under autonomic control, maintains the high-pressure zone or continence zone and, along with the EAS, keeps the anal canal closed.
- The EAS provides the voluntary squeeze pressure that prevents incontinence with increasing rectal or abdominal pressure. The EAS is innervated by the hemorrhoidal branch of the pudendal nerve from the S2-S4 nerve roots.
- A common cause of fecal incontinence is damage to the anal sphincter at the time of vaginal delivery, with or without neuronal injury. Prevention of these injuries is critical.
- The incidence of occult external anal sphincter disruption after vaginal delivery determined by endoanal ultrasound ranges from 11% to 35%. The chance of muscular injury is increased with midline episiotomy, instrumented delivery, and vaginal delivery of larger infants.
- Approximately 1 in 10 women will develop some fecal incontinence or fecal urgency after one vaginal delivery.
- At a tertiary colorectal referral clinic, a prospective study showed that further evaluation, including radiologic and physiologic tests, altered the final diagnosis or the cause of fecal incontinence in 19% of cases.
- Biofeedback for patients with fecal incontinence shows a similar reduction in incontinence episodes after intense education with a nurse specialist on the subjects of bowel care, medications, and dietary and fluid management. This highlights the importance of conservative management techniques.
- Overlapping anterior anal sphincteroplasty provides symptomatic control of incontinence in 60% to 80% of patients initially, but long-term outcomes are not nearly as successful.

## KEY REFERENCES

Baeten CG, Bailey HR, Bakka A, et al. Safety and efficacy of dynamic graciloplasty for fecal incontinence: report of a prospective, multicenter trial. Dynamic Graciloplasty Therapy Study Group. *Dis Colon Rectum.* 2000;43:743-751.

Bartolo DC, Roe AM, Locke-Edmunds JC, et al. Flap-valve theory of anorectal continence. *Br J Surg.* 1986;73:1012-1014.

Brouwer R, Duthie G. Sacral nerve neuomodulation is effective treatment for fecal incontinence in the presence of a sphincter defect, pudendal neuropathy, or previous sphincter repair. *Dis Colon Rectum.* 2010;53:273-278.

Danielson J, Karlbom U, Wester T, et al. Efficacy and quality of life 2 years after treatment for faecal incontinence with injectable bulking agents. *Tech Coloproctol.* 2013;17:389-395.

Frascio M, Mandolfino F, Imperatore M, et al. The SECCA procedure for faecal incontinence: a review. *Colorectal Dis.* 2014;16:167-172.

Gilliland R, Altomare DF, Moreira Jr H, et al. Pudendal neuropathy is predictive of failure following anterior overlapping sphincteroplasty. *Dis Colon Rectum.* 1998;41:1516-1522.

Graf W, Mellgren A, Matzel KE, et al. Efficacy of dextramomer in stabilised hyaluronic acid for treatment of faecal incontinence: a randomised, sham-controlled trial. *Lancet.* 2011;377:997-1003.

Hull T, Giese C, Wexner SD, et al. Long-term durability of sacral nerve stimulation therapy for chronic fecal incontinence. *Dis Colon Rectum.* 2013;56:234-245.

Johnson BL 3rd, Abodeely A, Ferguson MA, et al. Is sacral neuromodulation here to stay? Clinical outcomes of a new treatment for fecal incontinence. *J Gastrointest Surg.* 2015;19:15-19.

Jorge JM, Wexner SD. Etiology and management of fecal incontinence. *Dis Colon Rectum.* 1993;36:77-97.

Knowles CH, Horrocks E, et al. Percutaneous tibial nerve stimulation versus sham electrical stimulation for the treatment of faecal incontinence in adults (CONFIDeNT): a double-blind, multicenter, pragmatic, parallel-group, randomised controlled trial. *Lancet.* 2015;386(10004):1640-1648.

Maeda Y, Laurberg S, Norton C. Perianal injectable bulking agents as treatment for faecal incontinence in adults. *Cochrane Database Syst Rev.* 2013;2:CD007959.

Norton C, Chelvanayagam S, Wilson Barnett J, et al. Randomized controlled trial of biofeedback for faecal incontinence. *Gastrenterology*. 2003;125:1320-1329.
Paquette IM, Varma MG, Kaiser AM, et al. The American Society of Colon and Rectal Surgeons' Clinical Practice Guideline for the Treatment of Fecal Incontinence. *Dis Colon Rectum*. 2015;58:623-636.
Pickrell KL, Broadbent IR, Masters FW, et al. Constitution of a rectal sphincter and restoration of anal incontinence by transplanting the gracilis muscle; a report of four cases in children. *Ann Surg*. 1952;135:853-862.
Richter HE, Matthews CA, Muir T, et al. A vaginal bowel-control system for the treatment of fecal incontinence. *Obstet Gynecol*. 2015;125(3):540-547.
Ruiz Carmona MD, Alós Company R, Roig Vila JV, et al. Long-term results of artificial bowel sphincter for the treatment of severe faecal incontinence. Are they what we hoped for? *Colorectal Dis*. 2009;11:831-837.
Sultan AH, Kamm MA, Hudson CN, et al. Anal-sphincter disruption during vaginal delivery. *N Engl J Med*. 1993;329:1905-1911.
Thin NN, Horrocks EJ, Hotouras A, et al. Systematic review of the clinical effectiveness of neuromodulation in the treatment of faecal incontinence. *Br J Surg*. 2013;100:1430-1447.
Tjandra JJ, Chan MK, Yeh CH, et al. Sacral nerve stimulation is more effective than optimal medical therapy for severe fecal incontinence: a randomized, controlled study. *Dis Colon Rectum*. 2008;51:494-502.
Wong MT, Meurette G, Wyart V, et al. The artificial bowel sphincter: a single institution experience over a decade. *Ann Surg*. 2011;254:951-956.

Suggested Readings can be found on ExpertConsult.com.

# 23

# Genital Tract Infections

## Vulva, Vagina, Cervix, Toxic Shock Syndrome, Endometritis, and Salpingitis

*Carolyn Gardella, Linda O. Eckert, Gretchen M. Lentz*

For clarity of presentation, discussion of infectious diseases of the female genital tract is divided into those of the lower genital tract, the vulva, vagina, and cervix; and those of the upper genital tract, the endometrium and fallopian tubes. However, the female genital tract has anatomic and physiologic continuity, so infectious agents that colonize and involve one organ often infect adjacent organs. To understand the pathophysiology and natural history of infectious diseases of the genital tract, one must keep this continuity in mind.

The symptoms caused by infections of the lower genital tract produce the most common conditions seen by gynecologists. Therefore the initial focus of this chapter is on clinical presentation and the differential diagnosis of vulvitis, vaginitis, and cervicitis.

Toxic shock syndrome (TSS) and syphilis are also discussed in this chapter. Although the most devastating pathologic processes from these diseases occur in sites other than the genital tract, they often obtain entry into the body through the vulvar, rectal, vaginal, or cervical epithelium.

Many of the infections discussed in this chapter may be acquired through sexual contact and are termed *sexually transmitted infections* (STIs). STIs often coexist—for example, *Chlamydia trachomatis* and *Neisseria gonorrhoeae.* When one disease is suspected, appropriate diagnostic methods must be used to detect other infections.

The Centers for Disease Control and Prevention (CDC) regularly revises management protocols for STIs. Recommendations and medications in this edition are based on the 2015 CDC guidelines. Readers are urged to consult updates in the online CDC guidelines (http://www.cdc.gov) because bacterial sensitivities and epidemiologic concerns may lead to changes in treatment protocols.

## INFECTIONS OF THE VULVA

The skin of the vulva is composed of a stratified squamous epithelium containing hair follicles and sebaceous, sweat, and apocrine glands. The subcutaneous tissue of the vulva also contains specialized structures such as the Bartholin glands. Similar to skin elsewhere on the body, the vulvar area is subject to primary and secondary bacterial, viral, parasitic, or fungal infections and is sensitive to hormonal and allergic influences. Vulvar pruritus accounts for approximately 10% of outpatient gynecology visits. Vulvar itching or burning of acute onset and short duration suggests infection or contact dermatitis. Skin fissures and excoriation may be signs of infection, may be caused by the woman's scratching as a result of irritation from a vaginal discharge, or may be the manifestation of a primary dermatologic disease. Box 23.1 presents the differential diagnosis of vulvar pruritus and irritation (Prabhu, 2015).

**Box 23.1 Causes of Vulvar Pruritus and Irritation**

**Acute:**

**Contact Dermatitis**
Allergic
Irritant

**Infections**
Candidiasis
Scabies
Human papilloma virus
Molluscum contagiosum
Trichomoniasis

**Chronic:**

**Contact Dermatitis**
Allergic
Irritant

**Vulvar Dystrophies**
Lichen planus
Lichen sclerosis
Lichen simplex chronicus
Psoriasis

**Infections**
Candidiasis
Human papillomavirus

**Neoplasia**
Paget disease
Vulvar cancer

**Atrophy**

## INFECTIONS OF BARTHOLIN GLANDS

Bartholin glands are two rounded, pea-sized glands deep in the perineum that are not palpable unless enlarged. They drain via ducts approximately 2 cm long lined by transitional epithelium and located at the entrance of the vagina at 5 and 7 o'clock, in the groove between the hymen and the labia minora. Mucinous secretions from Bartholin glands provide moisture for the epithelium of the vestibule. Approximately 2% of adult women develop enlargements of one or both glands. The most common cause is cystic dilation of the Bartholin duct (Fig. 23.1), typically caused by distal obstruction secondary to non-specific inflammation or trauma. Following obstruction, there is continued secretion of glandular fluid, which results in the cystic dilation.

The differential diagnosis of vulvar cysts also includes mesonephric cysts of the vagina and epithelial inclusion cysts. Mesonephric cysts are generally more anterior and cephalad in the vagina, whereas epithelial inclusion cysts are more superficial. Rarely, a lipoma, fibroma, hernia, vulvar varicosity, or hydrocele may be confused with a Bartholin duct cyst.

Most women with Bartholin duct cysts are asymptomatic. The cysts may vary from 1 to 8 cm in diameter and are usually unilateral, tense, and nonpainful. Most cysts are unilocular. However, in chronic or recurrent cysts there occasionally are multiple compartments.

In contrast, an abscess of a Bartholin gland tends to develop rapidly over 2 to 4 days with significant symptoms, including difficulty in ambulation. Acute pain and tenderness can be severe and are secondary to rapid enlargement, hemorrhage, or secondary infection. The signs are those of a classic abscess: erythema, acute tenderness, edema and, occasionally, cellulitis of the surrounding subcutaneous tissue. Without therapy, most abscesses tend to rupture spontaneously by the third or fourth day. Unilateral or bilateral Bartholin gland infection in most cases is not caused by a sexually transmitted infection. Positive cultures from Bartholin gland abscesses are often polymicrobial and contain a wide range of bacteria similar to the normal flora of the vagina.

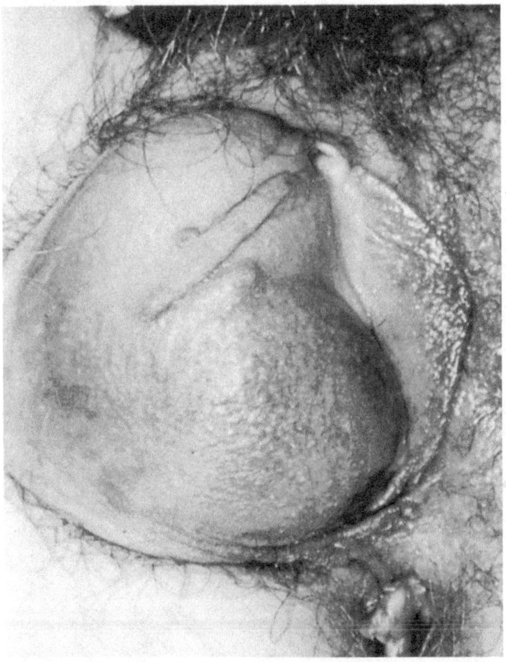

**Figure 23.1** Bartholin abscess. The mass is tender and fluctuant and is situated on the lower lateral aspect of labium minus at 5 o'clock. (From Kaufman RH. Cystic tumors. In: Kaufman RH, Faro S, eds. *Benign Diseases of the Vulva and Vagina.* 4th ed. St. Louis: Mosby-Year Book; 1994.)

The treatment of enlargement or infection of Bartholin glands depends on symptomatology. Asymptomatic cysts in women younger than 40 years do not need treatment. Simple incision and drainage of a Bartholin gland cyst or abscess is not recommended because recurrence after incision and drainage is frequent. Instead, the surgical treatment of choice is marsupialization to develop a fistulous tract from the dilated duct to the vestibule. An elliptical wedge of tissue is excised over the cyst just proximal to the hymenal ring. A cruciate incision is made into the cyst wall, and the edges of the duct or abscess are everted and sutured to the surrounding skin with interrupted absorbable sutures forming an epithelialized pouch that provides ongoing drainage for the gland. The recurrence rate following marsupialization is approximately 5% to 10%. An alternative surgical approach is to insert a Word catheter, a short catheter with an inflatable Foley balloon, through a stab incision into the abscess and leave it in place for 4 to 6 weeks (Fig. 23.2). During this period, a tract of epithelium will form. All the procedures mentioned may be performed with local anesthesia. Antibiotics are not necessary unless there is an associated cellulitis surrounding the Bartholin gland abscess.

Women older than 40 years with gland enlargement require a biopsy to exclude adenocarcinoma of the Bartholin gland. Excision of a Bartholin duct and gland is indicated for persistent deep infection, multiple recurrences of abscesses, or recurrent enlargement of the gland in women older than 40 years. Excision can be challenging because of the rich vascular supply to the region and may be accompanied by morbidity, including intraoperative hemorrhage, hematoma formation, fenestration of the labia, postoperative scarring, and associated dyspareunia. It is best to use regional block or general anesthesia for excision. Excision of a Bartholin gland for recurrent infection should be performed when the infection is quiescent (Heller, 2014; Kessous, 2013; Khanna, 2010; Li, 2011; Wechter, 2009).

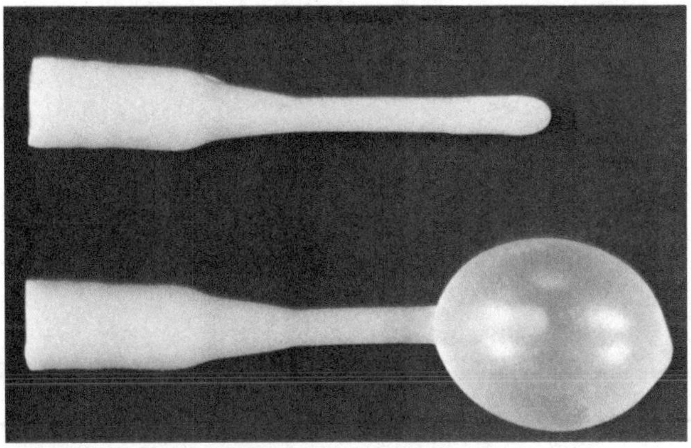

**Figure 23.2** Word catheters before and after inflation. They are used to develop a fistula from a Bartholin cyst or abscess to the vestibule. (From Friedrich EG. *Vulvar Disease.* 2nd ed. Philadelphia: WB Saunders; 1983.)

## *PEDICULOSIS PUBIS AND SCABIES*

The skin of the vulva is a frequent site of infestation by animal parasites, the two most common being the crab louse and the itch mite. Ideally, early diagnosis and treatment are of the utmost importance in controlling parasitic infection.

Pediculosis pubis is an infestation by the crab louse, *Phthirus pubis.* The crab louse is also called the *pubic louse* and is a different species from the body or head louse. Lice in the pubic hair are the most contagious of all STIs, with over 90% of sexual partners becoming infected following a single exposure. The louse is usually transmitted by close contact, although nonsexual transmission of pubic lice has been documented from towels or bedding. *P. pubis* is generally confined to the hairy areas of the vulva. It may occasionally be found in other areas, such as the eyelids. The major nourishment of the louse is human blood.

The louse's life cycle has three stages, egg (nit), nymph, and adult. The entire life cycle is spent on the host. Eggs are deposited at the base of hair follicles. The adult parasite is approximately 1 mm long and dark gray when its alimentary tract is not filled with blood (Fig. 23.3). Of clinical importance for diagnosis is the fact that the louse moves slowly. The incubation period for pediculosis is approximately 30 days.

The predominant clinical symptom of louse infestation is constant pubic pruritus caused by allergic sensitization. Usually, initial sensitization takes several weeks to develop but may be as rapid as 5 days following initial infection. Following a reinfection, pruritus may occur within 24 hours. Examination of the vulvar area without magnification demonstrates eggs and adult lice and pepper grain feces adjacent to the hair shafts (Fig. 23.4). The tiny rough spots visualized with the naked eye are the alimentary tracts of lice filled with human blood. The vulvar skin may become secondarily irritated or infected by constant scratching. For definitive diagnosis, one can make a microscopic slide by scratching the skin papule with a needle and placing the crust under a drop of mineral oil. The louse's body looks like that of a miniature crab, with six legs that have claws on them.

Scabies is a parasitic infection of the itch mite, *Sarcoptes scabiei.* Similar to the crab louse, it is transmitted by close contact. Unlike louse infestation, scabies is an infection that is widespread over the body, without a predilection for hairy areas. The adult female itch mite digs a burrow just beneath the skin. She lays eggs in this home during her life span of approximately 1 month. The adult itch mite is usually less than 0.5 mm long, approximately the size of a grain of sand. Unlike the crab louse, an itch mite travels rapidly over skin and may move up to 2.5 cm in 1 minute. Mites are able to survive for only a few hours away from the warmth of skin.

The predominant clinical symptom of scabies is severe but intermittent itching. Generally, more intense pruritus occurs at night when the skin is warmer and the mites are more active. Initial symptoms usually present approximately 3 weeks after primary infestation. Scabies may present as papules, vesicles, or burrows. However, the pathognomonic sign of scabies infection is the burrow in the skin. The burrow usually has the appearance of a twisted line on the skin surface, with a small vesicle at one end. Any area of the skin may be infected, with the hands, wrists, breasts, vulva, and buttocks being most commonly involved. A handheld magnifying lens is helpful for examining suspicious areas. Microscopic slides may be made using mineral oil and a scratch technique (Fig. 23.5). Mites lack lateral claw legs but have two anterior triangular hairy buds. Scabies has been termed the *great dermatologic imitator,* and the differential diagnosis includes almost all dermatologic diseases that cause pruritus. The treatment of pediculosis pubis or scabies involves an agent that kills both the adult parasite and the eggs.

The therapy currently recommended by the CDC's 2015 guidelines for pediculosis pubis involves the use of permethrin, 1% cream rinse, applied to affected areas and washed off after 10 minutes, or pyrethrins, with piperonyl butoxide applied to the affected area and washed off after 10 minutes. Alternative regimens include malathion, 0.5% lotion, applied for 8 to

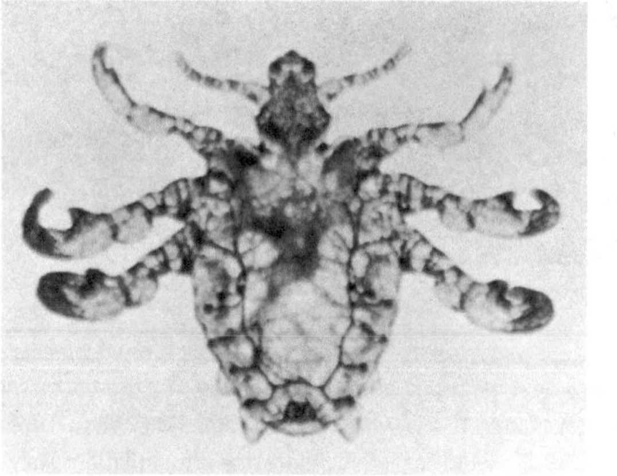

**Figure 23.3** Pubic louse, *Phthirus pubis,* after blood meal. (From Billstein S. Human lice. In: Holmes KK, Mårdh PA, Sparling PF, et al, eds. *Sexually Transmitted Diseases.* New York: McGraw-Hill; 1984.)

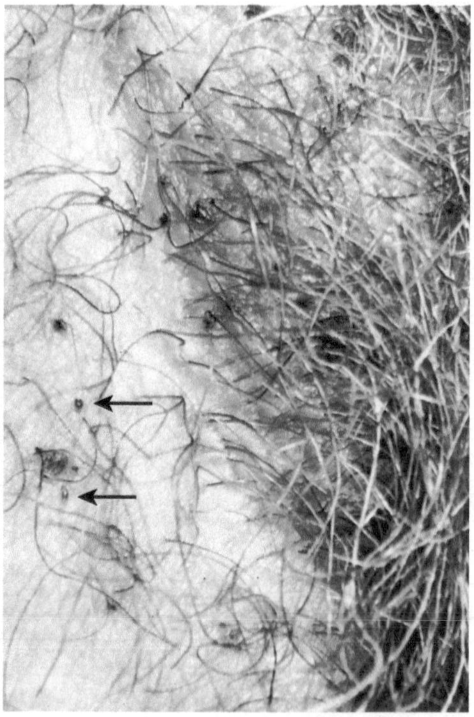

**Figure 23.4** Crab lice and nits of pediculosis pubis *(arrows).* (From Kaufman RH. Miscellaneous vulvar disorders. In: Kaufman RH, Faro S, eds. *Benign Diseases of the Vulva and Vagina.* 4th ed. St. Louis: Mosby-Year Book; 1994.)

12 hours and washed off, or ivermectin, 250 μg/kg, repeated in 2 weeks. None of these should be applied to the eyelids. Retreatment may be necessary if lice are found or if eggs are observed at the hair-skin junction. Patients with pediculosis pubis should be evaluated for other STIs and evaluated after 1 week if symptoms persist. Those who do not respond to one of the recommended regimens should be retreated with an alternative regimen.

To treat scabies, CDC recommends permethrin cream applied to all areas of the body from the neck down and washed off after 8 to 14 hours or ivermectin, 200 μg/kg orally, repeated in 2 weeks, if necessary. Alternative regimens include lindane, 1%, 1 oz of lotion or 30 g of cream applied thinly to all areas of the body from the neck down and thoroughly washed off after 8 hours. Resistance to lindane has been reported in some parts of the United States. Lindane is not recommended as first-line therapy because of toxicity. It should only be used as an alternative if the woman cannot tolerate other therapies or if they have failed. Lindane should not be used immediately after a bath or shower and should not be used by persons who have extensive dermatitis, women who are pregnant or lactating, or children younger than 2 years. Patients with scabies have intense pruritus that may persist for many days following effective therapy. An antihistamine will help alleviate this symptom. Similar to pediculosis pubis, women should be examined 1 week following initial therapy and retreated with an alternative regimen if live mites are observed (Hu, 2008).

To avoid reinfection by pediculosis pubis or scabies, treatment should be prescribed for sexual contacts within the previous 6 weeks and other close household contacts. Those with close physical contact should be treated at the same time as the infected woman, regardless of whether they have symptoms. Bedding and clothing should be decontaminated (i.e., machine washed, machine dried using the heat cycle, or dry cleaned) or removed from body contact for at least 72 hours. Fumigation of living areas is not necessary. Importantly, women and physicians should not confuse the 1% cream rinse of permethrin dosage recommended for pubic lice with the 5% permethrin cream recommended for scabies (Leone, 2007; Scott, 2011).

## MOLLUSCUM CONTAGIOSUM

Molluscum contagiosum is a poxvirus that replicates in the cytoplasm of cells and causes a chronic localized infection consisting of flesh-colored, dome-shaped papules with an umbilicated center. Like many viruses in the pox family, molluscum is spread by direct skin-to-skin contact. However, lesions can be spread by autoinoculation, during contact sports, or by fomites on bath sponges or towels. The incubation period is 2 to 7 weeks. In adults, it is primarily an asymptomatic disease of the vulvar skin, and, unlike most STIs, it is only mildly contagious. Widespread infection in adults is most closely related to underlying cellular immunodeficiency, such as during an HIV infection. It can also occur in the setting of chemotherapy or corticosteroid administration.

Diagnosis is made by the characteristic appearance of the lesions. The small nodules or domed papules of molluscum contagiosum are usually 1 to 5 mm in diameter (Fig. 23.6). Close inspection reveals that many of the more mature nodules have an umbilicated center. An infected woman will typically have 1 to 20 solitary lesions randomly distributed over the vulvar skin. A crop of new nodules will persist from several months to years. If the diagnosis cannot be made by simple inspection, the white waxy material from inside the nodule should be expressed on a microscopic slide. The finding of intracytoplasmic molluscum bodies with Wright or Giemsa stain confirms the diagnosis. The major complication of molluscum contagiosum is bacterial superinfection. The umbilicated papules may resemble furuncles when secondarily infected.

Molluscum contagiosum is usually a self-limiting infection and spontaneously resolves after a few months in immunocompetent individuals. However, treatment of individual papules will decrease sexual transmission and autoinoculation of the virus. After injection of local anesthesia, the caseous material is

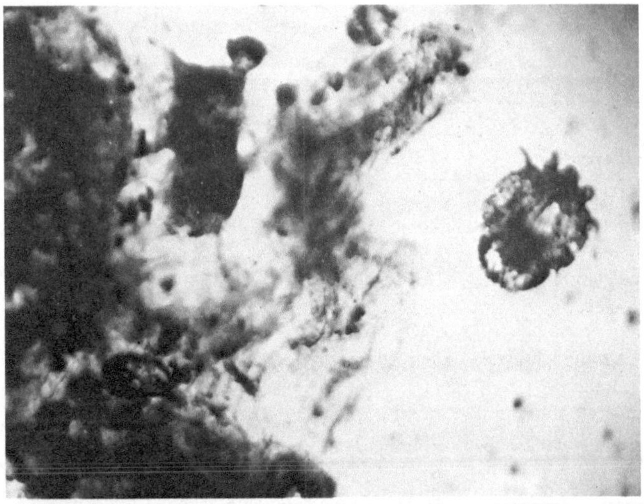

**Figure 23.5** Skin scrapings of unexcoriated papules fortuitously disclose adults, larvae, eggs, and fecal pellets, any of which would be diagnostic of scabies. (From Orkin M, Howard IM. Scabies. In: Holmes KK, Mårdh PA, Sparling PF, et al, eds. *Sexually Transmitted Diseases*. New York: McGraw-Hill; 1984.)

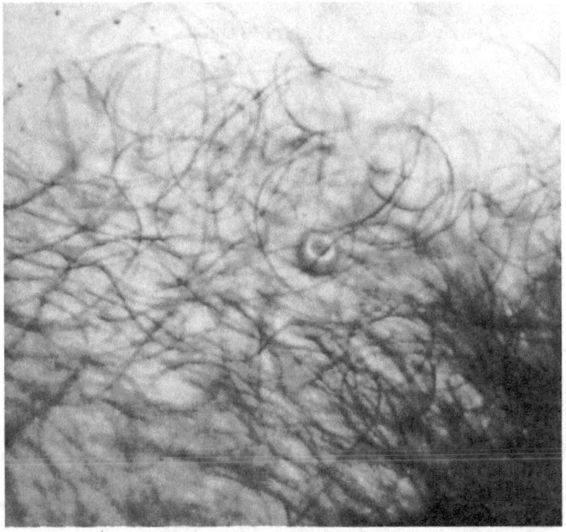

**Figure 23.6** Papule of molluscum contagiosum with umbilicated center. (From Brown ST. Molluscum contagiosum. In Holmes KK, Mårdh PA, Sparling PF, et al, eds. *Sexually Transmitted Diseases*. New York: McGraw-Hill; 1984.)

evacuated and the nodule excised with a sharp dermal curette. The base of the papule is chemically treated with ferric subsulfate (Monsel solution) or 85% trichloroacetic acid. Alternative methods are cantharidin, a chemical blistering agent, imiquimod, or cryotherapy (Al-Mutairi, 2010; Chen, 2013; Gamble, 2012; Mathes, 2010).

In immunocompromised individuals, treatment is more difficult. In the HIV-infected woman, there have been multiple reports of recalcitrant molluscum lesions resolving only after initiating highly active antiretroviral therapy (HAART).

## GENITAL ULCERS

Herpes, granuloma inguinale (donovanosis), lymphogranuloma venereum, chancroid, and syphilis may all present as ulcerations in the genital area. However, their causes, disease courses, and treatments are different. Table 23.1 lists some of their major characteristics. Physicians must always consider the possibility of more than one STI concurrently infecting an individual.

### Genital Herpes

Genital herpes is a recurrent viral infection that is incurable and highly contagious, with 75% of sexual partners of infected individuals contracting the disease. It is among the most frequently encountered STIs; a study of 5452 asymptomatic adults in private community-based clinics in six geographic regions in the United States found the seroprevalence of herpes simplex virus type 2 (HSV-2) was 25.5%. Approximately 80% of infected individuals are unaware that they are infected. Frequently, herpes is transmitted during episodes of asymptomatic shedding, which may occur as frequently as once in 5 days (Bernstein, 2013). It is important that the woman understand the natural history of disease with emphasis on the probability of recurrent attacks, effect of antiviral agents, and risks of neonatal infection. Although recurrent genital herpes is not a debilitating physical disease, it may present a psychological burden. Excellent online patient education and support can be found www.ashastd.org.

There are two distinct types of HSV, type 1 (HSV-1) and type 2 (HSV-2). In the past, a broad generalization was that HSV-1 tends to infect epithelium above the waist, and HSV-2 tends to cause ulceration below the waist. However, HSV-1 is the most commonly acquired genital herpes in women younger than 25 years and, in some series, HSV-1 may cause lower genital tract infection in 13% to 40% of patients. Genital HSV-1 is transmitted from orolabial lesions to the vulva during oral-genital contact or from genital to genital to genital contact with a partner with genital HSV-1.

In primary herpes, the incubation period is between 3 and 7 days (average, 6 days). Although subclinical primary herpes infection is common, both local and systemic disease manifestations occur when the primary infection is symptomatic. The woman typically experiences paresthesia of the vulvar skin followed by the eruption of multiple painful vesicles, which progress to shallow, superficial ulcers over a large area of the vulva. Patients experience multiple crops of ulcers for 2 to 6 weeks. The ulcers usually heal spontaneously without scarring (Fig. 23.7). Viral shedding may occur for 2 to 3 weeks after vulvar lesions appear and, during primary infections, positive cultures for herpesvirus may be obtained from lesions in 80% of women. Most symptomatic women have severe vulvar pain, tenderness, and inguinal adenopathy and simultaneous involvement of the vagina and cervix is common (Fig. 23.8).

Systemic symptoms, including general malaise and fever, are experienced by 70% of women during the primary infection. Rarely, there is central nervous system (CNS) infection, with the reported mortality rate from herpes encephalitis being approximately 50%. Primary infections of the urethra and bladder may result in acute urinary retention, necessitating catheterization. The symptoms of vulvar pain, pruritus, and discharge peak between days 7 and 11 of the primary infection. The typical woman experiences severe symptoms for approximately 14 days.

Recurrent genital herpes is a local disease with less severe symptoms. On average, a woman will have four recurrences during the first year and, in 50% of women, the first recurrence occurs within 6 months of the initial infection. The probability

**Table 23.1** Clinical Features of Genital Ulcers

| | Type | | | | |
|---|---|---|---|---|---|
| **Parameter** | **Syphilis** | **Herpes** | **Chancroid** | **Lymphogranuloma Venereum** | **Donovanosis** |
| Incubation period | 2-4 wk (1-12 wk) | 2-7 days | 1-14 days | 3 days-6 wk | 1-4 wk (up to 6 mo) |
| Primary lesion | Papule | Vesicle | Papule or pustule | Papule, pustule, or vesicle | Papule |
| Number of lesions | Usually one | Multiple, may coalesce | Usually multiple, may coalesce | Usually one | Variable |
| Diameter (mm) | 5-15 | 1-2 | 2-20 | 2-10 | Variable |
| Edges | Sharply demarcated Elevated, round or oval | Erythematous | Undermined, ragged, irregular | Elevated, round or oval | Elevated, irregular |
| Depth | Superficial or deep | Superficial | Excavated | Superficial or deep | Elevated |
| Base | Smooth, nonpurulent | Serous, erythematous | Purulent | Variable | Red and rough (beefy) |
| Induration | Firm | None | Soft | Occasionally firm | Firm |
| Pain | Unusual | Common | Usually very tender | Variable | Uncommon |
| Lymphadenopathy | Firm, nontender Pseudoadenopathy bilateral | Firm, tender, often bilateral | Tender, may suppurate, usually unilateral | Tender, may suppurate, loculated, usually unilateral | |

From Holmes KK, Mårdh PA, Sparling PF, et al, eds. *Sexually Transmitted Diseases*, 2nd ed. New York: McGraw-Hill, 1990.

and frequency of recurrence of herpes are related to the HSV serotype. Approximately 80% of women with an initial genital HSV-2 infection will experience a recurrence within 12 months. If her primary HSV-2 infection was severe, she will have recurrences approximately twice as often, with a shorter time to recurrence intervals compared with women with milder initial episodes of the disease. In contrast, if the initial pelvic infection was HSV-1, there is a 55% chance of a recurrence within 1 year, with the average rate of recurrence slightly less than one episode per year (Phipps, 2011; Tronstein, 2011).

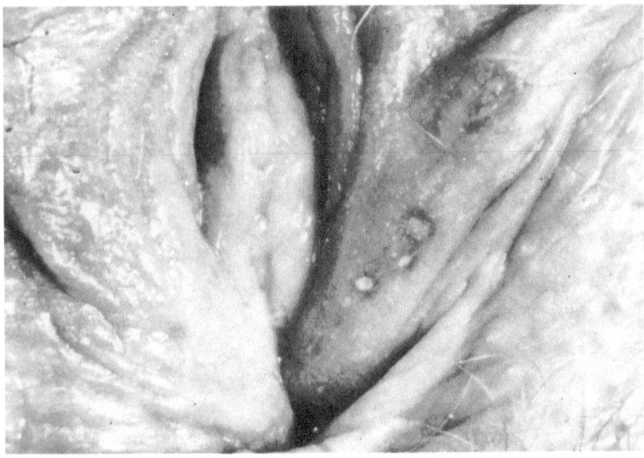

**Figure 23.7** Recurrent herpes genitalis. Superficial ulcers are noted following rupture of vesicles. (From Kaufman RH, Faro S. Herpes genitalis: clinical features and treatment. *Clin Obstet Gynecol.* 1985;28:152-163.)

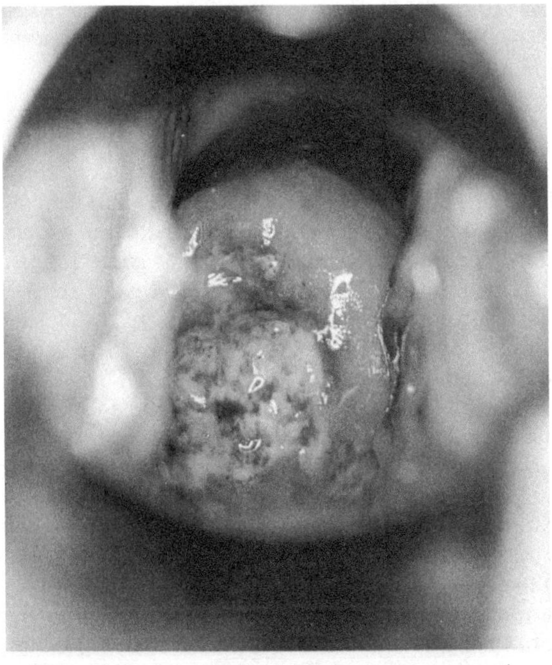

**Figure 23.8** Primary herpes involving the cervix. A necrotic exophytic mass is seen on posterior lip. This was clinically thought to be invasive carcinoma. Herpes simplex virus culture was positive. The lesion spontaneously disappeared. (From Kaufman RH, Faro S. Herpes genitalis: clinical features and treatment. *Clin Obstet Gynecol.* 1985;28:152-163.)

For recurrences, vulvar involvement is usually unilateral, attacks last an average of 7 days, and viral shedding occurs for approximately 5 days. The ability to culture herpesvirus successfully from recurrent herpetic ulcers is 40%. A common feature of recurrence is a prodromal phase of sacroneuralgia, vulvar burning, tenderness, and pruritus for a few hours to 5 days before vesicle formation. Extragenital sites of recurrent infection are common. The herpesvirus resides in a latent phase in the dorsal root ganglia of S2, S3, and S4.

The clinical diagnosis of genital herpes is often made by simple clinical inspection. Women come to their physician when they develop symptoms from vulvar ulcers. Herpetic ulcers are painful when touched with a cotton-tipped applicator, whereas the ulcers of syphilis are painless. Viral cultures are useful in confirming the diagnosis in primary episodes when culture sensitivity is 80%, but less useful in recurrent episodes. Most herpesvirus cultures will become positive within 2 to 4 days of inoculation. The most accurate and sensitive technique for identifying herpesvirus is the polymerase chain reaction (PCR) assay. Serologic tests are helpful in determining whether a woman has been infected in the past with herpesvirus. The Western blot assay for antibodies to herpes is the most specific method for diagnosing recurrent herpes, as well as unrecognized or subclinical infection. However, Western blot tests are not widely available and are difficult to perform. Type-specific HSV serologic assays might be useful in the following situations: (1) recurrent genital symptoms or atypical symptoms, with negative HSV cultures; (2) clinical diagnosis of genital herpes without laboratory confirmation; or (3) partner with genital herpes. HSV serologic testing should be considered for persons presenting for an STI evaluation, especially for those with multiple sex partners or HIV infection and at increased risk for HIV acquisition. Screening for HSV-1 or HSV-2 in the general population is not indicated.

Enzyme-linked immunoassay (ELISA) and immunoblot tests are available for HSV-1 and HSV-2. Rapid serologic point-of-care tests are available for HSV-2 antibodies. Appropriate screening tests for other STIs should be obtained, because they may coexist with herpes.

Treatment of HSV-1 or HSV-2 may be used for three different clinical scenarios:

1. Primary episode
2. Recurrent episode
3. Daily suppression

In primary episodes, the duration and severity of symptoms are lessened, and shedding is shortened with antiviral therapy. Antiviral therapy is recommended for in all patients with primary episodes.

Episodic therapy for recurrences can shorten the duration of the outbreak if started within 24 hours of prodromal symptoms or lesion appearance. Because of the necessity of starting antiviral therapy immediately after recognizing symptoms, it is important that the woman with HSV be given a prescription for antiviral therapy to have at home.

Patient-initiated therapy has been found to be superior to therapy ordered by a physician because patients initiate therapy earlier in the course of a recurrence. The antiviral medication should be started as early as possible during the prodrome, and definitely within 24 hours of the appearance of lesions. Daily suppressive therapy is recommended when the woman has six

Table 23.2 Antiviral Treatment for Herpes Simplex Virus in the Nonpregnant Patient

| Indication | Antiviral Agent: Valacyclovir | Acyclovir | Famciclovir |
|---|---|---|---|
| First clinical episode | 1000 mg bid, 7-10 days | 200 mg five times/day; or 400 mg tid, 7-10 days | 250 mg tid, 7-10 days |
| Recurrent episodes | 1000 mg daily, 5 days; or 500 mg bid, 3 days | 400 mg tid, 5 days; 800 mg bid, 5 days; or 800 mg tid, 2 days | 125 mg bid, 5 days<br>500 mg once then 250 mg bid, 2 days; 1000 mg bid, 1 day |
| Daily suppressive | 1000 mg daily (≥10 recurrences/year) or 500 mg daily (≤9 recurrences/year) | 400 mg bid | 250 mg bid |

Data from Workowski KA, Bolan GA, Centers for Disease Control and Prevention. Sexually transmitted diseases treatment guidelines, 2015. *MMWR Recomm Rep*. 2015; 64(RR-03):1-137. *bid*, Twice per day; *tid*, three times per day.

or more episodes annually or for psychological distress. It is important for patients to be aware that asymptomatic viral shedding can occur even when on daily suppressive therapy (Bavaro, 2008; Gupta, 2004).

In serodiscordant couples a prospective placebo-controlled randomized trial has demonstrated that daily use of valacyclovir for suppression in the seropositive partner results in significantly fewer cases of HSV acquisition in the seronegative partner. Regular use of condoms in serodiscordant couples also decreases transmission but is not 100% protective. HSV-seronegative women are three times as likely to acquire HSV infection from seropositive male partners compared with seronegative males acquiring HSV from infected female partners. A summary of CDC-recommended treatment regimens is presented in Table 23.2.

Acyclovir is a drug with relatively minimal toxicity and reports have documented its safety in patients receiving daily therapy with acyclovir for as long as 6 years and with valacyclovir or famciclovir for 1 year. However, the CDC recommends that acyclovir or other suppressive drugs be discontinued after 12 months of suppressive therapy to determine the subsequent rate of recurrence for each individual woman (Workowski, 2015). Even if herpes is not treated over time, clinical recurrences tend to dramatically decrease in number.

A vaccine would be the logical approach for optimum prevention of herpes. Research is ongoing.

### *Granuloma Inguinale (Donovanosis)*

Granuloma inguinale, also known as *donovanosis*, is a chronic, ulcerative, bacterial infection of the skin and subcutaneous tissue of the vulva. Rarely, the vagina and cervix are involved in advanced untreated cases. Granuloma inguinale is common in tropical climates such as New Guinea and the Caribbean Islands, but fewer than 20 cases are reported each year in the United States. This disease can be spread sexually and through close nonsexual contact. However, it is not highly contagious, and chronic exposure is usually necessary to contract the disease. The incubation period is extremely variable, from 1 to 12 weeks. It is caused by an intracellular, gram-negative, nonmotile, encapsulated rod, *Klebsiella granulomatis*, which is difficult to culture on standard media. There are no U.S. Food and Drug Administration (FDA)–approved molecular tests for the detection of *K. granulomatis* DNA. Serologic tests are nonspecific.

The initial growth of granuloma inguinale is a nodule that gradually progresses into a painless, slowly progressing ulcer surrounded by highly vascular granulation tissue. This gives the ulcer a beefy red appearance, and it bleeds easily when touched. Unless secondarily infected, the ulcers are painless and without regional adenopathy. Typically, multiple nodules are present, resulting in ulcers that grow and coalesce and, if untreated, will eventually destroy the normal vulvar architecture. If untreated, the chronic form of the disease is characterized by scarring and lymphatic obstruction, which produces marked enlargement of the vulva. In endemic areas, the disease is usually diagnosed by its clinical manifestations. The diagnosis may also be established by identifying Donovan bodies in smears and specimens taken from the ulcers (Fig. 23.9). Donovan bodies appear as clusters of dark-staining bacteria with a bipolar (safety pin) appearance found in the cytoplasm of large mononuclear cells. The differential diagnosis includes lymphogranuloma venereum, vulvar carcinoma, syphilis, chancroid, genital herpes, amebiasis, and other granulomatous diseases.

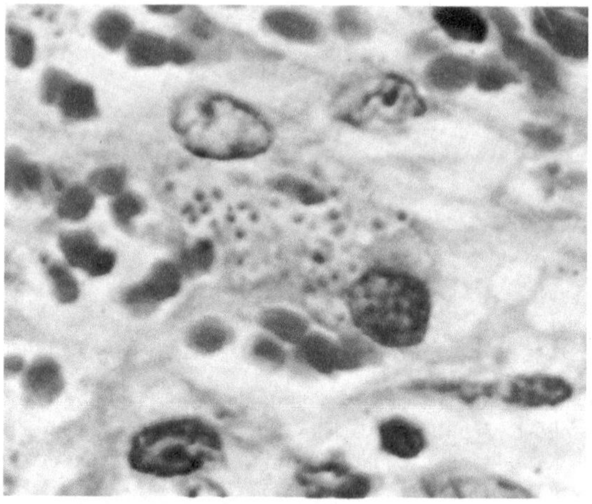

**Figure 23.9** Donovanosis. Biopsy specimen shows intracytoplasmic Donovan bodies (H&E stain). (From Hart G. Donovanosis. In: Holmes KK, Mårdh PA, Sparling PF, et al, eds. *Sexually Transmitted Diseases*. New York: McGraw-Hill; 1984.)

A wide range of oral broad-spectrum antibiotics may be used to manage granuloma inguinale. The CDC recommends azithromycin 1 g orally once a week or 500 mg daily for 3 weeks and until all lesions have healed. Alternative antibiotic regimens include the following: doxycycline, 100 mg orally, twice daily for a minimum of 3 weeks; ciprofloxacin, 750 mg orally twice daily; erythromycin base, 500 mg orally four times daily; or trimethoprim-sulfamethoxazole (TMP-SMZ), one double-strength tablet orally twice daily. Therapy should be continued until the lesions have healed completely. Alternative antibiotic therapy such as an aminoglycoside has been used in refractory cases. Rarely, medical therapy fails and surgical excision is required. Co-infection with another sexually transmitted pathogen is a distinct possibility. Sex partners of women who have granuloma inguinale should be examined if they have had sexual contact during the 60 days preceding the onset of symptoms (Workowski, 2015).

### *Lymphogranuloma Venereum*

Lymphogranuloma venereum (LGV) is a chronic infection of lymphatic tissue produced by *Chlamydia trachomatis.* It is found most commonly in the tropics. Cases occur infrequently in the United States, with fewer than 150 new cases being reported each year, most of which occur in men. In women, the vulva is the most frequent site of infection, but the urethra, rectum, and cervix may also be involved. This sexually transmitted infection is caused by serotypes L1, L2, and L3 of *C. trachomatis.* Serologic studies in high-risk populations have found that subclinical infection is common. The incubation period is between 3 and 30 days.

There are three distinct phases of vulvar and perirectal LGV. The primary infection is a shallow, painless ulcer that heals rapidly without therapy. It is typically located on the vestibule or labia but occasionally in the periurethral or perirectal region. One to 4 weeks after the primary infection, a secondary phase marked by painful adenopathy develops in the inguinal and perirectal areas. Two thirds of women have unilateral adenopathy and 50% have systemic symptoms, including general malaise and fever. When the disease is untreated, the infected nodes become increasingly tender, enlarged, matted together, and adherent to overlying skin, forming a bubo (tender lymph nodes). A classic clinical sign of LGV is the double genitocrural fold, or groove sign (Fig. 23.10), a depression between groups of inflamed nodes. Within 7 to 15 days, the bubo will rupture spontaneously and form multiple draining sinuses and fistulas. These are classic signs of the tertiary phase of the infection. Extensive tissue destruction of the external genitalia and anorectal region may occur during the tertiary phase. This tissue destruction and secondary extensive scarring and fibrosis may result in elephantiasis, multiple fistulas, and stricture formation of the anal canal and rectum.

Diagnosis is established by detecting *C. trachomatis* by culture, direct immunofluorescence, or nucleic acid detection from the pus or aspirate from a tender lymph node. *Chlamydia* serology (complement fixation titers >1:64) can support the diagnosis in the appropriate clinical context. However, the diagnostic usefulness of serologic methods other than complement fixation and some microimmunofluorescence procedures remains unclear. In the absence of specific LGV diagnostic testing, patients should be treated based on the clinical presentation, including proctocolitis or genital ulcer disease with lymphadenopathy. The differential diagnosis of LGV includes syphilis, chancroid, granuloma inguinale, bacterial lymphadenitis, vulvar carcinoma, genital herpes, and Hodgkin disease.

The CDC recommends doxycycline, 100 mg twice daily for at least 21 days, as the preferred treatment. An alternative therapy choice is erythromycin base, 500 mg four times daily orally for 21 days. Azithromycin, 1 g orally once weekly for 3 weeks, is probably effective, but clinical data are lacking.

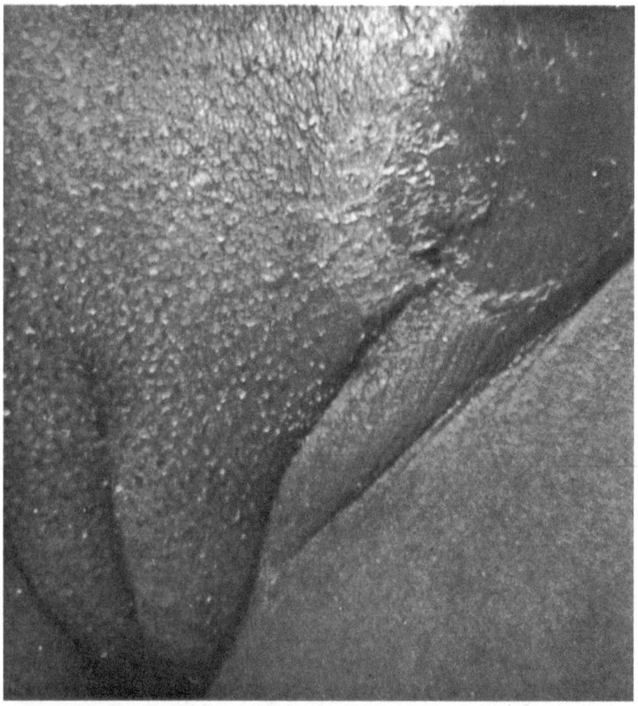

**Figure 23.10** Lymphogranuloma venereum bubo with groove sign. (From Friedrich EG. *Vulvar Disease.* 2nd ed. Philadelphia: WB Saunders; 1983.)

Fluoroquinolone-based treatments may also be effective, but extended treatment intervals are likely required (Workowski, 2015).

Antibiotic therapy cures the bacterial infection and prevents further tissue destruction. However, fluctuant nodes should be aspirated to prevent sinus formation. Rarely, incision and drainage of infected nodes are necessary to alleviate inguinal pain. The late sequelae of the destructive tertiary phase of LGV often require extensive surgical reconstruction. It is important to administer antibiotics during the perioperative period.

### *Chancroid*

Chancroid is a sexually transmitted, acute, ulcerative disease of the vulva caused by *Haemophilus ducreyi,* a highly contagious, small, nonmotile, gram-negative rod. Chancroid is a common disease in developing countries but infrequent in the United States. Epidemiologic studies have suggested that chancroid tends to occur in clusters and may account for a substantial portion of genital ulcer cases when present. However, difficulty in making the diagnosis may cause underreporting. The clinical importance of chancroid has been enhanced by reports that the genital ulcers of chancroid facilitate the transmission of HIV infection.

The soft chancre of chancroid is always painful and tender. In comparison, the hard chancre of syphilis is usually asymptomatic. On Gram stain, this facultative anaerobic bacterium exhibits a classic appearance of streptobacillary chains, or what has been described as an extracellular school of fish. The incubation period is short, usually 3 to 6 days. Tissue trauma and excoriation of the skin must precede initial infection because *H. ducreyi* is unable to penetrate and invade normal skin.

The initial lesion is a small papule. Within 48 to 72 hours, the papule evolves into a pustule and subsequently ulcerates.

The extremely painful ulcers are shallow, with a characteristic ragged edge, and usually occur in the vulvar vestibule and rarely in the vagina or cervix. The ulcers have a dirty, gray, necrotic, foul-smelling exudate and lack induration at the base (the soft chancre). Multiple papules and ulcers may be in different phases of maturation secondary to autoinoculation. Within 2 weeks of an untreated infection, approximately 50% of women develop acutely tender inguinal adenopathy, a bubo, which is typically unilateral. Fluctuant nodes should be treated by needle aspiration to prevent rupture or by incision and drainage if larger than 5 cm.

A definitive diagnosis of chancroid requires the identification of *H. ducreyi* on special culture media that are not widely available from commercial sources; even when these media are used, sensitivity is less than 80%. No FDA-approved PCR test for *H. ducreyi* is available in the United States, but this testing can be performed by clinical laboratories that have developed their own PCR test and conducted a Clinical Laboratory Improvement Amendments (CLIA) verification study. Sometimes, the clinical diagnosis is made in a woman with painful vulvar ulcers after excluding other common STIs that produce vulvar ulcers, including genital herpes, syphilis, LGV, and donovanosis.

Due to antibiotic resistance to tetracyclines and sulfonamides, the CDC recommends the following: azithromycin, 1 g orally in a single dose or ceftriaxone, 250 mg intramuscular (IM) in a single dose or ciprofloxacin, 500 mg orally twice daily for 3 days; or erythromycin base, 500 mg orally three times daily for 7 days. Sexual partners should be treated in a similar fashion. Successful antibiotic therapy results in symptomatic and objective improvement within 5 to 7 days of initiating therapy. Large ulcers may require 2 to 3 weeks to heal, with clinical resolution of lymphadenopathy slower than that of ulcers. Buboes respond at a slower rate than skin ulcers (Workowski, 2015). Approximately 10% of women whose ulcers initially heal have a recurrence at the same site. Women with HIV infection have an increased rate of failure to the standard treatments for chancroid and therefore often require more prolonged therapy. Co-infection with another ulcer causing an STI should be considered, especially in women lacking an appropriate response to treatment.

### Syphilis

Syphilis is a chronic, complex systemic disease produced by the spirochete *Treponema pallidum.* The infection initially involves mucous membranes. Syphilis remains one of the important STIs in the United States, and epidemiologists speculate that only one of four new cases of syphilis is reported. Early syphilis is a cofactor in the transmission and acquisition of HIV and, currently, 25% of new syphilis cases occur in persons co-infected with HIV. Even with mandatory screening, congenital syphilis continues to be a public health problem. Mothers who experience stillbirth or neonatal death from syphilis usually have not received prenatal care. Syphilis should be included in the differential diagnosis of all genital ulcers and cutaneous rashes of unknown origin, and all women diagnosed with syphilis should be screened for HIV.

*T. pallidum* is an anaerobic, elongated, tightly wound spirochete. Because of its extreme thinness, it is difficult to detect by light microscopy. Therefore the presence of spirochetes is diagnosed by use of specially adapted techniques, dark-field microscopy, or direct fluorescent antibody tests (Fig. 23.11). These organisms have the ability to penetrate skin or mucous

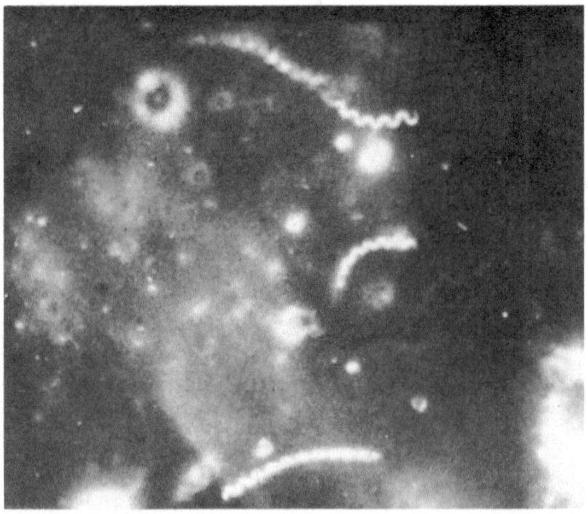

**Figure 23.11** Dark-field microscopic appearance of *Treponema pallidum*. (From Larsen SA, McGrew BE, Hunter EF, et al. Syphilis serology and dark field microscopy. In: Holmes KK, Mårdh PA, Sparling PF, et al, eds. *Sexually Transmitted Diseases*. New York: McGraw-Hill; 1984.)

membranes. The incubation period is from 10 to 90 days, with an average of 3 weeks. They replicate every 30 to 36 hours, which accounts for the comparatively long incubation period.

Syphilis is a moderately contagious disease. Approximately 3% to 10% of patients contract the disease from a single sexual encounter with an infected partner. Similar studies have documented that 30% of individuals become infected during a 1-month exposure to a sexual partner with primary or secondary syphilis. Patients are contagious during primary, secondary, and probably the first year of latent syphilis. Syphilis can be spread by kissing or touching a person who has an active lesion on the lips, oral cavity, breast, or genitals. Case transmission can occur with oral-genital contact.

The diagnosis of syphilis is complicated by the fact that the organism cannot be cultivated in vitro. Definitive diagnosis is via darkfield microscopy to detect *T. palladium* in lesion exudate or tissue. *T. palladium* detection kits are not commercially available, but some labs provide locally developed PCR tests. Therefore presumptive diagnosis and screening rely on serologic tests. There are two types of serologic tests, the nonspecific nontreponemal and the specific antitreponemal antibody tests. The nontreponemal tests, such as the Venereal Disease Research Laboratory (VDRL) slide test and the rapid plasma reagin (RPR) card test are inexpensive and easy to perform. They are used as screening tests for the disease, typically become positive 4 to 6 weeks after exposure, and also are a useful index of treatment response. These tests evaluate the woman's serum for the presence of reagin IgG and IgM antibodies as they react with an antigen from beef heart. Quantitative nontreponemal antibody titers usually correlate with the activity of the disease. Serologic testing is an indirect method of diagnosis because it relies on a humoral immune response to infection. As such, it has some inherent limitations. Approximately 1% of patients have technical or biologic false-positive results with the nonspecific tests. Many conditions produce biologic false-positive results, including a recent febrile illness, pregnancy, immunization, chronic active hepatitis, malaria, sarcoidosis, intravenous (IV) drug use, HIV infection, advancing age, acute herpes simplex, and

Table 23.3 Potential Causes of Biologic False-Positive Results in Syphilis Serology

| | Biologic False-Positive Reaction | |
|---|---|---|
| Cause | Acute | Chronic |
| Physiologic | Pregnancy | Advanced age, multiple blood transfusions |
| Infectious | Varicella, vaccinia, measles, mumps, infectious mononucleosis, herpes simplex, viral hepatitis, HIV seroconversion illness, cytomegalovirus, pneumococcal pneumonia, *Mycoplasma pneumoniae*, chancroid, lymphogranuloma venereum, psittacosis, bacterial endocarditis, scarlet fever, rickettsial infections, toxoplasmosis, Lyme disease, leptospirosis, relapsing fever, rat bite fever | HIV, tropical spastic paraparesis, leprosy,* tuberculosis, malaria,* lymphogranuloma venereum, trypanosomiasis,* kala-azar* |
| Vaccinations | Smallpox, typhoid, yellow fever | |
| Autoimmune disease | | Systemic lupus erythematosus, discoid lupus, drug-induced lupus, autoimmune hemolytic anemia, polyarteritis nodosa, rheumatoid arthritis, Sjögren syndrome, Hashimoto thyroiditis, mixed connective tissue disease, primary biliary cirrhosis, chronic liver disease, idiopathic thrombocytopenic purpura |
| Other | | IV drug use, advanced malignancy hypergammaglobulinemia, lymphoproliferative disease |

Data from Nandwani R, Evans DTP. Are you sure it's syphilis? A review of false-positive serology. *Int J STD AIDS*. 1995;6:241; Hook EW III, Marra CM. Acquired syphilis in adults. *N Engl J Med*. 1992;326:1062.
*Biologic false-positive reaction resolves with resolution of infection.
*HIV*, Human immunodeficiency virus.

autoimmune diseases such as lupus erythematosus or rheumatoid arthritis. Biologic false-positive serum tests usually are associated with extremely low titers (<1:8). A false-negative result is a possibility, occurring in approximately 1% to 2% of tests. This negative reaction occurs in women in whom there is an excess of anticardiolipin antibody in the serum, termed the *prozone phenomenon*. Women with immunocompromise also may have false-negative tests because of their inability to produce the antibodies detected by these screening tests.

If a nonspecific test result is positive, the significance of this result must be confirmed by a specific antitreponemal test. Antitreponemal tests are more sensitive; however, occasionally, they may produce false-positive results. Most false-positive results occur in women with lupus erythematosus (Table 23.3). The standard for antitreponemal tests are the fluorescent-labeled *Treponema* antibody absorption (FTA-ABS) test and the microhemagglutination assay for antibodies to *T. pallidum* (MHA-TP). The MHA-TP does not have as high a rate of false-positive results as the FTA-ABS. A woman with a positive reactive treponemal test usually will have this positive reaction for her lifetime, regardless of treatment or activity of the disease.

Clinically, syphilis is divided into primary, secondary, and tertiary stages. In primary syphilis, a papule, which is usually painless, appears at the site of inoculation 2 to 3 weeks after exposure. This soon ulcerates to produce the classic finding of primary syphilis, a chancre that is a painless ulcer, 1 to 2 cm, with a raised indurated margin and a nonexudative base (Fig. 23.12). Usually, the chancre is solitary, painless, and found on the vulva, vagina, or cervix, although extragenital primary lesions, including lesions of the mouth, anal canal, and breast nipple, have been reported in approximately 5% of patients. Nontender and firm regional adenopathy is present during the first week of clinical disease. Within 2 to 6 weeks, the painless ulcer heals spontaneously. Hence, many women do not seek treatment, a feature that enhances the likelihood of transmission. Confirmation that the ulcer is primary or secondary syphilis depends on the identification of *T. pallidum* by dark-field microscopy from wet smears of the ulcer. Special preparations must be made to obtain suitable smears. It is important to clean and abrade the ulcer with gauze before obtaining the serum for the slides. At the time of dark-field identification of *T. pallidum* from a primary chancre, approximately 70% of women will have a positive serologic test. If the serologic test result remains negative for 3 months, it is unlikely that the ulcer was syphilis. Syphilis is not frequently diagnosed in the primary stage in women.

If primary syphilis is untreated, approximately 25% of individuals develop secondary syphilis, which is the result of hematogenous dissemination of the spirochetes. Secondary syphilis is a systemic disease that develops between 6 weeks and 6 months (average, 9 weeks) after the primary chancre. The stages are not exclusive. Approximately 25% of women still have a primary chancre when the secondary lesions appear. An untreated attack of secondary syphilis will last 2 to 6 weeks, and a multitude of systemic symptoms may occur, depending on the major organs involved, such as rash, fever, headache, malaise, lymphadenopathy, and anorexia. The classic rash of secondary syphilis is red macules and papules over the palms of the hands and the soles of the feet (Fig. 23.13). Vulvar lesions of condyloma latum are large, raised, flattened, grayish white areas (Fig. 23.14). On wet surfaces of the vulva, soft papules often coalesce to form ulcers. These ulcers are larger than herpetic ulcers and are not tender unless secondarily infected. A woman with syphilis is most infectious during the first 1 to 2 years of disease, with decreasing infectivity thereafter.

The latent stage of syphilis follows the secondary stage and varies in duration from 2 to 20 years; it is characterized as positive serology without symptoms or signs of disease. Women with syphilis in the primary or secondary stages and during the first year of latent syphilis are believed to be infectious. Most women diagnosed with syphilis are detected via positive blood tests during the latent stage of the disease. Early latent syphilis is an infection of 1 year or less. All other cases are referred to as *late latent* or *latent syphilis of unknown duration*. Women who have been sexually active with latent syphilis should have a pelvic examination to discover potential lesions involving the vagina or cervix.

The tertiary phase of syphilis is devastating in its potentially destructive effects on the central nervous, cardiovascular, and musculoskeletal systems. Tertiary syphilis develops in approximately 33% of patients who are not appropriately treated during the primary, secondary, or latent phases of the disease (Fig. 23.15). The manifestations of late syphilis include optic atrophy, tabes dorsalis, generalized paresis, aortic aneurysm, and gummas of the skin and bones. A gumma is similar to a cold abscess, with a necrotic center and the obliteration of small vessels by endarteritis.

Parenteral penicillin G is the drug of choice for syphilis. *T. pallidum* is exquisitely sensitive to penicillin. However, because of the slow replication time of the spirochete, blood levels must be maintained for 7 to 14 days. The CDC recommends 2.4 million units of benzathine penicillin G IM in one dose for early syphilis (primary and early latent secondary syphilis). Patients who are allergic to penicillin should receive oral tetracycline,

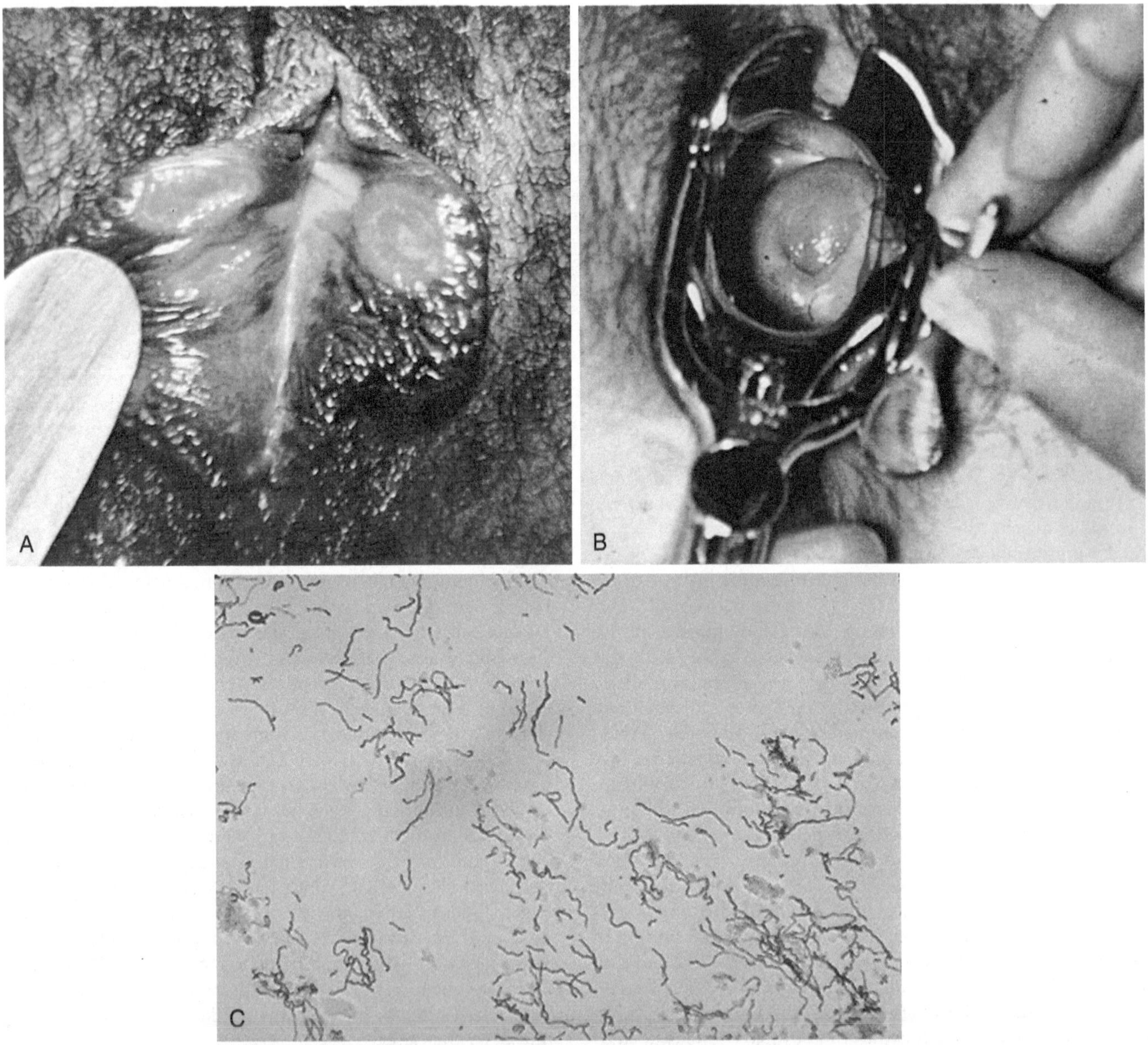

**Figure 23.12** Primary syphilis. **A** and **B**, Primary chancres of syphilis, which began as a papule, erode, and develop into painless ulcers with raised, firm, indurated borders and a clean smooth base. **C**, Microscopic spirochetes. These corkscrew-shaped organisms seen with Warthin-Starry silver staining are *Treponema pallidum* organisms, which cause syphilis. (*A* and *B*, From U.S. Public Health Service. *Syphilis: A Synopsis*. Washington, DC: U.S. Government Printing Office, 1967:47, 50. **C**, From Klatt EC. Blood vessels. In Klatt EC, ed. *Robbins and Cotran Atlas of Pathology*. 3rd ed. Philadelphia: Elsevier; 2015:1-26.)

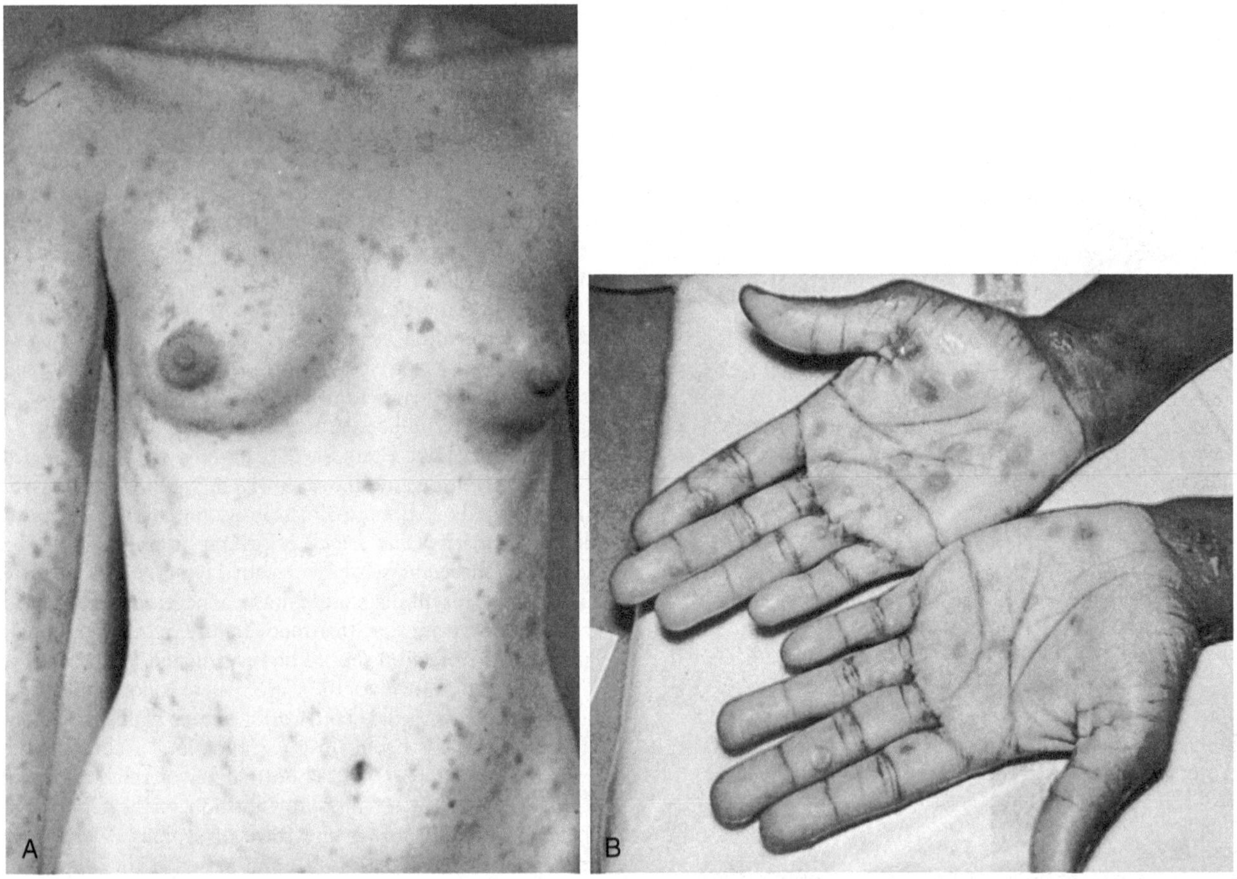


**Figure 23.13** Rash of secondary syphilis. **A,** Common presentation on the trunk and arms. **B,** Red maculopapular lesions involve palms and soles. (From Kissane JM. Bacterial diseases. In: Kissane JM, ed. *Anderson's Pathology.* St. Louis: Mosby-Year Book; 1985.)

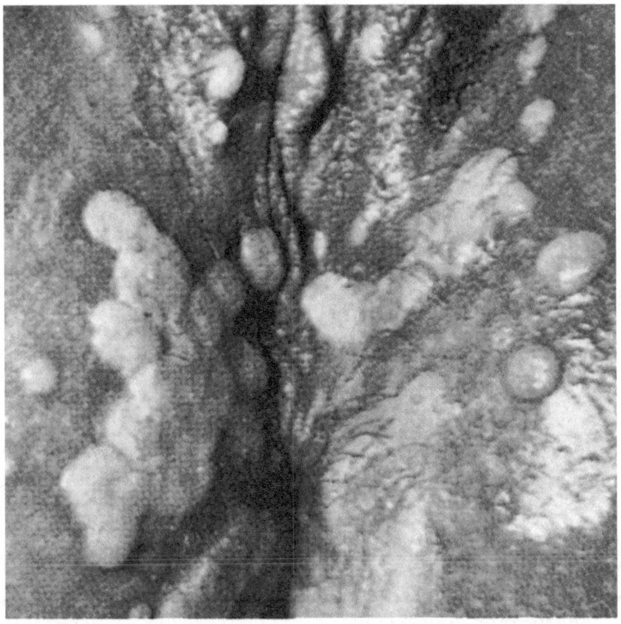

**Figure 23.14** Multiple lesions of condylomata lata on vulva and perineum. Dark-field microscopic findings were positive. (From Faro S. Sexually transmitted diseases. In: Kaufman RH, Faro S, eds. *Benign Diseases of the Vulva and Vagina.* 4th ed. St. Louis: Mosby-Year Book; 1994.)

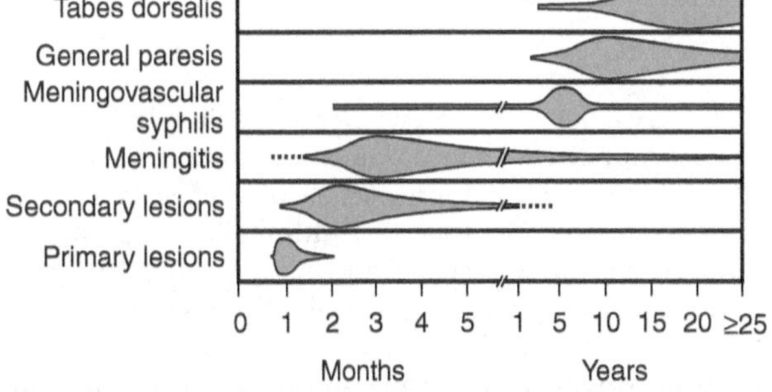


**Figure 23.15** Approximate time course of the clinical manifestations of early syphilis and neurosyphilis. *Shaded areas* corresponding to each syndrome represent the approximate proportion of patients with the syndrome specified and do not indicate the proportion of all patients with syphilis who have that syndrome. (From Hook EW 3rd, Marra CM. Acquired syphilis in adults. *N Engl J Med.* 1992;326[16]:1060-1069.)

**Box 23.2 Centers for Disease Control and Prevention Recommended Treatment of Syphilis (2014)**

**Early Syphilis (primary, secondary, and early latent syphilis of less than 1 year in duration)**

Recommended regimen: Benzathine penicillin G, 2.4 million U IM, one dose

Alternative regimen (penicillin-allergic nonpregnant patients): Doxycycline, 100 mg orally bid for 2 wk *or* tetracycline, 500 mg orally qid for 2 wk

**Late Latent Syphilis (>1 year in duration, gummas, and cardiovascular syphilis)**

Recommended regimen: Benzathine penicillin G, 7.2 million U total, administered as three doses of 2.4 million U IM at 1-wk intervals

Alternative regimen (penicillin-allergic nonpregnant patients): Doxycycline 100 mg orally 2 times a day for 2 wk if <1 year, otherwise, for 4 wk; *or* tetracycline, 500 mg orally qid for 2 wk if <1 year; otherwise, for 4 wk

**Neurosyphilis**

Recommended regimen: Aqueous crystalline penicillin G, 18-24 million U daily, administered as 3-4 million U IV every 4 hr, for 10-14 days

Alternative regimen: Procaine penicillin, 2.4 million U IM daily, for 10-14 days plus probenecid, 500 mg PO qid for 10-14 days

**Syphilis in Pregnancy**

Recommended regimen: Penicillin regimen appropriate for stage of syphilis. Some experts recommend additional therapy (e.g., second dose of benzathine penicillin, 2.4 million U IM) 1 wk after the initial dose for those who have primary, secondary, or early latent syphilis

Alternative regimen (penicillin allergy): Pregnant women with a history of penicillin allergy should be skin-tested and desensitized

**Syphilis in HIV-Infected Patients**

Primary and secondary syphilis: Benzathine penicillin G, 2.4 million U IM. Some experts recommend additional treatments, such as three weekly doses of benzathine penicillin G. Penicillin-allergic patients should be desensitized and treated with penicillin

Latent syphilis (normal CSF examination): Benzathine penicillin G, 7.2 million U as three weekly doses of 2.4 million U each

Data from Workowski KA, Bolan GA, Centers for Disease Control and Prevention. Sexually transmitted diseases treatment guidelines, 2015. *MMWR Recomm Rep.* 2015;64(RR-03):1-137.

*bid*, Twice per day; *CSF*, cerebrospinal fluid; *qid*, four times per day.

500 mg every 6 hours for 14 days, or doxycycline, 100 mg orally twice a day for 2 weeks. Standard treatment protocols for syphilis are detailed in Box 23.2. Approximately 60% of women develop an acute febrile reaction associated with flulike symptoms such as headache and myalgia within the first 24 hours after parenteral penicillin therapy for early syphilis. This response is known as the *Jarisch-Herxheimer reaction* (Workowski, 2015).

All women with early syphilis should be reexamined clinically and serologically at 6 and 12 months following therapy. With successful therapy in early syphilis, the titer should decline fourfold in 6 months and become negative within 12 months. Women with latent syphilis should have quantitative nontreponemal serologic tests 6, 12, and 24 months following therapy. During the first 3 to 4 years of the latent phase, a woman may experience relapses of secondary syphilis. Women who have a sustained fourfold increase in nontreponemal test titers have failed treatment or become reinfected. They should be retreated and evaluated for concurrent HIV infection. When women are retreated, the recommendation is three weekly injections of benzathine penicillin G, 2.4 million units IM. For long-term follow-up, the same serologic tests should be ordered. Optimally, the test should be obtained from the same laboratory. The VDRL and RPR tests are equally valid, but RPR titers tend to be slightly higher than VDRL titers. With successful treatment, the VDRL titer will become nonreactive or, at most, be reactive, with a lower titer within 1 year. There is a 1% to 2% chance that the woman will not exhibit a fourfold titer decline, and these cases are considered therapeutic failures. They should be retreated. Patients with syphilis lasting longer than 1 year should have quantitative VDRL titers for 2 years following therapy because their titers will decline more slowly. A specific test for syphilis, such as the FTA-ABS, remains reactive indefinitely. In summary, all women with a first attack of primary syphilis should have a negative nonspecific serology within 1 year, and women treated for secondary syphilis should have a negative serology within 2 years. If they are not, treatment failure, reinfection, and concurrent HIV infection should be investigated.

Syphilis often involves the CNS. There is no established diagnostic test that is a gold standard for neurosyphilis. The diagnosis of neurosyphilis is based on a combination of clinical findings, reactive serologic tests, and abnormalities of cerebrospinal fluid, serology, cell count, or protein. Infection of the CNS by spirochetes may occur during any stage of syphilis. Women should undergo a cerebrospinal fluid examination if they develop neurologic or ophthalmologic signs or symptoms, evidence of active tertiary syphilis, treatment failures, and HIV infection with late latent syphilis or syphilis of an unknown duration. To treat neurosyphilis, the CDC recommends aqueous crystalline penicillin G, 18 to 24 million units daily, administered as 3 to 4 million units IV every 4 hours for 10 to 14 days. An alternative regimen is procaine penicillin, 2.4 million units IM daily, plus probenecid, 500 mg orally four times daily for 10 to 14 days. The duration of both these regimens for neurosyphilis is shorter than that of the regimen used for late syphilis in the absence of neurosyphilis. Therefore some experts administer benzathine penicillin, 2.4 million units IM, after completion of either regimen to provide a comparable total duration of therapy (Workowski, 2015).

It is important for all women with syphilis to be tested for HIV infection. Simultaneous syphilis and HIV infections alter the natural history of syphilis, with earlier involvement of the CNS. Women with HIV infection may have a slightly increased rate of treatment failure with currently recommended regimens. Similarly, they may exhibit unusual serologic responses. Usually, serologic titers are higher than expected. However, false-negative serologic tests or delayed appearance of seroreactivity has been reported. Nevertheless, the CDC's recommendation for treating early syphilis in women is the same whether or not they are concurrently infected with HIV. Following penicillin treatment for syphilis, women with HIV should be followed with quantitative titers at more frequent intervals—for example, at 3, 6, 9, 12, and 24 months following therapy.

Sexual partners of women with syphilis in any stage should be evaluated clinically and serologically. The time intervals used to identify an at-risk sex partner are 3 months plus duration of symptoms for primary syphilis, 3 months plus duration of symptoms for secondary syphilis, and 1 year for early latent syphilis. Those who are exposed within the 90 days preceding the diagnosis of primary, secondary, or early latent syphilis in their sexual partners should be treated presumptively because they may be infected, even if seronegative.

## VAGINITIS

Vaginal discharge is the most common symptom in gynecology. Other symptoms associated with vaginal infection include superficial dyspareunia, dysuria, odor, and vulvar burning and pruritus. The three common causes of vaginitis are (1) a fungus (candidiasis), (2) a protozoon *(Trichomonas),* and (3) a disruption of the vaginal bacterial ecosystem leading to bacterial vaginosis. Relative prevalence differs depending on the population studied; in a group of middle-class women in the reproductive range, bacterial vaginosis represents approximately 50% of cases, whereas candidiasis and *Trichomonas* infection each constitute approximately 25% of cases.

The vaginal environment has been described as a dynamic ecosystem. The normal vaginal pH is approximately 4.0 in premenopausal women. The maintenance of an optimum pH balance involves a complex interplay of hormonal, microbiologic, and other unknown factors. In women of reproductive age, estrogen stimulates the glycogen content of vaginal epithelial cells. The glycogen is metabolized to lactic acid and other short-chain organic acids, principally by the lactobacilli but also by other vaginal bacteria and enzymes. *Lactobacillus,* an aerobic, gram-positive rod, is found in 62% to 88% of asymptomatic women and is the regulator of normal vaginal flora. Lactobacilli make lactic acid, which maintains the normal vaginal pH of 3.8 to 4.5 and inhibits the adherence of bacteria to vaginal epithelial cells. Approximately 60% of vaginal lactobacilli strains make hydrogen peroxide, which inhibits the growth of bacteria and destroys HIV in vitro. Estrogen improves lactobacilli concentration by enhancing the vaginal epithelial cell production of glycogen, which breaks down into glucose and acts as a substrate for the bacteria.

One of the most helpful diagnostic aids in the differential diagnosis of vaginitis is the measurement of vaginal acidity with pH indicator paper. A vaginal pH higher than 5.0 indicates bacterial vaginosis or *Trichomonas* infection, or possibly an atrophic vaginal discharge. A vaginal pH less than 4.5 represents a physiologic discharge or fungal infection, although fungal infection can occur concurrently with bacterial vaginosis or *Trichomonas.* Cervical mucus and semen have neutral or basic pH and may temporarily change the normal acidity. Semen has been found to buffer vaginal acidity for 6 to 8 hours following intercourse. The vaginal pH is slightly higher in postmenopausal than in premenopausal women.

Normal physiologic vaginal discharge consists of cervical and vaginal epithelial cells, normal bacterial flora, water, electrolytes, and other chemicals. The quantitative concentration of bacterial organisms is $10^8$ to $10^9$ colonies/mL of vaginal fluid. The concentrations of anaerobic and aerobic bacteria vary considerably during the menstrual cycle. Qualitatively, the number of bacterial species may vary from 17 to 29. Anaerobic bacteria are quantitatively the most prevalent, five times more common than aerobic bacteria.

**Table 23.4** Bacterial Vaginal Flora in Asymptomatic Women without Vaginitis

| Organism | Range of Recovery (%) |
|---|---|
| **Facultative Organisms** | |
| **Gram-Positive Rods** | |
| Lactobacilli | 50-75 |
| Diphtheroids | 40 |
| **Gram-Positive Cocci** | |
| *Staphylococcus epidermidis* | 40-55 |
| *Staphylococcus aureus* | 0-5 |
| Beta-hemolytic streptococci | 20 |
| Group D streptococci | 35-55 |
| **Gram-Negative Organisms** | |
| *Escherichia coli* | 10-30 |
| *Klebsiella* spp. | 10 |
| Other organisms | 2-10 |
| **Anaerobic Organisms** | |
| *Peptococcus* spp. | 5-65 |
| *Peptostreptococcus* spp. | 25-35 |
| *Bacteroides* spp. | 20-40 |
| *Bacteroides fragilis* | 5-15 |
| *Fusobacterium* spp. | 5-25 |
| *Clostridium* spp. | 5-20 |
| *Eubacterium* spp. | 5-35 |
| *Veillonella* spp. | 10-30 |

From Eschenbach DA. Vaginal infection. *Clin Obstet Gynecol.* 1983;26(1):186-202.

In addition to lactobacilli, other common aerobic bacteria found in the vagina are diphtheroids, streptococci, *Staphylococcus epidermidis,* and *Gardnerella vaginalis.* The most common gram-negative bacillus is *Escherichia coli.* Anaerobic bacteria have been detected in approximately 80% of women, with the most prevalent being *Peptococcus, Peptostreptococcus,* and *Bacteroides* spp. (Table 23.4). *Candida* spp. and mycoplasmas are also common inhabitants of asymptomatic women. Our knowledge of vaginal flora has traditionally relied on classic microbiology. Newer molecular techniques are demonstrating even greater complexity in vaginal flora.

The clinical diagnosis of vaginitis depends on the examination of the vaginal secretions under the microscope and measurement of the vaginal pH. Nevertheless, it is helpful to generalize about the characteristics of normal secretions and the three common vaginal infections (Table 23.5).

Normal vaginal secretions are white, floccular or curdy, and odorless. In a woman with a normal or physiologic discharge, it is important to note that the vaginal discharge is present only in the dependent portions of the vagina. Pathologic discharges usually involve the anterior and lateral walls of the vagina. It should be emphasized that vaginal discharge characteristics, especially the amount of discharge, are insensitive and nonspecific diagnostic criteria for vaginitis. However, thick, white, curdy, patchy discharge, when present, is highly associated with fungal infections. Gray-white discharges that are thin and usually profuse suggest a differential diagnosis of *Trichomonas* or bacterial vaginosis, as do vaginal discharges that have a foul odor.

Table 23.5 Typical Features of Vaginitis

| Condition | Symptoms and Signs* | Findings on Examination* | pH | Wet Mount | Comment |
|---|---|---|---|---|---|
| Bacterial vaginosis† | Increased discharge (white, thin), Increased odor | Thin, whitish gray, homogeneous discharge, cocci, sometimes frothy | >4.5 | Clue cells (>20%) shift in flora<br>Amine odor after adding potassium hydroxide to wet mount | Greatly decreased lactobacilli<br>Greatly increased cocci<br>Small curved rods |
| Candidiasis | Increased discharge (white, thick)‡<br>Dysuria<br>Pruritus<br>Burning | Thick, curdy discharge<br>Vaginal erythema | <4.5 | Hyphae or spores | Can be mixed infection with bacterial vaginosis, *T. vaginalis*, or both, and have higher pH |
| Trichomoniasis§ | Increased discharge (yellow, frothy)<br>Increased odor<br>Dysuria<br>Pruritus | Yellow, frothy discharge, with or without vaginal or cervical erythema | >4.5 | Motile trichomonads<br>Increased white cells | More symptoms at higher vaginal pH |

From Eckert LO. Clinical practice: acute vulvovaginitis. *N Engl J Med.* 2006;355(12):1244-1252.
*Although these features are typical, their sensitivity and specificity are generally inadequate for diagnosis.
†For a diagnosis of bacterial vaginosis, a report of increased discharge has a sensitivity of 50% and a specificity of 49%; odor, a sensitivity of 49% and a specificity of 20%; and pH >4.7, a sensitivity of 97%, and a specificity of 65%, compared with the use of a Gram stain.
‡Of patients presenting with symptoms of vaginitis, 40% report increased (white) discharge, but this discharge is not related to *Candida albicans* in many studies.
§A report of a yellow discharge has a sensitivity of 42% and a specificity of 80%; a frothy discharge on examination has a sensitivity of 8% and a specificity of 99%.

## BACTERIAL VAGINOSIS

Bacterial vaginosis is the most prevalent cause of symptomatic vaginitis, with a prevalence of approximately 15% to 50% (Allsworth, 2007). Bacterial vaginosis reflects a shift in vaginal flora from lactobacilli-dominant to mixed flora, including genital mycoplasmas, *G. vaginalis*, and anaerobes, such as peptostreptococci, and *Prevotella* and *Mobiluncus* spp. Although *Gardnerella* and anaerobic organisms can be found in women with normal vaginal flora, their concentration increases severalfold in women with bacterial vaginosis concurrent with a marked decrease in lactobacilli.

The origin of bacterial vaginosis remains elusive. No causative agent has been identified. Because of the inability to find a transmissible agent, bacterial vaginosis has not been classified as an STI. Currently, bacterial vaginosis is described as a "sexually associated" infection rather than a true sexually transmitted infection. Risk factors for bacterial vaginosis include new or multiple sexual partners. It also is prevalent in women who have sex with women; genotyping has revealed identical bacterial strains between monogamous lesbian partners. Also, bacterial vaginosis is more common in lesbian couples who share sex toys with each other without cleaning the toys between use (Bailey, 2004; Marrazzo, 2010a, 2010b). Molecular techniques have identified a cluster of noncultivable bacteria related to *Clostridium* in women with bacterial vaginosis (Fredricks, 2005; Hillier, 2005). As newer techniques analyzing vaginal flora evolve, it may be possible to determine a causal agent.

Other risk factors include douching as least monthly or within the prior 7 days, and social stressors (e.g., homelessness, threats to personal safety, insufficient financial resources). A lack of hydrogen peroxide–producing lactobacilli is also a recognized risk factor for bacterial vaginosis and may explain, in part, the higher prevalence of bacterial vaginosis in black women independent of other risk factors.

Histologically, there is an absence of inflammation in biopsies of the vagina—thus the term *vaginosis* rather than *vaginitis.* Bacterial vaginosis has been associated with upper tract infections, including endometritis, pelvic inflammatory disease, postoperative vaginal cuff cellulitis, and multiple complications of infection during pregnancy, such as preterm rupture of the membranes, endomyometritis, decreased success with in vitro fertilization, and increased pregnancy loss of less than 20 weeks' gestation.

In women with bacterial vaginosis, the most frequent symptom is an unpleasant vaginal odor, which patients describe as musty or fishy (Table 23.6). The odor is often stronger following intercourse, when the alkaline semen results in a release of aromatic amines.

The vaginal discharge associated with bacterial vaginosis is thin and gray-white. Speculum examination reveals that the discharge is mildly adherent to the vaginal walls, in contrast to a physiologic discharge, which is in the most dependent areas of the vagina. The vaginal discharge is frothy in approximately 10% of women, and it is rare to have associated pruritus or vulvar irritation.

Bacterial vaginosis is clinically diagnosed. The classic findings on wet smear are clumps of bacteria and clue cells, which are vaginal epithelial cells with clusters of bacteria adherent to their external surfaces (Fig. 23.16). Leukocytes are not nearly as frequent as epithelial cells underneath the microscope.

The four criteria for the diagnosis of bacterial vaginosis are (1) a homogeneous vaginal discharge is present; (2) the vaginal discharge has a pH of 4.5 or higher; (3) the vaginal discharge has an amine-like odor when mixed with potassium hydroxide, the whiff test; and (4) a wet smear of the vaginal discharge demonstrates clue cells more than 20% of the number of the vaginal epithelial cells. For the clinician, three of these four criteria are sufficient for a presumptive diagnosis. Fifty percent of women who have three of the four clinical criteria for bacterial vaginosis are asymptomatic. If available, Gram staining of vaginal secretion is an excellent diagnostic method. A colorimetric test that detects proline iminopeptidase has been developed for office use. Enzyme levels in vaginal fluid are elevated in women with bacterial vaginosis. Vaginal bacterial culture has no role in the evaluation of bacterial vaginosis.

Table 23.6 Diagnostic Tests Available for Vaginitis

| Test | Sensitivity (%) | Specificity (%) | Comments |
|---|---|---|---|
| **Bacterial Vaginosis** | | | |
| pH >4.5 | 97 | 64 | |
| Amsel's criteria | 92 | 77 | Must meet three of four clinical criteria (pH >4.5, thin watery discharge, >20% clue cells, positive whiff test), but similar results achieved if two of four criteria meet Nugent criteria; Gram stain morphology score (1-10) based on lactobacilli and other morphotypes; score of 1-3 indicates normal flora, score of 7-10 bacterial vaginosis; high interobserver reproducibility |
| Pap smear | 49 | 93 | |
| Point-of-care tests | | | |
| QuickVue Advance, pH + amines | 89 | 96 | Positive if pH >4.7 |
| QuickVue Advance, *G. vaginalis* | 91 | >95 | Tests for proline iminopeptidase activity in vaginal fluid; if used when pH >4.5, sensitivity is 95% and specificity is 99% |
| OSOM BV blue | 90 | <95 | Tests for vaginal sialidase activity |
| **Candida** | | | |
| Wet mount | | | |
| Overall | 50 | 97 | |
| Growth of 3-4 + on culture | 85 | | *C. albicans* a commensal agent in 15%-20% of women |
| Growth of 1 + on culture | 23 | | |
| pH ≤4.5 | Usual | | If symptoms present, pH may be elevated if mixed infection with bacterial vaginosis or *T. vaginalis* present |
| Pap smear | 25 | 72 | |
| ***Trichomonas vaginalis*** | | | |
| Wet mount | 45-60 | 95 | Increased visibility of microorganisms with a higher burden of infection |
| Culture | 85-90 | >95 | |
| pH >4.5 | 56 | 50 | |
| Pap smear | 92 | 61 | False-positive rate of 8% for standard Pap test and 4% for liquid-based cytologic test |
| Point-of-care test: OSOM | 83 | 98.8 | 10 min required to perform tests for *T. vaginalis* antigens |

From Eckert LO. Clinical practice: acute vulvovaginitis. *N Engl J Med.* 2006;355(12):1244-1252.

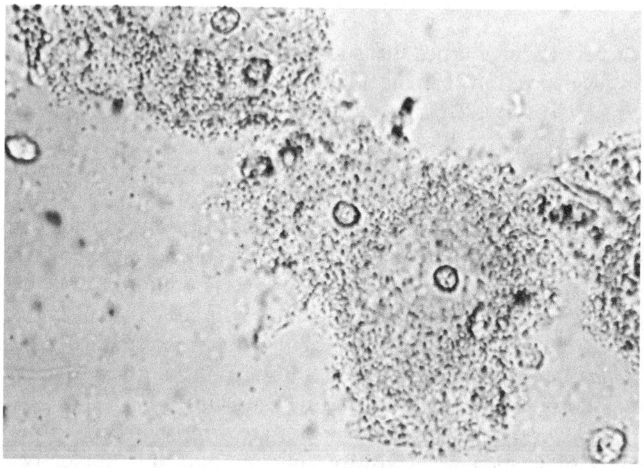

**Figure 23.16** Vaginal epithelial cells from woman with bacterial vaginosis. These are typical clue cells, heavily covered by coccobacilli, with loss of distinct cell margins (× 400). (From Holmes KK. Lower genital tract infections in women: cystitis/urethritis, vulvovaginitis, and cervicitis. In: Holmes KK, Mårdh PA, Sparling PF, et al, eds. *Sexually Transmitted Diseases.* New York: McGraw-Hill; 1984.)

Because there are no effective means of replacing lactobacilli, the treatment for bacterial vaginosis is to decrease anaerobes with antibiotic therapy and hope the woman will then regenerate her own lactobacilli. Table 23.7 provides treatment options. Cure rates are comparable; the agent used should depend on the woman's preference and cost factors. Treatment results in an 80% symptomatic and 70% microbiologic cure at 1 month. Single-dose oral therapy of 2 g of metronidazole is no longer recommended because of high failure rates. alternative regimens include the following: tinidazole, 2 g orally for 3 days or 1 g orally for 5 days; clindamycin, 300 mg orally, twice daily for 7 days; and clindamycin ovules, 100 mg intravaginally, once at bedtime for 3 days.

Recurrent bacterial vaginosis (three or more episodes in the previous year) is a common clinical problem. One double-blind, randomized, placebo-controlled trial demonstrated that after 10 days of daily induction therapy with vaginal metronidazole, the twice-weekly use of 0.75% metronidazole gel for 16 weeks maintains a clinical cure in 75% of patients at 16 weeks and 50% by 28 weeks.

Concurrent treatment of the male partner is not recommended at this time. Alternative therapies such as the use of oral or vaginal *Lactobacillus* are not efficacious.

Table 23.7 Centers for Disease Control and Prevention Recommendations for Treatment of Acute Vaginitis (2015)

| Disease | Drug | Dose | Cost† |
|---|---|---|---|
| Bacterial vaginosis* | Metronidazole (Flagyl) | 500 mg PO, bid for 7 days† | $ |
| | Tinidazole | 2-g dose PO daily for 2 days | $$$ |
| | Tinidazole | 1-g dose PO daily for 5 days | $$$ |
| | 0.75% metronidazole gel (Metrogel) | One 5-g application intravaginally daily for 5 days‡ | $$$ |
| | 2% clindamycin cream (Cleocin vaginal) | One 5-g application intravaginally every night for 7 days | $$$ |
| | Clindamycin | 300 mg PO, bid for 7 days | $ |
| | Clindamycin ovules | 100 mg intravaginally every night for 3 days | $$ |
| **Vulvovaginal Candidiasis, Uncomplicated** | | | |
| Intravaginal therapy‡ § | Azoles | | |
| | 2% butoconazole cream (Mycelex-3) | 5 g/day for 4 days§ | $$ |
| | 2% sustained-release butoconazole cream (Gynazole) | One 5-g dose | $$$ |
| | 1% clotrimazole cream (Mycelex-7) | 5 g for 7-14 days§ | $ |
| | Clotrimazole (Gyne-Lotrimin 3) | Two 100-mg vaginal tablets/day for 3 days; one 500-mg vaginal tablet | $<br>$ |
| | 2% miconazole cream | 5 g/day for 7 days§ | $$ |
| | Miconazole (Monistat-7) | One 100-mg vaginal suppository/day for 7 days§ | $$ |
| | Miconazole (Monistat-3) | One 200-mg vaginal suppository/day for 3 days | $$ |
| | Miconazole (Monistat-1) | One 1200-mg vaginal suppository§ | |
| | 6.5% tioconazole ointment (Monistat 1-day) | One 5-g dose§ | $ |
| | 0.4% terconazole cream (Terazol 7) | 5 g/day for 7 days | $$$ |
| | 0.8% terconazole cream (Terazol 3) | 5 g/day for 3 days | $$ |
| | Terconazole vaginal | One 80-mg vaginal suppository/day for 3 days | $$$ |
| Oral therapy | Fluconazole (Diflucan) | One 150-mg dose PO | $ |
| **Vulvovaginal Candidiasis, Complicated**†‖ | | | |
| Intravaginal therapy‡ | Azole | 7-14 days | $$ |
| Oral therapy¶ | Fluconazole (Diflucan) | Two 150-mg doses PO, 72 hr apart | $$$ |
| Trichomoniasis | Metronidazole (Flagyl) | One 2-g dose PO, 500 mg orally bid for 7 days | $ |
| | Tinidazole (Tindamax) | One 2-g dose PO** | $$ |

Modified from Eckert LO. Clinical practice: acute vulvovaginitis. *N Engl J Med*. 2006;355(12):1244-1252. *Bid*, Twice per day.
*†Oral therapy is recommended for pregnant women.
†‡Drug may cause gastrointestinal upset in 5% to 10% of patients; a disulfiram reaction is possible; alcohol should be avoided for 24 hr after ingestion.
‡§Vaginal treatments cause local vaginal irritation in 2% to 5% of patients.
§This agent is available over the counter.
‖Complicated vulvovaginitis refers to disease in women who are pregnant, women who have uncontrolled diabetes, women who are immunocompromised, or women who have severe symptoms, non-*Candida albicans* candidiasis, or recurrent episodes (four or more/year).
¶Oral therapy is not recommended for pregnant women.
**Drug may cause gastrointestinal upset in 2% to 5% of patients; disulfiram reaction is possible; alcohol should be avoided 72 hr after ingestion.

## TRICHOMONAS *VAGINAL INFECTION*

Trichomoniasis is caused by the anaerobic flagellated protozoon, *T. vaginalis* (Fig. 23.17), a unicellular organism that is normally fusiform in shape. Three to five flagella extend from one end of the organism and provide active movement of the protozoon.

It is estimated that there are 5 million new cases of trichomoniasis annually in the United States. The prevalence of the disease remains high, despite the availability of effective treatments since the early 1960s. *Trichomonas* vaginal infection is the cause of acute vaginitis in 5% to 50% of cases, depending on the population studied, and is the most prevalent nonviral, nonchlamydial STI of women.

This infection is a highly contagious STI; following a single sexual contact, at least two thirds of male and female sexual partners become infected. The protozoa are isolated from 30% to 40% of male partners of women with a positive culture and approximately 85% of female partners of a male with a positive culture. The incubation period is 4 to 28 days. *Trichomonas* is a hardy organism and will survive for up to 24 hours on a wet towel and up to 6 hours on a moist surface. However, experimental studies have established that successful vaginal infection depends on the deposition of an inoculum of several thousand organisms. Hence, it is unlikely that infection may be related to exposure from infected towels or swimming pools.

*Trichomonas* produces a wide variety of patterns of vaginal infection. The primary symptom of *Trichomonas* vaginal infection is profuse vaginal discharge. Patients often complain that the copious discharge makes them feel "wet." Approximately 50% of symptomatic women also detect an abnormal vaginal odor and experience vulvar pruritus; dysuria is a symptom in approximately one of five women with symptomatic *Trichomonas* infection. Women with chronic infection may have a malodorous discharge as their only complaint.

Many women with *Trichomonas* are symptom free. In one study of women with positive cultures, only one out of two women had symptoms of abnormal vaginal discharge, and only one out of six women complained of vulvar pruritus. Positive wet smears or cultures for *Trichomonas* are reported in 3% to 10% of asymptomatic gynecology patients, with a much higher percentage being found in women attending an STI clinic.

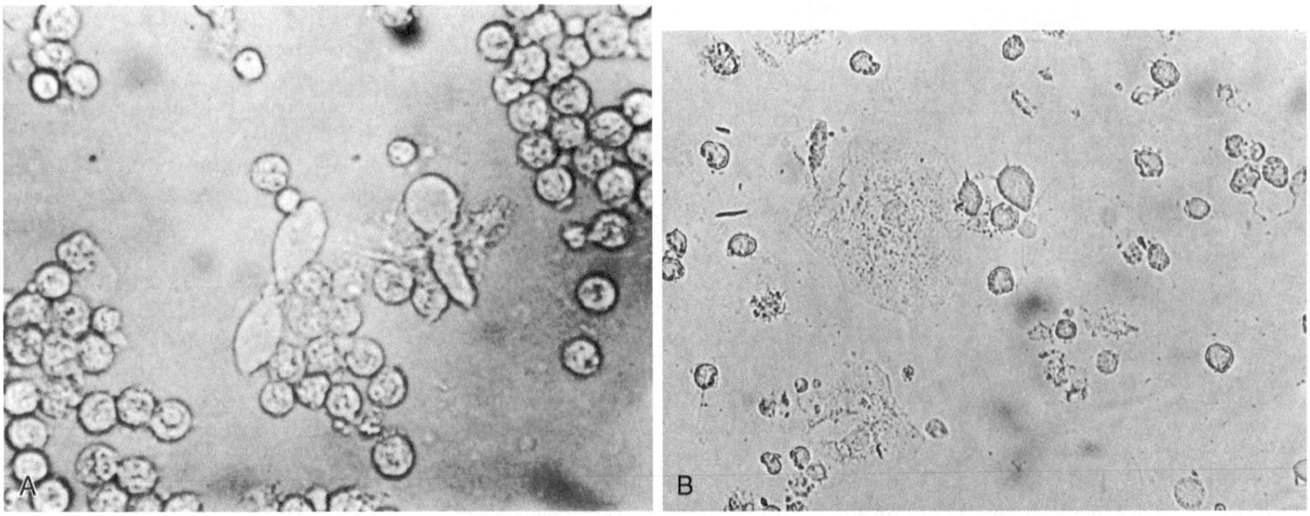


**Figure 23.17** **A** and **B,** Trichomonads in wet mount prepared with physiologic saline. (**A,** From Faro S. Trichomoniasis. In: Kaufman RH, Faro S, eds. *Benign Diseases of the Vulva and Vagina.* 4th ed. St. Louis: Mosby-Year Book; 1994. **B,** From Friedrich EG. *Vulvar Disease.* 2nd ed. Philadelphia: WB Saunders; 1983.)

On physical examination, a woman with *T. vaginalis* may have erythema and edema of the vulva and vagina. Vulvar skin involvement is limited to the vestibule and labia minora, which helps distinguish it from the more extensive vulvar involvement of *Candida* vulvovaginitis. The discharge color may be white, gray, yellow, or green, and the classic discharge of *Trichomonas* infection is termed *frothy* (with bubbles) and often has an unpleasant odor. The classic sign of a strawberry appearance of the upper vagina and cervix is rare and is noted in less than 10% of women.

The CDC encourages use of highly sensitive tests to detect *T. vaginalis* is both symptomatic and asymptomatic women. Nucleic acid amplification tests (NAATs) are three to five times more sensitive than wet prep. NAAT can be performed on vaginal secretions or urine. There are several FDA-approved point of care NAATs to detect *T. vaginalis* (Workowski, 2015).

Previously, culture was considered the gold standard to detect *T. vaginalis,* and wet prep was the most commonly performed diagnostic test (see Table 23.7). Under best conditions when samples are viewed within 10 minutes of collection and the swab does not dry out, wet prep is 80% sensitive to identify trichomonads.

Attempts to diagnose *T. vaginalis* infection by Papanicolaou (Pap) smear results in an error rate of at least 50%. There have been a large number of false-positive and false-negative reports.

Nitroimidazoles are the only class of drugs recommended for treatment of *Trichomonas* vaginitis. A single oral dose (2 g) of metronidazole or tinidazole is recommended. An alternate regimen is metronidazole, 500 mg orally, twice daily for 7 days. Tinidazole is a second-generation nitroimidazole and has a longer half-life of 24 hours. Metronidazole is safe in all trimesters of pregnancy. Tinidazole is categorized as a category C drug in pregnancy. Nausea is the most frequent complication and is experienced by 5% of women. Patients should be warned that nitroimidazoles inhibit ethanol metabolism. Women should avoid alcohol for 24 hours after metronidazole and 72 hours after tinidazole therapy to avoid a disulfiram-like reaction. Topical therapy for *Trichomonas* vaginitis is not recommended because it does not eliminate disease reservoirs in Bartholin and Skene glands. Data have shown that metronidazole, 2-g single oral dose, was not as effective as 500 mg twice daily for 7 days for trichomoniasis in HIV-infected women. Therefore a multidose treatment regimen for *T vaginalis* may be considered for HIV-infected women.

Patients should be rescreened with a NAAT in 3 months due to high reinfection rates. In most cases, women who have a recurrence have been re-infected or complied poorly with therapy. The prevalence of low-level metronidazole resistance in *T. vaginalis* is 2% to 5%; in case series, prolonged treatment with higher doses of metronidazole and tinidazole has been successful. Because *T. vaginalis* is sexually transmitted, treatment of the woman's partner is important and increases cure rates. If reexposure is not an issue, and the infection is not cleared after adequate therapy, one should consult the CDC treatment guidelines for further therapeutic options or for assistance in performing susceptibility testing (Workowski, 2015).

Asymptomatic women with *Trichomonas* identified in the lower genital urinary tract should be treated. Extended follow-up studies have shown that one of three asymptomatic women will become symptomatic within 3 months. Furthermore, HIV acquisition is increased in women with *Trichomonas* infection. Similar to bacterial vaginosis, *T. vaginalis* is associated with upper genital tract infections, including infections after delivery, surgery, abortion, pelvic inflammatory disease, preterm delivery, infertility, and cervical dysplasia treatment. Because all STIs have common epidemiologic backgrounds, finding one dictates carrying out appropriate studies to rule out colonization or infection with another STI.

## CANDIDA *VAGINITIS*

*Candida vaginalis* is produced by a ubiquitous, airborne, gram-positive fungus. In most populations, more than 90% of cases are caused by *Candida albicans* (Fig. 23.18), with 5% to 10%

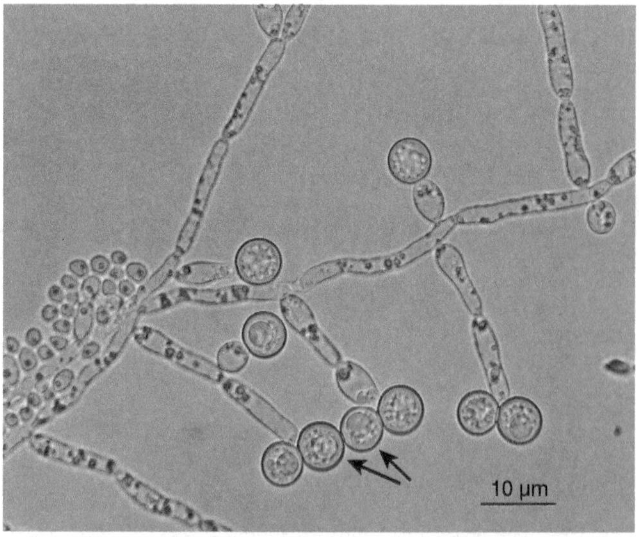


**Figure 23.18** High power microscopic view of *Candida albicans*. (From Marsh P, Lewis M, Williams D, et al, eds. *Oral Microbiology*. 5th ed. Edinburgh: Churchill Livingstone; 2010.)

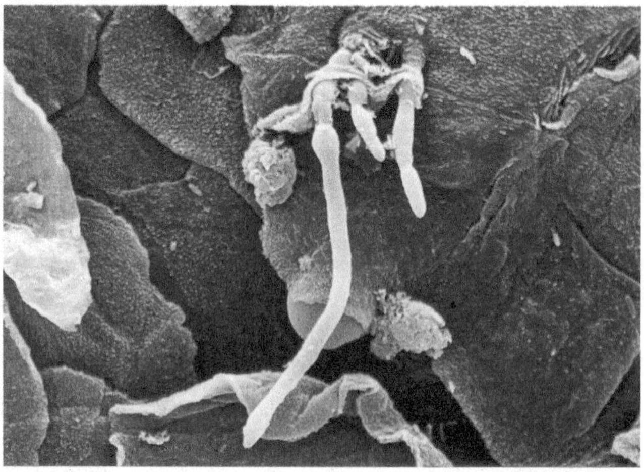

**Figure 23.19** Scanning electron micrograph of intraluminal debris of specimen of vaginal wall taken from patient with vaginal candidiasis (× 3500). The hyphae of *C. albicans* penetrate the epithelial layers of vaginal surface. (From Merkus JM, Bisschop MP, Stolte LA. The proper nature of vaginal candidosis and the problem of recurrence. *Obstet Gynecol Surv.* 1985;40:493-504.)

of vaginal fungal infections produced by *Candida glabrata* or *Candida tropicalis. Candida* spp. are part of the normal flora of approximately 25% of women, being a commensal saprophytic organism on the mucosal surface of the vagina. Its prevalence in the rectum is three to four times greater and in the mouth two times greater than in the vagina. *Candida* organisms develop filamentous (hyphae and pseudohyphae) and ovoid forms, termed *conidia, buds,* or *spores.* The filamentous forms of *C. albicans* have the ability to penetrate the mucosal surface and become intertwined with the host cells (Fig. 23.19). This results in secondary hyperemia and limited lysis of tissue near the site of infection. In contrast, *C. glabrata* does not produce filamentous forms.

When the ecosystem of the vagina is disturbed, *C. albicans* can become an opportunistic pathogen. Hormonal factors, depressed cell-mediated immunity, and antibiotic use are the three most important factors that alter the vaginal ecosystem. The hormonal changes associated with pregnancy and menstruation favor growth of the fungus. The prevalence of *Candida* vaginitis increases throughout pregnancy, probably as a result of the high estrogen levels. The literature was initially mixed with respect to the relationship between oral contraceptives and candidiasis. However, with the currently used low-dose estrogen oral contraceptives, there is no increase in the incidence of fungal vaginitis. Women tend to report recurrent episodes of vaginitis immediately preceding and immediately following their menstrual periods.

Lactobacilli inhibit the growth of fungi in the vagina. Therefore when the relative concentration of lactobacilli declines, rapid overgrowth of *Candida* spp. occurs. Broad-spectrum antibiotics, especially those that destroy lactobacilli (e.g., penicillin, tetracycline, cephalosporins), are notorious for precipitating acute episodes of *C. albicans* vaginitis. Obesity and debilitating disease are other predisposing factors.

Probably the most important host factor is depressed cell-mediated immunity. Women who take exogenous corticosteroids and women with AIDS often experience recurrent *Candida* vulvovaginitis. Altered local immune responses, such as hyper–IgE-mediated response to a small amount of *Candida* antigen, may occur in women with recurrent vulvovaginal candidiasis. Also, some women with recurrent vulvovaginal candidiasis have tissue infiltration with polymorphonuclear (PMN) leukocytes. This high density of PMNs correlates with symptomatology but does not result in clearance of *Candida.*

Vaginitis caused by fungal infection is primarily a disease of the childbearing years. It is estimated that three of four women will have at least one episode of vulvovaginal candidiasis during their lifetime. The greatest enigma of this condition is the recurrence rate after an apparent cure, varying from 20% to 80%. Approximately 3% to 5% of these women experience recurrent vulvovaginal candidiasis (RVVC), which is defined as four or more documented episodes in 1 year.

Fungal vaginitis usually presents as a vulvovaginitis. Pruritus is the predominant symptom. Depending on the degree of vulvar skin involvement, pruritus may be accompanied by vulvar burning, external dysuria, and dyspareunia. The vaginal discharge is white or whitish gray, highly viscous, and described as granular or floccular, with no odor. The amount of discharge is highly variable. The vulvar signs include erythema, edema, and excoriation. With extensive skin involvement, pustules may extend beyond the line of erythema. During speculum examination, a cottage cheese–type discharge is often visualized, with adherent clumps and plaques (thrush patches) attached to the vaginal walls. These clumps, or raised plaques, are usually white or yellow. The vaginal pH associated with this infection is below 4.5, in contrast to bacterial vaginosis and *Trichomonas* vaginitis, which are associated with an elevated pH.

The diagnosis is established by obtaining a wet smear of vaginal secretion and mixing this with 10% to 20% potassium hydroxide (Fig. 23.20). The alkali rapidly lyses red blood cells and inflammatory cells. Active disease is associated with filamentous forms, mycelia, or pseudohyphae, rather than spores. However, it may be necessary to search the slide and scan many different microscopic fields to identify hyphae or pseudohyphae. The average concentration of organisms is $10^3$ to $10^4$/mL. Although symptoms can be present at a low colony count, the ability to

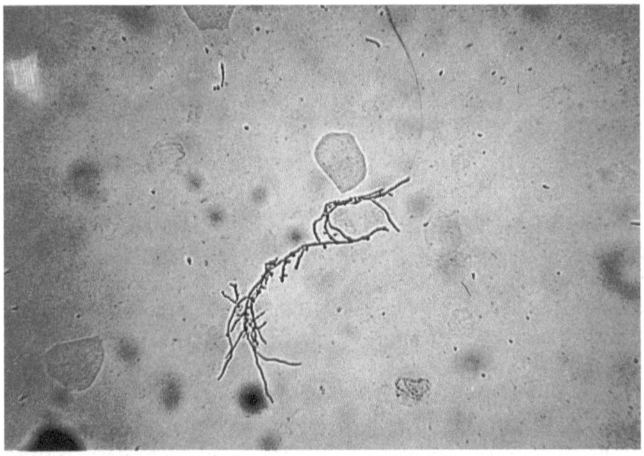

**Figure 23.20** Microscopic appearance of vaginal smear in a case of vaginal candidiasis (potassium hydroxide preparation, yeast cells and pseudomycelia; × 320). (From Merkus JM, Bisschop MP, Stolte LA. The proper nature of vaginal candidosis and the problem of recurrence. *Obstet Gynecol Surv.* 1985;40:493-504.)

detect *C. albicans* on a wet mount is 80% when semiquantitative culture growth is 3 to 4+, but only 20% when culture growth is 2+. Hence, a negative smear does not exclude *Candida* vulvovaginitis. The diagnosis can be established by culture with Nickerson or Sabouraud medium. These cultures will become positive in 24 to 72 hours. Vaginal culture for *Candida* is particularly useful when a wet mount is negative for hyphae, but the patients have symptoms and discharge or other signs suggestive of vulvovaginal candidiasis on examination. Fungal culture may also be useful for women who have recently treated themselves with an antifungal agent; up to 90% have a negative culture within 1 week after treatment. It should be stressed that obtaining a vaginal culture for bacteria is not useful because anaerobes, coliforms, and *G. vaginalis* all are part of normal vaginal flora. The differential diagnosis includes other common causes of vaginitis, such as bacterial vaginosis, *Trichomonas* vaginitis, and atrophic vaginitis. Also, one should consider noninfectious conditions such as allergic reactions, contact dermatitis, chemical irritants, and rare diseases such as lichen planus.

The over-the-counter (OTC) availability of vaginal antifungal therapy makes self-treatment an option for many women. However, it must be recognized that symptoms suggestive of uncomplicated vulvovaginal candidiasis may reflect an alternative diagnosis. One study of women seen at a clinic for STIs found that self-treatment of the symptoms listed on the package insert of an OTC medication for candidiasis would correctly treat only 28% of patients; 53% had bacterial vaginosis, infection with *T. vaginalis*, gonorrhea, or chlamydia. In another study involving women purchasing OTC antifungal therapy, only 34% had vulvovaginal candidiasis and no other vaginal infection. If a woman chooses self-treatment, she should be advised to come in for examination if the symptoms are not eliminated with a single course of OTC therapy.

For treatment of vulvovaginal candidiasis, the CDC recommends placing the woman into an uncomplicated or complicated category to guide treatment (Box 23.3). A number of azole vaginal preparations and a single oral agent, fluconazole, are approved for treatment. In patients with uncomplicated

**Box 23.3 Classification of Vulvovaginal Candidiasis (VVC)**

| **Uncomplicated VVC** | **Complicated VVC** |
|---|---|
| ▪ Sporadic or infrequent vulvovaginal candidiasis | ▪ Recurrent vulvovaginal candidiasis |
| *and* | *or* |
| ▪ Mild to moderate vulvovaginal candidiasis | ▪ Severe vulvovaginal candidiasis |
| *and* | *or* |
| ▪ Likely to be *C. albicans* | ▪ Non-*albicans* candidiasis |
| *and* | *or* |
| • Nonimmunocompromised women | ▪ Women with uncontrolled diabetes, debilitation, or immunosuppression |

Modified from Workowski KA, Bolan GA, Centers for Disease Control and Prevention. Sexually transmitted diseases treatment guidelines, 2015. *MMWR Recomm Rep.* 2015;64(RR-03):1-137.

vulvovaginal candidiasis, topical antifungal agents are typically used for 1 to 3 days, or a single oral dose of fluconazole. Patient preference, response to prior therapy, and cost should guide the choice of therapy (Workowski, 2015).

For patients with complicated vaginitis, topical azoles are recommended for 7 to 14 days. If using oral therapy, a second dose of fluconazole (150 mg) given 72 hours after the first dose is recommended.

In women with RVVC, the resolution of symptoms typically requires longer duration of therapy. Seven to 14 days of topical therapy or three doses of oral fluconazole 3 days apart (e.g., days 1, 4, and 7) are options. After this initial treatment, maintenance therapy will help prevent recurrence of symptoms. Oral fluconazole (e.g., 100-, 150-, or 200-mg dose) weekly for 6 months is typically first-line treatment. However, topical treatments used intermittently as a maintenance regimen may be considered. Women with recurrent vulvovaginitis should receive a vaginal fungal culture to determine species and sensitivities.

Infections with *Candida* spp. other than *C. albicans* are often azole resistant. However, one study of terconazole for non–*C. albicans* fungal vaginitis resulted in a mycologic cure in 56% of patients and a symptomatic cure in 44% of women. Vaginal boric acid capsules (600 mg in 0 gelatin capsules) are another option. In one study, treatment for a minimum of 14 days resulted in a symptomatic cure rate of 70% for women with non–*C. albicans* infection. Boric acid inhibits fungal cell wall growth. It may also be used for suppression in women with recurrent vulvovaginal candidiasis. Following 10 days of therapy, one 600-mg capsule intravaginally twice weekly for 4 to 6 months decreases symptomatic recurrences. Boric acid is toxic if ingested, so it should be stored in a safe manner (Sobel, 1995, 2001, 2003).

Studies of alternative therapies for vulvovaginal candidiasis (such as oral or vaginal *Lactobacillus*, garlic, or diet alterations such as yogurt ingestion) do not show efficacy. A summary of diagnostic tools for determining the cause of vaginitis and a list treatment options are provided in Tables 23.6 and 23.7.

## TOXIC SHOCK SYNDROME

Toxic shock syndrome (TSS) is an acute febrile illness produced by a bacterial exotoxin, with a fulminating downhill course involving dysfunction of multiple organ systems. The cardinal features of the disease are its abrupt onset and rapidity with which the clinical signs and symptoms may present and progress. It is not unusual for the syndrome to develop from a site of bacterial colonization rather than from an infection.

A woman with TSS may develop a rapid onset of hypotension associated with multiorgan system failure. TSS was first described in 1978 by Todd as a sometimes fatal sequela of *Staphylococcus aureus* infection in children. In the early 1980s, more than 95% of the reported cases of TSS were diagnosed in previously healthy, young (<30 years), menstruating females. *S. aureus* was isolated from the vagina in more than 90% of these cases.

Between 1979 and 1996, 5296 TSS cases were reported. Menstrual cases accounted for 74% of total cases, although the proportion has decreased over time (91% from 1979 to 1980, 71% from 1981 to 1986, and 59% from 1986 to 1996). The number of cases of menstrual TSS has declined from 9 of 100,000 women in 1980 to 1 of 100,000 women since 1986. The case-fatality rate has also declined; it was 1.8% from 1987 to 1996 after a high of 5.5% in 1979 to 1980. Most likely, the withdrawal of highly absorbent tampons and polyacrylate rayon–containing products from the market partially explains the decrease. However, tampon use remains a risk factor for TSS. Women who develop TSS are more likely to have used higher absorbency tampons, several cycle days of tampons, and kept a single tampon in for a longer period of time.

Approximately 50% of cases of TSS are not related to menses. Nonmenstrual TSS may be a sequelae of focal staphylococcal infection of the skin and subcutaneous tissue, often following a surgical procedure. It has been recognized that occasionally severe postoperative infections by *Streptococcus pyogenes* produce a similar streptococcal toxic shock–like syndrome. TSS related to a surgical wound occurs early in the postoperative course, usually within the first 48 hours. The proportion of cases following surgical procedures increased from 14% in 1979 to 1986 to 27% in 1987 to 1996.

There are three requirements for the development of classic TSS: (1) the woman must be colonized or infected with *S. aureus*, (2) the bacteria must produce TSS toxin 1 (TSST-1) or related toxins, and (3) the toxins must have a route of entry into the systemic circulation. Most strains of *S. aureus* are unable to produce TSS toxin 1. Interestingly, approximately 85% of women have antibodies against TSST-1.

If an individual woman continues to use tampons when the vagina is colonized with *S. aureus,* there is a significant chance of recurrence. It has been reported that one woman experienced five episodes of the disease. There appears to be no pattern to these recurrent episodes. Interestingly, women with menstrual-related TSS do not respond immunologically to TSST-1 as do women with non–menstrual-related TSS. It is rare for a woman with nonmenstrual TSS to have a recurrence.

The signs and symptoms of TSS are produced by the exotoxin named *toxin 1*. Toxin 1 is a simple protein with a molecular weight of 22,000 kDa and is accepted as the underlying cause of the disease. Thus toxins act as superantigens, molecules that activate up to 20% of T cells at once, resulting in massive cytokine production. Pathophysiologically, superantigens do not require processing by antigen-presenting cells. The primary effects of toxin 1 are to produce increased vascular permeability, thus resulting in profuse leaking of fluid (capillary leak) from the intravascular compartment into the interstitial space and an associated profound loss of vasomotor tone, causing decreased peripheral resistance.

Studies of the bacteriology of the vagina of normal menstruating females have documented that 5% to 17% of women are colonized with *S. aureus*. Approximately 5% test positive when the culture is obtained at midcycle, and the percentage increases to 10% to 17% during menses. Rarely are blood cultures positive for *S. aureus* in a woman with TSS. Thus the exotoxin is believed to be absorbed directly from the vagina. It is possible that microulcerations produced by use of tampons facilitate the toxin's entry into the systemic circulation. The risk of nonmenstrual TSS is definitely increased in women who use barrier contraceptives such as a diaphragm, cervical cap, or a sponge containing nonoxynol 9.

Because of the severity of the disease, gynecologists should have a high index of suspicion for TSS in a woman who has an unexplained fever and a rash during or immediately following her menstrual period. The syndrome has a wide range of symptoms. The varying degree of severity of symptoms and signs depends on the magnitude of involvement of individual organs. Most women experience a prodromal flulike illness for the first 24 hours. Between days 2 and 4 of the menstrual period, the patient experiences an abrupt onset of a high temperature associated with headache, myalgia, sore throat, vomiting, diarrhea, generalized skin rash, and often hypotension. It is important to consider that not all women with TSS experience the full-blown manifestations of the disease. The rigid criteria developed by the CDC are used for epidemiologic studies. Clinically, many women present with a forme fruste of TSS, with low-grade fever and dizziness rather than hypotension.

The most characteristic manifestations of TSS are the skin changes. During the first 48 hours, the skin rash appears similar to intense sunburn. During the next few days, the erythema will become more macular and resemble a drug-related rash. From days 12 to 15 of the illness, there is a fine, flaky desquamation of skin over the face and trunk, with sloughing of the entire skin thickness of the palms and soles. The vaginal mucosa is hyperemic during the initial phase of the syndrome. During pelvic examination, patients complain of tenderness of the external genitalia and vagina. More than 90% of women with TSS experience myalgia, vomiting, and diarrhea (Box 23.4). Many abnormal laboratory findings are associated with the disease and, again, they reflect the severity of involvement of individual organ systems (Box 23.5). The differential diagnosis of toxic shock syndrome includes Rocky Mountain spotted fever, streptococcal scarlet fever, and leptospirosis.

The management of a classic case of severe TSS demands an intensive care unit and the skills of an expert in critical care medicine. The first priority is to eliminate the hypotension produced by the exotoxin. Copious amounts of IV fluids are given while pressure and volume dynamics are centrally monitored. Mechanical ventilation is required for women who develop adult respiratory distress syndrome.

When the woman is initially admitted to the hospital, it is important to obtain cervical, vaginal, and blood cultures for *S. aureus*. Although there have been no controlled series documenting its efficacy, it is prudent to wash out the vagina with saline or dilute iodine solution to diminish the amount of exotoxin that may be absorbed into the systemic circulation.

**Box 23.4 Case Definition of Toxic Shock Syndrome**

1. Fever (temperature 38.9° C [102° F])
2. Rash characterized by diffuse macular erythroderma
3. Desquamation occurring 1-2 wk after onset of illness (in survivors)
4. Hypotension (systolic blood pressure ≤90 mm Hg in adults) or orthostatic syncope
5. Involvement of three or more of the following organ systems:
   a. Gastrointestinal (vomiting or diarrhea at onset of illness)
   b. Muscular (myalgia or creatine phosphokinase level twice normal)
   c. Mucous membrane (vaginal, oropharyngeal, or conjunctival hyperemia)
   d. Renal (BUN or creatinine level ≥ twice normal or ≥5 WBCs/HPF in absence of UTI)
   e. Hepatic (total bilirubin, SGOT, or SGPT twice normal level)
   f. Hematologic (platelets ≤100,000/mm$^3$)
   g. Central nervous system (disorientation or alteration in consciousness without focal neurologic signs when fever and hypotension are absent)
   h. Cardiopulmonary (adult respiratory distress syndrome, pulmonary edema, new onset of second- or third-degree heart block, myocarditis)
6. Negative throat and cerebrospinal fluid cultures (a positive blood culture for *Staphylococcus aureus* does not exclude a case)
7. Negative serologic test results for Rocky Mountain spotted fever, leptospirosis, rubeola

From Centers for Disease Control (CDC). Toxic-shock syndrome, United States, 1970-1982. *MMWR Morb Mortal Wkly Rep.* 1982;31:201.
*BUN*, Blood urea nitrogen; *HPF*, high-powered field; *SGOT*, serum glutamic-oxaloacetic transaminase; *SGPT*, serum glutamic-pyruvic transaminase; *UTI*, urinary tract infection; *WBC*, white blood cell count.

**Box 23.5 Laboratory Abnormalities in Early Toxic Shock Syndrome**

Present in >85% of patients
Coagulase-positive staphylococci in cervix or vagina
Immature and mature polymorphonuclear cells >90% of WBCs
Total lymphocyte count <650/mm$^3$
Total serum protein level <5.6 mg/dL
Serum albumin level <3.1 g/dL
Serum calcium level <7.8 mg/dL
Serum creatinine clearance >1 mg/dL
Serum bilirubin level >1.5 mg/dL
Serum cholesterol level ≤120 mg/dL
Prothrombin time >12 seconds
Present in >70% of patients
Platelet count <150,000/mm$^3$
Pyuria >5 WBCs/HPF
Proteinuria ≥2+
BUN >20 mg/dL
Aspartate aminotransferase (formerly SGOT) >41 U/L

From Chesney PJ, Davis JP, Purdy WK, et al. Clinical manifestations of toxic shock syndrome. *JAMA.* 1981;246:746.
*BUN*, Blood urea nitrogen; *HPF*, high-powered field; *SGOT*, serum glutamic-oxaloacetic transaminase; *WBCs*, white blood cells.
Results were available for at least 18 patients per category with the following exceptions: cervicovaginal cultures (12 patients), cholesterol level (15 patients), and prothrombin time (14 patients).

Women with TSS caused by methicillin-susceptible *S. aureus* should be treated with clindamycin, 600 mg IV every 8 hours, plus nafcillin or oxacillin, 2 g IV every 4 hours. Most experts recommend a 1- to 2-week course of therapy with an antistaphylococcal agent such as clindamycin or dicloxacillin, even in the absence of a positive *S. aureus* culture. In patients with TSS caused by methicillin-resistant *S. aureus* (MRSA), clindamycin plus vancomycin (30 mg/kg/day IV in two divided doses) or linezolid (600 mg oral or IV every 12 hours) is used. If the diagnosis is questionable, it is best to include an aminoglycoside to obtain coverage for possible gram-negative sepsis. Antibiotic therapy probably has little effect on the course of an individual episode of TSS. However, if the underlying cause of toxic shock syndrome is a skin infection, the infected site should be drained and débrided. Treatment with mupirocin to decrease colonization is recommended, applying half of the ointment from a single-use tube into one nostril and the other half into the other nostril twice daily for 5 days.

In summary, the treatment of TSS depends on the severity of involvement of individual organ systems. Not all patients develop a temperature higher than 38.9° C and hypotension. Thus clinicians should be aware of the forme fruste manifestations of the syndrome. The foundation of treatment of the disease is prompt and aggressive management because of the rapidity with which the disease may progress.

It is possible to decrease the incidence of TSS by a change in the use of catamenial products. Women should be encouraged to change tampons every 4 to 6 hours. The intermittent use of external pads is also good preventive medicine. Women will usually accept the recommendation to wear external pads during sleep. The incidence of TSS has decreased dramatically with the removal of super-absorbing tampons from the market. A study by Tierno and Hanna reported that all-cotton tampons are the safest choice to avoid menstrual TSS.

Finally, there are cases of streptococcal toxic shock–like syndromes that are secondary to life-threatening infections with group A streptococcus *(Streptococcus pyogenes)*. Several different exotoxins have been identified, and M types 1 and 3 are the two most common serotypes. In gynecology, most of these cases involve massive subcutaneous postoperative infections. One of the most distinguishing characteristics of a necrotizing skin infection is the intense localized pain in the involved area. Older women and women who are diabetic or immunocompromised are at much greater risk to develop invasive streptococcal infection and streptococcal toxic shock–like syndrome. The mortality rate is approximately 30% when TSS is secondary to group A streptococcal infections (Al-ajmi, 2012; LeRiche, 2012).

## CERVICITIS

Cervicitis, an inflammatory process in the cervical epithelium and stroma, can be associated with trauma, inflammatory systemic disease, neoplasia, and infection. Although it is clinically important to consider all causes of inflammation, this section focuses on infectious origins.

The cervix acts as a barrier between the abundant bacterial flora of the vagina and the bacteriologically sterile endometrial cavity and oviducts. Cervical mucus is much more than a simple physical barrier; it exerts a bacteriostatic effect. Mucus may also act as a competitive inhibitor with bacteria for receptors on the endocervical epithelial cells. Cervical mucus also contains antibodies and inflammatory cells that are active against various sexually transmitted organisms.

Often, the woman is asymptomatic, even though the cervix is colonized with organisms. The cervix is a potential reservoir for *Neisseria gonorrhoeae, Chlamydia trachomatis,* HSV, human papillomavirus, and *Mycoplasma* spp. Cervical infection can be ectocervicitis or endocervicitis. Ectocervicitis can be viral (HSV) or from a severe vaginitis (e.g., strawberry cervix associated with *T. vaginalis* infection) or *C. albicans.* Endocervicitis may be secondary to infection with *C. trachomatis* or *N. gonorrhoeae.* Bacterial vaginosis and *Mycoplasma genitalium* have also been associated with endocervicitis. Infection of the endocervix becomes a major reservoir for sexual and perinatal transmission of pathogenic microorganisms. Primary endocervical infection may result in secondary ascending infections, including pelvic inflammatory disease and perinatal infections of the membranes, amniotic fluid, and parametria.

The histologic diagnosis of chronic cervicitis is so prevalent that it should be considered the norm for parous women of reproductive age. The histopathology of endocervicitis is characterized by a severe inflammatory reaction in the mucosa and submucosa. The tissues are infiltrated with a large number of PMNs and monocytes and, occasionally, there is associated epithelial necrosis. Physiologically, there is a resident population of a small number of leukocytes in the normal cervix. Thus the emphasis is on a severe inflammatory reaction by a large number of PMNs. This section focuses on mucopurulent cervicitis and techniques to diagnose common cervical infections.

## MUCOPURULENT CERVICITIS

The diagnosis of cervicitis continues to rely on symptoms, examination, and microscopic evaluation. Two simple, definitive, objective criteria have been developed to establish mucopurulent cervicitis—gross visualization of yellow mucopurulent material on a white cotton swab (Fig. 23.21) and the presence of 10 or more PMN leukocytes per microscopic field (magnification, × 1000) on Gram-stained smears obtained from the endocervix. Alternative clinical criteria that may be used are erythema and edema in an area of cervical ectopy or associated with bleeding secondary to endocervical ulceration or friability when the endocervical smear is obtained. Women may also report increased vaginal discharge and intermenstrual vaginal bleeding.

The prevalence of mucopurulent cervicitis depends on the population being studied. Approximately 30% to 40% of women attending clinics for STIs and 8% to 10% of women in university student health clinics have the condition. More than 60% of women with this disease are asymptomatic. Symptoms that suggest cervical infection include vaginal discharge, deep dyspareunia, and postcoital bleeding. The physical sign of a cervical infection is a cervix that is hypertrophic and edematous.

*C. trachomatis* is the cause of cervical infection in many women with mucopurulent cervicitis (Fig. 23.22). Depending on the geographic region, gonorrhea is also an important cause of mucopurulent cervicitis. However, most women who have lower reproductive tract infections caused by *C. trachomatis* or *N. gonorrhoeae* do not have mucopurulent cervicitis. The corollary is that most women who have mucopurulent cervicitis are not infected by *C. trachomatis* or *N. gonorrhoeae.* Mucopurulent cervicitis is present in approximately 40% to 60% of women in whom no cervical pathogen can be identified. Thus this condition often persists following adequate broad-spectrum antibiotic therapy. The presence of active herpes infection is correlated with ulceration of the ectocervix but not with mucopus.

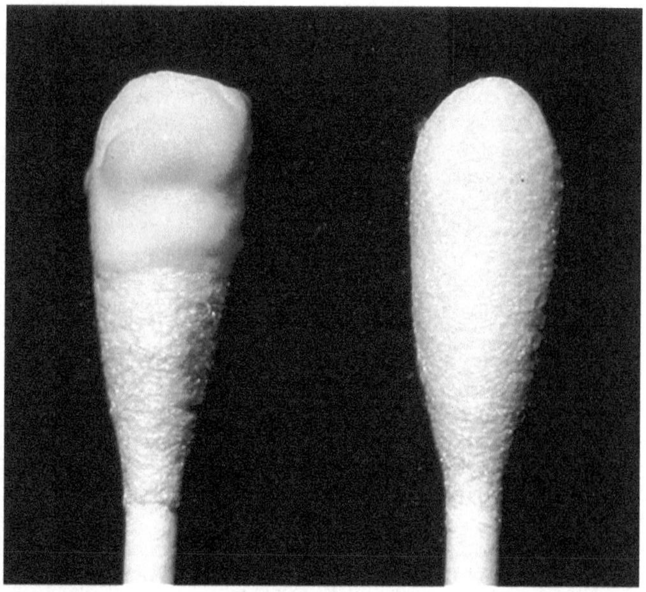

**Figure 23.21** Mucopurulent cervicitis demonstrated by a cotton swab test.

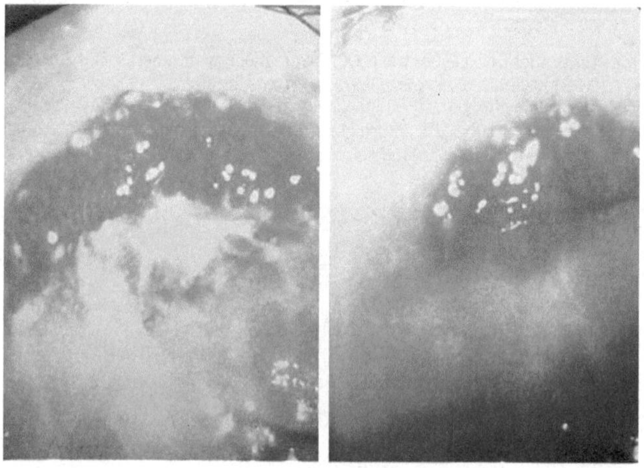

**Figure 23.22** Patient with *C. trachomatis* mucopurulent cervicitis with resolution post treatment.

When mucopurulent cervicitis is clinically diagnosed, empirical therapy for *C. trachomatis* is recommended for women at increased risk of this common STI (age <25 years, new or multiple sex partners, unprotected sex). If the prevalence of *N. gonorrhoeae* is more than 5%, concurrent therapy for *N. gonorrhoeae* is indicated. Concomitant trichomoniasis should also be treated if detected, as should bacterial vaginosis. If presumptive treatment is deferred, the use of a sensitive nucleic acid test for *C. trachomatis* and *N. gonorrhoeae* is needed.

Recommended regimens for presumptive cervicitis therapy include azithromycin, 1 g orally in a single dose, or doxycycline, 100 mg orally twice daily for 7 days, adding gonococcal treatment if the prevalence is over 5% in the population assessed. Women treated for chlamydia should be instructed to abstain from sexual intercourse for 7 days after single-dose therapy or until completion of the 7-day regimen (Workowski, 2015).

*Mycoplasma genitalium,* which is noncultivable, has been associated in women with mucopurulent cervicitis by DNA testing. Empiric treatment for *M. genitalium* in cases of persistent cervicitis after standard treatment may be considered but should be done in consultation with a specialist. There is no FDA-approved diagnostic test for *M. genitalium* in the United States. Some research laboratories may have PCR-based testing. Bacterial vaginosis has also been associated with mucopurulent cervicitis; cervicitis resolved with bacterial vaginosis treatment (Workowski, 2015).

## DETECTION OF PATHOGENIC CERVICAL BACTERIA

### Neisseria gonorrhoeae

Nucleic acid amplification testing (NAAT) of the urine or vaginal secretions is the most sensitive and specific diagnostic tool for identifying gonorrheal infections. Urine tests should be first void (either the first void in morning or at least 1 hour since last void). This technique allows for the sensitive detection of DNA particles originating from the urethra or endocervix, which fall into the vaginal pool and vestibule.

Most women who are colonized with *N. gonorrhoeae* are asymptomatic. Therefore it is important to screen women at high risk for gonorrheal infection routinely. Screening of high-risk individuals is the primary modality to control the disease. Gonorrheal NAAT results are over 95% sensitive and specific.

Antibiotic-resistant gonorrhea culture (GC) is problematic. CDC STD Treatment Guidelines (2015) recommend dual therapy with ceftriaxone 250 mg once IM and azithromycin 1 g orally in a single dose, preferably under direct observation, for all GC infections (Boxes 23.6 and 23.7). Routine co-treatment using two antimicrobials with different mechanisms of action, such as a cephalosporin plus azithromycin, may slow the selection and spread of antibiotic-resistant GC. Based on experience with other microbes that developed antimicrobial resistance rapidly, a theoretic basis exists for combination therapy using two antimicrobials with different mechanisms of action to improve treatment efficacy and potentially delay emergence and spread of resistance to cephalosporins. Azithromycin is preferred to doxycycline because of the convenience and compliance advantages of single-dose therapy and the substantially higher prevalence of gonococcal resistance to tetracycline than to azithromycin in tracked isolates.

If the woman is asymptomatic, the CDC no longer recommends follow-up testing for a test of cure for lower tract infections (uncomplicated gonorrhea). However, studies have shown a high rate of reinfection, so rescreening patients is prudent. Women with positive cultures for gonorrhea should have a serologic test for syphilis in 4 to 6 weeks, even though patients with incubating syphilis are usually cured by antibiotic combinations of ceftriaxone and tetracycline. Similarly, patients should be offered informed consent and testing for HIV infection.

It is important to remember that *N. gonorrhoeae* attaches to the columnar epithelium, so a vaginal cuff swab in women with prior hysterectomies is not recommended (Workowski, 2015).

### Chlamydia trachomatis

As with gonorrhea, the gold standard of techniques used to identify *C. trachomatis* infection is NAAT. *C. trachomatis* also attaches to the columnar epithelium. Hence, vaginal specimens should not be collected from women who have had a hysterectomy. When a culture is used for diagnosis, *C. trachomatis* is an obligatory intracellular organism; hence, it is mandatory to obtain epithelial cells to maximize the percentage of positive cultures. A Dacron, rayon, or calcium alginate swab is placed in the endocervical canal. It is rotated for 15 to 20 seconds to abrade the columnar epithelium gently. The Cytobrush, which was developed primarily to enhance sampling of endocervical cells for cytology, has been found to be the optimal instrument for appropriate sampling for *Chlamydia* culture as well. Chlamydial antigen detection is insensitive and nonspecific compared with NAAT and is no longer recommended.

*C. trachomatis* infection is frequently asymptomatic. Chlamydial screening programs have been successful at decreasing the prevalence of the disease. The CDC recommends annual screening of all sexually active women 25 years of age or younger and screening of older women with risk factors (e.g., those who have a new sex partner or multiple partners).

For all women with a chlamydial or gonorrheal infection, partners should be treated. Patients should be instructed to refer all sex partners of the past 60 days for evaluation and treatment and to avoid sexual intercourse until therapy is completed and they and their partner have resolution of symptoms.

If a woman is unsure whether her partner will be treated, delivery of antibiotic therapy (by prescription or medication)

**Box 23.6 Centers for Disease Control and Prevention Recommended Dual Treatment of Uncomplicated Gonococcal Infections of the Cervix, Urethra, and Rectum in Adults (2014)**

Ceftriaxone, 250 mg IM, single dose
*or, if not an option*
Cefixime, 400 mg PO, single dose
*plus*
Azithromycin 1 g orally in a single doses, preferably under direct observation

Modified from Workowski KA, Bolan GA, Centers for Disease Control and Prevention. Sexually transmitted diseases treatment guidelines, 2015. *MMWR Recomm Rep.* 2015;64(RR-03):1-137.

**Box 23.7 Recommended Regimens for Treatment of Chlamydial Infection**

Azithromycin, 1 g PO, single dose*
*or*
Doxycycline, 100 mg PO bid for 7 days

**Alternative Regimens**
Erythromycin base, 500 mg PO qid for 7 days
*or*
Erythromycin ethylsuccinate, 800 mg PO qid for 7 days
*or*
Ofloxacin, 300 mg PO bid for 7 days
or
Levofloxacin, 500 mg PO once daily for 7 days

Modified from Workowski KA, Bolan GA, Centers for Disease Control and Prevention. Sexually transmitted diseases treatment guidelines, 2015. *MMWR Recomm Rep.* 2015;64(RR-03):1-137. *bid*, Twice per day; *qid*, four times per day.
*Consider concurrent treatment for gonococcal infection if prevalence of gonorrhea is high in the patient population under assessment.

is an option. Studies have demonstrated that patient-delivered partner therapy results in lower rates of chlamydial persistence or recurrence. All women with *C. trachomatis, N. gonorrhoeae,* or mucopurulent cervicitis of unknown origin need evaluation to rule out pelvic inflammatory disease (Workowski, 2015).

## ENDOMETRITIS

Once an infection ascends through the cervix into the endometrium or into the salpinx, it is an upper genital tract infection. Nonpuerperal endometritis is infection of the uterine lining. Although endometritis commonly coexists with salpingitis, several studies have supported endometritis as a distinct clinical syndrome. In one large study of 152 women with suspected pelvic inflammatory disease (PID), all of whom underwent laparoscopy and endometrial biopsy, 43 (28%) had neither endometritis nor salpingitis, 26 (17%) had isolated endometritis, and 83 (55%) had acute salpingitis. Those with endometritis alone had distinct risk factors (douching in past 30 days, current intrauterine device [IUD] in place, and douching in days 1 to 7 of the menstrual cycle). Also, among those women with suspected PID, endometritis was associated with clinical manifestations (e.g., cervical motion tenderness, rebound, fever) and infection with *N. gonorrhoeae, C. trachomatis,* or both intermediate in frequency between women with salpingitis and those with neither salpingitis nor endometritis.

The gold standard diagnosis of endometritis is based on endometrial biopsy. At least one plasma cell/×120 field of endometrial stroma combined with five or more neutrophils in the superficial endometrial epithelium/×400 field is the histopathologic criterion for endometritis. In severe cases, diffuse lymphocytes and plasma cells in the endometrial stroma or stromal necrosis may be present.

The concept of subclinical endometritis has evolved, in part, because many women with tubal infertility have no history of clinical symptoms consistent with prior PID. Several large cross-sectional studies in various geographic regions have studied women with no symptoms or signs of acute salpingitis (no cervical motion or adnexal or uterine tenderness) to define subclinical endometritis further. Most of these studies were conducted in STI clinics or emergency rooms in women at risk for PID; endometritis is associated with young age (20 to 22 years old in most studies), abnormal uterine bleeding (menorrhagia or metrorrhagia), menstrual cycle day less than 14, douching in past 30 days, and a history of prior PID.

Lower genital tract infections with *C. trachomatis, N. gonorrhoeae,* bacterial vaginosis, *M. genitalium,* and *T. vaginalis* and mucopurulent cervicitis are associated with histologic endometritis with an odds ratio (OR) of 1.5 to 3.0, depending on the study. One study demonstrated that in women with current *N. gonorrhoeae* or *C. trachomatis* infection, endometritis was apparent in 43% of those with a history of prior PID and 23% of those without prior PID. This is suggestive of possible immunologic memory. Some women with endometritis do not have an isolated pathogen.

Because many of the symptoms and signs associated with endometritis are subtle, a clinician needs to have a low threshold for performing an endometrial biopsy to aid in the diagnosis.

Antimicrobial therapy for endometritis is effective. One study has demonstrated significant reduction in abnormal bleeding, cervicitis, uterine tenderness, and histologic endometritis following treatment with cefixime, 400 mg orally, azithromycin, 1000 mg, with or without metronidazole, 500 mg orally twice daily for 7 days. Endometritis in HIV-seropositive women has not been well characterized. One series of 42 seropositive women, none of whom had *C. trachomatis* or *N. gonorrhoeae,* has demonstrated a 38% prevalence of endometritis. Compared with the seropositive women without endometritis, the seropositive women with endometritis did not have increased uterine tenderness, lower counts of $CD4^+$ lymphocytes, or other findings. A small subset of those with endometritis had a repeat endometrial biopsy following antimicrobial therapy, and 50% of the endometritis had resolved histologically. The authors concluded that endometritis in HIV-infected women might be related to pathogens that were not evaluated, to prior infection, or to reduced immunity from HIV.

The sequelae of endometritis distinct from salpingitis are difficult to determine. In a series of 614 women in the PID evaluation and clinical health (PEACH) study, women with endometritis, upper genital tract infection with *N. gonorrhoeae* or *C. trachomatis,* or both were compared with women without endometritis or upper genital tract infection for outcomes of pregnancy, infertility, recurrent PID, and chronic pelvic pain. The women with endometritis or upper genital tract infection had higher age- and race-specific pregnancy rates than the national average after adjusting for age, race, education, PID history, and baseline infertility. In the group with clinically suspected mild PID treated with standard antimicrobial therapy, endometritis or upper genital tract infection was not associated with reproductive morbidity.

## PELVIC INFLAMMATORY DISEASE

PID is an infection in the upper genital tract not associated with pregnancy or intraperitoneal pelvic operations. Thus it may include infection of any or all of the following anatomic locations: endometrium (endometritis; see the previous section), oviducts (salpingitis), ovary (oophoritis), uterine wall (myometritis), uterine serosa and broad ligaments (parametritis), and pelvic peritoneum. Many authors prefer the term *salpingitis* because infection of the oviducts is the most characteristic and common component of PID. Importantly, most long-term sequelae of PID result from destruction of the tubal architecture by the infection. In most clinical situations, the terms acute *salpingitis* and *pelvic inflammatory disease* are used synonymously to describe an acute infection.

The incidence of PID in the United States is decreasing. However, the prevalence of STIs and corresponding PID is a major public health concern. The estimated number of cases in women 15 to 44 years of age was 189,662 in 2002 and 168,837 in 2003 (National Ambulatory Medical Care Survey [NAMCS]). The number of hospitalizations for acute PID steadily declined in the 1980s and 1990s, increased somewhat in the period from 2001 to 2004 but, by 2006, had dropped back to 50,000/year, levels consistent with those in 2000. Outpatient visits have also declined. From 2001 to 2008, the number of visits to physician's offices for PID declined from 244,000 to 104,000. Reduction of the medical impact of acute PID requires aggressive therapy for lower genital tract infection and early diagnosis and treatment of upper genital tract infection. Public health emphasis also must be placed on primary prevention involving attempts to prevent exposure and acquisition of STIs. This includes teaching adolescents safe sex practices and promoting the use of condoms and chemical barrier methods. Secondary prevention of PID involves the universal screening of women at high risk for chlamydia and gonorrhea, screening for active cervicitis, increasing use of sensitive tests to diagnose lower genital infection, treatment of sexual partners, and education to prevent recurrent infection.

Acute PID results from ascending infection from the bacterial flora of the vagina and cervix in more than 99% of cases. This ascending infection occurs along the mucosal surface, resulting in bacterial colonization and infection of the endometrium and fallopian tubes. The process sometimes extends to the surface of the ovaries and nearby peritoneum, and rarely into the adjacent soft tissues, such as the broad ligament and pelvic blood vessels. Acute PID is rare in the woman without menstrual periods, such as the pregnant, premenarcheal, or postmenopausal woman. In less than 1% of cases, acute PID results from transperitoneal spread of infectious material from a perforated appendix or intraabdominal abscess. Hematogenous and lymphatic spread to the tubes or ovaries is another remote possibility. Unlike an infection in many other areas of the body that may be caused predominantly by one species of microorganism, acute PID is usually a polymicrobial infection that is a mixture of aerobic and anaerobic bacteria, clinically appearing as a complex infection. More than 20 species of microorganisms have been cultured from direct tubal aspiration of purulent material. Therapeutic strategies and regimens are of a broad range, seeking to suppress aerobic and anaerobic organisms.

Annually, acute PID occurs in 1% to 2% of all young, sexually active women. It is the most common serious infection of women ages 16 to 25 years. Approximately 85% of infections are spontaneous in sexually active females. The other 15% of infections develop following procedures that break the cervical mucus barrier, allowing the vaginal flora the opportunity to colonize the upper genital tract. These procedures include endometrial biopsy, curettage, IUD insertion, hysterosalpingography, and hysteroscopy.

One in four women with acute PID experiences medical sequelae. Following acute PID, the rate of ectopic pregnancy increases 6- to 10-fold, and the chance of developing chronic pelvic pain increases 4-fold. In the United States, each year, 26,100 ectopic pregnancies and 90,000 new cases of chronic abdominal pain are directly related to PID. The incidence of infertility following acute PID varies widely (6% to 60%), depending on the severity of the infection, number of episodes of infection, and age of the woman. Weström reported that hospitalized patients have an incidence of infertility caused by tubal obstruction of 11.4% after one episode of PID, 23.1% after two episodes, and 54.3% after three or more episodes. Women with one episode of acute PID are also more susceptible to developing a subsequent infection. It is difficult to distinguish whether this tendency is related primarily to mucosal damage or to reinfection by a potentially infected mate.

The clinical symptoms and signs of acute PID vary considerably and are usually nonspecific. Importantly, some patients may have very little symptomatology, a condition called silent, or asymptomatic pelvic inflammatory disease. These women may have tubal infertility without a prior history of symptoms or signs consistent with an acute infection (see "Endometritis," presented earlier in the chapter).

Ideally, laparoscopy with direct visualization of the internal female organs not only improves the diagnostic accuracy but also affords the opportunity for direct culture of purulent material, which might help establish optimum therapy. However, most women do not undergo this procedure because of the expense and risk.

In summary, the CDC has emphasized that physicians should treat women aggressively if there is any suspicion of the disease because the sequelae are so devastating and the clinical diagnosis made from symptoms, signs, and laboratory data is often incorrect (Workowski, 2015).

## ETIOLOGY

As noted, acute PID is usually a polymicrobial infection caused by organisms ascending from the vagina and cervix along the mucosa of the endometrium to infect the mucosa of the oviduct. In many cases, no causative organism is found. The two classic sexually transmitted organisms associated with PID, *N. gonorrhoeae* and *C. trachomatis,* cause acute PID in many cases. These two organisms may frequently coexist in the same individual. Endogenous aerobic and anaerobic bacteria that originate from the normal vaginal flora are cultured from tubal fluid in approximately 50% of cases. In women with bacterial vaginosis (BV) and PID, BV-associated microorganisms have been isolated laparoscopically from the fallopian tubes, demonstrating ascension of these organisms. Direct cultures have shown that tubal infections are usually polymicrobial throughout the active infectious process. One investigator found an average of seven different species in intraabdominal cultures obtained via the laparoscope. Laparoscopic studies have demonstrated a correlation of no more than 50% between endocervical and tubal cultures. Thus endocervical cultures are, at best, a crude index of the specific cause of upper genital tract infection.

Approximately 15% of women with cervical infection by *N. gonorrhoeae* subsequently develop acute PID. The virulence of the strain or colony type of *N. gonorrhoeae* helps predict the incidence of upper genital tract infection. Transparent colonies of *N. gonorrhoeae* on culture medium attach more readily to epithelial cells and thus produce tubal infection more frequently than opaque-appearing colonies. Immunologic studies have demonstrated that an antibody against the outer membrane protein of the gonococcus develops in approximately 70% of women following severe pelvic infection. The lack of significant antibody titers may help explain why teenagers are more likely to develop upper genital tract disease than women in their late 20s.

There is an extremely wide variation in the recovery rates of *N. gonorrhoeae,* depending on the geographic location of the study (Table 23.8). However, the prevalence of *N. gonorrhoeae* cervicitis in young women is significantly increased in the South and southeastern regions of the United States. Therefore the proportion of patients with salpingitis from *N. gonorrhoeae* in these regions is likely much higher than in the Pacific Northwest or other geographic regions with a low gonorrhea prevalence.

Once the gonococcus ascends to the fallopian tube, it selectively adheres to nonciliated mucus-secreting cells. However, most damage occurs to the ciliated cells, most likely because of

Table 23.8 Comparison of *C. trachomatis* and *N. gonorrhoeae* Cervical Isolation and *N. gonorrhoeae* Tubal Isolation in Women with Acute Pelvic Inflammatory Disease

| | | Cervical Infection | | Tubal or Peritoneal Infection* |
|---|---|---|---|---|
| Author† | No. of Patients | *C. trachomatis* | *N. gonorrhoeae* | *N. gonorrhoeae* |
| Henry-Suchet | 17 | 6/16 (38%) | 0/4 | 1/4 (25%) |
| Møller | 166 | 37 (22%) | 9 (5%) | |
| Mårdh | 60 | 23 (38%) | 4 (5%) | |
| Gjønnaess | 65 | 26/56 (46%) | 5 (8%) | 0/65 |
| Mårdh | 63 | 19/53 (36%) | 11 (17%) | 1/14 (7%) |
| Adler | 78 | 4 (5%) | 14 (18%) | |
| Ripa | 206 | 52/156 (33%) | 39 (19%) | |
| Osser | 209 | 52/111 (47%) | 41 (20%) | |
| Paavonen | 106 | 27 (25%) | 27 (25%) | |
| Paavonen | 101 | 32 (32%) | 25 (25%) | |
| Paavonen | 228 | 69 (30%) | 60 (26%) | |
| Eilard | 22 | 6 (27%) | 7 (32%) | 1/22 (5%) |
| Bowi | 43 | 22 (51%) | 15 (35%) | |
| Eschenbach | 204 | 20/100 (20%) | 90 (44%) | 7/54 (13%) |
| Sweet | 39 | 2 (5%) | 18 (46%) | 8/35 (23%) |
| Cunningham | 104 | | 56 (54%) | 30/104 (29%) |
| Thompson | 30 | 3 (10%) | 24 (80%) | 10/30 (33%) |
| Total | 1741 | 400/1365 (29%) | 445/1728 (26%) | 58/328 (18%) |

From Eschenbach DA. Acute pelvic inflammatory disease, vol 1. In: *Gynecology and Obstetrics*. Philadelphia: Harper & Row; 1985:8.
*Isolation of *N. gonorrhoeae* from the peritoneum of the total number of women studied.
†Reference to studies appears in original source.

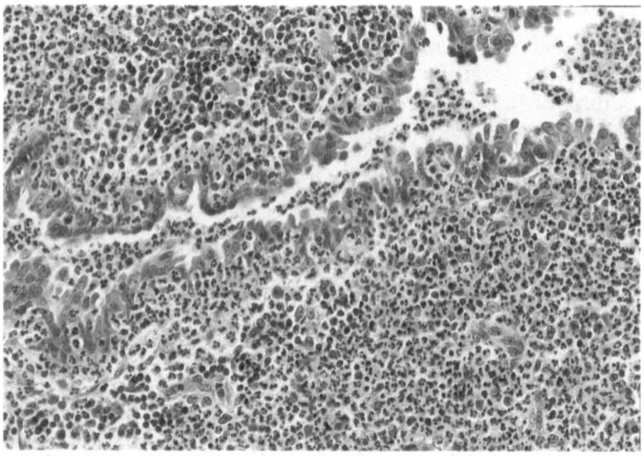

**Figure 23.23** Acute salpingitis with a mixture of neutrophils, lymphocytes, and plasma cells in the fallopian tube destroying some of the epithelial lining. (From Voet RL. *Color Atlas of Obstetric and Gynecologic Pathology*. St. Louis: Mosby; 1997:107.)

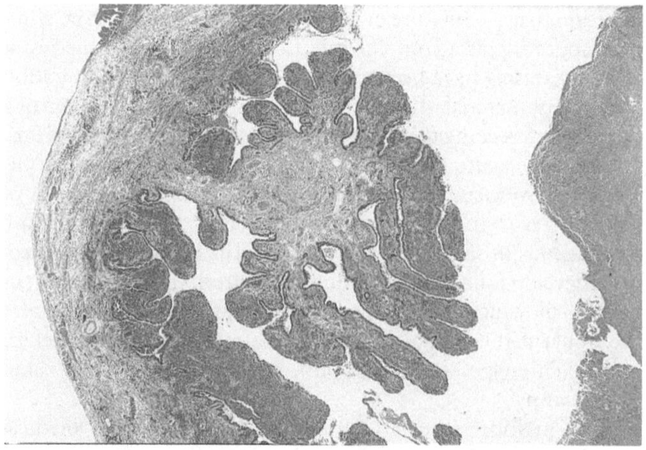

**Figure 23.24** Acute salpingitis showing dilation of the fallopian tube and blunting of the papillary fronds. (From Voet RL. *Color Atlas of Obstetric and Gynecologic Pathology*. St. Louis: Mosby; 1997:102.)

an acute complement-mediated inflammatory response with the migration of polymorphonuclear leukocytes, vasodilation, and transudation of plasma into the tissues (Figs. 23.23 and 23.24). This robust inflammatory response causes cell death and tissue damage. The process of repair with removal of dead cells and fibroblast presence results in scarring and tubal adhesions.

*C. trachomatis* is an intracellular, sexually transmitted bacterial pathogen. A report from Edinburgh has found a ratio of chlamydial-to-gonococcal PID diagnosed by laparoscopy of 4:1. However, there is a widespread difference in isolation rates (Table 23.9). Chlamydia has become more prevalent than gonorrhea. From 20% to 40% of sexually active women have antibodies against *C. trachomatis*. From 10% to 30% of women with acute PID who do not have cultures positive for *Chlamydia* have evidence of acute chlamydial infection by serial antibody titer testing. Approximately 30% of women with documented acute cervicitis secondary to chlamydia subsequently develop acute PID (Risser, 2007). Studies have shown that upper tract chlamydial infection increases the risk of an ectopic pregnancy by three to six times compared with women without chlamydial infection.

Whereas *N. gonorrhoeae* remains in the fallopian tubes for at most a few days in untreated patients, *Chlamydia* may remain in the fallopian tubes for months after initial colonization of the upper genital tract. Sophisticated PCR assays, in situ hybridization, and electron microscopy studies have demonstrated the persistence of the *C. trachomatis* in the fallopian tubes for years. Whether this represents persistent or recurrent infection of the upper genital tract is unknown.

**Table 23.9** *Chlamydia trachomatis* in Acute Pelvic Inflammatory Disease

| | | Isolation Rate of *C. trachomatis* | | |
|---|---|---|---|---|
| **Study*** | **Fourfold Rise in Number of Patients** | **Endocervix (%)** | **Peritoneal Cavity (%)** | **Serum Antibodies (%)** |
| Eilard et al | 22 (23) | 6 (27) | 2 (9)† | 5 |
| Mårdh et al | 53 | 19 (37) | 6/20 (30)† | |
| Treharne et al | 143 (62)‡ | | | 88 |
| Paavonen et al | 106 (26) | 27 (26) | | 19/72 |
| Paavonen | 228 (19) | 68 (30) | | 32/167 |
| Mårdh et al | 60 (40) | 23 (38) | | 24/60 |
| Ripa et al | 206 (57)§ | 52/156 (33) | | 118 |
| Gjønnaess et al | 56 (46) | 26 (46) | 5/42 (12)† | 26/52 |
| Møller et al | 166 (21) | 37 (22) | | 34 |
| Osser and Persson | 111 (51) | 52 (47) | | 37/72 |
| Eschenbach et al | 100 (20) | 20 (20) | 1/54 (2)ǁ | 15/74 |
| Sweet et al | 37 (23) | 2 (5) | 0† | 5/22 |
| Thompson et al | 30 | 3 (10) | 3 (10)¶ | |
| Sweet et al | 71 | 10 (14) | 17 (24)** | |
| Wasserheit et al | 22 | 10 (45) | 8 (36)** | |
| Kiviat et al | 55 | 12 (22) | 12 (22)** | |
| Brunham et al | 50 (40) | 7 (14) | 4 (8)¶ | 20 |
| Landers et al | 148 | 41 (28) | 32 (22)** | |
| Soper et al | 84 | 13 (15) | 1 (1)¶, 6 (7)** | |
| Kiviat et al | 69 | | 16 (23) | |

From Sweet RL, Gibbs RS. *Infectious Diseases of the Female Genital Tract*. 3rd ed. Baltimore: Williams & Wilkins; 1995.
*References appear in the original source.
†Fallopian tube.
‡Chlamydial immunoglobulin G (IgG) ≥1:64; 23% had IgM = 1:8.
§Chlamydial IgG ≥1:64; fourfold rise in 28/80 (35%).
ǁCuldocentesis.
¶Exudate from fallopian tube.
**Fallopian tube or endometrial cavity.

Cell-mediated immune mechanisms appear to be important in tissue destruction associated with *C. trachomatis* infection. Primary infection appears to be self-limited, with mild symptoms and little permanent damage. In animals, repeat genital exposures to *C. trachomatis* can induce a chronic hypersensitivity response to chlamydial antigens. Because chlamydial 57-kDa protein and human 60-kDa heat shock protein have homologous regions, repeat exposures to *Chlamydia,* such as may occur in asymptomatic untreated *C. trachomatis* cervical infection, may lead to an autoimmune response that causes severe tubal damage, even if *C. trachomatis* is no longer present. Immunologically sensitized studies have demonstrated that women with antibodies to chlamydial heat shock protein are more likely to have severe tubal scarring and Fitz-Hugh–Curtis syndrome (adhesions between the liver and diaphragm indicating prior peritonitis) than women who do not mount this antibody response. Basic research has demonstrated a genetic modulation of the immune response to *C. trachomatis* infection, with an increased risk in women with human leukocyte antigen (HLA)-1. Preliminary evidence has suggested that the specific chlamydial strain also may be an important variable.

Atypical, or silent, PID is an asymptomatic, or relatively asymptomatic, inflammation of the upper genital tract often associated with chlamydial infection. The sequelae of repeated asymptomatic chlamydial infections are tubal infertility and ectopic pregnancy. Some investigators believe that atypical PID may be the more common form of upper tract infection, and symptomatic PID may just be the tip of the iceberg. As many as 40% of women with cervicitis without upper tract symptoms will also have endometritis noted on endometrial biopsy. Studies of women with tubal infertility have found that many women, although not diagnosed as having had overt PID, have had symptoms of acute pelvic pain (see earlier, Endometritis).

The role of genital mycoplasmas as the cause of acute PID is unclear. Cervical cultures positive for *Mycoplasma hominis* and *Ureaplasma urealyticum* may be obtained from most young, sexually active women; the rate of isolation of genital mycoplasmas from the cervix is approximately 75% and similar in populations of women who are sexually active, with and without PID. Direct tubal cultures have demonstrated *M. hominis* in 4% to 17% and *U. urealyticum* in 2% to 20% of women with acute PID. However, serologic studies in women with acute PID have demonstrated that only one woman in four develops a significant rise in antibody titers to these organisms. Experimental inoculation of the cervix of the grivet monkey has demonstrated that the route of spread of mycoplasmas is via the parametria rather than the mucosa. Thus the primary upper genital tract infection is in the parametria and the tissue surrounding the tubes, not in the tubal lumen. This may help explain the low success rate of direct tubal cultures. Histologically, *Mycoplasma* does not appear to produce damage to the tubal mucosa. These organisms are not highly pathogenic. In summary, in vitro and in vivo studies have suggested that *Mycoplasma* may be a commensal bacterium rather than a pathogen in the oviducts.

However, *M. genitalium,* which is noncultivable and identified by PCR, has been associated with cervicitis, endometritis,

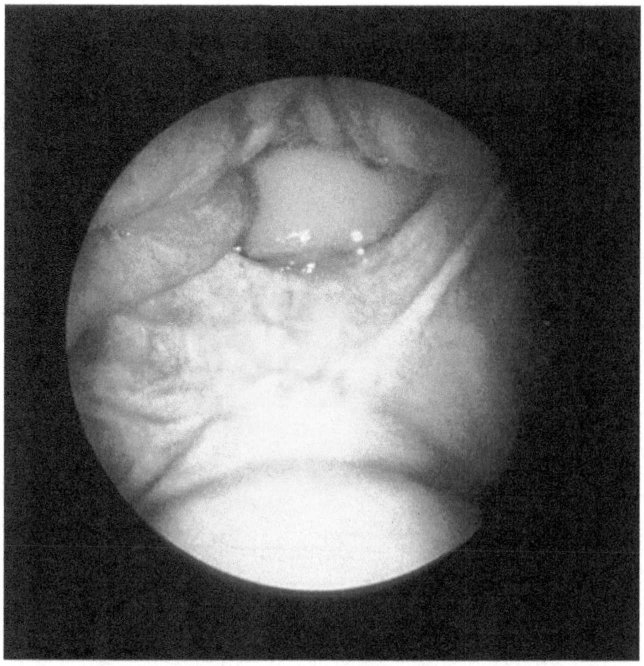

**Figure 23.25** Laparoscopic view of the pouch of Douglas with pus from acute PID.

and tubal factor infertility. In one study of 123 women with laparoscopically determined acute salpingitis, *M. genitalium* was detected in 9 (7%), including 1 woman with a positive fallopian tube specimen. In a different study, *M. genitalium* was detected in the cervix, endometrium, or both of 58 women with histologically confirmed endometritis (Workowski, 2015).

The endogenous aerobic and anaerobic flora of the vagina will frequently ascend to colonize and infect the upper reproductive tract. Direct cultures of purulent material (Fig. 23.25) from the tubal lumen or posterior cul-de-sac have demonstrated a wide range of organisms. The most common aerobic organisms are nonhemolytic *Streptococcus, E. coli,* group B *Streptococcus,* and coagulase-negative *Staphylococcus.* Anaerobic organisms tend to predominate over aerobes, and the most common anaerobic organisms are *Bacteroides* spp., *Peptostreptococcus,* and *Peptococcus.* Anaerobic organisms are almost ubiquitous in pelvic abscesses associated with acute PID. A tubo-ovarian complex and abscess are more common in women with concurrent bacterial vaginosis or HIV infection. The findings of concurrent bacterial vaginosis and PID, as well as the association of bacterial vaginosis with endometritis, emphasize the contributory role of these organisms in the pathogenesis of PID. Regardless of the initiating event, the microbiology of PID should be treated as mixed.

## RISK FACTORS

Risk factors are important considerations in the clinical management and prevention of upper genital tract infections. There is a strong correlation between the incidence of STIs and acute PID in any given population. In epidemiologic studies, age at first intercourse, marital status, and number of sexual partners are all gross indicators of the frequency of exposure to STIs and PID. Having multiple sexual partners increases the chance of acquiring acute PID by approximately fivefold. Social factors such as involvement with a child protective agency, prior suicide attempt, and alcohol use before intercourse have also been identified in case-control studies as risk factors for PID. The frequency of intercourse with a monogamous partner is not a risk factor.

The age distribution of uncomplicated STI is usually the same as that for acute PID. It is a condition of young women, with 75% of cases occurring in women younger than 25 years. The sexual behavior of teenagers, including lack of contraception, predisposes them to STIs and, correspondingly, acute PID. The incidence decreases with advancing age. The risk that a sexually active adolescent female will develop acute PID is 1 in 8, which decreases to 1 in 80 for women older than 25 years. For unknown reasons, young women with colonization of the cervix by *Chlamydia* have a higher incidence of upper genital tract infection than older women. A hypothesis to explain the increased infection rate in teenagers includes the comparative lack of antibody protection and the wider area of cervical columnar epithelium, which allows colonization by *C. trachomatis* and *N. gonorrhoeae.*

Stone and associates tabulated proved and hypothetical methods of preventing STIs and acute PID (Table 23.10). Clinical and laboratory studies have documented that the use of contraceptives changes the relative risk of developing acute PID. Barrier methods (e.g., condoms, diaphragms, spermicidal preparations) are effective as mechanical obstructive devices and as chemical barriers. Nonoxynol 9, the material ubiquitous in spermicidal preparations, is bactericidal and viricidal. Laboratory tests have demonstrated that nonoxynol 9 kills *N. gonorrhoeae,* genital *Mycoplasma* spp., *T. vaginalis, T. pallidum,* HSV, and HIV. However, doses of 100-mg gel, alone or in a contraceptive sponge, are associated with increased epithelial abrasions and ulcers. The porosity of latex in condoms is more than 1000 times smaller than viral particles. Thus routine condom use prevents the deposition and transmission of infected organisms from the semen to the endocervix. Many studies have found that women who frequently use a vaginal douche have a threefold to fourfold increased relative risk of PID over women who douche less frequently than once a month.

Multiple case-control studies carried out 20 to 30 years ago reported an increased risk of acute PID in women who were using an IUD. There has been just criticism of these early epidemiologic studies for their selection of control groups and the bias of including women with Dalkon shield IUDs in their statistics. The increase in risk for PID occurs only at the time of insertion of the IUD and in the first 3 weeks after placement. An analysis from the World Health Organization (WHO) has found the rate of PID to be 9.7/1000 woman-years for the first 20 days after insertion compared with 1.4/1000 woman-years for the next 8 years of follow-up. Studies evaluating the newer progesterone-containing IUD have not shown an increased risk of intrauterine infection. Many experts believe that IUDs may be considered in carefully selected nulliparous patients.

Acute salpingitis occurring in a woman with a previous tubal ligation is extremely rare and, when it does occur, the symptoms of the infection are less severe. Phillips and D'Ablaing reported the incidence of acute PID developing in the proximal stump of previously ligated fallopian tubes, occurring in 1 of 450 women hospitalized for acute salpingitis (Phillips, 1986).

Table 23.10 Methods of Preventing STDs, Mechanisms of Action, and Efficacy

| Method | Mechanism | Efficacy in Prevention of Sexually Transmitted Diseases |
|---|---|---|
| **Behavioral** | | |
| Monogamy<br>Reducing number of partners<br>Avoiding certain sexual practices<br>Inspecting and questioning partners | Decreases likelihood of exposure to infected persons<br>Decreases likelihood of contact with infectious agents | Not well studied; theoretic efficacy |
| **Barriers** | | |
| Condom | Protects partner from direct contact with semen, urethral discharge, or penile lesion<br>Protects wearer from direct contact with partner's mucosal secretions | Effective in vitro barrier to chlamydiae, CMV, and HIV, partial protection HSV<br>Appears to decrease risk of acquiring urethral/cervical GC, PID, and male urethral *Ureaplasma* colonization; partial HPV protection<br>Effect on risk of acquiring NGU not established |
| Spermicide | Chemically inactivates infectious agents | Nonvaginal use has not been studied<br>Inactivates gonococci, syphilis spirochetes, trichomonads, ureaplasmas, and HIV in vitro. In vivo studies disappointing<br>100 mg gel dose and contraceptive sponge associated with epithelial ulcers and abrasions |
| Diaphragm/spermicide | Mechanical barrier covers cervix<br>Used with spermicides | Diaphragm alone has not been studied<br>Appears to decrease risk of acquiring cervical GC and PID |
| Vaccines | Induce antibody response that renders host immune to disease | Commercially available hepatitis B vaccine is safe and effective<br>Results of clinical trials of gonococcal and herpes simplex vaccines ongoing<br>Gonococcal, HIV, and HSV vaccines research in progress<br>Effective quadrivalent HPV vaccine safe and effective |
| **Oral Antibiotics** | | |
| Penicillin | Kill infectious agent on or shortly after exposure before infection is established | No studies among women or civilian men |
| Sulfathiazole | | Appears to decrease risk of acquiring GC and hard and soft chancres, but use not recommended |
| **Local** | | |
| Postcoital urination<br>Postcoital washing | Flushes infectious agents out of urethra and washes infectious agents of genital skin and mucous membrane | Poorly studied |
| Postcoital antiseptic douching | Inactivates and washes infectious agents out of vagina | Poorly studied<br>Not recommended<br>Increases risk of endometritis |

From Stone KM, Grimes DA, Magder LS. Primary prevention of sexually transmitted diseases: a primer for clinicians. *JAMA*. 1986;255(13):1763-1766. Copyright 1986, American Medical Association.

*CMV*, Cytomegalovirus; *GC*, gonorrhea; *HIV*, human immunodeficiency virus; *HPV*, human papillomavirus; *HSV*, herpes simplex virus; *NGU*, nongonococcal urethritis; *PID*, pelvic inflammatory disease.

Epidemiologic studies have documented that previous acute PID is a definite risk factor for future attacks of the disease. Approximately 25% of women with acute PID subsequently develop another acute tubal infection. Direct cultures have proved that the disease is another primary infection. The microscopic tubal damage produced by the initial upper genital tract infection may facilitate repeat infection. It is possible that prior infection causes an immunologic priming effect, making upper genital tract infection more likely with repeated cervical exposure (see earlier discussion of *C. trachomatis* pathology). The increased risk may also be related to an untreated male partner.

Transcervical penetration of the cervical mucus barrier with instrumentation of the uterus is a risk factor because it may initiate iatrogenic acute PID. The incidence of upper genital tract infection associated with first-trimester terminations is approximately 1 in 200 cases. Recent practice has emphasized the use of prophylactic antibiotics to decrease the incidence of associated acute PID. Women with concurrent bacterial vaginosis have a higher risk for postabortal infection and thus should be treated with oral antibiotics with anaerobic coverage.

A growing area of research involves the identification of changes in the virulence of organisms and the host's response to the organisms. Virulence factors of an organism may explain why some lower tract infections progress to upper tract disease but others do not. The gonococcus has characteristics that may become activated in certain environments to increase the virulence of the organism. Similarly, other organisms that are usually of low virulence may have features that affect their virulence and pathogenicity. Both bacterial virulence factors, such as hemolysin enzymes and proteases, and bacterial defense mechanisms that inhibit host responses may become activated in varying microenvironments. Genetic variation may be another risk factor. Some women may be genetically predisposed to mount a robust inflammatory process that may lead to tubal scarring (e.g., chlamydial heat shock protein).

## SYMPTOMS AND SIGNS

Patients with acute PID present with a wide range of nonspecific clinical symptoms and signs. The severity of the clinical presentation of acute PID varies from lack of discernible symptoms to diffuse peritonitis and a life-threatening illness. Because the diagnosis is usually based on clinical criteria, there are high false-positive and high false-negative rates. The diagnosis of acute PID, even by experienced clinicians, is imprecise. The differential diagnosis of acute PID includes lower genital tract pelvic infection, ectopic pregnancy, torsion or rupture of an adnexal mass, acute appendicitis, gastroenteritis, and endometriosis.

Laparoscopic studies of women with a clinical diagnosis of acute PID have established the inadequacy of diagnosis by the usual criteria of history, and physical examination, and laboratory studies. In these studies, approximately 20% to 25% of women had no identifiable intraabdominal or pelvic disease. Another 10% to 15% of patients were found to have other pathologic conditions, such as ectopic pregnancy, acute appendicitis, or torsion of the adnexa (Tables 23.11 and 23.12). In one study of women in whom laparoscopy was performed because of clinically suspected acute PID, the clinical diagnosis was confirmed at laparoscopy in 532 women (65%). Laparoscopic studies also demonstrate a lack of correlation among the number and intensity of symptoms, signs, and degree of abnormality of laboratory values and the severity of tubal inflammation. Women with *C. trachomatis* infections may exhibit minor symptoms but have a severe inflammatory process visualized by laparoscopic examination. Criteria for establishing the severity of acute PID by laparoscopic examination are listed in Table 23.13.

Historically, the diagnosis of acute PID was not established unless the woman had the triad of fever, elevated erythrocyte sedimentation rate (ESR), and adnexal tenderness or a mass. Only 17% of laparoscopically identified cases have this classic triad. Thus reliance on these stringent clinical criteria generally results in most cases being overlooked and untreated. In practice, most women with acute PID do not undergo laparoscopy because of the expense of this invasive technique. Endometrial biopsy is more readily available as a diagnostic tool.

More recently, the PEACH trial found that for women with endometritis diagnosed on endometrial biopsy, the requirement of all three clinical criteria—lower abdominal tenderness, adnexal tenderness, and cervical motion tenderness—resulted in decreased sensitivity. Hence, in 2006, the CDC treatment guidelines were changed to state that empirical therapy for PID should be initiated in sexually active young women and other women at risk for STIs with pelvic or lower abdominal pain if cervical motion tenderness, uterine tenderness, or adnexal tenderness is present. The CDC 2015 diagnostic criteria are summarized in Box 23.8 (Workowski, 2015).

**Table 23.11** Laparoscopic Findings in Patients with False-Positive Clinical Diagnosis of Acute Pelvic Inflammatory Disease (PID) but with Pelvic Disorders Other than PID

| Laparoscopic Finding | Number |
|---|---|
| Acute appendicitis | 24 |
| Endometriosis | 16 |
| Corpus luteum bleeding | 12 |
| Ectopic pregnancy | 11 |
| Pelvic adhesions only | 7 |
| Benign ovarian tumor | 7 |
| Chronic salpingitis | 6 |
| Miscellaneous | 15 |
| Total | 98 |

From Jacobson LJ. Differential diagnosis of acute pelvic inflammatory disease. *Am J Obstet Gynecol*. 1980;138(7 Pt 2):1006-1011.

**Table 23.12** Preoperative Diagnoses in Patients with False-Negative Clinical Diagnosis of Acute Pelvic Inflammatory Disease Prior to Laparoscopy/Laparotomy

| Clinical Diagnosis | Visual Diagnosis: Acute PID (Number) |
|---|---|
| Ovarian tumor | 20 |
| Acute appendicitis | 18 |
| Ectopic pregnancy | 16 |
| Chronic salpingitis | 10 |
| Acute peritonitis | 6 |
| Endometriosis | 5 |
| Uterine myoma | 5 |
| Uncharacteristic pelvic pain | 5 |
| Miscellaneous | 6 |
| Total | 91 |

From Jacobson LJ. Differential diagnosis of acute pelvic inflammatory disease. *Am J Obstet Gynecol*. 1980;138(7 Pt 2):1006-1011.

**Table 23.13** Severity of Disease by Laparoscopic Examination

| Severity | Findings |
|---|---|
| Mild | Erythema, edema, no spontaneous purulent exudates*; tubes freely movable |
| Moderate | Gross purulent material evident; erythema and edema, marked; tubes may not be freely movable, and fimbria stoma may not be patent |
| Severe | Pyosalpinx or inflammatory complex abscess† |

From Hager WD, Eschenbach DA, Spence MR, et al. Criteria for diagnosis and grading of salpingitis. *Obstet Gynecol*. 1983;61:113-114.
*The tubes may require manipulation to produce purulent exudate.
†The size of any pelvic abscess should be measured.

The most frequent symptom of acute PID is new-onset lower abdominal and pelvic pain. Typically, the pain is diffuse, bilateral, and usually described as constant and dull. It may be exacerbated by motion or sexual activity and, on occasion, the pain may become cramping. The duration of pain is usually less than 7 days. If the pain has been present for longer than 3 weeks, it is unlikely that the woman has acute PID. Approximately 75% of patients with acute PID have an associated endocervical infection or coexistent purulent vaginal discharge. Abnormal uterine bleeding, especially spotting or menorrhagia, is noted in approximately 40% of patients.

**Box 23.8 Centers for Disease Control and Prevention Guidelines for Diagnosis of Acute Pelvic Inflammatory Disease: Clinical Criteria for Initiating Therapy**

**Minimum Criteria**

Empirical treatment of PID should be initiated in sexually active young women and others at risk for STIs if the following minimum criteria are present and no other causes(s) for the illness can be identified:

Lower abdominal tenderness *or*
Adnexal tenderness *or*
Cervical motion tenderness

**Additional Criteria for Diagnosing PID**

Oral temperature >38° C
Abnormal cervical or vaginal discharge (mucopurulent)
Presence of abundant WBCs on microscopy of vaginal secretions
Elevated erythrocyte sedimentation rate
Elevated C-reactive protein
Laboratory documentation of cervical infection with *N. gonorrhoeae* or *C. trachomatis*

**Definitive Criteria for Diagnosing PID**

Histopathologic evidence of endometritis on endometrial biopsy
Transvaginal sonography or MRI showing thickened fluid-filled tubes, with or without free pelvic fluid or tubo-ovarian complex
Laparoscopic abnormalities consistent with PID

Although initial treatment can be made before bacteriologic diagnosis of *C. trachomatis* or *N. gonorrhoeae* infection, such a diagnosis emphasizes the need to treat sex partners.

*PID*, Pelvic inflammatory disease; *STIs*, sexually transmitted infections; *WBCs*, white blood cells.
Data from Workowski KA, Bolan GA, Centers for Disease Control and Prevention. Sexually transmitted diseases treatment guidelines, 2015. *MMWR Recomm Rep*. 2015;64(RR-03):1-137.

Nausea and vomiting are relatively late symptoms in the course of the disease.

The symptoms of acute pelvic infection secondary to *N. gonorrhoeae* are of rapid onset, and the pelvic pain usually begins a few days after the start of a menstrual period. Acute pelvic infection caused by *C. trachomatis* alone often may have an indolent course with slow onset, less pain, and less fever. It is important to remember that up to 50% of women with tubal damage never experience any symptoms consistent with PID.

Five percent to 10% of women with acute PID develop symptoms of perihepatic inflammation, the Fitz-Hugh–Curtis syndrome (Fig. 23.26). Persistent symptoms and signs include right upper quadrant pain, pleuritic pain, and tenderness in the right upper quadrant when the liver is palpated. The pain may radiate to the shoulder or into the back. Liver transaminase levels may be elevated. The condition is often mistakenly diagnosed as pneumonia or acute cholecystitis. Fitz-Hugh–Curtis syndrome develops from transperitoneal or vascular dissemination of the gonococcal or *Chlamydia* organism to produce the perihepatic inflammation. Other organisms, including anaerobic streptococci and coxsackievirus, have also been associated with this syndrome. When laparoscopy is performed, the liver capsule will appear inflamed, with classic violin string adhesions to the parietal peritoneum beneath the diaphragm. Women with perihepatitis have a higher prevalence of moderate to severe pelvic adhesions and a higher prevalence and titers of antibodies to

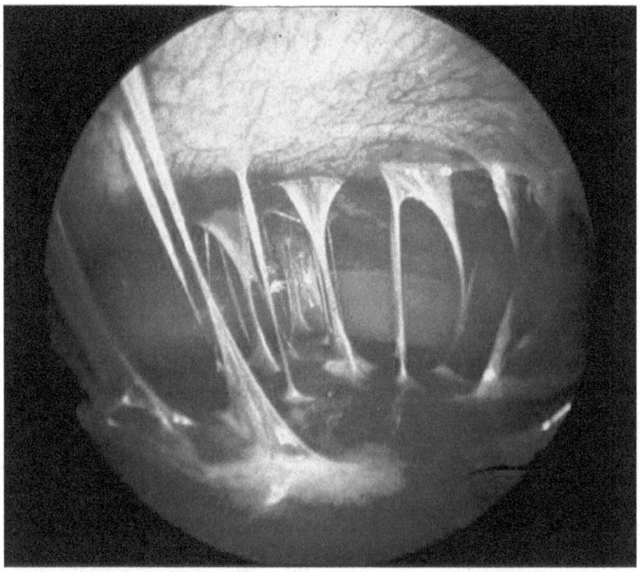

**Figure 23.26** Classic violin string sign of Fitz-Hugh–Curtis syndrome in PID.

chlamydial heat shock protein 60. Treatment is the same as the treatment for acute salpingitis.

Lower abdominal and pelvic tenderness during examination is the hallmark of acute PID. On abdominal examination, patients have tenderness to direct palpation in the lower abdomen, and occasionally rebound tenderness. On pelvic examination, bilateral tenderness of the parametria and adnexa is present and may be exacerbated with movement of the uterus or cervix during the pelvic examination. An ill-defined adnexal fullness is frequently noted, which may represent edema, inflammatory adhesions to the small or large intestine, or an adnexal complex or abscess. The incidence of true adnexal abscess is approximately 10% in women with acute PID.

## DIAGNOSIS

Direct visualization via the laparoscope is the most accurate method of diagnosing acute PID (Binstock, 1986). If the woman has impending septic shock, acute surgical abdomen, or a complicated differential diagnosis in a postmenopausal woman, laparoscopy or laparotomy is strongly indicated. The laparoscopy is diagnostic but also offers the additional advantage of concurrent operative procedures such as lysis of adhesions, potential drainage of an abscess, and irrigation of the pelvic cavity. To date, operative laparoscopy during acute infection has not been proved to reduce the prevalence of long-term sequelae. With the change in management toward outpatient therapy, laparoscopy is used less frequently. Acute PID should be included in the differential diagnosis of any sexually active young woman with pelvic pain.

Elevated temperature is an unreliable diagnostic sign because only one of three women with acute PID present with a temperature higher than 38° C. Laboratory tests may be ordered but are also insensitive and nonspecific. Less than 50% of women with acute PID have a white blood cell count higher than 10,000 cells/mL. Leukocytosis does not correlate with the need for hospitalization or the severity of tubal

Table 23.14 Diagnostic Test Characteristics of Laboratory Tests for the Diagnosis of Acute Upper Genital Tract Infection

| Test | Sensitivity (%) | Specificity (%) | Prevalence (%) 30% NPV | 30% PPV | 60% NPV | 60% PPV |
|---|---|---|---|---|---|---|
| **Entire Cohort (*N* = 120)** | | | | | | |
| ESR | 70 | 52 | 80 | 38 | 54 | 69 |
| CRP | 71 | 66 | 84 | 47 | 60 | 76 |
| WBC | 57 | 88 | 83 | 67 | 58 | 88 |
| Vaginal WBC | 78 | 39 | 80 | 35 | 54 | 66 |
| **Classical PID (*N* = 70)** | | | | | | |
| ESR | 72 | 53 | 82 | 40 | 56 | 70 |
| CRP | 76 | 59 | 85 | 44 | 62 | 74 |
| WBC | 66 | 80 | 85 | 59 | 61 | 83 |
| Vaginal WBC | 87 | 38 | 87 | 38 | 66 | 68 |
| **Nonclassical PID (*N* = 50)** | | | | | | |
| ESR | 64 | 51 | 77 | 36 | 49 | 66 |
| CRP | 58 | 73 | 80 | 48 | 54 | 76 |
| WBC | 38 | 97 | 78 | 84 | 51 | 95 |
| Vaginal WBC | 62 | 41 | 72 | 31 | 42 | 6 |

From Peipert JF, Boardman L, Hogan JW, et al. Laboratory evaluation of acute upper genital tract infection. *Obstet Gynecol.* 1996;87(5 Pt 1):730-736.
*CRP*, C-reactive protein; *ESR*, erythrocyte sedimentation rate; *NPV*, negative predictive value; *PID*, pelvic inflammatory disease; *PPV*, positive predictive value; *WBC*, white blood cell count.

inflammation. The ESR is elevated (>15 mm/hr) in approximately 75% of women with laparoscopically confirmed acute pelvic infection. However, 53% of women with pelvic pain and visually normal pelvic organs have an elevated ESR. C-reactive protein levels have been used but are not reliable enough to guide clinical management. Combinations of positive test results improve diagnostic specificity and positive predictive value. However, this results in a diminution of sensitivity and negative predictive value (Table 23.14). Women with acute PID should have a sensitive test for human chorionic gonadotropin to help in the differential diagnosis of ectopic pregnancy. Approximately 3 to 4 of every 100 women who are admitted to a hospital with a diagnosis of acute pelvic infection have an ectopic pregnancy.

Because most cases of upper genital tract infection are preceded by lower genital tract infection, it is important to examine the endocervical mucus for inflammatory cells and perform the NAAT for *N. gonorrhoeae* and *C. trachomatis*. The presence of an increased number of vaginal white blood cells is the most sensitive laboratory indicator of acute PID. If the cervical discharge appears normal and no white blood cells are found on the wet preparation of vaginal fluid, the diagnosis of PID is unlikely, and alternative causes of pain should be considered.

Because clinical symptoms and signs are nonspecific for the disease, the false-positive and false-negative rates are high when the diagnosis is based on clinical criteria. However, because of the long-term sequelae of the disease, most clinicians maintain a low threshold in entertaining a diagnosis of acute PID, readily accepting that they are treating many women who actually do not have pelvic infection so as not to omit treating those with early or mild disease. For the CDC guidelines for the diagnosis of acute PID, see Box 23.8 (Workowski, 2015).

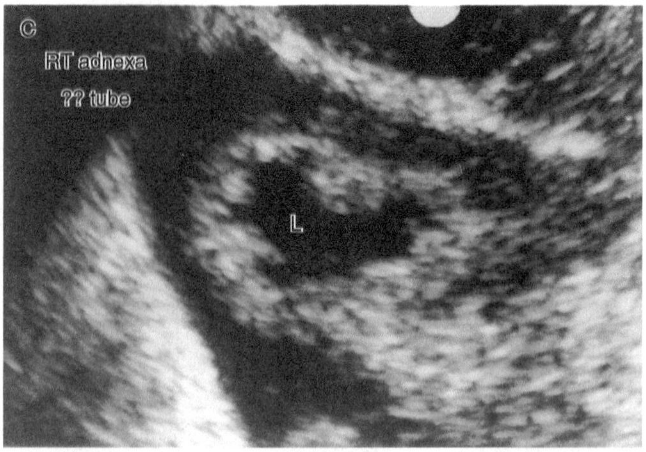


**Figure 23.27** Transvaginal sonographic image of acute salpingitis. The central sonolucent fluid in the lumen *(L)* and the thickened endosalpingeal folds give this a cogwheel appearance. (From Timor-Tritsch IE, Lerner JP, Monteagudo A, et al. Transvaginal sonographic markers of tubal inflammatory disease. *Ultrasound Obstet Gynecol.* 1998;12:56-66.)

An endometrial biopsy for evidence of endometritis can be a useful tool. This test only is used to help confirm clinical suspicion because of the time required to obtain the result. Although most women with acute salpingitis have coexisting endometritis, the converse—that most women with endometritis have salpingitis—has not been established. In one study of women with biopsy-proved endometritis, the accuracy of coexistent acute PID confirmed by laparoscopy had a sensitivity of 89% and a specificity of 87%.

Ultrasonography is of limited value for patients with mild or moderate PID because of its low sensitivity, but vaginal ultrasonography is helpful in documenting an adnexal mass. It is also a noninvasive diagnostic aid for patients who are so tender during pelvic examination that the physician cannot determine the presence or absence of a pelvic mass. Although ultrasonography is neither specific nor sensitive in distinguishing the cause of a pelvic mass, findings of dilated and fluid-filled tubes, free peritoneal fluid, and adnexal masses may confirm symptoms and physical signs (Figs. 23.27 to 23.30). Thus vaginal ultrasound has a high positive predictive value when used in a high-risk population (Romosan, 2014). Magnetic resonance imaging (MRI) is sensitive, but its expense and limited acute availability in some locations have restricted its role in PID diagnosis.

The percentage of American women with acute PID who also are infected with HIV has been estimated to be 6% to 22%. Women with acute PID and HIV infection have a higher incidence of adnexal masses. However, an acute pelvic infection responds to antibiotic therapy in a similar fashion to that in women who are not infected with HIV. The CDC continues to emphasize the importance of treating partners of women with STIs (Workowski, 2015).

## TREATMENT

Treatment of the woman with PID encompasses more than just prescribing the appropriate antimicrobial regimen. Determining the need for hospitalization, patient education, treatment of

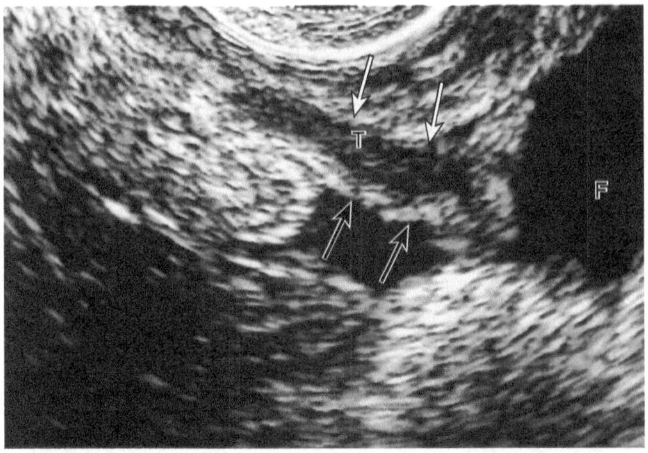


**Figure 23.28** Longitudinal section of a slightly dilated and fluid-filled tube *(T)*. Its walls are slightly thickened *(arrows)*. Endometrial biopsy showed plasma cell endometritis. *F*, Free fluid. (From Cacciatore B, Leminen A, Ingman-Friberg S, et al. Transvaginal sonographic findings in ambulatory patients with suspected pelvic inflammatory disease. *Obstet Gynecol.* 1992;80:912-916.)

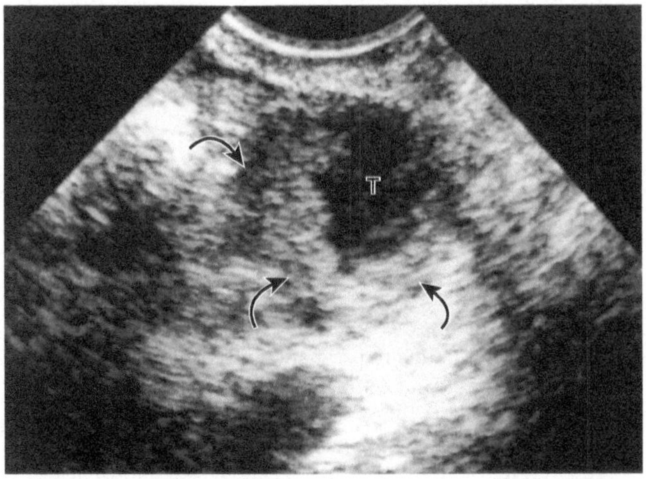


**Figure 23.29** Sonographic image of a cross section of a dilated and fluid-filled fallopian tube *(T)*. The wall is thickened and irregular in shape *(arrows)*. Endometrial biopsy revealed plasma endometritis. (From Cacciatore B, Leminen A, Ingman-Friberg S, et al. Transvaginal sonographic findings in ambulatory patients with suspected pelvic inflammatory disease. *Obstet Gynecol.* 1992;80:912-916.)

sexual partners, and careful follow-up are key issues. The two most important goals of the medical therapy of acute PID are the resolution of symptoms and preservation of tubal function. Antibiotic therapy should be started as soon STI screening results have been obtained and the diagnosis has been suggested. Early diagnosis and early treatment will help reduce the number of women who suffer from the long-term sequelae of the disease. Women who are not treated in the first 72 hours following the onset of symptoms are three times as likely to develop tubal infertility or ectopic pregnancy as those who are treated early in the disease process. Animal and human studies have suggested that early antibiotic treatment improves long-term fertility. In the management of acute PID, one should not forget the treatment and education of the male partner for the prevention of the disease, including the use of proper contraceptives, which help reduce the rate of upper genital tract infection.

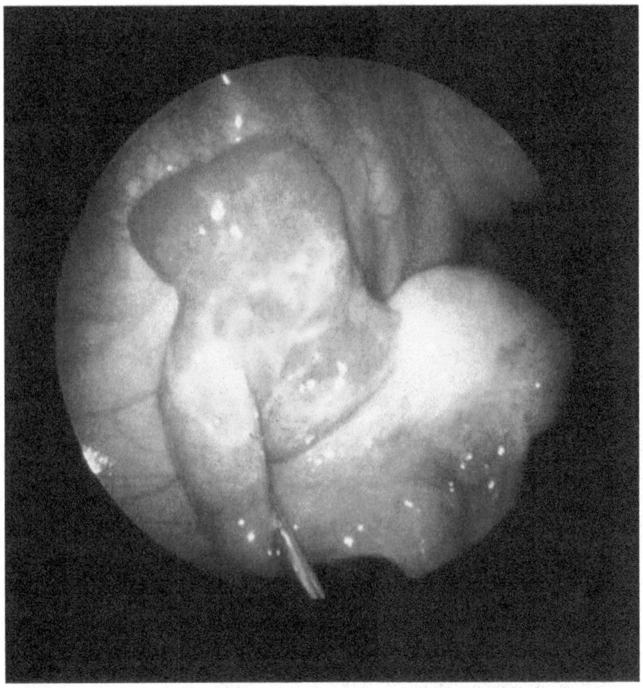

**Figure 23.30** Laparoscopic view of acute PID and a tubo-ovarian abscess.

Although the choice of antibiotic therapy for most infectious diseases is usually based on cultures and sensitivity of bacteria obtained directly from the site of the infection in PID, direct tubal cultures are not practical. Because most cases of PID are polymicrobial, broad-spectrum antibiotic coverage is indicated. Empirical antibiotic protocols should cover a wide range of bacteria, including *N. gonorrhoeae, C. trachomatis,* anaerobic rods and cocci, gram-negative aerobic rods, and gram-positive aerobes (Table 23.15). Selection of one antibiotic protocol over another may be influenced by the clinical history. For example, acute PID following an operative procedure is usually caused by endogenous flora of the vagina, whereas acute PID in a 19-year-old college student is likely secondary to *C. trachomatis.*

A failure of outpatient oral therapy may be related to noncompliance, reinfection, or inadequate antibiotic coverage for penicillinase-producing gonorrhea, chromosomally mediated resistant *N. gonorrhoeae,* or facultative or anaerobic organisms involved in upper genital tract infection that are resistant to the drug prescribed. It is important to know resistance profiles in your geographic region. Inpatient failure rates for resolution of acute symptoms with IV antibiotics are approximately 5% to 10%.

A variety of oral and parenteral antibiotic regimens have been effective in achieving short-term clinical and microbiologic cures in randomized clinical trials. However, there are limited data comparing the effect of various protocols on the incidence of long-term complications and elimination of bacterial infection in the endometrium and fallopian tubes. The CDC has published recommendations for the outpatient treatment of PID (Box 23.9) (Workowski, 2015). Ceftriaxone, 250 mg IM once, or cefoxitin, 2 g IM, plus probenecid, 1 g orally in a single

Table 23.15 Microorganisms Isolated from Fallopian Tubes of Patients with Acute Pelvic Inflammatory Disease

| Type of Agent | Organism |
|---|---|
| Sexually transmitted disease | *Chlamydia trachomatis*<br>*Neisseria gonorrhoeae*<br>*Mycoplasma hominis* |
| Endogenous agent aerobic or facultative | *Streptococcus* species<br>*Staphylococcus* species<br>*Haemophilus*<br>*Escherichia coli* |
| Anaerobic | *Bacteroides* species<br>*Peptococcus* species<br>*Peptostreptococcus* species<br>*Clostridium* species<br>*Actinomyces* species |

From Weström L. Introductory address: treatment of pelvic inflammatory disease in view of etiology and risk factors. *Sex Transm Dis.* 1984;11(4 Suppl):437-440.

**Box 23.9 Centers for Disease Control and Prevention Recommendations for Ambulatory Management of Acute Pelvic Inflammatory Disease**

Ceftriaxone, 250 mg IM, single dose
*or*
Cefoxitin, 2 g IM, single dose, and probenecid, 1 g PO administered concurrently in a single dose
*or*
Other parenteral third-generation cephalosporin (e.g., ceftizoxime, cefotaxime)
*plus*
Doxycycline, 100 mg PO bid for 14 days
*with or without*
Metronidazole, 500 mg PO bid for 14 days

Modified from Workowski KA, Bolan GA, Centers for Disease Control and Prevention. Sexually transmitted diseases treatment guidelines, 2015. *MMWR Recomm Rep.* 2015;64(RR-03):1-137.

dose, concurrently once, or another parenteral third-generation cephalosporin such as ceftizoxime or cefotaxime together with doxycycline, 100 mg orally twice daily for 14 days, is the recommended outpatient regimen. The optimal cephalosporin choice is not known. Ceftizoxime has unparalleled coverage against *N. gonorrhoeae;* cefotaxime has better anaerobic coverage. The clinician should individualize the choice of regimens depending on his or her estimate of the need for anaerobic coverage. Importantly, if the woman has bacterial vaginosis, adding prolonged coverage with metronidazole, 500 mg orally twice daily for 14 days, is preferable.

Other regimens with at least one trial include amoxicillin–clavulanic acid and doxycycline. However, this regimen may be difficult to tolerate because of adverse gastrointestinal symptoms. Azithromycin has demonstrated short-term effectiveness in one randomized trial; another trial used azithromycin combined with ceftriaxone, 250 mg IM single dose, with azithromycin, 1 g orally once weekly for 2 weeks. Also, with these regimens, consider the addition of metronidazole, because anaerobic organisms are suspected in the cause of PID and metronidazole will also treat BV, which is frequently associated with PID. Quinolone-containing regimens are no longer routinely recommended because of gonorrhea resistance. However, if parenteral cephalosporin therapy is not feasible, the use of fluoroquinolones (levofloxacin, 500 mg orally once daily, or ofloxacin, 400 mg twice daily for 14 days), with or without metronidazole, may be considered if the community prevalence and individual risk of gonorrhea are low, or if the diagnostic test result for gonorrhea performed prior to instituting therapy is negative.

**Box 23.10 Indications for Hospitalizing Patients with Acute Pelvic Inflammatory Disease**

Surgical emergencies (e.g., appendicitis) cannot be excluded.
The patient is pregnant.
The patient does not respond clinically to oral antimicrobial therapy.
The patient is unable to follow or tolerate an outpatient oral regimen.
The patient has severe illness, nausea and vomiting, or high fever.
The patient has a tubo-ovarian abscess.

Data from Workowski KA, Bolan GA, Centers for Disease Control and Prevention. Sexually transmitted diseases treatment guidelines, 2015. *MMWR Recomm Rep.* 2015;64(RR-03):1-137.

It is important to reexamine women within 48 to 72 hours of initiating outpatient therapy to evaluate the response of the disease to oral antibiotics. The woman should be hospitalized when the therapeutic response is not optimal. If the disease is responding well, approximately 4 to 6 weeks after therapy the woman should be reexamined to assess the resolution of clinical symptoms and establish a posttreatment baseline.

In the past, many practitioners preferred to hospitalize nulliparous women for the treatment of PID, but this is no longer recommended. A multicenter trial of 831 women has found no advantage to inpatient treatment of mild to moderate PID randomized to inpatient versus outpatient treatment. In over 84 months of follow-up, there were an equivalent number of pregnancies, live births, time to pregnancy, infertility, recurrent PID, chronic pelvic pain, and ectopic pregnancy in the inpatient and outpatient treatment groups. This was true even in teenagers and women without a previous live birth.

The CDC has established criteria for hospitalization (Box 23.10) (Workowski, 2015). These include unsure diagnosis, being too ill to tolerate oral therapy, no improvement with oral therapy, and presence of a tubo-ovarian abscess or pregnancy. Acute PID associated with the presence of an IUD may be more advanced at the time of diagnosis than infection without a foreign body. Patient and physician delays in diagnosis are not unusual. Often, women misinterpret the early signs and symptoms of an infection as being related to the IUD. Pelvic infections with an IUD in place and pelvic infections following operative or diagnostic procedures often are caused by anaerobic bacteria. Outpatient therapy leaving the IUD in situ may be attempted if close follow-up of the woman is possible. If the pelvic infection worsens or does not improve, the IUD should be removed. Concurrent immunodeficiency, especially HIV infection with a low $CD4^+$ count, is another reason to consider hospitalization. If a therapeutic response or compliance with oral medications has not been optimal or is questionable, or if follow-up in 72 hours is not possible, the woman should be admitted for IV antibiotic therapy.

The 2014 CDC guidelines for inpatient treatment of acute PID with parenteral therapy are listed in Box 23.11. The

**Box 23.11 Inpatient Management of Acute Pelvic Inflammatory Disease**

**Parenteral Regimen A**

Cefotetan, 2 g IV every 12 hr

*or*

Cefoxitin, 2 g IV every 6 hr

*plus*

Doxycycline, 100 mg PO or IV every 12 hr

Note: Because of pain associated with infusion, doxycycline should be administered orally when possible, even when the patient is hospitalized. PO and IV administration of doxycycline provide similar bioavailability.

**Parenteral Regimen B**

Clindamycin, 900 mg IV every 8 hr

*plus*

Gentamicin, loading dose IV or IM (2 mg/kg of body weight) followed by a maintenance dose (1.5 mg/kg) every 8 hr. Single daily dosing may be substituted.

**Alternative Parenteral Regimens**

Limited data support the use of other parenteral regimens. The following regimen has been investigated in a least one clinical trial, and has broad-spectrum coverage:

Ampicillin-sulbactam, 3 g IV every 6 hr

*plus*

Doxycycline, 100 mg PO or IV every 12 hr

One trial has demonstrated high short-term clinical cure rates with azithromycin, either as monotherapy for 1 wk (500 mg IV × one or two doses followed by 250 mg PO, 5-6 days) or combined with a 12-day course of metronidazole.

Modified from Workowski KA, Bolan GA, Centers for Disease Control and Prevention. Sexually transmitted diseases treatment guidelines, 2015. *MMWR Recomm Rep*. 2015;64(RR-03):1-137.

protocols stress the polymicrobial origin of acute pelvic infection, increasing importance of *C. trachomatis,* and emergence of penicillin-resistant *N. gonorrhoeae.* With IV protocols, the CDC recommends that IV antibiotics be continued for at least 24 hours after substantial improvement in the patient. When the woman has a mass, we add ampicillin to clindamycin and gentamicin. However, for patients without a mass, we switch to oral antibiotics when the symptoms have diminished and the woman has been afebrile for 24 hours. In both regimens, doxycycline is continued for a total of 14 days.

Regimen A is a combination of doxycycline and IV cefoxitin. It is excellent for community-acquired infection. Doxycycline and cefoxitin provide excellent coverage for *N. gonorrhoeae, C. trachomatis,* and penicillinase-producing *N. gonorrhoeae.* Cefoxitin is an excellent antibiotic against *Peptococcus* and *Peptostreptococcus* spp. and *E. coli.* The disadvantage of this combination is that the two drugs are less than ideal for a pelvic abscess or anaerobic infections. To date, cefotetan has been found to be as effective as cefoxitin. There is no clinically significant difference in the bioavailability of doxycycline whether it is given by the oral or IV route. Thus doxycycline should be administered orally whenever possible because of the marked superficial phlebitis produced by IV infusion.

Doxycycline should be included in the regimen of follow-up oral therapy. Sweet and associates have observed 17 women with PID who initially had endometrial cultures positive for *Chlamydia.* Clinically, 16 of 17 women responded to treatment with cephalosporins alone. However, posttreatment endometrial cultures remained positive for *Chlamydia* in 12 of 13 women. Therefore without tetracycline or erythromycin, a woman may appear free of symptoms but may still be harboring *Chlamydia.* Antibiotics active against *C. trachomatis* must be present in effective dosages for at least 7 days for clinical and microbiologic cures to occur. *C. trachomatis* has a 48- to 72-hour life cycle inside the mucosal cell. Thus prolonged therapeutic levels of the antichlamydial antibiotic are imperative.

Regimen B is a combination of clindamycin and an aminoglycoside (gentamicin). It has the advantage of providing excellent coverage for anaerobic infections and facultative gram-negative rods. Therefore it is preferred for patients with an abscess, IUD-related infection, and pelvic infection after a diagnostic or operative procedure. Studies have demonstrated that high IV levels of clindamycin, such as 900 mg every 8 hours, provide activity against 90% of bacterial strains of *Chlamydia.* Most infectious disease experts recommend the use of a single daily dose of gentamicin rather than a dose given every 8 hours. The initial once-daily aminoglycoside dosage is based on nomograms that take body weight into consideration. The advantages of a once-daily aminoglycoside program are decreased toxicity, increased efficacy, and decreased cost. Also, no serum drug levels must be measured. Aztreonam, a monobactam, has an antibiotic spectrum similar to that of the aminoglycosides but without renal toxicity but is much more expensive. It may be given in a dose of 2 g IV every 8 hours. Also, a third-generation cephalosporin may be used instead of an aminoglycoside in a woman with renal disease. Parenteral antibiotic therapy may be discontinued when the woman has been afebrile for 24 hours, and oral therapy with doxycycline (100 mg twice daily) should continue to complete 14 days of therapy.

Alternative inpatient regimens include ampicillin-sulbactam plus doxycycline because they have excellent anaerobic coverage and would be a good choice for women with a tubo-ovarian complex. The alternative regimen has less extensive clinical trials.

In summary, no regimen is uniformly effective for all patients. To date, there are insufficient clinical data to suggest the superiority of one regimen over another with respect to initial response or subsequent fertility.

Operative treatment of acute PID has decreased markedly since the 1990s. Operations are restricted to life-threatening infections, ruptured tubo-ovarian abscesses, laparoscopic drainage of a pelvic abscess, persistent masses in some older women for whom future childbearing is not a consideration, and removal of a persistent symptomatic mass. Because of the techniques of in vitro fertilization, every effort is made to perform conservative surgery and preserve ovarian and uterine function in women who are not done with childbearing. Unilateral removal of a tubo-ovarian complex or an abscess is a frequent conservative procedure for acute PID. Similarly, drainage of a cul-de-sac abscess via percutaneous drainage or a colpotomy incision results in preservation of the reproductive organs.

Rigorously defined, an abscess is a collection of pus within a newly created space. In contrast, a tubo-ovarian complex is a collection of pus within an anatomic space created by the adherence of adjacent organs. Abscesses caused by acute PID contain a mixture of anaerobes and facultative or aerobic organisms (Figs. 23.31 and 23.32). The environment of an abscess cavity results in a low level of oxygen tension. Therefore anaerobic organisms predominate and have been cultured from 60% to 100% of reported cases. Basic studies have discovered that clindamycin penetrates the human neutrophil, and it is possible that this property facilitates the level of clindamycin within the abscess. Clindamycin is also stable in the abscess environment, which is not true of many other antibiotics. Thus a combination of clindamycin and an aminoglycoside is considered the standard for treatment of a tubo-ovarian abscess. This combination does not treat *Enterococcus*, and ampicillin should be added if there is suspicion that this organism is involved. Metronidazole alone is an effective alternative to clindamycin for anaerobic infections but does not provide gram-negative coverage. If abscesses do not respond to parenteral broad-spectrum antibiotics, drainage is imperative.

Transvaginal or transabdominal percutaneous aspiration or drainage of pelvic abscesses may be accomplished under ultrasonic or computed tomography (CT) guidance. This technique has shown excellent results. In one small, randomized trial, early transvaginal drainage and intensive antibiotic therapy were compared with intensive antibiotic therapy alone. A favorable short-term outcome occurred in 90% of those who underwent ultrasound-guided transvaginal drainage in contrast to 65% of the control group. However, fertility and ectopic pregnancy rates after percutaneous drainage are unknown at this time. Long-term recurrence and sequelae must be evaluated before this technique is accepted as a therapeutic standard. A strong contraindication to percutaneous aspiration is any suspicion of an infected carcinoma in the differential diagnosis. Laparoscopic aspiration of tubo-ovarian complexes is another alternative. This procedure has shown good results but does not have greater benefit than percutaneous ultrasound-guided aspiration of abscess cavities. Laparoscopic aspiration obviously carries more operative risks than ultrasound-guided aspiration.

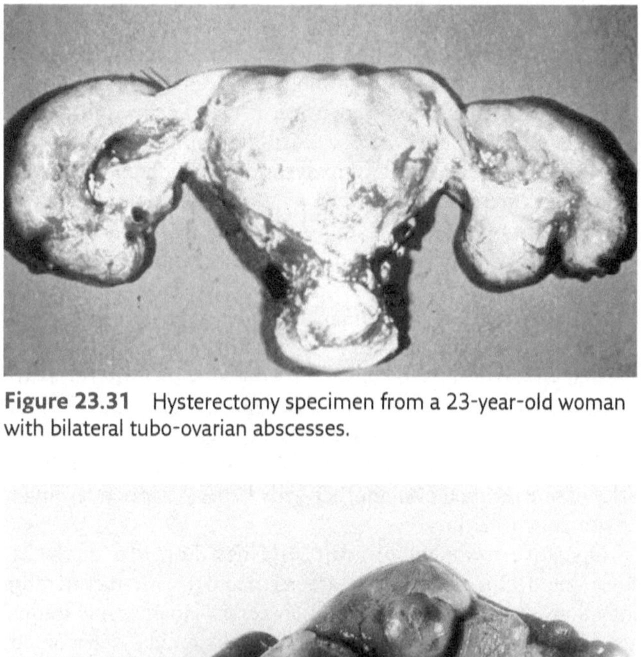

**Figure 23.31** Hysterectomy specimen from a 23-year-old woman with bilateral tubo-ovarian abscesses.

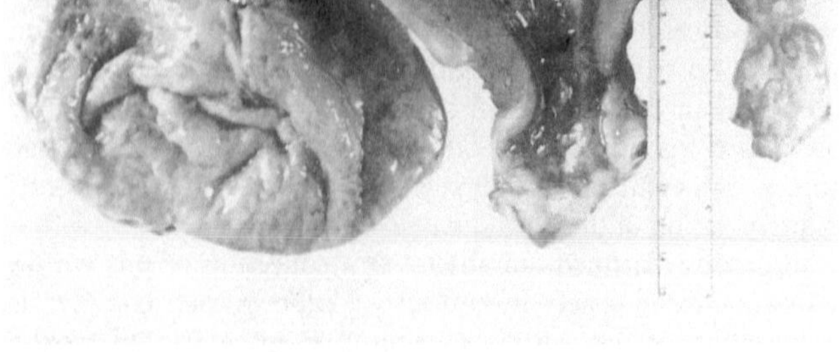

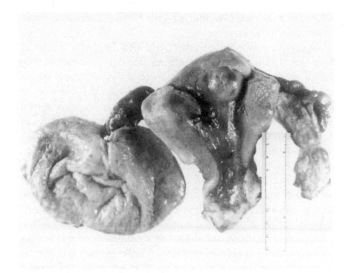

**Figure 23.32** Pyosalpinx. The right tube is markedly enlarged and contains 50 mL of creamy pus. The tubal wall is thickened. (From Janovski NA, ed. *Color Atlas of Gross Gynecologic and Obstetric Pathology*. New York: McGraw-Hill; 1969:131.)

Postmenopausal women with suspected PID should have appropriate imaging studies to rule out other concurrent diseases, especially malignancies. The bacterial cause in postmenopausal women does not usually include a sexually transmitted microorganism, but rather bacteria from the intestinal tract or normal vaginal flora. The disease process involves tubo-ovarian complexes and abscesses. Medical treatment should emphasize broad-spectrum antibiotic regimens with adequate anaerobic coverage. Operative intervention in a postmenopausal woman should be considered early in the disease, especially if the condition does not improve rapidly with medical treatment.

## SEQUELAE

Approximately 25% of women experience recurrent acute PID. Younger women become reinfected twice as often as older women. A great challenge to health care providers is to educate women with PID to reduce their chances of a second episode of infection. It is essential and imperative for preventive medicine to include treatment and education of the male partner. Liberal prescriptions for treatment of lower genital tract disease and selection of contraceptives that will reduce the chance of upper genital tract infections are also important for these women. Because sequelae to PID, overt and silent, are related to the number of infections, prevention cannot be overemphasized. Because most PID in the United States is related to STIs, increased attention to partner treatment and education is appropriate.

The morbidity, suffering, and cost of PID arise from the scarring and adhesion formation that accompany healing of damaged tissues after the infection itself is eradicated. These effects result in ectopic pregnancy, chronic pain, and infertility. Approximately 10% to 15% of pregnancies will be ectopic after laparoscopically mild to moderate PID, and almost 50% after severe PID. The number of hospitalizations for ectopic pregnancies peaked around 1989 at 90,000 and declined to 20,000 in 2009. This decline is partially a result of outpatient management of ectopic pregnancies but is mostly a result of successful chlamydia screening and prevention programs. One case-control study has suggested that chlamydia-associated PID alone causes almost half of all ectopic pregnancies (Table 23.16).

Studies have found that chronic pain is a common sequela of a symptomatic pelvic infection. In one study, the chance that a woman will develop chronic pelvic pain following acute salpingitis was four times greater than the risk for control subjects. Approximately 20% of women with acute pelvic infections subsequently developed chronic pelvic pain versus approximately 5% in controls without pelvic infection. Other studies have found similar results (Table 23.17). Among women with chronic pelvic pain, approximately two of three are involuntarily infertile, and a similar percentage of these women have deep dyspareunia. In a study from Oxford of 1355 women with PID and 10,507 controls, chronic abdominal pain developed 10 times more commonly in those who had PID (Table 23.18). Chronic pelvic pain may be caused by a hydrosalpinx, a collection of sterile watery fluid in the fallopian tube. A hydrosalpinx (Fig. 23.33) is the end-stage development of a pyosalpinx. Chronic pain often develops in a woman, even though she may have had a normal pelvic examination when examined 4 to 8 weeks following her acute infection. The pain may result from adhesions and the resultant fixation or tethering of organs intended to have freedom of movement during physical activity, coitus, and ovulation (Table 23.19). Women with chronic pelvic pain and a history of acute PID may benefit from laparoscopy to establish the diagnosis and rule out other diseases, such as endometriosis.

Acute pelvic infection is one of the major causes of female infertility. Epidemiologic studies have estimated that between 4% and 13% of women are infertile or undergo an operative procedure secondary to acute PID.

The sequelae of infections include a damaged yet patent oviduct, peritubular and periovarian adhesions that may hinder ovum pickup, and finally complete tubal obstruction. Tubal obstructions secondary to infection are commonly found at the fimbrial end or cornual region of the oviduct. An alarming factor that has been documented with chlamydial infection is the tubal damage from subacute PID. Patton and colleagues found almost equally severe tubal damage, adhesion, degeneration of endosalpingeal structures, and cilia dysfunction in women with acute chlamydial PID and women with silent chlamydial infection.

Infertility rates were significantly lower in younger women than in older women following a single episode of infection

**Table 23.16** Summary of Reproductive Events after Index Laparoscopy in the Total Sample of 1732 Patients and 601 Control Subjects

| Category | No. of Patients (%) | No. of Control Subjects (%) |
|---|---|---|
| Total no. followed | 1732 | 601 |
| Avoiding pregnancy | 370 (21.4) | 144 (24.0) |
| Not pregnant for unknown reasons* | 53 (3.1) | 6 (1.0) |
| Attempting pregnancy | 1309 | 451 |
| Pregnant | 1100 (80.8) | 439 (96.1) |
| First pregnancy ectopic | 100 (9.1) | 6 (1.4) |
| Not pregnant | 209 (16.0) | 12 (2.7) |
| Completely examined | 162 | 3 |
| With proved TFI | 141 | 0 |
| With nTFI (other cause of infertility) | 21 | 3 |
| Incompletely examined | 47 | 9 |

From Weström L, Joesoef R, Reynolds G, et al. Pelvic inflammatory disease and fertility: a cohort study of 1,844 women with laparoscopically verified disease and 657 control women with normal laparoscopic results. *Sex Transm Dis.* 1992;19(4):185-192.
*nTFI*, Nontubular factor infertility; *TFI*, tubal factor infertility.
*Reporting no use of contraceptive and not consulting for infertility.

**Table 23.17** Frequency and Predictors of Long-Term Sequelae of Acute Pelvic Inflammatory Disease

| | | | Univariate Analysis | | |
|---|---|---|---|---|---|
| Sequela | Frequency (No. and %) | Risk Factor | *P* | Relative Risk and 95% Confidence Interval | Multivariate Analysis *P* Value |
| Involuntary infertility | 17/42 (40%) | History of PID | 0.05 | 1.8 (1.0-3.3) | 0.05 |
| | | Age at time of first sex | 0.04 | 0.39 | 0.07 |
| | | ≥2 days of pain before therapy | 0.02 | 2.0 (1.1-3.6) | |
| Chronic pelvic pain | 12/51 (24%) | History of PID | 0.03 | 1.5 (1.0-2.2) | |
| PID after index episode | 22/51 (43%) | History of PID | 0.06 | 1.7 (0.9-3.1) | 0.02 |
| | | Mean no. of days of pain before therapy | 0.04 | — | 0.04 |
| | | Age at time of first sex | 0.0008 | — | 0.01 |
| Ectopic pregnancy | 2/51 (2.4%) | * | | | |

From Safrin S Schacter J, Dahrouge D, Sweet RL. Long-term sequelae of acute inflammatory disease: a retrospective cohort study. *Am J Obstet Gynecol.* 1992;166(4):1300-1305.
*Risk analysis not performed because of small numbers involved.
*PID*, Pelvic inflammatory disease.

**Table 23.18** Standardized (Indirect Standardization) First Event Rates per 1000 Woman-Years for Specified Outcomes*

| Outcome Condition | Women with PID (*N* = 1,200) | Women with Control Conditions (*N* = 10,507) | Relative Risk |
|---|---|---|---|
| Nonspecific abdominal pain | 16.7 (155) | 1.7 (158) | 9.8 |
| Gynecologic pain | 3.6 (38) | 0.8 (70) | 4.5 |
| Endometriosis | 2.2 (18) | 0.4 (34) | 5.5 |
| Hysterectomy | 18.2 (152) | 2.3 (204) | 7.9 |
| Ectopic pregnancy | 1.9 (19) | 0.2 (14) | 9.5 |

From Buchan H, Vessey M, Goldacre M, et al. Morbidity following pelvic inflammatory disease. *Br J Obstet Gynaecol.* 1993;100(6):558-562.
*After admission with acute pelvic inflammatory disease or a control event in cohorts of women in the Oxford Record Linkage Study followed from 1970 to 1985. Number of women shown in parentheses.

(Table 23.20). The milder the episode of acute PID, the less likely a woman was to suffer tubal obstruction and infertility. The infertility rate also increased directly with the number of episodes of acute pelvic infection. These data are not surprising because the prevalence of long-term sequelae is directly proportional to the number and severity of the episodes of acute PID. Lepine and coworkers reported additional data from the largest and longest prospective cohort study of women with acute PID. They found that increasing severity of the initial episode of acute pelvic infection correlates with a longer low-term probability of live birth. The cumulative proportion of women achieving a live birth after 12 years was 90% for women whose initial infection was mild, 82% for women with moderate disease, and 57% for women with severe PID. Subsequent episodes of pelvic infection had a greater effect on women whose initial episode was judged as severe as for those with milder disease.

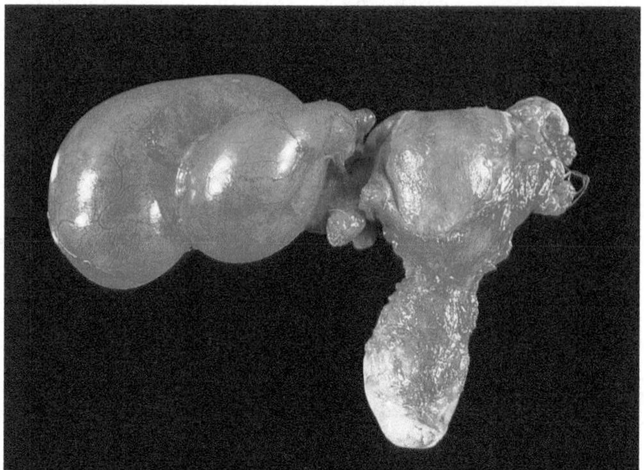

**Figure 23.33** Hydrosalpinx with marked dilation of the fallopian tube and blunting of the fimbriated end. (From Voet RL. *Color Atlas of Obstetric and Gynecologic Pathology*. St. Louis: Mosby; 1997:107.)

## ACTINOMYCES INFECTION

*Actinomyces* is a rare cause of upper genital tract infection. *Actinomyces israelii*, the most common species found, is a gram-positive anaerobic bacterium that is difficult to culture. To culture this organism successfully, an anaerobic environment must be maintained for 2 to 3 weeks.

*A. israelii* is discovered by histologic examination or culture from women with tubo-ovarian abscesses. There are many large series of tubo-ovarian abscesses without a single case of *A. israelii* described. Most cases described have been in women chronically wearing an IUD for an average of 8 years. Usually, *A. israelii* is part of a polymicrobial infection, and whether its role is primary or secondary in the infectious process is unknown.

There is controversy about the significance of discovering actinomycetes on a Pap smear of women wearing an IUD. The contrasting, relatively high detection rate of actinomycetes observed on Pap smears from IUD users, and extreme rarity of subsequent development of pelvic actinomycosis, has led most experts to conclude that progression to upper tract infection is

**Table 23.19** Associations among History of Acute Pelvic Inflammatory Disease and Adnexal Adhesions, Distal Tubal Occlusion, or Perihepatic Adhesions

| | Pelvic Inflammatory Disease | | | | |
|---|---|---|---|---|---|
| **Laparoscopic Findings** | **Yes (*N* = 22)** | **No (*N* = 90)** | **OR** | **95% CI** | ***P*** |
| Distal tubal occlusion | 4 (18.2%) | 7 (7.8%) | 2.6 | 0.7-10.0 | 0.14 |
| Tubal adhesions | 8 (36.4%) | 21 (23.3%) | 1.9 | 0.7-5.1 | 0.16 |
| Ovarian adhesions | 9 (40.9%) | 21 (23.3%) | 2.3 | 0.9-6.5 | 0.08 |
| Perihepatic adhesions | 3/21 (14.3%) | 2/84 (2.4%) | 6.8 | 1.1-43.9 | 0.05 |
| Any adhesions | 11 (50.0%) | 25 (27.8%) | 2.6 | 1.0-6.8 | 0.04 |

From Wølner-Hanssen P. Silent pelvic inflammatory disease: is it overstated? *Obstet Gynecol*. 1995;86(3):321-325.
*CI*, Confidence interval; *OR*, odds ratio.

**Table 23.20** Percentage and Number of Patients Attempting to Conceive*

| | Age (Years) | | |
|---|---|---|---|
| **No. of Episodes of PID** | **<25 % (*n*/*N*)** | **≥25 % (*n*/*N*)** | **Total % (*n*/*N*)** |
| One | 7.7 (59/771) | 9.1 (20/220) | 8.0 (79/991) |
| Mild | 0.8 (2/241) | 0.0 (0/71) | 0.6 (2/312) |
| Moderate | 6.4 (23/361) | 5.6 (5/89) | 6.2 (28/452) |
| Severe | 20.1 (34/169) | 25.0 (15/60) | 21.4 (49/229) |
| Two | 18.4 (29/158) | 25.9 (7/27) | 19.5 (36/185) |
| Three or more | 37.7 (23/61) | 75.0 (3/4) | 40.0 (26/65) |
| Total | 11.2 (111/990) | 12.0 (30/251) | 11.4 (141/1241) |

From Weström L, Joesoef R, Reynolds G, et al. Pelvic inflammatory disease and fertility: a cohort study of 1,844 women with laparoscopically verified disease and 657 control women with normal laparoscopic results. *Sex Transm Dis*. 1992;19(4):185-192.
*Women had tubal factor infertility by age, number of acute PID episodes, and severity of PID, excluding those with nontubal factor infertility and with incomplete infertility examinations.
*n*, Total number of cases followed; *N*, total number of evaluable cases; *PID*, pelvic inflammatory disease.

highly unlikely to be related. The decision to remove the IUD to treat a woman is influenced by the presence or absence of clinical symptoms. Unless there are associated symptoms, such as fever, abdominal pain, or abnormal uterine bleeding, the identification of the organism in any cervical smear should not prompt antibiotic therapy or IUD removal.

Actinomycetes may produce a chronic endometritis, with an associated foul-smelling discharge. The clinical infection may be manifest by widespread adhesions, induration, and fibrosis. The diagnosis of *Actinomyces* infection is usually not made until a tubo-ovarian abscess is examined by the pathologist. Then, the classic sulfur granules are observed histologically, along with gram-positive filaments.

Although much has been written about chronic draining sinuses with *Actinomyces* infection, this complication is unusual in gynecology. However, when this organism is present in a tubo-ovarian abscess, the woman should receive oral penicillin, doxycycline, or a fluoroquinolone for 12 weeks following an operative procedure (Evans, 1993).

## TUBERCULOSIS

Tuberculosis of the upper genital tract, primarily chronic salpingitis and chronic endometritis, is a rare disease in the United States. Most gynecologists may never encounter a single case. However, pulmonary tuberculosis has been steadily increasing in the United States and it is likely that the incidence of pelvic tuberculosis also may rise. Tuberculosis is a frequent cause of chronic PID and infertility in other parts of the world. Thus it should be suspected in immigrants, especially those from Asia, the Middle East, and Latin America. Although the disease is usually found in premenopausal women, it occurs in postmenopausal women 10% of the time.

Pelvic tuberculosis may be produced by *Mycobacterium tuberculosis* or *Mycobacterium bovis*. The primary site of infection for tuberculosis is usually the lung. Early in the course of pulmonary infection, the bacteria spread hematogenously and the infection becomes located in the oviducts, which are the primary and predominant site of pelvic tuberculosis. Subsequently, the bacilli usually spread to the endometrium and, less commonly, to the ovaries. In developing countries without pasteurization of milk, bovine tuberculosis produces primary infections in the human gastrointestinal tract. Subsequent lymphatic or hematogenous dissemination results in pelvic tuberculosis. Autopsy studies published 25 years ago demonstrated that 4% to 12% of women who died of pulmonary tuberculosis concurrently had evidence of upper genital tract infection. In a large study from India, 117 women had tubal blockage secondary to tuberculosis. When these women underwent laparoscopy, the findings were 50% simple tubal blockage, 15% tubo-ovarian masses, and 24% a frozen pelvis.

In general, extrapulmonary tuberculosis may present as an insidious or rapidly progressing disease. The clinical symptoms and signs of pelvic tuberculosis are similar to the chronic sequelae of nontuberculous acute PID. The predominant presentations of this chronic infection are infertility and abnormal uterine bleeding. Mild to moderate chronic abdominal and pelvic pain occur in 35% of women with the disease. Advanced cases are often accompanied by ascites. Some women may be asymptomatic. The findings at pelvic examination are normal in approximately 50% of cases. The remaining patients have mild adnexal tenderness and bilateral adnexal masses, with an inability to manipulate the adnexa because of scarring and fixation.

Tuberculous salpingitis may be suspected when a woman is not responding to conventional antibiotic therapy for acute bacterial PID. Results of a tuberculin skin test will be positive. However, approximately one in three women does not have evidence of pulmonary tuberculosis on chest radiographic films. The diagnosis may be established by performing an endometrial biopsy late in the secretory phase of the cycle. A portion of the endometrial biopsy should be sent for culture and animal inoculation and the remaining portion should be examined histologically. The findings of classic giant cells, granulomas, and caseous necrosis confirm the diagnosis (Fig. 23.34). Approximately two of three women with tuberculous salpingitis will have concomitant tuberculous endometritis. Pelvic tuberculosis may not be diagnosed until laparotomy or celiotomy, when the characteristic changes may be visualized. The distal ends of the oviduct remain everted, producing a tobacco pouch appearance. When the diagnosis has been established, the woman should have a chest radiographic examination, IV pyelography, serial gastric washings, and urine cultures for tuberculosis. Approximately 10% of women with pelvic tuberculosis have concomitant urinary tract tuberculosis.

The treatment of pelvic tuberculosis is medical. Not uncommonly, patients will be admitted to the hospital for initiation of therapy, for observation, and to ensure appropriate compliance. Initial therapy in a woman with newly diagnosed tuberculosis usually will include five drugs because of the emergence of multidrug-resistant organisms. Multidrug-resistant (MDR) tuberculosis is defined as infection from a strain of *M. tuberculosis* that is resistant to two or more agents, including isoniazid. The mortality rate in HIV-negative patients who develop MDR infection may be as high as 80%. Often, health care workers become infected during outbreaks of MDR tuberculosis. The CDC has recommended starting a woman on a

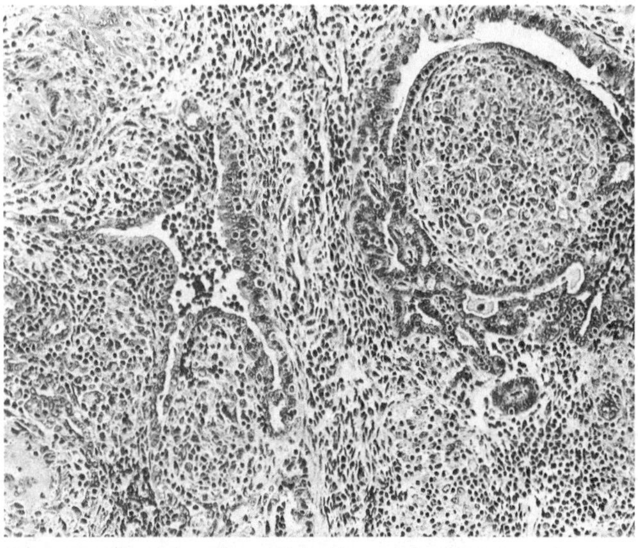

**Figure 23.34** Tuberculous salpingitis—Langerhans giant cell granuloma. (From Gompel C, Silverberg SG, eds. *Pathology in Gynecology and Obstetrics*. 2nd ed. Philadelphia: JB Lippincott; 1977:258.)

multidrug regimen until the culture results yield specific sensitivity. At that time, medications may be decreased to two or three agents. Patients who have infection from MDR strains are usually kept on a five-drug regimen. Operative therapy for pelvic tuberculosis is reserved for women with persistent pelvic masses, some women with resistant organisms, women older than 40 years, and women whose endometrial cultures remain positive. Although the major sequela of pelvic tuberculosis is infertility, occasionally a woman will become pregnant after medical therapy (Chow, 2002; Ilhan, 2004).

## KEY POINTS

- The CDC regularly revises its treatment protocols for STIs. This information may be accessed online at www.cdc.gov/publications.
- Pediculosis pubis, an infestation by the crab louse *Phthirus pubis,* is characterized by constant itching, predominantly vulvar involvement, and the finding of eggs and lice by visual inspection. It may be treated by topical application of 1% permethrin cream rinse (Nix) or 1% lindane shampoo (Kwell).
- Scabies, an infection by the itch mite *Sarcoptes scabiei,* is characterized by intermittent pruritus, most commonly in the hands, wrists, breasts, vulva, and buttocks. It may be treated by a topical application of 5% permethrin cream (Nix) or 1% lindane lotion or 30 g of cream.
- Genital herpes is a recurrent incurable STI. Approximately 80% of individuals are unaware that they are infected. It is usually transmitted by individuals who are asymptomatic and unaware that they have the infection at the time of transmission.
- Nonspecific tests for syphilis, the VDRL and RPR, have a 1% false-positive rate. Therefore specific tests such as the *Treponema pallidum* immobilization (TPI), FTA-ABS, and MHA-TP must be used when a positive nonspecific test result is encountered.
- In women in the reproductive age range, bacterial vaginosis represents approximately 50% of vaginitis cases and candidiasis and *Trichomonas* infection represent approximately 25% each. HIV acquisition is increased in women with bacterial vaginosis and *T. vaginalis* infection.
- *T. vaginalis* infection is a highly contagious STI. It is the most prevalent nonviral, nonchlamydial STI of women. An asymptomatic female who has *Trichomonas* identified in the lower female genital urinary tract should definitely be treated.
- Symptoms that suggest cervical infection include vaginal discharge, deep dyspareunia, and postcoital bleeding. Most women who have lower reproductive tract infections caused by *C. trachomatis* or *N. gonorrhoeae* do not have mucopurulent cervicitis. The corollary is that most women who have mucopurulent cervicitis are not infected by *C. trachomatis* or *N. gonorrhoeae.*
- Acute PID is usually caused by a polymicrobial infection of organisms ascending from the vagina and cervix, traveling along the mucosa of the endometrium to infect the mucosa of the oviduct. It should be diagnosed with a minimum of suspicion with the knowledge that overtreatment is preferable to missed diagnosis.
- Approximately one in four women with acute PID experiences further medical sequelae, including recurrent acute PID, ectopic pregnancy, and chronic pelvic pain.

## KEY REFERENCES


Al-ajmi JA, Hill P, O'Boyle C, et al. Group A Streptococcus toxic shock syndrome: an outbreak report and review of the literature. *J Infect Public Health.* 2012;5(6):388-393.

Al-Mutairi N, Al-Doukhi A, Al-Farag S, et al. Comparative study on the efficacy, safety, and acceptability of imiquimod 5% cream versus cryotherapy for molluscum contagiosum in children. *Pediatr Dermatol.* 2010;27(4):388-394.

Allsworth JE, Peipert JF. Prevalence of bacterial vaginosis: 2001-2004 National Health and Nutrition Examination Survey data. *Obstet Gynecol.* 2007; 109(1):114-120.

Bailey JV, Farquhar C, Owen C. Bacterial vaginosis in lesbians and bisexual women. *Sex Transm Dis.* 2004;31(11):691-694.

Bavaro JB, Drolette L, Koelle DM, et al. One-day regimen of valacyclovir for treatment of recurrent genital herpes simplex virus 2 infection. *Sex Transm Dis.* 2008;35(4):383-386.

Bernstein DI, Bellamy AR, Hook 3rd EW, et al. Epidemiology, clinical presentation, and antibody response to primary infection with herpes simplex virus type 1 and type 2 in young women. *Clin Infect Dis.* 2013;56(3):344-351.

Binstock M, Muzsnai D, Apodaca L, et al. Laparoscopy in the diagnosis and treatment of pelvic inflammatory disease: a review and discussion. *Int J Fertil.* 1986;31(5):341-351.

Chen X, Anstey AV, Bugert JJ. Molluscum contagiosum virus infection. *Lancet Infect Dis.* 2013;13(10):877-888.

Chow TW, Lim BK, Vallipuram S. The masquerades of female pelvic tuberculosis: case reports and review of literature on clinical presentations and diagnosis. *J Obstet Gynaecol Res.* 2002;28(4):203-210.

Evans DT. Actinomyces israelii in the female genital tract: a review. *Genitourin Med.* 1993;69(1):54-59.

Fredricks DN, Fiedler TL, Marrazzo JM. Molecular identification of bacteria associated with bacterial vaginosis. *N Engl J Med.* 2005;353(18):1899-1911.

Gamble RG, Echols KF, Dellavalle RP. Imiquimod vs cryotherapy for molluscum contagiosum: a randomized controlled trial. *Arch Dermatol.* 2012; 148(1):109-112.

Gupta R, Wald A, Krantz E, et al. Valacyclovir and acyclovir for suppression of shedding of herpes simplex virus in the genital tract. *J Infect Dis.* 2004;190(8):1374-1381.

Heller DS, Bean S. Lesions of the Bartholin gland: a review. *J Low Genit Tract Dis.* 2014;18(4):351-357.

Hillier SL. The complexity of microbial diversity in bacterial vaginosis. *N Engl J Med.* 2005;353(18):1886-1887.

Hu S, Bigby M. Treating scabies: results from an updated Cochrane review. *Arch Dermatol.* 2008;144(12):1638-1640. discussion 1640-1631.

Ilhan AH, Durmusoglu F. Case report of a pelvic-peritoneal tuberculosis presenting as an adnexial mass and mimicking ovarian cancer, and a review of the literature. *Infect Dis Obstet Gynecol.* 2004;12(2):87-89.

Kessous R, Aricha-Tamir B, Sheizaf B, et al. Clinical and microbiological characteristics of Bartholin gland abscesses. *Obstet Gynecol.* 2013;122(4):794-799.

Khanna G, Rajni, Azad K. Bartholin gland carcinoma. *Indian J Pathol Microbiol.* 2010;53(1):171-172.

Leone PA. Scabies and pediculosis pubis: an update of treatment regimens and general review. *Clin Infect Dis.* 2007;44(Suppl 3):S153-S159.

LeRiche T, Black AY, Fleming NA. Toxic shock syndrome of a probable gynecologic source in an adolescent: a case report and review of the literature. *J Pediatr Adolesc Gynecol.* 2012;25(6):e133-e137.

Li SF, Gennis P. Treatment of bartholin abscesses. *J Emerg Med.* 2011;41(2):187.
Marrazzo JM, Thomas KK, Agnew K, et al. Prevalence and risks for bacterial vaginosis in women who have sex with women. *Sex Transm Dis.* 2010a;37(5):335-339.
Marrazzo JM, Thomas KK, Fiedler TL, et al. Risks for acquisition of bacterial vaginosis among women who report sex with women: a cohort study. *PLoS One.* 2010b;5(6):e11139.
Mathes EF, Frieden IJ. Treatment of molluscum contagiosum with cantharidin: a practical approach. *Pediatr Ann.* 2010;39(3):124-128. 130.
Phillips AJ, d'Ablaing 3rd G. Acute salpingitis subsequent to tubal ligation. *Obstet Gynecol.* 1986;67(3 Suppl):55S-58S.
Phipps W, Saracino M, Magaret A, et al. Persistent genital herpes simplex virus-2 shedding years following the first clinical episode. *J Infect Dis.* 2011;203(2):180-187.
Prabhu A, Gardella C. Common vaginal and vulvar disorders. *Med Clin North Am.* 2015;99(3):553-574.
Risser WL, Risser JM. The incidence of pelvic inflammatory disease in untreated women infected with Chlamydia trachomatis: a structured review. *Int J STD AIDS.* 2007;18(11):727-731.
Romosan G, Valentin L. The sensitivity and specificity of transvaginal ultrasound with regard to acute pelvic inflammatory disease: a review of the literature. *Arch Gynecol Obstet.* 2014;289(4):705-714.
Scott GR, Chosidow O. IUSTI/WHO: European guideline for the management of pediculosis pubis, 2010. *Int J STD AIDS.* 2011;22(6):304-305.
Sobel JD, Brooker D, Stein GE, et al. Single oral dose fluconazole compared with conventional clotrimazole topical therapy of Candida vaginitis. Fluconazole Vaginitis Study Group. *Am J Obstet Gynecol.* 1995;172(4 Pt 1):1263-1268.
Sobel JD, Chaim W, Nagappan V, et al. Treatment of vaginitis caused by Candida glabrata: use of topical boric acid and flucytosine. *Am J Obstet Gynecol.* 2003;189(5):1297-1300.
Sobel JD, Kapernick PS, Zervos M, et al. Treatment of complicated Candida vaginitis: comparison of single and sequential doses of fluconazole. *Am J Obstet Gynecol.* 2001;185(2):363-369.
Tronstein E, Johnston C, Huang ML, et al. Genital shedding of herpes simplex virus among symptomatic and asymptomatic persons with HSV-2 infection. *JAMA.* 2011;305(14):1441-1449.
Wechter ME, Wu JM, Marzano D, et al. Management of Bartholin duct cysts and abscesses: a systematic review. *Obstet Gynecol Surv.* 2009;64(6):395-404.
Workowski KA, Bolan GA. Centers for Disease Control and Prevention: Sexually transmitted diseases treatment guidelines, 2015. *MMWR Recomm Rep.* 2015;64(RR-03):1-137.

# 24

# Preoperative Counseling and Management

## Preoperative Evaluation, Informed Consent, Perioperative Planning, Surgical Site Infection Prevention, and Avoidance of Complications

*Jamie N. Bakkum-Gamez, Sean C. Dowdy, Fidel A. Valea*

Preoperative evaluation can involve both the art and science of clinical medicine. Optimal preparation for the operation facilitates a successful result and protects the patient and the physician.

In regard to the task of obtaining preoperative information, there are two goals. The first is to ensure that the procedure is appropriate for the patient's diagnosis. The content of this part of the clinician's task is covered elsewhere in this text; the process of the task involves the physician-patient relationship. Just as crucial is the second goal, ensuring that the patient is safe for the procedure and that comorbidities are appropriately addressed. Some comorbidities will require further consultation with other specialists, and it is important for the gynecologic surgeon to recognize when consultation is needed.

The gynecologic surgeon, as leader of the surgical team, has a responsibility to prepare the patient, her family, and the surgical team for the surgical procedure. Even in emergency situations, preoperative preparation should be detailed and complete. Almost any surgical procedure is a major event in a patient's life that can be accompanied by anxiety and apprehension of the anticipated surgical procedure. Among elective procedures, there may also be ambivalence in deciding whether to have the operation. In all cases, it is important for the surgeon to outline the natural history of the gynecologic disease and options for management. The risks, benefits, and alternatives must be discussed. The impact of a surgical intervention on normal body function, sexuality, and cosmesis must also be addressed. If the patient is ambivalent concerning the need for a surgical procedure, a second opinion may be warranted and should be offered. Some third-party payer programs may require patients to obtain a second opinion before elective gynecologic operations.

It is the surgeon's responsibility to protect his or her patient's privacy and dignity throughout the perioperative period. The surgeon must appreciate that the preoperative period may be one of great psychological stress for the patient and her support team. Emotional responses may include vulnerability and helplessness, and grief associated with loss of a reproductive organ. The surgeon-patient relationship is far more than the legally described contractual one. An important aspect of the relationship is that the surgeon and patient partner in joint decision making. Trust in a surgeon's care is established via mutual respect and open communication.

Preoperative consultation with the surgeon is a crucial first step in successful surgery. Ideally, the surgeon, patient, and her selected support team meet for a confidential consultation.

A thorough and detailed history and physical examination should be performed during the surgical consultation. A number of studies have demonstrated that the most significant risk factors for postoperative morbidity are preoperative conditions. Known or unsuspected medical illnesses may affect the operation, anesthesia, and postoperative course and may preclude the procedure altogether. Also, it is important to evaluate the impact of the gynecologic diagnosis on other organ systems, such as a pelvic mass on the ureters or menorrhagia on hemoglobin level.

This chapter outlines the preoperative preparations for gynecologic surgery and perioperative management considerations. The preparations and plans for surgery extend into the postoperative period in a continuous spectrum. Thus several topics will be introduced here and discussed further in Chapter 25. Emphasis is placed on obtaining a standard complete history, performing an adequate physical examination, counseling the patient, establishing informed consent, and perioperative planning to reduce complications associated with gynecologic surgery.

## PREOPERATIVE HISTORY

A detailed complete history not only obtains information but may also help relieve the patient's fears and anxieties. When the history is obtained in an unhurried manner, the process can be reassuring. The extent and depth of the general history should be tailored to the age and general health of the woman and the surgical procedure that is being recommended. However, even minor operations may have major complications, so it is important to be prepared for all possibilities.

Obtaining a detailed and comprehensive preoperative history includes the use of open-ended questions as well as directed questions to complete the preoperative picture. A standardized historical questionnaire prior to the initial consultation is often requested by the surgeon or even required by the surgeon's institution. Each surgeon develops his or her method of preparation for consultation. Review of the patient's medical record, obtaining outside records and prior operative reports, and pertinent imaging and pathology can be done prior to the in-person consultation. This can allow for efficient evaluation, consultation, and preoperative referrals if needed.

Although this chapter does not review all the components of a complete history, which are discussed further in Chapter 7, it may be advantageous to group questions under the specific organ systems. Specific questions should be included to cross-check the review of symptoms. Questions should be included that address prior problems with surgery, anesthesia, or bleeding in the woman or her family. Medication allergies and current medications should be reviewed. Reconciliation of prescribed and over-the-counter (OTC) medications as well as vitamins, herbal medications, and supplements is critical, as some have the potential to affect surgery through coagulation, healing, and cross-reactivity with other medications. Approximately 0.5% of the general population and 1.5% of women older than 55 years are receiving continuous glucocorticoids. Thus a specific question about glucocorticoid therapy for chronic medical problems should be included. The patient's primary care physician should be involved in the decision to temporarily stop certain medications prior to surgery, and he or she may also be able to provide guidance regarding anticoagulation bridging and stress-dose steroid dosing, if either are needed.

Patients often do not consider aspirin or oral contraceptives as medication; therefore specific questions regarding these substances are needed. General questions regarding smoking, alcohol, exercise tolerance, and recent upper respiratory infections should also be included. Specific questions should be directed toward sensitivity to iodine or latex. Latex allergy is directly responsible for 12% of the perioperative anaphylactic reactions in adult women and for 70% in children. Health care workers are particularly prone to latex allergy. Women with spinal cord injuries, or those who have had to perform self-catheterization, are at higher risk for latex allergy.

The patient's contraceptive history, including any recent change, must be known. Ensuring that pregnancy is excluded either through the preoperative history or a pregnancy test is critical prior to gynecologic surgery. Included with the contraceptive history are key questions concerning possible exposure to viruses such as hepatitis B, hepatitis C, and human immunodeficiency virus (HIV). Also, the surgeon should discuss the possibility and risks of blood transfusion and learn whether there are religious objections if a blood transfusion is needed during surgery.

## PHYSICAL EXAMINATION

The preoperative physical examination should answer three basic questions:

1. Has the primary gynecologic disease process changed since the initial diagnosis?
2. What is the effect of the primary gynecologic disease on other organ systems?
3. What deficiencies in other organ systems may affect the proposed surgery and hospitalization?

Observations and findings in the physical examination may prompt further laboratory and diagnostic tests. One of the most important features of the preoperative physical exam is that it should be performed in a thorough and compulsive manner. One should use the same sequence every time to help focus attention on the evaluation of each organ system and to prevent omissions. Two important axioms should be stressed. First, even in emergency situations, it is imperative to perform a thorough physical examination. This should include an evaluation of blood pressure and pulse in the recumbent and sitting positions; orthostatic hypotension and tachycardia are crude indices of a decrease in circulating intravascular volume. Second, although it is important to perform a pelvic examination during the initial consultation, it can also be informative to perform a pelvic examination in the operating room immediately before the surgical incision. An exam while the patient is under anesthesia may provide additional information, help avoid intraoperative surprises, and affect the surgical plan.

## LABORATORY AND PREOPERATIVE DIAGNOSTIC PROCEDURES

The general purpose of preoperative laboratory testing is to identify conditions that will alter or aid in perioperative management. Screening tests are used to find unsuspected asymptomatic conditions that may affect the anticipated surgical procedure. Preoperative laboratory tests may also help establish the extent of known disease and may influence the scheduling of elective surgery. Being selective in ordering preoperative test avoids unnecessary costs associated with test results that would otherwise not affect the surgical plan. Additionally, special imaging procedures may be needed to determine the effects of pelvic disease on other organ systems.

Age-appropriate screening tests should be reviewed with each patient prior to gynecologic surgery. Papanicolaou (Pap) smears should be up to date prior to gynecologic surgery. Mammograms should at least be discussed with women ≥40 years of age, and colonoscopy, should be discussed with women older than 50 years.

Presently, there is debate over which preoperative laboratory procedures should be standard. Attention has been drawn to the cost-benefit ratio of preoperative screening. Although the cost of each individual test is usually low, the aggregate costs can be substantial. In a classic study, Kaplan and colleagues retrospectively studied the usefulness of preoperative laboratory procedures. They estimated that 60% of routinely ordered tests, such as differential cell count, platelet count, and 12-factor automated body chemistry analyses, would not have been performed if tests had been ordered only for an indication discovered by history or physical examination. Most important, only 0.22% of these tests demonstrated an abnormality that might influence perioperative management (Fig. 24.1). The final conclusion in their assessment of 2000 patients undergoing elective operations was that in the absence of specific indications, most routine preoperative laboratory tests do not significantly contribute to patient care and could be eliminated (Kaplan, 1985). Additionally, the current American Society of Anesthesiologists (ASA) Practice Advisory for Preanesthesia Evaluation states that routine preoperative tests, defined as a test ordered in the absence of a clinical indication or purpose, should not be ordered. Preoperative tests should be ordered for indicated purposes that guide or optimize perioperative care (Committee on Standards and Practice Parameters, 2012).

However, a preoperative complete blood count and blood type and antibody screen should be performed prior to most gynecologic surgeries. In the setting of anemia, the risks and benefits of proceeding with gynecologic surgery should be considered. It is important that the blood bank have the capability of providing cross-matched blood within a reasonable time period if serious intraoperative bleeding were to occur. Routine coagulation studies are not cost effective and rarely provide useful clinical information unless indicated by history and physical examination, as the patient's menstrual history should identify women with bleeding disorders.

Other individualized preoperative laboratory testing should be determined based on the age of the woman, extent of the surgical procedure, and findings at the time of complete history and physical examination. It may be indicated to order limited blood screening tests for women older than 40 years or who have positive family histories or questionable past histories of hepatic or renal disease. Determining the preoperative creatinine or blood urea nitrogen (BUN) level is especially important if the woman is going to be treated with antibiotics excreted by the kidneys. A pregnancy test may be appropriate, depending on contraceptive and sexual history, but it should almost always be performed if the patient is a teenager, as menstrual history is at best an imperfect indication of an early pregnancy. Serum electrolyte levels are ordered for women taking diuretics or those with a history of renal disease or heart disease. Also, serum electrolyte levels should be evaluated in women with vomiting, diarrhea, ileus, bowel obstruction, or any condition that affects electrolyte balance. Ideally, abnormal results from any laboratory test ordered preoperatively should result in some change in perioperative management.

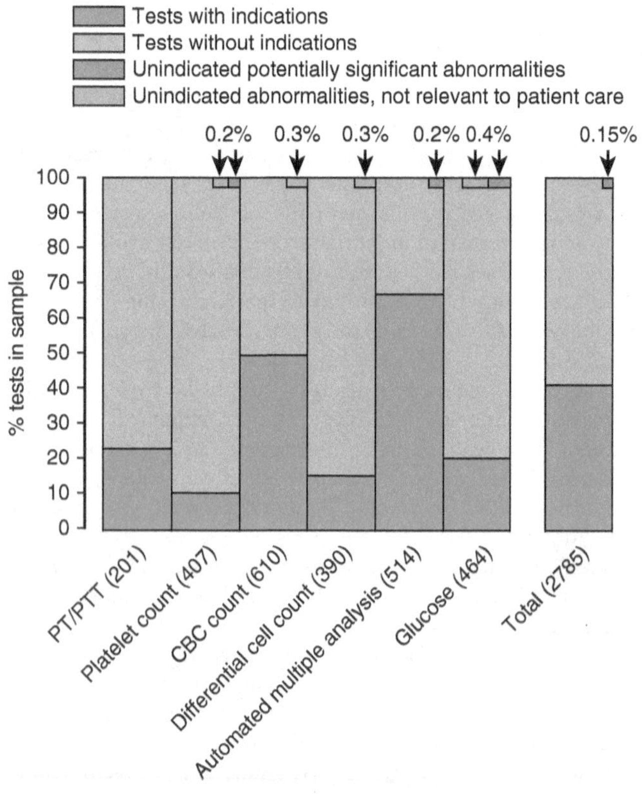


**Figure 24.1** Proportions of indicated and unindicated preoperative tests, drawn to scale. Numbers in parentheses represent sample sizes used. *CBC*, Complete blood count; automated multiple analysis is the sixth factor; *PT/PTT*, prothrombin time/partial thromboplastin time. (From Kaplan EB, Scheiner LB, Boeckmann AJ, et al. The usefulness of preoperative laboratory screening. *JAMA*. 1985;253[24]:3576-3581.)

Routine chest x-rays on all patients often do not affect perioperative management in elective gynecologic surgery. A history and physical examination are sufficient for screening, and chest x-rays should be obtained in patients with positive findings. A meta-analysis of studies of routine preoperative chest x-rays demonstrated that false-positive results leading to invasive procedures and associated morbidity are more frequent than the discovery of new findings leading to a change in management. However, chest films should be ordered for women who are 20-pack/year smokers, women with cardiac or pulmonary symptoms, immigrants who have not had a recent chest film, and women older than 70 years (Qaseem, 2006). Interestingly, there appears to be a great deal of institutional variability regarding the absolute age cutoff.

A baseline preoperative electrocardiogram (ECG) has been found to be cost effective in asymptomatic women ≥60 years without a history of cardiac disease or significant risk factors. An ECG may also be indicated in younger women with a history of smoking and those with diabetes or renal disease, depending on the severity.

Based on the complete history, physical examination, and preoperative testing, the gynecologic surgeon should determine whether consultation with other specialists is necessary. This decision should take into account the severity of comorbidities and the complexity of the proposed operation.

## PATIENT EDUCATION AND INFORMED CONSENT

One of the primary responsibilities of the gynecologic surgeon is to educate the patient and her support team about the anticipated surgical procedure, hospitalization, and recovery. Informed consent is an important principle to ensure that the patient's right to self-determination is respected. The ethical concept of the process of informed consent includes two components, comprehension and free consent. Throughout the educational process, questions from the patient or her support team should be welcomed. Educating the patient can also address anxiety. Written information, when available, can be helpful. Psychological preparation of the patient's support team is equally important, and arrangements for appropriate communication with the patient's family or support team during the operation should be made.

Few concepts bring more ambivalence and concern to the physician than the doctrine of informed consent. In the present medicolegal climate, the absence of informed consent is cited as a major problem in many lawsuits. Some of these issues are discussed further in Chapter 6. It is important to differentiate between the concepts of consent and informed consent. Consent involves a simple yes-no decision, but informed consent is an educational process. To obtain informed consent, the surgeon must explain the following to the patient in understandable terms: the nature and extent of the disease process; the nature and extent of the contemplated operation; the anticipated benefits and results of the surgery, including a conservative estimate of successful outcome; the risks and potential complications of the operative procedure; alternative methods of therapy; and any potential changes in sexual, reproductive, and other functions. The surgeon should also discuss with the patient what the operation will not accomplish. Questions from the patient should be encouraged and addressed. Any details specific to the situation should be clarified in the consent note in addition to stating that the procedure, alternative treatments, and risks have been discussed and questions have been answered. The possibility of unanticipated pathologic conditions should be discussed with the woman and permission obtained on the written consent form for the most extensive operative procedure that may be necessary.

One of the greatest dilemmas in the doctrine of informed consent is the extent and depth of discussions concerning potential complications of an operation. Attorneys who specialize in defending gynecologic surgeons in medical malpractice litigation strongly advise discussing all major complications, including death from surgery and rare, serious complications, such as urinary tract fistulas following hysterectomy. Studies have documented that approximately 70% of patients do not read the consent form before signing it. Ideally, to protect the surgeon, another member of the health care delivery team should witness the final discussion of the informed consent process. The surgeon should document critical highlights of this discussion in the patient's medical record.

The gynecologic surgeon must not only educate his or her patient but must be prepared to discuss other information that the patient has received, including information from the lay press and Internet. During the preoperative educational process, so much information may be given that it causes confusion. Studies have noted that the more information given, the less information is actually retained, much less correctly retained. A study by Sandberg and colleagues has noted that during the preoperative evaluation, information given by anesthesiologists and other health care providers vastly exceeds the short-term capacity of patients (Sandberg, 2008). Thus it is extremely helpful to provide written preoperative instructions and important information.

## PREOPERATIVE PREPARATION

Because of the increasing emphasis on same-day admission to the hospital, most procedures and orders are accomplished on an outpatient basis. Preoperative orders should be standardized to avoid omissions and electronic order sets are standard at most institutions. Orders individualized to a patient should be written in specific detail to avoid confusion by nursing and other hospital personnel.

Prior to presentation to the hospital, the patient should be provided with a list of specific instructions for the 24 hours before surgery. If an enhanced recovery pathway is being utilized, the patient can usually eat solid food up until midnight and clear liquids until 30 minutes prior to presenting to the hospital. To avoid hypoglycemia, most enhanced recovery after surgery protocols allow patients to eat solid food up to 6 hours before surgery. Clear liquids are emptied from the stomach within minutes; however, fatty foods delay gastric emptying. Incomplete preparation of the upper gastrointestinal tract increases the risk of aspiration. Studies have documented the safety of allowing inpatients and outpatients to ingest clear liquids up until two hours before elective surgery. Interestingly, the extent of preoperative anxiety does not influence gastric fluid volume or acidity.

## CONSULTATION WITH ANESTHESIOLOGY

Among patients with no or limited comorbidities, the consultation with their anesthesiologist may occur in the preoperative area on the day of surgery. During this time, the anesthesiologist reviews and obtains any additional medical information, evaluates the patient's airway, determines the American Society of Anesthesiologists (ASA) risk score for the patient, and writes any preoperative medication orders. Among patients with complex medical histories or comorbidities, prior complications with anesthesia, family history of anesthesia complications, or planned high complexity surgery, a preoperative evaluation with an anesthesiologist in an outpatient clinic a day or more prior to surgery is warranted. The goal for this evaluation is to ensure all preoperative assessments needed to optimize anesthesia safety have been performed.

Surgeons and anesthesiologists frequently have to determine whether to continue or interrupt medications during the perioperative period. If the medication is prescribed for a chronic medical illness, it is likely best to continue the drug throughout the perioperative period. However, it is essential to determine whether the drug will adversely affect the course of the anesthesia or surgery and whether it will interact with other drugs to be given during the procedure. It is acceptable for the patient to take oral medications the morning of surgery. The 30 to 60 mL of water needed to swallow the oral medication is negligible compared with gastric fluid volumes.

Anesthesiologists classify surgical procedures according to the patient's risk of mortality. In 1961, Dripps first published guidelines to determine the risk of death related to major operative procedures. This physical status scale (Table 24.1) has been

**Table 24.1** American Society of Anesthesiologists (ASA) Physical Status Classification

| ASA Physical Status Class | Description |
|---|---|
| 1 | A normal healthy patient |
| 2 | A patient with mild systemic disease |
| 3 | A patient with severe systemic disease |
| 4 | A patient with severe systemic disease that is a constant threat to life |
| 5 | A moribund patient who is not expected to survive without the operation |

From Koo CY, Hyder JA, Wanderer JP, et al. A meta-analysis of the predictive accuracy of postoperative mortality using the American Society of Anesthesiologists' Physical Status Classification System. *World J Surg*. 2015;39(1):88-103.

adopted by the ASA and has been revalidated many times over the years. With minor modifications, these anesthetic risk classes are still widely used. An emergency operation doubles the mortality risks for classes 1, 2, and 3; produces a slightly increased risk in class 4; and does not change the risk in class 5 (Koo, 2015).

## PERIOPERATIVE MANAGEMENT

### ENHANCED RECOVERY

Enhanced recovery refers to a bundled process with the aim of attenuating pathophysiologic changes and the stress response occurring with surgery. These processes replace traditional but untested practices of perioperative care with the primary goal of hastening recovery. This challenge to traditional surgical paradigms—such as mechanical bowel preparation, the overnight fasting rule, delayed postoperative feeding, hypervolemia, and intravenous narcotics—was first described in Europe in the 1990s (Kehlet, 1997). There has been widespread uptake of formalized evidence-based enhanced recovery after surgery (ERAS) protocols internationally, particularly in colorectal surgery. Adoption of enhanced recovery has resulted in an average reduction in length of stay of 2.5 days (Chambers, 2014; Varadhan, 2010) and a decrease in complications by as much as 50%. Similarities between gynecologic oncology procedures and those performed in surgical specialties such as colorectal surgery suggest that patients with gynecologic cancer may obtain comparable benefits.

In one investigation of patients undergoing gynecologic surgery, 241 (81 complex cytoreductive, 84 staging, and 76 vaginal surgery cases) were managed with an enhanced recovery protocol and compared with 235 historical controls matched by procedure (Kalogera, 2013). The protocol included omission of preoperative fasting (Brady, 2003), use of carbohydrate loading (Mathur, 2010; Nygren, 1995), omission of mechanical bowel preparation (Güenaga, 2011), use of preemptive analgesia, nausea and vomiting prophylaxis, and maintenance of perioperative euvolemia (Brandstrup, 2003). Laparotomy wounds were injected with bupivacaine, as epidural analgesia was not utilized for patients undergoing laparotomy in this series. Intrathecal analgesia was utilized in more than 40% of vaginal cases in this series. Nasogastric tubes (Nelson, 2007), surgical drains (Kalogera, 2012), and intravenous patient-controlled analgesia was avoided or omitted, whereas early feeding (Charoenkwan, 2007; Cutillo, 1999; Minig, 2009), laxative use, and early mobilization were encouraged (Table 24.2). Enhanced recovery achieved the greatest benefit in patients undergoing complex cytoreduction for ovarian cancer, of whom 57% underwent colonic or small bowel resection. Patient-controlled anesthesia use decreased from 99% to 33%, and total opioid use decreased by 80% in the first 48 hours with no increase in pain scores. Hospital stay was reduced by four days with 30-day cost savings of more than $7600 per patient (18.8% reduction). In benign vaginal cases, mean pain scores significantly improved and hospital stay was significantly reduced by one day with the use of intrathecal analgesia. Ninety-five percent of patients rated satisfaction with perioperative care as excellent or very good. Other investigations in patients undergoing gynecologic surgery have shown that enhanced recovery is safe and confers significant benefits in hospital length of stay, pain control, and overall recovery (Carter, 2012; Chase, 2008; Eberhart, 2008; Gerardi, 2008; Kalogera, 2013; Marx, 2006; Wijk, 2014).

The popularity of thoracic epidural anesthesia (TEA) following major open gynecologic surgery is due to its effectiveness in controlling pain and the quicker return of bowel function seen in patients with epidural anesthetics (Ferguson, 2009). However, the role of TEA in an ERAS care plan is less clear, as it can compete at times with some of the ERAS goals such as early ambulation and voiding. The use of TEA has been associated with more interventions to treat hypotension, longer length of hospital stay, as well as more complications in one series of early stage endometrial cancer patients (Belavy, 2013). The estimated length of stay in most ERAS pathways for simple hysterectomy is approximately 1 to 2 days. The use of TEA in this setting not only is a poor utilization of resources but also will likely interfere with the expected expedient discharge from the hospital. Further study is needed to determine if TEA or other local or regional analgesic approaches in radical abdominal procedures such as ovarian cancer debulking improve the return of bowel function or shorten hospital stay.

### GASTROINTESTINAL TRACT CONSIDERATIONS

If gastrointestinal symptoms are present prior to gynecologic surgery, preoperative endoscopy or imaging studies of the gastrointestinal tract should be considered to better understand the etiology of these symptoms. The effect of nausea, vomiting, or diarrhea on serum electrolyte levels and on the nutritional status of the patient also needs to be evaluated. The evaluation should be individualized to determine whether a primary gynecologic process is causing the gastrointestinal symptoms.

If a bowel preparation is felt to be necessary, a single day of an oral solution can be used. Magnesium citrate, sodium phosphate (Fleet phospho-soda), and polyethylene glycol (PEG; GoLYTELY) are the three most commonly used agents. Oliveria and colleagues reported a large randomized trial comparing sodium phosphate and PEG-based oral lavage solutions. The efficacy of the two preparations was similar. However, there was superior subjective patient tolerance to the 90-mL dose of sodium phosphate (Oliveira, 1997). Care must be taken in selecting patients who are to receive oral sodium phosphate as a bowel preparation because it may lead to hypokalemia, has been associated with acute phosphate nephropathy, and is contraindicated in women with hepatic, renal, or heart disease. As a result, the U.S. Food and Drug Administration (FDA) issued a warning in late 2008 regarding the use of all oral sodium phosphate preparations when used as a bowel cleanser. Special care must be taken in patients over the age of 55 or younger than 18, patients taking medications that can affect kidney function, or patients who are dehydrated.

## REDUCING POSTOPERATIVE COMPLICATIONS

#### *Site Marking and Universal Protocol*

Depending on the surgical procedure being performed, operative site marking may be required. Most institutions mandate site marking to be performed in the setting of surgical procedures that involve or remove one or both organs or structures that are paired. This is controversial in gynecologic surgery, as

Table 24.2 Evidence-Based Enhanced Recovery after Surgery (ERAS) Protocol for Gynecologic Surgery Patients

| | |
|---|---|
| **Preoperative** | |
| Diet | Evening before surgery: carbohydrate-loading drink; may eat until midnight<br>May ingest fluids up to 4 hours before procedure<br>Eliminate use of mechanical bowel preparation; rectal enemas still performed |
| **Intraoperative** | |
| Analgesia before OR entry | Celecoxib 400 mg PO once<br>Acetaminophen 1000 mg PO once<br>Gabapentin 600 mg PO once |
| Postoperative nausea and vomiting prophylaxis | Before incision (± 30 min): dexamethasone 4 mg IV once + droperidol 0.625 mg IV once<br>Before incision closure (± 30 min): granisetron 0.1 mg IV once |
| Fluid balance | Goal: maintain intraoperative euvolemia<br>Decrease crystalloid administration<br>Increase colloid administration if needed |
| Analgesia | Opioids IV at discretion of anesthesiologist supplemented with ketamine or ketorolac<br>After incision closure: injection of bupivacaine at incision site |
| Anesthesia in complex vaginal surgery | Subarachnoid block containing bupivacaine and hydromorphone (40-100 μg)<br>Sedation versus "light" general anesthetic at the discretion of the anesthesiologist<br>Ketorolac 15 mg at the end of the procedure for patients able to tolerate it<br>No wound infiltration with bupivacaine in this cohort |
| **Postoperative** | |
| Activity | Evening of surgery: out of bed greater than 2 hours, including 1 or more walks and sitting in chair<br>Day after surgery and until discharge: out of bed greater than 8 hours, including 4 or more walks and sitting in chair<br>Patient up in chair for all meals |
| Diet | No nasogastric tube (NGT); if NGT used intra operatively, remove at extubation<br>Patient encouraged to start low-residue diet 4 hours after procedure<br>Day of surgery: 1 box of liquid nutritional supplement. Encourage oral intake of at least 800 mL of fluid, but no more than 2000 mL by midnight.<br>Day after surgery until discharge: 2 boxes of liquid nutritional supplement. Encourage daily oral intake of 1500-2500 mL of fluids.<br>Osmotic diarrhetics: senna and docusate sodium; magnesium oxide; magnesium hydroxide prn |
| Analgesia | Goal: no IV patient-controlled analgesia (PCA)<br>Oral opioids<br>Oxycodone 5-10 mg PO every 4 hours as needed for pain rated 4 or greater or greater than patient stated comfort goal (5 mg for pain rated 4–6 or 10 mg for pain rated 7–10). For patients who received intrathecal analgesia start 24 hours after intrathecal dose given.<br>Scheduled acetaminophen*<br>Acetaminophen 1000 mg PO every 6 hours for patients with no or mild hepatic disease; acetaminophen 1000 mg PO twice daily for patients with moderate hepatic disease; maximum acetaminophen should not exceed 4000 mg per 24 hours from all sources.<br>Scheduled NSAIDs<br>Ketorolac 15 mg IV every 6 hours for 4 doses (start no sooner than 6 hours after last intra-operative dose); then, ibuprofen 800 mg PO every 6 hours (start 6 hours after last Ketorolac dose administered)<br>If patient unable to take NSAIDs<br>Tramadol 100 mg PO four times a day (start at 6 a.m. day after surgery) for patients less than 65 years of age and no history of renal impairment or hepatic disease; tramadol 100 mg PO twice daily (start at 6 a.m. day after surgery) for patients 65 years of age or older or creatinine clearance less than 30 mL/min or history of hepatic disease.<br>Breakthrough pain (pain greater than 7 more than 1 hour after receiving oxycodone)<br>Hydromorphone 0.4 mg IV once if patient did not receive intrathecal medications; may repeat once after 20 minutes if first dose ineffective.<br>IV PCA<br>Hydromorphone PCA started only if continued pain despite two doses of IV hydromorphone |
| Fluid balance | Operating room fluids discontinued upon arrival to floor<br>Fluids at 40 mL/hour until 8:00 a.m. on day after surgery, then discontinued<br>Peripheral lock IV when patient had 600 mL PO intake or at 8:00 a.m. on day after surgery, whichever came first. |

*PO*, Administered orally.
From Kalogera E, Bakkum-Gamez JN, Jankowski CJ, et al. Enhanced recovery in gynecologic surgery. *Obstet Gynecol*. 2013;122(2 Pt 1):319-328.
*Doses for patients greater than 80 kg and less than 65 years of age; doses adjusted as appropriate for patients less than 80 kg and/or 65 years of age or older.

the preoperative determination of adnexal laterality is not always reliable. If site marking is done, it should performed in the preoperative area while the patient is awake and nonsedated. The patient should participate in Universal Protocol and confirm which organ(s) will undergo surgery. Universal Protocol and site marking reduces the risk of wrong site, wrong procedure, and wrong person operations (Knight, 2010).

### Preoperative Briefing

It is now common practice to perform a preoperative briefing, or "huddle," prior to bringing the patient to the operating room. Usually performed in the preoperative area, the entire surgical team should be briefed on the patient's diagnosis, surgical plan, positioning, relevant comorbidities, intraoperative orders, and perioperative considerations. Medications to be administered, including antibiotics, prophylactic dose heparin, local analgesics, and specialty medications such as local or systemic dye injections or vasoactive medications should be discussed. The anesthesia plans and estimated blood loss for the procedure should be reviewed. Special equipment needed for the procedure should be noted so that it is immediately available when needed. The anticipated wound classification should be noted so that it is accurately documented in the patient's medical record. Ideally, the entire operating room team should be present for the briefing, including the surgeon, resident/fellow, nurse, surgical assistant and tech, and anesthesia team. All team members' questions should be answered prior to bringing the patient to the operating room.

### Positioning for Surgery

After anesthesia has taken effect and the abdominal wall is relaxed, a preoperative pelvic examination may be indicated depending on the surgical procedure planned. The findings may influence the choice of incision or operative approach. Additionally, the surgeon should supervise the positioning of the patient to ensure that she is properly positioned for the procedure being performed. Pressure points should be avoided to protect against neuromuscular and skin injury, especially over bony prominences (Irvin, 2004).

### Surgical Site Infection Prevention

The occurrence of a surgical site infection (SSI) is one of the most common complications after surgery. SSIs dissatisfy patients and providers, but they also increase the cost of surgical care, increase morbidity, and can increase mortality (Bakkum-Gamez, 2013; Tran, 2015). Additionally, SSIs associated with hysterectomies performed through abdominal incisions (laparotomy, laparoscopy, or robotics) are reported to the Centers for Medicare and Medicaid Services (CMS) and are utilized to compare hospitals to the national benchmark for surgical quality. Ultimately, the occurrence of an SSI after hysterectomy will likely influence third-party reimbursement. As such, there are multiple reasons to reduce SSI occurrences.

SSIs are multifactorial in etiology. There are host and endogenous flora factors that may or may not be modifiable. Additionally, surgical procedures, the surgical team, hospital practice factors, and prophylactic interventions will influence the risk of SSI (Fig. 24.2). SSIs are categorized into three classifications

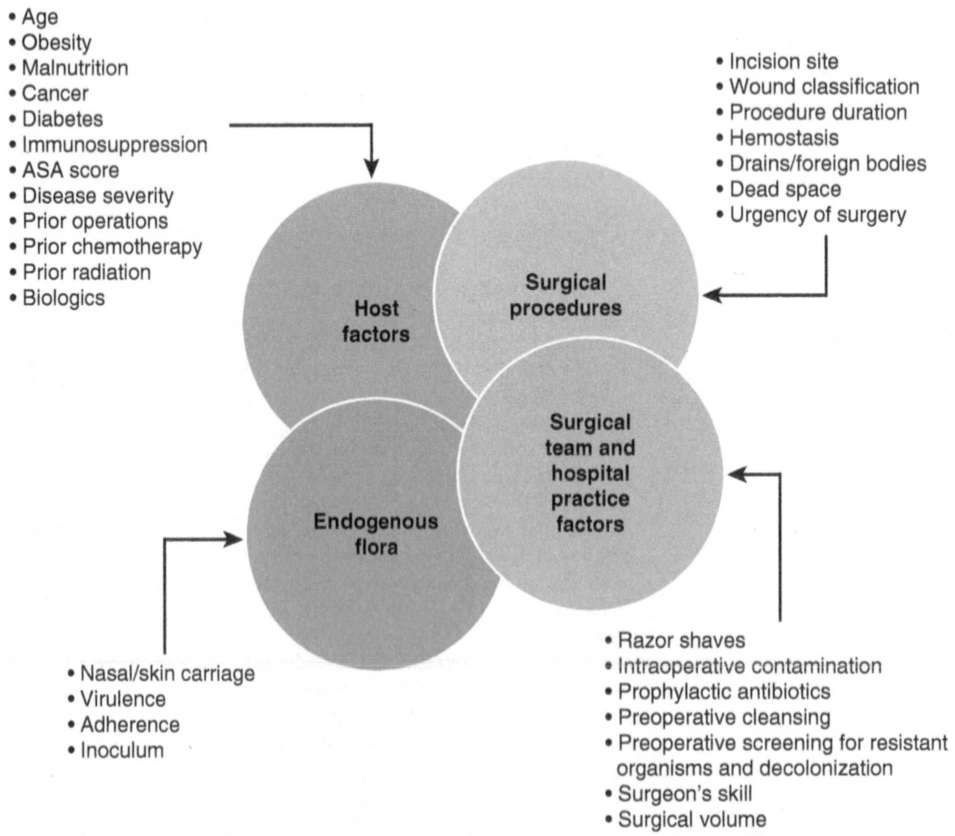


**Figure 24.2** Surgical site infections are multifactorial in etiology.

by the Centers for Disease Control and Prevention (CDC) and the American College of Surgeons National Surgical Quality Improvement Program (ACS NSQIP): (1) superficial incisional, (2) deep incisional, and (3) organ/space (ACS NSQIP, 2011) (Box 24.1); each has different risk factors (Bakkum-Gamez, 2013). Given the implications of an SSI diagnosis, it is important to ensure that if a wound complication occurs, the surgeon classifies it appropriately.

### *Surgical Site Infection Reduction Bundles*

In approaching the challenge of reducing SSIs, the combination of evidence-based medicine with consensus best practices into "bundles" of interventions has been shown to have some of the greatest impacts. The term *bundle* has been defined by the Institute for Healthcare Improvement (IHI) as a structured way of improving the processes of care and patient outcomes or a small, straightforward set of evidence-based practices that, when performed collectively and reliably, have been proved to improve patient outcomes. Elements shown to decrease SSI that are often included in reduction bundles include preoperative nicotine cessation (Sørensen, 2012), preoperative antiseptic showering (Webster, 2007) and chlorhexidine preparation (Darouiche, 2010), using hair clippers instead of a razor (Cruse, 1980; Kjønniksen, 2002), appropriate preoperative antibiotic selection (Bratzler, 2013), normothermia (Rajagopalan, 2008; Scott, 2006; Warttig, 2014), and glycemic control (Kwon, 2013). SSI reduction bundles that include various combinations of these elements as well as additional evidence-based and best practices have been shown to decrease SSI after hysterectomy by 40% (Revolus, 2014) and by more than 50% in general surgery and colorectal surgery (Cima, 2013; van der Slegt, 2013; Waits, 2014). The colorectal surgery SSI reduction bundle at the Mayo Clinic (Fig. 24.3) has been validated in the gynecologic surgery practice as well (Cima, 2013). Additionally, in at least one study of patients undergoing colorectal surgery, there was an inverse association with SSI and the number of bundle elements utilized (Waits, 2014), which suggests it is the combination of interventions rather than one element alone yielding the impact.

**Box 24.1 Classification of Surgical Site Infections (SSI) by the Centers for Disease Control and Prevention (CDC) and American College of Surgeons National Surgical Quality Improvement Program (ACS NSQIP)**

**Superficial Incisional SSI***
1. Purulent incisional drainage from above the fascia
2. Organisms isolated from an aseptically obtained culture of fluid or tissue from the superficial incision
3. Pain/tenderness, wound swelling, redness, or heat and the superficial incision is deliberately opened by the surgeon (unless it is culture negative)

**Deep Incisional SSI* (involves deep soft tissues, such as the fascia or muscle layers of the incision)**
1. Purulent drainage from the deep incision
2. Spontaneous dehiscence or deliberate opening of the fascia in the setting of fever or localized pain/tenderness (unless it is culture negative)
3. An abscess is found involving the deep incision via physical examination, reoperation, or radiologic examination

**Organ/Space SSI***
1. Purulent drainage from an intraperitoneal drain
2. Presence of organisms in culture of fluid obtained aseptically from an organ or space
3. Abscess or other infection involving an organ or space on physical examination, reoperation, histopathologic or radiologic examination

From ACS NSQIP. Classic, essential, small-rural, targeted, and Florida variables & definitions. *American College of Surgeons National Surgical Quality Improvement Program Operations Manual.* Chicago: ACS; 2011:24-26.
*Surgeon diagnosis of any of the three types of SSI also meets NSQIP criteria.

### *Prophylactic Antibiotics*

The use of prophylactic antibiotics in gynecologic surgical procedures has become standard. Rigidly defined, prophylactic antibiotic use involves the administration of antibiotics to patients without evidence of current infection to prevent postoperative morbidity related to infection. The goal of antibiotic therapy is to prevent SSI by the endogenous flora of the lower female reproductive tract. There is abundant literature supporting the use of prophylactic antibiotics in gynecology. The incidence of febrile morbidity may be reduced from 40% to 15%, and the incidence of pelvic infection decreased from 25% to 5%. The current guidelines for antimicrobial prophylaxis for vaginal or abdominal hysterectomy include the first- or second-generation cephalosporins of cefazolin, cefotetan, cefoxitin, or ampicillin-sulbactam. Among women with a β-lactam allergy, the recommended combinations are (1) clindamycin or vancomycin plus an aminoglycoside, or (2) aztreonam, or (3) a fluoroquinolone, metronidazole, and aminoglycoside, or (4) a fluoroquinolone alone (Bratzler, 2013).

Emphasis has focused on short duration of therapy for prophylactic antibiotics. Comparative studies have documented that single-dose therapy is as effective as 24 hours of antibiotics. No advantage exists to continuing prophylactic antibiotics beyond the immediate operative period. This short duration of administration also reduces cost and complications. The incidence of serious complications, such as drug allergy and resistant bacteria, is directly related to the length of administration of the antibiotic.

The Surgical Care Improvement Project (SCIP) implemented by CMS focused on appropriate antibiotic selection and timing of administration with the goal of reducing SSI rates by 25% between 2006 and 2010. Despite high compliance to SCIP measures, which later included normothermia, glucose control, and hair removal guidelines, SSI rates do not correlate with SCIP compliance (Hawn, 2011). So although antibiotic prophylaxis is an important element in SSI reduction, antibiotics alone cannot mitigate the SSI risk.

### *Minimally Invasive Surgery*

With the introduction of laparoscopy and robotic surgery, the armamentarium of minimally invasive gynecologic surgery approaches changed dramatically. Vaginal surgery continues to carry the lowest risks of SSI (Lake, 2013) and should remain the preferred surgical approach when feasible. However, when minimally invasive approaches to hysterectomy replace laparotomy, the risk of SSI can be reduced by up to 16-fold (Bakkum-Gamez,

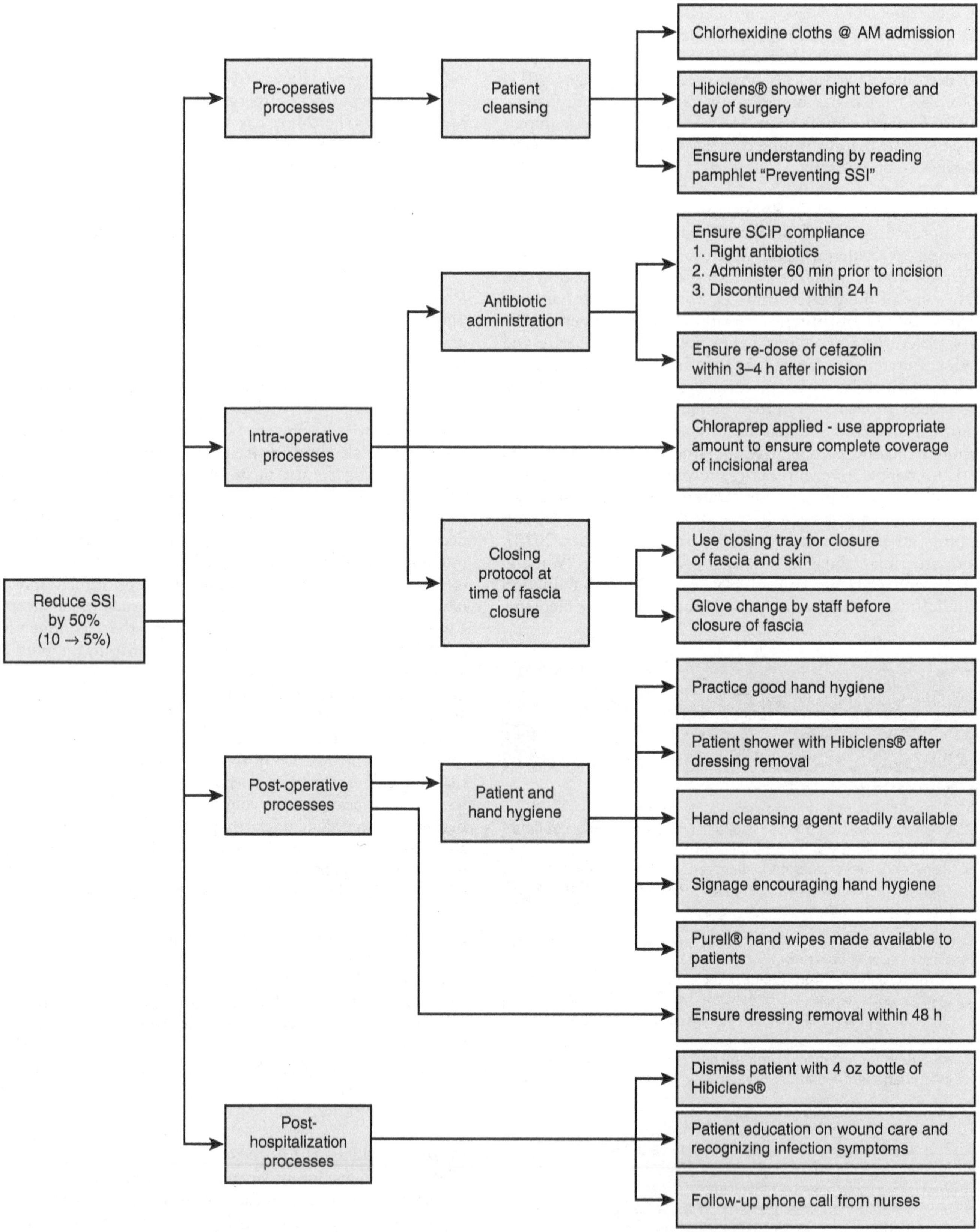


**Figure 24.3** Surgical site infection reduction bundle in colorectal surgery at Mayo Clinic. Surgical site infection was reduced by >50% with the implementation of this full bundle. (From Cima R, Dankbar E, Lovely J, et al. Colorectal surgery surgical site infection reduction program: a national surgical quality improvement program-driven multidisciplinary single-institution experience. *J Am Coll Surg*. 2013;216[1]:23-33.)

2013; Colling, 2015). As such, the utilization of minimally invasive surgery is a critical modifiable factor in the SSI prevention bundle.

### *Hair Removal*

Multiple studies have documented a two- to threefold increase in SSI rate directly related to perioperative shaving. Cruse and Foord studied approximately 63,000 operations over a 10-year period and found a 0.9% incidence of SSI when patients were not shaved as opposed to 2.5% when they were shaved (Cruse, 1980). Razors produce macroscopic and microscopic nicks and cuts that allow a protective environment for colonization by skin bacteria. Depilatory agents often produce intense burning if used on the perineum. A systematic review by Kjonniksen and associates has concluded that if the hair is mechanically in the way, it should be clipped just before the operation (Kjønniksen, 2002). Patients should also be advised not to shave themselves prior to surgery for this reason.

### *Chlorhexidine/Alcohol Skin Preparation*

A randomized trial comparing chlorhexidine gluconate with 70% isopropyl alcohol versus an aqueous solution of 10% povidone-iodine for skin cleansing showed a 40% reduction in SSIs in clean contaminated (type II) wound types (Darouiche, 2010). The solution is highly flammable, and care must be taken to ensure adequate drying time in order to avoid a fire when electrocautery is used.

### *Smoking*

The risk of an SSI is significantly increased in the setting of smoking (van Walraven, 2013). Ideally, patients should stop smoking for at least 8 weeks prior to surgery. However, abstinence from cigarettes for 2 to 4 weeks preoperatively is still beneficial. Providing nicotine replacement is helpful in alleviating the symptoms of acute nicotine withdrawal. Referral to preoperative smoking cessation programs not only decreases smoking around the time of surgery and related perioperative complications but also leads to an increased incidence of long-term smoking cessation. In one multicenter study, Lindström and associates noted that the patients in a smoking cessation program had perioperative complication rates of 21% versus 41% in controls (Lindström, 2008).

### *Normothermia*

Hypothermia, frequently defined as a core body temperature less than 36° C, has been shown to increase the incidence of wound infection and postoperative myocardial events, increase perioperative blood loss, impair drug metabolism, and prolong postoperative recovery (Rajagopalan, 2008; Scott, 2006; Warttig, 2014). Patients undergoing major surgery are at high risk of hypothermia due to prolonged periods with an open abdomen. Furthermore, general anesthesia induces peripheral vasodilation leading to accelerated heat loss. The use of esophageal probes is frequently used to monitor temperature. Methods to maintain normothermia include the use of forced air devices (Galvão, 2010), underbody warming mattresses (Perez-Protto, 2010), and warmed intravenous fluids (Campbell, 2015). Whichever method is used, it is important to understand that preventing intraoperative hypothermia improves surgical outcomes.

### *Glucose Control in the Diabetic and Nondiabetic*

The prevalence of diabetes is approximately 10% in women <65 years of age, and the incidence increases rapidly as women get older. The stress of surgery often produces changes in glucose tolerance and insulin resistance. Because pancreatic reserve is a continuum, even women who are not diabetic by standard blood glucose criteria may develop detrimental hyperglycemia secondary to the physiologic stresses of surgery. Glucose levels >180 mg/dL among diabetics and nondiabetics increase the risk of SSI by twofold (Kwon, 2013). Perioperative blood glucose levels among both diabetics and nondiabetics should be maintained at <200 mg/dL. Category 1A evidence has demonstrated that strict glucose control (80 to 130 mg/dL) in both diabetics and nondiabetics does not improve SSI rates over glucose levels <200 mg/dL (Chan, 2009), and strict control may have detrimental effects on postoperative outcomes (Gandhi, 2007).

In 2004, the American College of Endocrinology published a position paper, "Inpatient Diabetes and Metabolic Control," emphasizing not only the effects of elevated blood glucose levels but the beneficial effects of adequate insulin (Box 24.2). Insulin decreases lipolysis. Elevated free fatty acid levels are associated with arrhythmias. Insulin inhibits several inflammatory mediators, especially the proinflammatory cytokines. Adequate insulin also leads to an increase in nitric oxide levels in the endovasculature, inducing vasodilation.

The principal postoperative complications in diabetic women are increased risk of cardiac morbidity, SSI, and wound disruptions. The increase in SSI rate is believed to be secondary to a decrease in cellular and humoral responses to bacteria. Women with diabetes have approximately a fivefold increase in incidence of SSI compared with age-matched controls. The increased incidence of wound disruptions is caused by a decreased tensile strength during healing associated with insulin resistance and an elevated blood sugar level.

Important questions during the preoperative evaluation focus on the severity of the diabetes, types of medications, and recent diabetic control. Recent blood glucose and hemoglobin A1c (HbA1c) levels may be helpful predictors of perioperative

**Box 24.2 Mechanisms Causing Adverse Outcomes from Poorly Controlled Diabetes**

**Hyperglycemia**
Dehydration
Academia from keto acids and lactate
Nonenzymatic glycosylation of proteins central to immune function: complement, impaired IgG, inhibited neutrophil activity
Fatigue and muscle wasting from lipolysis and protein catabolism
Increased circulating fatty acids
Increased skeletal muscle breakdown
Cell membrane instability
Decline in myocardial contractility and increased cardiac arrhythmias
Inhibited endothelial function
Insulin resistance
Increased lipolysis
Presence of insulin inhibits inflammatory factors
Decreased endothelial-derived relaxing factor—nitric oxide
Insulin and glucose inhibit proinflammatory cytokines

Modified from the American College of Endocrinology. Position statement on inpatient diabetes and metabolic control. *Endocr Pract.* 2004;10(1):77-82.

Table 24.3 Caprini Score Risk Assessment Model for Venous Thromboembolism

| 1 Point | 2 Points | 3 Points | 5 Points |
|---|---|---|---|
| Age 41-60 | Age 61-74 | Age ≥75 | Stroke (<1 mo) |
| Minor surgery | Arthroscopic surgery | History of VTE | Elective arthroplasty |
| BMI >25 kg/m² | Major open surgery (>45 min) | Family history of VTE | Hip, pelvis, or leg fracture |
| Swollen legs | Laparoscopic surgery (>45 min) | Factor V Leiden | Acute spinal cord injury (<1 mo) |
| Varicose veins | Malignancy | *Prothrombin 20210A* mutation | |
| Pregnancy or postpartum | Confined to bed (>72 h) | Lupus anticoagulant | |
| History of unexplained or recurrent spontaneous abortion | Immobilizing plaster cast | Anticardiolipin antibodies | |
| Oral contraceptives or hormone replacement | Central venous access | Elevated serum homocysteine | |
| Sepsis (<1 mo) | | Heparin-induced thrombocytopenia | |
| Serious lung disease, including pneumonia (<1 mo) | | Other congenital or acquired thrombophilia | |
| Abnormal pulmonary function | | | |
| Acute myocardial infarction | | | |
| Congestive heart failure (<1 mo) | | | |
| History of inflammatory bowel disease | | | |
| Medical patient at bed rest | | | |

From Gould MK, Garcia DA, Wren SM, et al. Prevention of VTE in nonorthopedic surgical patients: *Antithrombotic Therapy and Prevention of Thrombosis*, 9th ed. American College of Chest Physicians Evidence-Based Clinical Practice Guidelines. *Chest*. 2012;141(2 Suppl):e227S-e277S.

morbidity, even if they are not modifiable. At the very least, their severity should be documented in the medical record to ensure accurate accounting of perioperative morbidity.

### *Screening for* Staphylococcus aureus

Approximately 25% of all SSIs are caused by *Staphylococcus aureus*. Patients at high risk for *S. aureus* SSI (previous *S. aureus* infection or colonization, obesity, or diabetes) likely benefit from preoperative *S. aureus* screening by nasal culture. If positive cultures are documented, eradication of colonization with chlorhexidine baths and twice-daily intranasal mupirocin has been shown to decrease the rate of SSI. Bode and colleagues demonstrated a decrease in SSI from 7.7% to 3.4% when *S. aureus* was detected and decolonization performed (Bode, 2010).

### *Venous Thromboembolism Prevention*

Venous thromboembolism (VTE) of the pelvic or leg veins is a frequent complication of gynecologic surgery. Studies using $^{125}$I-fibrinogen scanning techniques have documented that approximately 15% of women having gynecologic surgery for a benign disease and approximately 22% of women having surgery for malignant disease develop VTE (Bonnar, 1985). Most of these women will be asymptomatic. Several aspects of pelvic surgery predispose women to VTE, including venous stasis, surgical injury to the walls of large veins, associated anaerobic infection, and hormonal status. Gynecologic malignancy also increased the risk of VTE.

Approximately 40% of deaths following gynecologic surgery are related to pulmonary emboli. Although the initial venous injury most often occurs at the time of the operation, approximately 15% of symptomatic emboli cases do not present until the first week following discharge from the hospital. Because of the significant morbidity and mortality associated with a postoperative pulmonary embolus, every effort should be made to reduce the incidence of thrombophlebitis.

One method commonly used to determine the VTE risk for an individual patient is to calculate the Caprini score, which takes into consideration risk factors such as a history of previous VTE and personal or family history of hypercoagulability. The presence of such a history should also prompt an evaluation for a thrombophilia. Other risk factors for VTE include active malignancy, previous radiation therapy, congestive heart failure, chronic pulmonary disease, nephrotic syndrome, morbid obesity, venous disease, edema of the legs, active pelvic infection, age older than 40 years, current use of oral contraceptives or hormone replacement therapy up to the time of the operation, length of immobilization or preoperative hospitalization, and the length of the planned surgical procedure (Table 24.3). A Caprini score of 0 is very low risk for VTE, 1 to 2 is low risk, 3 to 4 is moderate risk, and ≥5 is considered high risk for VTE. Women in the very low-risk group have less than a 3% risk of VTE, women in the moderate group have a 10% to 30% risk, and women in the high-risk groups have a more than 30% risk of a VTE. The American College of Chest Physicians have published evidence-based clinical practice guidelines aimed at mitigating VTE risk in the setting of abdominal-pelvic surgery that vary by risk stratification (Table 24.4) (Gould, 2012). The utilization of an inferior vena cava (IVC) filter for primary VTE prevention is not recommended. (The use of IVC filters is currently limited to secondary prevention in patients who cannot be anticoagulated or in patients with a "breakthrough" pulmonary embolism on anticoagulation.) Additionally, surveillance with lower extremity Doppler ultrasound for asymptomatic VTE is not recommended (Gould, 2012). These guidelines are widely accepted for VTE prevention.

The main complication from heparin prophylaxis is bleeding. Some women are transiently anticoagulated by the heparin and may experience excessive bleeding during or following the operative procedure. This complication is rare and experienced by approximately 2% of women. The risk of bleeding is significantly lower with low-molecular-weight heparin (LMWH). Obese or extremely thin women should have their dosage of heparin adjusted accordingly.

**Table 24.4** Venous Thromboembolism Prophylaxis Recommendations for Abdominal-Pelvic Surgery

| Risk Stratification | Prophylaxis Measures |
|---|---|
| Very low risk (Caprini score 0) | Early ambulation |
| Low risk (Caprini score 1-2) | Mechanical prophylaxis with SCDs |
| Moderate risk (Caprini score 3-4)<br>Not at high risk for bleeding | Daily prophylactic dose LMWH or thrice-daily prophylactic dose LDUH or SCDs |
| Moderate risk (Caprini score 3-4)<br>High risk for bleeding or consequences of bleeding severe | Mechanical prophylaxis with SCDs |
| High risk (Caprini score ≥5)<br>Not at high risk for bleeding | Daily prophylactic dose LMWH or thrice-daily prophylactic dose LDUH + elastic stockings or SCDs |
| High risk (Caprini score ≥5)<br>Undergoing surgery for cancer | Daily prophylactic dose LMWH or thrice-daily prophylactic dose LDUH + elastic stockings or SCDs<br>Extended duration (4 weeks) daily prophylactic dose LMWH |
| High risk (Caprini score ≥5)<br>LMWH and LDUH contraindicated | Low-dose aspirin or fondaparinux or SCDs |

Data from Gould MK, Garcia DA, Wren SM, et al. Prevention of VTE in nonorthopedic surgical patients: *Chest*. 2012;141(2):e227S-e277S.
*LDUH*, Low-dose unfractionated heparin; *LMWH*, low-molecular-weight heparin; *SCDs*, sequential compression devices.

LMWH is superior to standard unfractionated heparin because it has a longer half-life, almost 100% bioavailability, dose-independent clearance, and a more consistent anticoagulation effect from dose to dose. Most studies have reported significantly fewer hemorrhagic complications with LMWH than with unfractionated heparin. Also, the incidence of heparin-induced thrombocytopenia is significantly lower in women given LMWH than in those receiving unfractionated heparin. In the gynecologic surgical community there are two major "protocols" for the timing of pharmacologic prophylaxis. One uses a dose 1 to 2 hours before surgery and postoperatively, and the other begins the pharmacologic prophylaxis between 6 and 12 hours after surgery. A meta-analysis of studies summarizing 1600 surgeries for elective hip repair, as high risk as gynecologic procedures, has found perioperative and postoperative LMWH administration to be equally effective. The rates of deep vein thrombosis were 12.4% and 14.4%, respectively. The risks of bleeding were higher in the perioperative protocol groups, 6.3% versus 2.5% for postoperative dosing. It was concluded that dosing may begin 12 hours after the procedure in most cases and no less than 6 hours after the procedure (Raskob, 2003).

## CHRONIC ANTICOAGULATION AND BLEEDING DISORDERS

In women who are currently taking full anticoagulation because of an active VTE or cardiac indication, short-term interruption of blood thinning is indicated for surgical procedures that pose a greater risk of bleeding than a dilation and curettage (D&C). Bridging with LMWH preoperatively and postoperatively may be indicated, and oral anticoagulants should be restarted shortly after surgery. The physician managing the patient's anticoagulation should be part of the team guiding bridging and oral agent interruption. In general, warfarin should be held for at least 5 days prior to surgery, and the international normalized ratio (INR) should be <1.5 prior to incision. Therapeutic dose aspirin should be held for 7 days prior to surgery. Once-daily dosing of baby aspirin (81 mg/day) can usually be continued. There are novel oral anticoagulants (NOACs) that are becoming more common; these are factor Xa inhibitors and direct thrombin inhibitors, such as fondaparinux, which inactivates factor Xa by binding antithrombin. Factor Xa inhibitors should be held for 2 to 3 days before surgery, depending on the individual drug's half-life. Direct thrombin inhibitors should be held for 2 to 4 days prior to surgery, depending on renal function. Depending on the indication for full anticoagulation, bridging with LMWH may be required, and this should be guided by the patient's primary prescribing physician. Factor Xa inhibitors and direct thrombin inhibitors should be resumed when the surgeon feels the patient is stable and at low risk for postoperative bleeding from full anticoagulation; these oral anticoagulants have a short half-life and effectively fully anticoagulate within a matter of hours (Robertson, 2015). Also of note, patients with an acute VTE who cannot have their surgery delayed may require placement of a temporary IVC filter.

Bleeding disorders usually cause symptomatic issues in most patients earlier in their lives, and it is estimated that approximately 1% to 2% of patients in the United States have some type of bleeding diathesis. The most common is von Willebrand disease. Patients who have had symptoms of easy bruising, frequent nosebleeds, anemia, menorrhagia, and excessive bleeding with surgical procedures should be considered for a hematologic assessment. Any positive test result should be followed by consultation with a hematologist, as supplementation with coagulation factors in the perioperative period may be required. Women with already confirmed bleeding problems should have a consultation for appropriate prophylaxis, and factor replacement should be guided by a hematologist.

## STRESS-DOSE STEROIDS

Glucocorticoids are prescribed for a variety of illnesses. Exogenous glucocorticoids will blunt the natural response of the hypothalamic-pituitary-adrenal (HPA) axis in the necessary response to stress. Steroid use for longer than a 2-week period within the year prior to surgery necessitates augmented steroid administration during the perioperative period. Even if the dosing was small (as little as 5 to 7.5 mg of daily prednisone), adrenal insufficiency may occur. In fact, any patient who has received the equivalent dose of 20 mg of daily prednisone for more than 5 days is at risk for HPA suppression (Axelrod, 2003). Supplemental stress-dose corticosteroids should be given at the time of surgery. Minor surgery will only necessitate one dose; major surgeries require dosing for the surgery and may require up to 24 hours of additional treatment postoperatively. If on chronic corticosteroids, the patient should resume preoperative dosing immediately after surgery.

### *Assessment of Cardiopulmonary Comorbidities*

Most healthy patients planning gynecologic surgery will not require extensive preoperative testing beyond a complete history, physical examination, and the basic preoperative testing described earlier. However, a patient with significant medical comorbidities will likely require more extensive testing and consultation with other specialties to optimize the patient's perioperative outcome. It is beyond the scope of this book to cover the full evaluation of the various medical comorbidities one will encounter in clinical practice, but a basic understanding of what the consulting physician will consider in his or her evaluation of the patient is important to help counsel the patient and set proper expectations.

### Pulmonary Disease

Pulmonary complications are a frequent form of postoperative morbidity experienced by approximately 5% of women following gynecologic surgery. The goals of the preoperative assessment of the respiratory system are to identify women at risk for developing postoperative pulmonary complications and prescribe appropriate preoperative therapy to reduce these risks. Similar to the evaluation of other organ systems, the history and physical examination are the most important parts of the pulmonary evaluation. Pulmonary function tests of lung volumes and flow rates are only indicated to evaluate women with a history or physical findings suggestive of restrictive or obstructive pulmonary disease. Pulmonary function tests help assess the pulmonary reserve and identify the extent to which the dysfunction is reversible. These tests measure lung volumes, forced vital capacity (FVC), and flow rates, forced expiratory volume in 1 second ($FEV_1$), to help distinguish restrictive defects from obstructive defects. Women who have compromised preoperative pulmonary function are especially susceptible to develop clinically significant postoperative atelectasis, which occurs following approximately 10% of gynecologic operations. Predisposing factors that increase the incidence of atelectasis include morbid obesity, smoking, pulmonary disease, and advanced age. Increased pain, the supine position, abdominal distention, impaired function of the diaphragm, and sedation also contribute to decreased lung volumes and reduced dynamic measurements of pulmonary function postoperatively. Women with chronic lung disease often have shunting of blood in the lungs and arterial hypoxemia. A preoperative arterial blood gas may be able to demonstrate if the patient is hypoxic or hypercarbic, a serious sign, as the patient's respiratory drive may be refractory to hypercarbia. Hence, oxygen therapy for women who are morbidly obese or with symptoms of sleep apnea should be done with care, as these conditions may further suppress respiratory drive.

Asthma increases the incidence of perioperative respiratory problems approximately fourfold. Asthmatic women are susceptible to perioperative respiratory complications secondary to bronchial hyperresponsiveness, airflow obstruction, and hypersecretion of mucus. Ideally, an asthmatic woman should have elective surgery when she is free of wheezing and her pulmonary function is optimal.

### Cardiovascular Disease

Cardiac complications are the leading cause of postoperative deaths. Approximately 1.5% of adults who undergo inpatient noncardiac surgery die in during the first 30 postoperative days. (Devereaux, 2015). Unstable angina of less than 3 months' duration is a strong contraindication to an elective operation. After a myocardial infarction, it is important to delay an elective operation for approximately 6 months. The excessive mortality rate associated with a noncardiac operative procedure within 3 months of an acute myocardial infarct is 27% to 37%. Following a 6-month interval, the chance of a reinfarction is 4% to 6% with elective operations.

The accurate assessment of cardiac risk is important for several reasons. First, it permits the patient to make an informed decision when weighing the risks and benefits of the proposed surgery. Second, the accurate estimation of cardiac risk can also guide preoperative interventions and postoperative care, including the intensity of monitoring. Finally, it allows for more accurate reporting of outcomes that are linked to the intensity of comorbid conditions. There are currently two cardiac risk indexes that are commonly used: the Revised Cardiac Risk Index (RCRI) is the most validated, and the National Surgical Quality Improvement Program risk index for Myocardial Infarction and Cardiac Arrest (NSQIP MICA) has the best predictive performance (http://www.surgicalriskcalculator.com/miorcardiacarrest). Both models assign points based on risk factors, but each defines a cardiac event a little differently, making direct comparisons difficult. For example, the RCRI assigns 1 point for each of the following: high-risk surgery; prior congestive heart failure, stroke, or transient ischemic attack; ischemic heart disease; use of insulin therapy; and creatinine level >2 mg/dL. The risk of a myocardial infarction is 0.5% with 0 points, 1.3% with 1 point, 3.6% with 2 points, and 9.1% with ≥3 points. Unfortunately, clinical risk indexes tend to underestimate risk in patients who are immobile prior to surgery, as they may lack some of the symptoms of cardiac disease simply because they are immobile. It is in this setting that noninvasive cardiac testing is used such as stress nuclear scintigraphy, which missed 30% of postoperative myocardial infarctions in one series or preoperative coronary computed tomographic angiography, which tends to overestimate cardiac risk.

One of the more common practices used to limit cardiac complications was the routine use of beta-blockers perioperatively as an attempt to blunt the sympathetic stress response. Unfortunately, the use of beta-blockers perioperatively reduced the risk of nonfatal myocardial infarction but increased the risk of death, nonfatal stroke, hypotension, and bradycardia. As a result, the common practice of perioperative beta-blockade has given way to its selective use to treat ischemia and tachycardia that can be safely and accurately identified by means of noninvasive cardiac monitoring.

## PROPHYLAXIS AGAINST INFECTIVE ENDOCARDITIS

The indications for prophylactic antibiotic use for the prevention of infective endocarditis (IE) have changed considerably since the American Heart Association guidelines were first published in 1955. In the most recent version of the guidelines, the indications for prophylaxis are very limited compared with prior guidelines (Wilson, 2007). The impetus behind the change is that the risk of IE is greater from random spontaneous bacteremias associated with daily activities than from invasive gastrointestinal (GI), genitourinary (GU), or even dental procedures.

There is a lack of published data convincingly demonstrating that prophylaxis actually prevents IE. In addition, the use of prophylactic antibiotics may prevent a very small number of IEs, at the expense of more adverse antibiotic-associated events, tilting the risk-benefit scale in the wrong direction. As a result, the guidelines no longer recommend IE prophylaxis based solely on an increased lifetime risk of acquisition of IE. They restrict the use of prophylactic antibiotics only for patients who are planning invasive, higher risk procedures (Wilson, 2007). They do not recommend any prophylaxis to prevent IE for elective, noninfected genitourinary GU or GI invasive procedures. They acknowledge that there may be a very small number of IE cases, if any, that could be prevented with prophylactic antibiotics use in this patient population. However, with no proved benefit, the administration of prophylactic antibiotics solely to prevent endocarditis is not recommended for patients who undergo GU or GI tract procedures.

## SUMMARY

In summary, it is the gynecologic surgeon's responsibility to ensure his or her patient is adequately informed of the risks, benefits, and alternative treatments for each recommended surgical procedure. Caring for the patient as a team by involving her primary care provider or other long-term specialty physicians to guide management of medical conditions and long-term medications that may affect the surgical procedure or anesthesia is essential. Early consultation with an anesthesiologist is important for patients with multiple comorbidities, prior anesthesia complications, or patients undergoing complex gynecologic operations, as this improves the preparation and safety of the procedure. Universal Protocol, guidelines to prevent VTE, pathways to enhance postoperative recovery, and surgical site infection prevention bundles improve the quality of gynecologic surgical care and should be used routinely.

## *KEY POINTS*

- Optimal preparation for an operation facilitates a successful result and protects the patient and physician.
- The most significant risk factors for postoperative morbidity are preoperative conditions. They may affect the operation, anesthesia, and postoperative course and may preclude the procedure altogether.
- Approximately 0.5% of the general population and 1.5% of women older than 55 years are receiving continuous glucocorticoids.
- Latex allergy is directly responsible for 12% of the perioperative anaphylactic reactions in adult women and for 70% in children. Health care workers, women with spinal cord injuries, or those who have had to perform self-catheterization are at higher risk for latex allergy.
- The preoperative physical examination should answer three basic questions:
  - Has the primary gynecologic disease process changed since the initial diagnosis?
  - What is the effect of the primary gynecologic disease on other organ systems?
  - What deficiencies in other organ systems may affect the proposed surgery and hospitalization?
- An exam while the patient is under anesthesia may provide additional information, help avoid intraoperative surprises, and affect the surgical plan.
- It is estimated that 60% of routinely ordered tests would not have been performed if tests had been ordered only for an indication discovered by history or physical examination.
- The American Society of Anesthesiologists (ASA) Practice Advisory for Preanesthesia Evaluation states that routine preoperative tests, defined as a test ordered in the absence of a clinical indication or purpose, should not be ordered.
- A preoperative complete blood count and blood type and antibody screen should be performed prior to most gynecologic surgeries.
- Other individualized preoperative laboratory testing should be determined based on the age of the woman, extent of the surgical procedure, and findings at the time of complete history and physical examination.
- Determining the preoperative creatinine or blood urea nitrogen (BUN) level is especially important if the woman is going to be treated with antibiotics excreted by the kidneys.
- A pregnancy test may be appropriate, depending on contraceptive and sexual history, but it should almost always be performed if the patient is a teenager, as menstrual history is at best an imperfect indication of an early pregnancy.
- Serum electrolyte levels are ordered for women taking diuretics or those with a history of renal disease or heart disease. Also, serum electrolyte levels should be evaluated in women with vomiting, diarrhea, ileus, bowel obstruction, or any condition that affects electrolyte balance.
- Routine chest x-rays on all patients often do not impact perioperative management in elective gynecologic surgery, but they should be ordered for women who are 20-pack/year smokers, women with cardiac or pulmonary symptoms, immigrants who have not had a recent chest film, and women older than 70 years.
- A baseline preoperative ECG has been found to be cost effective in asymptomatic women ≥60 years without a history of cardiac disease or significant risk factors.
- In the present medicolegal climate, the absence of informed consent is cited as a major problem in many lawsuits.
- Preoperative orders should be standardized to avoid omissions, and electronic order sets are standard at most institutions.
- If an enhanced recovery pathway is being utilized, the patient can usually eat solid food up until midnight and clear liquids until 30 minutes prior to presenting to the hospital.
- To avoid hypoglycemia, most enhanced recovery after surgery protocols allow patients to eat solid food up to 6 hours before surgery.
- Anesthesiologists classify surgical procedures according to the patient's risk of mortality using the ASA risk class stratification (classes 1-5).

*Continued*

## KEY POINTS—cont'd

- An emergency operation doubles the mortality risks for ASA classes 1, 2, and 3; produces a slightly increased risk in class 4; and does not change the risk in class 5.
- Enhanced recovery refers to a bundled process with the aim of attenuating pathophysiologic changes and the stress response occurring with surgery. These processes replace traditional but untested practices of perioperative care with the primary goal of hastening recovery.
- Adoption of enhanced recovery has resulted in an average reduction in length of stay of 2.5 days and a decrease in complications by as much as 50%.
- Enhanced recovery achieved the greatest benefit in patients undergoing complex cytoreduction for ovarian cancer, of whom 57% underwent colonic or small bowel resection.
- The popularity of TEA following major open gynecologic surgery is due to its effectiveness in controlling pain and the quicker return of bowel function seen in patients with epidural anesthetics.
- The role of TEA in an ERAS care plan is less clear, as it can compete at times with some of the ERAS goals and its use. TEA has been associated with more interventions to treat hypotension, longer length of hospital stay, and more complications in one series of early stage endometrial cancer patients.
- An SSI is one of the most common complications after surgery. SSIs dissatisfy patients and providers, but they also increase the cost of surgical care, increase morbidity, and can increase mortality.
- SSIs are categorized into three classifications by the CDC and the ACS NSQIP: (1) superficial incisional, (2) deep incisional, and (3) organ/space.
- Elements shown to decrease SSI that are often included in reduction bundles include preoperative nicotine cessation, preoperative antiseptic showering and chlorhexidine preparation, using hair clippers instead of a razor, appropriate preoperative antibiotic selection, normothermia, and glycemic control.
- There is abundant literature supporting the use of prophylactic antibiotics in gynecology. The incidence of febrile morbidity may be reduced from 40% to 15% and the incidence of pelvic infection decreased from 25% to 5%.
- The current guidelines for antimicrobial prophylaxis for vaginal or abdominal hysterectomy include the first- or second-generation cephalosporins of cefazolin, cefotetan, cefoxitin, or ampicillin-sulbactam.
- Among women with a β-lactam allergy, the recommended combinations are (1) clindamycin or vancomycin plus an aminoglycoside, or (2) aztreonam, or (3) a fluoroquinolone, metronidazole, and aminoglycoside, or (4) a fluoroquinolone alone.
- Comparative studies have documented that single-dose therapy is as effective as 24 hours of antibiotics. No advantage exists to continuing prophylactic antibiotics beyond the immediate operative period.
- Vaginal surgery continues to carry the lowest risks of SSI and should remain the preferred surgical approach when feasible. However, when minimally invasive approaches to hysterectomy replace laparotomy, the risk of SSI can be reduced by up to 16-fold.
- Multiple studies have documented a two- to threefold increase in the SSI rate directly related to perioperative shaving; if the hair is mechanically in the way, it should be clipped just before the operation.
- The use of chlorhexidine gluconate with 70% isopropyl alcohol as a skin preparation demonstrated a 40% reduction in SSIs in clean contaminated (type II) wound types compared with a 10% povidone-iodine solution.
- The risk of an SSI is significantly increased in the setting of smoking, and patients should be encouraged to stop as patients in a smoking cessation program had perioperative complication rates of 21% versus 41% in controls.
- Hypothermia has been shown to increase the incidence of wound infections, postoperative myocardial events, and perioperative blood loss; impair drug metabolism; and prolong postoperative recovery. Preventing intraoperative hypothermia improves surgical outcomes.
- Glucose levels >180 mg/dL among diabetics and nondiabetics increase the risk of SSI by twofold. Perioperative blood glucose levels should be maintained at <200 mg/dL for all patients.
- Category 1A evidence has demonstrated that strict glucose control (80 to130 mg/dL) in both diabetics and nondiabetics does not improve SSI rates over glucose levels <200 mg/dL. Strict control may have detrimental effects on postoperative outcomes.
- Approximately 25% of all SSIs are caused by *Staphylococcus aureus*.
- Approximately 40% of deaths following gynecologic surgery are related to pulmonary emboli. Although the initial venous injury most often occurs at the time of the operation, approximately 15% of symptomatic emboli do not present until the first week following discharge from the hospital.
- Using the "Caprini score," women in the very low risk group have less than a 3% risk of VTE, women in the moderate group have a 10% to 30% risk, and women in the high risk groups have a more than 30% risk of a VTE.
- LMWH is superior to standard unfractionated heparin because it has a longer half-life, almost 100% bioavailability, dose-independent clearance, and a more consistent anticoagulation effect from dose to dose.
- A meta-analysis of studies evaluating high-risk procedures found perioperative and postoperative LMWH administration to be equally effective.
- In general, warfarin should be held for at least 5 days prior to surgery and the INR should be <1.5 prior to incision.
- Therapeutic dose aspirin should be held for 7 days prior to surgery. Once-daily dosing of baby aspirin (81 mg/day) can usually be continued.
- Factor Xa inhibitors should be held for 2-3 days before surgery, depending on the individual drug's half-life. Direct thrombin inhibitors should be held for 2-4 days prior to surgery, depending on renal function.
- Patients with bleeding disorders usually present early in their lives with bleeding. It is estimated that approximately 1% to 2% of patients in the United States have some type of bleeding diathesis, the most common of which is von Willebrand disease.

## KEY POINTS—cont'd

- Steroid use for longer than a 2-week period within the year prior to surgery necessitates augmented steroid administration during the perioperative period.
- Pulmonary function tests of lung volumes and flow rates are only indicated to evaluate women with a history or physical findings suggestive of restrictive or obstructive pulmonary disease.
- Predisposing factors that increase the incidence of atelectasis include morbid obesity, smoking, pulmonary disease, and advanced age. Increased pain, the supine position, abdominal distention, impaired function of the diaphragm, and sedation also contribute to decreased lung volumes and reduced dynamic measurements of pulmonary function postoperatively.
- The excessive mortality rate associated with a noncardiac operative procedure within 3 months of an acute myocardial infarct is 27% to 37%. Following a 6-month interval, the chance of a reinfarction is 4% to 6% with elective operations.
- The routine use of beta-blockers perioperatively to reduce the risk of nonfatal myocardial infarction is no longer practiced due to the increased risk of death, nonfatal stroke, hypotension, and bradycardia. As a result, the common practice of perioperative beta-blockade has given way to its selective use.
- The administration of prophylactic antibiotics solely to prevent endocarditis is no longer recommended for patients who undergo GU or GI tract procedures.

## KEY REFERENCES


American College of Surgeons National Surgical Quality Improvement Program (ACS NSQIP). Classic, essential, small-rural, targeted, and Florida variables & definitions. *American College of Surgeons National Surgical Quality Improvement Program Operations Manual.* Chicago, IL: American College of Surgeons; 2011:24-26.

Axelrod L. Perioperative management of patients treated with glucocorticoids. *Endocrinol Metab Clin North Am.* 2003;32(2):367-383.

Bakkum-Gamez JN, Dowdy SC, Borah BJ, et al. Predictors and costs of surgical site infections in patients with endometrial cancer. *Gynecol Oncol.* 2013;130(1):100-106.

Belavy D, Janda M, Baker J, et al. Epidural analgesia is associated with an increased incidence of postoperative complications in patients requiring an abdominal hysterectomy for early stage endometrial cancer. *Gynecol Oncol.* 2013;131(2):423-429.

Bode LG, Kluytmans JA, Wertheim HF, et al. Preventing surgical-site infections in nasal carriers of Staphylococcus aureus. *N Engl J Med.* 2010;362(1):9-17.

Bonnar J. Venous thromboembolism and gynecologic surgery. *Clin Obstet Gynecol.* 1985;28(2):432-446.

Brady M, Kinn S, Stuart P. Preoperative fasting for adults to prevent perioperative complications. *Cochrane Database Syst Rev.* 2003;(4):CD004423.

Brandstrup B, Tønnesen H, Beier-Holgersen R, et al. Effects of intravenous fluid restriction on postoperative complications: comparison of two perioperative fluid regimens: a randomized assessor-blinded multicenter trial. *Ann Surg.* 2003;238(5):641-648.

Bratzler DW, Dellinger EP, Olsen KM, et al. Clinical practice guidelines for antimicrobial prophylaxis in surgery. *Am J Health-Syst Pharm.* 2013;70(3):195-283.

Campbell G, Alderson P, Smith AF, et al. Warming of intravenous and irrigation fluids for preventing inadvertent perioperative hypothermia. *Cochrane Database Syst Rev.* 2015;4:CD009891.

Carter J. Fast-track surgery in gynaecology and gynaecologic oncology: a review of a rolling clinical audit. *ISRN Surg.* 2012;2012:368014.

Chambers D, Paton F, Wilson P, et al. An overview and methodological assessment of systematic reviews and meta-analyses of enhanced recovery programmes in colorectal surgery. *BMJ Open.* 2014;4(5):e005014.

Chan RP, Galas FR, Hajjar LA, et al. Intensive perioperative glucose control does not improve outcomes of patients submitted to open-heart surgery: a randomized controlled trial. *Clinics (Sao Paulo).* 2009;64(1):51-60.

Charoenkwan K, Phillipson G, Vutyavanich T. Early versus delayed (traditional) oral fluids and food for reducing complications after major abdominal gynaecologic surgery. *Cochrane Database Syst Rev.* 2007;(4):CD004508.

Chase DM, Lopez S, Nguyen C, et al. A clinical pathway for postoperative management and early patient discharge: does it work in gynecologic oncology? *Am J Obstet Gynecol.* 2008;199(5):541.e1-541.e7.

Cima R, Dankbar E, Lovely J, et al. Colorectal surgery surgical site infection reduction program: a national surgical quality improvement program–driven multidisciplinary single-institution experience. *J Am Coll Surg.* 2013;216(1):23-33.

Colling K, Glover J, et al. Abdominal hysterectomy: reduced risk of surgical site infection associated with robotic and laparoscopic technique. *Surg Infect (Larchmt).* 2015;16(5):498-503.

Committee on Standards and Practice Parameters, Apfelbaum JL, Connis RT, et al. Practice advisory for preanesthesia evaluation: an updated report by the American Society of Anesthesiologists Task Force on Preanesthesia Evaluation. *Anesthesiology.* 2012;116(3):522-538.

Cruse P, Foord R. The epidemiology of wound infection. A 10-year prospective study of 62,939 wounds. *Surg Clin North Am.* 1980;60(1):27-40.

Cutillo G, Maneschi F, Franchi M, et al. Early feeding compared with nasogastric decompression after major oncologic gynecologic surgery: a randomized study. *Obstet Gynecol.* 1999;93(1):41-45.

Darouiche RO, Wall Jr MJ, Itani KM, et al. Chlorhexidine–alcohol versus povidone–iodine for surgical-site antisepsis. *N Engl J Med.* 2010;362(1):18-26.

Devereaux PJ, Sessler DI. Cardiac complications in patients undergoing major noncardiac surgery. *N Engl J Med.* 2015;373(23):2258-2269.

Eberhart LK, Ploger B, et al. Enhanced recovery after major gynaecological surgery for ovarian cancer - an objective and patient-based assessment of a traditional versus a multimodal 'fast track' rehabilitation programme. *Anasthesiol Intensivmed.* 2008;49:180-194.

Ferguson SE, Malhotra T, Seshan VE, et al. A prospective randomized trial comparing patient-controlled epidural analgesia to patient-controlled intravenous analgesia on postoperative pain control and recovery after major open gynecologic cancer surgery. *Gynecol Oncol.* 2009;114(1):111-116.

Galvão CM, Liang Y, Clark AM. Effectiveness of cutaneous warming systems on temperature control: meta-analysis. *J Adv Nurs.* 2010;66(6):1196-1206.

Gandhi GY, Nuttall GA, Abel MD, et al. Intensive intraoperative insulin therapy versus conventional glucose management during cardiac surgery: a randomized trial. *Ann Intern Med.* 2007;146(4):233-243.

Gerardi MA, Santillan A, Meisner B, et al. A clinical pathway for patients undergoing primary cytoreductive surgery with rectosigmoid colectomy for advanced ovarian and primary peritoneal cancers. *Gynecol Oncol.* 2008;108(2):282-286.

Gould MK, Garcia DA, Wren SM, et al. Prevention of VTE in nonorthopedic surgical patients: Antithrombotic Therapy and Prevention of Thrombosis, 9th ed: American College of Chest Physicians Evidence-Based Clinical Practice Guidelines. *Chest.* 2012;141(2 Suppl):e227S-e277S.

Güenaga K, Matos D, Wille-Jørgensen P. Mechanical bowel preparation for elective colorectal surgery. *Cochrane Database Syst Rev.* 2011;(9). CD001544.

Hawn MT, Vick CC, Richman J, et al. Surgical site infection prevention: time to move beyond the surgical care improvement program. *Ann Surg.* 2011;254(3):494-501.

Irvin W, Andersen W, Taylor P, et al. Minimizing the risk of neurologic injury in gynecologic surgery. *Obstet Gynecol.* 2004;103(2):374-382.

Kalogera E, Bakkum-Gamez JN, Jankowski CJ, et al. Enhanced recovery in gynecologic surgery. *Obstet Gynecol.* 2013;122(2 Pt 1):319-328.

Kalogera E, Dowdy SC, Mariani A, et al. Utility of closed suction pelvic drains at time of large bowel resection for ovarian cancer. *Gynecol Oncol.* 2012;126(3):391-396.

Kaplan EB, Sheiner LB, Boeckmann AJ, et al. The usefulness of preoperative laboratory screening. *JAMA*. 1985;253(24):3576-3581.
Kehlet H. Multimodal approach to control postoperative pathophysiology and rehabilitation. *Br J Anaesth*. 1997;78(5):606-617.
Kjønniksen I, Andersen BM, Søndenaa VG, et al. Preoperative hair removal–a systematic literature review. *AORN J*. 2002;75(5):928-938, 940.
Knight N, Aucar J. Use of an anatomic marking form as an alternative to the Universal Protocol for Preventing Wrong Site, Wrong Procedure and Wrong Person Surgery. *Am J Surg*. 2010;200(6):803-809.
Koo CY, Hyder JA, Wanderer JP, et al. A meta-analysis of the predictive accuracy of postoperative mortality using the American Society of Anesthesiologists' Physical Status Classification System. *World J Surg*. 2015;39(1):88-103.
Kwon S, Thompson R, Dellinger P, et al. Importance of perioperative glycemic control in general surgery: a report from the Surgical Care and Outcomes Assessment Program. *Ann Surg*. 2013;257(1):8-14.
Lake AG, McPencow AM, Dick-Biascoechea MA, et al. Surgical site infection after hysterectomy. *Am J Obstet Gynecol*. 2013;209(5):490.e1-490.e9.
Lindström D, Sadr Azodi O, Wladis A, et al. Effects of a perioperative smoking cessation intervention on postoperative complications: a randomized trial. *Ann Surg*. 2008;248(5):739-745.
Marx C, Rasmussen T, Jakobsen DH, et al. The effect of accelerated rehabilitation on recovery after surgery for ovarian malignancy. *Acta Obstet Gynecol Scand*. 2006;85(4):488-492.
Mathur S, Plank LD, McCall JL, et al. Randomized controlled trial of preoperative oral carbohydrate treatment in major abdominal surgery. *Br J Surg*. 2010;97(4):485-494.
Minig L, Biffi R, Zanagnolo V, et al. Early oral versus "traditional" postoperative feeding in gynecologic oncology patients undergoing intestinal resection: a randomized controlled trial. *Ann Surg Oncol*. 2009;16(6):1660-1668.
Nelson R, Edwards S, Tse B. Prophylactic nasogastric decompression after abdominal surgery. *Cochrane Database Syst Rev*. 2007;(3):CD004929.
Nygren J, Thorell A, Jacobsson H, et al. Preoperative gastric emptying. Effects of anxiety and oral carbohydrate administration. *Ann Surg*. 1995;222(6):728-734.
Oliveira L, Wexner SD, Daniel N, et al. Mechanical bowel preparation for elective colorectal surgery. A prospective, randomized, surgeon-blinded trial comparing sodium phosphate and polyethylene glycol-based oral lavage solutions. *Dis Colon Rectum*. 1997;40(5):585-591.
Perez-Protto S, Sessler DI, Reynolds LF, et al. Circulating-water garment or the combination of a circulating-water mattress and forced-air cover to maintain core temperature during major upper-abdominal surgery. *Br J Anaesth*. 2010;105(4):466-470.
Qaseem A, Snow V, Fitterman N, et al. Risk assessment for and strategies to reduce perioperative pulmonary complications for patients undergoing noncardiothoracic surgery: a guideline from the American College of Physicians. *Ann Intern Med*. 2006;144(8):575-580.
Rajagopalan S, Mascha E, Na J, et al. The effects of mild perioperative hypothermia on blood loss and transfusion requirement. *Anesthesiology*. 2008;108(1):71-77.
Raskob GE, Hirsh J. Controversies in timing of the first dose of anticoagulant prophylaxis against venous thromboembolism after major orthopedic surgery. *Chest*. 2003;124(6 Suppl):379S-385S.
Revolus T, Tetrokalashvilli M. Implementation of evidence-based innovative bundle checklist for reduction of surgical site infection. *Obstet Gynecol*. 2014;123(Suppl 1):32S.
Robertson L, Kesteven P, McCaslin JE. Oral direct thrombin inhibitors or oral factor Xa inhibitors for the treatment of deep vein thrombosis. *Cochrane Database Syst Rev*. 2015;6:CD010956.
Sandberg EH, Sharma R, Wiklund R, et al. Clinicians consistently exceed a typical person's short-term memory during preoperative teaching. *Anesth Analg*. 2008;107(3):972-978.
Scott EM, Buckland R. A systematic review of intraoperative warming to prevent postoperative complications. *AORN J*. 2006;83(5):1090-1104, 1107-1013.
Sørensen L. Wound healing and infection in surgery: the clinical impact of smoking and smoking cessation: a systematic review and meta-analysis. *Arch Surg*. 2012;147(4):373-383.
Tran CW, McGree ME, Weaver AL, et al. Surgical site infection after primary surgery for epithelial ovarian cancer: predictors and impact on survival. *Gynecol Oncol*. 2015;136(2):278-284.
van der Slegt J, van der Laan L, Veen EJ, et al. Implementation of a bundle of care to reduce surgical site infections in patients undergoing vascular surgery. *PLoS One*. 2013;18(8):e71566.
van Walraven C, Musselman R. The Surgical Site Infection Risk Score (SSIRS): a model to predict the risk of surgical site infections. *PLoS One*. 2013;8(6):e67167.
Varadhan KK, Neal KR, Dejong CH, et al. The enhanced recovery after surgery (ERAS) pathway for patients undergoing major elective open colorectal surgery: a meta-analysis of randomized controlled trials. *Clin Nutr*. 2010;29(4):434-440.
Waits SA, Fritze D, et al. Developing an argument for bundled interventions to reduce surgical site infection in colorectal surgery. *Surgery*. 2014;155(4):602-606.
Warttig S, Alderson P, Campbell G, et al. Interventions for treating inadvertent postoperative hypothermia. *Cochrane Database Syst Rev*. 2014;11:CD009892.
Webster J, Osborne S. Preoperative bathing or showering with skin antiseptics to prevent surgical site infection. *Cochrane Database Syst Rev*. 2007;(2):CD004985.
Wijk L, Franzen K, Ljungqvist O, et al. Implementing a structured Enhanced Recovery After Surgery (ERAS) protocol reduces length of stay after abdominal hysterectomy. *Acta Obstet Gynecol Scand*. 2014;93(8):749-756.
Wilson W, Taubert KA, Gewitz M, et al. Prevention of infective endocarditis: guidelines from the American Heart Association: a guideline from the American Heart Association Rheumatic Fever, Endocarditis, and Kawasaki Disease Committee, Council on Cardiovascular Disease in the Young, and the Council on Clinical Cardiology, Council on Cardiovascular Surgery and Anesthesia, and the Quality of Care and Outcomes Research Interdisciplinary Working Group. *Circulation*. 2007;116(15):1736-1754.

# 25

# Perioperative Management of Complications

## Fever, Respiratory, Cardiovascular, Thromboembolic, Urinary Tract, Gastrointestinal, Wound, and Operative Site Complications; Neurologic Injury; Psychological Sequelae

*Leslie Clark, Paola Alvarez Gehrig*

The goal of postoperative care is the restoration of a woman's normal physiologic and psychological health. The postoperative period includes the time from the end of the procedure in the operating room until the woman has resumed her normal routine and lifestyle.

Postoperative complications may occur at any time; however, early recognition and management will often preclude larger problems. Thus attention to postoperative details cannot be overemphasized. Complications increase the duration of the postoperative stay in the hospital. In a study of women readmitted for postoperative complications, approximately 40% had been discharged earlier than the mean length of stay for the corresponding operative procedure (Meeks, 1992). Because many procedures are now performed using minimally invasive techniques, patients will usually leave less than or close to 24 hours after surgery. Prior to discharge, it is important that the patient receive education regarding expectations, signs and symptoms of infection and other complications, and contact information.

Significant risk factors in any surgical population include underlying cardiac and pulmonary disease, smoking, obesity, prior or current abdominal/thoracic surgery, and type of anesthesia. General caveats of postoperative management emphasize attention to the particular needs of each woman. Studies conflict on whether age alone is an independent risk factor for perioperative morbidity and mortality. Older patients tend to have more underlying disease, placing them at higher risk for perioperative complications. Unfortunately, this alone does not completely account for their worse outcomes. In one large population-based study, even *healthy* elderly patients continued to have higher morbidity and mortality. It is likely that elderly patients respond differently to perioperative physiologic stressors and pharmacologic interventions. Individualization is especially important in the postoperative care of geriatric women. Special nursing attention and minimal doses of narcotics help prevent confusion and disorientation. Ongoing verbal communications with the nursing staff help eliminate misunderstandings that might result in less than ideal postoperative care.

Surgical stress invokes several physiologic responses meant as the body's defenses. Many of these responses may be more problematic than the actual surgery. For example, some women will respond to the insulin resistance of surgical trauma with severe hyperglycemia, which is detrimental to healing. Peri- and postoperative management strategies are aimed at minimizing or preventing these adverse effects, such as prevention of thromboembolism, or selective use of beta blockade in older patients to prevent cardiac complications (Fig. 25.1) (Kehlet, 2003).

This chapter discusses major issues of management during the period from the end of surgery until the return to normal physiologic and psychological function. However, much of the data regarding postoperative complications only involve the period up through postoperative day 30. Problems and complications arise over the whole spectrum of the postoperative time frame and are interrelated. Thus the clinician must be aware at all times of a woman's changing status during recovery. For simplicity, this chapter is organized around organ systems and their potential complications.

## POSTOPERATIVE FEVER

The exact definition of postoperative febrile morbidity varies greatly among authors. Diurnal fluctuations are characteristic of the normal daily body temperature patterns of humans. Most definitions use a temperature greater than 38° C 24 hours after surgery as the indicator of febrile morbidity. It is not unusual for gynecologic patients to have a mild temperature elevation during the first 72 hours of the postoperative period, especially during the late afternoon or evening. Up to 75% of patients develop a temperature greater than 37° C, which is usually not associated

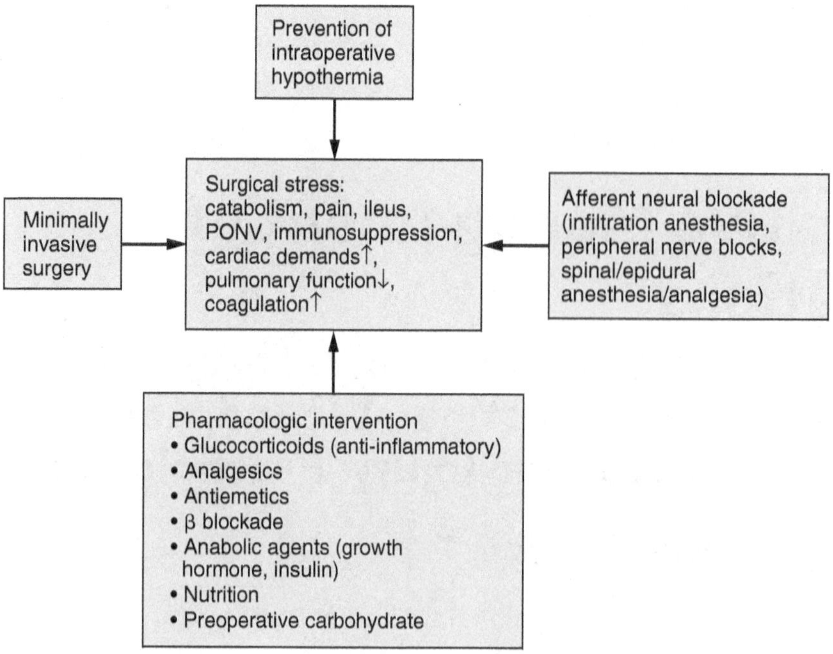


**Figure 25.1** Stresses of surgery and interventions to counteract adverse responses. (Modified from Kehlet H, Dahl JB. Anaesthesia, surgery, and challenges in postoperative recovery. *Lancet.* 2003;362[9399]:1921-1928.)

with an infectious process. The incidence of postoperative febrile morbidity following benign hysterectomy ranges from 14% to 16% (Kendrick, 2008; Peipert, 2004).

Fever is the most common morbidity in the postoperative patient. Common causes of a fever include atelectasis, pneumonia, urinary tract infection (UTI), nonseptic phlebitis, wound infection, and operative site infection. Two intraoperative factors that dramatically increase the risk of postoperative fever are an operative time longer than 2 hours and the necessity for intraoperative transfusion. Increased intraoperative blood loss is associated with a 3.5 relative risk (relative risk [RR]; 95% confidence interval [CI]: 1.8-6.8) of developing a postoperative fever (Peipert, 2004).

The physician's primary goal in examining the postoperative febrile patient is to determine the etiology of the fever. Approximately 20% of postoperative fevers are directly related to infection and 80% are related to noninfectious causes (Schey, 2005). Some conditions necessitate active intervention, whereas others are self-limiting. Thus it is imperative not to treat a postoperatively febrile patient empirically with broad-spectrum antibiotics. Protocols limiting antibiotic use to high-risk patients (bowel operation, preoperative infection, immunodeficiency, indwelling vascular access, mechanical heart valves, or intensive care unit [ICU] admission) or those with persistent fevers over 101° F for more than 48 hours have been shown to be safe (Kendrick, 2008).

The pathophysiology of postoperative fever is primarily related to the release of cytokines. The cause of a postoperative fever may be simple and common, such as atelectasis or dehydration, or unusual, such as malignant hyperthermia or septicemia. The temporal relationship of the onset of a woman's febrile response to common postoperative complications is depicted in Table 25.1.

Table 25.1 Onset of Fever for Various Postoperative Complications

| | Day | | | | | | |
|---|---|---|---|---|---|---|---|
| **Causes** | **1** | **2** | **3** | **4** | **5** | **6** | **1 Week or Longer** |
| Atelectasis | → | → | → | → | | | |
| Pneumonia | | | → | → | → | → | → |
| Wound infection | | | | | | | |
| Streptococcal or clostridial | → | → | → | | | | |
| Other bacterial | | | | | | | |
| Ovarian abscess | | | | | → | → | → |
| Cuff cellulitis | | | | | | | → |
| Phlebitis | | | | → | → | → | |
| Superficial | | | | → | → | → | |
| Deep | | | → | → | → | → | → |
| Urinary tract infection | | | → | → | → | → | → |
| Ureteral or bladder injury | | | | | | | → |

## *WORKUP FOR FEVER*

The initial workup for a postoperative fever should focus on the most common problems. Medical students memorize the "five Ws" in the differential diagnosis of a postoperative fever: ***w***ind (atelectasis), ***w***ater (UTI), ***w***ound (infection or hematoma), ***w***alk (superficial or deep vein phlebitis), and ***w***onder drugs (drug-induced fever). The proper workup of a postoperative fever, similar to that of any problem in medicine, involves the three classic steps of history, physical examination, and laboratory evaluations, with major emphasis placed on the physical examination. The physical examination emphasizes the following:

examination of the lungs for atelectasis and pneumonia; the wound and operative site for infection or hematoma formation; the costovertebral angles for tenderness, which may suggest pyelonephritis; and superficial veins in the arms for superficial phlebitis and deep veins in the legs for deep vein phlebitis.

The findings of the history and especially the physical examination will influence the extent of laboratory tests ordered. The three most commonly ordered laboratory tests are complete blood count, chest radiography, and urinalysis. A study by Schwandt and colleagues has emphasized that chest radiography and urine cultures are best ordered only for specific clinical signs not as reflex orders (Schwandt, 2001). Other common tests include culture and Gram stains of body fluids, including sputum, urine, and blood. One study of over 300 women who were febrile following hysterectomy did not identify a single positive blood culture, while another study found a 9.7% positive blood culture rate in over 500 patients, suggesting a role for judicious use of blood cultures (Kendrick, 2008; Schey, 2005). Women with persistent and undiagnosed fevers may need imaging studies, such as pelvic ultrasound or computed tomography (CT) to detect problems such as compromised ureters, abscesses, or foreign bodies.

Each major complication will be discussed in detail later in the chapter. However, several specific generalizations concerning the type and characteristics of fever patterns should be emphasized. Fever is a common postoperative finding and rarely is the cause of the fever a serious infection. Microatelectasis is thought to be the cause of approximately 90% of fevers occurring in the first 48 hours after operation. Patients who develop fever as a result of an indwelling catheter, such as intravenous (IV) lines or Foley catheters, are afebrile for several days and then experience an abrupt temperature spike. In contrast, wound or pelvic infections, which are usually clinically diagnosed from the fourth to seventh postoperative days, usually are associated with a low-grade fever that begins early in the postoperative period. An empiric trial of IV heparin for 72 hours is often a diagnostic and therapeutic trial for pelvic thrombophlebitis in refractory cases of postoperative fever of unknown origin.

Importantly, infection in the older woman will not always present with classic findings. The amount of temperature elevation may not reflect the severity of the infection. Not uncommonly, the first signs of infection in older adults will be mental status changes. Additionally, the degree of leukocytosis, being blunted or absent may not reflect infection.

A woman with a drug-induced fever feels better and does not look as ill as her temperature course indicates. The tachycardia associated with the elevated temperature is usually much less than usually anticipated with a similar temperature elevation secondary to inflammation or infection. The presence of eosinophilia suggests a drug-induced fever. However, drug fever is rare and is usually a diagnosis of exclusion. Presumptive evidence of a drug-induced fever is established when the fever disappears after discontinuation of the drug. The most commonly implicated drugs include allopurinol, carbamazepine, lamotrigine, phenytoin, sulfasalazine, vancomycin, minocycline, dapsone, and sulfamethoxazole. The risk of developing a drug-induced fever is higher in elderly and HIV-infected patients.

Superficial thrombophlebitis often produces an enigmatic fever. Often, there is tenderness at the IV site. IV catheters should be removed at the first sign of tenderness or erythema, but routine replacement to prevent thrombophlebitis is not indicated (Webster, 2013). Transfusion reactions can also cause febrile events. Leukocyte or platelet antibodies usually cause these reactions. As long as a major blood type incompatibility is not found, treatment is usually conservative.

It is common practice to repeat the basic fever workup at regular intervals until the diagnosis is established. The woman should be reexamined and selective laboratory tests reordered. Rare causes of postoperative fever include pulmonary embolism (PE), thyroid storm, and malignant neoplasms. These diagnoses usually present with other signs and symptoms as well as temperature elevation. It is important to consider that fever is a potentially beneficial physiologic response of the patient. Therefore unless the woman is symptomatic secondary to the elevated temperature, it is not necessary to order antipyretic medications. Cellular damage usually occurs when the core temperature exceeds 41° C. Active cutaneous cooling does not reduce core temperature effectively and may have undesirable effects, such as increasing the metabolic rate and activating the autonomic nervous system.

## MANAGEMENT OF FALLING HEMOGLOBIN

Bleeding is one of the most worrisome postoperative complications. Significant arterial bleeding in the first 24 hours often necessitates reoperation. This complication is discussed later in the chapter, along with the management of shock and pelvic hematoma.

Vital signs should be ordered at frequent intervals during the first 24 hours to detect hypovolemia. Most institutions have standard postoperative monitoring floor orders of at least every 4 hours. Most women will have sufficient intravascular volume to compensate (during the early phases of hemorrhage) through the redistribution of blood flow from less vital to more vital organs. As a result, low urine output may be the earliest sign of a decrease in intravascular volume. Thus following an operation, sizable amounts of unrecognized intraperitoneal or retroperitoneal bleeding are sometimes present without the woman having subjective symptoms or appreciable changes in her vital signs. This may be the case particularly in young, healthy women. Minimum urine output should be 0.5 mL/kg/hr. A consistent orthostatic decrease in blood pressure of more than 10 mm Hg may indicate a decrease of 20% of the blood volume. Thus measuring hemoglobin at two intervals during the postoperative course is helpful. Hemoglobin drawn 24 hours following an operation may not truly reflect postoperative blood loss, thus a repeat hemoglobin measurement could be evaluated at 48 to 72 hours postoperatively to identify the nadir if indicated.

The normal physiologic response to the stress of the operation and tissue destruction is a release of increased levels of aldosterone, cortisol, and antidiuretic hormone (ADH). The higher levels of aldosterone produce an increase in sodium and water retention, whereas increased levels of ADH promote free water retention. This has been called the *ebb phase* of postoperative physiology. It is common for women to have notable lower extremity edema for the first few postoperative days, because they are often given significant amounts of IV fluids. Depending on the type and amount of intraoperative and postoperative IV fluids, the hemoglobin on the first postoperative day may be

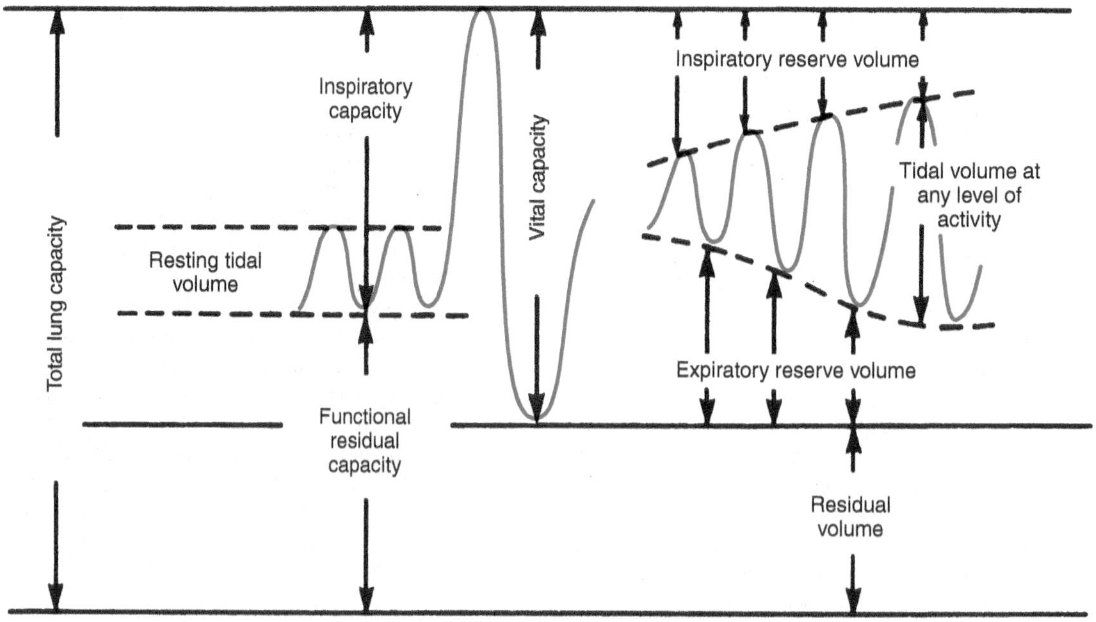


**Figure 25.2** Graphic illustration of lung volumes and capacities. (From Wellman JJ. Respiratory care in the surgical patient. In: Lubin MF, Walker HD, Smith RB, eds. *Medical Management of the Surgical Patient.* Stoneham, MA: Butterworth; 1982.)

misleading and reflect fluid changes rather than intraoperative or postoperative hemorrhage. The hemoglobin from the third postoperative day is a more accurate measurement of postoperative change. If the patient is doing well, stress hormone levels decline, and water retention stops, the patient will begin to experience a brisk diuresis beginning around the third postoperative day. Hemoglobin samples should be obtained in a standard fashion to eliminate sampling errors. For example, samples drawn from central lines or during blood gas determinations often give false values because of the heparin or saline flush solutions.

After the effects of the operative blood loss are subtracted from the preoperative hemoglobin, each further reduction in hemoglobin of 1 to 2 points reflects a postoperative hemorrhage of approximately 250 to 500 mL. The safe level of postoperative anemia is a controversial issue. Historically, patients were transfused to maintain hemoglobins greater than 10, but mounting evidence supported the role of individualized treatment in consideration for transfusion. In hemodynamically stable patients a hemoglobin of <7 is usually an indication for transfusion. Postoperative patients with a hemoglobin of 7 to 8 should be considered for transfusion if cardiovascular disease is present. In a patient with a hemoglobin of 8 to 10 transfusion is not indicated unless symptomatic anemia, ongoing bleeding, or concern for acute coronary syndrome is noted (Klein, 2007). The morbidity and mortality associated with a surgical procedure are directly related to the amount of intraoperative and postoperative blood loss and not the corresponding level of preoperative anemia.

## RESPIRATORY COMPLICATIONS

Alterations of pulmonary function are an expected physiologic change in women having general anesthesia and operations that enter the peritoneal cavity. Of importance, respiratory complications contribute to up to 25% of deaths in women who die during the first 7 postoperative days. Respiratory problems may arise secondary to inadequate ventilation by women as they try to minimize acute pain from the operative incision.

### *ATELECTASIS*

The term *atelectasis* is derived from two Greek words that mean "imperfect expansion." The severity of atelectasis ranges from lack of expansion of a small group of terminal bronchioles and alveoli to complete collapse of a lung. In most patients, atelectasis is the failure to maintain patency of the small pulmonary airways and alveoli. Atelectasis is the most common cause of postoperative temperature elevations. Studies have demonstrated that there is no association between fever and the amount of atelectasis seen radiographically. The incidence of atelectasis depends on the number of predisposing risk factors and the vigor with which the clinical diagnosis is established.

Of all postoperative respiratory complications, 90% are related to atelectasis. The immediate postoperative period is characterized by a decrease in functional residual capacity and lung compliance (Fig. 25.2). Thus the work of breathing is increased. Micro atelectasis is most common when small airways (<1 mm in diameter) become blocked by secretions. When small airways remain closed by a combination of mucous plugs and bronchospasm, the gas distal to the obstruction is absorbed. This process results in atelectasis. These changes occur during the first 72 hours following an operation. When atelectasis becomes progressive and involves a large area of lung tissue, there is an associated decrease in oxygen saturation and a decrease in arterial oxygen pressure ($Po_2$). This is associated with a normal to low arterial carbon dioxide pressure ($Pco_2$).

Pulmonary and nonpulmonary factors that favor premature airway closure and development of atelectasis are listed in

**Box 25.1 Nonpulmonary and Pulmonary Factors Favoring Premature Airway Closure and Atelectasis**

**Nonpulmonary Factors**

Supine position
Obesity
Increased abdominal girth (ileus, pneumoperitoneum)
Breathing at low lung volumes
- Bindings around the chest and abdomen
- Incisional pain
- Sedative narcotic drugs
- Prolonged effect of paralyzing drugs
- Immobility
- Excessively high concentrations of oxygen for prolonged periods

**Pulmonary Factors**

Interstitial edema
Loss of surfactant with air space instability
Airway obstruction
- Inflammatory with swelling of bronchial and interbronchial tissue
- Constriction of bronchial smooth muscle
- Retained secretions

From Wellman JJ. Respiratory care in the surgical patient. In: Lubin MF, Walker HK, Smith RB, eds. *Medical Management of the Surgical Patient*. Stoneham, MA: Butterworth; 1982.

Box 25.1. The supine position decreases the functional residual capacity by approximately 20% compared with the erect position. Obesity, smoking, age older than 60 years, prolonged operative time, presence of a nasogastric tube, and coexisting medical conditions, such as cardiac or lung disease and pulmonary infection, all predispose women to atelectasis. Insufflation of the abdomen for laparoscopic and robotic surgery also contributes to postoperative atelectasis by collapsing the dependent portion of the lung bases if adequate ventilation pressures are not used.

In normal breathing, periodic, involuntary, deep inspirations help expand all areas of the lung. Incisional pain, the supine position, narcotics, and abdominal distention contribute to a pattern of monotonous shallow breathing without spontaneous deep sighs in the postoperative period. As a result of the incisional pain, chest wall breathing dominates over abdominal breathing. The resultant decrease in the movement of the diaphragm contributes to the development of atelectasis. A further decrease in functional residual capacity, a decrease in surfactant, and a depression of mucociliary transport, all contribute to ventilation-perfusion ($\dot{V}/\dot{Q}$) mismatches and reduced $\dot{V}/\dot{Q}$ ratios. The results are gas trapping, atelectasis, and vascular shunting. In most individuals, microatelectasis is patchy and localized to small areas. However, the severity of atelectasis varies and may involve a complete lung. Distribution of pulmonary blood flow is influenced by gravity. A greater proportion of pulmonary blood flows to dependent areas of the lungs in the supine patient. This increased blood flow, combined with the atelectasis in dependent areas, results in an increased impairment of oxygenation, as well as a decrease in the elimination of carbon dioxide. Obese patients, in general, should be kept slightly upright, not prone, for the first 24 hours to improve vital capacity and ventilation, thus decreasing atelectasis.

Atelectasis may present as the classic triad of fever, tachypnea, and tachycardia developing within the first 72 hours following an operation. On physical examination, tubular breathing, decreased breath sounds, and moist inspiratory rales may be heard. These findings are most prominent over the bases of the lung. If the condition progresses, an increase in productive cough and leukocytosis results. Chest radiographic films may demonstrate a patchy infiltrate with elevations of the diaphragm.

Atelectasis usually resolves spontaneously by the third to fifth postoperative day. Nevertheless, major efforts are made to prevent atelectasis, especially in high-risk individuals. The foundations of prevention of atelectasis are the encouragement of uneven ventilation and the production of episodes of prolonged inspiration to increase functional residual capacity. Thus the patient is encouraged to walk, take deep breaths, cough, turn from side to side, remain semierect rather than supine, and use the incentive spirometer regularly. Early mobilization and ambulation have been documented to be as effective as chest physical therapy in the prevention of pulmonary complications. Keeping pain relief to a level at which the woman will be able to cooperate and not have monotonous shallow breathing is also helpful. Although the use of neither postoperative continuous positive airway pressure (CPAP) nor incentive spirometry has been shown to reduce postoperative pulmonary morbidity, simple bedside incentive spirometry can be used to prevent and reverse atelectasis (Nascimento, 2014; Ireland, 2014). Many women need encouragement by the hospital staff to use these devices effectively. The primary risk of atelectasis is progression to pneumonia.

## *PNEUMONIA*

Postoperative pneumonia is commonly associated with atelectasis because bacterial infections often begin in collapsed areas of the lungs. Predisposing factors to the development of pneumonia include chronic pulmonary disease, heavy cigarette smoking, alcohol abuse, obesity, advanced age, nasogastric tubes, long operative procedures, gram-negative bacterial infections, postoperative peritonitis, and debilitating illnesses.

The symptoms and signs of pneumonia are fever, cough, dyspnea, tachypnea, and purulent sputum. When pain occurs, it may be felt in the back or chest. The classic physical finding of pneumonia is coarse rales over the infected area. The patient usually has a higher temperature and more systemic toxicity than a woman with atelectasis. Leukocytosis is pronounced in most patients, although it may be delayed or attenuated in older women. Chest radiographs often demonstrate diffuse patchy infiltrates of the lung. Radiographic diagnoses are approximately 60% accurate for bacterial or viral pneumonia in women with laboratory-proved pneumonia. Gram staining of the sputum helps differentiate between bacterial colonization and infection. In cases of pneumonia, the smear contains a large number of inflammatory cells with both intracellular and extracellular bacteria.

The management of pneumonia is similar to the management of atelectasis, with the addition of parenteral antibiotics. Antibiotic choice is based on the type of pneumonia diagnosed. Most postoperative patients will fall into one of the following categories: hospital-acquired pneumonia (HAP) occurring 48 hours or more after hospital admission, ventilator-acquired pneumonia (VAP) developing 48 to 72 hours after endotracheal intubation, or health care–associated pneumonia (HCAP) occurring in a nonhospitalized patient with extensive health care contact. HCAP was added as a category in 2005, as individuals with extensive health care contact are at an increased risk for developing pneumonia with multidrug resistant bacteria. Patients meet the definition of HCAP if they are not hospitalized, develop pneumonia, and have one of the following: IV therapy, wound care, or IV chemotherapy in the prior 30 days; reside in a nursing facility or long-term care facility or have been hospitalized for 2 or more days in the past 90 days; or attended a hospital or hemodialysis clinic in the prior 30 days. Most patients with HAP, HCAP, and VAP who do not have significant risk factors for multidrug resistance and can be treated with empiric antibiotics using one of the following regimens: (1) ceftriaxone 2 gm IV daily, (2) ampicillin-sulbactam 3 gm IV every 6 hours, (3) levofloxacin or moxifloxacin 750 mg IV daily or 400 mg IV daily, or (4) ertapenem 1 gm IV daily. However, in the setting of risk factors for multidrug resistance (antibiotics in the past 90 days, current hospitalization >5 days, high frequency of resistance in the community or hospital unit, immunosuppression due to therapy or disease), one should choose one of the following: (1) an antipseudomonal cephalosporin (such as cefepime 2 gm IV every 8 hours or ceftazidime 2 gm IV every 8 hours), (2) an antipseudomonal carbapenem (such as meropenem 1 gm IV every 8 hours or imipenem 500-1000 mg every 6 hours), or (3) piperacillin-tazobactam 4.5 gm IV every 6 hours. In patients with severe penicillin allergies who cannot have these regimens, aztreonam 2 gm IV every 6 to 8 hours should be used. In addition, the provider should add either an antipseudomonal fluoroquinolone (ciprofloxacin or levofloxacin) or aminoglycoside (gentamycin, tobramycin, or amikacin). Finally, methicillin-resistant *Staphylococcus aureus* (MRSA) coverage should be provided with linezolid (600 mg every 12 hours), vancomycin (15 to 20 mg/kg IV every 8 to 12 hours), or telavancin (10 mg/kg IV every 24 hours).

Postoperative patients can also develop aspiration pneumonia due to loss of protective airway reflexes during intubation and extubation, or related to postoperative nausea and vomiting. The most common pathogens in aspiration pneumonia are upper airway pathogens such as *Streptococcus pneumonia, Haemophilus influenza, Staphylococcus aureus,* and gram-negative rods. Aspiration pneumonia is best treated with clindamycin 600 mg IV every 8 hours, followed by 300 mg PO four times daily or 450 mg PO three times daily. Alternative regimens include amoxicillin-clavulanate 875 mg twice daily or amoxicillin 500 mg three times daily with metronidazole 500 mg three times daily.

Approximately 1 in 3000 surgical procedures are complicated by aspiration pneumonitis produced by the aspiration of gastric fluid (sterile and highly acidic). The aspiration produces a severe chemical pneumonitis. Aspiration and its complications are a cause of approximately 30% of anesthetic mortalities. Risk factors for aspiration pneumonia include older age, obesity, hiatal hernia, or emergency surgery associated with a full stomach. The morbidity from aspiration is secondary to both particulate matter entering into the lungs and the caustic nature of gastric acid. The combination of these insults leads to a destructive inflammatory response. When aspiration is significant and severe, adult respiratory distress syndrome often develops. Secondary infection usually complicates aspiration pneumonitis, and broad-spectrum antibiotics should be given when this diagnosis is entertained. Preventive measures include early removal of nasogastric suction, antacid ingestion, and H2 blockers in the perioperative period, as well as careful use of narcotics and sedatives.

## SLEEP APNEA

Sleep apnea has become a significant concern because of the rising incidence of obesity and morbid obesity in the United States. The increased soft tissues of the head and neck can lead to airway compromise that leads to intermittent apnea and hypoventilation while a woman sleeps. The increased weight of the extra adipose tissue on the neck, chest, and abdominal wall lead to a decrease in pulmonary compliance. As a result, the relative hypoxia may induce systemic as well as pulmonary hypertension. Patients may also develop chronic hypercapnia as the respiratory drive shifts from a $CO_2$-driven response to a hypoxia-driven response in patients with sleep apnea. It is important to note that when morbidly obese patients are given higher levels of oxygen, as well as narcotics, they are at increased risk for apnea. These patients develop an increased sensitivity to narcotics that shuts down the respiratory drive. Patients with chronic hypoxia from any cause will often have an increased sensitivity to narcotics, but it is particularly problematic in the obese patient who is dependent on low levels of oxygen for respiratory stimulation. These patients should be given oxygen as needed. However, during the postoperative period, when narcotics are given, the goal should be to keep the oxygen saturation in the 94% range. At saturation levels of 96% to 99% these patients may lose respiratory drive and become hypercarbic and acidotic (Ahmad, 2008).

Preoperatively patients who are thought to be at risk for sleep apnea may be queried by asking them the "STOP-BANG" questions. These eight questions can predict sleep apnea with a high degree of sensitivity. The questions include the following: Do you ***s***nore? Do you often feel ***t***ired? Has anyone ***o***bserved you stop breathing? Are you being treated for high blood ***p***ressure? Is your ***b***ody mass index >35? Are you older than ***a***ge 50? Is your ***n***eck size >16 inches for a woman? ***G***ender-male? A "yes" answer to zero to two questions implies that one is low risk for obstructive sleep apnea (OSA); three to four "yes" answers places one at intermediate risk for OSA; six to eight "yes" answers places one at high risk for OSA (Chung, 2008).

## CARDIOVASCULAR PROBLEMS

### HEMORRHAGIC SHOCK

Shock is defined as a condition in which circulatory insufficiency prevents adequate vascular perfusion of vital organs. Systemic hypotension results in poor tissue perfusion and reduced capillary filling. If this pathophysiologic state is neglected, prolonged hypotension results in oliguria, progressive metabolic acidosis, and multiple organ failure. Shock may be produced by hemorrhage, cardiac failure, sepsis, and anaphylactic reactions. Hypovolemic shock is the most common cause of acute circulatory failure in gynecologic patients. Cardiogenic shock and septic shock are less common. Shock from postoperative hemorrhage is usually seen in the first several hours following surgery. In the perioperative period, hypovolemia may be secondary to several factors, including preoperative volume deficiency, underreplaced blood loss during surgery, extracellular fluid loss during surgery, inadequate fluid replacement and, most commonly, continued blood loss following the surgical procedure. Tachycardia is the classic cardiovascular physiologic response to hypotension. Progressive hypovolemia results in diminished urine output.

The majority of perioperative cases of shock are related to hemorrhage secondary to inadequate hemostasis. The development of shock from acute blood loss depends on the rate of bleeding; for example, slow venous oozing may produce a large amount of blood loss but not produce shock. Rapid loss of 20% of a woman's blood volume produces mild shock, whereas a loss of greater than 40% of blood volume results in severe shock. Even with the extensive use of suction equipment, the actual measurement of intraoperative blood loss is imprecise. Massive blood loss has been defined as hemorrhage that results in replacement of 50% of the circulating blood volume in less than 3 hours.

Hypotension in the immediate postoperative period may be secondary to the residual effects of anesthesia or over sedation. For example, older patients often experience prolonged vasodilation secondary to the sympathetic blockade produced by epidural or spinal anesthesia. The most common cause of postoperative bleeding is a less than ideal ligature or hemorrhage from a vessel that has retracted during the operation. Bleeding may come from an isolated artery or vein or may be more generalized when the bleeding is secondary to a clotting abnormality. The differential diagnosis of postoperative hemorrhagic shock includes conditions such as pneumothorax, PE, massive pulmonary aspiration, myocardial infarction, and acute gastric dilation. However, in the postoperative period the index of suspicion would be highest for bleeding.

The differential diagnosis of ineffective coagulation includes sepsis, fibrinolysis, diffuse intravascular coagulation, and a previously unrecognized coagulation defect, such as von Willebrand disease. Coagulopathies can also develop from excessive transfusion and dilution of fibrinogen and other clotting factors. The progressive acidosis associated with shock increases hemostatic problems by interfering with assembly of coagulation factor complexes. Hypothermia further complicates hemostasis because it produces platelet dysfunction and coagulopathy secondary to decreased activity of thromboxanes. Thrombocytopenia, impaired platelet function, and a decrease in factors V, VIII, and XI commonly occur with massive transfusions, of more than 5 units of packed red blood cells (PRBCs). Hypofibrinogenemia is the first to develop, followed by deficiencies of other coagulation factors. Thrombocytopenia is frequently the last defect to be recognized in the coagulopathy cascade. However, the timing of its development varies among individuals. Thus transfusion of platelets should be determined by serial platelet counts (Box 25.2). Similarly, preset formulas for the transfusion of fresh-frozen plasma (FFP), such as 2 units of FFP for every 5 units of PRBCs, should be replaced by selective transfusion of plasma as needed to match a clotting deficiency as measured by the prothrombin time (PT) and activated partial thromboplastin time (aPTT). Each unit of FFP can be expected to raise increase clotting protein levels by 2.5% to 10%.

Two early signs of hypovolemia caused by hidden internal bleeding include tachycardia and decreased urine output. The body's adrenergic response to hemorrhage includes perspiration, tachycardia, and peripheral vasoconstriction. Urine output decreases to less than 0.5 mL/kg/hr (20 to 25 mL/hr) as a result of poor perfusion of the kidneys. With further loss of blood, agitation, weakness, and skin pallor can appear, the extremities may feel cold and clammy, and, ultimately, systolic blood pressure drops below 80 mm Hg. Again, because of adaptive cardiovascular changes, it takes a rapid loss of approximately one third of the blood volume to produce significant hypotension.

**Box 25.2 Suggested Transfusion Guidelines for Platelets**

- Recent (within 24 hr) platelet count <10,000/mm$^3$ (for prophylaxis)
- Recent (within 24 hr) platelet count <50,000/mm$^3$ with demonstrated microvascular bleeding (oozing) or a planned surgical/invasive procedure
- Demonstrated microvascular bleeding and a precipitous fall in platelet count
- Adult patients in the operating room who have had complicated procedures or have required more than 10 units of blood *and* have microvascular bleeding. Giving platelets assumes that adequate surgical hemostasis has been achieved.
- Documented platelet dysfunction (e.g., prolonged bleeding time >15 min, abnormal platelet function tests) with petechiae, purpura, microvascular bleeding (oozing), or surgical or invasive procedure
- Unwarranted indications:
  - Empirical use with massive transfusion when patient is not having clinically evident microvascular bleeding (oozing)
  - Prophylaxis in thrombotic thrombocytopenic purpura, hemolytic-uremic syndrome, or idiopathic thrombocytopenic purpura
  - Extrinsic platelet dysfunction (e.g., renal failure, von Willebrand disease)

From Rutherford EJ, Skeet DA, Schooler WG. Hematologic principles in surgery. In: Townsend CM, Beauchamp RD, Evers BM, eds. *Sabiston Textbook of Surgery.* 17th ed. Philadelphia, Saunders; 2004.

**Box 25.3 Management Priorities in Massive Transfusion***

- Restore circulating blood volume.
- Maintain oxygenation.
- Correct coagulopathy.
- Maintain body temperature.
- Correct biochemical abnormalities.
- Prevent pulmonary and other organ dysfunction.
- Treat underlying cause of hemorrhage.

From Donaldson MDJ, Seaman MJ, Park GR. Massive blood transfusion. *Br J Anaesth.* 1992;69(6):621-630.
*The exact priority depends on the circumstances.

Postoperatively, occult intraperitoneal and retroperitoneal bleeding often occurs without significant local symptoms. Extraperitoneal bleeding may present as bleeding from the vaginal cuff. Abdominal distention, muscle rigidity, and shoulder pain are late signs of intraperitoneal hemorrhage. The diagnosis of clinically significant postoperative bleeding may be confirmed by serial changes in hemoglobin levels. However, it is important to caution that marked changes in hematocrit and hemoglobin levels require time to develop. Imaging studies may demonstrate hematomas or increased intraperitoneal free fluid.

The management goals of postoperative shock are to replace, restore, and maintain the effective circulating blood volume and establish normal cellular perfusion and oxygenation (Box 25.3). To accomplish this goal, an adequate cardiac output and appropriate peripheral vascular resistance must be maintained. The first priority is to provide adequate ventilation because poor respiratory gas exchange is the most frequent cause of death in these patients. The second, almost simultaneous, priority is rapid fluid replacement with adequate amounts of blood and crystalloid solution (normal saline or lactated Ringer solution). The 3:1 rule suggests a ratio of 3 mL of crystalloid solution for every 1 mL of blood loss. The optimal fluid replacement is a fluid evenly distributed throughout multiple body compartments. Randomized trials of crystalloid and colloid resuscitation solutions have shown no clear survival benefit to the use of colloids (albumin, gelatin, dextran, and hydroxyethyl starch), but a reduced rate of tissue edema, abdominal compartment syndrome, and hyperchloremic metabolic acidosis is demonstrated. The substantial cost of these agents should be weighed against potential benefits (Bougle, 2013). Crystalloids should be considered the initial resuscitation fluid of choice in hemorrhagic shock; colloids are appropriate for resuscitation in conjunction with crystalloids when blood products are not immediately available. Guidelines for transfusion of PRBCs are listed in Box 25.4.

**Box 25.4 Suggested Transfusion Guidelines for Red Blood Cells**

Hemoglobin <8 g/dL or acute blood loss in an otherwise healthy patient with signs and symptoms of decreased oxygen delivery with two or more of the following:
- Estimated or anticipated acute blood loss of >15% of total blood volume (750 mL in 70-kg man)
- Diastolic blood pressure <60 mm Hg
- Systolic blood pressure drop >30 mm Hg from baseline
- Tachycardia (>100 beats/min)
- Oliguria, anuria
- Mental status changes

Hemoglobin <10 g/dL in patients with known increased risk of coronary artery disease or pulmonary insufficiency who have sustained or are expected to sustain significant blood loss

Symptomatic anemia with any of the following:
- Tachycardia (>100 beats/min)
- Mental status changes
- Evidence of myocardial ischemia, including angina
- Shortness of breath or dizziness with mild exertion
- Orthostatic hypotension

Unfounded or questionable indications:
- To increase wound healing
- To improve the patient's sense of well-being
- 7 g/dL < hemoglobin < 10 g/dL (or 21% < hematocrit < 30%) in otherwise stable, asymptomatic patient
- Mere availability of predesignated autologous blood without medical indication

From Rutherford EJ, Skeet DA, Schooler WG. Hematologic principles in surgery. In: Townsend CM, Beauchamp RD, Evers BM, eds. *Sabiston Textbook of Surgery.* 17th ed. Philadelphia: Saunders; 2004.

The goals of fluid replacement are to obtain and maintain a systolic blood pressure that is similar to preoperative readings and maintain urine output greater than 0.5 mL/kg/hr (usually, >30 mL/hr). Table 25.2 lists types of blood components used for replacement therapy. Traditionally in massive hemorrhage replacement a ratio of 2 units of packed red blood cells to 1 unit of fresh-frozen plasma is desirable, but resuscitation should be tailored to the clinical scenario. For every 6 units of packed red blood cells, a six-pack of platelets may be required. Each unit or pack of platelets will raise the platelet level by 15,000/mm$^3$. The platelet count should be maintained above 50,000/mm$^3$ in a woman who is bleeding (Stroncek, 2007). The importance of adequate transfusion is not only support of intravascular volume but also supply of oxygen.

Coagulation studies, prothrombin time, and activated prothrombin time should be obtained regularly during the bleeding episode. The term *washout* is used to describe the loss of clotting factors as a woman uses up her blood volume and is replaced with PRBCs and crystalloid. Disseminated intravascular coagulation (DIC) is an intravascular consumption and is different than washout. However, both conditions require replacement and ongoing evaluation. Importantly, with continued severe bleeding, the use of recombinant factor VIIa (70 to 90 μg/kg) should be considered. Although expensive, factor VIIa initiates a rapid burst of thrombin production and stimulates the entire clotting cascade. Many studies have shown it to be very effective in situations of continued bleeding from small vessels (Bougle, 2013).

The decision to return to the operating room to control hemorrhage is commonly difficult to make as the offending artery or vein is often unable to be identified at the time or reoperation. Additionally, friable inflamed postoperative tissues can result in further bleeding. If ongoing postoperative bleeding requires reoperation, this decision should not be postponed. It should be performed expediently after volume replacement and sometimes concomitantly. During this second operation, excellent anesthesia, a full selection of surgical instruments, and the value of good assistance cannot be overemphasized. Proper exposure is paramount for the success of this operation. Initially the old clots are removed and further bleeding is reduced by direct pressure over the presumed bleeding vessels while a systematic search is conducted in an effort to identify the individual vessels that are bleeding.

Bilateral ligation of the anterior divisions of the hypogastric arteries distal to the posterior parietal branch is an effective

**Table 25.2** Indications for Administration of Various Blood Products

| | | Indication | |
|---|---|---|---|
| **Product** | **Content** | **Acceptable** | **Unacceptable** |
| Red blood cells | Red cells | To increase oxygen-carrying capacity in anemic women; for orthostatic hypotension secondary to blood loss | For volume expansion; to enhance wound healing; to improve general well-being |
| Platelet concentrates | Platelets | To control or prevent bleeding associated with deficiencies in platelet number or function | In patients with immune thrombocytopenic purpura (unless bleeding is life-threatening) |
| Fresh-frozen plasma | Plasma, clotting factors | To increase the level of clotting factors in patients with demonstrated deficiency | For volume expansion; as a nutritional supplement; prophylactically with massive blood transfusion |
| Cryoprecipitate | Factors I, V, VIII, XIII, von Willebrand factor, fibronectin | To increase the level of clotting factors in patients with demonstrated deficiency of fibrinogen, factor VIII, factor XIII, fibronectin, or von Willebrand factor | Prophylactically with massive blood transfusion |

From American Congress of Obstetricians and Gynecologists. *ACOG Tech Bull.* 1994;199:1.

operation to control persistent postoperative pelvic hemorrhage. This procedure results in a reduction of pulse pressure, which allows a stable clot to form at the site where the pelvic vessels are injured. Classically, two ligatures are placed and tied around each hypogastric artery (Fig. 25.3). The major potential complication of this procedure is injury to the hypogastric vein. If there is generalized oozing, thrombocytopenia, DIC, or factor VIII deficiency should be suspected. If these conditions are excluded, venous oozing from small vessels in the pelvis may be controlled by the local application of microfibrillar collagen compounds (e.g., Avitene, Gelfoam, FloSeal).

Intraoperative rapid autologous blood transfusion is a technique that is used extensively in cardiovascular and trauma surgery. Regretfully, it is underused or rarely performed by gynecologists. The major complication of rapid autologous transfusion is a 10% hemolysis rate. The risks of air embolism or infusion of particulate matter are minimal. Obviously, autologous blood does not contain platelets or clotting factors, so platelets and fresh-frozen plasma will have to be given concurrently for severe hemorrhage. Rapid autologous transfusion is contraindicated in advanced pelvic infection or malignancy.

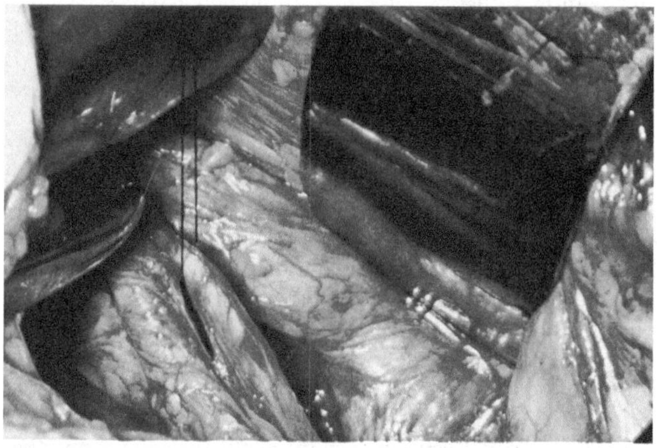

**Figure 25.3** Ligation of internal iliac artery. Double loop is being directed toward bifurcation of common iliac artery. (From Breen JL, Gregori CA, Kindzierski JA. Hemorrhage in gynecologic surgery. In: Shaefer G, Graber EA, eds. *Complications in Obstetric and Gynecologic Surgery*. Hagerstown, MD: Harper & Row, 1981.)

In many cases, angiographic embolization, instead of exploratory laparotomy, is preferable (Fig. 25.4). Introduction of digital road mapping technology has improved the rapid identification of bleeding vessels. Similarly, treatment of recurrent postoperative hemorrhage or hemorrhage late in the postoperative course (7 to 14 days) may be performed with angiographic arterial embolization. Absorbable gelatin sponges, which produce vascular occlusion for 10 to 30 days, or metal coils with Dacron fibers, which produce permanent occlusion, may be used.

## HEMATOMAS

This section describes the management of wounds or pelvic hematomas that develop slowly and are diagnosed after the first postoperative day. Proper management of postoperative hematomas is challenging and controversial. The incidence of hematomas is inversely related to the extent to which meticulous hemostasis is obtained intraoperatively. Women who are given low-dose heparin or who take aspirin chronically are at a slightly higher risk of hematoma formation. Women on antiplatelet medication or anticoagulation are also at risk. Hematomas result from intermittent or slow, continuous venous bleeding and are almost always self-limiting. Eventually, the pressure of the expanding hematoma will exceed the venous pressure and a stable clot will form.

The extent of the hematoma is determined partially by the potential size of the compartment into which the bleeding occurs. Retroperitoneal, or broad ligament, hematomas may

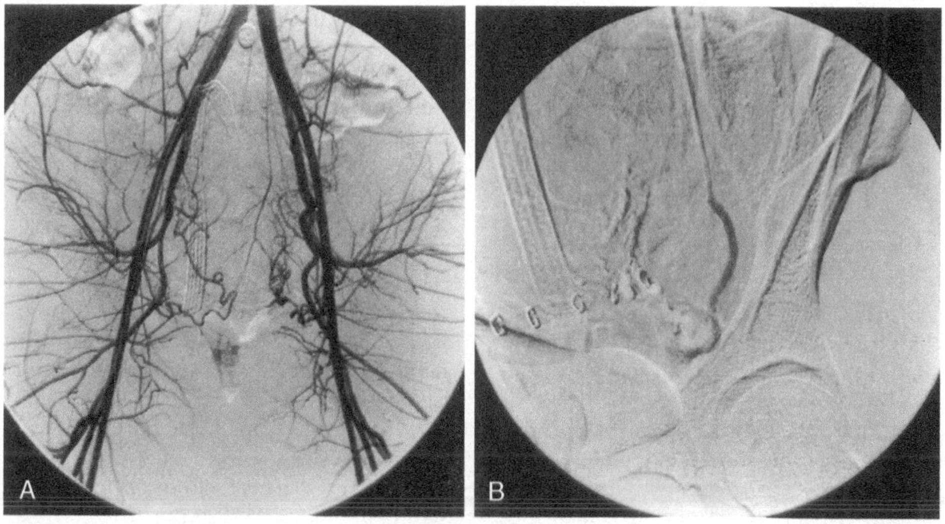


**Figure 25.4** **A,** Anteroposterior digital subtraction pelvic angiogram in 37-year-old woman with persistent pelvic bleeding after surgical myomectomy for uterine leiomyomas demonstrates contrast pooling *(arrows)* from branches of left uterine artery, consistent with active hemorrhage. **B,** Postembolization left uterine arteriogram shows occluded left uterine artery *(long arrows)* with no evidence of active bleeding. (From Vedantham S, Goodwin SC, McLucas B, et al. Uterine artery embolization: an underused method of controlling pelvic hemorrhage. *Am J Obstet Gynecol*. 1997;176[4]:938-948.)

contain several units of blood. The diagnosis of a wound, or pelvic, hematoma is usually suspected when the patient's hemoglobin on postoperative day 3 is unexpectedly low. The woman may have mild to moderate tenderness over the affected area. By the fifth postoperative day, the hematoma liquefies and may be easier to outline during bimanual examination. Distinguishing between an uninfected hematoma and a hematoma that has become secondarily infected is difficult before incision and drainage. Both clinical situations produce tenderness and fever secondary to the inflammation surrounding the hematoma. The diagnosis of a retroperitoneal hematoma may be made by physical examination; most helpful is a careful rectovaginal examination. However, radiologic imaging studies are indicated when a hematoma is suspected and cannot be palpated. Imaging is commonly used to make the diagnosis of a postoperative hematoma.

Hematomas smaller than 5 cm in diameter may be treated conservatively. Larger hematomas may be drained transcutaneously with CT or ultrasound guidance. If not treated, most large hematomas will become secondarily infected, even if treated with parenteral antibiotics. Effective drainage of most pelvic and broad ligament hematomas usually can be accomplished vaginally or radiographically. Small subcutaneous hematomas or fascial hematomas usually resolve. However, they are associated with an increased incidence of wound infection and pain.

## RETAINED FOREIGN BODY

With any operation there is the potential risk of an unrecognized retained foreign body, sponge, or laparotomy pad. The exact incidence of this worrisome complication is difficult to establish but is estimated to be from 1 in 1200 to 1500 laparotomies, typically with correct sponge counts at the time of surgery. When this complication is discovered during the first postoperative week, the woman usually has a tender pelvic mass that is infected. When this mass is discovered after the immediate postoperative course, patients are often asymptomatic or exhibit minimal tenderness. The possibility of a retained foreign body should be considered in the differential diagnosis of pelvic hematomas and abscesses. A retrospective study of retained sponges by Gawande and associates noted that retained foreign bodies are more commonly associated with a higher body mass index (BMI), emergency surgeries, and an intraoperative change in the type of procedure to be performed (Gawande, 2003).

## THROMBOPHLEBITIS AND PULMONARY EMBOLUS

Surgery is a time of hypercoagulability secondary to the stress response. As such, the surgeon must be aware of the potential complications of thromboembolism throughout the postoperative course. Prophylaxis against deep vein thrombosis (DVT) is discussed in Chapter 24. However, prophylaxis must be continued throughout the hospital stay and, in certain high-risk cases, even after discharge. For example, patients with malignancy who undergo laparotomy, patients with previous blood clot or personal history of thrombophilia, and those who will have decreased ambulation may benefit from up to 4 weeks of low-molecular-weight heparin (LMWH) after leaving the hospital. Studies in patients with hip replacements and with abdominal pelvic malignancies have shown significant reductions (50% to 66%) in the incidence of DVT with prolonged anticoagulation, up to 4 weeks postoperatively. Currently, there is insufficient evidence to make recommendations for prolonged thromboprophylaxis for routine gynecology patients, except in high-risk situations such as gynecologic cancer surgery (Guyatt, 2012). There is a reduced risk of venous thromboembolism (VTE) with minimally invasive hysterectomy compared with abdominal hysterectomy. Without specific guidelines, the length of time for thromboprophylaxis should be individualized. Prophylaxis will not prevent all DVTs; thus part of daily rounds includes assessments for this complication.

### *Superficial Thrombophlebitis*

Superficial thrombophlebitis is one of the most frequently occurring postoperative complications and is most commonly associated with IV catheters. Superficial thrombophlebitis is a benign disease. However, it is associated with deep vein thrombophlebitis in approximately 5% of cases. Superficial thrombophlebitis is frequently overlooked or disregarded as a cause of postoperative fever. Superficial tenderness and erythema outline the course of the veins. Women with established superficial varicosities in the lower extremities are especially susceptible because of localized stasis or pressure during the operative procedure and inactivity during the first 24 hours after operation. Patients with superficial thrombophlebitis of the legs may also have concomitant deep venous disease. Thus the finding of superficial thrombophlebitis does not eliminate the necessity to consider DVT as well. Some series have documented the association of inherited thrombophilias with superficial phlebitis, increasing the risk by 4- to 13-fold, with the more potent thrombophilias contributing to the higher risk. Recurrent superficial phlebitis, in varying anatomic sites, may be a sign of occult malignant disease. Detailed basic investigations have identified fibrin sheaths surrounding IV catheters in 60% to 100% of patients studied. The exact fate of the several inches of clot and fibrin sheath after the removal of the IV catheter is uncertain. Venography studies have found that these clots and fibrin sheaths do not break up on catheter removal but initially remain in situ. IV catheters are an important source of nosocomial infections. Approximately 30% of all hospital-acquired bacteremias are secondary to IV lines. The most serious complication of IV catheter use is infection of the thrombus, producing suppurative phlebitis or catheter sepsis.

The classic symptom of phlebitis is inflammation of the subcutaneous tissue along the course of a vein or over the area of merging varicosities. The woman develops a painful, tender, erythematous induration (nodule or core). In most severe cases, there is associated fever. The duration of phlebitis is prolonged if the catheter is not immediately removed when the diagnosis of superficial phlebitis is made. It has previously been recommended that the IV catheters be removed and replaced in intervals ranging from 72 to 96 hours, regardless of whether signs or symptoms of superficial phlebitis are present. However, a Cochrane review in 2013 showed no evidence to support routine catheter exchange without evidence of inflammation, infiltration, or blockage (Webster, 2013).

Although routine exchange is not indicated, venous catheters should be removed at the first sign of induration, erythema, or edema. Superficial phlebitis is a common cause of an enigmatic postoperative fever during the first postoperative week. The clinical management of mild superficial thrombophlebitis includes rest, elevation, and local heat. Moderate to severe superficial thrombophlebitis may be treated with a nonsteroidal anti-inflammatory drug (NSAID) such as ibuprofen or low-dose heparin. The rare case of proximal progression of the inflammatory process should be treated with therapeutic doses of IV heparin and antibiotics.

### *Deep Vein Thrombosis*

Fifty percent of thromboembolic complications occur within the first 24 hours and 75% occur within 72 hours. Approximately 15% occur after the seventh postoperative day. Diagnosis of deep vein thrombosis by physical examination is insensitive. Thus imaging studies are essential for establishing the correct diagnosis. Venous thrombosis and pulmonary embolism (PE) are the direct causes of approximately 40% of deaths in gynecologic cases. The incidence of fatal PE following gynecologic operations is approximately 0.2%. Because women often die within a few hours of the appearance of initial symptoms, emphasis must be placed on prevention rather than treatment of this complication. PE is not the only major consequence of deep venous thrombosis. Many women develop chronic venous insufficiency or postphlebitic syndrome of the legs as a major sequela following thrombophlebitis. The resulting damage to valves of the deep veins produces shunting of blood to superficial veins, chronic edema, pain on exercise, and skin ulceration.

The reported incidence of DVT with gynecologic operations without prophylaxis varies from 7% to 45%, with an average of approximately 15% (Walsh, 1974). In a review conducted since the institution of universal mechanical prophylaxis, VTE rates as low as 0.6% for open hysterectomies and 0.2% for minimally invasive hysterectomies were documented (Barber, 2015). The incidence of thrombosis is directly dependent on risk factors such as the type and duration of operation, age of the woman, history of thrombophilia, or deep vein thrombosis, peripheral edema, surgical blood loss, restrictions in preoperative ambulation, obesity, immobility, malignancy, sepsis, diabetes, current oral contraceptive or hormone use, and conditions that produce venous stasis, such as ascites and heart failure (Box 25.5) (Kyrle, 2005). Older and obese women have an increased incidence of thrombosis because of dilation of their deep venous system. There is a two- to fourfold increased risk for venous thrombosis in women taking postmenopausal estrogen therapy. The length of the surgical procedure also has an important influence on the development of thrombosis. If the operation is 1 to 2 hours in duration, approximately 15% of women develop the disease; if the surgery is longer than 3 hours, the risk is greater (Table 25.3).

The process of thrombosis usually begins in the deep veins of the calf. It is estimated that 75% of pulmonary emboli originate from a thrombus that began in the leg veins. If one leg is involved, the contralateral leg will have a thrombus in approximately 33% of women. Usually, the thrombus remains localized, it lyses spontaneously, and the local symptoms resolve. In approximately 1 in 20 cases the process extends centrally to the veins of the upper leg and pelvis. Involvement of the femoral vein often results in swelling caused by obstruction of this large vein. Pulmonary emboli from calf veins alone are rare, with only 4% to 10% of pulmonary emboli originating from this area. In contrast, there is a 50% risk of a PE if thrombosis of the femoral vein is not treated.

**Box 25.5 Conditions Associated with Increased Risk for Deep Vein Thrombosis**

- Active cancer
- Acute medical illness (e.g., acute myocardial infarction, heart failure, respiratory failure, infection)
- Advancing age
- Antiphospholipid syndrome
- Behçet syndrome
- Central venous catheter
- Chronic care facility stay
- Congenital venous malformation
- Dyslipoproteinemia
- Heparin-induced thrombocytopenia
- Hormone replacement therapy
- Immobilization
- Inflammatory bowel disease
- Intravenous drug abuse
- Limb paresis
- Long-distance travel
- Myeloproliferative diseases
- Nephrotic syndrome
- Obesity
- Oral contraceptives
- Other drugs
  - Antipsychotics
  - Chemotherapeutic agents
  - Tamoxifen
  - Thalidomide
- Paroxysmal nocturnal hemoglobinuria
- Pregnancy, puerperium
- Previous venous thromboembolism
- Prolonged bed rest
- Superficial vein thrombosis
- Surgery
- Trauma
- Varicose veins
- Vena cava filter

From Kyrle PA, Eichinger S. Deep vein thrombosis. *Lancet.* 2005;365(9465):1163-1174.

In 1854, Virchow described the three key predisposing or precipitating factors in the production of thrombi: an increase in coagulation factors, damage to the vessel wall, and venous stasis. Subsequent studies have documented that all three events occur with gynecologic operations. Blood flow in the iliac vein decreases by approximately 55% during an operation. During an operation, there are several normal physiologic changes that produce hypercoagulability, including increases in factors VIII, IX, and X, number of platelets, platelet aggregation and adherence, fibrinogen, and, lastly, thromboplastin-like substance from tissue necrosis.

Kakkar has described the cascade of events leading to the development of thrombosis. The initial event in the cascade is stasis. Stasis leads to localized anoxia with subsequent generation of thrombi at the anoxic site. This produces changes in the lining of the vessel, with exposure of the basement membrane, platelet adhesion, and local coagulation. Thus the most important event in thrombosis is the generation of thrombi in the presence of venous stasis. A thrombus may generate in an area of stasis or it may generate wherever a vessel wall is damaged, with resultant exposure of the subendothelial collagen, to which platelets will adhere.

Table 25.3 Risk Categories of Thromboembolism in Gynecologic Operations

| | Risk Level | | |
|---|---|---|---|
| **Risk Category** | **Low** | **Medium** | **High** |
| Age (yr) | 40 | 40 | 50 |
| **Contributing Factors** | | | |
| Operation | Uncomplicated or minor | Major abdominal or pelvic | Major, extensive |
| Weight | | Moderately obese—75 to 90 kg or >20% above ideal weight | Morbidly obese— >115 kg or >30% above ideal weight<br>Previous venous thrombosis<br>Varicose veins<br>Cardiac disease<br>Diabetes (insulin-dependent) |
| Calf vein thrombosis (%) | 2 | 10-35 | 30-60 |
| Iliofemoral vein thrombosis (%) | 0.4 | 2-8 | 5-10 |
| Fatal pulmonary emboli (%) | 0.2 | 0.1-0.5 | 1 |
| Recommended prophylaxis | Early ambulation | Low-dose heparin or intermittent pneumatic compression | Low-dose heparin or intermittent pneumatic compression |

From Mattingly RF, Thompson JD, eds. *Te Linde's Operative Gynecology*. 6th ed. Philadelphia: JB Lippincott; 1985.

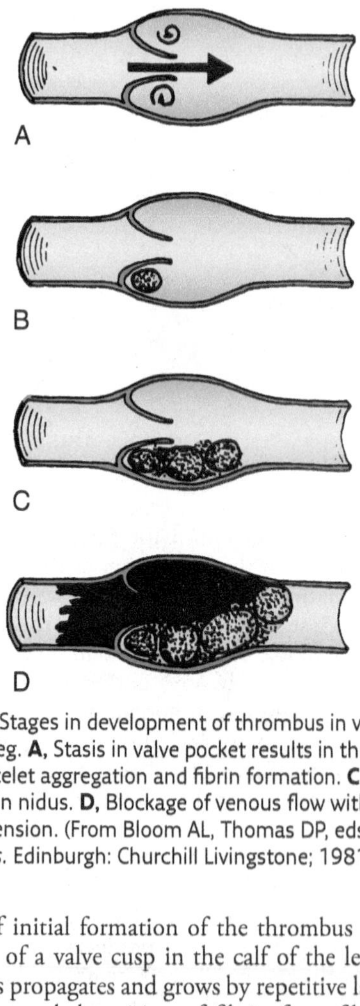

**Figure 25.5** Stages in development of thrombus in valve pocket of deep veins of leg. **A,** Stasis in valve pocket results in thrombin generation. **B,** Platelet aggregation and fibrin formation. **C,** Propagation of platelet-fibrin nidus. **D,** Blockage of venous flow with resultant retrograde extension. (From Bloom AL, Thomas DP, eds. *Haemostases and Thrombosis*. Edinburgh: Churchill Livingstone; 1981:684.)

The site of initial formation of the thrombus is most often near the base of a valve cusp in the calf of the leg (Fig. 25.5). The thrombus propagates and grows by repetitive layers of platelet aggregation and deposition of fibrin from fibrinogen. The most recently formed portion of the propagating thrombi are free-floating (not attached to the vein) and are most likely to become pulmonary emboli. The body attempts to repair the area of thrombosis through an invasion of fibroblasts from the vein wall to encompass the base of the thrombus. Eventually, the thrombus is attached to the vein wall, the area is reepithelialized, organization occurs, and symptoms resolve.

The signs and symptoms of deep vein thrombosis depend directly on the severity and extent of the process. Many localized cases of deep vein thrombosis in the calf are asymptomatic and are only recognized by a screening procedure such as duplex ultrasonography. However, even extensive areas of deep vein thrombosis may be asymptomatic; the first sign may be the development of a PE. In a woman who is asymptomatic, the pathophysiologic process may not totally obstruct the individual vein and drainage is obtained via associated competent collateral circulation.

Studies using $^{125}$I-labeled fibrinogen to screen the legs have documented that approximately one of two women who develop deep vein thrombosis following gynecologic surgery is totally free of symptoms (Walsh, 1974). Among women who develop signs and symptoms, approximately 68% have induration of the calf muscles, 52% have minimal edema, 25% have calf tenderness, and 11% develop a difference of more than 1 cm in diameter of the leg. The Homan sign is present in 10%, and differential pain over the calf with a blood pressure cuff is present in approximately 40%. The clinical diagnosis of iliofemoral thrombosis is much easier—the woman usually develops severe symptoms caused by obstruction of venous return. Usually, there is an acute onset of severe pain and swelling.

The clinician must maintain a high degree of suspicion to begin the diagnostic workup for deep vein thrombosis. The clinical symptoms and signs of DVT are nonspecific. A clinical clue is the persistence of a low-grade fever with unexplained tachycardia. The tachycardia is often more rapid than one would expect with a low-grade fever. The finding of a definite difference in leg circumference is supportive evidence of DVT. Physical examination of the legs produces false-positive findings in approximately 50% of cases. At the time of the initial bedside examination, the physician will develop a level of suspicion for DVT based on physical findings and clinical characteristics. If the likelihood were low, the next step would, in nonsurgical patients, be a D-dimer level; however in the postoperative patient, D-dimer is not as reliable. D-Dimer is a protein from cross-linked fibrin after it has been degraded by plasmin in the fibrinolytic process.

Table 25.4 Options for Initial Anticoagulant Treatment of Deep Vein Thrombosis

| Drug | Method of Administration | Dosage* | Reported Risks (no./total no. [%]) Heparin-Induced Thrombocytopenia† | Major Bleeding |
|---|---|---|---|---|
| Unfractionated heparin | IV | Loading dose, 5000 U or 80 U/kg of body weight with infusion adjusted to maintain aPTT within therapeutic range | 9/332 (2.7) | 35/1853 (1.9) |
| LMW heparin | | | 0/333 (0) | 20/1821 (1.1) |
| Dalteparin | Subcutaneous | 100 U/kg every 12 hr or 200 U/kg daily; maximum, 18,000 U/day | | |
| Enoxaparin | Subcutaneous | 1 mg/kg every 12 hr or 1.5 mg/kg daily; maximum, 180 mg/day | | |
| Tinzaparin | Subcutaneous | 175 U/kg daily; maximum, 18,000 U/day | | |
| Nadroparin | Subcutaneous | 86 U/kg every 12 hr or 171 U/kg daily; maximum, 17,100 U/day | | |

From Bates SM, Ginsberg JS. Treatment of deep-vein thrombosis. *N Engl J Med.* 2004;351(3):268-277.

*Doses vary in patients who are obese or who have renal dysfunction. Monitoring of antifactor Xa levels has been suggested for these patients, with dose adjustment to a target range of 0.6 to 1.0 U/mL 4 hr after injection for twice-daily administration or 1.0-2.0 U/mL for once-daily administration. Even though there are few supporting data, most manufacturers recommend capping the dose for obese patients at that for a 90-kg patient.

†The therapeutic range of activated partial thromboplastin time corresponds to heparin levels of 0.3 to 0.7 U/mL, as determined by antifactor Xa assay. High levels of heparin-binding proteins and factor VIII may result in so-called heparin resistance. In patients requiring more than 40,000 U/day to attain a therapeutic aPTT, the dosage can be adjusted on the basis of plasma heparin levels.

Thus D-dimer may be elevated because of trauma, surgery, intravascular hemolysis, pregnancy, and other inflammatory states. If the signs and symptoms are suggestive or the woman is at high risk, the next step should be imaging. Interestingly, the more symptomatic the disease, the more adherent the thrombus. The greater the symptoms, the less likely the development of a PE.

Ascending contrast venography (phlebography) is the most accurate method for detecting deep vein thrombosis with a diagnostic accuracy of more than 95% for peripheral disease and more than 90% for iliofemoral thrombosis. However, it is rarely if ever used. Duplex ultrasound, the combination of Doppler and real-time B-mode ultrasound, and color Doppler are the preferred methods for diagnosing deep vein thrombosis. Duplex ultrasonography has remarkably high sensitivity and specificity in symptomatic women. Real-time ultrasound imaging provides visualization of the larger veins, and sensitive Doppler ultrasound is focused simultaneously on the suspicious vessel. The technology depends on changes in venous flow for a positive diagnosis. The documented sensitivity of duplex ultrasonography in detecting proximal thrombi is 95% (95% CI: 92%-98%) and the specificity is 99% (95% CI: 98%-100%) (Wells, 1995). The advantages of this method are that it is noninvasive, easy to use, highly accurate, objective, simple, and reproducible. Color Doppler ultrasonography may improve the diagnostic accuracy in larger veins. The main disadvantage of duplex ultrasound is its limited accuracy when investigating small vessels in the calf. The inability to compress the deep vein by moderate pressure with the ultrasound probe is the most widely used criterion for the positive diagnosis of DVT.

A prospective study of 220 patients used compressibility of the vein as the sole criterion for diagnosis of DVT (Lensing, 1989). For all patients in their study, including both proximal vein and calf vein thrombosis, the sensitivity was 91% and the specificity was 99%. The objectives of the clinical management of deep vein thrombosis associated with gynecologic surgery are early detection and early therapy. In reality, antithrombotic therapy is preventive medicine, because the therapeutic agent interrupts progression of the disease (thrombus formation) but does not actively resolve the disease process. Anticoagulation with heparin (unfractionated or LMW) is the initial treatment of choice for the diagnosis of DVT or PE (Table 25.4). LMWH is as effective and is safer than unfractionated heparin. LMWH, although more expensive than unfractionated heparin, has several advantages and has effectively replaced unfractionated heparin as the gold standard for treatment of DVT. LMWH may be given subcutaneously once or twice daily using weight-based dosing, for example enoxaparin: 1.5 mg/kg daily or 1 mg/kg twice daily (Guyatt, 2012). LMWH does not require monitoring in women with normal and stable renal function. It induces significantly less heparin-induced thrombocytopenia and has a lower risk of inducing bleeding. Because blood levels are more reproducible, there is actually a lower incidence of complications noted in some studies in terms of progression from DVT to pulmonary emboli. Additionally, studies comparing LMWH with unfractionated heparin have shown a greater effect with thrombus regression within the veins themselves. Testing of levels of LMWH is based not on the activated partial thromboplastin time (aPTT) but on the antifactor Xa activity level. Levels are calculated specifically for each LMWH. An aPTT of 1.5 times normal corresponds approximately to an antifactor Xa activity level of 0.2. Therapeutic levels are found between 0.4 and 0.8. Bleeding usually occurs when levels of the antifactor Xa activity level rise more than 1.0 to 1.2. If needed in patients with unstable renal status, levels may be checked approximately 4 hours after dosing.

If unfractionated heparin is desired as an IV infusion, weight-adjusted or fixed dose infusions are acceptable. The weight-adjusted dose is 80 IU/kg/hr bolus followed by 18 IU/kg/hr. The fixed dose uses an initial loading dose of 5,000 IU, followed by a continuous infusion of 1000 IU/hr (Guyatt, 2012). The dosage of unfractionated IV heparin should be adjusted to prolong an aPTT to 2.5 times control values. Continuous heparin infusion is preferred over periodic bolus injections because there are fewer hemorrhagic complications (6% versus 14%). The average half-life of heparin is 1 to 2 hours after IV injection. Failure to achieve adequate anticoagulation in the first 24 hours of therapy increases the risk of recurrent venous thromboembolism 15-fold.

For women who are pregnant or have a malignancy, LMWH is the treatment of choice for long-term anticoagulation. Other women can be treated with unfractionated heparin in addition to the initiation of oral warfarin (Coumadin) with a goal international normalized ratio (INR) of 2.5 (range, 2 to 3). A loading dose of warfarin is 5 to 10 mg nightly for two doses followed by INR-guided doses. Heparin should be continued until the INR is greater than 2. The biologic half-life of warfarin is 2 to 3 days. In general, anticoagulation with warfarin should be continued for 3 to 6 months for adequate secondary prophylaxis of a provoked thrombus. The length of treatment should be adjusted based on the clinical scenario with provoked clots from reversible risk factors requiring the shortest duration of treatment. For example, a provoked clot following an abdominal hysterectomy without other risk factors should be managed with 3 months of therapy (Guyatt, 2012). Patients with large DVT, antiphospholipid antibody syndrome, or malignancy may require extended therapy beyond 6 months because of increased risks of recurrence.

The primary risk of chronic anticoagulation therapy is the potential for major bleeding complications. Major bleeding occurs in approximately 4% woman-years of therapy. Thus it is important to follow these women carefully with serial coagulation studies. Approximately 1% of patients on full-dose heparin develop thrombocytopenia (platelet count <100,000/mm$^3$). If thrombocytopenia develops, heparin should be discontinued because of the potential risk of paradoxic thrombosis.

Rarely, patients are not candidates for anticoagulation. In these patients, inferior vena cava filters may be used to protect against pulmonary emboli. Temporary vena cava filters may be placed with fluoroscopic guidance. In some patients with large DVT and other risk factors, such as compound thrombophilias and malignancy, consideration may be given to both anticoagulation and filter placement.

Routine screening for thrombophilia in all patients with VTE is not indicated. The presence of a hereditary thrombophilia does not alter therapeutic or prophylactic management of a patient and has not been associated with improved outcomes. Patients who may benefit from testing include those with recurrent thrombosis, patients with a family history of thrombosis, patients with thrombosis in unusual locations (hepatic vein, portal vein, mesenteric vein, or arterial), and possibly patients younger than 45 years of age. Patients with a provoked thrombosis from cancer, hormonal therapy, and surgery do not require testing for thrombophilias.

There is no evidence that bed rest is helpful for patients with DVT or that immobilization will prevent pulmonary embolism. Patients with confirmed DVT may receive NSAIDs, because coagulation factors will be monitored. Patients should also be prescribed support stockings, which should be worn for several months and for up to 2 years. The use of support stockings decreases the risks of postthrombotic syndrome. In a systematic review, women who used stockings up to 2 years after DVT had up to a 50% reduction in the incidence of postthrombotic syndrome (Segal, 2007).

### *Pulmonary Embolism*

The accurate diagnosis of PE is essential for the prevention of morbidity from lack of treatment or unnecessary anticoagulation therapy. Autopsy studies have documented that pulmonary emboli are undiagnosed clinically in approximately 50% of women who experience this complication. Approximately 10% of women with a PE die within the first hour. The mortality of women with correctly diagnosed and treated pulmonary emboli is 8%, in contrast to approximately 30% if the disease is not treated. Most pulmonary emboli in gynecologic patients originate from thrombi in the pelvic and femoral veins. Predisposing risk factors are found in most women with PE.

**Table 25.5** Symptoms and Signs of Pulmonary Embolism

| Symptoms | Patients with Finding (%) |
|---|---|
| Predisposing factors* | 94 |
| Dyspnea | 84 |
| Pleuritic chest pain | 74 |
| Apprehension | 59 |
| Cough | 53 |
| Hemoptysis | 30 |
| Syncope | 14 |
| **Signs** | |
| Tachypnea | 92 |
| Rales | 58 |
| Accentuation of pulmonic valve closure | 53 |
| Tachycardia | 44 |
| Cyanosis | 20 |

From Blinder RA, Coleman RE. Evaluation of pulmonary embolism. *Radiol Clin North Am*. 1985;23(3):391-405.

*Prolonged immobilization, postoperative state, congestive heart failure, carcinomatosis.

No combination of symptoms or signs is pathognomonic for PE. They are nonspecific and similar to symptoms caused by other forms of cardiorespiratory disease. Many patients with PE will be asymptomatic. Common conditions considered in the differential diagnosis of pulmonary embolism include pneumonia, cardiac failure, atelectasis, aspiration, acute respiratory distress syndrome, and sepsis. Although the differential diagnosis is broad in scope, the symptoms should alert the physician to the possibility of a PE, thus allowing a proper diagnostic workup to establish or rule out the disease. Chest pain, dyspnea, and apprehension are the most common symptoms. The dyspnea is often of abrupt onset. The classic triad of shortness of breath, chest pain, and hemoptysis is seen in less than 20% of women with proved PE. Tachycardia, tachypnea, rales, and an increase in the second heart sound over the pulmonic area are the most frequently found signs of pulmonary emboli (Table 25.5). Approximately 15% of women with pulmonary emboli have an unexplained low-grade fever associated with a PE. A high fever is rarely associated with a PE but may occur. The clinical manifestations of PE are produced primarily by occlusion of the large branches of the pulmonary arteries by embolic material with subsequent associated reflex bronchial constriction and vasoconstriction that intensify the symptomatology. More than 50% of clinically recognized pulmonary emboli are multiple. The most frequent location of pulmonary emboli is in the lower lobes of the right lung. Shock and syncope are associated with massive pulmonary emboli.

Although imaging techniques are the gold standard for establishing the diagnosis of pulmonary emboli, several studies have found that clinical assessment is almost as accurate (Goldhaber,

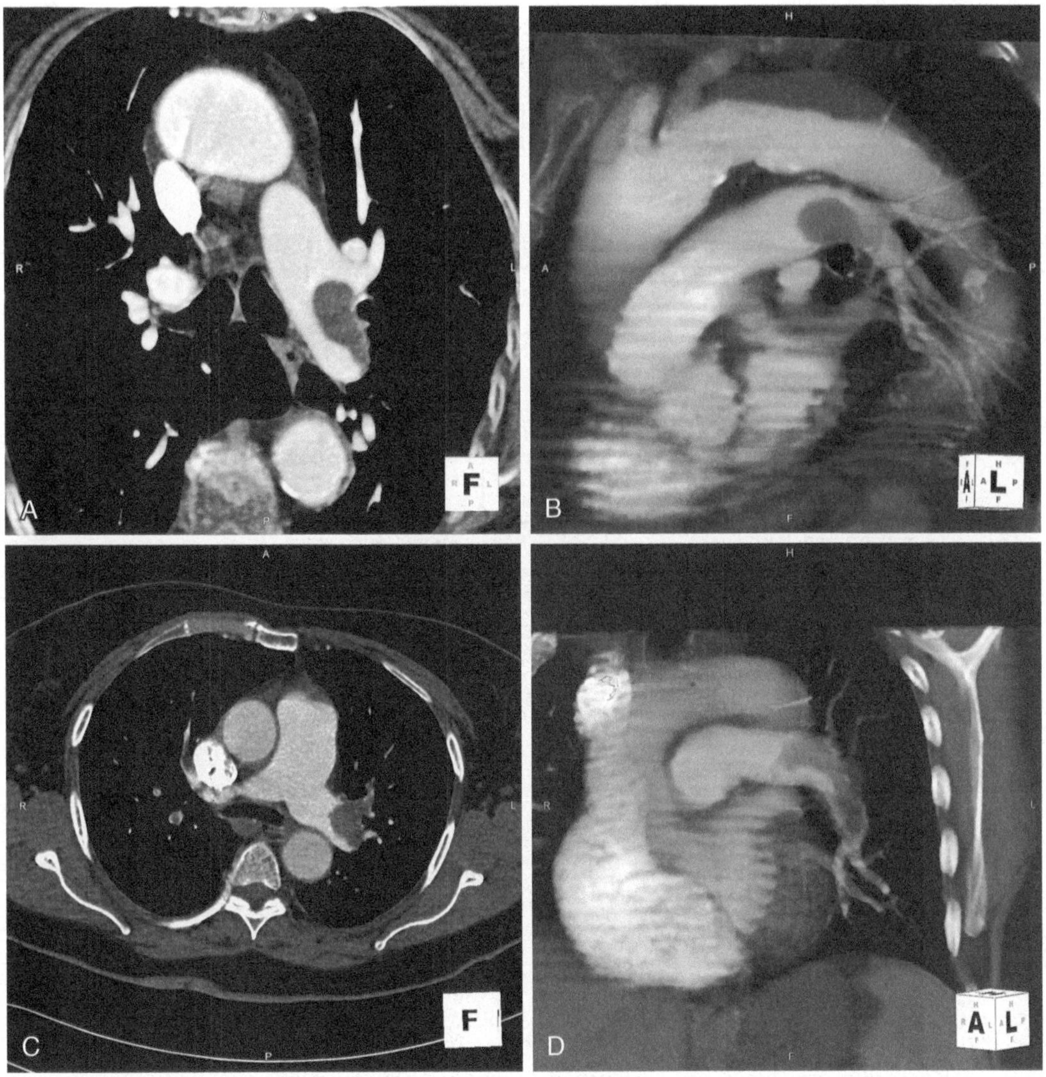


**Figure 25.6 A** to **D**, Helical CT of pulmonary embolism. The letters on the cube help orient the viewer as the three-dimensional image is rotated. *A*, Anterior; *F*, foot; *H*, head; *L*, left. (Courtesy of Dr. Charles McGlade, Sacred Heart Medical Center, Eugene, OR.)

2003a, 2003b). Laboratory studies that may help in diagnosis and management include electrocardiograms (ECGs), chest radiographs, blood gas analyses, assessment of troponin, d-dimer (not reliable in postoperative patients), and brain natriuretic peptide (BNP). Less than 15% of ECGs demonstrate significant changes of right ventricular strain, with T wave inversion in $V_1$ to $V_4$ with a PE. Most women with pulmonary emboli demonstrate hypoxemia on blood gas determinations, but as with other routine tests, these findings do not occur invariably. Diminished pulmonary vascular markings may be a suggestive finding on a chest film, but they are fairly nonspecific. The chest radiograph may be helpful in the differential diagnosis by demonstrating other pulmonary processes. The most common findings on chest film examination with a PE are infiltrate, pleural effusion, atelectasis, and enlargement of the heart or descending pulmonary artery.

In women who are in mild to moderate distress, IV heparin should be started while imaging studies are being ordered. If there is any question of severe distress or hemodynamic instability, thrombolytic therapy may be indicated for the appropriate patient. In stable patients, a stepwise approach is useful. Many clinicians will order Doppler studies of the lower extremities. If the Doppler studies are positive, the woman will be anticoagulated and no further workup for a thrombotic source is necessary. If the tests are negative, further imaging is still necessary, because in the postoperative patient, pelvic clots may be the origin of the pulmonary embolus, not lower extremity clots. The next two options are a ventilation-perfusion ratio ($\dot{V}/\dot{Q}$) scan or helical CT.

Helical CT has largely replaced ($\dot{V}/\dot{Q}$ scanning as the most common imaging technique to establish or exclude the diagnosis of PE (Fig. 25.6). Helical CT, also called spiral CT, uses imaging of the pulmonary vessels. Imaging of the pulmonary vessels is facilitated by the use of IV contrast media. The procedure is minimally invasive and provides a volumetric image of the lung by rotating the detector at a constant rate around the woman. A cost-effective analysis from Doyle and colleagues has found that helical CT is the most cost-effective first-line test to

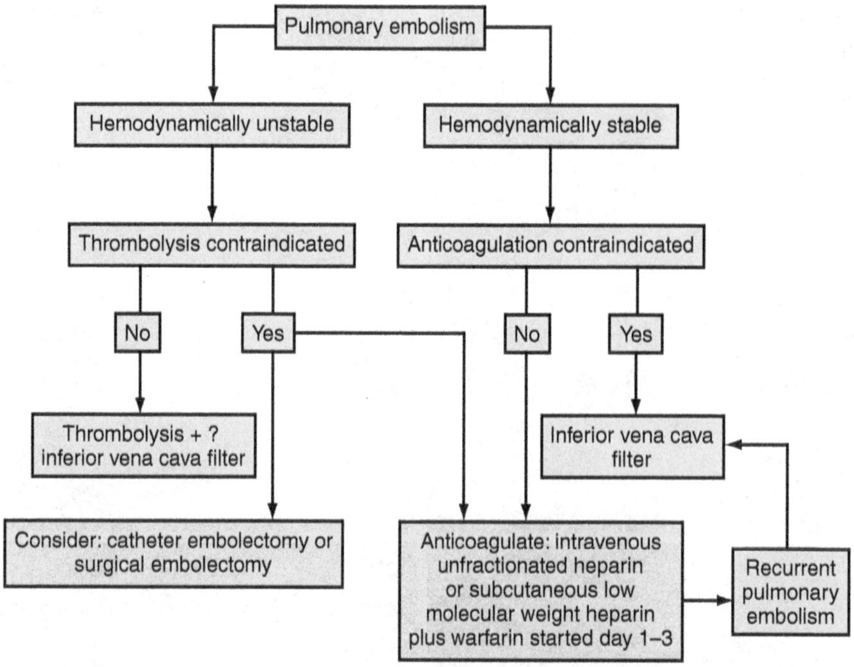


**Figure 25.7** Algorithm for treatment of pulmonary embolism. (From Taj MR, Atwal AS, Hamilton G. Modern management of pulmonary embolism. *Br J Surg.* 1999;86[7]:853-868.)

diagnose pulmonary embolus. A limitation of helical CT is a sixfold increase in radiation exposure compared with the $\dot{V}/\dot{Q}$ scan. This leads to a slight increased risk of breast cancer (<1%). Prior to $\dot{V}/\dot{Q}$ scanning, a chest x-ray should be obtained. If the chest x-ray shows other findings, such as atelectasis, the $\dot{V}/\dot{Q}$ scan has a much higher chance of being nondiagnostic and CT should be ordered instead.

The $\dot{V}/\dot{Q}$ scan is a safe and relatively easy-to-perform test. The scan involves the injection of small radiocolloid particles into the circulation. They are trapped in small vessels; their distribution depends on regional pulmonary blood flow. Ventilation scintigraphy uses radionuclides of technetium aerosol or xenon gas. The combination of lack of symmetry and a mismatch in the ventilation scan is the abnormality that leads to the diagnosis. Whereas a normal result effectively rules out the diagnosis of PE, 40% of patients with a suspected PE will have a normal scan. The multicenter Prospective Investigation of Pulmonary Embolism Diagnosis (PIOPED) found that 4% of patients with normal or near-normal perfusion lung scans subsequently were discovered to have pulmonary emboli. This study emphasized a high sensitivity of 98% but a low specificity of 10% for $\dot{V}/\dot{Q}$ scans in the diagnosis of PE. The authors noted that almost all patients with acute PE had abnormal scans, but so did most patients without emboli. $\dot{V}/\dot{Q}$ scans have a high sensitivity but a variable specificity for the diagnosis of PE. For example, other cardiorespiratory diseases such as asthma may result in regional areas of decreased perfusion. If the scan documents multiple segments or lobar perfusion defects with a ventilation mismatch, the probability of pulmonary emboli is more than 85%. $\dot{V}/\dot{Q}$ scans with less extensive perfusion abnormalities or matching ventilation defects do not reliably exclude the diagnosis of PE.

The management of the majority of pulmonary emboli is with anticoagulation with IV unfractionated heparin or full-dose LMWH, similar to the management of deep vein thrombosis (Fig. 25.7). Prompt and early therapy with heparin provides anticoagulation and inhibits the release of serotonin from platelets. Potentially, this results in a decrease in the associated bronchoconstriction. Some women are candidates for thrombolytic therapy (streptokinase-urokinase). The time window for effective use of thrombolysis is up to 14 days following the initial symptoms or signs of a PE, although it is rarely used beyond 48 to 72 hours. Thrombolytic therapy works by transforming plasminogen to plasmin. Use of thrombolytic therapy during the early postoperative period is contraindicated because of the increased risk of serious hemorrhage, except for unique circumstances. Recombinant human tissue-type plasminogen activator (TPA) has been shown to be more rapid in onset and safer than urokinase for thrombolytic therapy. Thrombolytic therapy is the method of choice in patients with massive pulmonary emboli (angiographically, >50% obstruction of the pulmonary arterial bed) with associated moderate to severe hemodynamic instability, lobular obstruction, or multiple segmental profusion defects. Random trials of heparin versus thrombolytic therapy have shown that emboli clear more rapidly with initial thrombolytic therapy.

The Management Strategies and Prognosis of Pulmonary Embolus–3 trial (MAPPET-3) found that in severely affected patients (but not those in shock), thrombolytic therapy was superior to heparin. However, for all patients, particularly those with small emboli, the increased risks of intracranial bleeding may outweigh the benefits (1% to 3% of patients). Trials have evaluated thrombolytic therapy with heparin and found the combination superior to heparin alone. A thrombolytic agent is infused IV for the first 12 to 24 hours and heparin therapy is continued for 7 to 10 days. The clinical assumption is that approximately 7 days are needed for the intravascular venous thrombus to become firmly attached to the vein's sidewall. In patients who have heparin allergies, or develop heparin-induced thrombocytopenia (HIT), thrombin inhibitors are an alternative therapy.

An adjunct for treatment is vena cava filters. The most widely accepted indication for vena cava filters is failure of medical management or a contraindication to heparin therapy. Approximately 35% of vena cava filters are placed for prophylactic indications. A randomized trial reported by Decousos and colleagues compared vena cava filters with LMWH or unfractionated heparin. They concluded that the initial beneficial effect of vena cava filters for the prevention of PE is counterbalanced by an excess of recurrent DVT, without any difference in mortality rates. Treatment of a massive PE in an unstable woman involves a choice of thrombolytic therapy, pulmonary artery embolectomy, transvenous catheter embolectomy, or filter placement in the inferior vena cava.

All patients with pulmonary emboli should have maintenance therapy with warfarin or LMWH for 3 or more months following assessment of the patient's bleeding risk (Guyatt, 2012). New oral medications are emerging, but their role is uncertain at this time, particularly in the oncologic population. The risk of a woman developing a subsequent fatal PE during the 3 months of anticoagulation therapy is approximately 1 in 70 to 100.

## URINARY TRACT PROBLEMS

### *INABILITY TO VOID*

Many women experience an inability to void or an incomplete emptying of the bladder during the immediate postoperative period. The cause is complex, but the inability to void is more frequent and lasts longer after an operation that involves the urethra or bladder neck. The major pathophysiologic change is the direct trauma and edema produced by the surgical procedure to the perivesical tissues. Other factors that contribute include the potential of overdistention from excessive hydration and dyssynchronous contractions from the bladder neck. The differential diagnosis includes anxiety, mechanical interference, obstruction by swelling and edema, neurologic imbalance, and drug-associated detrusor hypotonia.

Most voiding dysfunction resolves without medication and with time. If a mechanical obstruction is not suspected, intermittent straight catheterization is indicated to manage postoperative voiding dysfunction. This will result in a lower incidence of urinary tract infections (UTI) and facilitate a more rapid return to normal bladder function. Overdistention of the bladder produces a temporary paralysis of the detrusor activity that may take several days to resolve and should be avoided. Rarely, medications may be given to patients who experience prolonged periods of inability to void. Reflex urethral spasm is common after surgery to repair an enterocele or rectocele. Urethral spasm may be diminished by an α-adrenergic receptor blocking agent such as phenoxybenzamine. However, hypotension may be associated with this drug. Bladder hypotonia may occur as a result of overdistention, prolonged inactivity, or use of medications such as beta-blockers. Bladder hypotonia may be treated with bethanechol, 10 to 50 mg orally every 6-8 hours.

### *URINARY TRACT INFECTION*

The most commonly acquired infection in the hospital and the most frequent cause of gram-negative bacteremia in hospitalized patients is catheter-associated urinary tract infection (UTI). Approximately 40% of nosocomial infections are UTIs, and 60% of these are directly related to an indwelling urethral catheter. Of patients with infections from bladder catheters, 1% will develop bacteremia. Therefore indwelling catheters should only be used when absolutely necessary and for as short a period of time as possible.

The normal urothelium inhibits adherence of surface bacteria to the walls of the urethra and bladder. A bladder catheter disrupts this property and surface bacteria are able to colonize the lower urinary tract. Additionally, bacteria form a sheet or biofilm of microorganisms and bacterial bioproducts that adheres to the catheter. These biofilms protect bacteria from antibiotics. This characteristic of biofilms explains why antibiotic suppression is ineffective for patients with chronic catheterization and why replacement of a catheter is necessary in the treatment of systemic infection secondary to a colonized urinary tract. The incidence of a positive culture increases dramatically with time. After a Foley catheter has been in place for 36 hours, approximately 20% of women have bacterial colonization and, after 72 hours, more than 75% have positive cultures. If the catheter drains into an open system for longer than 96 hours, 100% develop bacteriuria. Women with an indwelling catheter in place with a closed drainage system develop UTIs at the rate of approximately 5%/24 hours; this increases to 50% after 7 days of continuous catheterization.

Catheter-related UTIs are related to the patient's age. In one study, 30% of women older than 50 years developed an infection, compared with 16% of postoperative women younger than age 50. Diabetes increased the incidence of catheter-related UTIs threefold. The incidence of infection is directly related to how long the catheter is in place. The incidence of a positive urine culture after a single in-and-out catheterization is approximately 1%. Sterile technique used during insertion, strict aseptic catheter care, and maintenance of a closed drainage system are all important steps for reducing the incidence of infection through reduced colonization. Bacteria ascend from the exterior to the bladder via the lumen of the catheter or around the outside of the catheter. A sterile, closed drainage system is another prophylactic measure to reduce the incidence of UTIs. In one study, strict closed drainage reduced the rate of infection from 80% to 23%. Studies have documented a lower risk of infection with a suprapubic, transabdominal urinary catheter. The latter technique also decreases patient discomfort and permits earlier spontaneous voiding. Systemic prophylactic antibiotics exert a short-term effect, decreasing the initial incidence of infection. However, the negative effect of prophylactic antibiotics has been an increased emergence of antibiotic-resistant bacteria. Therefore prophylactic antibiotics should not be used, except in immunocompromised patients. With catheterization for longer than 3 weeks, all patients have bacterial colonization, regardless of the use of prophylactic antibiotics and a closed system.

The symptoms of UTI usually develop 24 to 48 hours after the Foley catheter is removed. Patients with lower UTIs usually do not have fever but experience urinary frequency and mild dysuria, which are difficult to distinguish from normal postoperative discomfort. Older women may manifest mental status changes as the first sign of problems. Women with upper UTIs usually have a high fever, chills, and flank pain. If urinary tract symptoms persist after appropriate antibiotic therapy, one should obtain imaging studies to evaluate the possibility of obstruction in the urinary tract. Obstruction of the ureter without associated infection may be asymptomatic or produce only mild flank tenderness. No appreciable change may be noted in urinary output or serum creatinine with an isolated unilateral ureteral obstruction.

The diagnosis of UTI is established by urinalysis and urine culture. Women with high-volume urine output may demonstrate minimal findings on urinalysis but have a positive urine culture. In a catheterized specimen, a bacterial concentration of $10^2$ organisms/mL is significant. More than 95% of patients with $10^2$ colony-forming units (CFU)/mL subsequently developed the standard criterion of infection, which is 100,000 CFU/mL for a midstream culture (Stark, 1984).

A minimum of 3 days of antibiotic therapy for a woman who has developed cystitis after catheter use is the recommended treatment. One-day, single-dose antibiotic treatment is not an effective treatment for UTI.

## URETERAL INJURY AND URINARY FISTULA

Vesicovaginal and ureterovaginal fistulas are infrequent yet significant complications of operations for benign gynecologic conditions. In the United States, gynecologic operations are found to be the cause of approximately 75% of urinary tract fistulas. Surprisingly, it is not the difficult cancer operation but rather the simple total abdominal hysterectomy for benign disease, such as myomas or abnormal bleeding that is most frequently associated with this complication. Fistulas following gynecologic surgery are a result of abdominal hysterectomy in 75% of cases and vaginal surgery in the remaining 25%. A Cochrane database review by Aarts and coworkers noticed a higher incidence of urinary tract injuries with minimally invasive surgery (MIS) compared with traditional abdominal hysterectomy (Aarts, 2015). Unfortunately, the numbers for MIS are still too low and the data may still be affected by the learning curve of MIS. The exact incidence of injury to the ureter associated with gynecologic surgery is unknown because many patients do not exhibit symptoms. However, it has been estimated that ureteral injury occurs as frequently as 1/200 abdominal hysterectomies. Ibeanu and associates have performed concomitant cystoscopy on 839 women undergoing hysterectomies for benign disease (few laparoscopic procedures). They noted that 2.9% of patients had bladder injuries and 1.8% had ureteral injuries (Ibeanu, 2009). Other studies have reported similar results. The site of ureteral injury is usually near the uterine artery. Injuries may include transection, sutures that constrict or devascularize the ureter, and thermal injuries from cautery. Stanhope and coworkers have noted a mean increase of only 0.8 mg/dL in the serum creatinine level following unilateral ureteral obstruction secondary to gynecologic surgery (Stanhope, 1991).

The classic clinical symptom of a urinary tract fistula is the painless and almost continuous loss of urine, usually from the vagina. On occasion, the uncontrolled loss of urine may be related to change in position or posture. Urinary incontinence that presents within a few hours of the operative procedure is usually secondary to a direct surgical injury to the bladder or ureter that was not appreciated during the surgery. Most fistulas become symptomatic in 8 to 12 days and occasionally as late as 25 to 30 days after the operation. Damage to the blood supply from clamping, cautery, or figure-of-eight sutures produces

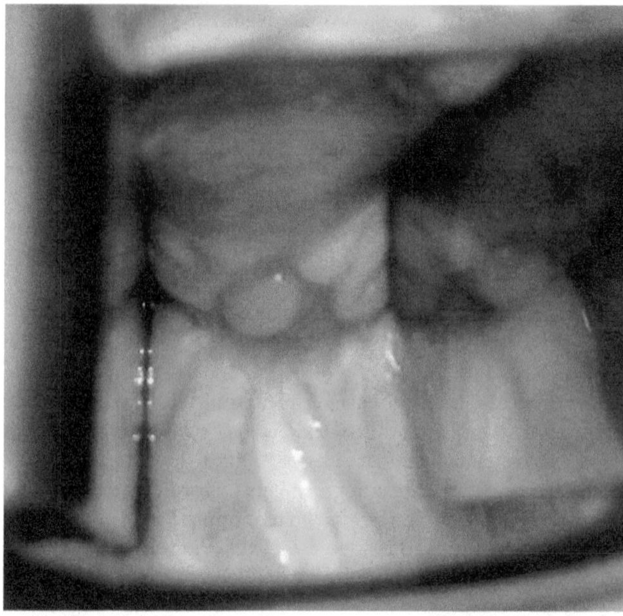

**Figure 25.8** Vesicovaginal fistula with the classic "rosette" of inflammatory tissue denoting the opening to the fistulous track. (From Badlani GH, De Ridder D, Mettu JR, et al. Urinary tract fistulae. In: Wein AJ, Kavoussi LR, Partin AW, et al, eds. *Campbell-Walsh Urology.* 11th ed. Philadelphia: Elsevier; 2016.)

avascular necrosis and subsequent sloughing of the urogenital tissue. Pelvic examination often reveals a small erythematous area of granulation tissue at the site of the fistula (Fig. 25.8).

A small fistula may be clinically identified by placing a tampon in the vagina and instilling a dilute solution of methylene blue dye into the urinary bladder. This will also help differentiate between a vesicovaginal fistula and ureterovaginal fistula. If the blue coloring is discovered on the tampon, the defect is most likely in the bladder. If the tampon is not colored, 3 to 5 mL of indigo carmine should be injected IV. The subsequent finding of blue coloring on the tampon is presumptive evidence of an ureterovaginal fistula. Oral phenazopyridine can also be used in lieu of indigo carmine, staining the tampon orange. An IV pyelogram or CT urogram should be obtained in either case to detect obstruction of the ureter and diagnose compound (ureter and bladder) fistulas.

As with most other postoperative complications, preventive medicine is paramount. The woman should have an empty bladder and the physician should obtain adequate exposure of the site. Sharp dissection should be made along tissue planes with proper traction and countertraction. When operating near the bladder or ureter, bleeding vessels should be secured individually. If possible, the ureter should not be completely detached from the overlying peritoneum. With extensive dissection of the periureteral tissue, care should be taken to avoid interference with the longitudinal vascular supply of the ureter, the Waldeyer sheath. In the most difficult cases, in which anatomic landmarks are obscure, opening of the dome of the bladder and palpation with the index finger and thumb may help identify the proper surgical plane. The urinary system, especially the bladder, is very forgiving if given a short period of rest to recover. If trauma to the bladder is suspected, continuous catheter drainage for 3 to 5 days usually results in spontaneous healing. Selective cystoscopy following complicated or difficult operative procedures can be considered, although universal cystoscopy after all hysterectomies misses less urinary injuries.

When leakage from the urinary tract is first discovered, the bladder should be drained with a large-bore Foley catheter. Ureteral injuries should be evaluated for treatment with retrograde ureteral catheters. Approximately 20% of bladder injuries and 30% of ureteral injuries that are drained and stented will heal spontaneously without further surgery. Ureteral injuries that occur secondary to cauterization or coagulation may present several days to a few weeks after surgery. Symptoms may vary from pain, bloating, ileus, leukocytosis, and urinary ascites. Serum creatinine levels may be normal or elevated with intraabdominal leaking of urine. If levels are elevated in the presence of fever or ileus, imaging studies should be considered. With the increase in laparoscopic and robotic surgery, the incidence of thermal injury to the urinary tract has significantly increased. There is a fourfold increase in urinary tract injury in laparoscopic hysterectomies compared with supracervical cases (Harmanli, 2009). Many injuries go unrecognized at the time of surgery, resulting in readmission. In cases in which the injury is seen at or around the time of surgery, immediate treatment facilitates healing of the defect before epithelialization of the aberrant tract occurs. Spontaneous healing usually occurs within the first 4 weeks. With a ureteral fistula, follow-up imaging should be considered to detect delayed ureteral strictures.

Operative repair of a vesicovaginal fistula is usually accomplished via a multilayered closure performed by the vaginal route. The principles for a successful operation include the following: adequate exposure, dissection, and mobilization of each tissue layer; excision of the fistulous tract; closure of each layer without tension on the suture line; and excellent hemostasis with closure of the dead space. Reliable bladder drainage is provided to avoid tension on the suture line for approximately 10 days. The Latzko operation is the simplest means of repairing a fistula at the vaginal apex. This technique of partial colpocleisis involves denudation of the vaginal mucosa surrounding the fistula and subsequent multilayer closure. The primary disadvantage of the procedure may be postoperative shortening of the vagina.

Many ureteral injuries discovered during the immediate postoperative period will heal when treated by percutaneous nephrostomy and ureteral catheters. Ureterovaginal fistulas that do not heal spontaneously are usually repaired 2 to 3 months after the original operation. Reimplantation of the ureter into the bladder is the preferred repair for an injury involving the lower third of the ureter.

## GASTROINTESTINAL COMPLICATIONS

### *POSTOPERATIVE DIET*

Most patients may be given a regular diet as soon as tolerated after elective gynecologic surgery, including patients that undergo bowel resection. This section discusses nausea and postoperative gastrointestinal (GI) complications, as well as glycemic control as it relates to postoperative nutrition. Part of the physiologic stress response to surgery is a drive for gluconeogenesis. This process is enhanced by a hormonally mediated insulin resistance. The resultant hyperglycemia is advantageous in the teleological sense of the fight-or-flight response, but it is detrimental for wound healing, cardiovascular function, and inflammatory processes. Several studies have correlated clinical outcomes with glucose levels. The American Association of Endocrinology has noted an 18-fold increase in hospital mortality in general medicine and general surgery patients with glucose levels above 200 mg/dL (Garber, 2004).

Glucose control begins preoperatively and is discussed in Chapter 24. Women who are given insulin infusions during surgery should have their infusions continued until they are tolerating regular meals. At this point, they may be given subcutaneous insulin, if necessary. Metformin is often avoided in the perioperative setting because of the potential risks of lactic acidosis. There is no clear consensus, but stopping metformin for 24 hours prior to surgery, with resumption when the patient resumes full oral intake, appears to adequately limit this risk. In women with a history of insulin resistance, women who are morbidly obese, and those older than 60 years, glucose levels should be checked at the bedside every 4 to 6 hours during the first postoperative day. If a woman's glucose rises above 150 mg/dL, she should be treated.

The American Diabetic Association recommendations suggest that critically ill patients have better outcomes with tighter glucose control—fasting levels less than 110 mg/dL and postprandial levels less than 140 mg/dL. Non–critically ill patients should have fasting levels less than 140 mg/dL and postprandial levels less than 180 mg/dL (Umpierrez, 2012). However, a study of 6100 critically ill patients (NICE-SUGAR) has suggested that tight control of 80- to 108-mg/dL fasting levels may actually be associated with worse outcomes because of complications from iatrogenic hypoglycemia (Finfer, 2009). Studies of non–critically ill patients, in contrast, have found that hyperglycemia is associated with more wound infections. Ramos and associates have noted an increased incidence of infection by 30% for every increase in glucose of 40 mg/dL over the recommended 110 mg/dL (Ramos, 2008).

Sliding scale insulin treatments, though less effective than intravenous infusions in the first 24 hours, are easier to manage. Sliding scale regular insulin is most appropriate for women without a previous history of diabetes and without risk factors, and those with short surgeries who will resume normal activity and diet within 24 hours. Infusions are preferable if glucose levels are elevated significantly, early in the postoperative course and for women with longer surgeries who will not resume regular eating and activity for a few days. Insulin infusions are begun with concomitant infusions of $D_5$ half-normal saline (5% dextrose in half-strength normal saline) with 10 mEq of KCl. The Portland Insulin Protocol allows for control of glucose levels and, with nursing support, can be effective (see Appendix A).

When transitioning off insulin infusions, it is reasonable to use the rule of thumb of 80% of the previous 24-hour total insulin dose. This amount may be divided into split doses of NPH insulin or longer acting glargine. Glargine is associated with less hypoglycemia. Initially, a bolus of fast-acting insulin, lispro, may be added with meals. The bedside glucose level is measured every 4 hours. In patients who go home at 24 hours, oral medications or insulin may be restarted at the time of discharge with the same dose as that which was used before the operative period.

## POSTOPERATIVE NAUSEA AND GASTROINTESTINAL FUNCTION

Minor disturbances in GI function are a normal consequence of anesthesia, perioperative medications, and surgical manipulation. Most women experience some nausea for approximately 12 to 24 hours, pass flatus some time during the first 48 hours, and have a spontaneous bowel movement by the third or fourth postoperative day after uncomplicated, benign gynecologic surgery.

**Table 25.6** Gastrointestinal Information

| Category | Clear Liquid (*N* = 107) | Regular Diet (*N* = 138) |
|---|---|---|
| **Morbidity** | | |
| Nausea | 21 (19.6) | 26 (18.8) |
| Vomiting | 10 (9.3) | 19 (13.8) |
| Abdominal distention | 10 (9.3) | 18 (13.0) |
| Nasogastric tube use | 1 (0.9) | 8 (5.8) |
| **Tolerance** | | |
| Diet on first attempt | 101 (94.4) | 121 (87.7) |
| Regular diet on first attempt | 103 (96.3) | |
| If intolerant, time to tolerance (days) | 5.3 ± 1.5 | 3.6 ± 1.5 |
| Flatus before discharge | 55 (51.4) | 69 (50.0) |
| **Intervals (days)** | | |
| Bowel sounds | 1.2 ± 0.5 | 1.2 ± 0.5 |
| Flatus | 2.8 ± 1.4 | 2.8 ± 1.0 |
| Regular diet* | 2.4 ± 2.5 | 1.1 ± 0.3 |
| Hospital stay | 3.6 ± 3.0 | 3.4 ± 1.7 |

From Pearl MI, Frandina M, Mahler L, et al. A randomized controlled trial of a regular diet as the first meal in gynecologic oncology patients undergoing intraabdominal surgery. *Obstet Gynecol*. 2002;100:232.
Data presented as mean ± standard deviation or *N* (%).
**P* <.05; no other significant differences between groups.

The current best practice for women after gynecologic surgery including cancer and bowel resections, regardless of age, is clear liquids within 6 hours of surgery and immediate advancement to a regular diet with cessation of nausea and as tolerated by the patient. Traditionally, patients were to have nothing by mouth until the passage of flatus and then given a gradual resumption of diet from clear liquid to full liquid to soft to regular diet, commonly called *step-up diets*. Several studies have shown that delayed feeding such as this is unnecessary and, in some ways, detrimental. Steed and colleagues, in a study of major gynecologic surgeries, including oncologic cases, compared restricted oral intake with step-up diets to early full diet and found no adverse effects, as well as a shorter length of stay in the early feeding group (Steed, 2002). Similarly, a low-residual diet at 6 hours postoperative followed by a regular diet compared with a traditional delayed feeding and a step-up diet after return of bowel function showed more nausea and emesis in the delayed feeding group, with a shorter length of stay in the early feeding group (Kalogera, 2013) (Table 25.6).

Approximately one third of adult women experience postoperative nausea and vomiting (PONV). Several factors affect the likelihood and severity of PONV, including preoperative anxiety, decreased threshold for nausea and vomiting, previous history of PONV, duration of surgery, drugs used for anesthesia, obesity, and postoperative pain medications. Gan and associates, in the 2014 Consensus Guidelines for the Management of Postoperative Nausea and Vomiting, have recommended certain preventive measures (Gan, 2014). These include avoiding general anesthesia with the use of more regional anesthesia, use of propofol for induction and maintenance, avoidance of nitrous oxide and other volatile anesthetics, adequate hydration, and minimizing the perioperative use of opioids. The list of recommended pharmacologic antiemetics for PONV prophylaxis can be seen in Table 25.7. Serotonin is the

**Table 25.7** Antiemetics Used for Postoperative Nausea and Vomiting (PONV)

| Drugs | Dose | Evidence | Timing | Evidence |
|---|---|---|---|---|
| Aprepitant | 40 mg per os | A2[113,115] | At induction | A2[113] |
| Casopitant | 150 mg per os | A3[117,118] | At induction | |
| Dexamethasone | 4-5 mg IV | A1[121] | At induction | A1[326] |
| Dimenhydrinate | 1 mg/kg IV | A1[152-154] | | |
| Dolasetron | 12.5 mg IV | A2[84,85] | End of surgery; timing may not affect efficacy | A2[85] |
| Droperidol* | 0.625-1.25 mg IV | A1[138,139] | End of surgery | A1[140] |
| Ephedrine | 0.5 mg/kg IM | A2[223,224] | | |
| Granisetron | 0.35-3 mg IV | A1[91-93] | End of surgery | A1[108-110] |
| Haloperidol | 0.5-<2 mg IM/IV | A1[146] | | |
| Methylprednisolone | 40 mg IV | A2[137] | | |
| Ondansetron | 4 mg IV, 8 mg ODT | A1[74,75] | End of surgery | A1[107] |
| Palonosetron | 0.075 mg IV | A2[105,106] | At induction | A2[105,106] |
| Perphenazine | 5 mg IV | A1[162] | | |
| Promethazine | 6.25-12.5 mg IV | A2[222,295] | | |
| Ramosetron | 0.3 mg IV | A2[102] | End of surgery | A2[102] |
| Rolapitant | 70-200 mg per os | A3[119] | At induction | |
| Scopolamine | Transdermal patch | A1[157,158] | Prior evening or 2 h before surgery | A1[157] |
| Tropisetron | 2 mg IV | A1[97] | End of surgery | Expert opinion |

From Gan TJ, Diemunsch P, Habib AS, et al. Consensus guidelines for the management of postoperative nausea and vomiting. *Anesth Analg*. 2014;118(1):85-113.
All references are from the original source article.
These recommendations are evidence based, and not all the drugs have an Food and Drug Administration (FDA) indication for PONV. Drugs are listed alphabetically.
*See FDA black box warning.

most important neurotransmitter and intestinal hormone affecting nausea. Serotonin affects the GI nerves and also central nervous system (CNS) receptors, specifically through the 5-hydroxytryptamine (5-HT3) receptors. It should be no surprise that (5-HT3) receptor antagonists are effective and perhaps the most studied, specifically ondansetron. However, there are other 5-HT3 receptor antagonist medications, as well as neurokinin-1 (NK-1) receptor antagonists, corticosteroids, butyrophenones, antihistamines, and anticholinergics, that have activity and are currently used in clinical practice.

A randomized clinical trial of 5199 patients by Apfel and colleagues has examined several regimens for the prophylaxis of PONV. This multicenter trial documented several important principles for postoperative management. The antiemetic interventions of dexamethasone, ondansetron, and droperidol were found to be equally effective for treating nausea. Droperidol is associated with a rare but problematic side effect of prolonged QT intervals and has subsequently led to most pharmacies removing this medication from their formularies. Dexamethasone, 2.5 to 5 mg, should be given at the beginning of surgery to be most effective. The repeat use of medications for rescue effects is less efficacious if an agent has been given previously (Apfel, 2004). Previous studies have found that agents such as metoclopramide are ineffective for prophylaxis. Antiemetics in the phenothiazine class, such as promethazine and prochlorperazine, are effective but have some limitations because of side effects of sedation, dry mouth, and extrapyramidal effects, which may be worse for older women. Although ondansetron is the gold standard to which other antiemetics are compared, it is less effective than aprepitant for reducing emesis and Palonosetron on the incidence of PONV.

Apfel and associates' study also looked at risk factors for PONV, and one of the strongest is female gender (RR, 3.13; 95% CI: 2.33-4.20). Thus all women should be considered for prophylactic measures. Other factors include 1.78 RR (95% CI: 1.35-2.95) for patients with hysterectomies, 1.57 RR (95% CI: 1.32-1.07) for nonsmokers, and 2.14 (95% CI: 1.75-2.61) for use of postoperative opioids (Apfel, 2004). With patients going home within 24 hours of surgery, the term *postdischarge nausea and vomiting* (PDNV) is used. Several small randomized controlled trial (RCTs) have demonstrated efficacy in preventing PDNV with orally disintegrating ondansetron tablets, acupoint stimulation of P6, and transdermal scopolamine patches.

## ILEUS

Ileus is a delay in the normal return of bowel function caused by an inhibition of the normal propulsive reflexes of the bowel that are regulated by the autonomic nervous system. Adynamic (paralytic) ileus is a misnomer, as it is a normal event defined as delayed bowel function of minor to moderate degree in the absence of a mechanical obstruction. It may be expected to follow any intraperitoneal or pelvic operation. Brief declines in the motility of the GI tract are normal responses after surgery, and the stomach returns to full motility within 24 hours. However, some gastric secretions will continually pass into the duodenum. The stomach secretes 500 to 1000 mL of fluid/day, making the total output from the upper tract approximately 1 to 1.5 L daily. The pancreas secretes an additional liter. The small intestine resumes peristalsis within 6 hours after surgery. The right colon resumes full motility in about 24 hours, but the left colon may take up to 72 hours. The incidence and duration of adynamic ileus are less following vaginal or laparoscopic hysterectomy than abdominal hysterectomy. If the delay in bowel function persists longer than 5 to 7 days, the patient has an ileus and one should also consider the possibility etiologies: either a mechanical cause such as a bowel obstruction or some other condition leading to an adynamic, or paralytic, ileus such as an infection or retained foreign body.

Ileus, or specifically adynamic ileus, is believed to result from a lack of coordinated motor activity of the intestine, which results in disorganized propulsive activity. Electrical activity is present, but the pathophysiologic problem is continuous activity of the intrinsic inhibitor neurons in the wall of the small intestine. Usually, the process is generalized, but occasionally may be localized, involving only an isolated loop of bowel. The cause of prolonged postoperative ileus is a subject of continued debate. Generally, the mechanisms include an increased neurologic inhibition of intestinal motility caused by sympathetic nerve activity, as well as an inflammation within the intestinal wall. Bauer and Boeckxstaens have described leukocytic infiltration secondary to cytokine production from manipulation of the bowel during surgery. The inflammation inhibits the appropriate neuromuscular reactions, which then decrease motility (Bauer, 2004). Postoperative narcotics also contribute to the problem by stimulating the opioid receptors increasing the dyssynchronous contractions that are the hallmark of an ileus, further decreasing motility and increasing pain.

The classic symptoms of a prolonged ileus include absence of flatus, abdominal distention, and obstipation. Often, these symptoms are associated with nausea and effortless vomiting. Bowel sounds may be hypoactive or absent. This condition may be associated with abdominal tenderness and the abdomen is usually tympanic to percussion. Nausea and vomiting that persist more than 24 hours after surgery are a cause for concern. Diagnostic films of the abdomen (supine, erect, lateral) may help establish the correct diagnosis but are frequently overutilized (Table 25.8). CT scanning has also been found to be a useful test for differentiating adynamic ileus from complete obstruction (Mattei, 2006).

**Table 25.8** Differential Radiographic Findings in Ileus and Mechanical Obstruction

| Adynamic Ileus | Mechanical Obstruction |
|---|---|
| Small and large bowel distended in proportion to each other | In small bowel obstruction, there is dilated small bowel proximal to site of obstruction; in colonic obstruction, the colon is distended and small bowel distention is present with an incompetent ileocecal valve |
| Air-fluid levels in small bowel infrequent; when present, they at the same levels | Air-fluid levels are common and at different levels in the bowel |
| Quantitative difference in small bowel distention | Greater small bowel distention than with ileus |
| Small bowel distention in central part of abdomen with colon in periphery | Small bowel distention present in central part of abdomen; no peripheral large bowel distention |

From Buchsbaum HJ, Mazer J. The gastrointestinal tract. In: Buchsbaum HJ, Walton LA, eds. *Strategies in Gynecologic Surgery*. New York: Springer-Verlag; 1986.

Table 25.9 Treatment Options for Postoperative Ileus

| Treatment | Potential Mechanism | Comments |
|---|---|---|
| **Nonpharmacologic Options** | | |
| Nasogastric tube | Gastric, small bowel decompression | No evidence nasogastric tubes reduce duration of POI<br>May increase pulmonary postoperative complications pulmonary postoperative complications |
| Early enteral nutrition | Stimulates gastrointestinal motility by eliciting reflex response and stimulating release of several hormonal factors | Appears safe, well tolerated<br>Some, but not all, studies suggest decrease in POI |
| Sham feeding | Cephalic-vagal reflex | Small clinical trials suggest some benefit |
| Early mobilization | Possible mechanical stimulation | No significant change in duration of POI but may decrease other postoperative complications |
| Laparoscopic surgery | Decreased opiate requirements, decreased pain, less abdominal wall trauma | Most studies find decreased duration of POI with laparoscopy |
| Psychological preoperative preparation | Improves bowel motility through visceral learning | One study found positive benefit in decreasing time to flatus and hospital discharge |
| **Pharmacologic Treatment Options** | | |
| Metoclopramide | Dopamine antagonist, cholinergic agent | |
| Cisapride | Dopamine antagonist, cholinergic agonist, serotonin receptor agonist | Possibly effective, withdrawn from U.S. market due to cardiovascular side effects |
| Erythromycin | Motilin agonist | Two RCTs suggest no benefit |
| Opiate antagonists | Block peripheral opiate receptors | One RCT shows ADL8-2698 decreases time to flatus, bowel movement, and hospital discharge, but not currently available outside of clinical trials<br>Other agents have not been evaluated in POI movement, and hospital discharge, but not currently available outside of clinical trials<br>Other agents have not been evaluated in POI |
| Epidural anesthesia | Inhibits sympathetic reflex at cord level, opioid-sparing analgesia | Several RCTs suggest benefit in decreasing POI, most effective when inserted at thoracic level |
| NSAIDs | Opiate-sparing analgesia, inhibits COX-mediated prostaglandin synthesis | Probable benefit. COX-2 selective medications need further evaluation |
| Laxatives | Stimulant, prokinetic effects | No RCTs<br>One nonrandomized, unblinded study suggests possible benefit |
| Antiadrenergic agents | Blocks sympathetic neural reflex | Little practical benefit in POI drugs often limited by cardiovascular side effects |
| Cholinergic agents | Acetylcholine modulation | Frequent systemic side effects<br>Neostigmine has possible benefit |
| Multimodality therapy | Combination therapy may work via multiple mechanisms | Possible benefit in reducing POI<br>No RCTs have been reported |

From Behm B, Stollman N. Postoperative ileus: etiologies and interventions. *Clin Gastroenterol Hepatol*. 2003;1(2):71-80.
*COX*, Cyclooxygenase; *NSAIDs*, nonsteroidal anti-inflammatory drugs; *POI*, postoperative ileus; *RCTs*, randomized controlled trials.

Oral administration of radiocontrast material may be both therapeutic and diagnostic. The osmolality of the radiocontrast material is approximately six times greater than that of normal saline. Thus a large amount of fluid enters the small bowel and acts as a direct stimulant of peristalsis. In one study, after preliminary abdominal films were obtained, a dosage of 120 mL of 66% diatrizoate meglumine, 10% diatrizoate sodium (Gastrografin), was administered orally or via nasogastric tube. Passage of liquid stool occurred within a few hours in patients with adynamic ileus. Gastrografin, unlike barium, is nontoxic if it accidentally contaminates the peritoneal cavity during an operation for bowel obstruction.

Early carbohydrate intake, as well as postoperative gum chewing, has demonstrated some efficacy in decreasing the rates of postoperative ileus and promoting the return of normal bowel function. In addition, a carbohydrate loading drink the night before surgery and allowing fluids up to 4 hours before surgery may assist with postoperative recovery as well (Kalogera, 2013). It is also known that early feeding decreases the incidence of postoperative ileus, most likely through stimulation of intestinal reflexes. The workup of postoperative ileus should include evaluation of serum electrolyte and magnesium levels, because hypokalemia and abnormal magnesium levels may contribute to the ileus. Narcotics, intraabdominal infection, urinary ascites, and retroperitoneal hematomas may all affect GI motility. The management of a postoperative ileus is controversial, with numerous remedies that are unproved but demonstrate isolated, anecdotal success (Table 25.9).

Severe adynamic ileus is a self-limiting condition that responds to GI rest, IV fluids, and time. During the period of watchful expectancy, adequate fluid and electrolyte replacement is necessary. Patients experience mild cramping and passage of flatus and regain their appetite with the return of normal peristalsis. If adequate bowel sounds are present, a rectal tube, a Fleet enema, or a rectal suppository may facilitate the initial passage of flatus. Some advocate the routine postoperative administration of a "wetting agent," such as simethicone, to reduce surface tension of intestinal mucus and liberate entrapped gas. Opinions

Table 25.10 Average Daily Volume and Electrolyte Concentrations of Gastrointestinal Secretions

| Secretion | Volume (mL/day) | Electrolyte Concentration (mEq/L) Na+ | K+ | Cl- |
|---|---|---|---|---|
| Saliva | 1000-1500 | 10-40 | 10-20 | 6-30 |
| Gastric juice | 2000-2500 | 60-120 | 10-20 | 10-30 |
| Hepatic bile | 600-800 | 130-155 | 2-12 | 80-100 |
| Pancreatic juice | 700-1000 | 150-155 | 5-10 | 30-50 |
| Duodenal secretions | 300-800 | 90-140 | 2-10 | 70-120 |
| Jejunal and ileal secretions | 2000-3000 | 125-140 | 5-10 | 100-130 |
| Colonic mucosal secretions | 200-500 | 140-148 | 5-10 | 60-90 |
| Total: | 8000-10,000 | | | |

Table 25.11 Composition of Intravenous Solutions

| Solution | Glucose (g/L) | Component (mEq/L) $Na^+$ | $Cl^-$ | $HCO_3^-$ | $K^+$ | $Ca^{2+}$ | $Mg^{2+}$ | $HPO_4^-$ | $NH_4^-$ |
|---|---|---|---|---|---|---|---|---|---|
| Extracellular fluid | 1000 | 140 | 102 | 27 | 4.2 | 5 | 3 | 0.3 | |
| 5% dextrose and water | 50 | | | | | | | | |
| 10% dextrose and water | 100 | | | | | | | | |
| 0.9% sodium chloride (normal saline) | | | 154 | 154 | | | | | |
| 0.45% sodium chloride (half normal saline) | | | 77 | 77 | | | | | |
| 0.21% sodium chloride (¼ normal saline) | | | 34 | 34 | | | | | |
| 3% sodium chloride (hypertonic saline) | | | 513 | 513 | | | | | |
| Lactated Ringer's solution | | | 130 | 109 | 28* | 4 | 2.7 | | |
| 0.9% ammonium chloride | | | 168 | | | | | | 168 |

From Miller TA, Duke JH. Fluid and electrolyte management. In: Dudrick SJ, Baue AE, Eiseman B, et al, eds, *Manual of Preoperative and Postoperative Care*, 3rd ed. Philadelphia: WB Saunders; 1983.

*Present in solution as lactate but is metabolized to bicarbonate.

are mixed as to whether such an agent reduces the incidence or intensity of adynamic ileus. Randomized trials of the prokinetic agents erythromycin and metoclopramide have shown these agents to be ineffective in relieving ileus. Importantly, prophylactic nasogastric suctioning will not prevent ileus. In many studies, prophylactic nasogastric suctioning is associated with an increased risk of aspiration as well as an increased rate of ileus—the very symptom the treatment is supposed to prevent (Nelson, 2007). However, if a severe ileus does not resolve, nasogastric suctioning is necessary. Nasogastric suction prevents progression of the intestinal distention. During periods when nasogastric suctioning is used, special attention should be given to correct replacement of fluid and electrolytes (Tables 25.10 and 25.11). A rare but worrisome complication of prolonged ileus is massive dilation of the cecum. Massive dilation of the colon related to a pseudo-obstruction produced by severe adynamic ileus in the absence of mechanical obstruction is known as Ogilvie syndrome. This condition may be treated medically by evacuating the air with colonoscopy or rectal tube, and in severe cases, cecostomy may be necessary. An alternative method of treating this condition is IV neostigmine.

## INTESTINAL OBSTRUCTION AND ADHESIONS

Adhesions are the most common cause of postoperative intestinal obstruction. During subsequent operations, up to 90% of women are found to have some adhesions following abdominal laparotomy, although most are filmy. In a large retrospective cohort study covering a 10-year period following laparotomy for gynecologic conditions, approximately one in three women had adhesion-related readmissions to the hospital (Ellis, 1999). Less common causes of intestinal obstruction are hernias, mesenteric defects, intussusception, volvulus, and neoplasm. Large raw areas of the pelvis with hypoxic tissue facilitate the attachment of small intestine following pelvic surgery. Previous gynecologic surgeries are the most common cause of small bowel obstruction in women. The incidence of operation for obstruction of the small intestine after an abdominal hysterectomy is estimated to be approximately 2%. Interestingly, in one series, adhesions involving the pelvic peritoneum were responsible for the intestinal obstruction in 85% of cases, and adhesions to the closure of the anterior abdominal wall accounted for the other 15%. Fortunately, the fibrous adhesions that form during the first 2 to 3 weeks after an operation are soft and filmy. Thus intestinal strangulation during the postoperative period is extremely rare. Dense adhesions may develop several months after surgery. Adhesion formation after surgical procedures appears to be related to irritation of the peritoneum. The reaction of injured peritoneum involves a reepithelialization by peritoneal cells to cover raw intra-abdominal surfaces. The process begins within 24 hours of surgery. Fibrin-rich exudates cover areas of denuded viscera and abdominal wall. Factors that increase adhesion formation include inflammation, infection, and trauma. Thus suturing of peritoneum should be kept to a minimum. The greatest risk, as noted by Dubuisson and colleagues in a series of 1000 consecutive laparoscopies, was in previous midline incisions, with more than 50% having adhesions, compared with less than 3% after a previous laparoscopy (Dubuisson, 2010). The incidence of intestinal obstruction depends on the type of gynecologic surgery performed. Approximately 2/1000 women develop an obstruction

Table 25.12 Differential Diagnosis between Postoperative Ileus and Postoperative Obstruction

| Clinical Features | Postoperative Ileus | Postoperative Obstruction |
|---|---|---|
| Abdominal pain | Discomfort from distention but not cramping pains | Cramping, progressively severe |
| Relationship to previous operation | Usually within 48-72 hr of operation | Usually delayed; may be 5-7 days for remote onset |
| Nausea and vomiting | Present | Present |
| Distention | Present | Present |
| Bowel sounds | Absent or hypoactive | Borborygmi with peristaltic rushes and high-pitched tinkles |
| Fever | Only if related to associated peritonitis | Rarely present unless bowel becomes gangrenous |
| Abdominal radiograph | Distended loops of small and large bowels; gas usually present in colon | Single or multiple loops of distended bowel, usually small bowel with air-fluid levels |
| Treatment | Conservative with nasogastric suction, enemas, cholinergic stimulation | Partial—conservative with nasogastric decompression, *or* Complete—surgical |

after a benign gynecologic operation, whereas approximately 8% develop intestinal obstruction after radical cancer surgery. Intestinal obstruction occurs in the small intestine in approximately 80% of cases and in the colon in the remaining 20%. As noted, differentiating between bowel obstruction and ileus can be difficult in the postoperative period (Table 25.12).

The acute symptoms of intestinal obstruction usually present between the fifth and seventh postoperative days. Most patients have a short period of normal intestinal function before the onset of symptoms. Women with bowel obstruction appear to have more acute distress than women with an ileus. The abdominal pain is intermittent, colicky, and may be sharp in nature. Episodes of colicky pain usually last from 1 to 3 min. Associated symptoms include vomiting, abdominal distention, and constipation. Bowel sounds are loud, high pitched, and rushing. Nasogastric drainage is usually more profuse than in patients with severe adynamic ileus.

Abdominal radiographs demonstrate a stepladder appearance—multiple air-fluid levels throughout the small intestine, with a paucity of gas in the colon and rectum. Pneumoperitoneum from an exploratory celiotomy usually persists for up to 7 days. Thus in the early postoperative period, free air under the diaphragm is not diagnostic of perforation of a hollow viscus. Obstruction of the colon may be diagnosed by retrograde infusion of contrast material or by flexible endoscopy.

The foundation of early treatment of postoperative intestinal obstruction is decompression of the small intestine and adequate replacement of fluids and electrolytes. Decompression may be accomplished by means of a nasogastric tube. Serial monitoring of white blood cell counts with differentials should be performed. Repeat physical examinations and abdominal radiographic examinations are used to assess the degree of intestinal distention. Expectant management is successful in the majority of patients. Historically, less than 40% of patients with small bowel obstruction caused by adhesions will require surgery. Some advocate for immediate administration of Gastrografin upon presentation for adhesive obstruction with conservative management of patients in whom Gastrografin dose not reach the colon in 24 hours. Patients in whom contrast reached the colon in 5 hours or less had a 90% success rate of conservative management (Gowen, 2003).

The major cause of morbidity and death with bowel obstruction is delay in diagnosis, with resultant strangulation, perforation and secondary sepsis. Women who develop strangulation experience a dramatic increase in the intensity of abdominal pain, and the pain becomes continuous. Strangulation of the small bowel is associated with localized peritoneal irritation, increase in temperature, and marked leukocytosis. Bowel obstruction may also lead to translocation of intestinal bacteria across the bowel wall, promoting sepsis. It has been shown that the more distal the obstruction, the greater the incidence of anaerobic septicemia.

Fecal impaction is most often seen in older patients. It results from loss of peristalsis in the colon, with an impaired perception of rectal fullness. This may result in diarrhea as intestinal contents pass around the impaction or obstipation. Treatment involves obtaining partial analgesia with lidocaine jelly and, subsequently, manually fragmenting and extracting the fecal mass.

## RECTOVAGINAL FISTULA

Rectovaginal fistulas and fecal incontinence secondary to perineal tears are usually obstetric complications and are only rarely associated with gynecologic surgery. In general, rectovaginal fistulas following hysterectomy or repair of an enterocele are usually located in the upper third of the vagina, whereas those secondary to a posterior colporrhaphy are in the lower third of the vagina. Other causes of rectovaginal fistula are carcinoma, radiation therapy, perirectal abscess, inflammatory bowel disease, lymphogranuloma venereum, and trauma.

The initial signs and symptoms associated with potential fistulous tracts between the rectum and vagina usually present 7 to 14 days after an operation. The first warning may be the rectal passage of several blood clots, indicating that a hematoma has ruptured into the rectum. Distressing symptoms include passage of gas from the vagina and, depending on the size of the opening, the passage of fecal material from the vagina. Associated with these classic symptoms and signs are a chronic, foul-smelling vaginal discharge and subsequent dyspareunia. Aside from the physical symptoms of the anatomic defect, fistulas cause severe emotional distress because they affect almost every aspect of the woman's daily life.

The diagnosis is not difficult to establish, and only very small openings present a diagnostic problem. What appears to be granulation tissue in the posterior aspect of the vagina is the dark red rectal mucosa, which stands out in contrast to the lighter vaginal mucosa. Usually, the defect may be successfully defined with a small, malleable metal probe. If this is not successful, a Foley catheter should be placed in the rectum. Methylene blue dye or milk may then be instilled into the rectum with a tampon in the vagina, similar to the procedure for establishing the diagnosis of

Table 25.13 Differences between Antibiotic-Associated Diarrhea from *Clostridium difficile* and Diarrhea from Other Causes

| | **Cause** | |
|---|---|---|
| **Characteristic** | ***C. difficile* Infection** | **Other Causes** |
| Most commonly implicated antibiotics | Clindamycin, cephalosporins, penicillins | Clindamycin, cephalosporins, or amoxicillin-clavulanate |
| History | Usually no relevant history of antibiotic intolerance | History of diarrhea with antibiotic therapy common |
| **Clinical Features** | | |
| Diarrhea | May be florid; evidence of colitis with cramps, fever, and fecal leukocytes common | Usually moderate in severity (i.e., nuisance diarrhea) without evidence of colitis |
| Findings on CT or endoscopy | Evidence of colitis (not enteritis) common | Usually normal |
| Complications | Hypoalbuminemia, anasarca, toxic megacolon, relapses with treatment with metronidazole or vancomycin | Usually none except occasional cases of dehydration |
| Results of assay for *C. difficile* toxin | Positive | Negative |
| Epidemiologic pattern | May be epidemic for endemic in hospitals or long-term care facilities | Sporadic |
| **Treatment** | | |
| Withdrawal of implicated antibiotic | May resolve but often persists or progresses | Usually resolves |
| Antiperistaltic agents | Contraindicated | Often useful |
| Oral metronidazole or vancomycin | Prompt response | Not indicated |

From Bartlett JG. Antibiotic-associated diarrhea. *N Engl J Med*. 2002;346(5):334-339. *CT*, Computed tomography.

a vesicovaginal fistula. Contrast enemas and colonoscopy may also be used in cases where there is a high degree of suspicion and the fistula cannot be identified by other means.

For initial treatment the woman should be obstipated with a low-residue diet and diphenoxylate hydrochloride (Lomotil). Approximately one in four anatomic defects heal spontaneously before epithelialization of the tract. A low-residue diet or hyperalimentation may be helpful in facilitating spontaneous closure of some anatomic defects. Timing of the operative repair is important. The gynecologist should inspect the area surrounding the fistula to ensure that the tissues are free of edema, induration, and infection. Preoperative evaluation includes visualization of the entire vagina and sigmoidoscopy of the rectal mucosa in an attempt to discover more than one opening. Imaging studies and endoscopy are important diagnostic tools if there is any suspicion of coexistence of Crohn disease.

The operative technique used depends on the size and location of the fistula. Standard operative principles include removal of the entire fistulous tract and closure of tissue layers without tension on the suture line. In the repair of large rectovaginal fistulas in the lower part of the vagina, it is usually easier to convert the rectovaginal fistula into a fourth-degree laceration. Diverting colostomy should be used for all radiation-induced fistulas, most fistulas associated with inflammatory bowel disease, and some large postoperative fistulas at the apex of the vagina. The stool should be kept soft with low-residue diets and stool softeners such as mineral oil for the first 2 weeks after the operative repair.

## ANTIBIOTIC-ASSOCIATED DIARRHEA

Patients may develop diarrhea in the postoperative period after exposure to antibiotics. Oral and parenteral antibiotics produce similar rates of diarrhea, with some studies noting that up to one third of patients receiving antibiotics will develop diarrhea. Antibiotic therapy, for prophylaxis or treatment, can disrupt the normal intestinal flora. The result is a disturbed breakdown of bile acids and carbohydrates that induce loose stools. Diarrhea may develop secondary to medications other than antibiotics, including oral contrast media, diabetic foods that contain artificial sweeteners, and many cardiac medications. If the woman is afebrile, the diarrhea is mild, and the abdominal examination is unremarkable, stopping or changing antibiotics and providing supportive care are all that is necessary. If the woman has a temperature higher than 38° C, a leukocytosis, abdominal tenderness, severe abdominal distention, bloody diarrhea, or persistent diarrhea, evaluation for *Clostridium difficile* infection is indicated (Table 25.13).

*C. difficile* is a species of spore-forming, gram-positive anaerobic bacteria found normally in 5% of healthy adults. However, after antibiotic treatment and disruption of normal enteric flora, up to 25% of hospitalized adults will become colonized with *C. difficile*. The organism is spread by nosocomial oral-fecal contamination. Persistence of the spores of *C. difficile* and contamination of the environment are primary factors in cross infection. After colonizing the intestine, the organism may secrete toxins, which produce a spectrum of clinical disease. Symptoms from the infection are varied and range from a mild diarrhea to colitis to a pseudomembranous colitis that in rare cases may be fatal (Bartlett, 2002). Almost any antibiotic has been associated with the development of *C. difficile* diarrhea, but second- and third-generation cephalosporins are the antibiotics associated with the highest risk of developing *C. difficile* diarrhea. Symptoms usually appear 5 to 10 days after the initiation of antibiotic therapy; however, they may appear from a few days to a few weeks after antibiotic exposure. Enzyme-linked immunosorbent assay (ELISA) testing for *C. difficile* cell cytotoxin B in the stool is the gold standard for diagnosis because it is the most sensitive and specific and is also relatively inexpensive. The results are usually available within 24 hours.

Use of drugs that slow intestinal transit time, such as diphenoxylate atropine (Lomotil) or narcotics, are definitely contraindicated because the toxins of *C. difficile* remain in the GI tract for a longer period. Therapy for the infection is metronidazole 500 mg PO three times daily or 250 mg PO four times daily. Alternatively, vancomycin PO 125 mg four times daily can be used. Metronidazole therapy has a lower cost and 90% clinical cure rate, so is often preferred as first-line treatment. Vancomycin has a higher cure rate, 98%, and should be used in cases not responsive to metronidazole. Gastrointestinal symptoms usually improve within the first 72 hours of therapy and complete resolution of symptoms occurs within 10 days. Host factors are involved in the pathogenesis of the disease; older and more chronically ill patients usually develop more severe symptoms. Up to 25% of women may develop a recurrence or relapse. Studies have confirmed that more than 50% of recurrences of symptoms after initial response to treatment are caused by reinfection rather by a relapse. Recurrences usually can be successfully treated with oral antibiotics using longer courses (Bartlett, 2002).

## WOUND COMPLICATIONS

### *INFECTION*

A major wound infection prolongs the hospital stay by approximately 2 to 6 days. In a historic review of 23,649 operations, the incidence of abdominal wound infection after abdominal hysterectomy was approximately 5%. Contemporary studies show rates of surgical site infection after hysterectomy of 3.9% for abdominal surgery and 1.8% for minimally invasive approaches ($P < .001$), with an odds ratio of 0.44 (CI 0.37-0.53) (Gandaglia, 2014). Hysterectomy is classified as a clean-contaminated operative procedure because the bacterial flora of the vagina is in continuity with the operative site during the surgery. The Centers for Disease Control and Prevention have revised their nomenclature describing incisional infection. They subdivide incisional infections into superficial infections that involve only the skin and subcutaneous tissue and deep infections that involve the deep soft tissues, including fascia and muscles. Although some infections are generally associated with specific organisms such as streptococcus or clostridia, most gynecologic infections are polymicrobial. Thus antibiotic treatments are aimed at providing broad-spectrum coverage for aerobic, anaerobic, and gram-negative organisms. A list of common antibiotics is found in Appendix B.

The pathophysiology of wound infection depends on an interaction between the number and virulence of bacterial contamination and the resistance of the woman. Inoculation of bacteria into the wound occurs in the operating room during the surgical procedure. A wide spectrum of common endogenous bacteria produce wound infections, including most gram-positive cocci and aerobic and anaerobic rods. Small numbers of bacteria are present in all surgical wounds; however, bacterial growth is facilitated by decreased tissue oxygen and excessive amounts of necrotic tissue. It takes from 100,000 to 1,000,000 bacteria/g of tissue to produce infection in a surgical wound of the skin and subcutaneous tissue. The incidence of superficial skin infection is directly related to the length of the operative procedure. Each additional hour of surgery results in a doubling of the incidence of superficial skin infections. The primary source of bacterial contamination of an abdominal wound may be exogenous to the woman (e.g., a break in sterile technique) or endogenous (e.g., purulent material from a pelvic abscess).

Local and systemic factors contribute to the level of host resistance and thus to the incidence of wound infections. Local factors are more significant and include the presence of hematomas, necrotic tissue, foreign bodies, dead space, use of cautery, and decreased local tissue perfusion. Systemic factors include obesity, diabetes, liver disease, malnutrition, immunosuppression, defects in the reticuloendothelial system, age, and duration of preoperative hospitalization (Box 25.6). The incidence of postoperative wound infection is increased eightfold when the woman's preoperative weight exceeds 200 pounds. In a series of women undergoing abdominal hysterectomy, the thickness of subcutaneous tissue was the greatest risk factor for wound infection (Soper, 1995). If an abdominal incision is more than 4 cm in depth, the risk of a superficial skin infection is increased approximately threefold. Multiple regimens and protocols have been studied to decrease rates of wound infection. Skin warming to improve circulation, supplemental oxygen, and antibiotics given before incision time have all been emphasized as techniques for infection prevention.

**Box 25.6 Factors Associated with Wound Infections**

- Preexisting skin and operative site infection
- Tissue with poor oxygenation
- Hematoma
- Necrotic tissue
- Foreign bodies
- Cauterized tissue
- Poor circulation from vascular disease
- Dead space within the wound
- Anemia
- Decreased perfusion from tension
- Obesity
- Long preoperative hospitalization
- Poor nutrition
    - Vitamin deficiencies
    - Mineral deficiencies (e.g., zinc)
- Glucocorticoids, other immunosuppressive medications
- Diabetes
- Liver disease
- Ionizing radiation
- Advanced age

The first symptom of most wound infections usually appears between the fifth and tenth postoperative days. Wound infection may occur as late as several months following surgery, but more than 90% of cases present within the first 2 weeks of the postoperative period. The first sign is usually fever, followed by tachycardia and varying degrees of increased incisional erythema, induration, tenderness, and pain. As the infection progresses, many wounds develop areas that are fluctuant or firm, and some develop crepitus. There may be associated spontaneous purulent drainage from the wound later in the course of the infection.

Fever during the first 24 to 48 hours is usually secondary to atelectasis. However, two rare types of wound infections are so virulent that they produce toxicity within the first 48 hours. Typically, these early infections are those produced by *Clostridium* spp. and acute β-hemolytic streptococcal infection. Clinically, wound infections secondary to β-hemolytic streptococci appear swollen and red and have an odorless discharge. In contrast, infections secondary to *Clostridium* are boggy and edematous and the discharge has a sweet odor.

Initial treatment of any wound infection consists of opening and draining the wound. Purulent material exhibits a wide range of consistency from the thin watery discharge typical of a streptococcal infection to the thick purulence associated with staphylococcal subcutaneous infections. Gram staining with aerobic and anaerobic cultures of the wound should be performed. These cultures are valuable in guiding treatment if the woman does not respond to initial management. In such cases, the differential diagnosis would be between infections involving deeper tissue planes and infection for which host resistance has failed, even after drainage of the wound. Once a wound infection has been opened and drained, care is directed toward initial packing of the wound with gauze to effect débridement and periodic irrigation. If necrotic tissue is seen, the tissue should be resected back to the point where vital tissue can be identified. If there is a distinct zone of diffuse erythema surrounding a wound infection, the most likely organism is a streptococcal infection, and IV antibiotics are indicated. If methicillin-resistant *Staphylococcus aureus* (MRSA) is cultured, the great majority of women will respond solely to débridement. If the woman does not respond or responds slowly, antibiotics specific for MRSA should be used, such as clindamycin or sulfamethoxazole-trimethoprim. Systemic antibiotics are always indicated for women with immunosuppression or concomitant disease with impaired defense mechanisms.

Most women with a wound infection will become afebrile within 48 to 72 hours after the wound has been opened and débrided. When the woman becomes afebrile and granulation tissue begins to form, consideration may be given to delayed secondary closure. If the incision is large and débridement has been extensive, closure may be facilitated with the use of vacuum-assisted devices. The vacuum promotes granulation, reduces edema in the subcutaneous tissue, and greatly speeds healing. The vacuum should be changed every 48 to 72 hours for wound evaluation. It may be used on an outpatient basis (Fig. 25.9).

Prevention is the foundation of any approach to the treatment of wound infections. Prevention involves consideration of local and systemic factors, which, if unattended, predispose to infection. Prophylactic antibiotics decrease the incidence of wound infection. These antibiotics are discussed in Chapter 24. If the wound is grossly contaminated, it should be left open after surgery. Delayed primary closure on the third or fourth postoperative day may be appropriate. Women who should be considered as candidates for delayed primary closure include those who are immunosuppressed or malnourished, have advanced malignancies, have a contaminated wound, or are morbidly obese. Delayed primary closure reduces the incidence of wound infection from 23% in a control group to 2%. When delayed primary closure is planned, sutures may be placed at the time of surgery and secured, but not tied. The incision should be packed loosely with gauze. If the wound is dry and without evidence of infection on postoperative day 3, the edges may be approximated with the preplaced sutures.

Delayed secondary closure may be accomplished in previously infected wounds after several days of drainage and débridement, and once the wound exhibits nice healthy granulation tissue. Delayed secondary closure markedly reduces the time necessary for eventual closure of the skin defect by secondary intention. The woman's satisfaction is dramatically increased with delayed secondary closure. If delayed closure does not appear to be a likely option, such as in women who have more than 3 cm of subcutaneous tissue, application of a closed vacuum system can be initiated.

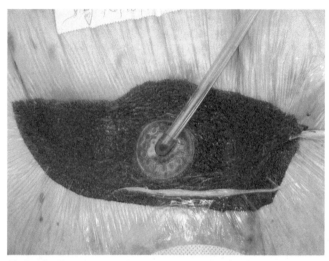

**Figure 25.9** Wound-Vac device on an abdominal wound. The *black area* is the sponge within the incision. (From Heridge RT, Leong M, Phillips L: Wound healing. In: Townsend CM, Beauchamp RD, Evers BM, Mattox KL, eds. *Sabiston Textbook of Surgery.* 18th ed. Philadelphia: Saunders; 2008:191-216.)

A virulent, rapidly progressing form of soft tissue wound infection is necrotizing fasciitis. Often, the diagnosis is not suspected during the early part of the infection because of the relative minor changes in the skin overlying the deeper infection. The early symptoms are local pain with systemic symptoms of tachycardia and fever, which are higher than would be expected with an uncomplicated wound infection. The woman may experience marked tenderness when the infected area is palpated. Conversely, necrotic tissue may become hypoesthetic, or completely numb. An appearance of an area that appears infected but is anesthetic should heighten the suspicion for the diagnosis of necrotizing fasciitis. As the disease progresses, the wound edges usually darken, with crepitance and bullae formation and anesthetic areas developing. Necrotizing fasciitis involves the subcutaneous tissue and superficial fascia. The infection rapidly expands in the subcutaneous spaces and often tracks far beyond the superficial margins of the involved skin.

This condition is a life-threatening surgical emergency and patients should have débridement as soon as possible. It is important for the gynecologist to have a high degree of suspicion for this condition because even with adequate surgical débridement, the mortality rate is 30% to 50%. Only 35% of patients with necrotizing fasciitis will display radiographic evidence of subcutaneous gas. If the diagnosis is questionable, a full-thickness core biopsy and frozen section of the tissue should be performed. This rare but potentially fatal condition necessitates wide débridement of all necrotic tissue, high levels of broad-spectrum antibiotics, and sometimes hyperbaric oxygen. Débridement to freely bleeding tissue helps determine the surgical margin. It is not unusual for the woman to need repetitive débridement. Women with diabetes, malnutrition, immunosuppression, malignancy, obesity, and poor tissue perfusion are most susceptible to this complication.

## DEHISCENCE AND EVISCERATION

Dehiscence is a failure of normal healing and refers to a disruption of any of the layers of a surgical incision. The physiologic, biochemical, and structural changes that characterize normal wound healing are complex and, at best, imperfectly understood. However, the most important fact for the clinician is that the strength of the wound increases over time (Fig. 25.10). The strength of a skin incision increases at a rapid and almost constant rate for the first 4 months and at a much slower rate for the first year. Clinically, a wound dehiscence refers to the separation of the skin, subcutaneous tissue, and fascia, but not peritoneum. This complication usually occurs during the first several days following an operation. Wound evisceration is a complete breakdown of the healing process through all levels of the abdominal incision, with omentum or bowel presenting through the fascia.

The incidence of wound dehiscence is approximately 1 in 200 gynecologic operations. The major short-term result of wound dehiscence is the prolongation of hospital stay. Over the long term, dehiscence predisposes to incisional hernias. Wound infection is present in approximately 50% of women with wound disruption. As with wound infections, preventive management is the most important therapeutic consideration. The incidence of dehiscence has decreased with the use of longer lasting and stronger sutures. Many clinicians prefer to use polydioxanone suture (PDS), a treated Vicryl, or a permanent suture such as polypropylene (Prolene) for greater strength and prolonged presence in the tissue. The rule of thumb is that the suture should remain strong in the tissue until the tissue can resume its original strength. In patients with a propensity for poor or prolonged healing, such as women with malignancy, diabetes, or immune suppression, the use of a permanent suture should be strongly considered. When infection is present, a monofilament suture is preferable to a braided or polyfilament suture (Tables 25.14 and 25.15).

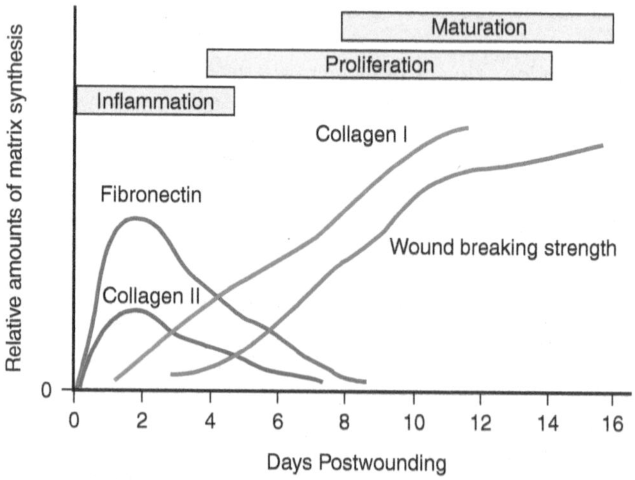


**Figure 25.10** Wound healing over time. (From Heridge RT, Leong M, Phillips L. Wound healing. In: Townsend CM, Beauchamp RD, Evers BM, Mattox KL, eds. *Sabiston Textbook of Surgery*. 18th ed. Philadelphia: Saunders; 2008:191-216.)

The consensus regarding fascial disruption is that local factors are much more important in the pathophysiology of wound disruption than systemic factors, although both should be considered. Important mechanical factors predisposing to disruption are conditions that increase the tension on the incision line, such as abdominal distention and chronic lung disease, or a technically inadequate closure of the wound. Other factors include obesity, advanced age, malignancy, uremia, liver failure, diabetes, hypoproteinemia, hematoma formation, sepsis, corticosteroids or chemotherapy, prior radiation therapy, and whether the incision is made through an area of a previous incision. Whether an incision is horizontal or vertical has little effect on the incidence of wound disruption. The pathophysiology of fascial dehiscence involves exaggerated collagen lysis in the wound. Clinically, the sutures tear through the fascia rather than dissolving or becoming untied. For example, approximating and tying sutures too vigorously, especially with a figure-of-eight suture, may lead to strangulation and necrosis of the tissue and subsequent wound dehiscence. Primary mass closure with a continuous monofilament, delayed absorbable suture, helps avoid this problem in high-risk patients.

The classic symptom and sign of wound disruption is the spontaneous passage of copious serosanguineous fluid from the abdominal incision. This usually occurs between the fifth and eighth postoperative days. Patients with uninfected wounds generally have been asymptomatic, but often report a "pop" after

**Table 25.14** Comparison of Absorbable Sutures

| Suture Reaction | Types | Raw Material | Tensile Strength Retention in Vivo | Tissue |
|---|---|---|---|---|
| Surgical gut suture | Chromic | Collagen derived from healthy beef and sheep | Individual patient characteristics can affect rate of tensile strength loss. | Moderate reaction |
| Monocryl suture (poliglecaprone 25) | Monofilament | Copolymer of glycolide and epsilon-caprolactone | ~50%-60% (violet, 60%-70%) remains at 1 wk; ~20%-30% (violet, 30%-40%) remains at 2 wk; lost within 3 wk (violet, 4 wk) | Minimal acute inflammatory reaction |
| Coated vicryl (polyglactin 910) | Braided | Copolymer of lactide and glycolide coated with 370 and calcium stearate | ~75% remains at 2 wk | Minimal acute inflammatory reaction |
| Suture | Monofilament | | ~50% remains at 3 wk, 25% at 4 wk | |
| PDS II suture (polydioxanone) | Monofilament | Polyester polymer | ~70% remains at 2 wk; ~ 50% remains at 4 wk; ~ 25% remains at 6 wk | Slight |

Modified from Neumayer L, Vargo D. Principles of perioperative and operative surgery. In: Townsend CM, Beauchamp RD, Evers BM, Mattox KL, eds. *Sabiston Textbook of Surgery*. 18th ed. Philadelphia: Saunders; 2008:251-279.

an episode of coughing or emesis. Patients who develop wound defects often lack the normal healing ridge of tissue that can be palpated in normal healing wounds.

Imperative for prevention of wound dehiscence is proper closure of the incision in a woman at high risk for less than optimum healing. Although there are many regional preferences for the choice of suture and method of closure, the most popular technique is some modification of the Smead-Jones closure with permanent suture (Fig. 25.11). Closure with the Smead-Jones technique results in a dehiscence rate of approximately 1 in 1000 operations. With this technique, it is important to place individual sutures at least 1 to 1.5 cm away from the adjacent sutures and include at least 2 cm of fascia on either side of the incision. The alternative technique is the more common, running mass closure using a monofilament permanent suture material such as nylon or Prolene.

Rarely, the vaginal cuff may separate, producing a dehiscence and possibly vaginal evisceration of abdominal contents. This complication often presents with sudden vaginal drainage, bleeding, and pain. The incidence of vaginal cuff dehiscence varies by mode of surgery and is lowest in vaginal hysterectomy (0.11%), followed by abdominal hysterectomy (0.38%), and highest in laparoscopic hysterectomy (range 0.75 to 4.93%) (Hurr, 2011). Risk factors for vaginal cuff dehiscence are summarized in Table 25.16. If there is no evidence of infection at the time of repair, the vaginal cuff may be closed primarily without opening the abdomen. If there is any concern about an intraabdominal complication, an abdominal approach allows for a better intraabdominal evaluation, although reports of laparoscopic evaluation of the abdomen, even in the setting of evisceration with vaginal closure of the cuff, have been successful. Most would also consider antibiotic treatment with broad-spectrum coverage because of the association of vaginal dehiscence with vaginal cuff cellulitis. Vaginal evisceration is uncommon but, when it occurs, it is usually several weeks after surgery and may follow intercourse. Reports have noted an increase in vaginal cuff disruption and evisceration with robotic surgery. This is postulated to be secondary to increased use of cauterization, leading to poor wound healing (Hurr, 2011). This complication may present up to 8 weeks or more after surgery. As a result, many gynecologists ask patients to refrain from intercourse for up to 12 weeks after surgery to allow time for the sutures to dissolve completely and for the tissue to heal.

The treatment of vaginal dehiscence is prompt reclosure in the operating room. Once the diagnosis is recognized, the wound and viscera should be covered with moist gauze and transported to the operating room supine and possibly in slight Trendelenburg position to help keep abdominal contents from eviscerating. Broad-spectrum antibiotics are usually begun, although there is no proof of their efficacy in this circumstance. Once the woman is anesthetized, the wound should be evaluated so that the full extent of the problem can be evaluated. The wound edges may have to be débrided and the wound closed with a wide mass closure, making sure not to incorporate the bladder or rectum in the closure.

## WOUND CARE FOR OBESE PATIENTS

Obesity is one of the most significant risk factors for wound infection and disruption. As noted, hyperglycemia is an associated risk factor in this population of patients. Optimal healing, collagen synthesis, and reepithelialization require good oxygenation. Adipose tissue is poorly vascularized and thus has suboptimal oxygenation. Poor ventilation after surgery in the obese woman further exacerbates this problem. Techniques to improve wound healing in obese patients have been summarized by Walsh and associates; these include maintaining normothermia in the operating suite, which decreases vasoconstriction, supplemental

**Table 25.15** Comparison of Nonabsorbable Sutures

| Suture | Types | Raw Material | Tensile Strength Retention in Vivo | Tissue Reaction |
|---|---|---|---|---|
| Perma-Hand—silk suture | Braided | Organic protein called *fibroin* | Progressive degradation of fiber may result in gradual loss of tensile strength over time | Acute inflammatory reaction |
| Ethilon—nylon suture | Monofilament | Long-chain aliphatic polymers nylon 6 or nylon 6,6 | Progressive hydrolysis may result in gradual loss of tensile strength over time | Minimal acute inflammatory reaction |
| Nurolon—nylon suture | Braided | Long-chain aliphatic polymers nylon 6 or nylon 6,6 | Progressive hydrolysis may result in gradual loss of tensile strength over time | Minimal acute inflammatory reaction |
| Mersilene—polyester fiber suture | Braided Monofilament | Polyethylene terephthalate | No significant change known to occur in vivo | Minimal acute inflammatory reaction |
| Ethibond *Excel*—polyester fiber suture | Braided | Polyethylene terephthalate coated with polybutilate | No significant change known to occur in vivo | Minimal acute inflammatory reaction |
| Prolene—polypropylene suture | Monofilament | Isotactic crystalline stereoisomer of polypropylene | Not subject to degradation or weakening by action of tissue enzymes | Minimal acute inflammatory reaction |
| Pronova—poly-vinylidene fluoride suture | Monofilament | Polymer blend of poly(vinylidene fluoride) and poly(vinylidene fluoride-cohexafluoropropylene) | Not subject to degradation or weakening by action of tissue enzymes | Minimal acute inflammatory reaction |

Modified from Neumayer L, Vargo D. Principles of perioperative and operative surgery. In: Townsend CM, Beauchamp RD, Evers BM, Mattox KL, eds. *Sabiston Textbook of Surgery*. 18th ed. Philadelphia: Saunders; 2008:251-279.

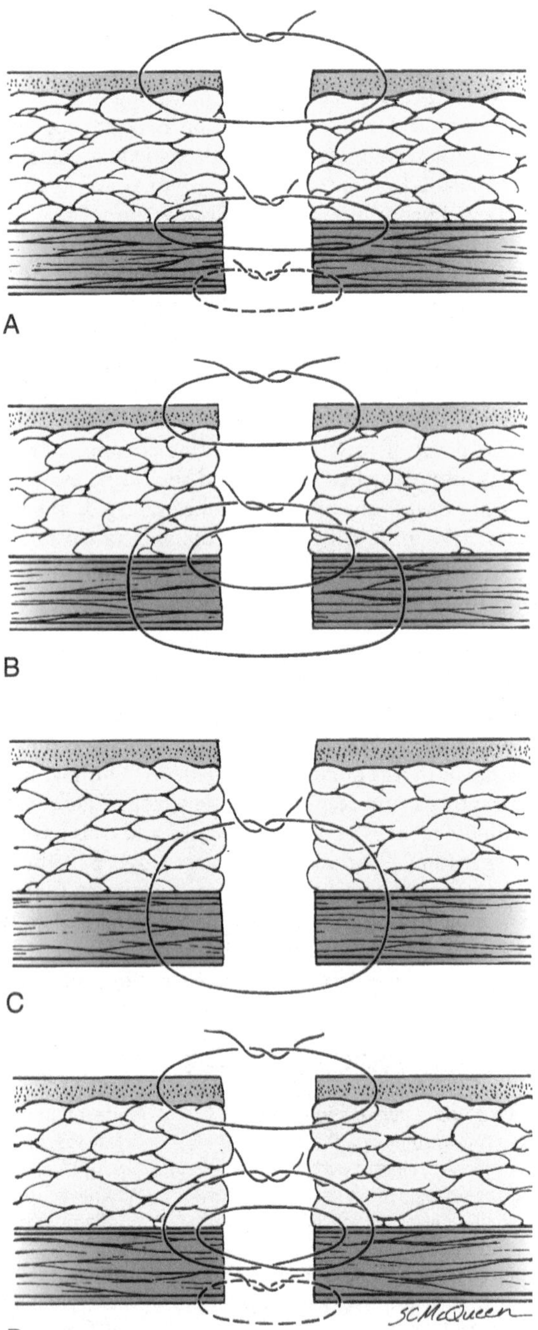


**Figure 25.11** Types of abdominal incision closures. **A,** Layered. **B,** Smead-Jones. **C,** Through and through. **D,** Far near. (From Braun TE. Wound dehiscence. In: Schaefer G, Graber EA, eds. *Complications in Obstetric and Gynecological Surgery.* Hagerstown, MD: Harper & Row; 1981.)

oxygen, and closure of the subcutaneous space if it is larger than 2 cm (Walsh, 2009). Subcutaneous drains do not decrease the infection or wound disruption rate. When patients weigh greater than 120 kg, prophylactic antibiotic dose should be increased (e.g., from 2 g of cefazolin to 3 g). However, extending the dosing beyond surgery is not helpful. Maintaining euglycemia is essential as previously discussed. See Box 25.7.

**Table 25.16** Predisposing Factors to Evisceration*

| Predisposition | Clinical No./No. with Data Reported (%) |
|---|---|
| Postmenopausal (age >51 yr) | 9/12 (75) |
| Prior pelvic surgery | 10/12 (83) |
| Postmenopausal with surgery | 9/12 (75) |
| Enterocele and vaginal vault | 10/12 (83) |
| Posterior enterocele | 6/12 (50) |
| Vaginal cuff defect | 4/12 (33) |
| Coital trauma | 1/12 (8) |
| Spontaneous | 7/12 (58) |
| Trauma | 1/12 (8) |

From Croak AJ, Gelshart JB, Kingele CJ, et al. Characteristics of patients with vaginal vault rupture and evisceration. *Obstet Gynecol.* 2004;103:573.
*Total numbers reported for each predisposition were limited by availability of data. Some patients had more than one predisposition.

**Box 25.7 Techniques to Decrease Wound Disruption and Infection in Obese Surgical Patients**

1. Chlorhexidine bath or shower the night before surgery
2. Women with BMI >35—double the dosage of prophylactic antibiotics
3. Maintain core normothermia during the operation
4. Close subcutaneous tissue if >2 cm in depth
5. Sterile dressing for 24-48 hours
6. Maintain euglycemia
7. Subcutaneous drains do not improve outcomes

## OPERATIVE SITE COMPLICATIONS

### *PELVIC CELLULITIS AND ABSCESS*

Infections of the contiguous retroperitoneal space immediately above the vaginal apex are common complications following abdominal or vaginal hysterectomy. However, the frequency of this postoperative complication has dramatically decreased in direct relation to the use of prophylactic antibiotics and MIS. These soft tissue infections range in severity from localized minor cellulitis to large pelvic abscesses and have many names, from cuff cellulitis to infected hematoma. Nevertheless, they are similar to soft tissue infections in other parts of the body. These infections prolong hospital stay and increase the cost of patient care. The bacterial spectrum that produces these infections includes aerobic and anaerobic bacteria from exogenous and endogenous sources. Most postoperative pelvic infections are polymicrobial, usually from endogenous vaginal flora, and approximately 60% to 80% involve anaerobic organisms.

The pathophysiology of the development of retroperitoneal infection is straightforward. The classic "clamp, crush, cut, and tie technique" used in pelvic surgery produces an abundance of hypoxic and anoxic tissue that helps establish an optimal environment for infection. In addition to this anoxic tissue, the retroperitoneal tissue produces an average of 40 mL of serosanguineous fluid daily during the first 72 postoperative hours. When the endogenous flora of the upper vagina colonize and multiply in this retroperitoneal serosanguineous fluid or pelvic hematoma, a pelvic cellulitis and possibly a pelvic abscess can form.

The major symptoms of an operative site infection are fever associated with lower quadrant abdominal and pelvic pain. The fever usually becomes prominent between the third and fifth postoperative days. As the infection becomes more severe, the fever becomes spiking in character, the pain intensifies, and the patient develops moderate leukocytosis.

The diagnosis of cuff cellulitis is confirmed by pelvic examination. Pelvic tenderness and induration are prominent during the bimanual examination. A subtle difference exists between normal postoperative pelvic tenderness and induration and the tenderness and induration produced by an infection. Postoperative infection is accompanied by an increase in suprapubic pain and lateral parametrial tenderness. Cuff cellulitis sometimes responds to drainage by opening the vaginal cuff. Persistent cellulitis, one encompassing a large area, or a pelvic abscess necessitates parenteral antibiotic therapy. Large or complex fluid collections may be present without adverse clinical consequences. CT-directed drainage and culture may aid in diagnosis.

Because of their polymicrobial origin, infections are usually treated with an aminoglycoside (gentamicin) and an antibiotic specific for anaerobic infection (clindamycin). Metronidazole (Flagyl) may be substituted for clindamycin. An alternative therapy is substitution of a third-generation cephalosporin or the monobactam agent aztreonam (Azactam) for the aminoglycoside. IV antibiotics should be continued until the patient is afebrile for 24 hours. Once afebrile, the patient can be transitioned to a 10- to 14-day course of oral antibiotics, although some authors question the utility of this practice. Alternatives to the aminoglycoside-clindamycin regimen include broad-spectrum antibiotics combined with β-lactamase inhibitors such as ampicillin-sulbactam, amoxicillin-clavulanate, piperacillin-tazobactam, or ticarcillin-clavulanate. These drugs have better coverage of *Enterobacteriaceae* spp. and *Enterococcus*. Ertapenem can also be used in this patient population.

Drainage of an abscess through surgical intervention or interventional radiology is a key component of treatment. The success rates seen with antibiotic therapy alone (without drainage) range from 345 to 87%, depending on the abscess size and location (Jaiyeoba, 2012). Abscesses over 5 cm would likely benefit from immediate drainage. Appropriate cultures should be obtained from the center of an abscess cavity when the abscess is operatively incised. If a woman does not become afebrile within 48 hours of adequate drainage of a retroperitoneal abscess, a concomitant complication of pelvic thrombophlebitis should be suspected. If pelvic thrombophlebitis is suspected, a 72-hour trial of IV heparin therapy with concurrent antibiotics should be instituted.

## GRANULATION TISSUE

Granulation tissue at the apex of the vaginal vault is a frequent complication following hysterectomy. Small areas of friable, red granulation tissue are seen at the 6-week postoperative pelvic examination in more than 50% of women. Granulation tissue is more common following abdominal than vaginal hysterectomy. In women undergoing total abdominal hysterectomy, polyglactin (Vicryl) has a reduced risk of developing granulation tissue compared with chromic catgut for closure of the cuff, 32% versus 68%.

Excessive granulation tissue is the result of an exaggerated healing response of the vascular-rich pelvic tissues. One of the causes is believed to be inversion of the vaginal epithelium between the margins of the edges of the incision at the apex of the vaginal vault. Some patients are asymptomatic, but many women experience spotting or a bloody discharge after intercourse. On speculum examination, the granulation tissue appears as a polypoid projection hanging from the vaginal suture line. The differential diagnosis includes a prolapsed fallopian tube and recurrent carcinoma in a woman with a pelvic malignancy. The polypoid mass is easily avulsed from the vaginal apex. The remaining area of granulation tissue should be treated with a chemical cautery (e.g., silver nitrate, Monsel solution) in the office or by cryocauterization or electrocauterization, if proper anesthesia is available.

## INCISIONAL HERNIA

Vertical midline incisions produce the highest rate of abdominal wall hernias, 10% to 15%. Most will present within 1 year of surgery. Diabetes, poor nutrition, and obesity are all predisposing factors for postoperative hernia. Transverse and Pfannenstiel incisions have a low rate, followed by laparoscopic incisions, with the lowest rate of hernia formation. In obese and diabetic patients, it is prudent to close the fascia if the laparoscopic incision extends beyond 1 cm. Studies have noted a 2% to 3% hernia rate in laparoscopic sites of 12 mm or larger. Studies performed since the institution of modern trocars have noted even lower rates of (1%) of trocar site hernias.

## PROLAPSED FALLOPIAN TUBE

Prolapse of the distal end of the fallopian tube is a rare complication of abdominal or vaginal hysterectomy. It is usually discovered during a routine visit during the first few months (up to 6 months) following surgery. Factors that may predispose a woman to develop prolapse of the fallopian tube include hematoma formation and postoperative pelvic infection.

Many women with this complication are free of symptoms, but others experience a watery discharge, postcoital spotting and pain, or moderate lower abdominal and pelvic pain. Differing from granulation tissue, the fallopian tube is not friable and is firmly attached. Grasping the fallopian tube with an instrument and applying traction produces much more pain than traction on granulation tissue. Treatment is the destruction of the segment of the fallopian tube protruding through the vaginal vault with cryocauterization or laser. Because the fallopian tube is well innervated, any destructive procedure must be performed with anesthesia. The fallopian tube may be removed during a subsequent outpatient procedure with adequate anesthesia. Most clinicians opt for a vaginal approach, with ligation of the fallopian tube as high as possible. The stump of the tube is buried retroperitoneally and the vaginal epithelium is closed. Some difficult cases can also be performed using MIS. An alternative treatment is coagulation of the segment of fallopian tube protruding through the vaginal apex with cryocauterization. Often, the vaginal wall reepithelializes over the area, thereby excluding the tube from any connection with the vaginal cavity.

## LYMPHOCYST

A lymphocyst is a local collection of lymphatic fluid within the retroperitoneal spaces of the pelvis resulting from retrograde drainage of lymph. It is a rare complication, discovered most frequently after pelvic node dissections. In the past, this complication occurred in approximately 20% of patients having undergone radical surgery. However, with meticulous attention to ligation of distal lymphatic channels and abandonment of the practice of reperitonealization, this complication is reported in less than 5% of these cases. A peritoneal opening, or peritoneal window, allows flow of the lymphatic fluid into the peritoneal cavity, with subsequent peritoneal resorption. The incidence is lower in series in which palpation alone is used to identify the cysts. If ultrasound examination is used postoperatively to screen for lymphocysts, the incidence is 10-fold greater. Conditions that predispose the woman to formation of a lymphocyst are previous radiation and anticoagulation.

Lymphocysts usually present during the first 6 postoperative weeks. They vary greatly in size and seldom become infected. The cyst usually begins anteriorly and medially to the iliac vessels. As it expands, it may produce pelvic pain, leg pain, fever, obstruction or angulation of the ureter, pressure symptoms on the bladder, or partial venous obstruction. Small lymphocysts (<4 cm in diameter) are usually asymptomatic and regress spontaneously within 8 weeks. Larger cysts may necessitate treatment by intermittent aspiration or marsupialization performed laparoscopically, or placement of an omental flap.

## POSTOPERATIVE NEUROPATHY

Postoperative neuropathy is an uncommon but significant and sometimes debilitating problem. The three most common causes of neuropathy in gynecologic surgery are self-retaining retractors, overly flexed thighs in the dorsal lithotomy position, and surgical resection.

The femoral nerve is the largest branch of the lumbar plexus and arises from the primary dorsal rami of L2, L3, and L4. It provides motor function to several leg muscles, including the quadriceps, and sensory fibers that innervate the anterior and medial surfaces of the thigh and leg. The vascular supply to the femoral nerve may be compromised during an abdominal or vaginal hysterectomy. The cause of this complication is usually related to continuous pressure, usually by a self-retaining retractor producing ischemic necrosis of the nerve. The vascular circulation of the nerve itself is compromised by diminished blood flow in the vasa nervorum. The most common site of nerve compression is 4 to 6 cm above the inguinal ligament where the nerve pierces the psoas muscle.

Factors that contribute to the development of this complication are thinness of the woman, long retractor blades, prolonged operative times, and systemic diseases such as diabetes mellitus, gout, alcoholism, and malnutrition. The classic woman who develops this complication is a short, thin, athletic woman who has a transverse incision in which a self-retaining retractor is used. A similar problem may develop after vaginal operations or laparoscopy in thin women who are placed into exaggerated hip flexion or abduction in the dorsal lithotomy position. Femoral neuropathy following vaginal surgery is believed to be secondary to compromise of the nerve by severe angulation of the woman, not secondary to pressure injury from retractors. Bohrer and associates found peripheral nerve injury in 1.8% of 616 patients with elective gynecologic procedures, with almost all related to positioning. Most of these could be related to exaggerated flexion

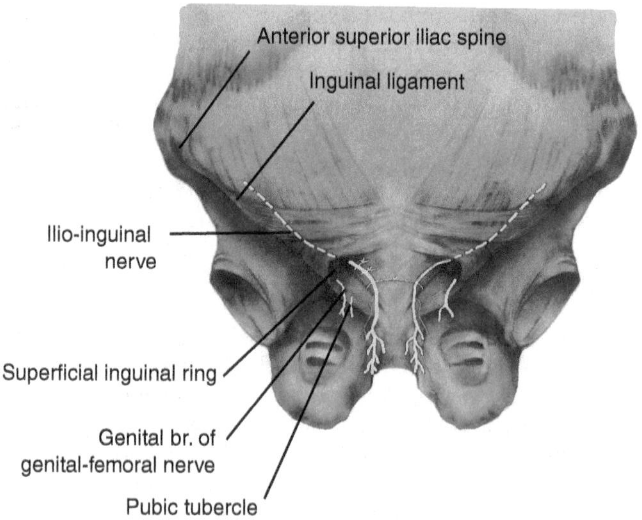


**Figure 25.12** Ilioinguinal nerve entrapment during needle suspension for stress incontinence. (From Miyazaki F, Shook G. Ilioinguinal nerve entrapment during needle suspension for stress incontinence. *Obstet Gynecol.* 1992;80[2]:246-248.)

for laparoscopic and vaginal surgeries. Two patients had motor and sensory losses. In this series, all but one woman had resolution of neuropathy with medical treatment (Bohrer, 2009).

Patients with this complication may experience numbness, paresthesias, and difficulty with their gait. Patients may have difficulty lifting the affected knee because of the involvement of the quadriceps. Symptoms may present with a spectrum of severity. Usually, the neurologic symptoms develop within the first 24 to 72 hours following surgery. Because of the inability to lift the leg, climbing stairs is a particular problem. Muscle and sensory function recover spontaneously over several weeks to several months. The woman should be seen by a physical therapist to facilitate ambulation and prevent muscle atrophy.

To prevent this complication, it is important to palpate the lateral pelvic wall after placement of a self-retaining retractor. In a thin woman, placing folded towels between the skin surface and self-retaining retractor helps prevent this complication by decreasing the depth of penetration of the lateral retractor blades. The ilioinguinal and iliohypogastric nerves pass in a transverse and diagonal course through the anterior lower abdominal musculature medial to the inguinal ligament and through the inguinal canal. The nerves supply sensory fibers to the labia, mons pubis, and medial thigh. The nerves may become injured during surgery with a Pfannenstiel incision or during a urinary incontinence procedure (Fig. 25.12). Pathophysiologically, the nerve may be transected or entrapped by suture or scar formation. Sharp or burning pain may develop immediately postoperatively or usually within a few days. The pain may radiate to the groin or vulva. Most symptoms will resolve spontaneously. Severe pain may necessitate nerve block, suture removal, or segmented removal of the involved nerve.

Several specific postoperative neuropathies are related to specific procedures. Uterosacral ligament suspension may affect the sacral plexus (S2 to S4) and produce pain and numbness in the posterior thigh and buttocks. Genitofemoral neuropathy and injury to the obturator nerve can be seen following pelvic lymphadenectomy. If the nerve was not cut, most will resolve in

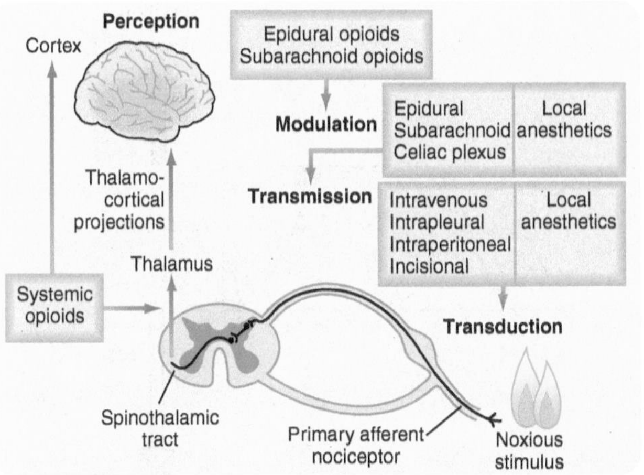


**Figure 25.13** Schematic drawing of the pathways for transmission of painful stimuli. (From Sherwood E, Williams CG, Prough DS. Anaesthesiology principles, pain management, and conscious sedation. In: Townsend CM, Beauchamp RD, Evers BM, et al, eds. *Sabiston Textbook of Surgery.* 17th ed. Philadelphia: Saunders; 2004.)

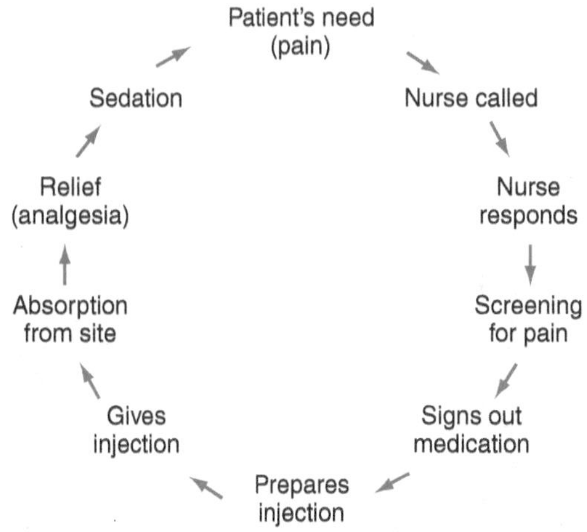


**Figure 25.14** Pain cycle. (From White PF. Pain management [special report]. *Postgrad Med.* 1986;80:8.)

time, although physical therapy is very helpful. Pudendal neuropathy has been reported with cystocele repairs and graft placement producing pain and numbness in the vulva and perineum. If symptoms are not relieved with analgesics and other medications, such as gabapentin, surgical removal of the sutures may be necessary.

## PSYCHOLOGICAL SEQUELAE

### PAIN RELIEF

The proper management of pain during the postoperative period should be an essential task and goal of all gynecologists. Most women experience moderate to severe pain during the first 36 to 48 hours following a gynecologic operation. Pain is initiated at the local level through the trauma of the surgery. Systemic and neurologic pathways are then activated (Fig. 25.13). The most effective pain management strategies involve inhibiting the initiation and activation of these broader pain reflexes. Such inhibition is also associated with the fewest side effects. Factors that predict postoperative pain and the use of pain medications include preoperative pain, mental state, and type of surgery. Age is inversely correlated with pain and pain medication usage (Vivian, 2009). Studies comparing types of hysterectomy, abdominal, vaginal, and laparoscopic have found a descending order of postoperative pain, as may be anticipated.

The current literature documents that pain relief is often treated inadequately in postoperative patients. Inadequate pain relief prolongs hospital stay and has adverse psychological consequences. Also, several investigators have noted that inadequately treated pain increases secondary morbidities, including atelectasis from decreased mobility, increased inflammatory response, and elevated glucose levels, with higher catecholamine levels. Studies have shown that epidural anesthesia has a significantly diminished effect on the immune response in patients undergoing laparotomy. Syndromes of chronic pain are presumed to begin with inadequate pain relief in the postoperative period.

A schematic representation of the pain cycle and the potential delays in pain relief with traditional as-needed analgesic regimens is shown in Fig. 25.14. Many studies have confirmed that regular-interval preventive pain relief is superior to conventional on demand analgesic medication during the first 36 to 48 hours after surgery. However, there is great variability in absorption. In addition, the therapeutic window—the range of effective blood concentration before undesired side effects occur—is narrow. Peak concentrations can vary as much as fivefold among different individuals, and the time to reach peak blood level can vary as much as sevenfold. Thus patient-controlled analgesia (PCA) systems became popular because they dramatically decrease patients' anxiety over pain control as the patient is in control, rather than the hospital staff (Fig. 25.15). PCA systems are safe and effective as long as there is a lockout period, and they help minimize individual differences in pharmacokinetics. Unfortunately, they also lead to a great deal of postoperative bowel dysfunction and, as a result, are frequently "de-emphasized" in most postoperative enhanced recovery after surgery (ERAS) protocols as discussed in Chapter 24. The current recommendations for postoperative pain relief is for multimodality therapy with NSAIDs, acetaminophen, and regional blocks with injection of long-acting local anesthetics such as bupivacaine and oral narcotics. In general, patients use PCA much less frequently in this setting. If a PCA is used, the patient should be given instructions about use of a PCA. Additionally, families need instruction in not pushing the medication for the patient to help alleviate pain. Sample dosing for PCA is listed in Appendix C.

Some patients can also benefit from the use of continuous postoperative thoracic epidural anesthesia, especially patients who are planning larger open cases with a more prolonged recovery. Perioperative intrathecal or epidural injections of opioids effectively relieve postoperative pelvic pain in most situations. Side effects are primarily itching and a small risk of hypotension. Continuous PCA epidurals may also be used. The advantages and disadvantages of PCA and epidural anesthesia are presented in Table 25.17.

In addition to narcotics, NSAIDs are valuable as adjunctive agents. NSAIDs are most effective when given as scheduled medications and as early as possible in the postoperative period. Their mechanism of action is the inhibition of prostaglandin

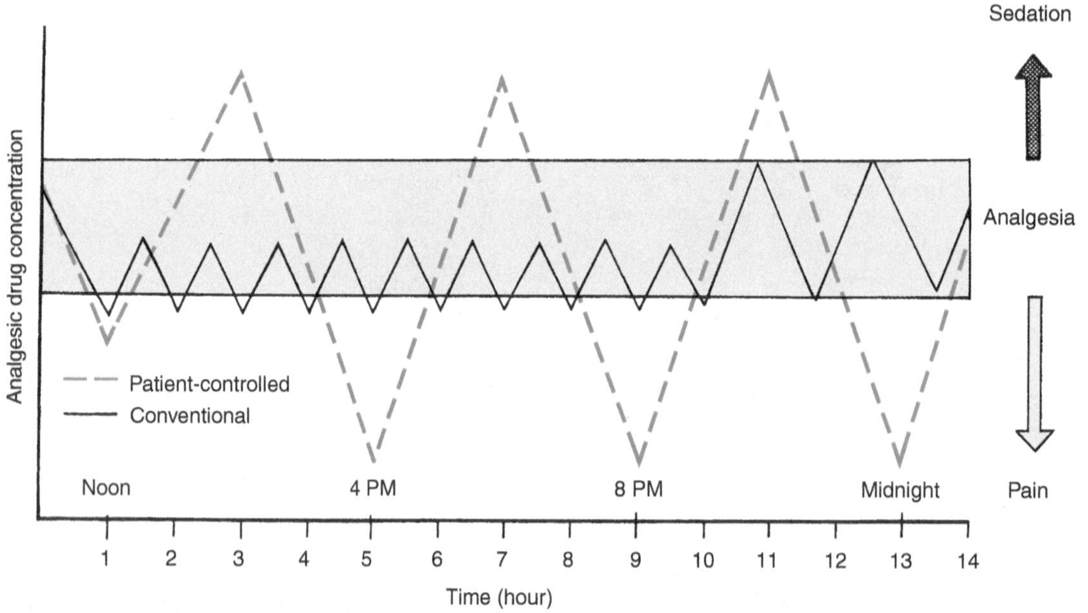


**Figure 25.15** Theoretic relationships among dosing interval, analgesic drug concentration, and clinical effects when comparing patient-controlled analgesia (PCA) system *(solid lines)* with conventional intramuscular therapy *(dashed lines)*. (Modified from White PF. Patient-controlled analgesia: a new approach to the management of postoperative pain. *Semin Anesth.* 1985;4:255-266.)

**Table 25.17** Advantages and Disadvantages of Epidural Analgesia and Patient-Controlled Analgesia

| Epidural Analgesia | Patient-Controlled Analgesia | Comments |
|---|---|---|
| Advantages | Immediate pain relief | Requires no special nursing or anesthesia support postoperatively |
| | May improve colon motility | Gives the patient personal control over administration of pain medication |
| | May improve postoperative pulmonary function after lower abdominal and pelvic surgery | |
| | Less sedating than patient-controlled analgesia | |
| Disadvantages | Requires a skilled anesthesiologist for correct placement | Patient may experience pain in the recovery room until an adequate serum level of medication is achieved |
| | May interfere with ambulation | |
| | May delay removal of Foley catheter | |

From Baker VV. Principles of postoperative care. In: Baker VV, Deppe G, eds. *Management of Perioperative Complications in Gynecology*. Philadelphia: WB Saunders; 1997.

production. Through inhibition of prostaglandins, pain is prevented rather than blocked centrally. NSAIDs have three potential side effects. The first is increased gastric acid, best treated by H2 blockers or proton pump inhibitors. The second is renal toxicity, which may be prevented by using set doses and prescribing only for women with normal renal function and adequate intravascular volume. The third is inhibition of platelet function with higher doses of NSAIDs. Some clinicians will wait 1 to 2 hours after surgery before giving these agents to avoid excessive bleeding, but there are no data to support this practice. Advantages of prostaglandin synthetase inhibitors are a lack of effect on gastrointestinal motility and a much smaller effect on sensorium than narcotic agents. Commonly used NSAIDs for postoperative pain include ibuprofen, naproxen, and ketorolac (Toradol). Ketorolac should not be used for more than 4 consecutive days because of GI side effects. In older adults, changes in GI function may limit the usefulness of these agents. Stomach colonization with *Helicobacter pylori* increases with increasing age. Of women older than 80 years, 80% are colonized. These bacteria increase sensitivity to GI irritation. Prophylactic H2 blockers or proton pump inhibitors should be considered when administering NSAID to older patients. Further NSAID use should be limited in patients with prior gastric bypass surgery due to risk of marginal ulcer development.

Many surgeons and anesthesiologists believe that giving preemptive analgesics in the perioperative period prior to the patient's sensation of pain leads to better pain control. Many studies have noted that the beneficial effects are significant when infiltration is given prior to the surgical incision. Because much pain arises from peritoneal irritation and fascial trauma, incisional infiltration is most effective with minimally invasive procedures such as laparoscopy. Infiltration is most commonly used with a local anesthetic, lidocaine 1%, or bupivacaine, 0.25%. Temporary indwelling infusion catheters that use local anesthetics have been shown in multiple studies and systematic reviews to benefit patients through decreased opioid use, earlier ambulation, and decreased PONV. Catheters are placed above and below the fascia and removed on day 3. In patients who are expected to require large amounts of opioid, such as those already on chronic narcotics for pain, the addition of gabapentin decreases narcotic use, perceived pain levels, and PONV. A meta-analysis has found a 35% reduction in pain (95% CI: 0.59-0.72). Most studies used 1200 mg/day.

Patients with persistent incisional pain, longer than 4 to 6 months, should be evaluated for incisional neuromas. Neuromas are thought to arise from damaged and transected peripheral nerves that develop a fibrous capsule. If a superficial small trigger area can be identified, an injection of 1% hydrocortisone with 2 to 3 mL of 0.25% bupivacaine may be attempted and is diagnostic if it helps. If this is unsuccessful, referral to a surgeon with expertise in peripheral nerves and chronic pain should be considered.

## POSTOPERATIVE CONCERNS IN OLDER SURGICAL PATIENTS

Patients older than 70 years, particularly those older than 80 years need special consideration in the perioperative period. Studies of older women undergoing gynecologic surgery have found that for elective procedures, the complication rates are no different from those of younger women after adjusting for comorbidities. Box 25.8 summarizes physical changes that should be kept in mind when caring for older surgical patients. The cardiovascular system is affected with increased systemic vascular resistance and a poorer response to systemic catecholamines. Many anesthetic agents decrease cardiac contractility. Atrial fibrillation and cardiac failure are the two most common cardiac complications, and attention to intravascular volume is important to maintain cardiac output. Many older women have decreased appetites and poor nutrition; this should be addressed prior to elective surgery. The nursing staff often is hesitant to give enough pain medications for fear of oversedation. However, inadequate pain relief can lead to worse sequela. Epidural PCA is a desirable postoperative tool for pain relief in this patient population.

Postoperative delirium and postoperative cognitive dysfunction (POCD) are examples of altered levels of mental function occurring after surgery. These conditions are more common in older adults. Prolonged and delayed mental status changes may be caused by decreased oxygen, decreased cardiac output, medications, and drug-drug interactions. In general, postoperative delirium occurs 24 to 72 hours after surgery. Disorientation, sleep deprivation, polypharmacy, and pain may all be contributing factors. The condition occurs in 5% to 15% of older patients and increases the risk of patient falls. Postoperative cognitive dysfunction may occur for a few months after surgery and has been noted to some degree in up to 5% of older surgical patients.

Postoperative disorientation and agitation are associated with higher risk of patient falls, as patients attempt to get out of bed without assistance.

**Box 25.8 Physiologic Changes in Older Adults That May Affect Surgery**

**Cardiovascular**
- Approximate 1% decrease in cardiac output/yr after age 30 yr
- Decreased vascular compliance and increased systemic vascular resistance (SVR)
- Increased cardiovascular disease
- Decreased cardiac output in response to stress
- Increased susceptibility to conduction abnormalities

**Pulmonary**
- Decreased pulmonary reserve
- Decreased mucus-producing cells, with increased susceptibility to infection
- Decreased elasticity in the lungs
- Decreased forced expiratory volume in 1 second ($FEV_1$)
- Decreased functional residual capacity (FRC), exacerbated with postoperative pain and atelectasis

**Renal**
- Decreased glomerular filtration rate (GFR), ≈ 1% decrease/yr after age 20
- Serum creatinine level not effective measure of renal function in this situation

**Skeletal**
- Increased osteoporosis, with increase in injury from falls
- Decreased rib expansion, so poorer response to need for postoperative lung expansion

**Nutritional**
- Poorer nutrition
- Greater incidence of vitamin deficiencies, including vitamin $B_{12}$

## PSYCHOSEXUAL PROBLEMS AND DEPRESSION

The time immediately before and after a surgical procedure is a stressful period for all women and their families. Anxiety and fear are normal responses and should be anticipated by health care providers. Any surgery on the female reproductive organs stimulates questions and conflicts concerning body image, feminine identity, sexuality, and possibly future childbearing. The period after a gynecologic operation is one of transition and is a unique psychological challenge to the woman. The reader should review Chapter 9 for a more detailed discussion of the problems of loss and grief. After gynecologic surgery, every woman needs support to deal with this challenge, and it is important to emphasize that it may take many months to complete the process.

Personal issues that relate to a woman's body image and sexuality are particularly affected by hysterectomy. Open discussions with the woman that allow her to discuss issues regarding sexuality are important during preoperative and postoperative visits. Psychological studies have confirmed that sexual function after a hysterectomy is related to a number of factors. Poor knowledge of reproductive anatomy, a negative expectation of sexual recovery after the operation, preoperative psychiatric morbidity, and a history of unsatisfactory sexual relationships are all associated with a poor outcome. The effect of hysterectomy on sexual function is an exceedingly complex topic, with both physical and psychological factors known to have varying and almost unquantifiable influences.

## MENTAL STATUS CHANGES

Anxiety and mental status changes are not uncommon in the postoperative period. Medications, hemodynamic changes, fever, and altered sleep patterns contribute to changes in sensorium. These changes are most pronounced in older adults. Multivariate analyses have correlated pain levels, hematocrit under 30%, smoking,

**Box 25.9 Causes of Acute Delirium**

Drug intoxication (alcohol, antihistamines, sedatives)
Drug withdrawal (alcohol, narcotics, anxiolytics)
Acute cerebral disorders (edema, transient ischemic attack stroke, neoplasm)
Metabolic disturbances (electrolyte, imbalance, hypoglycemia)
Hemodynamic disturbances (hypovolemia, myocardial infarction, congestive heart failure)
Infections (septicemia, urinary tract infection, pneumonia)
Respiratory disorders (respiratory failure, pulmonary embolism)
Trauma (head injury, burns)

From Dayton MT. Surgical complications. In: Townsend CM, Beauchamp RD, Evers BM, et al, eds. *Sabiston Textbook of Surgery.* 17th ed. Philadelphia: Saunders; 2004.

and a history of psychiatric disorders with postoperative mental status changes. Other than hematocrit levels, these factors are difficult to control. Mental status change does require evaluation (Box 25.9). Changes in oxygenation, electrolyte imbalance, sepsis, medication interactions, and acute anemia need to be excluded.

A syndrome of nausea, sweating, tachycardia, tremors, delirium, and even grand mal seizures postoperatively is often misdiagnosed as a drug or anesthetic reaction. This constellation of signs and symptoms is usually caused by alcohol withdrawal. The presence of a tremor should alert health care providers to the correct diagnosis. In the treatment of post–alcohol withdrawal symptoms, benzodiazepines are the drug of choice. In older women, especially after emergency surgery, postoperative confusion, anxiety, changes in personality, and memory impairment are frequent findings, and a large differential diagnosis must be considered.

## DISCHARGE INSTRUCTIONS AND POSTOPERATIVE VISITS

Simple but complete discharge instructions are an important component of postoperative care. The physician should anticipate the most common questions and give the woman explicit instructions. Particular attention should be given to limitations in physical activity, such as heavy lifting and resumption of sexual relations. Information should be given about vaginal spotting as sutures dissolve. Appropriate contact information should be provided in case of unanticipated complications and to schedule return appointments. Discharge instructions should not be given on the morning of discharge. Rather, patients should receive these instructions the day before discharge; this ensures that on the morning of discharge instructions can be reviewed and questions answered to ensure the patient understands. Instructions should be given in verbal and written format. Because an increasing number of procedures are performed as outpatient surgery or short stays, the physician must modify instructions to accommodate the gradual resumption of activity. The 24- to 48-hour postdischarge phone call to the recovering woman provides an excellent forum for answering questions and providing reassurance. Studies of outpatient surgeries have found this contact to be most important. Additionally, it is difficult for the woman and her significant others to remember instructions received during the first 24 hours after surgery. Written guidelines are extremely valuable for outpatient procedures. Careful training of nursing and triage staff in regard to postoperative questions cannot be overemphasized. Patients will usually be home when the first signs of complications occur. These signs and symptoms may in themselves be minor, but they may presage a more serious complication that could evolve. Thus a much higher index of suspicion should be used with these patients.

Most clinicians will see patients one or more times in the postoperative period as patients are transitioning back to routine activities. Questions about appropriate levels of activity can be answered in person or via a postdischarge phone call. Discussions of reestablishing sexual relations and physical activity are important to review at several time points. Unless there is a problem or a specific issue, a pelvic examination may be deferred until 5 to 6 weeks after the procedure. The discussion of surgical findings occurs at several points during the postoperative period. Initially, patients are drowsy after waking up from anesthesia or IV analgesics. Families may want to know the results prior to the patient hearing them. Preoperatively, it is important to clarify with the woman who in the family can know what information. During the early postoperative period, the gynecologist must judge how much information to provide. This should be tailored to what the patient can understand, depending on her level of wakefulness. By the end of the first few days, the discussion may move to details of surgical findings as well as treatment options, sequelae, and prognosis if a long-term problem has been found.

## KEY POINTS

- Postoperative febrile morbidity is related to infection in approximately 20% of cases and noninfectious causes in 80% of cases.
- Infection in older adults will not always present with classic findings. The amount of temperature elevation may not reflect the severity of the infection. Not uncommonly, the first signs of infection in older adults will be mental status changes. Also, the degree of leukocytosis may not reflect infection, being blunted or absent.
- Minimum urine output should be 0.5 mL/kg/hr. The use of a 20-mL/hr benchmark for all women is only an approximation and should be adjusted for the patient's weight.
- Because of the shifts in water balance, the postoperative hemoglobin at 72 hours is a more accurate measurement of operative and postoperative blood loss than a hemoglobin at 24 hours.
- After subtracting the effects of the operative blood loss from the preoperative hemoglobin, a further reduction in hemoglobin of 1 to 2 points reflects a postoperative hemorrhage of approximately 500 mL.
- Women should be transfused when their hemoglobin falls below 7, or sooner if they are symptomatic or have significant cardiac or pulmonary comorbidities.
- Microatelectasis is a common occurrence developing during almost all pelvic surgeries and is persistent 24 hours

## KEY POINTS—cont'd

postoperatively in approximately 50% of women. Current studies have demonstrated that there is no association between fever and the amount of atelectasis diagnosed radiologically.

- Radiographic diagnoses are approximately 60% accurate for bacterial or viral pneumonia in women with laboratory-proved pneumonia.
- Rapid loss of 20% of a woman's blood volume produces mild shock, whereas a loss of greater than 40% of blood volume results in severe shock.
- From 15% to 45% of surgical blood loss is absorbed onto drapes, pads, and other areas. Thus blood levels in the suction bottle are inaccurate markers of total operative blood loss.
- Massive blood loss has been defined as hemorrhage that results in replacement of 50% of circulating blood volume in less than 3 hours.
- Returning a patient to the operating room to control hemorrhage is often a difficult decision. However, when indicated this decision should not be postponed, and the patient should have an exploratory operation as soon as possible after volume replacement.
- The extent of wound or pelvic hematomas is determined by the potential size of the compartment into which the bleeding occurs. Retroperitoneal or broad ligament hematomas may contain several units of blood.
- Superficial phlebitis is the leading cause of an enigmatic postoperative fever during the third, fourth, or fifth postoperative day.
- The clinical management of mild superficial thrombophlebitis includes rest, elevation, and local heat. Moderate to severe superficial thrombophlebitis may be treated with nonsteroidal antiinflammatory agents.
- Venous thrombosis and PE are the direct causes of approximately 40% of deaths in gynecologic cases once the diagnosis is confirmed.
- Signs and symptoms of pulmonary emboli are nonspecific; however, the most common symptoms are chest pain, dyspnea, apprehension, tachypnea, rales, and an increase in the second heart sound over the pulmonic area.
- Intermittent in-and-out catheterization is preferable to continuous drainage with a Foley catheter for women with intermediate-term voiding dysfunction.
- Although symptoms of urinary incontinence may present within a few hours of the operative procedure, most fistulas usually present 8 to 12 days after operation, and occasionally as late as 25 to 30 days after the operation.
- If there is a suspicion that trauma to the bladder has occurred during an operative procedure, continuous catheter drainage for 3 to 5 days usually results in spontaneous healing.
- Approximately 25% of adult women experience postoperative nausea and vomiting.
- Normal return of bowel function after abdominal surgery can take 3 to 7 days. The left colon takes the longest to resume function, approximately 72 hours after surgery. If an ileus lasts for longer than 5 to 7 days, a diagnosis of mechanical bowel obstruction or another cause for the ileus should be considered.
- Postoperative oral feeding is safe and efficacious. This practice is preferred as it facilitates recovery and shortens hospital stay.
- The difference between small bowel obstruction and adynamic ileus is subtle, because adynamic ileus can be associated with partial obstruction of the small intestine. The use of Gastrografin contrast can be both diagnostic and therapeutic.
- Second- and third-generation cephalosporins are the antibiotics associated with the highest risk of developing *C. difficile* diarrhea.
- The incidence of postoperative wound infection is increased eightfold when the woman's preoperative weight exceeds 200 pounds. The thickness of subcutaneous tissue is the greatest risk factor for wound infection in women undergoing abdominal hysterectomy.
- Necrotizing fasciitis involves the subcutaneous tissue and superficial fascia. It rapidly expands in the subcutaneous spaces. This condition is a surgical emergency and patients should have operative débridement as soon as possible.
- The incidence of wound dehiscence is approximately 1 in 200 gynecologic operations. Wound infection is found in approximately 50% of women with wound disruption.
- The classic feature of an impending wound disruption is the spontaneous passage of copious serosanguineous fluid from the abdominal incision.
- Most postoperative pelvic infections are polymicrobial, usually from endogenous vaginal flora, and approximately 60% to 80% involve anaerobic organisms.
- Common causes of femoral neuropathy are continuous pressure from self-retaining retractors or exaggerated hip flexion or abduction in the dorsal lithotomy position in thin women.
- Discharge instructions should be given in verbal and written forms, and the gynecologist should anticipate the most common questions.

*Appendixes A, B, and C are available at* ExpertConsult.com.

## KEY REFERENCES


Aarts JW, Nieboer TE, Johnson N, et al. Surgical approach to hysterectomy for benign gynaecological disease. *Cochrane Database Syst Rev.* 2015;8:CD003677.

Ahmad S, Nagle A, McCarthy RJ, et al. Postoperative hypoxemia in morbidly obese patients with and without obstructive sleep apnea undergoing laparoscopic bariatric surgery. *Anesth Analg.* 2008;107(1):138–143.

Apfel CC, Korttila K, Abdalla M, et al. A factorial trial of six interventions for the prevention of postoperative nausea and vomiting. *N Engl J Med.* 2004;350(24):2441–2451.

Barber EL, Neubauer NL, Gossett DR. Risk of venous thromboembolism in abdominal versus minimally invasive hysterectomy for benign conditions. *Am J Obstet Gynecol.* 2015;212(5):609.e1–609.e7.

Bartlett JG. Antibiotic-associated diarrhea. *N Engl J Med.* 2002;346(5):334–339.

Bauer AJ, Boeckxstaens GE. Mechanisms of postoperative ileus. *Neurogastroenterol Motil.* 2004;16(Suppl 2):54–60.

Bohrer JC, Walters MD, Park A, et al. Pelvic nerve injury following gynecologic surgery: a prospective cohort study. *Am J Obstet Gynecol.* 2009;201(5):531.e1–531.e7.

Bougle A, Harrois A, Duranteau J. Resuscitative strategies in traumatic hemorrhagic shock. *Ann Intensive Care.* 2013;3(1):1.

Chung F, Yegneswaran B, Liao P, et al. Validation of the Berlin questionnaire and American Society of Anesthesiologists checklists and screening tools for obstructive sleep apnea in surgical patients. *Anesthesiology.* 2008;108(5):822–830.

do Nascimento Junior P, Módolo NS, Andrade S, et al. Incentive spirometry for prevention of postoperative pulmonary complications in upper abdominal surgery. *Cochrane Database Syst Rev.* 2014;2:CD006058.

Dubuisson J, Botchorishvili R, Perrette S, et al. Incidence of intraabdominal adhesions in a continuous series of 1000 laparoscopic procedures. *Am J Obstet Gynecol.* 2010;203(2):111.e1–111.e3.

Ellis H, Niran BJ, Thompson JN, et al. Adhesion-related hospital readmissions after abdominal and pelvic surgery: a retrospective cohort study. *Lancet.* 1999;353(9163):1476–1480.

Finfer S, Chittock DR, Su SY, et al. Intensive versus conventional glucose control in critically ill patients. *N Engl J Med.* 2009;360(13):1283–1297.

Gan TJ, Diemunsch P, Habib AS, et al. Consensus guidelines for the management of postoperative nausea and vomiting. *Anesth Analg.* 2014;118(1):85–113.

Gandaglia G, Ghani KR, Sood A, et al. Effect of minimally invasive surgery on the risk for surgical site infections: results from the National Surgical Quality Improvement (NSQIP) Database. *JAMA Surg.* 2014;149(10):1039–1044.

Garber AJ, Moghissi ES, Bransome Jr ED, et al. American College of Endocrinology Task Force on Inpatient Diabetes Metabolic Control: Position statement on inpatient diabetes and metabolic control. *Endocr Pract.* 2004;10(1):77–82.

Gawande AA, Studdert DM, Orav EJ, et al. Risk factors for retained instruments and sponges after surgery. *N Engl J Med.* 2003;348(3):229–235.

Goldhaber SZ, Elliot CG. Acute pulmonary embolism: part I. *Circulation.* 2003a;108(22):2726–2729.

Goldhaber SZ, Elliot CG. Acute pulmonary embolism: part II. *Circulation.* 2003b;108(23):2834–2838.

Gowen GF. Long tube decompression is successful in 90% of patients with adhesive small bowel obstruction. *Am J Surg.* 2003;185(6):512–515.

Guyatt GH, Akl EA, Crowther M, et al. Executive summary: Antithrombotic Therapy and Prevention of Thrombosis, 9th ed: American College of Chest Physicians Evidence-Based Clinical Practice Guidelines. *Chest.* 2012;141(2 Suppl):7S–47S.

Harmanli OH, Tunitsky E, Esin S, et al. A comparison of short-term outcomes between laparoscopic supracervical and total hysterectomy. *Am J Obstet Gynecol.* 2009;201(5):536.e1–536.e7.

Hurr HC, Donnellan N, Mansuria S, et al. Vaginal cuff dehiscence after different modes of hysterectomy. *Obstet Gynecol.* 2011;118(4):749–801.

Ibeanu OA, Chesson RR, Echols KT, et al. Urinary tract injury during hysterectomy based on universal cystoscopy. *Am Coll Obstet Gynecol.* 2009;113(1):6–10.

Ireland CJ, Chapman TM, Mathew SF, et al. Continuous positive airway pressure (CPAP) during the postoperative period for prevention of postoperative morbidity and mortality following major abdominal surgery. *Cochrane Database Syst Rev.* 2014;8:CD008930.

Jaiyeoba O. Postoperative infections in obstetrics and gynecology. *Clin Obstet Gynecol.* 2012;55(4):904–913.

Kalogera E, Bakkum-Gamez JN, Jankowski, et al. Enhanced recovery in gynecologic surgery. *Obstet Gynecol.* 2013;122(2 Pt 1):319–328.

Kehlet H, Dahl JB. Anaesthesia, surgery, and challenges in postoperative recovery. *Lancet.* 2003;362(9399):1921–1928.

Kendrick JE, Numnum TM, Estes JM, et al. Conservative management of postoperative fever in gynecologic patients undergoing major abdominal or vaginal operations. *J Am Coll Surg.* 2008;207(3):393–397.

Klein HG, Spahn DR, Carson JL. Red blood cell transfusion in clinical practice. *Lancet.* 2007;370(9585):415–426.

Kyrle PA, Eichinger S. Deep vein thrombosis. *Lancet.* 2005;365(9465):1163–1174.

Lensing AW, Prandoni P, Brandjes D, et al. Detection of deep-vein thrombosis by real-time B-mode ultrasonography. *N Engl J Med.* 1989;320(6):342–345.

Loftus T, Moore F, VanZant E, et al. A protocol for the management of adhesive small bowel obstruction. *J Trauma Acute Care Surg.* 2015;78(1):13–19.

Mattei P, Rombeau JL. Review of the pathophysiology and management of postoperative ileus. *World J Surg.* 2006;30(8):1382–1391.

Meeks GR, Waller GA, Meydrech EF, et al. Unscheduled hospital admission following ambulatory gynecologic surgery. *Obstet Gynecol.* 1992;80(3 Pt 1):446–450.

Nelson RL, Edwards S, Tse B. Prophylactic nasogastric decompression after abdominal surgery. *Cochrane Database Syst Rev.* 2007;(3):CD004929.

Peipert JF, Weitzen S, Cruickshank C, et al. Risk factors for febrile morbidity after hysterectomy. *Obstet Gynecol.* 2004;103(1):86–91.

Ramos M, Khalpey Z, Lipsitz S, et al. Relationship of perioperative hyperglycemia and postoperative infections in patients who undergo general and vascular surgery. *Ann Surg.* 2008;248(4):585–591.

Schey D, Salom EM, Papadia A, et al. Extensive fever workup produces low yield in determining infectious etiology. *Am J Obstet Gynecol.* 2005;192(5):1729–1734.

Schwandt A, Andrews SJ, Fanning J. Prospective analysis of a fever evaluation algorithm after major gynecologic surgery. *Am J Obstet Gynecol.* 2001;184(6):1066–1067.

Segal JB, Streiff MB, Hofmann LV, et al. Management of venous thromboembolism: a systematic review for a practice guideline. *Ann Intern Med.* 2007;146(3):211–222.

Soper DE, Bump RC, Hurt WG. Wound infection after abdominal hysterectomy: effect of the depth of subcutaneous tissue. *Am J Obstet Gynecol.* 1995;173(2):465–469.

Stanhope CR, Wilson TO, Utz WJ, et al. Suture entrapment and secondary ureteral obstruction. *Am J Obstet Gynecol.* 1991;164(6 Pt 1):1513–1517.

Stark RP, Maki DG. Bacteriuria in the catheterized patient. *N Engl J Med.* 1984;311(9):560–564.

Steed HL, Capstick V, Flood C, et al. A randomized controlled trial of early versus "traditional" postoperative oral intake after major abdominal gynecologic surgery. *Am J Obstet Gynecol.* 2002;186(5):861–865.

Stroncek DF, Rebulla P. Platelet transfusions. *Lancet.* 2007;370(9585):427–438.

Umpierrez GE, Hellman R, Korytkowski M, et al. Management of hyperglycemia in hospitalized patients in non-critical care setting: an endocrine society clinical practice guideline. *J Clin Endocrinol Metab.* 2012;97(1):16–38.

Vivian HY, Abrishami A, Peng PWH, et al. Predictors of postoperative pain and analgesic consumption. *Anesthesiology.* 2009;111(3):657–677.

Walsh JJ, Bomar J, Wright FW. A study of pulmonary embolism and deep leg vein thrombosis after major gynaecological surgery using labelled fibrinogen-phlebography and lung scanning. *J Obstet Gynaecol Br.* 1974;81:311.

Walsh C, Scaife C, Hopf H. Prevention and management of surgical site infections in morbidly obese women. *Obstet Gynecol.* 2009;113(2 Pt 1):411–415.

Webster J, Osborne S, Rickard CM, et al. Clinically-indicated replacement versus routine replacement of peripheral venous catheters. *Cochrane Database Syst Rev.* 2013;4:CD007798.

Wells PS, Hirsh J, Anderson DR, et al. Accuracy of clinical assessment of deep-vein thrombosis. *Lancet.* 1995;345(8961):1326–1330.

Suggested Readings can be found on ExpertConsult.com.

# 26

# Abnormal Uterine Bleeding

## Etiology and Management of Acute and Chronic Excessive Bleeding

*Timothy Ryntz, Roger A. Lobo*

**Abnormal uterine bleeding** (**AUB**) can present in many ways, from infrequent episodes, to excessive flow, or prolonged duration of menses and intermenstrual bleeding. Alterations in the pattern or volume of blood flow of menses are among the most common health concerns of women. Infrequent uterine bleeding is called **oligomenorrhea** if the intervals between bleeding episodes vary from 35 days to 6 months, and **amenorrhea** is defined by no menses for at least 6 months. These are discussed in Chapter 38. Excessive or prolonged bleeding will be discussed in this chapter. An overview of several therapeutic modalities being used to treat excessive uterine bleeding will also be discussed here.

To define excessive abnormal uterine bleeding, it is necessary to define normal menstrual flow. The mean interval between menses is 28 days (±7 days). Thus if bleeding occurs at intervals of 21 days or less or 35 days or more it is abnormal. The mean duration of menstrual flow is 4 days. Few women with normal menses bleed more than 7 days, so bleeding for longer than 7 days is considered to be abnormally prolonged. It is useful to document the duration and frequency of menstrual flow with the use of menstrual diary cards; however, it is difficult to determine the amount of menstrual blood loss (MBL) by subjective means. Several studies have shown that there is poor correlation between subjective judgment and objective measurement of MBL (Chimbira, 1980).

Although subjective methods are used in predicting blood loss, and some investigators have used a pictorial bleeding assessment chart, a more accurate system is the alkaline hematic method, which measures hematin. Average menstrual blood loss is 35 mL. Total volume, however, is twice this amount, being made up of endometrial tissue exudate. The amount of MBL increases with parity but not age in the absence of disease. An MBL of 80 mL or greater is defined as heavy menstrual bleeding, which occurs in 9% to 14% of women (Shapley, 2004).

Although mortality and serious complications of abnormal uterine bleeding are uncommon, their impact on health-related quality of life is burdensome. Direct costs are calculated at more than $1 billion annually in the United States, and indirect costs due to lost work, social function, and vitality has been estimated at more than $12 billion annually (Liu, 2007).

## CAUSES OF ABNORMAL UTERINE BLEEDING

The causes of AUB can be described by a universally accepted systematic nomenclature. This system was reported by the International Federation of Gynecology and Obstetrics (FIGO) in 2011 (Munro, 2011). It subdivides causes of AUB into nine main categories, which are arranged according to the acronym **PALM-COEIN**: polyp, adenomyosis, leiomyoma, malignancy and hyperplasia, coagulopathy, ovulatory dysfunction, endometrial, iatrogenic, and not yet classified. The etiologies that constitute the first group (**PALM**) are structural or histologic causes that are diagnosed through imaging or biopsy. Those that compose the second group (**COEIN**) are nonstructural (Fig. 26.1). The term *dysfunctional uterine bleeding (DUB)* is no longer favored and should be discarded. In the past, this term has represented causes of abnormal bleeding when structural causes and other specific defects, such as coagulation defects, had been excluded. Cases that previously would have been described as DUB are now referred to as AUB due to ovulatory dysfunction or endometrial causes.

According to FIGO, this classification system should be notated in a consistent and systematic manner. The acronym AUB is followed by the letters PALM-COEIN and a subscript 0 or 1 associated with each letter to indicate the absence or presence, respectively, of the abnormality. For example, a patient with abnormal bleeding due to a polyp would be described as AUB-$P_1A_0L_0M_0$-$C_0O_0E_0I_0N_0$. Because patients may have abnormal bleeding due to more than one condition, this notation allows for description of simultaneous factors. For example, a patient with abnormal bleeding that is both irregular and heavy may have endometrial hyperplasia due to anovulation. As such, this patient's bleeding would be described as AUB- $P_0A_0L_0M_1$-$C_0O_1E_0I_0N_0$.

What follows is an introduction to each of the pathologies described by the PALM-COEIN system. Following this discussion, a diagnostic approach for women with AUB will be outlined. Treatments for acute and chronic bleeding due to these conditions conclude this chapter.

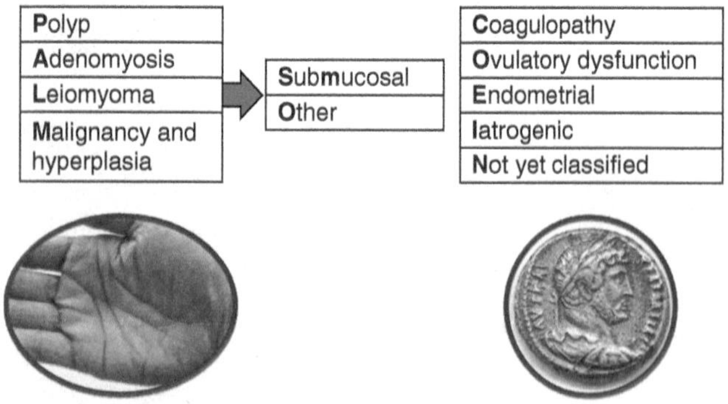


**Figure 26.1 PALM-COEIN Classification System for Abnormal Uterine Bleeding.** The basic system comprises four categories that are defined by visually objective structural criteria (PALM), four that are unrelated to structural anomalies (COEI), and one reserved for entities that are not yet classified (N). The leiomyoma category is subdivided into patients with at least one submucosal myoma ($L_{SM}$) and those with myomas that do not affect the endometrial cavity ($L_O$). (From Munro MG, Critchley HOD, Broder MS, Fraser IS. FIGO classification system [PALM-COEIN] for causes of abnormal uterine bleeding in nongravid women of reproductive age. *Int J Gynecol Obstet.* 2011;113[1]:3-13.)

## *ENDOMETRIAL POLYPS*

Endometrial polyps (AUB-P) are localized overgrowths of endometrial tissue, containing glands, stroma, and blood vessels, covered with epithelium (Peterson, 1956). Endometrial polyps are most commonly found in reproductive-age women, and estrogen stimulation is thought to play a key role in their development. As such, polyps are rarely found before menarche. Molecular mechanisms involving overexpression of endometrial aromatase and gene mutations in HMGIC and HMGI[Y] have also been proposed (Maia, 2006; Tallini, 2000).

The majority of endometrial polyps are benign. A systematic review of the oncogenic potential of endometrial polyps demonstrated that symptomatic vaginal bleeding and postmenopausal status are associated with an increased risk of malignancy. Among symptomatic postmenopausal women with endometrial polyps, 4.5% had a malignant polyp compared with 1.5% in asymptomatic women (Lee, 2010). A strong correlation exists for both tamoxifen use and obesity and the development of malignancy in endometrial polyps. Diabetes mellitus and hypertension have not been reliably shown to increase the risk for malignancy in an endometrial polyp.

The importance of small and asymptomatic endometrial polyps is less clear. Transvaginal ultrasound detected asymptomatic polyps in up to 12% of women undergoing routine gynecologic examination; small endometrial polyps smaller than 1 cm appear to regress spontaneously (Hamani, 2013). Endometrial polyps were discovered in 32% of 1000 patients on office hysteroscopy about to undergo in vitro fertilization, suggesting a possible association between endometrial polyps and infertility (Hinckley, 2004). Women with symptomatic polyps can be treated safely and effectively with operative hysteroscopy (Video 26.1).

## *ADENOMYOSIS*

Adenomyosis (AUB-A) is defined by the presence of endometrial glands and stroma in the uterine myometrium. The presence of ectopic endometrial tissue leads to hypertrophy of the surrounding myometrium. Adenomyosis can occur as focal (adenomyoma) or diffuse, with a peak incidence in the fifth decade of life. Multiparity is considered the most significant risk factor for developing adenomyosis, but any process that allows for penetration of endometrial glands and stroma past the basalis layer (e.g., dilation and curettage, cesarean delivery, spontaneous abortion) is thought to contribute. There also appears to be a positive correlation between overexpression of immunoproteins interleukin-6, interleukin-18, and cyclooxygenase-2 and the presence of ectopic endometrial tissue, though these may not be causative (Leyendecker, 2004; Huang, 2010). Adenomyosis is a histologic diagnosis, but findings of an enlarged, asymmetric uterus on ultrasound and magnetic resonance imaging (MRI) are indicative. Anechoic avascular cysts scattered throughout the myometrium on sonography are considered pathognomonic for adenomyosis on ultrasound. MRI, which is both more sensitive and specific than ultrasound, will demonstrate thickening of the junctional zone, the area between the endometrium and the myometrium, equal to or greater than 12 mm (Figs. 26.2 and 26.3) (Dueholm, 2007). Abnormal bleeding due to adenomyosis is thought to be a result of altered uterine contractility and is commonly associated with profound dysmenorrhea.

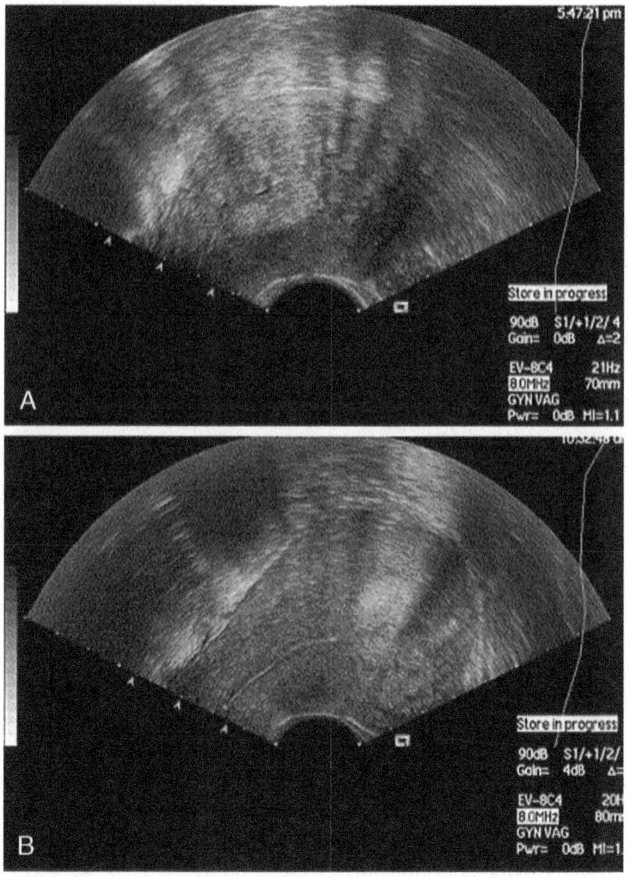


**Figure 26.2** Transvaginal sonography of uterus with adenomyosis: heterogeneous and hypoechogenic, poorly described areas in the myometrium with characteristic anechoic lacunae, and linear striations radiating out from the endometrium into the myometrium (**A**) and increased echo texture of the myometrium with an indistinct endomyometrial junction (**B**). (From Dueholm M. Transvaginal ultrasound for diagnosis of adenomyosis: a review. *Best Pract Res Clin Obstet Gynaecol.* 2006;20[4]:569-582.)

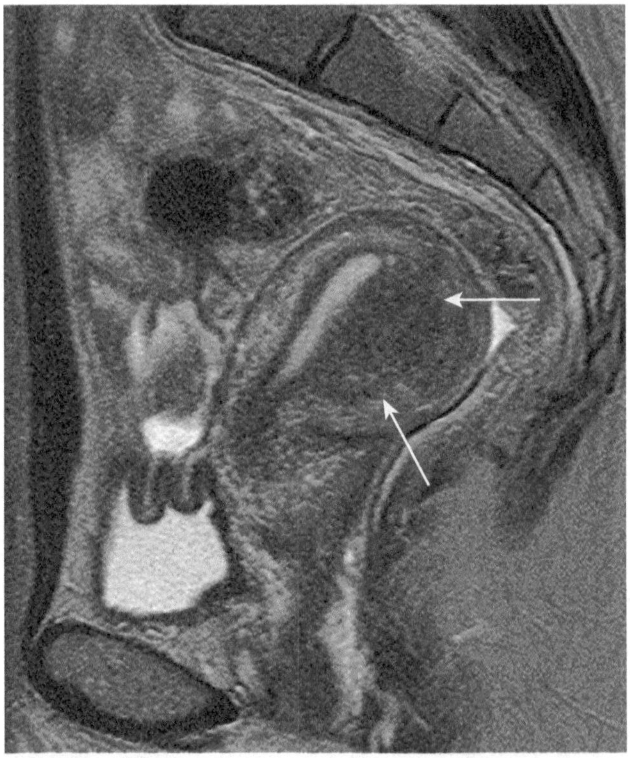

**Figure 26.3** Magnetic resonance image of asymmetric adenomyosis. (From Tamai K, Koyama T, Umeoka S, et al. Spectrum of MR features in adenomyosis. *Best Pract Res Clin Obstet Gynaecol.* 2006;20[4]:583-602.)

## LEIOMYOMA

Leiomyoma (AUB-L), or fibroids, are benign tumors of the uterine myometrium with a complex and heterogeneous clinical presentation as varied as their biologic origins. Various genetic mutations are described in leiomyoma, but the pathogenesis is thought to initiate from myometrial injury leading to cellular proliferation, decreased apoptosis, and increased production of extracellular matrix. Critical in this pathway is the overexpression of transforming growth factor beta that leads to fibrosis of these tumors (Laughlin, 2011). Transforming growth factor beta also contributes to implantation failure in women with fibroids who are subfertile.

Although the prevalence of fibroids among women is approximately 70%, as many as 50% of these will be symptomatic (Gupta, 2008). Mechanisms by which fibroids cause abnormal bleeding are varied and depend on size, location, and number. Subclassification of leiomyomas describes their location throughout the myometrium (Fig. 26.4). Intracavitary fibroids (type 0) and submucosal fibroids, where more than 50% are intracavitary (type 1) or less than 50% are intracavitary (type 2), as well as intramural fibroids, which are large, may increase the overall surface area of the endometrial cavity or alter uterine contractility. These effects in turn lead to abnormal and excessive uterine bleeding. Whereas hysterectomy for fibroids remains among the leading indications for the procedure in the United States, treatments are diverse including hormonal or surgical ablation of the endometrium, uterine artery embolization, radiofrequency ablation, and myomectomy through a variety of surgical approaches (Videos 26.2, 26.3, and 26.4).

According to the FIGO system, leiomyomas can be notated in the PALM-COEIN system with a subscript 0 in their absence or by the number 1 when present. Additionally, the letters *SM* can be inserted to indicate a fibroid's location as submucosal.

## MALIGNANCY

Malignancies (AUB-M) associated with the female reproductive tract include vulvar, vaginal, cervical, endometrial, uterine, and adnexal (ovarian or fallopian tube) cancers. Although vaginal cancers can cause abnormal bleeding, there are only approximately 3000 new cases reported annually in the United States. Bleeding from cervical malignancy classically presents as coital bleeding or intermenstrual bleeding; thus a thorough cervical evaluation is an important part of the workup of any woman with these symptoms. In a series of 73 women with coital bleeding referred for evaluation, squamous cell carcinoma of the cervix was present in 1.4% of patients, and 15% had cervical intraepithelial neoplasia (Havenga, 2013).

AUB is the most common presenting symptom of endometrial cancer. Although endometrial cancer presents most often in the seventh decade, 15% of cases are diagnosed in premenopausal women, and 3% to 5% present in women under the age of 40 (Haidopoulos, 2010). Conditions that lead to increased circulating levels of estrogen are risk factors. Obesity is associated with increased estrone levels due to peripheral conversion by aromatase in adipose tissue; but the primary source of estrogen in premenopausal women remains the ovary. Impaired ovulation and the absence of progesterone withdrawal can result in sustained exposure of the endometrium to estrogen. This hyperestrogenic state can lead to the pathologic progression from normal endometrium to hyperplasia and ultimately to adenocarcinoma.

Lynch syndrome, or hereditary nonpolyposis colorectal cancer, is an autosomal dominant disease caused by a disruption in the mismatch repair (MMR) genes. Lynch syndrome also carries a 40% to 50% lifetime risk of endometrial cancer, with a significant proportion of endometrial cancers occurring before the age of 45. In addition, estrogen-producing ovarian tumors may become manifest by abnormal uterine bleeding. Granulosa theca cell tumors are the most common tumors to have this presentation, although many ovarian tumors can produce estrogen.

## COAGULOPATHY

Systemic diseases, particularly disorders of blood coagulation (AUB-C) such as von Willebrand disease and prothrombin deficiency, may initially present as AUB (Minjarez, 2008). Routine screening for coagulation defects is mainly indicated for the adolescent who has prolonged heavy menses beginning at menarche. In adults, screening for these disorders is of little value unless otherwise indicated by clinical signs such as bleeding gums, epistaxis, or ecchymosis. Twenty percent of adolescent girls who require hospitalization for abnormal uterine bleeding have been reported to have coagulation disorders (Claessens, 1981). Coagulation defects are present in approximately 25% of those whose hemoglobin levels fall below 10 g/100 mL, in one third of those who require transfusions, and in 50% of those whose severe

| PALM | | | COEIN |
|---|---|---|---|
| Polyp | | | Coagulopathy |
| Adenomyosis | → | Submucosal | Ovulatory dysfunction |
| Leiomyoma | → | Other | Endometrial |
| Malignancy and hyperplasia | | | Iatrogenic |
| | | | Not yet classified |

**Leiomyoma subclassification system**

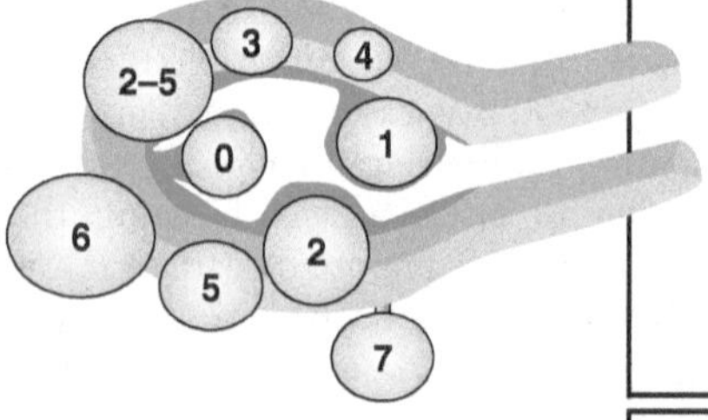


| | | |
|---|---|---|
| **SM - Submucosal** | 0 | Pedunculated intracavitary |
| | 1 | <50% intramural |
| | 2 | ≥50% intramural |
| **O - Other** | 3 | Contacts endometrium; 100% intramural |
| | 4 | Intramural |
| | 5 | Subserosal ≥50% intramural |
| | 6 | Subserosal <50% intramural |
| | 7 | Subserosal pedunculated |
| | 8 | Other (specify e.g., cervical, parasitic) |
| **Hybrid leiomyomas** (affect both endometrium and serosa) | Two numbers are listed separated by a hyphen. By convention, the first refers to the relationship with the endometrium while the second refers to the relationship to the serosa. One example is below. | |
| | 2–5 | Submucosal and subserosal, each with less than half the diameter in the endometrial and peritoneal cavities, respectively. |

**Figure 26.4** Tertiary classification system of fibroids including submucosal, intramural, and subserosal fibroids. (From Munro MG, Critchley HOD, Broder MS, Fraser IS. FIGO classification system [PALM-COEIN] for causes of abnormal uterine bleeding in nongravid women of reproductive age. *Int J Gynecol Obstet.* 2011;113[1]:3-13.)

menorrhagia occurred at the time of the first menstrual period. Others report that a coagulation disorder is found in only 5% of adolescents hospitalized for heavy bleeding (Falcone, 1994).

Both studies indicated that the likelihood of a blood disorder in adolescents with heavy menses is sufficiently high that all adolescents should be evaluated to determine whether a coagulopathy is present.

Disorders of platelets are most often quantitative, but defects in platelet membrane or storage granules can result in normal circulating levels with altered function. Hemophilias A and B are X-linked recessive deficiencies of factor VIII and factor IX, respectively. Women who are carriers for these disorders can have reduced levels of factors VIII and IX, some less than 30% of normal and enough to be considered to have mild hemophilia. Rare inherited coagulopathies of the other clotting factors (V, VII, X, XI, XIII) include menorrhagia as a potential symptom. Other disorders that produce platelet deficiency, such as leukemia, severe sepsis, idiopathic thrombocytopenic purpura, and hypersplenism, can also cause excessive bleeding.

Chronic anticoagulation as a result of heparin, low-molecular-weight heparin, direct thrombin inhibitors, and direct factor Xa inhibitors is necessary for prevention of thrombosis in women with inherited thrombophilias, those with mechanical heart valves, and those with rare anatomic disorders such as May-Thurner syndrome. In the absence of other gynecologic pathology, these patients present most often with heavy menstrual bleeding. Although it may seem that these patients could be considered as having iatrogenic abnormal bleeding due to prescribed medications, heavy bleeding is a result of a derangement in the coagulation cascade and is thus categorized here.

## OVULATORY DYSFUNCTION

The predominant cause of ovulatory dysfunction (AUB-O) in postmenarchal and premenopausal women is secondary to alterations in neuroendocrine function. In women with AUB-O, there is continuous estradiol production without corpus luteum formation and progesterone production. The steady state of estrogen stimulation leads to a continuously proliferating endometrium, which may outgrow its blood supply or lose nutrients with varying degrees of necrosis. In contrast to normal menstruation, uniform slough to the basalis layer does not occur, which produces excessive uterine bleeding.

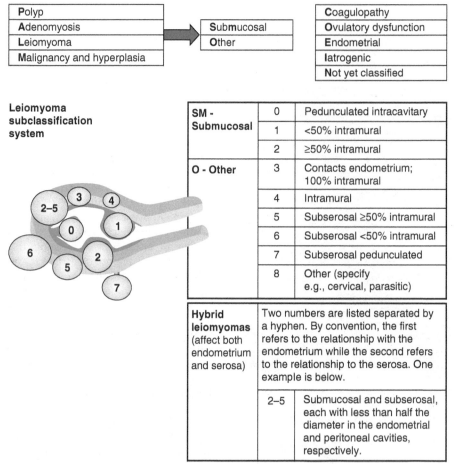

Anovulatory bleeding occurs most commonly during the extremes of reproductive life—in the first few years after menarche and during perimenopause. In the adolescent, the cause of anovulation is an immaturity of the hypothalamic-pituitary-ovarian (HPO) axis and failure of positive feedback of estradiol to cause a luteinizing hormone (LH) surge. In the perimenopausal woman, a lack of synchronization between the components of the HPO axis occurs as the woman approaches ovarian decline at menopause.

The pattern of anovulatory bleeding may be oligomenorrhea, intermenstrual bleeding, or heavy menstrual bleeding. Why different patterns of bleeding occur within a distinct entity of anovulatory bleeding is unclear but is probably related to variations in the integrity of the endometrium and its support structure. Up to 20% of women reporting normal menses may also be anovulatory.

What are the causes of anovulation? Apart from the extremes of reproductive life, as noted, women in their reproductive years often have a cause for anovulatory bleeding. This is most frequently because of polycystic ovary syndrome (PCOS), which may be suggested by other symptoms and signs, such as acne, hirsutism, and increased body weight (see Chapter 41). If not PCOS, anovulation can result from hypothalamic dysfunction, which could have no known cause or be related to weight loss, severe exercise, stress, or drug use. In addition, abnormalities of other nonreproductive hormones can lead to anovulation. The most common hormones involved are thyroid hormone, prolactin, and cortisol.

Hypothyroidism, evidenced by an elevated thyroid stimulating hormone (TSH) level, can lead to anovulatory bleeding. Unexplained causes of endometrial problems in the face of normal ovulation (discussed later) may also be explained by subtle hypothyroidism. Hyperprolactinemia (prolactin [PRL] level >20 ng/mL) can also lead to anovulatory bleeding, as can hypercortisolism. However, Cushing syndrome is rare and may be considered only if other signs are present (e.g., obesity, moon facies, buffalo hump, striae, weakness). Accordingly, TSH and PRL assays should be part of the normal workup of anovulatory women.

## IATROGENIC

Iatrogenic bleeding (AUB-I) is abnormal bleeding resulting from medications. The most common of these are hormonal preparations, including selective estrogen receptor modulators, and gonadotropic releasing hormone agonists and antagonists. All hormonal long-acting reversible contraceptives result in some degree of anovulation and irregular or intermenstrual bleeding. However with time, most patients become amenorrheic. The prevalence of amenorrhea with depomedroxyprogesterone acetate users at 90, 180, 270, and 360 days are 12%, 25%, 37%, and 46%, respectively, as determined by a systematic review (Hubacher, 2009). And chronic progestogen therapy of various types can lead to irregular spotting and bleeding. Similarly, irregular bleeding is an expected consequence of levonorgestrel intrauterine devices initially, but 20% of users are amenorrheic by 1 year. Implantable progestin devices have similar amenorrhea rates, but over 40% of patients have irregular or prolonged bleeding. This pattern of bleeding is the most common reason for discontinuation of the subdermal implants within the first year (Mark, 2013).

Hyperprolactinemia can result from central nervous system dopamine antagonism of certain antipsychotic drugs. The prevalence of hyperprolactinemia among women taking risperidone was 88%, and among women taking conventional antipsychotics it was 47% in one study. As previously described, elevations in prolactin are disruptive to the HPO axis and can contribute to anovulation, with 48% of those women on risperidone experiencing abnormal uterine bleeding (Kinon, 2003).

It is well known that commonly combined and progesterone-only oral contraceptives may result in breakthrough bleeding (BTB). BTB most likely reflects alterations in the structural integrity, vascular density, and vascular morphology of the endometrial vasculature due to alterations in the expression of steroid receptors and the integrity of the endometrial epithelial layer (Smith, 2005). Compliance issues and interactions between oral contraceptives and other medications, such as antibiotics and anticonvulsants may alter circulating levels of steroids, allowing follicular recruitment and increased endogenous levels of estrogen. These variations are a common cause of irregular bleeding in contraceptive users.

## ENDOMETRIAL

Women who present with heavy menstrual bleeding in the absence of other abnormalities are thought to have underlying disorders of the endometrium (AUB-E) or are otherwise unclassified. In the past, this category has been called "ovulatory dysfunctional uterine bleeding."

The primary line of defense to excessive bleeding during normal menses is the formation of the platelet plug. This is followed by uterine contractility, largely mediated by prostaglandin F2α (PGF2α). Thus prolonged and heavy bleeding can occur with abnormalities of the platelet plug or inadequate uterine levels of PGF2α. It has been shown that in some women with heavy menstrual bleeding, there is excessive uterine production of prostacyclin, a vasodilatory prostaglandin that opposes platelet adhesion and may also interfere with uterine contractility. Deficiency of uterine PGF2α or excessive production of PGE (another vasodilatory prostaglandin) may also explain ovulatory DUB (Smith, 1982). The ratio of PGF2α/PGE correlates inversely with menstrual blood loss (Fig. 26.5). In addition to these, other uterine factors affecting blood flow, such as the endothelins and vascular endothelial growth factor, which controls blood vessel formation, may be abnormal in some women with heavy menstrual bleeding. Unfortunately, no commercially available assays exist, and endometrial causes of AUB remain a diagnosis of exclusion in most cases.

Chronic inflammatory changes of the endometrium as evidenced by plasma cell infiltration indicate endometritis. However the causal relationship between inflammatory changes and abnormal bleeding is unclear, resulting from a variety of factors including infection, vascular endothelial damage, or alterations in vasculogenesis. Subclinical infection with *Chlamydia trachomatis* has also been associated with AUB.

## NOT OTHERWISE SPECIFIED

Abnormal bleeding not classified in the previous categories is considered AUB-N. Examples of such conditions may include foreign bodies or trauma. Treatment is tailored to the specific cause.

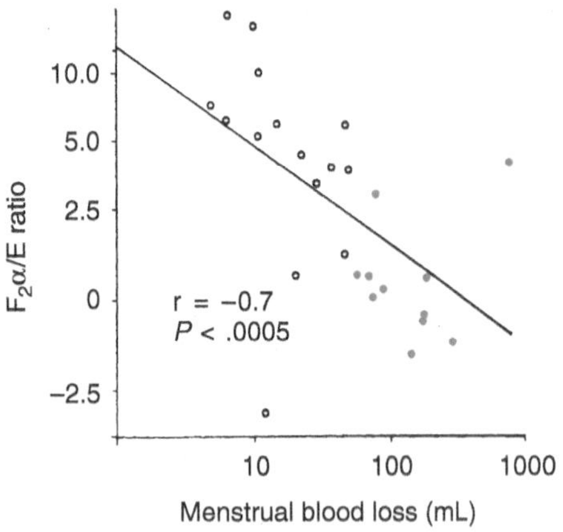


**Figure 26.5** Correlation between ratio of endogenous concentrations of prostaglandin F2alpha and prostaglandin E and menstrual blood loss (MBL); normal secretory endometrium; persistent endometrium. (From Smith SK, Abel MH, Kelly RW, et al. The synthesis of prostaglandins from persistent proliferative endometrium. *J Clin Endocrinol Metab.* 1982;55[2]:284-289.)

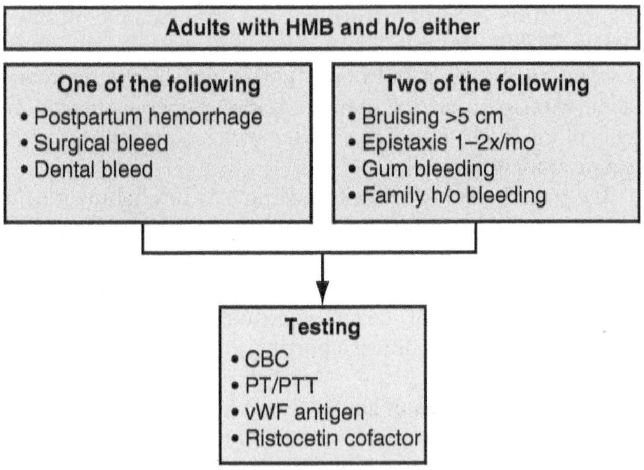


**Figure 26.6** Diagnostic approach to adults with abnormal uterine bleeding due to coagulopathy. (Data from Kouides PA, Conard J, Peyvandi F, et al. Hemostasis and menstruation: appropriate investigation for underlying disorders of hemostasis in women with excessive menstrual bleeding. *Fertil Steril.* 2005;84[5]:1345-1351.)

## DIAGNOSTIC APPROACH

When a woman presents with a complaint of abnormal bleeding, it is essential to take a thorough history regarding the frequency, duration, and amount of bleeding, as well as to inquire whether and when the menstrual pattern changed. This history is important for describing the menstrual abnormality as oligomenorrhea, polymenorrhea, heavy menstrual bleeding, or intermenstrual bleeding. History and physical examination provide clues about the diagnosis of ovulatory disorders and other systemic illnesses. Providing the woman with a calendar to record her bleeding episodes is a helpful way to characterize definitively the bleeding episodes. A number of commercially available smart phone applications exist to track abnormal bleeding conveniently, although none of these have been validated. Symptoms present for the majority of the preceding 6 months are considered chronic, but symptoms lasting 3 months sufficiently indicate the need for investigation.

Because there is a poor correlation between a woman's estimate of the amount of blood flow and the measured loss, as well as great variation in the amount of blood and fluid absorbed by different types of sanitary napkins and tampons (and by the same type in different women), objective criteria should be used to determine if menorrhagia (blood loss >80 mL) is present.

As direct measurement of MBL is not generally possible, indirect assessment by measurement of hemoglobin concentration, serum iron levels, and serum ferritin levels are useful. The serum ferritin level provides a valid indirect assessment of iron stores in the bone marrow. Additional useful laboratory tests include a sensitive β-hCG level determination and a sensitive TSH assay, as well as PRL. If PCOS is suspected, androgen level measurements may be considered but are not necessary.

For adolescent girls with heavy menstrual bleeding, as well as older women with the constellation of systemic disease, easy bruising and petechiae, a coagulation profile including platelet count, prothrombin time, von Willebrand factor, and ristocetin cofactor should be obtained to rule out a coagulation defect. Once thought to be extremely rare as a cause for abnormal bleeding, studies have found a fairly high prevalence of coagulation disorders in women presenting with heavy menstrual bleeding. Most abnormalities are platelet related. The single most common abnormality is a form of von Willebrand disease. It has been estimated that the prevalence of von Willebrand disease, the most common of these bleeding disorders, is 11% in women with heavy menstrual bleeding (Dilley, 2001). von Willebrand factor is responsible for proper platelet adhesion and protects against coagulant factor degradation. History is essential before a comprehensive hematologic workup is undertaken. This includes a history of menorrhagia, family history of bleeding, epistaxis, bruising, gum bleeding, postpartum hemorrhage, and surgical bleeding. In the absence of these clues, a comprehensive workup is probably unnecessary at the outset but should be considered in cases refractory to treatment. A hematologist should be consulted to assist in confirming the diagnosis and to suggest possible treatment (Fig. 26.6).

If the woman has regular cycles, it is helpful to determine whether she is ovulating. However, if bleeding is very irregular, it may be difficult to determine the phase of the cycle to document ovulatory function by means of serum progesterone level. Patients with chronic anovulation are at increased risk for endometrial hyperplasia and malignancy. If there is an enhanced risk for endometrial disease on the basis of history, endometrial sampling is indicated. Endometrial sampling is also recommended in patients with heavy menstrual bleeding over the age of 45 (NIH Clinical Excellence, 2007). Sampling is most often performed with a 3 mm Pipelle in the office, with little or no anesthesia. Sampling should include a measurement of the uterine length and subjective assessment of the quantity of tissue. When office endometrial biopsy is not possible or if the tissue sample is insufficient, dilation and curettage (D&C) should be performed under anesthesia. The sensitivity of endometrial biopsy was 68% when compared with hysterectomy specimens and was 78% when compared with D&C in one

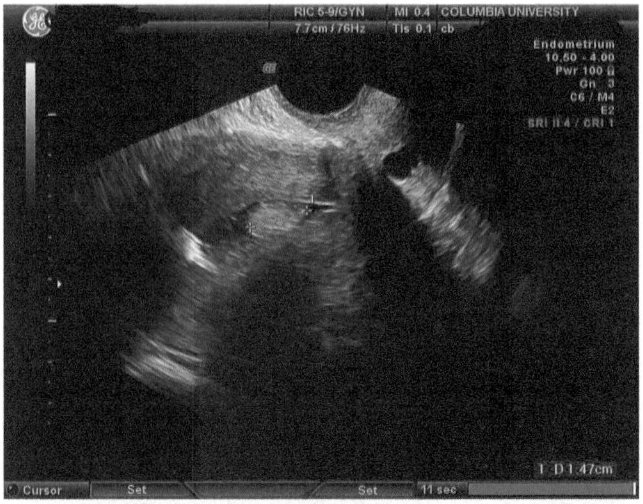


**Figure 26.7** Saline sonography demonstrating a 1.4-cm diameter endometrial polyp in a woman with heavy menstrual bleeding. (Courtesy of Dr. J. Lerner, Columbia University Medical Center, New York.)

meta-analysis, concluding that a sampling error occurred in 0% to 54% of cases (Rodriguez, 1993). It thus works best in cases where pathology is global. In cases of regular heavy menstrual bleeding, a biopsy at the time of bleeding can also help determine whether the bleeding is caused by ovulatory function if it reveals a secretory endometrium.

Apart from obtaining a careful history and physical examination, blood testing (as noted earlier), ultrasound, and endometrial biopsy (if indicated), it is often valuable to assess the uterine cavity through sonohysterogram (SHG) or flexible hysteroscopy. This is to rule out an intracavitary lesion before ascribing the diagnosis to endometrial disorders or ovulatory dysfunction.

For SHG, 10 to 15 mL of saline or sterile water is usually introduced through the cervix with an insemination catheter, or with a special catheter that has a balloon for inflation in the cervical canal, allowing continuous infusion. Office-based flexible hysteroscopy is an excellent diagnostic technique that provides direct visualization of the endometrium and has the potential advantage of being able to treat the abnormality at the same time, for example, as removal of a polyp. The sensitivity and specificity of SHG and hysteroscopy are equivalent in diagnosing intracavitary lesions, but both are superior to transvaginal pelvic ultrasound alone (Kelekci, 2005). Studies show that both studies are well accepted by patients (Van Dongen, 2008) (Fig. 26.7).

Evaluation of the myometrium includes imaging modalities capable of detecting leiomyomas and adenomyosis. Ultrasonography is a sensitive screening tool and performs similarly to MRI in the detection of uterine fibroids with a sensitivity of 99% (Dueholm, 2002). But with a wide array of treatment modalities available, assessment of the myometrium requires an exact understanding of fibroid position, size, and number. In most instances, MRI performs superiorly. Compared with findings at the time of hysterectomy, MRI, ultrasound and hysteroscopy perform equally well in the detection of submucous fibroids, but MRI performs superiorly in the evaluation of the extent of myoma invasion (Dueholm, 2001). In large uteri (>375 mL) or when fibroids number more than four, MRI is also superior to ultrasound in detecting and mapping fibroid location. However, hysteroscopy and sonohysterography continue to offer less expensive alternatives to MRI for adequate determination of endometrial distortion.

## TREATMENT OF ABNORMAL UTERINE BLEEDING

Treatment of abnormal bleeding requires an accurate diagnosis. Endometrial polyps that cause abnormal bleeding require surgical removal via hysteroscopy. The management of malignancy and hyperplasia is discussed elsewhere. Many of the following medical managements may be applied to leiomyoma, but large and complicated uteri or submucosal fibroids often require surgery. In the absence of an organic cause for excessive uterine bleeding, it is preferable to use medical instead of surgical treatment, especially if the woman desires to retain her uterus for future childbearing or will be undergoing natural menopause within a short time. There are several effective medical methods for the treatment of ovulatory or endometrial bleeding. These include estrogens, progestogen (systemic or local), nonsteroidal anti-inflammatory drugs (NSAIDs), antifibrinolytic agents, and gonadotropin-releasing hormone (GnRH) agonists. The type of treatment depends on whether it is used to stop an acute heavy bleeding episode or is given to reduce the amount of MBL in subsequent menstrual cycles. A definitive diagnosis is required before instituting long-term treatment, and should be made on the basis of hysteroscopy, sonohysterography, or directed endometrial biopsies, if indicated.

This section is organized into treatment options for chronic conditions followed by management of severe acute bleeding. Whereas these medical options treat the underlying pathology and manage the symptoms in patients with ovulatory dysfunction and endometrial causes, medical treatment options may be initiated in patients with adenomyosis or leiomyoma not severe enough to require surgery. Last, a brief overview of surgical options is presented.

### *ABNORMAL UTERINE BLEEDING: OVULATORY DYSFUNCTION*

In adolescents, after ruling out coagulation disorders, the main direction of therapy is to temporize because with time and maturity of the HPO axis, the problem will be corrected. A cyclic progestogen—for example, medroxyprogesterone acetate, 10 mg for 10 days each month for a few months—is all that is needed to produce reliable and controlled menstrual cycles. This may be continued for up to 6 months with the situation reevaluated thereafter. Alternatively, some clinicians prefer to use an oral contraceptive (OC), although this may not be necessary and does not allow the HPO to mature on its own. If the problem persists beyond 6 months, OCs become an option in that the condition may be more chronic.

In the perimenopausal woman who has dysregulation of the HPO axis, there is much variability and unpredictability of cycles because the HPO axis is in flux, moving toward ovarian failure. Although most of the bleeding in this setting is caused by anovulation, occasional ovulation can occur, with or without a normal luteal phase, which is highly variable and erratic. Here, it is more efficient to use a low-dose (20-μg) OC in a nonsmoking woman. Progestogens used cyclically, although preventing endometrial tissue from building up because of anovulation, will help the endometrium but will not reliably control bleeding, because of the unpredictability of the hormonal situation.

During reproductive life, chronic anovulatory bleeding is primarily caused by hypothalamic dysfunction or PCOS. OCs work well in this setting, although an alternative is cyclic progestogens, as noted previously. Some of these women may also wish to conceive, in which case ovulation induction is indicated.

## ABNORMAL UTERINE BLEEDING: ENDOMETRIAL

For women with heavy menstrual bleeding, for whom there is no known cause and anatomic lesions have been ruled out, the aim of therapy is to reduce the amount of excessive bleeding. As noted, some women with AUB-E have abnormal prostaglandin production and some have alterations of endometrial blood flow.

Options for treatment to reduce blood loss include a more prolonged regimen of progestogens (3 weeks each month); shorter cyclic therapy does not work here. Doses in excess of 10 mg daily of medroxyprogesterone acetate (MPA) have been used, but large doses can cause side effects and weight gain when used for several months and may not be necessary. OCs will reduce the blood loss by at least 35% in women with AUB-E (Shabaan, 2011). Another beneficial option is the use of the levonorgestrel intrauterine system (IUS), whereby menorrhagia can be substantially reduced (discussed later). It should be noted that in ovulatory heavy menstrual bleeding, although all obvious lesions have been ruled out, some anatomic abnormalities cannot be easily diagnosed. These include endometriosis and, in particular, adenomyosis, although the diagnosis may be improved with MRI. Thus other options also have to be considered for reducing blood loss.

### Local Progestogen Exposure

The levonorgestrel-releasing intrauterine system (LNG-IUS) has an effective duration of action of more than 5 years. Research on the use of this IUS as treatment for heavy menstrual bleeding found that at the end of 3 months, it caused an average 80% reduction in MBL, which increased to 100% at the end of 1 year. This reduction in MBL was significantly greater than that achieved with an antifibrinolytic agent or a prostaglandin synthetase inhibitor in studies by the same investigators (Milsom, 1991) (Fig. 26.8). Other studies have shown that the LNG-IUS reduces MBL by 74% to 97% and is effective in increasing hemoglobin levels, decreasing dysmenorrhea, and reducing blood loss caused by fibroids and adenomyosis.

Although endometrial ablation achieves a more rapid return to normal flow, studies comparing the LNG-IUS to endometrial ablation show similar bleeding profiles after 1 year, with similar patient satisfaction scores (Kaunitz, 2009). In addition, the LNG-IUS has also been compared with hysterectomy for menorrhagia and has been considered to be a viable alternative.

Patients with AUB due to coagulopathy, especially secondary to anticoagulation therapy, also can be managed successfully with the LNG-IUS. In one series of 23 patients, MBL was reduced in 59% of LNG-IUS users on oral anticoagulation (Pisoni, 2006). Similar results have been demonstrated in patients with von Willebrand disease (Kingman, 2004). Importantly, a systematic review has failed to answer whether the risk of thrombosis is decreased in hormonal contraceptive users while taking oral anticoagulation (Culwell, 2009). The World Health Organization states that combined oral contraceptives should not be used in patients with active deep venous thrombosis, but the benefits of progesterone-only methods outweigh the risks (Mohllajee, 2005). As such, the LNG-IUS has become an appropriate initial therapy in patients with heavy menstrual bleeding due to anticoagulation therapy.

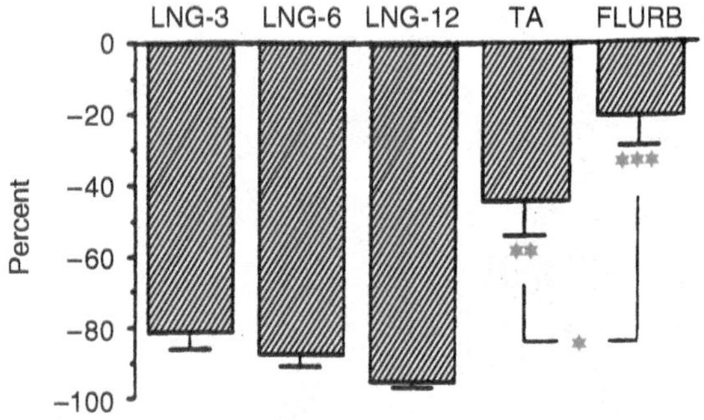


**Figure 26.8** Reduction in menstrual blood loss (MBL) expressed as a percentage of the mean of two control cycles for each form of treatment. Significance of difference between treatment with levonorgestrel-releasing intrauterine device (LNG-IUD) and tranexamic acid (TA) and flurbiprofen (FLURB), indicated by double asterisks ($P < .01$) and triple asterisks ($P < .001$), and between treatment with TA and FLURB indicated by a single asterisk ($P < .05$). (From Milson I, Andersson K, Andersch B, et al. A comparison of flurbiprofen, tranexamic acid, and a levonorgestrel-releasing intrauterine contraceptive device in the treatment of idiopathic menorrhagia. *Am J Obstet Gynecol.* 1991;164:879.)

## NONSTEROIDAL ANTI-INFLAMMATORY DRUGS

NSAIDs are prostaglandin synthetase inhibitors that inhibit the biosynthesis of the cyclic endoperoxides, which convert arachidonic acid to prostaglandins. In addition, these agents block the action of prostaglandins by interfering directly at their receptor sites. To decrease bleeding of the endometrium, it would be ideal to block selectively the synthesis of prostacyclin alone, without decreasing thromboxane formation, because the latter increases platelet aggregation. Presently, there are no NSAIDs that possess this ability. All NSAIDs are cyclooxygenase inhibitors and thus block the formation of both thromboxane and the prostacyclin pathway. Nevertheless, NSAIDs have been shown to reduce MBL, primarily in women who ovulate. However, the mechanisms whereby prostaglandin inhibitors reduce MBL are not yet completely understood, and their therapeutic action may take place through some as yet undiscovered mechanism. Several NSAIDs have been administered during menses to groups of women with menorrhagia and ovulatory DUB and have been found to reduce the mean MBL by approximately 20% to 50% (Vargyas, 1987). Drugs used in various studies have included mefenamic acid (500 mg, three times daily), ibuprofen (400 mg, three times daily), meclofenamate sodium (100 mg, three times daily), and naproxen sodium (275 mg, every 6 hours after a loading dose of 550 mg), as well as other NSAIDs. These drugs are usually given for the first 3 days of menses or throughout the bleeding episode. All appear to have similar levels of effectiveness.

Not all women treated with these agents have reduction in blood flow, but those without a decrease usually did not have excessive bleeding to begin with. The greatest amount of MBL reduction occurs in women with the greatest pretreatment blood loss. The treatment of heavy menstrual bleeding with mefenamic acid in 36 women for longer than 1 year resulted in a significantly sustained reduction in the amount of MBL and in a significant increase in serum ferritin levels (Fraser, 1983). Thus this approach can be used for long-term treatment because side effects, mainly gastrointestinal (GI), are mild.

Although NSAIDs have been studied as sole therapy to treat women with MBL who ovulate, they can also be given in combination with OCs or progestogens. With this combined approach, a reduction in MBL can be achieved more effectively than with the use of any of these agents alone.

### Antifibrinolytic Agents

ε-Aminocaproic acid (EACA), tranexamic acid (AMCA), and para-aminomethyl benzoic acid (PAMBA) are potent inhibitors of fibrinolysis and have therefore been used in the treatment of various hemorrhagic conditions. Nilsson and Rybo have compared the effect on blood loss of EACA, AMCA, and oral contraceptives in 215 women with menorrhagia. EACA was given in a dose of 18 g/day for 3 days and then 12, 9, 6, and 3 g daily on successive days. The total dose was always at least 48 g. AMCA was administered in a dose of 6 g/day for 3 days, followed by 4, 3, 2, and 1 g/day on successive days. The total dose of AMCA was at least 22 g. There was a significant reduction in blood loss after treatment with EACA, AMCA, and OCs, and use of each of these agents resulted in approximately a 50% reduction in MBL (Nilsson, 1971) (Table 26.1). Of interest was the finding that the greatest reduction in blood loss with antifibrinolytic therapy occurred in women who exhibited the greatest pretreatment MBL. Preston and colleagues have compared the effects of 4 g of AMCA daily for 4 days each cycle with 10 mg of norethindrone for 7 days each cycle in a group of women with ovulatory menorrhagia with a mean MBL of 175 mL. AMCA reduced MBL by 45%, but there was a 20% increase with norethindrone. The side effects of this class of drugs, in decreasing order of frequency, are nausea, dizziness, diarrhea, headaches, abdominal pain, and allergic manifestations. These side effects are much more common with EACA than with AMCA. Other investigators have compared the use of AMCA with placebo in double-blind studies and have found no significant differences in the occurrence of side effects. Renal failure, pregnancy, and history of thrombosis are contraindications to the use of antifibrinolytic agents.

Antifibrinolytic agents clearly produce a reduction in blood loss and may be used as therapy for women with menorrhagia who ovulate. However, their use is somewhat limited by side effects. These are mainly GI side effects and can be minimized by reducing the dose and limiting therapy to the first 3 to 5 days of bleeding. Antifibrinolytics may have value in treating bleeding due to structural causes as well. Tranexamic acid administered in doses of 3.9 g/day demonstrated a statistically significant reduction of MBL in women with fibroids, with greatest reductions on days 2 and 3 (Eder, 2013). Due to the increased risks of thrombosis and myocardial infarction, antifibrinolytic agents should not be combined with oral contraceptives. Combined treatment with tranexamic acid and the oral contraceptive pill has been implicated in coronary ulcerated plaque and acute myocardial infarction (Iacobellis, 2004).

**Table 26.1** Mean Menstrual Blood Loss and Reduction with Treatment

| | Mean Blood Loss (mL) | | |
|---|---|---|---|
| Agent Used | Before Treatment | After Treatment | Decrease (%) |
| EACA | 164 | 87 | 47 |
| AMCA | 182 | 84 | 54 |
| Oral contraceptives | 158 | 75 | 52 |
| Methylergobaseimmaleate | 164 | 164 | 0 |

Modified from Nilsson L, Rybo G. Treatment of menorrhagia. *Am J Obstet Gynecol.* 1971;110:713.

*AMCA*, Tranexamic acid; *EACA*, ε-aminocaproic acid.

### Gonadotropin-Releasing Hormone Agonists

GnRH agonists may be used to inhibit ovarian steroid production, as estrogen production is necessary for endometrial proliferation. In a small study of four women, daily administration of a GnRH agonist for 3 months markedly reduced MBL from 100 to 200 mL per cycle to 0 to 30 mL per cycle. Unfortunately, after therapy was discontinued, blood loss returned to pretreatment levels (Shaw, 1984) (see Fig. 26.8). Two other observational studies, one using sequential add-back in 20 women and another using goserelin in 60 women, also showed some benefit (Thomas, 1996; Cheung, 2005). Because of the expense and side effects of these agents, their use for heavy menstrual bleeding is limited to women with severe MBL who fail to respond to other methods of medical management and wish to retain their childbearing capacity. More commonly, GnRH agonists are an effective means of bridging patients to surgical treatment, allowing for correction of anemia. Use of an estrogen or progestogen (add-back therapy) together with the agonist will help prevent bone loss.

## MANAGEMENT OF ACUTE BLEEDING

In women who are bleeding heavily and are hemodynamically unstable, the quickest way to stop acute bleeding is with curettage. This should also be the preferred approach for older women and those with medical risk factors for whom high-dose hormonal therapy may pose a great risk.

## PHARMACOLOGIC AGENTS FOR ACUTE BLEEDING

To stop acute bleeding that does not require curettage the most effective regimen involves high-dose estrogen. This treatment, aimed at stopping acute bleeding, is diagnosis-independent and is merely a temporary measure.

There has also been some experience with using high dose progestogens alone for the management of acute bleeding (discussed later).

### Estrogens

The rationale for the therapeutic use of estrogen for the treatment of DUB is based on the fact that estrogen in pharmacologic doses causes rapid growth of the endometrium. This strategy is for the acute management of abnormal bleeding. The bleeding that results from most causes of abnormal bleeding will respond to this therapy because a rapid growth of endometrial tissue occurs over the denuded and raw epithelial surfaces. This effect is independent of the cause of abnormal bleeding. To control an acute bleeding episode, the use of oral conjugated equine estrogen (CEE) 10 mg/day, in four divided doses, is a therapeutic regimen that has been found to be clinically useful. It is possible that in addition to the rapid growth mechanism of action, these large doses of CEE may alter platelet activity, thus promoting platelet adhesiveness. Six hours after infusion of an average dose of 30 mg of CEE to individuals with a prolonged bleeding time caused by renal failure, the bleeding time was significantly shortened (Livio, 1986). In this study, measurements of various clotting factors were unchanged after CEE infusion. Acute bleeding from most causes is usually controlled, but if bleeding does not decrease within the first 24 hours, consideration must be given to an organic cause and curettage should be considered.

Intravenous (IV) administration of estrogen is also effective in the acute treatment of menorrhagia. Compared with women given a placebo, a significantly greater percentage of women had cessation of bleeding 2 hours after the second of two 25-mg doses of CEE was administered IV, 3 hours apart. There was no significant difference in cessation of bleeding between women administered estrogen and those given a placebo 3 hours after the first infusion (DeVore, 1982). This study indicated that at least several hours are required to induce mitotic activity and growth of the endometrium, whether the estrogen is administered orally or parenterally. Thus IV estrogen therapy accompanied by its rapid metabolic clearance does not appear to offer a significant advantage compared with a comparable dose of estrogen given orally as long as the oral dosing can be tolerated in terms of symptoms such as nausea. From a practical standpoint, if IV therapy is chosen, it usually requires that women remain in the office or clinical setting for 4 to 6 hours to receive at least a second dose.

Usually, estrogen therapy reduces the amount of uterine bleeding within the first 24 hours after treatment is initiated. However, because most women with an acute heavy bleeding episode bleed because of anovulation, progestogen treatment is also required. Therefore after bleeding has ceased, oral estrogen therapy is continued at the same dosage and a progestogen, for example, MPA, 10 mg once daily, is added. Both hormones are administered for another 7 to 10 days (or longer if desired and tolerated by the woman), after which treatment is stopped to allow withdrawal bleeding, which may have an increased amount of flow but is rarely prolonged. After the withdrawal bleeding episode, one of several other treatment modalities should be used. Before instituting long-term treatment, a definitive diagnosis should be made after reviewing the endometrial histology. Definitive treatment should be based on these findings. OCs are usually the best long-term treatment in the absence of contraindications.

A more convenient method to stop acute bleeding than the sequential high-dose estrogen-progestin regimen is the use of a combination oral contraceptive containing both estrogen and progestin. Four tablets of an oral contraceptive containing 30 to 35 µg of estrogen taken every 24 hours in divided doses will usually provide sufficient estrogen to stop acute bleeding and simultaneously provide progestin. Treatment is continued for at least 1 week after the bleeding stops. This regimen is successful and convenient and is thus the preferred method of some clinicians. Not well documented is the expectation that the IV regimen is more effective than using OCs. A theoretic reason for this suggestion may be that the combined use of estrogen and progestin does not cause as rapid endometrial growth as estrogen alone, because the progestin decreases the synthesis of estrogen receptors and increases estradiol dehydrogenase in the endometrial cell, thus inhibiting the growth-promoting action of estrogen.

It must be noted that high-dose estrogen, even for a short course, may be contraindicated for some women (e.g., those with prior thrombosis, certain rheumatologic diseases, estrogen-responsive cancer). In these cases, the options are therapy with progestogen alone given continuously or intermittently. Although invasive, curettage remains the fastest way to stop acute bleeding and should be used in women who are volume-depleted and severely anemic (hemodynamically unstable).

When ultrasound is available, it is more logical to use estrogen therapy if there is prolonged heavy bleeding in the setting of a thin endometrium (<5-mm stripe). Conversely, if the endometrium is thick (>10 to 12 mm) or if an anatomic finding is suspected, curettage should be considered. Unless bleeding is extremely heavy (where estrogen therapy is preferred), progestogens may be used initially and will help by organizing the endometrium. In the setting of a thickened irregular endometrium, if curettage is not performed, an endometrial biopsy should be obtained.

### *Progestogens*

Progestogens not only stop endometrial growth but also support and organize the endometrium so that an organized slough occurs after their withdrawal. In the absence of progesterone, erratic unorganized breakdown of the endometrium occurs. With progestogen treatment, an organized slough to the basalis layer allows a rapid cessation of bleeding. In addition, progestogens stimulate arachidonic acid formation in the endometrium, increasing the PGF2α/PGE ratio. Some studies support the efficacy of progestogens alone in the management of acute bleeding.

In one randomized trial, medroxyprogesterone acetate (MPA) at a dose of 60 mg daily (20 mg three times daily) for 7 days followed by 20 mg per day for 3 weeks stopped bleeding in 76% of women in 3 days and had equal efficacy to an OC given as three tablets a day for 7 days, followed by one tablet a day for 3 weeks (Munro, 2006). In another uncontrolled short-term study, Depo-MPA 150 mg intramuscularly followed by oral MPA 60 mg (20 mg three times daily) for 3 days stopped bleeding in all 48 women within 5 days (Ammerman, 2013).

High-dose progestogens in this setting may be expected to exert direct stabilizing effects on the endometrium in a rapid sequence. Similarly, large doses of norethindrone acetate (30 mg per day) may be expected to perform equally well. In addition, higher doses of norethindrone may be efficacious on the basis of some conversion to ethinyl estradiol (thus mimicking the use of a low-dose OC) (Chu, 2007). For longer-term management of abnormal bleeding, the mainstay of progestogen therapy is opposing the effects of estrogen in anovulatory women. For women with a history of bothersome intermenstrual bleeding, it is advisable to use intermittent progestogens for several months or an OC.

MPA 10 mg/day for 10 days each month is a successful therapeutic regimen that produces regular withdrawal bleeding in women with adequate amounts of endogenous estrogen to cause endometrial growth. 19-norprogestogens, such as norethindrone or norethindrone acetate (2.5 to 5 mg) may be used in the same regimen. Although more androgenic progestogens are less favorable for metabolic parameters (e.g., high-density-lipoprotein [HDL] cholesterol, carbohydrate tolerance), when used as prolonged therapy, short-term cyclic therapy is not harmful.

## ANDROGENS

Danazol is a synthetic androgen used in doses of 200 mg daily for the treatment of heavy menstrual bleeding (Hingham, 1993). A Cochrane review has noted that, although nine randomized controlled trials (RCTs) were identified with danazol, studies have been generally underpowered. Nevertheless, danazol appears to be more effective than placebo, oral progestogens, oral contraceptives, and NSAIDs. However, compared with NSAIDs, the side effects of weight gain and skin problems were sevenfold and fourfold greater, respectively, when compared with progestogens (Beaumont, 2002). Consequently, its use is limited.

### Surgical Therapy: Dilation and Curettage

The performance of a D&C can be diagnostic and is therapeutic for the immediate management of severe bleeding. For women with markedly excessive uterine bleeding who may be hypovolemic, a D&C is the quickest way to stop acute bleeding. Therefore it is the treatment of choice in women who suffer from hypovolemia. A D&C may be preferred as an approach to stop an acute bleeding episode in women older than 35 when the incidence of pathologic findings increases.

The use of D&C for the treatment of anovulatory bleeding has been reported to be curative only rarely. Temporary cure of the problem may occur in some women with chronic anovulation, because the curettage removes much of the hyperplastic endometrium; however, the underlying pathophysiologic cause is unchanged. D&C has not proved useful for the treatment of women who ovulate and have heavy menstrual bleeding. More than 1 month after D&C, there is no difference or an increase in MBL in women with menorrhagia who ovulate (Nilsson, 1971). Therefore D&C is only indicated for women with acute bleeding resulting in hypovolemia and for older women who are at higher risk of having endometrial neoplasia. All other women, after having an endometrial biopsy, sonohysterography, or diagnostic hysteroscopy to rule out organic disease, are best treated with medical therapy, as outlined earlier, without D&C.

### Surgical Therapy: Endometrial Ablation

Abnormal bleeding may be treated by endometrial ablation (EA) if medical therapy is not effective or is contraindicated. Exceptions are women who have very large uteri caused by fibroids or abnormal pathology, such as endometrial hyperplasia or cancer. Various endometrial ablation methods are available. These methods are an alternative to hysterectomy or to the use of the levonorgestrel IUS, which is also highly effective (discussed earlier).

Although the concept of EA was developed in 1937, the hysteroscopic technique was first used in 1981 with the introduction of the neodymium-yttrium-aluminum-garnet (Nd:YAG) laser. Laser-based approaches were largely replaced with resectoscopic techniques to resect, vaporize, or electrodesiccate the endometrium. Currently, most commonly, various global endometrial ablation (GEA) devices have been approved by the U.S. Food and Drug Administration (FDA) for this type of treatment.

Endometrial resection is usually carried out with a loop electrode, roller ball, or grooved or spiked electrode to vaporize the endometrium. Hysteroscopic surgical techniques have the advantage of dealing definitively with associated pathology (e.g., polyps, submucous fibroids), although they require greater surgical skill, have longer procedure times, and have higher complication rates compared with nonresectoscopic methods.

Various GEA methods are given in Table 26.2, which lists the success rates and limitations based on anatomy. Most systems, except the Hydro ThermAblator (Boston Scientific, Marlborough, MA), are carried out without hysteroscopic monitoring. Cryotherapy may be performed in approximately 10 minutes using a 4.5-mm disposable cryoprobe (Her Option, Cooper Surgical, Trumbull, CT), which is moved from one uterine cornual recess to the other. The Hydro ThermAblator uses heated normal saline delivered through a 7.8-mm sheath. The uterus is distended and causes a closed circuit process, heating the saline to 90° C and maintaining this temperature for 10 minutes, followed by a 1-minute cooling process. The closed system is automated to shut down if there is 10 mL or more leakage of fluid via the cervix or fallopian tubes. Microwave endometrial ablation is carried out with an 8-mm reusable or disposable probe. Once the port is inserted into the fundus, transmission of endometrial tissue temperature is available, and the microwave system is activated when the tissue temperature is 30° C. Movement within the uterus of the microwave probe allows endometrial destruct to occur within 2 to 4 minutes.

The NovaSure radiofrequency electricity system (Hologic, Bedford, MA) uses a 7.2-mm probe with a bipolar gold mesh electrode that opens to conform to the shape of the uterus. A fixed volume of $CO_2$ is injected and monitored to confirm the integrity of the endometrial cavity. Suction is carried out during the application of radiofrequency energy to remove debris stream. The vaporization and desiccation is carried out until a current resistance of 50 ohms is met or until 90 seconds have passed.

The ThermaChoice system (Ethicon, Somerville, NJ) uses a balloon-tipped catheter (5.5 mm) through which heated 5%

Table 26.2 Characteristics and Outcomes at 1 Year for Nonresectoscopic Endometrial Ablation

| Option | Maximum Uterine Size (cm) | Use with Fibroids (<3 cm) | Amenorrhea (%) | Diary Success (%)* | Satisfaction† |
|---|---|---|---|---|---|
| ThermaChoice III (balloon) | 10 | Yes | 37 | 81 | 96 |
| Her option (cryotherapy) | 10 | — | 22 | 67 | 86 |
| Hydro ThermAblator (heated fluid) | 10.5 | Yes | 35 | 68 | — |
| Microwave EA system | 14 | Yes | 55 | 87 | 99 |
| NovaSure (radiofrequency) | 10 | Yes | 36 | 78 | 93 |

*Score <75 using pictorial blood loss assessment chart (% patients).

†Similar rate of satisfaction as with levonorgestrel intrauterine system but both significantly better than medical therapy.

dextrose in water is injected up to a pressure of 160 to 180 mm Hg. A controller unit heats the fluid and monitors the pressure and treatment time. Destruction of the endometrium is carried out in approximately 8 minutes.

Prior to any EA techniques, endometrial sampling is required as part of the workup evaluation of the woman with abnormal bleeding. The uterine cavity should be evaluated for size and presence of pathology that may limit some of the techniques. With the possible exception of the use of the NovaSure system, a review by Sowter has confirmed the benefit of pretreatment with danazol or a GnRH agonist before an ablation. GEA is more successful when a thin endometrial lining is present. Most systems typically treat to a depth of 4 to 6 mm. In the evaluation, it is important to note that there is no thinning of the myometrium from some other cause, such as prior surgery, particularly with the microwave method. The myometrium should be no less than 10 mm anywhere in the uterus. Most methods of GEA, with the exception of the Her Option, may be beneficial in treating submucous fibroids up to 3 cm in size, with the strongest data coming from the use of the microwave and ThermaChoice systems (see Table 26.2). Complications are infrequent with GEA if adherence to the manufacturer's guidelines is maintained. Cervical lacerations and perforations occur more commonly with endometrial resection. Lower genital tract burns may occur, as well as endometritis (≈1%), and there is a syndrome of tubal pain post-EA caused by trapping of endometria at the cornual recesses. This is more likely in women with a tubal ligation. If pregnancy occurs unexpectedly, there is a high incidence of poor outcomes, including prematurity and placenta accreta. Contraception is recommended for all sexually active patients after GEA.

Use of GEA in patents with AUB-O should be judicious. Women with ovulatory dysfunction often have numerous risk factors for endometrial cancer. The length of time between ablation procedure and diagnosis of endometrial cancer was 6 months to 10 years in a systematic review (AlHilli, 2011). Although the length of time did not affect the ability to diagnose endometrial cancer and all cancers were stage 1, the issue remains that destruction of the uterine cavity may prevent early presentation of symptoms or impede accurate sampling of the lining for prompt diagnosis.

GEA procedures can be safely performed in an office setting with paracervical block and conscious sedation. Although amenorrhea may not always occur (only up to 55% of the time), bleeding is significantly improved for most women. Of note, the success is slightly worse in women with a retroverted uterus. Up to 20% of patients will pursue hysterectomy after endometrial ablation, with the most common reasons being persistent bleeding and pain. A history of dysmenorrhea, cesarean delivery, structural abnormalities, and office-based procedure increased the risk of subsequent hysterectomy (AlHilli, 2011).

### *Surgical Therapy: Hysterectomy*

The decision to remove the uterus should be made on an individual basis and should usually be reserved for the woman with other indications for hysterectomy, such as leiomyoma or uterine prolapse. Hysterectomy should only be used to treat persistent abnormal uterine bleeding after all medical therapy has failed, medical therapy is contraindicated, and the amount of MBL has been documented to be excessive by direct measurement. Although the number of hysterectomies performed for the treatment of fibroids, endometriosis, and other benign causes has declined from 1998 to 2010, the number of hysterectomies performed for the treatment of benign abnormal uterine bleeding has remained stable at 200,000 cases per year. AUB is now the leading cause of hysterectomy in the United States and elsewhere (Wright, 2013). A Cochrane review on the treatment showed medical and conservative surgical treatments have similar efficacy at 1 year, with more side effects in hormone users. Although hysterectomy can reliably provide complete cessation of bleeding and improved mental health at 6 months over conservative treatments, it is associated with greater number of serious complications (Marjoribanks 2006).

Uterine artery embolization is not particularly effective unless fibroids are the cause of excessive bleeding.

If hysterectomy is chosen, many options are available, including vaginal hysterectomy, laparoscopic-assisted vaginal hysterectomy (LAVH), laparoscopic or supracervical hysterectomy, laparoscopic total hysterectomy, robotic hysterectomy, and abdominal supracervical hysterectomy.

## *SUMMARY OF APPROACHES TO TREATMENT*

Having reviewed the various options, an important perspective is to approach the woman according to her acute and chronic needs or short-term and long-term therapy. Acute bleeding, which necessitates immediate cessation of bleeding, requires the use of pharmacologic doses of estrogen or curettage; the latter is used more liberally in older women with risk factors or in those who are hemodynamically compromised. This approach is not dependent on whether the woman is anovulatory or ovulatory. Although estrogen will be temporarily helpful, even if there are abnormal anatomic findings such as fibroids, it is preferable to perform curettage if pathology is suspected.

In our view, there is less experience with large doses of progestogens used acutely to stop bleeding. However, this is an option and may be preferable for some women who could be sensitive to, or have contraindications to, the use of estrogens.

After the acute episode, it is imperative to determine the exact cause or causes for a woman's abnormal bleeding. Causes most commonly are structural, hormonal, or both. Less common causes are coagulopathies, idiopathic, endometrial, or unclassified. In the adolescent, 10 mg of MPA, 10 days each month for at least 3 months, should be prescribed and observed carefully thereafter. In this group, additional diagnostic studies should be performed to detect possible defects in the coagulation process, particularly if bleeding is severe. For the woman of reproductive age, long-term therapy depends on whether she requires contraception, induction of ovulation, or treatment of anovulatory bleeding alone. In the latter case, oral OCs or MPA can be administered monthly for at least 6 months, whereas OCs and clomiphene citrate are used for the other indications. For the perimenopausal woman who characteristically has fluctuating amounts of circulating estrogen, use of cyclic progestogen alone is frequently not curative. In these women, abnormal bleeding is best treated by low-dose OCs.

The most difficult type of abnormal bleeding to treat is chronic ovulatory heavy menstrual bleeding due to an endometrial defect. If anatomic abnormalities are absent, long-term treatment is necessary to reduce MBL. For these women, NSAIDs, progestins, oral contraceptives, anti-fibrinolytics, and GnRH analogues are all useful therapeutic modalities. A combination of two or more of these agents is often required to obviate the need for endometrial ablation or hysterectomy. The LNG-IUS has become one of the most successful options and is the first-line therapy in patients with bleeding due to anticoagulation.

## KEY POINTS

- The mean amount of menstrual blood loss in one cycle in normal women was previously reported to be approximately 35 mL but may be as much as 60 mL, with an average loss of 13 mg of iron.
- Heavy menstrual bleeding occurs in 9% to 14% of healthy women, and most have a normal duration of menses.
- A systematic and standardized nomenclature exists for the characterization of abnormal uterine bleeding.
- Pregnancy should always be ruled out in women presenting with AUB.
- Diagnostic tests in women with menorrhagia include measurement of hemoglobin, serum iron, serum ferritin, β-hCG, TSH, and PRL levels, endometrial biopsy and hysteroscopy, sonohysterography, and hysterosalpingography. MRI may be helpful in the diagnosis of adenomyosis or surgical planning for leiomyoma but is not part of the initial evaluation.
- High doses of oral or IV estrogen will usually stop acute bleeding episodes in most cases of abnormal bleeding. An alternative regimen is high-dose oral progestogen for a week, with tapering of the dosage thereafter.
- Patients who are being treated for abnormal uterine bleeding due to endometrial causes (and who are ovulatory) may be given oral contraceptives, NSAIDs (antiprostaglandins), antifibrinolytics or a prolonged course of progestogens, or levo-norgestrel released locally from an IUS. Those treated with the LNG-IUS have similar outcomes at 1 year to those treated by surgery.
- NSAIDs administered during menses reduce MBL by 20% to 50% in women with ovulatory DUB.
- LNG-IUS is the first-line therapy for heavy menstrual bleeding due to anticoagulation or inherited bleeding disorders.
- D&C should be used to stop the acute bleeding episode in patients with hypovolemia or those older than 45 years. D&C only treats the acute episode of excess uterine bleeding, not subsequent episodes.
- Various endometrial ablation techniques achieve a 22% to 55% amenorrhea success rate at 1 year but an 86% to 99% satisfaction rate with regard to normalizing menstruation.
- Within 4 years after endometrial ablation, approximately 25% of women treated will have a hysterectomy.
- Abnormal uterine bleeding has become the leading cause for hysterectomy in the United States.

## KEY REFERENCES


AlHilli MM, Hopkins MR, Famuyide AO. Endometrial cancer after endometrial ablation: a systematic review of the literature. *J Minim Invasive Gynecol.* 2011;18(3):393–400.

Ammerman SR, Nelson AL. A new progestogens-only medical therapy for outpatient management of acute, abnormal uterine bleeding: a pilot study. *Am J Obstet Gynecol.* 2013;208(6):499.e1–499.e5.

Beaumont HY, Augood C, Duckitt K, et al. Danazol for heavy menstrual bleeding. *Cochrane Database Syst Rev.* 2002;(2). CD001017.

Cheung TH, Lo KW, Yim SF, et al. Dose effects of progesterone in add-back therapy during GnRHa treatment. *J Reprod Med.* 2005;50(1):35–40.

Chu MC, Zhang X, Gentzschein E, et al. Formation of ethinyl estradiol in women during treatment with norethindrone acetate. *J Clin Endocrinol Metab.* 2007;92(6):2205–2207.

Claessens EA, Cowell CA. Acute adolescent menorrhagia. *Am J Obstet Gynecol.* 1981;139:277–280.

Culwell KR, Curtis KM. Use of contraceptive methods by women with current venous thrombosis on anticoagulant therapy: a systematic review. *Contraception.* 2009;80(4):337–345.

DeVore GR, Owens O, Kase N. Use of intravenous Premarin in the treatment of dysfunctional uterine bleeding: a double-blind randomized control study. *Obstet Gynecol.* 1982;59(3):285.

Dilley A, Drews C, Miller C, et al. von Willebrand disease and other inherited bleeding disorders in women diagnosed with menorrhagia. *Obstet Gynecol.* 2001;97(4):630–636.

Peterson WF, Novak ER. Endometrial polyps. *Obstet Gynecol.* 1956;8(1):40–49.

Pisoni C, Cuadrado MJ, Khamashta MA, et al. Treatment of menorrhagia associated with oral anticoagulation: efficacy and safety of the levonorgestrel releasing intrauterine device (Mirena coil). *Lupus.* 2006;15(12):877–880.

Rodriguez GC, Yaqub N, King ME. A comparison of the Pipelle device and the Vabra aspirator as measured by endometrial denudation in hysterectomy specimens: the Pipelle device samples significantly less of the endometrial surface than the Vabra aspirator. *Am J Obstet Gynecol.* 1993;168(1 Pt 1):55–59.

Shabaan MM, Zakherah MS, El-Nashar SA, et al. Levonorgestrel-releasing intrauterine system compared to low dose combined oral contraceptive pills for idiopathic menorrhagia: a randomized clinical trial. *Contraception.* 2011;83(1):48–54.

Shaw RW, Fraser HM. Use of a superactive luteinizing hormone releasing hormone (LHRH) agonist in the treatment of menorrhagia. *Br J Obstet Gynaecol.* 1984;91(9):913–916.

Smith SK, Abel MH, Kelly RW, et al. The synthesis of prostaglandins from persistent proliferative endometrium. *J Clin Endocrinol Metab.* 1982;55(2):284–289.

Smith OP, Critchley HO. Progestogen only contraception and endometrial break through bleeding. *Angiogenesis.* 2005;8(2):117–126.

Tallini G, Vanni R, Manfioletti G, et al. HMGI-C and HMGI(Y) immunoreactivity correlates with cytogenetic abnormalities in lipomas, pulmonary chondroid hamartomas, endometrial polyps, and uterine leiomyomas and is compatible with rearrangement of the HMGI-C and HMGI(Y) genes. *Lab Invest.* 2000;80(3):359–369.

Thomas EJ. Add-back therapy for long-term use in dysfunctional uterine bleeding and uterine fibroids. *Br J Obstet Gynaecol.* 1996;103(Suppl 14):18–21.

van Dongen H, de Kroon CD, van den Tillaart SA, et al. A randomized comparison of vaginoscopic office hysteroscopy and saline infusion sonography: a patient compliance study. *BJOG.* 2008;115(10):1232–1237.

Vargyas JM, Campeau JD, Mishell Jr DR. Treatment of menorrhagia with meclofenamate sodium. *Am J Obstet Gynecol.* 1987;157(4 Pt 1):944–950.

Wishall KM, Price J, Pereira N, et al. Postablation risk factors for pain and subsequent hysterectomy. *Obstet Gynecol.* 2014;124(5):904–910.

Wright JD, Herzog TJ, Tsui J, et al. Nationwide trends in the performance of inpatient hysterectomy in the United States. *Obstet Gynecol.* 2013;122(2 Pt 1):233–241.


Suggested Readings can be found on ExpertConsult.com.

# 27

# Principles of Radiation Therapy and Chemotherapy in Gynecologic Cancer:

## Basic Principles, Uses, and Complications

*Judith Ann Smith, Anuja Jhingran*

This chapter describes the underlying concepts and principles of radiation therapy and chemotherapy as they pertain to the treatment of gynecologic malignancies. The rationale and logistics of individual cancer treatments are detailed separately in other chapters specifically dedicated to each gynecologic malignancy.

Included with the basic concepts of radiation physics are discussions of atomic and nuclear structure, particles, and nomenclature; radiation production; interactions of radiation with bodily tissues; the biologic effects of radiation on cells; and the factors that modify these effects. Common radiation sources and their properties are illustrated as they relate to the treatment of specific gynecologic malignancies. Basic principles of normal tissue tolerance and the complication risks of radiation therapy as they relate to gynecologic malignancies are also presented.

Cell growth, division, and metabolism are modified by cancer-related changes in gene expression and protein regulation and by chemotherapeutic alteration of cellular metabolism. Treating physicians must recognize the various classes of chemotherapeutic agents, their actions in gynecologic malignancies, and their treatment-related toxicities. General approaches are to be followed in administering chemotherapy, specifically including the monitoring of patients receiving these agents. This chapter reviews all of these factors.

## RADIATION THERAPY

### *RADIATION THERAPY PRINCIPLES*

Radiation therapy is the safe clinical application of radiation for the local treatment of abnormally proliferating benign or malignant tumors. The principles of radiation physics and radiobiology underlying treatment are discussed, but several key therapeutic goals deserve mentioning first. The dose response of tumor cells after radiation treatment follows a sigmoid curve, with increasingly effective tumor cell kill or arrest of division associated with increasing dose (Fig. 27.1). A similar treatment response exists for normal tissues, and the ability of radiation therapy to control malignancy depends on the greater tolerance of normal tissues to radiation exposure and a diminished capacity of cancer cells to recover from radiation-induced damage. Thus if one were to treat up to the total radiation dose that causes no normal tissue damage, only a small proportion of a tumor would be controlled by radiation-induced damage. Conversely, if one were to treat to a total dose that could eradicate almost the entire tumor, irreparable damage to normal tissue would often occur. This would lead to an unacceptable series of complications or even patient death after radiation treatment. The therapeutic goal of radiation therapy is to balance attempts at maximum local tumor control while minimizing adverse symptoms of treatment and normal tissue damage. Basic radiation therapy principles are detailed throughout the chapter but briefly include the following (Hall, 2000):

- *Fractional cell kill:* Each radiation dose kills a constant fraction of the tumor cell population. Tumor cell kill follows a linear-quadratic relationship with the potential for cell-mediated repair of radiation-induced damage between radiation dose fractions.
- *Radiation dose rate:* Large radiation doses per fraction produce the greatest number of tumor cell kills; these same large radiation doses also produce the greatest damage burden on normal tissues, leading to early and late adverse complications.
- *Radiation resistance:* Although all tumor cells are sensitive to the effects of radiation, select malignant tumor cells show reduced radiosensitivity, resulting in slow tumor regression or renewed tumor repopulation during or after radiation treatment. Radiation resistance is associated with (1) enhanced cell-mediated repair of radiation-induced damage, (2) active concentration of chemical radioprotectors, or (3) cellular hypoxia or nutritional deficiency.
- *Cell cycle dependency of cell kill:* Actively proliferating tumor cells are most often killed by radiation therapy. Ionizing radiation imparts its greatest cell kill effect during the mitotic phase (M phase) and, to a lesser extent, during the late Gap1 phase and early DNA synthesis phase (G1/S). Radiation has little effect during the late synthetic phase (S phase). Before each phase of the cell cycle, genomic integrity is monitored and, if found intact, a cell then progresses through the next

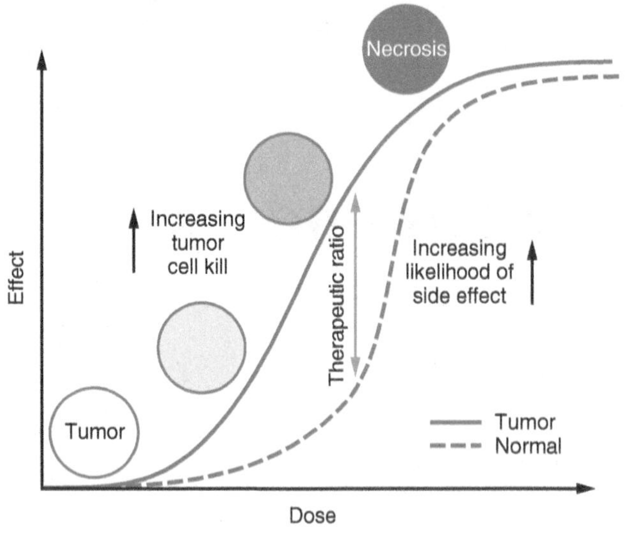


**Figure 27.1** Therapeutic ratio. The concept of the therapeutic ratio for radiation therapy compares the radiation dose-response curves for tumor control and normal tissue side effect rate. Optimally, the tumor control curve lies to the left of the normal tissue curve. For every incremental increase in total dose needed to control tumor, there is a corresponding increase in the likelihood of normal tissue side effects from treatment. The magnitude of the difference between effective tumor cell kill and the likelihood of treatment-related side effects corresponds to the therapeutic ratio *(gray arrow)*. Improved tumor-directed, image-guided radiotherapy planning, use of radiation sensitizers, and use of chemotherapeutic agents (which push the tumor control curve to the left) or the use of radioprotectors (which push the normal tissue curve to the right) can widen the therapeutic ratio.

phase. If, however, genomic damage is detected, a cell arrests the cell cycle so that the damage may be repaired. If the normal monitors of genomic integrity are faulty, as in the case of most cancers, then a cell traverses the cell cycle with radiation-induced damage, leading to mitotic cell death or loss of critical genomic information vital to future cell survival.

With these basic fundamental principles of radiation therapy discussed, it is important to examine in depth the effects of electromagnetic radiation on biologic systems as they pertain to the treatment of gynecologic malignancies.

## BASIC RADIATION PHYSICS

Matter is made up of subatomic particles bound together by energy to form atoms. The simplest representation of the atom consists of a central core of one or more positively charged protons (+1; 933 MeV [mega electron volt]) and zero or more uncharged neutrons (±0; 933 MeV) surrounded by a cloud of negatively charged orbital electrons (−1; 0.511 MeV). As Bowland described, four fundamental forces hold these subatomic particles together: the strong force ($10^1$ N), electromagnetic or coulomb force ($10^{-2}$ N), weak force ($10^{-13}$ N), and gravitational force ($10^{-42}$ N). The strong nuclear force acts over a short range ($10^{-14}$ m), keeping an atom's protons from repelling one another because of the similar electrostatic charge. The coulomb force of attraction binds orbital electrons to the nucleus so that the closer an electron is to the nucleus, the higher the binding energy of the electron. As described later, the strength of the binding energy of orbital electrons relates to the interaction of radiation on matter and its subsequent biologic effects. The chemical identity of an atom relates to its number of protons, and this number identifies the atom's atomic number (Z). The neutron number (N) varies among atoms and increases as the atomic number increases to stabilize the nucleus. An atom's atomic mass number (A) is approximately the sum of the proton number and the neutron number (A = Z + N). Radionuclides are represented by the following notation: $^{A}X$.

When an atom is neutral, it has no electric charge, meaning that the number of protons equals the number of electrons. If incident energy is transferred to an atom, an ionization event can occur whereby the atom acquires a positive or negative charge. When a charge is acquired, an atom is said to be ionized. Removal of an orbital electron results in an atom with a positive charge; the energy required to strip an electron off an atom must exceed the binding energy of that particular electron. Addition of an orbital electron results in an atom with a negative charge. This can occur when an electron passes close enough to an atom to experience a strong attractive force from the nucleus. Atoms can also undergo excitation, a process whereby an incident particle's energy is not sufficient to eject an atom's orbital electron but rather raises one or more electrons to a higher orbital energy state. It is through these types of interactions in atoms that radiation therapy elicits biologic consequences within tissues.

Radiation itself can be defined as the emission and propagation of energy through space or a physical medium. Radiation can be particulate, meaning that units of matter with discrete mass and momentum propagate energy (e.g., alpha particles, protons, neutrons, electrons), or it can be electromagnetic (photons), meaning that energy travels in oscillating electric and magnetic fields that have no mass and no charge, with a velocity of the speed of light ($c = 3.8 \times 10^8$ m/sec). Both particulate radiation and electromagnetic radiation can ionize atoms, events that occur randomly throughout the medium.

In the treatment of gynecologic malignancies, the most common source of radiation is electromagnetic (photon) radiation. Photons are generally referred to as *x-rays* (extranuclear or from the atom) or *gamma rays* (from the nucleus) based on their origin. Important properties of a photon include its wavelength ($\lambda$), frequency ($\nu$), speed $c = (\lambda\nu)$, and energy $E = (h\nu)$, where $h$ is Planck's constant. A photon's energy (E) is proportional to its frequency—that is, higher energies are transmitted at a higher frequency. Because the frequency of a photon is inversely proportional to the wavelength, electromagnetic radiation with a shorter wavelength has a higher frequency and thus a higher energy. As Kahn described in his textbook on the physics of radiation therapy, the energy that is produced is measured in electron volts, 1 eV = $1.6 \times 10^{-19}$ J, and it takes approximately 34 eV to generate one ion pair in water. The photons used to treat gynecologic malignancies can be generated externally at a distance from the woman's tumor (teletherapy) or internally, close to the woman's tumor (brachytherapy). Teletherapy x-ray radiotherapy units can deliver a range of photon energies from 50,000 eV (50 keV) to more than 30 MeV, depending on their radiation source or linear accelerator design. Nuclear decay of radioactive isotopes generates the gamma ray photons used in brachytherapy; such decay or disintegration was measured historically in a unit called a *curie (Ci)*. One Ci is defined as $3.7 \times 10^{10}$ disintegrations/

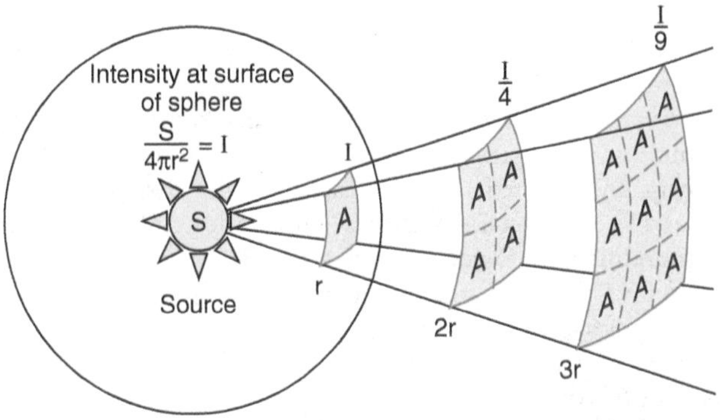


**Figure 27.2** Inverse square law. Radiation intensity decreases with the square of the distance away from a point source of radiation. The intensity *(I)* of radiation at any given radius *(r)* is the source strength *(S)* divided by the area *(A)* of the sphere. For example, the energy intensity three times as far from a point source is spread over nine times the area—hence, one ninth the intensity.

sec, which is equivalent to the rate of disintegration of 1 g of radium. The modern standard unit for activity is the becquerel (Bq), which is 1 disintegration/sec, or $2.7 \times 10^{-11}$ Ci.

Regardless of the source of electromagnetic or photon radiation, the transmitted energy diverges as the distance it travels from the source increases. This divergence causes a decrease in energy, a relationship described by the inverse square law. The inverse square law states that the energy dose of radiation per unit area decreases proportionately to the square of the distance from the site to the source ($1/r^2$). For example, the dose of radiation 3 cm from a point source is only one ninth of the value of the dose at 1 cm (Fig. 27.2) (Bowland, 2000; Kahn, 2003).

## THERAPEUTIC RADIATION PRODUCTION

In general, two techniques are used in radiation therapy treatment: teletherapy (external) and brachytherapy (internal). Teletherapy in the form of external beam radiation treatment produces ionizing radiation through radioactive decay of unstable radionuclides such as cobalt ($^{60}Co$) or, more commonly, through acceleration of electrons. In a typical $^{60}Co$ teletherapy unit, the shielded $^{60}Co$ source resides in a treatment head mounted to a gantry that has a 360-degree rotation around the patient. Collimators consisting of interleaved bars or custom-made blocks of high Z materials can shape the treatment beam to conform the dose to the target volume. With the decay of each $^{60}Co$ atom, two gamma ray photons are emitted at 1.17 and 1.33 MeV (average, 1.25 MeV). Over a specified time limit of exposure, these gamma ray photons deliver a specific radiation dose. Absorbed radiation dose is measured in a unit called a *gray* (1 Gy = 1 J/kg). Typical dose rates are 3 Gy/min at 80 cm from the source. The $^{60}Co$ source decays with a half-life of 5.263 years; thus the source must be replaced every 5 to 7 years.

In a typical linear accelerator teletherapy unit, electrons are "boiled" off a filament and accelerated under vacuum along an accelerating waveguide using alternating microwave fields. These accelerated electrons can be used to treat the patients themselves or can hit a high Z material transmission target to produce photons of various energies by an interaction known as *bremsstrahlung,* which means braking radiation. Currently, most treatment machines generate photon energies of 4 to 20 MeV and, similar to $^{60}Co$ teletherapy units, have 360-degree gantry rotation around a patient. Typical linear accelerator dose rates are 3 Gy/min at 100 cm from the source. It is important to realize key differences between these two types of treatment machines: (1) a $^{60}Co$ unit is always "on" when the source is not shielded because radioactive decay always occurs, whereas a linear accelerator is "on" only when energized because there is no radionuclide source; (2) the photon spectra are different in that $^{60}Co$ has a discrete average monoenergetic energy, whereas linear accelerators produce photons of variable energies and an average energy of one third the maximum generated energy; and (3) $^{60}Co$ produces treatment beams using only gamma ray photons, whereas a linear accelerator produces treatment beams of electrons or x-ray photons, depending on its treatment mode.

Alternate forms of teletherapy treatment are available, but they are rarely used to treat gynecologic malignancies. A teletherapy radiation dose can be delivered using alpha particles (helium nucleus), neutrons, or protons. Alpha particles produce a large number of ionizations over a short distance, but they have limited use as a mode of therapy because of their short range in tissue. Neutrons are highly penetrating into tissue because of their lack of charge; they cause high-energy collisions with atomic nuclei, principally of hydrogen, to produce recoil protons that then lose energy in surrounding tissues by ionization. Accelerated protons, as positively charged particles, used as therapy deposit a radiation dose sparingly along their path until near the end of their range, where the peak dose is delivered, the so-called *Bragg peak.* Neutron and proton therapies are used to treat cancer but are not used routinely in the treatment of gynecologic malignancies.

To produce a consequential radiobiologic effect in tissues or tumor, incident photons or other forms of radiation must interact with matter. Kahn has noted that there are five possible electromagnetic (photon) interactions with matter (Kahn, 2003):

1. *Coherent scattering* (<10 keV) occurs when an incident photon scatters off an atom's outer orbital electron without losing energy. This produces no radiobiologic effect.
2. *Photoelectric effect* (10 to 60 keV) occurs when an incident photon interacts with an inner orbital electron and the photon's energy is completely absorbed by that electron. If enough energy is transferred to the orbital electron to exceed the binding energy of the inner orbital electron, it is ejected, leaving a vacancy that an outer orbital electron fills. When an outer orbital electron fills the vacancy, a characteristic x-ray is produced with energy equal to the difference in binding energy between the two electron orbitals. The probability of a photoelectric effect event happening is proportional to $Z^3/E^3$. Diagnostic radiographic or computed tomography (CT) images that are acquired at relatively low photon energies have high tissue–bone contrast detail because the $Z^3/E^3$ ratio is maximized.
3. *Compton effect* (60 keV to 10 MeV) occurs when an incident photon ($E\gamma$) loses some or all of its energy to an outer orbital electron. The photon, if it remains, is scattered at some angle away from the atom. An electron that has acquired energy exceeding its binding energy ($E_{BE}$) leaves the atom with sufficient kinetic energy ($E_{KE} = E\gamma - E_{BE}$) to penetrate tissue and

produce molecular damage through downstream ionizations. For simplicity, at common therapeutic photon energies (4 to 18 MeV), the Compton effect is biologically most important in that incident photons interact predominantly with cellular water. Human and mammalian tissues are principally composed of water (≈90%) and functional biomolecules such as proteins and DNA (Fig. 27.3). Incident photons ionize water to produce an ion radical ($H_2O^+$) and a free electron ($e^-$). The ion radical is highly reactive (half-life of $10^{-10}$ second) and can interact with another molecule of water to form a hydroxyl radical (ĊOH). Hydroxyl radicals are also highly reactive (half-life of $10^{-9}$ second) and can break chemical bonds in target molecules such as proteins and DNA (ĊR). Breaks in the chemical bonds of DNA can lead to DNA base damage, DNA cross-links, DNA single-strand breaks, and DNA double-strand breaks. As discussed later, DNA strand breaks can result in the loss of vital genomic material during subsequent cell divisions, potentially leading to mitotic death of the damaged cell. In this way, therapeutic radiation leads to significant radiobiologic effects by functionally modifying cellular proteins and damaging DNA.

4. *Pair production* (>10 MeV) occurs when an incident photon has an energy greater than 1.022 MeV. This threshold is required because the photon disappears to form an electron-positron pair, with each particle having an energy of 0.511 MeV. Once formed, free electrons slow by nuclear attraction and are quickly stopped in tissue. However, the formed positron is highly reactive and short-lived in that it is annihilated with surrounding electrons to create two photons of 0.511 MeV, each traveling 180 degrees apart from one another. Positron emission tomography (PET) scanners build images based on the coincident detection of photons formed by this process.
5. *Photodisintegration* (>10 MeV) occurs when an energetic photon penetrates the nucleus of an atom and dislodges a neutron. Emitted neutrons cannot ionize tissue themselves because they have no charge; rather they collide with surrounding atomic nuclei to produce recoil, positively charged protons that elicit radiobiologic effects through subsequent ionizations.

## Radiation Biology

Munro has shown that nuclear DNA is unquestionably one essential target of therapeutic radiation (Munro, 1970). In his textbook on radiobiology, Hall reported that one third of radiation-induced DNA damage is from the direct interaction of incident photons ionizing atoms within DNA itself (Hall, 2000). Two thirds of radiation-induced DNA damage is a consequence of the indirect damage done by freely diffusing hydroxyl radicals (ĊOH). However, Hall and Hei described a bystander effect whereby lethal damage to cellular proteins, organelles, or the cell membrane in an irradiated cell can lead to neighboring cell death in cells that would not have died on their own (Hall, 2003). The bystander effect suggests that damage to cellular proteins or organelles in one cell may also result in cell lethality. Note that not all radiation damage is lethal to the cell; some damage to DNA can undergo repair—namely, sublethal DNA damage repair. Sublethal DNA damage repair occurs in normal cells and malignant cells, but it occurs much less so in malignant cells because these often have abnormal

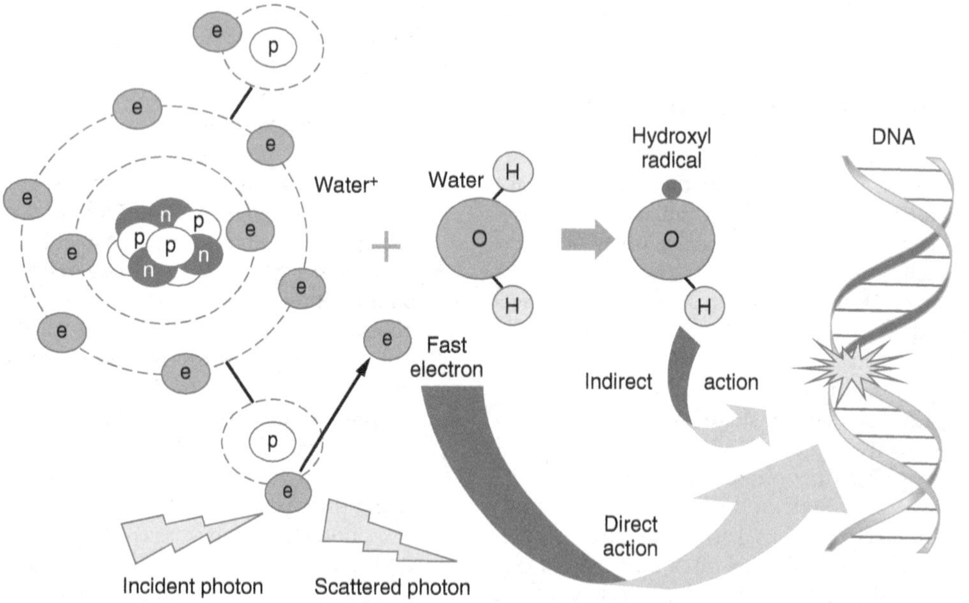


**Figure 27.3** Compton effect. Cells are composed of biomolecules dissolved in an aqueous solution (≈90% water by weight). Incident photons *(p)* randomly ionize *(left)* cellular water to produce an ion radical (water$^+$) and a free fast electron ($e^-$) that can damage biomolecules such as DNA. The water ion radical interacts with another molecule of water to form a hydroxyl radical (ĊOH). Most often (≈66%), formed hydroxyl radicals diffuse throughout the cell, breaking chemical bonds in target molecules such as proteins and DNA *(right)*. Breaks in the chemical bonds of DNA can lead to DNA base damage, DNA cross-links, DNA single-strand breaks, and DNA double-strand breaks, contributing to the loss of vital genomic material during subsequent cell divisions and possibly mitotic death of the damaged cell.

DNA repair mechanisms. A variety of complex and redundant repair mechanisms have been identified, including base excision repair and nucleotide excision repair for damage to the DNA base and deoxyribose backbone, homologous recombination repair for DNA single-strand breaks, and nonhomologous end-joining repair for DNA double-strand breaks. As the time interval between radiation doses lengthens, cell survival increases because of the prompt repair of radiation-induced damage. The repair process is usually complete within 1 to 2 hours, although this period may be longer in some slowly renewing cellular tissues. Before discussing the consequences of DNA damage, it is important to understand key factors that can modify the rate at which DNA damage accumulates.

Intracellular molecular oxygen importantly modifies radiation-induced DNA damage as it fixes damage done by free hydroxyl radicals. Palcic and Skarsgard reported that molecular oxygen, when present during or within microseconds of photon-induced ionization events, reacts with the altered chemical bonds of ionized molecules (ċR) to produce organic peroxides ($RO_2$), a nonreparable form of the target molecule (Palcic, 1984). Molecules fixed in this manner are permanently altered and may function abnormally. Thus tumor and tissue oxygenation have practical implications in radiation therapy insofar as a rapidly proliferating gynecologic malignancy may have a poor blood supply, which decreases tumor cell oxygenation, particularly at the center of large tumors. Tumor tissue hypoxia leads to radiation resistance, as reflected by increased cell survival after radiation treatment (Dunst, 2003). Laboratory experiments have shown that the radiation dose necessary to kill the same proportion of hypoxic cells as compared with aerated cells approaches 3:1 (Siemann, 2003). This ratio is commonly referred to the *oxygen enhancement ratio.* For oxygen to have its maximal effect, the dissolved oxygen concentration in a tumor must be approximately 3 mm Hg (venous blood is 30 to 40 mm Hg), according to Hall (Hall, 2000). In the treatment of gynecologic malignancies, Dunst and coworkers found that cervical cancer patients undergoing radiation therapy with a serum hemoglobin level greater than 10 mg/dL have improved tumor oxygenation, resulting in superior local control and superior clinical outcomes compared with patients whose hemoglobin level is less than 10 mg/dL (Dunst, 2003). Also, hypoxic cell sensitizers such as the nitroimidazoles, as studied by Adams and colleagues, and the bioreductive drug tirapazamine, as reported by Goldberg and coworkers, improve the radiosensitivity of hypoxic cells within tumors (Adams, 1991; Goldberg, 2001). The potential benefit of these agents in the treatment of gynecologic cancers has been explored in clinical trials.

The rate at which energy is lost per unit path length of medium, or linear energy transfer (LET), also has an effect on the accumulation of radiation-induced DNA damage. For photons, energy loss is infrequent along its path length, typical of low-LET radiation. Sparsely ionizing, low-LET radiation produces one or more sublethal events and thus multiple hits are needed to kill the cell. Heavy particulate radiation from alpha particles or protons is densely ionizing because energy is deposited more diffusely along its path length. This is typical of high-LET radiation. Because the probability of producing a lethal event in a cell is much higher with high- LET radiation, cell death in this case is independent of tumor oxygenation. Thus research efforts have been directed toward the development of heavy particle generators that can overcome the limitation of poor oxygenation of cancer cells.

Within the cell, molecules that have sulfhydryl moieties at one end and a strong base such as an amine at the other end are capable of scavenging free radicals produced by radiation-induced ionization events. These molecules can also donate hydrogen atoms to ionized molecules before molecular oxygen can fix the damage done by radiation-induced hydroxyl radicals. As Utley and associates reported, amifostine is a nonreactive phosphorothioate that accumulates (1) readily in normal tissues by active transport to be metabolized into an active compound to scavenge free radicals and (2) slowly in tumors by passive diffusion, with limited or no conversion to the active compound (Utley, 1976). It is reasonable to conclude that the presence of a radioprotector such as amifostine would decrease radiation-induced DNA damage and limit normal tissue radiation-related side effects. Clinical trials have been investigating the radioprotective effect of amifostine in gynecologic malignancies but, at present, amifostine has shown the most promise as a chemoprotectant and has been approved to reduce the renal toxicity associated with repeated administration of cisplatin chemotherapy in women with advanced ovarian cancer.

What constitutes cell death in the traditional sense—cessation of cellular respiration and vital function—is not the same in radiation biology. Death in radiation biology is the loss of reproductive integrity or the inability to maintain uninterrupted cellular proliferation with high fidelity. Thus radiation kills without the actual physical disappearance of malignant cells, although body macrophages often remove the dead cells, causing tumors to shrink in size. Malignant cells may remain a part of a tumor but have discontinued cellular metabolism and proliferation. Most cells, when exposed to radiation, die a mitotic death, meaning that cells die at the next or a subsequent cell division, with all progeny also dying. Inflammation can accompany mitotic cell death, potentially resulting in local adverse side effects. Jonathan and associates noted that alternative forms of loss in reproductive capacity caused by radiation include terminal differentiation, senescence, and apoptosis (Jonathan, 1999). In apoptosis, cells undergo a complex process of programmed cellular involution and phagocytosis by neighboring cells. There is no inflammatory response resulting from apoptosis. One remarkable example of apoptosis is the formation of the spaces between the digits of the hand during human fetal development.

Returning to radiation-induced DNA damage, electromagnetic radiation (x-ray or gamma) deposits energy in cells, which may damage DNA directly or indirectly through hydroxyl radicals (OH). In relative terms, more than 1000 DNA base-damaging events, 1000 DNA single-strand breaks, and 40 DNA double-strand breaks occur with each typical radiation dose fraction. Although base and DNA single-strand breaks must be repaired so that mutations are not propagated, DNA double-strand breaks are believed to be the most crucial radiobiologic effect of radiation therapy. There is an increased statistical probability that a cell will be unable to repair a DNA double-strand break, resulting in the loss of genetic material at cell division. Also, attempts by cells to repair the DNA double-strand breaks often result in bizarre chromosome arrangements that interfere with the normal division of the cell. Cell death ensues through loss of critical genes or impaired cell division.

Cell death following radiation therapy is modeled by a linear-quadratic relationship (Fig. 27.4). The initial slope of the cell survival curve is shallow and curvilinear, whereas the terminal slope is more linear. In the low-dose region of the survival curve typical of daily-dose fractions used in radiation therapy, the fraction of cells surviving is high because of the repair of single-event sublethal damage (e.g., multiple base damage or DNA single-strand breaks). In the high-dose region of the survival curve, the fraction of cells surviving is low because of multiple event damage in the form of DNA double-strand breaks or the accumulation of too many sublethal events that can be repaired before the next cell division. Capacity to repair sublethal damage depends on radiation quality (LET), tissue oxygenation, and cell cycle time.

As shown in Figure 27.5 and as described by Deshpande and associates and Pawlik and Keyomarsi, there are four highly regulated phases of the cell cycle (Deshpande, 2005; Pawlik, 2004). After completing mitosis, cells enter a gap phase (G1), variable in time span, in which the cell performs protein synthesis and other functional metabolic and biologic processes. Under the influence of complex, finely regulated intercellular and intracellular signaling, cells then enter the DNA replication phase (S phase) in which the cell must exactly replicate its DNA to produce an identical set of chromosomes. Entry into the S phase is controlled by sequentially activated, highly regulated cyclin-dependent kinases (CDKs) responsible for differentially recruiting and amplifying specific gene products necessary for DNA replication. Moreover, there are corresponding cell cycle inhibitory proteins (CDKIs) that negatively regulate cell cycle progression. After DNA replication, the cell enters a second gap phase (G2), in part to ensure high DNA replication fidelity in the newly formed chromosomes. At the completion of the G2 phase, cells undergo mitosis, whereby two identical daughter cells are produced.

To maintain genetic integrity through the cell cycle, the cell has multiple checkpoints through which it must pass, notably at the G1/S and G2/M transitions, as described by Pawlik and Keyomarsi (Pawlik, 2004). The G1/S checkpoint prevents the replication of damaged DNA, as in the case of radiation therapy. Malumbres and Barbacid have reported that proteins critical to the G1/S checkpoint include p53, p21, and the retinoblastoma protein (Rb), all of which modulate the activity of CDKs responsible for the transition to S phase (Malumbres, 2001). Briefly, Rb lacks phosphorylated subunits in its active form, binding to the E2F transcription factors and preventing E2F translocation to the nucleus to recruit genes needed for the S phase. Sequential phosphorylation of RB by CDK 4/6-cyclin D and CDK2-cyclin E complexes releases the E2F transcription factors. Radiation-induced DNA damage results in the accumulation of the G1 checkpoint regulatory protein p53, which in turn activates the CDKI p21; p21 inhibits the phosphorylation of RB, delaying the G1/S transition. The G2/M checkpoint prevents the segregation of aberrant chromosomes at mitosis. Two molecularly distinct checkpoints have been identified, one that is regulated by the ataxia-telangiectasia mutated gene product (ATM) and one that is ATM-independent. ATM has multiple phosphorylation products that modulate CDKs at the G2/M transition (Chk1 and Chk2) as well as p3 expression through modification of its degradation pathway. According to Xu and associates, phosphorylation of Chk1 and Chk2 inhibits the cdc2 protein kinase, blocking cells at the G2/M transition (Xu, 2002). ATM's essential role in DNA damage recognition is highlighted by the extreme radiosensitivity of patients with mutated ATM. Malignant cells that often have mutated cell cycle checkpoint proteins have an impaired ability to repair damage done to nuclear DNA

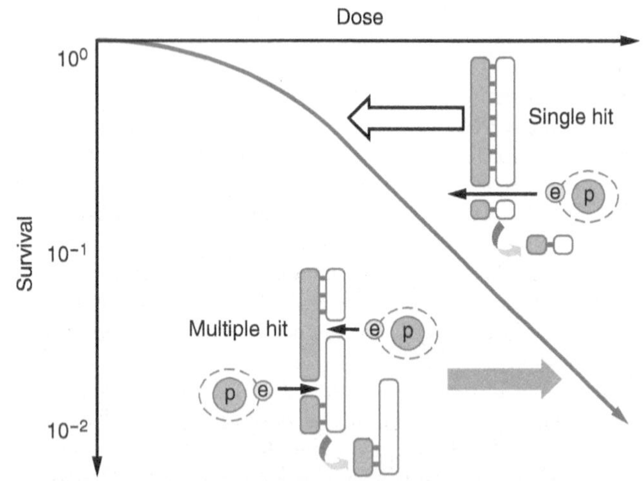


**Figure 27.4** Cell survival curves. A radiation survival curve plots cell survival on a logarithmic scale against radiation dose on a linear scale. Survival represents the number of cells retaining reproductive capacity to form approximately 50 cell colonies (i.e., approximately five to six cell divisions) after a specified radiation dose. The initial slope is shallow, forming a shoulder in the low-dose region (1 to 3 Gy/fraction) caused by repair of sublethal damage. Occasionally, a single hit will produce a DNA double-strand break, resulting in the loss of genetic material *(open arrow)*. In the high-dose region (>3 Gy/fraction), the slope steepens because of multiple damaging events leading to DNA double-strand breaks. If not repaired, significant vital genetic material may be lost at a subsequent cell division and the cell may die. *e*, Electron; *p*, photon.

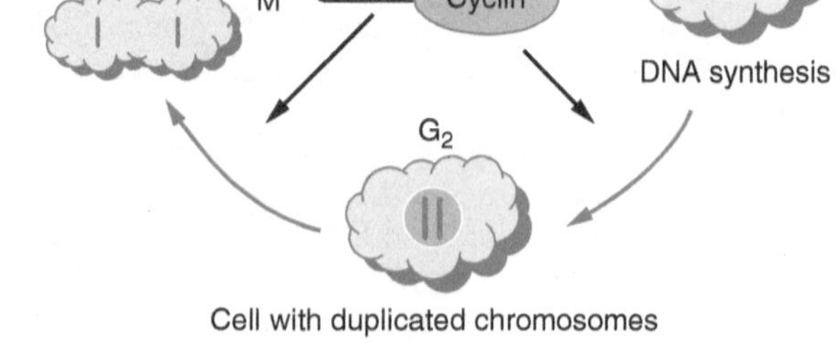

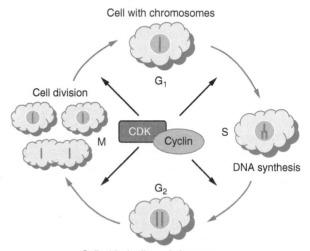


**Figure 27.5** Phases of the cell. After mitosis *(M)*, there is an interval of variable duration during which there is RNA and protein synthesis and a diploid DNA content (G1 [Gap1]). The cell may also enter a prolonged or resting phase (G0) and then reenter the cycle during DNA synthesis, the S phase, in which DNA is duplicated. During the G2 (Gap2) phase, there again is protein and RNA synthesis. During the M phase, the cell divides into two cells, each of which receives diploid DNA content. *CDK*, Cyclin-dependent kinase.

and thus accumulate lethal DNA-damaging events that lead to cell kill in a few cell cycles.

Cells show different radiosensitivities during the cell cycle. M-phase cells are particularly radiosensitive because the DNA is packaged tightly into chromosomes, so ionization events have a high likelihood of causing lethal DNA double-strand breaks. S-phase cells are particularly radioresistant because enzymes responsible for ensuring high-fidelity DNA replication are relatively overexpressed and recognize altered DNA bases or inappropriate strand breaks. Cells in the G1 or G2 phase of the cell cycle are relatively radiosensitive compared with the S phase. Chemotherapies that inhibit cell cycle–dependent pathways or impede DNA repair enhance the radiobiologic effect of radiation (Amorino, 1999; Lawrence, 2003).

## RADIATION TREATMENT: BRACHYTHERAPY AND TELETHERAPY

In general, two techniques are used in radiation treatment: brachytherapy (internal) and teletherapy (external). Brachytherapy involves the placement of radioacve sources within an existing body cavity (e.g., the vagina) in close proximity to the tumor. In the treatment of gynecologic malignant tumors, radioactive sources can be placed within hollow needles that are implanted directly into the tissue to be irradiated (interstitial implant) or within a hollow cylinder, or they can be inserted in tandem into the uterus through the cervical os, respectively. For the treatment of cervical cancer, two vaginal ovoids, one on each side of the tandem, are positioned in the vaginal fornices (intracavitary therapy). The most widely used intracavitary applicator is the Fletcher-Suit applicator, which is useful for the treatment of a cervical tumor or a tumor located near the cervix (Fig. 27.6). For interstitial and intracavitary brachytherapy, the radiation dose delivery to the tumor and surrounding tissues follows the inverse square law as modified by source and tissue photon attenuation. With the increased use of high-dose rate brachytherapy, a tandem and ring may be used where the ring replaces the ovoids (see Fig. 27.6). In the past, interstitial or intracavitary brachytherapy needles or applicators without radioactive sources are placed first in the operating room with the patient under anesthesia. After postanesthesia patient recovery, the position of the needles or applicators is confirmed by radiographic imaging. These radiographic images help guide radiotherapy planning. With the increased use of high-dose brachytherapy described later, the majority of patients are just sedated or spinal anesthesia is used during the procedure. The instruments are placed and then the patient undergoes imaging, usually a CT or magnetic resonance imaging (MRI) scans, and planning is done on these images instead of plain films. Once the plan is completed, the patient is treated in the radiation oncology department and then released to go home. The approximately time for the entire procedure varies from 3 to 5

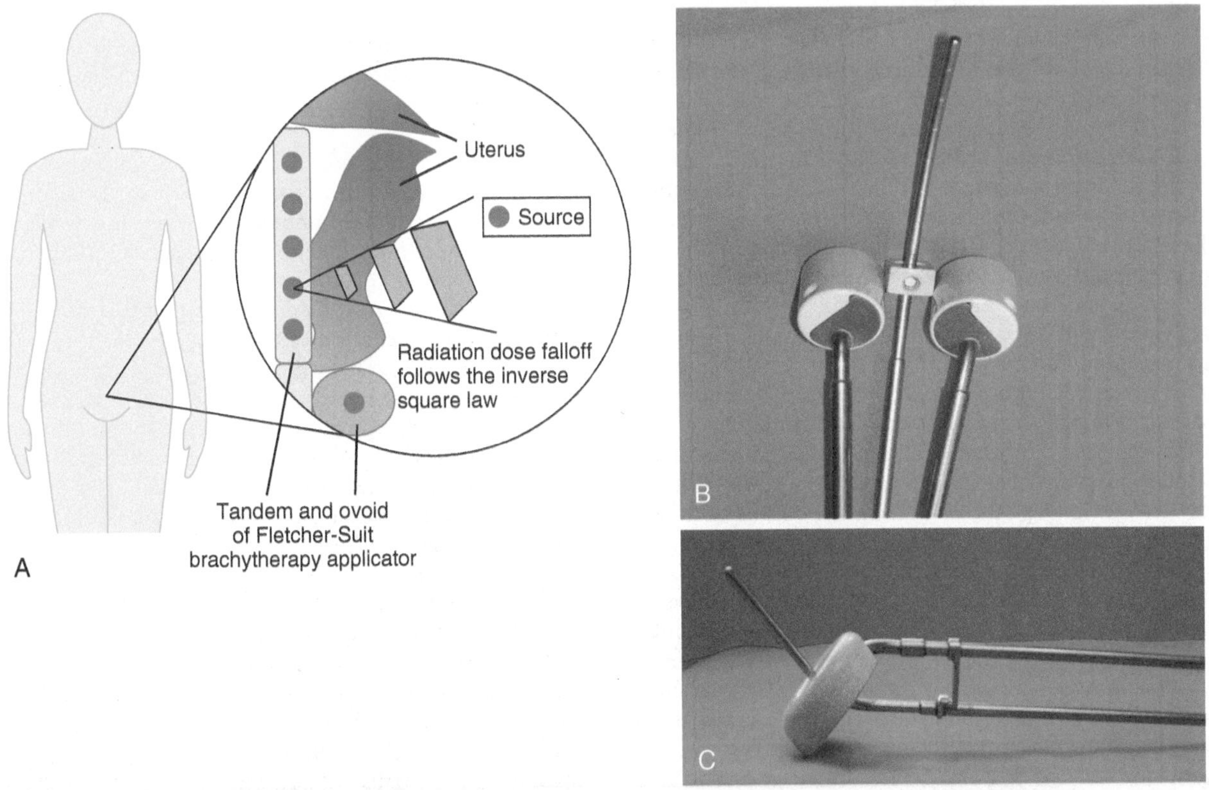


**Figure 27.6** Brachytherapy. For the treatment of gynecologic malignancies, brachytherapy usually consists of the placement of radiation sources *(dark circles)* in close proximity to the tumor (**A**). This can be accomplished by the intracavitary placement of hollow applicators such as the Fletcher-Suit applicator *(inset)* (**B**) or tandem and ring (**C**) placed within the uterine cavity and vaginal vault or by the interstitial placement of hollow needles through the tissues themselves. The radiation dose decreases as the square of the distance away from the radiation source.

hours. The entire procedure is done on an outpatient basis and is usually repeated three to six times, usually twice a week.

Several radioisotopes with various photon energies and half-lives are used in gynecologic brachytherapy. Although uncommon, radioisotopes with a short half-life (e.g., $^{198}$Au [gold]) may be placed within the woman and left permanently. Radioisotopes with a long half-life (e.g., $^{137}$Cs [cesium]) are placed temporarily within interstitial or intracavitary needles or applicators and are removed after a prescribed radiation dose has been administered. Historically, brachytherapy for most gynecologic malignancies consisted of temporary low-dose rate (40 to 70 centigray [cGy]/hr) sources in place for 1 to 3 days. A low-dose rate requires that the woman be in a shielded hospital room with medical personnel supervision, on bed rest, with prolonged analgesia and prophylactic anticoagulation, and limited family contact during radiation dose administration. High-dose rate, catheter-based brachytherapy has become popular because the procedure can be performed in 1 day on an outpatient basis. The high-dose rate uses a thin wire tipped with iridium ($^{192}$Ir) to deliver radiation doses at rates exceeding 200 cGy/min. Unlike low-dose rate therapy, high-dose rate therapy is performed in a shielded treatment room requiring patient immobilization for a short period and minimal patient analgesia and anesthesia. Table 27.1 indicates the half-lives of some of the isotopes commonly used in treating gynecologic cancers. It is also important that a uniform distribution of radiation be achieved in the adjacent tissues to avoid hot spots, which can damage normal tissue, as well as cold spots, which can lead to reduced dose delivery to the tumor.

Teletherapy in the form of external beam radiotherapy means that the source of radiation is at a distance from the woman, sometimes located at a distance 5 to 10 times more than the depth of the tumor being irradiated. This distance is referred to as the *source-to-surface distance (SSD)* and is used to calculate dose using the inverse square law. When using an SSD patient treatment setup, the SSD is used along with tumor depth, radiation beam energy, depth of the point of maximum dose, and output parameters for a given treatment field size to determine the daily radiation dose. Alternatively, with the use of different angles and ports of treatment, the concept of source-axis distance has been introduced; it denotes the distance from the radiation source to the central axis of machine rotation. The woman is positioned so that this axis passes through the center of the tumor, and treatment ports are arranged around this axis to optimize tumor dose. When using a source-axis distance patient treatment setup, the daily radiation dose is calculated using machine output and beam attenuation at the depth for a given treatment field size.

Conventional external beam radiation is delivered with beams of uniform intensity. Advances in computer-guided planning and treatment have made the use of beams of varying intensity more commonplace. This approach of planned dose intensification allows the high-dose region to be conformed precisely to the shape of the planned treatment volume, a technique called *intensity-modulated radiotherapy (IMRT)*. The advantage of this technique is that there may be more sparing of normal tissue, especially small bowel, and therefore hopefully decrease both short-term and long-term toxicity (Fig. 27.7). Advances in radiotherapy delivery systems have allowed linear accelerators to be coupled with helical CT scanners. Image-guided radiation therapy using this type of device is called *helical tomotherapy*. In conventional therapy, and in intensity-modulated radiotherapy and helical tomotherapy,

**Table 27.1** Half-Lives of Commonly Used Radioisotopes for Gynecologic Malignancies

| Radionuclide | Half-Life |
|---|---|
| Gold ($^{198}$Au) | 2.7 days |
| Phosphorus ($^{32}$P) | 14.3 days |
| Iridium ($^{192}$Ir) | 73.8 days |
| Cobalt ($^{60}$Co) | 5.26 years |
| Cesium ($^{137}$Cs) | 30 years |
| Radium ($^{226}$Ra) | 1620 years |

beams from the external radiation source can be sculpted using high electron-dense material collimators. Collimators limit scatter radiation and block portions of the treatment beam from delivering an intolerant radiation dose to critical tissues (Fig. 27.8). In general, the higher the energy source of the radiation, the deeper the beam can penetrate into tissue. Thus high-energy radiation has its predominant effect in deeper tissues and spares the surface of the skin of a radiation effect.

An isodose curve is a line that connects points in the tissue that receive equivalent doses of irradiation. Figure 27.8 contrasts the isodose curves for 6- and 22-MeV machines. For the 6-MeV machine, the maximum dose is near the surface, with a more rapid falloff in the deeper tissues. For the 22-MeV machine, the maximum dose is deep to the surface, sparing the effects of radiation on the overlying skin. In addition to the energy of the beam, the energy of radiation absorbed at various depths is affected by the size of the field being treated. Larger fields contain more scattered radiation, which leads to a greater dose at a given depth. Figure 27.8 shows the effect of increasing the size of the field with an increasing dose at a given depth for three different types of energy sources.

Thus the radiation dose delivered to the tumor is affected by the energy of the source, depth of the tumor beneath the surface, and size of the field undergoing irradiation. With external therapy, usually 180 to 200 cGy/day is given five times per week.

### Tissue Tolerance and Radiation Complications

Adverse radiation effects are commonly divided into two broad categories, early and late, which demonstrate markedly different patterns of response to radiation dose fractionation. It is important for the treating physician to understand critical tissues and organ systems at risk of radiation damage. Table 27.2 presents the approximate tolerance of tissues to radiation therapy.

Early or acute effects manifest as the result of death in a large population of cells and can occur within days to weeks after the initiation of radiation therapy. For early effects, the total dose of radiation and, to a lesser extent, the dose per fraction determine the severity of the side effect. Radiation acutely affects tissues undergoing rapid cell division to replace lost normal functioning cells. This is most pronounced in areas such as the skin, intestinal mucosa, mucosa of the vagina and bladder, and hematopoietic system, in which precursor stem cells are renewing functional mature cells. The radiation dose given in multiple small fractions reduces the untoward adverse effects of cell damage on normal tissue and allows normal healing to occur between treatment fractions through sublethal DNA damage repair (the shallow curvilinear portion of the cell survival curve). During the treatment of gynecologic malignancies, most adverse early treatment-related toxicities can be managed with medication. It is preferred practice that radiation treatment not be interrupted for treatment-related

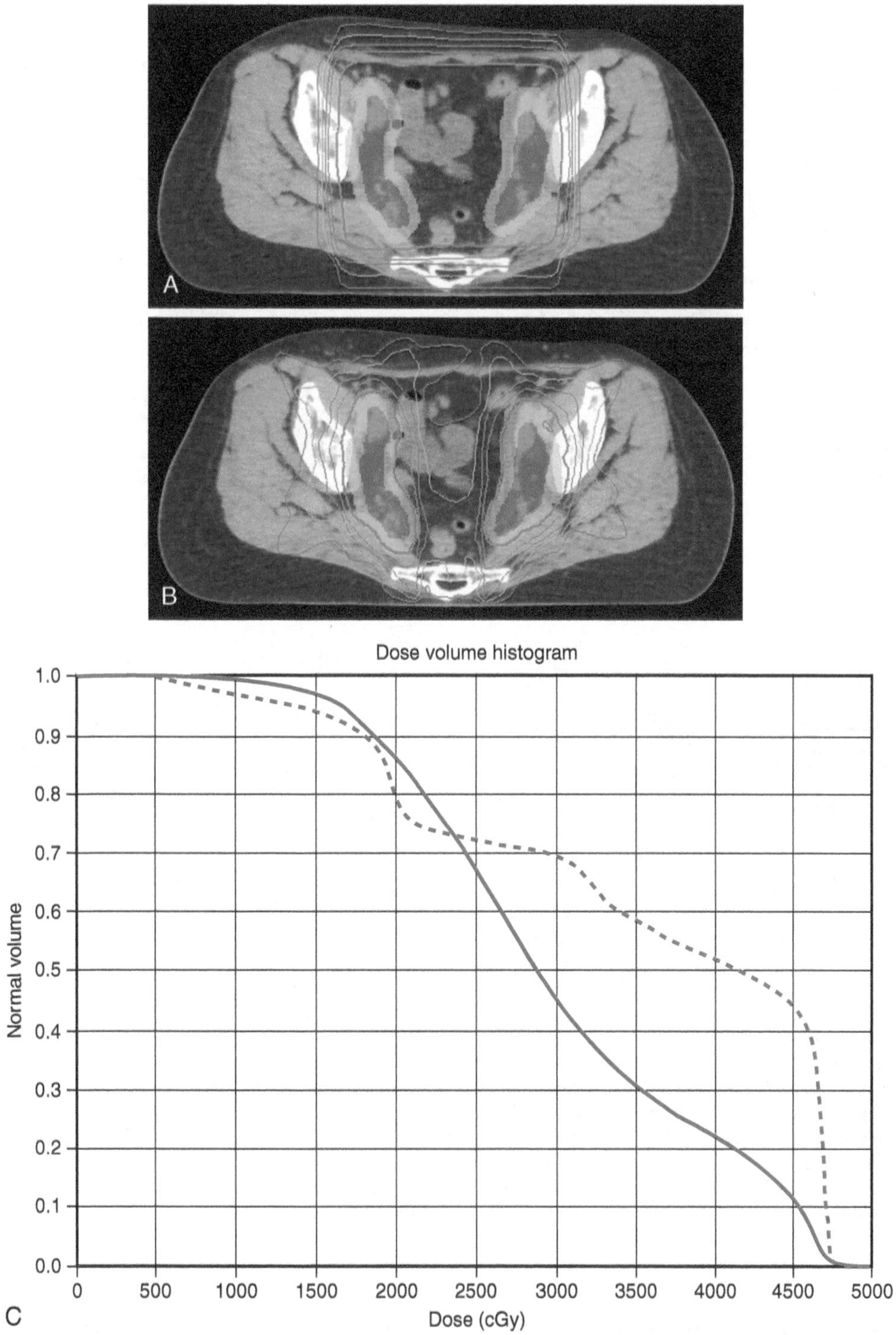


**Figure 27.7** Treatment plan. **A,** The distribution of dose with a standard three-dimensional (3D) plan. The red line is the 45 Gy isodose line and, as shown, everything within the red line gets 45 Gy, including all the bowel. **B,** The distribution of dose using IMRT. Again, the red line is the 45 Gy isodose line and what can clearly be seen is the sparing of bowel using IMRT. **C,** The dose to bowel—the dotted line is the bowel dose using the 3D plan and the solid line is the bowel dose using the IMRT plan. As shown, with IMRT, the bowel gets a less high dose compared to the 3D plan.

toxicities caused by radiation-induced tumor accelerated repopulation. Only rarely does a treatment program have to be temporarily discontinued for treatment-related toxicities.

Late effects occur after a delay of months or years after radiation therapy. Late effects are often the product of parenchymal connective tissue cell loss and vascular damage. Late effects may be seen in slowly renewing tissues such as the lung, kidney, heart, and liver and in the central nervous system. In the treatment of gynecologic malignancies, late adverse effects include tissue necrosis and fibrosis, as well as fistula formation and ulceration.

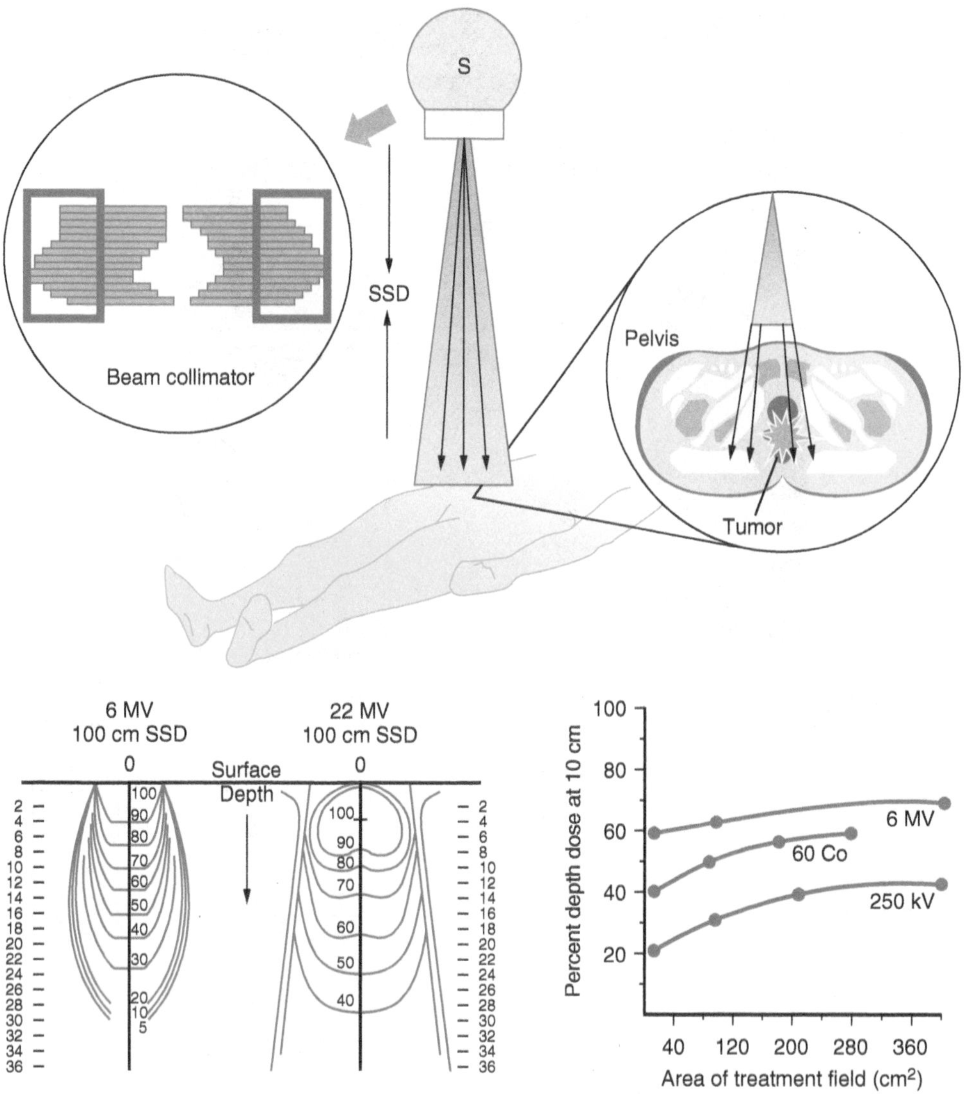


**Figure 27.8** Teletherapy. Conventional external beam radiotherapy is the delivery of radiation dose to tissues at a distance (SSD) away from the radiation source (S). As the beam emerges from the treatment machine, the beam diverges and can be shaped by high-Z material leaflets of a beam collimator *(top)* or custom blocks. As the treatment beam hits the patient, photon interactions occur, producing ionization events *(inset)*. Energy deposition within tissue creates isodose curves. Isodose curves and depth-dose distributions for 6- and 22-MV photons are shown *(bottom left)*. Note that the higher-energy machine delivers radiation to a greater depth for the same surface dose, resulting in skin sparing. As treatment field size varies, the dose delivered at a specified depth varies *(bottom right)*.

**Table 27.2** Normal Tissue Tolerance to Radiation Therapy

| Tissue | Tolerance (Gy) |
|---|---|
| Kidney | 20-23 |
| Liver | 25-35 |
| Small bowel | 45-50 |
| Rectum | 60-70 |
| Bladder | 60-70 |
| Vaginal mucosa | 70-75 |
| Cervix | >120 |

In contrast to early effects, late effects depend primarily on the dose per fraction. Fractionated radiation therapy using a daily radiation dose of 180 to 200 cGy minimizes the risk of late effects. Second cancers (mostly sarcomas) induced after radiation are rare (1 in 500 to 1000 cases) and do not usually appear until 15 to 20 years after radiation exposure. Arai and associates noted an excess of rectal cancer, bladder cancer, and leukemia in women with carcinoma of the cervix treated by radiation in comparison with those treated by surgery (Arai, 1991).

The skin overlying the tumor being treated visibly reveals the effects of radiation-induced normal tissue damage. Skin effects are manifest by reddening of the skin and loss of hair where the radiation treatment beam enters the body. Erythema may progress to dry or moist skin breakdown or desquamation caused by loss of the actively proliferating basal layer of the epidermis that renews the overlying epithelium. This is less common now than in prior years because higher energy radiation beams, which spare the surface dose, are used. However, during the treatment of vulvar malignancies, the skin surface and superficial groin nodes are the radiotherapeutic target, so desquamation is more commonly observed. Medical treatments consisting of non–metal-containing creams and emollients during therapy reduce discomfort and allow healing within 2 to 4 weeks after completion of radiation therapy. Late skin fibrosis may produce a rough, leathery texture to the skin in the irradiated field. Chiao and Lee as well as Gothard and coworkers have reported on the use of pentoxifylline and vitamin E to promote healing of late subcutaneous and deep tissue fibrosis after radiation (Chiao, 2005; Gothard, 2005).

In the treatment of gynecologic malignancies, other sites at risk of radiation-induced normal tissue damage are the bladder, rectum, and large and small bowel. The bladder epithelium consists of a basal layer of small diploid cells covered by large transitional cells. Radiation damage to the diploid cells results in slow renewal of the overlying transitional cells that are periodically sloughed off during urination. Radiation cystitis manifested as dysuria and urinary frequency results in bladder irritation. Treatment with analgesics such as phenazopyridine (Pyridium) can alleviate symptoms. Hematuria may also occur. Therapy with sclerosing solutions or fulguration through a cystoscope may be necessary. McIntyre and colleagues noted that ureteral stricture after radiation for stage I carcinoma of the cervix is 1% at 5 years and 2.5% at 20 years, a rare but important complication (McIntyre, 1995). In rare cases, urinary diversion may be required. Bladder fibrosis and reduced bladder capacity are late effects of pelvic radiation therapy.

In the intestine, the renewing stem cells are found at the bottom of the crypts of Lieberkuhn. Within 2 to 4 days after the start of radiation, these cells can become depleted, leading to atrophy of intestinal mucosa. Damage to the bowel usually occurs in the form of inflammation (sigmoiditis or enteritis), which commonly results in increased bowel motility or diarrhea but also, rarely, may be associated with severe bleeding and cramping pain. Less severe cases can often be controlled with a low-roughage diet and antispasmodic medications. Although uncommon, severe cases may require bowel resection or permanent bowel diversion through a colostomy. Covens and coworkers noted that those who require operation for radiation damage to the bowel have an approximately 25% risk of dying in 2 years, with ileal damage being the most risky (Covens, 1991). Those with complications not requiring surgery frequently have decreased vitamin $B_{12}$ and bile acid absorption. Late bowel toxicities include radiation proctitis caused by small vessel vascular damage in the epithelium, which may progress to intermittent rectal bleeding. Bowel stenosis or obstructions resulting from fibrosis and adhesion formation may occur, especially in patients who have had previous pelvic or abdominal surgery. Occasionally, enteric fistulas can develop, and bowel perforation may occur. In the latter case, surgical therapy is required, usually to bypass the affected area of the intestine. As a rule, extensive dissection of irradiated tissue is avoided. Montana and Fowler have shown that the risks of proctitis and cystitis are dose related (Montana, 1989). For example, they found severe proctitis and cystitis at doses of 6750 and 6900 cGy, respectively, whereas such complications were not observed in patients whose median dose was 6300 and 6500 cGy.

A lowering of circulating lymphocytes, granulocytes, platelets, and red blood cells can be seen with pelvic radiation therapy for gynecologic malignancies. The stem cells of the bone marrow in an adult reside in the axial skeleton (vertebrae, ribs, and pelvis). Usual external beam radiation therapy treatment fields for gynecologic malignancies encompass the sacrum and lower vertebrae and pelvis, thereby reducing precursor stem cells for circulating blood cells. This is an important consideration if the woman is to receive concurrent radiosensitizing chemotherapy or subsequent cytotoxic chemotherapy. Growth factor support with synthetic erythropoietin or granulocyte colony-stimulating factor (G-CSF) is often required for patients receiving multiagent chemotherapy following treatment with pelvic radiation therapy.

Finally, fistulas between the vagina and bladder or between the vagina and rectum may develop when there has been extensive radiation damage to the intervening tissues. This usually takes place during therapy for large carcinomas of the cervix. As a rule, such complications will occur 6 to 24 months after treatment, although they may occur many years after primary therapy. Diverting surgery or resection of the fistulas is often needed to correct these serious complications.

## CHEMOTHERAPY

Although many patients with gynecologic cancers present initially with a clinically appreciable mass or tumor, only a minority of patients have localized disease, curable with surgery or radiation treatment alone. More often, the cancer has spread to regional lymph nodes or disseminated to other organs, even though these sites may not be clinically appreciated at the time of initial diagnosis.

Chemotherapy regimens for gynecologic cancers have evolved since the 1940s. Initially, Li and colleagues demonstrated the first successful effort in gynecologic cancer using the antimetabolite methotrexate, which could cause permanent remission of metastatic trophoblastic disease (Li, 1956). Shortly thereafter, treatment regimens emerged with single-agent melphalan followed by single-agent cyclophosphamide. When cisplatin was introduced into clinical practice, it added significant improved activity to cyclophosphamide; this combination then became the standard of care. In the 1980s, clinical studies to evaluate paclitaxel for treatment of ovarian cancer were undertaken. Paclitaxel soon replaced cyclophosphamide and paclitaxel plus cisplatin became the standard of care for ovarian cancer and, since then, has become a popular treatment option for all gynecologic malignancies (McGuire, 1996; Piccart, 2003). Because of toxicity associated with cisplatin, numerous studies were conducted to justify substitution with carboplatin for cisplatin because of its improved toxicity profile, but controversy remains over which taxane or platinum agent is preferred (Ozols et al, 2003). Overall, the consensus is that primary chemotherapy should include a taxane and a platinum agent (Ozols, 2006).

**Box 27.1 Clinical Pearls**

- The use of intraperitoneal (IP) chemotherapy as first-line treatment of advanced ovarian cancer has been recommended by the National Comprehensive Cancer Network guidelines. The key lesson learned from the study by Armstrong and colleagues is that patient selection is critical for tolerability of this regimen. Those who are younger, with optimal tumor debulking, no significant bowel resection, and good organ function, will tolerate IP therapy better.
- Patient assessment prior to each regimen of chemotherapy is essential to minimize toxicity. This includes evaluation of complete blood count, liver function tests, and calculation of renal function. Consider the use of growth factors or dose adjustments as appropriate.

Historically, there has been no clear difference or advantage in regard to which taxane or platinum agent was used or which dose intensity was selected until the clinical trial by Katsumata and colleagues. This study suggested that there is an advantage with a weekly schedule or dose density compared with the standard platinum-taxane, every 3-week regimen (Katsumata, 2009). However, there are concerns about the toxicity associated with the dose-dense regimen; questions about the feasibility of this regimen have arisen with the typical older women seen in clinical practice, so a confirmatory Gynecologic Oncology Group (GOG 262) phase III study is ongoing.

In addition to dosing schedule, the route of chemotherapy administration has also been an area of research interest. For decades, many researchers have conducted numerous clinical trials of intraperitoneal (IP) chemotherapy. In 2006, Armstrong and colleagues published the first IP therapy clinical trial to demonstrate a survival advantage over the standard intravenous (IV) regimen (Box 27.1) (Armstrong, 2006). However, these advances in chemotherapy for the treatment of advanced ovarian cancer have not translated into major changes in overall 5-year survival, which remains less than 20%.

A number of general principles have been developed during the study of chemotherapeutic agents. These provide guidelines for their recommended use and administration (see Box 27.1).

## CHEMOTHERAPY PRINCIPLES AND GUIDELINES

Some of the concepts used in antibiotic therapy for infections have been applied to the chemotherapeutic approach to cancer management. However, major differences exist. Infections are frequently caused by a single virus or even multiple types of bacteria with specific growth patterns and sensitivities to antibiotics. Although it is believed that a cancer can originate from a single cell, clinically evident disease is composed of a heterogeneous population of cells with different cell cycle durations, varying growth fractions, and diverse expression of genes, potential mutations, and proteins responsible for cell proliferation and metastasis. Intrinsic and acquired drug resistance remains one of the daunting challenges in the treatment of gynecologic cancers.

Basic principles for cancer chemotherapy arose from experiments in murine tumor models, notably mice leukemias, conducted by Skipper and colleagues at the Southern Research Institute (Skipper, 1965). These principles include the following:

- *Fractional cell kill:* Each dose of chemotherapy kills a constant fraction of the tumor cell population. Tumor cell kill usually correlates in a linear relationship with the pharmacokinetic parameter of the area under the drug concentration curve (AUC).
- *Dose intensity:* High chemotherapy doses interspersed with short rest periods produce the greatest tumor cell kill in rapidly proliferating malignancies.
- *Drug resistance:* Single-agent chemotherapy administration selectively isolates drug-resistant tumor cells, leading to an outgrowth of hardy, resistant malignant cells. Chemotherapy drug resistance has been associated with the following: (1) cell-mediated modification of drug targets, (2) active drug transport out of the cell, and (3) alteration of drug activation or targeting.
- *Cell cycle dependency of cell kill:* Actively proliferating tumor cells are most often killed by chemotherapy agents; drugs inhibiting DNA processing act during the S phase and those impairing cell division act during the M phase. If the normal monitors of genomic integrity are intact, a cell may suspend the cell cycle to repair any detected damage. If, however, these monitors are abnormal, a cell may continue progression through the cell cycle, which may lead to unrecoverable cell cycle arrest or irreparable damage to critical genes vital for future cell survival. Malignant cancer cells often demonstrate abnormal monitors of genomic integrity, in part permitting their rapid proliferation but also increasing their sensitivity to chemotherapies.

## APPROACHES TO TREATMENT

The dose of an anticancer chemotherapy agent is usually calculated as a function of body surface area (square meters), which provides a better measure of potential toxicity than body weight. This is partly because of the observation that body surface area more closely reflects cardiac output and blood flow than body weight alone. Chemotherapeutic agents have varying toxicities (discussed later). A major problem with most agents is bone marrow toxicity, requiring careful monitoring of mature and stem cell turnover in the hematopoietic system. Most gynecologic cancer chemotherapy agents are administered intravenously in cycles varying from weekly to 3- or 4-week intervals between each cycle. If mature white blood cells (i.e., absolute neutrophil count) and platelets have not recovered adequately by the time the next cycle is due, treatment delay or a dose reduction is often considered. In patients with a history of prolonged myelosuppression or with regimens associated with significant myelosuppression, the proactive use of growth factor support is often helpful in allowing chemotherapy treatments to continue at full dose and on time, as scheduled.

Additional considerations about the toxicity of chemotherapeutic agents relate to hepatic metabolism or renal excretion. It may be necessary to modify the dose of the drug administered when renal or hepatic function is compromised. For example, consider the following:

- Doxorubicin (Adriamycin) and paclitaxel are metabolized in the liver, and dose reductions must be made if the drug is administered to a woman with hepatic dysfunction.

- Methotrexate and cisplatin effects are increased in patients with renal damage, necessitating dose reduction in these patients.
- Cisplatin not only has its effects intensified in patients with renal insufficiency but also is toxic to the kidney, requiring particular caution if administered to those with compromised renal function or those undergoing therapy with other renal toxic medications.

Plasma protein binding (PPB) can also alter toxicity profile. For example, paclitaxel and topotecan both are associated with PPB greater than 80%. When PPB drugs are displaced, the unbound or free fraction of drug increases, which may increase toxicity or the effects of chemotherapy. Furthermore, a low serum albumin level leads to an increase in the free fraction of the chemotherapeutic agent, which is one reason why malnourished patients have a heightened toxicity to chemotherapy.

Various chemotherapeutic agents can be differentially toxic to other organ systems of the body, including the gastrointestinal, nervous, pulmonary, and reproductive systems. The primary toxicities affecting gynecologic cancer patients are nausea and vomiting, prolonged myelosuppression, and neuropathies. Acute nausea and vomiting can usually be prevented with the combination of a serotonin antagonist with a steroid. Despite the introduction of newer agents such as aprepitant and palonosetron, delayed nausea and vomiting continue to constitute therapeutic challenges. Unfortunately there are limited options for the prevention and management of chemotherapy-induced neuropathy other than dose reduction or switching chemotherapy agents.

Myelosuppression is a manageable toxicity with most chemotherapy regimens. Prevention of myelosuppression with the use of a myeloid growth factor (e.g., G-CSF) has better efficacy than waiting until prolonged neutropenia develops. Although not often relevant for patients with gynecologic cancer, loss of ovarian function and fertility is often an important consideration when selecting adjuvant treatments for younger women with other cancers. The goal of treatment is to provide as high a dose of the chemotherapeutic agent at a planned frequency, as defined by clinical trial data to produce maximum chemotherapeutic effectiveness without causing unacceptable toxicity or side effects.

There are four ways in which chemotherapy is generally used for the treatment of gynecologic cancers: (1) as an induction treatment for advanced disease (neoadjuvant therapy) in a gynecologic setting, it is used to shrink tumor prior to surgery to improve the potential for optimal tumor debulking, which is followed by additional chemotherapy; (2) as an adjunct to radiation therapy; (3) as primary treatment for cancer in the gynecologic cancer setting, it is often administered after completion of tumor debulking surgery; or (4) as consolidation after a complete response is achieved to target undetectable microscopic disease.

In assessment of the effect of chemotherapeutic agents, a number of definitions are used to describe the response of the tumor being treated. Clinical response should be assessed on an individual basis, with tumors in some patients monitored by physical examination and in some patients through imaging, typically with CT or MRI. Other means of assessing response to therapy include serial assessment of specific tumor markers (e.g., cancer antigen 125 [CA-125] for ovarian cancer or β-human chorionic gonadotropin for gestational trophoblastic disease) or identification of changes in hypermetabolic foci by PET.

**Table 27.3** Response Evaluation Criteria in Solid Tumors (RECIST) Criteria to Assess Clinical Response to Therapy

| Criterion | Features |
|---|---|
| CR (complete response) | Disappearance of all target lesions |
| PR (partial response) | 30% decrease in sum of greatest diameters of target lesions |
| PD (progressive disease) | 20% increase in sum of greatest diameters of target lesions |
| SD (stable disease) | Small changes that do not meet the above criteria |

In 2000, an international committee endorsed a technique for measuring tumors by CT and MRI that is easy and highly reproducible. This is known as RECIST (***r***esponse ***e***valuation ***c***riteria ***i***n ***s***olid ***t***umors) and is applicable for subjects with at least one measurable target lesion. The greatest diameters of all target lesions are summed, and changes in this sum during treatment are used to assign response (Table 27.3).

## CHEMOTHERAPEUTIC AGENTS

A large number of chemotherapeutic drugs have been used in the treatment of gynecologic cancers (Fig. 27.9). In general, these agents can be classified into platinum compounds, taxanes, antitumor antibiotics, topoisomerase I inhibitors, alkylating agents, antimetabolites, vinca alkaloids, biologic and targeted therapy, and anticancer hormones. Agents currently used alone or in combination for the treatment of gynecologic cancer are discussed here.

### Platinum Analogues

Cisplatin and carboplatin are two of the most active and widely used chemotherapeutic agents in the treatment of gynecologic malignancies and are used in the primary treatment of ovarian, tubal, peritoneal, endometrial, cervical, and vulvar cancers, as well as some cases of metastatic gestational trophoblastic disease.

Platinum (PLT) analogues form PLT-DNA adducts that intercalate the DNA, interrupting DNA synthesis. Although its cell cycle specificity has not been clearly defined, cisplatin's radiosensitizing mechanisms include the formation of toxic intermediates in the presence of radiation-induced free radicals, radiation-induced increased cellular platinum uptake, inhibition of radiation-induced DNA repair, and cell cycle arrest at the G2-M transition. For the treatment of most gynecologic malignancies, cisplatin is given by an IV or IP infusion. Cisplatin is emetogenic but can be appropriately managed with serotonin antagonists. Hypomagnesemia is a problem in patients receiving cisplatin, often requiring frequent magnesium replacement. Because cisplatin is nephrotoxic, copious hydration and mannitol infusion usually accompany cisplatin administration to prevent renal tubular necrosis because the drug is excreted in the urine in its active form. Cisplatin also induces myelosuppression and high-frequency ototoxicity. Audiograms may be obtained before and during treatment to assess ototoxicity. Cisplatin induces severe peripheral neuropathy, which may improve somewhat after cessation of therapy but tends to be long lasting.

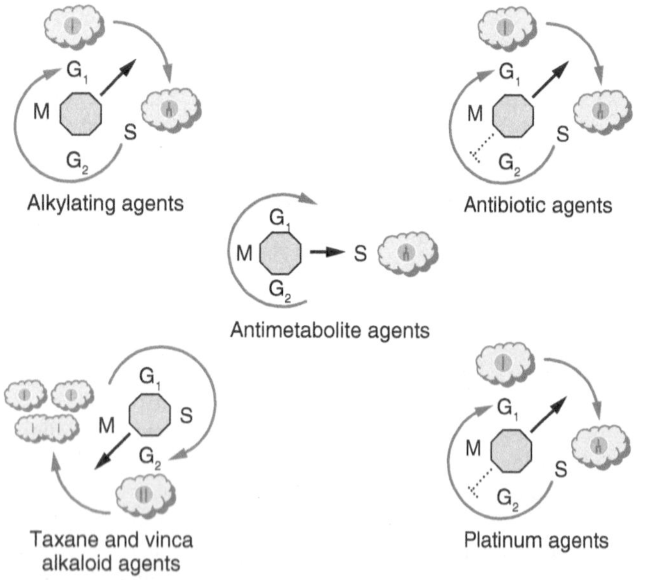


**Figure 27.9** Chemotherapy cell cycle activity. Chemotherapeutic agents demonstrate variable antitumor cytotoxic and radiosensitizing activities, depending on their mechanism of action during the cell cycle. Alkylating agents facilitate the transfer of alkyl groups to DNA, disrupting the G1/S transition *(top left)*. Agents derived from bacteria deregulate normal DNA and RNA processing, slowing progression through the G1/S and G2/M transitions *(top right)*. Antimetabolites result in faulty base insertion into replicated DNA or specifically inhibit rate-limiting enzymes such as ribonucleotide reductase that are needed to produce deoxyribonucleotides for DNA replication during the S phase *(center)*. Taxane and vinca alkaloid agents alter the mitotic spindle during mitosis, preventing cell division *(bottom left)*. Platinum agents show activity throughout the cell cycle and form DNA structural adducts, limiting progression at various cell cycle checkpoints. Chemotherapeutic agents themselves are cytotoxic but also increase tumor cell sensitivity to ionizing radiation during critical periods of the cell cycle in which radiation has a maximal effect. The safe combination of these various classes of chemotherapeutic agents and radiation is an area of active clinical research.

Carboplatin is an analogue of cisplatin; a study conducted by Ozols and colleagues has reported that it has activity in ovarian epithelial carcinoma comparable with that of cisplatin (Ozols, 2003). Its mechanism of action and antitumor activity throughout the cell cycle are similar to those of cisplatin, but carboplatin is less potent in producing DNA interstrand cross-links compared with cisplatin. Yang and coworkers found that the cellular uptake of carboplatin increases after ionizing radiation treatment with a concomitant increase in drug-DNA binding (Yang, 1995).

Carboplatin is dosed based on the woman's specific renal function. Often, the calculated creatinine clearance is used in place of the measured glomerular filtration rate (GFR) to estimate renal function. Carboplatin is dosed based on a target area under the curve (AUC) from 5 to 7 mg/mL *min; the dose is calculated using the Calvert formula:

$$\text{Dose (mg)} = \text{target AUC} \times (\text{GFR} + 25)$$

Although carboplatin is renally eliminated because of this dose algorithm, it is not associated with the degree of nephrotoxicity as cisplatin; thus rigorous prehydration is not required, allowing for it to be administered on an outpatient basis. The adverse drug effects associated with carboplatin include neurotoxicity, nausea, and vomiting, but to a lesser extent compared with cisplatin. Myelosuppression, primarily thrombocytopenia, is the dose-limiting toxicity (DLT) associated with carboplatin.

The DLT of carboplatin is myelosuppression, primarily thrombocytopenia, although neutropenia and anemia also occur. Typically, after dosing single-agent carboplatin, the nadir occurs between 15 and 20 days. Because carboplatin's typical dose is individualized based on the woman's specific renal function, it appears to have an improved toxicity profile. It is important to keep in mind that appropriate parameters must be used to estimate renal function to minimize toxicity. Less common toxicities include alopecia, hepatotoxicity, neurotoxicity, and ototoxicity.

Both platinum analogues can be associated with delayed hypersensitivity reactions. Because carboplatin is used more often in a recurrent setting, there are more hypersensitivity reactions reported with carboplatin. There is a high cross-sensitivity, so patients who react to one platinum agent will be at significant risk for another reaction if exposed to another platinum analogue. Desensitization protocols with complete histamine blockade (H1 and H2) and steroids have been successful and allow continuation of treatment with the platinum agent.

### *Taxanes*

Paclitaxel is a taxane that is naturally derived from the bark of the Pacific or Western yew *(Taxus brevifolia)*. Docetaxel are derived from the bark of the English yew *(Taxus baccata)*. Both chemotherapeutic agents promote microtubule assembly, stabilizing microtubules to prevent and inhibit depolymerization of tubulin during mitosis (M phase). By arresting cell division through a functional block of the M phase, paclitaxel and docetaxel are potent chemotherapeutic agents, with activity in most solid tumors. Although administration of both taxanes can be accompanied by severe hypersensitivity reactions and hypotension, these responses are more commonly observed with paclitaxel because of its diluent, polyethoxylated castor oil (Cremophor EL) and ethanol. Thus premedication with antihistamines and steroids are recommended to minimize infusion-related hypersensitivity reactions. Neutropenia is the major toxic side effect, but sensory peripheral neuropathy is also a serious problem. Bradycardia and severe cardiac problems have been reported with the administration of paclitaxel, but they are rare. A rare complication has been the report of bowel perforation in a few individuals while on paclitaxel therapy, as noted by Rose and Piver (Rose, 1995). In addition to its use in the treatment of ovarian cancer, paclitaxel or docetaxel is being used in the treatment of other cervical cancers, endometrial cancer, and uterine sarcomas.

### *Antitumor Antibiotics*

Antitumor antibiotics are derived from products of bacterial or fungal cultures. The chemotherapeutic agents generally used for gynecologic malignancies are actinomycin D (dactinomycin), doxorubicin, and bleomycin (Blenoxane).

Actinomycin D is derived from the bacteria *Streptomyces parvulus* and is used primarily in the treatment of gestational trophoblastic disease. It lodges between adjacent purine-pyrimidine (guanine-cytosine) base pairs, blocking DNA-dependent ribosomal RNA synthesis by RNA polymerase. Actinomycin D is

Table 27.4 Side Effects of Drugs Often Used or Being Tested in Gynecologic Oncology

| Agent | Common Toxicities |
|---|---|
| Altretamine | Nausea and vomiting, diarrhea, abdominal cramping, myelosuppression |
| Bevacizumab | Hypertension (DLT), proteinuria, congestive heart failure, increase risk of bleeding, thromboembolism, GI perforation |
| Bleomycin | Interstitial pneumonitis, pulmonary fibrosis (DLT), mucocutaneous toxicity, fever |
| Capecitabine | Diarrhea (DLT), paresthesias, palmar-plantar erythrodysesthesia (PPE), dermatitis, hyperbilirubinemia, fatigue, anorexia |
| Carboplatin | Nausea and vomiting, myelosuppression (DLT), nephrotoxicity, electrolyte wasting, diarrhea, stomatitis, hypersensitivity reactions |
| Cyclophosphamide | Hemorrhagic cystitis, SIADH, alopecia, myelosuppression (DLT) |
| Dactinomycin | Myelosuppression (DLT), hepatotoxicity, alopecia, fatigue, myalgia, pneumonitis, malaise, lethargy |
| Docetaxel | Myelosuppression, fluid retention, hyperlacrimation, nail disorders |
| Etoposide | Myelosuppression, nausea and vomiting, hypotension, anorexia, alopecia, headache, fever |
| 5-Flurouracil | Nausea and vomiting, diarrhea, anorexia, myelosuppression, PPE, cardiotoxicity |
| Gemcitabine | Myelosuppression (DLT), flulike symptoms, headache, somnolence, nausea and vomiting, stomatitis, diarrhea, constipation, rash |
| Letrozole | Nausea and vomiting, bone pain, arthralgias, hot flashes |
| Leuprolide acetate | Peripheral edema, gynecomastia, hot flashes, hyperphosphatemia, nausea and vomiting, weight gain |
| Liposomal doxorubicin | Myelosuppression, stomatitis, mucositis, alopecia, flushing, shortness of breath, hypotension, headaches, cardiotoxicity, hand-foot syndrome |
| Methotrexate | Stomatitis, nausea and vomiting, myelosuppression, nephrotoxicity, elevation in hepatic enzymes, interstitial pneumonitis |
| Paclitaxel | Hypersensitivity reactions, peripheral neuropathy (DLT), nausea and vomiting, alopecia |
| Tamoxifen | Thromboembolism, hot flashes, decreased libido, nausea and vomiting, thrombocytopenia, anemia |
| Topotecan | Myelosuppression (DLT), nausea and vomiting, diarrhea, stomatitis, abdominal pain, alopecia, SGOT and SGPT elevation |
| Vincristine | Neurotoxicity, constipation (DLT), alopecia |
| Vinorelbine | Myelosuppression (DLT), neurotoxicity, constipation, asthenia, fatigue |

*DLT,* Dose-limiting toxicity; *GI,* gastrointestinal; *SGOT,* serum glutamic pyruvic transaminase; *SGPT,* serum glutamic pyruvic transaminase; *SIADH,* syndrome of inappropriate antidiuretic hormone secretion.

maximally effective in the G1 phase of the cell cycle, but data suggest that this drug may act throughout the entire cell cycle. Because bound actinomycin D dissociates slowly from DNA, cells actively progressing through the cell cycle are stopped from doing so at the G1/S checkpoint for genomic integrity, leading to cell death. If radiation is delivered in the presence of the drug, treated cells show a radiosensitizing effect. The drug causes severe myelosuppression, often leading to leukopenia and thrombocytopenia (nadir, 7 to 10 days). Toxicity to the gastrointestinal mucosa is associated with vomiting within 20 hours, stomatitis, and nonbloody diarrhea. Reversible alopecia may also occur. Dermatitis resulting from radiation recall has also been noted, meaning that skin erythema and inflammation arise in skin areas previously irradiated.

Doxorubicin and its newer liposomal formulation (Doxil) are anthracyclines derived from the bacteria *Streptomyces peucetius,* var. *caesius.* Within the cell nucleus, doxorubicin wedges between stacked nucleotide pairs in the DNA helix and, because of its bulk, inhibits binding of enzymes needed for DNA-directed RNA and DNA transcription, as well as DNA replication. Doxorubicin therefore has maximal activity in the G1 and S phases of the cell cycle. A second mechanism of action noted for doxorubicin includes the inhibition of topoisomerase II in the G2 phase of the cell cycle. Topoisomerase II assists in the coiling and supercoiling of DNA prior to mitosis by facilitating enzymatic DNA double-strand breaks. Doxorubicin has been shown to stabilize the double-strand break generated by topoisomerase II, thereby promoting loss of genetic material during mitotic division. Doxorubicin must be administered carefully by IV injection because extravasation leads to soft tissue and skin necrosis and ulceration. Doxorubicin is metabolized by the liver, and dosages must be reduced in patients with compromised hepatic function. Myelosuppression occurs regularly with therapeutic doses. Complete but reversible alopecia is a side effect (Table 27.4). Because the doxorubicin metabolism creates free radicals that bind to cardiac myocytes, it can cause significant cardiac toxicity, leading to irreversible congestive heart failure. Therefore cardiac function is assessed routinely before administration, and cumulative doses are kept to less than 450 mg/m$^2$. Liposomal doxorubicin has a synthetic lipid-like membrane around the doxorubicin molecule that is proposed to promote tumor uptake and protect against cardiotoxicity. Cardiomyopathy is less common with liposome-encapsulated doxorubicin, but skin toxicity, notably palmar plantar erythrodysesthesia (PPE), is more common.

Bleomycin is derived from the bacteria *Streptomyces verticillus* and, when complexed with ferrous iron, is a potent oxidase, producing single-strand DNA breaks by hydroxyl radical formation. Bleomycin may be administered intravenously, intramuscularly, or subcutaneously. It is excreted via the kidney, and some dose reduction is made if renal function is compromised. The drug does not produce significant myelosuppression, in contrast to most of the other cytotoxic agents. It is, however, highly toxic to the lungs in that pneumonitis and pulmonary fibrosis occurs in 10% of patients. Thus particular care must be used in persons with compromised lung function. To prevent this complication, cumulative doses of less than 400 units are given. If pneumonitis develops, as evidenced by symptoms of low-grade fever and nonproductive cough, treatment is a tapered course of oral corticosteroid therapy. Bleomycin is also toxic to skin and can produce erythema, peeling, and pigmentation. It has been used as part of combination therapy, with particular effectiveness against ovarian germ cell tumors, and has been tried for a variety of other gynecologic malignancies, particularly carcinoma of the cervix.

### *Topoisomerase I and II Inhibitors*

As noted, topoisomerases are DNA enzymes that control the topology of DNA double-helix cellular functions during transcription and replication of genetic material. There are two classes of topoisomerases, I and II. Drugs that prevent these functions are referred to as *topoisomerase inhibitors*.

#### Topotecan

Topotecan is in the class of camptothecins and is used for the treatment of cervical and epithelial ovarian cancers. Camptothecins inhibit topoisomerase I, causing stabilization of the cleavable complex and resulting in an accumulation of single-strand and double-strand DNA breaks, and ultimately cell death. It has been approved by the U.S. Food and Drug Administration (FDA) to be used in combination with cisplatin for the treatment of platinum-sensitive recurrent cervical cancer.

Topotecan is a semisynthetic analogue of camptothecin, a chemical derived from the *Camptotheca acuminata* tree native to China. This drug stabilizes single-strand breaks made by topoisomerase I, an enzyme that relaxes DNA structural tension by facilitating single-strand breaks and subsequent relegation. Topotecan has the greatest activity during the G1/S phases of the cell cycle. Toxicities include bone marrow suppression, nausea and vomiting, alopecia, mucositis, and diarrhea.

#### Etoposide

Etoposide is an epipodophyllotoxin derived from the root of the mayapple or mandrake plant that stabilizes DNA strand breaks made by topoisomerase II during coiling and supercoiling of DNA during mitosis. The primary toxicity of etoposide is myelosuppression, leading to depression of leukocytes and platelets. Other common toxicities include anorexia, nausea and vomiting, stomatitis, and severe hypotension if infused in less than 30 minutes. Uncommon toxicities include cardiotoxicity, bronchospasm, and somnolence. It is important to recognize that oral etoposide has an erratic absorption, with significant interpatient variability, from 0 to 100% bioavailability. Oral etoposide is typically used in the recurrent setting after failure of other second-line agents. Oral etoposide should never be used in place of the IV formulation when there is a curative intent—that is, a BEP regimen (bleomycin sulfate, etoposide phosphate, and cisplatin) for germ cell tumors.

### *Alkylating Agents*

Alkylating agents are chemical compounds that facilitate the replacement of hydrogen for an alkyl group, potentially disrupting normal function of the altered molecule. As chemotherapeutic agents, alkylating agents interact directly with DNA by transferring positively charged alkyl groups to negatively charged chemical groups intrinsic to the DNA molecule. Examples of this class include cyclophosphamide and ifosfamide. In general, the effectiveness of these agents appears to be similar, but there are some variations in toxicity. As a drug class, alkylating agents affect rapidly dividing cells and are particularly toxic to bone marrow, leading to severe myelosuppression.

Cyclophosphamide and its structural analogue ifosfamide are bifunctional cyclic phosphamide esters of nitrogen mustard. Both drugs interact with the N7 position of guanine in the DNA helix to form cross-link bridges between the same strand of DNA (intrastrand), opposite strands of DNA (interstrand), and DNA and cellular proteins. By forming intrastrand and interstrand DNA bridges, cyclophosphamide and ifosfamide impair the functional binding of enzymes used to process and replicate DNA, disrupting the G1/S phase transition of the cell cycle. These drugs are inactivated in the liver and exclusively excreted by the kidney. Their urinary metabolite acrolein may accumulate within the urinary system, causing severe urothelial damage that may result in hemorrhagic cystitis within 24 hours or weeks after administration. Prophylactic hydration (3 L/day) to increase dilute urinary output and administration of 2-mercaptoethane sulfonate (mesna), a compound that binds to acrolein and prevents urotoxicity, can be used to prevent this complication. Administration of these agents also leads to leukopenia (nadir, 8 to 14 days) and thrombocytopenia (nadir, 18 to 21 days), alopecia, nausea and vomiting, and amenorrhea. Therapy with alkylating agents has been associated with a subsequent risk of developing acute leukemia. This risk may range from 2% to 10% and appears to be related to the dose of and duration of alkylating agent treatment. They may be administered intravenously or orally but are only rarely used in the primary treatment of gynecologic malignancies.

### *Antimetabolites*

Antimetabolites interfere with cell metabolism by competing with naturally occurring purines or pyrimidines, whose chemical structure they resemble. In this way, they interfere or prevent vital biochemical reactions.

5-Fluorouracil (5-FU) is a fluorinated pyrimidine analogue resembling the DNA nucleoside thymine; it differs from the RNA nucleoside uracil by a fluorinated carbon in the fifth position in the nucleoside ring, as described by Grem. Conversion of 5-FU into fluorodeoxyuridine monophosphate blocks DNA synthesis by covalently binding to thymidylate synthase. This inhibits the formation of de novo thymidylate, a necessary precursor of hymidine triphosphate essential for DNA synthesis and cell division. The conversion of 5-FU into fluorouridine triphosphate results in the erroneous incorporation of fluorouridine triphosphate into RNA strands, which interferes with RNA processing and protein synthesis. By these actions, 5-FU perturbs normal progression through the G1/S transition, bringing about impaired cell division caused by altered nucleotide pools and DNA repair. As such, 5-FU is a potent radiosensitizer. One advantage of the drug is that 5-FU can be administered as a bolus or continuous IV infusion or orally as a prodrug (e.g., capecitabine) that is metabolized to 5-FU. Common toxicities associated with 5-FU have been reported and include myelosuppression, stomatitis, diarrhea, alopecia, nail changes, dermatitis, acute cerebellar syndrome, cardiac toxicity, hyperpigmentation over the vein used for infusion, and PPE (see Table 27.4). The 5-FU given intravenously is normally used in conjunction with cisplatin as a radiation sensitizer in the treatment of advanced cervical and vulvar cancers. Oral 5-FU (capecitabine) is often used in the treatment of recurrent ovarian and endometrial cancers.

Methotrexate is a folic acid analogue that binds tightly to dihydrofolate reductase, which plays a critical role in intracellular folate metabolism. This prevents the metabolic transfer of one carbon unit within the cell and thereby arrests DNA, RNA, and protein synthesis. Cells exhibit sensitivity to this drug predominantly in the S-phase portion of the cell cycle. The effects of methotrexate can be overcome by the administration of folinic acid (citrovorum factor) 24 hours after methotrexate, which replenishes the tetrahydrofolate. Some chemotherapeutic protocols have used very high doses of methotrexate to treat the tumor, followed by citrovorum rescue to avoid severe toxic side effects (see Table 27.4). Methotrexate is administered intravenously, intramuscularly, or orally using a variety of dose regimens. It is excreted in the urine and dose adjustments must be made if there is decreased renal function. Methotrexate results in severe myelosuppression (nadir, 6 to 13 days). Stomatitis, nausea, and vomiting are reported. Hepatotoxicity resulting in liver enzyme elevation may be seen within 12 hours after high-dose treatment. Therapeutic serum methotrexate levels are evident long after treatment in patients with ascites or pleural effusion because these act as a reservoir for the drug. The predominant use of the drug for gynecologic malignancies has resulted in the effective treatment of trophoblastic disease.

Gemcitabine, a synthetic deoxycytidine nucleoside analogue, targets ribonucleotide reductase (RR), the rate-limiting enzyme in deoxyribonucleotide metabolism during the S phase. Gemcitabine is triphosphorylated in tumor cells by the enzyme deoxycytidine kinase, inhibiting DNA polymerase activity and interrupting DNA replication. As a nucleoside analogue, gemcitabine is incorporated as a fraudulent base pair in DNA; as a diphosphate, it inhibits the regulatory subunit of the RR enzyme, which leads to the depletion of deoxyribonucleotide pools needed for DNA synthesis in the S phase of the cell cycle. Reported treatment toxicities include myelosuppression, transient elevation of liver enzyme levels, nausea, vomiting, flulike symptoms, and fatigue (see Table 27.4). Gemcitabine is used in the treatment of recurrent ovarian cancer, endometrial cancer, and uterine sarcomas.

### *Vinca Alkaloids*

The vinca alkaloids bind to the β-tubulin subunits of the mitotic spindles, blocking polymerization of the microtubules in mitosis. For gynecologic malignancies, the vinca alkaloids used most often include vinorelbine and vincristine. Vincristine is derived from the periwinkle plant *(Vinca rosea)* and acts in a cell cycle–dependent manner, blocking the assembly of tubulin and causing toxic destruction of the mitotic spindle, which arrests cellular mitosis. Vinorelbine is a semisynthetic vinca alkaloid derived from vinblastine. By affecting the late G2 and M phases of the cell cycle, these drugs are potent cytotoxins and increase cell radiosensitivity by slowing the G2/M transition in which radiation effects are maximal. Vincristine is severely neurotoxic and can produce numbness, motor weakness, and constipation as a result of its autonomic effects. The DLT of vinorelbine is myelosuppression (see Table 27.4).

### *Altretamine*

Altretamine has been used for a number of years but in recent years has been replaced with more active agents. The exact mechanism of action of altretamine is not known. It does not act as an alkylating agent in vitro but is possibly activated to one in vivo. Altretamine is metabolized by cytochrome P450 (CYP450) and the reduced form of nicotinamide adenine dinucleotide phosphate (NADPH) to N-hydroxymethyl pentamethylmelamine, which has been shown to bind covalently to DNA. Additional N-methylmelamines formed may also mediate some of the cytotoxicity of this agent.

It is an oral agent that is usually given in four divided doses. Altretamine therapy may be associated with some nausea, vomiting, diarrhea, abdominal cramping, and myelosuppression (see Table 27.4). In addition, a pharmacist should monitor for potential CYP450-drug interactions in patients on multiple prescriptions and alternative medications.

### *Biologic and Targeted Agents*

Since the early 2000s, there have been major efforts toward the incorporation of monoclonal antibodies such as bevacizumab and cetuximab and small-molecule tyrosine inhibitors such as sunitinib, gefitinib, and sorafenib into first-line and recurrent treatment regimens for gynecologic cancers. Although as single-agent therapy the biologic agents have not demonstrated significant activity against gynecologic cancers, there are mounting clinical data to support the implementation of agents such as bevacizumab into first-line and maintenance regimens to improve progression-free survival, specifically for ovarian cancer.

#### Bevacizumab

Bevacizumab is a recombinant humanized monoclonal antibody that targets and inactivates vascular endothelial growth factor (VEGF) to inhibit the angiogenesis pathway. As a single agent in the recurrent ovarian cancer setting, bevacizumab has had only a moderate response ranging from 16% to 21% (Cannistra, 2007; Monk, 2006). However, in combination with chemotherapy, bevacizumab has had promising response rates, ranging from 15% to 80% (Micha, 2007; Penson, 2009). There are significant limitations to incorporating bevacizumab with chemotherapy regimens because of the high risk of bowel perforation in ovarian cancer patients that was first observed in phase II studies. Hence, the current recommendation is that patients should not have had recent bowel surgery or a history of significant bowel resections.

Bevacizumab has been evaluated in combination with oral cyclophosphamide, paclitaxel, and gemcitabine for the treatment of recurrent ovarian cancer. The integration of bevacizumab into a first-line treatment regimen has focused on the benefits with paclitaxel plus carboplatin followed by maintenance with bevacizumab alone. Based on the encouraging results of ICON7 that incorporated bevacizumab into front-line therapy, the GOG initiated a confirmatory phase III study comparing six cycles of standard paclitaxel plus carboplatin to six cycles of the same regimen with bevacizumab to determine whether bevacizumab improves efficacy of front-line treatment (Oza, 2015). However, the duration of maintenance bevacizumab remains an area of therapeutic and pharmacoeconomic controversy.

#### Targeted Agents

Tyrosine kinase inhibitors (TKIs) such as sorafenib, sunitinib, pazopanib, and cediranib also target the VEGF angiogenesis pathway via inhibition of the VEGF receptor (VEGFR). Current research efforts have been focused on combination regimens of these TKIs with cytotoxic agents for first-line treatment and also for the treatment of recurrent ovarian cancer. Another agent of interest is aflibercept (VEGF Trap), which is a fusion protein that targets VEGF-A. Initial studies have demonstrated that it is beneficial in the treatment of malignant ascites. Unfortunately, the popular epidermal growth factor receptor (EGFR) agents such as erlotinib, which have had so much benefit in the treatment of other cancers, have not demonstrated activity alone or in combination with chemotherapy or with bevacizumab for the treatment of gynecologic cancers. Finally, the newer classes of targeted therapies, such as latelet-derived growth factor (PDGF) inhibitors and poly (ADP-ribose) polymerase (PARP) inhibitors, are being incorporated into numerous clinical studies in an attempt to improve progression-free and overall survival. Olaparib, a PARP inhibitor was recently approved for treatment of recurrent, platinum sensitive ovarian cancer patients who express the breast cancer gene *BRCA-1*; however, emerging data suggest there will be benefit in patients with "*BRCA*-ness" like pathology (Ledermann, 2012).

### Anticancer Hormone Therapy

Hormone therapy has been effectively developed for the treatment of breast cancer. Estrogen and progesterone receptors have been clearly identified in endometrial carcinomas and have been found in other types of gynecologic cancers, particularly ovarian epithelial carcinomas. Progestins such as megestrol (Megace), depot medroxyprogesterone acetate (Depo-Provera), and 17-hydroxyprogesterone caproate (Delalutin), as well as antiestrogens such as tamoxifen and raloxifene, have been used in the treatment of endometrial carcinomas and seem to have their best effects against well-differentiated tumors.

## DRUG RESISTANCE

A daunting challenge is overcoming drug resistance, which occurs fairly often in the recurrent setting of all gynecologic malignancies. Platinum sensitivity is defined by a disease-free interval longer than 6 months after treatment with a platinum agent. If platinum-sensitive, patients can be retreated with a platinum agent, which usually will be single-agent carboplatin because it is tolerated better. Platinum resistance is present when there is tumor progression while receiving a platinum agent or disease relapse within less than 6 months after the completion of chemotherapy, and alternative agents must be considered. Taxane resistance follows the same parameters.

The optimal chemotherapeutic agent or regimen in the treatment of platinum-resistant disease is currently unknown. Ideally, the agent should be active in gynecologic cancer and should be non–cross-resistant with taxanes or platinum agents. Overall, regardless of the agent, the response rate is low for all the agents in platinum-refractory (resistant) cancer. Typically, it is recommended to give three cycles prior to evaluation for response to the new agent unless there is a more than 50% doubling of CA-125. Because tumor regression is so rare in the recurrent setting, even achieving stable disease is considered a treatment success. If no response is observed after three cycles, an alternative chemotherapy regimen may be selected.

## EVALUATION OF NEW AGENTS

In the development of new oncology drugs, serial evaluations are necessary to assess the effectiveness of the drug and ascertain its toxicity. A number of trials are necessary to move a new agent from the point of evaluation to allow it to be used in regular medical practice. Unlike other areas of drug development, clinical trials for cytotoxic agents can only be conducted in those with active cancer, often those who have already failed current standard therapy treatment options.

Table 27.5 Assessment of Performance Status

| Score | Karnofsky Performance Status Scale |
|---|---|
| 100 | Normal, no complaints; no evidence of disease |
| 90 | Able to carry on normal activity; minor signs or symptoms of disease |
| 80 | Normal activity with effort; some signs or symptoms of disease |
| 70 | Cares for self but unable to carry on normal activity or do active work |
| 60 | Requires occasional assistance but is able to care for most personal needs |
| 50 | Requires considerable assistance and frequent medical care |
| 40 | Disabled; requires special care and assistance |
| 30 | Severely disabled; hospitalization indicated, although death not imminent |
| 20 | Very sick; hospitalization necessary; active support treatment necessary |
| 10 | Moribund; fatal process progressing rapidly |
| 0 | Dead |
| **Grade** | **Gynecologic Oncology Group Performance Status Scale** |
| 1 | Fully active, able to carry on all predisease performance without restriction |
| 2 | Restricted in physically strenuous activity but ambulatory and able to carry out work of a light or sedentary nature (e.g., light housework, office work) |
| 3 | Capable of only limited self-care, confined to bed or chair >50% of waking hours |
| 4 | Completely disabled; cannot carry on any self-care; totally confined to bed or chair |
| 5 | Dead |

A standard method frequently used to measure a patient's general functional condition before enrollment in clinical chemotherapy trials of new agents is the Karnofsky Performance Status Scale (Table 27.5). In general, patients are poor candidates from clinical trials if their score is 50 or less. Cooperative research groups, such as the GOG, have modified the Karnofsky scoring system to reflect a five-point graded classification.

After extensive preclinical evaluation, investigational new drug (IND) applications are filed to move new drugs into human studies. The human clinical trial process is a fairly rigorous and costly process to determine not only safety and efficacy but also improvement over the current standard of care for each new agent proposed, sometimes alone or in various combination regimens. A general outline of phase trials is as follows:

- *Phase I trial:* A phase I trial tests new drugs at various doses to evaluate toxicity and determine tolerance to the drug. At the various doses tested, some therapeutic effects may be observed, although this is not the primary aim of the trial.
- *Phase II trial:* A phase II trial tests the therapeutic effectiveness and extent of toxicity of the drug at doses expected to be effective against a specific tumor type.

- *Phase III trial:* A phase III trial compares new treatment therapies against the current treatment standard of care. For example, this trial design assesses whether a new drug therapy is superior, equivalent, or inferior to the chemotherapeutic agent currently used.

Numerous programs have been implemented to facilitate drug approval and access to investigational drugs, such as the Fast Track Drug Approval Program and Orphan Drug Approval. Special consideration for either program requires preapplication and approval by the FDA. Often, in the gynecologic oncology setting, FDA approval for new gynecologic indications is not sought because of small patient populations and the inability to conduct phase III studies in a timely fashion. Compendia listings are often granted based on peer-reviewed published literature, which expands reimbursement for treatment recommendations.

Progress has been slow and unsuccessful in finding a cure for ovarian cancer and recurrent endometrial or cervical cancers. In the absence of a curative treatment for recurrent disease, selecting an investigational trial treatment still remains the best option for ovarian cancer patients. Research is needed to identify and develop new approaches for preventing recurrence and new options for treating advanced primary and recurrent disease. Efforts should especially focus on agents to modulate or overcome drug resistance or new molecular targets to optimize chemotherapy outcomes.

## KEY POINTS

- Electromagnetic radiation is a form of energy that has no mass or charge and travels at the speed of light.
- The inverse square law states that the energy measured from a radiation source is inversely proportional to the square of the distance from the radiation source.
- Each delivered radiation dose kills a constant fraction of tumor cells irradiated. Oxygen can render radiation-induced DNA damage permanent.
- The effect of photon radiation (low LET) on tissues is altered by tissue oxygenation, whereas neutron radiation (high LET) is independent of oxygenation.
- The cell replication cycle consists of M (mitosis), G1 (Gap1 = RNA and protein synthesis), S (DNA synthesis), and G2 (Gap2 = RNA and protein synthesis). When the cell is not in the replication cycle, it is in the G0 phase.
- The dose of radiation delivered to a tumor depends on the energy of the source, the size of the treatment field, and the depth of the tumor beneath the surface. Increasing the dose increases the depth of maximum dose beneath the skin surface.
- Radiation acts on cells primarily in the M phase, making rapidly proliferating cells the most radiosensitive.
- Normal tissues repair the radiobiologic effects of radiation more effectively than tumor tissue.
- Radiation side effects usually involve erythema of the skin, without desquamation and mild fatigue.
- Uncommon side effects include lowering of the circulating blood cells, dysuria and urinary frequency, diarrhea, bowel injury, and fistula formation.
- Cytotoxic chemotherapeutic agents act on various phases of the cell cycle, primarily affecting rapidly proliferating cells, and at a given dose destroy a constant fraction of tumor cells.
- Growth factors or G-CSF are used to limit the hematologic toxicity of chemotherapy.
- After the completion of the staging and primary surgical treatment, the current standard of care is six cycles of a taxane–platinum-containing chemotherapy regimen.
- If recurrence is less than 6 months after completion of chemotherapy, the tumor is defined to be platinum or taxane resistant.
- The antitumor activity of second-line chemotherapy regimens is similar; the choice of treatment for recurrent disease depends on residual toxicities, physician preference, and patient convenience. Participation in a clinical trial is also a reasonable option for these patients.

## KEY REFERENCES


Adams GE, Stratford IJ, Bremner JC, et al. Nitroheterocyclic compounds as radiation sensitizers and bioreductive drugs. *Radiother Oncol.* 1991;20(Suppl 1):85–91.

Amorino GP, Freeman ML, Carbone DP, et al. Radiopotentiation by the oral platinum agent, JM216: Role of repair inhibition. *Int J Radiat Oncol Biol Phys.* 1999;44:399–405.

Arai T, Nakano T, Fukuhisa K, et al. Second cancer after radiation therapy for cancer of the uterine cervix. *Cancer.* 1991;67:398–405.

Armstrong DK, Bundy B, Wenzel L, et al. Intraperitoneal cisplatin and paclitaxel in ovarian cancer. *N Engl J Med.* 2006;354:34–43.

Bowland JD. Radiation oncology physics. In: Gunderson LL, Tepper JE, eds. *Clinical Radiation Oncology.* New York: Churchill Livingstone; 2000:64–118.

Cannistra SA, Matulonis UA, Penson RT, et al. Phase II study of bevacizumab in patients with platinum-resistant ovarian cancer or peritoneal serous cancer. *J Clin Oncol.* 2007;25:5180–5186.

Chiao TB, Lee AJ. Role of pentoxifylline and vitamin E in attenuation of radiation-induced fibrosis. *Ann Pharmacother.* 2005;39:516–522.

Covens A, Thomas G, DePetrillo A, et al. The prognostic importance of site and type of radiation-induced bowel injury in patients requiring surgical management. *Gynecol Oncol.* 1991;43:270–274.

Deshpande A, Sicinski P, Hinds PW. Cyclins and CDKS in development and cancer: A perspective. *Oncogene.* 2005;24:2909–2915.

Dunst J, Kuhnt T, Strauss HG, et al. Anemia in cervical cancers: impact on survival, patterns of relapse, and association with hypoxia and angiogenesis. *Int J Radiat Oncol Biol Phys.* 2003;56:778–787.

Goldberg Z, Evans J, Birrell G, et al. An investigation of the molecular basis for the synergistic interaction of tirapazamine and cisplatin. *Int J Radiat Oncol Biol Phys.* 2001;49:175–182.

Gothard L, Cornes P, Brooker S, et al. Phase II study of vitamin E and pentoxifylline in patients with late side effects of pelvic radiotherapy. *Radiother Oncol.* 2005;75:334–341.

Hall EJ. *Radiobiology for the Radiologist.* ed 5 Philadelphia: Lippincott Williams & Wilkins; 2000.

Hall EJ, Hei TK. Genomic instability and bystander effects induced by high-LET radiation. *Oncogene.* 2003;22:7034–7042.

Jonathan EC, Bernhard EJ, McKenna WG. How does radiation kill cells? *Curr Opin Chem Biol.* 1999;3:77–83.
Kahn FM. *The Physics of Radiation Therapy.* ed 3 Philadelphia: Lippincott Williams & Wilkins; 2003.
Katsumata N, Yasuda M, Takahashi F, et al. Dose-dense paclitaxel once a week in combination with carboplatin every 3 weeks for advanced ovarian cancer: a phase 3, open-label, randomized controlled trial. *Lancet.* 2009;374:1331–1338.
Lawrence TS, Blackstock AW, McGinn C. The mechanism of action of radiosensitization of conventional chemotherapeutic agents. *Semin Radiat Oncol.* 2003;13:13–21.
Ledermann J, Harter P, Gourley C, et al. Olaparib maintenance therapy in platinum-sensitive relapsed ovarian cancer. *N Engl J Med.* 2012;366:1382–1392.
Li MC, Hertz R, Spencer DB. Effect of methotrexate therapy upon choriocarcinoma and chorioadenoma. *Proc Soc Exp Biol Med.* 1956;93:361–366.
Malumbres M, Barbacid M. To cycle or not to cycle: a critical decision in cancer. *Nat Rev Cancer.* 2001;1:222–231.
McGuire WP, Hoskins WJ, Brady MF, et al. Cyclophosphamide and cisplatin compared with paclitaxel and cisplatin in patients with stage III and stage IV ovarian cancer. *N Engl J Med.* 1996;334:1–6.
McIntyre JF, Eifel PJ, Levenback C, et al. Ureteral stricture as a late complication of radiotherapy for stage IB carcinoma of the uterine cervix. *Cancer.* 1995;75:836–843.
Micha JP, Goldstein BH, Rettenmaier MA, et al. A phase II study of outpatient first-line paclitaxel, carboplatin, and bevacizumab for advanced-stage epithelial ovarian, peritoneal, and fallopian tube cancer. *Int J Gynecol Cancer.* 2007;17:771–776.
Monk BJ, Han E, Josephs-Cowan CA, et al. Salvage bevacizumab (rhuMAB VEGF)-based therapy after multiple prior cytotoxic regimens in advanced refractory epithelial ovarian cancer. *Gynecol Oncol.* 2006;102:140–144.
Montana GS, Fowler WC. Carcinoma of the cervix: analysis of bladder and rectal radiation dose and complications. *Int J Radiat Oncol Biol Phys.* 1989;16:95–100.
Munro TR. The relative radiosensitivity of the nucleus and cytoplasm of the Chinese hamster fibroblasts. *Radiat Res.* 1970;42:451–470.
Oza AM, Cook AD, Pfisterer J, et al. Standard chemotherapy with or without bevacizumab for women with newly diagnosed ovarian cancer (ICON7): overall survival results of a phase 3 randomised trial. *Lancet Oncol.* 2015; 16:928–936.
Ozols RF. Systemic therapy for ovarian cancer: current status and new treatments. *Semin Oncol.* 2006;33(Suppl 6):S3–S11.
Ozols RF, Bundy BN, Greer BE, et al. Phase III trial of carboplatin and paclitaxel compared with cisplatin and paclitaxel in patients with optimally resected stage III ovarian cancer: a Gynecologic Oncology Group study. *J Clin Oncol.* 2003;21:3194–3200.
Palcic B, Skarsgard LD. Reduced oxygen enhancement ratio at low doses of ionizing radiation. *Radiat Res.* 1984;100:328–329.
Pawlik TM, Keyomarsi K. Role of cell cycle in mediating sensitivity to radiotherapy. *Int J Radiat Oncol Biol Phys.* 2004;59:928–942.
Penson RT, Dizon DS, Cannistra SA, et al. Phase II study of carboplatin, paclitaxel, and bevacizumab with maintenance bevacizumab as first-line chemotherapy for advanced mullerian tumors. *J Clin Oncol.* 2009;28:154–159.
Piccart MJ, Bertelsen K, Stuart G, et al. Long-term follow-up confirms a survival advantage of the paclitaxel-cisplatin regimen over the cyclophosphamide-cisplatin combination in advanced ovarian cancer. *Int J Gynecol Cancer.* 2003; 13(Suppl 2):144–148.
Rose PG, Piver MS. Intestinal perforation secondary to paclitaxel. *Gynecol Oncol.* 1995;57:270–272.
Siemann DW, Shi W. Targeting the tumor blood vessel network to enhance the efficacy of radiation therapy. *Semin Radiat Oncol.* 2003;13:53–61.
Skipper HE. The effects of chemotherapy on the kinetics of leukemic cell behavior. *Cancer Res.* 1965;25:1544–1550.
Utley JF, Marlowe C, Waddell WJ. Distribution of 35S-labeled WR-2721 in normal and malignant tissues of the mouse. *Radiat Res.* 1976;68:284–291.
Xu B, Kim S-T, Lim D-S, et al. Two molecularly distinct G(2)/M checkpoints are induced by ionizing irradiation. *Mol Cell Biol.* 2002;22:1049–1059.
Yang LX, Douple EB, Wang HJ. Irradiation enhances cellular uptake of carboplatin. *Int J Radiat Oncol Biol Phys.* 1995;33:641–646.

Suggested Readings can be found on ExpertConsult.com.

# 28

# Intraepithelial Neoplasia of the Lower Genital Tract (Cervix, Vagina, Vulva)

## Etiology, Screening, Diagnosis, Management

*Mila Pontremoli Salcedo, Ellen S. Baker, Kathleen M. Schmeler*

Cervical cancer is a leading cause of cancer and cancer-related deaths among women worldwide, with more than 500,000 new cases and 250,000 deaths annually. More than 85% of these cases and deaths occur in low- and middle-income countries (LMICs), primarily due to a lack of organized screening programs (Torre, 2015). Cervical cancer was previously the leading cause of cancer-related death among women in the United States. However, the incidence and mortality has decreased by approximately 70% since the 1970s. This decline is largely due to the introduction in 1941 of the Papanicolaou (Pap) smear, which has led to a systemic effort to detect early cervical cancer and precancerous lesions (Papanicolaou, 1941). In stark comparison, cervical cancer continues to be one of the leading causes of cancer and cancer-related death among women in LMICs and many underserved parts of the United States due to the lack of organized screening and early detection programs. Cervical cancer is a preventable disease, with excellent tools for prevention (vaccination) and screening (Pap and human papillomavirus testing). Furthermore, there is a treatable preinvasive phase that lasts several years before progressing to invasive cancer.

## ETIOLOGY: THE HUMAN PAPILLOMAVIRUS

It is now known that virtually all cases of cervical cancer are caused by persistent infection with high-risk types of the human papillomavirus (HPV) (Walboomers, 1999). HPV is the most common sexually transmitted disease, and it is estimated that 80% of women will be infected with HPV at some point in their lifetime. The initial infection usually occurs during adolescence or early adulthood, with the majority of women clearing the infection within 18 to 24 months (Wheeler, 1996; Moscicki, 1998; Moscicki, 2004; Moscicki, 2008). However, in 3% to 5% of women, the HPV infection persists and they develop significant preinvasive disease, and in <1% invasive cancer develops. HPV infection is therefore necessary but not sufficient for cervical cancer development. HPV infection is also the causative agent of other malignancies, including cancer of the oropharynx, anus, penis, vulva, and vagina.

HPV is a double-stranded DNA virus that replicates within epithelial cells (Chang, 1990; Wolf, 2001). To date, more than 120 HPV types have been identified, and approximately 40 HPV viruses are known to infect the genital tracts of men and women. Of these, approximately a dozen are considered high-risk types, with HPV 16 and 18 being responsible for more than 70% of cervical cancers. High-risk HPV causes neoplastic cellular changes when viral DNA becomes integrated into the host cell genome. When this happens, certain repressor areas of the viral genome are lost. Consistently, the loss of these control mechanisms allows for the expression of the viral E6 and E7 genes. The production of oncoproteins results in the inactivation of the p53 and retinoblastoma tumor suppressors (Munger, 2004). These changes are believed to lead to cell immortalization and rapid cell proliferation. However, in most cases, the transformed cells are managed by the individual's immune system, and the infection clears or intraepithelial neoplasia regresses. In some women, the transformed cells replicate and, if left untreated, a cancer can develop after a period of several years.

## RISK FACTORS

The mean age at diagnosis of cervical cancer in the United States is 48 years. The lifetime risk of developing cervical cancer by age 74 is 0.9% in developed countries compared with 1.6% in LMICs. Similarly, the lifetime risk of death from cervical cancer is 0.3% in developed countries compared with 0.9% in LMICs (Torre, 2015). Despite widespread infection with HPV, most women do not develop cervical cancer (Fig. 28.1). The search for a predictive measure to distinguish between women who are infected and will clear the virus and those in whom the infection will persist and who will develop cancer has been difficult. Although it is clear that women who have a compromised immune system from any cause (e.g., genetic, iatrogenic, infectious) have a greater risk of developing a persistent HPV infection (Aldieh, 2001), there is no way to predict which healthy women are unable to clear the virus spontaneously. The majority of risk factors associated with cervical cancer are those associated with acquiring HPV infection and include early onset of sexual activity, multiple sexual partners, history of sexually transmitted infections, oral contraceptive use, and a history of vulvar or vaginal dysplasia, which is also associated with HPV infection (International Collaboration of Epidemiological Studies of Cervical Cancer, [ICESCC] 2007). Smoking has

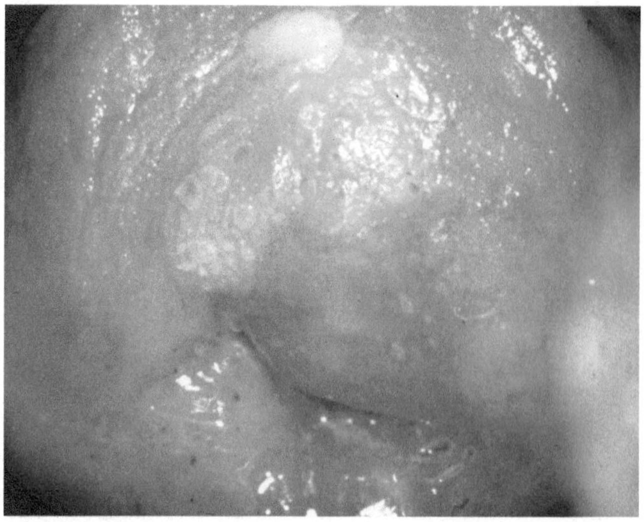

**Figure 28.1** Image of a cervix with an active human papillomavirus infection. The patient had a cytology sample reported as a low-grade squamous intraepithelial lesion. She was followed without treatment, and the lesions regressed over the next year.

been associated with the development of squamous cell carcinoma of the cervix but not adenocarcinoma (McIntyre-Seltman, 2005; ICESCC, 2006; ICESCC, 2007).

## PRIMARY PREVENTION: HUMAN PAPILLOMAVIRUS VACCINATION

Three very effective preventive vaccines are currently commercially available. The bivalent vaccine (Cervarix) targets two high-risk HPV types (16 and 18), which account for 70% of the cervical cases worldwide. The quadrivalent vaccine (Gardasil) targets high-risk HPV types 16 and 18, as well as two low-risk HPV types (6 and 11), which cause genital warts. The nonvalent vaccine (Gardasil-9) has been approved for use in the United States and targets the same HPV types as the quadrivalent vaccine (6, 11, 16, and 18) as well as types 31, 33, 45, 52, and 58 (FUTURE II Study Group, 2007; Paavonen, 2009; Joura, 2015). All three vaccines have been shown in randomized clinical trials to have 93% to 98% efficacy in the prevention of cervical dysplasia (and presumably cervical cancer) in women not previously infected with HPV 16 and 18. In addition, several studies have shown the vaccines to be safe with no scientific evidence that HPV vaccination increases the risk of serious adverse events. The vaccines do not work on existing infection or associated preinvasive or invasive disease, and it is therefore most effective if given prior to sexual debut and exposure to HPV.

The Centers for Disease Control and Prevention (CDC) recommend that the HPV vaccine be given to both boys and girls between the ages of 11 and 12 years, but it can be administered as early as 9 years. Catch-up vaccination should be offered for females aged 13 to 26 years who have not been previously vaccinated (Markowitz, 2014). Unfortunately, the uptake of HPV vaccination in the United States has been poor, with only about one third of eligible children completing the three vaccine series. The uptake in other developed countries (Canada, Australia, the United Kingdom) has been much higher at approximately 70%, likely due to government supported school-based programs. Several LMICs have instituted HPV vaccination programs as the Global Alliance for Vaccination and Immunization (GAVI) has made the HPV vaccine available to low-income countries for US$4 to $5 per dose (compared with $150 per dose in the United States). However, economic, political, and logistical barriers in many low-income countries have limited universal mass vaccination programs. Studies are underway to determine whether two doses of the vaccine provide sufficient protection. In addition, it is not yet known whether vaccination protection is lifelong or whether a booster dose will be required. Because the vaccines currently available do not provide protection against all cancer-associated HPV types, and because the duration of immunity is not yet known, routine screening is still recommended in vaccinated women.

## SECONDARY PREVENTION

### *CERVICAL CYTOLOGY TESTING*

Cervical cytology testing (Pap test) became available in the 1950s after the studies of Papanicolaou demonstrated that cancer and its precursors could be identified by examining a properly prepared and stained cellular sample scraped from the uterine cervix (Papanicolaou, 1941). The 1941 monograph by Papanicolaou and Traut remains one of the sentinel breakthroughs in the history of preventive medicine. Their work led to the demonstration that local therapy of precancerous lesions can prevent the development of cancer. Despite the fact that Pap testing has a low sensitivity, widespread Pap testing has reduced the incidence of cervical cancer by 50% to 70%. In part, the success of this screening technique relies on the fact that it takes many years for invasive cancer to develop following a persistent HPV infection and development of dysplasia, and that most women are tested repeatedly. Generally, in the United States, women who develop invasive cervical cancer have never been screened or have not been screened for many years.

The Pap test is performed by placing a speculum into the vagina and scraping cervical cells using a spatula and endocervical brush (Figs. 28.2 and 28.3). Cells are sampled from the transformation zone, which is the area of the cervix where cervical cancer can develop. The transformation zone includes the squamocolumnar junction, which is the area where the squamous epithelium of the ectocervix meets the columnar epithelium of the endocervix. The transformation zone is dynamic throughout a woman's lifetime, and the squamocolumnar junction migrates from the ectocervix into the endocervical canal as woman ages and reaches menopause. In the past, the collected sample was placed on a glass slide and fixed with alcohol. This method has been replaced by a liquid-based approach. The sample is now placed in a liquid medium for transport to the laboratory where the slide is prepared. The transport medium also can be used for HPV DNA testing.

### *PRIMARY HUMAN PAPILLOMAVIRUS TESTING*

There is increasing evidence that HPV testing is effective for cervical cancer screening. A number of studies have demonstrated that HPV testing is more sensitive than Pap testing, with only a small loss in positive predictive value (PPV) (Dillner, 2008; Huh, 2015; Monsonego, 2015). Although the Pap test is still the most widely used screening test in developed countries, co-testing with HPV is now also recommended. Furthermore, primary HPV testing alone is gaining acceptance. In addition, the World Health Organization (WHO) recommends HPV testing as the

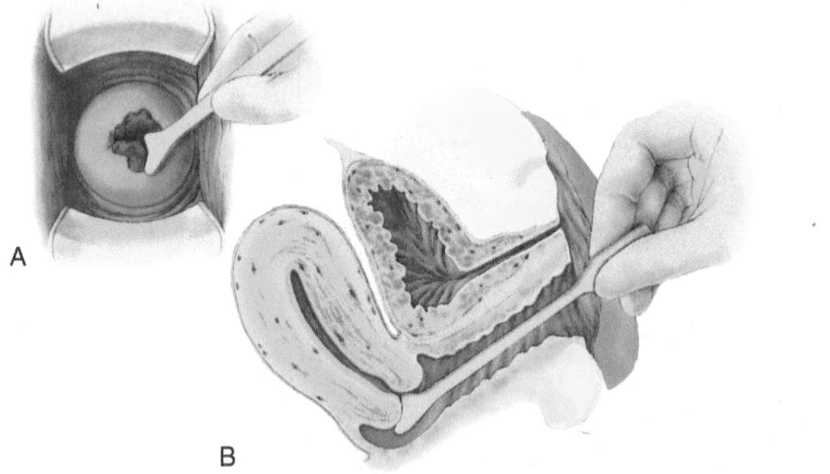


**Figure 28.2** A spatula is often used to obtain a specimen from the exocervix. It must be used with an instrument that samples the endocervix. **A,** Cervix as seen through a speculum, with the spatula being used to obtain a cell sample. **B,** Longitudinal view at the same point in the procedure.

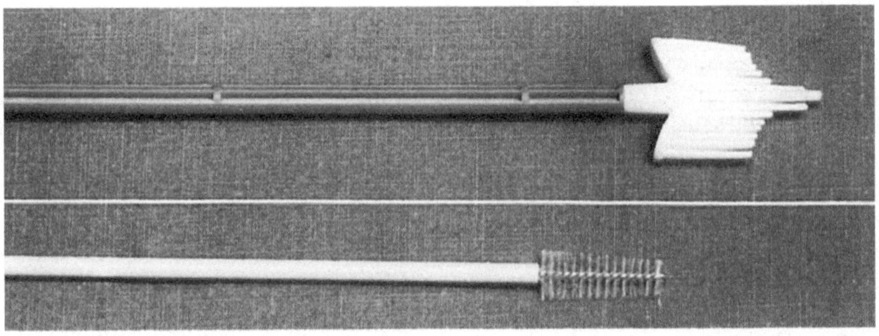

**Figure 28.3** A cervical broom (*top*, Unimar) and Cytobrush (*bottom*, Cooper Surgical) can be used to obtain a cytologic sample from the endocervix.

preferred screening method in countries where Pap testing is not feasible and HPV testing is available (WHO, 2015).

## CERVICAL CANCER SCREENING GUIDELINES

The current guidelines in the United States recommend screening women for cervical cancer between the ages of 21 and 65 (Saslow, 2012). Cervical cancer screening should not be performed in women younger than 21 years of age, regardless of age of onset of sexual activity. The screening guidelines are as follows:

- 21 to 29 years: Pap testing every 3 years. No HPV testing.
- 30 to 65 years: Co-testing with Pap and HPV every 5 years (preferred) or Pap testing alone every 3 years.
- Screening is *not* recommended for women >65 years of age who have had three consecutive negative Pap tests or two consecutive negative HPV tests, provided they have had no history of high-grade dysplasia (CIN2/3) or cancer (CIN2+) in the past 20 years. However, women presenting at age 65 years of age or older who have not had previous screening should undergo Pap and HPV testing.
- Screening with Pap test or HPV testing is *not* recommended for women who have had a hysterectomy with removal of the cervix and who do not have a history of CIN2+.

Of note, these guidelines do not apply to those special populations with additional risk factors and other complicating history.

## CERVICAL CYTOLOGY REPORTING: THE BETHESDA SYSTEM

In 1988, the National Cancer Institute convened a conference in Bethesda, Maryland, to develop a uniform terminology for the reporting of Pap test results, the Bethesda System (TBS) (Solomon, 2002). Almost all laboratories in the United States and many in countries throughout the world use this terminology. Figure 28.4 shows how TBS, CIN, and dysplasia categories correspond to tissue changes.

The first part of a TBS report states whether the sample is satisfactory or unsatisfactory. A sample may be unsatisfactory if there is lack of a label, loss of transport medium, scant cellularity, and contamination by foreign material. Few samples are reported as unsatisfactory if a liquid-based technique is used. The report next indicates whether the cellular material is normal. If other than normal, the abnormalities are further divided into squamous and glandular. The cytologist may also comment on whether there is evidence of infection, such as yeast, or changes consistent with a diagnosis of bacterial vaginosis.

## ATYPICAL SQUAMOUS CELLS

The most common squamous abnormality is atypical squamous cells (ASC) of undetermined significance (ASC-US). This finding indicates that a few cells may show features associated with

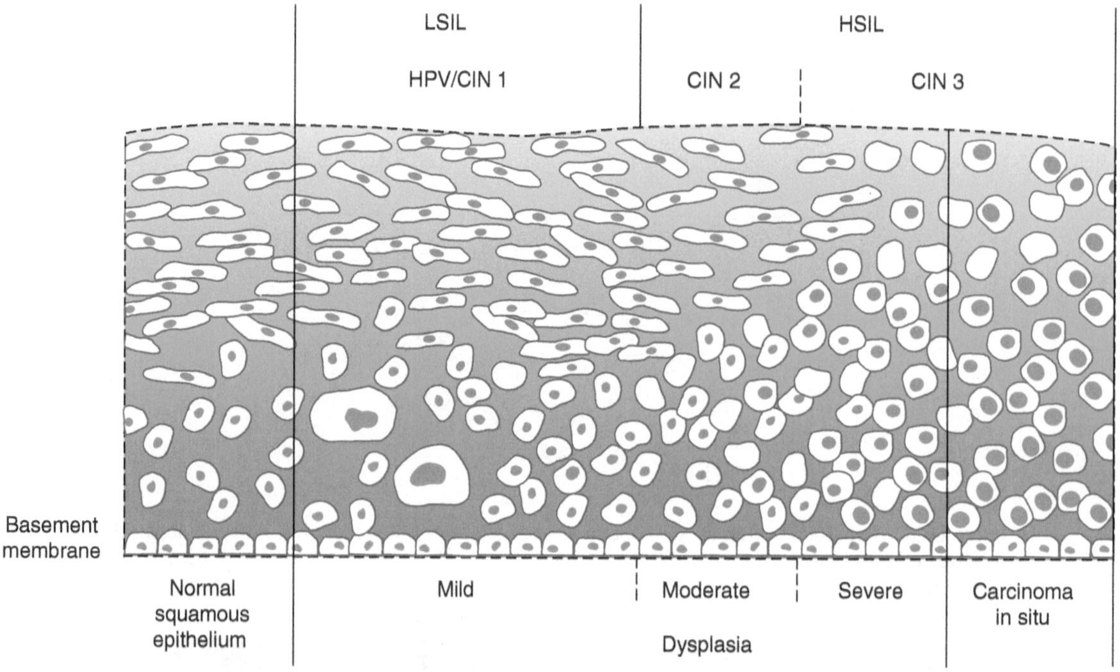


**Figure 28.4** Diagram of cervical epithelium showing various terminologies used to characterize progressive degrees of cervical neoplasia. *CIN*, Cervical intraepithelial neoplasia; *HPV*, human papillomavirus; *HSIL*, high-grade squamous intraepithelial lesion; *LSIL*, low-grade squamous intraepithelial lesion.

squamous intraepithelial lesions, but there are few of these cells present or the changes are not consistent with a more precise diagnosis. ASC-US changes are reported in approximately 3% to 5% of all Pap samples. The management of ASC-US and other Pap abnormalities is based on the recommendations of the American Society of Colposcopy and Cervical Pathology (ASCCP), with the most recent guidelines published in 2012 (Solomon, 2001; Massad, 2013). Patients with ASC-US Pap result can undergo repeat cytology at 12 months or reflex HPV testing. If HPV testing is positive, colposcopy is performed. If HPV testing is negative, return to routine screening is recommended.

The second ASC abnormality is ASC-H (atypical squamous cells, cannot exclude a higher-grade lesion). Approximately 5% to 10% of ASC cases are classified at ASC-H. Women with this diagnosis should be evaluated with colposcopy because there is a higher likelihood that a significant lesion, such as CIN 2/3, is present (Massad, 2013).

## *LOW-GRADE SQUAMOUS INTRAEPITHELIAL LESION*

Low-grade squamous intraepithelial lesion (LSIL) is often found to be consistent with histology reports of low-grade dysplasia or cervical intraepithelial neoplasia 1 (CIN 1) (Fig. 28.5, *A* and *B*). LSIL may resolve spontaneously or progress to more severe dysplasia and should be managed according to the ASCCP guidelines (Massad, 2013). If HPV testing is negative, both Pap and HPV testing should be repeated in 1 year. If no HPV testing is performed or HPV testing is positive, the patient should undergo colposcopy.

## *HIGH-GRADE SQUAMOUS INTRAEPITHELIAL LESION*

A diagnosis of high-grade squamous intraepithelial lesion (HSIL) indicates more severe dysplasia or CIN 2/3 (Figs. 28.6 and 28.7). If unmanaged, approximately 20% of patients with HSIL will progress to cervical cancer. All patients with HSIL should be evaluated with colposcopy, according to ASCCP guidelines, and the majority treated with excision or ablation, depending on age and colposcopy and biopsy results (Massad, 2013).

## *ATYPICAL GLANDULAR CELLS*

Atypical glandular cells (AGC) are noted in approximately 3 out of every 1000 Pap tests, and the risk of underlying invasive cancer is 3% to 17% (Zweitig 1997; ACOG, 2013). The atypical cells can sometimes be classified by the site of origin (e.g., endometrium, endocervix, ovary); however, this is not always possible. Per the ASCCP guidelines, it is recommended that all women with AGC undergo colposcopy with endocervical sampling (Massad, 2013). Endometrial sampling should also be performed in women who are older than 35 years or at risk for endometrial cancer (unexplained vaginal bleeding, obese, conditions suggesting chronic anovulation such as infertility or polycystic ovarian syndrome, or family history suggestive of Lynch syndrome/hereditary nonpolyposis colorectal cancer [HNPCC]).

# COLPOSCOPY

Colposcopy is often the first step in evaluation of women with abnormal cytology. The colposcope is a low-power binocular

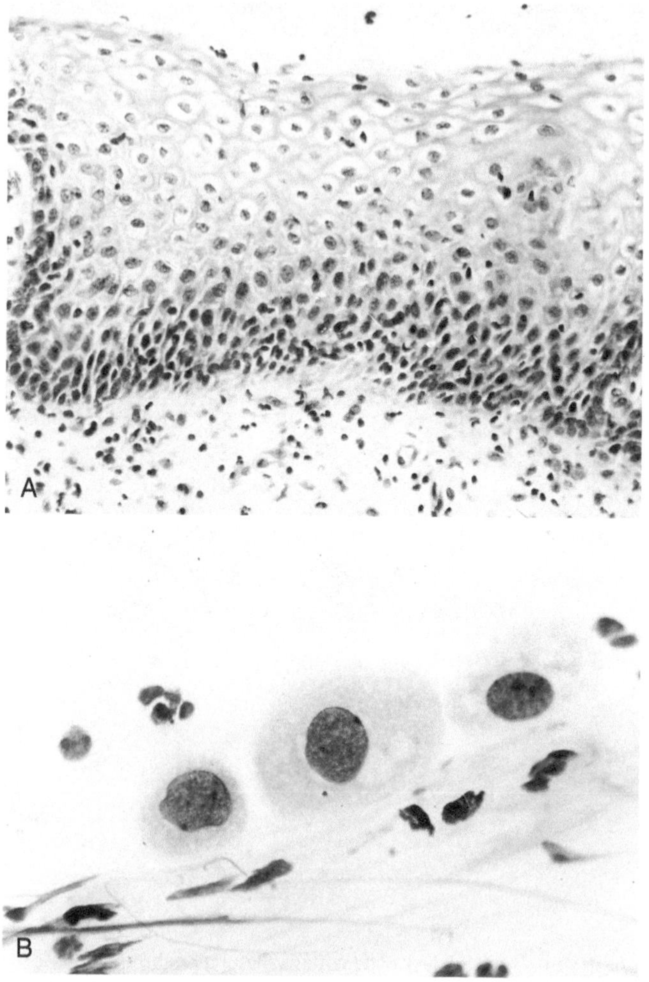


Figure 28.5 **A,** Cervical intraepithelial neoplasia 1 (mild dysplasia). Atypical cells are present in the lower one third of the epithelium (H&E stain, ×250). **B,** Low-grade squamous intraepithelial lesion cytology. These cells show an altered nuclear-to-cytoplasmic ratio with enlargement and have granular chromatin (Pap stain, ×800).

microscope with a powerful light source that is used to carefully examine the cervix. The instrument is placed just outside the vagina after a speculum has been inserted and the cervix brought into view. After any obscuring mucus is removed with a swab, the cervix is carefully examined for the presence of lesions. Dilute acetic acid (3% to 5%) is applied to the cervix, and after 30 to 60 seconds the cervix is again examined. Acetic acid dehydrates the epithelial cells and dysplastic cells with large nuclei will reflect light and appear white. An experienced colposcopist can distinguish those tissue patterns associated with cervical dysplasia from normal epithelium (Fig. 28.8).

For a thorough and complete exam, the entire transformation zone must be assessed ("satisfactory" colposcopy). If some portions of the transformation zone cannot be visualized as they extend into the endocervical canal or for other reasons, the colposcopy is considered "unsatisfactory" as the examiner is unable determine the presence or extent of abnormal tissue. In the case of abnormal cytology and an unsatisfactory colposcopy, it is recommended that an endocervical curettage (ECC) be performed. Cervical biopsies should be performed of any acetowhite lesions noted (Fig. 28.9). It is common for a small amount of bleeding to occur after biopsy, and this can be controlled with ferric subsulfate (Monsel's solution) or silver nitrate sticks. Cervical biopsy specimens are very small and the biopsy site usually heals within a few days (Fig. 28.10).

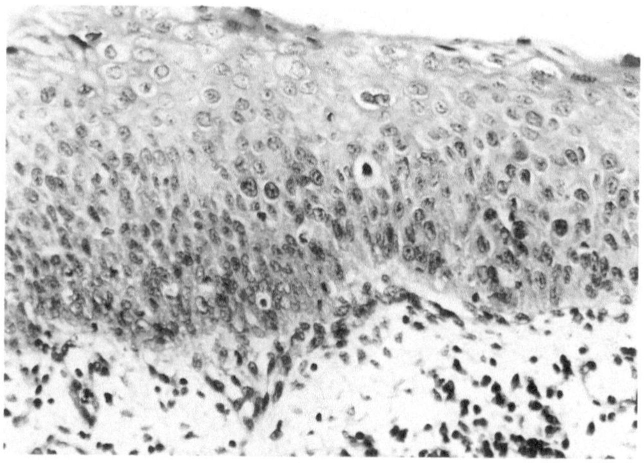

**Figure 28.6** Cervical intraepithelial neoplasia 2 (moderate dysplasia). The atypical cells extend approximately halfway through to the epithelium (H&E, ×300).

## CERVICAL DYSPLASIA IN PREGNANCY

In pregnancy, the cervix becomes larger, the blood supply to the cervix is increased, and decidual changes in the epithelium can be confused with CIN. The ASCCP provides guidelines for the management of abnormal cytology in pregnancy (Massad, 2013). Colposcopy is safe in pregnancy. However, biopsies should only be performed if there is suspicion for invasive disease. It is highly unlikely for dysplasia to progress significantly during pregnancy, and in the majority of patients further evaluation can be postponed until 6 to 8 weeks after delivery. If invasive cancer is suspected, cervical biopsies are indicated and can be performed safely during pregnancy. However, ECC should never be performed during pregnancy. If CIN2/3 is diagnosed, further evaluation and treatment can be delayed until the postpartum period. If there is significant concern for a dysplastic lesion, a follow-up with colposcopy or repeat cytology is acceptable at intervals no more frequent than every 12 weeks. If invasive cancer is diagnosed, a conization procedure under anesthesia can be performed.

## NATURAL HISTORY OF CERVICAL INTRAEPITHELIAL NEOPLASIA

Cervical intraepithelial neoplasia (CIN), the precancerous lesion of the squamous epithelium of the cervix, is a histologic (versus cytologic) diagnosis based on tissue examination of a cervical biopsy specimen. CIN is graded as 1, 2, or 3 depending on the how much of the epithelial layer contains atypical cells. CIN 1, or mild dysplasia, frequently spontaneously regresses, often within weeks to months. When cellular atypia involves two thirds of the thickness of the epithelium, it is designated as CIN 2. The process still remains reversible at this stage, with approximately 40% regressing spontaneously without treatment. When the cellular atypia involves more than two thirds of the epithelium, it

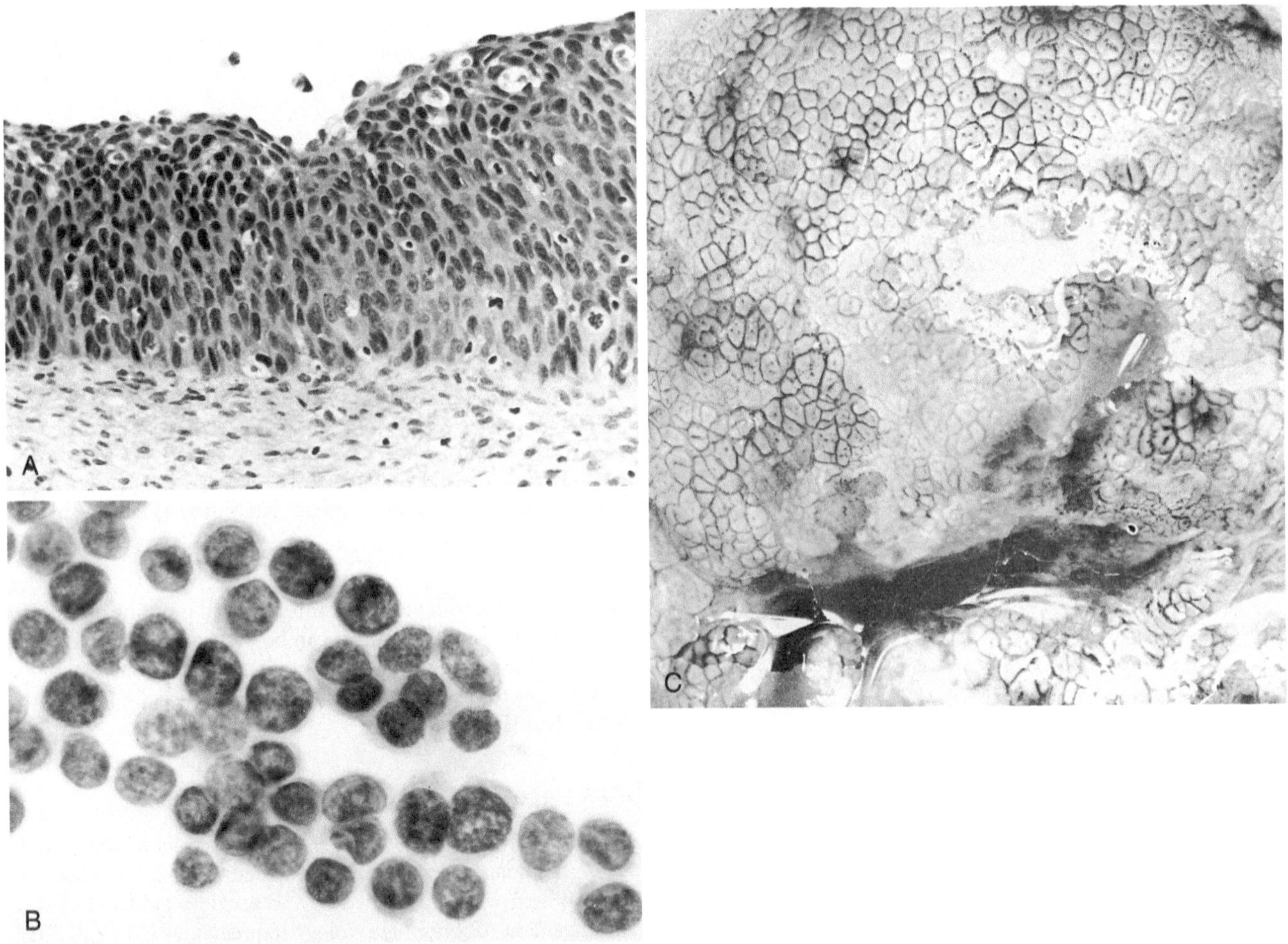

**Figure 28.7** **A,** Cervical intraepithelial neoplasia 3 (severe dysplasia, carcinoma in situ). There is a lack of squamous maturation throughout the thickness of the epithelium. Almost all the cells have enlarged nuclei with granular chromatin. Note that the basement membrane is intact, showing that this process is confined to the epithelial layer only. **B,** High-grade squamous intraepithelial lesion. These cells exhibit large nuclei with granular chromatin. Very little cytoplasm can be seen (Pap stain, ×800). **C,** Extensive cervical intraepithelial neoplasia 3 (CIN 3) lesion covering most of the epithelium visible in this image. The predominant feature is a mosaic pattern. There is umbilication of many of the tiles with a punctate vessel, a common feature of CIN 3. Although this large lesion must be examined carefully for evidence of atypical vessels, a hallmark of invasive cancer, none are seen in this view (×8). (**C,** From Kolstad P, Stafl A. *Atlas of Colposcopy.* Baltimore: University Park Press; 1972.)

is designated as CIN 3. This term encompasses what was once called severe dysplasia and carcinoma in situ. CIN 3 is a precursor to invasive cancer, and treatment is recommended. However, approximately one third of these lesions may spontaneously disappear.

Among women screened in the United States, the incidence of CIN 1 is approximately 4% and the incidence of CIN 2/3 is approximately 5%.

## MANAGEMENT OF CERVICAL DYSPLASIA

The approach to treatment of CIN lesions since the 1970s has changed and continues to evolve. Many low-grade lesions disappear spontaneously, and treatment is indicated for lesions that have demonstrated a potential for further progression. The ASCCP provides regularly updated guidelines for the management of cervical dysplasia (Massad, 2013).

### CERVICAL INTRAEPITHELIAL NEOPLASIA 1

In almost all cases, CIN 1 is a manifestation of a transient HPV infection, and the regression rates are high. Patients with CIN 1 require follow-up to ensure that the lesion regresses.

#### Cervical Intraepithelial Neoplasia 1 with Low-Grade Squamous Intraepithelial Lesion Cytology

Given the high rates of spontaneous regression, CIN 1 with LSIL cytology is usually managed with observation. These patients should undergo co-testing with cytology and HPV testing at 12 months or repeat cytology alone at 12 months in patients 21 to 24 years old. If CIN 1 persists for more than 2 years, a definitive excisional procedure can be considered.

#### Cervical Intraepithelial Neoplasia 1 with High-Grade Squamous Intraepithelial Lesion Cytology

If the diagnosis of CIN 1 is preceded by cytology showing HSIL or AGC, there is a higher chance of underlying CIN

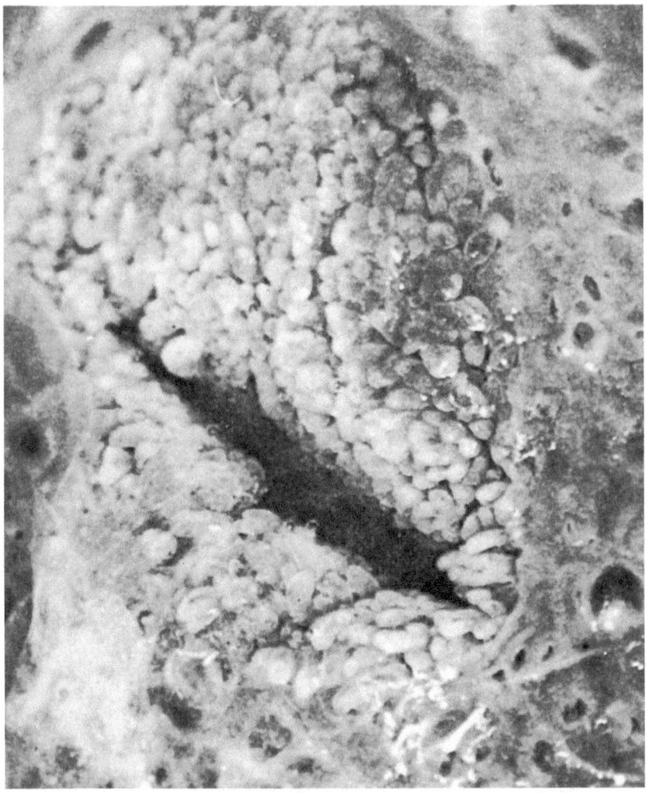

**Figure 28.8** Normal cervix as seen through a colposcope at approximately 6× magnification. The central grapelike structures are covered with columnar epithelium. The tissue outside this area represents squamous metaplasia. There are multiple gland openings in this area, indicating that columnar epithelium is being replaced by squamous epithelium. This area between the columnar and squamous epithelia is known as the *transformation zone*. (From Coppleson M, Pixley E, Reid B. *Colposcopy: A Scientific and Practical Approach to the Cervix in Health and Disease*. Springfield, IL: Charles C. Thomas; 1971.)

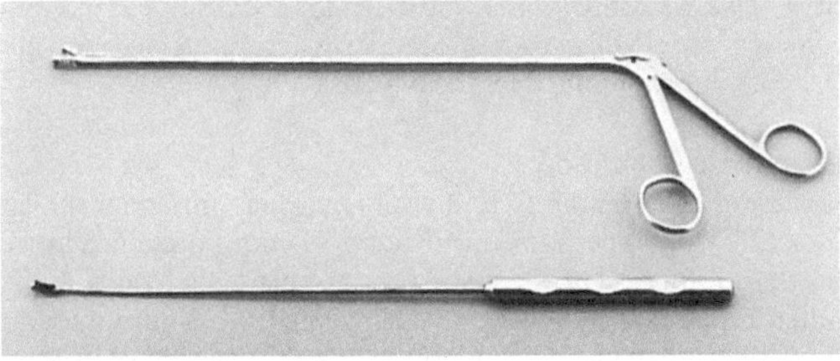

**Figure 28.9** Cervical biopsy instruments: biopsy *(top)*; endocervical curette *(bottom)*.

2/3, and more aggressive management should be considered. In patients who have completed childbearing, an excisional procedure is recommended. In women who desire future fertility, close follow-up with cytology and colposcopy at 6 months is recommended. A small percentage of CIN 1 lesions progress to CIN 2 or 3, but it is not possible to determine which lesions have this potential, so continued follow-up is recommended.

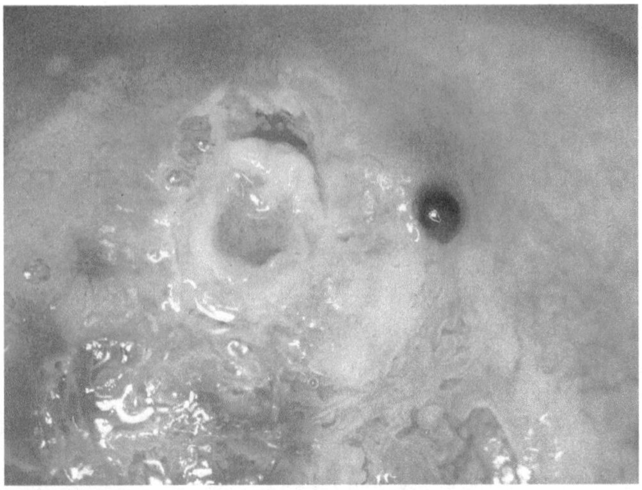

**Figure 28.10** Image (≈ ×12) of a cervical biopsy site 72 hours after the procedure. The eschar is already beginning to separate from the cervix.

## CERVICAL INTRAEPITHELIAL NEOPLASIA 2/3

It is difficult to distinguish CIN 2 from CIN 3 pathologically, so the two diagnoses are often grouped together as CIN 2/3 and managed similarly. Approximately 40% of CIN 2 lesions and 30% of CIN 3 lesions regress spontaneously (Castle 2009). However, 22% of CIN 2 will progress to CIN 3 and 5% will progress to cancer. Furthermore, 12% to 40% of CIN 3 will progress to cancer. Most women with CIN 2/3 should be treated with an ablative or excisional procedure. Young women and those desiring future fertility may be managed with careful observation, including cytology and colposcopy initially every 6 months with long-term follow-up depending on findings. Pregnant women with CIN 2/3 and no evidence of invasion may be observed during the pregnancy, with evaluation delayed until 6 weeks postpartum. Women with a history of CIN 2/3 are more likely to develop another lesion in the future. Therefore long-term follow-up for at least 20 years is recommended, even if this extends screening past age 65 (Massad, 2013).

## TREATMENT OF CERVICAL DYSPLASIA

Treatment of CIN can be accomplished by ablation or excision, with these methods having first-treatment success rates of greater than 90% in properly selected patients. (Ostör, 1993; Soutter, 1997; Mitchell, 1998; Martin-Hirsch, 2013; Massad, 2013). Ablative methods include cryotherapy and $CO_2$ laser ablation. Excisional procedures include the loop electrosurgical excision procedure (LEEP), cold knife conization (CKC), and $CO_2$ laser conization. The choice of treatment modality depends on the availability of equipment and the experience and expertise of the clinician. Hysterectomy is not recommended as the initial treatment of cervical dysplasia, as it is usually unnecessary for the treatment of CIN. Furthermore, if high-grade dysplasia is present, conization must first be performed to rule out underlying invasive cancer that may require more advanced procedures such as radical hysterectomy, radical trachelectomy, and lymph node dissection.

### *Ablative Methods*

Ablative procedures treat CIN but do not provide further diagnostic information. To qualify for ablative therapy, there should be no suspicion of glandular involvement or invasive cancer. Specific criteria for ablative therapies include the following:

- Satisfactory colposcopy with visualization of entire cervical squamocolumnar junction
- Biopsy confirming presence of CIN; abnormal cytology alone is not sufficient
- Lesion does not involve the endocervical canal and negative endocervical curettage (if available)

#### Cryotherapy

Cryotherapy is a commonly used treatment for CIN lesions that is safe, effective, and relatively simple to perform. However, it does not provide a specimen for pathology review and in many high-resource settings has been replaced by LEEP. Contraindications to cryotherapy include large lesions (those covering >75% of the cervix or those that cannot be covered by the cryoprobe) and lesions that extend into the endocervical canal. In addition, if the patient had an endocervical curettage performed and it shows evidence of dysplasia, cryotherapy is contraindicated.

The procedure includes performing colposcopy to confirm that the lesion is confined to the exocervix. A probe is selected that will cover the entire lesion. In most systems, $N_2O$ is used as the refrigerant. The cervix will freeze quickly, but the probe must remain in place until the ice ball extends to at least 5 mm beyond the edge of the instrument. In most cases, this takes 3 minutes. The refrigerant is then turned off, and the probe is allowed to thaw and separate from the cervix. It is recommended that a 3-5-3 double freeze–thaw cycle is performed with 3 minutes of freezing, followed by 5 minutes of thawing and another 3 minutes of freezing. Most patients experience little discomfort during the procedure. Because the tissue that was destroyed remains on the cervix, the patient will experience vaginal discharge within a few hours. As the tissue sloughs, the amount of discharge increases and malodor is common. It may take as long as 3 weeks for the discharge to stop. The patient should be cautioned to place nothing in the vagina for at least 3 weeks after the procedure to avoid dislodgment of the eschar.

#### $CO_2$ Laser Ablation

This technique became available in the 1980s but has largely been replaced by LEEP in the United States. A focused $CO_2$ laser beam is directed at the cervical epithelium, where water in the tissue absorbs the laser energy and the tissue is destroyed by vaporization. The lesion is typically ablated to a depth of 5 mm. Several safety procedures must be followed, including the use of protective eyewear by all personnel in the procedure room, the use of a blackened or brushed speculum to avoid damage to surrounding tissues by misdirected laser beams, and using wet towels and cloth drapes to prevent fire. Because little devitalized tissue is left after the procedure, there is no prolonged vaginal discharge as there is with cryotherapy. The success rate is similar to that for cryotherapy and excisional procedures. The advantages of this technique are that the area of tissue destruction can be minimized and there is no prolonged vaginal discharge as there is with cryotherapy. Similar to cryotherapy, there is no specimen for pathologic evaluation. Treatment success depends on the correct choice of laser energy delivered and proper depth and extent of treatment.

### *Excisional Methods*

Excisional procedures have the advantage over ablative procedures of providing a pathologic specimen for further diagnostic information. The specific indications for an excisional procedure over an ablative procedure include the following:

- Suspected microinvasion
- Adenocarcinoma in situ or other glandular abnormalities
- Unsatisfactory colposcopy in which the transformation zone is not fully visualized
- Lack of correlation between cytology and colposcopy/biopsies
- Unable to rule out invasive disease
- Lesion extending into the endocervical canal
- Endocervical curettage showing CIN or a glandular abnormality
- Recurrence after an ablative or previous excisional procedure

#### Loop Electrosurgical Excision

The loop electrosurgical excision procedure (LEEP), also called *large loop excision of the transformation zone (LLETZ),* is currently the most common method for the treatment of CIN 2/3 in the United States. It involves the removal of the transformation zone of the cervix under local anesthesia and can be performed safely in the office. The cervix is infiltrated with an anesthetic/vasoconstrictor solution, and a cone-shaped piece of the cervix inclusive of the transformation zone is removed (Martin-Hirsch, 2013). The LEEP procedure utilizes a thin wire in the shape of a loop and an electrosurgical generator, providing a cutting current to remove the tissue. The loops are available in a variety of shapes and sizes, allowing selection of a loop best fit to the patient's lesion (Fig. 28.11). Bleeding areas can be cauterized with a ball electrode attached to the current generator set to cautery.

The removed tissue is examined histologically for diagnosis and evaluation of margin status. Management guidelines for positive margins are provided by the ASCCP and include reexcision versus follow-up cytology and endocervical sampling, depending on pathology results, patient age, and the desire for future fertility.[25] Hysterectomy is rarely indicated for the treatment of CIN, unless a repeat diagnostic procedure is recommended but not feasible due to minimal remaining cervix.

#### Cold Knife Conization

Cold knife conization (CKC) is an excisional procedure similar to a LEEP but is performed with a scalpel under anesthesia in the operating room. For the evaluation of squamous lesions, CKC offers little advantage over LEEP. However, CKC is advantageous in patients with glandular abnormalities or suspicion of invasive cancer, as CKC uses a scalpel and avoids the thermal artifact sometimes seen at the margins of specimens obtained by LEEP. Once the specimen is removed, bleeding can be controlled with cauterization and the application of ferrous subsulfate (Monsel's solution). Sutures to control bleeding are rarely necessary.

## *FOLLOW-UP AFTER TREATMENT OF CERVICAL DYSPLASIA*

The rate of recurrent or persistent disease following excisional or ablative treatment for CIN 2/3 is 5% to 17%, with no significant differences in outcomes between the different treatment

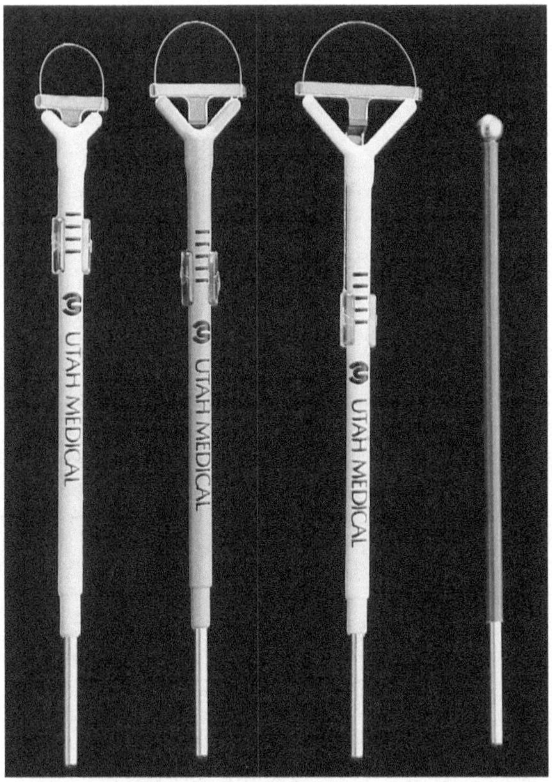


**Figure 28.11** Electrodes (Utah Medical) used for a loop electroexcision procedure. The width of the excised tissue specimens can range from 1 to 2 cm, and the specimen depth can be adjusted by sliding the guard attached to the electrode shaft. Following excision, the base of the cervix is often gently cauterized with a ball electrode. (Courtesy of Dr. Steven E. Waggoner, University of Chicago, Chicago, IL.)

modalities. Factors associated with recurrent/persistent disease include the following:

- Large lesion size
- Endocervical gland involvement
- Positive margins

The current ASCCP recommendations for surveillance following excision of CIN 2/3 with negative margins consist of co-testing with cervical cytology and HPV at 12 and 24 months. If both co-tests are negative, the woman can return to routine screening (Massad, 2013). If any test is abnormal, colposcopy with endocervical sampling is recommended.

## CERVICAL CANCER PREVENTION IN LOW- AND MIDDLE-INCOME COUNTRIES

Although the screening and diagnosis algorithms described earlier are effective, they are expensive and require high-level infrastructure and well-trained personnel. In addition, they require three separate patient visits with communication of test results between visits. There is therefore a significant need for alternative solutions, particularly in low-resource settings in the United States and in low- and middle-income countries (LMICs) where there is often a lack of trained personnel, infrastructure, and pathology services.

One commonly used approach in low-resource settings is visual inspection with acetic acid (VIA), in which acetic acid is applied to the cervix and, if there is whitening of the epithelium indicating a precancerous lesion, immediate treatment with cryotherapy is performed (See & Treat). VIA and cryotherapy can be performed by nonphysicians, such as community health workers. Such a program using VIA has been shown to decrease cervical cancer mortality by more than 30% in unscreened communities in India (Shastri, 2014). Several additional low-cost innovative screening options are also under development for LMICs.

## VAGINAL INTRAEPITHELIAL NEOPLASIA

Vaginal intraepithelial neoplasia (VaIN) is similar to CIN and is defined as squamous atypia without invasion. The true incidence of vaginal intraepithelial neoplasia (VaIN) is unknown but is estimated to be approximately 0.2/100,000 in the United States. It is most commonly diagnosed in women between 43 to 60 years of age. Classification is similar to CIN and reflects the depth of involvement of the epithelial layer (VaIN 1, 2, and 3). Risk factors for VaIN include current or previous neoplasia elsewhere in lower genital tract (cervix, vulva) and persistent HPV infection. Previous studies have shown 50% to 90% of patients with VaIN had prior or concurrent intraepithelial neoplasia or carcinoma of the cervix or vulva (Aho, 1991; Sillman, 1997; Cheng, 1999). Most cases of VaIN are discovered incidentally during colposcopy due to abnormal cytology. Presenting symptoms of postcoital discharge or spotting are rare. Suspicious lesions should be biopsied to confirm the diagnosis. The upper third of the vagina is the most common site of VaIN (Boonlikit, 2010).

Patients with VaIN 1 are followed with surveillance similar to patients with CIN 1 due to the low risk of progression to invasive cancer. However, it is recommended that patients with VaIN 2 or VaIN 3 undergo treatment, as the risk of progression to vaginal cancer is estimated to be 2% to 5%. Treatment options include excision, ablation, and topical therapy with 5-fluorouracil or imiquimod (Audet-Lapointe, 1990; Cardosi, 2001). There is a high recurrence rate of 20% to 30% regardless of the treatment modality used, and these patients should be carefully followed long term. There are no standard guidelines for the follow-up of patients with VaIN 2/3, but it is reasonable to perform cytology and colposcopy every 6 to 12 months for 2 years (Zeligs 2013). The role of HPV testing in patients with VaIN is still unknown.

## VULVAR INTRAEPITHELIAL NEOPLASIA

Vulvar intraepithelial neoplasia (VIN) is defined as squamous atypia of the vulva (Fig. 28.12). The incidence of VIN 3 is approximately 2.86 per 100,000 women in the United States (Judson, 2006). VIN is classified as (1) VIN, usual type, or (2) VIN, differentiated type (Sideri, 2005; ACOG, 2011). VIN, usual type, is the most common form of VIN and is an HPV-associated condition. It occurs in younger women, may be multifocal, and is associated with cervical and vaginal dysplasia. VIN, differentiated type, is less common and unrelated to HPV infection, but it is associated with chronic inflammatory conditions such as lichen sclerosus and lichen planus. Symptoms of VIN include pruritus, pain, and burning; however, many patients

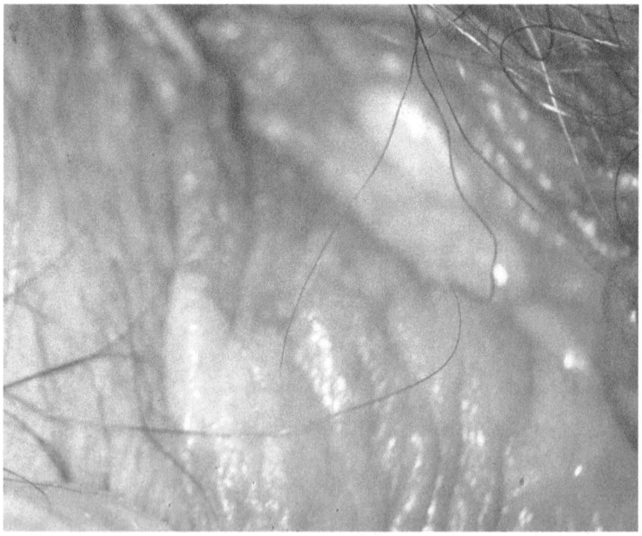

**Figure 28.12** Vulvar intraepithelial neoplasia (VIN) 3 lesion as seen through a colposcope after the application of acetic acid. A second lesion is out of focus but can be seen in the background. VIN is often multifocal.

are asymptomatic and VIN is incidentally discovered during a thorough pelvic exam. Punch biopsies should be performed of any lesions noted on the vulva, particularly those that persist or are not responsive to therapy for other conditions. Furthermore, colposcopy of the vulva (vulvoscopy) with biopsies of any lesions should be performed in all patients with CIN or VaIN due to the association with these other HPV-related conditions.

VIN 1 is a benign entity, and treatment for asymptomatic disease is not necessary. However, patients with VIN 2/3 should undergo treatment due to the risks of underlying cancer and progression of disease. Treatment modalities include excision, ablation, and topical therapies (Jones, 2005; ACOG, 2011). All modalities have similar effectiveness (Wallbillich 2012). The modality used depends on the risk of invasive disease, location of the lesion, and the extent of disease and symptoms. If underlying invasive disease is suspected, patients with VIN 2/3 should undergo wide local excision. Other options for diffuse disease include $CO_2$ laser ablation and topical therapies. The most commonly used topical therapy is imiquimod, a topical immune response modifier that is applied to vulvar lesions three times per week for 16 weeks. Small studies have shown imiquimod to be very effective with a complete response rate of 51%, a partial response rate of 25% and a recurrence rate of 16% (van Seters, 2008; Mahto, 2010). Similar to VaIN, VIN recurrence rates are high. There are no standard guidelines for the follow-up of patients with VIN 2/3, but it is reasonable to perform vulvoscopy every 6 to 12 months for 2 years. The role of HPV testing in patients with VIN is unknown.

## KEY POINTS

- HPV infection is the cause of virtually all cases of cervical cancer.
- Almost all HPV infections regress spontaneously, but if the infection persists, dysplasia and cancer may develop.
- Smoking increases the likelihood that an HPV infection will persist or progress.
- Vaccines are available that prevent HPV infection and the development of dysplasia and cancer.
- When Pap testing is used widely, it decreases the incidence of cervical cancer by approximately 70%.
- The Bethesda System (TBS) terminology is used for the reporting of cervical cytology specimens.
- The colposcope is used to evaluate women with abnormal Pap tests.
- In some cases, an HPV infection can lead to a precancer of the cervix, called *CIN*. CIN is graded as 1, 2, or 3, depending on the depth of the epithelial thickness involved.
- CIN 1 should be observed rather than treated because it usually regresses spontaneously.
- CIN 2/3 can be treated by ablation with cryotherapy or excision with LEEP or cold knife conization.

## KEY REFERENCES


ACOG Committee Opinion No. 509: Management of vulvar intraepithelial neoplasia. Committee on Gynecologic Practice of American College Obstetricians and Gynecologists. *Obstet Gynecol.* 2011;118(5):1192–1194.

ACOG Practice Bulletin - Clinical Management Guidelines for Obstetrician-Gynecologists: No. 140: Management of Abnormal Cervical Cancer Screening Test Results and Cervical Cancer Precursors. Committee on Practice Bulletin. *Obstet Gynecol.* 2013;122(6):1338–1367.

Aho M, Vesterinen E, Meyer B, Purola E, Paavonen J. Natural history of vaginal intraepithelial neoplasia. *Cancer.* 1991;68(1):195–197.

Aldieh L, Klein RS, Burk R, et al. Prevalence, incidence and type-specific persistence of human papillomavirus in human immunodeficiency virus (HIV)-positive and HIV-negative women. *J Infect Dis.* 2001;184:682–690.

Audet-Lapointe P, Body G, Vauclair R, et al. Vaginal intraepithelial neoplasia. *Gynecol Oncol.* 1990;35:232–239.

Boonlikit S, Noinual N. Vaginal intraepithelial neoplasia: a retrospective analysis of clinical features and colpohistology. *J Obstet Gynaecol Res.* 2010;36(1):94–100.

Cardosi RJ, Bomalaski JJ, Hoffman MS. Diagnosis and management of vulvar and vaginal intraepithelial neoplasia. *Obstet Gynecol Clin North Am.* 2001;28:685–702.

Castle PE, Schiffman M, Wheeler CM, et al. Evidence for frequent regression of cervical intraepithelial neoplasia-grade 2. *Obstet Gynecol.* 2009;113:18–25.

Chang F. Role of papillomaviruses. *J Clin Pathol.* 1990;43:269–276.

Cheng D, Ng TY, Ngan HY, Wong LC. Wide local excision (WLE) for vaginal intraepithelial neoplasia (VAIN). *Acta Obstet Gynecol Scand.* 1999;78(7):648–652.

Dillner J, Rebolj M, Birembaut P, et al. Long term predictive values of cytology and human papillomavirus testing in cervical cancer screening: joint European cohort study. *BMJ.* 2008;337:a1754.

FUTURE II Study Group: Quadrivalent vaccine against human papillomavirus to prevent high-grade cervical lesions. *N Engl J Med.* 2007;356(19):1915–1927.

Huh W, Ault K, Chelmow D, et al. Use of primary high-risk human papillomavirus testing for cervical cancer screening: interim clinical guidance. *Obstet Gynecol.* 2015;125(2):330–337.

International Collaboration of Epidemiological Studies of Cervical Cancer (ICESCC). Carcinoma of the cervix and tobacco smoking: collaborative reanalysis of individual data on 13,541 women with carcinoma of the cervix and 23,017 women without carcinoma of the cervix from 23 epidemiological studies. *Int J Cancer.* 2006;118(6):1481–1495.

International Collaboration of Epidemiological Studies of Cervical Cancer (ICESCC). Comparison of risk factors for invasive squamous cell carcinoma and adenocarcinoma of the cervix: collaborative reanalysis of individual data on 8,097 women with squamous cell carcinoma and 1,374 women with adenocarcinoma from 12 epidemiological studies. *Int J Cancer.* 2007;120(4):885–891.

Jones RW, Rowan DM, Stewart AW. Vulvar intraepithelial neoplasia: aspects of the natural history and outcome in 405 women. *Obstet Gynecol.* 2005;106(6):1319–1326.

Joura EA, Giuliano AR, Iversen OE, et al. A 9-valent HPV vaccine against infection and intraepithelial neoplasia in women. *N Engl J Med.* 2015;372(8): 711–723.

Judson P, Hammerman E, Baxter N, et al. Trends in the incidence of invasive and in-situ vulvar carcinoma. *Obstet Gynecol.* 2006;107(5):1018–1022.

Mahto M, Nathan M, O'Mahony C. More than a decade on: review of the use of imiquimod in lower anogenital intraepithelial neoplasia. *Int J STD AIDS.* 2010;21(1):8–16.

Markowitz LE, Dunne EF, Saraiya M, et al. Human Papillomavirus vaccination: recommendations of the Advisory Committee on Immunization Practices (ACIP). *MMWR Recomm Rep.* 2014;63(RR-05):1–30. Available online at htt p://www.cdc.gov/mmwr/preview/mmwrhtml/rr6305a1.htm.

Martin-Hirsch PP, Bryant A. Interventions for preventing blood loss during the treatment of cervical intraepithelial neoplasia. *Cochrane Database Syst Rev.* 2013a;12. CD001421.

Martin-Hirsch PP, Paraskevaidis E, Bryant A, et al. Surgery for cervical intraepithelial neoplasia. *Cochrane Database Syst Rev.* 2013b;12. CD001318.

Massad LS, Einstein MH, Huh WK, et al. 2012 updated consensus guidelines for the management of abnormal cervical cancer screening tests and cancer precursors. *J Low Genit Tract Dis.* 2013;17(5 Suppl 1):S1–S27.

McIntyre-Seltman K, Castle PE, Guido R, et al. Smoking is a risk factor for cervical intraepithelial neoplasia grade 3 among oncogenic human papillomavirus DNA-positive women with equivocal or mildly abnormal cytology. *Cancer Epidemiol Biomarkers Prev.* 2005;14:1165–1170.

Mitchell MF, Tortolero-Luna G, Cook E, et al. A randomized clinical trial of cryotherapy, laser vaporization, and loop electrosurgical excision for treatment of squamous intraepithelial lesions of the cervix. *Obstet Gynecol.* 1998;92(5):737–744.

Monsonego J, Cox JT, Behrens C, et al. Prevalence of high-risk human papilloma virus genotypes and associated risk of cervical precancerous lesions in a large U.S. screening population: data from the ATHENA trial. *Gynecol Oncol.* 2015;137(1):47–54.

Moscicki AB. Management of adolescents with abnormal cytology and histology. *Obstet Gynecol Clin North Am.* 2008 Dec;35(4):633–643.

Moscicki AB, Shiboski S, Broering J, et al. The natural history of human papillomavirus infection as measured by repeated DNA testing in adolescent and young women. *J Pediatr.* 1998;132(2):277–284.

Moscicki AB, Shiboski S, Hills NK, et al. Regression of low-grade squamous intra-epithelial lesions in young women. *Lancet.* 2004;364(9446):1678–1683.

Munger K, Baldwin A, Edwards KM, et al. Mechanisms of human papillomavirus-induced oncogenesis. *J Virol.* 2004;78(21):11451–11460.

Ostör AG. Natural history of cervical intraepithelial neoplasia: a critical review. *Int J Gynecol Pathol.* 1993;12(2):186–192.

Papanicolaou GN, Traut HF. The diagnostic value of vaginal smears in carcinoma of the uterus. 1941.

Sideri M, Jones RW, Wilkinson EJ, et al. Squamous vulvar intraepithelial neoplasia: 2004 modified terminology, ISSVD Vulvar Oncology Subcommittee. *J Reprod Med.* 2005 Nov;50(11):807–810.

Solomon D, Schiffman M, Tarone R, et al. Comparison of three management strategies for patients with atypical squamous cells of undetermined significance: baseline results from a randomized trial. *J Natl Cancer Inst.* 2001;93(4):293–299.

Soutter WP, de Barros Lopes A, Fletcher A, et al. Invasive cervical cancer after conservative therapy for cervical intraepithelial neoplasia. *Lancet.* 1997;349(9057):978–980.

van Seters M, van Beurden M, ten Kate FJ, et al. Treatment of vulvar intraepithelial neoplasia with topical imiquimod. *N Engl J Med.* 2008;358(14):1465–1473.

Wheeler CM, Greer CI, Becker TM, et al. Short-term fluctuations in the detection of cervical human papillomavirus DNA. *Obstet Gynecol.* 1996;88(2):261–268.

Wolf JK, Ramirez PT. The molecular biology of cervical cancer. *Cancer Invest.* 2001;19(6):621–629.

Zeligs K, Byrd K, Tarney C, Howard RS, et al. A clinicopathologic study of vaginal intraepithelial neoplasia. *Obstet Gynecol.* 2013;122(6):1223–1230.

Zweitig S, Noller K, Reale F, et al. Neoplasia associated with atypical glandular cells of undetermined significance on cervical cytology. *Gynecol Oncol.* 1997;65:314–318.

# 29

# Malignant Diseases of the Cervix

## Microinvasive and Invasive Carcinoma: Diagnosis and Management

*Anuja Jhingran, Larissa A. Meyer*

The majority of cervical malignancies are carcinomas; a summary of the more common histologic types is shown in Box 29.1. Approximately 80% to 85% of these tumors are squamous cell carcinomas, and 15% to 20% are adenocarcinomas. The incidence of adenocarcinomas has increased in most developing countries, particularly among younger women. Carcinoma of the cervix is closely associated with early and frequent sexual contact and cervical viral infection, particularly human papillomavirus (HPV) as detailed in Chapter 28. According to the American Cancer Society, the frequency of cervical cancer has been steadily decreasing, in part because of the effect of widespread screening for premalignant cervical changes by cervical cytology (Pap smear). In the United States, there will be an estimated 12,900 new cases of invasive cervical cancer diagnosed in 2015 with 4100 related deaths (Siegel, 2015). The incidence of cervical carcinoma in the United States is higher among the Hispanic population (10.5%) compared with whites (7.1%) and African Americans (10.2%) (Siegel, 2015). However, the mortality rate from cervical cancer is the highest among African Americans compared with other races, partly because African Americans tend to be diagnosed at a later stage. Invasive cervical cancers are diagnosed at a localized stage in 51% of white women and 43% of African American women. This chapter details the various types of cervical carcinoma and considers the natural history, methods of diagnosis and evaluation, and details of therapy. Primary sarcomas and melanomas of the cervix are extremely rare and are not considered separately (Fig. 29.1).

## HISTOLOGIC TYPES

Varieties of squamous cell carcinoma of the cervix are illustrated in Figure 29.2. An early form, microinvasive carcinoma, is considered separately in the next section. Most squamous cell carcinomas of the cervix are reported to be of the large cell, nonkeratinizing type, but some are keratinized, and squamous pearls may be seen. The degree of differentiation of the tumors is usually designated by three grades: G1, well differentiated; G2, intermediate; and G3, undifferentiated. However, there is no consensus on the value of tumor grade as a major prognostic factor for squamous cell carcinoma of the cervix.

A rare variety of squamous cell carcinoma is the so-called verrucous carcinoma, which is morphologically similar to that found in the vulva (see Chapter 30). These warty tumors appear as large bulbous masses (Fig. 29.3). They rarely metastasize but unfortunately may be admixed with the more virulent, typical squamous cell carcinomas, in which case metastatic spread is more likely.

Adenocarcinomas may have a number of histologic varieties. The typical variant often contains intracytoplasmic mucin and is related to the mucinous cells of the endocervix (endocervical pattern; Fig. 29.4). However, on occasion, the cells contain little or no mucin, and then the tumor may resemble an endometrial carcinoma (endometrioid pattern). It may be difficult histologically to ascertain whether these carcinomas arise in the cervix or endometrium. Although not independently diagnostic, the immunohistochemical panel that is recommended to assist in differentiating endocervical from endometrial primary malignancies includes estrogen receptor (ER), vimentin, monoclonal carcinoembryonic antigen (CEA), and p16. Typically, an

**Box 29.1 Summary of Major Categories of Cervical Carcinoma**

**Squamous Cell Carcinomas**
Large cell (keratinizing or nonkeratinizing)
Small cell
Verrucous

**Adenocarcinomas**
Typical (endocervical)
Endometrioid
Clear cell
Adenoid cystic (basaloid cylindroma)
Adenoma malignum (minimal deviation adenocarcinoma)

**Mixed Carcinomas**
Adenosquamous
Glassy cell carcinoma

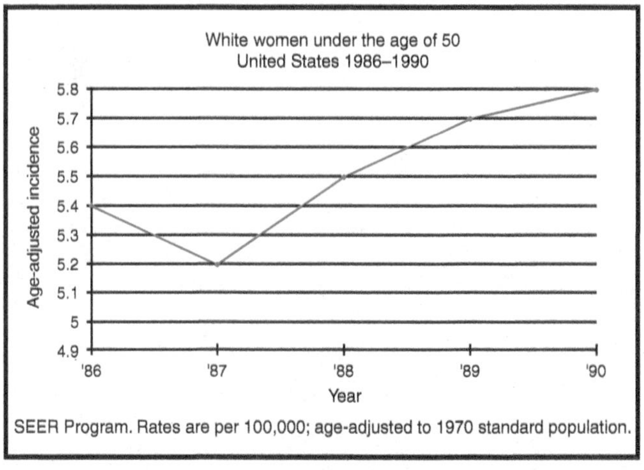


**Figure 29.1** Incidence rates of invasive carcinoma. (From Ries ALG, Miller BA, Hankey BF, et al. *SEER Cancer Statistics Review, 1973-1991* [NIH Publ. No. 94-2789]. Bethesda, MD: National Institutes of Health; 1994:136-144.)

endocervical carcinoma will stain diffusely positive for p16 and CEA and will be negative for ER and vimentin.

A rare but important virulent variety of adenocarcinoma is adenoma malignum. These microscopically innocuous-appearing tumors consist of well-differentiated mucinous glands (Fig. 29.5) that vary in size and shape and infiltrate the stroma. Despite their bland histologic appearance, they tend to be deeply invasive and metastasize early. The term *minimal deviation adenocarcinoma* is applied to these tumors.

Clear cell adenocarcinomas of the cervix are histologically identical to those of the ovary (see Chapter 33) and vagina (see Chapter 31). They are uncommon in the cervix and can be associated with intrauterine diethylstilbestrol exposure, although they also may develop spontaneously in the absence of diethylstilbestrol exposure.

Adenoid cystic carcinomas are rare. Berchuk and Mullin have summarized 88 cases reported in the literature (Berchuk, 1985). These tumors are aggressive and may resemble cylindromas of salivary gland or breast origin and histologically may resemble

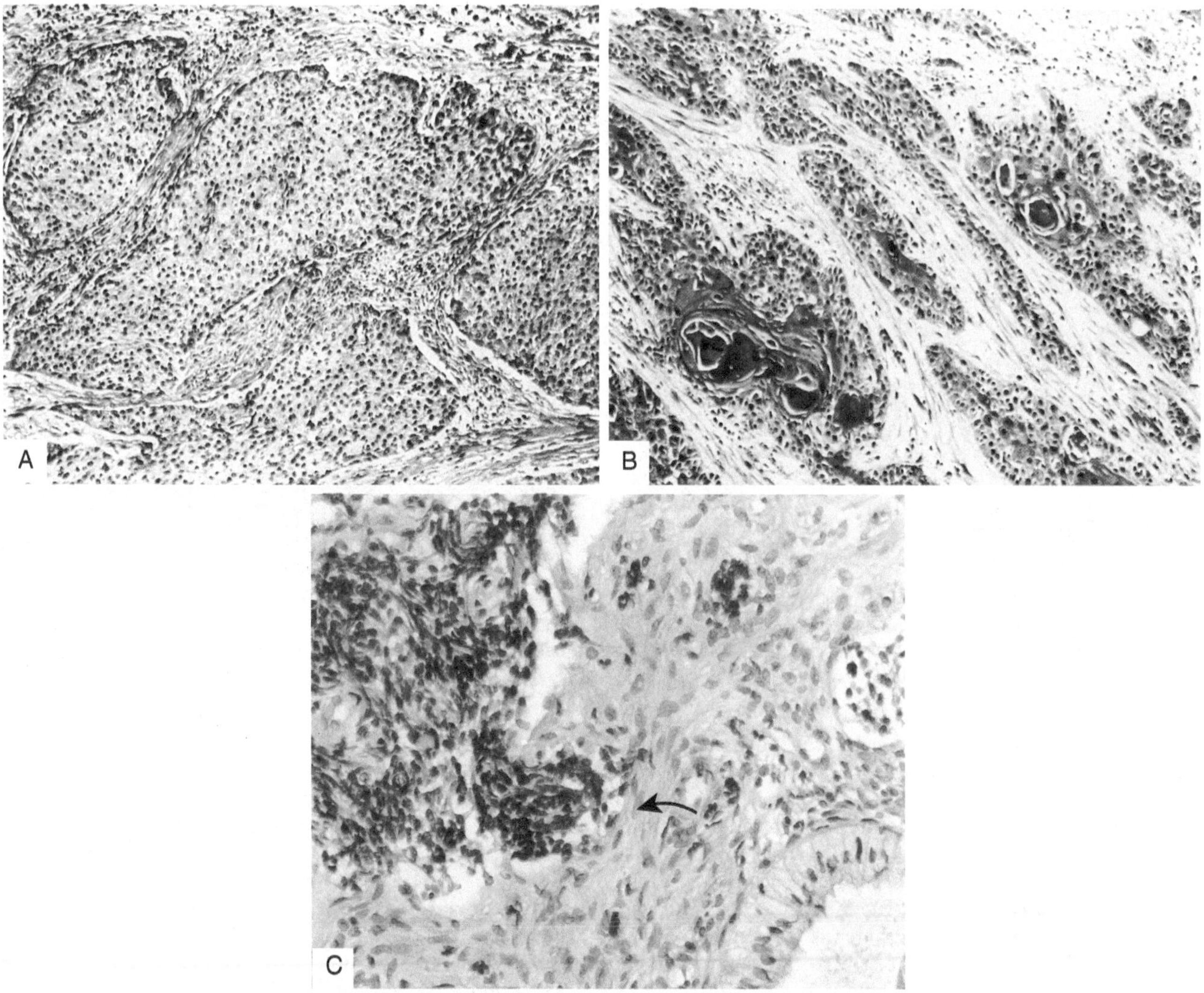


**Figure 29.2** ***A,*** Large-cell, nonkeratinizing squamous cell carcinoma. Discrete islands of uniform, large cells with abundant cytoplasm are separated by fibrous stroma (× 160). ***B,*** Keratinizing squamous cell carcinoma. Irregular nests of squamous cells forming several pearls are separated by fibrous stroma. The nests have pointed projections (× 160). ***C,*** Small cell neuroendocrine carcinoma of the cervix *(arrow)* infiltrating between normal endocervical glands (H&E, × 240). (***A*** and ***B,*** From Clement PB, Scully RE. Carcinoma of the cervix: histologic types. *Semin Oncol.* 1982;9:251-264; ***C,*** Courtesy of Dr. Anthony Montag, Department of Pathology, University of Chicago, Chicago.)

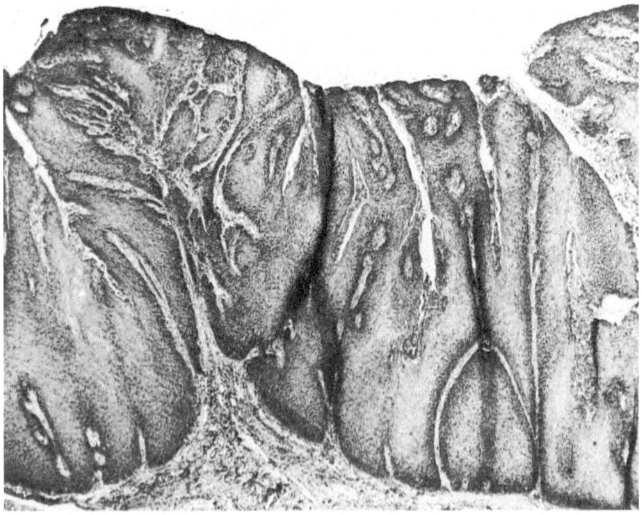

**Figure 29.3** Verrucous carcinoma. Downgrowths of papillae have broad bases. Tumor cells are well differentiated (× 34). (From Clement PB, Scully RE. Carcinoma of the cervix: histologic types. *Semin Oncol.* 1982;9:251-264.)

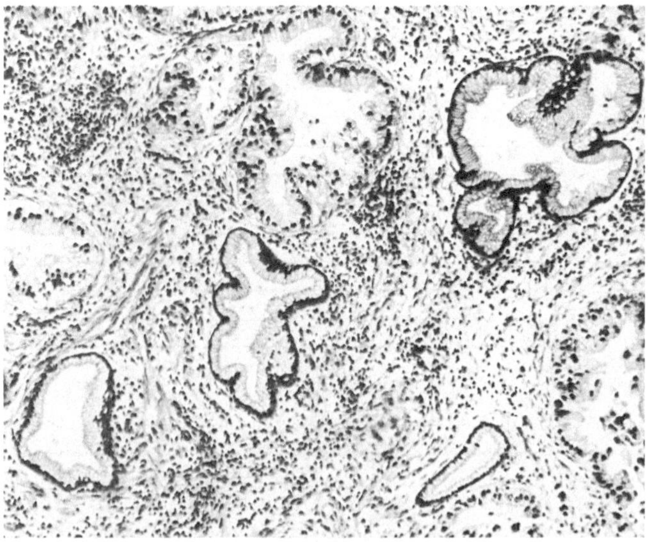

**Figure 29.5** Adenoma malignum. Glands are mostly well differentiated, appearing normal except for their irregular shapes. A few obviously malignant glands are also present (× 160). (From Clement PB, Scully RE. Carcinoma of the cervix: histologic types. *Semin Oncol.* 1982;9:251-264.)

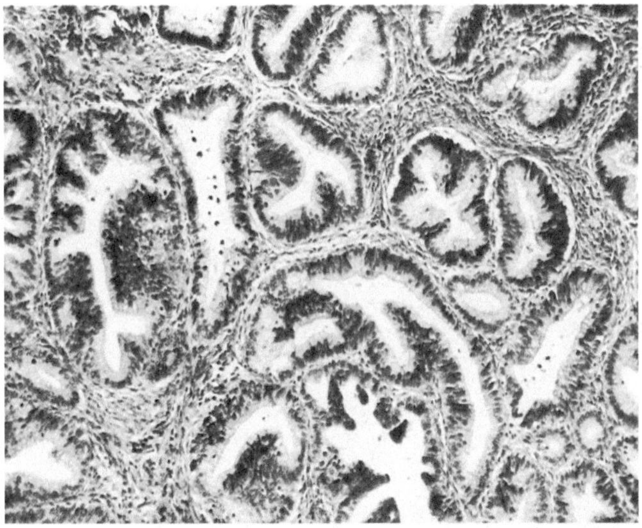

**Figure 29.4** Typical adenocarcinoma. Irregular glands are lined by stratified mucin-containing epithelium. Mitotic figures are numerous (× 160). (From Clement PB, Scully RE. Carcinoma of the cervix: histologic types. *Semin Oncol.* 1982;9:251-264.)

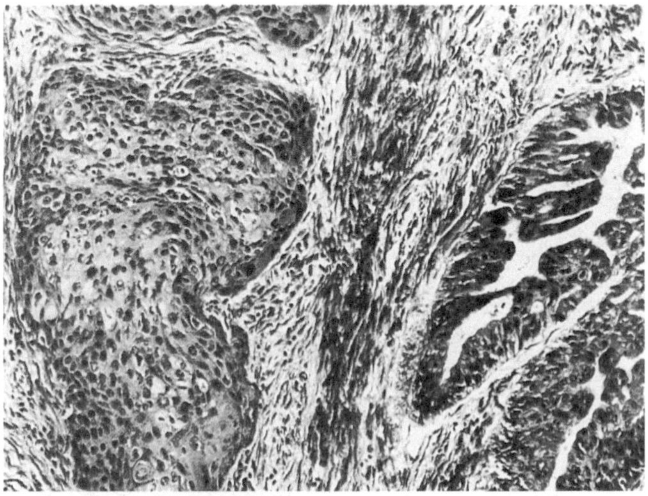

**Figure 29.6** Well-differentiated adenosquamous carcinoma. Glandular structure lies adjacent to a nest of nonkeratinizing large squamous cells (× 400). (From Clement PB, Scully RE. Carcinoma of the cervix: histologic types. *Semin Oncol.* 1982;9:251-264.)

basal cell carcinomas of the skin (adenoid basal, or basaloid, carcinomas). Most patients with these tumors are older than 60 years. The basaloid variety appears to be less aggressive.

Adenosquamous carcinomas, as the name implies, consist of squamous carcinoma and adenocarcinoma elements in varying proportions (Fig. 29.6). They occur frequently in pregnant women. A particularly virulent variety is termed *glassy cell carcinoma* (Fig. 29.7). This is an undifferentiated tumor consisting of large cells containing cytoplasm, with a ground-glass appearance. Glassy cell carcinomas tend to metastasize early to lymph nodes as well as to distant sites and usually have a fatal outcome.

Small cell carcinoma of the cervix is rare, comprising less than 5% of all carcinomas of the cervix. Women with small cell carcinoma are likely to be 10 years younger than those with squamous cell carcinoma. The cells are small anaplastic cells with scant cytoplasm. They behave aggressively and are frequently associated with widespread metastasis to multiple sites, including bone, liver, skin, and brain. Efforts to treat these cancers with approaches typically used for small cell carcinoma of the lung have had mixed results.

Another variant that is not in the World Health Organization (WHO) classification is non–small cell neuroendocrine tumors. These tumors contain intermediate to large cells, high-grade nuclei, and eosinophilic cytoplasmic granules of the type seen in neuroendocrine cells. Reported survival rates for patients with these aggressive carcinomas are similar to those of patients with small cell tumors, and optimal therapy has yet to be established.

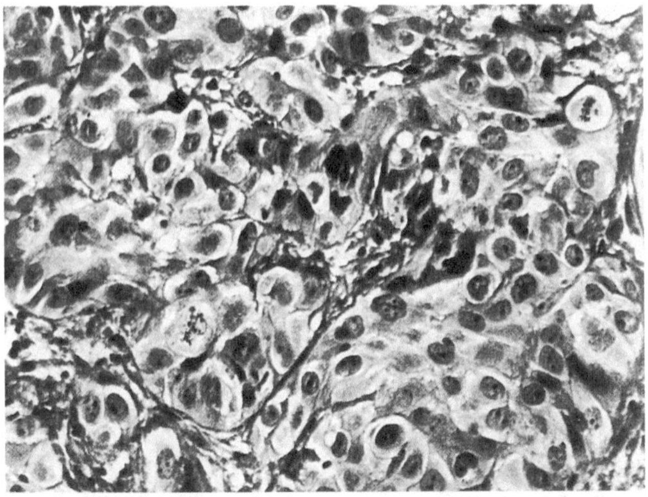

**Figure 29.7** Glassy cell carcinoma. Cells have sharp borders, ground-glass-type cytoplasm, and nuclei containing prominent nucleoli (× 1000). (From Clement PB, Scully RE. Carcinoma of the cervix: histologic types. *Semin Oncol.* 1982;9:251-264.)

# CARCINOMA OF THE CERVIX

## CLINICAL CONSIDERATIONS

Patients with carcinoma of the cervix characteristically present with abnormal bleeding or brownish discharge, frequently noted following douching or intercourse and also occurring spontaneously between menstrual periods. These patients often have a history of not having had a cytologic (Pap) smear for many years. Other symptoms, such as back pain, loss of appetite, and weight loss, are late manifestations and occur when there is extensive spread of cervical carcinoma. The patients tend to be in their 40s to 60s, with a median age of 52 years. Preinvasive intraepithelial carcinoma of the cervix (see Chapter 28) occurs primarily in women in their 20s and 30s and has become more common in those in their 20s, leading to a gradual increase in the incidence of invasive carcinoma in younger patients.

The diagnosis is established by biopsy of the tumor; a specimen can easily be obtained during an office examination. A Kevorkian, Eppendorf, Tischler, or similar punch biopsy instrument is convenient to use. Occasionally, it is necessary to biopsy nodularity or indurations in the vagina near the cervix to ascertain the limit of tumor spread and define a correct tumor stage. If the woman's cytologic smear suggests invasive carcinoma, with no gross lesion visible, and endocervical curettage does not demonstrate carcinoma, or if an adequate biopsy specimen to establish carcinoma cannot be obtained, cervical conization should be performed.

## STAGING

The staging of carcinoma of the cervix depends primarily on the pelvic examination; the designation may be modified by general physical examination, chest radiographic examination, intravenous pyelography (IVP), or computed tomography (CT) and is not changed based on operative findings. Table 29.1 describes the four stages of cervical carcinoma according to the International Federation of Gynecology and Obstetrics (FIGO; revised in 2009) (Pecorelli, 2009). The types of tumor distribution that may be observed in the various stages are illustrated in Figure 29.10.

**Table 29.1** Clinical Stages of Carcinoma of the Cervix Uteri

| Stage | Characteristics |
|---|---|
| I | Carcinoma is strictly confined to the cervix (extension to the corpus should be disregarded) |
| IA | Invasive cancer that can be diagnosed only by microscopy, with deepest invasion ≤5 mm and largest extension ≥7 mm (Fig. 29.8) |
| IA1 | Measured stromal invasion ≤3 mm in depth and extension of ≤7 mm (Fig. 29.9) |
| IA2 | Measured stromal invasion of >3 mm and not >5 mm, with an extension of not >7 mm |
| IB | Clinically visible lesions limited to the cervix uteri or preclinical cancers greater than IA* |
| IB1 | Clinically visible lesion ≤4 cm in greatest dimension |
| IB2 | Clinically visible lesion >4 cm in greatest dimension |
| II | Cervical carcinoma invades beyond the uterus, but not to the pelvic wall or lower third of vagina |
| IIA | No obvious parametrial involvement |
| IIA1 | Clinically visible lesion ≤4 cm in greatest dimension |
| IIA2 | Clinically visible lesion >4 cm in greatest dimension |
| IIB | Obvious parametrial involvement |
| III | The tumor extends to the pelvic wall or involves lower third of the vagina or causes hydronephrosis or nonfunctioning kidney† |
| IIIA | Tumor involves lower third of the vagina, with no extension to the pelvic wall |
| IIIB | Extension to the pelvic wall or hydronephrosis or a nonfunctioning kidney |
| IV | The carcinoma has extended beyond the true pelvis or has involved (biopsy-proven) mucosa of the bladder or rectum; a bullous edema, as such, does not permit a case to be allotted to stage IV |
| IVA | Spread of growth to adjacent pelvic organs |
| IVB | Spread to distant organs |

Modified from Pecorelli S. Revised FIGO staging for carcinoma of the vulva, cervix, and endometrium. *Int J Gynaecol Obstet.* 2009;105:103.

All cases with hydronephrosis or a nonfunctioning kidney are included, unless they are known to be from another cause.

*All macroscopically visible lesions, even with superficial invasion, are allotted to stage IB carcinomas. Invasion is limited to a measured stromal invasion, with a maximum depth of 5 mm and a horizontal extension of not >7 mm. Depth of invasion should not be >5 mm taken from the base of the epithelium of the original tissue, superficial or glandular. The depth of invasion should always be reported in millimeters, even in those cases with early (minimal) stromal invasion (minus 1 mm). The involvement of vascular or lymphatic spaces should not change the stage allotment.

†On rectal examination, there is no cancer-free space between the tumor and the pelvic wall.

## NATURAL HISTORY AND SPREAD

Carcinoma of the cervix is initially a locally infiltrating cancer that spreads from the cervix to the vagina and paracervical and parametrial areas. Grossly, the tumors may be ulcerated (Fig. 29.11), similar to carcinomas occurring elsewhere in the female genital tract, and may have an exophytic growth pattern or cauliflower-like appearance extruding from the cervix. Alternatively, they may be endophytic, in which case they are asymptomatic, particularly in the early stage of development, and tend to be deeply invasive when diagnosed. These usually start initially from an endocervical location and often fill the cervix and lower uterine segment, resulting in a barrel-shaped cervix. The latter tumors tend to metastasize to regional pelvic nodes and, because of the tendency of late diagnosis, are often more advanced than the exophytic variety. The primary

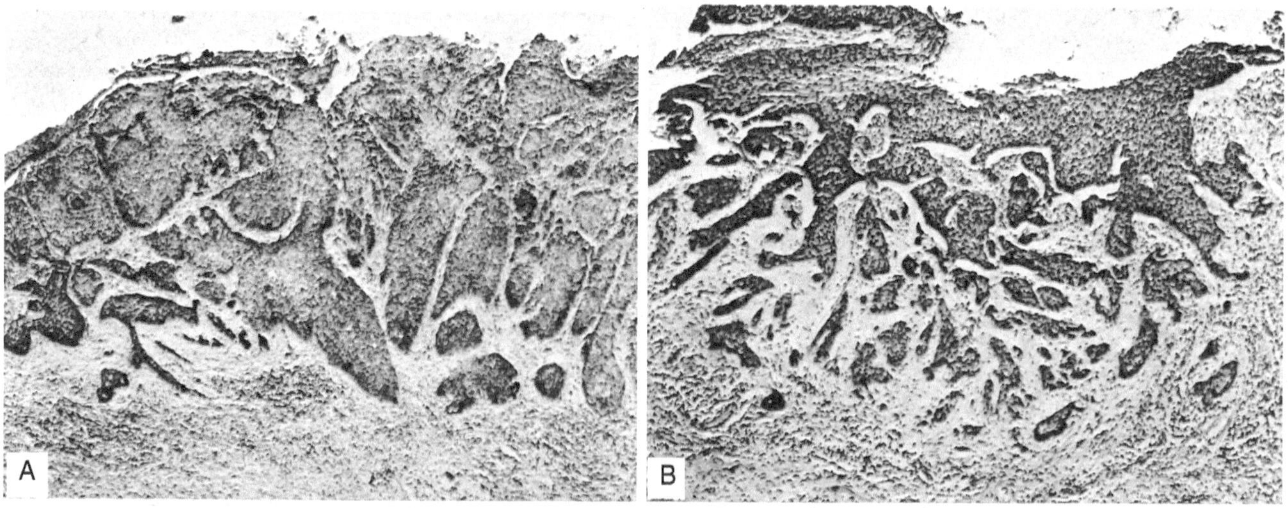

Figure 29.8 **A,** Tumor with only 0.5 mm of invasion (× 40). **B,** Example of so-called *spray pattern* with multiple invasive nodules in stroma. Invasion is only 1 mm (× 50). (From Creasman WT, Fetter BF, Clarke-Pearson DL, et al. Management of stage IA carcinoma of the cervix. *Am J Obstet Gynecol.* 1985;153:164-172.)

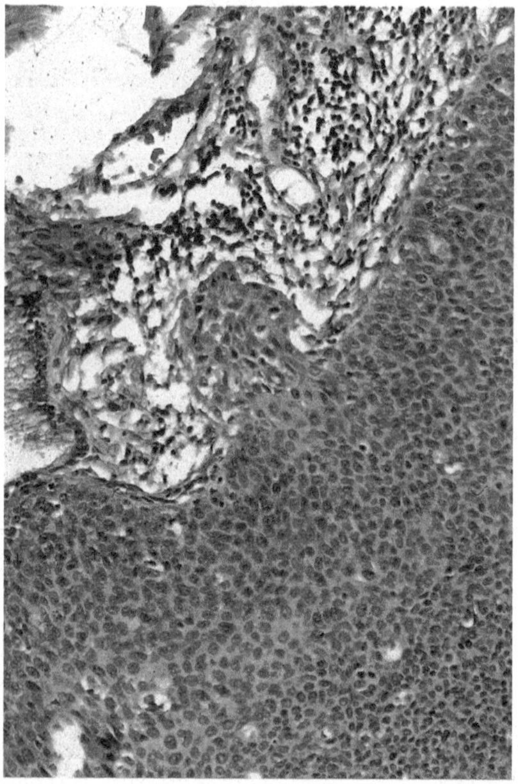

**Figure 29.9** Photomicrograph showing early stromal invasion. (Courtesy of Dr. Anthony Montag, Department of Pathology, University of Chicago, Chicago.)

path for distant spread is through lymphatics to the regional pelvic nodes. Bloodborne metastases from cervical carcinomas do occur but are less frequent and are usually seen late in the course of the disease.

Initially, cervical carcinoma spreads to the primary pelvic nodes, which include the pericervical node; presacral, hypogastric (internal iliac), and external iliac nodes; and nodes in the obturator fossa near the vessels and nerve. From this primary group, tumor spread proceeds secondarily to the common iliac and paraaortic nodes. Rarely, the inguinal nodes are involved; however, if the lower third of the vagina is involved, the median inguinal nodes should be considered a primary node. The distribution of lymph node involvement in 26 cases of untreated carcinoma of the cervix was studied in detail by Henriksen (Fig. 29.12) (Henriksen, 1949). A series studying the incidence and distribution pattern of retroperitoneal lymph node metastases in 208 patients with stages IB, IIA, and IIB cervical carcinomas who underwent radical hysterectomy and systemic pelvic node dissection reported that 53 patients (25%) had node metastasis. The obturator lymph nodes were the most frequently involved, with a rate of 19% (39 of 208), and the authors proposed them as sentinel nodes for cervical cancers. An important distal node that becomes involved after the paraaortic group is the left scalene node—that is, the left supraclavicular node. A biopsy of this node may be performed in the assessment of advanced cervical carcinoma to clarify whether the tumor has spread outside the abdomen. In addition to nodal spread, hematogenous spread of cervical carcinoma occurs primarily to the lung, liver and, less frequently, bone (see Recurrence later in the chapter).

## PROGNOSTIC FACTORS

FIGO stage is the most important determinant of prognosis for carcinoma of the cervix (Table 29.2); however, there are other factors, including tumor and patient characteristics that are prognostic and are not included in the FIGO staging system. One of the most important predictors is tumor size for local recurrence and death for patients treated with surgery or radiation therapy (Eifel, 1994). The FIGO staging classification for stage I disease has been modified to include tumor diameter (i.e., ≤4 cm, stage IB1; >4 cm, stage IB2). Another important prognostic factor is involvement of lymph nodes, which also is not part of the clinical staging system. In several surgical series, after a radical hysterectomy, patients with positive pelvic lymph nodes had a 35% to 40% lower 5-year survival rate than patients with negative nodes. Patients with positive paraaortic nodes have a survival rate that is approximately 50% that of patients

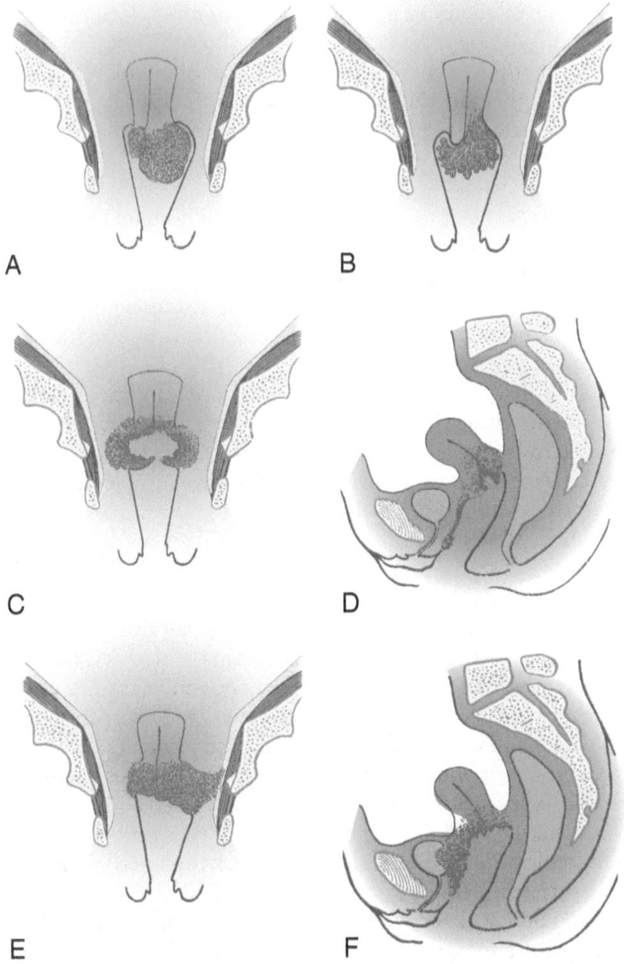


**Figure 29.10** Staging of cervical carcinoma. **A,** Stage IB, nodular cervix. **B,** Stage IIA, carcinoma extending into left vault. **C,** Stage IIB, parametrium involved on both sides, but carcinoma has not invaded pelvic wall; endocervical crater. **D,** Stage IIIA, submucosal involvement of anterior vaginal wall and small papillomatous nodule in its lower third. **E,** Stage IIIB, parametrium involved on both sides; at left, carcinoma has invaded pelvic wall. **F,** Stage IVA, involvement of bladder. (From Pettersson F, Bjorkholm E. Staging and reporting of cervical carcinoma. *Semin Oncol.* 1982;9:287-298.)

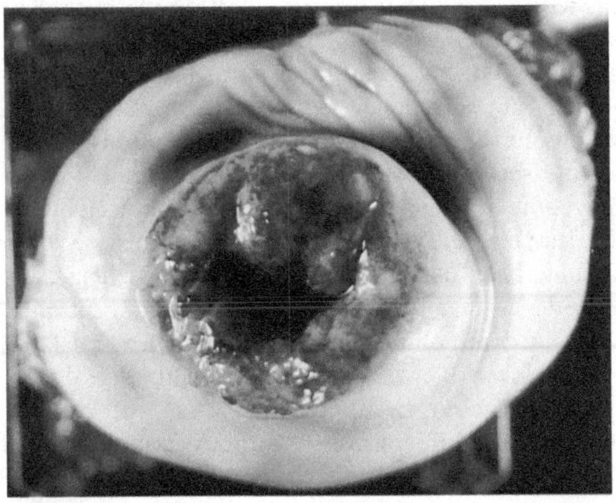

**Figure 29.11** Carcinoma of the cervix (gross specimen).

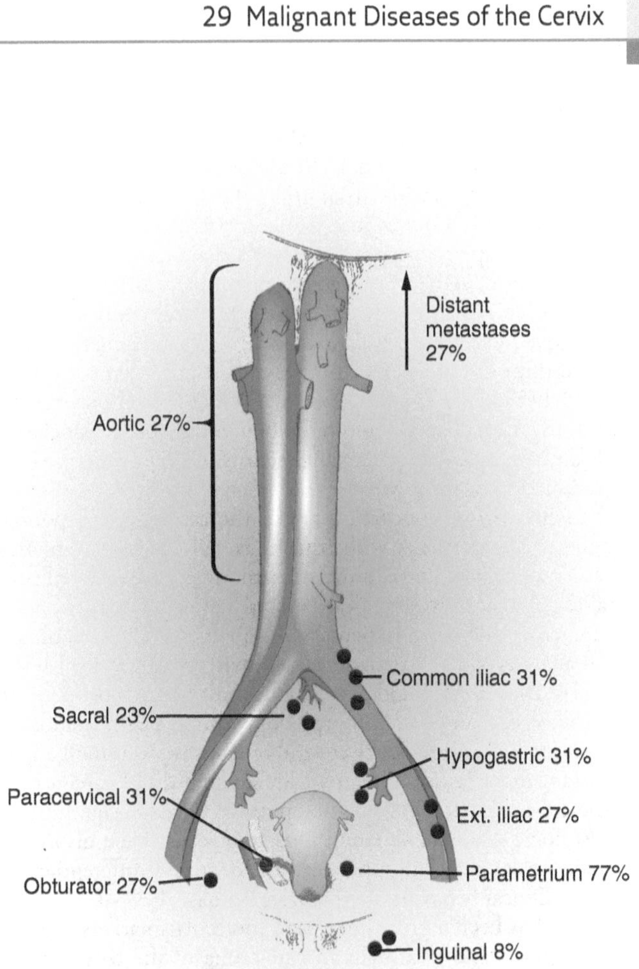


**Figure 29.12** Frequency of lymph node metastases in cervical carcinoma. Shown is the incidence of node group involvement in 26 nontreated cases of cervical carcinoma. (From Henriksen E: The lymphatic spread of carcinoma of the cervix and of the body of the uterus. *Am J Obstet Gynecol.* 1949;58:924-942.)

**Table 29.2** Carcinoma of the Uterine Cervix: Distribution by Stage and 5-Year Survival Rates for Patients Treated in 1990-1992 (*n* = 11,945)

| Stage | No. of Patients (*n*) | 5-Year Survival |
|---|---|---|
| Ia | 902 | 95.01% |
| Ib | 4657 | 80.1% |
| II | 3364 | 64.2% |
| III | 2530 | 38.31% |
| IV | 492 | 14% |

Modified from Pecorelli S, Creasman WT, Pettersson F, et al. *FIGO Annual Report on the Results of Treatment in Gynaecological Cancer,* vol 23. Milan, Italy: International Federation of Gynecology and Obstetrics; 1998.

with similar stage disease and negative paraaortic nodes. With extended-field radiation therapy, patients with positive paraaortic nodes have approximately a 40% to 50% 5-year survival rate. There is a strong correlation between positive nodes and positive lymph–vascular space invasion (LVSI) in the tumor specimen in patients with cervical carcinoma. However, LVSI may be an independent predictor of prognosis as shown in a number of larger surgical series.

In patients who have had a radical hysterectomy, histologic evidence of extracervical spread (≥10 mm), deep stromal invasion (>70% invasion), and LVSI are associated with a poorer prognosis. A randomized trial from the Gynecologic Oncology Group (GOG) compared observation versus adjuvant radiation therapy in patients after radical hysterectomy with a combination of two of the factors mentioned earlier; patients who received radiation therapy had better local control as well as improved overall survival (Sedlis, 1999). Involvement of the parametrium in the hysterectomy specimen has been correlated with higher rates of lymph node involvement, local recurrence, and death from cancer. Uterine body involvement is associated with an increased rate of distant metastases in patients treated with radiation or surgery.

Patients with adenocarcinomas of the cervix have a poorer prognosis than patients with squamous cell carcinomas of the cervix. Investigators have found that among patients treated surgically, patients with adenocarcinomas have high relapse rates compared with rates in patients with squamous cell carcinomas. In an analysis of 1767 patients treated with radiation for FIGO stage IB disease, Eifel and associates found that independent of age, tumor size, and tumor morphology, patients with adenocarcinomas had the same pelvic control rate but twice as high a rate of distant metastasis as patients with squamous cell carcinomas of the cervix (Eifel, 1994). Although the prognostic significance of histologic grade for squamous carcinomas has been disputed, there is a clear correlation between the degree of differentiation and the clinical behavior of adenocarcinomas.

There has been a great interest in molecular markers regarding prognosis and treatment in carcinoma of the cervix. One of the most studied markers is the serum squamous cell carcinoma antigen. Studies have shown that pretreatment levels of this antigen correlate well with stage of disease, tumor histology, grade, type of tumor (exophytic vs. infiltrative), microscopic depth of invasion, and risk of lymph node metastases in patients with early stage disease. Possible clinical applications of this antigen may be to predict clinical outcome as well as a marker for monitoring the course of disease and response to treatment in patients with cervical cancer. Several investigators have reported significantly lower survival rates in patients with elevated values compared with patients with normal baseline levels, independent of stage. For detection of tumor recurrence, serial squamous cell carcinoma antigen testing has proved to be more specific than sensitive, with specificities ranging from 90% to 100% and sensitivities ranging from 60% to 90%. Further investigation is needed in these areas. Some investigators have found a higher rate of recurrence in patients with HPV-positive nodes (although negative for malignancies) and poor prognosis with the presence of HPV mRNA in the peripheral blood of cervical cancer patients. Other markers that have been investigated include epidermal growth factor receptor, cyclooxygenase-2, DNA-ploidy, tumor vascularity, and S-phase fraction.

## TREATMENT

### Pretherapy Evaluation

Once a woman has been diagnosed as having an invasive carcinoma, a pretreatment evaluation is conducted to determine the extent of disease, arrive at an accurate clinical staging, and plan the program of therapy. The usual evaluation consists of a thorough history and physical examination, routine blood studies, IVP or CT, and chest radiography. Demonstration of an obstructed ureter or nonfunctioning kidney caused by tumor automatically assigns the case at least to stage III (see Table 29.1). A barium enema test or flexible sigmoidoscopy, as well as a cystoscopy, is sometimes performed in the case of large tumors or for patients who will be receiving radiation treatment.

The best radiographic imaging technique for detecting lymph node metastases is unclear. CT and magnetic resonance imaging (MRI) are good for identifying enlarged nodes; however, the accuracy of these techniques in the detection of positive nodes is compromised by their failure to detect small metastases, and many enlarged nodes are caused not by metastases but by inflammation associated with advanced disease. The accuracy of MRI in the detection of lymph node metastases (72% to 93%) is similar to that of CT but better than CT and physical examination for the evaluation of tumor location, tumor size, depth of stromal invasion, vaginal extension, and parametrial extension of cervical cancer. However, with regard to detecting lymph node metastases or other distant disease, positron emission tomography (PET) shows promise. Several studies from a single institution have shown that $^{18}$F-fluorodeoxyglucose PET (FDG-PET) detects abnormal lymph nodes more often than CT, and those findings with PET are a better predictor of survival than those with CT or MRI in patients with carcinoma of the cervix. Medicare has approved PET/CT as part of the initial staging evaluation for patients with cervical carcinoma, and most insurance companies approve PET/CT for a 3-month follow-up.

Surgical sampling of lymph nodes is the most sensitive method of evaluating whether regional lymph nodes contain metastases; however, it is invasive, expensive, and delays treatment to the primary lesions. Laparoscopic lymph node dissection may decrease the time between surgery and the start of treatment and may be associated with less late radiation-related morbidity than open transperitoneal staging. Laparoscopic extraperitoneal paraaortic lymphadenectomy has also been described and may further decrease radiation-related bowel morbidity by avoiding entrance into the peritoneal cavity. In a study by Ramirez and colleagues, 22% of patients who had positive pelvic but negative paraaortic nodes on PET/CT had histopathologically positive paraaortic nodes (Ramirez, 2011).

### Treatment for Stage I

#### Stage IA

The term *microinvasion* has been used for years to describe patients with minimally invasive cervical cancer, but this term is not part of the FIGO staging system. Microinvasion was used to describe patients with 3-mm invasion or less and essentially no risk of metastatic spread. Several investigators went a step further to measure not only the depth of invasion but also tumor volume by measuring lateral spread. Volumetric measurements are generally more difficult and have not been embraced by pathologists (at least not in North America). Nevertheless, volumetric measurements are used in the FIGO staging scheme. There is ample evidence that patients with small-volume tumors measured only by depth of invasion or by two-dimensional measurement have a low risk of relapse and death with radical surgery or more conservative surgical approaches.

The diagnosis of microinvasive tumor cannot be made based on a biopsy specimen alone; a cervical conization must be performed. If the margin of the cervical cone specimen contains neoplastic epithelium, the risk of invasive tumor in the remaining uterus is increased. Decisions on treatment should be based on an adequate cone biopsy specimen. If a woman has positive margins, the cone can be repeated. Sometimes, deeper invasion will be uncovered and more radical treatment will be required. In some patients, conization alone is adequate.

Stage IA1 tumors measured stromal invasion is 3 mm or less, with lateral extension of 7 mm or less. These measurements are determined on a cone biopsy, which also determines other prognostic factors (e.g., lymph vascular space involvement, histologic subtype, grade). These factors do not alter the stage assignment, in spite of their adverse prognostic significance. In the absence of LVSI or high-risk histologic subtypes, the risk of lymph node metastases is remote and nonradical surgery is adequate. This may include cone biopsy, simple trachelectomy, or simple hysterectomy, depending on the circumstances and patient preference.

Patients with stage 1A2 tumors have a measured stromal invasion of 5 mm or less. Patients in this category, even without LVSI, are at a low risk of nodal involvement. Thus radical or modified radical approaches are usually recommended, which include modified radical hysterectomy or trachelectomy and pelvic lymph adenectomy. Stage IA1 patients who have LVSI are treated in the same manner as stage IA2 patients.

There continues to be interest in determining the necessity of treating the parametrium in patients with low-stage cervical cancer. Several investigators have noted that the risk of parametrial involvement is 1% or less in patients undergoing radical hysterectomy in low-risk situations. Parametrial resection contributes significant short-term and long-term morbidity to surgery. Lymphatic mapping techniques suggest that parametrial sentinel lymph nodes can be identified and resected without a radical dissection. In the future, we expect that the indications for surgery that omits the parametrial resection will grow.

### Stage IB

Stage IB encompasses tumors that are larger than stage IA, meaning 5 mm or larger in measured stromal invasion or more than 7-mm lateral spread. Stage IB also includes all visible lesions, even if the invasion is superficial (<5 mm). Clinicians should be aware of low-grade squamous cancers that can be easily visualized without magnification and have very superficial invasion. In our judgment, these patients should be treated similarly to stage IA patients.

Stage IB1 patients have tumor limited to the cervix that is 4 cm or less in diameter. These patients have equally good outcomes with radical surgery or radiotherapy. A major factor in favor of radical surgery is younger age, especially premenopausal patients for whom ovarian preservation is an option. In addition, there is now increasing availability of ovum transfer and pregnancy surrogates. Other factors favoring radical surgery are smaller size, desire to preserve fertility, and absence of other comorbidities that escalate the risk of surgery. Factors that favor radiotherapy are the presence of indicators that would result in postoperative radiotherapy if surgery were the primary therapy. These include larger size, extensive LVSI, suspicious findings on preoperative imaging, high-risk histologic subtypes, and deep stromal invasion on imaging or examination that increases the risk of close margins.

The decision regarding radical surgery or radiotherapy should be made with the active involvement of the woman, gynecologic oncologist, and radiation oncologist. Both modalities are associated with the potential for significant short- and long-term complications. Some complications such as bladder atony, food intolerance, or loss of sexual function are not easy to measure and can persist for years following treatment. Long-term survival data are similar for well-selected patient populations. Some data suggest more long-term patient satisfaction with outcomes related to surgery than radiotherapy.

Most gynecologic oncologists and radiation oncologists recommend concurrent chemoradiation for patients with stage IB2 cervical cancer. Reports demonstrate that up to 80% of stage IB2 patients who have undergone a radical hysterectomy will have clear indications for postoperative radiotherapy. Our experience is that postoperative radiotherapy results in greater toxicity than treatment with the cervix intact. The counterargument is that radical hysterectomy obviates the need for high-dose brachytherapy that is associated with the most severe and difficult to manage complications, notably pelvic fistulas. A number of innovations in treatment targeting techniques appear to be having a beneficial impact on reducing post-treatment fistula. Concurrent chemoradiation is our primary recommendation for stage IB2 patients and is discussed later in this chapter.

### *Operative Therapy: Radical Hysterectomy and Pelvic Node Dissection*

Radical hysterectomy and bilateral pelvic lymphadenectomy are effective for the treatment of stage IB and some early stage IIA cancers. It is important that the surgery removes the same volume of tissue that has received tumoricidal doses of radiation in patients for whom radiation is the sole therapy. The amount of tissue removed, particularly in the paracervical and parametrial areas near the ureter, depends on the extent and location of the tumor. Piver and colleagues defined five classes to describe the extent of the operation (Piver, 1974). Class I guarantees the removal of the entire cervix and uterus. The ureter is not disturbed from its bed. In many cases, this is described as an extrafascial hysterectomy, the type used after preoperative radiation for treatment of a barrel-shaped cervix (discussed later). A class II operation (Fig. 29.13) removes more paracervical tissue than class I; the ureters are retracted laterally but are not dissected from their attachments distal to the uterine artery, and the uterosacral ligaments are ligated approximately halfway between the uterus and rectum. The operation is usually performed with pelvic lymphadenectomy and is often termed a *modified radical hysterectomy*. The operation is useful to treat small microscopic carcinomas of the cervix. Magrina and colleagues used modified radical hysterectomy primarily for tumors smaller than 2 cm (median, 1.1 cm), with 5-year survival of 96% (Magrina, 1999). This procedure may occasionally be used to treat small, central cervical recurrences of carcinoma that are diagnosed following radiation therapy of the primary tumor. For a class III operation, the uterine artery is ligated at its origin from the anterior division of the hypogastric artery and the uterosacrals are ligated deep in the pelvis near the rectum (see Fig. 29.12). This operation is usually termed a *radical hysterectomy* (Meigs-Wertheim hysterectomy) and is performed for stage IB and, rarely, for stage IIA carcinomas of the cervix.

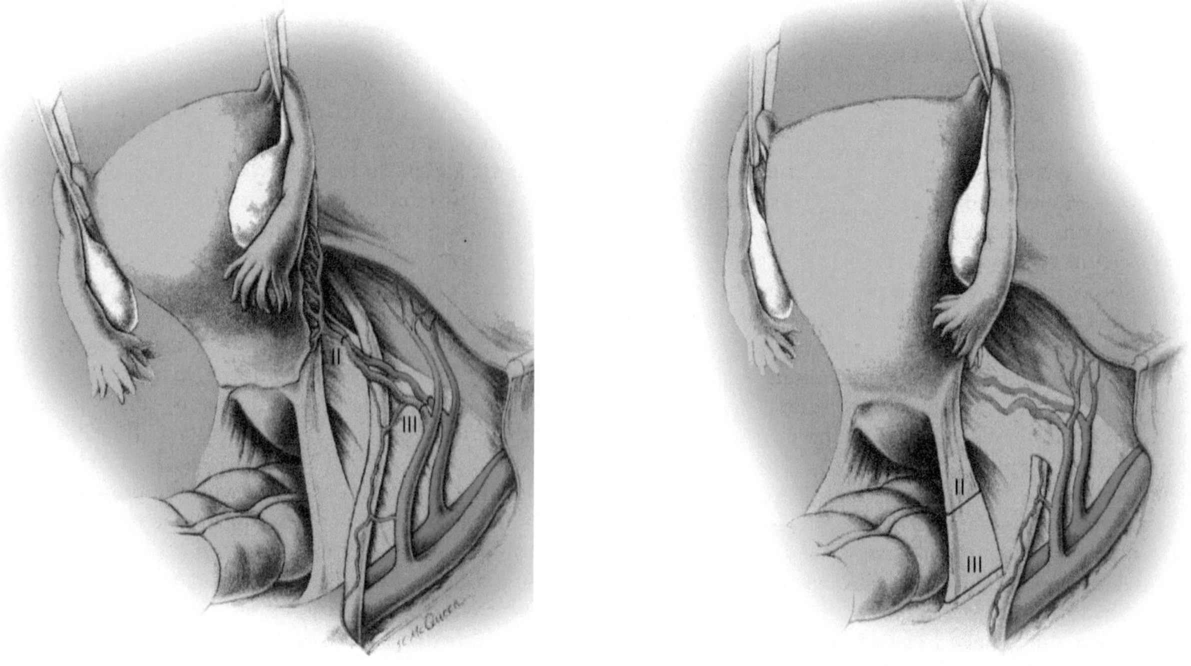


**Figure 29.13** Classes I and II radical hysterectomy with points of dissection shown (see text).

Class IV and V operations are infrequently performed. A class IV procedure involves a complete dissection of the ureter from its bed and sacrifice of the superior vesical artery. A class V operation involves resection of the distal ureter, bladder, or both, with reimplantation of the ureter into the bladder (ureteroneocystostomy). Both are designed to remove small, central recurrent disease and would be attempted to avoid an anterior exenteration (see later). Extensive data are not available, but the latter two procedures appear to have high complication rates.

Other classification systems for radical hysterectomy exist. Querleu and Morrow described a classification that is principally based on the lateral extent of resection (four types, A through D) with subtypes that address nerve preservation and paracervical lymphadenectomy (Querleu, 2008). Within this classification, four levels of lymph node dissection (1-4) are also defined according to arterial anatomy and overall radicality of the procedure.

Preoperative preparation for a woman who is to undergo a radical hysterectomy includes the same basic considerations for anyone undergoing a major operative procedure. Graduated compression, below-the-knee leg stockings and perioperative prophylactic doses of heparin or other low-molecular-weight heparin formulations are used to reduce the risk of thromboembolism. Prophylactic antibiotics are also frequently prescribed. During the course of the operation, care is taken not to grasp the ureters with instruments such as forceps to avoid damaging the periureteral capillary blood supply.

An important complication of pelvic lymphadenectomy is lymphocyst formation. Most gynecologic oncologists have abandoned the use of closed suction drains in radical hysterectomy patients and leave the pelvic peritoneum open to allow lymph fluid to drain internally in the peritoneal cavity.

Ovarian function may be preserved in younger patients if there is little likelihood of postoperative radiation. If intraoperative findings suggest that radiotherapy will be given postoperatively, the ovaries may be transposed superior and lateral to preserve their function. This technique has some liabilities, including early loss of ovarian function and abdominal pain from ovarian cysts.

In stage I cases treated by radical hysterectomy and node dissection, the results obtained are related primarily to the status of the pelvic nodes, as well as the surgical resection margins around the primary tumor (ideally, >1 cm). If the pelvic nodes are free of tumor, the 5-year survival rate can be expected to exceed 90%, whereas if the nodes are found to contain tumor, the 5-year survival rate drops to 45% to 50%. If the woman is found to have extensive spread of gross disease to the pelvic nodes, the studies of Potter and coworkers (Potter, 1990) have suggested that it is preferable to cease the operation and complete radiation therapy to improve pelvic control of tumor. However, Hacker and associates reported an estimated 5-year survival of 80% for 34 patients whose tumor-positive pelvic or paraaortic nodes were resected and the areas subsequently radiated (Hacker, 1995). In a GOG study, Sedlis and coworkers evaluated disease-free survival for patients treated with radical hysterectomy who have negative lymph nodes and surgical margins but with intermediate risk factors, including more than one third stromal invasion, capillary lymphatic space involvement, adenocarcinoma, and large tumor diameter by randomizing patients to pelvic radiotherapy or observation (Sedlis, 1999). Survival was improved in those who received postoperative pelvic radiation; however, there were radiation complications, including bowel obstruction and death.

Nerve-sparing radical hysterectomy is an innovation described by Hockel and others (Hockel, 2003). Bladder atony is a difficult-to-study outcome of radical hysterectomy. The incidence of complete bladder atony requiring self-catheterization or nerve stimulators is low, but milder forms are common. The severity of bladder atony is directly related to the trauma inflicted on the hypogastric nerves that may be traumatized during radical hysterectomy. The impact of the nerve-sparing approach on sexual function is not known.

### Fertility-Sparing Surgery

Dargent developed a combined laparoscopic and vaginal technique for removal of the pelvic lymph nodes, cervix, parametrium, and upper vagina (Dargent, 1995). Dargent trained gynecologic oncologists from around the world to perform radical vaginal trachelectomy and laparoscopic pelvic lymphadenectomy (Dargent, 1995). Long-term outcomes reported by Plante, Diaz, and others have confirmed that in well-selected patients, oncologic outcomes are identical to radical hysterectomy outcomes (Plante, 2005; Diaz, 2008). First-trimester pregnancy loss rates are approximately the same for radical trachelectomy patients as for the general population. Second-trimester pregnancy loss is approximately doubled in trachelectomy patients compared with the general population presumably because of the loss of cervical stroma. Approximately two thirds of patients have a successful pregnancy following radical trachelectomy.

When fertility-sparing surgery was first described, the assumption was that it would be offered to only a small proportion of patients. Sonoda and colleagues determined from a cohort of over 400 radical hysterectomy patients that approximately 50% of those younger than 40 years have low-risk histologic types and tumor size smaller than 2 cm, making them candidates for radical trachelectomy (Sonoda, 2004).

In spite of the contribution of radical vaginal surgery to fertility preservation, the technique has been difficult for gynecologic oncologists in the United States to master. Vaginal surgical skills are diminishing and there are no other indications for radical vaginal surgery. American gynecologic oncologists, unlike their counterparts in Canada and Europe, appear to have been discouraged by the long learning curve and have not invested the time to master the approach. Gynecologic oncologists in the United States have described abdominal radical trachelectomy as an alternative to the vaginal approach. Although smaller numbers have been published, it is anticipated that oncologic and fertility outcomes will be similar to the laparoscopic-vaginal approach. In addition, performance of robotic radical trachelectomy continues to rise and we anticipate will further advance use of the abdominal approach.

Patient selection is important when considering fertility-sparing surgery. Preoperative pelvic MRI is recommended for all patients with a visible lesion. Patients should have a desire to preserve fertility, no evidence of metastatic disease to lymph nodes or distant metastases, age <45, stage IAI with LVSI or IA2 or IB1 disease, and lesion size less than or equal to 2 cm with limited endocervical extension assessed by colposcopy and MRI.

### Minimally Invasive Surgery

Minimally invasive techniques for treatment of cervical cancer are attractive for several reasons. The tumor itself can be removed through the vagina, so an abdominal incision is not needed for this purpose. Lymph nodes can be removed safely through laparoscopic ports, especially if removed in a protective bag prior to pulling through the port. Minimally invasive surgery reduces postoperative adhesions. This is important, because these adhesions play a role in the severity of bowel complications if postoperative radiotherapy is given. Minimally invasive surgery is associated with shorter length of stay, less pain, few postoperative infections, fewer thromboembolic complications, and reduced blood loss compared with abdominal procedures.

Laparoscopic radical surgery has become more popular in North America because of faculty in major training programs who have embraced the concept and trained their associates. For gynecologic oncologists in practice, the long learning curve associated with laparoscopy has been an impediment to advancement. The most recent minimally invasive technique, robotic laparoscopic surgery, offers new advantages. The robot more closely replicates the wristed motions that surgeons use during open cases, offers three-dimensional imaging, and completely eliminates the tremor of the surgeon and the assistant holding the camera. Many gynecologic oncologists who have not had the time or inclination to master traditional laparoscopic surgery can master robotics relatively quickly. Radical pelvic surgery (e.g., radical prostatectomy, hysterectomy) is an ideal application for robotic surgery and will continue to become increasingly available in the United States.

### Sentinel Node Biopsy

Cervical cancer, like most solid tumors, spreads primarily by lymphatic spread. Surgical management of solid tumors, as pioneered more than 100 years ago by Halsted, is based on the resection of all regional lymph nodes and lymphatic channels connecting the lymph nodes to the primary tumor. Implicit in this approach is that all regional lymph nodes have the same risk of containing metastatic disease. Morton, working in patients with cutaneous melanoma, has demonstrated that there are sentinel lymph nodes that are the first nodes to receive lymphatic drainage from the primary tumor and are therefore the first site of metastases (Morton, 2001). Experience with thousands of melanoma and breast cancer patients has validated this concept, which has been successfully extended to other disease sites, notably vulvar cancer.

Cervical cancer is an excellent target for the sentinel lymph node concept because the tumor is easy to inject and the regional lymph nodes can be reached through an incision. Lymphatic drainage of the cervix is complex; however, most sentinel lymph nodes of the cervix are found along the external iliac artery or vein, obturator space, or parametrium. A number of investigators have reported their experience with sentinel lymph node biopsy in radical hysterectomy patients. So far, the procedure has shown great promise; however, the false-negative rates have been higher for cervical cancer patients than for those with, for example, vulvar cancer. Improving techniques and patient selection should correct this problem. It is likely that sentinel lymph node biopsy will ultimately be incorporated into the surgical management of cervical cancer.

### Surgical Complications

Following radical hysterectomy, many patients experience long-term complications. Montz and associates noted a 5% frequency of small bowel obstruction, which increases to 20% if radiation is used postoperatively (Montz, 1994). Fistulas from the urinary tract, particularly ureterovaginal fistulas, have been reported to occur in approximately 1% of cases. The low rate appears to result from the administration of antibiotics, prevention of retroperitoneal serosanguineous collections, and avoidance of direct manipulation of the ureter to avoid injury to the periureteral blood supply. Most gynecologic oncologists do not reperitonealize the pelvis, which allows direct drainage of lymphatic fluid to the peritoneal cavity, where it is reabsorbed.

Many women suffer postoperative bladder dysfunction. In part, this appears to be caused by disruption of the sympathetic nerve supply to the bladder. However, the dysfunction may be temporary. Low and associates noted an increase in bladder pressure with a decrease in urethral pressure following radical hysterectomy (Low, 1981). There was reduced bladder compliance with detrusor instability. The bladder can develop hypotonicity, and overdistention can then become a problem. If overdistention of the bladder and infection are avoided, progressive improvement of bladder function usually occurs. Forney correlated the degree of bladder dysfunction after radical hysterectomy with the extent of resection of the cardinal ligament (Forney, 1980). Those who had a complete resection of cardinal ligaments could void satisfactorily at an average of 51 days compared with 20 days for those with only partial resection of the ligaments. All patients experienced a decrease in bladder sensation. In a few patients, the decrease in bladder sensation can be permanent. For patients in whom it is temporary, recovery usually occurs after continuous drainage of the bladder with an indwelling catheter. Westby and Asmussen observed that by 1 year after surgery, a slight decrease in urethral pressure persists but that the decrease is not as great as that noted immediately after the operation (Westby, 1985). After 1 year, the postoperative changes and bladder function usually recover. Newer nerve-sparing surgical techniques where the uterosacral ligament is transected after separation of the hypogastric nerve and preservation of the bladder branches of the pelvic plexus have been associated with improved bladder function without compromising oncologic outcomes and survival.

In a 1999 study from Sweden, Bergmark and coworkers noted compromised sexual activity, decreased lubrication, and shortened vagina in women treated for cervical cancer by surgery or radiation (Bergmark, 1999). During the consent process, patients should be informed regarding the potential impact of radical hysterectomy on their sexual function.

Lymphedema is another complication of radical pelvic surgery that can affect quality of life. The areas most affected are the mons, lower abdomen, and upper thighs. Lymphedema massage may help reduce this problem, but treatment options are limited and of only modest effectiveness.

#### Outcomes After Surgical Treatment

Reported 5-year survival rates for women with stage IB cervical cancer treated with radical hysterectomy and pelvic lymphadenectomy are approximately 80% to 90%. Patients with positive or close margins or positive lymph nodes have the highest risk of recurrence and poor outcome. In large prospective studies, 3-year disease-specific survival rates of 85.6% in patients with negative nodes and 50% to 74% in patients with positive nodes were reported. A randomized study has shown that postoperative chemoradiation improves survival in patients with positive lymph nodes and positive surgical margins (Peters, 1999).

### *Radiation Treatment*

Most patients with carcinoma of the cervix are treated by radiation. The principles of external megavoltage treatment (teletherapy) and local implants (brachytherapy) are reviewed in Chapter 26. External beam radiation is administered in fractions, usually 180 cGy/day, 5 days/week, to destroy the tumor without causing permanent damage to normal tissues. This delivers uniform doses to the entire pelvis, including the regional pelvic nodes. The local implant delivers its highest energy locally to the cervix, surface of the vagina, and paravaginal and paracervical tissues. The radiation from the implant diminishes according to the inverse square law. The uterus and cervix serve as a receptacle for arranging and holding the intracavitary applicator stem (tandem) and accompanying vaginal applicators (ovoids) in a fixed and optimal position for delivering the desired radiation dosimetry. Usually, the tandem and ovoids or a tandem and ring are inserted with in the woman, and a pack is placed into the vagina to stabilize the apparatus and increase the distance from the mucosa of the bladder and rectum. After the position of the applicator has been confirmed to be satisfactory by imaging, the radioactive source, such as cesium-137 or Iridium 192, is inserted (afterloading technique). Other types of applicators are available, but the principle of delivering intense radiation to the cervix and paracervical areas is the same. The goal is to increase the total dose of radiation to the maximum allowable to achieve tumor control without introducing a major risk of complications and injury to adjacent normal tissue. The specific protocols followed in various treatment centers differ; individualization for specific patients is often needed depending on the stage and size of the cervical tumor as well as the patient's local anatomy. In general, external therapy is given first to treat the regional pelvic nodes and shrink the central tumor mass, which then is more amenable for a local implant. In some patients, external therapy can lead to excessive shrinkage of the vaginal apex, making safe, effective implantation of local radiation sources difficult. This can be a problem, particularly in older or postmenopausal patients. Occasionally, in those patients, the implantation is done first, especially for smaller stage I tumors. Intraoperative ultrasounds may be helpful especially in difficult cases for optimal implant positioning. In some cases, the central pelvis is shielded during external radiation therapy to allow for subsequent higher doses from the implant. Occasionally, interstitial therapy in the form of needles implanted into the area of the tumor is needed to achieve effective local tumor control. Although criteria differ, patients with stage III disease or poor vaginal anatomy are most often considered candidates for interstitial brachytherapy.

Intracavitary radiation therapy may be delivered at either a low-dose rate or a high-dose rate. The advantage of high-dose-rate brachytherapy is that it is given on an outpatient basis and can be done with 3 to 4 hours. High-dose-rate brachytherapy and low-dose-rate brachytherapy have similar survival and toxicity and high-dose-rate brachytherapy has become the most common type of brachytherapy available throughout the world. The number of fractions varies from two to five; the most common one in the United States is 5.5 Gy to 6 Gy to point A in five fractions.

In calculating the doses of radiation, two reference points, A and B, are used (Fig. 29.14). Point A is 2 cm above the external os and 2 cm lateral to the cervical canal. Point B is 5 cm lateral to the cervical canal and 3 cm lateral to point A, which places

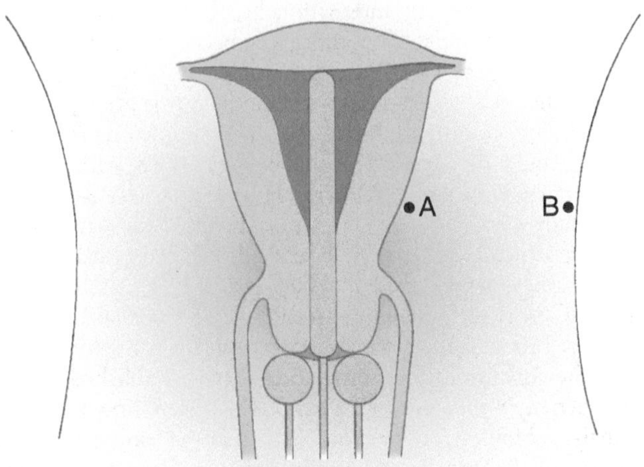


**Figure 29.14** Points A and B with central stem (tandem) and two ovoids in place.

point B in the vicinity of the lateral pelvic wall (see Fig. 29.14). The total dose administered depends on tumor stage but, in general, at the pelvic wall, it is in the range of 50 to 65 Gy, with the higher doses used for high-stage disease. At point A, it varies, but approximately 80 Gy is given for small IB1 lesions and doses higher than 85 Gy for larger lesions. The normal cervix is particularly resistant to radiation and can tolerate doses as high as 200 to 250 Gy over 2 months, whereas the adjacent bladder and, in particular, the rectum are much more sensitive, and their exposure in general should be limited at the point of maximal radiation to 80 Gy to the bladder and 70 Gy to the rectum, with overall average doses in the range of 65 to 70 Gy. The small bowel can be damaged at doses above 45 to 50 Gy, especially if adhesions limit intestinal mobility and a large volume is treated.

There has been increased interest in the use of image-based three-dimensional treatment planning for intracavitary and interstitial brachytherapy. Among the many potential advantages of image-based planning are its ability to provide a better sense of the actual doses delivered to critical structures and possibly a more solid basis for comparisons among institutions. Studies have used CT- and MRI-based images; at present, a large multi-institutional study of image-based brachytherapy is ongoing in Europe and worldwide.

### Outcomes

Radical radiation therapy achieves excellent survival and pelvic disease control rates in patients with stage IB or IIA cervical cancer. Eifel and associates reported 5-year disease-specific survival of 90%, 86%, and 67% in patients with stage IB tumors with cervical diameters less than 4 cm, 4 to 4.9 cm, and larger than 5 cm, respectively (Eifel, 1994). In 1961, a report suggested that adjuvant hysterectomy improved local control in patients with stage IB disease with tumors larger than 6 cm; however, several studies since then have shown no improvement in local control but an increase in toxicity (Keys, 1999). One of these studies was a large GOG study in which patients were randomized to a trial of radiation, with or without extrafascial hysterectomy; results showed no difference in survival or local control but a higher complication rate (Keys, 1999). Therefore there is no clear evidence that adjuvant hysterectomy improves outcome in patients with early stage disease and large tumor size. The 5-year survival for patients with stage IIA disease is similar to that for patients with stage IB disease. For patients with more advanced disease, 5-year survival rates of 65% to 75%, 35% to 50%, and 15% to 20% have been reported for stages IIB, IIIB, and IV tumors, respectively. The addition of chemotherapy has further improved local control and survival for stage IB2 and higher (discussed later).

### Chemoradiation

In 1999, prospective randomized trials involving concurrent cisplatin-containing chemotherapy to standard radiotherapy showed such improved survival that the trials were preliminarily halted to release the results, which changed clinical practice. In one of the studies by GOG, Rose and colleagues treated patients with advanced squamous cell, adenosquamous, or adenocarcinoma of the cervix (stages IIB, III, or IVA) (Rose, 1999). The patients received external radiation therapy (40.8 to 51 Gy) followed by one or two brachytherapy implants. The patients were randomized to receive one of three concomitant chemotherapy regimens: hydroxyurea; cisplatin, 5-fluorouracil, and hydroxyurea; or cisplatin alone. The best results were obtained with the cisplatin-containing regimens, with the least complications seen with weekly cisplatin (40 mg/m$^2$) alone. Progression-free survival at 24 months was an impressive 67% for this very high-risk group of patients.

In another collaborative trial, Keys and associates studied 369 women with bulky stage IB carcinoma (>4 cm) in diameter (Keys, 1999). They were randomized to receive radiation alone or with concomitant weekly cisplatin (40 mg/m$^2$). Adjuvant extrafascial hysterectomy was performed 3 to 6 weeks after conclusion of the chemoradiation treatments. The therapeutic results were markedly better in the chemoradiation group, with a 3-year 83% disease-free survival compared with 74% in the radiation group alone ($P$ = .008), and they noted no added benefit with the addition of extrafascial hysterectomy. At the same time, the Radiation Therapy Oncology Group also conducted a trial comparing paraaortic–pelvic radiation therapy with concurrent chemotherapy and pelvic radiation in patients with stages IB to IVA tumors and also found a significant improvement in outcome for all stages of disease with concurrent chemotherapy compared with radiation therapy alone (Eifel, 2004). Another trial studied concurrent chemotherapy with radiation therapy in patients who had undergone a radical hysterectomy for cervical cancer and were found to have pelvic lymph node metastases, positive margins, or parametrial involvement. In this trial, patients who received chemoradiation had a better disease-free survival rate than patients who received radiation therapy alone (Peters, 1999).

Only one large randomized trial has failed to demonstrate a significant advantage from concurrent cisplatin-based chemotherapy in cervical cancer patients. This trial, in Canada, was the smallest of six trials of concurrent cisplatin and radiation therapy (Pearcey, 2002).

In North America, the primary focus has been on cisplatin-based chemotherapy regimens, but international trials have evaluated others. In a large trial from Thailand, patients were randomized into four arms: radiation therapy alone, radiation therapy with concurrent mitomycin and oral fluorouracil, radiation therapy with adjuvant fluorouracil, or radiation with concurrent and adjuvant chemotherapy (Lorvidhaya, 2003). Patients in the two treatment groups that included concurrent chemotherapy had higher disease-free survival rates and lower rates of local recurrence than patients in the other two groups. More recently, Dueños-Gonzales published a trial comparing cisplatin-radiation therapy to cisplatin-gemcitabine-radiation therapy followed by two courses of cisplatin-gemcitabine (Dueñas-Gonzales, 2011). Patients who received gemcitabine had better overall survival and disease-free survival compared with patients who did not.

A meta-analysis review of trials that included a comparison of chemotherapy plus radiation to radiation therapy alone found a 6% improvement in 5-year survival with chemoradiotherapy (Chemoradiotherapy for Cervical Cancer Meta-Analysis Collaboration 2008). A larger survival benefit was seen for the two trials in which chemotherapy was administered after chemoradiotherapy. There was a significant survival benefit for the group of trials that used platinum-based and non–platinum-based chemoradiotherapy but no evidence of a difference in the size of the benefit by radiotherapy or chemotherapy dose or scheduling was seen. Chemoradiotherapy also reduced local and distant recurrence and progression and improved disease-free survival.

### Neoadjuvant Chemotherapy

Neoadjuvant chemotherapy may be given before surgery or before radical radiation therapy. Advantages of chemotherapy before surgery include the potential for reducing tumor volume, increasing resectability, and helping to control micrometastatic disease. Neoadjuvant chemotherapy may also have the potential to provide a viable alternative when access to radiotherapy is poor or if there are unavoidable delays in delivering radiotherapeutic treatment. In one study by Sardi and coworkers, 205 patients with stage IB1 were randomized to neoadjuvant chemotherapy plus radical hysterectomy or to radical hysterectomy alone (Sardi, 1993).[32] They reported that the patients who received neoadjuvant chemotherapy had more resectable tumors and better overall survival than patients who did not receive neoadjuvant chemotherapy. In the United States, the GOG closed a trial with 258 patients with stage IB2 cervical tumors who were randomized to neoadjuvant chemotherapy plus radical hysterectomy or to radical hysterectomy alone. They found no difference in the two arms in the rate of surgery performed (79% chemotherapy + surgery vs. 54% surgery) in the surgical-pathologic findings, specifically in progression-free survival (56% chemotherapy + surgery vs. 54% surgery) and overall survival (63% chemotherapy + surgery vs. 61% surgery) at 5 years. A meta-analysis of six randomized trials of neoadjuvant chemotherapy plus surgery compared with surgery alone found that although progression-free survival was improved with neoadjuvant chemotherapy, there was no significant survival benefit, and distant recurrence and rates of resection only tended to favor the neoadjuvant chemotherapy (Rydzewska, 2010). The authors observed heterogeneity in the trials but concluded that it remains unclear whether neoadjuvant chemotherapy consistently offers a benefit over surgery alone for women with early stage or locally advanced cervical cancer. In the United States, neoadjuvant chemotherapy is rarely used; however, internationally, there is much interest in using neoadjuvant chemotherapy, especially in countries in which radiotherapy is not easily accessible.

The other use of neoadjuvant chemotherapy is prior to radiation therapy. Seven randomized trials have studied neoadjuvant chemotherapy plus radiation therapy compared with radical radiation therapy alone. Other randomized trials have studied neoadjuvant chemotherapy plus surgery compared with radical radiation therapy in locally advanced cervical cancer. A meta-analysis published in 2004 evaluated 21 of these trials (NACCCMA Collaboration, 2004); however, all the trials that were included in this analysis were carried out before 1999, when the concurrent chemotherapies were all published. Much heterogeneity was found in the trials, which made them difficult to analyze. However, it was concluded that the timing and dose intensity of cisplatin-based neoadjuvant chemotherapy appeared to have an important impact on whether it benefited women with locally advanced cervical cancer; further exploration was recommended. Presently, two trials of this issue are ongoing in Europe and India, and in both trials the standard arm is concurrent chemoradiation.

### Para aortic Node Involvement

Numerous small series of patients having documented paraaortic node involvement have demonstrated that some patients have long-term disease-free survival. Patients with microscopic involvement have a better survival duration than those with gross involvement; however, even patients with gross involvement have a 15% to 20% survival rate with aggressive management. Laparoscopy and laparotomy using the extraperitoneal approach allow the removal of positive nodes and sampling of other paraaortic nodes, which may enhance control with radiation therapy and help design the treatment field.

Patients with paraaortic lymph node involvement can be treated effectively with extended-field radiation. The superior boundary of the extended field is usually placed at the T12 vertebral body to cover the paraaortic nodes. Patients are treated with a combination of external beam radiation therapy and brachytherapy. The 5-year survival rates range from 25% to 50%. At present, the standard treatment for patients with positive paraaortic nodes is extended-field radiation therapy with concurrent weekly cisplatin.

### Radiation Complications

Complications following radiation therapy are related to dose, volume treated, and sensitivity of the various tissues receiving radiation. The patient's habitus and presence of diseases that affect circulation, such as diabetes and high blood pressure, increase the risk, as does previous intra-abdominal surgery. Acute minor complications, such as diarrhea and nausea, subside after radiation therapy is completed. Complications usually develop in 1 to 2 years but can occur as early as 6 months or as late as many years after radiation therapy has been completed. Scarring of normal tissues can lead to severe radiation fibrosis. The rare development of a second primary cancer after radiation for cervical cancer was reported by Kleinerman and associates from 13 population-based European registries (Kleinerman, 1995). With 30 years of survival, there was approximately a doubling of the risk of a new primary in an irradiated pelvic organ, including the ovaries and bladder, as well as the vagina and vulva.

The treatment of radiation complications depends on the symptoms and location of the complication. Vaginal or cervical ulcerations occasionally occur, and local treatment with topical antibiotics and estrogen creams is usually satisfactory. Postradiation cystitis may manifest itself as urinary frequency or dysuria. After infection has been ruled out, symptomatic treatment is undertaken with drugs such as antispasmodics or urinary analgesics (e.g., phenazopyridine [Pyridium], 100 mg three times daily); these are prescribed until the symptoms clear. Occasionally, hemorrhagic cystitis develops, which may require hospitalization for continuous bladder irrigation or instillation of agents to control bleeding, such as silver nitrate or possibly fulguration of the bleeding points. In cases of hematuria, recurrent tumor should first be ruled out. Periureteral fibrosis can lead to ureteral obstruction and loss of kidney function. McIntyre and coworkers studied 1784 patients with stage IB carcinomas who were treated by radiation therapy and found 29 cases of ureteral stenoses, which increased from a frequency of 1% at 5 years to 2.5% at 20 years (McIntyre, 1995). Although tumor recurrence was the most common cause of early ureteral obstruction, radiation fibrosis can be a rare but occasionally fatal late complication.

Bowel complications tend to be more frequent than urinary complications. Proctosigmoiditis can lead to diarrhea, severe pain on defecation, or gastrointestinal bleeding. Conservative therapy with stool softeners and a low-roughage diet may suffice; occasionally, local corticosteroids (e.g., cortisone enema) are of assistance. Fistulas or rectal ulcerations are occasionally seen in the area adjacent to the tip of the cervix, which is also the area maximally radiated during local vaginocervical implantation. If a fistula develops, or in cases of ulceration or severe bleeding and pain, a diverting colostomy is required. Serious small bowel complications may occur, leading to obstruction, fistula formation, or necrosis. The use of parenteral nutrition and intravenous hyperalimentation are excellent measures to help deal with these problems. Follow-up studies by Klee and colleagues have shown that bladder and bowel symptoms tend to be chronic in some patients, but long-term fatigue is also reported. In most patients, it regresses in a few months (Klee, 2000).

Compromise of sexual function because of inelastic vaginal walls and decreased utilization was noted in the studies by Bergmark and associates (Bergmark, 1999). In a randomized trial of experimental psychoeducational intervention involving regular vaginal dilation, Robinson and coworkers noted a reduced fear of sexual activity posttreatment in the experimental group (Robinson, 1999).

## SPECIAL CONSIDERATIONS

### Cervical Stump Tumors

Some patients undergo supracervical hysterectomy for nonmalignant disease. Carcinomas that subsequently develop in the cervical stump pose special problems because of the shortness of the cervical canal and absence of the uterus, both of which curtail the effective use of brachytherapy, especially insertion of an intracervical tandem. There is also the risk that bowel adhesions to the apex of the vagina and cervix will increase the chances of radiation complications; a pretherapy barium study of the small and large bowel may be helpful to identify loops that adhere to the cervical apex. For patients with small stage IB tumors, an operative approach similar to radical hysterectomy can be considered. However, most patients are treated with radiation. External treatment is emphasized because of the difficulty of an optimal intracavitary implant. A transvaginal cone may also be used to supplement external pelvic therapy. Effective treatment of cervical stump carcinoma can be achieved, resulting in overall 5-year survival rates ranging from 45% to 60%. However, because of the previous supracervical hysterectomy, there is an increased risk of complications compared to patients treated with a supracervical hysterectomy. Results of chemoradiation studies of these tumors are not available but, based on data already presented, radiation, combined with weekly cisplatin, appears to be optimal.

### Carcinoma of the Cervix Inadvertently Removed at Simple Hysterectomy

Unfortunately, the situation occasionally arises in which a woman undergoes a simple total hysterectomy and an invasive carcinoma of the cervix is found after operation. Patients with unsuspected invasive cervical carcinoma detected after simple hysterectomy have been classified into five groups according to the amount of disease and presentation: (1) microinvasive cancer, (2) tumor confined to the cervix with negative surgical margins, (3) positive surgical margins but no gross residual tumor, (4) gross residual tumor by clinical examination documented by biopsy, and (5) patients referred for treatment more than 6 months after hysterectomy (usually for recurrent disease).

The treatment plan is based on the amount of residual disease. Sometimes, the surgeon can subsequently perform a radical operation, removing the tissues that would normally be removed at radical hysterectomy, including the regional pelvic nodes. Such an approach has been used, particularly in younger patients, especially those with small tumors. However, most women are usually treated with some sort of radiation therapy. Patients with minimal or no known residual disease at most require brachytherapy to the vaginal apex; patients with gross disease at the specimen margin require full-intensity therapy. Patients with minimal or no gross residual disease (groups 1 to 3) have excellent 5-year survival rates (59% to 79%), whereas rates for patients with gross residual disease (groups 4 and 5) are poorer (in the range of only 41%).

### Carcinoma of the Cervix in Pregnancy

Rarely, an invasive carcinoma of the cervix is discovered in a pregnant woman. Within each stage, survival statistics are similar in pregnant and nonpregnant women. A concern has been that the delivery of a fetus through a cervix replaced by carcinoma might worsen the prognosis because of tumor dissemination, but there is no clear evidence to indicate that the birth process causes tumor dissemination. However, tumor recurrence in episiotomy sites following vaginal delivery has been reported in some studies. The major risk to the patient of delivery through a cervix containing invasive carcinoma is that of hemorrhage as a result of tearing of the tumor during cervical dilation and delivery.

A problem arising in pregnancy is whether a woman with an abnormal cytologic smear has intraepithelial neoplasia or invasive cancer. In general, if the cytologic and histologic findings of colposcopically directed biopsies are comparable and suggest intraepithelial neoplasia or carcinoma in situ, the woman is observed and delivered, with final evaluation and therapy completed approximately 6 weeks after delivery. Even if there is a question of microinvasion, a woman so diagnosed in the last trimester of pregnancy is usually followed and evaluated further after delivery. Cervical conization during pregnancy can lead to severe complications, particularly hemorrhage and loss of the fetus. If it is necessary to perform a conization or preferably a wedge resection of the cervix during pregnancy, it is probably best to perform this procedure during the second trimester, when the risks of fetal loss and hemorrhage are minimal. For patients in whom invasive cancer is diagnosed, a therapeutic plan must be developed to deliver appropriate care, with regard also for the outcome of the pregnancy.

The therapy of carcinoma during pregnancy is influenced by the stage of the disease, time in pregnancy when the cancer is diagnosed, and beliefs and desires of the woman in terms of initiating therapy that can terminate the pregnancy, as opposed to postponing therapy until fetal viability is achieved. If carcinoma is diagnosed in the first trimester or early in the second trimester (before 20 weeks), treatment may be undertaken immediately because of the concern that a delay could lead to tumor progression or spread. If the woman has resectable tumor (stage IB or early IIA), effective treatment consists of radical hysterectomy and node dissection (class III). This procedure can usually be carried out without difficulty on a pregnant woman. Increased uterine motility and edema of the pelvic tissue planes help simplify the procedure for the experienced surgeon, but pregnancy does increase the risk of blood loss. For higher-stage tumors, therapy begins with external beam radiation (teletherapy) and, usually in 4 to 6 weeks, this leads to spontaneous abortion. The dose of external therapy prescribed varies depending on the stage of the tumor, but approximately 40 to 50 Gy is given. Although the results of a published series are not available, it would appear preferable to augment the radiation with weekly cisplatin because the pregnancy in this case would be terminated. Following abortion, the uterus involutes and an implant (brachytherapy) is placed. If the pregnancy does not spontaneously abort, dilation and curettage, prostaglandin-assisted delivery or, rarely, hysterotomy may be necessary to empty the uterus before brachytherapy. Alternatively, if the initial tumor was small and has completely regressed, an extrafascial hysterectomy or modified radical hysterectomy may be performed.

For patients beyond the 20th week of gestation, therapy is often delayed until fetal viability. The health and maturity of the fetus are determined by appropriate ultrasound studies and amniotic fluid analysis to ensure fetal lung maturity. Delivery is usually accomplished by cesarean section; after this, therapy is completed by surgery or radiation with the usual considerations of tumor stage and size. Overall, treatment results in pregnant patients are similar to those in nonpregnant patients, stage for stage. It should be noted that many published studies dealing with carcinoma of the cervix in pregnancy include cases treated as long as 1 year postpartum, which assumes that the carcinoma was present during pregnancy. Hacker and coworkers summarized the results of 1249 cases reported in various series in the literature (Hacker, 1982). Overall, a 5-year survival rate of 49.2% was recorded for pregnant patients compared with 51% for nonpregnant patients treated during the same period. Their statistics included not only patients treated during pregnancy, but also those treated up to 6 months after delivery, and the postpartum group had the poorest survival statistics. Survival was most closely related to stage, as expected, and those diagnosed during the first trimester had a better prognosis than those diagnosed during the third trimester.

## RECURRENCE

Approximately one third of patients treated for cancer of the cervix will experience tumor recurrence, which is defined as the reappearance of tumor 6 months or more after therapy. Metastases can occur anywhere, but most are in the pelvis—centrally in the vagina or cervix, or laterally near the pelvic walls—or, less frequently, distally in the periaortic nodes, lung, liver, or bone. It should be noted that liver, lung, and distal bone metastases outside the pelvis likely result from hematogenous tumor spread.

The symptoms caused by recurrence depend on the site and extent of metastatic disease. Vaginal discharge and abnormal bleeding are often symptoms of an early central pelvic recurrence. Malaise, loss of appetite, and general symptoms associated with widespread metastatic disease are late manifestations of recurrence. Lateral pelvic recurrences often have a retroperitoneal component, which can lead to sciatic nerve irritation and cause severe pain around the distribution of the sciatic nerve in back of the leg, as well as loss of muscle strength, causing the woman to walk with a limp. Unilateral leg edema frequently accompanies such metastases, or leg swelling may occur from fibrosis of lymphatics following surgery or radiation. In addition, tumor recurrence can also cause ureteral obstruction, leading to unilateral or bilateral compromise of kidney function. Low back pain frequently occurs.

Patients treated for carcinoma of the cervix are examined according to the same schedule as patients with other malignancies—every 3 months the first 2 years, every 6 months from years 3 to 5, and yearly thereafter. More frequent examinations are done if abnormal symptoms or signs develop. Examination consists of physical and pelvic examination at every visit and Pap smear annually unless an abnormality is detected on the Pap smear. Generally, a PET/CT is repeated at the 3 to 6 months post chemoradiation therapy and chest x-rays are done annually. Other imaging tests are only ordered if the patient has symptoms or there are other indications. Renal function tests may be indicated because ureteral fibrosis can occur more than 5 years after the completion of radiation therapy. Once recurrent disease is suspected, verification is usually obtained by biopsy of an accessible mass or CT-directed thin-needle aspiration, depending on the location of the tumor recurrence.

### *PELVIC RECURRENCE*

Approximately 50% of recurrences will develop in the pelvis. In addition to clinical assessment and CT, a vaginal ultrasound scan is often useful to document pelvic recurrence. Recurrences of adenocarcinoma are less frequent in the pelvis and are more likely to be at distant sites, such as the lung or supraclavicular areas. For patients who were initially treated by surgery, radiation is usually prescribed for pelvic recurrences; approximately 45- to 50-Gy whole-pelvis irradiation is given. Supplemental interstitial or intracavitary radiation is also prescribed, depending on the size and location of recurrence in the pelvis. As noted, chemoradiation is preferable. Patients who have isolated central recurrences without pelvic wall fixation or regional metastasis can be cured in as many as 60% to 70% of cases. The prognosis is much poorer when the pelvic wall is involved; usually, 10% to 20% of patients survive 5 years after radiation therapy. For patients who were initially treated with radiation who have developed a localized pelvic recurrence, surgical eradication of the tumor should be considered because further effective radiation is not possible and limited surgical resection of the pelvic recurrence may not lead to a cure but will often cause severe complications of wound healing and intestinal and urinary fistulas. However, in rare, carefully selected patients initially treated with primary radiation therapy, radical hysterectomy may be a feasible alternative to exenterative surgery. Coleman and associates reported on 50 patients who underwent a radical hysterectomy for persistent or recurrent disease and found 5- and 10-year survival rates of 72% and 60%, respectively, with complication rates of 64% for severe complications and 42% for permanent complications (Coleman, 1994). The authors concluded that a radical hysterectomy was an alternative to exenteration in patients with small, centrally recurrent cervical cancer, but that it should be used only in carefully selected patients. If neither surgery nor radiation is a feasible alternative, palliative chemotherapy is considered.

### *Pelvic Exenteration*

Exenterative therapy for central pelvic tumor recurrence is an extensive operative procedure used only if the preoperative evaluation suggests that the patient's condition has the potential be cured by this procedure. Exenteration is not performed for palliation. Three types of procedures may be used. Anterior pelvic exenteration is removal of the bladder, uterus, cervix, and all or part of the vagina. Posterior pelvic exenteration is removal of the anus and rectum and resection of the uterus, cervix, and all or part of the vagina. Total exenteration removes all the pelvic contents. Shepherd and coworkers noted that patients older than 69 years, those who had a recurrence within 3 years, or those who had persistent disease or positive resection margins had a poorer prognosis for the procedure (Shepherd, 1994). Rarely, select patients with recurrence involving the sidewall that would not be standard candidates for total pelvic exenteration secondary to concern for a positive surgical margin may be considered for an extended pelvic resection, or the laterally extended endopelvic resection (LEER procedure) (Hockel, 2003, 2008). This procedure requires multidisciplinary advanced surgical support and carries high risk of surgical morbidity, but it may be contemplated as a possible curative option for very select patients.

Before an exenterative operation is undertaken, the patient is thoroughly evaluated for any evidence of disease spread outside the pelvis. At operation, abdominal exploration is carried out to ensure that the tumor is resectable. Biopsy specimens of any enlarged lymph nodes or suspicious areas outside the pelvis are taken, and frozen-section studies are performed, including evaluation of the operative margins. Usually, total exenteration is performed.

Several surgical innovations have expanded the reconstruction options. The introduction of continent urinary diversion provides an alternative incontinent urinary conduit. Generally, the urinary stoma is located in the abdomen on the right side and the intestinal stoma on the left side. The use of intestinal stapling devices sometimes allows preservation of the rectal sphincter and anal function and avoids a permanent colostomy. Long-term complications are usually ureteral stricture or difficulty catheterizing the intestinal reservoir.

Continent conduits require the woman to catheterize the pouch every 4 hours, but no external appliance is required. Goldberg and colleagues reported long-term dissatisfaction among women with continent conduits and, in our practice, we have been doing an increasing number of incontinent diversions (Goldberg, 2006).

Transverse rectus abdominis myocutaneous (TRAM) flaps have provided a welcomed alternative to gracilis flaps. TRAM flaps, even small ones, as described by Sood and associates, are reliable and provide patients with the option of intercourse (Sood, 2005).

Severe postoperative and intraoperative complications can occur with this extensive procedure and perioperative mortalities as high as 10% to 20% have been reported in the past. Infection and bowel obstruction are the major risks. However, current surgical techniques of preoperative bowel preparation, use of antibiotics, careful intraoperative fluid and volume monitoring, and use of parenteral nutrition have reduced the immediate postoperative mortality to less than 5%. The use of a peritoneal graft or an omental flap, created from the right or left side of the omentum and placed in the pelvis to protect the denuded pelvic floor, can help avoid bowel obstruction and reduce postoperative morbidity. Occasionally, gracilis myocutaneous grafts are used to create a new vagina and bring a new blood supply to the previously irradiated pelvis, which aids in wound healing. Morley and associates reported on a 5-year survival rate of 61% in 100 patients aged 21 to 74 years (Morley, 1989). No patients with positive nodes in the operative specimen survived.

## *NONPELVIC RECURRENCE*

Recurrences outside of the pelvis can be treated with radiation, surgery, or chemotherapy. Localized recurrences in areas not previously irradiated are occasionally treated by radiation. Resection of the metastasis is rarely done; it is usually restricted to a localized lesion that occurs 3 to 4 years after primary therapy on the assumption that such a solitary metastasis can be effectively treated with local resection. However, in general, distant metastases are usually manifestations of systemic disease and are not cured with local therapy.

## *CHEMOTHERAPY AS TREATMENT FOR RECURRENCE*

Patients with advanced, recurrent, or persistent cervical cancer are the most difficult to treat and, for this patient population, chemotherapy offers the best hope. Cisplatin is the single most active drug in the treatment of cervical cancer. Several phase II studies have evaluated novel single agents or the combination of cisplatin with other agents, including mitolactol, ifosfamide, gemcitabine, topotecan, paclitaxel, and vinorelbine, and all have shown promising results. This has led to several phase III studies evaluating chemotherapy in patients with recurrent, advanced, or persistent cervical cancer.

The GOG has published results from four randomized phase III trials (protocols 110, 149, 169, and 179) trying to find the optimal platinum doublet to treat women with metastatic disease. The first of these trials to be published was GOG protocol 110, which compared single-agent cisplatin with cisplatin-mitolactol and cisplatin-ifosfamide (Omura, 1997). Despite the fact that overall response rates were 17.8% in the cisplatin-only arm, 21.1% in the cisplatin-mitolactol, and 31.1% in the cisplatin-ifosfamide arm ($P$ = .004), there was no significant difference in overall survival and greater toxicity with the cisplatin-ifosfamide regimen. GOG protocol 149 demonstrated that the addition of bleomycin did not enhance the activity of the cisplatin-ifosfamide doublet (Bloss, 2002), and GOG protocol 169 showed that the addition of paclitaxel to cisplatin or increasing the dose of cisplatin only improved response rate and prolonged progression-free survival but not overall survival (Moore, 2004).

GOG protocol 179 was a notable trial that demonstrated a significant improvement in overall survival (Long, 2005). In this trial, patients were randomized to single-agent cisplatin versus cisplatin and topotecan. There was a 2.9-month improvement in median survival in patients receiving the combination of cisplatin-topotecan versus cisplatin alone with no increase in toxicity. The result of this trial led to GOG protocol 204, which compared cisplatin-paclitaxel with cisplatin-topotecan, cisplatin-gemcitabine, and cisplatin-vinorelbine in patients with advanced, recurrent, or persistent disease in an attempt to find the optimal platinum doublet (Monk, 2009). The trial was closed early due to futility; however, in 513 patients, there was no difference in overall survival among the four arms but there was a trend in response rate, progression-free survival, and overall survival that favored the cisplatin-paclitaxel arm, and the conclusion of the study was that cisplatin-paclitaxel should be considered the standard treatment for patients with stage IVB or metastatic cervix cancer.

There has been a major step forward in the treatment of patients with recurrent or metastatic cervix with the addition of targeted therapy. In GOG 240, patients were randomized to treatment with one of two chemotherapy regimens (cisplatin plus paclitaxel vs. paclitaxel plus topotecan) and to bevacizumab versus no bevacizumab (Tewari, 2014). There was no difference in outcomes between the two chemotherapy regimens; however, the addition of bevacizumab significantly improved overall survival (17 months vs. 13.3), progression-free survival (8.2 months versus 5.9 months), and response rate (48% vs. 36%) compared to chemotherapy alone. Cisplatin-paclitaxel-bevacizumab triplet has been listed as category 2A in the National Comprehensive Cancer Network (NCCN) Clinical Practice Guidelines for cervical cancer (NCCN, 2014).

Despite the results of 240, the prognosis of patients with stage IVB or recurrent disease cervical cancer remains poor and represents an urgent unmet need worldwide. In addition to more robust prevention and screening strategies, better therapeutic strategies must be explored, including determining prognostic factors, the administration of novel agents that may improve the therapeutic index of definitive chemoradiation, and various immunotherapeutic approaches.

## KEY POINTS

- Carcinomas of the cervix are predominantly squamous cell carcinomas (85% to 90%), and approximately 10% to 15% are adenocarcinomas.
- Squamous cell carcinomas appear to have a viral and venereal association, particularly with HPV. In the United States, squamous cell carcinoma is more frequent in blacks than in whites.
- Cervical carcinoma is the third most frequent malignancy of the lower female genital tract, after endometrial and ovarian cancer, and the second most frequent cause of death, after ovarian cancer.
- Definitive diagnosis of microinvasive carcinoma is established only by means of cervical conization, not biopsy. The margins of the cone should be free of neoplastic epithelium before conservative therapy is undertaken.
- Microinvasive carcinoma of the cervix can be effectively treated by total hysterectomy, with a 5-year survival rate of almost 100%, but recurrent neoplasia can develop after 5 years. However, a precise and reliable definition of microinvasion is controversial.
- Prognosis in squamous cell cancer of the cervix is related to tumor stage and lesion volume (size), depth of invasion, and spread to lymph nodes.
- The prognosis of adenocarcinoma of the cervix is related to tumor stage, size, grade, and depth of invasion. Large adenocarcinomas tend to be poorly differentiated.
- Metastases to regional pelvic nodes in stage I squamous carcinomas correlate with lesion size, depth of invasion, and the presence of capillary lymphatic space involvement, and correlate inversely with patient age.
- Cervical carcinomas are locally invasive tumors that spread primarily to the pelvic tissues and then to the pelvic and paraaortic lymph nodes. Less frequently, hematogenous spread to the liver, lung, and bone occurs.
- The risk of the spread of cervical carcinoma to pelvic nodes is approximately 15% for stage I, 29% for stage II, and 47% for stage III. For the paraaortic nodes, the figures are 6% for stage I, 19% for stage II, and 33% for stage III.
- Stage IB carcinomas of the cervix may be treated equally effectively by radical hysterectomy and pelvic node dissection or radiation. The 5-year survival rate is approximately 80%. If lymph nodes are free of tumor, the 5-year survival rate is approximately 90%; if the nodes contain metastatic tumor, the rate is 50%. Improved overall survival rates have been reported for patients with tumors smaller than 4 cm in diameter treated by preliminary brachytherapy followed by radical hysterectomy.
- Surgery is often used for treating stage IB and early stage IIA carcinomas of the cervix, particularly for smaller tumors and for younger patients to preserve their ovarian function. Surgery produces less scarring and vaginal fibrosis than radiation and is preferred for women with a pelvic mass, pelvic infection, or history of conditions such as inflammatory bowel disease, which increase the risk for radiation complications.

## KEY POINTS—cont'd

- High-stage tumors are treated by chemoradiation. Current programs usually use cisplatin, 40 $mg/m^2$ weekly, during external treatment and with brachytherapy.
- Most cancers of the cervix are treated by radiation therapy (teletherapy and brachytherapy). Radiation doses vary with tumor size and stage but are approximately 50 to 65 Gy at point B and 80 to 85 Gy at point A. Current practice is to combine radiation with simultaneous chemotherapy to optimize the results.
- Improved cure rates of cervical cancers are obtained with increased doses, which also lead to an increased frequency of complications. Large increments in dose may increase complications without increasing cure rates.
- Complications following radiation are related to dose and volume of tissue treated; these include radiation inflammation of the bladder or bowel, which may lead to pain, bleeding, or, infrequently, fistula formation. The normal cervix is resistant to radiation, and the dose can be as high as 200 to 250 Gy over 2 months. The rectum should be limited to doses of 70 GY or less and the bladder to doses of 80 GY or less. Overall, the rate of moderate to severe radiation complications for treatment of all stages is approximately 10%.
- Worldwide 5-year survival rates reported for patients with carcinomas of the cervix are as follows: stage IA, 95%; stage IB, 80%; stage II, 70%; stage III, 50%; and stage IV, 20% with radiation therapy alone.
- Pregnancy does not adversely affect the survival rate for women with carcinoma of the cervix, stage for stage.
- Approximately one third of patients treated for cervical carcinoma develop tumor recurrence, and approximately 50% of these recurrences are located in the pelvis; most occur within 2 years.
- Patients whose recurrences occur more than 3 years after primary therapy have a better prognosis than those with earlier recurrence.
- Pelvic exenteration in carefully selected patients with central pelvic recurrence can lead to a 5-year survival rate of 50% or better.
- Chemotherapy of recurrent squamous cell carcinoma of the cervix does not produce long-term cures, but recent results suggest that cisplatin-paclitaxel-bevacizumab should be considered the standard treatment for patients with stage IVB recurrent or metastatic cervix cancer.
- Leg pain following the distribution of the sciatic nerve or unilateral leg swelling is often an indication of pelvic recurrence of carcinoma of the cervix.

## KEY REFERENCES


Berchuk A, Mullin TJ. Cervical adenoid cystic carcinoma associated with ascites. *Gynecol Oncol.* 1985;22:201.

Bergmark K, Avall-Lundqvist E, Dickman PW, et al. Vaginal changes and sexuality in women with a history of cervical cancer. *N Engl J Med.* 1999;340:1383.

Bloss JD, Blessing J, Behrens R, et al. Randomized phase III trial of cisplatin and ifosfamide with or without bleomycin in squamous carcinoma of the cervix: a Gynecology Oncology Group study. *J Clin Oncol.* 2002;20:1832.

Chemoradiotherapy for Cervical Cancer Meta-Analysis Collaboration. Reducing uncertainties about the effects of chemoradiotherapy for cervical cancer: a systematic review and meta-analysis of individual patient data from 18 randomized trials. *J Clin Oncol.* 2008;26:5802-5812.

Coleman RL, Keeney ED, Freedman RA, et al. Radical hysterectomy after radiotherapy for recurrent carcinoma of the uterine cervix. *Gynecol Oncol.* 1994;55:29-35.

Dargent D, Mathevet P. Schauta's vaginal hysterectomy combined with laparoscopic lymphadenectomy. *Baillieres Clin Obstet Gynaecol.* 1995;9:691.

Diaz JP, Sonoda Y, Leitas MM, et al. Oncologic outcome of fertility-sparing radical trachelectomy versus radical hysterectomy for stage IB1 cervical carcinoma. *Gynecol Oncol.* 2008;111:255.

Dueñas-Gonzales A, ZarbaJJ Patel F, et al. Phase III, open label, randomized study comparing concurrent gemcitabine plus cisplatin and radiation followed by adjuvant gemcitabine and cisplatin versus concurrent cisplatin and radiation in patients with stage IIB to IVA carcinoma of the cervix. *J Clin Oncol.* 2011;29:1678-1685.

Eifel PJ, Morris M, Wharton JT, et al. The influence of tumor size and morphology on the outcome of patients with FIGO stage IB squamous cell carcinoma of the uterine cervix. *Int J Radiat Oncol Biol Phys.* 1994;29:9.

Eifel PJ, Winter K, Morris M, et al. Pelvic irradiation with concurrent chemotherapy versus pelvic and para-aortic irradiation for high-risk cervical cancer: an update of radiation therapy oncology group trial (RTOG) 90-01. *J Clin Oncol.* 2004;22:872.

Forney JP. The effect of radical hysterectomy on bladder physiology. *Am J Obstet Gynecol.* 1980;138(4):374-382.

Goldberg GL, Sukumvanich P, Einstein MH, et al. Total pelvic exenteration: the Albert Einstein College of Medicine/Montelior Medical Experience (1987 to 2003). *Gynecol Oncol.* 2006;101(2):261-268.

Hacker NF, Berek JS, Lagasse LD, et al. Carcinoma of the cervix associated with pregnancy. *Obstet Gynecol.* 1982;59(6):735-746.

Hacker NF, Wain GV, Nicklin JL. Resection of bulky positive lymph nodes in patients with cervical carcinoma. *Int Gynecol Cancer.* 1995;5:250-256.

Henriksen E. The lymphatic spread of carcinoma of the cervix and of the body of the uterus. *Am J Obstet Gynecol.* 1949;58:924-942.

Hockel M. Laterally extended endopelvic resection (LEER)-principles and practice. *Gynecol Oncol.* 2008;111(2 Suppl):S13-S17.

Hockel M, Horn LC, Hentschel B, et al. Total mesometrial resection: high resolution nerve-sparing radical hysterectomy based on developmentally defined surgical anatomy. *Int J Gynecol Cancer.* 2003;13(6):791-803.

Keys HM, Bundy BN, Stehman FB, et al. Cisplatin, radiation, and adjuvant hysterectomy compared with radiation and adjuvant hysterectomy for bulky stage IB cervical carcinoma. *N Engl J Med.* 1999;340:1154-1161.

Klee M, Thranov I, Machin D. The patients' perspective on physical symptoms after radiotherapy for cervical cancer. *Gynecol Oncol.* 2000;76:14-23.

Kleinerman RA, Boice JD, Storm HH, et al. Second primary cancer after treatment for cervical cancer. *Cancer.* 1995;76:442-452.

Long 3rd HJ, Bundy B, Grendys EC, et al. Randomized phase III trial of cisplatin with or without topotecan in carcinoma of the uterine cervix. A Gynecologic Oncology Group study. *J Clin Oncol.* 2005;23:4626-4633.

Lorvidhaya V, Chitapanarux I, Sangruchi S, et al. Concurrent mitomycin C, 5-fluorouracil, and radiotherapy in the treatment of locally advanced carcinoma of the cervix: a randomized trial. *Int J Radiat Oncol Biol Phys.* 2003;55:1226-1232.

Low JA, Mauger GM, Carmichael JA. The effect of the Wertheim hysterectomy upon bladder and urethral function. *Am J Obstet Gynecol.* 1981;139:826-834.

Magrina JF, Goodrich MA, Lidner TK, et al. Modified radical hysterectomy in the treatment of early squamous cervical cancer. *Gynecol Oncol.* 1999;72:183-186.

McIntyre JF, Eifel PJ, Levenback C, et al. Ureteral stricture as a late complication of radiotherapy for stage Ib carcinoma of the uterine cervix. *Cancer.* 1995;75:836-843.

Monk BJ, Sill MW, McMeekin DS, et al. Phase III trial of four cisplatin-containing doublet combinations in stage IVB, recurrent or persistent cervical carcinoma: a Gynecology Oncology Group study. *J Clin Oncol.* 2009;27:4649-4655.

Montz FJ, Holschneider CH, Solh S, et al. Small bowel obstruction following radical hysterectomy: risk factors, incidence, and operative findings. *Gynecol Oncol.* 1994;53:114-120.

Moore D, Blessing J, McQuellon R, et al. Phase III study of cisplatin with or without paclitaxel in stage IVB, recurrent or persistent squamous cell carcinoma of the cervix: a Gynecologic Oncology Group study. *J Clin Oncol.* 2004;22:3113-3119.

Morley GW, Hopkins MP, Lindenauer SM, et al. Pelvic exenteration, University of Michigan: 100 patients at 5 years. *Obstet Gynecol.* 1989;74:934-943.

Morton DL. Lymphatic mapping and sentinel lymphadenectomy for melanoma: past, present and future. *Ann Surg Oncol.* 2001;8(9suppl):22S-28S.

NCCN Clinical Practice Guidelines in Oncology (NCCN Guidelines). Cervical Cancer Version 1 ; 2014. NCCN.org.

Neoadjuvant Chemotherapy for Cervical Cancer Meta-Analysis (NACCCMA) Collaboration. Neoadjuvant chemotherapy for locally advanced cervical cancer. *Cochrane Database Syst Rev.* 2004;(2). CD001774.

Omura G, Blessing J, Vaccarello L, et al. Randomized trial of cisplatin versus cisplatin plus mitolactol versus cisplatin plus ifosfamide in advanced squamous carcinoma of the cervix: a Gynecologic Oncology Group study. *J Clin Oncol.* 1997;15:165-171.

Pearcey R, Brundage M, Drouin P, et al. Phase III trial comparing radical radiotherapy with and without cisplatin chemotherapy in patients with advanced squamous cell cancer of the cervix. *J Clin Oncol.* 2002;20:966-972.

Pecorelli S. Revised FIGO staging for carcinoma of the vulva, cervix and endometrium. *Int J Gynaecol Obstet.* 2009;105:103-104.

Peters WAI, Liu PY, Barrett R, et al. Cisplatin, 5-fluorouracil plus radiation therapy are superior to radiation therapy as adjunctive therapy in high-risk, early-stage carcinoma of the cervix after radical hysterectomy and pelvic lymphadenectomy. Report of a Phase III Intergroup Study. *Gynecol Oncol.* 1999;72:443.

Piver MS, Rutledge F, Smith JR. Five classes of extended hysterectomy for women with cervical cancer. *Obstet Gynecol.* 1974;44:265-272.

Plante M, Renaud MC, Roy M. Radical vaginal trachelectomy: a fertility-preserving option for young women with early stage cervical cancer. *Gynecol Oncol.* 2005;99(Suppl 1):S143-S146.

Potter ME, Alvarez RD, Shingleton HM, et al. Early invasive cervical cancer with pelvic lymph node involvement: to complete or not to complete radical hysterectomy? *Gynecol Oncol.* 1990;37:78.

Querleu D, Morrow CP. Classification of radical hysterectomy. *Lancet Oncol.* 2008;9(3):297-303.

Ramirez PT, Jhingran A, Macapinlac HA, et al. Laparoscopic extraperitoneal para-aortic lymphadenectomy in locally advanced cervical cancer: a prospective correlation of surgical findings with positron emission tomography/computed tomography findings. *Cancer.* 2011;117(9):1928-1934.

Robinson JW, Faris PD, Scott CB. Psychoeducational group increases vaginal dilation for younger women and reduces sexual fears for women of all ages with gynecologic carcinoma treated with radiotherapy. *Int J Radiat Oncol Biol Phys.* 1999;44:497-506.

Rose PG, Bundy BN, Watkins EB, et al. Concurrent cisplatin-based radiotherapy and chemotherapy for locally advanced cervical cancer. *N Engl J Med.* 1999;340:1144-1153.

Rydzewska L, Tierney J, Vale CL, et al. Neoadjuvant chemotherapy plus surgery versus surgery for cervical cancer. *Cochrane Database Syst Rev.* 2010;(1).CD007406

Sardi J, Sananes C, Giaroli A, et al. Results of a prospective randomized trial with neoadjuvant chemotherapy in stage IB bulky, squamous carcinoma of the cervix. *Gynecol Oncol.* 1993;49:156-165.

Sedlis A, Bundy BN, Rotman MZ, et al. A randomized trial of pelvic radiation therapy versus no further therapy in selected patients with stage IB carcinoma of the cervix after radical hysterectomy and pelvic lymphadenectomy: a Gynecologic Oncology Group study. *Gynecol Oncol.* 1999;73:177-183.

Shepherd JH, Ngan HYS, Neven P, et al. Multivariate analysis of factors affecting survival in pelvic exenteration. *Int J Gynecol Cancer.* 1994;4:361-370.

Siegel RL, Miller KD, Jemal A. Cancer statistics, 2015. *CA Cancer J Clin.* 2015;65(1):5-29.

Sonoda Y, Abu-Rustum NR, Gemignani ML, et al. A fertility-sparing alternative to radical hysterectomy: how many patients may be eligible? *Gynecol Oncol.* 2004;95:534-538.

Sood AK, Cooper BC, Sorsosky JI, et al. Novel modification of the vertical rectus abdominis myocutaneous flap for neovagina creation. *Obstet Gynecol.* 2005;105(3):514-518.

Tewari KS, Sill MW, Long 3rd HJ, et al. Improved survival with bevacizumab in advanced cervical cancer. *N Engl J Med.* 2014;370:734-743.

Westby M, Asmussen M. Anatomical and functional changes in the lower urinary tract after radical hysterectomy with lymph node dissection as studied by dynamic urethrocystography in simultaneous urethrocystometrics. *Gynecol Oncol.* 1985;21:261-276.

Suggested Readings can be found on ExpertConsult.com.

# 30

# Neoplastic Diseases of the Vulva

## Lichen Sclerosus, Intraepithelial Neoplasia, Paget Disease, and Carcinoma

*Michael Frumovitz, Diane C. Bodurka*

Cancer of the vulva accounts for approximately 5% of malignancies of the lower female genital tract, ranking it fourth in frequency after cancers of the endometrium, ovary, and cervix. Well-defined predisposing factors for the development of vulvar carcinoma have not been identified. In general, premalignant and malignant changes frequently arise at multifocal points on the vulva. Human papillomavirus (HPV) has been noted in almost 70% of patients with carcinoma of the vulva (Saraiya, 2015), and invasive carcinoma may arise from areas of carcinoma in situ, similar to the mechanism in cervical squamous cell carcinoma (see Chapter 29). However, some cases of squamous cell carcinoma of the vulva appear to develop in the absence of HPV or premalignant changes in the vulvar epithelium. Other factors, such as granulomatous disease of the vulva, diabetes, hypertension, smoking, and obesity, have all been suggested as causative factors, but data do not provide consistent evidence regarding their association with vulvar carcinoma. Carcinoma of the vulva occurs with increasing frequency in those who have been treated for squamous cell carcinoma of the cervix or vagina, presumably as a result of the increased risk of carcinogenesis in the squamous epithelium of the lower genital tract in these patients. It appears that HPV DNA is involved in the development of a subset of vulvar carcinomas that tend to occur in younger patients, as noted by Crum (Crum, 1987). Monk and colleagues demonstrated that not only were the HPV DNA–associated carcinomas found in younger patients but also that HPV-negative patients appear to have had a poorer prognosis with tumors that were more likely to recur and lead to patient death (Monk, 1995). As demonstrated by Hording and coworkers, HPV-positive tumors tend to have a warty or basaloid appearance, whereas HPV-negative tumors tend to be keratinized (Hording, 1994). The former tend to be associated with premalignant vulvar changes (vulvar intraepithelial neoplasia [VIN]). The incidence of vulvar carcinoma in situ has increased by over 400% since the 1980s, with most of the cases occurring in women under 50 years old (Judson, 2006).

Most vulvar malignancies are squamous cell carcinomas and most occur in women over 50 years old. In fact, although over 80% of patients with vulvar carcinoma in situ are under 50 years old, less than 20% of women with invasive carcinoma are under 50. The age-specific incidence of vulvar cancer increases with each decade of life but overall has remained relatively stable since the 1980s (Fig. 30.1). Although most patients with carcinoma of the vulva are older than 60, those with carcinoma in situ of the vulva are usually 10 to 15 years younger—that is, 40 to 55 years of age. Premalignant changes of the vulva have been seen with increasing frequency among younger patients, often in their 20s and 30s, possibly as a result of an increasing rate of multiple sexual contacts and increased exposure to venereal infections, particularly HPV, in this population. Carter and colleagues reported a link between immunosuppression and invasive squamous cell carcinoma of the vulva in women younger than 40 years (Carter, 1993). Similar to cervical cancer, HPV-related infections would presumably progress through dysplasia to invasive cancer in these immunocompromised women. This chapter reviews the clinical and pathologic aspects of premalignant vulvar lesions and vulvar atypias (Box 30.1). This is followed by consideration of the diagnosis, natural history, and management of invasive cancers of the vulva, which includes not only the squamous cell carcinomas but also the rarer melanomas and sarcomas.

## VULVAR ATYPIAS

### SPECIFIC CONDITIONS

#### *Vulvar Atypias: Intraepithelial Neoplasia*

Lichen sclerosus (Fig. 30.2) is a change in the vulvar skin that often appears whitish. Microscopically, the epithelium becomes markedly thinned, with a loss or blunting of the rete ridges. In some cases, there is also a thickening or hyperkeratosis of the surface layers (Fig. 30.3). Inflammation is usually present. Hart and associates studied 107 patients with lichen sclerosus, and only one followed for 12 years eventually developed vulvar carcinoma (Hart, 1975). Five patients had vulvar carcinoma when lichen sclerosus was diagnosed. Twelve other patients subsequently developed malignancies at other sites, such as the cervix, colon, breast, ovary, and endometrium. In the past, patients with lichen sclerosus were thought not to be at increased risk for the development of vulvar carcinoma. A study by Carlson and colleagues has supported a small premalignant potential of lichen sclerosus (Carlson, 1998). Their study, and a literature review, showed

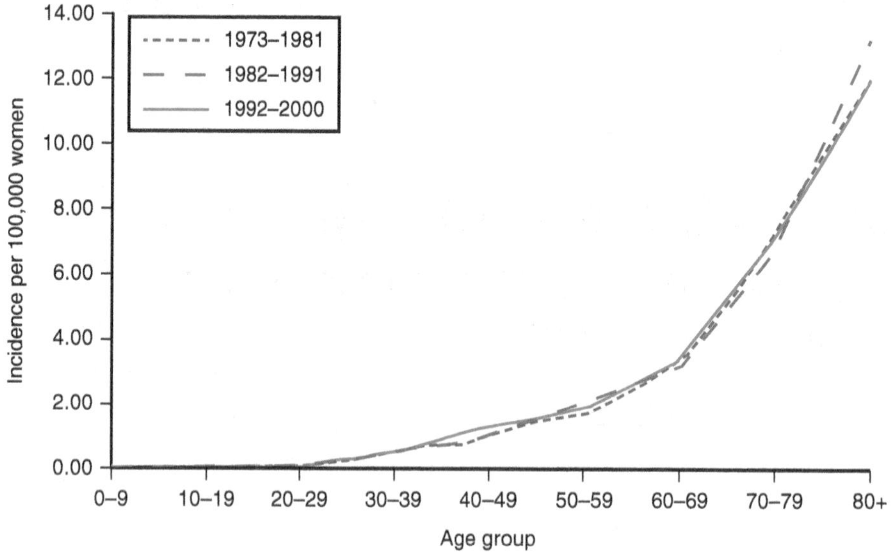


**Figure 30.1** Incidence of invasive vulvar cancer by age and diagnosis year. (Modified from Judson PL, Habermann EB, Baxter NN, et al. Trends in the incidence of invasive and in situ vulvar carcinoma. *Obstet Gynecol.* 2006;107[5]:1018-1022.)

**Box 30.1 Classification of Vulvar Atypias**

Squamous cell hyperplasia (formerly hyperplastic dystrophy)
Lichen sclerosus
Intraepithelial neoplasia
VIN I: Mild dysplasia
VIN II: Moderate dysplasia
VIN III: Severe dysplasia-carcinoma in situ
Others
  Paget disease
  Melanoma in situ (level 1)

*VIN*, Vulvar intraepithelial neoplasia.

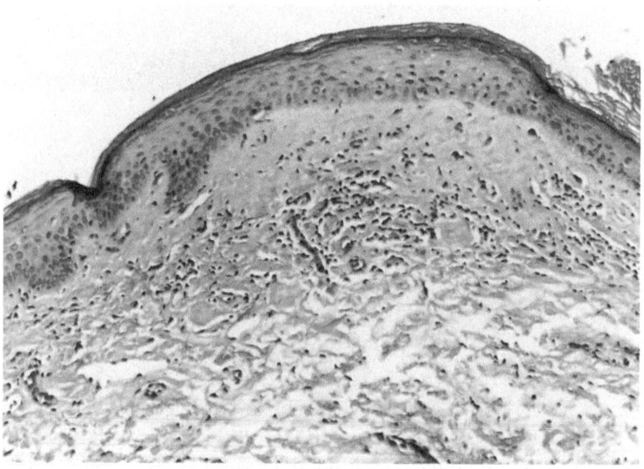

**Figure 30.2** Lichen sclerosus et atrophicus. Homogeneous collagen in the papillary dermis is accompanied by a scattered lymphocytic infiltrate and atrophy of the epithelium (H&E, ×80). (Courtesy of Dr. Anthony Montag, Department of Pathology, University of Chicago, Chicago.)

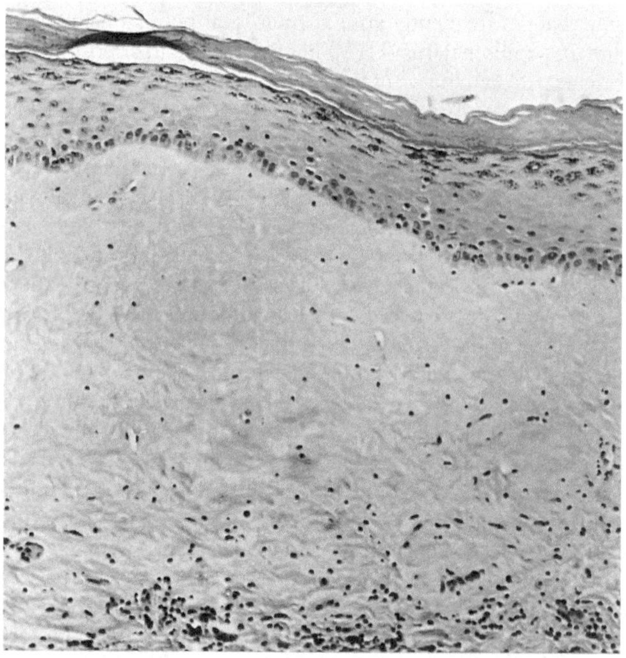

**Figure 30.3** Lichen sclerosus. Hyperkeratosis is occasionally present. (From Friedrich EG, Wilkinson EJ. The vulva. In: Blaustein A, ed. *Pathology of the Female Genital Tract.* New York: Springer-Verlag; 1982.)

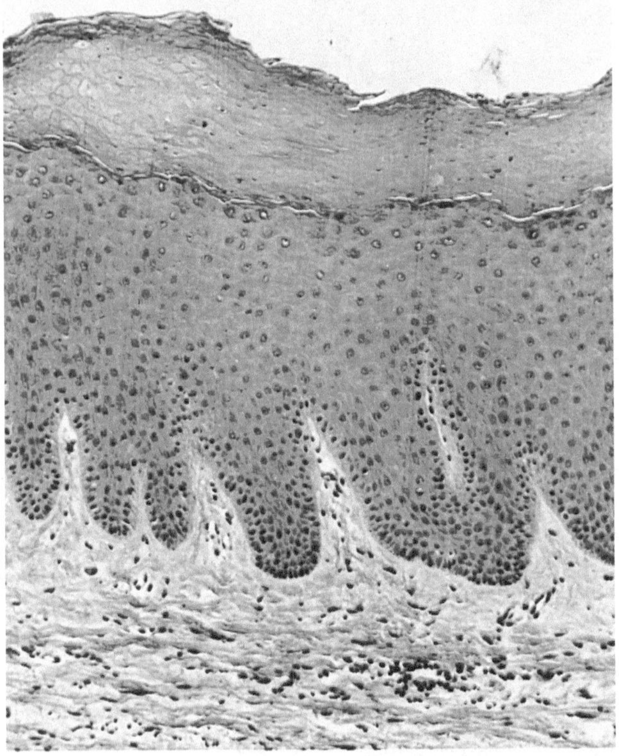

**Figure 30.4** Squamous hyperplasia (formerly hyperplastic dystrophy), benign. Hyperkeratosis, acanthosis, and mild inflammation are present. (From Friedrich EG, Wilkinson EJ. The vulva. In: Blaustein A, ed. *Pathology of the Female Genital Tract.* New York: Springer-Verlag; 1982.)

that a risk of lichen sclerosus and squamous cell carcinoma was 4.5%, with an average of 4 years latency between symptomatic lichen sclerosus and squamous cell carcinoma. The tumors that developed tended to be clitoral in location. For women who are compliant with topical corticosteroid therapy, the risk of developing vulvar dysplasia or carcinoma approaches 0% compared with noncompliant women, whose risk is 4.7% (Lee, 2015). Squamous hyperplasia (formerly, hyperplastic dystrophy) involves the elongation and widening of the rete ridges, which may be confluent (Fig. 30.4). There may also be hyperkeratotic surface layers, and the tissue grossly is often whitish or reddish.

Atypical changes may appear in the vulvar epithelium. These are usually marked by a loss of the maturation process usually seen in squamous epithelium, as well as an increase in mitotic activity and nuclear/cytoplasmic ratio (Fig. 30.5). Mild dysplasia (atypia) is diagnosed if these changes involve the lower third of the epithelium, moderate dysplasia (atypia) if half to two-thirds of the epithelium is involved, and severe dysplasia (atypia) if more than two-thirds of the epithelium is affected. Carcinoma in situ involves the full thickness of the epithelium. The term *VIN I* is used for mild atypia, *VIN II* for moderate atypia, and *VIN III* for severe atypia and carcinoma in situ. It is sometimes difficult to distinguish between squamous hyperplasia and intraepithelial neoplasia. Crum has suggested that VIN usually contains nuclei that are fourfold or greater different in size, whereas differences in the size of nuclei in condyloma or nonneoplastic epithelia are threefold or less (Crum, 1987). Furthermore, abnormal mitoses are usually observed in VIN.

### Carcinoma in Situ (Vulvar Intraepithelial Neoplasia III)

Carcinoma in situ is diagnosed if the full thickness of the epithelium is abnormal (Fig. 30.6, *A*). Occasionally, the process may histologically resemble carcinoma in situ of the cervix and, in many lesions, there are multinucleated cells, abnormal mitoses, an increased density in cells, and an increase in the nuclear-to-cytoplasmic ratio.

### Paget Disease

Paget disease is a rare intraepithelial disorder that occurs in the vulvar skin and histologically resembles Paget disease in the breast. Paget cells are large pale cells (Fig. 30.7). The cells often occur in nests and infiltrate upward through the epithelium. Frequently, histologic abnormalities of the apocrine glands of the skin may be noted in these lesions. There has been an increased association of Paget disease of the vulva with underlying invasive adenocarcinoma of the vulva, vagina, and anus, as well as distant sites, including the bladder, cervix, colon, stomach, and breast. Paget disease of the vulva tends to spread, often in an occult fashion, and recurrences are frequent after treatment.

## DIAGNOSIS

### Clinical Presentation

Atypias of the vulva present with a variety of symptoms and signs. Irritation or itching is common, although some patients do not report these symptoms. The vulva often has a whitish change because of a thickened keratin layer. In the past, the term *leukoplakia* was used. This term has been discarded, in part because abnormal lesions of the vulva require biopsy to establish a correct diagnosis. When lichen sclerosus is present, there is usually a diffuse whitish change to the vulvar skin (Fig. 30.8). The vulvar skin often appears thin and there may be scarring and contracture. In addition, fissuring of the skin is often present, accompanied by excoriation secondary to itching. Areas of squamous hyperplasias (formerly called *hyperplastic dystrophy without atypia*) also appear as whitish lesions in general, but the tissues of the vulva usually appear thickened and the process tends to be more focal or multifocal than diffuse (Fig. 30.9).

Abnormal areas of vulvar atypia or VIN may also appear as white, red, or pigmented areas on the vulva. However, the clinical appearance of VIN is variable. Friedrich and colleagues estimated that approximately one-third of patients with carcinoma in situ will present with pigmented lesions, emphasizing the importance of a biopsy to establish the diagnosis (Friedrich, 1980). The lesions tend to be discrete and multifocal and occur more frequently in those who have had squamous cell neoplasia of the cervix. In addition, reddish nodules may also be foci of Paget disease as well as of carcinoma in situ. Paget disease often has a reddish eczematoid appearance. It should be reemphasized that these conditions cannot be accurately diagnosed from their clinical appearance, and biopsies are needed.

### Diagnostic Methods

In general, cytologic evaluation (Pap smear) of the vulva has not proved helpful, in part because the vulvar skin is thick and keratinized and does not shed cells as readily as the epithelium of the vagina and cervix. However, in some cases, particularly if there

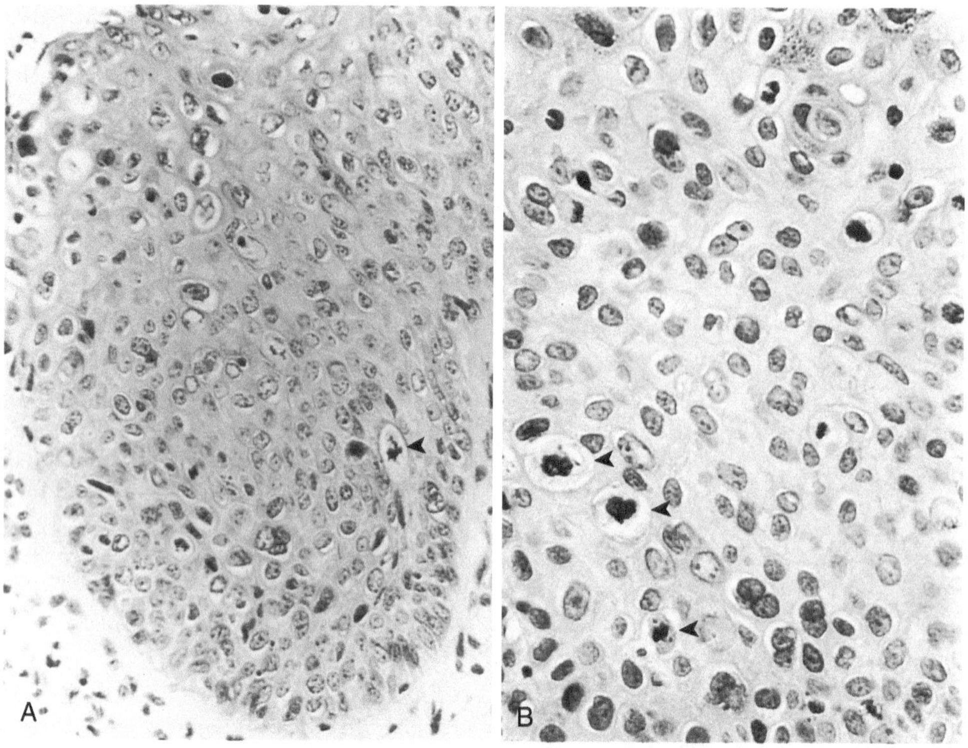


**Figure 30.5** **A,** Vulvar intraepithelial neoplasia from which human papillomavirus type 16 was isolated. Characteristic features displayed here include abnormal mitoses (a two-group metaphase is denoted by the *arrowhead*), a full-thickness population of abnormal cells, and abnormal differentiation. Superficial cells contain perinuclear halos, which in contrast to condylomata are small and concentric. **B,** The higher power photomicrograph of vulvar intraepithelial neoplasia illustrates the marked variability in nuclear size and staining, with both enlarged nuclei and multinucleated cells. Coarsely clumped mitoses *(small arrowheads)* and a three-group metaphase *(large arrowhead)* are present. (From Crum CP. *Pathology of the Vulva and Vagina.* New York: Churchill Livingstone; 1987.)

is ulceration of the vulva, a cytologic smear can be helpful diagnostically (see Fig. 32-6, *B*). A tongue depressor moistened with normal saline or tap water is scraped over the surface portion of the vulva to be sampled, and the specimen is placed on a glass slide and then fixed.

The toluidine blue test (1% toluidine blue applied for 1 minute, followed by 1% acetic acid) with biopsy of the retained blue-staining areas has generally been discarded because it appears to be very nonspecific.

Colposcopy of the vulva is difficult because the characteristic changes in vascular appearance and tissue patterns that are seen in the cervix are not present (see Chapter 28). Nevertheless, the magnification of the colposcope may be used to help follow patients with VIN as well as identify the discrete whitish or pigmented areas that warrant biopsy. The colposcope is not used for routine vulvar examination but is primarily used for those who are being evaluated or followed for vulvar atypia or VIN. The addition of 3% acetic acid highlights whitish areas for biopsy.

Biopsy of the vulva can be conveniently accomplished with a Keyes dermal punch biopsy (Fig. 30.10). Usually, a 3- to 5-mm diameter punch is used. Each area in which a biopsy sample is to be obtained is usually infiltrated with local anesthesia using a fine 25-gauge needle. The punch is then rotated and downward pressure applied so that a disk of tissue is circumscribed. When the entire thickness of the skin has been incised, the specimen is elevated with forceps and removed with a sharp scissors. Occasionally, a larger biopsy is needed, in which case a larger field is anesthetized and a small scalpel or cervical punch biopsy (see Fig. 30-14 later in the chapter) is used to obtain the specimen. Usually, little bleeding is encountered and it can generally be controlled by applying silver nitrate or ferrous subsulfate (Monsel's solution). Depending on the size of the atypical area and the variety of atypical-appearing areas, one or multiple biopsies may be needed.

## TREATMENT

### Vulvar Atypias

Most vulvar atypias have pruritus as the major symptom, so the relief of itching is often the woman's main concern. Once the correct diagnosis has been established by biopsy, appropriate therapy can be undertaken. Most whitish lesions will be benign, as lichen sclerosus is the most common condition encountered.

Topical steroids can be used for atrophic conditions of the vulva, particularly lichen sclerosus. The most commonly used option for the treatment of lichen sclerosus is 0.05% clobetasol propionate ointment. This can be used anywhere from nightly to twice weekly for up to 12 weeks and then used to re-treat,

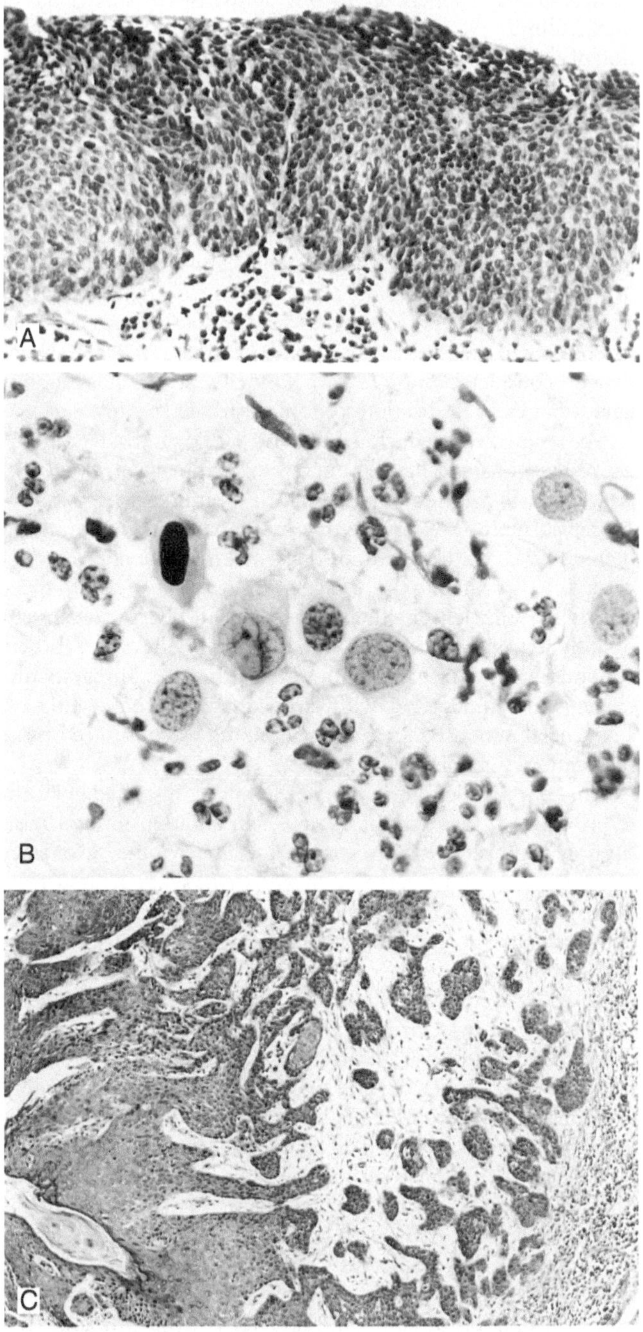


**Figure 30.6** **A,** Carcinoma in situ, histology. The full thickness of the epithelium is replaced by hyperchromatic cells with poorly defined cellular borders (×80). **B,** Carcinoma in situ, cytology. Cells derived from carcinoma in situ of the vulva may exhibit varying sizes and shapes, as depicted in this photomicrograph. Note variation in nuclear pattern from one nucleus to another. Degenerated polymorphonuclear leukocytes are present in the background (×800). **C,** Invasive squamous carcinoma, histology. Tumor nests and cords infiltrate stroma. The squamous nature of the tumor is more apparent on surface *(left)*, where cells have abundant dense cytoplasm. Keratin is also seen (×80).

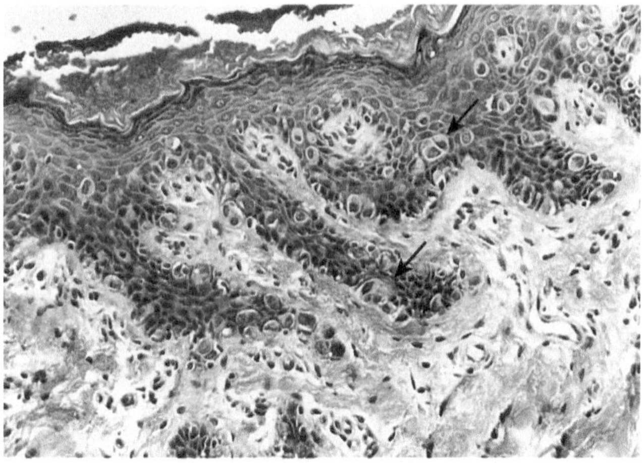

**Figure 30.7** Vulvar epidermis with Paget disease. Malignant cells *(arrows)* are seen infiltrating the epidermis and spreading along the dermal-epidermal junction (H&E, ×160). (Courtesy of Anthony Montag, MD, Department of Pathology, The University of Chicago.)

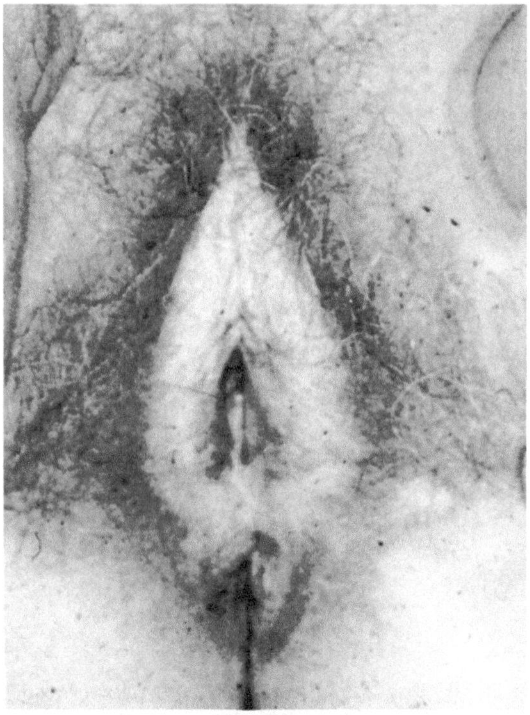

**Figure 30.8** Vulva, lichen sclerosus. The tissue of the labia minora and perineum have a white, brittle, cigarette paper appearance. (From Kaufman RH, Gardner HL, Merrill JA. Diseases of the vulva and vagina. In: Romney SL, Gray MJ, Little AB, et al, eds. *Gynecology and Obstetrics*. New York: McGraw-Hill; 1980.)

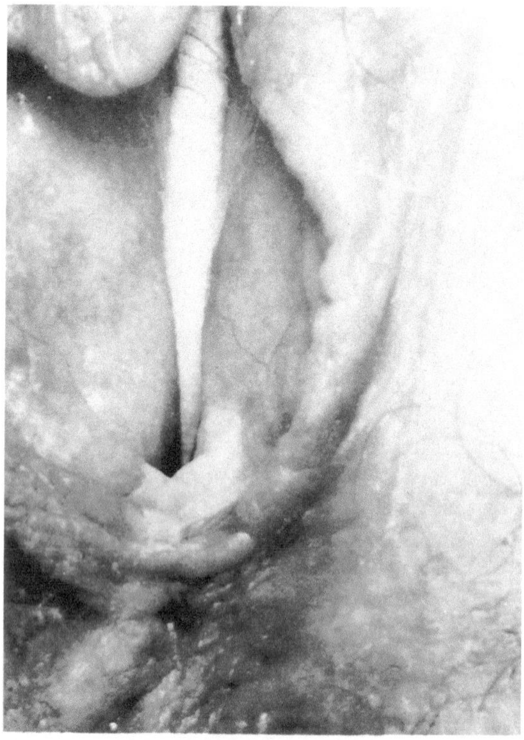

Figure 30.9 Vulva, hyperplastic dystrophy. A sharply demarcated, raised, white area is noted at lower tip of white pointer. (From Kaufman RH, Gardner HL, Merrill JA. Diseases of the vulva and vagina. In: Romney SL, Gray MJ, Little AB, et al, eds. *Gynecology and Obstetrics.* New York: McGraw-Hill; 1980.)

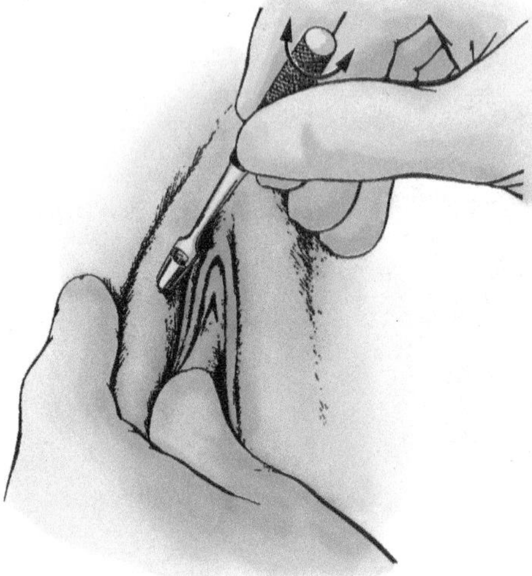

Figure 30.10 Diagnostic Keyes punch biopsy. (From Friedrich EG. *Vulvar Disease.* 2nd ed. Philadelphia: WB Saunders; 1983.)

as necessary. Although lichen sclerosus can be associated with the development of squamous cell carcinoma as described previously, use of a potent steroid cream may offer protection from malignant evolution.

A newer class of drug, topical calcineurin inhibitors (TCIs), has been evaluated as a nonsteroidal treatment of lichen sclerosis. Both of the TCIs pimecrolimus and tacrolimus have been compared with clobetasol. In one study, twice daily usage of pimecrolimus 1% cream was compared with once daily application of clobetasol 0.05% cream in 38 women with biopsy-proven vulvar lichen sclerosis (Goldstein, 2011). Although clobetasol was superior in improving inflammation, patients who used pimecrolimus did have some reduction in inflammation and showed equivalent improvement in pruritus and burning/pain. Another study compared nightly tacrolimus 0.1% ointment with nightly clobetasol 0.05% cream in 55 women with lichen sclerosis (Funaro, 2014). Both groups had significant improvement in disease-related symptoms, although the clobetasol group had a larger improvement. Most would agree that clobetasol should still be used as first-line therapy in the treatment of lichen sclerosis with consideration of TCIs in women who fail clobetasol or have other contraindications to topical steroid therapy.

For women who fail clobetasol and TCIs, some advocate the use of hormonal creams, although results from small clinical trials using testosterone and progesterone creams have been mixed. A preparation of 2% testosterone propionate in petrolatum can be used twice daily, with once-daily maintenance after the first week. Often, reducing the dosage of testosterone cream to twice weekly is a sufficient maintenance dose. Side effects, such as clitoral hypertrophy and increased hair growth, can occur. If there are undesirable side effects with testosterone, local progesterone cream is sometimes tried, with variable success. Those who have a beneficial response to testosterone should be continued on the medication indefinitely.

The control of local irritation of the vulva is discussed in Chapter 18 (Benign Gynecologic Lesions). In addition to local measures to diminish irritation (e.g., cotton underclothes, avoidance of strong soaps and detergents, avoidance of synthetic undergarments), topical fluorinated corticosteroids are helpful to control itching. Frequently used preparations are 0.025% or 0.1% triamcinolone acetonide (Aristocort, Kenalog), fluocinolone acetonide (Synalar), and 0.01% or 0.1% betamethasone valerate. These are usually applied twice daily to control the itching, which is often relieved in 1 to 2 weeks. Unfortunately, the prolonged use of fluorinated topical steroids can lead to vulvar atrophy and contraction. Thus once the symptoms of itching are controlled, the dose of topical corticosteroids is tapered off or, if long-term therapy is needed, a nonfluorinated compound such as 1.0% hydrocortisone is used to avoid vulvar contraction. Occasionally, 1% hydrocortisone is sufficient for initial therapy. In some cases, the corticosteroids are not successful, and numerous types of topical therapy must be tried to control symptoms. Gentle soaps are helpful. Burow's solution (5% solution of aluminum acetate) is frequently used as a wet dressing to help control irritation and itching. Doak tar, 3%, in petrolatum (USP) or in 1% hydrocortisone ointment is useful for severe cases.

In some patients with lichen sclerosus, severe contracture of the vulva, particularly in the area of the posterior fourchette, will occur with concomitant scarring and tenderness. Intercourse may then become painful for these patients. Woodruff and coworkers described a useful surgical technique to treat these vaginal outlet disorders by repair of the perineum (Woodruff, 1981). The contractured and fissured area in the posterior fourchette is excised, which results in an elliptic defect. This is then closed by undermining the distal 3 to 4 cm of the posterior vaginal mucosa and suturing the freed mucosa to the perineal skin (Fig. 30.11).

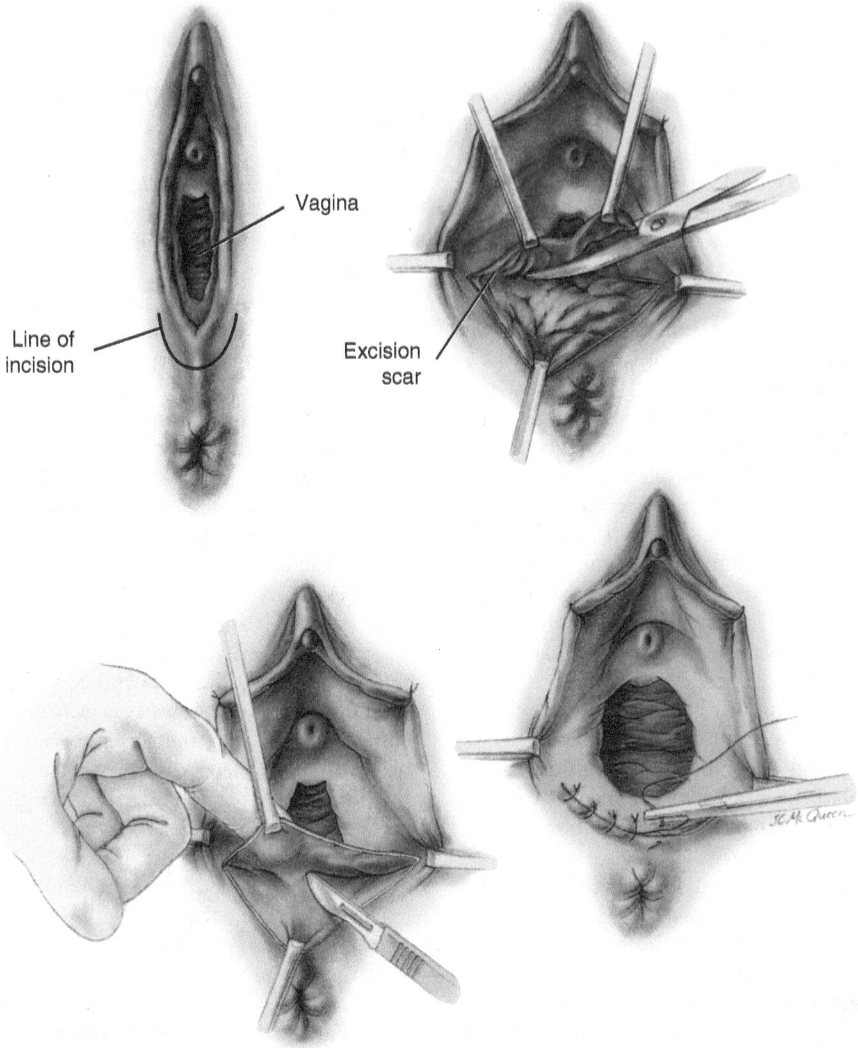


**Figure 30.11** Surgical correction of perineal scars. (From Woodruff JD, Julian C. Surgery of the vulva. In: Ridley JH, ed. *Gynecologic Surgery: Errors, Safeguards, Salvage.* Baltimore: Williams & Wilkins; 1974.)

### *Vulvar Intraepithelial Neoplasia*

Once the diagnosis of VIN has been established by biopsy, therapy is performed to eradicate the area containing the neoplasia. The clinician must be aware that the progress of vulvar atypia (mild dysplasia [VIN I]), to moderate dysplasia (VIN II), to severe dysplasia and carcinoma in situ (VIN III), and then to invasive carcinoma is not as well documented for vulvar neoplasia as it is for squamous cell neoplasia of the cervix. Moreover, vulvar neoplasia is frequently multifocal, requiring treatment of several areas. An additional complication is that some cases originally diagnosed as intraepithelial neoplasia have been reported to regress spontaneously.

In 1972, Friedrich reported bowenoid atypia (histologically similar to carcinoma in situ) in a pregnant woman that regressed spontaneously postpartum (Friedrich, 1972). Others also reported spontaneous regression of this lesion. These spontaneously regressing lesions tend to be discrete elevations in young women. Some may be explained by studies of the nuclear DNA content of vulvar atypias that suggest that not all lesions with this designation are premalignant. Fu and colleagues noted that only four of eight cases of vulvar atypia had an aneuploid (neoplastic) distribution. A polyploid distribution was noted in four of the cases, which is consistent with a benign process, whereas aneuploidy is consistent with intraepithelial neoplasia (Fu, 1981).

Although VIN has been diagnosed more commonly in younger women, the risk of progression to invasive cancer is higher for those who are older and for those who are immunosuppressed, such as women with AIDS or transplant recipients. Chafe and associates studied 69 patients with a diagnosis of VIN treated by surgical excision (Chafe 1988). Unsuspected invasion was found in 13 patients. The median age was 36 years for those without invasive carcinoma, whereas the median age was 58 years ($P = .003$) for those with invasion found in the excision specimen, emphasizing the increased risk of invasion in the older patients. Furthermore, the risk of invasion was higher in those who had raised lesions with irregular surface patterns. Thus patients who were older and those with irregular raised lesions had the greatest risk of unrecognized invasive carcinoma. A study by Modesitt and colleagues of 73 women, with a mean age of 45 years, found an invasive carcinoma in 22% of VIN III excision specimens (Modesitt, 1998). Not surprisingly, the risk of recurrence was almost 50% if the margins were positive, and only 17% if they were negative. The risk of progression from intraepithelial disease to invasive carcinoma appears to be less for vulvar cases than for cervical disease (see Chapter 28).

Women with HIV-AIDS are also more likely to develop vulvar carcinoma in situ and invasive cancer than the general population. In a large population-based study, Chaturvedi and colleagues found a relative risk (RR) of 1.59 for developing VIN III in the 28 to 60 months after the onset of AIDS and an RR of 4.91 for developing invasive carcinoma in this group (Chaturvedi, 2009).

Studies have suggested that the potential of VIN to develop into invasive cancer is low. Buscema and coworkers followed 102 patients with vulvar carcinoma in situ for 1 to 15 years without treatment; 4 patients developed invasive disease, 2 of whom were immunosuppressed (Buscema,1980). Unfortunately, current techniques do not allow precise prediction of which lesions of VIN are at the greatest risk of progression to invasive disease. A population-based study from Norway has confirmed an increasing frequency of VIN III that nearly tripled from the mid-1970s to 1988 to 1991 but, during the same period, the age-adjusted frequency of invasive vulvar carcinomas remained almost constant (Iversen, 1998). Iversen and Tretli further noted an estimated conversion rate of VIN III to invasive carcinoma of approximately 3.4% for these in situ lesions (Iversen, 1998).

HPV types 6 and 11 have generally been recognized as being found most often in benign vulvar warts, whereas primarily HPV types 16, 18, 31, 33, and 35 are more frequently associated with intraepithelial neoplasia or invasive carcinoma (see Chapter 28). The Centers for Disease Control and Prevention (CDC) has estimated that 80% of women aged 50 will have acquired a genital HPV infection at some point in their lives. Beutner and associates have predicted that as many as 1 million new cases of perineal warts will occur annually in the United States (Beutner, 1998). An additional complication is that HPV type 16 infection is not always accompanied by histologic evidence of VIN. Moreover, HPV types 6, 11, and 16 can be recovered from a single site, including those that show only condyloma as well as those that show carcinoma. Thus a unique role for HPV types in VIN has not been elucidated. With current data, therapy should be based on histologic findings and not on the presence or absence of HPV infection or specific HPV types. Studies by Buscema and associates have suggested that HPV type 16 is frequently found in vulvar neoplasia and, as noted, HPV 16 has been frequently associated with some vulvar carcinomas (Buscema, 1980).

### Human Papillomavirus Therapy

The problem of the management of vulvar HPV infection is particularly complicated because it is extremely prevalent and the risk of progression from HPV infection to VIN is small. Planner and Hobbs evaluated 148 women with cytologic evidence of vulvar HPV infection and found that two-thirds of them had pruritus and dyspareunia (Planner, 1988). Results of the biopsy revealed that only 11 of the 148 women had VIN. Follow-up showed spontaneous regression of HPV infection in 56 patients, whereas VIN III developed in 2 and invasive cancer eventually developed in 1. It appears that the best approach is to restrict therapy to those with clinically bothersome symptoms such as warts or to eradicate lesions with VIN, particularly VIN II and III. Cytologic or histologic evidence of an asymptomatic HPV infection, such as koilocytosis, is not an indication for therapy. Riva and colleagues treated lower genital tract HPV infection with laser to include the cervix, vagina, and vulva; 25 patients had proved subclinical HPV infection, and their male partners were also evaluated and treated (Riva, 1989). All 25 patients suffered severe pain and many required hospitalization. At 3 months after therapy, 24 of 25 again had evidence of subclinical HPV infection and 22 had persistent histologic evidence of koilocytosis, indicating the futility of trying to eradicate HPV infection by this method.

Many VIN lesions tend to be posterior, predominantly in the perineal area. Surgical removal has been effectively used, but the type of operation has been changing. In the past, simple vulvectomy was widely practiced to treat carcinoma in situ of the vulva, but this disfiguring operation is now infrequently used, particularly because the disease is occurring in younger women. To improve the cosmetic result and sexual function, Rutledge and Sinclair introduced the method of skinning vulvectomy (Rutledge, 1968). This removes the superficial vulvar skin, preserving the clitoris, and replaces the removed skin with a split-thickness vulvar graft. In many cases, however, such extensive surgery is not needed. Often, the abnormal area of the vulva can be removed only with wide local excision. Of the patients in the series reported by Buscema and coworkers, 62 were treated with local excision; 68% showed no recurrence (Buscema, 1980). For comparison, in 28 patients treated by vulvectomy, 70% showed no recurrence. The risk of recurrence is higher if neoplastic epithelium is found at the resection margin. Friedrich has noted a 10% risk of recurrence if the surgical margins are free of disease compared with a 50% risk if the surgical margins are involved with neoplasia (Friedrich, 1980). However, because recurrence may develop even if the resection margins are negative, long-term follow-up is mandatory.

The carbon dioxide laser has been used to treat VIN, usually to a depth of 1 to 3 mm, with a deeper depth being used for areas that contain hair. This results in eradication of the abnormal vulvar tissue and healing without scarring. Most patients require a single treatment but some require more, particularly those with large or multiple lesions. Usually, patients can be treated on an outpatient basis with local, regional, or general anesthesia. The laser is particularly useful for younger patients. It is essential to be certain that the woman does not have invasive disease before using the laser, so a biopsy of any suspicious lesions should be performed before laser ablation. The surgeon should be experienced in the diagnosis and treatment of vulvar disease before using laser ablation. Older patients or those with raised lesions should be treated by surgical excision. Treatment is usually carried out to a depth of 3 to 4 mm, and healing is usually complete within 2 to 3 weeks. Leuchter and associates treated 142 patients with carcinoma in situ of the vulva (Leuchter, 1982). Of the 42 treated by laser, 17% had recurrence; 4 of the 16 treated with vulvectomy (25%) and 15 of 45 treated by local excision (33%) also had recurrence. In view of the risk of unsuspected carcinoma in older patients, as noted by the studies of Chafe and colleagues (1988), those older than 45 years and those with raised or irregular lesions should have an excision performed and the entire tissue submitted for histologic evaluation. Posterior lesions near the anus require particular attention because the anal canal is often involved and this abnormal tissue also should be removed.

5-Fluorouracil (5-FU) cream has been tried to treat carcinoma in situ of the vulva, but it causes severe burning and is generally not used. Investigators have explored using 5% imiquimod cream as primary treatment for VIN III, with promising results. Van Seters and coworkers performed a randomized control study of 5% imiquimod topical cream versus placebo in 52 women with VIN II and III (van Seters, 2008). Most women included in the study (96%) were positive for HPV prior to initiation of therapy. In the treatment group, 81% had at least a reduction in the size of the primary lesion by over 25% at 20 weeks, and 35% had a complete response. In the placebo group, there were no patients with partial or complete responses. At 12 months after enrollment, 3 patients (6%), however, had progressed to microinvasive vulvar carcinoma (1 in treatment group, 2 in placebo group).

Therapeutic vaccines using HPV peptides have also been explored for the treatment of VIN III. Kenter and colleagues combined long peptides from the E6 and E7 oncoproteins of HPV 16 into a vaccine and immunized 20 women with HPV 16–positive VIN III (Kenter, 2009). At 12 months after last vaccination, 79% had a clinical response, with 47% achieving complete response. Of note, all the women who had a complete response by 12 months also remained disease free at 24 months.

#### *Paget Disease of the Vulva*

Paget disease is generally seen in postmenopausal women and typically appears grossly as a diffuse erythematous eczematoid lesion that has usually been present for a prolonged time. Itching is a common problem. The disease is primarily seen in white women and the average age is approximately 65 years. The major importance of Paget disease of the vulva is the frequent association with other invasive carcinomas. Squamous cell carcinoma of the vulva or cervix or an adenocarcinoma of the sweat glands of the vulva or Bartholin gland carcinoma may be present. Cases of adenocarcinoma of the gastrointestinal (GI) tract and breast accompanying Paget disease have also been reported. Once a diagnosis of Paget disease of the vulva is made, it is important for the gynecologist to rule out the presence of breast and GI malignancy. In a review by Fanning and associates, 20% of patients with vulvar Paget had nonvulvar malignancies including cancers of the breast, uterus, pancreas, lung, stomach, thyroid, and skin. In addition, 12% had invasive Paget disease of the vulva and 4% had invasive adenocarcinoma of the vulva (Fanning, 1999).

If no local or distant primary malignancy is uncovered, a wide excision of the affected area can be performed. It is important to remove the full thickness of the skin to the subcutaneous fat to ensure that all the skin adnexal structures are excised, because they may have a subclinical malignancy. Bergen and coworkers evaluated 14 patients with Paget disease of the vulva treated by surgery, usually vulvectomy, skinning vulvectomy with graft, or hemivulvectomy (Bergen, 1989). With a median follow-up of 50 months, all patients were free of disease, although 2 with positive margins and 1 with negative margins required treatment for recurrence. Fishman and colleagues studied 14 patients treated by various surgical procedures for Paget disease (Fishman, 1995). Frozen-section or gross visual inspection was used to judge the operative margins. In this series, visual estimation was as useful as frozen section insofar as the error rate for judging margins by the final pathology report was approximately 35%. In addition, 2 of 5 patients with positive margins had a recurrence after the initial operation compared with 3 of 9 with negative margins. This small series therefore suggests that gross visual inspection may be as useful as frozen section when judging the extent of surgical operation. Other small series evaluating Mohs micrographic surgery for treating vulvar extramammary disease have failed to reduce recurrence significantly. A conservative approach involving removal of gross Paget disease with approximately a 1-cm margin appears to be the most appropriate, with the understanding that reexcision may be required for recurrence in the future. The full thickness of the vulvar skin to the adipose layer should be removed.

Even if resection margins are free of Paget disease at the time of surgical excision, local recurrence remains a risk. Women who have been treated for Paget disease of the vulva should have as part of their routine follow-up an annual examination of the breast, cytologic evaluation of the cervix and vulva, and screening for GI disease, at least by testing for occult blood in the stool. Progression of Paget disease of the vulva to invasive adenocarcinoma has been rarely reported.

Investigators have also explored using topical imiquimod cream as a nonsurgical therapy for extramammary Paget disease of the vulva. In one retrospective study, 21 women with Paget disease were treated with imiquimod cream and 11 (52%) had a complete response to therapy, whereas an additional 6 (29%) had a partial response with no cases of progressive disease (Luyten, 2014). As treatment of Paget disease not associated with underlying malignancies is largely for symptom control, trial of imiquimod may be a reasonable approach for patients who do not desire surgery or are not surgical candidates. In addition, as achieving negative margins with surgical resection is rare, some may consider using a course of imiquimod adjuvantly after surgical resection in an effort to reduce recurrence.

## MALIGNANT CONDITIONS

### *SQUAMOUS CELL CARCINOMA*

Squamous cell carcinomas comprise approximately 90% of primary vulvar malignancies, but a variety of other vulvar cancers are encountered; the major types are listed in Box 30.2. Melanomas account for approximately 4% to 5%, and the other types make up the remainder.

#### *Morphology and Staging*

Grossly, vulvar carcinomas usually appear as raised, flat, ulcerated, plaquelike, or polypoid masses on the vulva (Fig. 30.12, *A*). Biopsy sample of the lesion reveals the characteristic histologic appearance of squamous cell carcinoma (see Fig. 30.6, *C*).

Four clinical stages are defined for carcinoma of the vulva according to the International Federation of Gynecology and Obstetrics (FIGO), similar to the system used for other gynecologic malignancies. In addition, many centers use the TNM

**Box 30.2 Primary Vulvar Malignancies**

- Squamous cell carcinoma
- Adenocarcinoma (including Bartholin gland)
- Verrucous carcinoma
- Basal cell carcinoma
- Melanoma
- Sarcoma

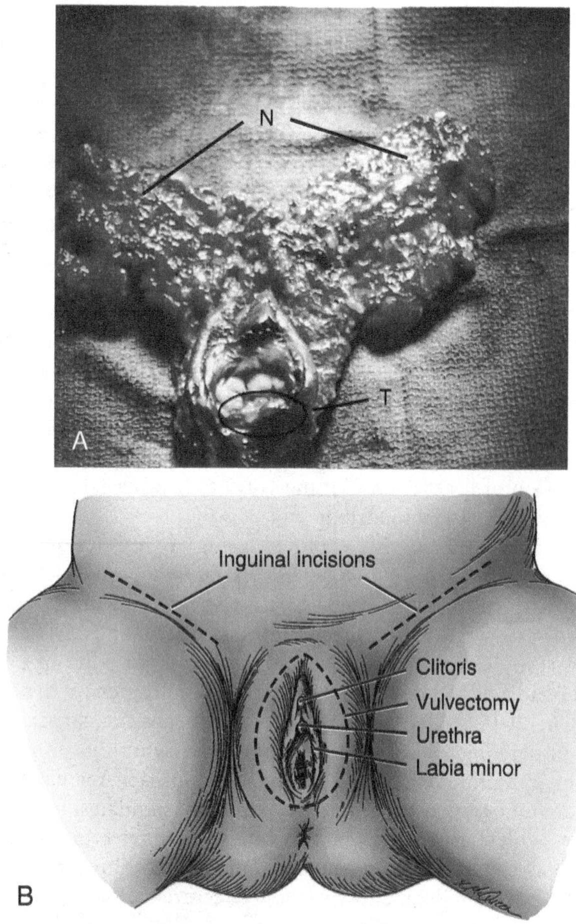


**Figure 30.12** **A,** Radical vulvectomy specimen. **B,** Vulvectomy with operative incision lines shown. Note groin incisions.

system (tumor, nodes, metastases) for classification; *T* denotes the size and extent of the tumor, *N* the clinical status of the nodes, and *M* the presence or absence of metastatic disease.

In the clinical staging system, lymph node status was assessed clinically and incorporated into the stage. Enlarged or clinically suspicious lymph nodes were assigned a higher stage, regardless of disease status documented at surgery. Clinically negative nodes were assigned an earlier stage, which was upheld even if they were found to harbor metastasis after surgical removal and pathologic examination. Therefore in 1988, the FIGO staging was modified to a surgical staging of vulvar cancer system to reflect lymph node status more accurately. In addition, a location on the perineum is no longer assigned to stage III. This system, with the modifications introduced in 2009 for new definitions of stages I to III, is shown in Box 30.3.

**Box 30.3 TNM and Staging Classifications of Carcinoma of the Vulva**

**TNM**

T: Primary tumor
Tis: Preinvasive carcinoma (carcinoma in situ)
T1: Tumor confined to the vulva or perineum, ≤2 cm in diameter
T2: Tumor confined to the vulva or perineum, >2 cm in diameter
T3: Tumor of any size with adjacent spread to the urethra, vagina, anus, or all of these
T4: Tumor of any size infiltrating the bladder mucosa, rectal mucosa, or both, including the upper part of the urethral mucosa or fixed to the anus
N: Regional lymph nodes
N0: No nodes palpable
N1: Unilateral regional lymph node metastases
N2: Bilateral regional lymph node metastases
M: Distant metastases
M0: No clinical metastases
M1: Distant metastases (including pelvic lymph node metastases)

**Staging (FIGO), Modified 2009**

Stage I—T1/2, N0, M0: Tumor confined to vulva or perineum
- IA: Lesions ≤2 cm in size, confined to the vulva or perineum and with stromal invasion ≤1 mm; no nodal metastasis
- IB: Lesions >2 cm in size or with stromal invasion >1.0 mm, confined to the vulva or perineum, with negative nodes

Stage II—T3, N0, M0: Tumor of any size with extension to adjacent perineal structures (one third lower urethra, one third lower vagina, anus) with negative nodes

Stage III—T1-3, N1/2, M0: Tumor of any size with or without extension to adjacent perineal structures (one third lower urethra, one third lower vagina, anus), with positive inguinofemoral lymph nodes
- IIIA: (i) With one lymph node metastasis (≥5 mm) or (ii) one or two lymph node metastasis(es) (<5 mm)
- IIIB: (i) With two or more lymph node metastases (≥5 mm) or (ii) three or more lymph node metastases (<5 mm)
- IIIC: With positive nodes with extracapsular spread

Stage IV—any T, any N, M1: Tumor invades other regional (two thirds upper urethra, two thirds upper vagina) or distant structures
- IVA: Tumor invades any of the following: (i) upper urethral or vaginal mucosa, bladder mucosa, rectal mucosa, or fixed to pelvic bone; or (ii) fixed or ulcerated inguinofemoral lymph nodes
- IVB: Any distant metastasis including pelvic lymph nodes

Modified from FIGO Committee on Gynecologic Oncology, European Institute of Oncology, Milan, Italy: Revised FIGO staging for carcinoma of the vulva, cervix, and endometrium. *Int J Gynecol Obstet.* 2009;105:103.
*FIGO*, International Federation of Gynecology and Obstetrics; *TNM*, tumor-node-metastasis.

### *Natural History, Spread, and Prognostic Factors*

The vulvar area is rich in lymphatics, with numerous cross connections. The main lymphatic pathways are illustrated in Figure 30.13. Tumors located in the middle of either labium tend to drain initially to the ipsilateral inguinofemoral nodes, whereas perineal tumors can spread to the left or right side. Tumors in the clitoral or urethral areas can also spread to either side. From the inguinofemoral nodes, the lymphatic spread of tumor is cephalad to the deep pelvic iliac and obturator nodes. Although there has been concern in the past that tumors in the clitoral-urethral area would spread directly to the deep pelvic nodes, this rarely, if ever, occurs. The characteristics of lymph drainage of the vulva have been evaluated by Iversen and Aas, who injected technetium-99 m colloid subcutaneously into the anterior and posterior labia majora, anterior and posterior labia minora, clitoral area, and perineum (Iversen, 1983). They then measured the radioactivity in the pelvic lymph nodes, which were surgically removed 5 hours later. More than 98% of the radioactivity was found in the ipsilateral node and less than 2% on the contralateral side. The anterior labial injections resulted in a 92% concentration of radioactivity in the ipsilateral side, with 8% on the

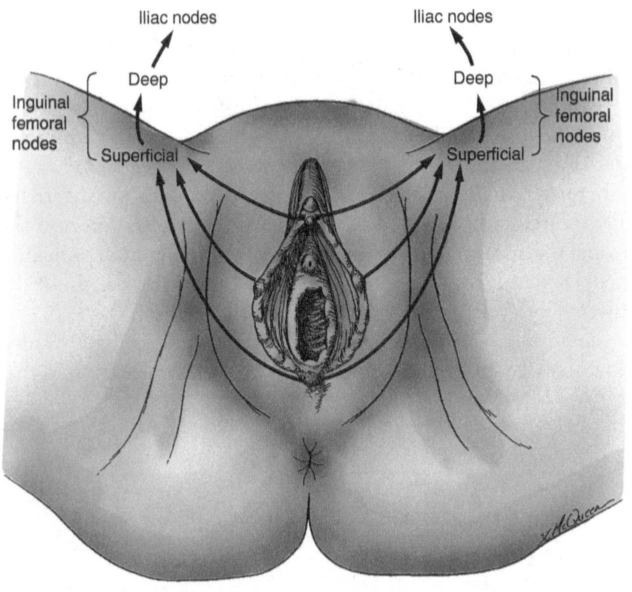


**Figure 30.13** Vulvar lymph drainage is shown in this general schematic representation of major drainage channels of vulva.

contralateral side. The clitoral and perineal injections developed a bilateral nodal distribution of radioactivity in all the patients. It is of interest that two-thirds of the patients with labial injections had a small amount of detectable radioactivity in the contralateral nodes. Thus anastomoses of the lymphatics do exist, but a direct connection from the clitoris to the deep nodes was not demonstrated.

The prognosis of a woman with vulvar carcinoma is related to the stage of the disease (Fig. 30.14), lesion size, and the presence or absence of cancer in regional nodes.

The status of the regional lymph nodes is the most important factor prognostically and therapeutically. Numerous studies, including a multicenter collaborative investigation from the Gynecologic Oncology Group (GOG), have indicated that tumor stage, location on the vulva, microscopic differentiation, presence or absence of vascular space involvement, and tumor thickness are all important prognostic factors. In a GOG study of 588 patients reported by Homesley and colleagues, the risk of lymph node metastases was related to lesion size (19% for <2 cm and 42% for >2 cm) (Homesley, 1991). Additional independent predictors of positive nodes were as follows: (1) tumor grade; (2) suspicious, fixed, or ulcerated lymph nodes; (3) lymphovascular

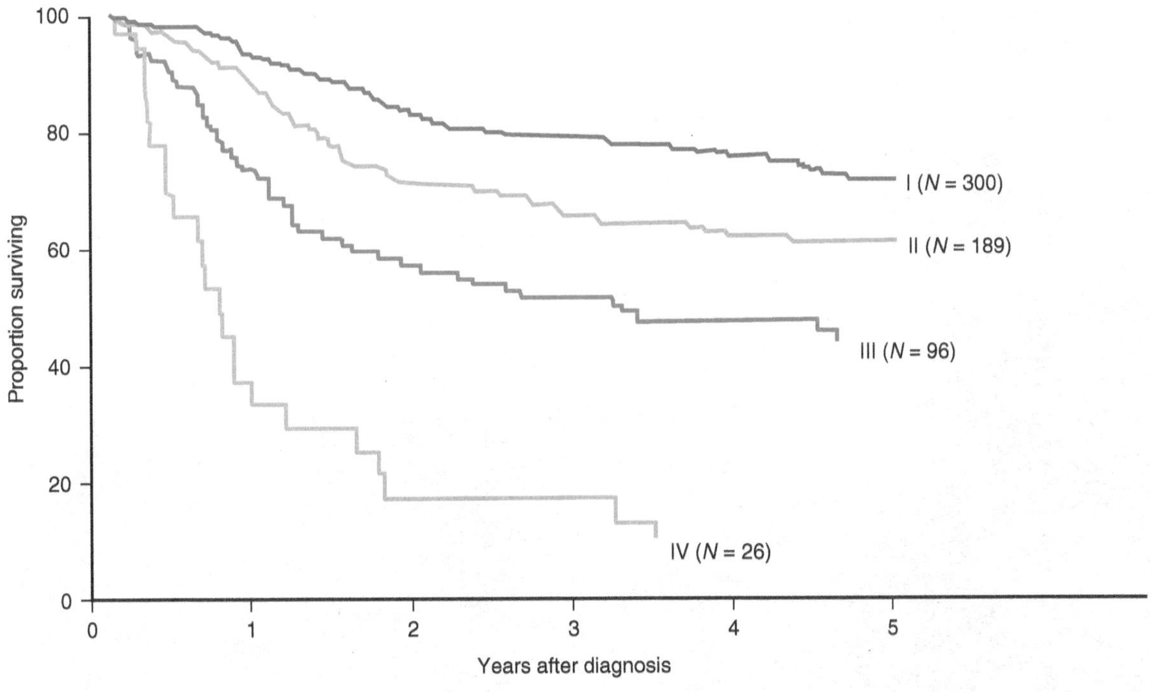


| Strata | Patients (N) | Mean age (years) | 1 year | Overall survival at 2 year | 3 year | 4 year | 5 year | Hazards ratio[a] (95% Confidence intervals) |
|---|---|---|---|---|---|---|---|---|
| I | 300 | 64.7 | 92.3% | 82.3% | 78.7% | 75.7% | 71.4% | Reference |
| II | 189 | 67.4 | 86.5% | 71.0% | 65.8% | 62.2% | 61.3% | 1.94 (1.36–2.75) |
| III | 96 | 69.4 | 72.0% | 57.2% | 51.3% | 47.5% | 43.8% | 3.84 (2.55–5.78) |
| IV | 26 | 72.8 | 33.3% | 16.7% | 16.7% | 8.3% | 8.3% | 12.2 (7.08–21.2) |

**Figure 30.14** Carcinoma of the vulva, patients treated from 1990 to 1992; survival by International Federation of Gynecology and Obstetrics stage (epidermoid invasive cancer only; N = 611). [a]Hazards ratio and 95% confidence intervals obtained from a Cox model adjusted for country. (From Pecorelli S, Creasman WT, Pettersson F, et al. *FIGO Annual Report on the Results of Treatment in Gynaecological Cancer*, vol 23. Milan, Italy: International Federation of Gynecology and Obstetrics; 1998.)

space involvement; (4) older age of the woman; and (5) tumor thickness. Table 30.1 summarizes these factors.

Lymphovascular space invasion also appears to be a prognostic factor in vulvar tumors, as it is in cervical carcinoma (see Chapter 28). In a small study of 22 patients, Rowley and associates noted no metastases in 20 patients without lymphovascular space invasion and in 2 patients with lymphovascular space invasion (Rowley, 1988).

## Stage IA: Carcinoma of the Vulva (Early or Microinvasive Carcinoma)

### Definition and Clinicopathologic Relationships

The term *microinvasive carcinoma of the vulva* typically refers to a lesion considered to be stage IA definition—that is, smaller than 2 cm, with less than 1 mm invasion—and is used to identify early tumors unlikely to spread to regional nodes. However, varying clinicopathologic results are reported when this definition is used.

Part of the confusion is because of different reference points from which the depth of invasion is measured—that is, from the surface or basement membrane. Dvoretsky and coworkers carefully analyzed the microscopic aspects of 36 cases of superficial vulvar carcinoma (Dvoretsky, 1984) Tumor penetration into the stroma was measured from the surface of the squamous epithelium (neoplastic thickness; Fig. 30.15, *A*) and also from the tip of the adjacent epithelial ridge (stromal invasion; see Fig. 30.15, *B*). Six of the 36 cases had spread to regional nodes, and all had invaded more than 3 mm from the surface. Yoder and associates found that

**Table 30.1** Factors Related to Positive Inguinal Nodes (588 Cases)

| GOG Grade | % Positive Nodes | Tumor Thickness (mm) | % Positive Nodes | Age (yr) | % Positive Nodes | LVSI | % Positive Nodes |
|---|---|---|---|---|---|---|---|
| 1 | 2.8 | ≤1 | 2.6 | <55 | 25.2 | + | 75 |
| 2 | 15.1 | 2 | 8.9 | 55-64 | 25.4 | — | 27 |
| 3 | 41.2 | 3 | 18.6 | 65-74 | 36.4 | | |
| 4 | 59.7 | 4 | 30.9 | >75 | 46 | | |
| | | ≥5 | 43 | | | | |

Modified from Homesley H, Bundy BN, Sedlis A, et al. Prognostic factors for groin node metastasis in squamous cell carcinoma of the vulva (a Gynecologic Oncology Group study). *Gynecol Oncol*. 1993;49:279.
*GOG*, Gynecologic Oncology Group; *LVSI*, lymphovascular space invasion.

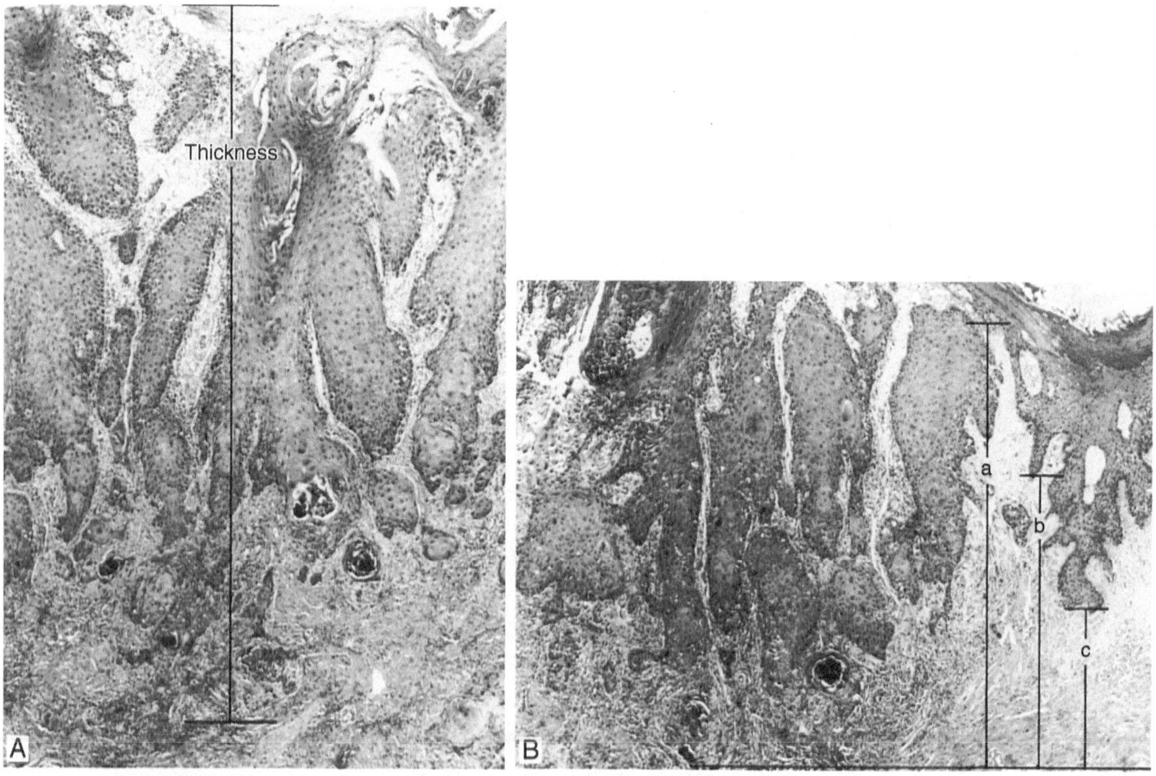


**Figure 30.15** **A,** Measurement of neoplastic thickness in squamous cell carcinoma (×35). **B,** Superficially invasive squamous cell carcinoma. The reference point used to measure the depth of stromal invasion is demonstrated by line b. Note the striking variation in the measurement of stromal invasion, depending on which reference point is chosen (line a, b, or c; ×35). (From Dvoretsky PM, Bonfiglio TA, Helkamp BF, et al. The pathology of superficially invasive thin vulva squamous cell carcinoma. *Int J Gynecol Pathol*. 1984;3:331.)

no women with squamous cell carcinoma of the vulva invading <1 mm had nodal disease. For women with lesions invading 1 to 3 mm, the risk of nodal spread was 6% and for those with lesions invading 3 to 5 mm, the risk of nodal spread increased to 20%. Furthermore, none of the patients with tumors invading <1 mm had local recurrence at 258 months' follow-up (Yoder, 2008).

The presence of carcinoma in situ in the primary lesion decreases the risk of node involvement in these cases. Ross and Ehrman have noted that only 1 of 35 patients with adjacent carcinoma in situ had nodal metastases, and this tumor penetrated the stroma 1.7 mm (Ross, 1987). In contrast, 5 of 27 superficial stage I patients (2.1 to 5.0 mm penetration) without adjacent carcinoma in situ had positive nodes. Thus spread to regional lymph nodes in stage IA carcinoma of the vulva is unlikely, particularly if the tumor is well differentiated (grade 1), invades less than 3 mm measured from the surface, or has a depth of invasion measured from the adjacent rete pegs of less than 1 mm and is without vascular space involvement. The presence of carcinoma in situ is a favorable factor. Less well-differentiated tumors or those with vascular involvement or confluence and with greater depths of invasion have an increased risk of lymph node involvement by cancer.

**Treatment**

Based on available evidence, it would appear prudent that most patients with stage IA carcinoma of the vulva by the criteria described earlier should be treated at least with a wide excision to give a margin of 1 to 2 cm. Depending on the location of the tumor, a hemivulvectomy may be needed. The lymph node dissection may be omitted or deferred, depending on the final pathologic evaluation of the tumor in the surgical specimen. For younger patients, especially with tumors that involve the labia or perineum at a distance from the clitoris, an operation that spares the clitoris should be used. Even if the criteria for stage IA are rigorously applied, a rare nodal metastasis may occur, as reported by Van der Velden and associates (Van der Velden, 1992). However, a report by Magrina and coworkers on 40 patients with T1 lesions (less than 2 cm in diameter) and less than 1 mm invasion indicated that they could be effectively treated with wide excision (Magrina, 2000). No nodal metastases were noted in this small group, and excision appeared to be as effective as a more radical operation in preventing recurrent disease.

## INVASIVE CARCINOMA OF THE VULVA

Figure 30.12, *A*, shows a typical carcinoma of the vulva, which usually appears as a polyploid mass. The woman frequently reports a sore that has not healed. She may also report bleeding, but this does not usually occur early in the course of the disease. Unfortunately, the delay in diagnosis is common because older patients frequently fail to seek prompt medical attention and, often when they do, a biopsy is not initially performed. For example, some patients with symptoms of irritation or itching are treated with various medications to eradicate the symptoms. It is vital that a biopsy sample be taken of any vulvar lesion before undertaking therapy, as was emphasized earlier. A biopsy of a tumor such as that shown in Figure 30.12, *A*, can easily be obtained on an outpatient basis using local anesthesia and biopsy forceps such as a Kevorkian punch as illustrated in Chapter 28, Intraepithelial Neoplasia of the Lower Genital Tract.

Effective therapy of clinical stage I or II and early stage III vulvar carcinoma can be accomplished with a wide radical excision and inguinofemoral node dissection. Lesions located more than 2 cm from the midline typically need only an ipsilateral inguinofemoral lymphadenectomy, whereas midline lesions necessitate bilateral groin dissections. Because the deep pelvic nodes are almost never involved unless the inguinal nodes are also involved, only the inguinofemoral nodes are removed at the time of the primary operation and the deep pelvic nodes subsequently treated with external radiation if the superficial nodes are involved with tumor. The inguinofemoral node dissection is performed through separate inguinal incisions followed by the vulvectomy portion. Figure 30.12, *A*, shows the type of specimen that can be obtained through separate groin incisions. The operative incisions are shown in Figure 30.12, *B*. It appears that an adequate surgical dissection with decreased wound complications can be accomplished by this technique. It is advisable to use suction drainage in the inguinal area until all drainage is complete, which usually takes 7 to 10 days, and drains are also frequently used in the vulvar area. It is important that an adequate margin, usually 1 to 2 cm, be obtained around the primary tumor at the time of surgery. Grimshaw and colleagues reported on 100 cases operated on through separate incisions and noted superb results with a corrected 5-year survival rate in stage I of 96.7% and stage II of 85% (Grimshaw, 1993). Similar excellent results for separate skin incisions were reported by Farias-Eisner and associates on 74 patients, with 5-year survival rates of 97% and 90% for stages I and II, respectively (Farias-Eisner, 1994). Tumor recurrence has occurred rarely in the skin bridge over the symphysis when separate groin incisions are used, without an en bloc dissection of the vulva and intervening lymph tissue.

In treating clinical stage I and stage II tumors of the vulva, the results of histologic evaluation of the inguinofemoral nodes are important. Many initially treat the superficial nodes above the cribriform fascia (Fig. 30.16). If these nodes are negative, the deep nodes are spared. The procedure can usually be accomplished with preservation of the saphenous vein, which was traditionally sacrificed. These modifications reduce the risk of leg edema. If the lymph nodes, particularly the upper femoral group, are involved with tumor, the deep pelvic nodes require treatment. Homesley and coworkers reported improved survival for those who received radiation (4500 to 5000 rad) to the deep pelvic nodes in comparison with those who had a pelvic node dissection (Homesley, 1986).

The results of therapy in clinical stages I and II disease relate not only to the stage of the disease but also to the status of the regional pelvic nodes. If the nodes do not contain metastatic tumor and the woman can be successfully treated by radical vulvectomy and bilateral node dissection, 5-year survival rates of approximately 95% have been reported. Iversen and associates, in a series of 424 patients, noted lymph node metastasis in 10.5% of clinical stage I cases, 30% of clinical stage II, 66% of clinical stage III, and 100% of clinical stage IV (Iversen, 1980). The number of positive nodes in the radical vulvectomy specimen correlates with the size of the primary tumor and also with the woman's survival. In a study of T1 and T2 tumors, Andrews and coworkers noted that only unilateral inguinal node metastases occurred and, furthermore, the deep nodes were involved only if the superficial nodes were positive (Andrews, 1994). However, there was a small (2% to 3%) risk of contralateral node involvement of the larger T2 lesions. In a study of 113 patients, Hacker and colleagues noted an actuarial 5-year survival rate of 96% for those with negative nodes, but there was a progressive decrease in the survival rate to 94% for those having one positive node, 80% for two positive nodes, and 12% for three or

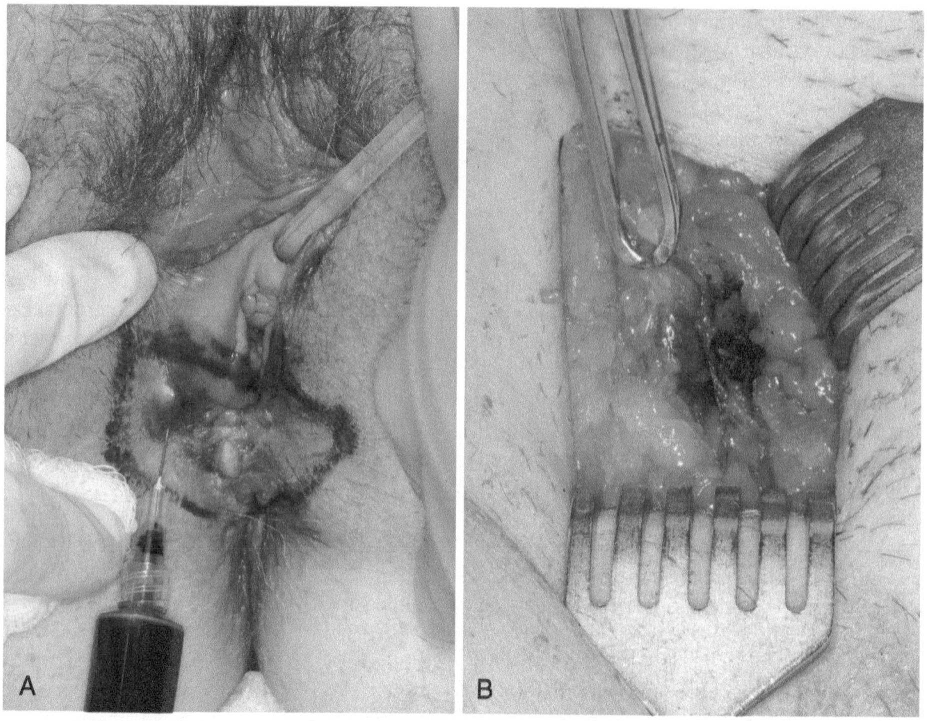


**Figure 30.16** **A** and **B**, Injection of blue dye into vulvar lesion and identification of sentinel node in inguinofemoral triangle.

more positive nodes (Hacker, 1983). In the various cases that have been studied, the deep pelvic nodes do not contain tumor unless the upper inguinofemoral nodes contain metastatic disease. The number of nodes involved and the size of the metastasis are both important. Hoffman and associates noted that 14 of 15 patients with inguinal lymph node metastases smaller than 36 $mm^2$ survived free of disease at 5 years compared with 12 of 29 whose lymph node metastases measured more than 100 $mm^2$ (Hoffman, 1985). These results should be taken into consideration when planning additional therapy for patients with positive nodes.

If tumor spread to the regional inguinofemoral nodes is identified, further treatment should be considered. If only one node is microscopically involved with tumor and the woman has undergone a complete lymph node dissection of the groin, no further therapy is usually needed, particularly if only a small volume is present. However, if one node is microscopically positive and the woman has undergone a superficial inguinofemoral lymph node dissection, many clinicians would be uncomfortable not treating the groin with adjuvant radiation therapy. If three or more nodes are involved, pelvic radiation as outlined is usually prescribed. For patients with only two nodes involved, the decision for further therapy will depend on the location of the nodes, extent of groin dissection performed, and size of the metastatic deposit of tumor, although most clinicians would opt for radiotherapy in such cases.

## ADVANCED VULVAR TUMORS

Large tumors of the vulva, particularly those that encroach on the anal-rectal area or urethra, may require more extensive treatment than radical vulvectomy to achieve effective tumor control. In such cases, it may be necessary to remove the anus or urethra as part of a primary operative procedure, in which case diversion of the urinary or fecal stream is required (see the discussion of exenterative surgery for carcinoma of the cervix in Chapter 29, Malignant Diseases of the Cervix).

For tumors that encroach on the urethra or anus, making procurement of negative margins improbable, multidisciplinary organ-sparing approaches may be used in an effort to reduce the morbidity of exenterative procedures. A useful therapeutic approach has been to treat large vulvar tumors with external radiation and then, after the tumor has been reduced in size, to remove the residual tumor surgically, usually by radical vulvectomy. External radiation is used to deliver approximately 4000 cGy to the tumor and 4500 cGy to the pelvis and inguinal nodes. The operation is usually performed approximately 5 weeks after the completion of radiation therapy. Although a large series of patients have not been treated by this technique, a sufficient number have been treated to demonstrate that marked tumor regression does occur. The primary cancer can be eradicated by a procedure that does not require diversion of the urine or feces. Boronow and associates initially summarized the treatment of 26 patients with primary carcinoma of the vaginal vulvar area with this technique and noted a 5-year survival rate of 80% (Boronow, 1987). Rotmensch and colleagues reported on 16 patients, 13 stage III and 3 stage IV, and achieved an overall 5-year survival rate of 45% with this technique, somewhat better than might be expected with stages III and IV (see Fig. 30.14) (Rotmensch, 1990). Recurrences are more likely if the resection margins were within 1 cm of the tumor.

Chemotherapy with radiation appears to offer a therapeutic advantage. Koh and coworkers studied 20 patients with stages III and IV disease and 3 with recurrence, using 5-FU with radiation (Koh, 1993). In addition, some patients also received cisplatin with concurrent radiotherapy. Actuarial 3- and 5-year survival rates in this small group were 59% and 49%, respectively. Similar results with 5-FU and radiation, occasionally with the addition of cisplatin, were also reported by Russell and associates in 25 patients (Russell, 1992). Moore and colleagues reported on a phase II GOG study and noted the need for a less extensive operation when chemotherapy with cisplatin and 5-FU were combined with preoperative radiation (Moore, 1998). Multiple chemoradiation programs are available, but a convenient outpatient regimen consists of weekly intravenous (IV) cisplatin with radiation, usually to 4500 cGy. Other complications reported include stenosis of the introitus, urethral stenosis, and rectovaginal fistula, but this technique is an effective alternative to primary exenteration for large vulvar vaginal carcinomas and is preferred in most treatment centers, although success with exenteration can occasionally be achieved.

### *Radiation Therapy and Recurrences*

In a few cases, the medical condition of the woman precludes surgery, and radiation therapy may be used as the sole treatment. However, the vulvar skin is prone to radiation dermatitis, fibrosis, and ulceration, making irradiation as the sole form of therapy a less desirable treatment. Therefore irradiation is seldom used as the sole treatment of carcinoma of the vulva. To manage recurrences, reoperation is often tried. Piura and colleagues analyzed 73 patients whose disease recurred only on the vulva (Piura, 1993). Salvage was achieved with wide radical local excision, which appeared to be successful in 30 patients in whom the recurrence was only on the vulva.

As may be expected, the risk of recurring carcinoma rises as the stage of the disease increases. In an analysis of 224 patients with vulvar carcinoma, Podratz and associates noted a recurrence rate of 14% in stage I and 71% in stage IV (Podratz, 1983) Local vulvar recurrences were the most common and occurred in 40 of 74 cases of recurrence (54%). The remaining recurrences were in the groin, pelvis, or distant sites. Radiation therapy or additional operations for local vulvar recurrences usually provide effective control and yield 5-year survival rates of approximately 50%. The risk of recurrence of the disease in the vulva requires careful attention to the surgical resection margins at the time of initial operation.

Combined chemotherapy and radiation has been used for primary treatment of late-stage advanced vulvar tumors, as noted. It has also been applied to recurrences, especially those near the anus or urethra. Radiation alone may also be used for vulvar recurrences, although chemoradiation would appear to be a more effective choice.

Treatment of patients with disseminated disease requires chemotherapy but, unfortunately, no chemotherapeutic regimen has been successful for treatment of this disease. Squamous cell carcinomas of the female genital tract have generally not been responsive to cytotoxic chemotherapy; the protocols followed are similar to those described for recurrent squamous cell carcinomas of the cervix (see Chapter 29).

### *Quality of Life and Vulvar Carcinoma*

There have been few studies regarding quality of life in patients with vulvar cancer. Body image disturbance is significant and may account for decreased or absent sexual activity in women who have undergone vulvectomy. Interestingly, Green and colleagues noted that the extent of surgery or type of vulvectomy performed does not correlate well with the degree of sexual dysfunction (Green, 2000). They demonstrated a significant need to address sexual problems with all women undergoing any type of vulvectomy. The Functional Assessment of Cancer Therapy–Vulvar (FACT-V) is a valid and reliable instrument to assess quality of life in women with vulvar cancer. Perhaps this tool can be used to help assess quality of life and also facilitate vital communication about quality-of-life issues in women with this disease.

### *Lymphatic Mapping and Sentinel Lymph Node Biopsy*

As noted, regional lymph node dissections are routinely performed in the surgical treatment of vulvar cancer because the status of regional lymph nodes is essential for therapeutic planning and overall prognosis. More than 80% of women with clinical stages I and II disease, however, will have no metastatic disease found in the lymph nodes, therefore making an extensive lymphadenectomy unnecessary while increasing postoperative morbidities, such as lymphedema and lymphocyst formation. Lymphatic mapping and sentinel lymph node biopsy, as used for the treatment of patients with melanoma and breast cancer, are appealing techniques for patients with vulvar cancer. The sentinel nodes are those that directly drain the primary tumor and are thought to predict the metastatic status of the upper echelon or nonsentinel nodes in the groin. If the sentinel node is negative, in theory, all the other groin nodes would also be negative and surgeons could abandon full groin dissections, thereby greatly reducing the associated morbidities of lymphocyst, lymphedema, and wound separation (see Fig. 30.16).

Van der Zee and colleagues performed a prospective observational study in 403 women with clinical stage I squamous cell carcinoma of the vulva smaller than 4 cm (GROningen INternational Study on Sentinal nodes in Vulvar cancer [GROINSS-V]) (Van der Zee, 2008). Women enrolled in this study underwent a sentinel node biopsy, with omission of complete inguinofemoral lymphadenectomy if no metastatic disease was found. Patients with negative sentinel nodes were triaged to no further therapy and observed for recurrence. With a median follow-up of 35 months, only six groin recurrences (2.3%) have been noted in patients without multifocal disease. In a validation study, Levenback and colleagues set out to determine the true sensitivity and negative predictive value of the sentinel node technique in 453 women with vulvar cancer (GOG 173) (Levenback, 2012). In contrast to GROINSS-V, all women in GOG 173 underwent a sentinel node biopsy followed by a complete inguinofemoral lymphadenectomy. They found a sensitivity of 90.1% and a negative predictive value of 95.7%. Therefore if the sentinel node was negative, there was only a 4.3% chance that disease was present in that groin (false negative predictive value). In an accumulation of data from smaller studies on the subject, Frumovitz and colleagues reviewed the combined data on 279 patients with vulvar cancer who had undergone lymphatic mapping and sentinel lymph node identification (Frumovitz, 2008). They found the overall sensitivity of the sentinel node for detecting metastatic disease in patients with vulvar cancer to be 97.7% and the false-negative rate for the procedure to be 2.3%. The overall negative predictive value was 99.3%. Although these numbers are promising, at this time, lymphatic mapping and sentinel lymph node biopsy are considered experimental, with the standard of care remaining full inguinofemoral node dissection.

## *OTHER VULVAR MALIGNANCIES*

### *Bartholin Gland Carcinoma*

Bartholin gland carcinomas are adenocarcinomas that constitute approximately 1% to 2% of vulvar carcinomas. An enlargement of Bartholin gland in a postmenopausal woman should raise suspicion for this malignancy. These tumors are treated similarly to primary squamous cell carcinoma of the vulva; radical vulvectomy with bilateral inguinofemoral lymphadenectomy is the treatment of choice. If the regional lymph nodes are free of tumor, the prognosis is good.

### *Basal Cell Carcinoma*

Basal cell carcinoma can arise in the vulva, as it can arise in the skin elsewhere in the body. It is rare and comprises approximately 2% of vulvar carcinomas. Therapy consists of wide local excision of the lesion, which is generally ulcerated. If the surgical resection margins are free of tumor, the disease is cured.

### *Verrucous Carcinoma*

Verrucous carcinomas of the vulva are also rare. They are a special variant of squamous cell cancer, with distinctive histologic features. Clinically, they appear as a large condylomatous mass on the vulva. Histologically, they consist of mature squamous cells and extensive keratinization, with nests that invade the underlying vulvar tissue. It is often necessary to perform multiple biopsies of the condylomatous lesion to establish a diagnosis of malignancy. Radiation therapy is ineffective and can worsen the prognosis by causing anaplastic changes in the tumor and is therefore contraindicated. The treatment of an authentic verrucous carcinoma is wide excision.

In 24 cases of verrucous carcinoma, Japaze and coworkers noted no lymph node metastases (Japaze, 1982). Some of the primary tumors were as large as 10 cm in diameter. Recurrences developed in nine patients, five of whom had previous radiation therapy. Wide local excision is effective therapy. Depending on the size and location of the tumor, simple vulvectomy may be needed, but a radical vulvectomy or inguinal node dissection is not indicated. The 17 patients treated surgically and reported by Japaze and colleagues had a 5-year survival rate of 94%. It is important to take a large biopsy specimen to establish the diagnosis. This is particularly important when dealing with a malignant-appearing tumor from a biopsy specimen that has been reported as benign, which can lead to incorrect therapy for condyloma acuminatum. Conversely, too shallow a biopsy may fail to show areas of squamous cell carcinoma that can coexist with verrucous carcinoma, but in the presence of areas of squamous cell carcinoma, local excision is inadequate therapy. Verrucous tumors with squamous cell carcinoma elements can metastasize to regional nodes; these tumors should not be treated as true verrucous carcinomas.

### *Melanoma*

Melanoma is the most frequent nonsquamous cell malignancy of the vulva. It comprises approximately 5% of primary cancers of this area. As is true elsewhere in the body, melanomas arise from junctional or compound nevi. Pigmented lesions of the vulva are usually junctional nevi and all such lesions should be removed by excision.

Patients with malignant melanoma of the vulva vary widely in age, from the late teens to women in their 80s. The average age is approximately 50 years. Clinically, melanomas appear as brown, black, or blue-black masses on the vulva. The lesion can be flat or ulcerated; occasionally, it is nodular, and small, darkly pigmented areas (satellite nodules) may surround the primary lesion. Some melanomas may be without pigment and can grossly resemble squamous cell carcinoma of the vulva. Most melanomas of the vulva occur on the labia minora or the clitoris (Fig. 30.17).

Vulvar melanomas, if staged, use the same FIGO classification used for squamous carcinomas. However, staging is not as useful a prognostic indicator as is the depth of invasion. A staging system for vulvar melanoma analogous to that used by Clark for cutaneous melanomas has been adopted. Five levels (I to V) have been defined based on the Clark classification. Figure 30.18 shows the depth of invasion for each level of superficial

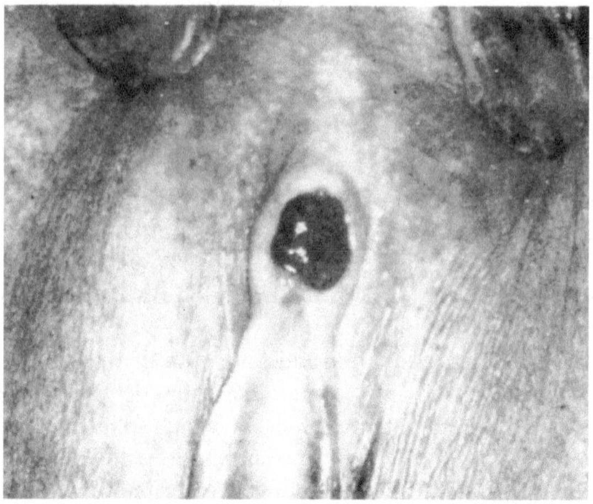

**Figure 30.17** Nodular melanoma arising directly from glans clitoris. (Courtesy of Dr. J.M. Morris [deceased], Yale University School of Medicine, New Haven, CT.)

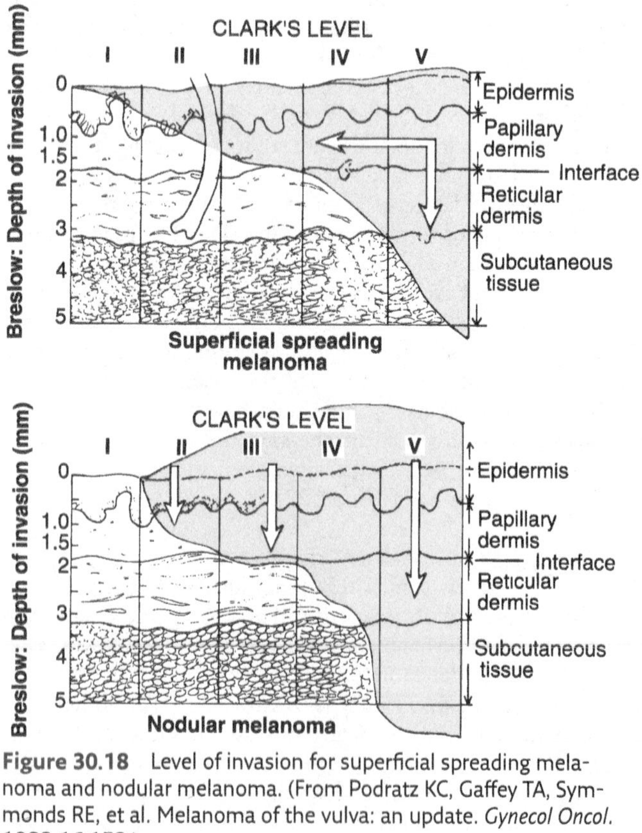


**Figure 30.18** Level of invasion for superficial spreading melanoma and nodular melanoma. (From Podratz KC, Gaffey TA, Symmonds RE, et al. Melanoma of the vulva: an update. *Gynecol Oncol.* 1983;16:153.)

spreading melanoma and nodular melanoma, the two most common varieties of melanomas that occur on the vulva. Superficial spreading melanoma is more common and, fortunately, has a better prognosis, with a 5-year survival rate of 71% reported in the series by Podratz and associates (Podratz, 1983). The 5-year survival for nodular melanoma, which is more invasive, was only 38%. The level of invasion correlates with survival, which varies from 100% for level II, to 83% for level IV, to 28% for level V.

Tumor thickness is also useful to evaluate the tumor. Breslow has reported that overall prognosis is excellent, and spread to a regional node is not likely for melanomas whose thickness is less than 0.76 mm, measured from the surface epithelium to the deepest point of penetration (Breslow, 1970). Most of these lesions would correspond to level I or II penetration by the modified Clark system. Stefanon and coworkers, in a study of 28 patients, noted no lymph node metastasis if melanoma thickness was less than 3 mm; the 5-year survival rate in this group was 50% compared with 25% for those whose melanomas were more than 3 mm thick (Stefanon, 1987). In a comprehensive long-term study of 219 Swedish women, Ragnarsson-Olding and coworkers noted that tumor thickness and ulceration are prognostic factors (Ragnarsson-Olding, 1999). In addition, gross amelanosis and advanced age worsened the prognosis. They further noted that amelanotic tumors were seen in approximately 25% of patients and that overall the vulvar melanomas were approximately 2.5 times more frequent than cutaneous melanomas. A preexisting nevus was not necessary; de novo melanoma development does appear to occur on the vulva, particularly in the glabrous (hairless) skin.

The standard therapy for vulvar melanoma is a wide excision of the primary tumor. Because the tumors are rare, a large clinical experience is not available. It was believed that melanoma of the vulva could metastasize to pelvic nodes, bypassing the inguinofemoral nodes, but it is now thought that there is no pelvic node involvement without previous inguinal node involvement. A further therapeutic consideration is that patients with melanoma whose pelvic nodes are involved with tumor usually do not survive the disease.

Excision margins have been extensively studied for cutaneous melanomas. Veronesi and colleagues found that cutaneous melanomas less than 2 mm thick could be adequately treated with a 1-cm margin, which was as effective as a 3-cm margin for these thin lesions (Veronesi, 1988). Although comparable data do not exist for vulvar melanomas, evidence from studies of cutaneous melanomas has suggested that a 1-cm margin may be used for very thin vulvar melanomas. In a report of 36 melanoma cases, Rose and associates noted that wide excision was as effective as radical vulvectomy (Rose, 1988). They found that the prognosis was improved in younger patients, presumably because most of them had superficial spreading (good prognosis) rather than nodular (poor prognosis) melanomas. Although firm recommendations from available data are not possible, a reasonable approach would be to excise a melanoma with a 2-cm margin without node dissection for tumors that are smaller than 0.76 mm thick. An excision with a 2- to 3-cm margin combined with node dissection would be carried out for more advanced melanomas.

For lesions that correspond to Clark's level 1 or 2—that is, less than 0.76 mm thick—a wide local excision results in 5-year survival rates of approximately 100%. The prognosis is poor for patients with melanomas more than 3 mm thick. If the regional nodes are negative, the survival rate is greater than 60% but decreases to less than 30% if the regional nodes are involved with tumor. Most series of malignant melanoma have reported overall survival rates of approximately 50%. Although metastases of melanoma to regional inguinal nodes are usually fatal, isolated prolonged survivals have been observed.

Distant metastases are frequently noted, and no effective program of chemotherapy has been described. Regressions (but not cures) have been reported with various multiagent cytotoxic programs. Current efforts are devoted to developing an effective program of bioimmunotherapy.

### *Sarcoma*

Sarcomas of the vulva are extremely rare, accounting for less than 3% of vulvar cancers. Leiomyosarcomas are the most common histologic subtype found, followed by liposarcomas, neurofibrosarcomas, angiosarcomas, and epithelioid sarcomas. Surgical removal of the primary tumor is the treatment of choice. Chemotherapeutic considerations are the same as those for sarcomas of other sites in the female genital tract.

### *Granular Cell Myoblastomas*

Granular cell myoblastoma is also an extremely rare tumor that is almost invariably benign but morphologically shows pleomorphism. Local excision is generally sufficient therapy. The tumor appears as a solitary, firm, nontender, slowly growing nodule in the subcutaneous tissue of the vulva.

## *KEY POINTS*

- Squamous cell carcinomas constitute 90% of primary vulvar malignancies. More than 80% of patients are older than 50 years at the time of diagnosis.
- Cancer of the vulva accounts for approximately 4% of malignancies of the lower female genital tract and occurs less frequently than uterine, ovarian, and cervical cancers.
- Paget disease generally occurs in postmenopausal women and is usually treated by wide excision. Invasive carcinomas at other sites should be ruled out.
- Prolonged use of fluorinated corticosteroids to treat itching accompanying vulvar dystrophy can lead to vulvar contraction.
- Topical testosterone is sometimes beneficial to treat lichen sclerosus but is absorbed systemically and occasionally can produce masculinizing symptoms.
- Studies have indicated that symptomatic lichen sclerosus is a premalignant condition preceding carcinoma by a mean of 4 years. The tumors that develop tend to be clitoral in location and identified in patients older than age 40 years.
- HPV vulvar infection is common. Intraepithelial neoplasia occurs much less frequently.
- HPV-positive tumors tend to occur in younger patients, and these tumors tend to have a better prognosis than HPV-negative tumors.

*Continued*

## KEY POINTS—cont'd

- A clear progression of dysplasia–carcinoma in situ (VIN I, II, and III) to invasive carcinoma in the vulva has not been clearly established. VIN may spontaneously regress. VIN III has an approximately 3.4% risk of progression to invasive carcinoma.
- Intraepithelial neoplasia of the vulva is usually treated by local excision. Laser therapy of the atypical area may be used for younger patients who do not have raised lesions.
- Vulvar carcinomas less than 2 cm in diameter and depth of invasion less than 1 mm (3-mm thickness) rarely metastasize to regional nodes.
- Unilateral vulvar tumors (>2 cm from midline) usually metastasize to ipsilateral inguinofemoral nodes only.
- Prognosis in vulvar cancer is primarily related to lesion size, lymph node status, and stage.
- The risk of lymph node groin metastases is related to tumor differentiation, lesion thickness, lymphovascular space involvement, patient age, and tumor size.
- The deep pelvic nodes do not become involved with metastatic vulvar cancer unless the inguinofemoral nodes are affected.
- The 5-year survival rate of vulvar carcinoma with negative nodes is more than 95%. With one positive node, the 5-year survival is approximately the same, 94%; with two nodes, it decreases to 80% and with three or more to 12%.
- Advanced vulvar tumors encroaching on the urethra or anus may be treated by radiation followed by wide radical excision rather than exenteration. Enhanced results have also been reported with the combined use of chemotherapy and radiation.
- Verrucous carcinomas are a variant of squamous cancer that do not metastasize to regional nodes. Radiation therapy is contraindicated, and local surgical excision is the treatment of choice.
- Melanomas constitute 5% of vulvar cancers and are the most frequent nonsquamous cell malignancies.
- The overall 5-year survival of patients with vulvar melanoma is approximately 50%.
- Superficial spreading melanomas tend to occur in younger patients and have a better prognosis than nodular melanomas.
- Prognosis of vulvar melanoma is related to tumor invasion (Clark's level) and to tumor thickness.
- Basal cell carcinoma of the vulva is treated by wide local excision.

## KEY REFERENCES


Andrews SJ, Williams BT, DePriest PD, et al. Therapeutic implications of lymph nodal spread in lateral T1 and T2 squamous cell carcinoma of the vulva. *Gynecol Oncol.* 1994;55:41.

Bergen S, DiSaia PJ, Liao SY, et al. Conservative management of extramammary Paget's disease of the vulva. *Gynecol Oncol.* 1989;33:151.

Beutner KR, Reitano MV, Richwald GA, et al. External genital warts: report of the American Medical Association consensus conference. *Clin Infect Dis.* 1998;27:796.

Boronow RC, Hickman BT, Reagan MT, et al. Combined therapy as an alternative to exenteration for locally advanced vulvovaginal cancer. *Am J Clin Oncol.* 1987;10:1711.

Breslow A. Thickness, cross-sectional areas, and depth of invasion in the prognosis of cutaneous melanoma. *Ann Surg.* 1970;172:908.

Buscema J, Woodruff JD, Parmley TH, et al. Carcinoma in situ of the vulva. *Obstet Gynecol.* 1980;55:225.

Carlson JA, Ambros R, Malfetano J, et al. Vulvar lichen sclerosus and squamous cell carcinoma: A cohort, case control, and investigational study with historical perspective; implications for chronic inflammation and sclerosus in the development of neoplasia. *Hum Pathol.* 1998;29:932.

Carter J, Carlson J, Fowler J, et al. Invasive vulvar tumors in young women—a disease of the immunosuppressed? *Gynecol Oncol.* 1993;51:307.

Chafe W, Richards A, Morgan L, et al. Unrecognized invasive carcinoma in vulvar intraepithelial neoplasia (VIN). *Gynecol Oncol.* 1988;31:154.

Chaturvedi AK, Madeleine MM, Biggar RJ, et al. Risk of human papillomavirus-associated cancers among persons with AIDS. *J Natl Cancer Inst.* 2009;101:1120.

Crum CP. Vulvar intraepithelial neoplasia: histology and associated viral changes. In: Wilkinson EJ, ed. *Pathology of the Vulva and Vagina.* New York: Churchill Livingstone; 1987.

Dvoretsky PM, Bonfiglio TA, Helkamp BF, et al. The pathology of superficially invasive thin vulva squamous cell carcinoma. *Int J Gynecol Pathol.* 1984;3:331.

Fanning J, Lambert HC, Hale TM, Morris PC, Schuerch C. Paget's disease of the vulva: prevalence of associated vulvar adenocarcinoma, invasive Paget's disease, and recurrence after surgical excision. *Am J Obstet Gynecol.* 1999;180(1 Pt 1):24–27.

Farias-Eisner R, Cirisano FD, Grouse D, et al. Conservative and individualized surgery for early squamous carcinoma of the vulva: the treatment of choice for stage I and II (T1-2 N0-1 M0) disease. *Gynecol Oncol.* 1994;53:55.

Fishman DA, Chambers SK, Schwartz PE, et al. Extramammary Paget's disease of the vulva. *Gynecol Oncol.* 1995;56:266.

Friedrich Jr EG. Reversible vulvar atypia: a case report. *Obstet Gynecol.* 1972;39:173.

Friedrich EG, Wilkinson EJ, Fu YS. Carcinoma in situ of the vulva: a continuing challenge. *Am J Obstet Gynecol.* 1980;136:830.

Frumovitz M, Levenback CF. Lymphatic mapping and sentinel node biopsy in vulvar, vaginal, and cervical cancers. *Oncology (Williston Park).* 2008;22(5):529–536.

Fu YS, Reagan JW, Townsend DE, et al. Nuclear DNA study of vulvar intraepithetial and invasive squamous neoplasms. *Obstet Gynecol.* 1981;57:643.

Funaro D, Lovett A, Leroux N, Powell J. A double-blind, randomized prospective study evaluating topical clobetasol propionate 0.05% versus topical tacrolimus 0.1% in patients with vulvar lichen sclerosus. *J Am Acad Dermatol.* 2014;71(1):84–91.

Goldstein AT, Creasey A, Pfau R, Phillips D, Burrows LJ. A double-blind, randomized controlled trial of clobetasol versus pimecrolimus in patients with vulvar lichen sclerosus. *J Am Acad Dermatol.* 2011;64(6):e99–e104.

Green MS, Naumann RW, Elliot M, et al. Sexual dysfunction following vulvectomy. *Gynecol Oncol.* 2000;77:73.

Grimshaw RN, Murdoch JB, Monaghan JM. Radical vulvectomy and bilateral inguinal-femoral lymphadenectomy through separate incisions: experience with 100 cases. *Int J Gynecol Cancer.* 1993;3:18.

Hacker NF, Berek JS, Lagasse LD, et al. Management of regional lymph nodes and their prognostic influence in vulvar cancer. *Obstet Gynecol.* 1983;61:408.

Hart WR, Norris HJ, Helwig ED. Relation of lichen sclerosus et atrophicus of the vulva to development of carcinoma. *Obstet Gynecol.* 1975;45:369.

Hoffman JS, Kumar NB, Morley GW: Prognostic significance of groin lymph node metastases of squamous carcin

Rotmensch J, Rubin SJ, Sutton HG, et al. Preoperative radiotherapy followed by radical vulvectomy with inguinal lymphadenectomy for advanced vulvar cancer. *Gynecol Oncol.* 1990;36:181.

Rowley KC, Gallion HH, Donaldson ES, van Nagell JR, Higgins RV, Powell DE, Kryscio RJ, Pavlik EJ. Prognostic factors in early vulvar cancer. *Gynecol Oncol.* 1988;31(1):43–49.

Russell AH, Mesic JB, Scudder SA, et al. Synchronous radiation and cytotoxic chemotherapy for locally advanced or recurrent squamous cancer of the vulva. *Gynecol Oncol.* 1992;47:14.

Rutledge F, Sinclair M. Treatment of intraepithelial carcinoma of the vulva by skin excision and graft. *Am J Obstet Gynecol.* 1968;102:807.

Saraiya M, Unger ER, Thompson TD, Lynch CF, Hernandez BY, Lyu CW. US assessment of HPV types in cancers: implications for current and 9-valent HPV vaccines. *J Natl Cancer Inst.* 2015;107(6). djv086.

Stefanon B, Clemente C, Lupi G, et al. Malignant melanoma of the vulva: a clinicopathologic study of 28 cases. *Cervix IFGT.* 1987;5:223.

Van der Velden J, Kooyman CD, Van Lindert ACM, et al. A stage Ia vulvar carcinoma with an inguinal lymph node recurrence after local excision: a case report and literature review. *Int J Gynecol Cancer.* 1992;2:157.

Van der Zee AG, Oonk MH, De Hullu JA, et al. Sentinel node dissection is safe in the treatment of early-stage vulvar cancer. *J Clin Oncol.* 2008;26(6):884–889.

van Seters M, van Beurden M, ten Kate FJ, et al. Treatment of vulvar intraepithelial neoplasia with topical imiquimod. *N Engl J Med.* 2008;358(14):1465–1473.

Veronesi V, Cascinelli N, Adams J, et al. Thin stage I primary cutaneous malignant melanomas: comparison of excision with margins of 1 or 3 cm. *N Engl J Med.* 1988;318:1159.

Woodruff JD, Genadry R, Poliakoff S. Treatment of dyspareunia and vaginal outlet distortions by perineoplasty. *Obstet Gynecol.* 1981;57:750.

Yoder BJ, Rufforny I, Massoll NA, Wilkinson EJ. Stage IA vulvar squamous cell carcinoma: an analysis of tumor invasive characteristics and risk. *Am J Surg Pathol.* 2008;32(5):765–772.

# 31

# Malignant Diseases of the Vagina

## Intraepithelial Neoplasia, Carcinoma, Sarcoma

*Diane C. Bodurka, Michael Frumovitz*

This chapter focuses on premalignant and malignant diseases of the vagina. Premalignant changes in the vagina occur less frequently than comparable lesions in the cervix and vulva. However, the histologic appearance of intraepithelial neoplasia of the vagina is similar to that described for the cervix (see Chapter 28). These changes are also similarly designated as dysplasia (mild, moderate, or severe) and carcinoma in situ. The term *VAIN* (***va****gaginal* ***i****ntraepithelial* ***n****eoplasia*) has been used to describe these histologic changes; the comparable categories are VAIN-1 (mild dysplasia), VAIN-2 (moderate dysplasia), and VAIN-3 (severe dysplasia to carcinoma in situ). VAIN-1 is classified as a low-grade squamous intraepithelial lesion, whereas VAIN-2 and VAIN-3 are grouped as high-grade squamous intraepithelial lesions (Audet-Lapointe, 1990). The cytologic and histologic features of these changes are illustrated in Figure 31.1.

VAIN occurs more commonly in patients previously treated for cervical intraepithelial neoplasia. The frequency of vaginal premalignancy in these patients is approximately 1% to 3%. Similarly, there is an increased risk of VAIN in those previously treated for squamous cell neoplasia of the vulva. The tendency to develop premalignant changes in the lower genital tract is known as a *field defect* and denotes the increased risk of squamous cell neoplasia arising anywhere in the lower genital tract in such individuals. Most VAIN cases are related to infection with human papillomavirus (HPV). Additional risk factors include HIV infection, cigarette smoking, previous radiation therapy of the genital tract, and immunosuppressive therapy. In situ and invasive vaginal neoplasias have many of the same risk factors as cervical cancer, including a strong association with HPV infection. Women who have previously been treated for anogenital cancer, particularly for cervical cancer, have a high relative risk of being diagnosed with vaginal cancer (Shrivastava, 2015).

Primary cancer of the vagina is rare and constitutes less than 2% of gynecologic malignancies. Most vaginal malignancies are metastatic, primarily from the cervix and endometrium. Less commonly, ovarian and rectosigmoid carcinomas, as well as choriocarcinoma, metastasize to the vagina. The most common histologic type of primary vaginal cancer is squamous cell carcinoma, which is usually seen in women older than 60 years. Other types of carcinoma, including melanomas and adenocarcinomas, occur less commonly. Malignant transformation of endometriosis has been described in the vagina and rectovaginal septum. Clear cell adenocarcinoma, historically associated with young women exposed in utero to diethylstilbestrol (DES), may also occur in unexposed women. Primary vaginal sarcomas are rare and are usually a disease of children. Table 31.1 summarizes the major primary malignancies of the vagina arranged according to age at occurrence.

## PREMALIGNANT DISEASE OF THE VAGINA

### *DETECTION AND DIAGNOSIS*

Because premalignant disease of the vagina is generally asymptomatic, detection depends primarily on cytologic screening (see Fig. 31.1, *B* and *D*). Usually, the changes will be observed in patients who have undergone previous therapy for intraepithelial disease of the cervix. This fact underscores the importance of continued examinations and Pap smears for women, even after hysterectomy for dysplastic conditions. VAIN usually occurs in the upper half of the vagina or along the vaginal cuff suture line. Once an abnormal smear from vaginal epithelium is identified, a biopsy is required for histologic identification (see Fig. 31.1, *A* and *C*). A colposcopic examination is usually performed to identify the areas requiring biopsy. As in the case of cervical neoplasia, a repeat Pap smear is often taken before the colposcopic examination. Vaginal colposcopic techniques are similar to those described for the cervix. A large speculum is used to aid in visualizing the entire vaginal wall. Although the abnormal colposcopic findings resemble those of the cervix (see Chapter 28), full visualization of the entire vaginal wall is often difficult and time consuming. A useful adjunct to colposcopy for identifying an area in which to perform a biopsy is to stain the vaginal epithelium with Lugol's solution and to take a biopsy sample from the nonstaining areas. The vaginal epithelium must be adequately estrogenized so that sufficient epithelial glycogen is present for the normal tissue to stain dark brown. The more rapidly dividing dysplastic epithelium uses up its glycogen and thus does not pick up the iodine stain. Vaginal estrogen cream used for 1 to 2 weeks before examination is helpful for evaluating postmenopausal women and those with atrophic vaginitis who present with cytologic atypia. The estrogen cream will not only increase epithelial glycogen but also helps mature the squamous epithelium, reducing the number of parabasal cells at the surface. Parabasal cells,

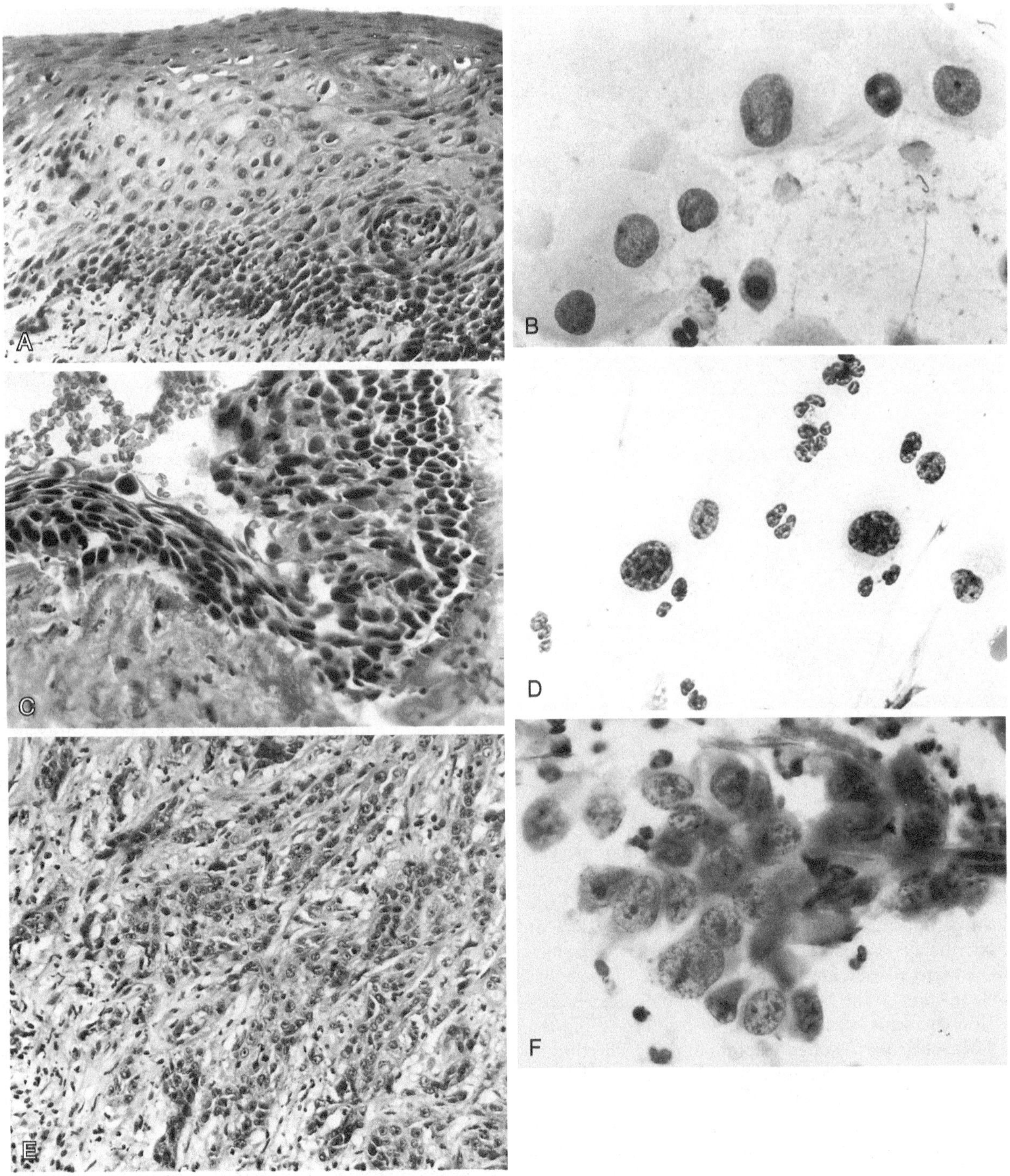


**Figure 31.1** **A,** Section of a vagina showing dysplasia. The epithelium appears thickened and shows abnormal maturation. Immature hyperchromatic cells occupy the lower two to four layers. The middle and upper thirds of mucosa show evidence of cytoplasmic differentiation with well-defined cellular borders. Nuclei in these areas are enlarged and pleomorphic. Parakeratosis is apparent on the surface. Because immature cells are confined to the lower third of the mucosa, dysplasia is classified as mild (hematoxylin and eosin [H&E] stain, × 250). **B,** Cytologic specimen showing mild dysplasia. Note the sheet of dysplastic cells. Cells show well-defined cytoplasmic borders. Nuclei are enlarged, and the nuclear contour is smooth. Chromatin is uniformly and finely granular. Focal condensations of chromatin (chromocenters) are present in some nuclei. Nucleoli are not present (Pap stain, × 1000). **C,** Section showing severe dysplasia to carcinoma in situ. The entire epithelial thickness is occupied by hyperchromatic dysplastic cells. Marked nuclear variation and mitoses are seen. Because of occasional cells with squamous differentiation (spindle-shaped cells, cells with well-defined cytoplasmic borders) in superficial layers, this lesion is sometimes classified as severe dysplasia. In carcinoma in situ, immature cells replace the full thickness, and there is no evidence of squamous differentiation on the surface (H&E stain, × 400). **D,** Cytologic specimen showing carcinoma in situ. Several isolated immature cells with a high nuclei-to-cytoplasm ratio and poorly defined cytoplasmic borders can be seen. Chromatin is coarsely granular, and no nucleoli are present. In the background are several polymorphonuclear leukocytes and strings of mucus (Pap stain, × 1000). **E,** Section showing invasive squamous carcinoma. Cords and sheets of poorly differentiated tumor cells infiltrate the stroma. Nuclei are pleomorphic and nucleoli are distinct. The mitotic rate is high. Squamous differentiation (keratin pearl formation, single-cell keratinization) was present in other areas of tumor (H&E stain, × 200). **F,** Cytologic specimen showing invasive squamous cell carcinoma. Note aggregate of tumor cells. Cellular boundaries are poorly defined, and nuclear orientation is lacking. Chromatin is irregularly distributed and has areas of clumping and clearing. Note nucleoli in some cells, which were absent in cells of patients with dysplasia and carcinoma in situ (Pap stain, × 800).

Table 31.1 Common Primary Vaginal Cancers

| Tumor Type | Predominant Age (Years) | Clinical Correlations |
|---|---|---|
| Endodermal sinus tumor (adenocarcinoma) | <2 | Extremely rare, α-fetoprotein secretion, often fatal, multimodality therapy |
| Sarcoma botryoides | <8 | Aggressive malignancy, multimodality therapy |
| Clear cell adenocarcinoma | >14 | Associated with intrauterine exposure to diethylstilbestrol |
| Melanoma | >50 | Very rare, poor survival |
| Squamous cell carcinoma | >50 | Most common primary vaginal cancer |

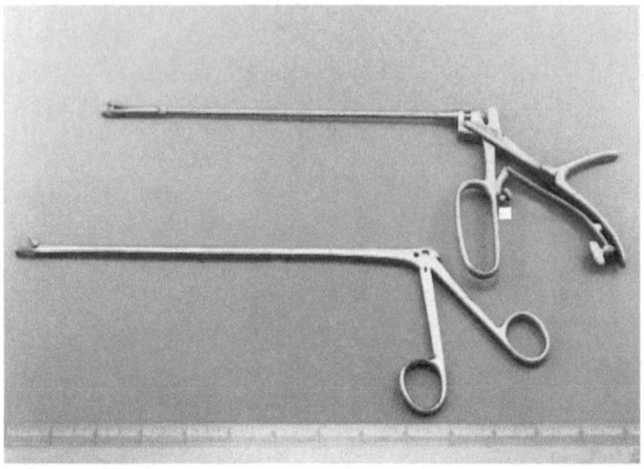

**Figure 31.2** Eppendorf *(upper)* and Kevorkian *(lower)* punch biopsy instruments.

with their large nuclei, are a common cause of false-positive Pap tests in this age group.

A biopsy is performed with small instruments, such as the Kevorkian or Eppendorf punch biopsy forceps (Fig. 31.2) or similar instruments that are also used for the cervix. Occasionally, it is necessary to use a fine instrument, such as a nerve hook, to provide traction on the vaginal epithelium to obtain a biopsy sample. Most patients experience some discomfort during the biopsy. Local anesthesia is often helpful, although injection of the anesthetic may be as uncomfortable as the biopsy itself. Vaginal neoplasia is often multifocal. Although the process is most often located in the vaginal apex, it can occur anywhere along the vaginal canal, necessitating examination of the vagina in its entirety (Jentschke, 2015).

## TREATMENT

There is limited information regarding the natural history of VAIN. The risk of progression to invasive cancer is thought to be low, approximately 9%. Those at highest risk of progression are women with high-risk strains of HPV, those with VAIN-3, cigarette smokers, and immunocompromised women (Gadducci, 2015). Significantly, Aho and colleagues have found that 28% of women undergoing evaluation for VAIN-3 have an underlying invasive carcinoma (Aho, 1991). This has led many to recommend surgical excision rather than destructive procedures for the treatment of VAIN-3.

The principles of managing VAIN are to rule out and prevent invasive disease and preserve vaginal function. As is true for cervical dysplasia, biopsy-proved VAIN-1, particularly those lesions associated with low-risk strains of HPV, can be observed, provided that the woman is compliant with follow-up. VAIN-2 and VAIN-3 are generally treated. Treatment options include $CO_2$ laser vaporization, topical 5-fluorouracil (5-FU) cream, and wide local excision. The choice of treatment depends largely upon the number of lesions, their location, and the level of concern for possible invasion. Radiation therapy, previously used to treat VAIN-2 and VAIN-3, often leads to scarring and fibrosis and is generally not recommended for the treatment of noninvasive disease. Because of the proximity of the bladder and rectum, cryotherapy is generally not used.

The main advantage of the $CO_2$ laser is that it vaporizes the abnormal tissue without shortening or narrowing the vagina, thereby preserving vaginal function. Criteria for $CO_2$ laser vaporization include a lesion that is discrete and easily visible and proof that invasive cancer has been ruled out. The beam is directed colposcopically. Iodine staining of the vagina can help outline those areas requiring therapy. Treatment is occasionally performed on an outpatient basis with a local anesthetic and an analgesic. More frequently, general or regional anesthesia is required. The intensity of therapy is regulated by adjusting the wattage of the laser, most commonly 15 to 20 W carried to a depth of 1.5 to 2 mm. Care must be taken not to apply the laser too deeply because of the proximity of the bladder and bowel, particularly in older women whose vaginal epithelium may be quite thin. The woman will experience a discharge for 1 to 2 weeks after therapy. Healing usually requires a few weeks. The success rates of laser in treating VAIN vary in the literature but are generally in the range of 60% to 85% (Petrilli, 1980). Regular follow-up every 4 months, including a Pap smear and colposcopy, is required during the first year and usually 6 to 12 months thereafter. The primary disadvantages of laser treatment are the lack of a pathologic specimen for evaluation of the adequacy of margins and the fact that the procedure can be tedious and difficult because of the many folds and crevices at the vaginal apex. It is often difficult to obtain a uniform depth of destruction in these areas (Piovano, 2015).

Topical chemotherapy, 5% 5-FU cream, can be self-administered to cover the entire area at risk. It is most often used for widespread multifocal lesions of HPV-associated VAIN-1 or VAIN-2. Half of a vaginal applicator (approximately 5 g) is inserted into the vagina at bedtime for 7 days. Because the cream is irritating, protective ointment such as zinc oxide should be applied to the vulva. If excess leakage occurs, less than half of an applicator should be used. In addition, the treatment should be discontinued before the 7-day course is completed if the woman notes excessive irritation. A cycle of therapy should be repeated in 3 to 4 weeks if intraepithelial neoplasia persists. In some cases, the application of 5-FU is continued for 10 to 14 days, in which case the nontherapy interval is increased to 2 or 3 months. In contrast, many postmenopausal women tolerate only small doses of 5-FU, presumably because of relatively thin vaginal epithelium. In one study, patients used one third of an applicator of 5% 5-FU weekly for 10 weeks. Seventeen of 20 patients with vaginal condyloma were free of disease at 3 months. Three patients received a second cycle, and 16 of 18 were free of disease at 10 to 20 months. Success rates of 80% to 90% for patients with VAIN after multiple treatment cycles have been reported. The disadvantage of topical therapy with 5-FU cream is related to the high level of motivation required to complete therapy. The 5-FU cream causes exfoliation and erosion of the vaginal mucosa and can be extremely painful. Only a small percentage of patients are able to complete a full course. Thus use of this topical therapy is limited. Imiquimod has been evaluated for the treatment of vaginal intraepithelial neoplasia. Complete regression of neoplasia has been reported in 26% to 100% of patients, whereas 0 to 60% have partial regression. Recurrence of neoplasia was identified in 0 to 37% of the patients. The most commonly reported side effects were local burning and tenderness, although not severe enough to discontinue treatment. Because patients who experience disease partial regression will require less extensive excision, this treatment may prove to be a promising option (de Witte, 2015).

Wide local excision (upper vaginectomy) is the treatment of choice for VAIN-3, especially for lesions occurring at the cuff after hysterectomy. Excision gives the surgeon the ability to excise the specimen to rule out invasion and ascertain margin adequacy. Excision also has a high success rate (84%). Upper vaginectomy, however, can result in vaginal shortening, which can be ameliorated by the use of topical estrogen cream and a vaginal dilator (or frequent intercourse) once healing is complete (Ait Menguellet, 2007).

## MALIGNANT DISEASE OF THE VAGINA

### *SYMPTOMS AND DIAGNOSIS*

Primary vaginal cancers usually occur as squamous cell carcinomas in women older than 60 years. To be considered a primary vaginal tumor, the malignancy must arise in the vagina and not involve the external os of the cervix superiorly or the vulva inferiorly. If this occurs, the tumor is classified as cervical or vulvar. Biopsies are mandatory if the cervix is intact in order to rule out primary carcinoma of the cervix. This is also an important therapeutic consideration, insofar as the same management techniques apply to small tumors of the upper third of the vagina and cervical carcinomas. Tumors of the lower third of the vagina are treated similarly to vulvar cancers (see Chapter 32). Table 31.2 lists the staging criteria for vaginal cancers according to the International Federation of Gynecology and Obstetrics (FIGO), which are illustrated in Figure 31.3 (Rajaram, 2015).

Delay in the diagnosis of these cancers frequently occurs, in part due to their rarity. Lack of recognition that abnormal symptoms may be caused by malignancy can also contribute to a delay. The most common symptom of vaginal cancer is abnormal bleeding or discharge. Pain is usually a symptom of an advanced tumor. Urinary frequency is also reported occasionally, particularly in the case of anterior wall tumors, whereas constipation or tenesmus may be reported when the tumors involve the posterior vaginal wall. In general, the longer the delay in diagnosis, the poorer the prognosis and the more difficult the therapy. Vaginal cancer is usually diagnosed by direct biopsy of the tumor mass (see Fig. 31.1, *E*). Abnormal cytologic findings (see Fig. 31.1, *F*) may prompt a thorough pelvic examination that will lead to diagnosis of vaginal cancer. It is important during the course of the pelvic examination to inspect and palpate the entire vagina and to rotate the speculum carefully to visualize the entire vagina, because a small tumor may occupy the anterior or posterior vaginal wall.

**Table 31.2** International Federation of Gynecology and Obstetrics Staging Classification for Vaginal Cancer

| Stage | Characteristics |
|---|---|
| I | Carcinoma limited to vaginal wall |
| II | Carcinoma involves subvaginal tissue but has not extended to pelvic wall |
| III | Carcinoma extends to pelvic wall |
| IV | Carcinoma extends beyond true pelvis or involves mucosa of bladder or rectum (bullous edema as such does not assign a patient to stage IV) |

## TUMORS OF THE ADULT VAGINA

### *SQUAMOUS CELL CARCINOMA*

Squamous cell carcinoma is the most common vaginal malignancy and accounts for 90% of primary vaginal cancers. Although reported in women in their 30s, the disease occurs primarily in women older than 60, and 20% are older than 80 years. Most squamous cell carcinomas occur in the upper third of the vagina, but primary tumors in the middle and lower thirds may also occur. Grossly, the tumor appears as a fungating, polypoid, or ulcerating mass, often accompanied by a foul smell and discharge related to secondary infection. Microscopically (see Fig. 31.1, *E*), the tumor demonstrates the classic findings of an invasive squamous cell carcinoma infiltrating the vaginal epithelium.

Treatment of these tumors is based on the size, vaginal tumor stage, and location of the lesion. Therapy is limited by the proximity of the bladder anteriorly and the rectum posteriorly. It is also influenced by the location of the tumor in the vagina, which determines the area of lymphatic spread (Fig. 31.4).

The lymphatics of the vagina envelop the mucosa and anastomose with lymphatic vessels in the muscularis. Those of the mid to upper vagina communicate superiorly with the lymphatics of the cervix and drain into the pelvic nodes of the obturator and internal and external iliac chains. In contrast, the lymphatics of the distal third of the vagina drain to the inguinal nodes and pelvic nodes, similar to the drainage of the vulva. The posterior wall lymphatics anastomose with the rectal lymphatic system and then to the nodes that drain the rectum, such as the inferior gluteal, sacral, and rectal nodes.

#### Treatment

Once the diagnosis of vaginal malignancy is established, a thorough bimanual and visual examination documenting the size and location of the tumor and assessment of spread to adjacent structures (submucosa, vaginal sidewall, bladder, rectum) should be performed to determine the clinical stage. Cystoscopy or proctoscopy may be helpful, depending on clinical concern, to rule out bladder or rectal invasion. Distant spread may be evaluated by computed tomography (CT) of the chest, abdomen, and pelvis or positron emission tomography (PET).

Similar to cervical carcinoma, early stage vaginal carcinoma, without lymph node involvement (stage I or II), may be treated with surgery or radiation. Young patients with early stage disease and upper vaginal lesions may be treated with radical upper vaginectomy, parametrectomy, and pelvic lymphadenectomy (Davis, 1991). Radiation therapy is the most frequently used mode of treatment and can be used for early and advanced

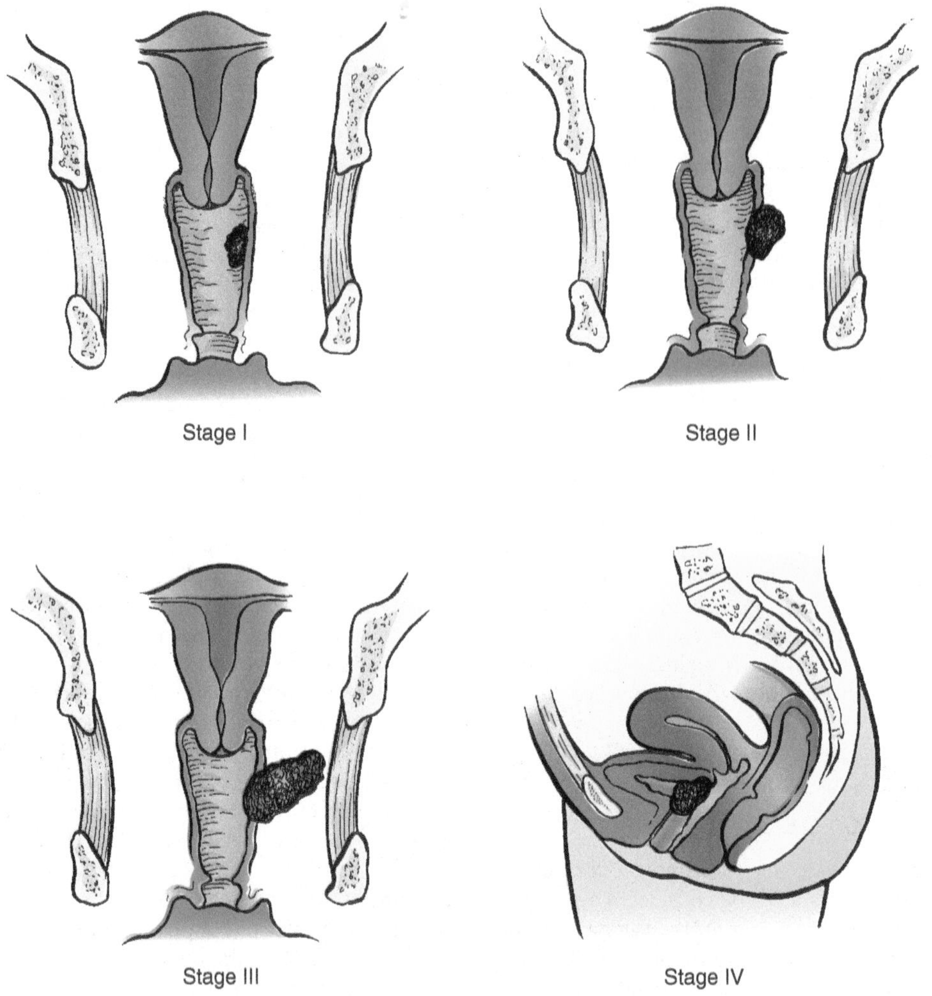


**Figure 31.3** Staging of vaginal cancer.

disease. Radiation is the most common therapy because most women with vaginal carcinoma are older and have a poorer surgical risk; radiation is highly effective. Pelvic exenteration can be used primarily to treat advanced disease in the absence of lymph node metastasis, but it is usually reserved for patients with localized recurrence after radiation. Cisplatin-based chemotherapy administered concurrently with radiation has been used with increasing frequency for squamous cell carcinomas of the vagina because of the well-documented improvements in outcomes for patients with squamous lesions of the cervix treated in this fashion. Although there have been no randomized prospective trials proving its effectiveness in this disease, the numerous similarities in pathophysiology between squamous lesions of the cervix and vagina would lead to the logical conclusion that concurrent chemotherapy with radiation will have increased efficacy over radiation alone in the treatment of vaginal carcinoma.

Stage I vaginal carcinoma may be treated with brachytherapy alone, without external beam therapy. Grigsby has recommended vaginal brachytherapy using vaginal cylinders, in one or two applications, delivering a dose of 65 to 80 Gy to the entire length of the vagina (Grigsby, 2002). For more advanced lesions, a combination of external beam and brachytherapy is used. External radiation therapy with megavoltage equipment is initially used to shrink the tumor. The size and extent of the radiation field will be determined by the presence or absence of nodal disease, as determined by the pretreatment PET or CT scan. The whole pelvis is generally treated to a dose of approximately 5040 cGy. This is followed by a local cesium or radium implant placed interstitially with needles or by intracavitary radiation using a vaginal cylinder or tandem and ovoids, if the cervix is still present. The brachytherapy will bring the total dose to between 7000 and 8500 cGy. The prognosis appears to improve if the interval from the end of external therapy to the initiation of brachytherapy is less than 28 days (Gadducci, 2015).

DiSaia and coworkers have reported using a fixed perineal template (Syed-Neblett applicator) to achieve reproducible isodose delivery to a large vaginal tumor volume (DiSaia, 1990). For lesions of the upper vagina after hysterectomy, a laparoscopy may be performed to remove any bowel loops from the vaginal apex. The omentum may be used to provide additional layer of separation of the bowel from the vaginal apex. Paley and associates have reported using a retropubic approach in a small series of six patients to achieve direct visualization of needle placement (Paley, 1998). Treatment is individualized, depending on tumor size and stage. For larger lesions, the dose of the external component of radiation therapy is increased, with a concomitant reduction in the local vaginal component of treatment of the primary tumor. Usually, a total tumor dosage of approximately 7500 cGy

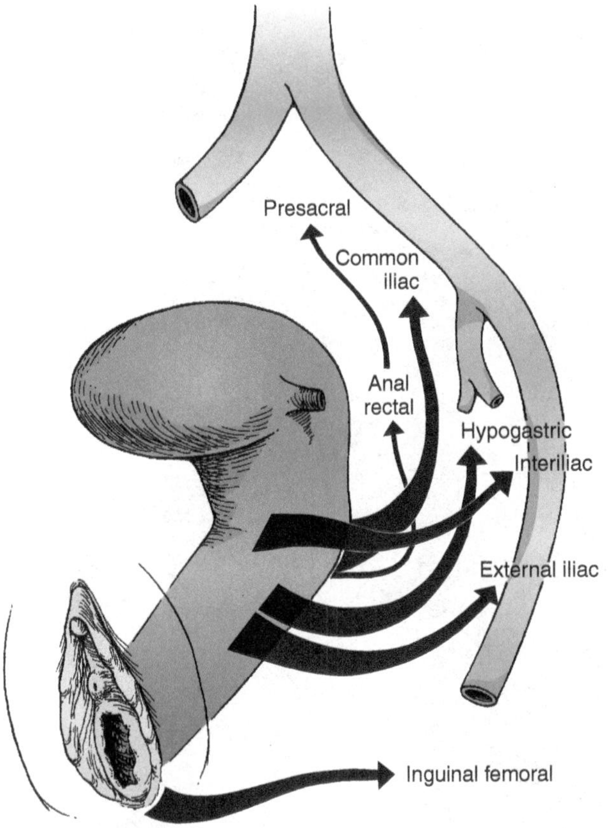


**Figure 31.4** Lymphatic drainage of the vagina. Predominant pathways from various parts of the vagina are shown.

is administered. Implants cannot be used in some patients with stage III or IV carcinoma; in such cases, only external therapy can be used, and a central boost is given after an initial 5000-cGy whole-pelvis treatment. Severe complications have been noted if the vaginal dose exceeds 9800 cGy. Kucera and Vavra, in a series of 434 patients treated with irradiation, noted that results were best for low-stage tumors, those in the upper third of the vagina, and when the tumor was well-differentiated (Kucera, 1991). Kirkbride and colleagues have reported that stage, tumor size, and tumor grade are prognostic and that the tumor dose must reach at least 7000 cGy, consistent with other studies (Kirkbride, 1995). Treatment time is also important; as noted by Lee and colleagues, it is preferable to complete the radiation therapy within 9 weeks (Lee, 1994).

### *Survival*

Overall 5-year survival rates for patients with primary carcinoma of the vagina have been reported to be approximately 45%. The stage of the tumor is the most important predictor of prognosis. In one series of 89 patients treated with surgery or irradiation, 5-year survival rates were 82% and 53%, respectively, for stage I and stage II disease. The use of concomitant chemotherapy with radiation can be expected to produce improved survival rates (Creasman, 1998).

## *CLEAR CELL ADENOCARCINOMA*

Clear cell adenocarcinomas in young women have been seen more frequently since 1970 as a result of the association of many of these cancers with intrauterine exposure to DES (Herbst, 1971). Therapeutic considerations are similar to those for squamous cell carcinoma, taking into account the young age of the patients undergoing therapy. Cervical clear cell adenocarcinomas are treated in the same manner as primary cervical carcinomas. The results of therapy for vaginal and cervical clear cell adenocarcinoma in young women are discussed together in this section. These tumors are also staged according to FIGO classification (see Table 31.2). Most tumors (80%) have been diagnosed as stage I or II. The overall results of therapy, based on the stage of the tumor at the time of treatment, are shown in Table 31.3. The survival rate is related directly to the stage of the tumor, similar to other gynecologic malignancies at these sites.

**Table 31.3** 5- and 10-Year Survival Rates for 588 Patients with Clear Cell Adenocarcinoma of the Vagina and Cervix

| Stage | 5-Year Survival (%) | 10-Year Survival (%) |
|---|---|---|
| I | 91 | 85 |
| IIA | 80 | 67 |
| IIB | 56 | 47 |
| II (vagina) | 82 | 67 |
| III | 37 | 25 |
| IV | 0 | 0 |

Modified from Registry Data, University of Chicago; Herbst A; Anderson D. Clear cell adenocarcinoma of the vagina and cervix secondary to intrauterine exposure to diethylstilbestrol. *Semin Surg Oncol.* 1990;6(6):343-346.

In general, surgery is the primary treatment modality because of the young age of the patients. For stage I and early stage II tumors, radical hysterectomy with partial or complete vaginectomy, pelvic lymphadenectomy, and reconstruction of the vagina with split-thickness skin grafts has been the most common approach. In most cases, ovarian function is preserved. In addition, efforts have been made to preserve fertility in patients who have small tumors of the vagina by the use of local irradiation of the primary tumor and immediate adjacent tissues to spare the ovaries. Because metastases to regional pelvic nodes can occur, even with small stage I tumors, retroperitoneal lymph node dissections are usually performed before local therapy.

Local excision of the tumor can be performed before irradiation to facilitate local application. Senekjian and associates have noted that the survival of patients with small vaginal tumors treated by local excision and then local irradiation is comparable with that obtained with conventional extensive therapy (Senekjian, 1989). The best candidates are those with tumors smaller than 2 cm in diameter, a predominant tubulocystic pattern (Fig. 31.5, *A*), and depth of invasion less than 3 mm. After wide local excision, the pelvic nodes are sampled to rule out tumor spread. If these are negative, local irradiation can then be given. Patients treated in this manner have become pregnant. Patients with larger tumors, however, receive full pelvic irradiation, in addition to an intracavitary implant. In a few cases, exenterative surgery has been successfully performed. This procedure is preferably applied to central recurrences that develop after primary irradiation. Local vaginal excision as the sole therapy is not usually adequate for small tumors because the tumor frequently recurs.

Three predominant histologic patterns are found in patients with clear cell adenocarcinoma (see Fig. 31.5). In addition, a number of prognostic factors have been identified. Older patients

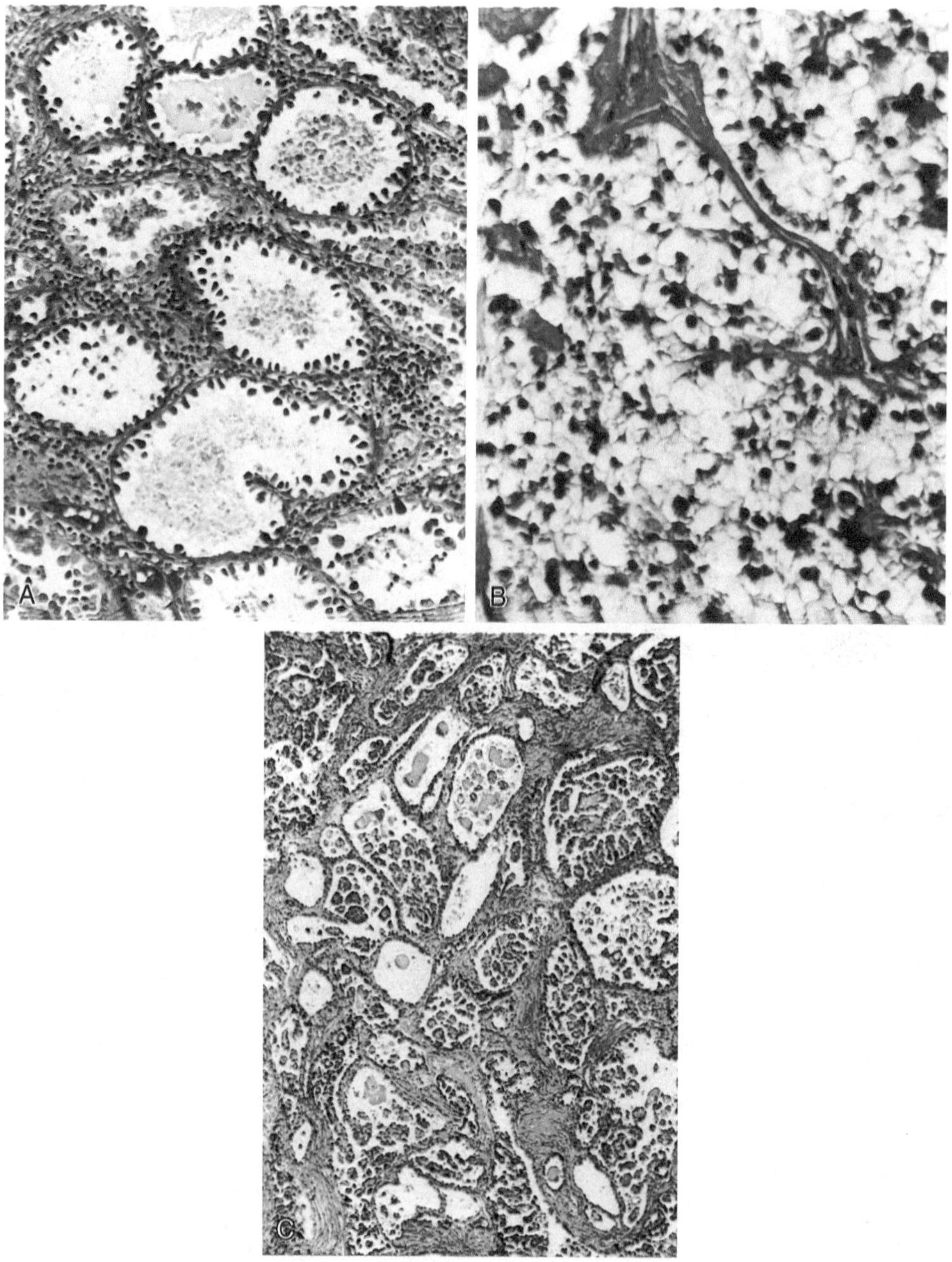


**Figure 31.5** **A,** Tubulocystic cell pattern. Note hobnail cells extruding into the lumina of tubular structures (H&E stain, × 180). **B,** Solid pattern (H&E stain, × 300). **C,** Papillary pattern (H&E stain, × 50). (**A** and **B,** from Scully RE, Robboy SJ, Herbst AL. Vaginal and cervical abnormalities, including clear cell adenocarcinoma, related to prenatal exposure to stilbestrol. *Ann Clin Lab Sci.* 1974;4[4]:222-233. **C,** from Scully RE, Robboy SJ, Welch WR. Pathology and pathogenesis of diethylstilbestrol-related disorders of the female genital tract. In: Herbst AL, ed. *Intrauterine Exposure to Diethylstilbestrol in the Human.* Washington, DC: American College of Obstetricians and Gynecologists; 1978.)

(>19 years) have been found to have a more favorable prognosis in comparison to younger patients (<15 years). This difference is associated with a more favorable outcome for those with the tubulocystic pattern of clear cell adenocarcinoma, the most frequent histologic pattern found in older patients. In addition, smaller tumor diameter and superficial depth of invasion correlate with improved patient survival. Waggoner and coworkers have shown that patients with clear cell adenocarcinoma and a maternal history of DES use survive longer than those without a maternal history of DES use (Waggoner, 1994). If the regional pelvic nodes are free of tumor, the prognosis is also more favorable. It is more likely that the regional pelvic lymph nodes will be free of tumor if other factors are favorable.

Clear cell adenocarcinomas can spread locally, as well as via lymphatics and blood vessels. Metastases to regional pelvic nodes are found in approximately one sixth of stage I cases. Spread to regional pelvic nodes becomes more frequent in higher stage tumors. Depending on the location of the tumor recurrence, therapy has consisted of additional radical surgery or extensive radiation in localized pelvic disease and systemic chemotherapy in cases of metastatic disease. Unfortunately, no single agent or combination of chemotherapeutic agents has emerged as an effective therapy. Prolonged follow-up is necessary for these patients because recurrences have been reported as long as 20 years after primary therapy, particularly in the lungs and supraclavicular areas. Data from the Registry on Hormonal Transplacental Carcinogenesis (Herbst, 1990) indicate that ovarian preservation with concomitant estrogen stimulation does not adversely affect survival in patients with clear cell adenocarcinoma of the vagina.

### MALIGNANT MELANOMA

Vaginal melanomas are rare and highly malignant. Only approximately 2% to 3% of primary vaginal cancers are melanomas. The most common presenting symptoms are vaginal discharge, bleeding, and a palpable mass. These lesions appear as darkly pigmented, irregular areas and may be flat, polypoid, or nodular. The average age of affected women is 57 years. Vaginal melanomas tend to metastasize early, via the bloodstream and lymphatics, to the iliac or inguinal nodes, lungs, liver, brain, and bones. Patients with vaginal melanoma have a poorer prognosis than those with vulvar melanoma, in part probably because of delay in diagnosis in comparison with vulvar carcinomas and in part because of their mucosal location, which seems to predispose patients to developing early metastasis (Kirschner, 2013).

Treatment usually consists of surgery with wide excision of the vagina and dissection of the regional nodes (pelvic, inguinal-femoral, or both), depending on the location of the lesion. Improved outcomes have been associated with the removal of all gross disease (Buchanan, 1998). Therapy is usually tailored to the extent of disease. Surgery, radiation, chemotherapy, and immunotherapy have all been described, but no single therapy or combination treatment is uniformly successful.

Local and distant recurrences are common, and the disease is usually fatal. Even with local control, distant failure is common in patients with melanoma. The overall 5-year survival rate is 8.4%, with an overall median survival of 20 months. Prognostic indicators include tumor size, mitotic index, and Breslow tumor thickness. Improved survival has been noted for patients whose tumors had fewer than six mitoses/10 high-power fields (HPF). Van Nostrand and associates have reported a 2-year survival for three of four patients with tumors smaller than 10 $cm^2$—that is, approximately 3 cm in diameter (Van Nostrand, 1994). However, Neven and coworkers have noted that among nine patients, all those with melanomas more than 2 mm thick died or had a recurrence regardless of type of therapy, emphasizing the importance of tumor thickness in melanoma prognosis (Neven, 1994).

### VAGINAL ADENOCARCINOMAS ARISING IN ENDOMETRIOSIS

The malignant transformation of extraovarian endometriosis is rare but has been reported with increasing frequency. The reason for this increase is not known. The rectovaginal septum is the most common extragonadal location (Yazbeck, 2005). When these tumors occur in the vagina or rectovaginal septum, the typical clinical presentation is pain, vaginal bleeding, or the presence of a vaginal mass in a woman who has previously undergone prior extirpative surgery for endometriosis. Risk factors include use of unopposed estrogen and tamoxifen use. The most common histology is endometrioid adenocarcinoma, followed by sarcomas (25%) and other tumors of müllerian differentiation. Treatment usually includes surgery plus radiation or chemotherapy. Leiserowitz and colleagues have reported a relatively favorable prognosis for women with endometriosis-related malignancies, with 70% alive at a mean follow-up of 31 months (2003).

## VAGINAL TUMORS OF INFANTS AND CHILDREN

### ENDODERMAL SINUS TUMOR (YOLK SAC TUMOR)

Endodermal sinus tumor, a type of adenocarcinoma, is a rare germ cell tumor that usually occurs in the ovary. This tumor secretes α-fetoprotein, which provides a useful tumor marker to monitor patients treated for these neoplasms. Approximately 69 cases of this unusual malignancy originated in the vagina of infants, predominantly those younger than 2 years of age. This tumor is aggressive, and most patients have died (Anderson, 1985). Young and Scully reported on six patients who were free of disease 2 to 9 years after surgery, irradiation, or both, who also received ***v***incristine, ***actinomycin*** D, and ***c***yclophosphamide (VAC) chemotherapy (Young, 1984). Copeland and colleagues have reported similar good results with combination chemotherapy and excision (Copeland, 1985). The combination of bleomycin, etoposide, and cisplatin (BEP) has also been used to treat this disease (Tao, 2012).

### SARCOMA BOTRYOIDES (EMBRYONAL RHABDOMYOSARCOMA)

Sarcoma botryoides is an uncommon vaginal sarcoma that is usually diagnosed in young girls. Rarely does it occur in a young child older than 8 years, although cases in adolescents have been reported. The most common symptom is abnormal vaginal bleeding, with an occasional mass present at the introitus (Fig. 31.6). The tumor grossly resembles a cluster of grapes forming multiple polypoid masses (Copeland, 1985).

These tumors are believed to begin in the subepithelial layers of the vagina and expand rapidly to fill the vagina. They are often multicentric. Histologically, they have a loose myxomatous stroma with malignant pleomorphic cells and occasional eosinophilic rhabdomyoblasts that often contain characteristic cross-striations (strap cells; Fig. 31.7).

Sarcoma botryoides lesions were treated in the past by radical surgery, such as pelvic exenteration. However, effective control with less radical surgery has been achieved with a multimodality approach consisting of multiagent chemotherapy (VAC) combined with surgery. Radiation therapy has also been used. Andrassy and associates have reported 21 patients with vaginal rhabdomyosarcomas who received chemotherapy (1995). Seven relapsed, five of whom had residual disease after incomplete resection. One had disseminated disease. In 17 patients who received chemotherapy for 8 to 48 weeks, a delayed excision could be performed. Long-term survival data for a large number of patients are not available, but such a combined approach appears to result in effective

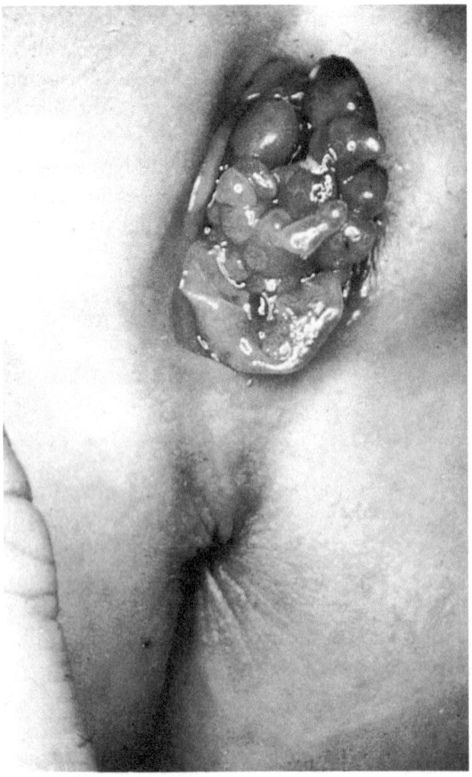

**Figure 31.6** Sarcoma botryoides protruding through the vaginal introitus. (From Herbst AL. Cancer of the vagina. In: Gusberg SB, Frick HC, eds. *Gynecologic Cancer.* 5th ed. Baltimore: Williams & Wilkins; 1978.)

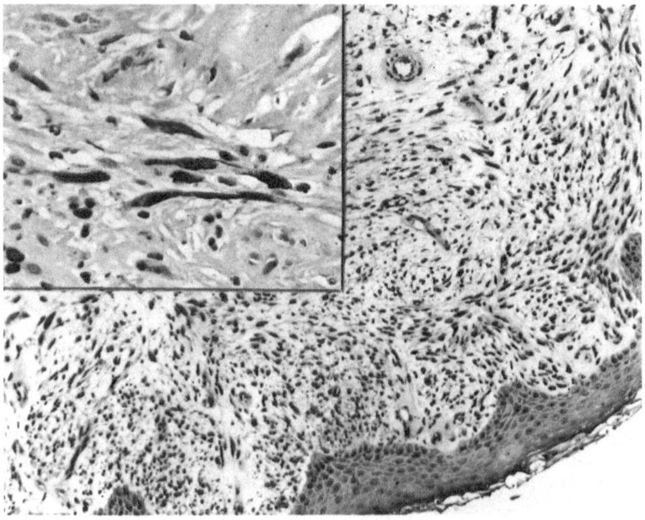

**Figure 31.7** Vaginal mucosa with sarcoma botryoides showing condensation of malignant cells under the epithelium (H&E, × 100). *Insert,* Immunohistochemical stain for desmin illustrating strap cells (× 240). (Courtesy of Dr. A. Montag, University of Chicago.)

treatment with less mutilating surgery (Piver, 1988). A multimodality approach, including chemotherapy, was used by Flamant and coworkers in 17 females with rhabdomyosarcoma of the vagina or vulva (Flamant, 1990). At the time of their report, 15 appeared cured; 11 of 12 pubescent females had experienced menses, whereas 2 had successfully conceived and delivered healthy children. This was emphasized in a report from the Intergroup Rhabdomyosarcoma Study by Andrassy and colleagues (1995). They found VAC chemotherapy to be effective for disease confined to the vagina without nodal spread. This therapy was effective without irradiation for disease that was locally resected, suggesting that for these patients, chemotherapy plus surgery can be effective therapy.

### PSEUDOSARCOMA BOTRYOIDES

Pseudosarcoma botryoides refers to a rare, benign vaginal polyp that resembles sarcoma botryoides and is found in the vagina of infants and pregnant women. Although large atypical cells may be present microscopically, strap cells are absent. Grossly, these polyps resemble the grapelike appearance of sarcoma botryoides and are therefore called "pseudosarcoma botryoides." Treatment by local excision is effective (Lin, 1995).

## KEY POINTS

- Predisposing factors associated with the development of vaginal intraepithelial neoplasia include infection with HPV, previous radiation therapy to the vagina, immunosuppressive therapy, and HIV infection.
- The tendency of intraepithelial squamous neoplasia to develop anywhere in the lower female genital tract is termed a *field defect* and describes the increased risk of premalignant changes occurring in the cervix, vagina, or vulva.
- Most cases of VAIN occur in the upper third of the vagina.
- VAIN can be treated by excision, laser, 5-FU, or imiquimod. Excision is often used for VAIN-3. Laser treatment is generally used for discrete lesions once invasion has been ruled out, and 5-FU and imiquimod cream are used to treat diffuse, multicentric, low-grade disease.
- The most common primary vaginal malignancy is squamous cell carcinoma (90%).
- Most cancers occurring in the vagina are metastatic.
- Vaginal cancers constitute less than 2% of gynecologic malignancies.
- Tumors of the upper vagina have a lymphatic drainage to the pelvis similar to cervical tumors. Tumors of the lower third of the vagina drain to the pelvic nodes and also to the inguinal nodes, similar to vulvar tumors.
- Radical surgery may be used to treat low-stage tumors, primarily of the upper vagina, in younger patients.
- Radiation therapy is the most frequently used modality for the treatment of squamous cell carcinoma of the vagina. Ideally, at least 7000 to 7500 cGy is administered in less than 9 weeks. Concurrent chemoradiation should strongly be considered.
- The overall 5-year survival rate of patients treated for squamous cell carcinoma of the vagina is approximately 45%.

## KEY POINTS—cont'd

- Clear cell adenocarcinoma is often associated with prenatal DES exposure. Prognosis is improved if the patient is older than 19 years, the tumor has a predominant tubulocystic tumor pattern, and the disease is low stage. Those with a positive DES maternal history have a better prognosis.
- Local therapy for small, stage I clear cell adenocarcinoma of the vagina is best considered if the tumor is smaller than 2 cm in diameter, invades less than 3 mm, and is predominantly of the tubulocystic histologic type. Pelvic nodes should be sampled and be free of tumor.
- The overall 5-year survival rate of patients treated for clear cell adenocarcinoma is approximately 80%, partially because of the high proportion of low-stage cases.
- Vaginal melanomas are usually fatal. They occur primarily in patients older than 50 years.
- Endometrioid adenocarcinomas of the vagina may occur through the malignant transformation of endometriosis, often associated with the use of unopposed estrogen or tamoxifen.
- Endodermal sinus tumors occur in children younger than 2 years. They secrete α-fetoprotein and are usually treated by multiagent chemotherapy, followed by surgical excision.
- Sarcoma botryoides occurs primarily in children younger than 8 years. It is treated by a multimodality approach using multiagent chemotherapy with surgical removal and occasionally irradiation.

## KEY REFERENCES


Aho M, Vesterinen E, Meyer B, et al. Natural history of vaginal intraepithelial neoplasia. *Cancer.* 1991;68:195-197.

Ait Menguellet S, Collinet P, Houfflin Debarge V, et al. Management of multicentric lesions of the lower genital tract. *Eur J Obstet Gynecol Reprod Biol.* 2007;132(1):116-120.

Anderson WA, Sabio H, Durso N, et al. Endodermal sinus tumor of the vagina. *Cancer.* 1985;56(5):1025-1027.

Andrassy RJ, Hays DM, Raney RB, et al. Conservative surgical management of vaginal and vulvar pediatric rhabdomyosarcoma: a report from the Intergroup Rhabdomyosarcoma Study III. *J Pediatr Surg.* 1995;30(7):1034-1036.

Audet-Lapointe P, Body G, Vauclair R, et al. Vaginal intraepithelial neoplasia. *Gynecol Oncol.* 1990;36(2):232-239.

Buchanan DJ, Schlaerth J, Kurosaki T. Primary vaginal melanoma: thirteen-year disease-free survival after wide local excision and review of recent literature. *Am J Obstet Gynecol.* 1998;178(6):1177-1184.

Copeland LJ, Gershenson DM, Saul PB, et al. Sarcoma botryoides of the female genital tract. *Obstet Gynecol.* 1985a;66(2):262-266.

Copeland LJ, Sneige N, Ordonez NG, et al. Endodermal sinus tumor of the vagina and cervix. *Cancer.* 1985b;55(11):2558-2565.

Creasman WT, Phillip JL, Menck HR. The National Cancer Database report on cancer of the vagina. *Cancer.* 1998;83(5):1033-1040.

Davis KP, Stanhope CR, Garton GR, et al. Invasive vaginal carcinoma: analysis of early-stage disease. *Gynecol Oncol.* 1991;42(2):131-136.

de Witte CJ, van de Sande AJ, van Beekhuizen HJ, et al. Imiquimod in cervical, vaginal and vulvar intraepithelial neoplasia: a review. *Gynecol Oncol.* 2015;139(2):377-384.

DiSaia PJ, Syed AMN, Puthawala AA. Malignant neoplasia of the upper vagina. *Endocr Hypertherm Oncol.* 1990;6:251.

Flamant F, Gerbaulet A, Nihoul-Fekete C, et al. Long-term sequelae of conservative treatment by surgery, brachytherapy, and chemotherapy for vulva and vaginal rhabdomyosarcoma in children. *J Clin Oncol.* 1990;8(11):1847-1853.

Gadducci A, Fabrini MG, Lanfredini N, et al. Squamous cell carcinoma of the vagina: natural history, treatment modalities and prognostic factors. *Crit Rev Oncol Hematol.* 2015;93(3):211-224.

Grigsby PW. Vaginal cancer. *Curr Treat Options Oncol.* 2002;3(2):125-130.

Herbst AL, Anderson D. Recent advances in clear cell adenocarcinoma of the vagina and cervix secondary to intrauterine exposure to DES. *Semin Surg Oncol.* 1990;6(6):343-346.

Herbst AL, Ulfelder H, Poskanzer DC. Adenocarcinoma of the vagina. Association of maternal stilbestrol therapy with tumor appearance in young women. *N Engl J Med.* 1971;284(15):878-881.

Jentschke M, Hoffmeister V, Soergel P, et al. Clinical presentation, treatment and outcome of vaginal intraepithelial neoplasia. *Arch Gynecol Obstet.* 2015. [Epub ahead of print].

Kirkbride P, Fyles A, Rawlings GA, et al. Carcinoma of the vagina – experience at the Princess Margaret Hospital (1974-1989). *Gynecol Oncol.* 1995;56(3):435-443.

Kirschner AN, Kidd EA, Dewees T, et al. Treatment approach and outcomes of vaginal melanoma. *Int J Gynecol Cancer.* 2013;23(8):1484-1489.

Kucera H, Vavra N. Radiation management of primary carcinoma of the vagina: clinical and histopathological variables associated with survival. *Gynecol Oncol.* 1991;40(1):12-16.

Lee WR, Marcus RB, Sombec MD, et al. Radiotherapy alone for carcinoma of the vagina: the importance of overall treatment time. *Int J Radiat Oncol Biol Phys.* 1994;29(5):983-988.

Leiserowitz GS, Gumbs JL, Oi R, et al. Endometriosis-related malignancies. *Int J Gynecol Cancer.* 2003;13(4):466-471.

Lin J, Lam SK, Cheung TH. Sarcoma botryoides of the cervix treated with limited surgery and chemotherapy to preserve fertility. *Gynecol Oncol.* 1995; 58(2):270-273.

Neven P, Shepherd TH, Masotina A, et al. Malignant melanoma of the vulva and vagina: a report of 23 cases presenting in a 10-year period. *Int J Gynecol Cancer.* 1994;4(6):379-383.

Paley PJ, Koh W-J, Stelzer KJ, et al. A new technique for performing Syed template interstitial implants for anterior vaginal tumors using an open retropubic approach. *Gynecol Oncol.* 1998;73(1):121-125.

Petrilli ES, Townsend DE, Morrow CP, et al. Vaginal intraepithelial neoplasm: biologic aspects and treatment with topical 5-flurouracil and the carbon dioxide laser. *Am J Obstet Gynecol.* 1980;138(3):321-328.

Piovano E, Macchi C, Attamante L, et al. CO2 laser vaporization for the treatment of vaginal intraepithelial neoplasia: effectiveness and predictive factors for recurrence. *Eur J Gynaecol Oncol.* 2015;36(4):383-388.

Piver MS, Rose PG. Long-term follow-up and complications of infants with vulvovaginal embryonal rhabdomyosarcoma treated with surgery, radiation therapy, and chemotherapy. *Obstet Gynecol.* 1988;71(3 Pt 2):435-437.

Rajaram S, Maheshwari A, Srivastava A. Staging for vaginal cancer. *Best Pract Res Clin Obstet Gynaecol.* 2015;29(6):822-832.

Senekjian EK, Frey KW, Herbst AL. Pelvic exenteration in clear cell adenocarcinoma of the vagina and cervix. *Gynecol Oncol.* 1989;34(3):413-416.

Shrivastava S, Agrawal G, Mittal M, et al. Management of vaginal cancer. *Rev Recent Clin Trials.* 2015;10(4):289-297.

Tao T, Yang J, Cao D, et al. Conservative treatment and long-term follow up of endodermal sinus tumor of the vagina. *Gynecol Oncol.* 2012;125(2):358-361.

Van Nostrand KM, Lucci III JA, Schell M, et al. Primary vaginal melanoma: improved survival with radical pelvic surgery. *Gynecol Oncol.* 1994;55(2): 234-237.

Waggoner SE, Mittendorf R, Biney N, et al. Influence of in utero diethylstilbestrol exposure on the prognosis and biologic behavior of vaginal clear cell adenocarcinoma. *Gynecol Oncol.* 1994;55(2):238-244.

Yazbeck C, Poncelet C, Chosidow D, Maldelenat P. Primary adenocarcinoma arising from endometriosis of the rectovaginal septum: a case report. *Int J Gynecol Cancer.* 2005;15(6):1203-1205.

Young RH, Scully RE. Endodermal sinus tumor of the vagina: a report of nine cases and review of the literature. *Gynecol Oncol.* 1984;18(3):380-392.


Suggested Readings can be found on ExpertConsult.com

# 32

# Neoplastic Diseases of the Uterus

## Endometrial Hyperplasia, Endometrial Carcinoma, Sarcoma: Diagnosis and Management

*Pamela T. Soliman, Karen H. Lu*

Endometrial carcinoma is the most common malignancy of the lower female genital tract in the United States. Approximately 54,870 new cases develop in the United States each year, according to 2015 figures from the American Cancer Society. This is approximately two times the frequency of ovarian cancer and more than four times the number of new cases of cervical cancer. Approximately 10,000 deaths occurred annually from uterine cancer, more than for cervical cancer (4100) and fewer than the estimated 14,000 for ovarian cancer. Overall, approximately 3 women in 100 in the United States will develop this disease during their lives.

This chapter reviews the clinical and pathologic features of endometrial hyperplasias and carcinomas, the factors that contribute to the development of these diseases, and the appropriate methods of management. Sarcomas of the uterus and their clinical behavior and therapy are also presented.

## EPIDEMIOLOGY

Adenocarcinoma of the endometrium affects women primarily in the perimenopausal and postmenopausal years and is most frequently diagnosed in those between the ages of 50 and 65. However, these cancers can also develop in young women during their reproductive years. Approximately 5% of the cases are diagnosed in women younger than 40 and approximately 10% to 15% in women younger than age 50. Women diagnosed under the age of 50 years are also at risk for having a synchronous ovarian cancer (Soliman, 2004). Figure 32.1 plots a typical age–incidence curve for cancers of the endometrium. The curve rises sharply after age 45 and peaks between 55 and 60; then there is a gradual decrease.

Complex atypical hyperplasia results from increased estrogenic stimulation of the endometrium and is a precursor to endometrioid endometrial cancer. Some endometrial cancers develop without previous hyperplasia. These non-estrogen-related carcinomas including serous histology tend to be poorly differentiated and clinically more aggressive (see the later discussion).

Multiple factors increase the risk of developing endometrial carcinoma (and hyperplasia) (Box 32.1). Obesity is a strong risk factor for endometrial cancer. Women who are obese (body mass index >30) have a two- to threefold increased risk, and this risk increased with increasing weight (Brinton, 1992). The association is believed to be due in part to increased circulating estrogen levels that result from conversion of androstenedione to estrone in the adipose tissue, decreased sex hormone-binding globulin, and other factors including insulin resistance. Although more historical than clinically relevant, unopposed estrogen stimulation is strongly associated with endometrial cancer, increasing the risk four to eight times for a woman using estrogen alone for menopausal replacement therapy. The risk increases with higher doses of estrogen (>0.625 mg conjugated estrogens), and more prolonged use but can be markedly reduced with the use of progestin (see Chapter 14). Similarly, combination (progestin-containing) oral contraceptives decrease the risk. As noted by Grimes and Economy, combination oral contraceptives protect against endometrial cancer, with most studies showing a relative risk reduction to approximately 0.5. The protection begins after 1 year of use and lasts approximately 15 years after discontinuation. Other conditions leading to long-term estrogen stimulation of the endometrium, including the polycystic ovary syndrome (Stein-Leventhal syndrome) and the much more rare feminizing ovarian tumors, are also associated with increased risk of endometrial carcinoma.

Patients who receive the selective estrogen receptor modulator (SERM) tamoxifen are also at increased risk of developing endometrial carcinoma. In the National Surgical Adjuvant Bowel and Breast B-14 trial examining tamoxifen as adjuvant therapy in women with breast cancer, risk of endometrial cancer was elevated 7.5-fold. This may be an overestimate as the risk of endometrial cancer in the control group was lower than expected. In the National Surgical Adjuvant Bowel and Breast P-1 trial examining tamoxifen as a chemopreventive agent, risk of endometrial cancer was elevated 2.5-fold. Risk increased with duration of use. The majority of endometrial cancers that developed in tamoxifen users were endometrioid histology and low grade and stage. However, high-grade endometrial cancers and sarcomas have also been reported in women taking tamoxifen. Screening strategies including transvaginal ultrasound and

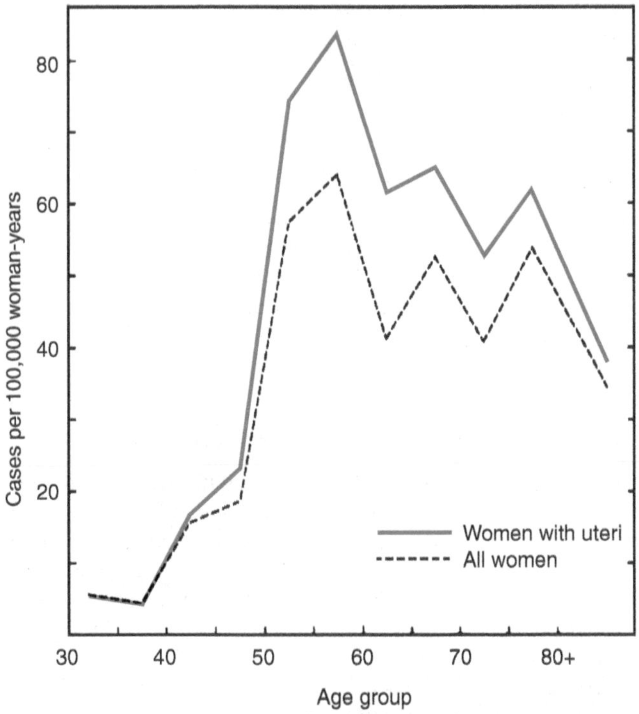


**Figure 32.1** Incidence curve for carcinoma of the endometrium by age. (From Elwood JM, Cole P, Rothman KJ, Kaplan SD. Epidemiology of endometrial cancer. *J Natl Cancer Inst.* 1977;59:1055.)

**Box 32.1 Endometrial Carcinoma Risk Factors**

**Increases the Risk**
Unopposed estrogen stimulation
Unopposed menopausal estrogen (4-8×) replacement therapy
Menopause after 52 years (2.4×)
Obesity (2-5×)
Nulliparity (2-3×)
Diabetes (2.8×)
Insulin resistance
Estrogen secreting ovarian tumors
Polycystic ovarian syndrome
Tamoxifen therapy for breast cancer

**Diminishes the Risk**
Ovulation
Progestin therapy
Combination oral contraceptives
Menopause before 49 years
Multiparity

office endometrial sampling have been studied in this cohort. There is a high false-positive rate with transvaginal ultrasonography because tamoxifen causes subendometrial cyst formation, which makes the endometrial stripe appear abnormally thick. Barakat and colleagues performed endometrial Pipelle sampling on a large cohort of women taking tamoxifen. They found very few cancers and concluded that women do not benefit from endometrial screening. Rather women should be counseled that tamoxifen increases the risk of endometrial cancer, and all women on tamoxifen who have irregular vaginal bleeding (if premenopausal) or any vaginal bleeding (if postmenopausal) should undergo endometrial sampling or dilation and curettage (D&C).

Various other factors increase the risk of endometrial cancer. Nulliparity is associated with a 2-fold increased risk in endometrial cancer. Diabetes increases the risk by 2.8-fold and has been found to be an independent risk factor. Hypertension is often related to obesity and diabetes but is not considered an independent risk factor. Insulin resistance or metabolic syndrome has also been recognized as a risk factor for endometrial cancer (Burzawa, 2011). Regarding racial factors, the incidence of endometrial cancer among white women is approximately twice the rate in black women. However, studies of Hill and coworkers demonstrated that black women tend to develop a much higher percentage of poorly differentiated tumors. The National Cancer Database report by Partridge and colleagues confirmed that patients who are black and have a low income do present at an advanced stage and have a poor survival compared with non-Hispanic whites (Partridge, 1996). The difference in survival between blacks and non-Hispanic whites does not appear to be solely based on access to care issues, and there are likely biologic differences that account for the disparity in survival.

Lynch syndrome, or hereditary nonpolyposis colorectal cancer syndrome (HNPCC), is an autosomal dominant hereditary cancer susceptibility syndrome caused by a germline defect in a DNA mismatch repair gene (MLH1, MSH2, or MSH6). Women with Lynch syndrome have a 40% to 60% lifetime risk for developing endometrial cancer, a 40% to 60% lifetime risk of developing colon cancer, and a 12% lifetime risk of developing ovarian cancer. This contrasts sharply with the general population risk of 3% for endometrial cancer, 5% for colon cancer, and 1.7% risk of ovarian cancer. Endometrial cancers in Lynch syndrome can be of any histology and grade. Broaddus and Lu reported that although most endometrial cancers in women with Lynch syndrome were in the early stage, approximately one fourth were high grade, high stage, or poor histology. Given that there are few longitudinal cohort studies, screening recommendations for gynecologic cancers are based on expert opinion and include annual endometrial biopsy and transvaginal ultrasound to evaluate the ovaries. Schmeler reported on the efficacy of prophylactic hysterectomy and salpingo-oophorectomy to decrease endometrial and ovarian cancer risk. Women with Lynch syndrome should be offered this option after childbearing is complete. Lynch syndrome is likely to account for approximately 2% of all endometrial cancers. Women with endometrial cancer and a family history of colon, endometrial, or ovarian cancer should be referred for genetic evaluation and colonoscopy. In addition, women who have a personal history of both endometrial and colon cancer have a significant risk for Lynch syndrome and should be referred. Although synchronous endometrial and ovarian cancers are fairly common, Soliman and colleagues estimated the risk of Lynch syndrome in this cohort to be less than 10%.

The molecular alterations present in endometrial cancer are well documented and are related to histologic cell type. PTEN mutations are frequently seen in endometrioid endometrial cancer and have also been seen in complex endometrial hyperplasia. Microsatellite instability occurs in approximately 25% to 30% of all endometrial cancers and is the result of either germline mutations in DNA mismatch repair proteins (MLH1, MSH2, or MSH6) or more frequently from the somatic methylation of the MLH1 promoter. In contrast to endometrioid endometrial cancers, uterine serous carcinomas have a high frequency of p53 mutations. HER-2/neu amplification is seen in 10% to 20% of uterine serous carcinomas and is likely associated with advanced stage and poor prognosis. Future studies will continue to elucidate our understanding of the molecular alterations of endometrial cancer.

## ENDOMETRIAL HYPERPLASIA

The normal morphologic changes that occur in the endometrium during the menstrual cycle are reviewed in Chapter 4. Endometrial hyperplasia is believed to result from an excess of estrogen or an excess of estrogen relative to progestin, such as occurs with anovulation. Kurman and Norris introduced terminology that the World Health Organization has adopted to describe endometrial hyperplasias and their premalignant potential. There are two important separate categories: atypical hyperplasia and hyperplasia without atypia. In these categories, two subgroups are recognized: simple hyperplasia and complex hyperplasia (Table 32.1).

### SIMPLE HYPERPLASIA

This term defines an endometrium with dilated glands that may contain some outpouching and abundant endometrial stroma (Fig. 32.2). The term *cystic hyperplasia* has been used to describe dilation of the endometrial glands, which often occurs in a hyperplastic endometrium in a menopausal or postmenopausal woman (cystic atrophy). It is considered to be weakly premalignant.

Table 32.1 Classifications of Endometrial Hyperplasias

| World Health Organization |
|---|
| Simple hyperplasia |
| Complex hyperplasia |
| Atypical simple hyperplasia |
| Atypical complex hyperplasia |

### COMPLEX HYPERPLASIA (WITHOUT ATYPIA)

In this condition, glands are crowded with very little endometrial stroma and a complex gland pattern and out-pouching formations (Fig. 32.3). In traditional terminology, this is a variant of adenomatous hyperplasia with moderate to severe degrees of architectural atypia but with no cytologic atypia. These hyperplasias have a low malignant potential.

### COMPLEX ATYPICAL HYPERPLASIA

This term refers to hyperplasias that contain glands with cytologic atypia and are considered premalignant. There is an increase in the nuclear/cytoplasmic ratio with irregularity in the size and shape of the nuclei (Fig. 32.4). Cytologic atypia occurs primarily with complex hyperplasia. Simple hyperplasia with atypia is rarely seen. Complex atypical hyperplasia has the greatest malignant potential.

A study from the Gynecologic Oncology Group highlighted the challenge in making the diagnosis of complex atypical hyperplasia. In this large prospective study, a gynecologic pathologist reviewed cases with a diagnosis of complex hyperplasia with atypia. One third of the cases were confirmed as complex atypical hyperplasia, one third were deemed to be "less than" complex atypical hyperplasia, and one third were considered endometrial cancers. This variability in diagnosis should be considered when determining treatment for these patients.

### NATURAL HISTORY

The rate at which endometrial hyperplasia progresses to endometrial carcinoma has not been accurately determined,

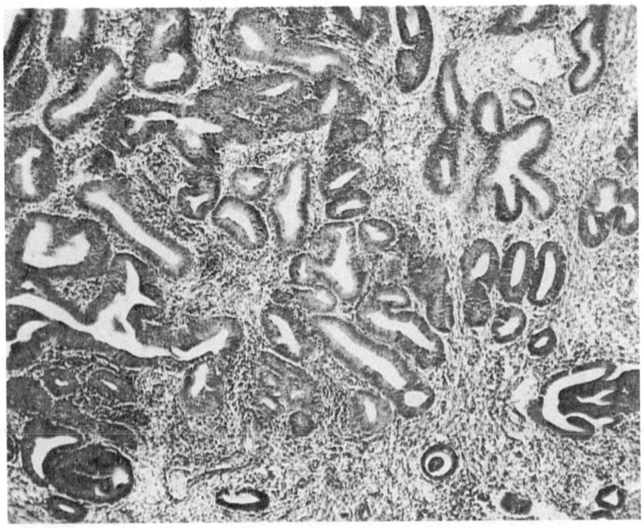

**Figure 32.2** Benign simple hyperplasia. (From Kurman RJ, Kaminski PF, Norris HJ. Behavior of endometrial hyperplasia: a long-term study of "untreated" hyperplasias in 170 patients. *Cancer.* 1985;56:403.)

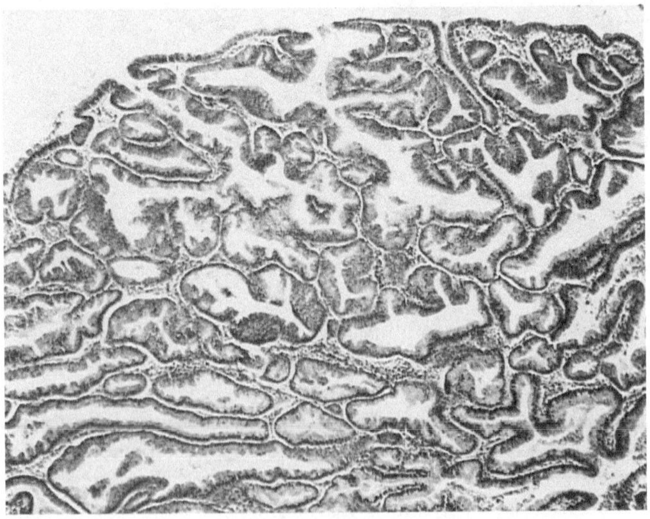

**Figure 32.3** Complex hyperplasia characterized by crowded back-to-back glands with complex outlines. (From Kurman RJ, Kaminski PF, Norris HJ. Behavior of endometrial hyperplasia: a long-term study of "untreated" hyperplasias in 170 patients. *Cancer.* 1985;56:403.)

as many of the studies have been retrospective. Kurman and associates studied 170 patients with endometrial hyperplasia diagnosed by D&C at least 1 year before hysterectomy (Kurman, 1985). Table 32.2 shows the results of their study. Overall, complex atypical hyperplasias had the highest risk of progression to carcinoma. Simple hyperplasia had a 1% rate of progression to cancer, complex hyperplasia without atypia had a 3% rate of progression to cancer, and complex atypical hyperplasia had a 29% rate of progression to cancer. In addition to possible progression to cancer, 40% of women who undergo hysterectomy for complex atypical hyperplasia have a concurrent endometrial cancer in their hysterectomy specimen. This high rate of cancer suggests that complex atypical hyperplasia may frequently be present with low-grade endometrial cancer and that endometrial sampling may not identify an endometrial cancer when admixed with a complex atypical hyperplasia. Clearly, there is a spectrum of histology that makes a definitive diagnosis of complex atypical hyperplasia difficult, and the clinician must be aware of this fact when planning management strategies.

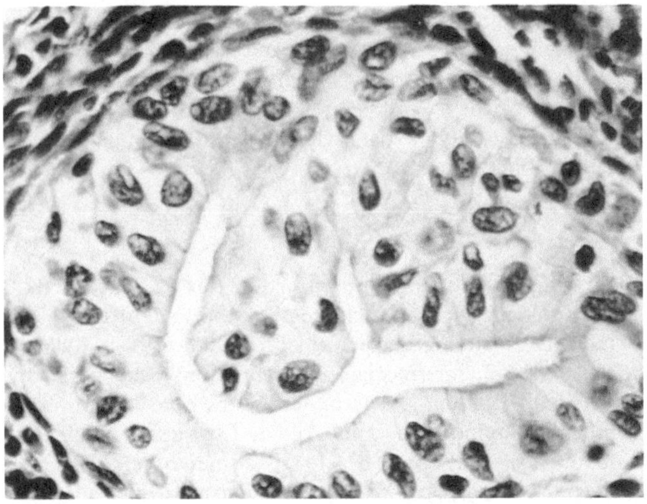

**Figure 32.4** Severely atypical hyperplasia (complex) of the endometrium with marked irregularity of nuclei (×720). (From Welch WR, Scully RE. Precancerous lesions of the endometrium. *Hum Pathol.* 1977;8:503.)

## DIAGNOSIS AND ENDOMETRIAL SAMPLING

Abnormal vaginal bleeding is the most frequent symptom of endometrial hyperplasia. In younger patients, hyperplasia may develop during anovulatory cycles and may even be detected after prolonged periods of oligomenorrhea or amenorrhea. It can occur at any time during the reproductive years but is most common with abnormal bleeding in the perimenopausal period. Premenopausal women with irregular vaginal bleeding and postmenopausal women with any vaginal bleeding should be evaluated with an office endometrial sampling or a D&C. The office sampling instruments, such as a thin plastic Pipelle, are introduced through the cervical os into the endometrial cavity and can provide very accurate information (see Chapter 10). Many patients tolerate office endometrial sampling without an analgesic agent, but paracervical block can be an effective anesthetic aid, particularly in nulliparous women. Some patients benefit from an oral nonsteroidal antiinflammatory drug taken approximately 30 minutes before biopsy.

Transvaginal ultrasonography has been evaluated as an adjunct for the diagnosis of endometrial hyperplasia and cancer. These studies have been performed in different populations, including asymptomatic postmenopausal women, women taking tamoxifen, and women presenting with postmenopausal bleeding. Langer and associates, in a study of 448 asymptomatic postmenopausal women, found a threshold of 5-mm endometrial thickness had only a 9% predictive value for detecting endometrial abnormalities (Langer, 1997). Its greater use was eliminating the diagnosis of neoplasia for those with thickness less than 5 mm (negative predictive value of 99%). These findings were confirmed in a literature review by Smith-Bindman and colleagues, who found that 96% of women with carcinoma had an abnormal ultrasound scan (endometrial thickness >5 mm). Conversely, 8% of postmenopausal women with an abnormal scan had no histologic abnormality, and the percentage grew to 23% for those on hormone replacement therapy. However, both of these studies were conducted in postmenopausal asymptomatic women.

Cecchini and coworkers performed biopsies on 108 postmenopausal patients on long-term tamoxifen with endometrial

**Table 32.2** Endometrial Hyperplasia Follow-up

| Type | Number of Patients | Age Range (Mean) | Regressed* | Progressed to Carcinoma: No. of Cases | Progressed to Carcinoma: Mean (Years) | Follow-up (Years) |
|---|---|---|---|---|---|---|
| Simple hyperplasia† pregnancies | 93 | 17-71 (42) | 74 (80%) | 1 | 11 | 1-26.7 |
| Complex hyperplasia‡ pregnancies | 29 | 20-67 (39) | 23 (79%) | 1 | 8.3 | 2-26 |
| Atypical hyperplasia pregnancies | 48 | 20-70 (40) | 28 (58%) | 11 | 4.1 | 1-25 |
| Atypical simple hyperplasia | 13 | | 9 | 1 | | |
| Atypical complex hyperplasia | 35 | | 20 | 10 | | |

Modifed from Kurman RJ, Kaminski PF, Norris HJ. *Cancer* 1985;56:403; and Kurman RJ, Norris HJ. Endometrial hyperplasia and related cellular changes. In: *Blaustein's Pathology of the Female Genital Tract*. 4th ed. New York: Springer-Verlag; 1994.

*A total of 34 patients with simple hyperplasia, 7 with complex hyperplasia and 15 with atypical hyperplasia, had no further therapy.

†Benign proliferation of the glands.

‡Greater crowding of glands, no cytologic atypia present.

thickness greater than 6 mm. One case of hyperplasia and one of carcinoma were found, and most patients had atrophic endometrium. The authors concluded that the false-positive rate of transvaginal ultrasonography in this population was too high to warrant its use as a screening modality, and they recommended using irregular vaginal bleeding as an indication for endometrial sampling (Cecchini, 1996). Similarly, Love and associates found that endometrial thickness is not necessarily a useful guide for biopsy in tamoxifen. In the study by Barakat and colleagues, routine screening with transvaginal ultrasonography was not of value, and they concluded that sampling should be done if the patient experiences bleeding.

In postmenopausal women with any vaginal bleeding, Gull and colleagues found that an endometrial stripe of less than 4 mm had a 100% negative predictive value (Gull, 2000). A finding of endometrial thickness less than 4 mm is a reasonable predictor of lack of endometrial pathology, even in a postmenopausal patient with bleeding. However, persistent vaginal bleeding should lead to endometrial sampling regardless of the ultrasound findings.

Endometrial ablation is sometimes undertaken to control severe uterine bleeding (see Chapter 26). However, pathologic evaluation of the endometrium should be performed before ablation in order to rule out an underlying endometrial hyperplasia or cancer.

### MANAGEMENT

The therapy employed for endometrial hyperplasia depends on the patient's age and the degree of atypia. For women with simple hyperplasia or complex hyperplasia without atypia, the risk of developing endometrial cancer is low, 1% and 3%, respectively. A diagnostic D&C can also be therapeutic, and progestins or combination oral contraceptive agents will likely be effective.

For complex atypical hyperplasia, the risk of developing endometrial cancer may be 29%, and, as stated previously, a concurrent endometrial cancer may be present. Women who desire preservation of childbearing function are treated with high-dose progestin therapy, usually megestrol acetate 40 mg three times daily to four times daily. The patient should have long-term follow-up and periodic sampling, the first at 3 months and at least every 6 months thereafter (Fig. 32.5, *A*). In these patients, the risk factors that led to the development of complex atypical hyperplasia are likely to remain. Therefore once the complex atypical hyperplasia is cleared, consideration should be given to periodic progestin treatment or oral contraception until the patient chooses to attempt pregnancy.

For older patients with complex atypical hyperplasia, the risk of carcinoma may be increased. Kurman and associates studied the uteri of patients after curettage had been performed, and atypical hyperplasia was found in the curettings. In their study, 11% of those younger than age 35, 12% of those 36 to 54, and 28% of those older than age 55 with atypical hyperplasia were found to have carcinoma in their uterus. Thus in older patients with moderate or severe atypical hyperplasia generally a hysterectomy is recommended. In addition, those who fail progestin therapy and especially those with severe cytologic atypia should also be considered for hysterectomy (see Fig. 32.5, *B*). If hysterectomy is not medically advisable, long-term high-dose progestin therapy can be used (megestrol acetate 160 mg/day or its equivalent depending on the endometrial response). Studies are being performed to evaluate the role of the progesterone containing intrauterine device. Periodic sampling of the endometrium is also performed. Figure 32.5 displays a flowchart guide to the management of endometrial hyperplasia. It is important to emphasize that the diagnoses are not distinct and these proliferative disorders are a continuum from mild abnormalities to malignant change.

## ENDOMETRIAL CARCINOMA

### SYMPTOMS, SIGNS, AND DIAGNOSIS

Postmenopausal bleeding, abnormal premenopausal bleeding, and perimenopausal bleeding are the primary symptoms of endometrial carcinoma. The diagnosis of endometrial carcinoma is established by histologic examination of the endometrium. Initial diagnosis can frequently be made on an outpatient basis, with an office endometrial biopsy. If endometrial carcinoma is found, endocervical curettage may be performed to rule out invasion of the endocervix. A routine cytologic examination (Pap smear) from the exocervix, which screens for cervical neoplasia, detects endometrial carcinoma in only approximately 50% of the cases.

If adequate outpatient evaluation cannot be obtained or if the diagnosis or cause of the abnormal bleeding is not clear from the tissue obtained, a hysteroscopy and fractional D&C should be performed. The endocervix is first sampled to rule out cervical involvement by endometrial cancer, hysteroscopy is done to visualize the endometrial cavity, and then a complete uterine curettage is performed.

### HISTOLOGIC TYPES

The various histologic types are listed in Box 32.2. Figure 32.6 illustrates typical adenocarcinomas of the endometrium and demonstrates varying degrees of differentiation (G1, well differentiated; G2, intermediate differentiation; G3, poorly differentiated). Grading is determined by the percentage of solid components found in the tumor: grade 1 has less than 5% solid components, grade 2 has 6% to 50% solid components, and grade 3 has more than 50% solid components.

Squamous epithelium commonly coexists with the glandular elements of endometrial carcinoma. Previously, the term *adenoacanthoma* was used to describe a well-differentiated tumor and *adenosquamous carcinoma* to describe a poorly differentiated carcinoma with squamous elements. More recently, the term *adenocarcinoma with squamous elements* has been used with a description of the degree of differentiation of both the glandular and squamous components. Zaino and colleagues, in a Gynecologic Oncology Group (GOG) study of 456 cases with squamous elements, showed that prognosis was related to the grade of the glandular component and the degree of myometrial invasion. They suggested the term *adenocarcinoma with squamous differentiation*, and this has been generally adopted.

Uterine serous carcinomas are a highly virulent and a less common histologic subtype of endometrial carcinomas (5% to 10%). These tumors histologically resemble papillary serous carcinomas of the ovary (Fig. 32.7). Slomovitz and associates evaluated 129 patients with uterine serous carcinoma (USC) and found a high rate of extrauterine disease even in cases without myometrial invasion (Slomovitz, 2003). They recommended a thorough operative staging (see next section) in all cases of these tumors because of the high risk of extrauterine disease even in cases admixed with other histologic types (endometrial or clear cell).

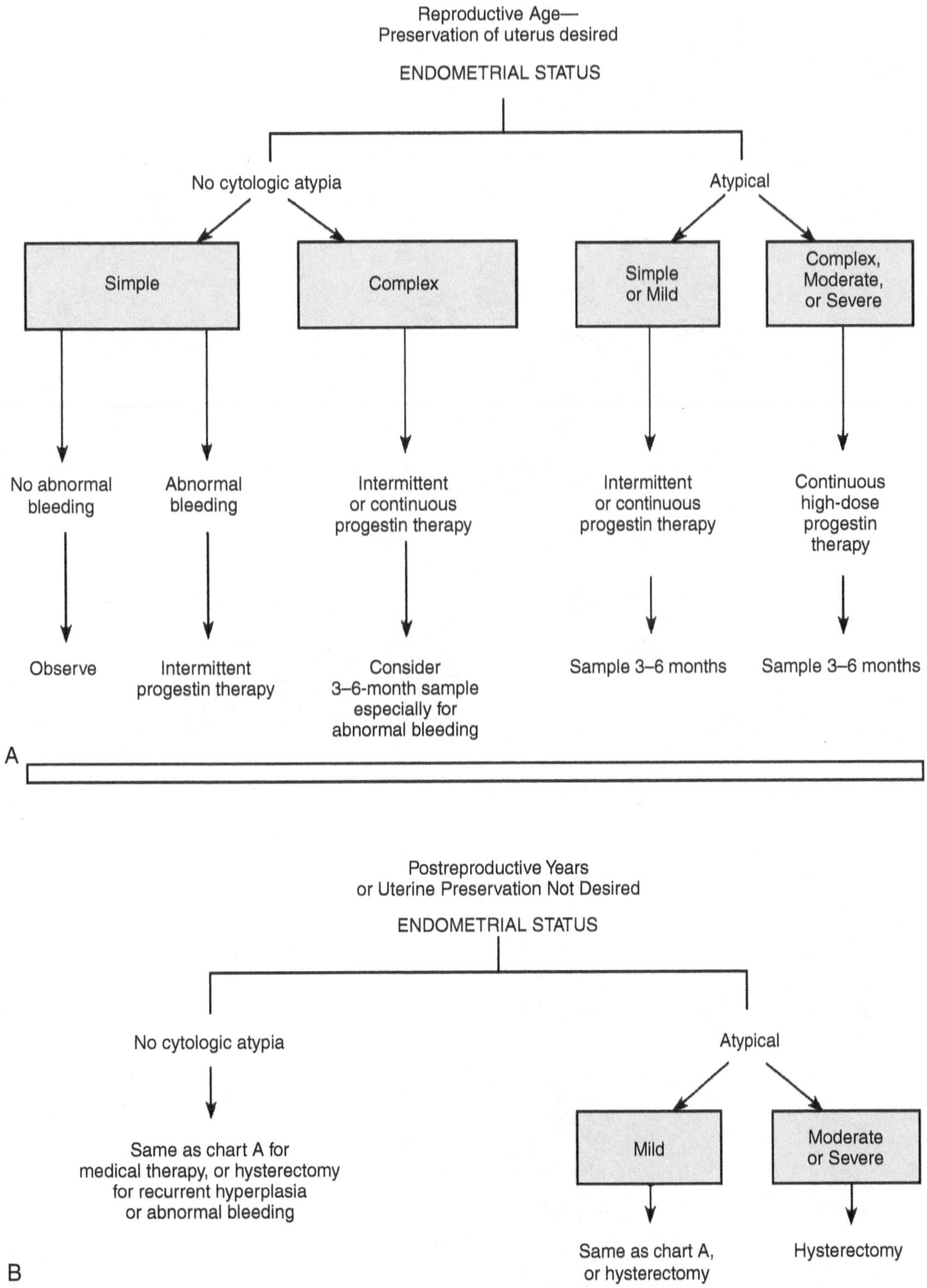


**Figure 32.5** Schematic diagram of endometrial hyperplasia management for reproductive (**A**) and postreproductive (**B**) patients.

**Box 32.2 Endometrial Primary Adenocarcinomas**

Typical endometrioid adenocarcinoma
Adenocarcinoma with squamous elements*
Clear cell carcinoma
Serous carcinoma
Secretory carcinoma
Mucinous carcinoma
Squamous carcinoma

*Previously termed *adenoacanthoma* or *adenosquamous carcinoma*.

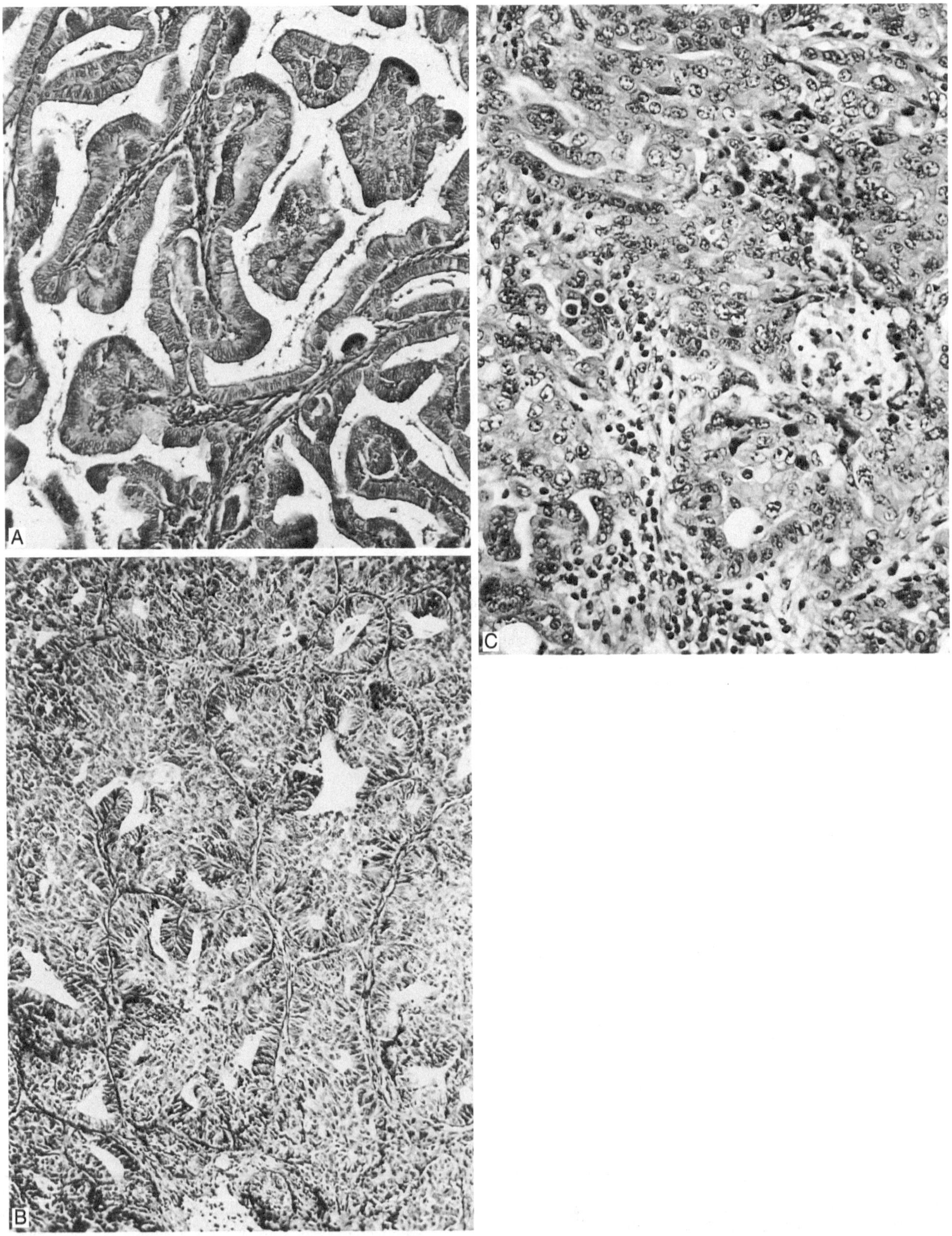


**Figure 32.6** **A,** Well-differentiated adenocarcinoma of the endometrium. The glands are confluent (×130). **B,** Moderately differentiated adenocarcinoma of the endometrium. The glands are more solid, but some lumens remain (×100). **C,** Poorly differentiated adenocarcinoma of the endometrium. The epithelium shows solid proliferation with only a rare lumen (×100). (From Kurman RJ, Norris HJ. Endometrial neoplasia: hyperplasia and carcinoma. In: Blaustein A, ed. *Pathology of the Female Genital Tract.* 2nd ed. New York: Springer-Verlag; 1982.)

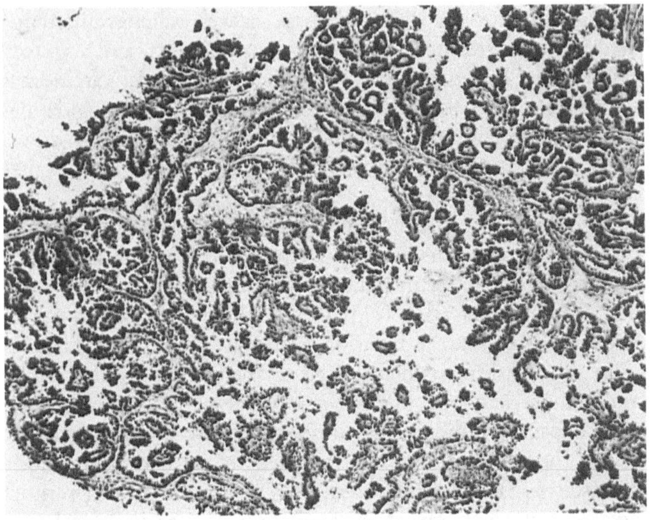

**Figure 32.7** Serous carcinoma characterized by a complex papillary architecture resembling serous carcinoma of the ovary. (From Kurman RJ. *Blaustein's Pathology of the Female Genital Tract.* 3rd ed. New York: Springer-Verlag; 1987.)

Clear-cell carcinomas of the endometrium are less common (<5%). Histologically, they resemble clear-cell adenocarcinomas of the ovary, cervix, and vagina. Clear-cell tumors tend to develop in postmenopausal women and carry a prognosis much worse than typical endometrial adenocarcinomas. Survival rates of 39% to 55% have been reported, much less than the 65% or better usually recorded for endometrial carcinoma. Abeler and Kjorstad reviewed 97 cases and noted the best prognosis (90%) for those without myometrial invasion. Patients whose tumors had vascular invasion experienced a 15% 5-year survival (Abeler, 1991). Carcangiu and Chambers reviewed 29 cases and found 5-year survival rates for stages I and II of 72% and 59%, respectively (Carcangiu, 1995).

## STAGING

In 2009, a revised International Federation of Gynecology and Obstetrics (FIGO) surgical staging classification was introduced (Table 32.3). The surgical staging was modified to better define clinically relevant risk strata based on the FIGO annual report and other supporting publications.

## PROGNOSTIC FACTORS

Many variables affect the behavior of endometrial adenocarcinomas. These variables can be conveniently divided into clinical and pathologic factors. The clinical determinants are patient age at diagnosis, race, and clinical tumor stage. The pathologic determinants are tumor grade, histologic type, tumor size, depth of myometrial invasion, microscopic involvement of vascular spaces in the uterus by tumor, and spread of tumor outside the uterus to the retroperitoneal lymph nodes, peritoneal cavity, or uterine adnexa.

## CLINICAL FACTORS

Older patients have tumors of a higher stage and grade when compared to younger patients. White patients have a higher survival rate than black patients, a finding partially explained by higher-stage and higher-grade tumors among black women. In addition, black women are more likely to develop uterine serous cancers. The 10-year survival of 136 black patients in the series of Aziz and coworkers was 40% compared with 72% for 135 white patients.

Table 32.3 Revised FIGO Staging for Endometrial Cancer (Adopted 2009)

| Stages* | Characteristic |
|---|---|
| I | Tumor confined to the corpus uteri |
| IA | No or less than half myometrial invasion |
| IB | Invasion equal to or more than half of the myometrium |
| II | Tumor invades cervical stroma but does not extend beyond the uterus† |
| III | Local or regional spread of the tumor |
| IIIA | Tumor invades serosa of the corpus uteri or the adnexa‡ |
| IIIB | Vaginal or parametrial involvement‡ |
| IIIC | Metastases to pelvic or paraaortic lymph nodes‡ |
| IIIC1 | Positive pelvic nodes |
| IIIC2 | Positive paraaortic lymph nodes with or without positive pelvic lymph nodes |
| IV | Tumor invades bladder or bowel mucosa, or distant metastasis |
| IVA* | Tumor invasion of bladder or bowel mucosa |
| IVB | Distant metastases, including intraabdominal or inguinal lymph nodes |

*G1, G2, or G3.
†Endocervical glandular involvement only should be considered as stage I and no longer as stage II.
‡Positive cytology has to be reported separately without changing the stage.

Table 32.4 Carcinoma of the Corpus Uteri: Patients Treated in 1990-1992: Survival by 1988 FIGO Surgical Stage, *N* = 5562

| Stage | 5-Year Survival Rate |
|---|---|
| IA | 90.9% |
| IB | 88.2% |
| IC | 81.0% |
| II | 71.6% |
| III | 51.4% |
| IV | 8.9% |

Modified from Pecorelli S, Creasman WT, Pettersson F, et al. FIGO annual report on the results of treatment in gynaecological cancer. Milano, Italy. *J Epidemiol Biostat.* 1998;23.

## PATHOLOGIC FACTORS

Tumor stage is a well-recognized prognostic factor for endometrial carcinoma (Table 32.4). Fortunately, most cases are diagnosed in stage I, which provides a favorable prognosis.

The histologic grade of the tumor is a major determinant of prognosis. Endometrial carcinomas are divided into three grades: grade 1, well differentiated; grade 2, intermediate differentiation; and grade 3, poorly differentiated. Figure 32.8 shows the survival of 895 patients studied by the GOG that relates endometrial carcinoma survival to tumor grade and demonstrates the worsening of prognosis with advancing grade.

The histologic type of the endometrial carcinoma (Fig. 32.9) is also related to prognosis, with the best prognosis associated

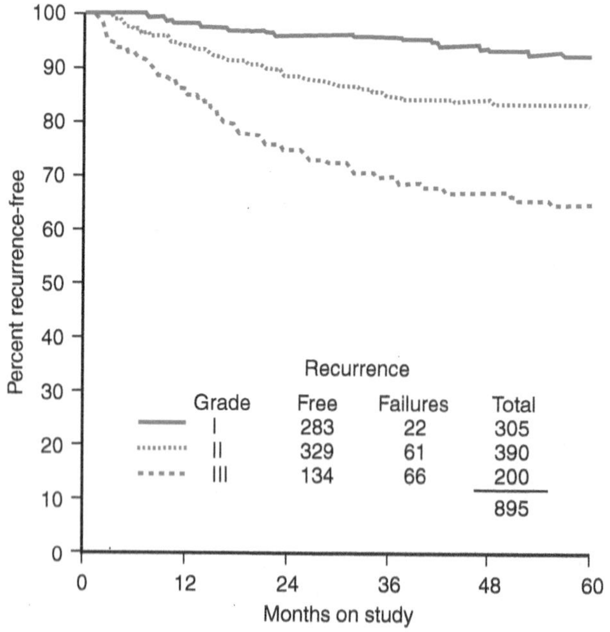


**Figure 32.8** Recurrence-free interval by histologic grade. (Modified from Morrow CP, Bundy BN, Kurman RJ, et al. Relationship between surgical-pathologic risk factors and outcome in clinical stage I and II carcinoma of the endometrium: a Gynecologic Oncology Group study. *Gynecol Oncol.* 1991;40:55.)

with endometrioid adenocarcinomas, as well as better differentiated tumors with or without squamous elements, and secretory carcinomas. Approximately 80% of all endometrial carcinomas fall into the favorable category. Poor prognostic histologic types are serous carcinomas, clear-cell carcinomas, and poorly differentiated carcinomas with or without squamous elements, as previously noted.

The degree of myometrial invasion correlates with the risk of tumor spread outside the uterus, but the higher grade and higher stage tumors in general are more likely to have deep myometrial penetration (Fig. 32.10). The importance of tumor grade and myometrial invasion is also illustrated by a study of their relationship to their spread to the retroperitoneal pelvic and paraaortic lymph nodes. Studies of 142 patients by Schink and colleagues indicate that tumor size is also prognostic. Only 4% of those with tumors 2 cm or less in size had lymph node metastases. The rate increased to 15% for those with tumors greater than 2 cm to 35% when the entire endometrial cavity was involved (Schink, 1991). Table 32.5 summarizes the clinical and pathologic factors affecting outcome in early stage tumors. Peritoneal cytology has been studied as a prognostic factor, and the results are conflicting. In a study of 567 surgical stage I cases, Turner and associates found that positive peritoneal cytology was an independent prognostic factor. In contrast, Grimshaw and coworkers evaluated 322 clinical stage I cases and found that positive peritoneal cytology was an

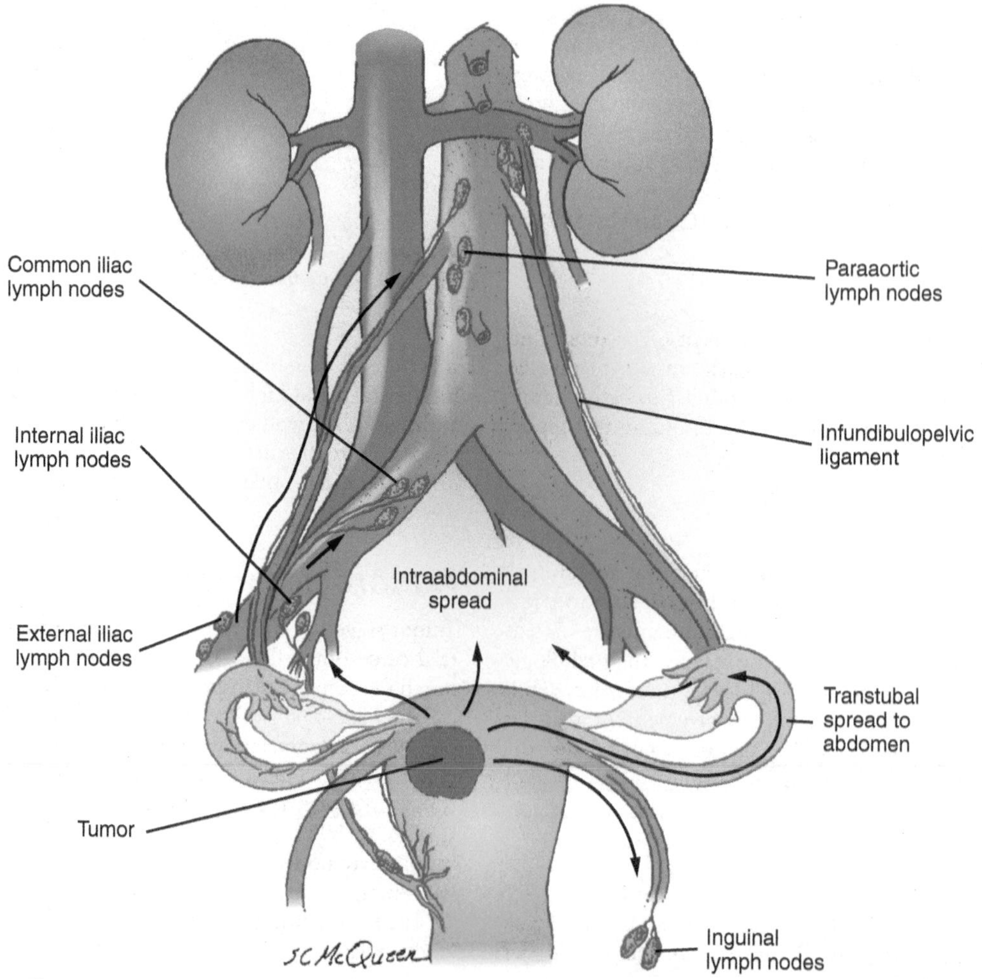


**Figure 32.9** Spread of Endometrial Carcinoma. The major pathways of tumor spread are illustrated (see text).

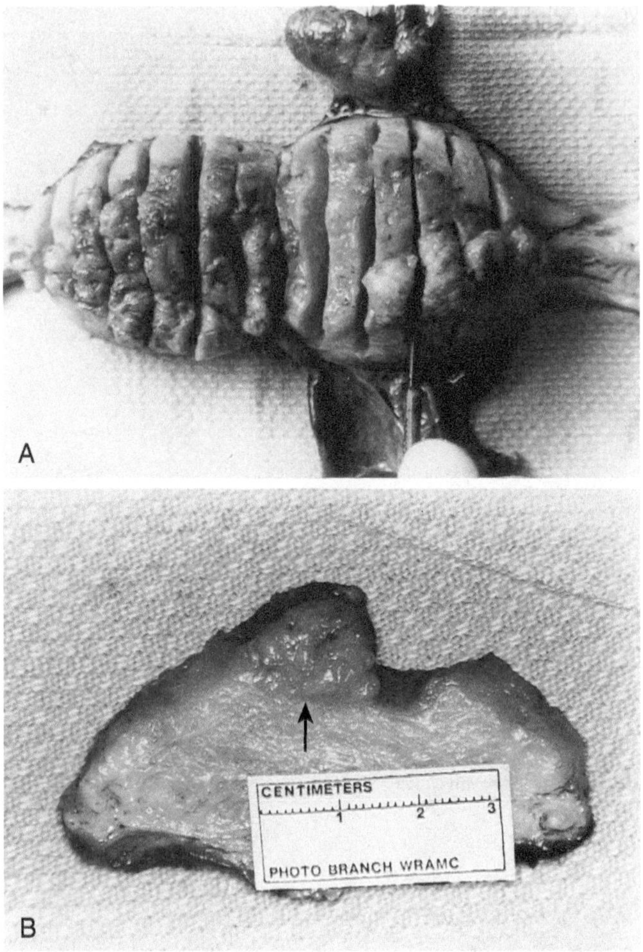


**Figure 32.10** **A,** Technique for intraoperative assessment of the depth of myometrial invasion. **B,** Cross section of uterine wall demonstrating superficial myometrial invasion. *Arrow* shows the tumor-myometrial junction. (From Doering DL, Barnhill DR, Weiser EB, et al. Intraoperative evaluation of depth of myometrial invasion in stage I endometrial adenocarcinoma. *Obstet Gynecol.* 1989;74:930.)

adverse prognostic factor, but they did not find it to be an independent risk factor when other variables were considered. More recently, Kadar and associates and Lurain and colleagues noted that positive peritoneal cytology was associated primarily with adverse features such as extrauterine disease and that therapy (see the following discussion) for positive peritoneal cytology as an isolated finding did not appear to improve survival. In the revised FIGO surgical staging (2009), positive cytology is no longer classified as stage IIIA.

### Patterns of Spread of Endometrial Carcinoma

Plentl and Friedman noted four major channels of lymphatic drainage from the uterus that serve as sites for extrauterine spread of tumor: (1) a small lymphatic branch along the round ligament that runs to the inguinal femoral nodes, (2) branches from the tubal and (3) ovarian pedicles (infundibulopelvic ligaments), which are large lymphatics that drain into the paraaortic nodes, and (4) the broad ligament lymphatics that drain directly to the pelvic nodes. The pelvic and paraaortic node drainage sites (2, 3, and 4) are the most important clinically. In addition, direct peritoneal spread of tumor can occur through the uterine wall or via the lumen of the fallopian tube. Clinically, therefore the clinician must assess the retroperitoneal nodes, the peritoneal cavity, and the uterine adnexa for the spread of endometrial carcinoma (see Fig. 32.9).

Extensive studies by the GOG have elucidated both the frequency of lymph node metastases in endometrial carcinoma and the pathologic factors that modify this risk in stage I disease. Tumor grade, size of the uterus, and degree of myometrial invasion were studied (Creasman, 1999). Table 32.6 illustrates the frequency of lymph node metastases according to uterine size and tumor grade. There are differences in the proportion of positive nodes between stages IB and IA (pre-1988 staging) cases as well as tumor grade. Table 32.7 shows the effects of tumor grade and depth of myometrial invasion. The frequency of nodal involvement becomes much greater with higher-grade tumors and with greater depth of myometrial invasion. The risk of lymph node involvement appears to be negligible for endometrial carcinoma involving only the endometrium. With invasion of the inner third of the myometrium, there is negligible risk of node involvement for grade 1 and 2 cases. If the outer third of the myometrium is involved, the risk of nodal metastases is greatly increased. These data emphasize the importance of myometrial invasion and tumor spread, providing the basis for the FIGO Surgical Staging System. Table 32.8 summarizes the risk of nodal metastases based on the GOG studies published by Creasman and colleagues. In a more recent GOG study cited previously, Morrow and coworkers noted that for patients without metastases at operation, the greatest risk of future recurrence was grade 3 histology. Furthermore, among 48 patients with histologically documented aortic node metastases, 47 were found to have positive pelvic nodes, adnexal metastases, or tumor invasion to the outer one third of the myometrium, emphasizing the poor prognostic aspects of these three findings. Mariani and colleagues at the Mayo Clinic found that tumor size can also be incorporated into a staging paradigm to identify patients at highest risk for nodal spread. They found that in grade 1 and 2 tumors with less than 50% invasion and tumor size less than 2 cm, the risk of lymph node involvement was virtually none (Mariani 2000a).

## EVALUATION

In addition to the usual routine preoperative evaluation, the patient should have a chest radiographic examination or a chest and abdominal pelvic computed tomography scan. However, a study by Connor and associates noted that preoperative computed tomography scan had only a 50% positive predictive value for nodal disease. Furthermore, postoperative computed tomography monitoring did not appear to improve survival. The measurement of cancer antigen 125 (CA 125), usually used in cases of ovarian carcinoma, may occasionally be useful. An elevated CA125 preoperatively can often indicate extrauterine disease (Sood, 1997). It may be a particularly useful marker for those with serous carcinoma of the endometrium.

## MANAGEMENT

### Stage I

Surgery is the primary treatment modality for patients with endometrial carcinoma. Complete surgical staging includes hysterectomy with or without bilateral salpingo-oophorectomy,

Table 32.5 Surgical Stage I and II Tumors: The Proportional Hazards Modeling of Relative Survival Time

| Variable | Regression Coefficient | Relative Risk | Significance Test* (*P* value) |
|---|---|---|---|
| **Endometrioid** | | | |
| Grade 1 | — | 1.0 | — |
| Grade 2 | 0.28 | 1.3 | 2.7 (0.1) |
| Grade 3 | 0.56 | 1.8 | |
| **Endometrioid with Squamous Differentiation** | | | 0.1 (0.7) |
| Grade 1 | 0.20 | 1.2 | |
| Grade 2 | -0.01 | 1.0 | 0.3 (0.6) |
| Grade 3 | 0.22 | 0.8 | |
| **Villoglandular** | | | 2.2 (0.1) |
| Grade 1 | -4.91 | 0.01 | |
| Grade 2 | -0.59 | 0.5 | 10.4 (0.001) |
| Grade 3 | 3.73 | 41.9 | |
| **Myometrial Invasion** | | | |
| Endometrium only | — | 1.0 | |
| Superficial | 0.39 | 0.5 | |
| Middle | 1.20 | 3.3 | 19.6 (0.0002) |
| Deep | 1.53 | 4.6 | |
| Age | 0.17 | — | |
| $Age^2$ | -0.000837 | — | 20.7 (0.0001) |
| 45 (arbitrary reference) | — | 1.0 | |
| 55 | 0.85 | 2.3 | |
| 65 | 1.52 | 4.6 | |
| 75 | 2.03 | 7.6 | |
| Vascular space involvement | 0.32 | 1.4 | 1.2 (0.3) |

Modified from Zaino RJ, Kurman RJ, Diana KL, Morrow CP. Pathologic models to predict outcome for women with endometrial adenocarcinoma. *Cancer.* 1996;77:1115.
*P* value for grading is for overall grade within cell type.
*Wald $x^2$ test.

Table 32.6 Grade, Depth of Myometrial Invasion, and Node Metastasis: Stage I

| Depth of Invasion | G1 *n* = 180 | G2 *n* = 288 | G3 *n* = 153 |
|---|---|---|---|
| **Pelvic** | | | |
| Endometrium only (*n* = 86) | 0 (0%) | 1 (3%) | 0 (0%) |
| Inner (*n* = 281) | 3 (3%) | 7 (5%) | 5 (9%) |
| Middle (*n* = 115) | 0 (0%) | 6 (9%) | 1 (4%) |
| Deep (*n* = 139) | 2 (11%) | 11 (19%) | 23 (34%) |
| **Aortic** | | | |
| Endometrium only (*n* = 86) | 0 (0%) | 1 (3%) | 0 (0%) |
| Inner (*n* = 281) | 1 (1%) | 5 (4%) | 2 (4%) |
| Middle (*n* = 115) | 1 (5%) | 0 (0%) | 0 (0%) |
| Deep (*n* = 139) | 1 (6%) | 8 (14%) | 15 (23%) |

Modified from Creasman WT, Morrow CP, Bundy BN, et al: Surgical pathologic spread patterns of endometrial cancer. *Cancer.* 1987;60:2035.
*G*, Grade.

Table 32.7 FIGO Staging and Nodal Metastasis

| | Metastasis | |
|---|---|---|
| **Staging** | **Pelvic** | **Aortic** |
| IA G1 (*n* = 101) | 2 (2%) | 0 (0%) |
| G2 (*n* = 169) | 13 (8%) | 6 (4%) |
| G3 (*n* = 76) | 8 (11%) | 5 (7%) |
| IB G1 (*n* = 79) | 3 (4%) | 3 (4%) |
| G2 (*n* = 119) | 12 (10%) | 8 (7%) |
| G3 (*n* = 77) | 20 (26%) | 12 (16%) |

From Creasman WT, Morrow CP, Bundy BN, et al. Surgical pathologic spread patterns of endometrial cancer. *Cancer.* 1987;60:2035.
*FIGO*, International Federation of Gynecology and Oncology; *G*, grade.

Table 32.8 Risk Factors for Nodal Metastases: Stage I

| Factor | Pelvic | Aortic |
|---|---|---|
| **Low Risk**<br>Grade 1<br>Endometrium only<br>No intraperitoneal spread | 0/44 (0%) | 0/44 (0%) |
| **Moderate Risk**<br>Grade 2 or 3<br>Invasion to middle third | 15/268 (6%) | 6/268 (2%) |
| **High Risk**<br>Invasion to outer third | 21/116 (18%) | 17/118 (15%) |

Modified from Creasman WT, Morrow CP, Bundy BN, et al. Surgical pathologic spread patterns of endometrial cancer. *Cancer.* 1987;60:2035.

and pelvic and paraaortic lymphadenectomy. According to Orr and Chamberlin, the exceptions include women with significant medical comorbidities and young, premenopausal women who desire future fertility with grade 1 endometrial adenocarcinoma associated with endometrial hyperplasia.

Surgical staging allows accurate surgical and histologic assessment of (1) tumor spread within the uterus, (2) degree of penetration into the myometrium, and (3) extrauterine spread to retroperitoneal nodes, adnexa, or the peritoneal cavity. This approach is used for cases that are staged according to the 2009 FIGO system (see Table 32.3).

Minimally invasive surgery in the treatment of early stage endometrial cancer has become standard of care. The GOG published a phase III randomized trial of surgical staging for

Table 32.9 Summary of Randomized Trials of Adjuvant Radiotherapy in Stage I Endometrial Carcinoma

| Trial | Surgery | Randomization | Locoregional Recurrences | Survival |
|---|---|---|---|---|
| Norwegian 1968-1974 | TAH-BSO | Brachytherapy vs. brachy and pelvic RT | 7% vs. 2% at 5 years, $P < .01$ | 89% vs. 91% at 5 years, $P$ = NS |
| PORTEC | TAH-BSO | Obs vs. pelvic RT | 14% vs. 4% at 5 years, $P < 0.001$ | 85% vs. 81% at 5 years, $P = .31$ |
| GOG | TAH-BSO, nodes | Obs vs. pelvic RT | 12% vs. 3% at 2 years, $P < .01$ | 86% vs. 92% at 4 years, $P = .56$ |

*GOG*, Gynecologic Oncology Group; *PORTEC*, Post Operative Radiation Therapy in Endometrial Carcinoma; *TAH-BSO*, total abdominal hysterectomy-bilateral salpingo oophorectomy; *Obs*, Obstetric; *RT*, radiotherapy.

endometrial car cinoma comparing the laparoscopic approach to the more traditional abdominal approach (Walker, 2009). The pathologic outcomes were the same, and a majority of patients in the laparoscopy arm were able to have the surgery completed. There were some benefits in the minimally invasive arm, including shorter hospital stay and improved quality of life in the postoperative period. Minimally invasive surgery can be used particularly for patients who are incompletely staged at the time of initial operation and require a second staging procedure.

The role of sentinel lymph node (SLN) mapping in the staging of endometrial cancer is currently being defined. The use of SLN could potentially maximize the identification of positive lymph nodes while minimizing the risks of full lymphadenectomy. A number of studies have described SLN detection rates as greater than 80% for any SLN and greater than 50% for bilateral sentinel lymph nodes (Barlin, 2012). Several authors have shown high sensitivity and a high negative predictive value. Although the data are promising, validation studies that require a comprehensive surgical staging are ongoing.

For patients with significant medical comorbidities, radiation therapy alone can be used. However, radiation as the sole method of therapy yields inferior results, as Bickenbach and colleagues noted, with an 87% 5-year survival rate for patients with stage I carcinoma treated by surgery alone, in comparison with a 69% survival rate for those treated with radiation therapy alone. For those who cannot tolerate surgery or external beam therapy, treatment by intracavitary radiation alone offers some benefit. Lehoczky and associates reported on 170 elderly patients treated with brachytherapy alone with uncorrected 5-year survival rates for stages IA and IB of 46% and 30%, respectively. For patients with grade 1 cancers, progesterone therapy could also be considered if patients are not medically fit for surgery or radiation therapy.

Occasionally, morbidly obese patients are encountered for whom an abdominal operation is risky. Sood and coworkers noted that for stage I patients with preoperative CA 125 less than 20 U/mL, the risk of extrauterine disease was only 3%, making vaginal hysterectomy a therapeutic option. Dotters reported CA 125 more than 35 U/mL usually predicted extrauterine disease, although approximately one third of patients needing full operative staging were not identified by an elevated CA 125 for grade 1 or 2 cases, whereas for grade 3, the sensitivity increased to 88%. However, a few false positive cases were noted, making the results a useful guide but not sufficiently precise to be the sole criterion for performing lymphadenectomy.

### Stage I, Grade 1

The risk of spread of a grade 1 tumor to pelvic nodes is extremely small (see Table 32.7). At the time of surgery, the abdomen is explored, peritoneal cytology is obtained, and an extrafascial total abdominal hysterectomy with bilateral salpingo-oophorectomy is performed. Pelvic and paraaortic lymph node dissection should be considered in cases at risk for lymph node involvement. In patients with stage I, grade 1 tumors, postoperative radiation (vaginal brachytherapy or external beam irradiation) may be considered if there is deep myometrial invasion.

### Stage I, Grades 2 and 3

Patients considered at risk of lymph node involvement (grade 1/2 tumors greater than 2 cm in size and any grade 3 tumor) should undergo complete surgical staging. Mariani and coworkers reported improved survival in patients at high risk of nodal disease who underwent paraaortic lymphadenectomy in compared with those who did not have this procedure. Use of postoperative irradiation depends on the pathologic findings (Mariani, 2000b).

Three phase III randomized trials evaluating the use of adjuvant radiotherapy in patients with high-risk stage I endometrial cancer have shown no improvement in overall survival (Table 32.9). In a Norwegian study comparing brachytherapy to brachytherapy and pelvic radiation, local recurrences were decreased in the group of patients receiving pelvic radiation. In the Post Operative Radiation Therapy in Endometrial Carcinoma (PORTEC) trial from The Netherlands, Creutzberg and colleagues reported on 714 patients with presumed stage I disease (Creutzberg, 2000). Patients received full pelvic radiotherapy or observation. Although locoregional control was better in the treatment arm, there was no difference in overall survival. In a GOG trial, Keys and associates randomized almost 400 patients who underwent complete surgical staging to whole pelvic radiation versus observation. Similar to the PORTEC trial, there was a decrease in local recurrences in the radiation arm with no difference in overall survival (Keys, 2004).

## *Stage II*

Three therapeutic options have been employed for the treatment of stage II carcinoma of the endometrium that also involves the endocervix: (1) primary operation (radical hysterectomy and pelvic and paraaortic lymph node dissection), (2) primary radiation (intrauterine and vaginal implant and external irradiation) followed by an operation (extrafascial hysterectomy), and (3) simple hysterectomy followed by external beam irradiation.

Radical hysterectomy and pelvic dissection have been used as effective therapy. Mariani and colleagues reported on 57 patients with endocervical involvement at the time of diagnosis (Mariani, 2001). Of these, 61% underwent radical hysterectomy and staging. There were no recurrences in the radical hysterectomy group if their nodes were negative at the time of surgery. Five-year disease-related survival and recurrence-free survival in the radical hysterectomy patients were 76% and 71%.

Another option for patients with stage II carcinoma of the endometrium is treatment with a combination of radiation and extrafascial hysterectomy. A protocol includes external radiation (45 Gy) and a single brachytherapy implant usually followed by extrafascial total abdominal hysterectomy, bilateral salpingo-oophorectomy, and paraaortic node sampling. Podczaski and coworkers noted that those with gross cervical tumor had a poor prognosis and were likely to have extrauterine disease at operation. For patients with cervical involvement on biopsy but no gross tumor, Trimble and Jones found radiation treatment by a single implant alone followed by a hysterectomy to be effective, and they added external therapy depending on the nodal findings and myometrial invasion. Andersen reported on 54 patients with stage II tumors and found a 70.6% survival rate in patients treated by abdominal hysterectomy followed by radiation.

Comparable outcomes have been reported using high-dose-rate brachytherapy approaches in stage I–II patients unable to undergo surgery. Nguygen and coworkers reported a 3-year disease-free survival rate of 85% in 36 stage I patients treated with definitive radiation therapy (Nguyen, 1998). Nineteen patients were considered inoperable due to morbid obesity, and the remainder had significant medical problems precluding anesthesia. All patients were treated as outpatients with five weekly Brach-therapy applications performed under conscious sedation. At a median follow-up of 32 months, the 3-year actuarial uterine-control rate was 88%.

### Adjuvant Systemic Therapy for Early Stage Endometrioid Endometrial Cancer

In addition to radiation therapy, adjuvant chemotherapy is being explored for patients with endometrial cancer and high-risk features. Although the addition of postoperative radiation to high-risk patients does reduce the local recurrence rate, distant metastasis continues to be problematic. In approximately 25% of patients with low-stage, grade 3 lesions, the disease will recur at a distant site. In addition, 20% of clinical stage II patients and at least 30% of patients who present with extrauterine disease recur at distant sites even after patients have received adjuvant pelvic radiation.

Adjuvant chemotherapy may also be useful in this group of patients. The Japanese GOG compared pelvic radiation to combination chemotherapy in high-risk early stage patients and found an improvement in both progression-free and overall survival in the chemotherapy arm. A GOG study evaluating the role of vaginal brachytherapy and chemotherapy versus pelvic radiation as adjuvant treatment in patients with high intermediate-risk disease recently completed accrual. Preliminary results show no difference in survival between the two treatment arms.

### *Stage I or II Uterine Serous Carcinoma*

The best treatment for early stage uterine serous cancers is still unknown. Even with minimal disease within the uterus, patients with USC often have extrauterine spread of disease. In a retrospective, multi-institutional study, Huh and associates reported on 60 patients with stage I USC who underwent comprehensive surgical staging. The investigators found that recurrence rates were lower than previously reported and inferred that complete staging may provide a potential benefit. In their study, none of the seven patients who received chemotherapy had a recurrence. In a multi-institutional retrospective study of early stage USC, Dietrich and colleagues found that the combination of carboplatin and paclitaxel in the adjuvant setting was effective in improving survival and limiting recurrences (Dietrich, 2005).

Combined chemotherapy and radiation therapy may play a role in the management of patients with early stage disease. Turner and associates reported the application of vaginal irradiation at a high-dose rate in combination with chemotherapy in surgical stage I patients. The 5-year survival rate was 94%, which is higher than that of most other studies for patients with stage I disease.

### *Management of Stage III/IV or Recurrent Endometrial Cancer*

Because of the hematogenous and lymphatic spread of endometrial cancer, patients with recurrent or advanced disease often present with tumor outside of the pelvis. Systemic therapy therefore plays an important role in the management of these patients. Both hormonal and cytotoxic agents have activity in patients with advanced or recurrent endometrial cancer. In addition, there continues to be a role of radiation therapy to obtain local control or to treat disease in the pelvis.

In stage III carcinoma, the disease has spread outside the uterus but remains confined to the pelvis or the retroperitoneal nodes. Patients with stage IIIA disease include those with disease spread to the adnexa or the serosa of the uterus. Stage IIIB involves the vagina and stage IIIC includes spread to the retroperitoneal lymph nodes. In the revised FIGO staging, stage IIIC has been further divided into those with positive pelvic nodes only (stage IIIC1) and those with positive paraaortic nodes (stage IIIC2). Stage III accounts for approximately 7% of all endometrial carcinomas and occur in patients who are older than those with lower stage tumors and often medically less able to undergo an operation. Adjuvant treatment is often a combination of tumor-directed radiation and systemic chemotherapy.

Approximately 3% of endometrial carcinomas are stage IV, and many of these patients have tumor metastases outside the pelvis. If possible, optimal surgical debulking has been associated with a prolonged survival. Bristow and coworkers reported that the amount of residual disease after cytoreductive surgery, age, and performance status appear to be important determinants of survival in patients with stage IVB endometrial carcinoma (Bristow, 2000).

Several chemotherapeutic agents or combinations have demonstrated activity in patients with endometrial cancer. Combination therapy is more effective than single-agent therapy in treating this disease. Doxorubicin was one of the first drugs identified with good activity against endometrial cancer. Single-agent doxorubicin has a response rate of approximately 25% with a median duration of response of less than 1 year. Single-agent cisplatin also has demonstrated response rates between 20% and 42% when used as a first-line agent. The duration of response was again very short (3 to 5 months). In several phase II studies, adding cisplatin to doxorubicin resulted in response rates between 45% and 60%. In a GOG randomized phase III study, cisplatin and doxorubicin in combination had a higher response rate compared with single-agent doxorubicin (45% versus 27%), but there was no difference in overall survival. The European Organisation for Research and Treatment of Cancer (EORTC) performed a similar trial comparing the same two regimens. Again, the combination arm had a higher response rate than doxorubicin alone. In this study, there was a modest survival advantage in those patients who received the combination regimen. The median overall survival in cisplatin- and doxorubicin-treated patients was 9 months compared with 7 months in the patients who received doxorubicin alone ($P = .065$).

Single agent paclitaxel has shown significant activity in chemo-naive patients with recurrent endometrial cancer with a response rate of 36%. The antitumor effect of single-agent paclitaxel led to the incorporation of paclitaxel into combination therapy regimens. In a phase II study, the combination of cisplatin and paclitaxel demonstrated a 67% response rate. In a phase III study, the GOG found similar activity between the combination of cisplatin and doxorubicin versus doxorubicin and paclitaxel. Following this study, the GOG performed a phase III trial evaluating doxorubicin and cisplatin compared with doxorubicin, cisplatin, and paclitaxel (TAP) with granulocyte-colony-stimulating factor (Miller, 2012). The TAP regimen yielded a superior response rate (57% versus 34%, $P < .001$), longer progression-free survival (8.3 versus 5.3 months, $P < .001$), and longer overall survival (15.3 versus 12.3 months, $P = .037$).

In an attempt to decrease the toxicity related to cisplatin therapy, carboplatin has been investigated. Single-agent carboplatin demonstrates modest activity in chemo-naive patients with little or no activity in patients pretreated with chemotherapy. In a phase II study, the combination of paclitaxel and carboplatin was evaluated in patients with advanced and recurrent disease. In patients with advanced endometrioid endometrial cancer, there was a 78% response rate to this combination. The median failure-free survival time was 23 months, and the 3-year overall survival rate was 62%. In patients with recurrent disease, the response rate was 56%, and the median failure-free interval was 6 months.

The combination of carboplatin and paclitaxel has a more favorable toxicity profile than TAP. The GOG completed accrual to a phase III randomized, noninferiority study to compare TAP with carboplatin and paclitaxel. The preliminary results showed that paclitaxel and carboplatin were not inferior to TAP in terms of progression-free and overall survival. As a result, paclitaxel and carboplatin are now considered first-line standard of care for advanced and recurrent endometrial cancer.

Prognosis is very poor for patients who fail first-line chemotherapy. The response rates for second- and third-line agents are often less than 10%, and the overall survival is less than 9 months. Paclitaxel may have better activity than other agents in this setting. In patients who have failed previous chemotherapy, paclitaxel has response rates up to 27%. In particular, in a cohort of patients who were refractory to platinum, paclitaxel was shown to have a 22% response rate. Preliminary data suggest that retreatment with a platinum/paclitaxel-based regimen may be effective in patients who previously responded to these agents. Clinical trials and in particular targeted therapies should be considered in women who fail first-line chemotherapy.

For patients with an isolated recurrence in the pelvis, radiotherapy can be useful. Ackerman and coworkers treated 21 patients with pelvic relapse and found radiation achieved pelvic control of disease in 14 (67%) (Ackerman, 1996). The best results were with recurrences in the vaginal mucosa. Similarly, Sears and colleagues treated 45 patients with vaginal recurrence of endometrial cancer with radiation and achieved a 44% 5-year survival rate (Sears, 1994). Carey and associates salvaged 15 of 17 patients with vaginal recurrence initially treated by operation alone. The addition of chemotherapy at the time of radiation is currently being evaluated. In patients who have had previous irradiation, pelvic exenteration can be considered for those with an isolated central recurrence.

### Chemotherapy for Advanced and Recurrent Uterine Serous Carcinoma

The majority of information available for patients with USC is from retrospective, nonrandomized case series. In addition, response rates to therapy often come from subset analysis of studies of all types of advanced or recurrent endometrial cancer, including phase III GOG studies. Levenback and associates reported 20 patients with recurrent or advanced USC treated with cyclophosphamide, doxorubicin, and cisplatin. Fifty-eight percent of the patients were alive without disease after 24 months. However, this regimen was highly toxic. Price and coworkers also evaluated cyclophosphamide, doxorubicin, and cisplatin in 19 patients with advanced disease and 11 patients with recurrent disease. Of the patients treated in the adjuvant setting for advanced disease, 58% were alive without evidence of disease with a median follow-up of 24 months. In the patients with recurrent disease, the response rate was 27%. In addition, all the patients developed treatment-related toxicities.

More favorable results using paclitaxel with and without carboplatin have been demonstrated. In a phase II study evaluating carboplatin and paclitaxel, the response rate was 60% in 20 patients with high-stage USC. The progression-free survival time was 18 months, and the 3-year overall survival rate was 39%. Two of four patients with recurrent USC demonstrated a response to carboplatin and paclitaxel. Zanotti and colleagues evaluated 24 patients with measurable disease (either progressive disease after initial surgery or recurrent disease). There was an 89% response rate in patients treated after initial surgery and a 64% response rate for patients with recurrent disease. At the University of Texas MD Anderson Cancer Center, single-agent paclitaxel demonstrated a 77% response rate in patients with recurrent disease. Despite this activity, the duration of response in these studies is less than 1 year (Ramondetta, 2001). Other agents are under investigation for the treatment of USC.

## HORMONE THERAPY

### Progestins for Advanced or Recurrent Disease

Since the 1960s, progestational agents have been valuable in the armamentarium against endometrial cancer, particularly in patients with recurrent disease. Progestins are generally well tolerated. Side effects are usually minor and include weight gain, edema, thrombophlebitis, headache, and occasional hypertension. In patients with medical comorbidities, use of hormonal agents may be preferable to cytotoxic chemotherapy. Initial clinical trials in patients with advanced or recurrent endometrial cancer demonstrated response rates of 30% to 50%. Larger studies with more specific response criteria demonstrate more modest response rates, usually between 11% and 24%. Podratz and colleagues treated 155 patients with advanced or recurrent endometrial cancer with progesterone. The objective response rate was 11%. Overall, survival after initiation of hormone therapy was 40% at 1 year, 19% at 2 years, and 8% at 5 years. In a GOG phase II study, patients who had no previous exposure to chemotherapy or hormonal agents were treated with megestrol acetate (800 mg/day) (Lentz, 1996). The overall response rate was 24%. The progression-free survival and overall survival were 2.5 months and 7.6 months, respectively.

Current recommendations for progestin therapy include oral medroxyprogesterone acetate (Provera), intramuscular medroxyprogesterone acetate (Depo-Provera), and megestrol acetate (Megace). Although there are no randomized studies that have directly compared different formulations of progestins, response rates are similar. In addition, although a dose-response effect of progestin therapy has been reported in breast cancer, there is no evidence of this effect in patients with endometrial cancer. In a randomized trial of oral medroxyprogesterone acetate, patients receiving the low-dose regimen (200 mg/day) had a higher response to therapy than those receiving the high-dose regimen (1000 mg/day).

There are a number of tumor characteristics that increase the likelihood of response to hormone therapy. These include low-grade tumors, the presence of steroid hormone receptors (i.e., progesterone-receptor [PR] and estrogen-receptor [ER]-positive), and a longer disease-free interval. The GOG demonstrated a response rate of 8% in women whose tumors were PR negative and 37% for women whose tumors were PR positive. In addition, there was a 7% response rate in women with ER-negative tumors compared with a 26% response rate in women with ER-positive tumors. Patients with poorly differentiated tumors or hormone-receptor-negative tumors have significantly lower response rates to progestin therapy.

Because of the low toxicity profile and modest efficacy, progestins should be considered in patients with recurrent endometrial cancer. In particular, all patients not eligible for clinical trials with well-differentiated hormone receptor positive recurrent or advanced disease can be given a trial of progestin therapy. If the patient has an objective response, the progestin may be continued indefinitely until there is disease progression.

### Selective Estrogen Receptor Modulators and Aromatase Inhibitors

Selective estrogen receptor modulators (SERMs) with antiestrogenic effects in the uterus have been used to treat women with recurrent endometrial cancer. First-generation SERMs such as tamoxifen have mixed estrogenic agonist and antagonist activity. Early response rates for tamoxifen in advanced or recurrent endometrial cancer were between 20% and 36%. However, in a GOG phase II study of tamoxifen given at a dose of 20 mg twice daily, only 10% of patients demonstrated an objective response. Grade 1 and 2 tumors were more likely to respond to tamoxifen than grade 3 tumors.

Short-term administration of tamoxifen can cause an increase in the progesterone receptor levels in postmenopausal women with endometrial cancer. Studies with alternating tamoxifen and progestins have been performed to determine whether this up-regulation increases the response to progestin therapy. Phase II trials of tamoxifen plus alternating cycles of progestin demonstrated a 27% to 33% response rate (Whitney, 2004). The Eastern Cooperative Oncology Group found no difference in response rates between patients treated with progestin alone and those treated with progestin in combination with tamoxifen (Pandya, 2001).

The U.S. Food and Drug Administration has approved anastrozole, an oral nonsteroidal aromatase inhibitor, for postmenopausal women with progressive breast cancer following tamoxifen therapy. Aromatase is elevated in the stroma of endometrial cancer. In a phase II trial by the GOG, anastrozole was found to have minimal activity (9% response rate) in an unselected population of patients with advanced or recurrent endometrial cancer. More than 25% of the patients in this study had nonendometrioid histologic subtypes, and only 22% of the patients had ER- and PR-positive tumors or demonstrated a response to previous therapy. In the subset of women with FIGO grade 1 and 2 tumors with endometrioid histology, the response rate was 30%.

## *TARGETED THERAPY*

There are a number of molecular aberrations commonly seen in endometrioid adenocarcinomas, the most common being abnormalities in the PTEN/AKT pathway. A number of clinical trials exploiting this pathway have shown promising results in women with recurrent endometrial cancer. Several studies have shown efficacy of mTOR inhibitors including temsirolimus, everolimus, and ridaforolimus in endometrial cancer recurrence (Slomovitz, 2010). In the first-line setting, response rates have been 9% to 24% with clinical benefit rates up to 90%. Combining agents such as everolimus and letrozole have a reported response rate of 31% with a median duration of response of 12.5 months. The GOG has an ongoing study comparing this combination to tamoxifen alternating with Megace, which is considered the standard hormonal regimen.

# SARCOMAS

Sarcomas account for less than 5% of uterine malignancies and are much less frequent than endometrial carcinomas, particularly in Western countries. Numerous terms have been used to describe the many histologic types. One useful classification is based on determination of the resemblance of the sarcomatous elements to mesenchymal tissue normally found in the uterus (homologous sarcomas) in contrast to tissues foreign to the uterus (heterologous sarcomas). Homologous types include leiomyosarcoma, endometrial stromal sarcoma (ESS), and, rarely, angiosarcoma. Heterologous types include rhabdomyosarcoma, chondrosarcoma, osteosarcoma, and liposarcoma. These sarcomas may exist exclusively or may be admixed with epithelial adenocarcinoma, in which case the term *carcinosarcoma* (malignant mixed müllerian tumor) is applied. Box 32.3 shows a morphologic classification for uterine sarcomas. A study by Zelmanowicz and colleagues suggests risk factors for these tumors are similar to those of endometrial carcinoma—that is, estrogens and obesity increase the risk and oral contraceptive use decreases the risk. No uniformly defined staging criteria exist for these tumors, and the most widely used definitions are similar to those for endometrial carcinoma: stage I, confined to the corpus; stage II, corpus and cervix involved;

**Box 32.3 Modified Classification of Uterine Sarcomas**

I. Pure sarcoma
  A. Homologous
    1. Smooth muscle tumors
      a. Leiomyosarcoma
      b. Leiomyoblastoma
      c. Metastasizing tumors with benign histologic appearance
        i. Intravenous leiomyomatosis
        ii. Metastasizing uterine leiomyoma
        iii. Leiomyomatosis peritonealis disseminata
    2. Endometrial stromal sarcomas
      a. Low grade: endolymphatic stromal myosis
      b. High grade: endometrial stromal sarcoma
  B. Heterologous
    1. Rhabdomyosarcoma
    2. Chondrosarcoma
    3. Osteosarcoma
    4. Liposarcoma
  C. Other sarcomas
II. Carcinosarcoma: malignant mixed müllerian tumors
  A. Homologous (carcinosarcoma): carcinoma + homologous sarcoma
  B. Heterologous: carcinoma + heterologous sarcoma
III. Müllerian adenosarcoma
IV. Lymphoma

Modified from Clemet P, Scully RE. Pathology of uterine sarcomas. In: Coppleson M, ed. *Gynecologic Oncology*. New York: Churchill Livingstone; 1981:591.

stage III, spread outside the uterus but confined to the pelvis or retroperitoneal lymph nodes; and stage IV, spread outside the true pelvis or into the mucosa of the bladder or rectum. Similar to endometrial adenocarcinoma, operative stage is the most important predictor of survival (Zelmanowicz, 1998).

## LEIOMYOSARCOMA

Leiomyosarcomas represent 1% to 2% of uterine malignancies and approximately one third of uterine sarcomas (Fig. 32.11). Although the exact cause is unknown, leiomyosarcomas are not thought to arise from benign leiomyomas. Leibsohn and coworkers noted that among 1423 patients who had hysterectomies for presumed leiomyomas with a uterine size comparable with a 12-week pregnancy or larger, the risk of sarcoma increased with age, from 0.4% for those in their 30s to 1.4% for those in their 50s. The determination of malignancy is made in part by ascertaining the number of mitoses in 10 hpf as well as the presence of cytologic atypia, abnormal mitotic figures, and nuclear pleomorphism (see Fig. 32.11). Vascular invasion and extrauterine spread of tumor are associated with worse prognoses. A finding of more than 5 mitoses per 10 hpf with cytologic atypia leads to a diagnosis of leiomyosarcoma; when there are four or fewer mitoses per 10 hpf, the tumors usually have a more benign clinical course. The prognosis worsens for tumors with more than 10 mitoses per 10 hpf. The presence of bizarre cells may not necessarily establish the diagnosis because they can occasionally be seen in benign leiomyomas and in patients receiving progestational agents. Furthermore, it is important to note that an increase in mitotic

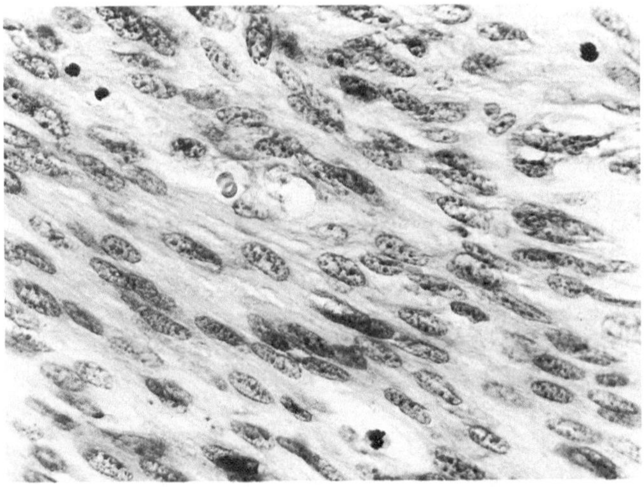

**Figure 32.11** Leiomyosarcoma. Nuclear hyperchromatism and mitotic figures are present (×660). (From Clement PB, Scully RE. Pathology of uterine sarcomas. In: Coppleson M, ed. *Gynecologic Oncology*. Edinburgh: Churchill Livingstone; 1981.)

count in leiomyomas occurs in pregnancy, as well as during oral contraceptive use. This can occasionally cause confusion in the histologic diagnosis.

Usually, the patient has an enlarged pelvic mass, occasionally accompanied by pain or vaginal bleeding. Leiomyosarcomas are suspected if the uterus undergoes rapid enlargement, particularly in patients in the perimenopausal or postmenopausal age group. Approximately 85% of women diagnosed with a leiomyosarcoma have clinical stage I or II disease (i.e., disease that is limited to the uterus and cervix). The risk of lymph node involvement is very low. Primary treatment includes total hysterectomy, bilateral salpingo-oophorectomy, and staging. Despite the low incidence of high-stage disease, approximately 50% of patients will have a recurrence within 2 years. The recurrence in most of these patients is outside the pelvis.

The GOG evaluated the role of adjuvant radiation therapy in patients ($N$ = 48) with clinical stage I and II disease (see Table 32.9). There was no difference in the progression-free interval, absolute 2-year survival rate, or site of first recurrence between patients who received pelvic radiation ($N$ = 11) and those who did not ($N$ = 37). This is not surprising because most recurrences were outside the pelvis (83%). There was recurrence in 48% of the patients, and most of these patients had a recurrence within 17 months of diagnosis. In the adjuvant chemotherapy trial by the GOG, patients treated with Adriamycin had a recurrence less frequently than those in the observation arm (44% versus 61%); however, this difference was not statistically significant. There is no known benefit to adjuvant radiation or chemotherapy in women with leiomyosarcoma limited to the uterus.

Several studies have evaluated treatment of advanced or recurrent leiomyosarcoma. Hannigan and colleagues used vincristine, actinomycin D, and cyclophos phamide (Cytoxan) and noted a 13% complete response rate and 16% partial response rate in 74 patients with advanced metastatic uterine sarcomas. A large collaborative trial was conducted by the GOG and reported by Omura and associates. The best responses were obtained for patients with lung metastases who received doxorubicin and dacarbazine (DTIC). Current evidence suggests that a multidrug program offers the greatest response for these patients. Cisplatin, Adriamycin, paclitaxel (Taxol), ifosfamide, and etoposide (VP-16) all appear to have some effectiveness. Gemcitabine and docetaxel have been evaluated in a phase II study for patients with recurrent leiomyosarcoma (Hensley, 2002). In this study, 34 patients with leiomyosarcoma were treated. Overall response rate was 53%; however, the duration of response was only 5.6 months. This regimen is used commonly for advanced and recurrent disease. A phase III study completed by the GOG failed to show any additional benefit to the addition of bevacizumab to gemcitabine and docetaxel in the treatment of this disease (Hensley, 2014).

## ENDOMETRIAL STROMAL SARCOMA

Overall, stromal tumors comprise approximately 10% of uterine sarcomas. Their behavior correlates primarily with the mitotic rate. Although these tumors were once divided into low grade and high grade, more recently all ESSs are considered low grade. If high-grade elements are present, these tumors would be classified as undifferentiated high-grade sarcomas. Undifferentiated sarcomas have a greater degree of anaplasia and lack the branching vasculature characteristic of ESSs. ESSs have a peak incidence in the fifth decade of life. There is no association with previous radiation nor are risk factors of endometrial carcinoma associated with the development of ESS. Histologically, ESS most resembles proliferative endometrial stroma. Prognosis depends on the extent of disease and ability to remove the entire tumor at the time of surgery. In general, ESSs are indolent, slowly progressing tumors.

Recurrent disease may be diagnosed as many as 30 years after diagnosis. ESS tends to recur locally in the pelvis or peritoneal cavity and frequently spreads to the lungs. In treating metastatic disease, it should be remembered that these tumors contain estrogen and progestin steroid hormone receptors and are often sensitive to hormone therapy. Complete resolution has been reported with megestrol acetate (Megace), medroxyprogesterone (Provera), letrozole (Femara), tamoxifen, and 17α-hydroxyprogesterone caproate (Delalutin).

There are reports of radiation in the treatment of pelvic recurrence, with resolution of all residual tumors, but extensive experience with radiation therapy is not available. Systemic chemotherapy with cytotoxic agents has not been reported to be effective, although good responses to doxorubicin (Adriamycin) have been reported.

## UNDIFFERENTIATED SARCOMAS

These high-grade tumors behave aggressively and have a poor prognosis. These tumors must be evaluated carefully as they are often confused with other large cell undifferentiated tumors (lymphoma, leukemia, high-grade endometrial cancer, carcinosarcoma).

Microscopically, more than 10 mitoses per 10 hpf are present, and frequently 20 or more mitoses per 10 hpf are present. Some series have reported 100% fatalities, although Vongtama and coworkers reported survival of more than 60% for 24 patients with stage I and 1 patient with stage II disease. Recurrences are common in the pelvis, lung, and abdomen. If there has not been previous radiation treatment and the recurrence is confined to the pelvis, usually pelvic irradiation is prescribed. If there is disseminated disease, multiple-agent chemotherapy is used.

## CARCINOSARCOMA (MALIGNANT MIXED MÜLLERIAN TUMORS)

As shown in Box 32.3, these tumors consist of both carcinoma and sarcoma elements native to the uterus that may resemble the endometrial stroma of smooth muscle (homologous) or of sarcomatous tissues foreign to the uterus (heterologous). Spanos and colleagues reviewed 188 patients with mixed mesodermal tumor and found both the prognosis and the pattern of survival to be similar for both homologous and heterologous tumors. The study of George and coworkers showed that patients with these tumors had a markedly worse prognosis than patients with high-grade endometrial carcinomas. Unlike patients with endometrial stromal sarcoma or leiomyosarcoma, those with carcinosarcoma tend to be older and primarily postmenopausal, usually beyond the age of 62 years. Previous pelvic irradiation has been identified as an occasional predisposing factor and was experienced by 17 of the 136 patients reviewed by Norris and Taylor. The heterologous and homologous tumors occur with approximately equivalent frequency. These tumors can spread locally into the myometrium and pelvis, or distally to the abdominal cavity, lungs, and pleura, a pattern similar to the spread of endometrial carcinoma.

A common symptom is postmenopausal bleeding, often accompanied by an enlarged uterus. Occasionally, the diagnosis is made in tissue removed with D&C, and the tumor may appear to be a polypoid excrescence from the cervix; diagnosis may be made also by vaginal ultrasound examination.

As is true for other sarcomas, the primary treatment is surgical removal of the uterus. The extent of the tumor and the depth of myometrial invasion are important prognostic factors. Those with deep myometrial invasion are more likely to have spread to pelvic or paraaortic nodes. Patients with tumors confined to the uterus and little or no myometrial spread have the best prognosis. A comprehensive surgical staging procedure is recommended for all patients with this diagnosis. Nielsen and coworkers reported a 5-year survival rate of 58% for these patients when the disease was confined to the uterus.

In a phase I/II study of ifosfamide and cisplatin as adjuvant therapy in patients with high-stage carcinosarcoma, the GOG found this combination to be tolerable (Sutton, 2000). Progression-free and overall survival rates at 2 years were 69% and 82%, respectively. This study lacked appropriate controls, so the impact of this regimen on improving survival could not be evaluated. For patients with advanced or recurrent disease, the GOG evaluated ifosfamide versus ifosfamide and cisplatin in a phase III randomized study (Sutton, 2005). The response rate to the combination therapy was superior (54% versus 36%); however, the toxicity was significantly higher. In addition, no significant difference in overall survival was seen. A follow-up study compared ifosfamide to ifosfamide and paclitaxel in a phase III randomized study. Response rates in the combination arm were superior (45% versus 29%), but importantly there was a significant difference in overall survival (13 months versus 8 months) (Homesley, 2006). Finally, a phase II study showed efficacy of paclitaxel and carboplatin in women with advanced or recurrent carcinosarcoma with an overall response rate of 54% using this well-tolerated regimen (Powell, 2010). Paclitaxel and carboplatin are the current standard treatments for women with carcinosarcoma.

## MÜLLERIAN ADENOSARCOMA

Müllerian adenosarcoma is a rare low-grade malignancy composed of both a sarcomatous stroma (homologous) and a proliferation of benign glandular elements that are intimately associated. It occurs predominantly in women older than 60 years. Total abdominal hysterectomy with bilateral salpingo-oophorectomy is the treatment of choice. Mitotic index and sarcomatous overgrowth are related to prognosis.

## KEY POINTS

- Endometrial carcinoma is the most common malignancy of the female genital tract. In the United States, the lifetime risk of endometrial cancer is 3%.
- Most women who develop endometrial cancer are between 50 and 65 years of age.
- Women with Lynch syndrome (hereditary nonpolyposis colorectal cancer syndrome) have a 40% to 60% lifetime risk of endometrial cancer, which is similar to their lifetime risk of colon cancer.
- Chronic unopposed estrogen stimulation of the endometrium leads to endometrial hyperplasia and in some cases adenocarcinoma. Other important predisposing factors include obesity, nulliparity, late menopause, and diabetes.
- The risk of a woman developing endometrial carcinoma increases three times if her body mass index is greater than 30 $kg/m^2$.
- Tamoxifen use increases the risk of endometrial neoplasia two- to threefold.
- The primary symptom of endometrial carcinoma is postmenopausal bleeding. Women with abnormal bleeding should undergo an endometrial sampling to rule out endometrial pathology.
- Cytologic atypia in endometrial hyperplasia is the most important factor in determining malignant potential.
- Simple hyperplasia will develop into endometrial cancer in 1% of patients, whereas complex hyperplasia will develop into cancer in 29% of patients.
- Studies have found that there is a 40% concurrent rate of endometrial cancer in patients with a preoperative diagnosis of complex atypical hyperplasia.
- Prognosis in endometrial carcinoma is related to tumor grade, tumor stage, histologic type, and degree of myometrial invasion.
- Older patients with atypical hyperplasia are at increased risk of malignant progression compared with younger patients.
- A key determinant of the risk of nodal spread of endometrial carcinoma is depth of myometrial invasion, which is often related to tumor grade.
- Well-differentiated (grade 1) endometrial carcinomas usually express steroid hormone receptors, whereas poorly differentiated (grade 3) tumors usually do not express receptors.
- Uterine serous carcinoma is an aggressive histologic subtype associated with metastatic disease even in the absence of myometrial invasion.
- Ninety percent of recurrences of adenocarcinoma of the endometrium occur within 5 years.
- Overall survival rates for patients with adenocarcinoma of the endometrium by stage are as follows: stage I, 86%; stage II, 66%; stage III, 44%; stage IV, 16% (overall there is a 72.7% 5-year survival rate combining clinical and operative staging systems).
- Histologic variants of endometrial carcinoma with a poor prognosis include uterine serous carcinoma and clear-cell carcinoma.
- Patients with uterine serous or clear-cell carcinoma of the endometrium should have a full staging laparotomy similar to that for ovarian carcinoma.
- The most frequent sites of distant metastasis of adenocarcinoma of the endometrium are the lung, retroperitoneal nodes, and abdomen.
- Primary treatment of endometrial cancer includes hysterectomy, bilateral salpingo-oophorectomy, pelvic cytology, bilateral pelvic and paraaortic lymphadenectomy, and resection of all disease. The exceptions include young premenopausal women with stage I and grade 1 endometrial carcinoma associated with endometrial hyperplasia, and women with increased risk of mortality secondary to medical comorbidities.
- Postoperative adjuvant radiation has not been shown to improve overall survival.
- Patients with high-stage or recurrent disease should be treated in a multimodality approach including chemotherapy, radiation, or hormone therapy.
- Uterine sarcomas make up less than 5% of uterine malignancies.
- Uterine sarcomas are treated primarily by operation including removal of the uterus, tubes, and ovaries.
- Endometrial stromal sarcomas are low-grade sarcomas with an indolent course.
- Multiagent chemotherapeutic regimens are usually prescribed for metastatic sarcomas; complete responses are rare and usually temporary.

## KEY REFERENCES


Abeler VM, Kjørstad KE. Clear cell carcinoma of the endometrium: a histopathological and clinical study of 97 cases. *Gynecol Oncol.* 1991;40(3):207–17.

Ackerman I, Malone S, Thomas G, et al. Endometrial carcinoma: relative effectiveness of adjuvant irradiation vs therapy reserved for relapse. *Gynecol Oncol.* 1996;60:177–183.

Barakat RR, Wong G, Curtin JP, et al. Tamoxifen use in breast cancer patients who subsequently develop corpus cancer is not associated with a higher incidence of adverse histologic features. *Gynecol Oncol.* 1994;55:164–168.

Barlin JN, Koury-Callado F, Kim CH, et al. The importance of applying a sentinel lymph node mapping algorithm in endometrial cancer staging: beyond removal of the blue nodes. *Gynecol Oncol.* 2012;125(3):531–535.

Brinton LA, Berman ML, Mortel R, et al. Reproductive, menstrual, and medical risk factors for endometrial cancer: results from a case-control study. *Am J Obstet Gynecol.* 1992;167:1317–1325.

Bristow RE, Zerbe MJ, Rosenshein NB, et al. Stage IVB endometrial cancer: the role of cytoreductive surgery and determinants of survival. *Gynecol Oncol.* 2000;78:85–91.

Burzawa JK, Schmeler KM, Soliman PT, et al. Prospective evaluation of insulin resistance among endometrial cancer patients. *Am J Obstet Gynecol.* 2011;204(4):355.e1-e7.

Carcangiu ML, Chambers JT. Early pathologic stage clear cell carcinoma and uterine papillary serous carcinoma of the endometrium: comparison of clinicopathologic features and survival. *Int J Gynecol Pathol.* 1995;14(1):30–8.

Cecchini S, Ciatto S, Bonardi R, et al. Screening by ultrasonography for endometrial carcinoma in postmenopausal breast cancer patients under adjuvant tamoxifen. *Gynecol Oncol.* 1996;60:409–411.

Creasman WT, DeGeest K, DiSaia PJ, et al. Significance of true surgical pathologic staging: A Gynecologic Oncology Group Study. *Am J Obstet Gynecol.* 1999;181:31–34.

Creutzberg CL, van Putten WLJ, Kiper PCM, et al. Surgery and postoperative radiotherapy versus surgery alone for patients with stage-1 endometrial carcinoma: multicentre randomised trial. *Lancet.* 2000;355:1404–1411.

Dietrich CS 3rd, Modesitt SC, DePriest PD, et al. The efficacy of adjuvant platinum-based chemotherapy in Stage I uterine papillary serous carcinoma (UPSC). *Gynecol Oncol.* 2005;299:557–563.

Hensley ML, Maki R, Venkatraman E, et al. Gemcitabine and docetaxel in patients with unresectable leiomyosarcoma: results of a phase II trial. *J Clin Oncol.* 2002;20:2824–2831.

Hensley ML, Miller A, O'Malley DM, et al. A randomized phase III trial of gemcitabine + docetaxel + bevacizumab or placebo as first-line treatment for metastatic uterine leiomyosarcoma (uLMS): a Gynecologic Oncology Group study. *Gynecol Oncol.* 2014;133: 3(SGO #2) (Abstract).

Homesly HD, Filiaci VL, Bitterman, et al. Phase III trial of ifosfamide versus ifosfamide plus paclitaxel as first line treatment of advanced or recurrent uterine carcinosarcoma (mixed mesodermal tumors): a Gynecologic Oncology Group study. *Gynecol Oncol.* 2006;101(SGO#66):S31 (Abstract).

Keys HM, Roberts JA, Brunetto VL, et al. A phase III trial of surgery with or without adjunctive external pelvic radiation therapy in intermediate risk endometrial adenocarcinoma: a Gynecologic Oncology Group study. *Gynecol Oncol.* 2004;92:744–751.

Kurman RJ, Kaminski PF, Norris HJ. Behavior of endometrial hyperplasia: a long-term study of "untreated" hyperplasias in 170 patients. *Cancer.* 1985;56:403–412.

Langer RD, Pierce JJ, O'Hanlan KA, et al. Transvaginal ultrasonography compared with endometrial biopsy for the detection of endometrial disease. *N Engl J Med.* 1997;337:1792–1798.

Lentz SS, Brady MF, Major FJ, et al. High-dose megestrol acetate in advanced or recurrent endometrial carcinoma: a Gynecologic Oncology Group Study. *J Clin Oncol.* 1996;14:357–361.

Mariani A, Sebo TJ, Katzmann JA, et al. Pretreatment assessment of prognostic indicators in endometrial cancer. *Am J Obstet Gynecol.* 2000a;182:1535–1544.

Mariani A, Webb MJ, Galli L, Podratz KC. Potential therapeutic role of para-aortic lymphadenectomy in node-positive endometrial cancer. *Gynecol Oncol.* 2000b;76:348–356.

Mariani A, Webb MJ, Keeney GL, et al. Role of wide/radical hysterectomy and pelvic lymph node dissection in endometrial cancer with cervical involvement. *Gynecolo Oncol.* 2001;83(1):72–80.

Miller D, Filiaci V, Fleming G

Sears JD, Greven KM, Hoen HM, Randall ME. Prognostic factors and treatment outcome for patients with locally recurrent endometrial cancer. *Cancer.* 1994;74(4):1303–8.

Slomovitz BM, Burke TW, Oh JC, et al. Clinical and pathologic characteristics of uterine papillary serous carcinoma: A single institution review of 129 cases. *Gynecol Oncol.* 2003;91:463–469.

Slomovitz BM, Jiang Y, Yates MS, et al. Pahse II study of everolimus and letrozole in patients with recurrent endometrial carcinoma. *J Clin Oncol.* 2015;33(8):930–936.

Slomovitz BM, Lu KH, Johnston T, et al. A phase 2 study of the oral mammalian target of rapamycin inhibitor, everolimus, in patients with recurrent endometrial carcinoma. *Cancer.* 2010;116(23):5415–5419.

Soliman PT, Broaddus RR, Schmeler KM, et al. Women with synchronous primary cancers of the endometrium and ovary: do they have Lynch Syndrome? *J Clin Oncol.* 2005;23(36):9344–9350.

Soliman PT, Slomovitz BM, Broaddus RR, et al. Synchronous primary cancers of the endometrium and ovary: a single institution review of 84 cases. *Gynecol Oncol.* 2004;94:456–462.

Sood AK, Buller RE, Burger RA, et al. Value of preoperative CA 125 level in the management of uterine cancer and prediction of clinical outcome. *Obstet Gynecol.* 1997;90:441–447.

Sutton G, Brunetto VL, Kilgore L, et al. A phase III trial of ifosfamide with or without cisplatin in carcinosarcoma of the uterus: a Gynecologic Oncology Group Study. *Gynecol Oncol.* 2000;79:147–153.

Sutton G, Kauderer J, Carson LF, et al. Adjuvant ifosfamide and cisplatin in patients with completely resected stage I or II carcinosarcomas (mixed mesodermal tumors) of the uterus: a Gynecologic Oncology Group study. *Gynecol Oncol.* 2005;96:630–634.

Walker JL, Piedmonte MR, Spirtos NM, et al. Laparoscopy compared with laparotomy for comprehensive surgical staging of uterine cancer: Gynecologic Oncology Group Study LAP2. *J Clin Oncol.* 2009;27(32):5331–5336.

Westin SN, Broaddus RR. Personalized therapy in endometrial cancer: challenges and opportunities. *Cancer Biol Ther.* 2012;13(1):1–13.

Whitney CW, Brunetto VL, Zaino RJ, et al. Phase II study of medroxy-progesterone acetate plus tamoxifen in advanced endometrial carcinoma: Gynecologic Oncology Group study. *Gynecol Oncol.* 2004;92:4–9.

Zelmanowicz A, Hildescheim A, Sherman ME, et al. Evidence for a common etiology for endometrial carcinomas and malignant mixed mullerian tumors. *Gynecol Oncol.* 1998;69:253–257.


Suggested Readings can be found on ExpertConsult.com.

# 33

# Neoplastic Diseases of the Ovary

## Screening, Benign and Malignant Epithelial and Germ Cell Neoplasms, Sex-Cord Stromal Tumors

*Robert L. Coleman, Pedro T. Ramirez, David M. Gershenson*

Ovarian cancer is the second most common malignancy of the lower part of the female genital tract, occurring less frequently than cancers of the endometrium but more frequently than cancers of the cervix. However, it is the most frequent cause of death from gynecologic neoplasms in the United States. Cancer Statistics 2015 has reported that approximately 21,290 new cases of ovarian cancer will be diagnosed yearly in the United States, and there will be 14,180 deaths. A major contributing factor to the high death rate from the relatively few cases stems from the frequent detection of the disease after metastatic spread when symptoms direct clinical investigation or raise clinical concern. Surprisingly, most women diagnosed with ovarian cancer do report symptoms for months before diagnosis. As detailed later, only the severity and duration of symptoms differentially segregate cancer patients from noncancer patients. The incidence of ovarian cancer (Fig. 33.1) increases with age, becoming most marked beyond 50 years, with a gradual increase continuing to age 70 years followed by a decrease for those older than 80. Moreover, Yancik and associates noted that those older than 65

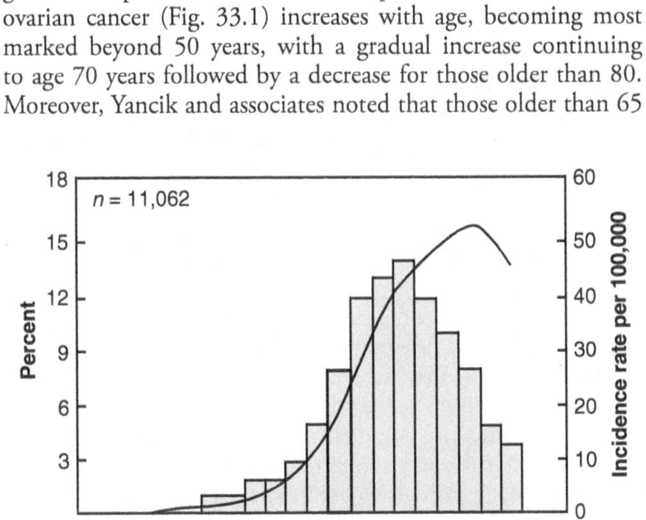


**Figure 33.1** Ovarian cancer incidence rates by age, 1973 to 1982. (From Yancik R, Ries LG, Yates JW. Ovarian cancer in the elderly: an analysis of Surveillance, Epidemiology, and End Results Program data. *Am J Obstet Gynecol.* 1986;154[3]:639-647.)

are more likely to have their cancers diagnosed at an advanced stage, leading to a worse prognosis and poorer survival compared with those younger than 65 years.

Despite numerous epidemiologic investigations, a clear-cut cause of ovarian cancer has not been defined. A number of theories have been advanced. It is thought that these malignancies are related to frequent ovulation, and therefore women who ovulate regularly appear to be at higher risk. Included are those with a late menopause, history of nulliparity, or late childbearing. Conversely, women who have had several pregnancies or who have used oral contraceptives appear to have some protection against ovarian cancer. Casagrande and colleagues related the development of ovarian cancer to ovulatory age—that is, the number of years during which the woman has ovulated. This number would be reduced by pregnancy, breast-feeding, or oral contraceptive use. Schildkraut and associates correlated overexpression of mutant p53 protein in ovarian cancers with reproductive histories and found that overexpression was more likely in those who had high ovulatory cycle histories. In addition, talcum powder used on the perineum has been postulated to increase the risk but, as noted by Cramer and coworkers, it is a weak association. The use of oral contraceptives decreases the risk by approximately 50% after 5 years of use (approximately 10% to 12%/year). The protection increases with duration of use to 10 years and appears to last for approximately 15 years after discontinuation of use. Schlesselman has calculated a decrease of 369 ovarian cancer cases/100,000 women for 8 years of use. Given that the approximate occurrence of ovarian cancer cases in this group would be expected to be1400, such a decrease approximates 25%. Breast-feeding, pregnancy, tubal ligation, and, to a lesser extent, hysterectomy with ovarian preservation also lower the risk of ovarian cancer. It has been suggested that ovulation-inducing drugs such as clomiphene citrate increase the risk of ovarian cancer, as noted by Whittemore and colleagues. Rossing and coworkers reported an increase in risk from a population-based study that suggested that the risk is associated with prolonged use of clomiphene insofar as no association was noted with less than 1 year of use. The study was significant but had wide 95% confidence limits, and only 11 cancer cases occurred in the clomiphene group among 3837 women studied in the infertility clinic. However, Venn and associates from Australia have not demonstrated an increase in ovarian cancer for those using fertility drugs for in vitro fertilization. Mahdavi and colleagues assembled a review of cohort and case-control studies evaluating the relationship of fertility agents to ovarian cancer. In this report, little evidence supported the hypothesis that ovulation induction substantially increases cancer risk. Furthermore, a large population-based Danish cohort study also failed to demonstrate any increased risk of ovarian cancer among 54,362 women seeking consultation relating to fertility problems. Agents evaluated in this study were gonadotropins, clomiphene citrate, human chorionic gonadotropin, and gonadotropin-releasing hormone. Additionally, no associations were found between these agents and the number of cycles of use, parity, or length of follow-up. However, three reports specifically evaluating the association of these agents and the development of borderline tumor or low malignant potential tumors have suggested that a relationship may exist. The frequent presence of hormone receptors in these lesions, as well as the hyperestrogenic microenvironment, may support this observation.

Cramer and coworkers found women with ovarian cancer to have a diet high in animal fat in compared with control subjects, and studies of Risch and associates suggested that saturated fat increases the risk of ovarian cancer, whereas vegetable fiber may reduce it. Table 33.1 shows the various factors that alter the risk of ovarian cancer. The familial or inherited aspects of the disease are considered subsequently.

There are geographic and racial differences in the distribution of ovarian cancers. These cancers occur most frequently in industrialized and affluent countries such as the United States and Western Europe and less frequently in Asia and Africa. The disease is more frequent among white than black women. Finally, patients with ovarian carcinoma have an increased risk of developing breast and endometrial cancer. Notwithstanding the familial syndromes, major factors appear to be related to the frequency of ovulation and residence in an industrialized country.

## FAMILIAL OVARIAN CANCER

In a case-control study, Hartge and colleagues showed that a familial history of breast cancer and a personal history of breast cancer are ovarian cancer risk factors. Lynch and associates reported on families with these hereditary ovarian cancers and noted that they tend to occur at a younger age than in the general population. It appears that germline mutations of the *BRCA* tumor suppressor gene on chromosome 17q are responsible for a large proportion of hereditary cancers (discussed later). However, these are a small proportion of all ovarian carcinomas. Risk alteration in these patients through oral contraceptive use is of uncertain impact. Narod and coworkers suggested that it might be possible to reduce incident risk by their administration. However, Modan and colleagues conducted a case-control study of Jewish women in whom *BRCA* founder mutational analysis was performed; they evaluated the risk of cancer development based by parity and oral contraceptive use. They were able to establish a protective effect by oral contraceptive use in the cohort, but subanalysis by carrier status demonstrated no effect in those harboring a *BRCA* founder mutation (odds ratio [OR], 1.07; 95% confidence interval [CI], 0.63-1.83). Further studies are needed.

**Table 33.1** Putative Associations of Increasing and Decreasing Risks of Ovarian Epithelial Carcinoma

| Increases | Decreases |
|---|---|
| Age | Breast-feeding |
| Diet | Oral contraceptives |
| Family history | Pregnancy |
| Industrialized country | Tubal ligation and hysterectomy, with ovarian conservation |
| Infertility | |
| Nulliparity | |
| Ovulation | |
| Ovulatory drugs | |
| Talc (?) | |

From Herbst AL. The epidemiology of ovarian carcinoma and the current status of tumor markers to detect disease. *Am J Obstet Gynecol*. 1994;170(4):1099-1105.

Hereditary ovarian cancers are uncommon, accounting for approximately 10% to 15% of all incident cases. However, identification of affected or unaffected women with significant familial risk is important, given their accelerated risk of ovarian and other cancers. In addition, these patients are frequently diagnosed at a younger age (median, 50 years), and unaffected individuals are able to consider prophylactic procedures that can affect their lifetime risk. The term *familial ovarian cancer* denotes an inherited trait that predisposes to ovarian cancer development. It has been widely studied and two definitions are important:

1. A first-degree relative is a mother, sister, or daughter of an affected individual.
2. A second-degree relative is a maternal or paternal aunt or grandmother.

As noted in the review by Kerlikowske and colleagues, previous studies suggested an increase from approximately 1.5% to 5% in the lifetime risk of ovarian cancer with one first-degree relative; with two or more, the risk reaches may exceed 7% to 12%. Because contemporary family size may preclude disease penetrance, careful attention to *BRCA*-associated cancers in either gender should be performed in a multigenerational history. Furthermore, the high association of fallopian tube cancer and underlying *BRCA* mutation has prompted some to call for routine *BRCA* testing in all such cases.

Most ovarian cancers develop sporadically. For the woman with a familial history of ovarian cancer (not the dominant genetic hereditary type), periodic surveillance with transvaginal ultrasonography 6 months after the age of 35 years has been suggested (see the ultrasonography discussion presented later in this chapter). Unfortunately, such a strategy has not been shown to be worthwhile or cost effective in disease prevention and may, on occasion, lead to additional tests or unnecessary procedures when a questionable ultrasound result is. The use of prophylactic oophorectomy in patients whose mothers had ovarian cancer has been a controversial topic. Kerlikowske and colleagues and Herbst have provided reasons opposing the widespread use of this practice. However, the use of prophylactic oophorectomy to reduce the risk of ovarian or peritoneal cancer in mutation carriers may have validity. Finch and associates studied 1828 women enrolled in an international registry over an 11-year period ending in 2003. In this cohort, 575 (30%) had undergone oophorectomy before enrollment, 490 (27%) underwent the procedure after study entry, and 783 (43%) did not undergo the procedure. After a median follow-up of 3.5 years, 50 incident cases were identified, 18 in women undergoing oophorectomy and 32 in women with intact ovaries. The protective effect was 80% (hazard ratio [HR], 0.2; 95% CI, 0.02-0.58; $P = .003$). It is reasonable that for patients with a significant family history in whom an operation such as hysterectomy is required, removal of both tubes and ovaries at the time of operation is appropriate. Similarly, mutation carriers who have finished childbearing may reduce their subsequent cancer risk by salpingo-oophorectomy. The recommendation for hysterectomy at this time is controversial but has been advocated by some to ensure complete removal of the fallopian tube (cornual segment). The woman must be aware that peritoneal carcinomatosis, a process resembling serous carcinoma of the ovary, can develop (rarely) despite the removal of both ovaries.

Because evidence has suggested a significant proportion of ovarian carcinomas arise for preinvasive intraepithelial carcinomas in the fallopian tube, interest in a two-step approach to removal of the adnexa has arisen. Preserving ovarian function in high-risk women while mitigating risk via removal of the fallopian tubes has appeal for maintaining quality of life and avoidance of the risks from premature castration. Nevertheless, much is unknown regarding the efficacy and safety of this approach, including how strong is the risk mitigation and to what degree does retaining the ovary increase risk of breast cancer in these at-risk women. Finally, the timing for oophorectomy is unknown. Fortunately, several prospective clinical trials are under way to address this novel approach to risk reduction surgery (Daly, 2015).

The following describes the classification and histology of the major ovarian neoplasms. Pertinent microscopic findings, clinical behavior, and appropriate therapy are presented.

## CLASSIFICATION OF OVARIAN NEOPLASMS

The most widely used classification of ovarian neoplasms is that of the World Health Organization (WHO). This classification, along with frequency of occurrence of the primary ovarian neoplasms, is shown in Table 33.2.

Epithelial stromal tumors (common epithelial tumors) are the most frequent ovarian neoplasms. They are believed to arise from the surface (coelomic) epithelium. Germ cell tumors are the second most frequent and are the most common among young women. Histologically, they may be composed of extraembryonic elements or may have features that resemble any or all of the three embryonic layers (ectoderm, mesoderm, or endoderm). Germ cell tumors are the main cause of ovarian malignancy in young women, particularly those in their teens and early 20s. Sex cord–stromal tumors are the third most frequent and contain elements that recapitulate the constituents of the ovary or testis. These tumors may secrete sex steroid hormones or may be hormonally inactive. Lipid (lipoid) cell tumors are extremely rare and histologically resemble the adrenal gland. Gonadoblastomas consist of germ cells and sex cord–stromal elements. They occur in individuals with dysgenetic gonads, particularly when a Y chromosome is present. All these ovarian neoplasms are discussed later in this chapter.

Soft tissue tumors not specific to the ovary, such as a hemangioma or lipoma, are extremely rare and are categorized according to the criteria for soft tissue tumors arising elsewhere in the body. Unclassified tumors, as the name implies, cannot be placed in any of the preceding categories. One example is small cell carcinoma, which is a highly virulent cancer affecting primarily young women (discussed later). Metastatic tumors to the ovary may arise elsewhere in the reproductive tract or from distant sites such as the bowel or stomach (Krukenberg tumors). Tumor-like conditions refer to enlargements of the ovary, such as extensive edema, pregnancy luteoma, endometriomas, and follicular or luteal cysts, none of which are true neoplasms. With the exceptions of metastatic tumors and small cell carcinoma of the ovary, none of these are considered further in this chapter.

**Table 33.2** World Health Organization Classification: Frequency of Ovarian Neoplasms

| Class | Approximate Frequency (%) |
|---|---|
| Epithelial stromal (common epithelial) tumors | 65 |
| Germ cell tumors | 20-25 |
| Sex cord–stromal tumors | 6 |
| Lipid (lipoid) cell tumors | <0.1 |
| Gonadoblastoma | <0.1 |
| Soft tissue tumors (not specific to ovary) | |
| Unclassified tumors | |
| Secondary (metastatic) tumors | |
| Tumor-like conditions (not true neoplasm) | |

## EPITHELIAL OVARIAN NEOPLASMS

According to Scully, two thirds of ovarian neoplasms are epithelial tumors; malignant epithelial tumors account for approximately 85% of ovarian cancers, probably arising from inclusion cysts lined with surface (coelomic) epithelium within the adjacent ovarian stroma. Table 33.3 summarizes the five cell types that most commonly constitute epithelial ovarian tumors, indicating their relative frequency.

Epithelial tumors can be categorized as benign (adenoma), malignant (adenocarcinoma), or of an intermediate form, known as borderline tumor or tumor of low malignant potential. The term *papillary* or the prefix *cyst-* (as in cystadenoma) is used when the tumor has, respectively, papillae or cystic

**Table 33.3** Epithelial Ovarian Tumor Cell Types

| | Approximate Frequency (%) | |
|---|---|---|
| Cell Type | All Ovarian Neoplasms | Ovarian Cancers |
| Serous | 20-50 | 35-40 |
| Mucinous | 15-25 | 6-10 |
| Endometrioid | 5 | 15-25 |
| Clear cell (mesonephroid) | <5 | 5 |
| Brenner | 2-3 | Rare |

Modified from Scully RE. Tumors of the ovary and maldeveloped gonads. In Scully RE. *Atlas of Tumor Pathology*. Fascicle 16. Series 2. Washington, DC: Armed Forces Institute of Pathology; 1979.

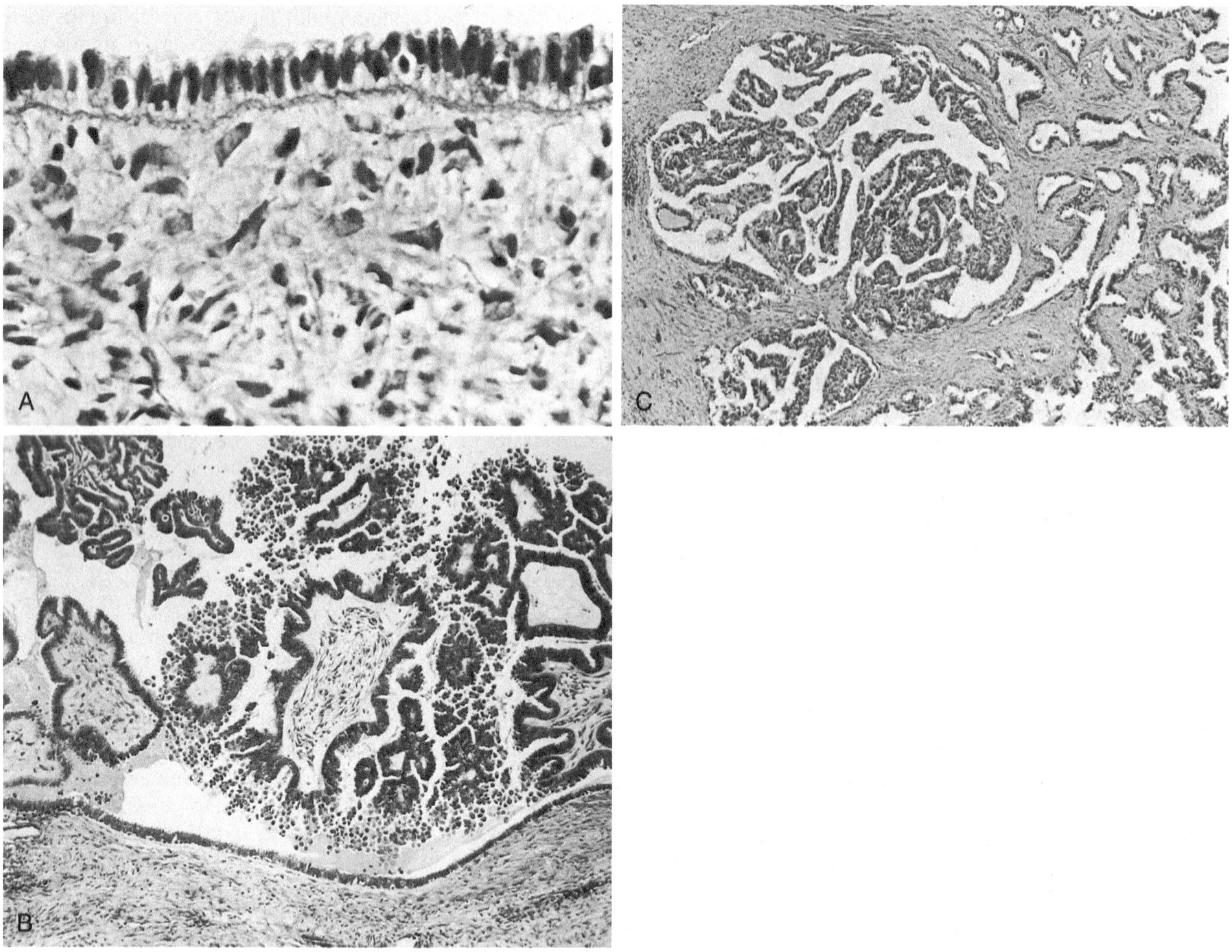


**Figure 33.2** **A,** Ciliated epithelium of a well-differentiated serous tumor (×800). **B,** Serous papillary cystadenoma of borderline malignancy. The epithelium resembles that of the fallopian tube, and a well-developed papillary pattern is present (×80). **C,** Serous papillary adenocarcinoma (×50). The neoplastic epithelium invades the stroma. (**A** and **C,** From Serov SF, Scully RE, Sobin LH. *Histologic Typing of Ovarian Tumors*. Geneva: World Health Organization; 1973. **B,** Courtesy of Dr. R. E. Scully.)

structures. The suffix *-fibroma* (as in adenofibroma) is added when the ovarian stroma predominates, with the exception of a Brenner tumor, which normally contains a large amount of ovarian stroma.

Low-grade (formerly well-differentiated) serous tumors (Fig. 33.2, *A* and *B*) consist of ciliated epithelial cells that resemble those of the fallopian tube. Serous tumors (Fig. 33.2, *C*) are the most frequent ovarian epithelial tumors. The malignant forms account for 40% or more of ovarian cancers, benign forms (serous cystadenomas) occur primarily during the reproductive years, borderline tumors occur in women 30 to 50 years of age, and carcinomas typically occur in women older than 40 years. Molecular investigation of genetic changes associated with low-grade serous tumors support the reclassification of serous ovarian cancers into low- or high-grade binaries. Currently, a popular theory hypothesizes that high-grade serous carcinoma may arise from fallopian tube epithelium.

Mucinous tumors (Fig. 33.3, *A* and *B*) consist of epithelial cells filled with mucin; most are benign. These cells resemble cells of the endocervix or may mimic intestinal cells, which can pose a problem in the differential diagnosis of tumors that appear to originate from the ovary or intestine. Benign mucinous tumors are found primarily during the reproductive years, and mucinous carcinomas (Fig. 33.3, *C*) usually occur in those in the 30- to 60-year age range. Overall, they can account for approximately 25% of ovarian tumors and as many as 10% of ovarian cancers.

Endometrioid tumors (Fig. 33.4), as the name implies, consist of epithelial cells resembling those of the endometrium. In the ovary, these neoplasms are less frequent (approximately 5%) than serous or mucinous tumors, but the malignant variety accounts for approximately 20% of ovarian carcinomas. Endometrioid carcinomas usually occur in women in their 40s and 50s. They may be seen in conjunction with endometriosis and ovarian endometriomas, although an origin from endometriosis is rarely demonstrated. Most endometrioid carcinomas arise directly from the surface epithelium of the ovary, as do the other epithelial tumors.

Clear cell tumors (mesonephromas) contain cells with abundant glycogen (Fig. 33.5, *A*) and so-called *hobnail cells* (Fig. 33.5, *B*),

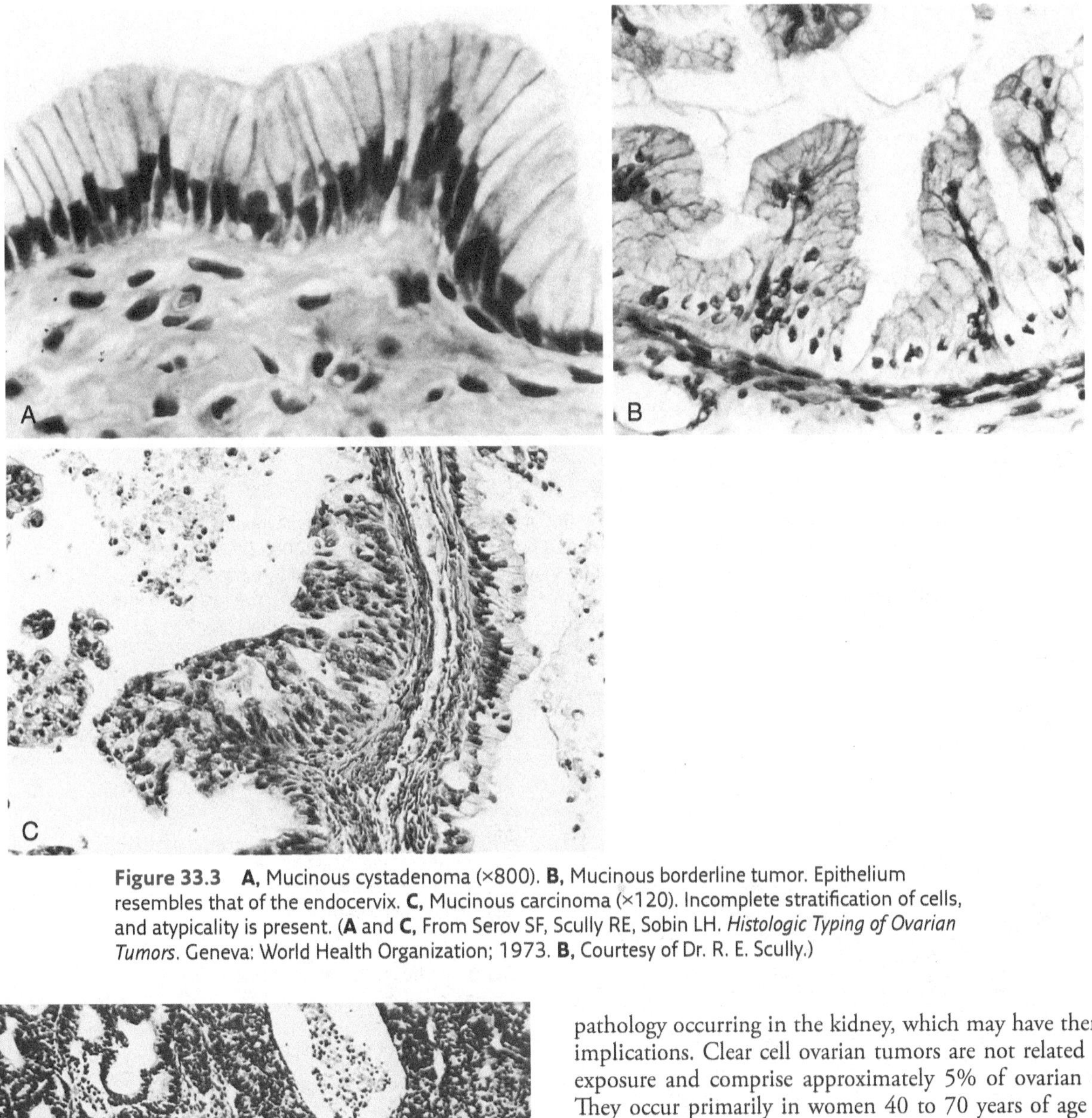


**Figure 33.3** **A,** Mucinous cystadenoma (×800). **B,** Mucinous borderline tumor. Epithelium resembles that of the endocervix. **C,** Mucinous carcinoma (×120). Incomplete stratification of cells, and atypicality is present. (**A** and **C,** From Serov SF, Scully RE, Sobin LH. *Histologic Typing of Ovarian Tumors*. Geneva: World Health Organization; 1973. **B,** Courtesy of Dr. R. E. Scully.)

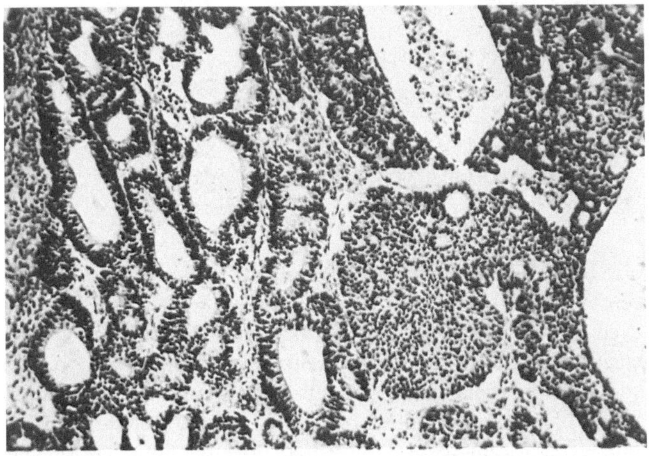

**Figure 33.4** Endometrioid carcinoma. Tubular glands are lined by stratified endometrium (×80). (Courtesy of Dr. R.E. Scully.)

in which the nuclei of the cells protrude into the glandular lumen. Tumors with identical histologic features are found in the endometrium, cervix, and vagina, the latter two often associated with intrauterine diethylstilbestrol (DES) exposure. Molecular evaluation of these tumors suggests a homology to similar pathology occurring in the kidney, which may have therapeutic implications. Clear cell ovarian tumors are not related to DES exposure and comprise approximately 5% of ovarian cancers. They occur primarily in women 40 to 70 years of age and are highly aggressive.

The major cell types of ovarian epithelial tumors recapitulate the müllerian duct–derived epithelium of the female reproductive system (serous-endosalpinx, mucinous-endocervix, endometrioid-endometrium). This differentiation occurs even though the ovary is not derived directly from the müllerian ducts (see Chapter 2). The clear cell tumors also mimic this müllerian tendency, frequently being admixed with endometrioid carcinomas and with ovarian endometriomas.

Brenner tumors (Fig. 33.6) consist of cells that resemble the transitional epithelium of the bladder and Walthard nests of the ovary. There is abundant stroma. These tumors constitute only 2% to 3% of all ovarian tumors.

In addition to the cell types shown in Table 33.3, epithelial tumors may be classified as undifferentiated if the tumor consists of poorly differentiated epithelial cells that are not characteristic of any particular cell type. They may be considered unclassifiable if they cannot be placed in any of the categories shown in this table.

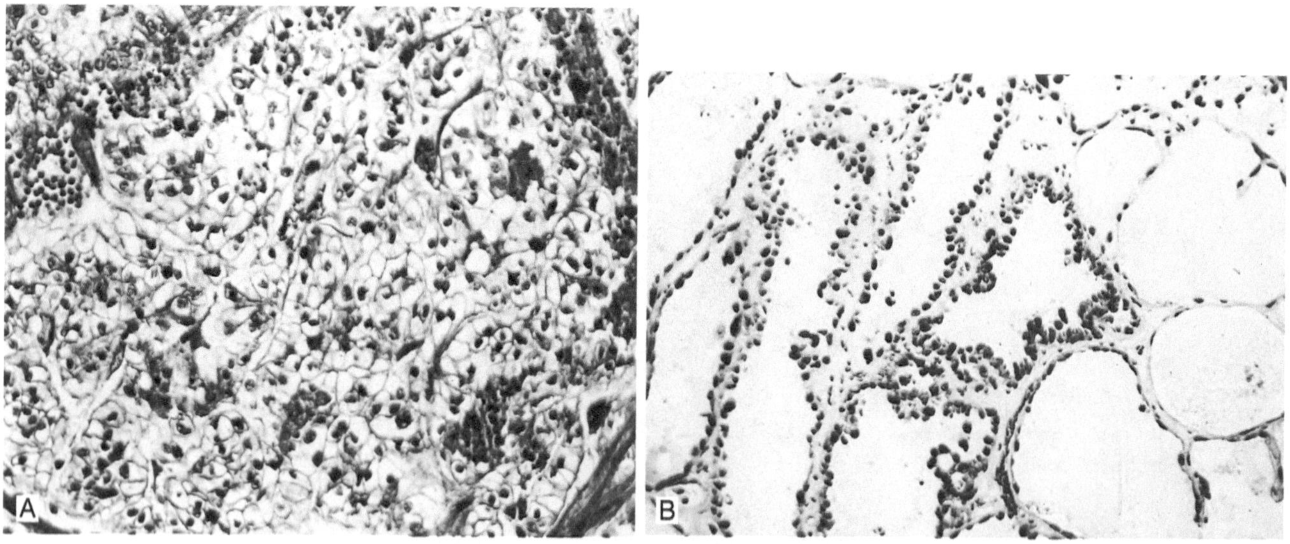

**Figure 33.5** **A,** Clear cell adenocarcinoma (×200). A solid pattern of abundant polyhedral tumor cells containing abundant clear cytoplasm is present. **B,** Clear cell adenocarcinoma (×200). *Left:* Hobnail cells with scant cytoplasm; protruding nuclei line shows tubules. *Right:* Cysts lined by flattened tumor cells. (**A,** From Barlow JF, Scully RE. "Mesonephroma" of ovary: tumor of müllerian nature related to the endometrioid carcinoma. *Cancer.* 1967;20[9]:1405-1417. **B,** Courtesy of Dr. R.E. Scully.)

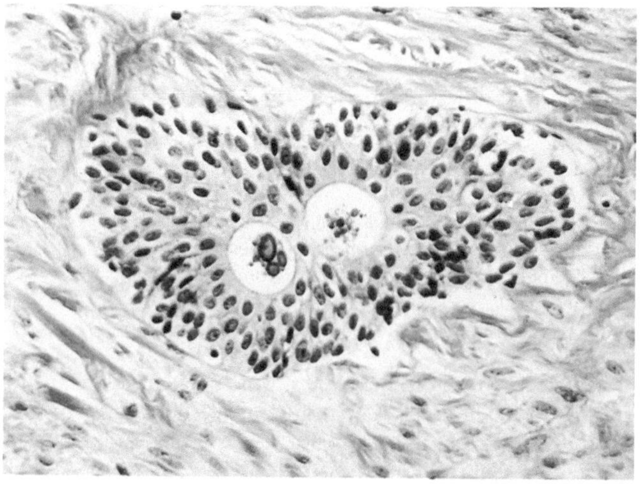

**Figure 33.6** Brenner tumor (×350). Note the nest of transition-like epithelium containing spaces with eosinophilic material. (From Scully RE. *Atlas of Tumor Pathology,* fascicle 16, series 2. Washington, DC: Armed Forces Institute of Pathology; 1979.)

**Table 33.4** Bilaterality of Ovarian Tumors

| Type of Tumor | Occurrence (%) |
|---|---|
| **Epithelial Tumors** | |
| Serous cystadenoma | 10 |
| Serous cystadenocarcinoma | 33-66 |
| Mucinous cystadenoma | 5 |
| Mucinous cystadenocarcinoma | 10-20 |
| Endometrioid carcinoma | 13-30 |
| Benign Brenner tumor | 6 |
| **Germ Cell Tumors** | |
| Benign cystic teratoma (dermoid) | 12 |
| Immature teratoma (malignant) | 2-5 |
| Dysgerminoma | 5-10 |
| Other malignant germ cell tumors | Rare |
| **Sex Cord-Stromal Tumors** | |
| Thecoma | Rare |
| Sertoli-Leydig cell tumor | Rare |
| Granulosa-theca cell tumor | Rare |

Many epithelial ovarian tumors can be bilateral, and the risk of bilaterality is an important consideration in therapy, particularly when an ovarian tumor is discovered in a young woman of reproductive age. Widely varying percentages have been reported for bilaterality in ovarian tumors; the most widely quoted are summarized in Table 33.4. Malignant epithelial tumors tend to involve both ovaries more frequently than benign epithelial tumors. Serous tumors also tend to be bilateral more frequently than mucinous tumors.

## BENIGN EPITHELIAL OVARIAN TUMORS: THE ADNEXAL MASS

As noted in Chapter 7, enlargement of the ovary beyond 5 cm is considered abnormal. However, age and menstrual status must also be considered before the appropriate course of action is chosen. A 5- to 8-cm ovarian mass in a woman with regular menses, even if she is in her 40s, is frequently a functioning ovarian cyst, such as a follicular or corpus luteum cyst. It will usually regress spontaneously during a subsequent menstrual cycle. Enlargements of this type in young patients in their 20s or early 30s do not automatically require immediate operative intervention and can be observed for two menstrual cycles. A potential exception would be a mass in a woman who is taking oral contraceptives. Because the principal mechanism of contraception is anovulation, the index of suspicion for neoplastic growth should be raised. However, contemporary oral contraceptives have lower sex steroid levels and may permit follicular development. Careful observation or immediate evaluation (discussed earlier) is warranted. Shushan and colleagues reported on ovarian cysts detected by ultrasonography in pre- and postmenopausal women

**Box 33.1 Cancer Antigen 125 Associations**

**Cancer**
Ovarian, primary peritoneal, fallopian tube
Uterine
Colon
Breast
Stomach
Liver

**Disease**
Leiomyomata
Endometriosis
Pelvic infection
Liver, heart, kidney failure
Alcoholism
Peritonitis
Pancreatitis

**Condition**
Pregnancy
Mild menstrual cycle

taking tamoxifen for breast cancer. Unilocular 5- to 8-cm cysts are likely to be functional (see Chapter 18), whereas multilocular or partially solid tumors are more likely to be neoplastic. After the age of 40, the risk of malignancy rises. The ovary shrinks during menopause and is approximately 1.5 to 2 cm in size. A transvaginal ultrasound scan can reliably detect an ovary larger than 1 cm in diameter. Higgins and associates estimated the upper limit of the volume of a postmenopausal ovary to be approximately 8 $cm^3$ compared with 18 $cm^3$ for the premenopausal ovary. Ten of their patients who exceeded these criteria and had solid or complex echo patterns had neoplastic tumors, and one carcinoma was discovered. An ultrasound examination, preferably with a vaginal probe, helps differentiate these adnexal masses (discussed later).

Occasionally, it is discovered that the adnexal mass is paraovarian. In a study of 168 paraovarian tumors, Stein and coworkers noted that only three (2%) were malignant. The three cysts all had solid components; the cysts were 8 to 12 cm size in patients 19 to 48 years of age.

### *Adnexal Mass and Ovarian Cancer*

Cancer antigen 125 (CA-125) was described by Bast and colleagues in the 1980s. It is expressed by approximately 80% of ovarian epithelial carcinomas but less frequently by mucinous tumors. The marker is increased in endometrial and tubal carcinoma, in addition to ovarian carcinoma, and in other malignancies, including those originating in the lung, breast, and pancreas. A level higher than 35 U/mL is generally considered to be increased. Box 33.1 lists some of the benign conditions for which the CA-125 level also has frequently been found to be increased.

As can be seen, many of these are frequently found in women of childbearing age. This lack of specificity must be remembered when one is interpreting increased CA-125 levels in younger women with adnexal masses or when screening is being considered (discussed later). In addition, there are rare individuals who have no disease but are found to have levels of CA-125 as high as 200 to 300 U/mL as a consequence of developing idiopathic antibodies to mouse IgG.

One must also be cautious in the interpretation of an increased CA-125 level, particularly in a premenopausal woman with an adnexal mass. The specificity appears to be better for increased values in the postmenopausal woman. In a study of 182 patients, Vasilev and coworkers (1988) have noted that the CA-125 level is increased in 22% of cases of benign masses, but for postmenopausal patients an increased level usually indicates malignancy. This was also shown in the CA-125 vaginal ultrasound study of 290 postmenopausal patients by Maggino and colleagues.

In addition to CA125 and transvaginal ultrasound, other biomarkers have been evaluated for their ability to preoperatively discriminate between benign disease and cancer. Currently, one test, OVA1, has been approved to aid this decision by providing a probability estimate of cancer based on a proprietary mathematical algorithm of five independent biomarkers: CA-125, $\beta_2$-microglobulin, transferrin, apolipoprotein A1, and transthyretin. OVA1 was the first blood test cleared by the U.S. Food and Drug Administration (FDA) to help evaluate the likelihood that a woman's ovarian mass is malignant or benign prior to a planned surgery. The OVA1 test, when performed in 516 women with adnexal masses deemed appropriate for surgical excision, improved the sensitivity of cancer versus noncancer discrimination in a double-blind clinical study from 72% to 92% when using the biomarker panel. Among gynecologic oncologists, the sensitivity increased from 86% to 99%. Although not approved for surveillance or diagnosis, the test may complement clinical decision making, particularly if a gynecologic oncologist is not available to perform appropriate staging should cancer be identified.

#### Evaluation of the Adnexal Mass

Ultrasound has helped define criteria to allow conservative follow-up and the risk of malignancy of some adnexal masses. Goldstein and associates studied 42 postmenopausal patients whose ultrasound scans have shown unilocular cysts smaller than 5 cm in diameter; 28 were explored, and none had malignancy, and 14 were followed for as long as 6 years, with no change in ultrasound appearance. Finkler and colleagues noted that the addition of a CA-125 serum assay to their ultrasound criteria in postmenopausal women increases the accuracy of preoperative evaluation. In a clinicopathologic study to define ultrasound criteria of malignancy, Granberg and associates (1989) studied the ovarian tumors in 1017 women. Of 296 with unilocular cysts, only one was malignant and had visible papillary formations on the cyst wall; 60% of these women were older than 40 years. In contrast, malignancy rates were 8% (20 of 229) for multilocular cysts, 65% (147 of 201) for multilocular solid tumors, and 39% (31 of 80) for solid ovarian masses. In a follow-up study of 180 women, the authors noted that 45 of 45 unilocular cysts were benign. In an ultrasound study of cystic ovarian masses in women older than 50 years, Bailey and coworkers noted that unilocular cysts smaller than 10 cm in diameter are rarely malignant, whereas complex cysts or those with solid areas are at high risk of malignancy.

Several scoring systems have been proposed to try to determine the risk of an ovarian mass being malignant. They usually include the following:

1. Is the finding a simple (unilocular) or complex (multicystic or multilocular with solid components) cyst?
2. Are there papillary projections?
3. Are the cystic walls or septa regular and smooth?
4. What is the echogenicity (tissue characterization)?

These terms, definitions, and measurements have been standardized under a consensus opinion from the International

Ovarian Tumor Analysis (IOTA) group and help refine the likelihood of malignancy. Shalev and coworkers combined transvaginal ultrasonography and normal CA-125 values in 55 postmenopausal women with simple cystic or septate cystic ovarian masses; all 55 had benign disease. Although this was a small study, it suggests the potential of applying stringent ultrasound criteria with CA-125 evaluation of ovarian masses in postmenopausal women.

Others have advocated using transvaginal pulsed Doppler color-enhanced flow studies to differentiate benign from malignant masses. The resistance index, which measures resistance to flow in the vessels, has been used and presumably is low in the presence of neovascularization that is seen with malignant tumors. The vessels of neoangiogenesis are abnormal in their distribution, with disorganized branching and a loss of the muscularis layer, all of which contribute to the decreased resistance to flow. A resistance of 0.40 or less was found useful by Kurjak and coworkers in a study of 254 women. In contrast, Bromley and colleagues, in a study of 33 postmenopausal women, used a cutoff of 0.6, which did not greatly add to their specificities; they relied on morphologic criteria (e.g., solid elements, papillary projections) to diagnose malignancy.

Valentin and associates evaluated the characteristics of 1066 adnexal masses; 266 were malignant (55 borderline ovarian tumors, 144 primary invasive epithelial cancers, 25 nonepithelial ovarian cancers, 42 metastatic cancers). A scoring system was used as well as information from color Doppler studies. They reported that borderline and stage I ovarian cancers shared similar morphology but had different characteristics from more advanced-stage tumors. They were larger, contained more papillary projections, and were more often multilocular, without solid components, but were less often purely solid and less likely to be associated with ascites. Significant variation was noted, however. Similarly, Twickler and colleagues described a scoring model to create an ovarian tumor index for women with adnexal disease. Of 244 women with follow-up, 214 had nonmalignant findings and 30 had cancer. In addition to age, transvaginal ultrasound variables, including ovarian volume, the Sassone morphology scale, and Doppler determination of angle-corrected systole, diastole, and time-averaged velocity, were evaluated. An ovarian tumor index was created from discriminant variables (continuous and weighted) correctly classifying the two cohorts. The area under the receiver operator characteristic curve (AUC) was highly significant (AUC = 0.91). Unfortunately, scoring systems such as these, developed from data produced by highly skilled and proficient sonographers, are difficult to generalize and, although promising, are highly operator dependent. The IOTA group has temporally and externally validated the diagnostic performance of two logistic regression models containing clinical and ultrasound variables for malignancy identification. In this study, the prevalence of invasive cancer was 3%. The likelihood of cancer from a positive screen exceeded 6 for both models; a negative likelihood ratio was under 0.1, suggesting that the criteria may be of use for evaluating women with an adnexal masses.

It should be noted that there is a difference in using ultrasonography to screen for ovarian cancer as opposed to using different modalities of ultrasonography to characterize an ovarian mass as benign or malignant. For example, the addition of color Doppler sonography, which measures blood flow and direction of flow, and power Doppler sonography, which can detect slow flow in small vessels, can add useful information. These permit visualization of flow location (peripheral, central, or within a septum). Most malignant tumors have a central flow (75% to 100%) compared with only 5% to 40% of benign ovarian tumors. Schelling and colleagues studied transvaginal B-mode and color Doppler sonography for the diagnosis of malignancy in 257 adnexal masses with unclear malignant status. They achieved 92% sensitivity and 94% specificity. The development of three-dimensional ultrasonography may allow more accurate volume assessments. In addition, color Doppler with three-dimensional ultrasonography may permit better detection of vessel irregularity, coiling, and branching. Another possibility is the use of contrast media to quantify and permit earlier detection of abnormal angiogenesis, as noted by Abramowicz. Contrast-enhanced (microbubble) power three-dimensional Doppler sonography has been investigated to evaluate the efficacy of antiangiogenic biologic in serial scanning.

### *Ovarian Cancer Screening*

Although ovarian cancer is characterized by advanced-stage disease at diagnosis and high mortality, early-stage disease is often curable. The greatest impact on these statistics, other than prevention, would be screening to identify early-stage disease. Three modalities, used individually or in combination, have been the common theme of this effort: physical examination, biomarkers (e.g., CA-125), proteomics-genomics (experimental) and sonography. For a disease to be amenable to screening, it should be sufficiently severe (high mortality) and have a natural history from latency to overt disease that is well characterized, and there should be a successful outcome if early disease is treated. The screening modality should have high positive and negative predictive values, and high sensitivity and specificity, and be acceptable to the population, cost-effective, and widely available. The screening population should be identifiable and, for those in whom early disease is identified, effective therapy should be available. Although ovarian cancer satisfies many of these mandates, it is rare in the general population and not readily characterized by an identifiable precursor, thus producing a high bar for any modality.

Of the three most commonly used modalities, the least sensitive and specific is physical examination. It is estimated that just one early ovarian cancer will be identified in 10,000 physical examinations. Although the easiest to implement, poor sensitivity limits this intervention as an effective strategy.

Biomarkers such as CA-125 are of great interest because they are easy to obtain and serial evaluation can be tracked. CA-125 has been used most consistently since being discovered as a reliable biomarker for epithelial nonmucinous ovarian cancer. Early, large, population-based studies highlighted its limitation as a sole strategy for ovarian cancer screening. Einhorn and associates screened 5550 women and, in 1992, reported that only two stage I cancers in 175 women with elevated CA-125 values were identified. As noted, a differential effect would be expected between pre- and postmenopausal women. Using the modality in women with a pelvic mass (in whom prevalence is increased) has substantial effects on test characteristics but overlooks the obvious need for cancer identification before gross ovarian enlargement. This has led to the development of combined evaluation (sonography) described here.

Ultrasonography as an isolated modality has also been advocated for screening. Although more expensive and less amenable to population screening, it has become increasingly accurate in identifying early changes within the ovary, as noted. Campbell and coworkers screened 5479 patients and obtained 338 abnormal scans. Five early-stage ovarian cancers were identified. The positive predictive value was only 1.5%. Similarly, van Nagell screened 1300 patients and obtained 33 abnormal scans. Two early-stage ovarian cancers were identified. As with single-modality testing, sonography is too insensitive to be widely used for screening.

Population-based ovarian cancer screening programs have been difficult to recommend and implement because poor sensitivity and positive predictive value characteristics accompany expensive and inefficient testing methodology and triage algorithms. Menon and colleagues approached this problem by evaluating a prospectively based algorithm in a population-based screening program in the United Kingdom. The population cohort used to evaluate this screening strategy involved 13,582 menopausal women 50 years or older with at least one ovary, of whom 6532 randomized women completed a first screen; the remainder served as controls. The screening strategy was a staged process in which each CA-125 sample drawn underwent a calculation for risk of ovarian cancer (ROCA). The calculation was based on the woman's age and CA-125 value relative to her personal baseline. In this trial, an estimated risk of less than 1 in 2000 was considered normal, whereas a risk of more than 1 in 500 was considered increased; those in between were considered intermediate and required repeat testing. Those not considered normal were referred for a second stage of screening that incorporated a transvaginal ultrasound scan and repeat CA-125 testing. A transvaginal ultrasound scan was considered normal, abnormal, or equivocal based on ovarian volume and morphology. From the combination of CA-125 risk estimation and transvaginal ultrasound scan, a follow-up recommendation was made that could be a gynecologic oncology referral, repeat CA-125 testing, or transvaginal ultrasound scan or annual screening. In the screened group, almost 80% continued with annual screening; 91 (1.4%) were considered at increased risk. Among the intermediate group, repeat testing was normal in 92%, leaving 188 (2.9% of the initial population) to undergo second-stage evaluation. Of the 144 who stayed in the program, 95 were returned to annual screening based on CA-125 and transvaginal ultrasound scan findings, 6 were found to have nongynecologic malignancies, 43 were referred to a gynecologic oncologist, of whom 27 were returned to annual screening, and 16 women underwent surgery. From this group, five ovarian cancers were identified (four malignant epithelial and one borderline); the 11 remaining women had benign ovarian neoplasms. Compared with the authors' previous algorithm based on flat CA-125 values (normal = 30 U/mL), the new process referred less than 50% to secondary screening. It was concluded that this algorithm increases screening precision.

Two other prospective trials of general population screening deserve mention: the Prostate, Lung, Colorectal and Ovarian (PLCO) study and the United Kingdom Collaborative Trial of Ovarian Cancer Screening (UKCTOCS). The primary objective of the PLCO study is to evaluate the impact of annual screening with transvaginal ultrasound (TVUS) and CA-125 on ovarian cancer mortality. The study is following a cohort of more than 34,000 largely postmenopausal women with intact ovaries prospectively with an algorithm indicating that an abnormal CA-125 level (≥35 U/mL) or an abnormality on TVUS is considered a positive screen. Follow-up procedures of a positive screen are not prespecified but have been tracked, as well as any surgical interventions resulting from these findings. Compliance over four rounds of screening decreased slightly over the 3 years of postbaseline evaluation but remained above 75%. In contrast to CA-125, screen-positive TVUS decreased over the interval from 4.6% at baseline to 3.4% at year 3. Almost 90 ovarian cancers have been diagnosed so far; 60 were identified by screening abnormalities. Overall, the ratio of screen-positive ovarian cancers relative to benign disease decreased from 30:1 to almost 20:1. Of the ovarian cancers identified, 72% were advanced stage. The study continues to mature, with relatively good compliance. However, the impact of screening on the primary end point (mortality) is unknown.

The UKCTOCS was designed to assess the effect of ovarian cancer screening on mortality definitively, as well as comprehensively address the cost, acceptance, physical and psychosocial morbidity, and performance characteristics of multimodal screening and ultrasound-based screening. Between 2001 and 2005, a total of 202,638 postmenopausal women 50 to 74 years of age were randomly assigned to control (no screening), annual CA-125 screening (based on risk of ovarian cancer [ROC] algorithm), and second-line ultrasound testing (multimodal screening [MMS]) or annual transvaginal ultrasound (USS) alone in a 2:1:1 ratio. In the prevalence screen, 50,078 women (98.9%) underwent MMS and 48,230 (95.2%) underwent USS. Overall, 9% of the MMS cohort and 12% of the USS cohort required repeat testing. Surgery was undertaken in a small proportion of both cohorts but was significantly more likely following USS. Ovarian neoplasms, benign and malignant, were identified in both screening cohorts. The proportion of stage I and II cases was 48.3% and was balanced between the two screening algorithms. However, specificity was significantly higher for the MMS strategy (99.8%) relative to USS (98.2%). The performance of both screening modalities is encouraging and establishes feasibility (Table 33.5). The impact of stage migration following screening, as reflected in disease-specific mortality, is pending study completion, expected in 2014.

Successful prediction of cancer in the general public is limited by the low prevalence of disease. Creasman and DiSaia have estimated that if vaginal ultrasound scanning and CA-125 testing were performed annually on all women older than 45 years in the United States, the cost would exceed $10 billion annually.

One strategy to improve the predictive index is to address a population in which prevalence is increased. A number of studies have been undertaken using transvaginal ultrasonography to screen for ovarian malignancy in higher risk women. Bourne and colleagues screened 775 women who had at least one first-degree ($n$ = 677) or second-degree ($n$ = 98) relative with ovarian cancer. Overall, 43 women were referred for surgery with abnormal-appearing ovaries and 39 underwent surgery, with three stage IA ovarian carcinomas discovered (3.9 of 1000 screened); one of these was a borderline tumor. One screened patient was found to have peritoneal carcinomatosis 11 months after a normal screening study. The remainder had

Table 33.5 Screening Performance of Multimodal and Transvaginal Ultrasound in the United Kingdom Collaborative Trial of Ovarian Cancer Screening Prevalence Study

| | Screening Modality | |
|---|---|---|
| Parameter | Multimodal Screening | Transvaginal Ultrasound |
| Repeat testing | 9% | 12% |
| Clinical evaluation | 0.3% | 3.9% |
| Surgery | 0.2% | 1.8% |
| Number of ovarian cancers | 42 | 45 |
| Borderline cancers | 8 | 20 |
| Stage I and II cancers (48.3% of cancers identified) | 16 | 12 |
| Sensitivity | 89.5% | 75% |
| Specificity | 99.8% | 98.2% |
| Positive predictive value | 35.1% | 2.8% |

nonmalignant findings. DePriest and associates screened 6470 asymptomatic postmenopausal women and defined abnormality as an ovary with a volume larger than 10 $cm^3$ or papillary projections in a cystic ovarian tumor. Ninety patients who had persistent findings by repeat ultrasound scanning at 4 to 6 weeks had an operation, with the finding of five early (stage IA; see later) and one advanced (stage IIIB) carcinomas. There were 37 serous cystadenomas and 20 assorted benign ovarian conditions. One woman with a normal scan was found to have peritoneal carcinomatosis 11 months later. These investigators noted that normal ovarian volume in a postmenopausal woman is smaller than 10 $cm^3$ and, in a premenopausal woman it is as much as 20 $cm^3$, as reported by Pavlik and colleagues.

Clinicopathologic studies of Bell and Scully, as well as ultrasound screening trials by Crayford and colleagues, have provided an explanation for the lack of success with ultrasound screening for detecting low-stage ovarian carcinomas. Bell and Scully proposed the term *early de novo carcinoma* to explain their findings of 14 carefully studied cases. None of these patients had clinical evidence of ovarian carcinoma at the time of operation. All had microscopic foci of carcinoma in their ovaries, and three cases were detected only years later postoperatively, when the patients were discovered to have widespread carcinoma consistent with what was found in their ovaries on retrospective study. Crayford and colleagues screened 5479 self-referred asymptomatic women by vaginal ultrasonography and removed all persistent ovarian cysts in an attempt to reduce the frequency of ovarian cancer. Of these, 88 patients had cysts removed. A slight nonsignificant increase in ovarian cancer deaths for this group was found 12 years after the conclusion of the study. Therefore it appears that most ovarian carcinomas (particularly serous) arise from a tiny cancer of the surface of the ovary, from which it can spread rapidly before the ovary enlarges. Some ovarian tumors, such as endometrioid carcinoma, may have their origin in endometriosis. These carcinomas, as well as mucinous, tend to be detected more frequently at earlier stages. Therefore they appear more likely to have a cystic rather than a de novo origin. These observations strongly suggest that current strategies to use vaginal ultrasound screening to detect early ovarian carcinoma will have only limited success, as noted by Herbst.

### Nonmalignant Neoplasms

Most nonmalignant epithelial ovarian tumors are asymptomatic unilateral adnexal masses that can be treated by oophorectomy or occasionally cystectomy (see Benign Cystic Teratomas [Dermoids,] presented later). In the past, some recommended bisecting the opposite ovary to rule out bilaterality in the case of benign epithelial ovarian tumors (see Table 33.4), but in view of the risk of adhesions and infertility as well as the availability of vaginal ultrasonography, this is no longer done. In a woman beyond her reproductive years, especially in the presence of a serous cystadenoma, which tends to be bilateral, hysterectomy and bilateral salpingo-oophorectomy are usually performed.

Mucinous tumors can become particularly large and reach sizes of 30 cm or larger. Possible complications of mucinous cystadenoma are perforation and rupture, which can lead to the deposit and growth of mucin-secreting epithelium in the peritoneal cavity (pseudomyxoma peritonei; discussed later).

Adenofibromas consist of fibrous and epithelial elements. The epithelial component may be serous, mucinous, clear cell, or endometrioid, the architectural subtypes of these benign ovarian tumors. Their appearance will depend on the predominant histologic features, epithelial or fibrous. These tumors are also managed by simple excision. Endometriomas are considered in Chapter 19.

Brenner tumors (see Fig. 33.6) are rare and often incidental findings when oophorectomy is performed for an indication other than ovarian enlargement. Usually these tumors occur in women in their 40s and 50s, but younger and older patients have been found to have them. Brenner tumors are almost always benign and can usually be managed by oophorectomy. When the ovary is palpably enlarged, approximately 5% of Brenner tumors will prove to be malignant. These tumors often occur in perimenopausal and postmenopausal women, in which case, hysterectomy and bilateral salpingo-oophorectomy are indicated. Unfortunately, malignant Brenner tumors appear to have a poor prognosis despite this operative therapy, and an effective program of chemotherapy has not been developed.

The differential diagnosis for and approach to an adnexal mass in women of various ages are discussed in Chapter 7. Ovarian enlargement in the premenarchal female is usually the result of a germ cell tumor, which may be malignant but is usually benign (discussed later). During the reproductive years, ovarian neoplasms are usually benign. For the woman in her 20s or 30s, most ovarian enlargements can be approached surgically through a lower abdominal transverse (Pfannenstiel) incision or by laparoscopy. However, contingency plans in the setting of an unanticipated malignancy should be considered preoperatively and discussed with the woman. Larger masses usually require a vertical skin incision to ensure intact removal and safe dissection. Although the diagnosis of cancer can only be verified in tissue, patient characteristics (e.g., age, family history), preoperative ovarian morphology (e.g., exophytic or endophytic masses, masses with large solid components, size), and biomarker studies (e.g., CA-125, HE4) may modulate risk assessment and thus the surgical approach.

The liberal use of intraoperative frozen-section assessment should be exercised, particularly in menopausal women. For women of reproductive age desiring fertility, if the diagnosis of malignancy is suspected but uncertain even after a frozen section is obtained, the operation should be terminated after removal of the ovarian tumor. A second procedure can be performed if malignancy is confirmed after detailed histologic study of the permanent sections. This is preferable to risking an unnecessary hysterectomy or bilateral salpingo-oophorectomy in a woman who desires to preserve childbearing function. Women who do not desire childbearing should undergo careful counseling to describe the potential need for a staging procedure in case a documented or suspected malignancy is identified from the frozen section.

## CARCINOMAS

### Diagnosis, Staging, Spread, Preoperative Evaluation, and Prognostic Factors

Ovarian carcinomas are usually diagnosed by detection of an adnexal mass on pelvic or abdominal examination. Occasionally, the diagnosis is made from a radiographic survey carried out for the evaluation of nonspecific gastrointestinal symptoms. Unfortunately, the diagnosis is frequently made only after the disease has spread beyond the ovary, as noted earlier when we described the de novo origin of these tumors. Scully has estimated that the risk of malignancy in a primary ovarian tumor increases to approximately 33% in a woman older than 45, whereas it is less than 1 in 15 for women who are 20 to 45 years of age. In general, more than 50% of ovarian carcinomas occur in women older than 50. In a hospital-based study of ovarian neoplasms in 861 women, Koonings and associates noted that the risk of malignancy was 13% in premenopausal women but rose to 45% in postmenopausal women. In their study, benign ovarian neoplasms were most common in those 20 to 29 years of age.

More than 90% of women diagnosed with ovarian cancer report symptoms before diagnosis. Unfortunately, these symptoms are vague and not specific for early-stage disease or even ovarian cancer. Goff and colleagues conducted a prospective survey of women seeking medical care. The case patients were those about to undergo surgery for a known or suspected pelvic or ovarian mass; the controls were women presenting to one of two primary care clinics, in which approximately two thirds were being seen for a specific problem. The voluntary questionnaire instrument administered to both cohorts asked the respondents to score the severity, frequency, and duration of 20 symptoms generally reported by ovarian cancer patients. In both groups, recurring symptoms were common and nonspecific. Symptomatology in control patients was related to the purpose of their visit (general checkup vs. specific complaint), underlying disease comorbidities, and menopausal status. Not surprisingly, women with the final diagnosis of ovarian cancer generally reported numerically more symptoms and of greater severity but of shorter duration of onset compared with the clinic controls or patients with benign ovarian tumors. Ovarian cancer patients were also statistically more likely to report increased abdominal size, bloating, urinary urgency, and pelvic pain. Because the combination of increased abdominal size, bloating, and urinary urgency was reported five times more often and had greater severity in cancer patients than in controls, the authors recommended further clinical investigation when identified. The diagnosis is established by histologic examination of tumor tissue removed at operation. Occasionally, the initial diagnosis is suggested by malignant cells found in ascitic or pleural fluid obtained at paracentesis or thoracentesis, respectively.

The staging of ovarian cancer (Table 33.6) is designed according to the criteria of the International Federation of Gynecology and Obstetrics (FIGO). It is based on the results of operative exploration. Before surgical exploration for suspected ovarian carcinoma, the woman has a preoperative workup that is standard for a major abdominal operation (see Chapter 24). Additional diagnostic studies may include a computed tomography (CT) scan of the abdomen to search for disease that would preclude a surgical intervention. Involvement of certain sites in the abdominal or pelvic cavity would be considered inoperable to achieve an optimal cytoreduction (<1 cm residual disease). These sites include retroperitoneal suprarenal lymph node enlargement, mesenteric disease, porta hepatis disease, or bilateral parenchymal liver metastases.

A few studies have evaluated the role of combined positron emission tomography (PET) and CT in the treatment of primary epithelial ovarian cancer. Risum and associates prospectively analyzed the diagnostic value of PET-CT for detecting a malignant tumor in 97 patients with no previous cancer history who presented with a pelvic mass. All the patients included in the study had PET-CT scans prior to surgery; the average serum CA-125 level was 784 U/mL. The sensitivity and specificity of PET-CT in diagnosing a malignant pelvic tumor were 100% and 92.5%, respectively.

Occasionally, a barium enema or colonoscopy is performed to evaluate pelvic or gastrointestinal symptoms. Consideration of gastrointestinal pathology is of importance for the potential of a primary colon carcinoma, which may present initially as an adnexal mass in the older woman. Approximately 4% of colon cancers have metastatic involvement of the ovary at diagnosis. Determination of the serum carcinoembryonic antigen level may be useful in this setting and is recommended as part of the preoperative evaluation of a pelvic mass. An endoscopic or gastrointestinal radiographic examination is performed if there is evidence of gastrointestinal bleeding or the suggestion of any gastrointestinal pathology.

A CA-125 sample is obtained and, if the level increased at the time of operation, is useful for following the progress of the woman during and after treatment and for demonstrating the response to therapy or detecting tumor progression. Buller and associates studied the regression slope for CA-125 during chemotherapy and found the slope of the regression curve to be predictive of therapeutic outcome. Other investigators have shown that patients whose CA-125 values decrease from increased to normal rapidly while undergoing primary chemotherapy have an improved prognosis over those whose values decrease more slowly. Markman has evaluated the survival impact of CA-125 levels reaching 50% of pretreatment baseline at 8 weeks after surgery and cisplatin-based chemotherapy. Survival was 21 months for those achieving this decrease versus only 10 months for those not achieving a 50% decrease. Clearly, this imperfect marker has prognostic significance in many situations. The serum inhibin level

Table 33.6 Staging of Ovarian Carcinomas*

| Stage | Characteristics |
|---|---|
| I | Tumor confined to the ovaries |
| IA | Growth limited to one ovary (capsule intact); no tumor on ovarian surface; no malignant cells in the ascites or peritoneal washings |
| IB | Tumor limited to both ovaries (capsule intact); no tumor on ovarian surface; no malignant cells in the ascites or peritoneal washings |
| IC | Tumor limited to one or both ovaries |
| 1C1 | Surgical spill |
| 1C2 | Capsule ruptured before surgery or tumor on ovarian surface |
| 1C3 | Malignant cells in the ascites or peritoneal washings |
| II | Tumor involves one or both ovaries with pelvic extension |
| IIA | Extension or metastases to the uterus or fallopian tubes |
| IIB | Extension to other pelvic intraperitoneal tissues |
| III | Tumor involving one or both ovaries with cytologically or histologically confirmed spread to the peritoneum outside the pelvis or metastasis to the retroperitoneal lymph nodes |
| IIIA1 | Positive retroperitoneal lymph nodes only (cytologically or histologically proved) |
| IIIA1 (i) | Metastasis up to 10 mm in greatest dimension |
| IIIA1 (ii) | Metastasis more than 10 mm in greatest dimension |
| IIIA2 | Microscopic extrapelvic (above the pelvic brim) peritoneal involvement with or without positive retroperitoneal lymph nodes |
| IIIB | Macroscopic peritoneal metastasis beyond the pelvis up to 2 cm in greatest dimension, with or without metastasis to the retroperitoneal lymph nodes |
| IIIC | Macroscopic peritoneal metastasis beyond the pelvis more than 2 cm in greatest dimension, with or without metastasis to the retroperitoneal lymph nodes (includes extension of tumor to capsule of liver and spleen without parenchymal involvement of either organ) |
| IV | Distant metastases excluding peritoneal metastases |
| IVA | Pleural effusion with positive cytology |
| IVB | Parenchymal metastases and metastases to extra-abdominal organs (including inguinal lymph nodes and lymph nodes outside of the abdominal cavity) |

*According to the International Federation of Gynecology and Obstetrics (FIGO), 2014.

has been reported to be elevated in mucinous carcinomas and may serve as a marker, according to the studies of Healy and associates. Frias and coworkers reported pretreatment levels of inhibin A to be a prognostic factor for survival in postmenopausal women with ovarian cancer. However, inhibin levels are not routinely determined in the woman with an epithelial ovarian malignancy.

Preoperatively, the use of routine bowel preparation prior to major abdominal surgery for advanced ovarian cancer is no longer consider routine standard of care. In fact, this practice has been shown to increase patient dissatisfaction and may cause dehydration. In a systematic review of 18 randomized clinical trials (5805 patients), Guenaga and colleagues found no statically significant evidence that patients benefit from either bowel preparation or rectal enemas; specifically, the infection and anastomotic leak rates in patients with a bowel preparation was 9.6% and 4.4%; respectively, compared with 8.5% and 4.5% for those without. Venous thromboembolism prophylaxis is of particular importance in patients with ovarian cancer because a large tumor burden is associated with venous stasis and prolonged operation times. Treatment with variable compression leg support stockings and heparin (fractionated and unfractionated) appears to reduce the risk of thromboembolism in gynecologic oncology patients undergoing surgical tumor extirpation. A study by Einstein and colleagues evaluated the usefulness of a dual prophylaxis protocol using sequential compression devices and heparin three times daily (or daily low-molecular-weight heparin) until discharge for patients with gynecologic malignancies. A dual prophylaxis protocol was shown to be associated with a significant reduction in the rate of venous thromboembolism without increasing bleeding complications.

Ovarian carcinomas infiltrate the peritoneal surfaces of the parietal and intestinal areas, as well as the undersurface of the diaphragm, particularly on the right side (Fig. 33.7). This is particularly important because tumors that appear at operation to be confined to the ovary may have small areas of diaphragmatic involvement as the sole site of extraovarian spread. As noted earlier, most ovarian carcinomas, particularly the serous type, appear to arise from microscopic ovarian sites and do not become clinically evident until there is widespread metastatic disease. Lymphatic dissemination is also a prominent part of disease spread (Fig. 33.8), and it is particularly important to note that the para-aortic nodes are at risk through lymphatics that run parallel to the ovarian vessels. Knapp and Friedman have noted that of 26 patients with ovarian cancer apparently limited to the ovary, 19% had para-aortic involvement, and all had poorly differentiated tumors. In a study of 180 patients, Burghardt and coworkers observed that the proportion of positive nodes increases with higher-stage tumors—24% in stage I, 50% in stage II, and 73.5% in stages III and IV. A study conducted by Schmeler and colleagues has evaluated the prevalence of lymph node involvement in women with primary mucinous ovarian carcinomas. A total of 107 patients were identified. Of the patients with tumor grossly confined to the ovary at surgical exploration who underwent lymphadenectomy, none had metastatic disease to the pelvic or para-aortic lymph nodes. In addition, the authors found no significant differences in progression-free survival or overall survival between patients who underwent lymphadenectomy and those who did not.

The prognosis for patients with ovarian carcinoma is related to tumor stage, tumor grade, cell type, and amount of residual tumor after resection. Worldwide results for patients treated from 1990 to 1992 are summarized in Table 33.7. Data from

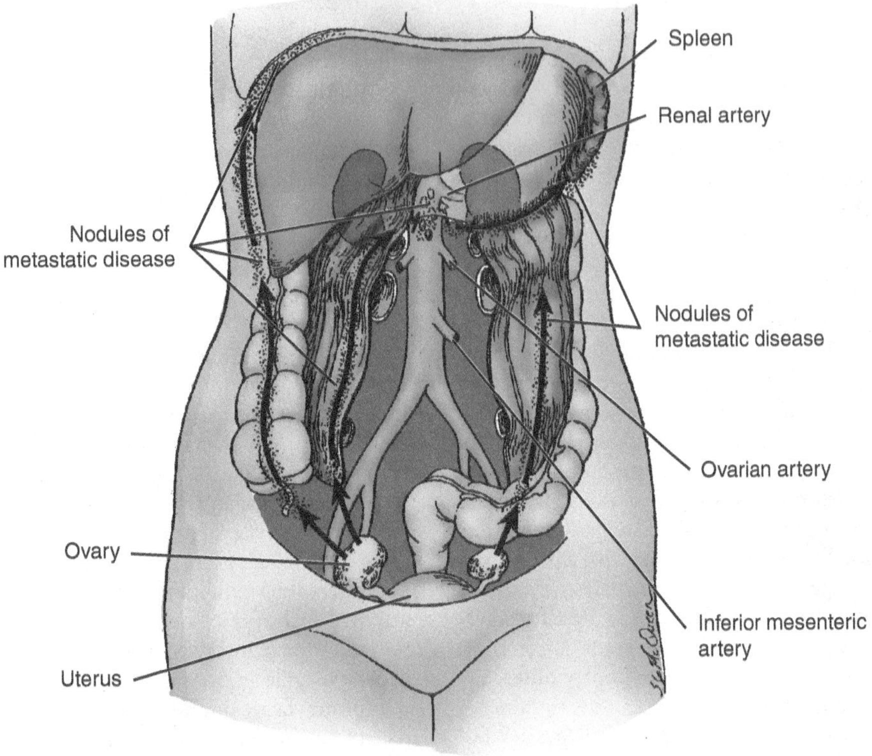


**Figure 33.7** Peritoneal spread of ovarian cancer. Portions of the omentum, small intestine, and transverse colon have been resected. (From Knapp RC, Berkowitz RS, Leavitt T Jr. Natural history and detection of ovarian cancer. In: *Gynecology and Obstetrics*. vol 4. Philadelphia: JB Lippincott; 1986.)

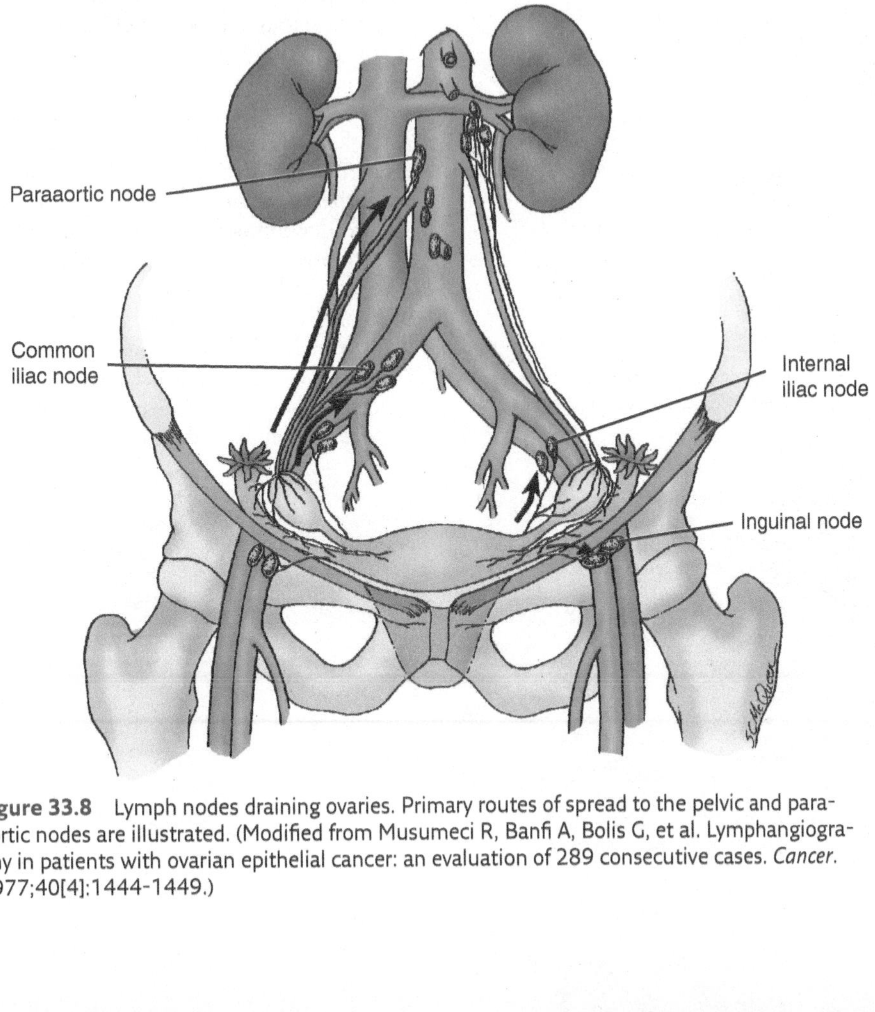


**Figure 33.8** Lymph nodes draining ovaries. Primary routes of spread to the pelvic and para-aortic nodes are illustrated. (Modified from Musumeci R, Banfi A, Bolis G, et al. Lymphangiography in patients with ovarian epithelial cancer: an evaluation of 289 consecutive cases. *Cancer*. 1977;40[4]:1444-1449.)

the Survey Epidemiology and End Results (SEER) database are presented in Table 33.8.

Cell type has been reported to be an important factor in prognosis, as shown in Figure 33.9, which summarizes the 20-year survival rate of a group of patients. The most common invasive epithelial cancers, serous carcinomas, have the worst prognosis; prognosis may be better for mucinous and endometrioid tumors. A variant of papillary serous carcinoma termed *transitional cell carcinoma* is thought by some to be a rare but more chemosensitive tumor. However, this has not been established in multi-institutional studies. Endometrioid carcinoma may be associated with endometriosis and, according to McMeekin and colleagues, such cases more commonly occur in younger women and have a better prognosis than typical endometrioid carcinomas of the ovary. Clear cell cancers have a worse prognosis, but Kennedy and associates noted that mitotic activity and tumor stage are important prognostic features of this tumor in their series. Tubulocystic pattern did not appear to affect prognosis, as earlier studies by Aure and colleagues had suggested (see Fig. 33.9). Nonetheless, these are aggressive tumors with a propensity for recurrence, even in stage I. In a follow-up analysis, Kennedy and associates noted a survival probability of only 50% for stages I and II. It should be noted that stage and grade affect these observations. Serous tumors tend to be more poorly differentiated and discovered at a higher-stage than mucinous tumors.

In some cases, patients are found to have small ovaries (<4 cm in diameter) and widespread papillary serous carcinoma in the abdomen. In such cases, the term *serous surface papillary carcinoma of the ovary* is applied. Fromm and coworkers reported on 74 patients and found that survival improves if the patients were treated postoperatively with combination chemotherapy (discussed later).

Another variety of serous carcinoma is primary peritoneal carcinoma. In these cases, the ovaries may be of normal size with surface metastatic tumor deposits. There is widespread intra-abdominal spread of carcinoma of serous histology. These cases can be associated with *BRCA1* and *BRCA2* mutations, as shown by the studies of Karlan and colleagues. The cloning of the *BRCA1* gene has advanced our knowledge of the molecular genetics of ovarian cancer, but the role of this gene, which resides on chromosome 17q21, is not clear. It appears to be a tumor suppressor gene that is highly expressed in ovarian borderline carcinoma. Mutations in *BRCA1* are strongly associated with an increased risk of breast and ovarian cancer, and a similar increase in risk occurs with mutations in *BRCA2*. These mutations are seen in approximately 2% to 2.5% of Ashkenazi Jewish women, who appear to be an appropriate target group for testing whether breast cancer is diagnosed before age 50 in the woman or a close relative, according to Warner and associates. Prophylactic oophorectomy reduces the risk of ovarian cancer in those with a mutation but does not eliminate the problem because of the potential for primary peritoneal carcinoma. The study of Rebbeck and colleagues of *BRCA1* mutation carriers has suggested that prophylactic oophorectomy may also reduce the subsequent risk of breast cancer. Boyd and coworkers reported that stage for stage, the hereditary ovarian cancer group may have a better prognosis than those with spontaneously occurring tumors. Lu and associates noted a high proportion of microscopic carcinomas in apparently normal ovaries removed from patients with *BRCA* mutations, an observation consistent with the de novo origin of serous and poorly differentiated carcinomas.

In addition to stage, the grade of the tumor is a major determinant of patient prognosis. Figure 33.10 demonstrates the survival of 442 patients with ovarian carcinoma by grade, with a markedly worse prognosis for poorly differentiated tumors (grade 3). The relationship between grade and survival also exists when the results are examined separately for each stage of disease.

The development of gene expression profiling has enabled a more precise evaluation of clinical behavior in some tumors. Bonome and coworkers studied the gene expression of low malignant potential (LMP) serous neoplasms and invasive low-grade and high-grade serous tumors. A distinct and separate clustering was observed between LMP tumors and high-grade cancers. Low-grade serous tumors generally clustered with LMP neoplasms. High-grade tumors differentially expressed genes

**Table 33.7** Carcinoma of the Ovary: Survival by International Federation of Gynecology and Obstetrics (FIGO) Stage*

| Stage | 5-Year Survival (%) |
|---|---|
| IA | 94% |
| IB | 92% |
| IC | 85% |
| IIA | 78% |
| IIB | 73% |
| IIIA | 59% |
| IIIB | 52% |
| IIIC | 39% |
| IV | 17% |

*Data from the American Cancer Society. Information is based on patients diagnosed from 2004 to 2010 and obtained from National Cancer Institute and SEER Database.

**Table 33.8** Summary of Primary End Points in Randomized Phase III Studies

| | Alberts et al (1996) (*n* = 546) | | Markman et al (2001) (*n* = 462) | | Armstrong et al (2006) (*n* = 415) | |
|---|---|---|---|---|---|---|
| **Outcome** | **IV** | **IP** | **IV** | **IP** | **IV** | **IP** |
| Pathologic CR | 36% | 47% | | | 41% | 57% |
| *P* value | — | | | | | |
| PFS (mo) | — | — | 22 | 28 | 18 | 24 |
| *P* value | | — | | .01 | | .05 |
| OS (mo) | 41 | 49 | 52 | 63 | 50 | 66 |
| *P* value | | .02 | | .05 | | .03 |

*CR*, Complete response; *OS*, overall survival; *PFS*, progression-free survival.

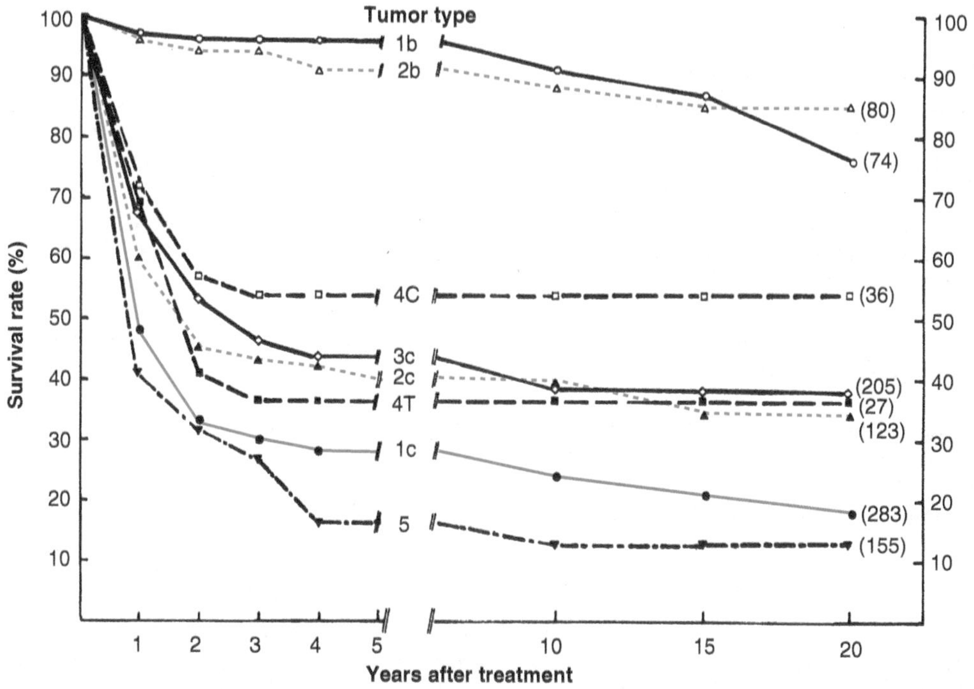


Figure 33.9 Survival rates for 983 patients with all stages of ovarian cancer by histologic type. *1b*, Serous, low malignant potential (74 cases); *2b*, mucinous, low malignant potential (80 cases); *1c*, serous carcinoma (283 cases); *2c*, mucinous carcinoma (123 cases); *3c*, endometrioid carcinoma (205 cases); *4C*, clear cell (36 cases); *4T*, tubulocystic pattern of clear cell (27 cases); *5*, undifferentiated (155 cases). (Modified from Aure JC, Hoeg K, Kolstad P. Clinical and histologic studies of ovarian carcinoma: long-term follow-up of 990 cases. *Obstet Gynecol.* 37[1]:1-9, 1971.)

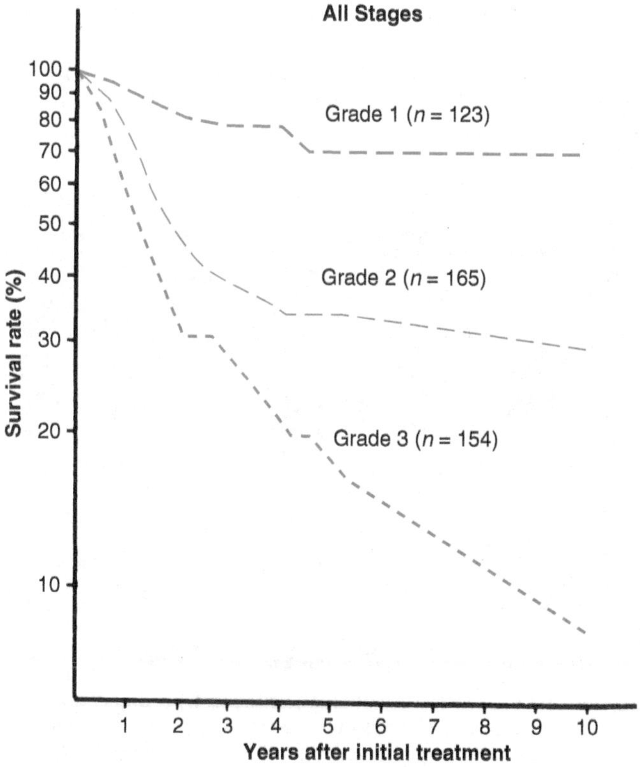


Figure 33.10 Survival rates for patients with ovarian cancer by tumor grade. Survival curves for the complete series according to the histologic degree of differentiation. All differences between curves are highly significant. (From Kosary CL. Ovarian carcinoma clinical trial. *Semin Surg Oncol.* 1994;10[1]:31-46.)

linked to cell proliferation, chromosomal instability, and epigenetic silencing. Based on these findings, high-grade epithelial cancers appear to have a distinct profile relative to LMP neoplasms. Low-grade serous tumors are remarkably similar to LMP serous neoplasms. These observations have ushered in the consideration of reclassifying invasive malignant cancers into two categories, low grade and high grade.

Studies of flow cytometry have indicated that the ploidy of the tumor is also prognostic, with aneuploidy being a negative prognostic factor. Klemi and colleagues noted an independent prognostic association with the DNA index and S-phase fraction. A better prognosis was observed if the proportion of S-phase cells was less than 11% or if the DNA index (the relative DNA content of aneuploid cells compared with diploid) was less than 1.3. Genetic studies by Slamon and coworkers showed that the *HER2/neu* oncogene is amplified in ovarian and breast cancers. As noted in a review by Berchuck and associates, the overexpression of *HER2/neu* was suspected to occur in approximately 30% of epithelial ovarian cancers and appears to be associated with a worse prognosis. However, a Gynecologic Oncology Group (GOG) study of trastuzumab (a monoclonal antibody to the extracellular domain of *HER2*) in patients with recurrent ovarian cancer has suggested that the incident overexpression by fluorescence in situ hybridization is much lower. In this study, 837 samples were screened for immunohistochemistry overexpression (2+ or 3+) or fluorescence in situ hybridization positivity. Only 95 patients (11.4%) met criteria for therapy. It is likely that this prospective trial more accurately represents the incidence of this factor in ovarian cancer. The *p53* tumor suppressor gene is mutated in approximately 50% of ovarian epithelial cancers studied, whereas the *C-myc* oncogene is overexpressed more commonly in serous cases and the *K-ras* oncogene has been identified more frequently in borderline ovarian cancers. The molecular genetic events surrounding ovarian carcinoma development and biologic behavior are incompletely understood.

The size of residual nodules and presence or absence of tumor after surgery has been related to the survival of patients treated for ovarian carcinoma. Chi and colleagues analyzed survival by diameter of residual disease (grouped in five categories) to determine the optimal goal of primary cytoreduction for patients with stage IIIC epithelial ovarian cancer. The median overall survival (OS) by diameter of residual disease were as follows: 106 months for no gross residual disease, 66 months for 0.5 cm or less, 48 months for 0.6 to 1 cm, 33 months for 1 to 2 cm, and 34 months for larger than 2 cm. Aure and colleagues noted a 5-year survival rate of more than 30% for stage III tumors that were completely resected compared with 10% when resection was incomplete. The impact of cytoreduction for advanced-stage disease is discussed next.

## TREATMENT

### Borderline Ovarian Tumors: Ovarian Carcinomas of Low Malignant Potential

Approximately 20% of ovarian epithelial cancers are tumors of LMP and usually have an excellent prognosis, regardless of stage. Most studies have been confined to borderline tumors of the serous (see Fig. 33.2*B*) and mucinous (see Fig. 33.3*B*) varieties, which are the most common histologies; however, other epithelial types (see Table 33.3) can occur. The cells of these epithelial tumors do not invade the stroma of the ovary. It is extremely important that the ovarian tumor be thoroughly sampled by the pathologist to ensure that a borderline tumor is not mixed with invasive elements. Numerous studies have confirmed that borderline tumors have a slower growth rate than invasive ovarian carcinomas, manifested by prolonged survival (see Fig. 33.9).

Surgery is the primary treatment for women with borderline ovarian tumors. The principal objectives of surgery are as follows: (1) diagnosis, (2) fertility-sparing surgery for patients who have not completed childbearing or who are young and have only unilateral ovarian involvement, (3) surgical staging for apparent early-stage disease, and (4) cytoreductive surgery for the minority of patients who have obvious advanced-stage disease.

The typical scenario is surgery for an adnexal mass of unknown type. One of the initial considerations in planning surgery for a pelvic mass is the surgical approach—minimally invasive or open technique. Factors to be considered in the selection of minimally invasive surgery (laparoscopic or robotic) include size of the ovarian mass(es), extent of tumor metastasis, number and type of previous operations, and body habitus. Several reports have documented the feasibility and safety of the minimally invasive approach when appropriately used (Romagnolo, 2006).

Once the mass is excised, frozen-section examination is a key element in assuring appropriate decision making. If the frozen section suggests a borderline ovarian tumor, considerations for fertility-sparing surgery include the woman's age, her desire for future childbearing, and the degree of involvement of the ovaries—unilateral versus bilateral disease. Options for fertility-sparing surgery include ovarian cystectomy and unilateral adnexectomy. Even with bilateral borderline ovarian tumors, bilateral ovarian cystectomies may be performed, depending on the extent of ovarian disease. Lim-Tan and associates reported on 33 cases of stage I serous borderline tumors initially treated by cystectomy. Only 3 of 33 patients undergoing cystectomy had recurrence or persistence of borderline tumor, and these patients had positive resection margins or multiple cysts present in the ovary, emphasizing the effectiveness of conservative operation. However, for most stage IA cases, unilateral adnexectomy is performed and, if the opposite ovary looks normal, no biopsy or wedge resection is done.

Surgical staging for borderline ovarian tumors remains somewhat controversial. The most compelling reason for surgical staging in a woman with borderline tumor on frozen-section examination is the risk of invasive carcinoma on final pathology. For women with pathologically confirmed borderline tumors, the incidence of lymph node involvement is only approximately 5%. Therefore most investigators have recommended against routine pelvic and para-aortic lymphadenectomy. However, omental and peritoneal biopsies are recommended because peritoneal implants are usually small or microscopic (Harter, 2014).

For stage I serous borderline tumors, surgery alone is the standard of care because the cure rate associated with this treatment approaches 100% (see Fig. 33.9). On the other hand, approximately 30% of women will have peritoneal implants, which are classified as noninvasive (Fig. 33.11) or invasive (Fig. 33.12). For these women, the recurrence rate associated with noninvasive implants is 20% to 40% and the recurrence rate with invasive implants is 50% to 70%. Unfortunately, no studies to date have convincingly demonstrated any benefit to postoperative therapy for women with stages II to IV disease. Although no standard exists, some oncologists recommend postoperative treatment—paclitaxel-carboplatin chemotherapy or hormonal therapy—only for patients with invasive implants based on the very high risk of relapse.

Outcome is influenced by several factors, including pathologic and clinical factors. Pathologic factors that may be associated with an increased risk of relapse include the presence of

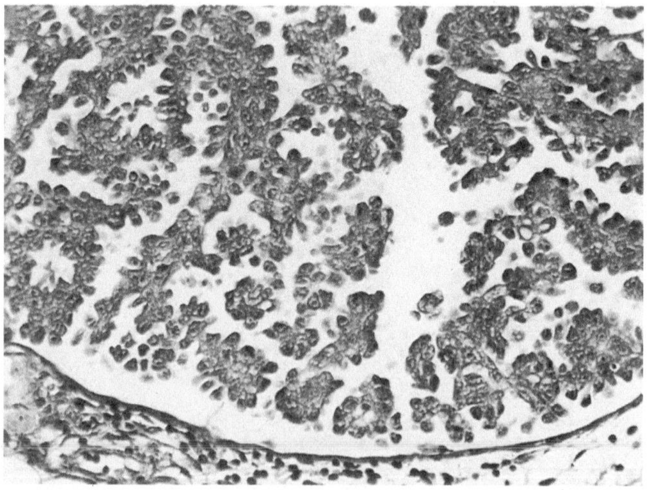

**Figure 33.11** Noninvasive implant, epithelial type. Branching papillae and detached clusters of polygonal cells showing moderate cytologic atypicality are present (H&E, ×313). (From Bell DA, Weinstock MA, Scully RE. Peritoneal implants of ovarian serous borderline tumors: histologic features and prognosis. *Cancer.* 1988;62[10]:2212-2222.)

the micropapillary/cribriform pattern or microinvasion in the primary ovarian serous LMP tumor or the presence of peritoneal implants (Longacre, 2005).

Mucinous borderline tumors also are associated with an excellent prognosis (see Fig. 33.9). Hart and Norris reviewed 97 patients with stage I tumors who were 9 to 70 years of age (median, 35 years). More than 10% of the tumors were discovered during pregnancy or in the immediate postpartum period. Follow-up data were available on 87 of the patients, and there were only three tumor-related deaths during the 5- to 10-year follow-up. The actuarial survival was 98% at 5 years and 96% at 10 years. This was also noted by Bostwick and colleagues, who reported on 109 borderline tumors, 33 of which were mucinous and all of which were stage I, contributing to the good prognosis.

Mucinous borderline tumors include two distinct subtypes, gastrointestinal and seromucinous or endocervical. In the seromucinous type, the association of endometriosis is high (≈40%). They also may have associated microinvasion and lymph node involvement. The prognosis associated with the seromucinous type is excellent. Conversely, the gastrointestinal type may rarely be associated with the condition known as *pseudomyxoma peritonei,* consisting of widespread growth of mucin-producing cells in the peritoneum. The result may be the accumulation of large amounts of mucinous material, which is sometimes associated with recurrent episodes of bowel obstruction. Studies by Young and coworkers suggested that pseudomyxoma peritonei usually arises in the appendix. The review of Ronnett and coworkers supports a primary appendiceal origin for these tumors and, therefore appendectomy is indicated for women with an intraoperative diagnosis of a mucinous ovarian tumor. The disease tends to recur and is frequently characterized by repeated laparotomy to relieve bowel obstruction. Chemotherapy and mucolytic agents have been tried but are usually not successful.

### Invasive Epithelial Carcinomas

The primary treatment of ovarian epithelial carcinoma is removal of all resectable gross disease. The woman's abdomen

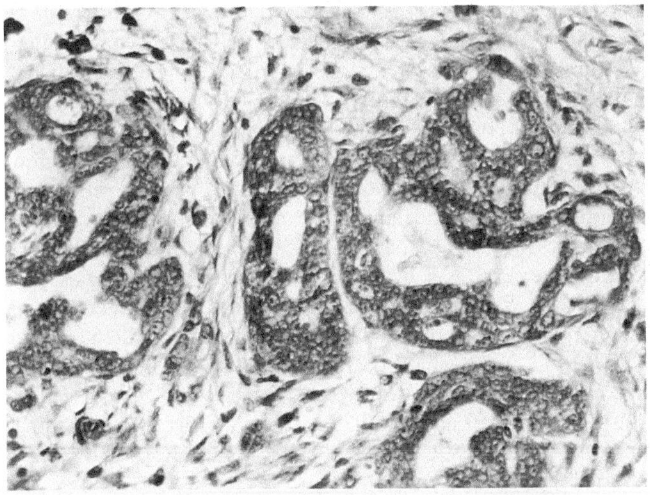

**Figure 33.12** Invasive implant. Glands with an irregular contour lined by severely atypical epithelial cells with extensive intraglandular bridging are present (H&E, ×313). (From Bell DA, Weinstock MA, Scully RE. Peritoneal implants of ovarian serous borderline tumors: histologic features and prognosis. *Cancer.* 1988;62[10]:2212-2222.)

is explored through a vertical incision. If ascitic fluid is present, it is sent for cytologic evaluation; if ascites is not present, 200 to 400 mL of normal saline solution is used to obtain cytologic samples from the peritoneum by irrigating at least the pelvis, upper abdomen, and right and left paracolic gutters before any resection is done. The diaphragm can be cytologically sampled by scraping the undersurface with a sterile tongue depressor and the sample placed on a glass slide and sprayed with a fixative. Biopsy or, preferably, excision of any suspicious nodules is performed. A total abdominal hysterectomy, bilateral salpingo-oophorectomy, and infracolic omentectomy are performed if technically possible. When there is no gross disease outside the pelvis, para-aortic and pelvic lymph node sampling is recommended, with care taken to remove enlarged nodes. Although the impact of systematic lymphadenectomy has been addressed in one randomized clinical trial by Benedetti-Panici and associates, without significant effect on overall survival, it is reasonable to explore these areas because inspection by palpation is notoriously inaccurate. Evidence suggests that if all gross disease can be resected, the duration of patient survival is enhanced. Although randomized clinical trials have not been performed to document this effect, a meta-analysis of 6885 patients gathered from 81 cohorts has suggested a linear relationship between the degree of cytoreduction and overall survival. In this report, Bristow and colleagues noted that for each 10% increase in cytoreduction, a 5.5% increase in survival was observed. The surgical procedures required to achieve maximal cytoreduction may be extensive and involve splenectomy, diaphragmatic stripping-resection, and posterior exenteration. It may occasionally be necessary to resect bowel to relieve impending obstruction or remove a tumor nodule, thereby eliminating all gross disease from the peritoneal cavity. Heintz and coworkers noted that prognosis is improved for younger patients (<50 years), those with good initial performance status (Karnofsky score >80), and those whose disease could be cytoreduced to less than 1.5 cm. Adverse factors were large before initial operation, ascites, and peritoneal carcinomatosis. In a small collaborative GOG study, Hoskins and colleagues found that those who started with large-volume disease did worse than those who initially had small-volume disease; no survival advantage could be demonstrated for the debulking operation in the large-volume disease group. Chi and associates noted that those with advanced disease and a preoperative CA-125 level higher than 500 U/mL had less than a 20% chance of an optimal surgical debulking (discussed later).

One exception to the required removal of the uterus and opposite ovary occurs in the case of well-differentiated (grade 1) ovarian tumors confined to one ovary (stage IA). DiSaia and coworkers outlined criteria for preserving childbearing function in a young woman with stage IA, grade 1 ovarian epithelial carcinoma, as follows:

1. Tumor confined to one ovary
2. Tumor well differentiated (grade 1), with no invasion of capsule, lymphatics, or mesovarium
3. Peritoneal washings negative
4. Omental biopsy specimen negative
5. Young woman of childbearing years with a strong desire to preserve reproductive function

These criteria can be applied to all types of epithelial ovarian tumors but are more likely to be satisfied in the case of mucinous tumors, which are more frequently well differentiated and unilateral than serous carcinomas. Wedge resection of a normal-appearing contralateral ovary is unlikely to uncover an occult tumor. In these cases, it is reasonable to follow the woman closely with vaginal ultrasonography for any evidence of future ovarian enlargement.

## *Early-Stage Ovarian Carcinomas*

### Stage I

The standard therapy for all patients with early-stage ovarian cancer (EOC) includes hysterectomy (usually performed via celiotomy) with bilateral salpingo-oophorectomy. In patients interested in preserving fertility, unilateral salpingo-oophorectomy with preservation of the contralateral ovary and uterus is often feasible. In addition, all patients with early-stage disease should undergo pelvic washings, omental biopsy, cytologic sampling of the surface of the diaphragm, complete bilateral pelvic and para-aortic lymphadenectomy or lymph node sampling, and bilateral biopsies of the paracolic gutters and pelvic peritoneal surfaces. It is important to emphasize that careful assessment of the subdiaphragmatic areas and inspection of the entire peritoneum and the retroperitoneal para-aortic and pelvic nodes are important, particularly in view of the risk of diaphragmatic and nodal spread in higher-grade tumors that initially appear to be at stage I, particularly those on frozen section that appear to be less well differentiated than grade 1.

Le and colleagues compared a group of patients who underwent minimal staging performed by a general gynecologist with a group of patients who underwent comprehensive staging performed by a gynecologic oncologist. They found the risk of recurrence to be increased for patients operated on by the general gynecologist. Another study by Mayer and associates showed that patients operated on by a gynecologic oncologist had a 24% improvement in 5-year overall survival.

### Rupture of Ovary

Occasionally, during removal, a stage I ovarian carcinoma is inadvertently ruptured (stage IC, see Table 33.6). There are conflicting opinions as to the potential adverse effects on prognosis. In an analysis of 394 patients, Sjövall and associates found that rupture during surgery did not affect survival, whereas there was marked reduction in survival in that study among those whose ovarian rupture occurred *before* the operation. In general, the spilled fluid and all residual tumor should be removed promptly from the operative field after a rupture (discussed later). Presumably higher-grade and larger tumors are most prone to rupture.

A study by Dembo and colleagues of 519 stage I patients found that adverse factors were grade of tumor, dense pelvic adherence (no invasion but adhesion), or more than 250 mL of ascites. Patients without these features had a 98% 5-year survival rate. It appears that patients with stage I grade 3 tumors should have postoperative therapy, but data are unclear for stage I grade 2 patients.

### Minimally Invasive Surgical Staging of Early-Stage Ovarian Cancer

An estimated 15% of women with EOC have early-stage disease at diagnosis. In these patients, comprehensive surgical staging is required to provide accurate prognostic information and plan treatment options. Frequently, the diagnosis of EOC is made incidentally during adnexal surgery for other indications. Because minimally invasive surgical procedures are becoming more common in gynecology and more in demand by the public at large, determining the feasibility and safety of these procedures for the staging of presumed early-stage EOC has become a necessity.

Laparoscopy often leads to a shorter hospital stay, less intraoperative blood loss, and a shorter recovery period than laparotomy. However, surgical staging for EOC requires meticulous inspection of the peritoneal cavity and careful dissection of lymph nodes, vessels, and other abdominal and pelvic structures. Thus to assess the feasibility of minimally invasive surgical staging, several issues must be considered, such as the frequency of complications, frequency of conversion to laparotomy, and recurrence rate following laparoscopic staging.

Nezhat and associates performed a retrospective review of 36 patients who underwent laparoscopic staging for presumed early-stage ovarian and fallopian tube carcinoma from 1995 to 2007. Of the 36 patients, 20 were diagnosed with invasive EOC, 11 with borderline ovarian tumors (BOT), and 5 with nonepithelial tumors. There were no intraoperative complications, but there were four postoperative complications (one partial small bowel obstruction managed conservatively, two lymphoceles, and one lymphocele cyst requiring drainage). The mean number of pelvic lymph nodes obtained was 14.8, and the mean number of para-aortic lymph nodes obtained was 12.2. Of the 9 patients who underwent completion staging, 7 (77.8%) had their disease upstaged. During a mean follow-up of 55.9 months, there were three recurrences in patients who underwent conservative surgery, and the overall survival rate was 100%. Jung and coworkers conducted a retrospective review to evaluate the feasibility and efficacy of laparoscopically assisted staging surgery for ovarian cancer in 24 patients with ovarian or fallopian tube cancer. There were no conversions to laparotomy and no intraoperative complications. The only postoperative complication was a port site metastasis. Ten patients (41.7%) had their disease upstaged. The mean number of pelvic lymph nodes obtained was 22.5 and the mean number of para-aortic lymph nodes obtained was 11. Interestingly, the mean hospital stay was 10.6 days, which was attributed to differences in practice patterns in Korea.

In a study by Gallota and colleagues, the authors evaluated the safety and perioperative outcomes of laparoscopic staging of patients with apparent early stage ovarian cancer (Gallota, 2014). A total of 300 patients were selected: 150 had been submitted to immediate laparoscopic staging (group 1), whereas 150 had undergone delayed laparoscopic staging (group 2). No significant differences of postoperative complications were observed between the two groups. Histologic data revealed more frequently serous tumors (0.06), grade 3 ($P = .0007$) and final up-staging ($P = .001$) in group 1. Recurrence and death of disease were documented in 25 (8.3%), and 10 patients (3.3%), respectively. The 3-year disease-free survival (DFS) and overall survival (OS) rates were 85.1%, and 93.6%, respectively, in the whole series. There was no difference between group 1 and group 2 in terms of DFS ($P$ value = 0.39) and OS ($P$ value = 0.27). The authors concluded that laparoscopic management of early ovarian cancer is safe and feasible.

In summary, it appears that minimally invasive surgical staging of presumed EOC is safe and effective when performed by a trained gynecologic oncologist.

### Adequacy of Minimally Invasive Surgery Compared with Laparotomy for Staging of Ovarian Neoplasms

Important concerns have been raised about laparoscopic staging for ovarian neoplasms, including concerns about the adequacy of the lymph node dissection, differences between laparoscopy and laparotomy in operative time, postoperative complications, and postoperative recovery. In one meta-analysis of laparoscopic staging surgery in patients with presumed early-stage ovarian cancer, Park and colleagues identified 11 observational studies (Park, 2013). The combined results of three retrospective studies showed that the estimated blood loss in laparoscopy was significantly lower than that for laparotomy ($P < .001$). The overall upstaging rate after laparoscopic surgery was 22.6% (95% CI, 18.1-27.9) without significant heterogeneity among all study results. The overall incidence of conversion from laparoscopy to laparotomy was 3.7% (95% CI, 2.0-6.9). The overall rate of recurrence in studies with a median follow-up period of ≥19 months was 9.9% (95% CI, 6.7-14.4). The authors concluded that the operative outcomes of a laparoscopic approach in patients with early-stage ovarian cancer could be compatible with those of laparotomy.

Data on the application of robotic surgery for ovarian cancer staging are scant. In a study by Brown and associates, the authors evaluated the safety and feasibility of robotic-assisted systematic lymph node staging in the management of early-stage ovarian cancer. A total of 26 early-stage ovarian cancer patients were identified. The mean operating time was 2.90 hours, and the estimated blood loss was 63 mL; there were no intraoperative complications, although one patient's surgery was significantly prolonged due to pelvic adhesions. The mean number of pelvic and para-aortic lymph nodes removed was 14.6 (2.3% incidence of pelvic lymph node metastases) and 5.8 (3.3% incidence of para-aortic lymph node metastases), respectively. The patients' mean duration of hospital stay was 18.4 hours, and 2 patients were readmitted for either a postoperative wound infection or vaginal dehiscence. The authors concluded that robotic-assisted surgical staging was feasible and safe; however, there was a low incidence of lymph node metastasis (2.3%) and the authors stressed the value of a systematic lymph node dissection.

### Stage II

Stage II ovarian cancer is initially treated by removal of all gross disease, including the uterus, tubes, and ovaries, and an omentectomy (infracolic) is performed. The pelvic and para-aortic nodes are sampled.

### Postoperative Management for Stages I and II

Recommendations for postoperative or adjuvant therapy generally have evolved around the identification of patients in whom a sufficient risk of recurrence is observed. The precision to make this assessment is low and has been based on morphologic features such as grade, histology, and presence of rupture and residuum. Historically, several modalities have been evaluated alone and in combination by prospective studies of unselected patients, including chemotherapy, radiation therapy, intraperitoneal (IP) radiocolloids, and immunotherapy. Guthrie and coworkers evaluated 656 patients treated for epithelial ovarian carcinomas that had been totally excised. Most carcinomas were stage I or II, and patients were randomly assigned to receive postoperative treatment of radiation therapy alone, chemotherapy alone, radiation therapy and chemotherapy, or no postoperative therapy. Follow-up was for at least 2 years. Approximately 20% of the tumors were borderline malignancies and the rest were invasive carcinomas. Perhaps surprisingly, the lowest frequency of death or recurrence was noted in the group receiving no postoperative therapy (2%), whereas in the other groups, the death or recurrence incidence was 14% to 17%. Thus this study has shown no benefit for adjuvant therapy and highlights the need for careful case selection and pathologic review. In addition, because survivorship of low-stage cancer is better, long-term follow-up is necessary to tease out the merits of intervention.

Two large multicenter trials have been conducted and were combined for analytic purposes to address this issue. The International Collaborative Ovarian Neoplasm 1 (ICON1) and Adjuvant ChemoTherapy in Ovarian Neoplasm (ACTION) trials compared platinum-based chemotherapy with observation in patients after surgery with EOC. The two trials differed somewhat in patient eligibility with ICON1 predominantly enrolling postoperative stages I and II patients with limited staging and ACTION enrolling postoperative stage IA and IB, grades 2 and 3, stages IC to IIA, all grades, and clear cell tumor patients. Overall, 925 patients were collectively enrolled (477 in ICON1 and 448 in ACTION) and followed for a median 4 years. The overall survival rate at 5 years was 82% in the chemotherapy arm and 74% in the observation arm (HR, 0.67; 95% CI, 0.5-0.9; $P = .001$). Recurrence-free survival at 5 years was also significantly higher in the chemotherapy arm compared with observation (HR, 0.64; 95% CI, 0.5-0.82). In select patients, platinum-based therapy appears to improve survival and lower recurrence at 5 years over observation. In all, three randomized clinical trials have addressed platinum-based chemotherapy versus observation in EOC. These three trials were evaluated via meta-analysis to assess the role of adjuvant chemotherapy. As expected, the combined data mirror the results of the two larger studies with regard to the impact of adjuvant chemotherapy (HR, 0.71; 95% CI, 0.53-0.93) on 5-year survival. However, when subcategorized by surgical staging, this benefit retained significance only in the group in whom nonoptimal staging was performed. An update from ICON1 with a median follow-up of 10 years confirmed the impact of adjuvant chemotherapy in this cohort (Collinson, 2014). These data highlight the importance of accurate surgical staging information when devising an appropriate postoperative treatment plan.

Young and colleagues conducted two randomized studies of adjuvant therapy for patients with stage I disease. The first study showed that those with stage IA, grades 1 and 2, had 5-year survival rates more than 90% and did not benefit from adjuvant alkylating agent chemotherapy. The second study showed comparable results for adjuvant $^{32}P$ and platinum-based therapy for a higher risk cohort, including stage I, grade 3, as well as completely resected stage II cases. The assessable cohort included 229 randomized patients. The cumulative incidence of recurrence at 10 years was 29% lower for those receiving chemotherapy compared with $^{32}P$ (28% vs. 35%; $P = .15$) but was not statistically significant. The recurrence risk in this cohort of patients was substantial—all stage I, 27%, and stage II, 44%. Inadequate distribution and small bowel perforation are cited as reasons that $^{32}P$ is less desirable as adjuvant therapy. Piver and associates reported 93% 5-year survival for stage IC or stage I, grade 3, patients who received multiagent chemotherapy containing cisplatin. Vergote and coworkers analyzed 313 patients treated with $^{32}P$ after the primary operation or second-look operation (discussed later). Bowel complications occurred in 22 (7%) and 13 required operation. Bolis and colleagues reported on two randomized trials comparing $^{32}P$ and chemotherapy with cisplatin, 50 mg/m$^2$, for six cycles. Stages IA and IB grades 2 to 3 and stages IC showed significantly reduced relapse rates in the cisplatin arms. Unfortunately, a survival advantage was not demonstrated, and those who had a recurrence after receiving chemotherapy did worse than those who received $^{32}P$.

When indicated, the most frequently used modality is now chemotherapy, although the ideal regimen and number of courses needed are still debated. Bell and associates reported the results of a GOG randomized study comparing three and six cycles of adjuvant paclitaxel and carboplatin for women with stages IA and IB, grade 3, all stage IC, clear cell tumor, and completely resected stage II epithelial ovarian cancer. The study was powered for a 50% or greater decrease in recurrence for six cycles of therapy. A total of 457 patients were recruited; 344 were alive a median of 6.8 years since entry. The overall treatment effect is a nonsignificant 24% reduction in recurrence for the six-cycle arm (HR, 0.76; 95% CI, 0.51-1.13; $P$ = .18). The improved impact on estimated recurrence at 5 years was 5%, and there was no difference in overall survival between the arms. Approximately one third of patients in both arms had stage II disease. Forest plot analysis by stage did not demonstrate any alteration in the study's conclusions in this cohort. Although no difference was observed in this trial, many investigators have questioned the pretreatment statistical goals and have continued to recommend six cycles of therapy in patients with early-stage disease requiring treatment. A post hoc analysis of the survival results by histology raises the hypothesis that six cycles of therapy may benefit patients with serous histology to a different degree than the others included in the trial. It also should be noted that the carboplatin dose used in this trial was AUC 7.5.

A follow-up study by the GOG (protocol, 0175) addressed the role of maintenance therapy in this setting. Women with the same eligibility as GOG 157 were randomized to three cycles of paclitaxel and carboplatin (AUC 6) followed by normal surveillance or 24 infusions of low-dose (40 mg/m$^2$) weekly paclitaxel. The study was powered to address a 43% reduction in the risk of recurrence and enrolled 542 patients. The stage distribution was 71% stage I; 80% of patients randomized to the maintenance arm received all assigned therapy. Toxicity was similar between the two arms. The HRs for progression-free survival (PFS) and OS were 0.81 (95% CI, 0.56-1.15) and 0.78 (95% CI, 0.52-1.17), respectively. Subgroup analysis demonstrated no effect by stage, histology, or grade. There was remarkable consistency between the two GOG studies in the 5-year survival recorded by the three-cycle cohort. Although the optimal treatment is still not known, high-risk, early-stage patients clearly benefit from therapy.

### Primary Cytoreductive Surgery

Most patients with ovarian cancer present with disease that has spread beyond the pelvis and into the upper abdomen. The routine recommendation for patients with advanced disease who are surgical candidates is to perform a total abdominal hysterectomy, bilateral salpingo-oophorectomy, complete omentectomy, and resection of all visible tumor. Bristow and colleagues performed a retrospective population-based study of consecutive patients diagnosed with epithelial ovarian cancer (Bristow, 2015). A total of 9933 patients were identified (stage I, 22.8%; stage II, 7.9%; stage III, 45.1%; stage IV, 24.2%), and 8.1% of patients were treated at comprehensive cancer centers (National Cancer Institute Comprehensive Cancer Center [NCI-CCC]). Overall, 35.7% of patients received National Comprehensive Cancer Network (NCCN) guideline adherent care, and NCI-CCC status (odds ratio [OR] 1.00) was an independent predictor of adherence to treatment guidelines compared with high-volume hospitals (HVHs) (OR, 0.83; 95% CI, 0.70-0.99) and low-volume hospitals (LVHs) (OR, 0.56; 95% CI, 0.47-0.67). The median ovarian cancer-specific survivals according to hospital type were NCI-CCC 77.9 (95% CI, 61.4-92.9) months, HVH 51.9 (95% CI, 49.2-55.7) months, and LVH 43.4 (95% CI, 39.9-47.2) months ($P$ < .0001). National Cancer Institute Comprehensive Cancer Center status (hazard ratio [HR] 1.00) was a statistically significant and independent predictor of improved survival compared with HVH (HR 1.18; 95% CI, 1.04-1.33) and LVH (HR 1.30; 95% CI, 1.15-1.47).

Aletti and associates sought to estimate the effect of aggressive surgical resection on the survival of epithelial ovarian cancer patients. They found that the 5-year disease-specific survival rate was markedly better for patients operated on by surgeons who were most likely to use radical procedures than for patients operated on by surgeons who were least likely to use radical procedures (44% vs. 17%; $P$ < .001). Also, the rate of optimal resection was 84% for the surgeons most likely to use radical procedures compared with 51% for the surgeons least likely to use radical procedures, highlighting the value of extensive surgical effort.

Zivanovic and colleagues evaluated the impact of upper abdominal disease (UAD) cephalad to the greater omentum on surgical outcomes for 490 patients with stage IIIC ovarian, fallopian tube, and primary peritoneal cancers. Patients were divided into three groups according to the amount of disease in the upper abdomen. Group 1 was defined as no disease in the upper abdomen, group 2 as having tumors smaller than 1 cm, and group 3 as having bulky disease, larger than 1 cm. The authors found that optimal cytoreduction was achieved in 81%, 63%, and 39% of patients in groups 1, 2, and 3, respectively. In the largest study of postoperative tumor residuum and outcome, resection to no visible intraperitoneal disease was substantially related to progression-free and overall survival. The study population ($n$ = 3126) was generated from three randomized phase III trials assessing primary chemotherapy regimens in advanced stage disease patients. Median overall survival was 99.1 months for patients with no postoperative tumor residua compared with 36.2 months for those with visible disease 1 cm or smaller and 29.6 months in those with more than 1 cm of tumor residua.

Chang and associates sought to quantify the impact of complete cytoreduction to no gross residual disease on overall survival among patients with advanced-stage ovarian cancer treated during the platinum-taxane era (Chang, 2013). A total of 18 relevant studies (13,257 patients) were identified for analysis. After controlling for other factors on multiple linear regression analysis, each 10% increase in the proportion of patients undergoing complete cytoreduction to no gross residual disease was associated with a significant and independent 2.3-month increase (95% CI, 0.6-4.0, $P$ = .011) in cohort median survival compared with a 1.8-month increase (95% CI, 0.6-3.0, $P$ = .004) in cohort median survival for optimal cytoreduction (residual disease ≤1 cm). Each 10% increase in the proportion of patients receiving intraperitoneal chemotherapy was associated with a significant and independent 3.9-month increase (95% CI, 1.1-6.8, $P$ = .008) in median cohort survival time. The authors found that the proportions of patients left with no gross residual disease and receiving intraperitoneal chemotherapy are independently significant factors associated with the most favorable cohort survival time.

### Role of Laparoscopy in Assessing Resectability to R0 in Advanced Ovarian Cancer

A number of studies have evaluated the use of serologic markers, such as CA-125, and imaging modalities, such as computed tomography (CT) or positron emission tomography/CT (PET/CT), to determine which patients are ideal candidates for primary cytoreductive surgery. More recently, laparoscopy has been proposed as a reliable predictor of R0 resection. In this chapter, we review the existing literature on the proposed criteria to predict the outcome of cytoreductive surgery and the role of laparoscopy-based scores in the management of advanced ovarian cancer.

Gómez-Hidalgo and colleagues published a comprehensive review of the evolution of laparoscopy as a tool to help identify ideal patients with advanced ovarian cancer for optimal cytoreduction (R0) (Gómez-Hidalgo, 2015). The authors concluded that existing studies point to a highly valuable role for laparoscopy for objectively assessing the feasibility of optimal primary and interval cytoreductive surgery for patients with advanced-stage ovarian cancer (FIGO stages III and IV). They went on to suggest that the Fagotti laparoscopy-based score is a useful predictor of optimal cytoreduction.

Nick and colleagues published an algorithm that identifies patients in whom complete gross resection at primary surgery is likely to be achieved (Nick, 2015). Such an algorithm is currently being used to ensure that the rate of optimal cytoreduction (R0) increases and the rate of patients unnecessarily undergoing neoadjuvant chemotherapy decreases. In addition, the algorithm allows surgeon to obtain tissue prior to the initiation of therapy, thus targeting molecular pathways in a much more precise and personalized strategy.

### Utility of Video-Assisted Thoracoscopy

Unfortunately, no tools are available that allow surgeons to predict with high confidence whether there is disease in the pleural cavity. Video-assisted thoracoscopic surgery (VATS) allows surgeons, through a minimally invasive approach, to not only drain the pleural cavity of fluid but also evaluate whether pleural disease is present.

In 2010, Diaz and coworkers published on a total of 42 patients who underwent VATS prior to cytoreduction. VATS was performed for right-sided effusions in 30 patients (71%). Macroscopic pleural disease was found in 29 patients (69%); the other 13 patients (31%) had no evidence of intrathoracic disease. Of the 29 patients with macroscopic disease, 17 underwent primary abdominal cytoreduction, and 12 went on to receive neoadjuvant chemotherapy. Eighteen patients (62%) had nodules larger than 1 cm. Twelve of these patients went on to receive neoadjuvant chemotherapy, and 6 patients underwent intrathoracic cytoreduction. Of the 27 patients with positive pleural cytology, 12 had macroscopic disease larger than 1 cm, 9 had macroscopic disease smaller than 1 cm, and 6 had no macroscopic disease. Of the 11 patients with negative pleural cytology, 4 had macroscopic disease (larger than 1 cm in 2 patients), and 7 had no macroscopic disease. The authors concluded that 31% of all patients who met the inclusion criteria and underwent VATS had no evidence of intrathoracic disease and that VATS altered primary management in 43% of patients.

### Diaphragmatic Stripping or Resection

At initial surgical exploration, diaphragmatic disease may be the largest volume metastatic disease. Unfortunately, the presence of diaphragmatic disease is one of the most common factors precluding optimal tumor reduction surgery. Large diaphragmatic metastases were cited as a significant barrier to optimal tumor-reductive surgery by 76% of the members of the Society of Gynecologic Oncologists in a study reported by Eisenkop and associates. In that same study, only 24% of those surveyed used diaphragm resection and 30% reported not being experienced with the procedure. Aletti and coworkers evaluated the therapeutic value of diaphragmatic surgery in patients with advanced ovarian cancer and found that patients who underwent diaphragmatic surgery (stripping of the diaphragm peritoneum, full- or partial-thickness diaphragm resection, or excision of nodules) had an improved 5-year overall survival rate relative to patients who did not undergo diaphragmatic surgery (53% vs. 15%, $P < .0001$).

A study by Pathiraja and colleagues compared the surgical morbidity of diaphragmatic peritonectomy versus full-thickness diaphragmatic resection with pleurectomy at radical debulking. A total of 42 patients were eligible for the study; 21 underwent diaphragmatic peritonectomy (DP, group 1) and 21 underwent diaphragmatic full thickness resection (DR, group 2). Forty patients out of 42 (93%) had complete tumor resection with no residual disease. Histology confirmed the presence of cancer in the diaphragmatic peritoneum of 19 patients out of 21 in group 1 and all 21 patients of group 2. The overall complications rate was 19% in group 1 versus 33% in group 2. The pleural effusion rate was 9.5% versus 14.5%, and the pneumothorax rate was 14.5% only in group 2. Two patients in each group required postoperative chest drains (9.5%). The authors concluded that patients in the pleurectomy group experienced pneumothorax and a higher rate of pleural effusion, but none had long-term morbidity or additional surgical interventions.

### Splenectomy

For optimal cytoreductive surgery, a splenectomy may be required if there is disease involving the hilum, capsule, or parenchyma of the spleen. Magtibay and colleagues evaluated 112 patients who underwent splenectomy as part of primary or secondary cytoreductive surgery. They found that the most common indications for splenectomy were direct metastatic involvement (46%), facilitation of an en bloc resection of perisplenic disease (41%), and intraoperative trauma (13%). In that same study, the authors found that 65% of patients had hilar involvement, 52% capsular involvement, and 16% parenchymal metastases. Interestingly, patients with disease directly involving the splenic parenchyma did not have a worse prognosis than patients with disease involving the splenic hilum or capsule.

### Hepatic Resection

The clinical significance of hepatic parenchymal metastasis on survival in patients with advanced ovarian cancer has been studied. Lim and coworkers reported on a series of patients with hepatic parenchymal metastases. In this series, patients underwent wedge resection, segmentectomy, or hemihepatectomy as part of their tumor reductive surgery. The 5-year PFS and OS rates for patients with stage IIIC disease and patients with stage IV disease and hepatic parenchymal metastasis from peritoneal seeding were 25% and 23% and 55% and 51%, respectively. The authors advocated that complete hepatic resection should be attempted for patients with hepatic parenchymal metastasis.

### Bowel Resection

Because ovarian cancer often presents with confluent tumor in the cul de sac, rectosigmoid resection—along with or en bloc with hysterectomy and bilateral salpingo-oophorectomy—is often necessary to achieve complete tumor resection in the pelvis. This results in high rates of optimal cytoreduction, with acceptable morbidity. An average of 26% of women with ovarian cancer undergo colon resection as part of their primary cytoreductive operation according to a study by Aletti and colleagues. Peiretti and associates aimed to determine the impact of rectosigmoid resection, at the time of primary cytoreductive surgery, on morbidity and survival of patients with advanced ovarian cancer. A total of 238 patients were identified; 180 (75%) had stages IIC to IIIC and 58 (25%) had stage IV. Complete cytoreduction was achieved in 41% of the cases. Stapled coloproctostomy was performed in 98%, whereas hand-sewn coloproctostomy was performed in only 2%; a protective ileostomy and colostomy were necessary (constructed) in 2 (0.8%) and 5 (2%) cases, respectively. The complications associated to rectosigmoid resection were anastomotic leakage in 7 (3%) patients and pelvic abscess in 9 (3.7%). Fifty percent of patients recurred during the study period, but only 5% of them showed a relapse at the level of the pelvis, whereas 8% presented with abdominal recurrence associated with pelvic disease as well. The median overall survival time among patients with complete cytoreduction was 72 months compared with 42 months among the rest of patients ($P = .002$). The authors concluded that rectosigmoid colectomy may significantly contribute to a complete primary cytoreduction for advanced stage ovarian, tubal, and peritoneal cancers and that pelvic complete debulking accomplished by rectosigmoid resection could be associated with a lower rate of pelvic recurrence as well.

### Retroperitoneal Lymphadenectomy

Whether systematic removal of retroperitoneal lymph nodes should be part of optimal cytoreductive surgery had been a topic of debate for many years. We now have evidence that systematic lymphadenectomy in patients with grossly uninvolved lymph nodes provides no benefit to the woman. A prospective randomized trial by Benedetti-Panici and colleagues showed that systematic lymphadenectomy improves PFS but not OS in women with optimally debulked advanced ovarian cancer. In addition, the median operating time was longer (300 vs. 210 minutes; $P < .001$) and the percentage of patients requiring blood transfusions was higher (72% vs. 59%; $P = .006$) in the systematic lymphadenectomy arm. An ongoing randomized trial of systematic lymphadenectomy versus no further dissection is being conducted in stages II to IV patients in whom complete cytoreduction has been otherwise achieved at the point of primary cytoreduction. The primary end points of the LION (Lymphadenectomy in Ovarian Neoplasms) study are OS, PFS, and quality of life.

## *Postoperative Therapy for Advanced Epithelial Carcinomas (Stages III and IV)*

For historical interest, early adjuvant therapy attempts in advanced disease included single-agent and combination chemotherapy regimens based on the alkylating agents. A limited number of responses were observed, and treatment frequently continued for 1 to 3 years. With the discovery of cisplatin (and carboplatin, subsequently), several randomized trials were conducted comparing platinum and platinum combinations with nonplatinum regimens. These pivotal trials secured platinum as the agent of choice in primary adjuvant therapy, which continues to this day. In addition, several clinical trials have established that little additional benefit to treatment is observed beyond four cycles of therapy. Most recently, the development of the taxanes has documented the importance of this agent (discussed later). By convention, six to eight cycles of combination platinum- and taxane-based therapy are now recommended as adjuvant therapy for most patients with advanced disease.

The pivotal trial establishing the importance of paclitaxel in primary ovarian cancer management was reported by McGuire and associates on behalf of the GOG. They conducted a randomized trial comparing cisplatin, 75 mg/m$^2$, with cyclophosphamide, 750 mg/m$^2$, or paclitaxel, 135 mg/m$^2$, over 24 hours and demonstrated a survival advantage in the paclitaxel arm. All patients had residual tumors larger than 1 cm after the primary operation. Response rates improved with paclitaxel relative to control in patients with measurable disease (73% vs. 60%). The median PFS was 18 months in the paclitaxel arm compared with 13 months in the platinum arm ($P < .001$). OS was similarly improved (38 vs. 24 months; HR = 0.6; 95% CI, 0.5-0.8; $P < .001$).

The results of this study were confirmed in similar randomized clinical trials conducted worldwide. The taxane-platinum combination was generally considered to be the recommended first-line therapy for ovarian cancer. The platinum analogue carboplatin was found to be less nephrotoxic and neurotoxic and easily administered without prehydration, thus shortening the time of infusion. After several randomized clinical studies demonstrating the equivalence of this agent to cisplatin in ovarian cancer, carboplatin was substituted for cisplatin in taxane-based regimens. In addition, paclitaxel infused over 3 hours was found likely to be equivalent to paclitaxel infused over 24 hours and, in combination with carboplatin, enabled the combination to be given on an outpatient basis. Phase III studies by Ozols and coworkers showed that paclitaxel-carboplatin is a feasible outpatient regimen with less toxicity than paclitaxel-cisplatin and is associated with equivalent survival.

It should be noted that carboplatin is quantitatively excreted by the kidney and its effective serum concentration can be calculated from a formula based on the woman's glomerular filtration rate (GFR). This can be determined by various methods but is generally estimated by calculating the creatinine clearance. The Calvert formula is most commonly used and determines a total dose by this formula:

$$\text{Carboplatin, total dose} = \text{Desired AUC} \times (\text{GFR} + 25)$$

AUC-based dosing is preferred for carboplatin because the AUC most accurately reflects observed dose-specific toxicity and is more reliable across patients than dosing based on the body mass index. A usual dose for carboplatin is calculated for AUC values of 5 to 7.5. Both paclitaxel and platinum compounds are neurotoxic, as noted by Warner, and this is often the dose-limiting toxicity. The taxane, docetaxel, was found to be potentially less neurotoxic than paclitaxel. Vasey and colleagues reported on a large phase III study comparing docetaxel and carboplatin with paclitaxel and carboplatin in patients with stages IC to IV ovarian cancer. Almost identical survival parameters were observed between the two agents. The docetaxel arm was significantly less neurotoxic; however, it was associated with more myelosuppression. Neurotoxicity, as evaluated by several objective measures, returned to parity several months after treatment. Granulocyte colony-stimulating factor is occasionally needed to reduce the duration of significant neutropenia in these regimens. A commonly used regimen is paclitaxel, 175 mg/m$^2$ over 3 hours, or docetaxel, 75 mg/m$^2$ over 1 hour, and carboplatin (AUC = 5 to 6) given as a 1-hour infusion every 3 weeks. Premedication is required for both taxanes to combat hypersensitivity reactions, which have been attributed to the taxane itself and the carrier vehicle required to make these agents water soluble. In addition, steroid administration is necessary after treatment for docetaxel to combat fluid retention and effusion, a complication that may occur in as many as 25% of patients without prophylaxis.

### *Alterations in Frontline Treatment Strategies*

Although the preferred sequence in primary advanced ovarian cancer management is surgery followed by chemotherapy, several authors have attempted to take advantage of the disease's intrinsic chemosensitivity to improve outcomes in patients with extensive disease. Two avenues have been pursued:

- Neoadjuvant chemotherapy, in which, following biopsy or limited surgery, chemotherapy is administered for a reduced number of cycles (usually three to four) and an operation is planned for removal of the primary tumor (if present) and residual metastases
- Interval cytoreduction, when an unsuccessful maximal attempt at cytoreduction is followed by a reduced number of chemotherapy cycles (usually three to four), followed by a second cytoreduction attempt

Both strategies are followed by three to four cycles of chemotherapy after surgery. This latter strategy has been evaluated in randomized clinical trials with conflicting results; the former was evaluated in a randomized evaluation.

#### Neoadjuvant Chemotherapy

Neoadjuvant chemotherapy is practiced as an alternative for patients thought to have substantial operative risk or preoperative disease distribution that could preclude optimal cytoreduction. Several authors have noted the potential benefits to this strategy, including the opportunity to allow for an improvement in performance status, decreasing operative morbidity through less extensive surgery, and increasing the opportunity to achieve an optimal result. Each of these goals has been demonstrated in small, single-institution retrospective and prospective studies. For example, in a series of 85 women treated with either neoadjuvant chemotherapy ($n$ = 57) or primary cytoreduction ($n$ = 28), Morice and associates reported a significant decrease in major morbidity, defined as morbidity requiring a second operation (7% vs. 36%; $P$ = .01). Survival in this trial was similar between the cohorts, although with wide confidence limits.

Schwartz and colleagues reported on 59 women undergoing neoadjuvant chemotherapy and compared their surgical morbidity with 206 patients treated in the same time period by a standard approach. They found that patients in the former group had a shorter intensive care unit stay and postoperative hospital stay compared with conventional patients. Both groups received platinum-based chemotherapy. Because patients in these small trials are selected for treatment based on presenting disease volumes or medical status, it has been difficult to determine whether there is a detriment to survival by this approach. Clearly, patients too infirm to be operated on gain from this approach because if they have chemoresistant disease, surgery would have little value and likely would hasten an adverse outcome. Conversely, patients able to undergo the procedure could have a poorer outcome because there could be further expansion of a large population of resistant clones by delaying cytoreductive disease.

Loizzi and coworkers reported a case-control study of neoadjuvant chemotherapy in 60 patients (30 in each group). Patients were matched 1:1 based on date of diagnosis, histology, and stage. They documented that although the neoadjuvant cohort was older and represented a poorer performance status, these patients underwent optimal cytoreduction at a favorable rate (76% vs. 60%) and, following platinum-based chemotherapy, had similar PFS and OS compared with the control cohort. A critical question to be answered in this methodology is one of biology, which can only be addressed in a prospective clinical study of potentially operable patients. Fortunately, two trials are ongoing to address this question, one of which was recently reported. In this prospective multi-institutional study, 668 evaluable patients were randomized to primary cytoreduction followed by six cycles of platinum-taxane chemotherapy or three cycles of neoadjuvant platinum-based therapy followed by interval cytoreduction and three additional cycles of therapy. Patients were diagnosed by biopsy before randomization. Only 10% of patients randomized to interval surgery did not undergo the procedure because of the uncommon event of primary platinum and taxane resistance. Optimal cytoreduction (to <1 cm or to no visible disease) was statistically higher in the neoadjuvant therapy arm. This arm was also associated with lower postoperative morbidity. However, no difference was observed in PFS (HR, 0.99; 95% CI, 0.87-1.13) or OS (HR, 0.98; 95% CI, 0.85-1.14). Low rates of primary optimal cytoreduction and relatively low absolute median survivals observed in this study have been raised as criticisms. In 2010, Vergote and colleagues published a prospective trial randomizing patients with stage IIIC or IV epithelial ovarian carcinoma, fallopian tube carcinoma, or primary peritoneal carcinoma to primary debulking surgery followed by platinum-based chemotherapy or to neoadjuvant platinum-based chemotherapy followed by debulking surgery (Vergote, 2010). Of the 670 patients randomly assigned to a study treatment, 632 (94.3%) were eligible and started the treatment. The majority of these patients had extensive stage IIIC or IV disease at primary debulking surgery (metastatic lesions that were larger than 5 cm in diameter in 74.5% of patients and larger than 10 cm in 61.6%). The largest residual tumor was 1 cm or less in diameter in 41.6% of patients after primary debulking and in 80.6% of patients after interval debulking. Postoperative rates of adverse effects and mortality tended to be higher after primary debulking than after interval debulking. The hazard ratio for death (intention/treat analysis) in the group assigned to neoadjuvant chemotherapy followed by interval debulking, as compared with the group assigned to primary debulking surgery followed by chemotherapy, was 0.98 (90% CI, 0.84-1.13; $P = .01$ for noninferiority), and the hazard ratio for progressive disease was 1.01 (90% CI, 0.89-1.15). Complete resection of all macroscopic disease (at primary or interval surgery) was the strongest independent variable in predicting overall survival. The authors concluded that neoadjuvant chemotherapy followed by interval debulking surgery was not inferior to primary debulking surgery followed by chemotherapy as a treatment option for patients with bulky stage IIIC or IV ovarian carcinoma in this study. They went on to suggest that complete resection of all macroscopic disease, whether performed as primary treatment or after neoadjuvant chemotherapy, remains the objective whenever cytoreductive surgery is performed.

An additional phase III trial comparing primary cytoreduction to the neoadjuvant chemotherapy (NACT) approach has been published (Kehoe, 2015). In this trial 552 women with stage III or IV ovarian cancer were randomized 1:1 to either primary surgery followed by six 3-week cycles of a carboplatin regimen (usually in combination with paclitaxel) or to 3 induction cycles of chemotherapy followed by surgery followed by 3 adjuvant cycles of chemotherapy. The primary end point was OS, which was similar (primary debulking surgery [PDS]: 22.6 months vs. NACT: 24.1 months, upper bound of the one-sided 90% CI, 0.98), favored the NACT arm. High-grade adverse events related to surgery, including mortality, were higher in the PDS arm. However, like the European Organization for Research and Treatment of Cancer (EORTC) trial, overall survival in the trial (both cohorts) was much lower than expected, reflecting low rates of complete cytoreduction (PDS: 17%, NACT: 39%) and heterogeneity in treatment care (76% of both arms receiving paclitaxel and carboplatin). Criticisms for both trials lie in patient selection and surgical effort potentially confounding the interpretation of contemporary management.

### Interval Cytoreduction

Cytoreductive surgery performed after an initial failed attempt or in patients who were initially not considered candidates for cytoreductive surgery is referred to as interval cytoreductive surgery. Rose and colleagues published a prospective trial in 2004 evaluating the role of interval cytoreduction. In this trial, GOG conducted a randomized phase III study involving 550 patients with stage III and IV EOC who had residual disease of more than 1 cm after an initial attempt at primary cytoreductive surgery. All patients received three cycles of initial chemotherapy in the form of cisplatin and paclitaxel. Eligible patients were randomly assigned to undergo interval cytoreductive surgery followed by chemotherapy ($n = 216$) or chemotherapy alone ($n = 208$). Protocol compliance was good; only 7% of the patients who were randomly assigned to undergo interval cytoreductive surgery did not undergo surgery. Among patients who were randomly assigned to receive chemotherapy alone, 3% had interval cytoreductive surgery. It was found that PFS did not significantly differ between the two groups (HR, 1.07; 95% CI, 0.87-1.31; $P = .54$). In addition, there was no significant difference in the relative risk (RR) of death for patients undergoing interval cytoreductive surgery compared with chemotherapy alone (RR, 0.99; 95% CI, 0.79-1.24; $P = .92$).

### Additions to the Paclitaxel and Carboplatin Backbone

It has been postulated that agents with nonoverlapping cross resistance mechanisms or alternative mechanisms of action may be complementary opportunities in primary ovarian cancer patients to improve the therapeutic index. Several trials have been completed, with mixed results. The prevalent strategy has been to add to platinum and taxane therapy or substitute another agent for paclitaxel. The largest trial reported to date is GOG-182, which randomized 4312 patients to one of four experimental arms against paclitaxel and carboplatin (Bookman, 2009). Two of the experimental arms involved a three-drug strategy (adding gemcitabine or pegylated liposomal doxorubicin to paclitaxel and carboplatin, with the latter triplet given every other course) and two others substituted topotecan or gemcitabine for paclitaxel for four of the eight planned cycles in a sequential administration design (Fig. 33.13).

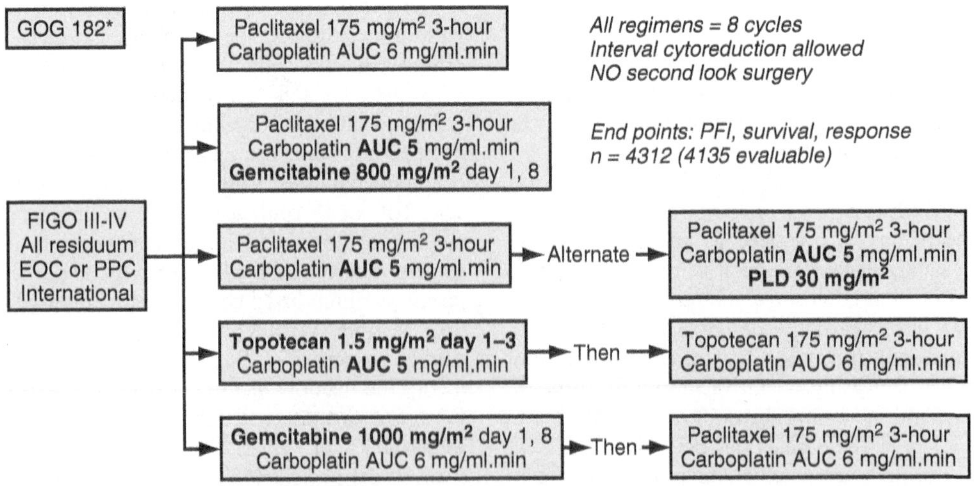


**Figure 33.13** GOG-182 trial that randomized 4312 patients to one of four experimental arms against paclitaxel and carboplatin. (Modified from Bookman MA, Brady MF, McGuire WP, et al. Evaluation of new platinum-based treatment regimens in advanced-stage ovarian cancer: a phase III trial of the Gynecologic Cancer Intergroup. *J Clin Oncol.* 2009;27[9]:1419-1425.)

Although considered a highly successful trial in terms of global participation and recruitment, the trial failed to improve outcomes by any parameter (response, PFS, or OS). However, as anticipated, the three-drug regimens were more toxic. Two other trials, the MITO-2, which randomized patients to an experimental regimen with carboplatin and pegylated liposomal doxorubicin, and OVAR9, which randomized patients to an experimental arm of paclitaxel, carboplatin, and gemcitabine, also failed to demonstrate superiority to this strategy. It is unclear whether the addition or substitution of available cytotoxic agents in this setting will improve outcomes in primary disease, given the probability for overlapping toxicities.

Based on emerging efficacy data regarding angiogenesis inhibition on ovarian cancer response and prevention of progression, several trials were launched with the agent bevacizumab. GOG 218 included two experimental arms with bevacizumab—one arm also administered bevacizumab as a maintenance agent for 16 21-day cycles following primary therapy and the other experimental arm administered only placebo in maintenance (Burger, 2011). ICON7 is a two-armed trial in which bevacizumab is administered with chemotherapy at half the dose of GOG 218 (7.5 mg/kg), but for 12 cycles in maintenance after administration with paclitaxel and carboplatin for five or six cycles (Perren, 2013). The trials have important differences (Table 33.9). Both have reported meeting their primary end point, PFS, but OS data are immature. In GOG 218, the improvement in PFS over controlled paclitaxel and carboplatin was seen only for arm 3, in which bevacizumab was administered with chemotherapy and in the maintenance setting. There was no difference in PFS for arm 2 compared with the control. The HR for PFS arm 3 versus arm 1 was 0.717 ($P < .001$); the HR for PFS, arm 2 versus arm 1, was 0.908 ($P = .16$) and corresponded to median durations of 10.3, 11.2, and 14.1 months, respectively. The anticipated HR for ICON7 was 0.78, which was observed, but details of this study have not been released.

Additional studies of other molecules targeting one or more processes of angiogenesis as well as novel targets, such as the folate receptor, are being pursued in this setting.

### Intraperitoneal Therapy

One promising but relatively old strategy that has been investigated is chemotherapy given by the IP route. Ovarian cancer appears to be IP-friendly because the distribution of disease is largely confined to this space, the pharmacokinetics of drug delivery are favorable, and the tumor is considered chemosensitive. Early experience with IP administration of chemotherapy has documented that it could be used to control ascites. Pharmacologic studies in the 1970s and 1980s demonstrated favorable profiles of relatively high direct drug exposure (high $C_{max}$ and AUC) for a number of agents subsequently identified to be important for ovarian cancer treatment. In this regard, platinum (cisplatin and carboplatin) and taxanes (paclitaxel and docetaxel) have been shown to have superior pharmacokinetic profiles when delivered into the peritoneum directly compared with IV administration.

Currently, administration is done principally via an implantable vascular access device placed during surgery or subsequent minilaparotomy (Fig. 33.14). A number of phase I and II clinical studies have been performed since the 1980s to document the safety of the strategy and to suggest efficacy. This has led to the performance and reporting of more than eight randomized clinical studies formally evaluating the efficacy of IP-based chemotherapy compared with IV-based chemotherapy in patients with advanced-stage ovarian cancer. A meta-analysis of these studies has been published and concluded that the route of administration "has the potential to improve cure rates from ovarian cancer." Similarly, the National Cancer Institute has issued a clinical announcement accompanying the publication of a large GOG study stating that the IV and IP regimen "conveys a significant survival benefit among women with optimally debulked epithelial ovarian cancer, compared with intravenous administration alone." In this latter study, patients with stage III epithelial ovarian cancer rendered optimal (defined as postsurgical disease residual <1 cm) were eligible for randomization to standard IV cisplatin and paclitaxel (24-hour infusion) or to IV paclitaxel (135 mg/m$^2$ on day 1), IP cisplatin (100 mg/m$^2$ on day 2), and IP paclitaxel (60 mg/m$^2$ on day 8) (Armstrong, 2006). This was the first phase III study to include IP paclitaxel in primary ovarian cancer therapy. Both cohorts were to undergo repeat cycles every 21 days for six total infusions. The primary end points were PFS and OS, and reassessment operations, if planned, were indicated at randomization.

This study was also the first to evaluate formally the impact of treatment on health-related quality of life. Assessment was made at baseline after the third cycle, after treatment completion, and 12 months after treatment completion. Overall, 415 eligible patients made up the study population. Both PFS and OS were significantly improved in the intent to treat the IP

**Table 33.9** Comparison of Gynecologic Oncology Group (GOG)-0218 and International Collaborative Ovarian Neoplasm (ICON)7 Study Characteristics

| | Trial | |
|---|---|---|
| **Parameter** | **GOG-0218** | **ICON7** |
| Setting and design | Double blinded, placebo controlled<br>Three-arm study<br>Bevacizumab for 16 cycles (maintenance)<br>Bevacizumab dose, 15 mg/kg/3 wk | Open label<br>Two-arm study<br>Bevacizumab for 12 cycles<br>Bevacizumab dose, 7.5 mg/kg/3 wk |
| Patient population | Stage III (suboptimal)<br>Stage III (optimal, visual or palpable)<br>Stage IV | Stage I or IIA (grade 3/clear cell histology)<br>Stages IIB-IV (all) |
| Additional end point | OS analysis (formal testing at time of PFS)<br>IRC | Defined final OS analysis (end, 2012)<br>No IRC |

*IRC*, Independent radiology review; *OS*, overall survival; *PFS*, progression-free survival.

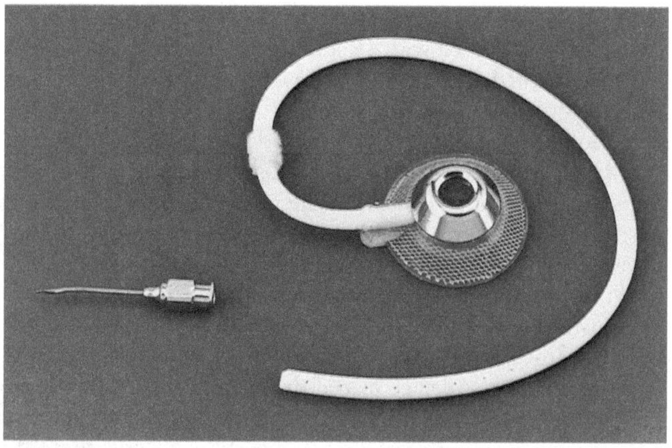

**Figure 33.14** Peritoneal catheter with access port for infusion of drugs. (Port-A-Cath, Pharmacia Deltec, St. Paul, MN.)

cohort ($HR_{PFS}$ = 0.80; 95% CI, 0.64-1.00; $HR_{Death}$ = 0.75; 95% CI, 0.58-0.97, respectively). The recorded median overall survival of 65.6 months is among the longest ever observed in an adjuvant therapy phase III ovarian cancer study. The results are even more impressive given that most (58%) randomized IP patients did not complete all six cycles of their assigned therapy via IP administration. This was largely because of significant differences in hematologic and nonhematologic toxicities associated with the IP regimen. Leukopenia and thrombocytopenia were significantly more common in the IP arm, as were pain (11-fold increase), fatigue (fourfold increase), fever (2.5-fold increase), and metabolic (fourfold increase), renal (threefold increase), infection (2.5-fold increase), neurologic (twofold increase), and gastrointestinal (twofold increase) events, among others. In addition, almost one in five (40 of 205 patients) randomized IP patients experienced a catheter failure necessitating treatment discontinuation. A detailed assessment of IP catheter complications in this trial has been published. A clear profile for catheter malfunction risk was not identified, although timing and accompanying surgical procedures were closely scrutinized. In a reflection of these observed adverse events, health-related quality-of-life assessments were significantly lower throughout the trial but returned to parity 12 months after therapy. It was concluded that the IP regimen provides superior survival efficacy and is associated with significant but manageable toxicity. The authors encouraged the use of IP therapy in clinical practice.

Lesnock and colleagues reported on the impact of somatic or germline *BRCA* mutation status relative to IP (vs. IV) therapy (Lesnock, 2013). In this trial just under half (48%) of the population had aberrant *BRCA* expression in the tumor. Patients with tumors harboring aberrant *BRCA* expression who received IP therapy had substantially longer PFS and OS relative to patients with aberrant *BRCA* expression receiving IV chemotherapy. This highlights the important role *BRCA* alterations have on outcomes, particularly in those receiving IP therapy. Unfortunately, toxicity concerns and a number of unanswered fundamental questions regarding efficacy (e.g., optimal agent, schedule, future trial designs) and the impact of alternative agents such as biologic therapies (e.g., vascular endothelial growth factor and epidermal growth factor targeting) have limited the general acceptance of this strategy in the clinical community without subsequent information. Clinical investigation with alternative agents such as docetaxel and carboplatin have completed phase I feasibility studies; phase III studies with the antiangiogenesis agent bevacizumab are ongoing.

### Dose-Dense Chemotherapy

One additional strategy, dose-dense and dose-intense chemotherapy, has received attention based on positive results reported in primary ovarian cancer patients (Katsumata, 2009). The trial, conducted by the Japanese Gynecologic Oncology Group (JGOG) and published in 2009, randomized 631 patients to standard paclitaxel (180 mg/m$^2$) and carboplatin (AUC 6), or weekly paclitaxel (80 mg/m$^2$/wk) and carboplatin (AUC 6), for six to nine cycles. The dose density (measured in mg/m$^2$/wk) was 33% greater in the experimental arm. Despite just 62% of patients receiving six or more cycles of the dose-dense strategy (vs. 73% in the control arm), the median PFS was 28 versus 17.2 months (HR, 0.714; $P$ = .0015). OS, although early, also demonstrated a significant difference, with 3-year OS in the experimental arm at 72.1% versus 65.1% in the control arm (HR, 0.75; $P$ = .03). Another trial evaluating dose dense strategy was GOG-262, which was conducted in women with suboptimal (defined as postoperative tumor residuum of greater than 1 cm) cytoreduction or undergoing NACT (Chan, 2014). In this phase III trial, 692 women were randomized 1:1 to dose dense paclitaxel (80 mg/m$^2$, weekly) plus carboplatin AUC 6 or standard 3-weekly paclitaxel/carboplatin. Bevacizumab could be added at the discretion of the physician and, if chosen, was to be administered in maintenance until progression. Overall, 84% of patients received bevacizumab and over 87% underwent a primary debulking attempt. In contrast to the JGOG trial, no significant difference was observed between the arms for PFS or OS. However, looking at just the cohort who opted not to receive bevacizumab, the dose-dense strategy was more effective on PFS. When bevacizumab was added, this effect was lost. This strategy is the subject of ongoing phase III studies with similar designs, addressing IP infusion, and with the addition of bevacizumab (e.g., IPocc, GOG-252).

### Evaluation of Chemotherapy Results

Chemotherapy is usually administered every 3 weeks. The patient is monitored with careful physical examination; blood tests to measure hematologic, liver, and kidney function; and radiographic studies, such as chest radiography, ultrasound, or, usually, CT of the abdomen and pelvis. Granulocyte colony-stimulating factor is added as needed to combat neutropenia. Mild neutropenia after chemotherapy can be managed expectantly, but for the patient who develops severe neutropenia with fever and an absolute neutrophil count of less than 500 cells/mL, antibiotics are prescribed to prevent septic complications.

If tumor is suspected on CT scan, fine-needle biopsy can frequently document the presence of persistent or recurrent disease. A negative CT scan, however, does not guarantee complete clinical response. Goldhirsch and coworkers noted that 5 of 26 patients with tumor nodules larger than 1 cm have negative CT scans, and the examination is most effective (80%) for detecting metastasis in retroperitoneal nodes. In 1989, Reuter and colleagues reported improved results of 8% false-negatives using newer equipment, with CT slices at 10- to 15-mm intervals. Patsner has reported that 24 of 60 patients with negative CT scans have a positive second-look operation, calling into question the value of this imaging study. Vaginal ultrasonography is particularly useful to assess the pelvis. CA-125 levels are used to monitor the course of the woman with carcinoma. As noted, Buller and colleagues calculated that the CA-125 level follows an exponential regression curve in successfully treated patients. This provides the possibility of mathematically estimating the patient's response to chemotherapy early in treatment. Bridgewater and associates reported that a greater than 50% decrease in the CA-125 level is a good sign of clinical response.

### *Second-Look Procedures*

Second-look laparotomy was introduced in the late 1940s as a method of assessing disease status after primary therapy in patients with colon cancer. In the 1970s, the same procedure was introduced for the treatment of epithelial ovarian cancer. In the field of gynecologic oncology, the rationale for using second-look surgery was that the optimal duration of chemotherapy was unknown (at the time) and the second-look procedure allowed surgeons to decide the optimal duration of exposure to alkylating agents for their patients. The primary concern with prolonged exposure to alkylating agents was the potential for secondary malignancies. Ideally, a second-look procedure would be able to identify the presence or absence of disease, which would help guide subsequent management.

Greer and coworkers performed a nonrandomized comparison in patients undergoing second-look laparotomy or clinical follow-up after receiving six cycles of combination chemotherapy with paclitaxel plus cisplatin or carboplatin. In that study, all patients were required to undergo optimal cytoreduction surgery prior to trial entry. The researchers demonstrated that second-look surgery was not associated with longer survival (in the context of a nonrandomized study). Therefore second-look surgery should only be performed in the setting of a clinical trial. If a second-look laparotomy is performed, it is important to extensively sample the peritoneal surfaces and lymph nodes. Particular attention is paid to areas that contained residual disease at the conclusion of the initial surgical procedure.

#### Maintenance Therapy

Unfortunately, many patients develop recurrent disease, even after a negative second-look operation. Rubin and associates noted a high rate of recurrence (45%) in patients with a negative second-look laparotomy. Those who initially have higher-stage and higher-grade tumors are more likely to have a recurrence after a negative second-look operation. However, those who were disease free at 5 years are likely to remain disease free by the subsequent follow-up period. Nonetheless, this high recurrence risk has prompted several authors to consider additional treatment at the identification of a complete response to primary treatment. This is often termed *maintenance* or *consolidation therapy*, although the former term is favored, given that the decision for treatment is based on the effect of primary therapy. Several randomized and nonrandomized clinical trials have been conducted in this arena, including hormones, vitamins, radiation therapy, chemotherapy, radioimmunoconjugates, immunotherapy, vaccines, gene therapy, biologic therapy, complementary medicines, and holistic approaches. Unfortunately, all have been negative in regard to improving overall survival. However, one randomized study did show an improvement in PFS. Markman and coworkers studied whether 3 or 12 additional months of paclitaxel could influence the time until progression in women who had achieved a complete clinical remission after primary treatment. The trial was designed to accrue 450 patients; however, at a planned interim analysis (after 277 patients were randomized), a statistically significant benefit for the longer treatment was demonstrated, which closed the trial to further accrual. The initial report demonstrated a 7-month improvement in median PFS (28 vs. 21 months; $P = .0035$); a later report with a long follow-up confirmed these earlier results (median PFS, 21 vs. 14 months; $P = .006$). No effect on survival was demonstrated, however. As noted, the addition of a maintenance biologic agent such as bevacizumab improved PFS relative to placebo, but the effect on overall survival remains to be seen.

Several additional biologic agents have entered phase III in this setting with mixed results. Pazopanib, an oral tyrosine kinase inhibitor (TKI) of vascular endothelial growth factor receptor (VEGFR), platelet-derived growth factor receptor (PDGFR) c-Kit, and fibroblast growth factor receptor (FGFR), was studied in women without evidence of progression on primary chemotherapy (du Bois, 2014). In all, 940 women were randomized and given either placebo or pazopanib for up to 24 months. The primary end point was PFS, which was extended by 5.6 months on the median (HR: 0.77; 95% CI, 0.64-0.91, $P = .0021$). Unfortunately, no difference was seen in OS, and the regimen was associated higher rates of hepatotoxicity, hypertension, and gastrointestinal adverse events. Further, among Asians, much lower dosages were required radioimmunoconjugates and there was a potential survival detriment in that cohort for patients taking pazopanib. Another TKI targeting the epidermal growth factor receptor (EGFR) pathway, erlotinib, was studied as a primary maintenance intervention in a phase III randomized trial (Vergote, 2014). In this trial, 835 patients achieving complete clinical response (CR) to six to nine cycles of platinum-based chemotherapy were randomized to either erlotinib (150 mg/day) for 24 months or observation. The primary end point was PFS, which was similar between the two arms (erlotinib: 12.7 months, observation 12.4 months; $P = .91$). Similarly, OS was no different between the arms. Of interest, a mutational analysis of EGFR, Ras, Raf, and PI3K was performed in 318 (38%) patients. The mutational rate in these genes was low ($n = 24$, 8%), and although PFS was significantly better in this cohort (positive prognostic factor), there was no difference in PFS based on mutation status (nonpredictive factor).

Another strategy that has been tried and continues to be of great interest is immunotherapy. Work from the Cancer Genome Atlas (TCGA) has demonstrated that ovarian cancers have a mutational load and thus the possibility for a high degree of expressed neoantigens, making them a prime target for immune targeted therapy (Bell, 2011). Although multiple vaccination strategies such as oregovomab, abagovomab, and agents targeting Muc-1 and Muc-16 have been conducted without direct effects, the appearance of the immune checkpoint inhibitors provides renewed interest in leveraging long-term immunosurveillance for ovarian cancer patients. Given the high stakes for patients at this point in their treatment, the effort to incorporate new knowledge of biology (e.g., poly-ADP [ribose] polymerase [PARP] inhibitors, discussed later) for treatment continues.

#### Cancer Antigen125 Surveillance after Primary Therapy

Because patients with advanced ovarian cancer frequently have CA-125 values that pace tumor response and progression during therapy, a common practice for monitoring patients following therapy involves serial CA-125 level determinations. The supposition is that earlier identification of recurrent disease can be better controlled by earlier initiation of therapy. To formally address this hypothesis, the European Organization for Research and Treatment of Cancer (EORTC) has conducted a randomized phase III trial in which women in complete clinical remission following primary surgery and chemotherapy were enrolled into a blinded surveillance program. Follow-up visits were scheduled every 3 months, when an examination was performed and blood was taken for CA-125 level assessment. All registrants were blinded to their CA-125 values during this time. However, when an individual's CA-125 level rose to twice the upper limit of normal, the patient was randomized 1:1 to unblinding of the result (early) or continued blinded surveillance (delayed). In this latter group, intervention was determined by the development of clinical or symptomatic relapse. Postprogression therapy was determined by local standards of care. The primary end point of the study was overall survival. In all, 1442 patients were registered, of whom 529 were randomly assigned to the treatment groups. Patients unblinded and made aware of their rising CA-125 values generally started treatment immediately, 4.8 months (median) before those in the delayed group. After a median follow-up of almost 57 months from randomization and 370 deaths, there was no difference in overall survival between the arms (HR, 0.98; 95% CI, 0.8-1.2). Median survival in the early treatment group was 25.7 months compared with 27.1 months in the delayed group. For patients receiving third-line therapy, the time differential to initiation was almost the same as the time differential to initiation of second-line therapy (median 4.6 months). Interestingly, a first deterioration in Global Health score occurred significantly sooner in the early treatment group. The authors concluded that no benefit in survival is gained by treatment dictated solely by an asymptomatic rise in CA-125 level and challenge the practice of routine biomarker surveillance in this setting.

Although practice standards may individually change on the basis this new information, counseling patients to watchful waiting is a challenge in the setting of rising CA-125 level without measurable recurrent disease. An alternative approach in this setting has been the use of hormonal therapy, such as tamoxifen. GOG completed a randomized clinical trial (GOG protocol 198) to address the impact of tamoxifen and thalidomide in women with significantly elevated CA-125 levels in the absence of measurable recurrent disease following primary therapy. Eligible patients had stage III or IV histologically confirmed epithelial ovarian, fallopian tube, or peritoneal primary cancer and a posttreatment CA-125 level exceeding twice the upper limit of normal in the absence of Response Evaluation Criteria in Solid Tumors (RECIST) 1.0 measurable disease. The primary end point of the trial was to compare PFS and OS between the two treatment arms and assess toxicity. At study closure, 139 women were randomized to oral thalidomide, 200 mg daily, with escalation to a maximum of 400 mg or tamoxifen, 20 mg orally twice daily. High-grade toxicities (grades 3 and 4) were experienced more frequently in the thalidomide arm (55% vs. 3%), with randomized patients experiencing more constitutional, somnolence, and pulmonary toxicities. There were more venous thromboembolism and gastrointestinal toxicities in the tamoxifen arm, but these were infrequent (<1.5%). The risk for progression was similar between the cohorts (HR, 1.31; 95% CI, 0.92-1.85), but the risk for death was significantly higher in the thalidomide arm (HR, 1.76; 95% CI, 1.16-2.68). Of interest, the time to measurable progression on tamoxifen was 4.5 months (vs. 3.2 months for thalidomide), which mirrors the lead time to symptomatic progression in patients blinded to their rising CA-125 level observed in the EORTC trial (4.8 months). Appropriate therapy for patients with rising CA-125 levels in the absence of measurable disease has yet to be determined.

### Recurrent Ovarian Cancer Management

Unfortunately, as many as 70% of patients who present with advanced staged disease will exhibit recurrent or persistent disease after primary treatment. These women may have prolonged survival despite developing recurrence; however, they are rarely cured. For this reason, treatment is generally considered palliative and must balance efficacy with toxicity. The choice of therapy is largely empirical; the treatment plan usually involves several agents in sequence, depending on treatment history, observed and expected toxicity, and performance status. Surgery, chemotherapy, immunotherapy, radiation therapy, biotherapy, and hormone therapy are options, alone and in combination, in this cohort of patients. It is not uncommon for a woman to undergo five or more different chemotherapy regimens, including cycles of retreatment with one or more agents. This characteristic reflects the increasing number of agents available for use, short duration of response, and general health of those receiving therapy.

Although there are few specific treatment guidelines as to how recurrence should be approached, initial consideration is most often guided by the interval of time until recurrence is identified. Patients are categorized as potentially platinum sensitive, platinum resistant, or platinum refractory based on the length of time from the completion of primary therapy until recurrence is identified. By convention, patients exhibiting a treatment-free interval of 6 months or longer are considered as having potentially platinum-sensitive disease. Those who achieved a complete response and were identified with recurrence under this benchmark are considered platinum resistant, and those who did not achieve a complete response or had disease progression during frontline therapy are considered platinum refractory. In reality, the probability for subsequent chemotherapy response likely represents a continuum based on this interval of time. However, clinically, the arbitrary division is used frequently to make treatment decisions.

#### *Platinum-Refractory Disease*

Patients who fall into this designation have a difficult disease to treat because their objective response to almost all available agents is low and the duration of any individual therapy is short. The choice of therapy depends on the woman's wishes and comorbidities. Because expectations for response to standard agents are low, these women are good candidates for investigative clinical studies, in which new agents with alternative mechanisms of action or targets are being evaluated. Under these expectations, some patients may opt to continue active treatment, whereas others may choose supportive care.

#### Platinum-Resistant Disease

Patients demonstrating an abbreviated initial response to frontline therapy represent cohorts who are unlikely to respond well to platinum retreatment. This is not to imply that some of these patients would not respond to retreatment with a platinum compound, just that the probability of response would be no greater than with any other agent and potentially lower. A current recommendation for most of these patients is to consider an alternative nonplatinum agent for the first treatment of recurrence. Table 33.10 lists the potential agents for treating these patients, their respective response rates, and significant common toxicities. Patients achieving stable disease or better are usually treated until the agent no longer demonstrates a clinical benefit or toxicity precludes further infusion.

Because expected overall survival is shorter in patients with this phenotype, a number of clinical trials with novel agents have been completed or are ongoing (see "Targeted Therapy," presented later in the chapter).

### Platinum-Sensitive Disease

Patients in whom disease recurrence is identified more than 6 months after the completion of front-line treatment are considered potentially platinum sensitive. These patients are good candidates for retreatment with platinum or a platinum-based combination regimen. In many cases, this combination is similar to that received in front-line treatment, paclitaxel and carboplatin. However, other two-drug and three-drug combinations have been investigated. A limited number of phase III studies have been conducted in this setting, but only one has demonstrated an overall survival advantage for the use of a taxane- and platinum-based regimen. The ICON4-AGO-OVAR 2.2 study randomized 802 women with recurrent ovarian cancer to paclitaxel and platinum or a nontaxane platinum regimen. Objective response was 66% in the taxane arm compared with 54% in the conventional arm ($P = .06$). PFS was significantly improved (12 vs. 9 months; HR, 0.76; 95% CI, 0.66-0.89), as was OS (29 vs. 24 months; HR, 0.82; 95% CI, 0.69-0.97). Approximately 75% of women in both groups had a treatment-free interval of at least 12 months, and 64% were taxane naïve at randomization. These are important factors when considering the study's conclusions. In all, six phase III clinical trials in platinum-sensitive patients have been completed. They differ substantially by agents investigated, sample size, use of measurable patients, prior exposure to paclitaxel and platinum in front-line therapy, and median progress-free interval prior to registration. Each of these factors has important consequences in regard to the data reported, making cross-trial comparisons among experimental groups hazardous. Table 33.11 summarizes the key features of these trials. It is noteworthy that two of these efforts included the use of nonplatinum agents in potentially platinum-sensitive patients, according to the definition provided earlier. These are important trials to consider given the high rate of drug hypersensitivity (platinum or taxane), intolerance, and lack of a clear benefit between platinum-containing and nonplatinum-containing agents in patients with moderate platinum-sensitive disease, such as those recurring between 6 and 12 months after primary therapy. Currently, only the combination of gemcitabine and carboplatin is approved for use in patients with platinum-sensitive recurrent disease in the United States.

Similar to work being conducted in platinum-resistant disease, investigation into improving the outcomes of these patients continues (see "Targeted Therapy," presented later in the chapter).

### Secondary Cytoreduction

The recurrence rate in patients with advanced epithelial ovarian cancer ranges from 50% to 90%. Therefore secondary cytoreductive surgery might be a viable treatment option for a select group of patients. Because patients with long treatment-free intervals have disease that is considered potentially chemotherapy sensitive, investigators have evaluated the role of surgery in this setting as well. Although there is some inconsistency in the definition of secondary cytoreduction procedures, the specific intent in this setting is resection of disease at recurrence, with the intent of debulking. The treatment of recurrent epithelial ovarian cancer is variable and dependent on a number of important criteria, which are evaluated at the time the recurrence is diagnosed. These include but are not limited to the time from completion of initial adjuvant therapy, site of disease, number of disease sites, and the woman's performance status. Most studies in the literature suggest that patients with platinum-resistant disease (recurrent disease within 6 months of completing platinum-based treatment) do not benefit from secondary cytoreductive surgery. However, others have argued for a role of surgery in this patient population. Musella and colleagues evaluated the role of secondary cytoreductive surgery in platinum-resistant recurrent ovarian cancer patients. Patients considered susceptible of cytoreductive surgery (group A) were compared with a historical series of patients with similar characteristics but not eligible for surgery (group B). Of 122 platinum-resistant patients, 18 met the inclusion criteria for the study and were enrolled. They

**Table 33.10** Clinical Efficacy of Cytotoxic Agents in Platinum-Resistant and Platinum-Sensitive Ovarian Cancer Toxicity

| | Response Rate (%) | | |
|---|---|---|---|
| **Agent** | **Platinum-Resistant** | **Platinum-Sensitive** | **Principal Toxicity** |
| PLD | 14-20 | 28 | PPE, mucositis |
| Topotecan | 14-18 | 33 | Myelosuppression |
| Hexamethylmelamine | 10-18 | 27 | Nausea, vomiting |
| Gemcitabine | 16 | | Myelosuppression |
| Etoposide | 27 | 35 | Myelosuppression, leukemia |
| Ifosfamide | 12 | | Hemorrhagic cystitis, CNS |
| Tamoxifen | 10-15 | 10-15 | Hot flashes, thromboembolic |
| Docetaxel | 22-25 | 38 | Myelosuppression |
| Paclitaxel | 12-33 | 20-41 | Myelosuppression |
| Vinorelbine | 21 | 29 | Myelosuppression |

*CNS*, Central nervous system neurotoxicity; *PLD*, pegylated liposomal doxorubicin; *PPE*, palmar-plantar erythrodysesthesia.

were compared with a historical series of 18 patients not surgically treated with analogous clinical and pathologic features. The most frequent sites of relapse included pelvic and aortic lymph nodes (39%), peritoneum (33%), bowel (28%), and pelvis (22 %). A low rate of intraoperative and postoperative complications was reported. No deaths were recorded. Overall survival was significantly longer in the cytoreductive group when compared with the control group (*P* = .035). Median overall survival was 44 months. Estimated 5-year overall survival rates were 57 versus 23.5 % for groups A and B, respectively.

No randomized trials have been conducted to identify a clinical benefit in this setting. However, several prospective and retrospective reports have suggested that only patients with extended treatment-free intervals and those who achieve a complete resection (no visible residual) benefit from the procedure.

In a study by Zang and colleagues, the authors aimed to identify prognostic factors and to develop a risk model predicting survival in patients undergoing secondary cytoreductive surgery (SCR) for recurrent epithelial ovarian cancer (Zang, 2011). Individual data of 1100 patients with recurrent ovarian cancer of a progression-free interval at least 6 months who underwent SCR were pooled and analyzed. Complete SCR was strongly associated with the improvement of survival, with a median survival of 57.7 months, when compared with 27 months in those with residual disease of 0.1 to 1 cm and 15.6 months in those with residual disease of >1 cm, respectively (*P* < .0001). Progression-free interval (≤ 23.1 months vs. >23.1 months, hazard ratio [HR]: 1.72; score: 2), ascites at recurrence (present vs. absent, HR: 1.27; score: 1), extent of recurrence (multiple vs. localized disease, HR: 1.38; score: 1) as well as residual disease after SCR (R1 vs. R0, HR: 1.90, score: 2; R2 vs. R0, HR: 3.0, score: 4) entered into the risk model.

In the AGO study, researchers also reported their efforts in establishing (DESKTOP I trial) and validating (DESKTOP II trial) a panel of features that would reliably predict optimal (no visible disease) secondary surgical outcomes in women with platinum-sensitive disease. The researchers found, as did others, that only complete surgical cytoreduction was associated with an improved OS and that this could be reliably achieved (>67% of the time) in patients who had a performance status of 0 or 1, were in the early stage, or had no visible tumor residuum following initial surgical cytoreduction and the absence of ascites.

Al Rawahi and coworkers evaluated the effectiveness and safety of optimal secondary cytoreductive surgery for women with recurrent epithelial ovarian cancer (Al Rawahi, 2013). The authors also aimed to assess the impact of various residual tumor sizes, ranging from 0 cm to 2 cm, on overall survival. The authors found nine nonrandomized studies that reported on

**Table 33.11** Phase III Trials in Patients with Platinum-Sensitive Recurrent Disease

| Control | Experimental | No. of Patients | TTP/PFS (wk) | *P* value | OS (wk) | *P* value | Comments |
|---|---|---|---|---|---|---|---|
| Carboplatin† | Carboplatin<br>Epirubicin | 190 | 65 vs. 78 | NS | 109 vs. 122 | NS | TFI = 17 mo; grade 4 ANC, 45%;T RBC, 30%, Plt, 25% |
| Platinum‡ | Platinum<br>Paclitaxel | 802 | 43 vs. 52; HR, 0.76 | <.001 | 104 vs. 130<br>HR, 0.82 | .023 | TFI = 75% >12 mo; neuro 1% vs. 20%; infection, 17%; hematologic, 46% vs. 29% |
| Carboplatin§ | Carboplatin<br>Gemcitabine | 356 | 23 vs. 35<br>HR, 0.72 | <.001 | 75 vs. 78 | NS<br>.0016 | TFI =60% >12 mo; RR: 31% vs. 47%<br>ANC, Plt more common in combination |
| Carboplatin, Paclitaxel‖ | Carboplatin<br>PLD | 976 | 41 vs. 49<br>HR, 0.82 | .001 (noninferiority)<br>.005 (superiority) | 30.7 vs 33.0 | .94 | TFI: Nonhematologic, 37% vs. 29%; HSR, 19% vs. 6%; grade 2-3 PPE, 2% vs. 12% |
| Topotecan¶ | Topotecan/etoposide<br>Topotecan-gemcitabine | 502 | HR, 0.84<br>HR, 0.84 | NS<br>NS | HR, 1.13<br>HR, 1.07 | NS<br>NS | TFI 64% >12 mo<br>More hematologic toxicity, less alopecia in topotecan-gemcitabine arm |
| PLD** | PLD<br>Trabectedin | 672 | 25 vs. 32<br>HR, 0.79 | 0.019 | 82 vs. 97<br>HR, 0.86 (*P* = .08) | PLD | TFI (32% >12 mo); effect seen only in PS cohort; PPE less in combination; ANC, LFT |

†Bolis G, et al. Carboplatin alone vs carboplatin plus epidoxorubicin as second-line therapy for cisplatin- or carboplatin-sensitive ovarian cancer. *Gynecol Oncol.* 2001;81:3-9.

‡Parmar MK, et al. Paclitaxel plus platinum-based chemotherapy versus conventional platinum-based chemotherapy in women with relapsed ovarian cancer: the ICON4/AGO-OVAR-2.2 trial. *Lancet.* 2003;361:2099-2106. This arm was mostly single agent platinum; however, platinum combinations were also allowed.

§Pfisterer J, et al. Gemcitabine plus carboplatin compared with carboplatin in patients with platinum-sensitive recurrent ovarian cancer: an intergroup trial of the AGO-OVAR, the NCIC CTG, and the EORTC GCG. *J Clin Oncol.* 2006;24:4699-4707.

‖Pujade-Lauraine E, et al. Pegylated liposomal doxorubicin and carboplatin compared with paclitaxel and carboplatin for patients with platinum-sensitive ovarian cancer in late relapse. *J Clin Oncol.* 2010;28:3323-3329.

Wagner U, Marth C, Largillier R, et al. Final overall survival results of phase III GCIG CALYPSO trial of pegylated liposomal doxorubicin and carboplatin vs paclitaxel and carboplatin in platinumsensitive ovarian cancer patients. *Br J Cancer.* 2012 Aug 7;107(4):588-91.

¶Sehouli J, et al. Nonplatinum topotecan combinations versus topotecan alone for recurrent ovarian cancer: results of a phase III study of the North-Eastern German Society of Gynecological Oncology Ovarian Cancer Study Group. *J Clin Oncol.* 2008;26:3176-3182.

**Monk BJ, et al. Trabectedin plus pegylated liposomal doxorubicin (PLD) versus PLD in recurrent ovarian cancer: overall survival analysis. *Euro J Cancer.* 2012;48:2361-2368.

*ANC,* Absolute neutrophil count; *HR,* hazard ratio; *HSR,* hypersensitivity reaction; *LFT,* liver function tests; *NA,* not available; *NS,* not significant; *OS,* overall survival; *PFS,* progression-free survival; *PLD,* pegylated liposomal doxorubicin; *Plt,* platelet count; *PPE,* palmar-plantar erythrodysesthesia; *RR,* response rate; *TFI,* treatment-free interval; *T RBC,* blood transfusion; *TTP,* time to treatment progression.

1194 women with comparison of residual disease after secondary cytoreduction using a multivariate analysis that met inclusion criteria. All of the studies included at least 50 women and used statistical adjustment for important prognostic factors. One study compared suboptimal (>1 cm) vs. optimal (<1 cm) cytoreduction and demonstrated benefit to achieving cytoreduction to less than 1 cm, if microscopic disease could not be achieved (HR 3.51; 95% CI, 1.84-6.70). Similarly, one study found that women whose tumor had been cytoreduced to less than 0.5 cm had less risk of death compared with those with residual disease greater than 0.5 cm after surgery (HR not reported; $P$ value < .001). Adverse events, quality of life, and cost effectiveness were not reported in any of the studies. The investigators concluded that in women with platinum-sensitive recurrent ovarian cancer, the ability to achieve surgery with complete cytoreduction (no visible residual disease) is associated with significant improvement in overall survival. However, in the absence of randomized controlled trial evidence, it is not clear whether this is solely due to surgical effect or due to tumor biology.

Two phase III trials are currently under way to address this question in patients with platinum-sensitive disease. GOG protocol 213 is evaluating the role of secondary cytoreductive surgery in patients with recurrent, platinum-sensitive ovarian cancer and the merit of adding an antiangiogenic agent (bevacizumab) to a combination of carboplatin and paclitaxel. In addition, this study will evaluate the usefulness of maintenance bevacizumab until progression relative to control. DESKTOP III is using the triage tool discussed earlier to identify patients likely to undergo complete surgical resection and randomizing them to surgery versus no surgery. Adjuvant therapy is not specified in this trial, but both are focused on overall survival as their primary end point.

### Targeted Therapy

The processes that govern cell transformation and immortalization, tumor growth, and metastases for ovarian cancer are complex and nonuniform. Nonetheless, several critical targets have been identified that appear to be differentially expressed in tumors cells relative to normal cells. Novel agents that target disruption or inhibition of these specific processes have been incorporated into the care of ovarian cancer patients. The most developed of these are agents that disrupt the signals to engender new vessel growth and development or angiogenesis. This process appears critical for a tumor to continue its growth beyond 8 $mm^3$. A number of cytokines have been described that tip the balance to sustained angiogenesis, but the most potent is vascular endothelial growth factor (VEGF). Prognostically, VEGF expression has been documented in all stages of ovarian cancer and has been correlated with impaired survival. VEGF overexpression has also been directly associated with ascites formation. This clinical feature is the result VEGF-induced endothelial hyperpermeability. The compound furthest in development for the treatment for ovarian cancer is bevacizumab, which has been investigated for primary and recurrent ovarian cancers (discussed earlier). However, a number of agents targeting VEGF, its receptors, angiopoietin, the epidermal growth factor receptor family, the phophatidylinositol-3-kinase (PI3K)/Akt/mTor pathway, and other cellular signaling pathways are also under investigation. In addition, new cytotoxics with alternative mechanisms of action, such as the tubulin poisons, and new topoisomerase inhibitors, agents that bind the minor groove of DNA (trabectedin), have been under phase III investigation. A summary of the outcomes of these trials is provided in Table 33.12. A detailed discussion of these trials is beyond the scope of this chapter; however, one trial deserves mention as it provided the background for the first approval of a biologically targeted agent in platinum-resistant disease. The AURELIA trial was a phase III open-label randomized trial comparing standard chemotherapy (weekly paclitaxel, pegylated liposomal doxorubicin, topotecan) to standard chemotherapy with bevacizumab (Pujade-Lauraine, 2014). The designation of chemotherapy was left to physician's choice, but each cohort was capped to provide equal representation in the randomization strata. The trial's primary end point was PFS. In the overall population, the addition of bevacizumab to chemotherapy significantly improved PFS (median 6.7 months vs. 3.4 months, HR: 0.48; 95% CI, 0.38-0.60, $P$ < .001). The observation was consistent in each chemotherapy stratum; in addition, objective response was significantly improved, both of which may have contributed to the increased frequency of adverse events. However, quality-of-life indicators demonstrated improvement in global symptoms despite these observations. No difference was seen in OS. These data, along with a substantial

**Table 33.12** Randomized Phase III Trials of Combination Chemotherapy in Platinum-Resistant Ovarian Cancer Patients

| Control | Experimental | N | PFS (mo) | *P* Value | OS (mo) | *P* Value | Comment |
|---|---|---|---|---|---|---|---|
| PLD* | PLD + trabectedin | 228 | 3.7 vs. 4 | NS | 14.2 vs. 12.4 | NS | RR: 16 vs. 23% |
| Paclitaxel weekly† | Paclitaxel + trebananib | 480 | 5.6 vs. 3.8 | HR, .65 | NA | NA | OS: effect in ascites |
| Chemotherapy (paclitaxel weekly, gemcitabine, topotecan)‡ | Chemotherapy + bevacizumab | 361 | 3.4 vs. 6.7 | <.001 | 16.6 vs. 13.3 | NS | RR: 12% vs. 27% (RECIST) |
| Chemotherapy + placebo (paclitaxel weekly, gemcitabine, topotecan)§ | Chemotherapy + pertuzumab | 156 | 4.3 vs. 2.6 | NS | 10.3 vs. 7.9 | NS | Similar to AURELIA except all low Her3 (64%) Placebo-controlled |

*Monk BJ, et al. Trabectedin plus pegylated liposomal doxorubicin in recurrent ovarian cancer. *J Clin Oncol.* 2010;28:3107-3114.
†Monk BJ, et al. Anti-angiopoietin therapy with trebananib for recurrent ovarian cancer (TRINOVA-1): a randomised, multicentre, double-blind, placebo-controlled phase 3 trial. *Lancet Oncol.* 2014;15:799-808.
‡Pujade-Lauraine E, et al. Bevacizumab combined with chemotherapy for platinum-resistant recurrent ovarian cancer: the AURELIA open-label randomized phase III trial. *J Clin Oncol.* 2014;32:1302-1308.
§Kurzeder C, et al. Efficacy and safety of chemotherapy (CT) ± pertuzumab (P) for platinum-resistant ovarian cancer (PROC): AGO-OVAR 2.20/ ENGOT-ov14/ PENELOPE double-blind placebo-controlled randomized phase III trial. *J Clin Oncol.* 2015;33.
*HR*, Hazard ratio; *NA*, not available; *NS*, not significant; *OS*, overall survival; *PFS*, progression-free survival; *PLD*, pegylated liposomal doxorubicin; *RR*, response rate.

Table 33.13 Summary of Phase III Trials Using Antiangiogenesis Targeted Agents in Patients with Ovarian Cancer

| Study | Agent | Target | HR-PFS (95% CI) | HR-OS (95% CI) |
|---|---|---|---|---|
| GOG 218* | Bevacizumab | VEGF Ligand | 0.72 (0.63-0.82) | 0.89 (0.75-1.04) |
| ICON7† | Bevacizumab | | 0.81 (0.70-0.94) | 0.99 (0.85-1.14) |
| AURELIA‖ | Bevacizumab | | 0.48 (0.38-0.60) | 0.85 (0.66-1.08) |
| OCEANS** | Bevacizumab | | 0.53 (0.41-0.70) | 0.96 (0.76-1.21) |
| GOG-213‡‡ | Bevacizumab | | 0.61 (0.52-0.72) | 0.83 (0.68-1.005)* |
| AGO-OVAR12‡ | Nintedanib | VEGFR, FGFR, PDGFR | 0.84 (0.72-0.98) | NR |
| AGO-OVAR16§ | Pazopanib | | 0.77 (0.64-0.91) | 0.99 (0.75-1.32) |
| ICON6†† | Cediranib | VEGFR | 0.57 (0.44-0.74) | 0.70 (0.51-0.99) |
| TRINOVA-1¶ | Trebananib | Ang ligand | 0.66 (0.57-0.77) | 0.86 (0.69-1.08) |

Modified from Coleman RL. Angiogenesis Inhibitors as a Therapeutic Strategy in Ovarian Cancer. http://fundaidc.org/Documentos/Simposio%20Cancer%20Ovario/Angiogenesis%20Columbia%20copy%20-%20copia.pdf.
*Burger R, et al. Incorporation of Bevacizumab in the Primary Treatment of Ovarian Cancer. *N Engl J Med.* 2011;365(26):2473-2483.
†Perren T, et al. A Phase 3 Trial of Bevacizumab in Ovarian Cancer. *N Engl J Med.* 2011;365(26):2484-2496..
‡du Bois A, et al. *J Clin Oncol.* 2013;31(18 suppl) LBA5503.
§du Bois A, et al. LBA ESGO. Liverpool, UK: 2013.
‖Pujade-Lauraine E. Bevacizumab and oral metronomic cyclophosphamide in platinum-resistant ovarian cancer. *J Gyn Oncol.* 2013;24(3):209.
¶Monk BJ, et al. LBA ESGO, Liverpool, UK.
**Aghajanian C, et al. OCEANS: A Randomized, Double-Blind, Placebo-Controlled Phase III Trial of Chemotherapy With or Without Bevacizumab in Patients With Platinum-Sensitive Recurrent Epithelial Ovarian, Primary Peritoneal, or Fallopian Tube Cancer. *J Clin Oncol.* 2012;30(17):2039-2045.
††Ledermann JA, et al. *Eur J Cancer.* 2013;49(suppl):LBA.
‡‡Coleman RL: SGO LBA3, 2015.
*Ang*, Angiopoietin; *FGFR*, fibroblast growth factor receptor; *HR*, hazard ratio; *OS*, overall survival; *PDGFR*, platelet derived growth factor receptor; *PFS*, progression-free survival; *VEGF*, vascular endothelial growth factor; *VEGFR*, vascular endothelial growth factor receptor.

database of bevacizumab use in ovarian and other cancers, led to the approval of bevacizumab in combination with chemotherapy for patients with recurrent platinum-resistant disease who have received one or two prior regimens.

Similarly, investigative efforts continue with novel therapies in patients with platinum-sensitive disease. A summary of the outcomes from these trials is presented in Table 33.13. Each of these trials has demonstrated a significant effect in improving PFS, but the impact on OS has been less robust and may directly relate to the opportunities for treatment cross-over and factors associated with long posttreatment survival. This effect is amplified in a woman with a long pretreatment interval. As mentioned previously, patients with a high likelihood for chemosensitivity and recurrent disease amenable to complete cytoreduction are potentially most likely to benefit from the interaction of surgery and novel therapeutic chemotherapy combinations. Although this hypothesis has not been confirmed, it is being prospectively studied in GOG-213.

### Poly (ADP-Ribose) Polymerase Inhibitors

Preclinical data have demonstrated the extreme sensitivity of *BRCA*-deficient cells to inhibition of the single-strand repair enzyme poly (ADP-ribose) polymerase (PARP). Inhibition of the PARPs leads to an accumulation of single-strand DNA breaks, which can lead to double-strand breaks at replication forks. Normally, these breaks are repaired through homologous recombination, in which the *BRCA* genes play a major role. However, synthetic lethality occurs when these genes themselves function improperly because of mutation or silencing. This has prompted the clinical development of a new class of novel therapeutics, the PARP inhibitors, which theoretically hold promise for patients whose tumors rely on PARP for continued cell growth.

To test this hypothesis and to evaluate the safety of the first drug in this class, olaparib, a phase I dose escalation clinical trial was conducted to examine the pharmacokinetic and pharmacodynamic effects in patients with cancers refractory to standard therapy. Given the mechanism of action of olaparib, the population was enriched for patients with *BRCA1* or *BRCA2* mutations. Overall, 60 patients were recruited to the trial, including 22 who carried a *BRCA1* or *BRCA2* mutation and one with a strong family history of *BRCA*-related cancer. The dose of olaparib (capsule formulation) ranged from 10 mg daily, administered for 2 or 3 weeks, to 600 mg twice daily, continuously. At the two highest dose levels, dose-limiting toxicities were observed. This led to a compromised dose of 200 mg twice daily, which was studied in a second cohort of *BRCA1* and *BRCA2* patients only. In general, the agent was well tolerated, with primary toxicities of somnolence, mood alteration, and fatigue. The toxicity profile was not increased in the *BRCA* subpopulation. Analysis of PARP function by pharmacodynamic studies has demonstrated rapid and high-level inhibition within the recommended dosing levels. In support of the hypothesis, objective antitumor activity (63% complete or partial response plus stable disease) was seen only in *BRCA* mutation carriers.

Olaparib has few side effects relative to conventional chemotherapy, inhibits PARP, and has antitumor activity only in patients with *BRCA* germline mutations. A phase II study in *BRCA* carriers has also been conducted, enrolling patients into two consecutive dosing cohorts. Overall, response rates were similar to those observed in the phase I study, with notable activity (>25%) in patients with platinum-resistant disease (Fong, 2009). Rates of discontinuation caused by adverse events were uncommon in both dosing cohorts. This promising degree of clinical activity was confirmed in a larger study of patients with multiple solid tumors including ovarian cancer ($n$ = 60) (Kaufman, 2015). Objective responses to single agent olaparib 400 mg twice daily, orally, continuously were observed in 31% (95% CI, 25% to 38%). This is favorably referenced to expected responses from chemotherapy in a similar setting. These data along an extensive safety database led to an accelerated regulatory approval of olaparib in *BRCA*-mutation carriers with three or more lines of prior therapy. Further perhaps clinical activity has been seen in the secondary maintenance setting. In a large randomized phase II trial of olaparib compared with placebo, PFS was significantly longer when patients with recurrent high-grade serous ovarian cancer were randomized to olaparib (vs. placebo) after achieving a response to platinum-based chemotherapy. In this study, patients taking olaparib (400 mg twice per day, orally continuously capsule formulation) had a median time to treatment progression of 8.4 months versus 4.8 months (HR: 0.35; 95% CI, 0.25-0.49); a post hoc analysis of patient carrying the *BRCA1/2* mutation demonstrated an even greater effect (Ledermann, 2012).

Currently, a number of PARP inhibitors are entering clinical investigation and are expanding eligibility to include patients whose tumors may harbor *BRCA* deficiency (the so-called *BRCA*-like state). Next-generation sequencing studies to identify patients with germline or somatic *BRCA* mutations as well as other alterations promoting a homologous recombination deficient stat in tumor tissue are being used in these trials and, if validated, may greatly expand the number of patients for whom PARP inhibitors may be helpful. Another active area of contemporary research are PARP inhibitor combinations, particularly with other biologic agents such as antiangiogenesis inhibitors, immune checkpoint inhibitors, cell cycle checkpoint inhibitors, cyclin dependent kinases, MAPK pathway inhibitors, and PI3K pathway inhibitors (Dalton, 2015; Liu, 2014).

### *Complications and Other Considerations*

#### Malignant Effusions

Pleural effusions are a common and devastating complication of advanced malignancies. Women with ovarian cancer frequently develop ascites, hydrothorax, or both, requiring repeated drainage by paracentesis or thoracentesis. In the majority of cases, malignant pleural effusion is associated with an incurable disease, with high morbidity and mortality. For the same reason, several studies have argued in favor of a palliative approach, rather than a conventional curative approach for treatment of this condition. Occasionally, sclerosing solutions are used in the thoracic cavity to prevent the reaccumulation of fluid, with resultant adherence of the pleural surfaces. New modalities, such as pleuroscopy and long-term indwelling pleural catheters, offer cost-effective outpatient or minimal hospital stay and less discomfort.

In a review by Musani and associates, it was reported that several mechanisms have been proposed to explain the development of malignant effusion. The inability of the parietal pleura to reabsorb pleural fluid because of the involvement of mediastinal lymph nodes by tumor is likely the most common cause of malignant pleural effusion. Therefore tumors that involve the mediastinal lymph nodes, such as lung cancer, breast cancer, and lymphoma, are responsible for most malignant pleural effusions. Other possible mechanisms include direct tumor invasion, as is sometimes seen in lung cancer, chest wall neoplasms, breast cancer, and ovarian cancer, as well as hematogenous spread to the parietal pleura.

There are several options for therapy, such as thoracentesis, chemical pleurodesis with chest tubes, video-assisted thoracoscopy (VATS), pleuroperitoneal shunts, and chronic indwelling pleural catheters. The advantage of a thoracentesis largely relies on the rapid relief of symptoms; however, it is unfortunately often associated with reaccumulation of fluid, multiple procedures and hospital visits, and associated complications, such as pneumothorax or reexpansion pulmonary edema. The option of chemical pleurodesis offers the advantage that it is highly effective; however, this treatment may be associated with required hospitalization and high cost. The VATS procedure is also highly effective and can be a diagnostic procedure in addition to a therapeutic procedure. The disadvantages are its cost, invasiveness, and its contraindication for patients who cannot tolerate single-lung ventilation. A pleuroperitoneal shunt may be considered in patients who have recurrent reaccumulation of fluid and those who have failed pleurodesis. However, this approach is not practical for patients with advanced or recurrent ovarian cancer because disease in these patients often also causes significant ascites. The option of a chronic indwelling catheter is ideal for patients who have recurrent episodes of reaccumulation of the pleural effusion. This approach is minimally invasive, cost effective, and successful. One of the major disadvantages is the risk for infection and the fact that the woman must be motivated to learn how to drain; otherwise, a family member or visiting nurse is required for home drainage.

A number of strategies have been studied in prospective trials. Most efficacious for problematic pleural effusion is pleurodesis with a sclerotic agent (e.g., talc slurry, antibiotic), decortication, or placement of an infusion catheter that can be operated by the woman. Tan and coworkers conducted a systematic review. Symptomatic ascites can also be problematic because few sclerodesis or surgical decortication-type procedures are available for long-term care. It is also not uncommon for patients to develop implants of tumor in the subcutaneous tissues after aspiration. Numnum and colleagues reported some success using bevacizumab as an adjuvant for this problem.

#### Malignant Bowel Obstruction

Intestinal obstruction is a common complication in patients with advanced epithelial ovarian cancer and is estimated to occur in 25% to 50% of patients. The onset of bowel obstruction is rarely an acute event. In cancer patients, compression of the bowel lumen develops slowly and often remains partial. Obstruction can result from partial or total occlusion of the bowel lumen or from alteration of the normal peristaltic motion. The initial symptoms are often abdominal cramps, nausea, vomiting, and abdominal distension that present periodically and resolve spontaneously.

Contrast radiography may help in defining the site and extent of the obstruction. Although barium may provide excellent radiographic definition, it is not absorbed well and may cause severe impaction. Diatrizoate meglumine and diatrizoate sodium solution (Gastrografin) is ideal for this type of contrast radiography because it offers similar radiographic definition and, in certain cases, may restore the intestinal transit. Abdominal CT is usually recommended because it can provide information about the location of the obstruction and the extent of disease. Surgical options may be offered to the woman, depending on a number of factors that dictate the success of surgical management. These include the site of obstruction, number of obstructions along the small or large bowel, number of prior chemotherapy regimens, prior episodes of bowel obstruction, nutritional status of the woman, and her overall functional status.

Pothuri and colleagues reviewed a series of patients undergoing surgery for intestinal obstruction caused by recurrent epithelial ovarian cancer and found that the mean time from original diagnosis of epithelial ovarian cancer to obstruction was 2.8 years. Surgical correction (intestinal surgery performed to relieve the obstruction) was achieved in 84% of cases, and successful palliation (the ability to tolerate a regular or low-residue diet by 60 days after surgery) was achieved in 71% of cases. The median survival in patients with successful palliation was 11.6 versus 3.9 months for all other patients. Major surgical morbidity was documented in 22% of patients. Interestingly, postoperative chemotherapy was administered to 79% of patients for whom surgical correction was possible. The authors noted that with respect to quality of life, it is important to consider that 56% of patients undergoing surgery for bowel obstruction had a colostomy or permanent gastrostomy tube. They also recommended that patients are not ideal surgical candidates if they have bulky carcinomatosis, rapidly progressive disease, multiple sites of obstruction, poor performance status, or heavy pretreatment with chemotherapy and radiation.

In patients who refuse palliative surgery or are considered poor surgical candidates, a percutaneous endoscopic gastrostomy (PEG) tube may offer symptomatic relief without the discomfort or complications of a nasogastric tube. The study by Pothuri and associates has shown that symptomatic relief (defined as the absence of nausea or vomiting) is achieved in 91% of patients with advanced epithelial ovarian cancer and bowel obstruction within 7 days of placement of a PEG tube. Only 13% of patients had resolution of obstruction and removal of the PEG tube after chemotherapy was administered. The median survival from the date of PEG tube placement was 8 weeks. The complication rate was 18%, and the most common complication was leakage. This study also demonstrated that the administration of total parenteral nutrition after PEG tube placement was not associated with a survival benefit. It is important to note that PEG tube placement is feasible for patients with a tumor encasing the stomach, diffuse carcinomatosis, or ascites.

Another potential nonsurgical option for the management of bowel obstruction is the use of metallic stents. These stents are flexible and self-expanding and can be inserted using radiologic or endoscopic techniques. The most important reported complications include local pain, gastric ulceration, gastroesophageal reflux, bleeding, and bowel perforation. Metallic stents are contraindicated in patients with multiple obstructions and peritoneal carcinomatosis. The literature on the usefulness of metallic stents for bowel obstruction in patients with gynecologic cancers is limited.

## Immunotherapy

Immunotherapy agents, such as *Corynebacterium parvum* and bacille Calmette–Guérin, have been administered to try to augment the immunologic response and promote tumor resistance in the host. These agents have also been used in combination with cytotoxic chemotherapy; preliminary improved results have been reported. IP immunotherapy approaches have been evaluated with agents such as interferon, lymphokine-activated killer cells, interleukin-2, and tumor necrosis factor. Berek and coworkers conducted a phase I and II trial of IP cisplatin (60 mg/m$^2$) and interferon-α (25 × $10^6$ IV) given every 4 weeks. Among 18 patients, there were three complete and four partial responses. Unfortunately, a randomized trial comparing interferon-α with no further treatment in women achieving complete response after primary chemotherapy has shown no benefit. A front-line phase III study of adding interferon-γ to paclitaxel and carboplatin was terminated early when an interim analysis of OS demonstrated a detrimental effect from the intervention.

The use of monoclonal antibodies as a form of site-directed therapy has been investigated. Epenetos and colleagues used tumor-associated antigens linked to $^{131}$I to treat recurrent ovarian carcinoma. After IP administration to 24 patients, responses were noted primarily in those with small-volume disease, with some responses lasting as long as 3 years evaluated by follow-up laparoscopy. Canevari and associates noted responses in 3 of 26 patients treated with autologous T lymphocytes targeted with a bispecific monoclonal antibody. Berek and coworkers reported a phase III study of oregovomab in women achieving a complete clinical response after primary therapy. This novel, murine-derived, immunotherapeutic agent targets the CA-125 antigen. In a placebo-controlled randomized trial, 145 women underwent infusion. The time to relapse was 13.3 months in the treatment arm and 10.3 months in the placebo arm ($P$ = .71). Although no benefit was observed, an exploratory analysis suggested that patients with "successful front-line therapy" were designated by patients with less than 2 cm residual postoperative tumor residuum and CA-125 reduction to ≤ 65 U/mL by cycle 3 of platinum and taxane chemotherapy and no clinical evidence of disease following primary therapy. These characteristics served as eligibility criteria for a follow-up phase III trial of oregovomab versus placebo. Unfortunately, this trial failed to meet its primary end point of extending time to progression. A third trial with an anti-idiotypic antibody to OC125 was conducted randomizing 888 patients, 2:1 to abagovomab or placebo (Sabbatini, 2013). The primary end point was relapse-free survival; there was no difference in this end point or in OS with treatment intervention.

Despite the many setbacks of immune-based therapy in ovarian cancer, the field is in a renaissance with the discovery of mechanisms providing immune escape. The development of various immune checkpoint inhibitors has begun to be explored in ovarian cancer, and is summarized in Table 33.14.

## Gene Therapy

The therapeutic impact of gene therapy in ovarian cancer has yet to be totally explored. Although the IP nature of this disease makes it well suited for this approach, various gene- or virus-based gene therapy programs have yielded mixed results at best. Several therapeutic models have been used in early investigations, including replacement of a tumor suppressor gene (e.g., *BRCA* and *p53*), suicide gene therapy, and inhibition of growth factor suppressors and regulators. As noted by Berchuck and Bast, there are a number of obstacles to developing this type of therapy to clinical usefulness. However, intensive investigation has been underway in a few centers to develop efficient and efficacious therapeutic programs.

## Chemotherapy Sensitivity Assays

A chemotherapy sensitivity and resistance assay (CRSA) is a laboratory algorithm wherein a sample of human tumor is subjected, under experimental conditions, to various chemotherapeutic agents and concentrations to assess response

Table 33.14 Ovarian Cancer

| Study (PD-1/PD-L1) | *n* | RR | Disease Control Rate | Prior Treatment |
|---|---|---|---|---|
| Nivolumab | | | | |
| Cohort 1: 1 mg/kg every 2 weeks | 10 | 1 (PR)/10 (10%) | 5/10 (50%) | ≥ 2 priors regimens |
| Cohort 2: 1 mg/kg every 2 weeks | 10 | 2 (CR)/10 (20%) | 4/10 (40%) | Platinum-resistant |
| Avelumab | 75 | 8 (PR)/75 (11%) | 41/75 (55%) | No limit on priors (median 4, range 1-11) |
| 10 mg every 2 weeks | | **2/2 clear cell** | | Platinum-resistant |
| Pembrolizumab | 26 | 3 (1 CR, 2PR)/26 (12%) | 9/26 (35%) | No limit on priors (>80% ≥4 priors) |
| 10 mg/kg every 2 weeks | | | | PD-L1 IHC positive (49/96, 51%) |

(tumor survival). Two broad categories of assay intent separate the available technologies: those that evaluate the inhibition of cell growth and those that address chemotherapy-associated cell death. Although these appear similar, they are different in laboratory protocol and may produce vastly disparate results. In most cases, several agents alone and in combination are evaluated. Theoretically, the most active agent or combination could be picked (sensitivity assay) or eliminated (resistance assay) from an empirical program, offering a more precise decision tool. The hypothesis is that differential selection will improve outcome. Although the concept is simplistic and rational, the effects of chemotherapy response and survival are complex and sometimes counterintuitive. It is frequently noted that a limited sample of tissue obtained from the primary or a metastatic site, at primary diagnosis or in recurrence and after previous chemotherapy or radiation exposure, would not necessarily be representative of active disease at any one time. However, Tewari and colleagues reviewed 119 synchronous and 334 metachronous ovarian primary, metastatic, and recurrent samples and found remarkable consistency in the tumor's drug-resistance profile. However, efficacy requires clinical correlation. Loizzi and coworkers reported a case-control study on 100 recurrent ovarian cancer patients treated by assay or empirical therapy. Overall response (65% vs. 35%; $P = .02$), PFS (15 vs. 7 months; $P = .0002$), and OS (38 vs. 21 months; $P = .005$) were all improved using the assay. Similarly, however, inherent selection bias and treatment overlap necessitate validation by a randomized clinical trial. In 2004, the American Society of Clinical Oncology issued a statement based on an extensive review of global literature; it concluded that this technology needs further investigation before widespread adoption. This was reiterated in 2011, and CRSAs remain an area of active research.

### Radiation Therapy

As presented earlier, radiation has been used for curative intent in women with early stage cancer, with some success. At least one report has suggested ovarian clear cell cancer may be responsive to radiotherapy, providing a potential treatment option for patients with this chemoresistant disease (Hoskins, 2012). Treatment planning involves a field that treats the entire abdomen as well as higher doses to the pelvis. Long-term efficacy must be balanced against uncommon toxicities of therapy, which include gastrointestinal stricture and fistulas and compromise of the bone marrow if chemotherapy is needed subsequently. The modality has also been used to treat recurrent disease. Cmelak and Kapp treated 41 patients with platinum-refractory ovarian cancer who had undergone secondary cytoreduction. They treated the whole abdomen with 28 Gy and a pelvic boost to 48 Gy. For 28 patients with residual disease smaller than 1.5 cm, the 5-year survival rate was 53%, which is better than would be expected with chemotherapy. However, no large-scale trial data are available for this technique and, because of the risk of complications and lack of extensive data regarding its effectiveness, whole abdominal radiation has generally not been used in these cases. However, localized radiation can be of use in select patients with isolated recurrences or persistent disease after chemotherapy or to manage localized symptomatic disease, such as bone metastases. The development of intensity-modulated radiation therapy has widened the therapeutic index by reducing toxicity to surrounding unaffected tissues.

### *Summary*

Therapy for epithelial ovarian carcinoma is based on the removal of all gross disease and sampling of areas at high risk of spread in the peritoneal cavity and retroperitoneal nodes. Postoperative therapy is used according to the stage and grade of the primary tumor. Multiagent platinum- and taxane-based chemotherapy is frequently used as adjunctive treatment for poorly differentiated tumors, such as stage I, grade 3, or for stage II cases without residual tumor.

For high-stage tumors and for patients with residual disease after initial operation, multiagent chemotherapy, usually paclitaxel and carboplatin, is used. It is accompanied by a number of short- and long-term toxic side effects, but initial response rates in stage III cases may exceed 90%. Five-year survival rates decrease to 30% or less. Long-term randomized trials and the development of new agents will be needed to improve rates of salvage and optimize therapy for epithelial ovarian carcinomas. Currently, second-line chemotherapy offers remission to some patients, but the best response rates are achieved with initial chemotherapy.

## RARE EPITHELIAL OVARIAN CANCER SUBTYPES

### *CLEAR CELL CARCINOMA*

Clear cell carcinoma is an aggressive subtype and accounts for approximately 5% to 10% of all epithelial ovarian cancers. It appears to be more prevalent in Japan. Over 50% are diagnosed in the stage I-II category, and outcomes are similar to those of women with high-grade serous carcinoma (Okamoto, 2014). For women with stage III or IV disease, however, the outcomes are worse than those associated with high-grade serous carcinoma (Mackay, 2010). A proportion of clear cell carcinomas appear to arise from endometriosis. The prevailing thought is that clear cell carcinomas are relatively resistant to conventional platinum/taxane chemotherapy. The most frequent alterations include mutations in *ARID1A* and the *PI3K/AKT/mTOR* pathway (Kuo, 2009; Wiegand, 2010). The angiogenesis pathway and *MET* amplification appear to be good potential targets as well (Mabuchi, 2010; Yamashita, 2013).

### LOW-GRADE SEROUS CARCINOMA

Low-grade serous carcinoma is a rare subtype constituting approximately 10% of all serous carcinomas. The stage distribution is very similar to that of high-grade serous carcinoma, with over 70% of cases in the stage III or IV category. Compared with high-grade serous carcinoma, low-grade serous carcinoma is characterized by young age at diagnosis, relative chemoresistance, and prolonged survival (Gershenson, 2015). Hormonal therapy has excellent activity for some patients (Gershenson, 2012). Likewise, antiangiogenic therapy appears to be active as well (Grisham, 2014). Translational research investigations have indicated that *K-ras* mutations occur in these tumors with a frequency of 20% to 40%, and *BRAF* mutations occur with a frequency of approximately 5%. MEK inhibitor therapy has demonstrated promising activity in the recurrent setting, and second-generation clinical trials are ongoing (Farley, 2013).

### MUCINOUS CARCINOMA

Mucinous carcinoma accounts for approximately 5% of epithelial ovarian cancers and is frequently confused histologically with mucinous tumors of the gastrointestinal tract. It is usually unilateral and is diagnosed in the stage I category in over 50% of cases. Stage I is associated with an excellent prognosis. Women with advanced stage mucinous carcinoma have a worse outcome than those with advanced stage serous carcinoma, and standard platinum/taxane chemotherapy does not appear to be active in this subtype. Consequently, colorectal cancer-type regimens have been administered in some patients; however, no systematic information is yet available. Although information on the biology of mucinous carcinoma is somewhat limited, potential genes or pathways for therapeutic targeting include *HER2/neu* amplification, *KRAS*, *src*, and the angiogenesis pathway.

## SMALL CELL CARCINOMA

Dickersin and colleagues described a virulent type of ovarian malignancy that occurs in young women, usually between the ages of 15 and 30 years. Because of its histologic appearance, it has been designated a small cell carcinoma. The tumor is often but not always accompanied by hypercalcemia, as noted by Young and associates in an analysis of 150 cases. Most patients have died, although a few stage I survivors have been reported, some of whom have been treated with adjuvant multiagent chemotherapy. Reed has reported a patient with stage IC disease treated with cisplatin, etoposide, and bleomycin who survived 5 years. Benrubi and coworkers treated a patient with stage II small cell carcinoma with debulking and multiagent chemotherapy followed by radiation; the woman was disease free for 4 years at the time of the report. Other isolated stage I 5-year survivals have been reported with multiagent chemotherapy programs augmented with subsequent pelvic radiation. However, for advanced-stage disease, and even in most stage I cases, the course of the tumor has been fatal. Harrison and colleagues reported the findings of the combined experience of the Gynecological Cancer Intergroup, which included 17 patients with small cell carcinoma of the ovary, hypercalcemic type. All *patients* were initially treated with surgery and platinum-based chemotherapy. Seven also received adjuvant radiotherapy with pelvic and para-aortic radiotherapy or pelvic and whole-abdomen radiotherapy. For 10 stage I patients, 6 received adjuvant radiotherapy, and 5 were alive and disease free at the time of the report. All but one of the 7 patients with stage III or unknown stage had died.

The molecular biology of this tumor, small cell carcinoma of the ovary, hypercalcemic type (SCCOHT), has been elucidated. Germline and somatic *SMARCA4* mutations have been identified in a high proportion of these patients, and this information coupled with recent pathology review have led to the conclusion that these neoplasms are actually malignant rhabdoid tumors (Jelinic, 2014).

### CARCINOSARCOMA

These are extremely rare ovarian malignancies that histologically resemble comparable tumors in the uterus. Treatment involves operation for cytoreduction, as noted by Muntz and associates, with added therapy, usually in the form of multiagent chemotherapy. Stage is a prognostic factor, and those with advanced stages usually do not survive.

As noted by Hellstrom and coworkers, approximately 500 of these rare tumors have been reported. In their series of 36 of these cases over 20 years, the median survival was 16.6 months, with a 5-year actuarial survival rate of only 18%. Low-stage tumors and those treated with multiagent chemotherapy (cyclophosphamide, doxorubicin [Adriamycin], cisplatin) had an improved survival. Although there remains some question about the efficacy of postoperative platinum-based chemotherapy for treatment of these tumors, as noted by Bicher and colleagues, this approach continues to be the standard. The most commonly used regimens include the combination of cisplatin plus ifosfamide and the combination of paclitaxel and carboplatin. Two reports have suggested that carcinosarcomas have a worse prognosis than high-grade serous carcinomas of the ovary.

**Box 33.2 Benign Conditions in Which Cancer Antigen 125 (CA-125) Level Is Elevated**

Endometriosis
Peritoneal inflammation, including pelvic inflammatory disease
Leiomyoma
Pregnancy
Hemorrhagic ovarian cysts
Liver disease

## GERM CELL TUMORS

These tumors are derived from the germ cells of the ovary. As a group, they are the second most frequent type of ovarian neoplasms and account for approximately 20% to 25% of all ovarian tumors. The classification of germ cell tumors, according to the WHO designation, is shown in Box 33.2.

The most frequent germ cell tumor is the benign cystic teratoma (dermoid); overall, only 2% to 3% of germ cell tumors are malignant. Of the malignant germ cell tumors, the most frequent is the dysgerminoma, which accounts for approximately 45% of malignant germ cell tumors. Next in frequency are immature teratomas and then yolk sac tumors (endodermal sinus tumors). In women younger than 30 years, germ cell tumors are the most frequent ovarian neoplasm, and approximately one third of the germ cell tumors found in those younger than 21 years are malignant.

The histogenesis of germ cell tumors has been extensively studied and summarized by Talerman. Figure 33.15 shows the theoretic histogenesis of these tumors. They are thought to originate from the primitive germ cell and gradually differentiate to mimic the developmental tissues of embryonic origin (ectoderm, mesoderm, or endoderm) and extraembryonic tissues (yolk sac and trophoblast). Germ cell tumors that originate in the ovary have homologous counterparts in the testes—that is, dysgerminoma and seminoma. Germ cell tumors are usually unilateral, except for teratomas and dysgerminomas (see Table 33.4). The morphologic and clinical aspects of each of the various types of germ cell tumors are considered separately.

### TERATOMAS

Teratomas consist of tissues that recapitulate the three layers of the developing embryo (ectoderm, mesoderm, and endoderm). One or more of the layers may be represented, and the tissues can be mature (benign) or immature (malignant). Chromosomal studies indicate that teratomas appear to arise from a single germ and have an XX karyotype. In the older literature, terms such as *malignant teratoma* and *teratocarcinoma* were used to denote the malignant variety of these tumors, but these terms have been replaced by the nomenclature shown in Box 33.3.

#### *Benign Cystic Teratomas (Dermoids)*

Benign cystic teratomas are the most common germ cell tumors and account for 25% of all ovarian neoplasms. They primarily occur during the reproductive years but may occur in postmenopausal women and in children. The risk of malignant transformation (discussed later) is markedly increased if these tumors are found in postmenopausal women. One of the interesting facets of teratomas is their ability to produce adult tissue, including skin, bone, teeth, hair, and dermal tissue. The presence of calcified bone or teeth allows the tumor to be diagnosed preoperatively by ultrasonography or radiography (Fig. 33.16).

Dermoids are usually unilateral, but 10% to 15% are bilateral. The outside wall of the tumor tends to be smooth, with a yellowish appearance caused by the sebaceous fatty material that fills the tumor. Hair is also a prominent feature once the cyst is opened (Fig. 33.17). Usually, the tumors are asymptomatic but can cause severe pain if there is torsion or if the sebaceous material perforates the cyst wall, leading to a reactive peritonitis. This rare complication is severe and can occur during pregnancy. Microscopically, a number of adult tissues are seen (Fig. 33.18).

Treatment of the reproductive-age woman or child consists of cystectomy or unilateral oophorectomy. In most cases, it should be possible to remove only the cyst and preserve normal ovarian tissue. The technique at open laparotomy is demonstrated in Figure 33.19. The opposite ovary should be inspected. If it is grossly normal, nothing further needs to be done. Current treatment involves preservation of the contralateral ovary without any biopsy if it grossly appears normal. In women beyond childbearing years, therapy for a dermoid usually consists of removal of the uterus, both tubes, and the ovaries.

Occasionally, teratomas may be solid and may consist only of adult tissues, leading to the diagnosis of a solid mature teratoma. These benign germ cell tumors are rare.

A cystic teratoma can undergo malignant degeneration, usually after menopause. Generally, it occurs in the squamous

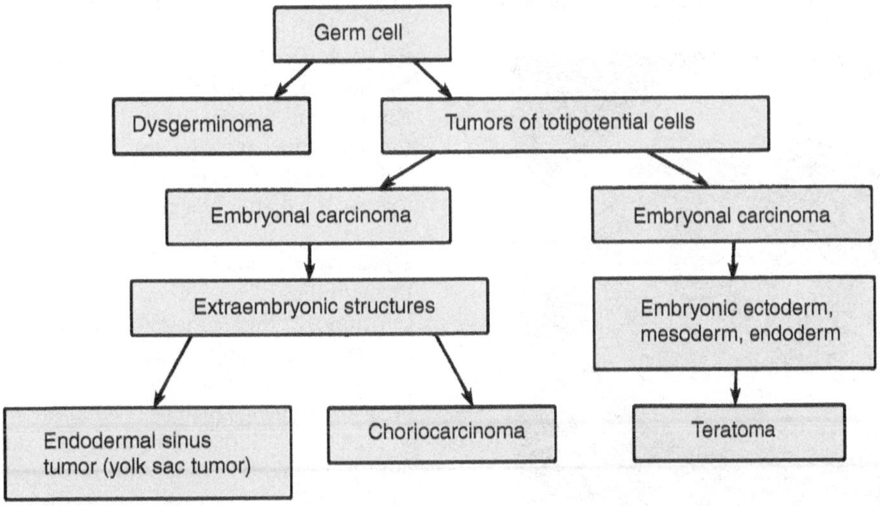


**Figure 33.15** Histogenesis of germ cell tumors. (Modified from Talerman A. Germ cell tumors of the ovary. In: Blaustein A, eds. *Pathology of the Female Genital Tract.* New York: Springer-Verlag; 1982.)

**Box 33.3 World Health Organization Classification of Germ Cell Tumors**

Dysgerminoma
- Endodermal sinus tumor
- Embryonal carcinoma
- Polyembryoma
- Choriocarcinoma
- Teratomas
- Immature
- Mature
  - Solid
  - Cystic

Dermoid cyst (mature cystic teratoma)
Dermoid cyst with malignant transformation
- Monodermal and highly specialized
  - Struma ovarii
  - Carcinoid
  - Struma ovarii and carcinoid
  - Others
- Mixed forms

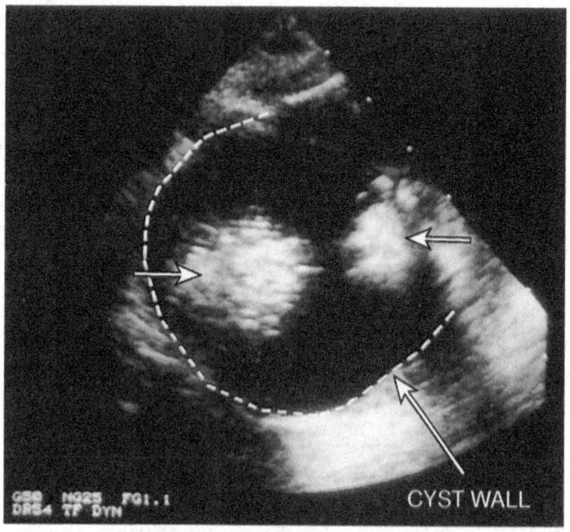


**Figure 33.16** Transvaginal ultrasound image of an ovarian dermoid cyst. *Arrows* indicate balls of hair. (Courtesy of Dr. Zubie Sheikh, Department of Obstetrics and Gynecology, University of Chicago, Chicago.)

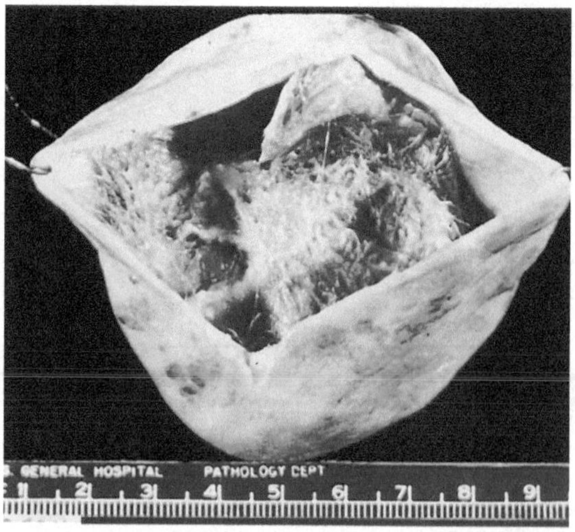


**Figure 33.17** Gross specimen of a dermoid cyst that was filled with sebaceous material and hair. (Courtesy of Dr. R.E. Scully.)

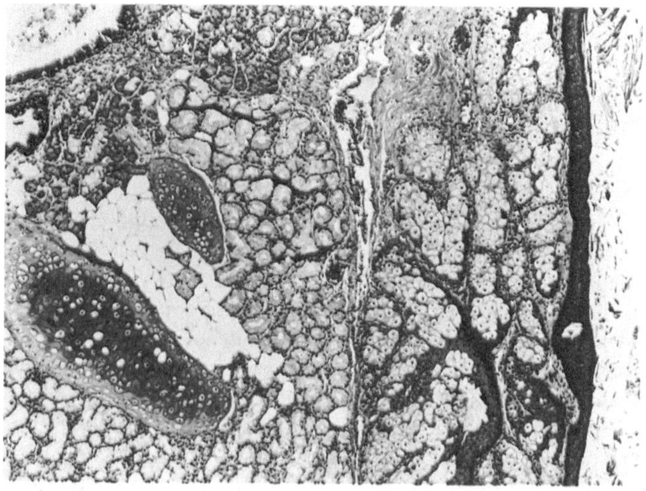

**Figure 33.18** Photomicrograph of a dermoid. Cartilage is shown *(right)* lined by epidermis and accompanying appendages *(left)* (×50). (From Serov SF, Scully RE, Sobin LH. *Histologic Typing of Ovarian Tumors*. Geneva: World Health Organization; 1973.)

epithelial elements of the dermoid, producing a squamous cell carcinoma. It is a rare complication, estimated to occur in less than 2% of these tumors. If the malignant tissue has spread beyond the confines of the ovary, the prognosis is poor. In such cases, additional therapy for squamous cell carcinoma with radiation therapy, chemotherapy, or both is used.

### *Immature Teratomas*

Immature teratomas are malignant and account for as many as 20% of the malignant ovarian tumors found in women younger than 20 years, but less than 1% of all ovarian cancers. They rarely occur in women after menopause. They consist of immature embryonic structures that can be admixed with mature elements. Approximately one third of immature teratomas express serum α-fetoprotein.

The prognosis for patients with immature teratomas is related to the stage (FIGO) and grade of the tumor. The grade of the tumor is based on the degree of immaturity of the various tissues. Grade 3 tumors consist of the most immature tissues and often have a high proportion of immature neuroepithelium. Figure 33.20 shows the survival of patients with immature teratomas by stage and grade before the advent of modern chemotherapy. Kurman and Norris reported that patients with stage IA immature teratoma have a 10-year actuarial survival rate of 70% after unilateral salpingo-oophorectomy; this rate is comparable with that recorded after bilateral salpingo-oophorectomy.

### *Dysgerminomas*

Dysgerminomas are the most common type of malignant germ cell tumors. They consist of primitive germ cells with stroma infiltrated by lymphocytes (Fig. 33.21). They are analogous to seminoma in the male testis and constitute approximately 1% of ovarian malignancies. Dysgerminomas occur primarily in women younger than 30 years. The tumor can be discovered during pregnancy. Some arise in dysgenetic gonads (discussed later). Unlike other malignant germ cell tumors, dysgerminomas are bilateral in approximately 10% of cases (see Table 33.4). Approximately 15% of dysgerminomas produce human chorionic gonadotropin related to areas of syncytiotrophoblast tissue.

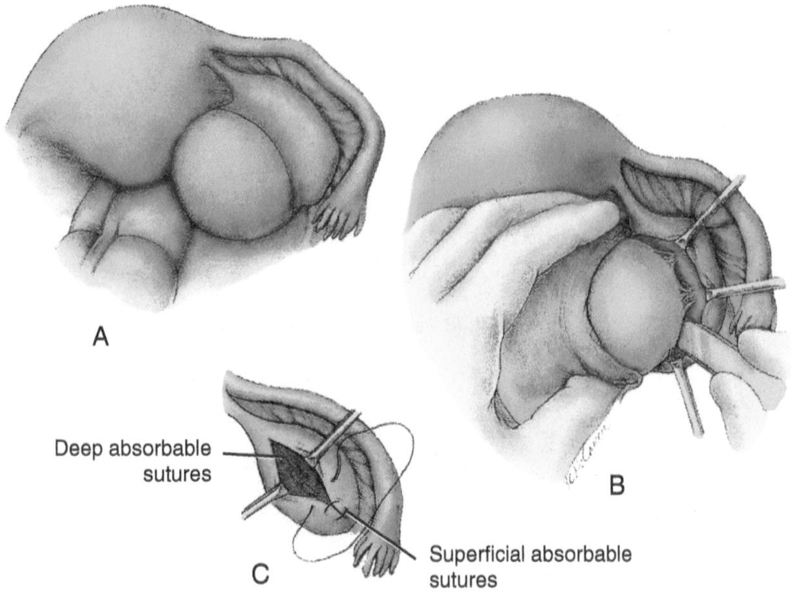


**Figure 33.19** Shelling out of teratoma. **A,** Scalpel incision in ovary at intersection of dermoid and normal ovary. **B,** Dermoid being separated. Note how the upper part peels away. **C,** Reconstruction of normal ovary.

### *Yolk Sac Tumors (Endodermal Sinus Tumors)*

The endodermal sinus tumor, or yolk sac tumor, which comprises 10% of malignant germ cell tumors, in part resembles the yolk sac of the rodent placenta, thus recapitulating extraembryonic tissues (see Fig. 33.15). One typical histologic pattern is shown in Figure 33.22. The tumor secretes α-fetoprotein, which is a specific marker useful for identifying and following these tumors clinically. These rapidly growing tumors occur in females between 13 months and 45 years of age. Kurman and Norris noted a median age of 19 years at diagnosis. The yolk sac tumor is the prototype for α-fetoprotein production.

### *Choriocarcinomas*

Nongestational choriocarcinoma is a highly malignant rare germ cell tumor resembling extraembryonic tissues. Like gestational choriocarcinoma (see Chapter 35), it consists of malignant cytotrophoblasts and syncytiotrophoblast; human chorionic gonadotropin is a useful tumor marker. This tumor mostly develops in women younger than 20 years, primarily in the ovary. The disease was usually fatal in the past and did not appear to respond to single-agent chemotherapy (e.g., methotrexate, actinomycin D) with the same frequency as gestational trophoblastic disease. This lack of response may be caused in part by the occurrence of these tumors in combination with other malignant germ cell tumors (mixed germ cell tumor) and, occasionally, the other germ cell elements may not be histologically recognized.

### *Embryonal Carcinomas*

Embryonal carcinoma is a rare malignant germ cell tumor composed of primitive embryonal cells. It occurs in young females between the ages of 4 and 28 years. Kurman and Norris summarized 15 cases. Trophoblastic elements may be present; both human chorionic gonadotropin and α-fetoprotein have also been reported to be present.

### *Polyembryomas*

Polyembryomas are exceedingly rare tumors that are usually found in the testes. They can occur in the ovary and consist of embryonal bodies that resemble early embryos. Trophoblastic elements with human chorionic gonadotropin and placental lactogen secretion have been reported.

### *Mixed Germ Cell Tumors*

Mixed germ cell tumors are combinations of any of the germ cell tumors of the ovary described earlier. They can be bilateral if dysgerminoma elements are involved; otherwise, they are unilateral.

## *TREATMENT OF MALIGNANT GERM CELL TUMORS*

Current treatment modalities result in cure rates approaching 100% for patients with stage I malignant germ cell tumors and more than 75% for patients with advanced-stage disease (stages III and IV). Because most patients are young and most of these tumors are unilateral, fertility-sparing surgery consisting of unilateral salpingo-oophorectomy with preservation of the contralateral ovary and the uterus is appropriate. After unilateral adnexal excision, frozen-section examination should be performed to confirm the diagnosis preliminarily. Once a malignant ovarian germ cell tumor is documented, routine biopsy of a normal contralateral ovary should be avoided because such an intervention could lead to future infertility related to peritoneal adhesions or ovarian failure. If bilateral ovarian masses are encountered at surgery, a unilateral salpingo-oophorectomy of the more suspicious side is appropriate. If the opposite ovary contains tumor or is dysgenetic, bilateral salpingo-oophorectomy is generally indicated. In the case of bilateral ovarian dysgerminomas in nondysgenetic ovaries, although not proved to be entirely safe, unilateral salpingo-oophorectomy and contralateral ovarian cystectomy may be considered in an effort to preserve

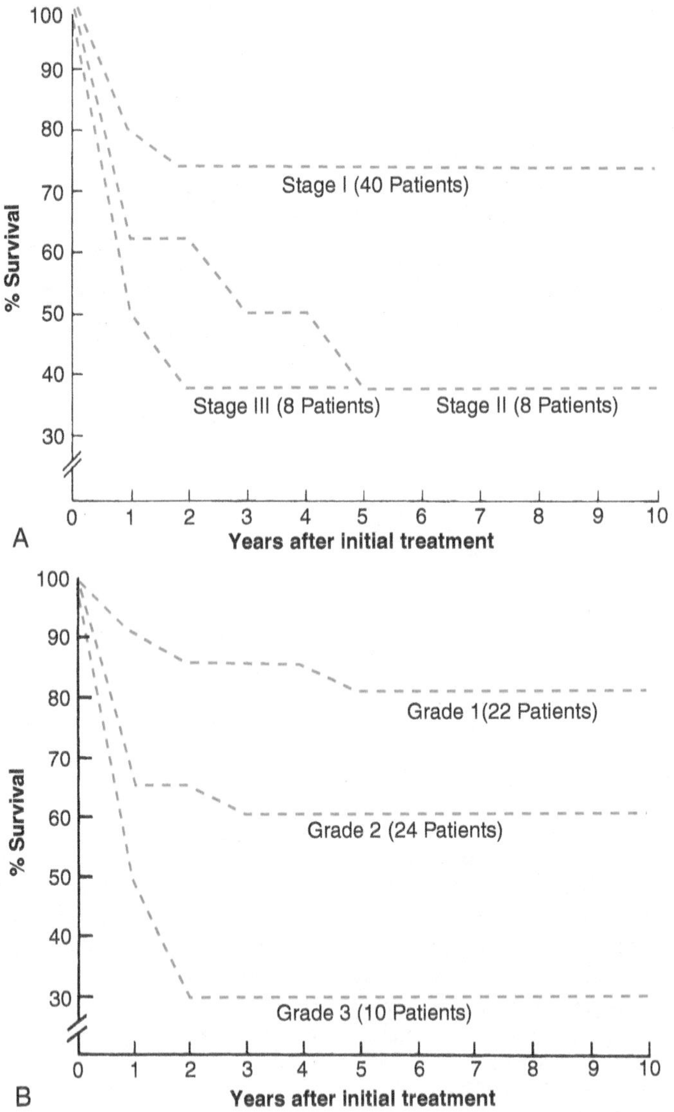


**Figure 33.20** **A,** Actuarial survival of 56 patients with malignant teratoma by neoplasm stage. **B,** By neoplasm grade. (From Norris HJ, Zirkin JH, Benson WL: Immature [malignant] teratoma of the ovary: a clinical and pathologic study of 58 cases. *Cancer*. 1976;37[5]:2359-2372.)

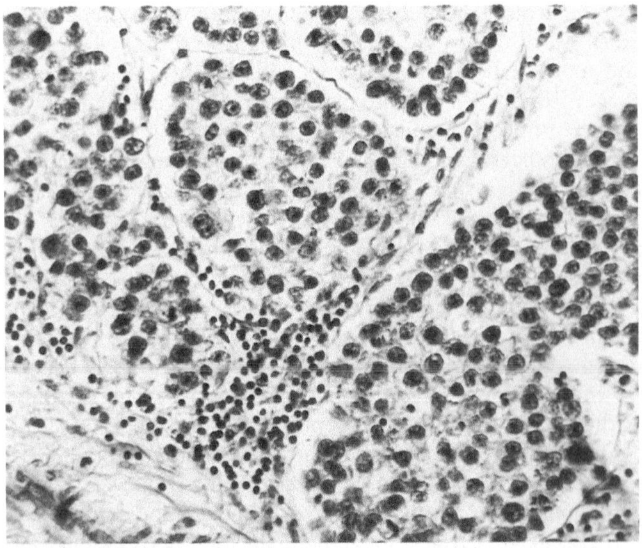

**Figure 33.21** Dysgerminoma (×300). Dysgerminoma cells are demonstrated as well as infiltration of stroma by lymphocytes. (From Scully RE: Germ cell tumors of the ovary and fallopian tube. In Meigs JV, Sturgis SH, eds. *Progress in Gynecology*. Vol 4. New York: Grune & Stratton; 1963.)

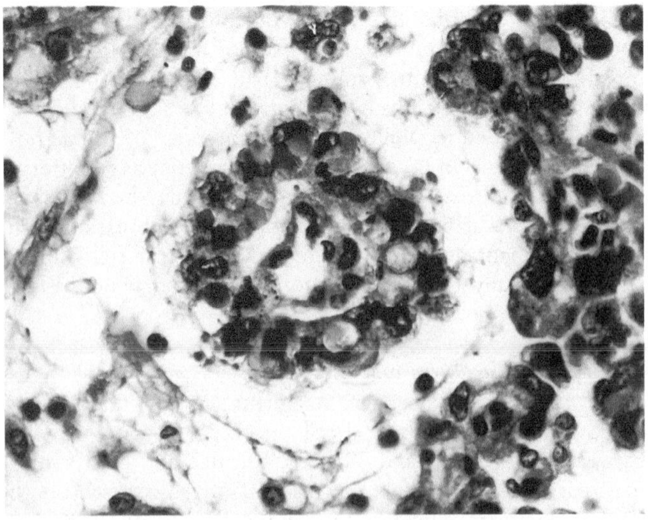

**Figure 33.22** Schiller-Duvall body associated with numerous hyaline droplets in an endodermal sinus tumor (×350). (From Kurman RJ, Norris HJ. Malignant germ cells of the ovary. *Hum Pathol*. 1977;8[5]:551-564.)

fertility. Conversely, if a contralateral ovary contains a mature cystic teratoma, which is more likely because it is present in 10% to 15% of cases, ovarian cystectomy is indicated.

If the tumor appears to be grossly confined to the ovary, comprehensive surgical staging is recommended, with cytologic washings, omentectomy, peritoneal biopsies, and bilateral pelvic and para-aortic lymphadenectomy. If obvious extraovarian metastases are present, the guiding principle is maximum cytoreductive surgery. The philosophy regarding comprehensive surgical staging for patients with malignant ovarian germ cell tumors is based primarily on that for common epithelial ovarian cancers and may or may not apply. For example, a very different perspective prevails in the pediatric surgery community. Based on an intergroup study report in which deviations from standard surgical guidelines did not adversely influence survival, Billmire and colleagues proposed a different set of surgical guidelines: collection of ascites or cytologic washings, examination of peritoneal surfaces with biopsy or excision of any nodules, examination and palpation of retroperitoneal lymph nodes and sampling of any firm or enlarged nodes, inspection and palpation of omentum with removal of any adherent or abnormal areas, biopsy or excision of any other abnormal areas, and complete resection of the tumor-containing ovary with sparing of the fallopian tube if not involved.

Historically, for most patients with malignant ovarian germ cell tumors, postoperative chemotherapy has been recommended. Notable exceptions include patients with stage IA pure dysgerminoma and patients with stage IA, grade 1, immature teratoma; these patients have a high cure rate with surgery alone. In the 1970s, the VAC regimen (vincristine, 1.5 mg/m$^2$ IV weekly for 8 to 12 weeks, and actinomycin D, 300 mcg/m$^2$/day for 5 days every 4 weeks, with cyclophosphamide [cytoxan] 150 mg/m$^2$/day for 5 days every 4 weeks) was the first effective combination chemotherapy regimen for patients with malignant germ cell tumors. VAC was the most widely used regimen during the 1970s and early 1980s and produced a relatively high proportion of cures in stage I disease (82%), but in patients with metastatic disease, the cure rate was less than 50%. During the VAC era, conversion of an immature teratoma to a mature teratoma under the influence of chemotherapy, so-called retroconversion, was observed.

By the late 1970s, based on the experience in testicular cancer, the combination of vinblastine, bleomycin, and cisplatin (VBP) was beginning to be used for malignant ovarian germ cell tumors, with superior outcomes compared with those achieved with the VAC regimen, particularly for patients with advanced-stage disease. By the mid-1980s, the VBP regimen was replaced by the combination of bleomycin, etoposide, and cisplatin (BEP) because of the latter's superior toxicity profile. The BEP regimen remains the standard today. Generally, most patients require three to four cycles of therapy. In 1990, Gershenson and colleagues reported that 25 of 26 patients treated with BEP for malignant germ cell tumors were in sustained remission. Subsequently, Williams and associates, reporting the GOG experience, noted that 89 of 93 patients (96%) with completely resected stage I, II, or III disease remained continuously disease free.

Special note should be made regarding dysgerminoma. Historically, for patients with metastatic dysgerminoma, the traditional postoperative treatment was radiotherapy. Although dysgerminoma is exquisitely radiosensitive and survival rates with this treatment were excellent, most patients suffered loss of fertility. With the advent of successful combination chemotherapy, such as BEP, chemotherapy has almost exclusively supplanted radiotherapy, with a high rate of fertility preservation. In a GOG report, adjuvant chemotherapy with etoposide and carboplatin for 39 patients with completely resected stage IC-III dysgerminoma resulted in no relapses.

Although second-look surgery was part of standard management for patients with malignant germ cell tumors until the mid-1980s, reports from the University of Texas M.D. Anderson Cancer Center and the GOG called into question the value of this procedure. Gershenson and coworkers reported their experience with second-look surgery, with negative findings in 52 of 53 patients; only 1 of the 52 negative patients relapsed and died of tumor. Subsequently, the GOG experience confirmed that the value of second-look surgery in patients with completely resected malignant germ cell tumors and incompletely resected malignant germ cell tumors not containing an immature teratoma element was negligible. For patients with incompletely resected malignant germ cell tumors with an immature teratoma element, however, second-look surgery appeared to have some impact. Advances in imaging technology may further minimize the need for second-look surgery, even in the latter group.

There has been a trend toward surveillance, with careful follow-up after surgery as an alternative to chemotherapy in select patients. Bonazzi and colleagues treated 32 patients with operation alone for stage I or II, grade 1 or 2, tumors. All patients with grade 3 or stage III tumors, or those with tumor recurrence, received cisplatin, etoposide, and bleomycin. Most patients underwent fertility-sparing surgery, and 10 received chemotherapy. All patients were free of disease with a median follow-up of 47 months, and 5 had delivered healthy infants. A Pediatric Oncology Group Study reported by Cushing and associates has indicated that patients younger than 15 years with a pure immature teratoma could be followed without chemotherapy; however, more than 90% of the tumors in their series were grade 1 or 2. Patterson and associates reported on surveillance in patients with stage IA malignant ovarian germ cell tumor. Relapses were reported in 8 of 22 (36%) patients with nondysgerminomatous tumors and 2 of 9 (22%) patients with dysgerminomas. All relapses occurred within 13 months of diagnosis, and one patient was not salvaged with chemotherapy. Mangili and colleagues reported 28 patients with stage I immature teratoma (9 grade 1, 12 grade 2, and 7 grade 3), 19 of whom were treated with surgery alone. Twenty-four of the patients underwent fertility-sparing surgery. Four patients treated with surgery alone relapsed—2 with mature teratoma and 2 with immature teratoma. All were salvaged with secondary surgery, with the 2 patients with immature teratoma receiving chemotherapy as well.

The Children's Oncology Group has conducted a clinical trial in the pediatric population. This trial included surveillance of a low-risk cohort, consisting of all patients with apparent stage I disease with close follow-up of serum markers and initiation of chemotherapy only if relapse occurred (Billmire, 2014). Twenty-five girls were enrolled in the trial. After a median follow-up of 42 months, 12 patients had persistent or recurrent disease. Eleven of the 12 patients were successfully salvaged with chemotherapy.

There is no standard surveillance for patients with malignant ovarian germ cell tumors after completion of primary therapy. For patients who have completed standard surgery plus chemotherapy, we generally recommend evaluation of serum tumor marker every 3 months for up to 2 years and then every 6 months until 5 years from diagnosis. Patients treated with fertility-sparing surgery should be closely followed with periodic transvaginal ultrasound or CT evaluations. Office visits, with a physical examination, are generally recommended every 3 months for the first 2 years and less frequently thereafter.

With the success of cure in a high proportion of young patients with malignant ovarian germ cell tumors has come an increasing focus on the late effects of therapy, particularly fertility preservation. In a report of 40 patients, Gershenson and colleagues noted that 27 had normal menses after multiagent chemotherapy for germ cell tumors, and 11 of 16 patients who attempted pregnancy were successful in bearing 22 children. Most of these patients received nonplatinum-based chemotherapy. Peccatori and associates reported on 139 patients with malignant germ cell tumors, 108 of whom had fertility-sparing operations. Multiagent platinum-containing chemotherapy was used, with a 96% survival rate and a mean follow-up of 55 months. In a GOG study, Williams and associates reported on 93 patients treated adjuvantly with cisplatin, etoposide, and bleomycin for three cycles. Of 93 patients, 91 were free of disease 4 to 90 months after treatment, although leukemia developed in one patient and lymphoma in a second patient. Brewer and coworkers reported on 26 patients treated with BEP, with 25 alive and disease-free and a median follow-up of 89 months. They reported that 71% resumed normal menstrual function and 6 patients conceived. Three additional large studies from Australia, Italy, and the United States have provided further support for the concept of preservation of fertility in most treated with fertility-sparing surgery and chemotherapy. In a GOG matched control study of 132 survivors (all of whom were treated with surgery and platinum-based chemotherapy) and 137 controls, 71 (54%) survivors underwent fertility-sparing surgery. Of the fertile survivors, 87% reported having normal menstrual function and 24 survivors had 37 offspring after cancer therapy. However, compared with controls, cancer survivors had significantly greater reproductive concerns and less sexual pleasure.

Several nonrandomized studies have suggested that the gonadotropin-releasing hormone agonist prophylaxis may be worthwhile to preserve ovarian function in young patients receiving chemotherapy. Blumenfeld and coworkers administered gonadotropin-releasing hormone agonist during chemotherapy for nongynecologic tumors to women of reproductive age, and 15 of 16 surviving patients (93.7%) resumed menses and ovulation. However, randomized trials are needed to validate this approach. In a randomized trial for breast cancer patients, a GnRH analogue appeared to reduce the incidence of chemotherapy-induced premature menopause.

### *SPECIALIZED GERM CELL TUMORS: STRUMA OVARII AND CARCINOIDS*

Specialized ovarian germ cell tumors are rare; two types are commonly recognized (see Box 33.3): the struma ovarii and carcinoids. Struma ovarii are dermoids with thyroid tissue exclusively or with thyroid tissue as a major component. The thyroid tissue can be functional, leading to clinical hyperthyroidism. Most of these tumors are benign, but malignant changes are possible. Metastatic disease, if present, has been reported to be effectively treated with $^{131}I$, as for primary thyroid carcinoma.

Carcinoids are ovarian teratomas that histologically resemble similar tumors in the gastrointestinal tract. Carcinoids are rare and are unilateral in the ovary. In approximately 30% of cases, a true carcinoid syndrome will develop, and 5-hydroxyindoleacetic acid can be detected and used to monitor the tumor postoperatively. These tumors occur primarily in older women and tend to grow slowly; the prognosis after hysterectomy and bilateral salpingo-oophorectomy is excellent. For a young woman desiring preservation of childbearing function, a stage IA carcinoid can be treated by unilateral salpingo-oophorectomy.

## GONADOBLASTOMAS (GERM CELL SEX CORD-STROMAL TUMORS)

The term *gonadoblastoma* was introduced by Scully in 1953 to describe a tumor that consists of germ cell and sex cord–stromal elements. Approximately 100 cases have been reported. The germ cells usually resemble dysgerminoma, whereas the sex cord–stromal elements may consist of immature granulosa and Sertoli cells. Leydig cells and luteinized cells may be present. The tumor usually occurs in patients with abnormal (dysgenetic) gonads. Most patients have a female phenotype but may be virilized. These patients have a Y chromosome detected in their karyotype, and patients with gonadal dysgenesis and a Y chromosome are at risk for the development of gonadoblastoma or malignant germ cell tumors, predominantly dysgerminoma, which may occur in those as young as 6 months. Removal of these gonads is indicated when they are discovered. Both gonads should be removed; if the presence of pure gonadoblastoma is confirmed, the prognosis is excellent because these tumors have not been reported to metastasize.

## SEX CORD-STROMAL TUMORS

Sex cord–stromal tumors are derived from the sex cords of the ovary and the specialized stroma of the developing gonad. The elements can have a male or female differentiation, and some of these tumors are hormonally active. This group accounts for approximately 6% of ovarian neoplasms and most hormonally

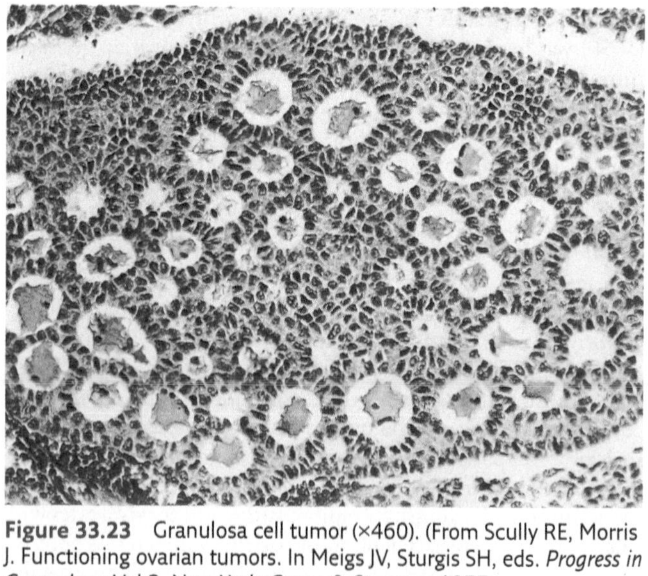

**Figure 33.23** Granulosa cell tumor (×460). (From Scully RE, Morris J. Functioning ovarian tumors. In Meigs JV, Sturgis SH, eds. *Progress in Gynecology*. Vol 3. New York: Grune & Stratton; 1957.)

functioning ovarian tumors. For the female derivatives, the sex cord component is the granulosa cell and the stromal component is the theca cell or fibroblast. For the male counterpart, the similar components are the Sertoli cell and Leydig cell. Granulosa–theca cell tumors and Sertoli-Leydig cell tumors tend to behave as low-grade malignancies. Their clinical and morphologic aspects considered separately.

## GRANULOSA-THECA CELL TUMORS

Granulosa cell tumors consist primarily of granulosa cells and a varying proportion of theca cells, fibroblasts, or both. One characteristic microscopic pattern is shown in Figure 33.23, which demonstrates the so-called *Call-Exner bodies,* eosinophilic bodies surrounded by granulosa cells. Functional granulosa cell tumors are primarily estrogenic. Approximately 5% occur before puberty and they can be one cause of precocious puberty, but the tumors have been described in women of all ages. In postmenopausal women, these tumors can produce increased levels of blood estrogens, uterine bleeding, and occasionally endometrial carcinoma. It is estimated that approximately 5% of the granulosa cell tumors in adults are associated with endometrial carcinoma. In menstruating women, the functional granulosa cell tumor can produce abnormal menstrual patterns, menorrhagia, and even amenorrhea.

These tumors can become large and may present as a ruptured mass, leading to laparotomy for an acute abdomen with hemoperitoneum. Because of the low-grade malignant character of these tumors, recurrences are frequently more than 5 years after primary therapy. In general, prognosis does not correlate with the histologic pattern of the tumor. A total of 90% of granulosa cell tumors present as stage I. Advanced clinical stage, the presence of tumor rupture, a large primary tumor (>15 cm), and a high mitotic rate have been associated with a poorer prognosis. Overall 10-year survival rates of 90% have been reported. Studies by Klemi and colleagues and others have suggested that most granulosa cell tumors have a diploid pattern and a low (<60%) S-phase fraction when analyzed by flow cytometry. Those with an aneuploid pattern had a worse prognosis. A variant found predominantly in females younger than 20 years is known as *juvenile granulosa cell tumor*. It was described by Young and coworkers and has an excellent prognosis, particularly if the tumor is confined to one ovary.

Molecular profiling investigations have found that almost all granulosa cell tumors have a *FOXL2* mutation (Shah, 2009). *FOXL2* is a member of the forkhead-winged-helix family of transcription factors and one of the earliest markers of ovarian differentiation.

The primary therapeutic approach is surgery. Because these tumors are rarely bilateral (<5%), young patients with stage IA tumors can be treated by unilateral adnexectomy. Lack and colleagues reported on 10 cases of granulosa cell tumors in premenarchal female patients, all of whom were treated by unilateral salpingo-oophorectomy. Two tumors were ruptured. All 10 of the patients were alive with no evidence of disease 2 to 33 years after therapy. Evans and associates noted a higher recurrence rate in women who were treated by unilateral salpingo-oophorectomy for stage IA cases compared with those treated with bilateral salpingo-oophorectomy. This finding has led to the recommendation that women of reproductive age treated for granulosa cell tumor by unilateral salpingo-oophorectomy have close follow-up. For women who have completed childbearing, abdominal hysterectomy and bilateral salpingo-oophorectomy are recommended. Regardless of the treatment of the pelvic organs, if a granulosa cell tumor is diagnosed on frozen-section examination, comprehensive surgical staging is recommended. Whether complete pelvic and para-aortic lymphadenectomy is indicated remains unresolved; there is some information that the incidence of lymph node metastases associated with this tumor type is low. Brown and coworkers evaluated the risk of lymph node metastasis in patients with sex cord–stromal tumors. A total of 262 patients were included in that study; of these, 178 patients were diagnosed with granulosa cell tumors. It was noted that none of the patients who underwent lymphadenectomy had evidence of lymph node metastasis.

Tumor markers may be helpful for monitoring the clinical course of granulosa cell tumors. Studies by Lappohn and colleagues have suggested that the peptide hormone inhibin is secreted by some granulosa cell tumors and serum measurements could serve as a tumor marker. In addition, serum CA-125, serum estradiol, or serum testosterone levels may occasionally serve as markers that should be followed serially.

Historically, radiotherapy, the VAC regimen (discussed earlier), or the combination of cisplatin, doxorubicin, and cyclophosphamide have been used for the treatment of metastatic granulosa cell tumors, but none of these options are currently recommended for general application. Many questions remain regarding recommendations for postoperative treatment. For patients with stage IA granulosa cell tumors, surgery alone is recommended. The recommendation for those with stage IC disease remains controversial, but consideration can be given to adjuvant therapy based on the probable increased risk of relapse. Postoperative therapy is recommended for all patients with stages II to IV disease, as well as for those patients with recurrent tumor.

Because of the rarity of granulosa cell tumors, no standard regimen exists. The GOG has reported the largest series of women treated with the BEP regimen. Homesley and associates reported on 57 eligible patients; 41 had recurrent disease and 16 had primary metastatic disease. Of these patients, 48 had granulosa cell tumors. Overall, 11 of 16 primary disease patients and 21 of 41 recurrent disease patients remained progression free at a median follow-up of 3 years. However, toxicity was fairly severe, with two bleomycin-related deaths reported.

Brown and coworkers reported the M.D. Anderson Cancer Center experience with taxane-based chemotherapy in a study of 44 patients with sex cord–stromal tumors of the ovary treated for primary metastatic or recurrent disease. The response rate for 30 patients treated with a taxane plus platinum for recurrent measurable disease was 42%. Thus the combination of paclitaxel and carboplatin is also an option for these patients. NRG Oncology (GOG) is conducting a randomized phase II study comparing BEP with the combination of paclitaxel and carboplatin for women with newly diagnosed or chemonaïve recurrent sex cord–stromal ovarian tumors. In general, however, the value of chemotherapy for ovarian sex cord-stromal tumors has been questioned (Meisel, 2015; van Meurs, 2014a). The rarity of these tumors and the indolent nature of some subtypes are features that complicate the assessment of the efficacy of chemotherapy.

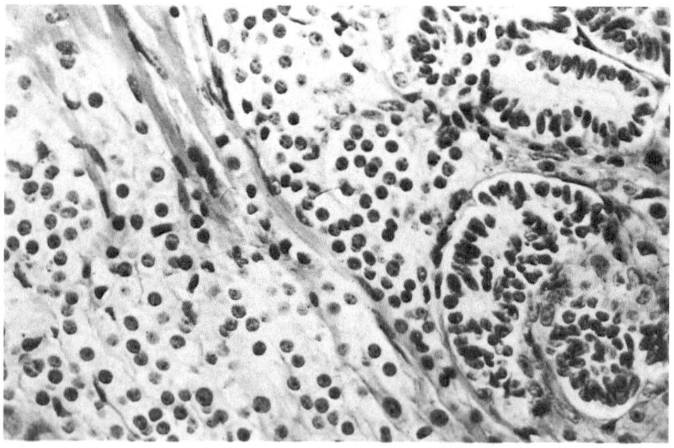

**Figure 33.24** Sertoli-Leydig cell tumor. Tubules of Sertoli cells *(right)* and Leydig cells *(left)* are shown (×250). (Courtesy of Dr. R.E. Scully.)

Hormonal therapy may also be considered for patients with metastatic granulosa cell tumors. Responses of these tumors to medroxyprogesterone acetate and gonadotropin-releasing hormone antagonists have been reported. Fishman and colleagues treated six patients with recurrent or persistent granulosa cell tumors with leuprolide acetate; of five patients with assessable disease, two had partial responses and three had stable disease. More recently, van Meurs and associates reviewed the literature and made a case for hormonal therapy as a good treatment alternative for granulosa cell tumors (van Meurs, 2014b). In addition, a phase II trial of bevacizumab in patients with recurrent sex cord-stromal tumors showed an objective response rate of 16.7% (Brown, 2014).

## *THECOMAS AND FIBROMAS*

A thecoma is a benign tumor that consists entirely of stroma (theca) cells. It predominantly occurs in women in their perimenopausal and menopausal years. These tumors can be associated with estrogen production but not as frequently as granulosa cell tumors. Removal of the tumor alone is adequate treatment for women in their reproductive years. For older women, total abdominal hysterectomy and bilateral salpingo-oophorectomy are performed. Rarely, thecomas have been reported to be malignant, and these are most likely fibrosarcomas. A closely related tumor is the fibroma, which is the most common benign solid ovarian tumor and accounts for 4% of all ovarian tumors. Like the thecoma, it can occur at any age but is more common in older women; it does not secrete hormones. These tumors contain spindle cells, and the tumors can grow to a large size. They are benign, and excision is adequate treatment. They are associated with ascites in approximately 40% of cases if the tumor is larger than 10 cm, according to Samanth and Black. They can also be responsible for hydrothorax with a benign ascites (Meigs syndrome), which regresses following tumor removal.

## *SERTOLI-LEYDIG CELL TUMORS (ANDROBLASTOMAS)*

Sertoli-Leydig cell tumors are very rare. Sertoli (sex cord) and Leydig (stromal) cells are present in varying amounts, and the tumor may consist almost entirely of Sertoli or Leydig cells (Fig. 33.24). These tumors tend to occur in young women of reproductive age and frequently are the cause of masculinization and hirsutism. The symptoms of virilization usually regress after tumor removal, but temporal hair recession and a deeper voice tend to remain. Rarely, they have also been reported to have estrogenic activity, leading to the same symptoms and signs as those of granulosa cell tumors. The tumors tend to behave as low-grade malignancies and the 5-year survival rate can vary from 70% to 90%. Poorly differentiated types tend to have a poor prognosis, as do higher-stage tumors. Young and Scully reviewed 207 cases; 75% were in those 30 years of age or younger and less than 10% were older than 50 years. One third of patients had evidence of androgen excess. Both ovaries were involved in only three cases. The well-differentiated tumors behaved clinically as benign tumors, whereas recurrence or extrauterine spread was noted occasionally in women with intermediate differentiation (11%) and frequently in those with poor differentiation (59%). Of 164 patients available for follow-up, 18% had metastasis or recurrence.

Studies have established that *DICER1* mutations are found in a relatively high percentage of patients with Sertoli-Leydig cell tumors (Heravi-Moussavi, 2012; Schultz, 2011). These mutations may be either germline or somatic and may be associated with familial pleuropulmonary blastoma.

Treatment of metastatic Sertoli-Leydig cell tumors is similar to that for granulosa cell tumors. In addition, because the prognosis for patients with stage I poorly differentiated Sertoli-Leydig cell tumors is so poor, consideration should be give to adjuvant treatment. However, it should be emphasized that there are no therapeutic data in this setting, and if treatment is recommended the optimal regimen remains unclear. The BEP regimen or the combination of paclitaxel and carboplatin may be considered for these patients.

## *OTHER SEX CORD-STROMAL TUMORS*

### *Gynandroblastomas*

Gynandroblastomas are rare sex cord–stromal tumors consisting of female (granulosa cells) and male (Sertoli cells) cell types. Theca or Leydig cells may also be present. Patients with this tumor typically present with androgenic manifestations, but stigmata associated with hyperestrogenism may also be observed. These tumors are usually unilateral and generally considered to be of low malignant potential.

### *Sex Cord Tumors with Annular Tubules*

Sex cord tumors with annular tubules are unusual. As suggested by the name, there is a prominent tubular pattern. Features of both Sertoli and granulosa cell tumors are present. Young and colleagues reviewed 74 cases; 27 were associated with mucocutaneous pigmentation and gastrointestinal tract polyposis (Peutz-Jeghers syndrome). The tumors may have estrogenic manifestations. Those associated with Peutz-Jeghers syndrome are benign and those not associated with this syndrome can be malignant. It is of interest that 4 of these 74 cases were associated with a virulent form of cervical adenocarcinoma (adenoma malignum).

### *Leydig Cell and Hilus Cell Tumors*

Leydig cell and hilus cell tumors are rare. They are composed of Leydig cells or cells of the ovarian hilus. Their cytoplasm contains hyaline bodies known as *crystalloids of Reinke*. They usually cause virilization and are benign. They tend to be small (<6 cm) and develop primarily in perimenopausal women.

## LIPID (LIPOID) TUMORS

Lipid tumors are infrequently occurring ovarian tumors composed of large cells that resemble Leydig cells, luteinized cells, or cells that arise in the adrenal cortex. Approximately 100 tumors have been reported. These tumors usually cause virilization but have also been associated with excess cortisol production. There is not enough experience with them to delineate an effective form of treatment. However, metastases of lipid cell tumors have been reported.

## METASTATIC OVARIAN TUMORS

Tumors from distant primary sites can metastasize to the ovary. Frequently, metastases are from primary tumors that originate elsewhere in the female reproductive tract, particularly from the endometrium and fallopian tube. Distant sites of origin occur most frequently from the breast and gastrointestinal tract. Metastatic tumors from the gastrointestinal tract to the ovary can be associated with sex hormone production, which usually leads to estrogenic manifestations. One special type of metastatic ovarian tumor is known as a Krukenberg tumor, which histologically consists of nests of mucin-filled signet ring cells in a cellular stroma (Fig. 33.25). The most common gastrointestinal tract origin for these tumors is the stomach, and the next frequent is the large intestine. However, breast metastases to the ovary can on occasion reveal the same histologic picture. A few cases of Krukenberg tumors have been described, with no apparent distant primary malignancy, suggesting the rare possibility of a primary ovarian tumor with the histologic features of a Krukenberg tumor.

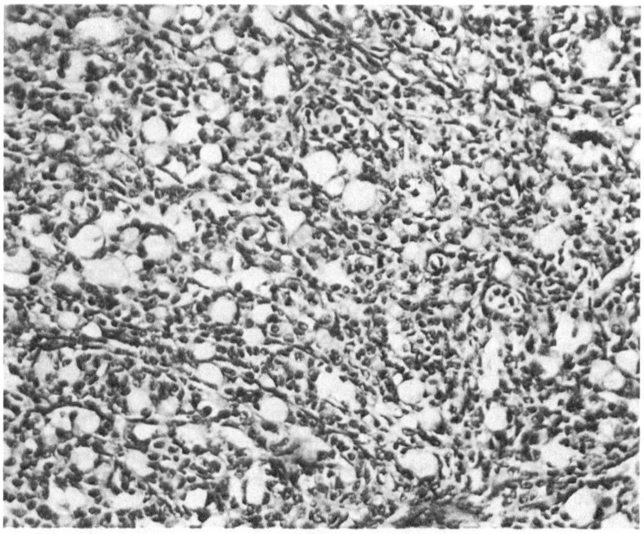

**Figure 33.25** Krukenberg's tumor (×256). Mucin-filled signet-ring cells are present. (Courtesy of Dr. R.E. Scully.)

A primary gastrointestinal tract malignancy should be considered in older women with an adnexal mass, particularly if it is bilateral and solid. A pretherapy evaluation to rule out a gastrointestinal tract or breast primary tumor is indicated. The tumor should be removed when discovered, and the primary site should be treated. The prognosis is poor; it is rare for a woman to survive for 5 years or longer after treatment.

## KEY POINTS

- Ovarian cancer is the leading cause of death from gynecologic cancer, but it occurs less frequently than endometrial cancers.
- Ovarian cancers in women older than 50 years are diagnosed at a more advanced stage, leading to a worse prognosis than for younger women.
- The risk of ovarian cancer is decreased by oral contraceptive use. Tubal ligation and hysterectomy also appear to decrease the risk.
- Most ovarian carcinomas are diagnosed in stage III or IV.
- Ovarian cancer risk rises from approximately 1.4% in general to 5% to 7% if the woman has one or two first- or second-degree relatives with ovarian cancer.
- Patients with ovarian cancer are at increased risk of developing breast cancer and endometrial cancer.
- It is important that the follow-up of ovarian cancer patients includes monitoring for breast cancer.
- Epithelial tumors are the most frequent ovarian neoplasm. They account for two thirds of all ovarian neoplasms and 85% of ovarian cancers.
- The major ovarian epithelial tumor cell types recapitulate müllerian-type epithelium (serous, endosalpinx; mucinous, endocervix; endometrioid, endometrium).
- Serous ovarian neoplasms are the most common type of epithelial tumors. Serous adenocarcinomas tend to be high grade, are the most virulent, and have the worst prognosis of epithelial adenocarcinomas. They are bilateral in 33% to 66% of cases.
- A cystic adnexal mass smaller than 8 cm in diameter in a menstruating female is most frequently functional.
- The normal postmenopausal ovary is approximately 1.5 to 2 cm in diameter.
- The risk of an ovarian tumor being malignant is approximately 33% in a woman older than 45, whereas it is less than 1 in 15 for those 20 to 45 years of age. More than 50% of ovarian cancers occur in women older than 50.
- There are three types of ovarian tumors with a serous histology: traditional serous adenocarcinomas, surface papillary tumors (ovary <4 cm), and primary peritoneal carcinomas (serous carcinomas metastatic to the ovary, with normal ovarian size).
- Most ovarian carcinomas start from small microscopic foci and spread throughout the peritoneum before becoming clinically evident (de novo origin), especially serous and poorly differentiated tumors.
- Ovarian carcinomas having a cystic origin are primary mucinous or endometrioid and are more likely to be discovered at a low stage.
- A vaginal ultrasound finding of a unilocular cyst of 5 cm or smaller in a perimenopausal woman can usually be followed without surgical intervention.

*Continued*

## KEY POINTS—cont'd

- Vaginal ultrasonography may detect early ovarian carcinoma but has not been proved to be a cost-effective screening technique.
- The primary distribution spread of epithelial carcinoma is transcoelomic to the visceral and parietal peritoneum, diaphragm, and retroperitoneal nodes.
- The risk of retroperitoneal node spread of epithelial carcinoma in apparent stage I cases is greatest for poorly differentiated tumors, for which the risk can reach 10% to 20%. The risk of retroperitoneal node spread increases in higher-stage cases.
- The prognosis of a patient with ovarian epithelial carcinoma is related primarily to tumor stage and tumor grade, and to the amount of residual tumor remaining after primary resection.
- Laparoscopic or robotic staging of early ovarian cancers appears to be feasible and comprehensive, without compromising survival
- The 5-year survival rate for patients with borderline epithelial ovarian carcinoma (grade 0) is close to 100% for stage I cases and more than 90% for all stages.
- The overall 5-year survival rate for patients with stage I ovarian carcinoma is 65%. For stage I, grade 1, the survival rate is reported to be more than 80%.
- Optimal surgical debulking (R0-microscopic residual) appears to confer a survival advantage in cases of stages III and IV ovarian carcinoma.
- Interval cytoreduction has little additional effect on overall survival if a maximal attempt is made at primary surgery.
- Neoadjuvant chemotherapy can reduce surgical morbidity; a randomized trial has indicated that this strategy may be equivalent to standard treatment for advanced-stage patients with surgery followed by chemotherapy.
- IP chemotherapy appears to benefit patients with optimal cytoreduction more than conventional IV chemotherapy, but with greater toxicity.
- CT scanning for patients with ovarian cancer can be approximately 80% to 90% effective for detecting tumor in retroperitoneal nodes, but it is much less successful in detecting intra-abdominal disease.
- Assessing the ovarian CA-125 level is useful to help monitor patients with ovarian carcinoma. Reaction to the antigen is positive in approximately 80% of cases.
- A rapid decrease in CA-125 values after treatment indicates a more favorable prognosis.
- The initial response rate of ovarian epithelial carcinomas multiagent chemotherapy is more than 90%, but the proportion of patients who survive decreases to approximately 30% in 5 years. Initial treatment is usually with platinum and taxane agents.
- Recurrent ovarian cancer is difficult to cure.
- Factors determining response to recurrent chemotherapy regimens include time to treatment progression, distribution and volume of disease, and performance status.
- Combination chemotherapy for platinum-sensitive recurrent disease improves response rates, with a less clear effect on survival.
- Secondary cytoreduction appears to benefit patients with limited recurrent disease who undergo complete tumor removal. The benefit may be most evident before chemotherapy for recurrence.
- Germ cell tumors are the second most common type of ovarian neoplasms and account for approximately 20% to 25% of all ovarian tumors.
- In women younger than 30 years, the most frequent ovarian neoplasm is a germ cell tumor; approximately one third of these germ cell tumors are malignant in those younger than 21. For women younger than 30 years, the most common ovarian neoplasm is the dermoid.
- The most common germ cell tumor is the benign cystic teratoma (dermoid). It is bilateral in 10% to 15% of the cases. Approximately 30% are calcified.
- Malignant germ cell tumors are usually unilateral except dysgerminomas, which are bilateral in approximately 10% to 15% of patients.
- Dysgerminomas are the most common malignant germ cell tumors and account for 1% to 2% of ovarian cancers.
- The prognosis for a patient with an immature teratoma is related to tumor grade and tumor stage. These tumors are the second most common type of malignant germ cell tumor.
- The 5-year survival rate of stage IA pure dysgerminoma treated by unilateral salpingo-oophorectomy is more than 90%.
- Pure dysgerminomas are radiocurable. However, multiagent chemotherapy, particularly with etoposide and platinum, with or without bleomycin, will frequently result in complete remission. Approximately two thirds of cases present as stage IA.
- Most patients with malignant ovarian germ cell tumors can be treated successfully with fertility-sparing surgery followed by BEP chemotherapy. Patients who do not require postoperative chemotherapy include those with stage IA dysgerminoma and stage IA, grade 1, immature teratoma. However, there has been a trend toward surveillance rather than chemotherapy for patients with stage I tumors of any histologic subtype.
- Multiagent chemotherapy has improved survival in patients with malignant germ cell tumors, preserving childbearing function in most cases. Standard chemotherapy consists of the BEP regimen.
- Gonadoblastomas are sex cord–stromal germ cell tumors that usually arise in dysgenetic gonads in patients with a Y chromosome; these are cured by removal.
- Granulosa cell tumors and Sertoli-Leydig tumors usually behave as low-grade malignancies, but there may be late recurrences.
- For patients with primary metastatic or recurrent sex cord–stromal tumors of the ovary, platinum-based chemotherapy is the treatment of choice. Commonly used regimens include BEP and paclitaxel-carboplatin.
- Some metastatic granulosa cell tumors may respond to hormone therapy, such as leuprolide acetate, tamoxifen, or aromatase inhibitors.
- Fibroma is the most common benign solid ovarian tumor.
- The most frequent sites of origin of tumors metastatic to the ovary are the lower reproductive tract, gastrointestinal tract, and breast.

## KEY REFERENCES


Al Rawahi T, Lopez AD, Bristow RE, et al. Surgical cytoreduction for recurrent epithelial ovarian cancer. *Cochrane Database Syst Rev.* 2013;2. CD008765.

Armstrong DK, Bundy B, Wenzel L, et al. Intraperitoneal cisplatin and paclitaxel in ovarian cancer. *N Engl J Med.* 2006;354(1):34-43.

Bell D, Berchuck A, Birrer M, et al. Integrated genomic analyses of ovarian carcinoma. *Nature.* 2011;474(7353):609-615.

Billmire DF, Cullen JW, Rescorla FJ, et al. Surveillance after initial surgery for pediatric and adolescent girls with stage I ovarian germ cell tumors: report from the Children's Oncology Group. *J Clin Oncol.* 2014;32(5):465-470.

Bookman MA, Brady MF, McGuire WP, et al. Evaluation of new platinum-based treatment regimens in advanced-stage ovarian cancer: a Phase III trial of the Gynecologic Cancer InterGroup. *J Clin Oncol.* 2009;27(9):1419-1425.

Bristow RE, Chang J, Ziogas A, et al. Impact of national cancer institute comprehensive cancer centers on ovarian cancer treatment and survival. *J Am Coll Surg.* 2015;220:940-950.

Bromley B1, Goodman H, Benacerraf BR. Comparison between sonographic morphology and Doppler waveform for the diagnosis of ovarian malignancy. *Obstet Gynecol.* 1994;83(3):434-437.

Brown J, Brady WE, Schink J, et al. Efficacy and safety of bevacizumab in recurrent sex cord-stromal ovarian tumors: results of a phase 2 trial of the Gynecologic Oncology Group. *Cancer.* 2014;120(3):344-351.

Burger RA, Brady MF, Bookman MA, et al. Incorporation of bevacizumab in the primary treatment of ovarian cancer. *N Engl J Med.* 2011;365(26):2473-2483.

Chan JK, Brady MF, Penson RT, et al. Weekly vs. every-3-week paclitaxel and carboplatin for ovarian cancer. *N Engl J Med.* 2016 Feb 25;374(8):738-748.

Chang SJ, Hodeib M, Chang J, Bristow RE. Survival impact of complete cytoreduction to no gross residual disease for advanced-stage ovarian cancer: a meta-analysis. *Gynecol Oncol.* 2013;130:493-498.

Collinson F, Qian W, Fossati R, et al. Optimal treatment of early-stage ovarian cancer. *Ann Oncol.* 2014;25:1165-1171.

Dalton HJ, Coleman RL. New biologic frontiers in ovarian cancer: olaparib and PARP inhibition. *Am J Hematology/Oncology.* 2015;11(5):5-12.

Daly MB, Dresher CW, Yates MS, et al. Salpingectomy as a means to reduce ovarian cancer risk. *Cancer Prev Res (Phila).* 2015;8(5):342-348.

du Bois A, Floquet A, Kim JW, et al. Incorporation of pazopanib in maintenance therapy of ovarian cancer. *J Clin Oncol.* 2014;32(30):3374-3382.

Farley J, Brady WE, Vathipadiekal V. A phase II trial of selumetinib (Azd6244) in women with recurrent low-grade serous carcinoma of the ovary or peritoneum. *Lancet Oncol.* 2013;14(2):134-140.

Fong PC, Boss DS, Yap TA, et al. Inhibition of poly(ADP-ribose) polymerase in tumors from BRCA mutation carriers. *N Engl J Med.* 2009;361(2):123-134.

Gallota V, Ghezzi F, Vizza E, et al. Laparoscopic staging of apparent early stage ovarian cancer: results of a large, retrospective, multi-institutional series. *Gynecol Oncol.* 2014;135:428-434.

Gershenson DM, Bodurka DC, Lu KH, et al. Impact of age and primary disease site on outcome in women with low-grade serous carcinoma of the ovary or peritoneum: results of a large single-institution registry of a rare tumor. *J Clin Oncol.* 2015;33(24):2675-2682.

Gershenson DM, Sun CC, Iyer RB, et al. Hormonal therapy for recurrent low-grade serous carcinoma of the ovary or peritoneum. *Gynecol Oncol.* 2012;125(3):661-666.

Gómez-Hidalgo NR, Martinez-Cannon BA, Nick AM, et al. Predictors of optimal cytoreduction in patients with newly diagnosed advanced-stage epithelial ovarian cancer: time to incorporate laparoscopic assessment into the standard of care. *Gynecol Oncol.* 2015;137(3):553-558.

Granberg S1, Wikland M, Jansson I. Macroscopic characterization of ovarian tumors and the relation to the histological diagnosis: criteria to be used for ultrasound evaluation. *Gynecol Oncol.* 1989;35(2):139-144.

Grisham RN, Iyer G, Sala E, et al. Bevacizumab shows activity in patients with low-grade serous ovarian and primary peritoneal cancer. *Int J Gynecol Cancer.* 2014;24(6):1010-1014.

Harter P, Gershenson D, Lhomme C, et al. Gynecologic Cancer InterGroup (GCIG) consensus review for ovarian tumors of low malignant potential (borderline ovarian tumors). *Int J Gynecol Cancer.* 2014;24(9 Suppl 3):S5-S8.

Heravi-Moussavi A, Anglesio MS, Cheng SWG, et al. Recurrent somatic DICER1 mutations in nonepithelial ovarian cancers. *N Engl J Med.* 2012;366(3):234-242.

Hoskins PJ, Le N, Gilks B, et al. Low-stage ovarian clear cell carcinoma: population-based outcomes in British Columbia, Canada, with evidence for a survival benefit as a result of irradiation. *J Clin Oncol.* 2012;30(14):1656-1662.

Jelinic P, Mueller JJ, Olvera N, et al. Recurrent SMARCA4 mutations in small cell carcinoma of the ovary. *Nat Genet.* 2014;46(5):424-426.

Katsumata N, Yasuda M, Takahashi F, et al. Dose-dense paclitaxel once a week in combination with carboplatin every 3 weeks for advanced ovarian cancer: a phase 3, open-label, randomised controlled trial. *Lancet.* 2009;374(9698):1331-1338.

Kaufman B, Shapira-Frommer R, Schmutzler RK, et al. Olaparib monotherapy in patients with advanced cancer and a germline BRCA1/2 mutation. *J Clin Oncol.* 2015;33(3):244-250.

Kehoe A, Hook J, Nankivell M, et al. Primary chemotherapy versus primary surgery for newly diagnosed advanced ovarian cancer (CHORUS): an open-label, randomised, controlled, non-inferiority trial. *Lancet.* 2015;386:249-257.

Kuo K-T, Mao T-L, Jones S, et al. Frequent activating mutations of PIK3CA in ovarian clear cell carcinoma. *Amer J Pathol.* 2009;174(5):1597-1601.

Ledermann J, Harter P, Gourley C, et al. Olaparib maintenance therapy in platinum-sensitive relapsed ovarian cancer. *N Engl J Med.* 2012;366(15):1382-1392.

Lesnock JL, Darcy KM, Tian C, et al. BRCA1 expression and improved survival in ovarian cancer patients treated with intraperitoneal cisplatin and paclitaxel: a Gynecologic Oncology Group Study. *Br J Cancer.* 2013;108(6):1231-1237.

Liu JF, Barry WT, Birrer M, et al. Combination cediranib and olaparib versus olaparib alone for women with recurrent platinum-sensitive ovarian cancer: a randomised phase 2 study. *Lancet Oncol.* 2014;15(11):1207-1214.

Longacre TA, McKenney JK, Tazelaar HD, et al. Ovarian serous tumors of low malignant potential (borderline tumors): outcome-based study of 276 patients with long-term (> or =5-year) follow-up. *Am J Surg Pathol.* 2005;29(6):707-723.

Mabuchi S, Kawase C, Altomare DA, et al. Vascular endothelial growth factor is a promising therapeutic target for the treatment of clear cell carcinoma of the ovary. *Mol Cancer Ther.* 2010;9(8):2411-2422.

Mackay HJ, Brady MF, Oza AM, et al. Prognostic relevance of uncommon ovarian histology in women with stage III/IV epithelial ovarian cancer. *Int J Gynecol Cancer.* 2010;20(6):945-952.

Meisel JL, Hyman DM, Jotwani A, et al. The role of systemic chemotherapy in the management of granulosa cell tumors. *Gynecol Oncol.* 2015;136(3):505-511.

Nick AM, Coleman RL, Ramirez PT, Sood AK. A framework for a personalized surgical approach to ovarian cancer. *Nat Rev Clin Oncol.* 2015;12:239-245.

Okamoto A, Glasspool RM, Mabuchi S, et al. Gynecologic Cancer InterGroup (GCIG) consensus review for clear cell carcinoma of the ovary. *Int J Gynecol Cancer.* 2014;24:S20-S25.

Park HJ, Kim DW, Yim GW, et al. Staging laparoscopy for the management of early-stage ovarian cancer: a metaanalysis. *Am J Obstet Gynecol.* 2013;209:58.e1-e8.

Perren TJ, Swart AM, Pfisterer J, et al. A phase 3 trial of bevacizumab in ovarian cancer. *N Engl J Med.* 2011;365(26):2484-2496.

Pujade-Lauraine E, Hilpert F, Weber B, et al. Bevacizumab combined with chemotherapy for platinum-resistant recurrent ovarian cancer: The AURELIA open-label randomized phase III trial. *J Clin Oncol.* 2014;32(13):1302-1308.

Reuter KL, Griffin T, Hunter. Comparison of abdominopelvic computed tomography results and findings at second-look laparotomy in ovarian carcinoma patients. *Cancer.* 1989;63(6):1123-1128.

Romagnolo C, Gadducci A, Sartori E, et al. Management of borderline ovarian tumors: results of an Italian multicenter study. *Gynecol Oncol.* 2006;101(2):255-260.

Sabbatini P, Harter P, Scambia G, et al. Abagovomab as maintenance therapy in patients with epithelial ovarian cancer: a phase III trial of the AGO OVAR, COGI, GINECO, and GEICO-The MIMOSA Study. *J Clin Oncol.* 2013;31(12):1554-1561.

Schultz KAP, Pacheco MC, Yang J, et al. Ovarian sex cord-stromal tumors, pleuropulmonary blastoma and DICER1 mutations: a report from the International Pleuropulmonary Blastoma Registry. *Gynecol Oncol.* 2011;122(2):246-250.

Shah SP, Köbel M, Senz J, et al. Mutation of FOXL2 in granulosa-cell tumors of the ovary. *N Engl J Med.* 2009;360(26):2719-2729.

van Meurs HS, Buist MR, Westermann AM, et al. Effectiveness of chemotherapy in measurable granulosa cell tumors. *Int J Gynecol Cancer.* 2014a;24(3):496-505.

van Meurs HS, van Lonkhuijzen LRCW, Limpens J, et al. Hormone therapy in ovarian granulosa cell tumors: a systematic review. *Gynecol Oncol.* 2014b;134(1):196-205.

Vasilev SA1, Schlaerth JB, Campeau J, et al. Serum CA 125 levels in preoperative evaluation of pelvic masses. *Obstet Gynecol.* 1988;71(5):751-756.

Vergote IB, Jimeno A, Joly F, et al. Randomized phase III study of erlotinib versus observation in patients with no evidence of disease progression after first-line platin-based chemotherapy for ovarian carcinoma: a European Organization for Research and Treatment of Cancer-Gynaecological Cancer Group, and Gynecologic Cancer Intergroup Study. *J Clin Oncol.* 2014;32(4):320-326.

Vergote I, Trope CG, Amant F, et al. Neoadjuvant chemotherapy or primary surgery in stage IIIC or IV ovarian cancer. *N Engl J Med.* 2010;363:943-953.

Wiegand KC, Shah SP, Al-Agha OM, et al. ARID1A mutations in endometriosis-associated ovarian carcinomas. *N Engl J Med.* 2010;363(16):1532-1543.

Yamashita Y, Akatsuka S, Shinjo K, Yatabe Y. Met is the most frequently amplified gene in endometriosis-associated ovarian clear cell adenocarcinoma and correlates with worsened prognosis. *PLoS One.* 2013;8(3):e57724.

Zang RY, Harter P, Chi DS, et al. Predictors of survival in patients with recurrent ovarian cancer undergoing secondary cytoreductive surgery based on the pooled analysis of an international collaborative cohort. *Br J Cancer.* 2011;105:890-896.

Suggested Readings can be found on ExpertConsult.com.

# 34

# Fallopian Tube and Peritoneal Carcinoma

*Kathleen M. Schmeler, David M. Gershenson*

Fallopian tube and peritoneal cancers have similar clinical characteristics, patterns of spread, response to treatment, and survival rates when compared with ovarian cancer. In addition, the most common histologic type for all three malignancies is high-grade serous adenocarcinoma. However, fallopian tube and peritoneal cancers have several distinct clinical and pathologic findings. This chapter reviews current information on fallopian tube and peritoneal cancer, with particular emphasis on diagnosis, natural history, and clinical management.

## CAUSES

### FALLOPIAN TUBE CANCER

Fallopian tube carcinoma is rare, accounting for approximately 0.2% of cancers among women. The estimated incidence of fallopian tube cancer in the United States is 0.41 per 100,000 women (Stewart, 2007). However, it has been suggested that many cases of ovarian carcinoma may actually arise from the epithelial lining of the fallopian tube fimbria, thereby grossly underestimating the incidence of primary fallopian tube carcinoma (Kindelberger, 2007; Carlson, 2008a).

Similar to ovarian cancer, the primary risk factor for fallopian tube cancer is an inherited mutation in the *BRCA1* and *BRCA2* tumor suppressor genes associated with hereditary breast and ovarian cancer syndromes. Women with *BRCA1* and *BRCA2* mutations have a 40% to 60% and 20% to 30% lifetime risk, respectively, for developing ovarian, fallopian tube, or peritoneal cancer (Chen, 2007; Mavaddat, 2013). Furthermore, previous reports have shown that approximately 15% to 45% of women with fallopian tube cancers have a *BRCA* mutation (Levine, 2003; Cass, 2005). Risk-reducing bilateral salpingo-oophorectomy (rrBSO) is therefore recommended for women with a *BRCA* mutation once they have completed childbearing (Kauff, 2002; Rebbeck, 2002; Rebbeck, 2009; Domchek, 2010). However, in women without a *BRCA* mutation, the cause of fallopian tube carcinoma remains unclear. Similar to ovarian cancer, associated risk factors for fallopian tube and peritoneal cancer include infertility, low parity, early menarche, and late menopause (Gates, 2010). Protective factors include oral contraceptive use, multiparity, breastfeeding, and tubal ligation (Cibula, 2011; Tsilidis, 2011).

### PERITONEAL CARCINOMA

Peritoneal carcinoma (previously known as *primary peritoneal carcinoma*) was first described in 1959 by Swerdlow (Swerdlow, 1959). It diffusely involves the peritoneal surfaces while sparing or minimally involving the ovaries and fallopian tubes. The incidence of peritoneal carcinoma in the United States has been estimated to be 0.46 per 100,000 women (Goodman, 2009); with a 1:10 ratio of peritoneal cancer to ovarian cancer cases. Peritoneal cancer is histologically indistinguishable from epithelial ovarian cancer and has similar clinical characteristics, patterns of spread, response to treatment, and survival rates (Fromm, 1990; Halperin, 2001). Risk factors for primary peritoneal carcinoma are similar to those for ovarian and fallopian tube cancer, including *BRCA* mutation and low parity. However, peritoneal cancer has also been associated with older age at diagnosis and increased rates of obesity when compared with ovarian cancer (Barda, 2004; Jordan, 2008).

The pathogenesis of peritoneal carcinoma is not well characterized. The germinal epithelium of the ovary and mesothelium of the peritoneum arise from the same embryonic origin, and it was previously suggested that primary peritoneal cancer may develop from a malignant transformation of these cells (Lauchlan, 1972). Another proposed theory was a field effect, with the coelomic epithelium lining the abdominal cavity (peritoneum) and ovaries (germinal epithelium) manifesting a common response to an oncogenic stimulus (Parmley, 1974; Truong, 1990). Molecular studies have been inconclusive in determining whether the tumor arises from the ovarian surface epithelium and spreads throughout the peritoneum or if a multifocal malignant transformation process occurs. Peritoneal carcinoma has therefore become a diagnosis of exclusion when a primary ovarian or fallopian tube carcinoma cannot be identified.

### SEROUS TUBAL INTRAEPITHELIAL CARCINOMA

There is increasing evidence that many cases of ovarian and peritoneal carcinoma may actually arise from the fallopian tube (Kindelberger, 2007; Carlson, 2008a). This hypothesis is supported by studies of women with *BRCA* mutations who have undergone risk-reducing bilateral salpingo-oophorectomy (rrBSO). Between 5% and 15% of women undergoing rrBSO have been reported to have occult serous cancers (Lu, 2000; Leeper 2002; Finch, 2006; Callahan, 2007; Reitsma, 2013). A large number of these early cancers involve the fallopian tube as invasive fallopian tube carcinoma or as a precursor lesion known as serous tubal intraepithelial carcinoma (STIC). In most cases, the tumor involves the fimbriated end of the fallopian tube. These studies have suggested that the fallopian tube may be the primary source of ovarian and peritoneal serous carcinomas in women with *BRCA* mutations. It is therefore recommended that the ovarian and fallopian tube specimens following rrBSO undergo careful examination for neoplasm. This consists of serial sectioning and extensively examining the fimbrial end of the fallopian tube using the sectioning and extensively examining the fimbriated end (SEE-FIM) protocol (Powell, 2005; Mehrad, 2010).

Studies of unselected women with ovarian and peritoneal cancer have also shown a significant number of cases to coexist with a STIC. Kindelberger and colleagues reported that a STIC was present in 47% of 43 tumors classified as primary ovarian cancers (Kindelberger, 2007). Similarly, Carlson and coworkers found a STIC present in the fallopian tube of 47% of 19 women with serous peritoneal cancers (Carlson, 2008a). In addition, *p53* mutational analyses have shown the same mutations in STIC and distant tumors, providing a genetic link between the two (Kuhn, 2012).

## CLINICAL FINDINGS

### FALLOPIAN TUBE CANCER

The mean age at diagnosis of fallopian tube carcinoma is 58 years, with a range of 26 to 85 years. However, in women with *BRCA*-associated fallopian tube carcinoma, the age at diagnosis is considerably younger. Cass and colleagues reported the median age at diagnosis to be 57 years in *BRCA* mutation carriers compared with 65 years in sporadic cases (Cass, 2005). Fallopian tube cancer is more common among white women (age-adjusted incidence rate, 0.41), compared with Black (0.27), Hispanic (0.27), and Asian and Pacific Islander women (0.25) (Stewart, 2007).

The presenting symptoms of fallopian tube carcinoma are largely related to the degree of obstruction of the distal tube. Many women are asymptomatic; however, the most commonly reported signs and symptoms include abnormal vaginal bleeding or serosanguineous vaginal discharge (35% to 60%), a palpable adnexal mass (10% to 60%), and crampy lower abdominal pain caused by tubal distention and forced peristalsis (20% to 50%). *Hydrops tubae profluens* is the term used to describe intermittent expulsion of clear or serosanguineous fluid from the vagina caused by contraction of a distended, distally occluded fallopian tube (Sinha, 1959). The discharge may be followed by shrinkage or resolution of the adnexal mass. The triad of intermittent serosanguineous discharge, colicky pain, and a mass (Latzko's triad) is considered to be pathognomonic of fallopian tube cancer but occurs in only approximately 15% of patients. In addition, approximately 10% to 40% of women with fallopian tube carcinoma have abnormal cervical cytology results, including adenocarcinoma or atypical glandular cells (AGUS). Evaluation with a cancer antigen 125 (CA-125) level and transvaginal ultrasound to rule out ovarian and fallopian tube cancer should be considered in women with these cytologic findings who have a negative workup for endocervical and endometrial carcinoma.

### PERITONEAL CANCER

Patients with peritoneal cancer tend to be older than women with ovarian or fallopian tube cancer, with the median age at diagnosis reported to range from 63 to 66 years. Similar to those with ovarian cancer, women with peritoneal cancer typically present with pain, abdominal distention, pressure, or gastrointestinal symptoms. A small proportion of patients are asymptomatic. Occasionally, primary peritoneal cancer is detected during exploratory surgery for other reasons.

## DIAGNOSIS

Similar to ovarian cancer, the diagnosis of fallopian tube or peritoneal cancer may be suspected based on imaging studies, CA-125 level, or symptoms, as well as physical examination findings. However, a definitive diagnosis is usually made at the time of surgery.

### ULTRASOUND

The classic ultrasound findings for fallopian tube cancer include a fluid-filled, tubular or ovoid mass—with internal papillary areas, mural nodules, or septations—that is separate from the uterus and ovaries. In peritoneal and fallopian tube cancers, ascites or peritoneal implants may be present. With both malignancies, the ovaries are often normal in appearance.

### OTHER IMAGING MODALITIES

Computed tomography (CT), magnetic resonance imaging (MRI), and positron emission tomography (PET) scans may provide additional information in women with suspected fallopian tube or peritoneal cancer. These studies can provide information regarding the extent of disease and sites of metastatic spread, allowing the physician to plan appropriate intervention and treatment.

### CA-125 LEVEL

The CA-125 level is elevated in more than 80% of women with fallopian tube and peritoneal cancer. CA-125 value is useful for monitoring response to treatment or evaluating a woman in whom the disease is suspected.

### STAGING

Both fallopian tube and peritoneal carcinomas are surgically staged. In 2014, the International Federation of Gynecology and Obstetrics (FIGO) revised and combined the staging for ovarian, fallopian tube and peritoneal cancer (Table 34.1) (Mutch, 2014). The updated system uses the same staging for all three entities due to the similar patterns of spread, surgical approach, treatment, and prognosis. However, the staging does require that the site of origin be noted if known (ovary, fallopian tube, peritoneum).

## PATHOLOGIC FINDINGS

### FALLOPIAN TUBE CARCINOMA

Fallopian tube carcinomas arise in either tube with similar frequency and are bilateral in 3% to 8% of cases. The fimbriated end of the fallopian tube is grossly occluded in approximately 50% of patients, resulting in a dilated lumen filled with tumor

Table 34.1 2014 FIGO Staging of Ovarian, Fallopian Tube, and Peritoneal Cancer

| Stage | Features |
|---|---|
| I | Tumor confined to ovaries or fallopian tube(s) |
| IA | Tumor limited to one ovary (capsule intact) or fallopian tube; no tumor on ovarian or fallopian tube surface; no malignant cells in the ascites or peritoneal washings |
| IB | Tumor limited to both ovaries (capsules intact) or fallopian tubes; no tumor on ovarian or fallopian tube surface; no malignant cells in the ascites or peritoneal washings |
| IC | Tumor limited to one or both ovaries or fallopian tubes, with any of the following:<br>IC1: surgical spill<br>IC2: capsule ruptured before surgery or tumor on ovarian or fallopian tube surface<br>IC3: malignant cells in the ascites or peritoneal washings |
| II | Tumor involves one or both ovaries or fallopian tubes with pelvic extension (below pelvic brim) or primary peritoneal cancer |
| IIA | Extension and/or implants on uterus and/or fallopian tubes and/or ovaries |
| IIB | Extension to other pelvic intraperitoneal tissues |
| III | Tumor involves one or both ovaries or fallopian tubes, or primary peritoneal cancer, with cytologically or histologically confirmed spread to the peritoneum outside the pelvis and/or metastasis to the retroperitoneal lymph nodes |
| IIIA1 | Positive retroperitoneal lymph nodes only (cytologically or histologically proven):<br>IIIA1(i): Metastasis up to 10 mm in greatest dimension<br>IIIA1(ii): Metastasis more than 10 mm in greatest dimension |
| IIIA2 | Microscopic extrapelvic (above the pelvic brim) peritoneal involvement with or without positive retroperitoneal lymph nodes |
| IIIB | Macroscopic peritoneal metastasis beyond the pelvis up to 2 cm in greatest dimension, with or without metastasis to the retroperitoneal lymph nodes |
| IIIC | Macroscopic peritoneal metastasis beyond the pelvis more than 2 cm in greatest dimension, with or without metastasis to the retroperitoneal lymph nodes (includes extension of tumor to capsule of liver and spleen without parenchymal involvement of either organ) |
| IV | Distant metastasis excluding peritoneal metastases |
| IVA | Pleural effusion with positive cytology |
| IVB | Parenchymal metastases and metastases to extra-abdominal organs (including inguinal lymph nodes and lymph nodes outside of the abdominal cavity) |

From Mutch DG, Prat J. 2014 FIGO staging for ovarian, fallopian tube and peritoneal cancer. *Gynecol Oncol*. 2014;133(3):401-404.

or fluid (Figs. 34.1 and 34.2). Histologically, 80% to 90% of fallopian tube carcinomas are adenocarcinomas (Figs. 34.3 and 34.4). Most of these are serous carcinomas, followed by endometrioid and clear cell adenocarcinomas. Other rare histologic subtypes include sarcomas, carcinosarcomas, germ cell tumors, and gestational trophoblastic tumors.

Similar to ovarian cancer, most patients with fallopian tube cancer have grade 2 or 3 tumors, with less than 5% being grade 1

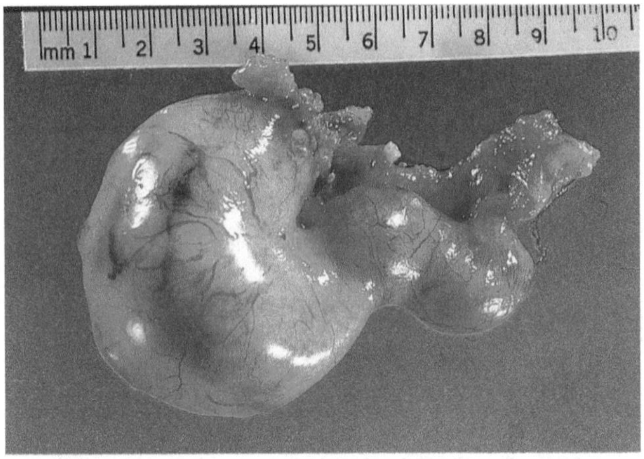

**Figure 34.1** Adenocarcinoma of the fallopian tube revealing a dilated fallopian tube with an obstructed fimbriated end. (From Voet RL. *Color Atlas of Obstetric and Gynecologic Pathology*. St. Louis: Mosby-Wolfe; 1997.)

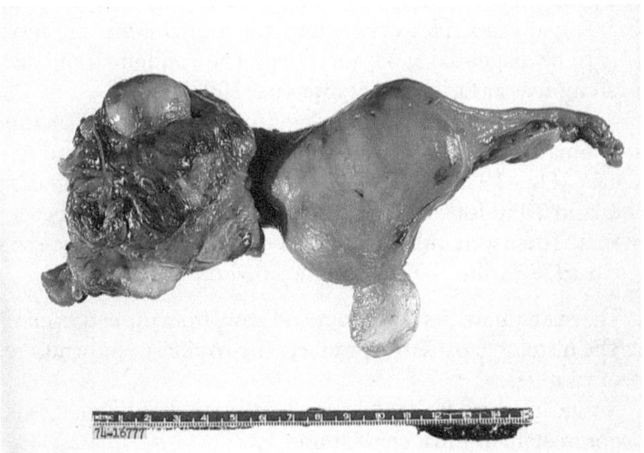

**Figure 34.2** Adenocarcinoma of the fallopian tube. (From Anderson MC, Robboy SJ, Russell P. The fallopian tube. In: Robboy SJ, Anderson MC, Russell P, eds. *Pathology of the Female Reproductive Tract*. Edinburgh: Churchill Livingstone; 2002.)

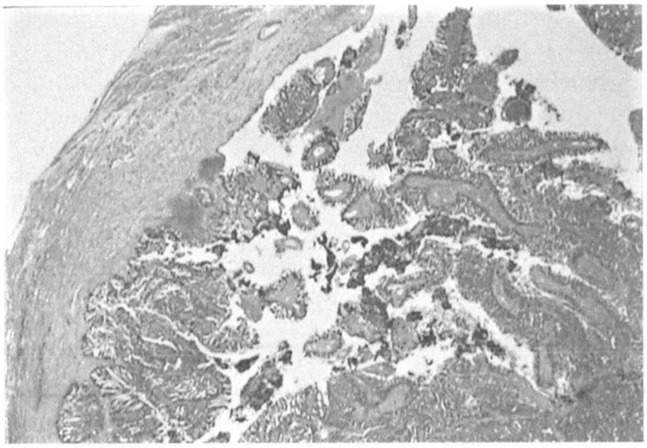

**Figure 34.3** Microscopic appearance of an adenocarcinoma of fallopian tube confined to the endosalpinx, with minimal invasion into the muscular wall. (From Voet RL. *Color Atlas of Obstetric and Gynecologic Pathology*. St. Louis: Mosby-Wolfe; 1997.)

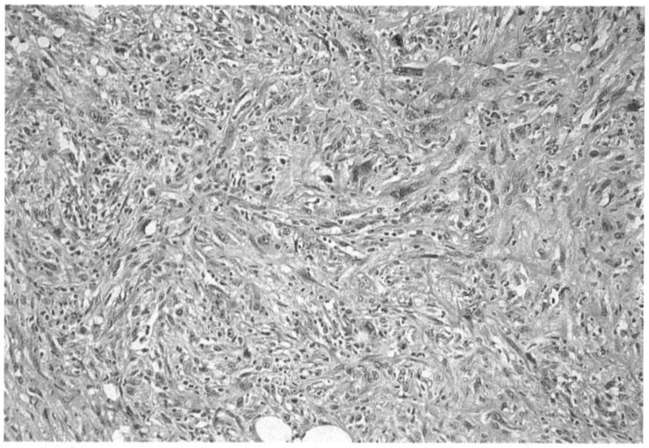

**Figure 34.4** Poorly differentiated tubal carcinoma. (From Anderson MC, Robboy SJ, Russell P. The fallopian tube. In: Robboy SJ, Anderson MC, Russell P, eds. *Pathology of the Female Reproductive Tract*. Edinburgh: Churchill Livingstone; 2002.)

tumors. Previous reports have shown stage at diagnosis to be evenly distributed among localized disease, regional spread, and distant metastases. However, serous adenocarcinomas are more likely to be diagnosed at advanced stages and endometrioid adenocarcinomas at earlier stages (Stewart, 2007).

It can be challenging to distinguish primary fallopian tube carcinoma from ovarian or peritoneal carcinomas. Hu and colleagues (Hu, 1950) initially developed pathologic diagnostic criteria in 1950 for the diagnosis of primary fallopian tube carcinoma. These were subsequently modified by Sedlis and associates in 1978 (Sedlis, 1978), and included the following:

1. The main tumor lies in the tube and arises from the endosalpinx.
2. The histologic pattern reproduces the papillary epithelium of tubal mucosa.
3. A transition can be demonstrated between the malignant and nonmalignant tubal epithelium.
4. The ovaries and uterus are normal or contain less tumor than the fallopian tube.

Data also suggest that if a STIC is present and there is minimal involvement of the ovary, a primary fallopian tube origin should be assigned. In contrast, if the majority of the tumor is in the ovary and no STIC is present, then an ovarian origin is considered (Carlson, 2008b).

The patterns of spread of fallopian tube carcinoma are largely related to the degree of obstruction of the distal tube. If the fimbriated end of the tube is obstructed by tumor, previous injury, or infection, the by-products of tumor growth, such as blood and increased serous fluid, distend the tube and are discharged intermittently through the vagina. If the distal portion of the fallopian tube is patent, the malignancy spreads more easily out the distal end of the tube, resulting in tumor seeding of the peritoneal cavity, ascites, and omental caking. Intraperitoneal spread may also occur as the tumor grows through the muscular wall of the tube. The peritoneum is therefore the most frequent site of metastatic spread. However, lymphatic spread also occurs to the pelvic and paraaortic lymph nodes. Occult lymph node metastases may be present in patients with tumor that grossly appeared to be confined to the fallopian tube.

### PERITONEAL CARCINOMA

Peritoneal carcinoma tends to involve the abdominal and pelvic surfaces diffusely. The most common histologic type is high-grade serous carcinoma, but cases of endometrioid, clear cell, mucinous, and carcinosarcoma have also been reported. Given the difficulty in distinguishing primary peritoneal carcinoma from ovarian carcinoma, the Gynecologic Oncology Group (GOG) previously developed the following pathologic criteria for the diagnosis of primary peritoneal carcinoma:

1. Both ovaries must be physiologically normal in size or enlarged by a benign process.
2. Involvement in the extraovarian sites must be greater than involvement on the surface of either ovary.
3. Microscopically, the ovarian component must be one of the following:
   - Nonexistent
   - Confined to the ovarian surface epithelium with no evidence of cortical invasion
   - Involving ovarian surface epithelium and underlying cortical stroma but with any given tumor size smaller than 5 × 5 mm
   - Tumor smaller than 5 × 5 mm within the ovarian substance, with or without surface disease
4. The histologic and cytologic characteristics of the tumor must be predominantly of the serous type that is similar or identical to ovarian serous papillary adenocarcinoma of any grade.

## TREATMENT

The treatment of fallopian tube and peritoneal carcinoma is similar to that of ovarian carcinoma. In most cases, it includes a combination of surgery and chemotherapy.

### SURGERY

Surgery for fallopian tube and primary peritoneal carcinoma generally includes collection of peritoneal washings or ascites, if present, followed by hysterectomy and bilateral salpingo-oophorectomy. A staging operation should be performed in patients with apparent early stage disease. This includes omentectomy, pelvic and paraaortic lymph node dissection, and peritoneal biopsies. In cases of advanced disease, cytoreductive surgery with removal of as much visible tumor as possible should be performed. Similar to ovarian cancer, improved survival rates are associated with optimal cytoreduction for fallopian tube and peritoneal cancers. Optimal cytoreduction may be more difficult to achieve in women with widespread peritoneal disease without a predominant pelvic or ovarian mass.

### CHEMOTHERAPY

The chemotherapeutic regimens used for fallopian tube and peritoneal cancers are the same as those used for ovarian cancer. Patients with advanced-stage disease are typically treated with a combination of carboplatin and paclitaxel. Many clinical trials for ovarian cancer include fallopian tube and peritoneal cancers because of their similar clinical and pathologic findings, as well as response to chemotherapeutic agents. Similar to ovarian cancer, neoadjuvant chemotherapy may be considered for patients with fallopian tube cancer and peritoneal cancer who have unresectable disease, a large tumor burden, or medical comorbidities precluding surgery. Given the limitations of existing imaging modalities to adequately assess the extent of disease, diagnostic laparoscopy is often used to determine resectability and decide whether primary surgery or neoadjuvant chemotherapy is more appropriate (Nick, 2015).

### *RADIATION THERAPY*

Similar to ovarian cancer, radiation therapy is not routinely recommended for fallopian tube or peritoneal cancer. Because of the tendency of these cancers to spread throughout the abdominal cavity, external beam radiation therapy cannot be administered in therapeutic doses without causing excessive side effects, thereby minimizing its usefulness.

## SURVEILLANCE

Surveillance following completion of treatment for fallopian tube and peritoneal cancer is identical to that for ovarian cancer. Follow-up visits are performed every 2 to 4 months for the first 2 years, every 3 to 6 months for the following 3 years, and then annually after 5 years. Visits include a physical examination with pelvic examination, as well as consideration of the measurement of the CA-125 level if initially elevated. Imaging studies are not routinely performed unless clinically indicated because of the woman's symptoms, physical examination findings, or increasing CA-125 level. Pap tests are generally not indicated as part of the surveillance for ovarian, fallopian tube, or peritoneal cancer.

## PROGNOSIS

As with ovarian cancer, the prognosis for patients with fallopian tube cancer is strongly related to the stage of disease. The 5-year survival rates are 81% for stage I disease, 67% for stage II disease, 41% for stage III disease, and 33% for stage IV disease (Heintz, 2006). Other prognostic factors for early stage disease include the degree of invasion of the fallopian tube wall, as well as the location of the tumor within the tube (fimbrial versus nonfimbrial). Similar to ovarian cancer, improved survival has been seen if the tumor can be completely removed at the time of surgery. In addition, patients with a *BRCA* mutation have been shown to have higher survival rates. Most studies have reported a better survival for patients with advanced-stage fallopian tube cancer compared with primary ovarian cancer. In contrast, retrospective case-control studies have shown no difference in survival rates between patients with peritoneal cancer and patients with ovarian cancer. This favorable prognosis for patients with fallopian tube cancer may be the result of a higher rate of *BRCA* mutation carriers among women with fallopian tube cancer compared with ovarian and peritoneal cancers. However, if a subset of ovarian and peritoneal carcinomas actually arises from the fallopian tube, the prognosis for women with fallopian tube, peritoneal, and ovarian cancer may actually be similar.

## *KEY POINTS*

- There is increasing evidence that many cases of ovarian and peritoneal carcinoma may actually arise from the fallopian tube, thereby underestimating the incidence of fallopian tube carcinoma.
- Fallopian tube and peritoneal cancers are similar entities to epithelial ovarian cancer.
- Fallopian tube and peritoneal cancers have similar clinical characteristics, patterns of spread, and response to treatment compared with ovarian cancer.
- The primary risk factor for fallopian tube and peritoneal cancer is an inherited mutation in the *BRCA1* or *BRCA2* tumor suppressor gene.
- The most common histologic subtype of fallopian tube and peritoneal carcinoma is high-grade serous carcinoma.
- The treatment of fallopian tube and peritoneal cancer is identical to that for ovarian cancer and typically includes a combination of surgery and chemotherapy.
- Prognosis for ovarian and peritoneal cancer is most strongly related to the stage of disease and amount of residual tumor following the initial tumor reduction surgery.
- Fallopian tube cancer has been shown to have a better prognosis compared with ovarian and peritoneal cancer, but this may be because of a higher rate of *BRCA* mutation carriers in women with fallopian tube cancer.

## KEY REFERENCES

Barda GJ, Menczer A, Chetrit F, et al. Comparison between primary peritoneal and epithelial ovarian carcinoma: a population-based study. *Am J Obstet Gynecol.* 2004;190(4):1039–1045.

Callahan MJ, Crum CP, Medeiros F, et al. Primary fallopian tube malignancies in BRCA-positive women undergoing surgery for ovarian cancer risk reduction. *J Clin Oncol.* 2007;25(25):3985–3990.

Carlson JW, Miron A, Jarboe EA, et al. Serous tubal intraepithelial carcinoma: its potential role in primary peritoneal serous carcinoma and serous cancer prevention. *J Clin Oncol.* 2008a;26(25):4160–4165.

Carlson J, Roh MH, Chang MC, et al. Recent advances in the understanding of the pathogenesis of serous carcinoma: the concept of low- and high-grade disease and the role of the fallopian tube. *Diagn Histopathol (Oxf).* 2008b;14(8):352–365.

Cass I, Holschneider C, Datta N, et al. BRCA-mutation-associated fallopian tube carcinoma: a distinct clinical phenotype? *Obstet Gynecol.* 2005;106(6):1327–1334.

Chen S, Parmigiani G. Meta-analysis of BRCA1 and BRCA2 penetrance. *J Clin Oncol.* 2007;25(11):1329–1333.

Cibula D, Widschwendter M, Majek O, et al. Tubal ligation and the risk of ovarian cancer: review and meta-analysis. *Hum Reprod Update.* 2011;17(1):55–67.

Domchek SM, Friebel TM, Singer CF, et al. Association of risk-reducing surgery in BRCA1 or BRCA2 mutation carriers with cancer risk and mortality. *JAMA.* 2010;304(9):967–975.
Finch A, Shaw P, Rosen B, et al. Clinical and pathologic findings of prophylactic salpingo-oophorectomies in 159 BRCA1 and BRCA2 carriers. *Gynecol Oncol.* 2006;100(1):58–64.
Fromm GL, Gershenson DM, Silva EG. Papillary serous carcinoma of the peritoneum. *Obstet Gynecol.* 1990;75(1):89–95.
Gates MA, Rosner BA, Hecht JL, et al. Risk factors for epithelial ovarian cancer by histologic subtype. *Am J Epidemiol.* 2010;171(1):45–53.
Goodman MT, Shvetsov YB. Rapidly increasing incidence of papillary serous carcinoma of the peritoneum in the United States: fact or artifact? *Int J Cancer.* 2009;124(9):2231–2235.
Halperin RS, Zehavi R, Langer E, et al. Primary peritoneal serous papillary carcinoma: a new epidemiologic trend? A matched-case comparison with ovarian serous papillary cancer. *Int J Gynecol Cancer.* 2001;11(5):403–408.
Heintz AP, Odicino F, Maisonneuve P, et al. Carcinoma of the fallopian tube. FIGO 26th Annual Report on the Results of Treatment in Gynecological Cancer. *Int J Gynaecol Obstet.* 2006;95(Suppl 1):S145–160.
Hu CY, Taymor ML, Hertig AT. Primary carcinoma of the fallopian tube. *Am J Obstet Gynecol.* 1950;59(1):58–67, illust.
Jordan SJ, Green AC, Whiteman DC, et al. Serous ovarian, fallopian tube and primary peritoneal cancers: a comparative epidemiological analysis. *Int J Cancer.* 2008;122(7):1598–1603.
Kauff ND, Satagopan JM, Robson ME, et al. Risk-reducing salpingo-oophorectomy in women with a BRCA1 or BRCA2 mutation. *N Engl J Med.* 2002;346(21):1609–1615.
Kindelberger DW, Lee Y, Miron A, et al. Intraepithelial carcinoma of the fimbria and pelvic serous carcinoma: Evidence for a causal relationship. *Am J Surg Pathol.* 2007;31(2):161–169.
Kuhn E, Kurman RJ, Vang R, et al. TP53 mutations in serous tubal intraepithelial carcinoma and concurrent pelvic high-grade serous carcinoma–evidence supporting the clonal relationship of the two lesions. *J Pathol.* 2012;226(3):421–426.
Lauchlan SC. The secondary Mullerian system. *Obstet Gynecol Surv.* 1972;27(3):133–146.
Leeper K, Garcia R, Swisher E, et al. Pathologic findings in prophylactic oophorectomy specimens in high-risk women. *Gynecol Oncol.* 2002;87(1):52–56.
Levine DA, Argenta PA, Yee CJ, et al. Fallopian tube and primary peritoneal carcinomas associated with BRCA mutations. *J Clin Oncol.* 2003;21(22):4222–4227.
Lu KH, Garber JE, Cramer DW, et al. Occult ovarian tumors in women with BRCA1 or BRCA2 mutations undergoing prophylactic oophorectomy. *J Clin Oncol.* 2000;18(14):2728–2732.
Mavaddat N, Peock S, Frost D, et al. Cancer risks for BRCA1 and BRCA2 mutation carriers: results from prospective analysis of EMBRACE. *J Natl Cancer Inst.* 2013;105(11):812–822.
Mehrad M, Ning G, Chen EY, et al. A pathologist's road map to benign, precancerous, and malignant intraepithelial proliferations in the fallopian tube. *Adv Anat Pathol.* 2010;17(5):293–302.
Mutch DG, Prat J. 2014 FIGO staging for ovarian, fallopian tube and peritoneal cancer. *Gynecol Oncol.* 2014;133(3):401–404.
Nick AM, Coleman RL, Ramirez PT, et al. A framework for a personalized surgical approach to ovarian cancer. *Nat Rev Clin Oncol.* 2015;12(4):239–245.
Parmley TH, Woodruff JD. The ovarian mesothelioma. *Am J Obstet Gynecol.* 1974;120(2):234–241.
Powell CB, Kenley E, Chen LM, et al. Risk-reducing salpingo-oophorectomy in BRCA mutation carriers: role of serial sectioning in the detection of occult malignancy. *J Clin Oncol.* 2005;23(1):127–132.
Rebbeck TR, Lynch HT, Neuhausen SL, et al. Prophylactic oophorectomy in carriers of BRCA1 or BRCA2 mutations. *N Engl J Med.* 2002;346(21):1616–1622.
Reitsma W, de Bock GH, Oosterwijk JC, et al. Support of the 'fallopian tube hypothesis' in a prospective series of risk-reducing salpingo-oophorectomy specimens. *Eur J Cancer.* 2013;49(1):132–141.
Sedlis A. Carcinoma of the fallopian tube. *Surg Clin North Am.* 1978;58(1):121–129.
Sinha AC. Hydrops tubae profluens as a presenting symptom in primary carcinoma of the fallopian tube: report of two cases and review of literature. *Br Med J.* 1959;2(5158):996–1001.
Stewart SL, Wike JM, Foster SL, et al. The incidence of primary fallopian tube cancer in the United States. *Gynecol Oncol.* 2007;107(3):392–397.
Swerdlow M. Mesothelioma of the pelvic peritoneum resembling papillary cystadenocarcinoma of the ovary; case report. *Am J Obstet Gynecol.* 1959;77(1):197–200.
Truong LD, Maccato ML, Awalt H, et al. Serous surface carcinoma of the peritoneum: a clinicopathologic study of 22 cases. *Hum Pathol.* 1990;21(1):99–110.
Tsilidis KK, Allen NE, Key TJ, et al. Oral contraceptive use and reproductive factors and risk of ovarian cancer in the European Prospective Investigation into Cancer and Nutrition. *Br J Cancer.* 2011;105(9):1436–1442.

# 35

# Gestational Trophoblastic Disease

## Hydatidiform Mole, Nonmetastatic and Metastatic Gestational Trophoblastic Tumor: Diagnosis and Management

*Geneviève Bouchard-Fortier, Allan Covens*

The most curable of all gynecologic malignancies, gestational trophoblastic disease (GTD), represents an oncologic success story attributable primarily to early disease recognition, effective chemotherapy regimens, and accurate assessment of disease status with sensitive β-human chorionic gonadotropin (β-hCG) assays. Understanding the disease process cannot be overstated to the general gynecologist, who is usually responsible for the initial diagnosis and management of GTD, as well as the timely referral to gynecologic oncology for further management of gestational trophoblastic neoplasia (GTN). A structured approach to diagnosis and management will result in cure for most patients, even in the setting of advanced disease, without adversely affecting future fertility.

GTD describes a heterogeneous spectrum of diseases of abnormal trophoblastic proliferation ranging from benign to malignant, with varying predilections toward local invasion and distant metastasis. Historically, the various terminology and classification systems surrounding GTD have created confusion and complicated a thorough understanding of the disease. In 2000, the International Federation of Gynecology and Obstetrics (FIGO) released a new staging for GTD incorporating the modified World Health Organization (WHO) Prognostic Scoring System, which has standardized the method for reporting the disease (FIGO, 2009). GTD is classified according to histopathologic, cytogenetic, and clinical features, using the WHO classification of GTD. The various histologic categories of GTD include benign trophoblastic lesions (placental site nodule and exaggerated placental reaction), hydatidiform mole (HM), which includes complete hydatidiform mole (CHM) and partial hydatidiform mole (PHM), and gestational trophoblastic neoplasia encompassing persistent and invasive mole, gestational choriocarcinoma, placental site trophoblastic tumor (PSTT), and epithelioid trophoblastic tumor (ETT) (Box 35.1). GTN is diagnosed based on clinical, laboratory, and histologic criteria, and those tumors have a tendency to invade and metastasize.

## HYDATIDIFORM MOLE

### *EPIDEMIOLOGY*

Marked regional variations in the incidence of GTD are seen worldwide. The precise estimate of the incidence of GTD is difficult to establish due to a number of factors such as low prevalence of the disease, inconsistencies between hospital- and population-based data, and disparity in access to centralized pathology review (Lurain, 2010). Prior estimates based on hospital data overestimated the incidence as deliveries (as opposed to pregnancies) were used in the denominator. Nonetheless, with the introduction of census data, true denominators have added validity to reported incidence rates. Similarly, improvements in central reporting through tumor registries have increased the certainty of case ascertainment. Other factors leading to the improved accuracy of incidence estimations include standardized definitions of GTD variants, improvements in cytogenetics, and recognition of rare variants, such as PSTT and ETT.

Population-based studies suggest that the incidence of HM is higher in Asia than in North America or Europe. The incidence of PHM in the United Kingdom, where all GTD cases are registered in a national database, is 3/1000 pregnancies, and that of CHM ranges from 1 to 3/1000 pregnancies (Seckl, 2010). Ethnic groups such as Native American Indians, Inuits, Hispanics, and African American continue to have an increased incidence of GTD, and this has not been explained by looking at genetic traits, cultural factors, or difference in reporting. The geographic risk association reflects the distribution of different ethnic groups with a higher incidence of HM rather than environmental or climatic factors.

### *RISK FACTORS*

#### *Age*

Pregnancy occurring at extremes of maternal age (<16 and >45 years) is a well-established risk factor for HM, with

**Box 35.1 World Health Organization Classification of Gestational Trophoblastic Disease**

**Benign Trophoblastic Lesions**
Placental site nodule
Exaggerated placental reaction

**Hydatidiform Moles**
Complete hydatidiform mole
Partial hydatidiform mole

**Gestational Trophoblastic Neoplasia**
Invasive mole
Choriocarcinoma
Placental site trophoblastic tumor
Epithelioid trophoblastic tumor

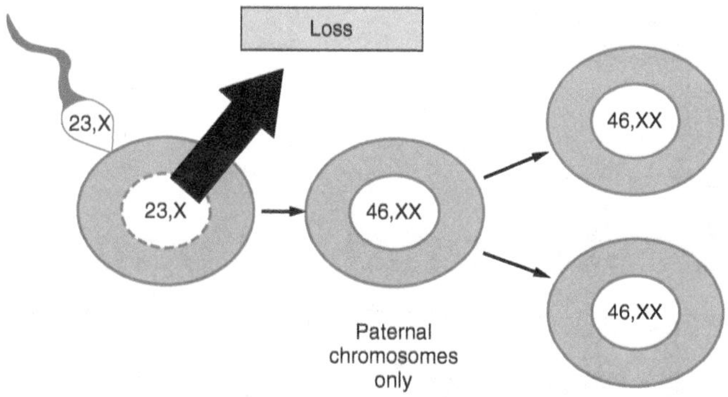


**Figure 35.1** Paternal chromosomal origin of a complete classic mode (46,XX). *Left to right:* Entry of normal sperm with haploid set of 23,X into an egg whose 23,X haploid set is lost. The egg is taken over by paternal chromosomes, which duplicate (without cell division) to reach the requisite complement of 46. Observe that almost the same result can be obtained through fertilization by two sperm gaining entry into an empty egg (dispermy). (From Szulman AE, Surti UL. The syndromes of partial and complete molar gestation. *Clin Obstet Gynecol.* 1984;27:172-180.)

incidence rates following a J-shaped distribution curve (Sebire, 2002). Risk increases after age 35, and a five- to tenfold fold increase is seen in women conceiving after age 40, rising precipitously thereafter. This increase is accounted for by abnormal gametogenesis or abnormal fertilization with advanced maternal age. However, due to the decreased fecundity in this cohort, the overall effect on incidence rates is low. Teenagers have a 1.5- to twofold increased risk of GTD. The risk between maternal age and HM is best established for CHM, with studies showing no risk or only a small increase in PHM. Studies on the impact of advancing paternal age have been inconsistent.

### *Reproductive History*

A reproductive history including HM is another risk factor, increasing the risk in future pregnancies by 5- to 40-fold that of the general population. Subsequent pregnancies have an approximate 1% risk, increasing to 25% when the number of previous HM is two or more (Seckl, 2013). The risk is not affected by changing partners. Bagshawe has shown that the risk following the first mole is 1 in 76 pregnancies, increasing to 1 in 6.5 pregnancies if more than one prior mole existed (Bagshawe, 1976). Patients with recurrent molar pregnancies are also at increased risk for the malignant sequelae of GTN. The impact of parity and prior abortion on HM risk is unclear, with studies showing conflicting results.

### *Diet*

Dietary risk factor analyses have shown conflicting results. Several case control studies have shown an increased risk of CHM with decreasing consumption of animal fat and beta-carotene (precursor to vitamin A) (Berkowitz, 1985). Vitamin A deficiency is more prevalent in countries where the incidence of GTD is higher. Dietary factors may somewhat explain geographic variations in the incidence of CHM; however, other studies detailing food intake have failed to show a decreased incidence with increasing consumption of dietary protein or fat.

### *Genetics*

A rare autosomal recessive disorder known as *familial recurrent HM* has been identified on chromosome 19q (Wang, 2009; Murdoch, 2006). Affected women have a mutation of *NLRP7* gene and, more rarely, *KHDC3L* gene, and they are predisposed to abnormal pregnancies characterized by CHM. CHM cases with familial recurrent HM are genetically normal with chromosome from each parent (diploid biparental CHM) as opposed to sporadic cases of CHM, which are androgenic in origin. Those women are unlikely going to achieve a normal pregnancy, and egg donation with in vitro fertilization is often necessary.

## *HISTOPATHOLOGY AND CYTOGENETIC FEATURES*

During early embryonic differentiation, trophoblasts are derived from the outer blastocyst layer, with three distinct trophoblasts recognized: cytotrophoblasts, syncytiotrophoblasts, and intermediate trophoblasts. Cytotrophoblasts are the trophoblastic stem cells that differentiate along a villous and extravillous pathway. The villous trophoblast forms the interface between maternal and fetal tissues (chorionic villi) and is composed of cytotrophoblasts and syncytiotrophoblasts. This layer is responsible for molecular exchange across compartments and, in the case of syncytiotrophoblasts, production of the pregnancy-associated hormones β-hCG and human placental lactogen (HPL). Along the extravillous pathway, they differentiate into intermediate trophoblasts in the placental bed at the implantation site. This layer is responsible for establishing the maternal-fetal circulation and infiltrating the decidua, myometrium, and spiral arteries.

In HM, chromosomal abnormalities differentiate the disease, with complete and partial moles having distinct chromosomal profiles (Figs. 35.1 and 35.2). CHMs are completely derived from paternal origin, with greater than 90% having a 46,XX genotype, produced by fertilization of an empty (anuclear) ovum by a single haploid (23,X) sperm, which then duplicates in the ovum. A small percentage of CHMs have a 46,XY genotype, produced by dispermy, in which a 23,X sperm and a 23,Y sperm fertilize an empty ovum. Rarely, complete moles may be triploid or aneuploid. The mechanism for production of the empty ovum is unknown.

In contrast, PHMs are derived from paternal and maternal chromosomes, resulting in a triploid genotype. A haploid ovum is fertilized by two haploid spermatozoa, with 69,XXX or 69,XXY being the most common karyotypes. Although a triploid karyotype is usually seen in PHM, not all triploid

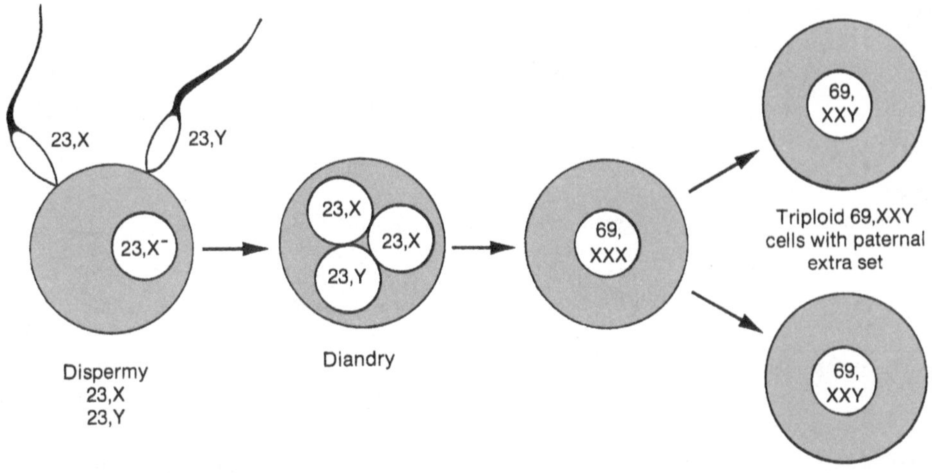


**Figure 35.2** Triploid chromosomal origin of partial mole (69,XXY dispermy). Fertilization of an egg equipped with a normal 23,X complement by two independently produced sperm (dispermy) to give a total of 69 chromosomes. Observe that triploidy can also result through fertilization by sperm carrying father's total complement of 46,XY. (From Szulman AE, Surti UL: The syndromes of partial and complete molar gestation. *Clin Obstet Gynecol* 1984;27:172-180.)

pregnancies will show histologic changes consistent with a partial mole. In addition, PHM may present in conjunction with a viable fetus, showing signs of triploidy such as multiple congenital anomalies or severe growth retardation. Conditions that may be confused pathologically with PHM include Beckwith-Wiedemann syndrome, placental angiomatous malformation, twin gestation with complete mole and an existing fetus, early complete mole, and hydropic complete mole.

The histopathologic differences between CHM and PHM are well defined. The gross appearance of CHM may be impressive, with a large volume of grapelike vesicles made up of edematous enlarged villi (Fig. 35.3). Histopathologic characteristics include the following: (1) lack of fetal or embryonic tissues, (2) hydropic (edematous) villi, (3) diffuse trophoblastic hyperplasia, (4) marked atypia of trophoblasts at the implantation site, and (5) absence of trophoblastic stromal inclusions. In comparison, the gross appearance of PHM may only show subtle abnormalities, with generally a smaller volume of hydropic villi and the possible presence of a fetus or fetal tissue. The histopathologic features are the following: (1) presence of fetal or embryonic tissues; (2) less diffuse, focal hydropic swelling of villi; (3) focal trophoblastic hyperplasia; (4) less pronounced trophoblastic atypia at the molar implantation site; and (5) presence of trophoblastic scalloping and stromal inclusions.

Differentiation between CHM and PHM in early first-trimester abortions can be difficult due to less pronounced trophoblastic proliferation and only subtle hydropic swelling of the villi. Absence of the immunohistochemical nuclear stain p57 (a paternally imprinted, maternally expressed gene) suggests paternal origin and can be used to differentiate between CHM from PHM or nonmolar pregnancies. Further studies such as flow cytometry, ploidy analysis by in situ hybridization, or molecular genotyping have been described to differentiate PHM (triploid) from CHM and nonmolar hydropic abortions. A summary of the genetic and histopathologic differences between CHM and PHM is presented in Table 35.1.

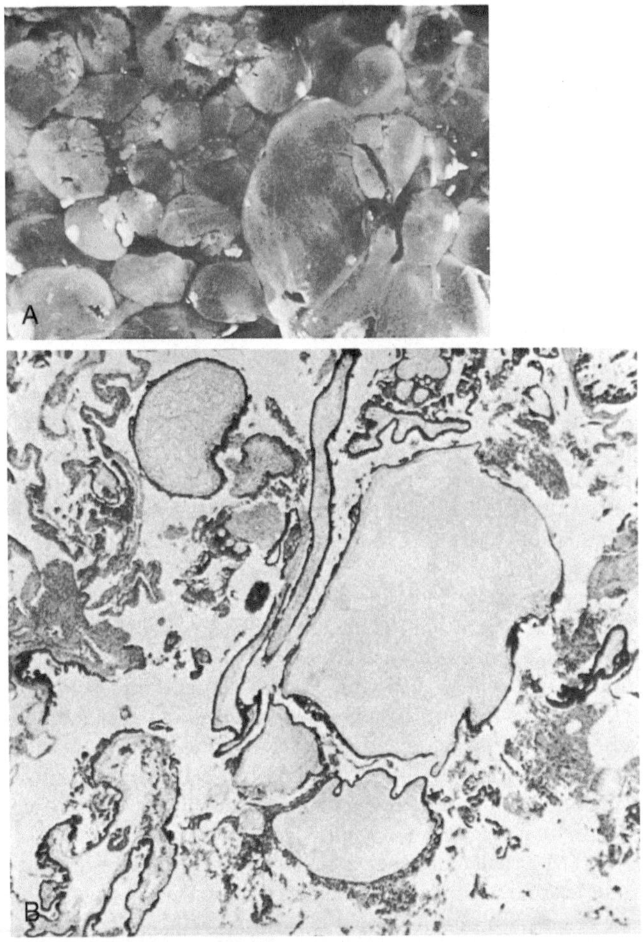


**Figure 35.3** **A,** Hydatidiform mole. A few vesicles approach 1 cm in diameter. The background is formed by smaller vesicles. **B,** Hydatidiform mole aborted by suction curettage. A large intact vesicle is near the center. Many vesicles, however, have been ruptured and have collapsed. (From Bigelow B. Gestational trophoblast disease. In: Blaustein A, ed. *Pathology of the Female Genital Tract,* 2nd ed. New York: Springer-Verlag; 1982.)

Table 35.1 Features of Complete and Partial Hydatidiform Moles

| Feature | Complete Moles | Partial Moles |
|---|---|---|
| Fetal or embryonic tissue | Absent | Present |
| Hydatidiform swelling of chronic villi | Diffuse | Focal |
| Trophoblastic hyperplasia | Diffuse | Focal |
| Trophoblastic stromal inclusions | Absent | Present |
| Genetic parentage | Paternal | Bipaternal |
| Karyotype | 46,XX; 46,XY | 69,XXY; 69,XYY |
| Persistent human chorionic gonadotropin | 20% of cases | 0.5% of cases |

From Eifel PJ, Gershenson DM, Kavanagh JJ, Silva EG. *Gynecologic Cancer.* New York: Springer-Verlag; 2006:230.

Table 35.2 Changing Clinical Presentation of Complete Hydatidiform Mole at the New England Trophoblastic Disease Center (%)

| Symptom or Sign | 1988-1993 (*N* = 74) | 1965-1975 (*N* = 306) |
|---|---|---|
| Vaginal bleeding | 84 | 97 |
| Size greater than dates | 28 | 51 |
| Anemia | 5 | 54 |
| Preeclampsia | 1.3 | 27 |
| Hyperemesis | 8 | 26 |
| Hyperthyroidism | 0 | 7 |
| Respiratory distress | 0 | 2 |
| Asymptomatic | 9 | 0 |

From Valena S-W, Bernstein M, Goldstein DP, Berkowitz R. The changing clinical presentation of complete molar pregnancy. *Obstet Gynecol.* 1995;86:775-779.

## CLINICAL FEATURES

Dramatic presentations of advanced HMs have become less common in the developed world, largely due to the increased use of ultrasonography and improvements in the sensitivity of β-hCG assays, both leading to earlier detection. The average gestational age of diagnosis of CHM today is 9.6 weeks versus 17 weeks in the 1960s. Following a delayed menses, CHM typically presents in the first trimester as vaginal bleeding, with or without the passage of molar vesicles. Other classic signs of CHM include a large-for-date uterus, absence of fetal movement, anemia secondary to occult hemorrhage, gestational hypertension before 20 weeks' gestation, presence of theca lutein cysts, hyperemesis, hyperthyroidism, and respiratory distress from trophoblastic emboli to the lungs.

When uterine enlargement is more than 14 to 16 weeks, 25% of patients will have medical complications related to the high levels of β-hCG commonly seen in CHM and proportional to the volume of trophoblastic hyperplasia. β-hCG is homologous to thyrotropin-releasing hormone, and the β-hCG isoforms seen in CHM may have a greater affinity for the thyrotropin-stimulating hormone receptor than normal β-hCG, causing excessive thyroid stimulation in some patients. Similarly, β-hCG is homologous to luteinizing hormone (LH), the purported mechanism whereby ovarian stimulation leads to the formation of theca lutein cysts in some patients.

Despite the possible medical complications associated with the disease, data from the New England Trophoblastic Disease Center have revealed the changing clinical presentation over time of HM (Table 35.2). This change in clinical presentation of HM was also recently demonstrated in China and Thailand, suggesting a worldwide phenomenon. Presently, patients are more likely to present with minimal symptoms. Nonetheless, if medical complications are present, the woman should be stabilized, followed by evacuation of the HM as soon as possible.

PHM usually presents incidentally following histopathologic examination of the products of conception from uterine evacuation of a suspected missed or therapeutic abortion. Medical complications such as gestational hypertension, hyperthyroidism, theca lutein cysts, and respiratory distress are rare with PHM. With a low clinical suspicion for PHM, underdiagnosis is a risk, reflecting the importance of a thorough histopathologic examination of curettage specimens to ensure quality care.

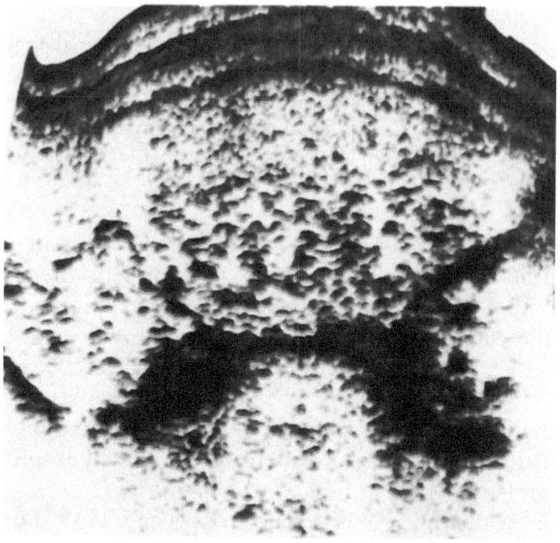

**Figure 35.4** Ultrasound scan of uterus demonstrating snowstorm appearance of hydatidiform mole.

## DIAGNOSIS

The various symptoms associated with HM such as vaginal bleeding or a uterus large for dates often prompts an ultrasound (US) examination to determine if a pregnancy is viable. US is the standard imaging modality for the diagnosis of a mole. CHMs are easier to diagnose by US than PHM, which are difficult to differentiate from incomplete or missed abortion. A CHM has the appearance on US of an echogenic endometrial mass accompanying an enlarged uterus, the so-called "snowstorm appearance" (Fig. 35.4). As the molar pregnancy progresses into the second trimester, the anechoic spaces of the molar vesicles become more evident. A transvaginal US may show the interface between molar tissue, endometrium, and dilated vesicles in the first trimester better, but it can worsen vaginal bleeding in the setting of metastatic disease to the vagina. Features suggestive of CHM on US are (1) absence of fetal or embryonic tissue, (2) absence of amniotic fluid, (3) enlarged placenta with multiple cysts, and (4) ovarian theca lutein cysts. Features suggestive of PHM on US are (1) presence of fetal or embryonic tissue, (2) presence of amniotic fluid, (3) abnormal placenta with multiple cysts or increased echogenicity of chorionic villi, (4) increased transverse diameter of gestational sac, and (5) absence of theca lutein cysts (Benson, 2000).

Although US may be the imaging modality of choice, Fowler and associates reviewed 859 cases of histologically proven HM and have shown that only 44% of cases had a pre-evacuation US suggesting HM, reinforcing the importance of histology for diagnosis (Fowler, 2006). The accuracy was higher for CHM (79%) than for PHM (29%).

### *Human Chorionic Gonadotropin*

The anterior pituitary produces a series of glycoproteins that differ only in their beta subunits, including hCG, follicle-stimulating hormone, LH, and thyroid-stimulating hormone. Outside of pregnancy, an elevated β-hCG level signifies the following: (1) GTN, (2) nongestational tumors secreting hCG, (3) false positives, and (4) menopause (secondary to LH elevation and cross reactivity of assays).

An unexpectedly elevated β-hCG level during pregnancy may suggest the diagnosis of CHM. β-hCG typically plateaus in pregnancy at approximately 10 weeks' gestation, with levels peaking at 100,000 IU/L and then falling thereafter. Genest and coworkers have shown that 46% of patients with CHM managed over a 10-year period had pretreatment β-hCG levels higher than 100,000 IU/L (Genest, 1991). Conversely, Berkowitz and colleagues have shown in one series that PHM presented with an elevated β-hCG above 100,000 IU/L in only 6% (2 of 30 cases) (Berkowitz, 1985).

## *TREATMENT*

Pre-evacuation diagnosis of HM allows for optimal treatment planning, but the diagnosis of most patients will be made histologically after surgery. If HM is suspected preoperatively, a chest x-ray should be performed, as evacuation may transiently shower the lungs with trophoblastic emboli, complicating the interpretation of a post-evacuation chest x-ray. A complete blood count, blood type with antibody screen, β-hCG level, and liver function testing should also be performed. As the RhD factor is expressed on the trophoblasts, patients who are Rh negative with an Rh positive or Rh unknown partner should be treated with Rho(D) immune globulin post-evacuation.

### *Suction Dilation and Curettage*

The preferred method of uterine evacuation of HM is suction dilation and curettage (D&C) under general anesthetic. The cervix is serially dilated and then a large suction curette is advanced just past the endocervix into the endometrial canal. After activating the suction device, a solution of crystalloid and oxytocin (20 U/L) is infused to increase uterine tone; this is continued postoperatively to reduce bleeding. A gentle sharp curettage may be performed to complete the procedure. Care must be taken during D&C to avoid perforation of the enlarged soft uterus in HM.

### *Hysterectomy*

For patients diagnosed with HM preoperatively for whom continued fertility is not an issue, hysterectomy with preservation of the adnexa is a treatment option. This decreases local (myometrial) persistence, but it does not eliminate the risk of distant metastases. For women older than 40 years with HM, hysterectomy is reasonable as the risk of developing GTN is 53% in women older than 40 and 60% in women older than 50 (Elias, 2010; Elias, 2012). Following hysterectomy, the risk of postmolar GTN is 3% to 5%, emphasizing the need for continued β-hCG monitoring.

### *Prophylactic Chemotherapy*

Following surgical evacuation, postmolar GTN, usually in the form of a locally invasive mole, occurs in 15% to 20% of CHM cases (>50% when the woman is older than 50 years) and only rarely (<5%) following PHM (Curry, 1975). Figure 35.5 outlines a treatment algorithm for GTD. If post-evacuation follow-up is anticipated to be compromised, patients with high-risk CHM may be considered for treatment with prophylactic chemotherapy. In a nonrandomized clinical trial by Uberti and associates, prophylactic single-dose actinomycin D (ActD) at the time of surgical evacuation decreased the frequency of persistent HM in high-risk patients (determined at the time of evacuation) from 34.3% to 18.4% with, at worst, mild side effects reported in 21.5% of patients treated (Uberti, 2006). In the prophylactic ActD group, the relative risk for development of postmolar GTN was 0.54, and the number needed to treat (NNT) to prevent one case of GTN was 7. A 2012 Cochrane review evaluated the evidence for the effectiveness and safety of prophylactic chemotherapy to prevent GTN after molar pregnancy (Fu, 2012). Three randomized controlled trials including 613 women diagnosed with CHM showed that prophylactic chemotherapy (ActD or methotrexate) reduces the risk of GTN by 63% (relative risk [RR] 0.37, 95% confidence interval [CI] 0.24 to 0.57). Nonetheless, the authors are reluctant to support routine use of prophylactic chemotherapy given the poor methodologic quality and small size of studies available for analysis.

Therefore prophylactic chemotherapy is an option in high-risk patients who have limited access to follow-up; however, its routine use is not recommended due to the morbidity associated with even a single dose of chemotherapy, requirement for surveillance regardless, and ultimate high cure rates eventually achieved in GTN.

#### Surveillance Following Hydatidiform Mole Evacuation

Following evacuation of a HM, surveillance with serial β-hCG serum measurements are required to ensure a timely diagnosis of postmolar malignant GTN (discussed later in the section Gestational Trophoblastic Neoplasia, Clinical Features). Within 48 hours of evacuation, a baseline β-hCG level should be obtained and repeated weekly until the level returns to normal (<5 mIU/mL). Most cases of postmolar GTN will occur within 6 months of evacuation, so monthly β-hCG monitoring is recommended following normalization for an additional 6 to 12 months.

Although the minimum conventional period for observation is 6 months, such a long duration of follow-up has been questioned, particularly for women with a narrow window of fertility due to advanced age. Wolfberg and coworkers reviewed 1029 cases of CHM and found that when a β-hCG titer of less than 5 mIU/mL was used, no cases of invasive mole were encountered in patients who reached a negative titer (Wolfberg, 2004). Thus discontinuing surveillance after two negative β-hCG titers 1 week apart may spare patients unnecessary anxiety, limit resource expenditure, and obviate the problems of noncompliance inherent with prolonged follow-up. In a separate analysis, Wolfberg and associates found the risk of GTN to be 1.1% or less when the β-hCG dropped below 50 mIU/mL at any point during their follow-up (Wolfberg, 2005).

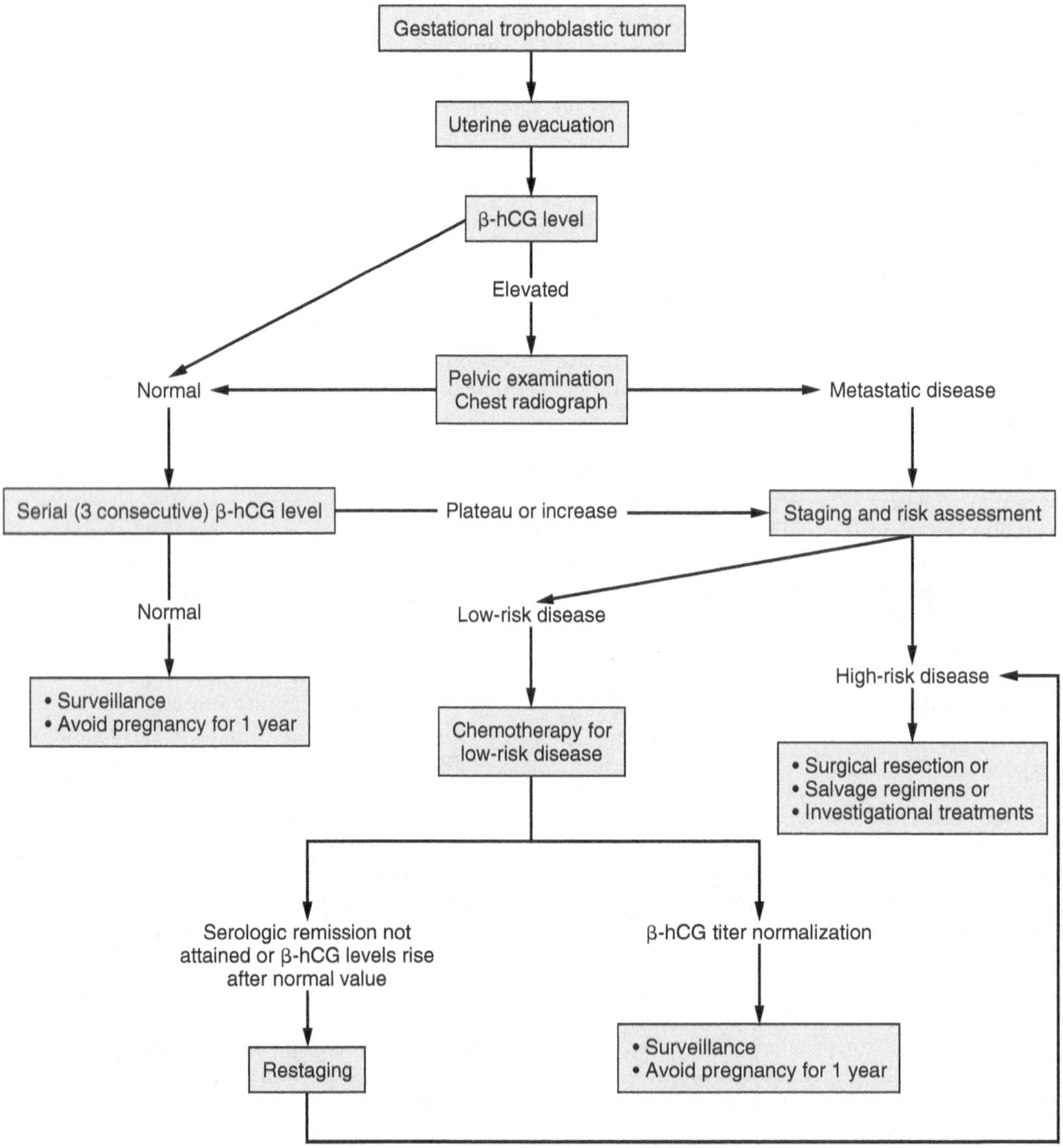


**Figure 35.5** Treatment algorithm. This is a diagnostic and therapeutic approach to gestational trophoblastic disease as practiced at the University of Texas M.D. Anderson Cancer Center. *hCG*, Human chorionic gonadotropin. (Modified from Eifel PJ, Gershenson DM, Kavanagh JJ, Silva EG. *Gynecologic Cancer*. New York: Springer-Verlag; 2006:235.)

In another analysis of 320 patients who achieved one undetectable β-hCG titer, none developed relapse as GTN. In this cohort, the mean time to achieve nondetectable β-hCG levels was 5.8 weeks. Analysis of the Hydatidiform Mole Registry in Melbourne, Australia, has revealed no cases of persistent disease in the setting of CHM if the β-hCG level normalizes within 8 weeks, and no cases with PHM if the β-hCG level normalizes (Wielsma, 2006). Schmitt and coworkers published a large prospective cohort study of more than 2000 patients with a diagnosis of HM to evaluate the risk of GTN after the β-hCG level normalizes (Schmitt, 2013). They found that the risk of GTN was 0.36% (4 of 1122) following a CHM and 0 (0 of 593) following PHM. Therefore monitoring can be stopped after normalization of β-hCG level following PHM; however, after CHM they still recommend follow-up for 6 months after normalization of β-hCG level. Despite these reports, most institutions still recommend a follow-up period of 6 months following normalization of β-hCG level.

During this period of surveillance, use of reliable contraception is strongly recommended to ensure that a rise in β-hCG level represents postmolar GTN and not a new pregnancy. One randomized controlled trial (RCT) has shown that use of the oral contraceptive pill (OCP) versus barrier methods of contraception results in 50% of the number of pregnancies during the surveillance period (Curry, 1989). In the past, there was concern that the OCP increased the risk of GTN, but two RCTs have shown no association between OCP use during postmolar surveillance and the incidence of GTN (Costa, 2006).

Prognostic factors associated with the development of GTN have been identified in various reports. The timing of molar evacuation was once felt to be a poor prognostic factor for the development of GTN; however, studies have demonstrated that advanced gestations do not contribute to an increased risk of invasive mole. As noted, advanced maternal age (>45 years) increases the risk of invasive mole, as does a history of HM. In addition, a β-hCG level higher than 100,000 IU/L on presentation may increase the risk of invasive mole. Other factors associated with persistent disease include uterine size large for date and bilateral ovarian enlargement (>8-cm theca lutein cysts) at the time of initial presentation. Ultrasound findings of uterine invasion may also be predictive of the development of GTN. In a retrospective analysis, Garavaglia and coworkers have shown that the presence of hyperechoic lesions (nodules) within the myometrium or increased signal intensity suggesting hypervascularization at baseline ultrasound was associated with an odds ratio (OR) of 17.57 for the development of GTN ($P < .001$) (Garavaglia, 2009).

**Phantom β-Human Chorionic Gonadotropin**

Persistent low levels of β-hCG must be evaluated to rule out false-positive assay results or phantom hCG, a rare finding that is secondary to heterophilic antibodies or proteolytic enzymes that mimic hCG. The diagnosis is made when a serum β-hCG is positive but a corresponding urine β-hCG samples taken at the same time tests negative. Alternatively, despite serial dilutions of serum, the test result will usually remain positive if heterophilic antibodies are the cause. Finally, physicians can test against multiple β-hCG assays, when available; heterophilic antibodies may cause a positive result in one test and a negative result in another. The reason for the negative urine β-hCG test is that heterophilic antibodies are large glycoproteins unable to cross the glomeruli and thus are not excreted in the urine. These antibodies—typically derived from exposure to mouse, rabbit, goat, or sheet antigens—are acquired through immunizations or time spent in agricultural settings, and they persist over time.

**Quiescent Gestational Trophoblastic Disease**

Following a hydatidiform mole, choriocarcinoma, or spontaneous abortion, the persistence of low levels (range, 1 to 212 IU/L) of β-hCG for 3 months or longer with no obvious increase or decrease in the β-hCG level trend along with the absence of clinical or radiologic evidence of GTN is termed *quiescent gestational trophoblastic disease*. This process is more common following a CHM but may occur after PHM, invasive mole, or choriocarcinoma and has been identified in patients treated with single-agent or multiagent chemotherapy. It is best described as a premalignant condition given that 25% of these cases progress to GTN-choriocarcinoma over a time frame ranging from 6 months to 10 years. Cole and colleagues have shown that the incorporation of hyperglycosylated hCG (hCG-H), a marker of invasive cytotrophoblasts, will detect 100% of quiescent GTD cases that require no further treatment, and 96% of self-resolving HM cases that require ongoing surveillance, differentiating these from GTN-choriocarcinoma cases that require further treatment (Cole, 2006; Cole, 2010). This methodology, however, requires validation in a prospective fashion.

## GESTATIONAL TROPHOBLASTIC NEOPLASIA

This category includes invasive mole/postmolar GTN, choriocarcinoma, placental site trophoblastic tumor (PSTT), and epithelioid trophoblastic tumor (ETT).

### CHARACTERISTICS

#### Histopathology and Cytogenetic Features

Invasive moles are HMs characterized by syncytiotrophoblast or cytotrophoblast hyperplasia, with the presence of villi. The presence of these villi extending into the myometrium constitutes invasion, and hence the name. Most of these tumors, as in HM, are diploid; anaplastic tumors are the exception.

The dominant histology in metastatic GTN is gestational choriocarcinoma following an HM or normal pregnancy and occurs in approximately 1 to 50 000 pregnancies (Smith, 2003). The characteristic appearance of choriocarcinoma is sheets of anaplastic trophoblastic tissue containing cytotrophoblast and syncytiotrophoblast cells without chorionic villi. These cells invade adjacent tissues with a propensity for vascular infiltration. Primary gonadal (nongestational) choriocarcinomas, a type of ovarian germ cell tumors, can develop without pregnancy and the estimated incidence is 1 in 369,000,000. They are highly aggressive, secrete β-hCG, and share the same histologic appearance as gestational choriocarcinoma. Nongestational choriocarcinomas are derived from differentiation of malignant germ cells into trophoblastic structures. The absence of paternal DNA within the tumor using DNA analysis differentiates nongestational choriocarcinomas from gestational choriocarcinomas. Furthermore, metastatic GTN must be distinguished from extragonadal germ cell tumors. Those rare tumors originating from midline locations such as anterior mediastinum and retroperitoneum have no primary tumor in the ovaries but do secrete β-hCG. The fluorescence in situ hybridization (FISH) method for identifying single-nucleotide variants in exons and introns on individual RNA transcripts is used to differentiate gestational choriocarcinoma from extragonadal germ cell tumors by quantifying allelic expression and differentiating maternal from paternal chromosomes.

PSTT is a rare tumor composed almost entirely of intermediate trophoblasts, lacking the syncytiotrophoblasts and cytotrophoblasts seen in other forms of GTD. PSTT has an infiltrative pattern, with nests or sheets of cells invading between myometrial cells and fibers. Compared with choriocarcinoma, PSTT is less prone to vascular invasion, necrosis, and hemorrhage. Immunohistochemical staining is positive in 50% to 100% for HPL and in less than 10% for β-hCG.

ETT was recognized by World Health Organization (WHO) tumor classification in 2003. It is considered a rare variant of PSTT and is also derived from intermediate trophoblasts. Similar to PSTT, these cells are arranged in sheets or nests and form tumor nodules in the myometrium. Immunohistochemical staining is positive for multiple markers such as cytokeratin and inhibin A.

#### Clinical Features

Symptoms associated with invasive mole include irregular vaginal bleeding, uterine subinvolution, and theca lutein cysts. Most GTN is identified in patients undergoing surveillance following evacuation of HM on the basis of β-hCG criteria, as outlined by FIGO (Box 35.2). These include a plateau in β-hCG values (remain within ±10% of the previous results) over a 3-week period (four values day 1, 7, 14, and 21), a rising β-hCG value of 10% or more over a 2-week period (three values day 1, 7, 14), persistent β-hCG detectable for more than 6 months following evacuation for HM, a histologic diagnosis of choriocarcinoma or evidence of metastases (clinically or radiologically). Following surgical evacuation of HM, β-hCG values decrease exponentially, with an expected initial steep decline followed by a slower decrease in β-hCG levels. Observing low levels of β-hCG for longer than 2 to 3 weeks is permitted, as delay will not adversely affect the woman's survival. This is particularly helpful for physicians faced with a plateau or increase of a low β-hCG level, for which continued observation as opposed to initiation of chemotherapy may be warranted.

### Locally Invasive Gestational Trophoblastic Neoplasia

With an invasive mole, myometrial invasion may involve local capillaries and veins, with persistent vaginal hemorrhage as the most commonly reported symptom. Uterine perforation with intraperitoneal hemorrhage, and infection secondary to tumor necrosis, may also occur. Although most of these tumors will regress spontaneously following evacuation, chemotherapy treatment may be initiated to prevent the serious morbidity and even mortality, which might ensue (see "Prophylactic Chemotherapy," presented earlier).

### Malignant Gestational Trophoblastic Neoplasia

Most metastatic GTN results from choriocarcinoma. Nonetheless, PSTTs are associated with metastases at the time of initial diagnosis in 40% of cases with lung metastasis being the most common site and 50% of ETT present with metastases at time of diagnosis. Both choriocarcinomas, PSTT and ETT, may follow after any pregnancy event. Metastases result from hematogenous dissemination, with almost any site possible. These tumors tend to be hemorrhagic and necrotic. Local metastases may include the vagina, with distant metastasis to the lung, brain, liver, gastrointestinal (GI) tract, and kidney having been seen. The lungs usually represent the first organ involved, followed by dissemination via the systemic circulation. Metastatic lesions are highly vascularized with thin-walled fragile vessels. Symptoms of metastatic GTN, such as hemoptysis or headache, may be related to hemorrhage at involved sites. When metastases are suspected, image-guided biopsy is contraindicated due to the potential risk of uncontrollable hemorrhage.

**Box 35.2 International Federation of Gynecology and Obstetrics (FIGO) Criteria for Diagnosis of Gestational Trophoblastic Neoplasia**

The International Federation of Gynecologists and Obstetricians (FIGO) standardized criterion for diagnosing gestational trophoblastic neoplasia GTN following a HM are the following:

1. Four β-hCG values plateauing (±10%) over a 3-week period (days 1, 7, 14, 21)
2. A rising β-hCG value of 10% or greater seen on three values measured over a 2-week period (days 1, 7, 14)
3. Persistence of detectable β-hCG for more than 6 months following evacuation of a HM
4. Histologic diagnosis of choriocarcinoma
5. Evidence of metastases (clinically or radiologically)

*β-hCG*, Beta-human chorionic gonadotropin; *GTN*, gestational trophoblaatic neoplasia; *HM*, hydatidiform mole.

## CLASSIFICATION AND STAGING

In 2000, a revised FIGO-WHO Prognostic Scoring System was adopted to attain uniformity in reporting, while indicating the extent of disease spread and risk factors important for predicting persistent disease and therefore appropriate chemotherapy treatment (Table 35.3). The stage of the disease relates to tumor spread, with stage I disease confined to the uterus, stage II disease including spread to the adnexa, vagina, and broad ligament, stage III disease defined by lung metastases, and stage IV disease including all other sites of metastases. Prognostic factors included in the WHO Prognostic Scoring System are age, antecedent pregnancy, interval months from index pregnancy, pretreatment serum β-hCG levels, largest tumor size (cm), site of metastases, number of metastases, and previous failed chemotherapy. A WHO score of 6 or lower is considered low risk and 7 or greater is considered high risk. Generally, stage relates to risk scoring, with stage I patients usually low risk and stage IV patients high risk.

The WHO Prognostic Scoring System does not apply to patients with PSTT and ETT, but they are staged using FIGO stage I to stage IV. Therefore those tumors are not described as low or high risk.

**Table 35.3** International Federation of Gynecology and Obstetrics (FIGO) 2000 Classification for Gestational Trophoblastic Neoplasia

| Staging | Features |
|---|---|
| Stage I | Disease confined to uterus |
| Stage II | GTN extends outside uterus, but limited to genital structures (adnexa, vagina, broad ligament) |
| Stage III | GTN extends to lungs, with or without known genital tract involvement |
| Stage IV | All other metastatic sites |

| | Scoring | | | |
|---|---|---|---|---|
| **Parameter** | **0** | **1** | **2** | **4** |
| Age (yr) | <40 | ≥40 | — | — |
| Antecedent pregnancy | Mole | Abortion | Term | — |
| Interval from index pregnancy (mo) | <4 | 4 to <7 | 7 to <13 | >13 |
| Pretreatment β-hCG (IU/mL) | $<10^3$ | $10^3$ to $10^4$ | $10^4$ to $10^5$ | $>10^5$ |
| Largest tumor size (cm; including uterus) | — | 3 to <5 cm | ≥5 cm | — |
| No. of metastases | — | 1 to 4 | 5 to 8 | >8 |
| Previous failed chemotherapy | — | — | Single drug | Two or more drugs |

*β-hCG*, Beta-human chorionic gonadotropin; *GTN*, gestational trophoblastic neoplasia.

## DIAGNOSIS

Diagnosis of persistent disease via β-hCG monitoring should prompt a complete history and physical examination accompanied by quantitative β-hCG, complete blood count (CBC), and renal, liver, and thyroid function testing. Invasive mole and choriocarcinoma typically have a high β-hCG level ranging from 100 to 100,000 mIU/mL, whereas PSTT and ETT produce low levels of β-hCG (usually <1000 mIU/mL). As a diagnostic imaging test, US will rule out concurrent intrauterine pregnancy and provides superior visualization to computed tomography (CT) for discerning the interface between normal myometrium and trophoblastic tissue. Examination via Doppler US may show hypervascularity and areas of tumor necrosis. In addition, US will identify patients whose large-volume uterine disease is best treated surgically. Following US of the pelvis, FIGO recommends a chest x-ray as the test of choice to rule out lung metastases. If the chest x-ray is negative, CT of the thorax may demonstrate small-volume metastases, but the importance of these findings is unclear (Ngan, 1998). In high-risk cases, up to 41% of patients will have findings identified on CT but not chest x-ray. Identification of lung metastases necessitates further imaging with CT or US of the abdomen, which includes assessment of the spleen, kidneys, GI tract, and liver. Use of intravenous (IV) contrast will identify metastases as round enhanced masses, which are usually multiple, heterogenous, and hypoechoic in appearance. An assessment of central nervous system (CNS) involvement, typically found at the gray-white matter junction, is best done with magnetic resonance imaging (MRI). MRI is also preferred for assessment of vaginal or parametrial lesions. Extrauterine diseases are more common in patients with a diagnosis of choriocarcinoma, PSTT, or ETT; therefore those patients should be screened with pelvic ultrasound, CT of the abdomen, and brain MRI. The role of $^{18}$F-fluorodeoxyglucose positron emission tomography (FDG-PET) in GTN is undefined, but its high sensitivity and specificity in other disease sites may make it a useful test when other modalities are equivocal; studies to date are limited to small case series. For asymptomatic patients with a negative chest x-ray and CT scan of thorax, further investigation is not required to assign a risk score, as high-risk sites of metastasis are rarely seen without evidence of pulmonary metastases.

## TREATMENT

### Low-Risk Gestational Trophoblastic Neoplasia

Low-risk GTN includes localized and metastatic disease and is defined by a WHO prognostic score of 6 or lower. The management of malignant GTN is based more on clinical presentation than histologic diagnosis. For these patients, clinicians can expect an excellent outcome with single-agent chemotherapy consisting of either methotrexate (MTX) or actinomycin D (ActD). While on chemotherapy, patients require monitoring of β-hCG level as well as hematologic and metabolic studies to gauge treatment toxicity. In addition, patients require reliable contraception, preferably with OCP, to prevent intercurrent pregnancies that would be adversely affected by the teratogenic chemotherapy and confuse the evaluation of β-hCG follow-up.

For patients with localized disease for whom fertility preservation is not an issue, hysterectomy may be undertaken to decrease the total number of chemotherapy cycles. Even with surgery, chemotherapy may still be required to treat occult disease. There have been no RCTs of combined hysterectomy and chemotherapy but, if chemotherapy has been given preoperatively, it should be continued postoperatively until β-hCG levels are normal.

Some authors advocate for a second D&C in the setting of localized GTN. The purpose of this debulking is to decrease the percentage of patients requiring chemotherapy and limit the treatment volume of chemotherapy in patients for whom a second curettage is not curative. Many believe that it is more than a debulking effect and may involve an inflammatory or immune response that contributes to the clinical response. There have been patients in whom no tumor was found on a second D&C, and the woman's β-hCG level has decreased. The cohort analysis by von Trommel and associates compared 85 patients who underwent a second D&C for persistent low-risk GTN with 209 patients who proceeded directly to chemotherapy (van Trommel, 2005). Of those treated surgically, 9.4% required no further treatment. The therapeutic effect of a second curettage was also seen, with a median of six cycles of chemotherapy in the control group versus five cycles in the D&C cohort ($P$ = .036). Major complications were seen in 4.8% of patients in the D&C group, with two uterine perforations seen and patients experiencing blood loss of more than 1000 mL. Schlaerth and coworkers demonstrated a similar magnitude of benefit with a second D&C, with cure achieved in 16% of patients and an 8% uterine perforation rate (Schlaerth, 1990). Preliminary results from a prospective multicenter Gynecologic Oncology Group (GOG) cohort study exploring the response of a second D&C in patients with persistent low-risk nonmetastatic GTN found that second curettage resulted in β-hCG normalization for 6 months in 38% of patients. Interestingly, four patients (6.3%) had PSTT in the second curettage pathology suggesting that some low-risk, nonmetastatic GTN may undergo malignant de-differentiation later. Second curettage may allow earlier diagnosis of those patients. An analysis of predictor of surgical failure is under way. Nonetheless, the value of repeated D&C remains controversial given chemotherapy achieves exceptional cure rate (nearly 100%) without the additional surgical risks.

A review of first-line therapies in low-risk GTN cases has identified 14 different treatment regimens. The most commonly used first-line treatments are MTX and ActD, with various dosing schedules used. MTX can be given on a 5-day schedule, once weekly, or every 2 weeks on an 8-day schedule, with or without folinic acid rescue; ActD can be given on a 5-day schedule or every 2 weeks (pulsed ActD). There is no consensus on the optimal regimen given the lack of RCTs.

Worldwide, the most common first-line agent (regimen) for low-risk disease is 8-day MTX alternating with folinic acid rescue due to factors such as established activity, low toxicity, and low cost. MTX use requires normal liver and renal function due to altered hepatic metabolism followed by renal excretion of the drug. Depending on the regimen used, patients may experience cutaneous side effects, mucositis, serositis, GI toxicities, alopecia, or hematologic suppression. ActD side effects increase with more dose-intense regimens. The 5-day regimen side effects include alopecia, nausea, and myelotoxicity. It is a vesicant, causing tissue necrosis if IV extravasation occurs. The effectiveness of pulse ActD versus the 5-day regimen appears to be equivalent, with decreased toxicity, cost, and fewer patient visits with the pulsed regimen.

The use of MTX with folinic acid rescue has been reported by McNeish and associates in a series of 485 low-risk patients (McNeish, 2002). Administration of methotrexate, 50 mg IM on days 1, 3, 5, and 7 with folinic acid, 7.5 mg PO on days 2, 4, 6, and 8 achieved a primary remission in 67% of women. The same regimen was used by Chalouhi and coworkers on 142 low-risk patients, with 78% primary remission achieved and a mean time to β-hCG level normalization of 21 weeks (Chalouhi, 2009). A 2012 Cochrane review of 5 RCTs (517 women) compared the efficacy and safety of MTX and ActD. ActD was associated with improved primary cure rate (RR 0.64, 95% CI 0.54 to 0.76), whereas MTX had more treatment failure (RR 3.81, 95% CI 1.64 to 8.86) (Alazzam, 2012). No difference in toxicity was identified; however, the results are inconclusive given the heterogeneity and the limited number of complications. This meta-analysis was criticized, as the studies included in the analysis were underpowered and compared various chemotherapy regimens that are not commonly used presently. A phase III trial (GOG-174) comparing weekly MTX to pulsed ActD in 216 patients with low-risk GTN demonstrated that biweekly ActD is superior to MTX (Osborne, 2011). Complete response was achieved in 70% of patients treated with pulsed ActD compared with 53% of those treated with weekly MTX ($P$ = .01). One criticism is that the GOG-174 used a dose of weekly MTX (30 mg/m$^2$) that is lower than what is often used in clinical practice (MTX 50 mg/m$^2$), and this may explain the difference observed. The results of a large phase III GOG RCT of pulse ActD versus multiday MTX for the treatment of low-risk GTN should help standardize the treatment of low-risk GTN worldwide.

Traditionally, chemotherapy treatment of low-risk disease has been given on a fixed time interval. The New England Trophoblastic Disease Center treats low-risk GTN on the basis of the β-hCG regression curve (Berkowitz, 1986). Following administration of single-agent MTX, further doses are withheld provided that the β-hCG level falls progressively. Their indications for further chemotherapy include the following: (1) a β-hCG plateau for 3 or more consecutive weeks and (2) failure of the β-hCG level to be 10 times smaller within 18 days of the previous chemotherapy. Chan and colleagues used a similar treatment strategy, with 45% of patients in their low-risk cohort achieving complete remission following a single dose of methotrexate (Chan, 2006).

Although most women with low-risk GTN will be cured with a first-line chemotherapy regimen, tumor resistance and relapse do occur. Resistance is defined as a 20% rise of β-hCG level over two consecutive measurements or a β-hCG level plateauing or decreasing by less than 90% over a 3-week period. In patients treated with single-agent MTX, resistance requiring a change to alternative first-line treatment can be expected in 10% to 31% of patients. The experience from the Charing Cross Hospital GTD database reveals that relapse after attaining a normal β-hCG level occurs in 3% of cases.

Box 35.3 provides an overview of management for low-risk GTN. Following normalization of the β-hCG level, chemotherapy is usually continued to reduce the risk of recurrence. The number of recommended consolidation cycles varies between one and three cycles and depends largely on the slope of the serum β-hCG regression curve. A steadily falling β-hCG level in a patient treated with single-agent chemotherapy for low-risk GTN might require only one or two consolidation cycles, whereas three cycles are likely necessary if the shape of the β-hCG regression curve is flatter with a longer time to reach β-hCG normalization. The conventional period of observation with monthly β-hCG measurements before attempting pregnancy is 12 months, as most relapses will occur during this period. Irrespective of which first-line agent is used, cure rates approaching 100% can be achieved with diligent follow-up and salvage therapy for failures. Salvage therapy with pulsed ActD after failed MTX treatment in low-risk GTN achieved complete response in 74% with a median of four cycles in a phase III trial (GOG-176) (Covens, 2006).

**Box 35.3 Management of Low-Risk Gestational Trophoblastic Neoplasia**

Following metastatic evaluation and determination of low-risk disease:

1. Initiate single-agent methotrexate or actinomycin D; consider hysterectomy, if fertility is not desired.
   - Monitor hematologic, renal, and hepatic indices before each cycle of chemotherapy.
   - Monitor β-hCG levels while on treatment.
   - If severe toxicity or resistance develops, consider switching to the alternative single agent.

   If resistance to the alternative agent develops:
2. Repeat the metastatic evaluation.
3. Consider hysterectomy if disease confined to uterus.
4. Multiagent therapy with EMA/CO (see treatment of high-risk GTN).

Modified from Soper JT, Spillman M, Sampson JH, et al. High-risk gestational trophoblastic neoplasia with brain metastases: individualized multidisciplinary therapy in the management of four patients. *Gynecol Oncol.* 2007;104(3): 691-694. Remission is defined as three consecutive weekly β-hCG values in the normal range. Following the first normal β-hCG, continue with one or two cycles of maintenance or consolidation chemotherapy. Monitor β-hCG levels for 12 months, with reliable contraception used in this time period.
*β-hCG*, Beta-human chorionic gonadotropin; *EMA/CO*, etoposide, methotrexate, actinomycin D, cyclophosphamide, vincristine; *GTN*, gestational trophoblaatic neoplasia.

### High-Risk Gestational Trophoblastic Neoplasia

In the developed world, high-risk GTN cases are uncommon. The timely involvement of specialist teams with experience in treating high-risk disease is key to achieving optimal outcomes. Patients with high-risk GTN, defined as a WHO prognostic score of 7 or higher, are at increased risk of treatment failure with single-agent therapy, hence the use of combination chemotherapy for this group (Lurain, 1995). As for low-risk disease, multiple treatment regimens exist, but no quality RCTs have been conducted comparing regimens. A 2012 Cochrane review design to determine the efficacy and safety of combination chemotherapy in treating high-risk GTN found only one RCT (42 women) comparing MAC (MTX, ActD, and chlorambucil) or the modified CHAMOCA (cyclophosphamide, hydroxyurea, ActD, MTX, doxorubicin, melphalan, and vincristine) (Deng, 2013). Direct comparison is further complicated by the various scoring systems used to classify the disease over time.

The greatest experience with combination treatment for high-risk GTN is with EMA/CO (etoposide, methotrexate, actinomycin D, cyclophosphamide, vincristine); however, no RCTs have been done (Table 35.4) (Lurain, 2006). This intensive regimen consists of etoposide, MTX, and ActD alternating with cyclophosphamide and vincristine. A number of case series, the largest from the Charing Cross group, have reported complete response rates of

Table 35.4 Chemotherapy Regimens for Intermediate- and High-Risk Gestational Trophoblastic Disease

| Drug Regimen | Administration |
|---|---|
| **EMA/CO (Preferred Regimen)—Course I (EMA)*** | |
| **Day 1** | |
| Etoposide | 100 mg/m$^2$ IV over 30 min |
| Methotrexate | 100 mg/m$^2$ IV bolus |
| Methotrexate | 200 mg/m$^2$ IV as 12-hr continuous infusion |
| Actinomycin D | 0.5 mg IV bolus |
| **Day 2** | |
| Etoposide | 100 mg/m$^2$ IV over 320 min |
| Folinic acid | 15 mg IV/IM/PO every 6 hr for four doses |
| Actinomycin D | 0.5 mg IV bolus |
| Course II (CO) | |
| **Day 8** | |
| Cyclophosphamide | 600 mg/m$^2$ IV over 30 min |
| Vincristine | 1 mg/m$^2$ IV bolus (up to 2 mg) |

Modified from Kantarjian HM, Wolf RA, Koller CA: *M.D. Anderson Manual of Medical Oncology*. New York: McGraw-Hill; 2006.
*Cytokine support may be used.
*EMA/CO*, Etoposide, methotrexate, actinomycin D, cyclophosphamide, vincristine.

78% to 80% using primary treatment with EMA/CO (Newlands, 1991). In the Charing Cross cohort, 17% developed resistance to EMA/CO, but 70% of these were salvaged with the addition of platinum-based chemotherapy. Deaths from GTN occurred in 4% of patients, and two women developed acute myeloid leukemia following treatment with EMA/CO. Side effects include universal alopecia, stomatitis, and hematologic and gastrointestinal toxicities. Patients may require granulocyte colony-stimulating factor to prevent dose delays in the setting of neutropenia. The risk of secondary malignancies (e.g., acute myeloid leukemia, colon cancer, breast cancer), mainly related to cumulative etoposide dosing, is 50% greater than expected in a standardized nontreated cohort.

Although less than 5% of patients with low-risk disease will relapse following apparent remission, this increases to 25% in patients with high-risk disease. Consolidation therapy with at least three additional course of chemotherapy after normalization of β-hCG level is warranted to reduce risk of relapse. The approach to these patients is multimodality treatment, including surgical resection of chemotherapy resistance sites and salvage second-line (or third-line) chemotherapy. EMA/EP (substituting etoposide and cisplatin for cyclophosphamide and vincristine in EMA/CO) achieves complete response in 90% of recurrent patients, but alternative regimens, including TE-TP (taxol, etoposide, *cis*-platinum), BEP (bleomycin, etoposide, cisplatin), VIP (vinblastine, ifosfamide, cisplatin), and ICE (ifosfamide, carboplatin, etoposide), have also been used, with success.

## HIGH-RISK SITES OF METASTASES

### Central Nervous System Metastases

Brain metastases portend a poor prognosis. Favorable outcomes have been achieved using a combination chemotherapy, with select craniotomy in some cases, with 30 of 39 patients in one series in remission (Newlands, 2002). Whole-brain radiotherapy to achieve hemostasis and tumor shrinkage has been used in conjunction with chemotherapy for patients with brain metastasis, but given the high success with chemotherapy and the deleterious long-term effects on overall function in survivors, including global intellectual impairment, chemotherapy is the preferred option. Many authors initiate steroid treatment and use one dose of single-agent MTX as a first regimen prior to EMA/CO to limit massive tumor necrosis, which may precipitate an intracranial bleed. Anti-epileptic drugs are not routinely given. Others have used a modified EMA/CO regimen, including intrathecal MTX in the CO portion of scheduling. However, given the vascular nature of these tumors and the fact that they are not protected by the blood-brain barrier, intrathecal chemotherapy is probably unnecessary. Nonetheless, a study of 27 GTN patients with brain metastases used EMA/CO or EMA-EP with an enhanced CNS MTX dose combined with intrathecal MTX (Savage, 2015). Eighty-five percent (23 of 27) were long-term survivors with only 4 deaths. All the patients who died had chemotherapy refractive disease.

### Pulmonary Metastases

Respiratory failure secondary to pulmonary metastases is a concern in patients with chest pain, cyanosis, anemia, and more than 50% lung field opacification. Cao and associates reported on 62 patients who underwent lobectomy for pulmonary metastasis, with complete response (CR) seen in 89% of recurrent cases, 79% of drug-resistant cases, and 100% of cases in whom a satisfactory response to chemotherapy was seen in the setting of residual pulmonary lesion (Cao, 2009). They recommended operative treatment of pulmonary metastases for recurrent drug-resistant cases in patients with adequate performance status to tolerate surgery, no evidence of active tumor elsewhere, and pulmonary metastases limited to one lung.

### Liver Metastases

Patients with liver metastases are at increased risk of hemorrhage with chemotherapy initiation. In addition to high-risk chemotherapy regimens, other treatment modalities described include radiation therapy, embolization, and surgical resection.

### Vaginal Metastases

Patients with vaginal metastases are at high risk for hemorrhage. Embolization or surgery may be used to control acute bleeding.

## TREATMENT OF PLACENTAL SITE TROPHOBLASTIC TUMOR AND EPITHELIOID TROPHOBLASTIC TUMOR

PSTTs and ETTs are rare trophoblastic tumors occurring with a frequency of less than 1%, with clinical behavior ranging from relatively benign to highly malignant. Metastases are seen in 40% to 50% of patients at the time of diagnosis and develop in a further 10% during posttreatment follow-up. Those types of GTN are relatively chemoresistant compared with invasive mole and choriocarcinoma. In a descriptive study of patients with PSTT, 61% of patients initially treated with chemotherapy had no or only incomplete response. Therefore surgery is the cornerstone for the treatment of nonmetastatic PSTT and ETT, with hysterectomy being sufficient provided that the ovaries are normal. Patients with metastatic PSTT and ETT have a poor prognosis. A retrospective study found that 83% (5/6) stage IV PSTT died despite multiagent chemotherapy (Hyman, 2013). Despite the lack of strong evidence, surgery, followed by combination chemotherapy with

EMA/EP or TP-TE (alternating weekly paclitaxel-cisplatin and paclitaxel-etoposide), has been recommended in advanced disease. The International Society for the Study of Trophoblastic Diseases (ISSTD) is currently collecting all the cases of PSTT and ETT to establish the largest international database in order to further inform on management of those rare tumors.

## SURVEILLANCE FOLLOWING GESTATIONAL TROPHOBLASTIC NEOPLASIA

After β-hCG remission is achieved for three weekly cycles, patients with high-risk GTN require repeat testing every 2 weeks for 3 weeks and then monthly for 1 year. Stage IV patients are encouraged to maintain monthly testing for 24 months. The risk of relapse beyond the first year is less than 1%. In patients who relapse, sustained remissions are achieved in more than 50%, suggesting value to prolonged β-hCG monitoring every 6 months, extending as long as 5 years.

The heterogeneity of β-hCG molecules in GTN is increased compared with that in normal gestation, with higher proportions of nicked β-hCG, β core fragment, and free β-hCG, stressing the requirement of an assay that detects both β-hCG as well as its fragments and metabolites. An assay with poor sensitivity may fail to detect low levels of β-hCG, leading to incorrect clinical decisions regarding treatment effect and disease persistence.

Reliable contraception in the post-GTN period is required, and the OCP is the method of choice. Cross-reactivity of LH, and therefore false positives, may occur with some assays. Furthermore, patients treated with multiagent chemotherapy may develop ovarian dysfunction, either transient or eventually premature ovarian failure, particularly those in their 30s or 40s. OCP has been recommended for those patients with the thought that it may suppress the production of LH from the pituitary glands and therefore protect the ovaries, although it remains controversial due to lack of high-quality studies.

## RECURRENCE

Recurrences following remission relate to the initial stage of disease. Goldstein and coworkers reported recurrences in 3% for stage I disease, 8% for stage II, 4% for stage III, and 9% for stage IV (Goldstein, 2012). The mean time from the last detectable β-hCG to recurrence was 6 months. For all stages I, II, and III patients, remissions were achieved with additional chemotherapy, whereas all stage IV patients with recurrences died of their disease. Ngan and colleagues found no relationship between time to relapse and mortality, with an overall survival of 78% in relapsed patients (Ngan, 2007). In contrast, the reported recurrence rate of PSTT and ETT are ranging from 20% to 30%, and despite salvage treatment (chemotherapy or surgery), only 30% will achieve long-term remission.

## PREGNANCY FOLLOWING GESTATIONAL TROPHOBLASTIC NEOPLASIA

Following molar pregnancy or GTN, patients can expect normal reproductive outcomes. Garner and associates summarized pregnancy outcomes following GTD from multiple centers (Garner, 2002). In a total of 2657 pregnancies following treatment for persistent GTN, 77% had live births, with 72% term deliveries, 5% preterm births, 1% stillbirths, 14% spontaneous abortions, and 2% of children born with congenital anomalies—pregnancy outcomes similar to those of the general population.

Following a molar pregnancy, however, there is an increased risk of subsequent molar pregnancy, increasing from roughly 1 to 3/1000 pregnancies to 1 to 2/100. Following two molar pregnancies, the risk in a subsequent pregnancy may be as high as 20%. Changing partners has not been proved to decrease this risk.

## PSYCHOSOCIAL CONSIDERATIONS

Diagnosis and treatment for GTN may have long-lasting psychosocial sequelae for patients, including sadness with a sense of loss following pregnancy, low self-esteem, sexual dysfunction, and anxiety about future pregnancies. Petersen and coworkers used validated questionnaires to assess quality of life in patients following treatment for molar pregnancy and found that more than 50% showed psychological symptomatology suggestive of an underlying psychiatric disorder (Petersen, 2005). They recommended a multidisciplinary approach to care to address the emotional and social aspects of a woman's well-being following treatment for GTN.

## KEY POINTS

- Persistent abnormal bleeding following normal pregnancy, abortion, or ectopic pregnancy should lead to a consideration of the diagnosis of GTD. Pulmonary nodules present on chest x-ray after a normal pregnancy suggest GTD. β-hCG levels will be elevated in these situations.
- Investigation of a young woman with metastatic disease of unknown primary should include a β-hCG level measurement.
- The risk of GTN after CHM is 15% to 20%, and it is only 1% to 5% after PHM.
- Approximately 50% of cases of GTN follow molar pregnancy, 25% follow normal pregnancy, and 25% follow abortion or ectopic pregnancy.
- The major risk factors for molar pregnancy include maternal age (>45 and <16 years) and a history of prior HM.
- The risk of HM is approximately 0.75 to 1/1000 pregnancies in North America.
- The risk of a subsequent HM after a primary mole increases 5- to 40-fold.
- Complete moles are of paternal origin, are diploid, and carry a 20% risk of GTD sequelae.
- Partial moles are of maternal and paternal origin, are triploid, and are rarely (2% to 4%) followed by GTD. They nonetheless require follow-up for potential malignant sequelae, as done for a complete mole.
- The monitoring of trophoblastic disease and its follow-up is accomplished by measurement of the β-hCG level.

## KEY POINTS—cont'd

- The diagnosis of a molar pregnancy can be established with ultrasonography and may coexist with a normal pregnancy.
- Hydatidiform moles are effectively and safely evacuated from the uterus using suction D&C.
- Medical complications of HM are rare but may include anemia, gestational hypertension before 20 weeks, hyperthyroidism, hyperemesis gravidarum, cardiac failure, and, rarely, pulmonary insufficiency.
- Patients are classified into low- or high-risk categories. Low-risk patients are treated with single-agent methotrexate or actinomycin D; high-risk patients receive combination chemotherapy, usually with EMA/CO.
- The cure rate for low-risk patients approaches 100%.
- Patients with high-risk metastatic GTN are successfully treated with chemotherapy in more than 70% of cases.
- Surgery plays an important role in the treatment of PSTT and ETT. They are both relatively chemoresistant.
- Patients treated for GTD should not become pregnant for approximately 6 months after treatment to allow accurate follow-up of β-hCG levels.
- Fertility rates and pregnancy outcomes are similar in patients treated for GTD compared with those in the general population.
- Patients treated with the EMA/CO regimen have an increased rate of secondary malignancies, particularly hematologic malignancies.

## KEY REFERENCES


Alazzam M, Tidy J, Hancock BW, et al. First-line chemotherapy in low-risk gestational trophoblastic neoplasia. *Cochrane Database Syst Rev*. 2012;7:CD007102.

Bagshawe KD. Risk and prognostic factors in trophoblastic neoplasia. *Cancer*. 1976;38:1373–1385.

Benson CB, Genest DR, Bernstein MR, et al. Sonographic appearance of first trimester complete hydatidiform moles. *Ultrasound Obstet Gynecol*. 2000;16(2):188–191.

Berkowitz RS, Cramer DW, Bernstein MR, et al. Risk factors for complete molar pregnancy from a case-control study. *American journal of obstetrics and gynecology*. 1985;152(8):1016–1020.

Berkowitz RS, Goldstein DP, Bernstein MR. Natural history of partial molar pregnancy. *Obstet Gynecol*. 1985;66:677–681.

Berkowitz RS, Goldstein DP, Bernstein MR. Ten year's experience with methotrexate and folinic acid as primary therapy for gestational trophoblastic disease. *Gynecol Oncol*. 1986;23:111–118.

Cao Y, Xiang Y, Feng F, et al. Surgical resection in the management of pulmonary metastatic disease of gestational trophoblastic neoplasia. *Int J Gynecol Cancer*. 2009;19:798–801.

Chalouhi GE, Golfier F, Soignon P, et al. Methotrexate for 2000 FIGO low-risk gestational trophoblastic neoplasia patients: efficacy and toxicity. *Am J Obstet Gynecol*. 2009;200:643.e1–643.e6.

Chan KK, Huang Y, Tam KF, et al. Single-dose methotrexate regimen in the treatment of low-risk gestational trophoblastic neoplasia. *Am J Obstet Gynecol*. 2006;195:1282–1286.

Cole LA, Butler SA, Khanlian SA, et al. Gestational trophoblastic diseases: 2. Hyperglycosylated hCG as a reliable marker of active neoplasia. *Gynecol Oncol*. 2006;102:151–159.

Cole LA, Muller CY. Hyperglycosylated hCG in the management of quiescent and chemorefractory gestational trophoblastic diseases. *Gynecol Oncol*. 2010;116:3–9.

Costa HL, Doyle P. Influence of oral contraceptives in the development of post-molar trophoblastic neoplasia—a systematic review. *Gynecol Oncol*. 2006;100:579–585.

Covens A, Filiaci VL, Burger RA, et al. Phase II trial of pulse dactinomycin as salvage therapy for failed low-risk gestational trophoblastic neoplasia: a Gynecologic Oncology Group study. *Cancer*. 2006;107(6):1280–1286.

Curry SL, Hammond CB, Tyrey L, et al. Hydatidiform mole: diagnosis, management, and long-term followup of 347 patients. *Obstet Gynecol*. 1975;45:1–8.

Curry SL, Schlaerth JB, Kohorn EI, et al. Hormonal contraception and trophoblastic sequelae after hydatidiform mole (a Gynecologic Oncology Group Study). *Am J Obstet Gynecol*. 1989;160:805–809.

Deng L, Zhang J, Wu T, Lawrie TA. Combination chemotherapy for primary treatment of high-risk gestational trophoblastic tumour. *Cochrane Database Syst Rev*. 2013;1:CD005196.

Elias KM, Goldstein DP, Berkowitz RS. Complete hydatidiform mole in women older than age 50. *J Reprod Med*. 2010;55(5-6):208–212.

Elias KM, Shoni M, Bernstein M, et al. Complete hydatidiform mole in women aged 40 to 49 years. *J Reprod Med*. 2012;57(5-6):254–258.

FIGO Committee on Gynecologic Oncology. FIGO staging for uterine sarcomas. *Int J Gynecol Obstet*. 2009;104(3):179.

Fowler DJ, Lindsay I, Seckl MJ, Sebire NJ. Routine pre-evacuation ultrasound diagnosis of hydatidiform mole: experience of more than 1000 cases from a regional referral center. *Ultrasound Obstet Gynecol*. 2006;27(1):56–60.

Fu J, Fang F, Xie L, et al. Prophylactic chemotherapy for hydatidiform mole to prevent gestational trophoblastic neoplasia. *Cochrane Database Syst Rev*. 2012;10:CD007289.

Garavaglia E, Gentile C, Cavoretto P, et al. Ultrasound imaging after evacuation as an adjunct to beta-hCG monitoring in posthydatidiform molar gestational trophoblastic neoplasia. *Am J Obstet Gynecol*. 2009;200:417.e1–417.e5.

Garner EI, Lipson E, Bernstein MR, et al. Subsequent pregnancy experience in patients with molar pregnancy and gestational trophoblastic tumor. *J Reprod Med*. 2002;47:380–386.

Genest DR, Laborde O, Berkowitz RS, et al. A clinicopathologic study of 153 cases of complete hydatidiform mole (1980-1990): histologic grade lacks prognostic significance. *Obstet Gynecol*. 1991;78(Pt 1):402–409.

Goldstein DP, Berkowitz RS. Current management of gestational trophoblastic neoplasia. *Hematol Oncol Clin North Am*. 2012;26(1):111–131.

Hyman DM, Bakios L, Gualtiere G, et al. Placental site trophoblastic tumor: analysis of presentation, treatment, and outcome. *Gynecol Oncol*. 2013;129(1):58–62.

Lurain JR. Gestational trophoblastic disease I: epidemiology, pathology, clinical presentation and diagnosis of gestational trophoblastic disease, and management of hydatidiform mole. *Am J Obstet Gynecol*. 2010;203(6):531–539.

Lurain JR, Elfstrand EP. Single-agent methotrexate chemotherapy for the treatment of nonmetastatic gestational trophoblastic tumors. *Am J Obstet Gynecol*. 1995;172(Pt 1):574–579.

Lurain JR, Singh DK, Schink JC. Role of surgery in the management of high-risk gestational trophoblastic neoplasia. *J Reprod Med*. 2006;51:773–776.

McNeish IA, Strickland S, Holden L, et al. Low-risk persistent gestational trophoblastic disease: outcome after initial treatment with low-dose methotrexate and folinic acid from 1992 to 2000. *J Clin Oncol*. 2002;20:1838–1844.

Murdoch S, Djuric U, Mazhar B, et al. Mutations in NALP7 cause recurrent hydatidiform moles and reproductive wastage in humans. *Nat Genet*. 2006;38(3):300–302.

Newlands ES, Bagshawe KD, Begent RH, et al. Results with the EMA/CO (etoposide, methotrexate, actinomycin D, cyclophosphamide, vincristine) regimen in high risk gestational trophoblastic tumours, 1979 to 1989. *Br J Obstet Gynaecol*. 1991;98:550–557.

Newlands ES, Holden L, Seckl MJ, et al. Management of brain metastases in patients with high-risk gestational trophoblastic tumors. *J Reprod Med*. 2002;47:465–471.

Ngan HY, Chan FL, Au VW, et al. Clinical outcome of micrometastasis in the lung in stage IA persistent gestational trophoblastic disease. *Gynecol Oncol*. 1998;70:192–194.

Ngan S, Seckl MJ. Gestational trophoblastic neoplasia management: an update. *Curr Opin Oncol*. 2007;19:486–491.

Osborne RJ, Filiaci V, Schink JC, et al. Phase III trial of weekly methotrexate or pulsed dactinomycin for low-risk gestational trophoblastic neoplasia: a gynecologic oncology group study. *J Clin Oncol*. 2011;29(7):825–831.

Petersen RW, Ung K, Holland C, et al. The impact of molar pregnancy on psychological symptomatology, sexual function, and quality of life. *Gynecol Oncol.* 2005;97:535–542.

Savage P, Kelpanides I, Tuthill M, et al. Brain metastases in gestational trophoblast neoplasia: an update on incidence, management and outcome. *Gynecol Oncol.* 2015;137(1):73–76.

Schlaerth JB, Morrow CP, Rodriguez M. Diagnostic and therapeutic curettage in gestational trophoblastic disease. *Am J Obstet Gynecol.* 1990;162:1465–1470.

Schmitt C, Doret M, Massardier J, et al. Risk of gestational trophoblastic neoplasia after hCG normalisation according to hydatidiform mole type. *Gynecol Oncol.* 2013;130(1):86–89.

Sebire NJ, Foskett M, Fisher RA, et al. Risk of partial and complete hydatidiform molar pregnancy in relation to maternal age. *BJOG.* 2002;109:99–102.

Seckl MJ, Sebire NJ, Berkowitz RS. Gestational trophoblastic disease. *Lancet.* 2010;376(9742):717–729.

Seckl MJ, Sebire NJ, Fisher RA, et al. Gestational trophoblastic disease: ESMO Clinical Practice Guidelines for diagnosis, treatment and follow-up. *Ann Oncol.* 2013;24(Suppl 6):vi39–50.

Smith HO. Gestational trophoblastic disease epidemiology and trends. *Clin Obstet Gynecol.* 2003;46:541–556.

Uberti EM, Diestel MC, Guiaes FE, et al. Single-dose actinomycin D: efficacy in the prophylaxis of postmolar gestational trophoblastic neoplasia in adolescents with high-risk hydatidiform mole. *Gynecol Oncol.* 2006;102:325–332.

van Trommel NE, Massuger LF, Verheijen RH, et al. The curative effect of a second curettage in persistent trophoblastic disease: a retrospective cohort survey. *Gynecol Oncol.* 2005;99:6–13.

Wang CM, Dixon PH, Decordova S, et al. Identification of 13 novel NLRP7 mutations in 20 families with recurrent hydatidiform mole; missense mutations cluster in the leucine-rich region. *J Med Genet.* 2009;46(8):569–575.

Wielsma S, Kerkmeijer L, Bekkers R, et al. Persistent trophoblast disease following partial molar pregnancy. *Aust N Z J Obstet Gynaecol.* 2006;46:119–123.

Wolfberg AJ, Berkowitz RS, Goldstein DP, et al. Postevacuation hCG levels and risk of gestational trophoblastic neoplasia in women with complete molar pregnancy. *Obstet Gynecol.* 2005;106:548–552.

Wolfberg AJ, Feltmate C, Goldstein DP, et al. Low risk of relapse after achieving undetectable HCG levels in women with complete molar pregnancy. *Obstet Gynecol.* 2004;104:551–554.

# 36

# Molecular Oncology in Gynecologic Cancer

## Immunologic Response, Cytokines, Oncogenes, and Tumor Suppressor Genes

*Premal H. Thaker, Anil K. Sood*

Cancer develops because of the accumulation of successive and multiple molecular lesions that result in an altered cellular phenotype that is self-sufficient in growth signaling, is insensitive to antigrowth signals and capable of tissue invasion and metastasis, and has limitless replicative potential, sustained angiogenesis, and evading apoptosis (Hanahan, 2000). These molecular changes can include overexpression, amplification, or mutation of oncogenes; the failure of tumor suppressor gene function because of a mutation, deletion, or viral infection; and the inappropriate expression of cytokines, growth factors, or cellular receptors. Also, natural or induced immune responses may play a role in the modulation of cancer growth because immune cells such as tumor-associated macrophages may actually cause tumors to grow. Based on a growing understanding of the immune response, biologic pathways, and cancer development, new immunotherapy and targeted therapies to gynecologic malignancies are being developed and are reviewed and summarized in this chapter.

## IMMUNOLOGIC RESPONSE

The immune system has adapted to fight off bacterial or viral infections, but it also plays a role in the surveillance and control of cancer cell growth. The immune system has two types of responses, innate and adaptive. Innate responses are non–antigen-specific and rapid and do not increase with repetitive exposure to a given antigen. Components of the innate immune system include physical barriers such as epithelial surfaces, macrophages, natural killer (NK) cells, neutrophils, dendritic cells, and components of the complement system. Dendritic cells and macrophages are phagocytic cells that act as antigen-presenting cells (APCs). Macrophages also play an important role in the production of cytokines. Innate immune responses form the initial immune response to invading pathogens and contribute to adaptive immunity, which is composed of T lymphocytes (T cells) and B lymphocytes (B cells) that are involved in cell-mediated immunity and humoral immunity, respectively (Berek, 2005).

### *INNATE IMMUNITY*

In contrast to the adaptive immune system, which can recognize a variety of foreign substances, including tumor antigens, the innate immune system can only recognize microbial substances. For the most part, neutrophils, macrophages, NK cells, and dendritic cells are involved in the innate immune response and depend on the recognition of pattern recognition receptors (PRRs), which are encoded in the germline and identically expressed by effector cells. These receptors recognize pathogen-associated molecular patterns (PAMPs), which are expressed by microbes and trigger intracellular signaling cascades that result in inflammation and microbial death. PRRs are expressed constitutively in the host and are not dependent on immunologic memory (Fig. 36.1). Toll-like receptors (TLRs) are PRRs that stimulate type 1 interferon (IFN) production, which has antimicrobial, antiviral, and anticancer activity (Akira, 2006). TLR agonists are being evaluated in a phase II study of VTX-2337 and pegylated liposomal doxorubicin in platinum-resistant ovarian cancer patients based on promising phase I data of 13% partial response and 63% stable disease (Monk, 2013). NK cells are a subset of the lymphocyte population, can directly kill infected cells, and recognize cells that lack major histocompatibility complex (MHC) class I molecules, such as bacteria. Moretta and colleagues reported that NK cells are cytotoxic to tumor cells, probably because of a similar lack of MHC class I molecules.

The complement system plays an important role in the innate immune system and is a complex system, consisting of a large group of interacting plasma proteins. Activation by binding to antigen-complexed antibody molecules activates what is termed the *classical pathway*. In contrast, the alternative pathway is activated by recognition of microbial surface structures in the absence of antibody. Activation of these pathways leads to cleavage of C3 protein into a larger C3b fragment that is deposited on the microbial surface, leading to complement activation of C3a, which serves as a chemoattractant for neutrophils. Complexing of downstream complement proteins C6, C7, C8, and C9 produces a membrane pore in tagged cells that ultimately results in cell lysis. Unfortunately, tumor cells are often resistant

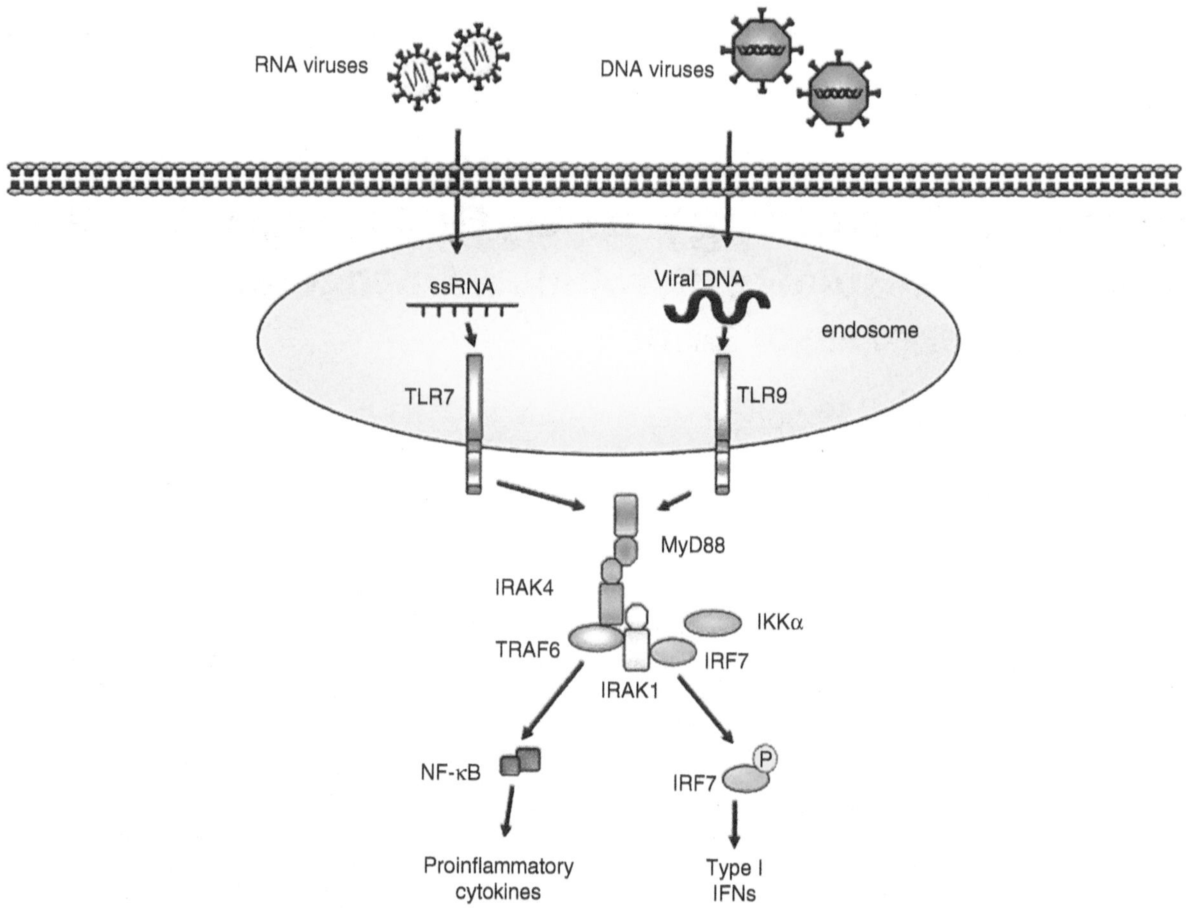


**Figure 36.1** Toll-like receptors (TLRs). TLRs are pattern recognition receptors that recognize microbes, viruses, and cancer cells. TLRs recruit MyD88, which is an adaptor protein that ultimately activates interferon and proinflammatory cytokines. *IKKα*, Inhibitor of nuclear factor-κB (IκB) kinase; IRAK1, interleukin-1R-associated kinase-1; *IRAK 4*, interleukin-1R-associated kinase-4; *IRF 7*, interferon regulatory factor-3; *TRAF6*, TNF receptor-associated factor 6. (From Takeuchi O, Akira S. Recognition of viruses by innate immunity. *Immunol Rev.* 2007;220:214-224.)

to complement-dependent cytotoxicity. The innate immune system is intricately linked to the adaptive immune system by activated macrophages that enhance T-cell activation and complement fragments that can activate B cells and antibody production.

## ADAPTIVE IMMUNITY

### Humoral Immunity: B Cells and Immunoglobulins

In humans, B cells are derived from hematopoietic stem cells and aggregate in the lymph nodes, gastrointestinal tract, or spleen. B lymphocytes synthesize antibodies in response to an activated $CD8^+$ cell or helper T cell (Th2). Then, the B lymphocytes differentiate into plasma cells that secrete large quantities of antibody (immunoglobulin) in response to an antigen. Unlike T cells, B cells recognize antigens in an unprocessed state. Each B cell is programmed to secrete a specific type of antibody, and it is estimated that more than $10^7$ different antibodies are capable of being produced in response to the presence of foreign antigens (Fig. 36.2).

Overall, antibodies have the same basic structure, except for extensive variability in the portion of the structure binding to the specific antigen. Two identical heavy and light chains constitute the basic immunoglobulin (Ig) structure. Each pair is connected by a disulfide bond. Both the heavy and light chains have a variable (V) region at the amino terminus and a constant region (C) at the carboxy terminus. The V region participates in antigen recognition and confers specificity, and the C region enables the antibody to bind to the phagocyte. Five immunoglobulin molecules (IgG, IgM, IgA, IgD, and IgE) exist and serve different effector functions. Early in the antibody response, IgM and IgD production occurs and the membrane-bound form of IgM and IgD binds antigen and activates naive B cells, leading to B-cell proliferation and clonal selection. Also, IgM is involved in the activation of the classical pathway of the complement system. Later in the antibody response the IgG response develops, which has a higher specificity for particular antigens. IgG is also responsible for neonatal immunity in the transfer of maternal antibodies across the placenta and gut. Also, IgG causes opsonization of the antigen for phagocytosis by macrophages and neutrophils, as well as activation of the classical pathway of the complement system. NK cells and other leukocytes can bind to IgG- and IgE-coated cells to facilitate antibody-dependent cytotoxicity. IgE mediates hypersensitivity reactions, and IgA is responsible for mucosal immunity.

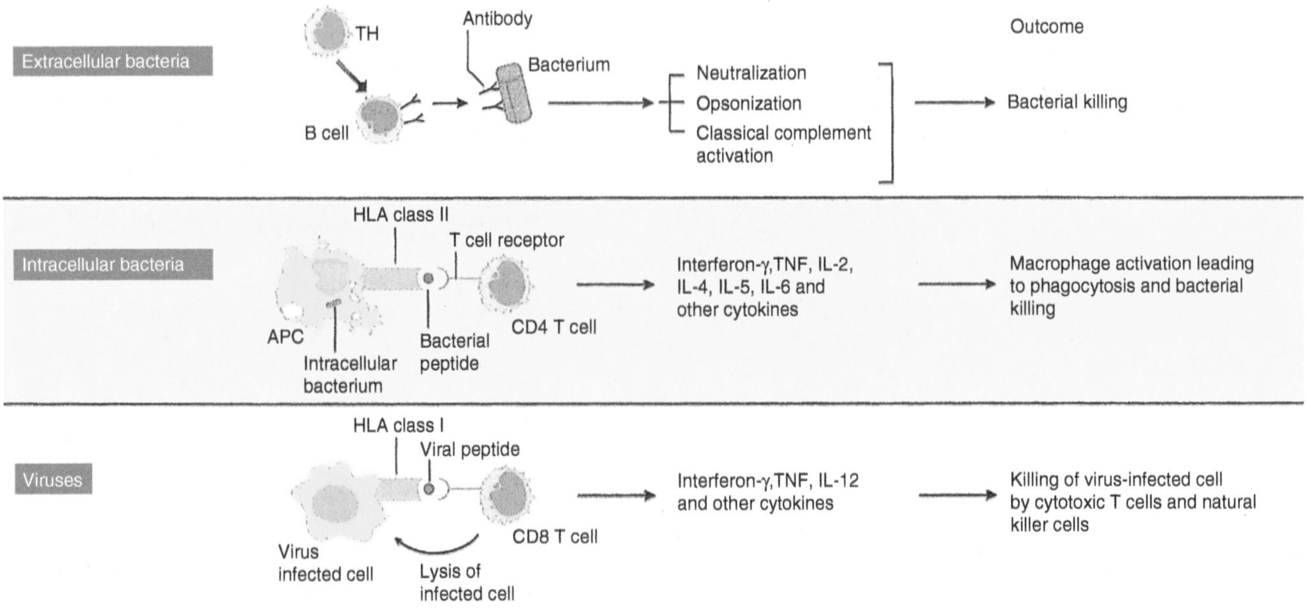


**Figure 36.2** Overview of specific immune responses. *Top row,* Humoral immunity. B lymphocytes eliminate microbes by secreting antibodies. *Middle and lower rows,* Cell-mediated immunity. Helper T lymphocytes activate macrophages or dendritic cells that kill phagocytosed molecules or cytotoxic T lymphocytes that eliminate infected cells. (From Chapel H, Haeney M, Misbah S, Snowden N. *Essentials of Clinical Immunology.* 5th ed. Malden, MA: Blackwell; 2006:35.)

### *Cellular Immunity: T Cells*

T cells originate in the bone marrow, differentiate in the thymus, and then circulate in the blood or are harbored in the lymph nodes, spleen, or Peyer patches of the intestine. In contrast to the humoral response, the cellular immune response (cellular immunity) depends on direct cell-cell contact. Although antibodies and B-cell receptors may recognize multiple types of antigens, T cells are restricted to peptide antigens and only recognize peptide sequences in the context of membrane-bound host proteins called *MHC molecules* (Fig. 36.3). There are two classes of MHC molecules. Each class presents antigens to different populations of T cells and is responsible for various functions in the cellular immune response. Th cells (which are $CD4^+$) respond to antigens bound to class II MHC molecules to secrete cytokines that stimulate the proliferation and differentiation of T cells as well as other B cells and macrophages. Class II MHC molecules are expressed primarily by professional APCs, which present phagocytosed and processed extracellular peptides to Th cells. There are two subsets of Th cells, which differ in their cytokine profiles and elicit different responses. Th1 cells secrete interleukin (IL)-2 and interferon-gamma (IFN-γ) to elicit a cell-mediated inflammatory response. Th2 cells secrete IL-4, IL-5, IL-6, and IL-10 to promote antibody secretion and the humoral response. Although both types are involved in most immune responses, they regulate the magnitude of each through mutual inhibition of cytokine production such that Th2 cell cytokines suppress production of Th1 cell cytokines and vice versa.

Unlike class II MHC molecules, class I MHC molecules are expressed by all nucleated cells in the body and are used to present intracellular peptides for surveillance to circulating cytotoxic T lymphocytes (CTLs). CTLs are also known as $CD8^+$ T cells and directly destroy cells that express foreign antigens that arise after a viral infection or are expressed as a result of tumorigenesis. Therefore CTLs are considered to be primarily responsible for the antitumor immune response. Zhang and colleagues reported that the presence of intratumoral T cells improves progression-free and overall survival in ovarian cancer patients. This effect was confirmed by Sato and colleagues, who documented a survival advantage in patients with a higher $CD8^+/CD4^+$ ratio of intratumoral cells in ovarian cancer patients compared with the lowest tertile of this cohort. Han and associates found that antigen-processing machinery component down-regulation and the subsequent lack of intratumoral T cells are independent prognostic factors for decreased survival of ovarian cancer patients.

A third class of T cells, regulatory T cells (Tregs), consists of $CD4^+$ T cells that are present in the peripheral circulation, inhibit immune responses, and prevent autoimmunity. Because most tumor-associated antigens are self-antigens, recognition by immune effector cells is regulated by Tregs through peripheral tolerance. High numbers of Tregs have been found in the peripheral blood of patients with epithelial ovarian cancer and Tregs preferentially accumulate in the tumor environment, such as ascites and ovarian tumor islets. Curiel and associates have shown that high levels of Tregs were found to predict poor overall survival in a cohort of 70 patients with ovarian cancer. Based on these data, a goal of immunotherapy is to eliminate Tregs in the hope of enhancing innate antitumor immunity. Denileukin diftitox (an engineered protein combining IL-2 with diphtheria toxin causing apoptosis of $CD25^+$ cells) selectively eliminates Tregs and has been investigated in ovarian cancer patients in a small phase I study. Results indicate that it induces tumor regression or stabilization, with low toxicity in about 50% of patients (Barnett, 2005).

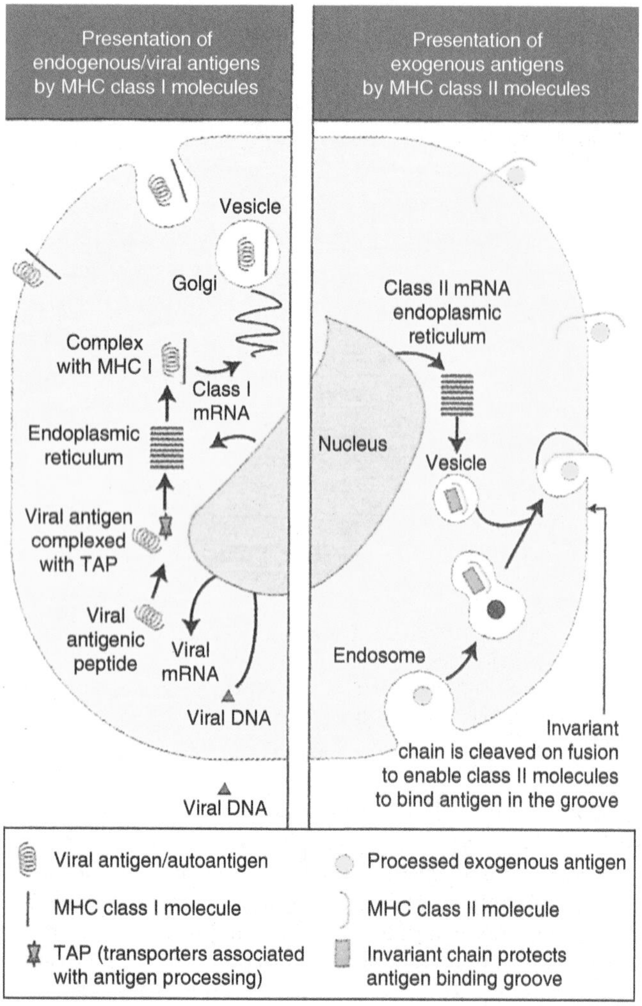


**Figure 36.3** Different routes of antigen presentation. After the antigen is processed into smaller fragments, the major histocompatibility complex class (I or II) and these fragments interact with the receptor on the surface of the T cell to activate cytotoxic or helper T cells. (From Chapel H, Haeney M, Misbah S, Snowden N. *Essentials of Clinical Immunology*. 5th ed. Malden, MA: Blackwell: 2006:7.)

## CYTOKINES

Cytokines are proteins secreted by immune cells that are produced in different phases of the immune response to control its duration and extent. During the activation phase of the immune response system, cytokines stimulate growth and differentiation of lymphocytes, whereas in the effector phase of the immune response, they activate other effector cells to help eliminate antigens and microbes. The major classes of cytokines include those that regulate innate immunity, regulate adaptive immunity, and stimulate hematopoiesis.

### Cytokines That Mediate Innate Immunity

#### Interleukins

Interleukins are potent cytokines produced by some leukocytes to affect other leukocytes. IL-1 is released in response to cell damage by macrophages, endothelial cells, and some epithelial cells. Although IL-1 has actions similar to those of tumor necrosis factor (TNF), it lacks the ability to cause septic shock symptoms. Macrophages can secrete a variety of ILs. M1 macrophages secrete IL-12, IL-18, IL-23, IFN-γ, and TNF-α and promote immune responses against tumors and intracellular microbes. IL-12 plays an important role in the transition between cell-mediated immunity and adaptive immunity. IL-12 stimulates NK cells and T cells to produce IFN-γ, which activates macrophages to kill phagocytosed foreign substances. Also, IL-12 increases cytolytic activity by stimulating $CD8^+$ cells. M2 macrophages produce vascular endothelial growth factor (VEGF), IL-6, IL-10, and prostaglandin E2, all of which have immunosuppressive functions and are found selectively in established tumors. The other ILs stimulate NK and T-cell activation and proliferation, as well as IFN-γ synthesis.

#### Chemokines

Chemokines are small secreted proteins that are part of the largest known cytokine family. The chemokines are subdivided based on the number and positioning of highly conserved cysteines. Functionally, chemokines released in response to inflammatory stimuli that cause leukocyte recruitment are considered to be inflammatory, whereas chemokines that cause migration of leukocytes to lymphoid organs are considered to be homeostatic. Chemokines affect tumor establishment in the following ways: determining the extent and type of leukocyte infiltration, promoting angiogenesis, controlling site-specific metastasis, and affecting tumor cell proliferation. The CXC chemokines (CXCL9, CXCL10, and CXCL11) are induced by IFN-γ and are typical chemoattractants of NK cells.[6] In ovarian cancer patients, the expression of CXCR4/CXCL12 correlates with decreased progression-free and overall survival. Because of the importance of chemokines in gynecologic and other malignancies, CXCR4 inhibitors such as peptide antagonists and neutralizing antibodies have been developed and are in clinical trial (Muralidhar, 2014).

#### Interferons

Type 1 IFN, IFN-α and IFN-β, are stimulated by intracellular TLRs and mediate the early innate immune response to viral infections. These cytokines inhibit viral replication, increase expression of class I MHC molecules, and promote a Th1 cell-mediated immune response by promoting T-cell proliferation and NK cell cytolytic activity. IFN-γ, a type II IFN, is principally responsible for macrophage activation and the effector functions of innate and adaptive immune responses.

### Cytokines That Mediate Adaptive Immunity

In addition to IFN-γ and transforming growth factor beta (TGF-β), IL-2, IL-4, IL-5, and IL-13 are all involved in the regulation of adaptive immunity. After T cells recognize the antigen, the T cells produce IL-2, which causes clonal expansion of activated T cells and additional production of cytokines such as IFN-γ and IL-4. IL-2 stimulates antibody synthesis and B cells by acting as a growth factor. IL-4 not only promotes IgE production from B cells but also stimulates the development of Th2 cells from naive T cells. IFN-γ is produced by T cells in response to antigen recognition or by NK cells in response to microbes or IL-12. IFN-γ activates the microbicidal function of macrophages, stimulates the expression of class I and II MHC and costimulatory molecules by antigen-presenting cells (APC), promotes the maturation of cells expressing CD4 into Th1 cells, and inhibits the Th2 cell pathway, thereby effectively promoting a cellular immune response. TGF-β inhibits the proliferation and differentiation of T cells and contributes to immune evasion of tumor cells by inhibiting antitumor host immune responses.

### *Cytokines That Mediate Hematopoiesis*

#### Colony-Stimulating Factors

IL-3 is a multilineage colony-stimulating factor that allows for the differentiation of cells into myeloid progenitor cells, granulocytes, monocytes, and dendritic cells. Granulocyte colony-stimulating factor (G-CSF) is a cytokine produced by macrophages, fibroblasts, and endothelial cells and promotes the mobilization of neutrophils from the bone marrow. Granulocyte-macrophage colony-stimulating factor (GM-CSF) is produced by T cells, macrophages, endothelial cells, and fibroblasts. GM-CSF stimulates the maturation of bone marrow cells into dendritic cells and monocytes. G-CSF and GM-CSF are available pharmacologically and are used in patients undergoing chemotherapy and bone marrow transplantation.

## *TUMOR CELL KILLING AND IMMUNOTHERAPY*

Immunotherapy has been developed to recognize and destroy tumor cells. Immune modulation, passive therapy, and active therapy are the three major classes of immunotherapy. Immune modulation relies on nonspecific means such as the administration of IL-2, IFNs, or bacille Calmette-Guérin to elicit an immune response. Passive therapy transfers components of the acquired immune system to the cancer patient (passive immunity). An example of passive therapy is the use of monoclonal antibodies directed toward tumor-specific antigens. Active therapy uses the woman's immune system to elicit a response; an example would be vaccines composed of peptides, proteins, DNA, or RNA.

Immune modulation has been used in ovarian cancer in the form of adjuvant IFN treatment after surgery and as consolidation therapy after surgery and standard chemotherapy. A phase III trial randomized patients with advanced ovarian cancer to IV cisplatin and cyclophosphamide chemotherapy versus the same regimen with intraperitoneal IFN-γ. Windbichler and colleagues have shown an improvement in progression-free but not overall survival in the IFN arm, with acceptable toxicity. Possible explanations for the improvement in the chemotherapy plus IFN include induction of cytotoxic T lymphocytes, stimulation of NK cells and macrophages, an antiangiogenic effect on tumor vasculature, and the direct inhibition of oncogene expression by high IFN-γ levels in the tumor microenvironment. This study was redone with the standard chemotherapy of carboplatin and paclitaxel with IFN-γ versus chemotherapy alone and showed a survival disadvantage in patients receiving IFN-γ, but no difference in progression-free survival (Alberts, 2008). Because of the mixed results, further trials investigating the potential synergistic effect of IFN administration and cytotoxic chemotherapy are needed to rigorously evaluate this approach for treatment.

Tumor cells have specific tumor-associated antigens or receptors on their surface that may distinguish them from normal cells. The antigen most often targeted in ovarian cancer is cancer antigen 125 (CA-125), a glycoprotein present at elevated levels in the serum of more than 80% of patients with epithelial ovarian cancer. A murine monoclonal antibody (MAb) to CA-125 (oregovomab) was investigated for its therapeutic usefulness as a consolidation treatment in ovarian cancer patients but did not demonstrate an overall survival advantage over controls. However, a subset of patients who had evidence of a robust antiantibody immune response in the form of antimurine antibodies had evidence of tumor protection after treatment (Berek, 2008). Trials of oregovomab, with or without chemotherapy, have also been conducted in patients with recurrent disease, and induction of anti–CA-125 T-cell responses may correlate with improved survival times in a minority of patients. Abagovomab (an anti-idiotypic MAb) stimulated human antimouse antibodies and an anti-anti-idiotypic as well as a CA125-specific cellular immune response in most patients, but it did not correspond into a prolonged progression-free or overall survival (Sabbatini, 2013). Bevacizumab (Avastin) is a monoclonal antibody directed against VEGF. In a phase II study of persistent or recurrent ovarian cancer patients, it showed an unprecedented 21% response rate, and 40% of patients did not have progression at 6 months. Two double-blind placebo-controlled phase III trials (GOG 218 and ICON7) enrolled over 3400 women to evaluate the benefit of bevacizumab to first-line intravenous chemotherapy of carboplatin and paclitaxel every 3 weeks and found an approximately 4-month improvement in progression-free survival in patients who received bevacizumab (Burger, 2011; Perren, 2011). Additionally, in the AURELIA open-label randomized phase III trial, 361 patients with platinum-resistant recurrent ovarian cancer received either weekly paclitaxel, weekly and/or five day topotecan, or pegylated doxorubicin per physician preference and were randomized to either chemotherapy alone and/or bevacizumab. The median progression-free survival in patients with chemotherapy alone was 3.4 months versus 6.7 months with a bevacizumab-containing therapy ($P < .001$) (Pujade-Lauraine, 2014). This trial did not show an overall survival benefit, as that was not the primary objective of the trial and crossover to the use of bevacizumab was allowed. The AURELIA trial led to U.S. Food and Drug Administration (FDA) approval of bevacizumab for ovarian cancer patients.

Adoptive T-cell immunotherapy uses the transfer of T cells expanded ex vivo in large numbers because of their ability to kill tumor cells specifically and to proliferate and persist for long periods after transfer. A strong rationale exists for the development of adoptive T-cell therapies in the treatment of ovarian cancer. First, tumor-specific T cells can be found in the peripheral circulation or in tumors in up to 50% of ovarian cancer patients. Second, the presence of intratumoral T cells being associated with improved survival suggests that administering adoptive immunotherapy could produce clinical results. Unfortunately, the advancement of adoptive T-cell therapies suffers from their complexity and labor-intensive manufacture, as well as toxicity from cross-reactivity and antigenic mimicry. Therefore trials in ovarian cancer are somewhat limited but ongoing using dendritic cells or naturally or genetically modified T-cell therapies (Kandalaft, 2011).

Targeting immune checkpoints, such as programmed cell death protein 1 (PD1), programmed cell death 1 ligand (PDL1), and cytotoxic T-lymphocyte antigen 4 (CTLA4), have shown clinical benefit in melanoma and lung cancer by blocking immunoinhibitory signals and enabling patients to mount an effective antitumor response. Varga and colleagues presented preliminary phase IB data in a heavily pretreated PDL1 positive ovarian cancer population and found that one patient had a complete response, two patients had a partial response, and six patients had stable disease by taking pembrolizumab. Clinical trials in all gynecologic malignancies are ongoing with these novel agents.

Another promising immunotherapy in gynecology has been the human papillomavirus vaccine (HPV) for the prevention of vulvar, vaginal, or cervical dysplasia and the corresponding cancers. A study conducted by Joura and workers has shown that the nine-valent vaccine against HPV 6, 11, 16, 18, 31, 33, 45, 52, and 58 decreases the incidence of dysplasia or cancer significantly; the vaccine was 96.7% effective (Joura, 2015). Currently, *Listeria monocytogenes*, which secretes the antigen HPV-16 E7 and is fused to a nonhemolytic listeriolysin O protein, has been used as a therapeutic vaccine for patients with advanced cervical cancer (Basu, 2014). The use of HPV vaccine therapy is efficacious and has tremendous implications for the treatment of gynecologic HPV-related dysplasias and cancers.

## MOLECULAR ONCOLOGY

Cancer development can be sporadic if it is caused by acquired mutations or can be hereditary if caused by inheritance of a mutated gene followed by acquisition of an acquired mutation in the other allele or loss of the other allele, also known as *loss of heterozygosity*. Genetic alterations occur in three major categories of genes—oncogenes, tumor suppressor genes, and DNA mismatch repair genes (MMRs). Knowledge of how these genes function is a rapidly expanding field and well beyond the scope of this chapter, but a general overview is provided here.

### ONCOGENES

An oncogene refers to a set of genes that when altered are associated with the development of a malignant cell. Functionally, oncogenes are involved in cell proliferation, signal transduction, and transcriptional alteration. Mechanisms of alteration in oncogene function include gene amplification (increase in the number of copies of the genes in the cell), translocation, or overexpression, which refers to excessive and abnormal protein production. Several classes of oncogenes such as peptide growth factors, cytoplasmic factors, and nuclear factors exist. Examples are described in the following section (Table 36.1).

#### Peptide Growth Factors

##### Epidermal Growth Factor Receptor Family

There are four types of *Erb*B receptors: *Erb*B1 (commonly known as *epidermal growth factor receptor [EGFR]*, human epidermal growth factor receptor [HER]1), *Erb*B2 (also known as *HER2/neu*), *Erb*B3 (also known as *HER3*), and *Erb*B4 (also known as *HER4*). All *Erb*B receptors share an extracellular domain that binds ligand, a transmembrane domain, and an intracellular tyrosine kinase domain. In the *Erb*B pathway, homodimers and heterodimers are formed from the various classes of receptors, resulting in activation of the Ras-Raf–mitogen-activated protein kinase (MAPK) pathway and the phosphoinositide 3-kinase (PI3K)–activated AKT pathway. Although *Erb*B3 lacks intrinsic kinase activity and *Erb*B2 has no specific ligand, the formation of heterodimers leads to activation of these classes of receptors.

The Ras-Raf-MAPK pathway is a major downstream target of the *Erb*B family of receptors and leads to the activation of Ras, causing the activation of MAPKs to regulate transcription of molecules linked to cell proliferation, survival, and transformation. Also, the PI3K-activated AKT pathway serves as another downstream target of the *Erb*B pathway; it drives tumor progression *via* cell growth, proliferation, survival, and motility. A number of mechanisms such as receptor gene amplification and overexpression, receptor mutations, and autocrine ligand production cause *Erb*B pathway disruption, leading to tumor formation. EGFR gene mutations have been found in glioblastomas, nonsmall cell lung cancer, and ovarian cancer. Slamon and colleagues reported that Her2/neu amplification is found in 20% to 30% of breast cancers and 10% of ovarian cancers. Because of the multitude of cancers with genetic alterations or changes in the ErbB family, several potential strategies exist for targeting EGFR, including monoclonal antibodies, low-molecular-weight tyrosine kinase inhibitors (TKIs), antisense oligonucleotides, and intracellular single-chain Fv fragments of antibodies, and many are used in clinical practice. Trastuzumab, a MAb that binds to HER2/neu, is currently used in the treatment of breast cancers that overexpress this receptor. Currently, monoclonal antibodies to the extracellular domain of EGFR such as cetuximab have been approved by the FDA for the treatment of metastatic colorectal cancer along with chemotherapy, as well as for the treatment of locally or regionally advanced head and neck cancer with radiation therapy.

Table 36.1 Classes of Genes Involved in Growth Stimulatory Pathways

| Peptide Growth Factors | Corresponding Receptors |
|---|---|
| Epidermal growth factor (EGF) and transforming growth factor-α (TGF-α) | EGF receptor (*erb*-B1), *erb*-B2 (Her-2/Neu), *erb*-B3, *erb*-B4 |
| Heregulin | |
| Vascular endothelial growth factor (VEGF) A, VEGF-B, VEGF-C, VEGF-D, VEGF-E, placental growth factor (PlGF) 1, PlGF2 | VEGFR-1, VEGFR-2, VEGFR-3, neuropilins |
| Insulin-like growth factors (IGF-I, IGF-II) | IGF-I and IGF-II receptors |
| Platelet-derived growth factor (PDGF) | PDGF receptor |
| Fibroblast growth factor (FGF) | FGF receptors |
| Macrophage colony-stimulating factor (M-CSF) | M-CSF receptor (FMS) |
| **Cytoplasmic Factors** | **Examples** |
| Tyrosine kinases | Eph family |
| G proteins | K-Ras, H-Ras, N-Ras |
| Serine-threonine kinases | AKT |
| Non receptor tyrosine kinases | Focal adhesion kinase (FAK), Src |
| **Nuclear Factors** | **Examples** |
| Transcription factors | C-myc, C-jun, C-fos |
| Cell cycle progression factors | Cyclins, E2F |

Modified from Boyd J, Berchuck A. Oncogenes and tumor suppressor genes. In: Hoskins WJ, Young RC, Markman M, et al, eds. *Principles and Practice of Gynecologic Oncology*. Philadelphia: Lippincott Williams & Wilkins; 2005:93-122.

##### Angiogenesis and Vascular Endothelial Growth Factor

Cancer growth requires a sufficient blood supply to extend beyond 1 $mm^3$ in size (Carmeliet, 2000). Angiogenesis occurs by sprouting (branching of new blood vessels from preexisting blood vessels) or by nonsprouting (requires the enlargement and splitting of preexisting blood vessels). The tumor vascular environment is characterized by vessels that are irregular in shape, dilated, tortuous, and disorganized. Angiogenesis is dependent on the relative increase of proangiogenic factors such as VEGF, platelet derived-growth factor (PDGF), and ephrins and their receptors. Also, endothelial cells are genetically stable, unlike tumor cells, thereby increasing the therapeutic value of targeting angiogenesis for cancer therapy.

VEGF is critical to endothelial cell survival, vascular permeability, cell fenestration, and vasodilation. There are seven proteins in this family: VEGF-A, VEGF-B, VEGF-C, VEGF-D, VEGF-E, placental growth factor (PlGF) 1, and PlGF2. Most human tumors, including those of the lung, thyroid, breast, gastrointestinal tract, female reproductive tract, and urinary tract, have marked expression of VEGF. There are three vascular endothelial growth factor receptors: VEGFR-1, VEGFR-2, and VEGFR-3. VEGFR-3 is expressed on the vascular and lymphatic endothelium, unlike the other two receptors, which are expressed only on the vascular endothelium. Also, there is a second class of VEGFRs known as the *neuropilins (NRPs),* which potentiate VEGF-A– and VEGFR-2–mediated actions. Similar to the EGFR family, there are many ligands to receptors in the VEGF family (Dvorak, 2002). Ultimately, activation of the VEGF receptors can lead to downstream effects on the mitogen-activated protein kinase (MAPK) pathway, v-src sarcoma viral oncogene homologue (SRC), PI3K-AKT, focal adhesion kinase (FAK), and Ras-Raf-MAPK (Ras-Raf-MAPK) superfamily. Because of the clinical significance of the VEGF pathway in many cancers, anti-VEGF antibodies such as bevacizumab, VEGFR tyrosine kinase inhibitors, and vascular targeting agents have been developed to target this critical pathway. In ovarian cancer, bevacizumab has been evaluated in conjunction with standard carboplatin and paclitaxel for first-line treatment, consolidation therapy, and in both platinum-sensitive and -resistant recurrent settings. A phase I/II study of docetaxel and aflibercept in 46 recurrent ovarian cancer patients with up to two previous chemotherapy regimens had an overall response rate of 54% without any gastrointestinal perforations or reversible posterior leukoencephalopathy, which can be serious side effects of bevacizumab (Coleman, 2011). The authors concluded that further evaluation is warranted. Another interesting phase II study evaluated the use of a polyadenosine diphosphate [ADP])-ribose polymerase (PARP) inhibitor olaparib with and without an antiangiogenic agent cediranib, which has activity against VEGFR1, VEGFR2, and VEGFR3 in recurrent platinum-sensitive ovarian cancer patients. The median progression-free survival was 17.7 months for the oral combination versus 9 months in the olaparib-only group ($P$ = .005) (Liu, 2014a). Additional clinical testing with this combination is underway.

### Ephrin Family of Ligands and Receptors

Tyrosine kinases provide a transfer of a phosphate from adenosine triphosphate (ATP) to tyrosine residues on specific cellular proteins; however, they can also play a role in the development of cancer and tumor progression. Attention has been given to elucidating the role of the ephrin receptor A2 (EphA2) in tumorigenesis and therapeutic targeting. EphA2 belongs to the largest known family of protein tyrosine kinase receptors, the Eph family, and there are two Eph receptors, A and B, that have corresponding ligands. The normal cellular function of EphA2 in epithelial tissue is not completely understood, but in cancer, EphA2 modulates cell growth, survival, migration, and angiogenesis (Pasquale, 2008). EphA2 overexpression has been correlated with disease severity and is predictive of a poor outcome in ovarian cancer patients (Thaker, 2004). There are several therapeutic approaches for targeting EphA2, including agonist monoclonal antibody, immunotherapy, soluble EphA receptors, and neutral liposomal small interfering RNA (siRNA), some of which are already in clinical trials (Ozcan, 2015).

### Phosphoinositide 3-Kinase Pathway

The PI3K family is composed of lipid and serine-threonine kinases that control second messengers through phosphorylation. AKT is the predominant downstream target of PI3K and has many targets, including mammalian target of rapamycin (mTOR), signal transducer and activation of transcription (STAT), MAPK, nuclear factor-κB, and protein kinase C. The activation of the PI3K-AKT pathway controls cell survival with inhibition of apoptosis, cell growth, cell metabolism, RNA translation, and cell proliferation. Also, this pathway has been implicated in chemotherapy resistance (Hennessy, 2005).

RAS is another cytoplasmic factor. It is a G protein involved in the transmission of growth stimulatory signals from the cell membrane to the nucleus. The RAS family of G proteins is positioned downstream of cell surface receptor tyrosine kinases and upstream of the cytoplasmic cascade of kinases, such as mitogen-activated protein (MAP) kinases. MAP kinases in turn activate nuclear transcription factors such as c-myc, c-jun, and c-fos. Currently, it is estimated that about one third of cancers have point mutations in RAS genes, such as *KRAS*, *HRAS*, and *NRAS*. Because RAS requires the posttranslational modification of the addition of a farnesyl group to the C terminus to move from the cytoplasm to the inner plasma membrane, inhibitors to farnesylation have been developed and clinical trials have been completed but results are still pending.

The RAF family of genes encodes serine-threonine kinases that interact with RAS proteins and continue signaling by activating MAP kinases, which translocate to the nucleus. Many cancers that lack a RAS mutation will have a *BRAF* mutation.

### Tumor Suppressor Genes

Tumor suppressor genes control cell growth and cellular proliferation and aberrations in tumor suppressor genes can cause malignancy. The retinoblastoma *(Rb)* gene was the first tumor suppressor gene to be identified and encodes a nuclear protein that regulates G1 phase cell cycle arrest. Knudson and colleagues have proposed the "two-hit" theory to explain the action of tumor suppressor genes. The first hit is the inheritance of the *Rb* mutated gene, and the second hit is the somatic mutation or loss that occurs later and leads to cancer (Amin, 2015).

In gynecologic malignancies, the most common tumor suppressor gene is *p53,* which is located on the short arm of chromosome 17. *p53* has key roles as a transcription factor and regulator of the cell cycle and apoptosis. Normal *p53* binds to transcriptional regulatory elements in the DNA and acts as a gatekeeper of the genome by responding to DNA damage with the activation of apoptotic effectors such as BAX, FAS, and bcl-2. Missense mutations that change a single amino acid in the encoded protein in exons 5 to 8 are the most common mutations of *p53.* The resultant mutant proteins can no longer bind to DNA but can bind to and inactivate any normal *p53* in a cell. Cells with mutant *p53* do not experience cell cycle arrest at the $G_1$-S checkpoint before DNA replication and at the $G_2$-M checkpoint prior to mitosis, nor do they undergo apoptosis.

Inactivation of the tumor suppressor gene TP53 is among the most frequent genetic events in endometrial cancers, and *p53* mutations are found in approximately 10% to 20% of endometrioid cancers, predominantly grade 3, and in 96% of late and sporadic ovarian cancers per the Cancer Genome Atlas Research Network (TCGA) (Cancer Genome Atlas Research Network, 2011; 2013). In cervical carcinogenesis, the E6 oncoprotein of HPV types 16 and 18 associates with *p53* and targets it for degradation, and the E7 oncoprotein of HPV type 16 binds to *Rb* in infected cells to upregulate proliferation (Asiaf, 2014). Although the *p53* mutation is one of the most common mutations in cancer, therapeutic targeting of *p53* has met with less than optimal results in several disease sites.

Phosphatase and tensin homologue (PTEN) is the regulatory counterpart of PI3K, and it does so by dephosphorylating proteins phosphorylated by PI3K. *PTEN* is a tumor suppressor gene and is found in approximately 20% of endometrial hyperplasia and 77.7% of endometrioid cancers per TCGA data (Cancer Genome Atlas Research Network, 2013). Mutations of *PTEN* occur in exons 3, 4, 5, 7, and 8 targeting the phosphatase domain and regions that control protein stability and localization. Decreased or absent expression of *PTEN* results in many of the mutations found in endometrioid cancers. Also, epigenetic mechanisms such as promoter hypermethylation and subcellular localization can affect *PTEN* function in the absence of intragenic mutations.

### *BRCA1* and *BRCA2*

Approximately 5% to 10% of breast and ovarian cancers arise in the setting of a genetic predisposition. The majority of these cases are associated with germline mutations in the *BRCA1* gene located on chromosome 17q21 and the *BRCA2* gene located on chromosome 13q12.3. The pattern of inheritance is autosomal dominant, and the prevalence of the mutated gene occurs more frequently in Ashkenazi Jewish and certain French Canadian women. The following women with no personal history of cancer but with a family history as listed here should be tested for a *BRCA* mutation (NCCN Guidelines, 2015).

- A known mutation in a cancer susceptibility gene within the family
- A woman with a family history of two or more women with breast cancer on the same side of the family
- A woman with greater than two breast cancer primaries in the same individual
- A first- or second-degree relative with breast cancer ≤45 years of age
- A woman with at least one family member with invasive ovarian, fallopian tube, or primary peritoneal cancers
- Male breast cancer
- Personal or family history of three or more of the following cancers: pancreatic cancer, prostate cancer, gastric cancer, melanoma, brain tumors

The cumulative risk of developing ovarian cancer by the age of 70 years is 40% to 50% for *BRCA1* mutation and 20% to 25% for *BRCA2* mutation carriers, but there is equal breast cancer penetrance in *BRCA1* or *BRCA2* mutation carriers. The *BRCA2* mutation is also associated with male breast cancer and pancreatic, urinary tract, and biliary tract cancers. Unfortunately, a woman with this mutation develops breast or ovarian cancer at a younger age than sporadic cancers.

*BRCA1* and *BRCA2* are tumor suppressor genes that encode for large proteins. Similar to other hereditary cancer syndromes, inheritance of a *BRCA* mutation confers an increased susceptibility to cancer, but not an absolute guarantee of developing cancer unless a second inactivation of the allele occurs. Both *BRCA1* and *BRCA* 2 encode proteins that are involved in the repair of DNA strand breaks. Most detected mutations are nonsense or frameshift alterations that lead to truncated proteins. *BRCA1* and *BRCA2* proteins are involved in the pathway mediated by RAD51, which is a protein important in repairing double DNA strand breaks. *BRCA1* is also involved in tumor suppression by transcriptional regulation of gene expression, such as being a *p53* independent transactivator of cyclin kinase inhibitor p-21. *BRCA2* has been identified as an FANCD1 gene, a member of the Fanconi anemia complex. Cells with deficient *BRCA1* or *BRCA2* are incapable of repairing DNA strand breaks, which leads to genetic instability and tumorigenesis. In *BRCA*-deficient cells, the defective maintenance of genomic integrity may not only accelerate cancer initiation and progression but may also render the cancer more susceptible to therapeutic agents whose cytotoxic potential is mediated through the induction of a specific type of DNA damage that *BRCA* normally functions to repair. For example, cisplatin and radiation cause DNA interstrand cross-links (Burgess, 2014). In a phase II study, PARP inhibitors such as olaparib have been used in the treatment of high-grade serous ovarian cancer patients with or without *BRCA1* and *BRCA2* mutations and were found to have an objective response rates of 41% for patients with *BRCA1/2* mutations and 24% for those without such mutations. The PARP inhibitors have an acceptable toxicity profile (Gelmon, 2011). The study that led to FDA approval for olaparib in the treatment of ovarian cancer evaluated olaparib as maintenance therapy in platinum-sensitive patients with unknown *BRCA* status who had received two or more platinum-based regimens and demonstrated a highly significant progression-free survival of 8.4 months versus 4.8 months upon completion of chemotherapy (Ledermann, 2012). PARPs are a family of multifunctional enzymes that repair DNA single-strand breaks through the repair of base excisions. The inhibition of PARPs leads to the accumulation of DNA double-strand breaks, which are normally repaired by *BRCA* proteins and thereby provide selectivity of treatment in this *BRCA* mutation population. Currently, clinical trials combining various PARP inhibitors and chemotherapy are ongoing in a *BRCA* mutation positive cancer population (Liu, 2014b), but the use of PARP inhibitors for therapy is a good example of how molecular oncology can be exploited for therapeutic value. Bolton and colleagues, as well as others, have demonstrated that women with *BRCA* mutations, especially *BRCA2* mutations, survive longer than their sporadic cancer counterparts (Bolton, 2012).

### DNA Mismatch Repair Genes

Hereditary nonpolyposis colorectal cancer (HNPCC), also known as *Lynch syndrome,* is an autosomal dominant cancer syndrome that predisposes an individual to colorectal, endometrial, gastric, biliary tract, urinary tract, or ovarian cancer. This syndrome is thought to account for all cases of hereditary endometrial cancer and up to 5% of hereditary ovarian cancers. The estimated lifetime risk for endometrial cancer in HNPCC gene carriers is 40% to 60%, corresponding to a relative risk of 13 to

20, whereas that of ovarian cancer is 6% to 20%, corresponding to a relative risk of 4 to 8. Linkage analysis of high-risk families led to the discovery of Lynch syndrome. It was found to be caused by germline mutations in genes responsible for recognizing and fixing errors in the DNA helix, resulting from incorrect pairings of nucleotides during replication or the formation of abnormal loops of DNA. *MSH2* (MutS homologue 2) and *MLH1* (Mut L homologue 1) are the most commonly mutated mismatch repair genes and are located on chromosomes 2p16 and 3p21, respectively. Other mismatch repair genes are *MSH6, MSH3, PMS1,* and *PMS2,* but these occur at a lower frequency. Cells with a defective mismatch repair system exhibit microsatellite instability (MSI). MSI occurs as DNA mismatches cause a shortening or lengthening of repetitive DNA sequences and these mismatches go unchecked. This results in the cancer containing a greater or lesser number of repeats than are present in the normal cells of the individual. There is a consensus panel of five microsatellite markers (D2S123, D5S346, D17S250, Bat 25, and Bat 26) that can be used to identify HNPCC-related cancers compared with sporadic ones. In endometrial cancer, MSI can occur from promoter methylation and must be distinguished from MSI caused by an inherited mismatch repair defect.

Taking a family history is the first step in identifying patients with HNPCC. The Bethesda criteria (Box 36.1) seem to be the most sensitive for predicting mismatch repair mutations, but the Amsterdam II criteria are more specific. Amsterdam II criteria include the following: colorectal carcinoma and/or endometrial cancer or transitional cell of the ureter or renal pelvis or carcinoma of the small bowel in at least three individuals, one of the patients is a first-degree relative of two other patients, disease occurs in at least two other family members, one of the diagnoses should be made before the age of 50 years, histologic confirmation of the diagnosis; and familial adenomatous polyposis has been excluded (NCCN Guidelines, 2014). However, many academic centers have gone to a universal screening protocol with immunohistochemistry in all endometrial cancer patients, which leads to a higher acceptance of genetic testing compared with referral based on risk factors alone (Frolova, 2015).

**Box 36-1 Bethesda and Amsterdam II Criteria for Hereditary Nonpolyposis Colorectal Cancer**

Any one of the following meet the Bethesda Criteria:

1. Colorectal cancer less than 50 years.
2. Presence of synchronous or metachronous HNPCC-related carcinomas regardless of age (colorectal, endometrial, stomach, ovarian, pancreas, ureter, renal pelvis, biliary tract, sebaceous gland, and small bowel).
3. Colorectal cancer with microsatellite instability high histology in individuals less than 60 years of age.
4. Colorectal cancer diagnosed in one or more first-colorectal-degree relatives with colorectal cancer or other HNPCC-related tumors. One of the cancers must have been diagnosed before the age of 50 years (this includes adenomas, which must have been diagnosed before the age of 40 years).
5. Colorectal cancer in two or more first- or second-degree relatives with a HNPCC-related tumor, regardless of age.

*Or*

All of the following meet the Amsterdam II Criteria:

1. Colorectal and/or endometrial cancer or transitional cancer of the ureter or renal pelvis or cancer of the small bowel in at least three individuals in the same family.
2. One of the patients is a first-degree relative of the other patients.
3. Disease occurs in at least two other family members in successive generations.
4. At least one of the diagnoses was made before the age of 50.
5. The diagnoses must be histologically confirmed.
6. Familial adenomatous polyposis is excluded in cases of colorectal cancer.

Data from National Comprehensive Cancer Network Guidelines, Version 2, 2015, Lynch Syndrome. Available at www.nccn.org.

## FUTURE DIRECTIONS

With the continued improved understanding of molecular oncogenesis and tumor progression, promising biologically targeted therapies will emerge. One such therapy is siRNA, which can be designed to target and silence oncogenes involved in all steps of cancer initiation, proliferation, and metastasis. Unlike small molecule inhibitors or fully humanized antibodies, siRNAs can aim at multiple downstream pathways or targets specifically and effectively based on direct, homology dependent, post-transcriptional gene silencing. The major challenges to the development of siRNA as a therapeutic tool have been its degradation by serum nucleases, poor cellular uptake, and rapid renal clearance following administration. However, the development of nuclease-resistant chemically modified siRNAs and neutral nanoliposomes such as 1,2-dioleoyl-*sn*-glycero-3-phosphatidylcholine (DOPC) for improved delivery should overcome these obstacles (Ozcan, 2015). Preclinically, neutral nanoliposomal EphA2 siRNA injection every 4 days decreased tumor growth in two ovarian cancer cell lines compared with control siRNA, and when EphA2-targeted siRNA was combined with paclitaxel there was a statistically significant decrease in tumor growth in both cell lines. Since the completion of safety studies, early stage clinical testing is under way.

Another potential therapeutic target is noncoding RNA (ncRNA). This includes a broad range of regulatory RNA molecules, such as ribozymes, antisense, siRNA, microRNA (miRNA), and aptamers. MiRNA negatively regulates protein expression in either cancer or normal cells. Changes in miRNA expression can occur by direct interaction between the stromal cells and cancer cells, by paracrine factors, or by direct communication between cells and secreted miRNAs. Once the miRNA communication pathways between the tumor microenvironment and the cancer cells can be decoded, miRNAs could be used for early detection, monitoring therapeutic responses, or targeted therapy with miRNA replacement (Kohlhapp, 2015). Small ncRNAs elicit at least four types of responses that trigger specific gene inactivation, which are important in a variety of cancers: destruction of homologous messenger RNA, inhibition of translation, de novo methylation of genomic regions that block transcription of target genes, and chromosomal rearrangement. These flexible molecules have proved to have enormous potential as diagnostic and therapeutic tools in cancer medicine.

## GYNECOLOGIC MALIGNANCIES

Cancer is a complex multistep process that requires self-sufficient growth signals, insensitivity to anti-growth signals, tissue invasion and metastasis, limitless replicative potential, sustained angiogenesis, and evasion of apoptosis. The clinical diversity of gynecologic cancers such as histologic type, stage, and outcome is probably attributable to molecular differences among cancers. The roles of oncogenes and tumor suppressor genes vary not only among cancers but also within a given type of cancer. With the data from TCGA, there is a better understanding of the molecular characterization of gynecologic cancers. This project sponsored by the National Institutes of Health carried out multiple "omics" studies including RNA, DNA, epigenetic, and protein analyses. With this improved characterization, TCGA identified four gene expression subtypes of high-grade ovarian cancer: mesenchymal, immunoreactive, differentiated, and proliferative. However, it is unclear whether these groupings will be clinically useful (Cancer Genome Atlas Research Network, 2011). Nevertheless, there are a number of findings that have increased our knowledge of the underpinnings of the cancers studied in TCGA. The following sections describe the roles of oncogenes and tumor suppressor genes that lead to the development of gynecologic cancers.

## ENDOMETRIAL CANCER

### Endometrial Cancer and Tumor Suppressor Genes

Endometrial cancer is divided into two types: type I, which is thought to be due to unopposed estrogen and develops in a background of endometrial hyperplasia, and type II, which comprises nonendometrioid and more aggressive cancers. Inactivation of tumor suppressor gene *p53* is among the most frequent genetic events in endometrial cancer occurring in about 20% to 30% of cases. Also, overexpression of *p53* occurs more frequently in advanced stage endometrial cancer and has been associated with worse survival after controlling for stage, suggesting that loss of *p53* tumor suppressor function leads to a more aggressive phenotype. There is a disproportionate frequency of *p53* mutations in 90% of serous and 33% of high-grade endometrioid cancers. In uterine sarcomas, overexpression of mutant *p53* occurs in the majority of malignant mixed mesodermal tumors (MMMTs) and in some leiomyosarcomas.

The *PTEN* gene is on chromosome 10q and encodes a phosphatase that functions by opposing the activity of PI3K. *PTEN* is the most commonly mutated gene in endometrial carcinoma. Mutations in this gene are usually deletions, insertions, or nonsense mutations that lead to truncated protein products and are associated with endometrioid histology, early stage, and favorable clinical behavior. Dellas and workers found that loss of *PTEN* and p27 protein expression in obese endometrial cancer patients is associated with a significantly better prognosis. Loss of *PTEN* in these cancers leads to increased activity of PI3K/AKT signaling cascade. Sometimes, *PTEN* mutation status can be used to differentiate an ovarian metastasis from an endometrial cancer *versus* synchronous primary cancers.

TCGA found other significantly mutated genes such as FBXW7, ARID1A, and PPP2R1A (Cancer Genome Atlas Research Network, 2013). FBXW7 regulates mTOR signaling and is mutated in about 30% of serous carcinomas. ARID1A, a large protein involved in chromatin remodeling, was initially reported to be mutated in ovarian endometrioid and clear cell tumors but now has been found to be mutated in 40% of endometrioid endometrial cancers. PP2R1A is a regulatory subunit of the protein phosphatase 2A and controls cell growth and division. Interestingly, it is mutated in uterine serous carcinomas but not ovarian carcinomas.

Germline mutations in DNA mismatch repair genes are essential to HNPCC. Endometrial cancer is the second most common malignancy observed in women with HNPCC after colon cancer. Unlike in colon cancer, loss of mismatch repair function in endometrial cancer has not been consistently associated with improved survival (see DNA Mismatch Repair Genes, presented earlier, for further details).

### Endometrial Cancer and Oncogenes

Unlike inactivation of tumor suppressor genes, fewer alterations in oncogenes have been found in endometrial cancer. *Her2/neu* has been found to be expressed in approximately 3% of endometrioid and 25% of serous carcinomas and was associated with aggressive phenotype and poor survival in a population-based series. Racial differences in the expression of *Her2/neu* have been found as well. Regardless, the levels of *Her2/neu* overexpression are much lower than in breast cancer (Engelsen, 2008). There have been clinical trials using trastuzumab (anti-*Her2/neu* antibody) for treatment of endometrial cancer, but without significant responses (Fleming, 2010).

*KRAS* mutations occur most often in type I endometrial cancers as well as in hyperplasias, suggesting that *KRAS* mutation is an early event in the development of type I endometrial cancers. The *BRAF* mutations were found in endometrial cancers with mismatch repair deficiency and have different frequencies in various populations (Feng, 2005).

The beta-catenin (β-catenin) gene maps to chromosome 3p21 and is important for cell differentiation, maintenance of normal tissue architecture, and signal transduction. Mutations in exon 3 of β-catenin result in stabilization of the protein, cytoplasmic and nuclear accumulation, and participation in signal transduction and transcriptional activation through the formation of complexes with DNA binding proteins. These mutations occur in approximately 15% to 50% of endometrial cancers and are independent of the presence of microsatellite instability and the mutational status of *PTEN* and *KRAS*. β-catenin exon 3 mutations were found to be a driver that characterizes an aggressive subset of low-grade and low-stage endometrioid adenocarcinomas in younger women, and this subset of patients may warrant more aggressive therapeutic management (Liu, 2014c).

The fibroblast growth factor receptor 2 *(FGFR2)* gene encodes one of a family of tyrosine kinase growth factor receptors that receive signals from a large family of ligands. Pollock and colleagues evaluated the *FGFR2* gene for activating mutations in a series of endometrial cancers and found them in approximately 10% of endometrioid cancers. The Gynecologic Oncology Group has completed a phase II trial evaluating an anti-*FGFR2* tyrosine kinase inhibitor brivanib in recurrent endometrial cancer; due to its tolerability and median PFS of 3.3 months, it warrants further development (Powell, 2014).

### Immunotherapy and Endometrial Cancer

Although endometrial cancer is the most frequent gynecologic cancer and the fourth most common cancer in women, immunotherapy is just emerging as a viable option for the treatment of endometrial cancer. Investigations have revealed that endometrial cancer is immunogenic and could be a reasonable target for immunotherapy. Santin and coworkers found that a strong in vitro tumor-specific response could be generated by tumor lysate–pulsed autologous dendritic cells in uterine papillary serous carcinoma. Although limited by few patients, a strong cytotoxic T-cell and Th1 response was characterized by enhanced IFN-γ and low IL-4 expression (Santin, 2002). In Belgium, a phase I/II clinical trial of six patients with recurrent uterine cancer who received autologous dendritic cell electroporated with Wilms tumor gene 1 showed feasibility of this approach, but the transient oncological responses were in human leukocyte antigen (HLA)-A2-positive patients (Coosemans, 2013). Immunotherapy for endometrial cancer is still in its infancy.

## OVARIAN CANCER

### Ovarian Cancer and Tumor Suppressor Genes

To date, alteration of the *p53* tumor suppressor gene is the most frequent genetic event in ovarian cancers. Advanced stage and serous cancers have a higher frequency of *p53* mutations than do early stage and nonserous cancers. Overall, 70% of advanced stage ovarian cancers have missense or truncation mutations in *p53*. Evidence suggests that inactivation of *Rb* greatly enhances tumor formation in ovarian cells with *p53* mutations.

Cyclin-dependent kinase inhibitors (CDKIs) also act as tumor suppressors because they inhibit cell cycle progression from the G1 to S phase. The *p16* gene (CDKN2A) undergoes homozygous deletion in approximately 15% of ovarian cancers. *BRCA1* and *p16* may be inactivated by transcriptional silencing because of promoter methylation rather than mutation or deletion. TCGA analysis found that only a small number of high-grade serous ovarian cases had deletions in PTEN and Rb, but endometrioid and clear cell ovarian cancers had higher mutation rates in ARID1A, PI3K, PTEN, and β-catenin (Cancer Genome Atlas Research Network, 2011).

### Oncogenes and Ovarian Cancer

Unlike in breast cancer, in which 30% express increased levels of *Her2/neu*, a minority of ovarian cancers have increased *Her2/neu* expression. The Gynecologic Oncology Group has conducted a trial to evaluate the response rate of ovarian cancer patients to single-agent anti-*Her2/neu* antibody therapy and found the rate of response to be approximately 7%. *KRAS* mutations are commonly found in borderline tumors of the ovary and mucinous ovarian cancers, but not in serous ovarian tumors. Additionally, in low-grade ovarian cancers, *BRAF* and *KRAS* mutations are found, and inhibitors of the *MEK 1/2* have been found to be active therapeutic agents with a 63% disease control in patients with recurrent low-grade serous carcinoma (Farley, 2013). PI3K and β-catenin are rarer mutations, but they are more likely to be found in endometrioid and clear cell tumors of the ovary.

### Immunotherapy and Ovarian Cancer

Because the clinical history of ovarian cancer entails periods of remission and relapse of sequentially shortened duration as chemotherapy resistance develops, immune-based strategies should be contemplated in women with minimal disease burden. The immune system protects the host against the development of cancer, but it also creates tumor immunogenicity. Immunotherapy trials generally focus on the effector phase of the immune response to elicit primarily an antibody response, produce humoral and cellular responses, or cause the activation or generation of antigen-specific CTLs and Th cells. The cancer-testis antigen NY-ESO-1 vaccines have been developed and used in a clinical trial of high-risk ovarian cancer patients in first clinical remission. Overall, these vaccines were found to have a low side effect profile and induced specific T-cell immunity, but they did not delay progression-free survival (Diefenbach, 2008). Also, anti-idiotype vaccines, which try to increase the immunogenicity of tumor-associated antigens by presenting the desired epitope to the host in a different molecular environment, have been used to increase antibody production. A phase I/II randomized trial of dendritic cell vaccination loaded with *Her2/neu*, human telomerase reverse transcriptase, and pan-DR epitope peptides with or without cyclophosphamide for consolidation therapy for advanced ovarian cancer patients in first or second remission demonstrated modest immunologic responses but was associated with a delayed progression-free survival and 3-year overall survival of 90% (Chu, 2012). In a phase I study utilizing intraperitoneal IL-12 plasmid formulated with the lipopolymer polyethyleneglycol-polyethyleneimine-cholesterol in combination with pegylated liposomal doxorubicin in patients with recurrent or persistent ovarian cancer, Thaker and colleagues found a clinical benefit of 57.1% and are developing additional clinical trials (Thaker, 2015). Check-point family members are involved in the Wnt, hedgehog, and Hippo pathway and modulate key regulatory proteins involved in tumorigenesis such as p53, β-catenin, and mouse double minute 2 homologue (MDM2). Clinical trials for check point inhibitors are in their infancy (Knippschild, 2014). Radionuclides conjugated with antibodies such as yttrium conjugated to the *MUC1* gene have been shown to have no difference in overall survival in ovarian cancer patients (Verheijen, 2006). Although, to date, numerous nonrandomized phase II immune targeted trials have shown benefit in terms of survival and presence of respective effectors, these have not been confirmed in phase III trials, but further investigation is warranted in ovarian cancer.

## CERVICAL CANCER: ONCOGENES, TUMOR SUPPRESSOR GENES, AND IMMUNOTHERAPY

Because only a small proportion of women with HPV develop cervical cancer, the inactivation of the TP53 tumor suppressor gene leads to genomic instability that results in secondary genetic alterations that lead to the development of cervical cancer. However, compared with other gynecologic cancers, the roles of oncogenes and tumor suppressor genes are not as well elucidated. The allelic loss of possible tumor suppressor genes at loci on chromosomes 3p, 11p, and others has been noted, but specific tumor suppressor genes remain unidentified. The RAS and MYC genes are key oncogenes in cervical carcinomas. Also, Mammas and colleagues found that the oncogenes *Hi* and *NRAS* are up-regulated in cervical cancer independently of HPV infection. Similar to endometrial and ovarian cancers, gene silencing caused by promoter hypermethylation may also be involved in cervical cancer development. The methylation status of the oncogene human telomerase reverse transcriptase and the tumor suppressor genes death-associated protein kinase and O6-methylguanine DNA methyltransferase could be used to distinguish the progression from normal to cervical dysplasia to invasive cancer. In terms of immunotherapy for the treatment of cervical cancer, ADXS11-001 is a live attenuated *Listeria monocytogenes* bioengineered to secrete an HPV-16 E7 fusion protein targeting HPV transformed cells. A prospective phase II study conducted in India with 110 recurrent cervical cancer patients receiving either three or four doses of the ADXS11-001 with cisplatin chemotherapy had a 12-month survival of 36% and 18-month survival of 28%. The total disease control rate was 43% in the patient population with very few options (Basu, 2014). This trial is also being conducted in the United States. Another approach is to use peptide-based vaccines, which have the advantages of relative tolerability, stability, and ease of production. However, they tend to have poor immunogenicity and require adjuvants to enhance vaccine potency. An ongoing clinical trial is utilizing ISA101, a HPV-16 E6/E7 long peptide vaccine, at varying doses with or without interferon alfa in combination with carboplatin and paclitaxel in women with HPV-16 positive advanced stage, metastatic or recurrent cervical cancer. Another exciting trial is the use of adoptive T-cell therapy in the treatment of nine patients with metastatic cervical cancer. All patients underwent isolation and ex vivo expansion of tumor-specific infiltrating T cells and three of six patients with HPV reactivity had objective tumor responses. This trial is being expanded for the recruitment of 35 patients. There are many other immunotherapy options in cervical cancer such as checkpoint inhibitors and using chimeric T-cell receptor antigens; the hope is that these trials will lead to durable cures (Eskander, 2015).

## CONCLUSION

Cancer pathogenesis is a complex process, but with the advent of high-throughput molecular technologies, a new understanding is rapidly advancing. This understanding of the biology and immunology of the disease offers hope for better means for prevention, early detection, and treatment.

## KEY POINTS

- The immune system consists of the innate and adaptive immune systems. The innate system is present at birth and consists of natural barriers, NK cells, macrophages, and the complement system. The adaptive immune system adapts to infection and consists of T and B cells.
- The cellular immune response occurs as a result of T lymphocytes reacting via a surface TCR that processes antigens presented to it by an APC in conjunction with MHC molecules.
- T-cell activation can result in activation of helper or inducer (Th) cells, cytotoxic or suppressor T cells, or cytokine production.
- Th cells recruit macrophages and cytotoxic or suppressor cells.
- Cytotoxic T cells have the ability to lyse infected cells or signal B cells to produce antibody.
- Humoral immunity results from antigenic stimulation of a B lymphocyte, which differentiates into a plasma cell and secretes antibody (immunoglobulin).
- The complement cascade provides a basis for the inflammatory response and can also mediate cytotoxicity.
- Cytokines (lymphokines) are regulatory substances of the immune system produced as a result of T-cell activation, cell damage by a virus, or other cells, such as macrophages and monocytes, involved in the immune response.
- Passive therapy transfers components of the acquired immune system to the recipient with cancer (e.g., monoclonal antibodies directed toward tumor-specific antigens).
- Active immunotherapy uses a patient's own immune system for protection against infection (e.g., vaccines).
- There are three types of genes associated with malignant development: oncogenes, tumor suppressor genes, and DNA mismatch repair genes.
- Malignant change is seen with point mutations, chromosomal aberration, gene amplification (increase in number of copies), or chromosomal translocation.
- *Ras* oncogenes are part of a group of signal transducer oncogenes that relay messages from the membrane to the cell nucleus. They are activated generally by point mutations.
- Growth factor genes include *C-erb-B2 (Her-2/neu),* which can be overexpressed and act as a tumor-specific target for monoclonal antibody therapy; these are especially useful in breast cancer therapy.
- Nuclear oncogenes include *myc* and *fos* and can activate other genes as well as stimulate DNA replication.
- Angiogenesis is the formation of new blood vessels in order for tumors to grow.
- Tumor suppressor genes such as *Rb* and *p53* restrain cell growth. They have two copies and, in general, alteration of both copies leads to a mutant expression, which allows tumorigenesis to occur.
- *BRCA1* and *BRCA2* mutations confer a high lifetime risk of breast or ovarian cancer. Mutation screening may be appropriate for women with family histories, suggesting a hereditary predisposition to breast or ovarian cancer.
- DNA mismatch repair genes act by recognizing and fixing errors in the DNA helix resulting from incorrect pairings of nucleotides. They prevent the accumulation of genetically damaged material in the cell.

## ACKNOWLEDGMENTS

Portions of this chapter were supported by grants from the National Institutes of Health (CA109298, P50CA083639, CA104825, P50 CA098258, and U54 CA151668, CA128797, P50CA134254), Ovarian Cancer Research Fund (Program Project Development Grant), Meyer and Ida Gordon Foundation 2, Foundation for Women's Cancer, and Betty Anne Asche Murray Distinguished Professorship.

## KEY REFERENCES


Akira S, Uematsu S, Takeuchi O. Pathogen recognition and innate immunity. *Cell.* 2006;124:783-801.

Alberts DS, Marth C, Alvarez RD, et al. Randomized phase 3 trial of interferon g-1b plus standard carboplatin/paclitaxel versus carboplatin/paclitaxel alone for first-line treatment of advanced ovarian and primary peritoneal carcinomas: results from a prospectively designed analysis of progression-free survival. *Gynecol Oncol.* 2008;109:174-181.

Amin AR, Karpowicz PA, Carey TE, Arbiser J, et al. Evasion of anti-growth signaling: a key step in tumorigenesis and potential target for treatment and prophylaxis by natural compounds. *Semin Cancer Biol.* 2015.

Asiaf A, Ahmad ST, Mohammad SO, Zargar MA. Review of the current knowledge on the epidemiology, pathogenesis, and prevention of human papillomavirus infection. *Eur J Cancer Prev.* 2014;23:206-224.

Barnett B, Kryczek I, Cheng P, et al. Regulatory T cells I ovarian cancer: biology and therapeutic potential. *Am J Reprod Immunol.* 2005;54:369-377.

Basu P, Mehta AO, Jain MM, et al. ADXS11–001 immunotherapy targeting HPV-E7: final results from a phase 2 study in Indian women with recurrent cervical cancer. *J Clin Oncol.* 2014;32. Abstract 5610.

Berek JS, Hacker NF. *Immunology and Biology: Practical Gynecologic Oncology.* ed 4. Philadelphia: Lippincott Williams, & Wilkins; 2005.

Berek JS, Taylor PT, McGuire W, et al. Oregovomab maintenance monoimmunotherapy does not improve outcomes in advanced ovarian cancer. *J Clin Oncol.* 2008;27:418-425.

Bolton KL, Chenevix-Trench G, Goh C, et al. Association between BRCA1 and BRCA 2 mutations and survival in women with invasive epithelial ovarian cancer. *JAMA.* 2012;307:382-390.

Burger RA, Brady MF, Bookman MA, et al. Incorporation of Bevacizumab in the Primary Treatment of Ovarian Cancer. *N Engl J Med.* 2011;365:2473-2483.

Burgess M, Puhalla S. BRCA1/2-mutation related and sporadic breast and ovarian cancer: more alike than different. *Front Oncol.* 2014;4:1-15.

Cancer Genome Atlas Research Network. Integrated genomic analysis of ovarian carcinoma. *Nature.* 2011;474:609–615.

Cancer Genome Atlas Research Network, Kandoth C, Schultz N, et al. Integrated genomic characterization of endometrial carcinoma. *Nature.* 2013;497: 67-73.

Carmeliet P. Mechanisms of angiogenesis and arteriogenesis. *Nat Med.* 2000;6:389-395.

Chu CS, Boyer J, Schullery DS, et al. Phase I/II randomized trial of dendritic cell vaccination with or without cyclophosphamide for consolidation therapy of advanced ovarian cancer in first or second remission. *Cancer Immunol Immunother.* 2012;61:629-641.

Coleman RL, Duska LR, Ramirez PT, et al. Phase 1-2 study of docetaxel plus aflibercept in patients with recurrent ovarian, primary peritoneal, or fallopian tube cancer. *Lancet Oncol.* 2011;12:1109-1117.

Coosemans AN, Vanderstraeten A, Tuyaerts S, et al. Wilms' tumor gene I (WT1)-loaded dendritic cell immunotherapy in patients with uterine tumors: a phaseI/II clinical trial. *Anticancer Res.* 2013;33:495-500.

Diefenbach CS, Gnjatic S, Sabbatini P, et al. Safety and immunogenicity study of NY-ESO-1b peptide and montanide ISA-51 vaccination of patients with epithelial ovarian cancer in high-risk first remission. *Clin Cancer Res.* 2008;14:2740-2748.

Dvorak HF. Vascular permeability factor/vascular endothelial growth factor: A critical cytokine in tumor angiogenesis and a potential target for diagnosis and therapy. *J Clin Oncol.* 2002;20:4368-4380.

Engelsen IB, Stefansson IM, Beroukhim R, et al. HER-2/neu expression is associated with high tumor cell proliferation and aggressive phenotype in a population-based patient series of endometrial carcinomas. *Int J Oncol.* 2008;32:307-316.

Eskander RN, Tewari KS. Immunotherapy: an evolving paradigm in the treatment of advanced cervical cancer. *Clin Ther.* 2015;37:20-38.

Farley J, Brady WE, Vathipadiekal V, et al. Selumetinib in women with recurrent low-grade serous carcinoma of the ovary or peritoneum: an open-label, single arm, phase 2 study. *Lancet Oncol.* 2013;14:134-140.

Feng YZ, Shiozawa T, Miyamoto T, et al. BRAF mutation in endometrial carcinoma and hyperplasia: Correlation with KRAS and p53 mutations and mismatch repair protein expression. *Clin Cancer Res.* 2005;11:6133-6138.

Fleming GF, Sill MW, Darcy KM, et al. Phase II of trastuzumab in women with advanced or recurrent HER-2 positive endometrial carcinoma: A Gynecologic Oncology Group study. *Gynecol Oncol.* 2010;116:15-20.

Frolova AI, Babb SA, Zantow E, et al. Impact of an immunohistochemistry-based universal screening protocol for Lynch syndrome in endometrial cancer on genetic counseling and testing. *Gynecol Oncol.* 2015;137:7-13.

Gelmon KA, Tischkowitz M, Mackay H, et al. Olaparib in patients with recurrent high-grade srous or poorly differentiated ovarian carcinoma or triple-negative breast cancer: a phase 2, multicentre, open-label, non-randomised study. *Lancet Oncol.* 2011;12:852-861.

Hanahan D, Weinberg RA. The hallmarks of cancer. *Cell.* 2000;100:57-70.

Hennessy BT, Smith DL, Ram PT, et al. Exploiting the PI3K/AKT pathway for cancer drug discovery. *Nat Rev Drug Discov.* 2005;4:988-1004.

Joura EA, Giuliano AR, Iversen OE, et al. A 9-valent HPV vaccine against infection and intraepithelial neoplasia in women. *N Engl J Med.* 2015;372:711-723.

Kandalaft LE, Powell Jr DJ, Singh N, Coukos G. Immunotherapy for ovarian cancer: what's next? *J Clin Oncol.* 2011;9:925-933.

Knippschild U, Kruger M, Richter J, et al. The CK1 family: contribution to cellular stress response and its role in carcinogenesis. *Front Oncol.* 2014;96:1-32.

Kohlhapp FJ, Mitra AK, Lengyel E, Peter ME. MicroRNAs as mediators and communicators between cancer cells and the tumor microenvironment. *Oncogene.* 2015 (Epub ahead of print).

Ledermann J, Harter P, Gourley C, et al. Olaparib maintenance therapy in platinum-sensitive relapsed ovarian cancer. *New Engl J Med.* 2012;366:1382-1392.

Liu JF, Barry WT, Birrer M, et al. Combination cediranib and olaparib versus olaparib alone for women with recurrent platinum-sensitive ovarian cancer: a randomized phase 2 study. *Lancet Oncol.* 2014a;15:1207-1214.

Liu JF, Konstantinopoulos PA, Matulonis UA. PARP inhibitors in ovarian cancer: current status and future promise. *Gynecol Oncol.* 2014b;133:362-369.

Liu Y, Patel L, Mills GB, et al. Clinical significance of CTNNB1 mutation and Wnt pathway activation in endometrioid endometrial carcinoma. *J Natl Cancer Inst.* 2014c;106:1-8.

Monk BJ, Brady WE, Lankes HA, et al. VTX-2337, a TLR8 agonist, plus chemotherapy in recurrent ovarian cancer: Preclinical and phase I data by the Gynecologic Oncology Group. *J Clin Oncol.* 2013 (suppl;abstr 3077).

Muralidhar GG, Barbolina MV. Chemokine receptors in epithelial ovarian cancer. *Int J Mol Sci.* 2014;15:361-376.

NCCN Clinical Practice Guidelines in Oncology. *Genetic/Familial High-Risk Assessment: Colorectal, Version 2*; 2014:1-66.

NCCN Clinical Practice Guidelines in Oncology. *Genetic/Familial High-Risk Assessment: Breast and Ovarian, Version 1*; 2015:1-82.

Ozcan G, Ozpolat B, Coleman RL, et al. Preclinical and clinical development of siRNA-based therapeutics. *Adv Drug Deliv Rev.* 2015.

Pasquale EB. Eph-ephrin bidirectional signaling in physiology and disease. *Cell.* 2008;133:38-52.

Perren TJ, Swart AM, Pfisterer J, et al. A phase 3 trial of bevacizumab in ovarian cancer. *N Engl J Med.* 2011;365:2485-2496.

Powell MA, Sill MW, Goodfellow PJ, et al. A phase II trial of brivanib in recurrent or persistent endometrial cancer: an NRG Oncology/Gynecologic Oncology Group Study. *Gynecol Oncol.* 2014;135:38-43.

Pujade-Lauraine E, Hilpert F, Weber B, et al. Bevacizumab Combined with Chemotherapy for Platinum-Resistant Ovarian Cancer: The AURELIA Open-Label Randomized Phase III Trial. *J Clin Oncol.* 2014;32:1302-1308.

Rainczuk A, Rao J, Gathercole J, et al. The emerging role of CXC chemokines in epithelial ovarian cancer. *Reproduction.* 2012;144:303-317.

Sabbatini P, Harter P, Scambia G, et al. Abagovomab as maintenance therapy in patients with epithelial ovarian cancer: a Phase III trial of AGO OVAR, COGI, GINECO, and GEICO-the MIMOSA study. *J Clin Oncol.* 2013;31:1554-1561.

Santin AD, Bellone S, Ravagii A, et al. Induction of tumour-specific CD8(þ) cytotoxic T lymphocytes by tumour lysate-pulsed autologous dendritic cells in patients with uterine papillary serous cancer. *Br J Cancer.* 2002;56:151-157.

Thaker PH, Brady W, Bradley W, et al. A phase I study of intraperitoneal EGEN-001 (IL-12 plasmid formulated with PEG-PEI-Cholesterol lipopolymer) administered in combination with pegylated liposomal doxorubicin in patients with recurrent or persistent epithelial ovarian, fallopian tube or primary peritoneal cancer. *ASCO abstract.* 2015;5541.

Thaker PH, Deavers M, Celestino J, et al. EphA2 expression is associated with aggressive features in ovarian carcinoma. *Clin Cancer Res.* 2004;10:5145-5150.

Verheijen RH, Massuger LF, Benigno BB, et al. Phase III trial of intraperitoneal therapy with yttrium-90-labeled HMFG1 murine monoclonal antibody in patients with epithelial ovarian cancer after a surgically defined complete remission. *J Clin Oncol.* 2006;24:571–578.


Suggested Readings can be found on ExpertConsult.com.

# Part V REPRODUCTIVE ENDOCRINOLOGY AND INFERTILITY

# 37

# Primary and Secondary Dysmenorrhea, Premenstrual Syndrome, and Premenstrual Dysphoric Disorder

## Etiology, Diagnosis, Management

*Vicki Mendiratta, Gretchen M. Lentz*

Dysmenorrhea, premenstrual syndrome, and premenstrual dysphoric disorder afflict a large percentage of women in their reproductive years. These conditions have a negative effect on the quality of these women's lives and the lives of their families, and they are also responsible for a huge economic loss as a result of the cost of medications, medical care, and decreased productivity. This chapter discusses current thinking with respect to the causes, pathophysiology, and management of these three conditions.

## DYSMENORRHEA

Dysmenorrhea is defined as a cyclic, painful cramping sensation in the lower abdomen often accompanied by other biologic symptoms, including sweating, tachycardia, headaches, nausea, vomiting, diarrhea, and tremulousness, all occurring just before or during the menses. The term *primary dysmenorrhea* refers to pain with no obvious pathologic pelvic disease. It is currently recognized that these patients are suffering from the effects of endogenous prostaglandins. The term *secondary dysmenorrhea,* on the other hand, is associated with pelvic conditions or pathology that causes pelvic pain in conjunction with the menses (Smith, 2016). Primary dysmenorrhea almost always first occurs in women younger than 20. Indeed, the woman will report pain as soon as she establishes ovulatory cycles. Secondary dysmenorrhea may, of course, occur in women younger than 20, but it is most often seen in women older than 20.

## INCIDENCE AND EPIDEMIOLOGY

A number of studies have attempted to determine the prevalence of dysmenorrhea; a wide range (16% to 90%) have been reported. These studies have been performed on students, teenagers and their mothers, and individuals from various specific populations, such as industrial workers or college students. The best estimate of the prevalence of primary dysmenorrhea is approximately 75%. Andersch and Milsom, 1982, surveyed all the 19-year-old women in the city of Gothenburg, Sweden. A total of 90.9% of these women responded to a randomly distributed questionnaire, and 72.4% of these stated that they suffered from dysmenorrhea. In addition, 34.3% of the total population reported mild menstrual symptoms, 22.7% cited moderate symptoms that required analgesia, and 15.4% stated that they had severe dysmenorrhea that clearly inhibited their working ability and that could not be adequately assuaged by general analgesia (Andersch, 1983) (Table 37.1). A 2005 Canadian study of 1546 menstruating women reported that 60% had primary dysmenorrhea and 60% reported their pain as moderate or severe (Burnett, 2005). Similarly, 17% missed school or work. Factors that may reduce the risk of developing dysmenorrhea include younger age at first childbirth, higher parity, and physical exercise. Women who have vaginally delivered a child are less likely to have dysmenorrhea. Pregnancy itself without actual birth does not seem to alleviate dysmenorrhea, because women who have had ectopic pregnancies or spontaneous or voluntary terminations of pregnancy are not relieved of their symptoms. Risk factors that have been reported to increase the risk of dysmenorrhea include age less than 30, body mass index (BMI) less than 20, premenstrual syndrome, pelvic inflammatory disease, sterilization, history of sexual assault, and heavy smoking (Latthe, 2006).

### *RELATIONSHIP TO MENSTRUATION AND THE MENSTRUAL CYCLE*

Andersch and Milsom, 1982 have demonstrated a significant positive correlation between the severity of dysmenorrhea and duration of menstrual flow, amount of menstrual flow, and early menarche. They showed no relationship with the actual duration of the menstrual cycle. In their series, 38.3% of patients reported that they had experienced dysmenorrhea for the first time during the first year after menarche, and only 20.8% reported that dysmenorrhea had not occurred until 4 years after menarche.

### *FAMILY HISTORY*

Dysmenorrhea has been reported to be increased significantly in mothers and sisters of women with dysmenorrhea.

Table 37.1 Severity of Primary Dysmenorrhea*

| Severity | Number of Women | Percentage of Total |
|---|---|---|
| None | 162 | 27.6 |
| Mild† | 201 | 34.3 |
| Moderate‡ | 133 | 22.7 |
| Severe§ | 90 | 15.4 |

Data from Andersch B, Milsom I: An epidemiologic study of young women with dysmenorrhea. *Am J Obstet Gynecol* 144:655, 1982.
*In a population of 586 19-year-old Swedish women.
†No systemic symptoms, medication rarely required, work rarely affected.
‡Few systemic symptoms, medication required, work moderately affected.
§Multiple symptoms, poor medication response, work inhibited.

## PRIMARY DYSMENORRHEA

### PATHOGENESIS

The pathogenesis of dysmenorrhea shows there is a close association between elevated prostaglandin F2α (PGF2α) levels in the secretory endometrium and the symptoms of dysmenorrhea, including uterine hypercontractility, complaints of severe cramping, and other prostaglandin-induced symptoms. Arachidonic acid, the precursor to prostaglandin production, has been found in increased amounts in the endometrium during ovulatory cycles. Arachidonic acid is converted to PGF2α, PGE2, and leukotrienes, which are involved in increasing myometrial contractions. During menses, these contractions decrease uterine blood flow and cause ischemia and sensitization of pain fibers (Fig. 37.1). Endometrial concentrations of PGF2α and PGE2 correlate with the severity of dysmenorrhea; cyclooxygenase inhibitors decrease menstrual fluid prostaglandin levels and decrease pain. In small studies, ultrasound and magnetic resonance imaging (MRI) have correlated dysmenorrhea with myometrial changes and decreased blood flow. PGF2α and PGE2 affect other organs such as the bowel and result in nausea, vomiting, and diarrhea.

### DIAGNOSIS

The diagnosis of primary dysmenorrhea is made largely by the history and physical exam. Patients typically complain of midline, crampy, lower abdominal pain, which begins with the onset of menstruation. The pain can be severe and can also involve the low back and thighs. The pain gradually resolves over 12 to 72 hours. Pain does not occur at times other than menses and only occurs in ovulatory cycles. Diarrhea, headache, fatigue, and malaise may be reported. Women with primary dysmenorrhea have a normal pelvic examination. There are no laboratory or imaging abnormalities associated with primary dysmenorrhea. In adolescents experiencing dysmenorrhea in the first 6 months from menarche, an obstructing malformation of the genital tract in the differential diagnosis should be considered.

### TREATMENT

Treatment for primary dysmenorrhea begins with providing patient education and reassurance. Individualized, supportive therapy can then be tailored to the patient's specific symptoms, degree of disability from those symptoms, and other health care considerations, such as need for contraception (Smith, 2016).

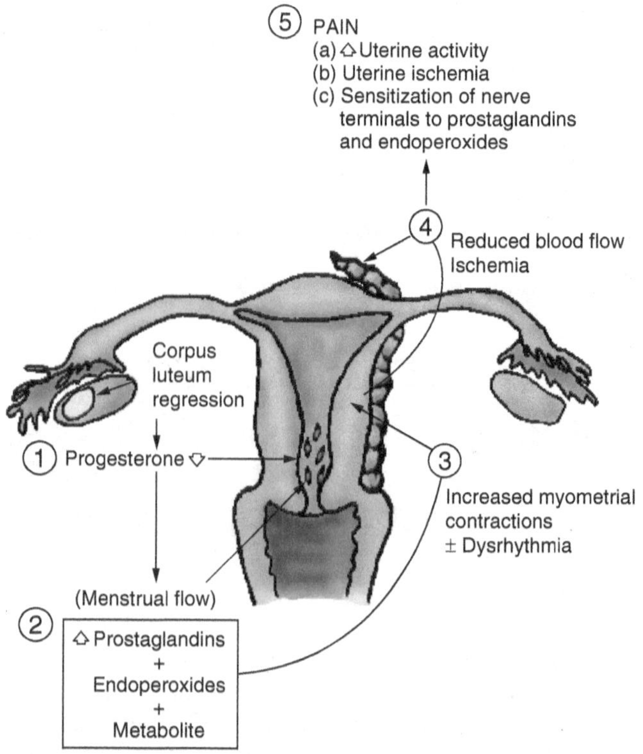


Figure 37.1 Mechanisms contributing to generation of pain in primary dysmenorrhea. (From Dawood MY. Nonsteroidal anti-inflammatory drugs and reproduction. *Am J Obstet Gynecol.* 1993;169:5.)

### NONPHARMACOLOGIC INTERVENTIONS

#### Exercise

Cochrane conducted a systematic review of the literature in 2010. Only one randomized controlled trial (RCT) was included that demonstrated efficacy of aerobic exercise in reducing dysmenorrhea. The many other benefits from exercise, however, warrant its recommendation as first-line therapy for women suffering from significant dysmenorrhea (Brown, 2010).

#### Heat

Two RCTs have shown that heat applied to the low abdomen, in the form of a patch or wrap, was effective in reducing dysmenorrhea. Unlike medications, this intervention has no side effects.

### BEHAVIORAL INTERVENTIONS

In 2007, a Cochrane review revealed some evidence from five RCTs that a variety of behavioral interventions may help to reduce cyclic menstrual pain. However, the authors cautioned that the data were of limited quality with a small sample size and suffered from some methodologic limitations. Interventions that have been utilized and studied include relaxation training, biofeedback, Lamaze exercises, hypnotherapy, imagery, coping strategies, and desensitization procedures (Proctor, 2007).

### VITAMINS AND DIET

Dietary and vitamin therapies may be beneficial but, to date, have not been studied in a rigorous fashion. A low-fat vegetarian diet decreased menstrual pain in one study, and vitamin E was more effective than placebo in reducing dysmenorrhea in adolescents. Vitamins $B_1$ and $B_6$, fish oil supplements, and a Japanese herbal combination have been helpful in reducing pain compared with placebo in small trials.

## MEDICATIONS

**Nonsteroidal anti-inflammatory drugs** (NSAIDs) are first-line therapies for primary dysmenorrhea. NSAIDs are prostaglandin synthetase inhibitors (PGSIs) that have been demonstrated to alleviate symptoms of dysmenorrhea. These substances are nonsteroidal and anti-inflammatory. They are generally divided into two chemical groups: the arylcarboxylic acids, which include acetylsalicylic acid (aspirin) and fenamates (mefenamic acid), and the arylalkanoic acids, including the arylpropionic acids (ibuprofen, naproxen, and ketoprofen) and the indoleacetic acids (indomethacin). The more specific cyclooxygenase (COX-2) inhibitors such as celecoxib have similarly been shown to alleviate the primary dysmenorrheal symptoms. COX-2 expression in the uterine glandular epithelium was maximal during menstruation in one trial of ovulatory women, suggesting a possible association with the cause. The increased expression of COX-2 was eliminated with continuous use of oral contraceptives (OCs), which also offer an effective treatment (discussed later). The specific effect of these agents on the uterine musculature is reduction of contractility, as measured by reduction of intrauterine pressure. COX-2 inhibitors may be considered for women with gastrointestinal toxicity due to NSAIDs; however, these agents carry a risk of serious adverse events and now contain a black box warning. These medications therefore should only be used with caution and full disclosure.

In 2010, Marjoribanks provided a review to the Cochrane Database of RCTs of NSAIDs in the treatment of dysmenorrhea. Seventy-three RCTs were included. NSAIDs were substantially more effective than placebo in pain reduction (odds ratio [OR] 4.50, 95% confidence interval [CI]: 3.85-5.27)(Marjoribanks, 2010).

Previously, in 1984, Owen reviewed the effectiveness of NSAIDs for the treatment of primary dysmenorrhea in 51 trials carried out in 1649 women. More than 72% of the women suffering from dysmenorrhea reported significant pain relief with NSAIDs, 18% reported minimal or no pain relief, and 15% showed a placebo response. Owen concluded that PGSI compounds were effective and safe for most women with primary dysmenorrhea (Owen, 1984). The fenamates seemed to be more effective in relieving pain than ibuprofen, indomethacin, or naproxen. All the compounds demonstrated minimal NSAID-associated side effects, with the exception of indomethacin. In trials with indomethacin, the dropout rate was higher, primarily because of symptoms involving the central nervous system (CNS) and gastrointestinal (GI) tract. Efficacy with the COX-2 inhibitors is similar, although several drugs in this class have been removed from the market because of serious adverse cardiovascular events.

Smith has demonstrated that the effectiveness of NSAIDs is related to tissue concentration. Using meclofenamate in 18 subjects who participated in a double-blind, placebo-controlled, crossover study, a parallel in time response curves was seen between the plasma levels of the drug and decrease in uterine contractility. Figure 37.2 demonstrates the average intrauterine pressure relationships between placebo-treated

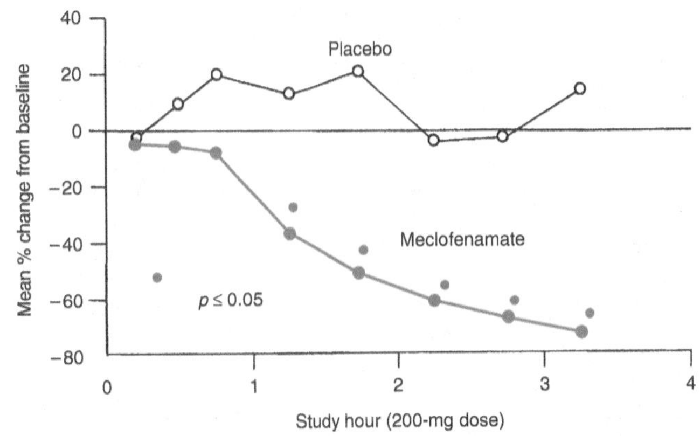


**Figure 37.2** Average pressure, meclofenamate versus placebo. (Modified from Smith RP. The dynamics of nonsteroidal anti-inflammatory therapy for primary dysmenorrhea. *Obstet Gynecol.* 1987;70:785.)

and drug-treated patients over time. Intrauterine pressure declined 20% to 56% in these patients during meclofenamate therapy (Smith, 1987).

NSAIDs should be given the day prior to the expected menses or at the onset of menses. If one NSAID is ineffective, switching to a different class of NSAIDs may be helpful. NSAIDs should not be given to patients who have shown previous hypersensitivity to such drugs. They are also contraindicated for women who have had nasal polyps, angioedema, and bronchospasm related to aspirin or NSAIDs. In addition, these agents are contraindicated for individuals with a history of chronic ulceration or inflammatory reaction of the upper or lower GI tract and for those with preexisting chronic renal disease. During the use of these agents, autoimmune hemolytic anemia, rash, edema and fluid retention, and CNS symptoms, such as dizziness, headache, nervousness, and blurred vision, can occur. In up to 15% of users, a slight elevation of hepatic enzyme levels may also be found. Table 37.2 lists some NSAIDs commonly used for the treatment of dysmenorrhea.

**Combined contraceptives** (CCs) containing estrogen and progesterone will relieve the symptoms of primary dysmenorrhea in approximately 90% of patients. This may be because CCs suppress ovulation and endometrial proliferation and the progestin component also blocks the production of the precursor to prostaglandin formation. The thinned endometrium from CCs then contains less arachidonic acid, which is the precursor to prostaglandins. If the woman also requires contraception, CC therapy may prove to be the treatment of choice.

In 2009, Wong and colleagues provided a review to the Cochrane Database of RCTs comparing combined oral contraceptives (COCs) with other COCs, placebo, and NSAIDs. Six studies revealed that COCs were significantly more effective than placebo for the treatment of dysmenorrhea (OR of 2.99, 95% CI: 1.76, 5.07) (Wong, 2009).

In small RCTs, low-dose OCs (with 20 μg ethinyl estradiol) were effective in reducing dysmenorrhea in adolescents and adult women. Continuous OC administration compared with traditional monthly cyclic dosing has been shown to reduce the menstrual pain symptoms. Breakthrough bleeding can be an undesirable side effect, although a review of RCTs reported bleeding and discontinuation rates to be similar. The extended-cycle

Table 37.2 Commonly Used Nonsteroidal Anti-inflammatory Drugs*

| Class | Brand Name | Generic Name | Usual Regimen (mg)* | Initial Dose | Subsequent Dose |
|---|---|---|---|---|---|
| Propionic acid | Motrin | Ibuprofen | 400 (qid)-800 (tid) | 500 | 250 tid-qid |
| | Naprosyn | Naproxen | 250 (qid)-500 (bid) | | |
| | Anaprox | Naproxen sodium | 275 (qid)-550 (bid) | | |
| | N/A | Ketoprofen | 25-75 (tid) | | |
| | Nalfon | Fenoprofen calcium | 200 (qid) | | |
| Fenamic acid | Ponstel | Mefenamic acid | 250 (qid) | 550 | 275 tid-qid |
| | N/A | Meclofenamate | 100 (qid) | | |
| Acetic acid | Indocin | Indomethacin | 25 (tid) | 50 | 25-50 tid-qid |
| | Voltaren | Diclofenac | 75 (bid) | | |
| | N/A | Tolmetin | 400 (tid) | | |
| | N/A | Diflunisal | 500 (bid) | | |
| | N/A | Etodolac | 400 (tid-qid) | | |
| | Toradol | Ketoralac | 10 (qid) | | |
| Oxicams | Feldene | Piroxicam | 20 (qd) | 500 | 250 qid |

*Maximum doses.

OCs available are also associated with less dysmenorrhea than are monthly cyclic OCs.

The vaginal ring CC has also been shown to reduce dysmenorrhea in a similar fashion as COCs. Dysmenorrhea was not, however, as well controlled in women using the transdermal CC patch as compared with COCs (Smith, 2016).

### *Progestin-Only Formulations*

Depot medroxyprogesterone, a long-acting injectable contraceptive, has not been studied specifically for primary dysmenorrhea. Trials in contraceptive studies report a reduction in dysmenorrhea in adolescents. Because this often causes a thinned endometrium and light menses or amenorrhea, it theoretically should be effective.

The 20 μg levonorgestrel-releasing intrauterine system (LNG-IUS) has been shown in randomized controlled trials to reduce menstrual pain. Levonorgestrel is a 19-nortestosterone derivative affecting endometrial progesterone receptors, leading to an atrophic endometrial lining. In 2013, a smaller a smaller LNG-IUS containing only 14 μg of levonorgestrel was approved by the U.S. Food and Drug Administration (FDA) and may represent another option for the management of dysmenorrhea (Smith, 2016). Of note, by comparison, the copper T380A intrauterine device (IUD) often increases dysmenorrhea.

The single-rod etonogestrel-releasing contraceptive (Implanon) has also been shown in clinical trials to reduce dysmenorrhea. This and the newer version, Nexplanon, represent additional progestin-only options.

### *Tocolytics*

Because of its ability to block uterine contractility, tocolytics may be beneficial in the treatment of dysmenorrhea. Studies using nifedipine at a dose of 20 to 40 mg orally have demonstrated pain relief. Moderate pain relief was noted in 36 of 40 women, but side effects of facial flushing, tachycardia, and headache can occur. Glyceryl trinitrate and magnesium have also been studied in limited fashion and have demonstrated effectiveness in reducing cyclic menstrual pain. Ongoing large-scale research is needed to assess safety and efficacy; therefore these medications are not often utilized for contemporary management of dysmenorrhea.

## *OTHER TREATMENTS*

Narcotic analgesics are often utilized in treating patients with chronic pain. Caution should be used, however, due to the very real potential for dependency or abuse. Short-term use may be considered as a bridge to other nonopioid options.

A meta-analysis of three trials has reported that transcutaneous electrical nerve stimulation (TENS) is more effective than placebo in relieving dysmenorrhea, although it is not as effective as analgesics. Milsom and colleagues, in Sweden, and Smith and Heltzel, in the United States, have noted that TENS relieves menstrual pain without reducing intrauterine pressure, suggesting that its mode of action may be in the CNS. High-frequency TENS provides more dysmenorrheal pain relief compared with placebo or low-frequency TENS. (Milsom, 1994; Smith, 1991).

Acupuncture and acupressure have been used for the management of dysmenorrhea. Several studies have evaluated the effectiveness of these complementary alternatives; however, they were of low quality. There is limited evidence that acupuncture may be of benefit.

A 2005 meta-analysis of eight RCTs of surgical interruption of nerve pathways concluded that there was insufficient evidence to advise laparoscopic uterine nerve ablation (LUNA) or laparoscopic presacral neurectomy (LPSN) for primary dysmenorrhea (Proctor, 2005).

## SECONDARY DYSMENORRHEA: CAUSES AND MANAGEMENT

Many other conditions cause or are associated with dysmenorrhea. Pelvic disease should be considered in patients who do not respond to NSAIDs or CCs or a combination of these agents for presumed primary dysmenorrhea. The diagnosis should also be considered when symptoms appear after many years of painless menses. Pelvic pathology may occur at any age and, in most cases, the pain experienced is secondary to the pathologic process of the condition or a specific result of it. These constitute the secondary dysmenorrhea group of problems and include cervical stenosis, endometriosis, adenomyosis, fibroids, pelvic inflammation, pelvic congestion, congenital obstructive müllerian

**Box 37.1 Causes of Secondary Dysmenorrhea**

**Gynecologic Pathology**
Cervical stenosis
Endometriosis and adenomyosis
Pelvic infection and adhesions
Uterine polyps or fibroids
Ovarian cyst or mass
Pelvic congestion
Congenital obstructed müllerian malformations

**Nongynecologic Disorders Causing Pelvic Pain**
Mental health issues/disorders
- Somatization
- Depression
- Drug-seeking behavior and opioid dependency
- History of physical or sexual abuse

Bowel disease
Irritable bowel syndrome
Inflammatory bowel disease
Celiac sprue
Lactose intolerance
Urinary tract disease
Ureteral obstruction
Interstitial cystitis
Nephrolithiasis

malformations, diseases of the gastrointestinal tract, and mental health conditions (Box 37.1)(Howard, 2013).

## CERVICAL STENOSIS

Severe narrowing of the cervical canal, particularly at the level of the internal os, may impede menstrual flow, causing an increase in intrauterine pressure at the time of menses. In addition, retrograde menstrual flow through the fallopian tubes into the peritoneal cavity may take place. Thus severe cervical stenosis may eventually be associated with pelvic endometriosis as well. The origin of cervical stenosis may be congenital or secondary to cervical injury, such as with electrocautery, cryocautery, or operative trauma (e.g., conization). The condition may also result from an inflammatory process caused by infection, the application of caustic substances, or hypoestrogenism. After any of these conditions, the cervical canal may narrow because of the contraction of scar tissue.

The possibility of cervical stenosis should be considered if there is a history of scant menstrual flow and if severe cramping continues throughout the menstrual period. Hematometra or pyometra may occur.

The diagnosis is suspected when the external os appears scarred or when it is impossible to pass a cervical Pap smear brush or uterine sound through the internal os during the proliferative stage of the menstrual cycle. Diagnosis is generally documented by the inability to pass a thin probe of a few millimeters' diameter through the internal os or by a hysterosalpingogram, which demonstrates a thin, stringy-appearing canal. If hysteroscopy and dilation and curettage (D&C) are performed, finding the passage through the internal os with a thin probe is often difficult but can frequently be accomplished with patience. Ultrasound guidance can be of great benefit to reduce the risk of making a false passage. Having the woman self-administer buccal or intravaginal misoprostol before the procedure may aid in the ease with which cervical dilation can be accomplished.

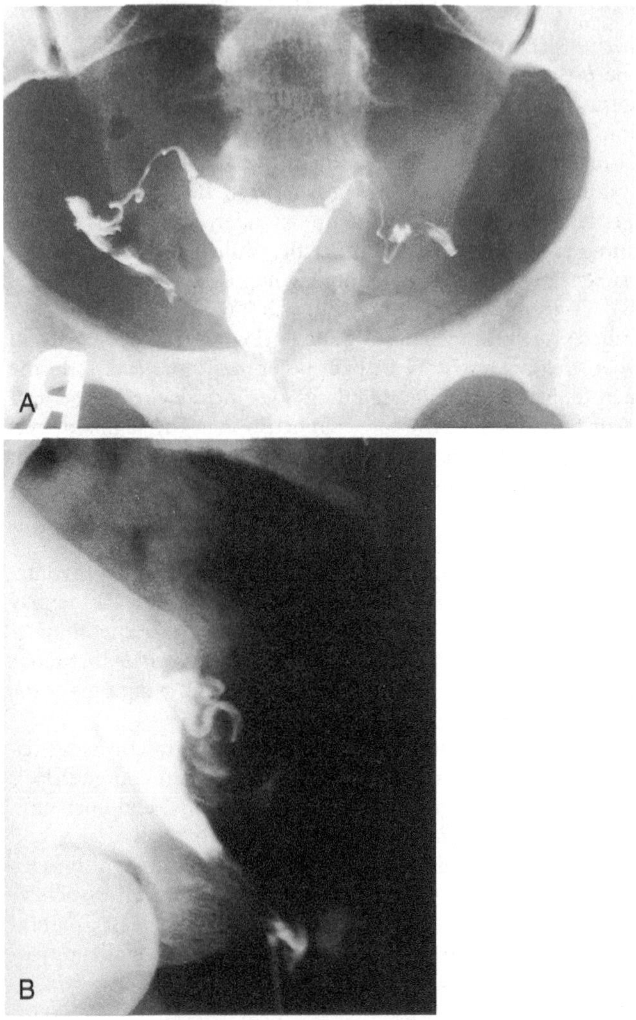


**Figure 37.3** Hysterogram. Anteroposterior (**A**) view and lateral (**B**) views of an 18-year-old patient with severe disabling dysmenorrhea. At hysteroscopy, she was found to have a tissue band across the internal os and an endocervical polyp at this site. Removal of the polyp and transection of the band completely relieved the dysmenorrhea.

Misoprostol is not FDA approved for this particular indication, but many studies have evaluated its effectiveness for procedures such as IUD insertion and hysteroscopy.

Treatment consists of dilating the cervix, which may be accomplished by D&C with progressive dilators or by the use of progressive *Laminaria* tents. Unfortunately, cervical stenosis often recurs after therapy, necessitating repeat procedures. Pregnancy and vaginal delivery often afford a more lasting cure.

Often other problems obstructing the cervix can have a similar presentation. Figure 37.3 shows anteroposterior and lateral views of a hysterogram in an 18-year-old nulliparous woman who had a 2-year history of severe disabling dysmenorrhea that usually required morphine therapy with each menstrual period. At hysteroscopy, she was found to have a tissue band across her internal os, at which site a large endocervical polyp had formed. Transecting the band and removing the polyp completely relieved the dysmenorrhea, and she had no further symptoms after 3 years.

## ECTOPIC ENDOMETRIAL TISSUE

### Endometriosis

The presence of endometrial glands and stroma outside of the uterus defines endometriosis. Endometriosis is a chronic condition that may manifest in generalized pelvic pain, cyclic pain, dysmenorrhea, dyspareunia, infertility, and bowel or bladder dysfunction. This condition affects 6% to 10% of reproductive age women and is found in approximately 70% to 80% with chronic pelvic pain (ACOG, Practice Bulletin #114). Approximately one third of women undergoing diagnostic laparoscopy due to chronic pelvic pain (CPP) will have endometriosis confirmed visually or by biopsy. Endometriosis should be considered when there is a history of pain becoming more severe during menses. Pertinent physical findings may include uterosacral ligament nodules, evidence for endometriosis in the vagina or cervix, and lateral displacement of the cervix. Treatment options for endometriosis are discussed in Chapter 19.

### Adenomyosis

The presence of endometrial glands and stroma in the myometrium defines adenomyosis. This ectopic endometrial tissue may induce hypertrophy and hyperplasia of the adjacent myometrium. It typically manifests in heavy, painful menses that tends to be progressive. Women may appreciate bulk symptoms as the uterus enlarges.

Koike and colleagues, in an in vitro experiment using tissue slices, found that the prostaglandin level in endometriosis implants is significantly higher than in normal endometrium, myometrium, leiomyomata, and normal ovarian tissue, and that adenomyosis implants produce larger amounts of 6-keto-PGF1 when the dysmenorrhea has been severe. They believe that prostaglandins in these conditions increase painful menstruation(Koike, 1994). Treatment options for adenomyosis are discussed in Chapter 18.

## PELVIC INFLAMMATION

Pelvic infections secondary to gonorrhea, chlamydia, or other microbes may cause pelvic inflammation or pelvic abscess and, with healing, may be associated with pelvic adhesions and tubal damage that may cause pelvic pain. Pelvic inflammatory disease (PID) can lead to chronic pelvic pain in up to 30% of women. This may often be aggravated during menses, causing dysmenorrhea. Infections secondary to other conditions, such as appendicitis or IUD use, may create a similar response. The pain may be secondary to the congestion and edema that occur normally at menses, which may subsequently be aggravated by the healed inflammatory areas and adhesions. Pelvic infections are further discussed in Chapter 23.

## PELVIC CONGESTION SYNDROME AND PELVIC VENOUS SYNDROMES

**Pelvic congestion syndrome** (PCS), which was first described by Taylor in 1949, results from the engorgement of pelvic vasculature. Controversy exists regarding whether this is an actual disorder because it has been difficult to prove. It is a poorly understood disorder of the pelvic venous circulation. PCS is defined by chronic pelvic discomfort (often burning or throbbing in nature) worsened by prolonged standing and intercourse in women who have periovarian varicosities on imaging studies. The etiology of PCS is unclear and the optimum treatment is uncertain. Development of an evidence-based approach to managing these patients has been limited by the absence of definitive diagnostic criteria.

Physical examination of the vagina and cervix may reveal vasocongestion, uterine enlargement and global tenderness of the cervix, uterus, and adnexa on palpation. Diagnosis is made by history and physical imaging, such as pelvic ultrasound, venography, computed tomography (CT), or magnetic resonance imaging (MRI), and by laparoscopy, which not only rules out other causes of pelvic pain but also demonstrates congestion of the uterus and engorgement or varicosities of the broad ligament and pelvic sidewall veins. If laparoscopy is used for diagnosis, it is important to observe the broad ligament vasculature as the pressure of the carbon dioxide or nitrous oxide is released. At full pressure during the procedure, these vessels may collapse as the pneumoperitoneal pressure exceeds venous pressure, but the dilated veins will reappear as pressure is released.

Other pelvic venous syndromes have been described that can cause pelvic pain and probably include what Taylor first described (Taylor, 1949). Vulvar varices, hypogastric vein insufficiency, and gonadal venous insufficiency have been described in a review of 57 female patients ages 24 to 48 years. Symptoms included pelvic pain, dysuria, dysmenorrhea, and dyspareunia. These disorders are poorly understood and poorly studied, so they often go undiagnosed. Diagnosis in this study was made by physical examination and a variety of radiologic investigations, including Doppler scans, duplex ultrasound scans, CT, MRI, and angiography. No standard therapeutic approach is available, so therapies range from ovarian hormone suppression, local sclerotherapy (for vulvar varices), and embolization of the hypogastric vein to resection of the gonadal vein to hysterectomy. A 2010 systematic review by Tu and coworkers has found 6 diagnostic and 22 treatment studies, but no consensus on diagnostic studies or treatment, although progestins and gonadotropin-releasing hormone (GnRH) agonists were effective in decreasing pain symptoms (Tu, 2010).

## MENTAL HEALTH CONDITIONS

In individuals with strong family histories of dysmenorrhea, or when a careful history demonstrates a possibility for societal reward or control because of the symptoms of pain, a conditioned behavior should be considered. It is important to obtain a careful medical and social history and to rule out all other causes of acquired dysmenorrhea. Conditions that may manifest in chronic pelvic pain including dysmenorrhea include somatization, opiate dependency, history of physical or sexual abuse, and depression. Women with chronic pelvic pain often have psychological issues, so careful evaluation of the patient's past and present social situation, administering a depression screen, and performing a mental status exam may be revealing. Referral to a mental health provider may be beneficial for further diagnostic testing, counseling, or medical therapy.

## RELATION TO FUNCTIONAL BOWEL DISEASE

Crowell and coworkers studied 383 women ages 20 to 40 using a Neuroticism-Extraversion-Openness (NEO) Personality Inventory on entry into the program, a Moos' Menstrual Distress Questionnaire, and a bowel symptom inventory every 3 months for 12

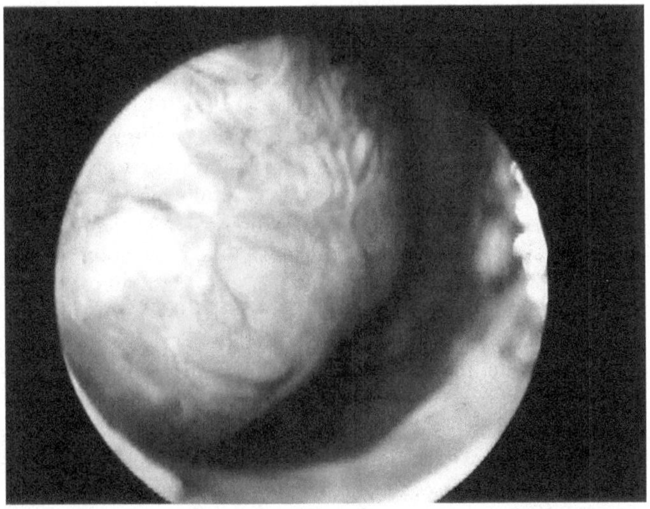

**Figure 37.4** Submucous myoma blocking the internal os causing secondary dysmenorrhea.

months. Dysmenorrhea was diagnosed in 19.8% of these women. Functional bowel disorder, defined as abdominal pain with altered bowel function, occurred in 61% of the women with dysmenorrhea but in only 20% of the others ($P < .05$) (Crowell, 1994). Bowel symptoms were significantly correlated with dysmenorrhea, even after controlling for the effects of neuroticism. Prostaglandin levels in vaginal fluid were elevated in patients with dysmenorrhea but did not consistently differentiate the diagnostic groups. It was concluded that there was a strong covariance of menstrual and bowel symptoms, along with an overlap in their diagnosis, suggesting a common physiologic basis.

In a study of women with irritable bowel syndrome (IBS) and menstrual cycle symptoms, dysmenorrhea was twice as prevalent among women with IBS than controls (21% versus 10%; $P = .09$), although this was not statistically significant. Women with IBS on OCs had significantly less dysmenorrhea than women in the control group who were not on OCs (11% versus 28%, $P = .02$). One case report found an association of celiac sprue and dysmenorrhea, but little is known about this finding.

### OTHER CAUSES

At times, dysmenorrhea may be related to unusual pathologic findings. These include small leiomyomas or polyps at the junction of the internal os and lower uterine segment (Fig. 37.4). Such a condition may produce a valvelike effect at the os at the time of menses. Frequently, myomas or polyps become engorged or edematous at the time of menses, accentuating the problem. Diagnosis is generally made by history and by saline infusion sonohysterography, hysterosalpingography, or hysteroscopy. Therapy consists of excising the pathologic tissue. In the case of a myoma, a myomectomy or hysterectomy may be necessary.

There are nongynecologic causes for pain during menses that should be considered in the differential diagnosis. These include appendicitis, lactose intolerance, celiac sprue, abdominal mass, and a number of urinary tract conditions (e.g., urinary tract infection, interstitial cystitis, nephrolithiasis, ureteral obstruction).

## PREMENSTRUAL SYNDROME AND PREMENSTRUAL DYSPHORIC DISORDER

Premenstrual syndrome (PMS) is defined as a group of mild to moderate symptoms, physical and behavioral, that occur in the second half of the menstrual cycle and that may interfere with work and personal relationships. Common physical complaints include breast tenderness, bloating, and headache. Common behavioral symptoms may include irritability, anxiety, and depression. These are followed by a period entirely free of symptoms. Frank first described the condition in 1931 and attempted to relate symptoms of then so-called *premenstrual tension* with hormonal changes of the menstrual cycle (Frank, 1931). The term *premenstrual syndrome* was first used by Dalton in 1953. The symptoms vary from woman to woman, and more than 150 symptoms have been linked with the disorder.

Premenstrual dysphoric disorder (PMDD) represents a more severe disorder, with marked behavioral and emotional symptoms. This condition is included in the American Psychiatric Association *Diagnostic and Statistical Manual,* fifth edition (DSM-V) (APA, 2014). PMDD differs from PMS in the severity of symptoms and the fact that women with PMDD must have one severe affective symptom. These include markedly depressed mood or hopelessness, anxiety or tension, affective lability, or persistent anger, which occur regularly during the last week of the luteal phase in most menstrual cycles. A number of physical symptoms may also be present. PMDD also differs from PMS because there is substantial impairment in personal functioning (Box 37.2). PMS and PMDD are similar in that the symptoms manifest in the luteal phase of the menstrual cycle and resolve during menses.

### INCIDENCE AND EPIDEMIOLOGY

Premenstrual symptoms occur in 75% of women at some point in their reproductive lives. The incidence of clinically relevant PMS occurs in 3% to 8% of women. Using DSM-V diagnostic criteria, 2% of reproductive-age women will suffer from PMDD (Yonkers, 2016). The average age of onset is 26 years. Likely risk factors for PMS include family history of PMS in the mother, personal past or current psychiatric illness involving mood or anxiety disorders, history of alcohol abuse, and history of postpartum depression. Some studies have found that nulliparity, earlier menarche, higher alcohol and caffeine intake, more stress, and higher body mass index are risk factors for certain PMS symptoms. Studies have supported earlier reports that familial and stress factors play a role in the syndrome. Younger women may experience more severe symptoms of PMDD. Some racial and ethnic differences have been reported, but PMS appears consistently in all cultures studied. Data from a California HMO PMS severity study of 1194 women found that Hispanics reported greater severity of symptoms than whites and blacks, and Asian women reported less (Sternfeld, 2002). Similar to PMS, PMDD prevalence is noted in many countries studied, including Croatia, Italy, Iceland, and Japan. A Japanese study found a 1.2% prevalence of PMDD, suggesting a cultural difference in prevalence or reporting (Gehlert, 2009).

In the Harvard Study of Moods and Cycles by Cohen and colleagues, a population-based, cross-sectional sample of 4164

**Box 37.2 Premenstrual Dysphoric Disorder, DSM-V**

**Diagnostic Criteria**
**625.4 (N94.3)**

A. In the majority of menstrual cycles, at least five symptoms must be present in the final week before the onset of menses, start to *improve* within a few days after the onset of menses, and become *minimal* or absent in the week postmenses.
B. One (or more) of the following symptoms must be present:
   - Marked affective lability (e.g., mood swings; feeling suddenly sad or tearful, or increased sensitivity to rejection).
   - Marked irritability or anger or increased interpersonal conflicts.
   - Marked depressed mood, feelings of hopelessness, or self-deprecating thoughts.
   - Marked anxiety, tension, and/or feelings of being keyed up or on edge.
C. One (or more) of the following symptoms must additionally be present, to reach a total of *five* symptoms when combined with symptoms from Criterion B above.
   - Decreased interest in usual activities (e.g., work, school, friends, hobbies).
   - Subjective difficulty in concentration.
   - Lethargy, easy fatigability, or marked lack of energy.
   - Marked change in appetite; overeating; or specific food cravings.
   - Hypersomnia or insomnia.
   - A sense of being overwhelmed or out of control.
   - Physical symptoms such as breast tenderness or swelling, joint or muscle pain, a sensation of "bloating," or weight gain.

   *Note:* The symptoms in Criteria A–C must have been met for most menstrual cycles that occurred in the preceding year.
D. The symptoms are associated with clinically significant distress or interference with work, school, usual social activities, or relationships with others (e.g., avoidance of social activities; decreased productivity and efficiency at work, school, or home).
E. The disturbance is not merely an exacerbation of the symptoms of another disorder, such as major depressive disorder, panic disorder, persistent depressive disorder (dysthymia), or a personality disorder (although it may co-occur with any of these disorders).
F. Criterion A should be confirmed by prospective daily ratings during at least two symptomatic cycles. (**Note:** The diagnosis may be made provisionally prior to this confirmation.)
G. The symptoms are not attributable to the physiological effects of a substance (e.g., a drug of abuse, a medication, other treatment) or another medical condition (e.g., hyperthyroidism).

From American Psychiatric Association (APA). Premenstrual dysphoric disorder. In: *Diagnostic and Statistical Manual of Mental Disorders.* 5th ed (DSM-V). American Psychiatric Association: Arlington, VA; 2014.

premenopausal women was studied retrospectively regarding PMDD prevalence. A PMDD diagnosis was made in 6.4% of the women, and PMDD was associated with lower education, a history of major depression, and current smoking (Cohen, 2002). This confirms the results of earlier studies reporting a significant lifetime comorbidity of PMDD and affective disorders. Past sexual abuse has been reported more frequently in women attending PMS clinics compared with women in the general population.

## SYMPTOMS

In a review by O'Brien, a number of common somatic and affective symptoms were enumerated (see Box 37.2). The most common somatic symptoms relate to abdominal bloating, breast tenderness, and various pain constellations, such as headache. Psychological symptoms vary from fatigue, irritability, and tension to anxiety, labile mood, and depression (O'Brien, 1982). In Sternfeld and associates' severity of PMS symptoms study in a health maintenance organization (HMO) population of 1194 women, consistency of symptoms was found over two consecutive cycles, especially for emotional symptoms (Sternfeld, 2002).

Depression is a common complaint in the population in general and also in PMS-PMDD sufferers during the luteal phase. Mortola and coworkers have shown that 16 PMS patients had marked worsening of scores on the Profile of Mood States and Beck Depression Inventory during the luteal phase compared with 16 controls. However, six patients suffering from endogenous depression had scores threefold higher on both indices than PMS patients who were in the luteal phase. Also, the amplitude of cortisol secretion pulses was higher in the depressed patients than in the PMS patients or control patients (Mortola, 1989). The data demonstrate that PMS patients have more episodes of depression during the luteal phase compared with controls, but these episodes are distinctly different from those suffered by patients with endogenous depression. The National Institute of Mental Health's Sequenced Treatment Alternatives to Relieve Depression (STAR-D) trial of clinically depressed women found that 64% of 433 subjects not on OCs reported worsening of their depressive symptoms before menses (Kornstein, 2005). Therefore it can be challenging to differentiate women with PMS from women with depression and premenstrual exacerbations of depressive symptoms.

In addition, Rapkin and colleagues have demonstrated that PMS patients show no deficit in cognitive processing and performance, as well as no loss in ability to concentrate and sustain attention and motivation. No such alterations were seen in 10 PMS patients during the luteal phase. Their performance was similar to nine controls when tested in these areas (Rapkin, 1989). In a later study, this group studied 30 patients with PMS and 31 controls during the follicular and luteal phases. Despite feelings of inadequacy, patients showed no statistically significant differences from controls in tests for attention, memory, cognitive flexibility, and overall mental agility.

A PMS diagnosis not only affects quality of life but also economic issues. Slight increases in direct costs (medical expenses) have been noted. Indirect costs to the employer in work absence and lost productivity amount to $4333/patient annually.

## CAUSES

When Frank first described the syndrome, it was attributed to estrogen excess. Others have offered theories that the disorder is related to an imbalance of estrogen and progesterone, endogenous hormone allergy, hypoglycemia, vitamin $B_6$ deficiency, prolactin excess, fluid retention, inappropriate prostaglandin activity, elevated monoamine oxidase (MAO) levels, endorphin malfunction, and a number of psychological disturbances. In 1981, Reid and Yen reviewed the subject and concluded that PMS was a multifactorial psychoendocrine disorder (Reid, 1981). Figure 37.5 shows a schematic of the proposed causes. Studies indicate that cyclic gonadal hormonal alterations and serotonergic neuronal mechanisms in the CNS may interact and be major causative factors for PMS in susceptible women. Evidence for this conclusion is indirect but includes successful clinical trials with selective serotonin

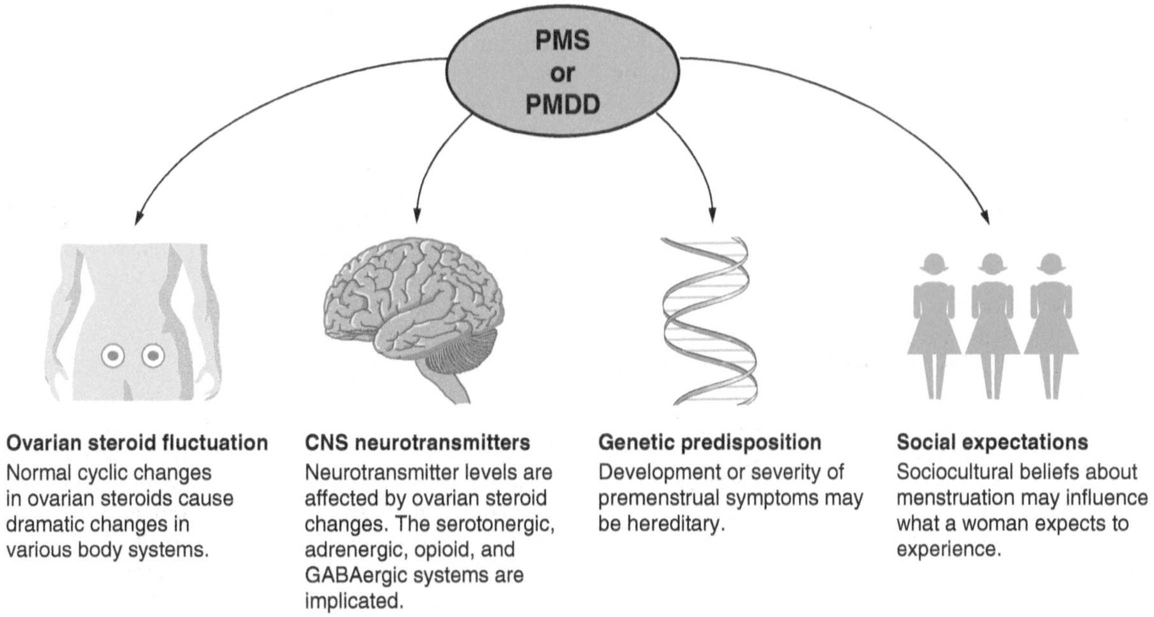


**Figure 37.5** Proposed causes of premenstrual syndrome and premenstrual dysphoric disorder. *GABA*, γ-Aminobutyric acid. (From Ling F, Mortola J, Pariser S, et al. *Premenstrual Syndrome and Premenstrual Dysphoric Disorder: Scope, Diagnosis, and Treatment.* Crofton, MD: Association of Professors of Gynecology and Obstetrics; 1998.)

reuptake inhibitors (SSRIs) and other neurotropic agents thought to affect the serotonin pump mechanism between CNS neurons. Other indirect evidence includes the fact that platelet tritium-labeled, imipramine-binding sites are thought to be reduced in patients suffering from depression and are believed to represent receptor sites that label for a presynaptic serotonin transporter on the presynaptic nerve terminal. In some studies, binding sites returned to normal several months after clinical remission of depression or during the response to psychotropic medications or electroconvulsive therapy. These platelet-binding sites have therefore been used as an indirect measure of the neuron receptor site. Steege and coworkers have demonstrated lower platelet tritium-labeled imipramine binding in women with late luteal phase dysphoric disorder (now called *PMDD*); they believe that this result supported the hypothesis that such patients suffer from alterations of the central serotonergic systems (Steege, 1992). More recently, beta-endorphin and gamma-aminobutyric acid (GABA) neurotransmitters have been implicated. Estrogen has been found to modulate neurotransmitters such as GABA and dopamine, which may serve as inhibitory or excitatory agents in the brain.

That ovarian steroids and, in particular, ovulation and therefore progesterone production are important in this syndrome has been known for some time. Studies related to the relationship of estrogen and progesterone in the circulation and the severity of the symptoms have not been fruitful. There are no consistent differences between estrogen and progesterone levels in PMS sufferers and those in controls. These women may have an abnormal response to normal cyclic ovarian steroid changes. Although symptom relief has been noted in several studies using GnRH agonists to block ovulation completely, no relief was found in a study by Chan and colleagues, who blocked progesterone receptors with the progesterone antagonist RU-486 (Chan, 1994). Rapkin and colleagues have evaluated the anxiolytic 3α, 5α reduced progesterone metabolite allopregnanediol during the luteal phase of 35 women with PMS and 36 controls (Rapkin, 1997). Serum progesterone and allopregnanediol levels were measured on days 19 and 26 of the cycles as determined by luteinizing hormone (LH) kits. Allopregnanediol levels were significantly lower in the PMS patients than controls on day 26, but there were no significant differences with respect to progesterone itself. They concluded that because PMS patients had lower levels of this anxiolytic metabolite during the luteal phase, they could be at greater susceptibility for various mood symptoms such as anxiety, tension, and depression. Allopregnanediol enhances GABA-A receptor function. Chuong and associates have demonstrated that beta-endorphin levels throughout the periovulatory phase are lower in PMS patients than in controls, especially in postovulatory days 0 to 4 (Chuong, 1994). Similarly, Halbreich and coworkers have demonstrated that PMS patients treated with 200 mg/day of danazol for 90 days have complete relief of symptoms in 23 anovulatory cycles, but relief of symptoms occurred in only 6 of 32 ovulatory cycles. They concluded that the beneficial effect of danazol in the treatment of PMS was achieved only when the anovulatory state eliminated the hormonal cyclicity of the normal cycle and not because of action of the drug per se (Halbreich, 1991). O'Brien and Abukhalil have advanced further evidence for this conclusion. They studied 100 women with PMS and premenstrual breast pain using a randomized, double-blind, placebo-controlled study of three menstrual cycles, using danazol, 200 mg/day, as the active drug. Treatment was given only during the luteal phase. Danazol did not effectively reduce the general symptoms of PMS, but it did relieve mastalgia (O'Brien, 1999). Severe PMS has been shown to be relieved by total abdominal hysterectomy and bilateral salpingo-oophorectomy, even with hormone replacement therapy using an estrogen, but some women on cyclic estrogen and progesterone therapy postmenopausally continue to complain of PMS symptoms. A 2003 study by Roca and colleagues has suggested that women with PMS may have an abnormal response to progesterone. Women with PMS failed to show a normal increased luteal phase hypothalamic-pituitary-adrenal axis response to exercise stress testing compared with controls

(Roca, 2003). This response is distinctly different in PMS patients compared with women with major depression.

Another potential causative factor is a genetic contribution. Twin studies have demonstrated a high heritability of PMS symptoms; the concordance rate is twice as high in monozygotic twins than in dizygotic twins.

Concerning other possible causes, most dietary and vitamin deficiency theories have been difficult to prove and have not been found to be a major cause of this syndrome. However, data from Bertone-Johnson and associates' case-control study involving the Nurses' Health Study II cohort (2005) have suggested that a high intake of calcium and vitamin D may reduce the risk of PMS, so further research is needed. Several studies have looked for prolactin excess because some of the women complain of breast tenderness, but no positive findings have been found. Although some of the symptomatology seems to relate to prostaglandin activity, and these symptoms are often reduced with treatment with NSAIDs, a direct cause and effect has not been established.

In summary, the cause of PMS and PMDD is associated with ovarian steroids and ovulation, which seem to produce alterations in neurohormones and neurotransmitters that lead to a reduction of serotonergic function during the luteal phase. The most effective evidence-based treatment for moderate to severe PMS and PMDD symptoms are SSRIs and agents that block ovulation. The temporal relationship between menstrual phase PMS and PMDD symptoms suggests a role of the reproductive hormones—not a direct linear role, but a more complex vulnerability to these cyclic hormonal shifts. Only 60% of women with PMDD respond to SSRI treatment, so serotonergic dysfunction may not be the only pathway involved. Beta-endorphin, GABA, the autonomic nervous system, and social expectations may all play a role in these complex disorders.

## DIAGNOSIS

The diagnosis of PMS and PMDD is made by the history of two consecutive menstrual cycles demonstrating luteal phase symptoms of PMS and PMDD. The facts given by the woman may allow the physician to construct a specific, individualized treatment regimen. It is important that the physician have a clear understanding of the woman's symptoms before undertaking therapy. After a complete history and physical examination, the physician should rule out any medical problems that could be influencing the symptomatology. There is limited utility in blood tests; however, it is reasonable to screen for thyroid disease with a serum thyroid-stimulating hormone (TSH). The physician should then ask the woman to keep a diary of her symptoms throughout two menstrual cycles. Although she and her physician may focus on the second half of the menstrual cycle, the woman should be encouraged to keep track of all symptoms, regardless of the stage of the menstrual cycle. A number of validated tools with diary sheets and symptom checklists are available. The Daily Record of Severity of Problems (DRSP) is most commonly utilized. It can be useful to have the woman write the symptoms that she perceives in her own words using validated visual analog scales rather than give her clues to specific response patterns. It is necessary to track symptoms for a full 2 months in order to compare follicular phase symptoms to luteal and menstrual phase data. At the end of two cycles, the physician should review the symptom diary with the woman and carefully discuss those symptoms that seem to be causing her the most difficulty. A change in the symptom severity score between 30% and 50% between the follicular and luteal phases suggests PMS and PMDD. It can be challenging for women to complete a diary with 2 months of symptoms.

The American College of Obstetricians and Gynecologists (ACOG) defines PMS as the presence of at least one symptom during the luteal phase of the cycle leading to significant impairment in functioning. It is important to differentiate PMS from other illnesses with similar symptomatology. Women with depression and anxiety disorders may present believing that they have PMS. A differentiating aspect is that PMS patients suffer their symptoms only during the luteal phase. Diagnosis can be difficult because women with depression and anxiety disorders can have premenstrual exacerbation of their symptoms, and PMS and PMDD can coexist with psychiatric disorders.

Many women who do not actually have PMS may be self-referred to a facility that treats this condition. In one study, Plouffe and coworkers carefully analyzed 100 consecutive women prospectively entering the uniform diagnostic and treatment protocol for PMS and found that 38 women had PMS, 24 had premenstrual magnification syndrome (i.e., other conditions that were magnified during the luteal phase), and 13 had affective or other psychiatric disorders. Only 44% of the women previously given a diagnosis of PMS were found to have this syndrome. Overall, in this study, 84% of the women with PMS and premenstrual magnification syndrome responded to treatment (Plouffe, 1993). A variety of currently accepted therapies were used.

Other conditions to consider based on patient symptoms include anemia, diabetes, endometriosis, autoimmune disorders, chronic fatigue syndrome, collagen vascular disorders, and many psychiatric disorders (e.g., depression, anxiety, dysthymia, bipolar disorder).

The diagnosis of PMS is therefore made by symptom diary and by the elimination of other diagnoses.

The diagnosis of PMDD is made following the DSM-V criteria, which require 5 of 11 symptoms of PMS, including one affective symptom (APA, 2014). These symptoms should be occurring for most of the preceding year. Affective symptoms include feeling sad or hopeless or having self-deprecating thoughts, anxiety or tension, mood lability and crying, and persistent irritability, anger, and increased interpersonal conflicts. Prospective menstrual cycle charting is required for the diagnosis. Box 37.3 lists physical and psychiatric disorders that should be considered in the differential diagnosis of PMDD.

**Box 37.3 Considerations in the Differential Diagnosis of Premenstrual Dysphoric Disorder**

Premenstrual syndrome
Endometriosis
Dysmenorrhea
Physical disorders with premenstrual exacerbations
Autoimmune disorders
Diabetes mellitus
Anemia
Hypothyroidism
Psychiatric disorders with luteal phase exacerbation
Depression
Anxiety
Dysthymic disorder
Bipolar disorder

## TREATMENT

### Diet, Supplements, Exercise, and Lifestyle Changes

Reassuring women with mild PMS without serious coexisting gynecologic disorders that this is a common problem should be part of the counseling. Thus the selection of medications and lifestyle changes should be tailored to the symptomatic needs of the patient. Lifestyle modifications can be recommended for 2 months while the woman completes the prospective diary for diagnosis.

Several dietary studies have been performed, but most were not rigorously controlled. Two trials have studied increasing complex carbohydrate intake, which reduced the severity of PMS mood symptoms. Complex carbohydrates may increase tryptophan availability and thereby increase serotonin. Because food cravings or increased appetite, mood changes, sleep disturbances and irritability, and fluid retention are listed among the key 17 symptoms, symptom severity may be affected by reducing or eliminating sugar, alcohol, caffeine, salty foods, and red meat.

A multicenter RCT of 466 women has shown that 1200 mg of calcium/day for three cycles reduces PMS symptoms significantly compared with placebo (48% versus 30%; $P < .001$) (Thys-Jacobs, 1998). This is a treatment to cautiously consider, as some amount of calcium supplementation is helpful for bone health. Caution must be taken, however, as higher supplementation may be linked to heart disease.

Vitamin $B_6$ (pyridoxine) deficiency in PMS patients has been suggested because vitamin $B_6$ is a coenzyme in the biosynthesis of dopamine and serotonin, and neurotransmitters have been implicated in the cause of PMS. A review of nine RCTs of vitamin $B_6$ for the treatment PMS found no high-quality trials, although several suggested relief of PMS symptoms over placebo (Wyatt, 1999). A double-blind placebo-controlled trial of 94 women with PMDD found a greater decrease in psychiatric symptoms with 80 mg of vitamin $B_6$ (Kashanian, 2007). Vitamin $B_6$ supplement at the rate of 50 mg/day can be tried for mild PMS symptoms. Higher doses of pyridoxine should be administered with caution because neuropathy can occur in patients treated with as little as 200 mg/day. Other side effects, such as sensory deficit, paresthesia, numbness, ataxia, and muscle weakness, may occur.

There is inconclusive evidence from four RCTs that magnesium (200 to 400 mg/day) reduces PMS symptoms (Canning, 2006)

Patients should be encouraged to regularly exercise for general health reasons. A general recommendation is exercise for at least 30 minutes, on most days of the week, including during the luteal phase when symptoms are present. Small trials have suggested aerobic exercise to be beneficial for PMS sufferers, and one trial found high-intensity aerobic exercise to be superior to low-intensity aerobic exercise for PMS treatment.

Many other adjunct treatments as well as complementary and alternative medicines (CAMs) have been studied. These therapies include massage, biofeedback, yoga, acupuncture, chiropractic manipulation, evening primrose oil, and Chinese herbal medicines. A 2009 Cochrane review concluded that there is insufficient evidence to recommend the use of Chinese herbal therapies for this condition (Jing, 2009). A systematic review of several trials has suggested that of all the alternative therapies, bright light therapy, which may increase serotonin, may be a reasonable option for PMDD. Avoiding stressful activities in the luteal phase and having enough sleep may also alleviate PMS and PMDD symptoms.

### Cognitive Behavioral Therapy

Studies in the 1950s showed that 50% of patients improved with psychotherapy alone. More recently, Lustyk and coworkers reviewed seven studies, three of which were RCTs, and reported efficacy of cognitive behavioral therapy for the management of PMS and PMDD (Lustyk, 2009). If patients have obvious psychiatric problems, as detected by history, psychotherapy should be added, but it is less effective as a primary therapy. Group psychoeducation in managing symptoms of PMS has been efficacious. Relaxation therapy may benefit patients with significant stress and anxiety components.

### Pharmacologic Agents

#### Psychoactive Drugs

SSRIs have been shown to be extremely effective for treating PMS and have become first-line treatment for PMDD. In 2013, a Cochrane review included 31 RCTs studying 4372 women affected with PMS. Included studies compared paroxetine, sertraline, escitalopram, fluoxetine, or citalopram versus placebo. The authors concluded that both continuous and luteal phase SSRIs were effective for PMS (Marjoribanks, 2013). Medication dosages are generally lower than those used for depression. The onset of action can be rapid, within 1 to 2 days, unlike when SSRIs are used for depression (for dosing, see Table 37.3). Some patients may prefer a luteal phase regimen as it is less expensive and has fewer side effects. This is started on cycle day 14 and continues until the onset of menses or for a few more days thereafter. Even for PMDD, using the psychoactive drugs in only the luteal phase of the menstrual cycle can be effective. However, Shah and colleagues' 2008 meta-analysis of 20 RCTs and 2964 women found that SSRIs are effective for treating PMS and PMDD (OR 0.40; 95% confidence interval [CI]: 0.31-0.51), but intermittent dosing was less effective (OR 0.55) than continuous dosing (OR 0.28) (Shah, 2008). If luteal phase treatment is not effective after 3 months, a trial of continuous SSRIs is warranted. No SSRI was demonstrably better than another. If one SSRI is ineffective, other agents may still be effective. SSRIs are effective in approximately 60% of PMS sufferers. Venlafaxine, a serotonin and norepinephrine reuptake inhibitor, has also been found in RCTs to be more effective than placebo (Freeman, 2001). This medication may be helpful for patients who have side effects or no benefit on other SSRIs. After three cycles of SSRI treatment for PMDD, symptoms recurred with the first cycle after drug discontinuation, suggesting that prolonged therapy may be necessary. Serious adverse effects can occur and must be weighed against the severity of the woman's symptoms.

Approximately 15% of women on SSRIs have significant side effects, including sexual dysfunction (anorgasmia), sleep alterations, GI distress (including nausea), and CNS complaints such

**Table 37.3** SSRIs for Premenstrual Dysphoric Disorder

| SSRI | Effective Doses |
|---|---|
| Fluoxetine hydrochloride | 20 mg/day |
| Sertraline hydrochloride | 50-150 mg/day |
| Paroxetine hydrochloride | 20-30 mg/day |
| Paroxetine controlled release (CR) | 25 mg/day |
| Citalopram | 20-30 mg/day |
| Escitalopram | 10-20 mg/day |

as headache and jitteriness. Some SSRIs can precipitate anxiety reactions, so caution should be used if anxiety symptoms predominate. Increased suicide rates have been observed with some SSRIs, so caution is needed if significant depressive symptoms are noted. This should be a low risk, given the low dose and intermittent luteal phase dosing.

In a carefully performed double-blind, placebo-controlled, crossover study of 19 patients suffering from PMS using alprazolam (Xanax), Smith and coworkers noted that the drug significantly relieved the severity of premenstrual nervous tension, mood swings, irritability, anxiety, depression, fatigue, forgetfulness, crying, cravings for sweets, abdominal bloating, cramps, and headaches compared with the placebo. They prescribed alprazolam, 0.25 mg three times/day, on days 20 to 28 of each cycle and then tapering to 0.25 mg twice daily on day 1 and 0.25 mg on day 2 (Smith 1987). Several RCTs have shown that doses higher than 0.75 mg/day are necessary to reduce PMS symptoms significantly. Alprazolam may be more effective for depressive and anxiety symptoms than for other PMS complaints. However, approximately 50% of women complain of drowsiness and sedation on these doses. Patients with a strong tendency to habituation should not be treated with this regimen. Therefore alprazolam is considered second-line treatment. Buspirone has less addictive potential than alprazolam and has been found in two RCTs to reduce symptoms. Continuous use of psychoactive drugs, such as tricyclics and lithium, has not yielded good PMS symptom relief.

Before using psychoactive drugs, it is extremely important to be sure of the diagnosis, because these drugs may not be effective and may actually be contraindicated in other psychiatric conditions that mimic PMS.

### Hormonal Suppression

**Progesterone**

Although a common treatment previously, many studies to date have shown progestogens to have mixed results in the treatment of PMS and PMDD. In 2012, a Cochrane review concluded that progestin therapy did not show a significant improvement for patients with PMS (Ford, 2009).

**Oral Contraceptives**

Early RCTs and descriptive studies using cyclic OCs have shown mixed results for the treatment of PMS, but OCs are likely beneficial because they inhibit ovulation. OCs mainly help physical symptoms such as breast pain, bloating, acne, and appetite. If used, monophasic OCs appear to be better. In Sulak and associates' retrospective review of 220 patients using an extended OC regimen and shortened hormone-free interval (3 to 4 days), 45% of patients chose this regimen for control of PMS symptoms and 40% for dysmenorrhea and pelvic pain symptoms (Sulak, 2004). Continuous combined OCs should suppress ovulation and provide symptom relief. A 2005 review found that few studies have reported on premenstrual symptoms on continuous- or extended-use OCs, but relief was noted in headaches, tiredness, bloating, and menstrual pain (Edelman, 2005). Finally, a prospective 2006 study by Coffee and colleagues has shown that an extended regimen of 30 μg of ethinyl estradiol with 3 mg of drospirenone for 168 days significantly reduces PMS symptoms compared with typical 21-day cyclic OCs. The FDA has approved a 20-μg ethinyl estradiol and 3-mg drospirenone combination OC for the treatment of PMDD, although limiting use to women with PMDD who also need contraception was mentioned. Because of drospirenone's antimineral corticoid and antiandrogenic properties, it has been hypothesized to be more effective (Coffee, 2006). A 2012 Cochrane systematic review supported its efficacy (Lopez, 2012). For women with PMS/PMDD who also desire contraception, this OC is a reasonable first therapy.

### Nonsteroidal Anti-inflammatory Drugs

For patients who complain of cramping or other systemic symptoms—such as aches, diarrhea, or heat intolerance—a trial with an NSAID may be useful. RCTs with mefenamic acid and naproxen have shown improvement in pain, mood, and somatic symptoms. It should be noted, however, that a toxic complication of NSAID use is nonoliguric renal failure. Because it is more likely to occur with NSAID use associated with severe dehydration, the agent should be discontinued if severe diarrhea is present and should not be used with diuretics.

### Diuretics

Historically, potassium-sparing diuretics were included in treatment consideration if the woman's complaints involve bloating, fluid retention, and a perceived change in body habitus during the luteal phase of the cycle. Study results on efficacy of this treatment, however, have been mixed. Spironolactone (100 mg/day) has been studied in four RCTs; three trials demonstrated moderate efficacy for breast tenderness and fluid retention, and two found reduced irritability symptoms. Diuretics should be avoided in patients with chronic renal disease or in those who are suffering from diarrhea or other fluid loss.

### Bromocriptine

Bromocriptine may be used for patients with cyclic mastalgia and may be helpful for some other symptoms of PMS, although its use in any individual case will need to be evaluated. A dose of 5 mg/day during the luteal phase is appropriate.

### Gonadotropin-Releasing Hormone Agonists

At least 10 RCTs have shown GnRH agonists (leuprolide, 3.75 mg IM monthly) to be effective for ovulation suppression and treatment of PMS and the physical symptoms of PMDD. GnRH agonists are less effective in treating the psychiatric symptoms of PMDD. However, they are expensive, can have marked side effects, and are limited in duration of use because of hypoestrogenism and osteoporosis. Using add-back estrogen and progesterone has been studied to offset the hypoestrogenic side effects without aggravating PMS and PMDD symptoms. The optimal add-back regimen is unclear from existing studies if GnRH agonists are to be used long term. Minimizing hormonal fluctuations with continuous estrogen and progesterone or minimizing the periods of exposure to progesterone seems prudent.

## *Surgical Treatment: Bilateral Oophorectomy with or without Hysterectomy*

For women with severe, disabling symptoms who have been refractory to other medical therapies, surgical management may be considered. Three observational studies found bilateral oophorectomy, typically with hysterectomy, to be effective in this group of rare patients. Although this approach is not offered as standard therapy for severe PMS, it may be a reasonable alternative for select patients for whom all other treatment regimens have failed. The use of a GnRH analogue for 3 to 6 months, with or without estrogen add-back, demonstrating efficacy is important prior to determining if the patient may benefit from surgical treatment.

The physician should be cautious when determining a treatment regimen for any individual patient and should attempt to verify the patient's symptoms and add medications only when relief has not been achieved. Because of the myriad of PMS symptoms, it is not surprising that individualization of treatment is essential. Many of the therapies mentioned, however, offer relief of most symptoms and hope for many sufferers.

## KEY POINTS

- Primary dysmenorrhea almost always occurs before the age of 20 years. Secondary dysmenorrhea may occur at any time during the menstrual years.
- Approximately 75% of all women complain of primary dysmenorrhea. Approximately 15% have severe symptoms.
- Education, supportive therapy, and NSAIDs are the treatments of choice for primary dysmenorrhea. Seventy-two percent of women suffering from dysmenorrhea report significant pain relief with this treatment strategy.
- COCs reduce the prevalence and severity of dysmenorrhea. They can be used in extended cycles for better relief. This is also a reasonable first-line treatment, especially if contraception is desired.
- If dysmenorrhea symptoms are not relieved with NSAIDs, OCS, or their combination, additional evaluation for pelvic pathology should be considered.
- Approximately 3% to 8% of all women suffer from clinically relevant PMS, with 2% demonstrating PMDD.
- PMS patients often suffer depression during the luteal phase, but it is not as severe as the depression noted by patients with endogenous depression when measured by standard depression scales. It can be difficult to distinguish PMS from depression with luteal phase exacerbation.
- The most useful diagnostic tool in caring for PMS and PMDD patients is a prospective symptom diary.
- Educating patients about the diagnosis of PMS or PMDD is critical. Exercise along with consideration for judicious calcium or vitamin $B_6$ supplementation may relieve PMS symptoms.
- Therapy with psychoactive drugs, particularly the SSRIs, has been demonstrated in RCTs to relieve PMS and PMDD symptoms. These medications should be considered first-line therapy. Specific cautions for the use of these agents must be followed. For women who also desire contraception, COCs are a valid option with demonstrated improvement in PMS/PMDD symptoms.

## KEY REFERENCES


ACOG practice bulletin no. 114: management of endometriosis. *Obstet Gynecol.* 2010;116(1):223-236.

American Psychiatric Association (APA). Premenstrual dysphoric disorder. In: *Diagnostic and Statistical Manual of Mental Disorders.* 5th ed. Arlington, VA: (DSM-V). American Psychiatric Association; 2014. Available at: http://dsm.psychiatryonline.org/doi/full/10.1176/appi.books.9780890425596.dsm04#BCFIEGFF.

Andersch B. Bromocriptine and premenstrual symptoms: A survey of double-blind trials. *Obstet Gynecol Surv.* 1983;38:643.

Andersch B, Milsom I. An epidemiologic study of young women with dysmenorrhea. *Am J Obstet Gynecol.* 1982;144:655.

Bertone-Johnson ER, Hankinson SE, Bendich A, et al. Calcium and vitamin D intake and risk of incident premenstrual syndrome. *Arch Intern Med.* 2005;165:1246.

Brown J, Brown S. Exercise for dysmenorrhoea. *Cochrane Database Syst Rev.* 2010;(2). CD004142.

Burnett MA, Antao V, Black A, et al. Prevalence of primary dysmenorrhea in Canada. *J Obstet Gynaecol Can.* 2005;27(8):765.

Canning S, Waterman M, Dye L, . Dietary supplements and herbal remedies for premenstrual syndrome (PMS): a systematic research review of the evidence for their efficacy.. *J Reprod Infant Psyc.* 2006;24(4):363-378.

Chan AF, Mortola JF, Wood SH, et al. Persistence of premenstrual syndrome during low-dose administration of the progesterone antagonist RU 486. *Obstet Gynecol.* 1994;84:1001.

Chuong CJ, Hsi BP, Gibbons WE. Periovulatory beta-endorphin levels in premenstrual syndrome. *Obstet Gynecol.* 1994;83:755.

Coffee AL, Kuehl TJ, Willis S, et al. Oral contraceptives and premenstrual symptoms: Comparison of a 21/7 and extended regimen. *Am J Obstet Gynecol.* 2006;195:1311.

Cohen LS, Soares CN, Otto MW, et al. Prevalence and predictors of premenstrual dysphoric disorder (PMDD) in older premenopausal women. The Harvard Study of Moods and Cycles. *J Affect Disord.* 2002;70:125.

Crowell MD, Dubin NH, Robinson JC, et al. Functional bowel disorders in women with dysmenorrhea. *Am J Gastroenterol.* 1994;89:1973.

Edelman AB, Gallo MF, Jensen JT, et al. Continuous or extended cycle vs cyclic use of combined oral contraceptives for contraception. *Cochrane Database Syst Rev.* 2005;(3). CD004695.

Ford O, Lethaby A, Roberts H, Mol BW. Progesterone for premenstrual syndrome. *Cochrane Database Syst Rev.* 2009;(2). CD003415.

Frank RT. The hormonal causes of premenstrual tension. *Arch Neurol Psychol.* 1931;126:1052.

Freeman EW, Rickels K, Yonkers KA, Kunz NR, McPherson M, Upton GV. Venlafaxine in the treatment of premenstrual dysphoric disorder. *Obstet Gynecol.* 2001;98(5 Pt 1):737.

Gehlert S, Song IH, Chang CH, et al. The prevalence of premenstrual dysphoric disorder in a randomly selected group of urban and rural women. *Psychol Med.* 2009;39:129.

premenstrual syndromes. *Fertil Steril.* 1991;56:1066.

Halbreich U, Rojansky N, Palter S. Elimination of ovulation and menstrual cyclicity (with danazol) improves dysphoric premenstrual syndromes. *Fertil Steril.* 1991;56:1066.

Howard F. Causes of chronic pelvic pain in women; 2013. Available at http://www.uptodate.com/contents/treatment-of-chronic-pelvic-pain-in-women.

Jing Z, Yang X, Ismail KM, Chen X, Wu T. Chinese herbal medicine for premenstrual syndrome. *Cochrane Database Syst Rev.* 2009;(1). CD006414.

Kashanian M, Mazinani R, Jalalmanesh S. Pyridoxine (vitamin $B_6$) therapy for premenstrual syndrome. *Int J Gynaecol Obstet.* 2007;96:43.

Koike H, Ikenoue T, Mori N. Studies on prostaglandin production relating to the mechanism of dysmenorrhea in endometriosis. *Nihon Naibunpi Gakkai Zasshi.* 1994;20:43.

Kornstein SG, Harvey AT, Rush AJ, et al. Self-reported premenstrual exacerbation of depressive symptoms in patients seeking treatment for major depression. *Psychol Med.* 2005;35:683.

Latthe P, Mignini L, Gray R, Hills R, Khan K. Factors predisposing women to chronic pelvic pain: systematic review. *BMJ.* 2006;332(7544):749.

Lopez LM, Kaptein AA, Helmerhorst FM. Oral contraceptives containing drospirenone for premenstrual syndrome. *Cochrane Database Syst Rev.* 2012;(2). CD006586.

Lustyk MK, Gerrish WG, Shaver S, Keys SL. Cognitive-behavioral therapy for premenstrual syndrome and premenstrual dysphoric disorder: a systematic review. Archives of women's mental health. *Arch Womens Ment Health.* 2009;12(2):85-96.

Marjoribanks J, Brown J, O'Brien PM, Wyatt K. Selective serotonin reuptake inhibitors for premenstrual syndrome. *Cochrane Database Syst Rev.* 2013;(6). CD001396.

Marjoribanks J, Proctor M, Farquhar C, Derks RS. Nonsteroidal anti-inflammatory drugs for dysmenorrhoea. *Cochrane Database Syst Rev.* 2010;(1). CD001751.

Milsom I, Hedner N, Mannheimer C. A comparative study of the effect of high-intensity transcutaneous nerve stimulation and oral naproxen on intrauterine pressure and menstrual pain in patients with primary dysmenorrhea. *Am J Obstet Gynecol.* 1994;170:123.

Mortola JF, Girton L, Yen SSC. Depressive episodes in premenstrual syndrome. *Am J Obstet Gynecol.* 1989;161:1682.

O'Brien PM. The premenstrual syndrome: A review of the present status of therapy. *Drugs.* 1982;24:140.

O'Brien PM, Abukhalil IEH. Randomized controlled trial of the management of premenstrual syndrome and premenstrual mastalgia using luteal phase-only danazol. *Am J Obstet Gynecol.* 1999;180:18.

Owen PR. Prostaglandin synthetase inhibitors in the treatment of primary dysmenorrhea: Outcome trials reviewed. *Am J Obstet Gynecol.* 1984;148:96.

Plouffe Jr L, Stewart K, Craft KS, et al. Diagnostic and treatment results from a southeastern academic center-based premenstrual syndrome clinic: The first year. *Am J Obstet Gynecol.* 1993;169:295.

Proctor ML, Latthe PM, Farquhar CM, et al. Surgical interruption of pelvic nerve pathways for primary and secondary dysmenorrhoea. *Cochrane Database Syst Rev.* 2005;(4). CD001896.

Proctor ML, Murphy PA, Pattison HM, Suckling J, Farquhar CM. Behavioural interventions for primary and secondary dysmenorrhoea. *Cochrane Database Syst Rev.* 2007;(3). CD002248.

Rapkin AJ, Chang LI, Reading AE. Mood and cognitive style in premenstrual syndrome. *Obstet Gynecol.* 1989;74:644.

Rapkin AJ, Morgan M, Goldman L, et al. Progesterone metabolite allopregnanediol in women with premenstrual syndrome. *Obstet Gynecol.* 1997;90:709.

Reid RL, Yen SSC. Premenstrual syndrome. *Am J Obstet Gynecol.* 1981; 139:85.

Roca CA, Schmidt PJ, Altemus M, et al. Differential menstrual cycle regulation of hypothalamic-pituitary-adrenal axis in women with premenstrual syndrome and controls. *J Clin Endocrinol Metab.* 2003;88:3057.

Shah NR, Jones JB, Aperi J, et al. Selective serotonin reuptake inhibitors for premenstrual syndrome and premenstrual dysphoric disorder: A meta-analysis. *Obstet Gynecol.* 2008;111:1175.

Smith P, Kaunitz M. Primary dysmenorrhea in adult women: Clinical features and diagnosis; 2016. Available at http://www.uptodate.com/contents/primary-dysmenorrhea-in-adult-women-clinical-features-and-diagnosis.

Smith RP. The dynamics of nonsteroidal anti-inflammatory therapy for primary dysmenorrhea. *Obstet Gynecol.* 1987;70:785.

Smith RP, Heltzel JA. Interrelation of analgesia and uterine activity in women with primary dysmenorrhea: A preliminary report. *J Reprod Med.* 1991;36:260.

Smith S, Rinehart JS, Ruddock VE, et al. Treatment of premenstrual syndrome with alprazolam: Results of a double-blind, placebo- controlled, randomized crossover clinical trial. *Obstet Gynecol.* 1987;70:37.

Steege JR, Stout AL, Knight DL, et al. Reduced platelet tritium-labeled imipramine binding sites in women with premenstrual syndrome. *Am J Obstet Gynecol.* 1992;167:168.

Sternfeld B, Swindle R, Chawla A, et al. Severity of premenstrual symptoms in a health maintenance organization population. *Obstet Gynecol.* 2002;99:1014.

Sulak PJ, Carl J, Gopalakrishnan I, et al. Outcomes of extended oral contraceptive regimens with a shortened hormone-free interval to manage breakthrough bleeding. *Contraception.* 2004;70:281.

Taylor HC. Vascular congestion and hyperemia: Their effect on the structure and function in the female reproductive system. *Am J Obstet Gynecol.* 1949;57:211.

Thys-Jacobs S, Starkey P, Bernstein D, et al. Premenstrual Syndrome Study Group: Calcium carbonate and the premenstrual syndrome: Effects on premenstrual and menstrual symptoms. *Am J Obstet Gynecol.* 1998;179:444.

Tu FF, Hahn D, Steege JF. Pelvic congestion syndrome-associated pelvic pain: A systematic review of diagnosis and management. *Obstet Gynecol Surv.* 2010;65:332.

Wong CL, Farquhar C, Roberts H, Proctor M. Oral contraceptive pill for primary dysmenorrhoea. *Cochrane Database Syst Rev.* 2009;(4). CD002120.

Wyatt KM, Dimmock PW, O'Brien PMS. Efficacy of vitamin B-6 in the treatment of premenstrual syndrome: systematic review. *Br Med J.* 1999;318:1375.

Yonkers K, Casper R. Epidemiology and pathogenesis of premenstrual syndrome and premenstrual dysphoric disorder; 2016. Available at http://www.uptodate.com/contents/epidemiology-and-pathogenesis-of-premenstrual-syndrome-and-premenstrual-dysphoric-disorder.

Suggested Readings can be found on ExpertConsult.com.

# 38

# Primary and Secondary Amenorrhea and Precocious Puberty

## Etiology, Diagnostic Evaluation, Management

*Roger A. Lobo*

**Amenorrhea** is defined as the absence of menstrual bleeding and may be primary (never occurring) or secondary (cessation sometime after initiation). **Cryptomenorrhea** is another condition caused by anatomic disorders interfering with the outflow of menses, such as an imperforate hymen or transverse vaginal septum, although these women are actually menstruating. These disorders are discussed in Chapter 11, so they will not be discussed here.

**Primary amenorrhea** is defined as the absence of menses in a woman who has never menstruated by the age of 15 years (Practice Committee, American Society for Reproductive Medicine, 2008.) Another definition includes girls who have not menstruated within 5 years of breast development, if occurring by age 10. Breast development (thelarche) should occur by age 13 or otherwise requires evaluation as well. The incidence of primary amenorrhea is less than 0.1%. **Secondary amenorrhea** is defined as the absence of menses for an arbitrary period, usually longer than 6 to 12 months. The incidence of secondary amenorrhea of more than 6 months' duration in a survey of a general population of Swedish women of reproductive age was found to be 0.7% but has been cited to be as high as 3%. (Practice Committee, American Society for Reproductive Medicine, 2008.) The incidence is significantly higher in women younger than 25 years and those with a prior history of menstrual irregularity.

Outside the United States, it is common to see women who have been categorized according to the World Health Organization (WHO) classification. WHO type I usually refers to women with low estrogen levels and low follicle-stimulating hormone (FSH) and prolactin (PRL) levels without central nervous system (CNS) lesions; type II refers to a normal estrogen status with normal FSH and PRL levels; WHO type III refers to low estrogen levels and a high FSH level, denoting ovarian failure.

## DELAYED MENARCHE

Before the onset of menses, the normal female goes through a progressive series of morphologic changes produced by the pubertal increase in estrogen and androgen production. In 1969, Marshall and Tanner defined five stages of breast development and pubic hair development (Marshall, 1969; Carel, 2008) (Fig. 38.1, Table 38.1). These changes sometimes are combined and called *Tanner,* or *pubertal,* stages 1 through 5. The first sign of puberty is usually the appearance of breast budding followed within a few months by the appearance of pubic hair.

Thereafter, the breasts enlarge, the external pelvic contour becomes rounder, and the most rapid rate of growth occurs (peak height velocity). These changes precede menarche. Thus breast budding is the earliest sign of puberty and menarche the latest. The mean ages of occurrence of these events in American women are shown in Table 38.2 and the mean intervals (with standard deviation [SD]) between the initiation of breast budding and other pubertal events are shown in Table 38.3 (Frisch, 1971). The mean interval between breast budding and menarche is 2.3 years, with an SD of approximately 1 year. Some individuals can progress from breast budding to menarche in 18 months, and others may take 5 years. As stated previously, if thelarche has not occurred by age 13, a diagnostic evaluation should be performed.

The mean time of onset of menarche was previously thought to occur when a critical body weight of approximately 48 kg (106 lb) was reached. However, it is now believed that body composition is more important than total body weight in determining the time of onset of puberty and menstruation. Thus the ratio of fat to both total body weight and lean body weight is probably the most relevant factor that determines the time of onset of puberty and menstruation. Individuals who are moderately obese, between 20% and 30% above the ideal body weight, have an earlier onset of menarche than nonobese women. Malnutrition, such as occurs with **anorexia nervosa** or starvation, is known to delay the onset of puberty.

One of the major links between body composition and the hypothalamic-pituitary-ovarian axis, and thus menstrual cyclicity, is the adipocyte hormone **leptin**. Leptin is produced by adipocytes and correlates well with body weight. Leptin is also important for feedback involving gonadotropin-releasing hormone (GnRH) and luteinizing hormone (LH) pulsatility and also binds to specific receptor sites on the ovary and endometrium. Leptin administration has been shown to affect LH pulsatile activity (Laughlin, 1997), and to restore cyclicity in women

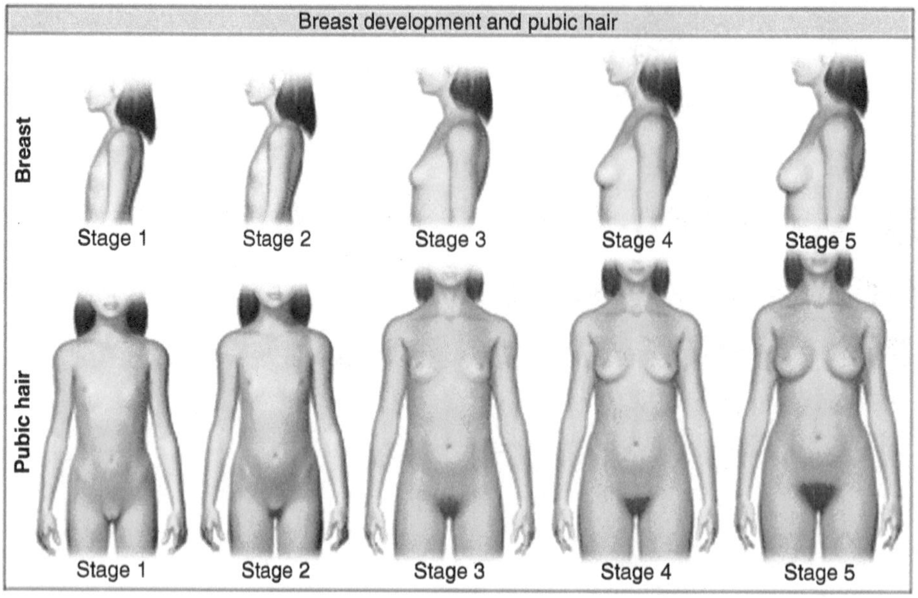


**Figure 38.1** Pubertal rating according to Tanner stage. **Top row,** Breast development in girls is rated from 1 (prepubertal) to 5 (adult). Stage 2 breast development (appearance of the breast bud) marks the onset of gonadarche. **Bottom row,** For girls, pubic hair stages are rated from 1 (prepubertal) to 5 (adult). Stage 2 marks the onset of adrenarche. (From Herring JA. *Tachdjian's Pediatric Orthopedics: From the Texas Scottish Rite Hospital for Children*. 5th ed. Philadelphia: Elsevier; 2014.)

**Table 38.1** Classification of Breast Growth and Pubic Hair Growth

| Classification | Description |
|---|---|
| **Breast Growth** | |
| B1 | Prepubertal: elevation of papilla only |
| B2 | Breast budding |
| B3 | Enlargement of breasts with glandular tissue, without separation of breast contours |
| B4 | Secondary mound formed by areola |
| B5 | Single contour of breast and areola |
| **Pubic Hair Growth** | |
| PH1 | Prepubertal—no pubic hair |
| PH2 | Labial hair present |
| PH3 | Labial hair spreads over mons pubis |
| PH4 | Slight lateral spread |
| PH5 | Further lateral spread to form inverse triangle and reach medial thighs |

**Table 38.2** Mean Ages of Girls at the Onset of Pubertal Events (United States)

| Event | Mean Age ± SD (yr) |
|---|---|
| Initiation of breast development | 10.8 ± 1.10 |
| Appearance of pubic hair | 11.0 ± 1.21 |
| Menarche | 12.9 ± 1.20 |

Modified from Frisch RE, Revelle R. Height and weight in menarche and a hypothesis of menarche. *Arch Dis Child*. 1971;46:695.
*SD*, Standard deviation.

with amenorrhea (Welt, 2004). Another hormone, a gastric peptide, ghrelin, interacts with leptin in this regard particularly when menstrual function is perturbed (Schneider, 2006).

Body weight and body fat content have been shown to be important for menstruation; a fatness nomogram is depicted in Figure 38.2 (Frisch, 1971). Well-nourished individuals

**Table 38.3** Pubertal Intervals

| Interval | Mean Age ± SD (Years) |
|---|---|
| B2—peak height velocity | 1.0 ± 0.77 |
| B2—menarche | 2.3 ± 1.03 |
| B2-PH2 | 3.1 ± 1.04 |
| B2-B5 (average duration of puberty) | 4.5 ± 2.04 |

Modified from Frisch RE, Revelle R. Height and weight in menarche and a hypothesis of menarche. *Arch Dis Child*. 1971;46:695.
*B2*, Initiation of breast development; *PH2*, appearance of pubic hair; *SD*, standard deviation.

with prepubertal strenuous exercise programs resulting in less total body fat have also been shown to have a delayed onset of puberty. Warren and colleagues have reported that ballet dancers, swimmers, and runners have menarche delayed to approximately age 15 if they began exercising strenuously before menarche (Warren, 1980) (Fig. 38.3). It is greater in those athletic activities requiring lower body weight, and where success is more subjective (ballet, gymnastics) as compared with swimming. It was also determined that stress per se is not the cause of the **delayed menarche** in these exercising girls, because girls of the same age with stressful musical careers did not have a delayed onset of menarche (Warren, 1980). Young women with strenuous exercise programs have sufficient estrogen to produce some breast development and thus do not need extensive endocrinologic evaluation if concern arises about the lack of onset of menses. Frisch and coworkers have reported that for girls engaged in premenarchal athletic training, menarche is delayed 0.4 year for each year of training. Individuals who exercise strenuously should be counseled that they will usually have a delayed onset of menses, but it is not a health problem. They should be told that they will most likely have regular ovulatory cycles when they stop exercising or become older.

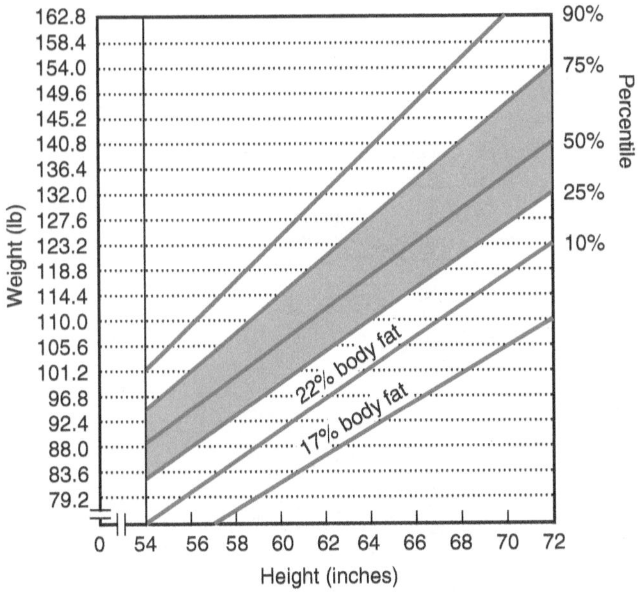


**Figure 38.2** Fatness index nomogram. (Modified from Frisch RE, Revelle R. Height and weight in menarche and a hypothesis of menarche. *Arch Dis Child.* 1971;46:695.)

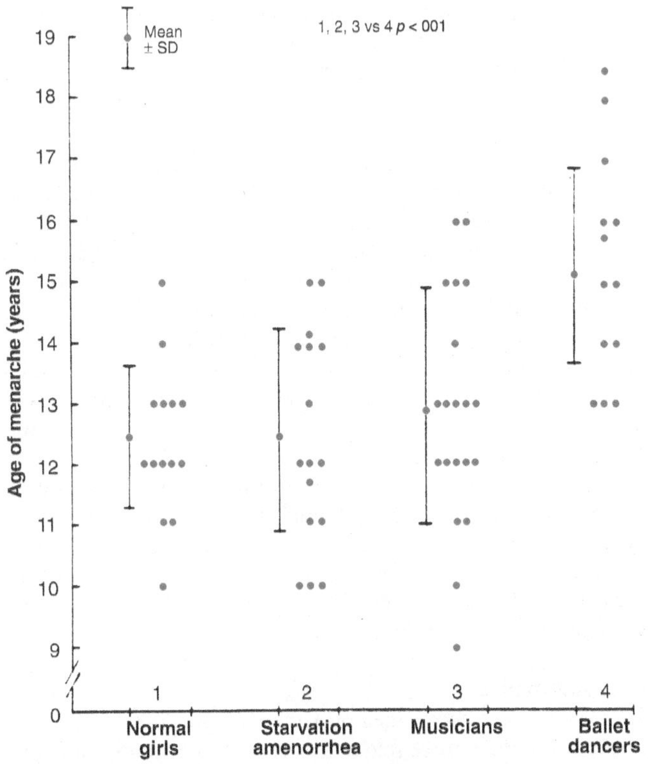


**Figure 38.3** Ages of menarche in ballet dancers compared with those of three other groups. (From Warren MP. The effects of exercise on pubertal progression and reproductive function in girls. *J Clin Endocrinol Metab.* 1980;51:1150.)

The metabolic features of amenorrheic athletes, who are considered to be in a state of negative energy balance, are fairly characteristic. These include elevated serum FSH, insulin-like growth factor-binding protein 1 (IGFBP-1), and lowered insulin insulin-like growth factor (IGF) levels.

Emotional stress can lead to inhibition of the GnRH axis. The mechanism involves an increased secretion of corticotropin-releasing hormone (CRH), releasing adrenocorticotropic hormone (ACTH), opioid peptides such as β-endorphin, and cortisol. CRH itself is known to inhibit GnRH.

Before puberty, circulating levels of LH and FSH are low with an FSH/LH ratio >1. The CNS–hypothalamic axis is extremely sensitive to the negative feedback effects of low levels of circulating estrogen. As the critical weight or body composition is approached, the CNS–hypothalamic axis becomes less sensitive to the negative effect of estrogen and GnRH is secreted in greater amounts, causing an increase in LH and, to a lesser extent, FSH levels. This release from the prepubertal "brake" on GnRH secretion is depicted in Figure 38.4, which also illustrates the integral role of neuropeptides such as kisspeptin (Terasawa, 2013). The initial endocrinologic change associated with the onset of puberty is the occurrence of episodic pulses of LH occurring during sleep (Boyar, 1974) (Fig. 38.5). These pulses are absent before the onset of puberty. After menarche, the episodic secretions of LH occur during sleep and while awake. The last endocrinologic event of puberty is activation of the positive gonadotropin response to increasing levels of $E_2$, which results in the midcycle gonadotropic surge and ovulation.

## PRIMARY AMENORRHEA

It is important that the clinician understand the sequential endocrinologic and morphologic chronologic changes taking place during normal puberty so as to make the differential diagnosis between delayed menarche and primary amenorrhea. Although the former condition requires only reassurance, the latter requires an endocrinologic evaluation.

### *CAUSES OF PRIMARY AMENORRHEA*

Although numerous classifications have been used for the various causes of primary amenorrhea, it has been found useful to group causes on the basis of whether secondary sexual characteristics (breasts) and female internal genitalia (uterus) are present or absent (Box 38.1). Thus the findings on a physical examination can alert the clinician to possible causes and indicate which laboratory tests should be performed. In a series of 62 individuals reported by Mashchak, the largest subgroup with primary amenorrhea (29) were those in whom breasts were absent but where a uterus was present; the second largest subgroup (22) had both breasts and a uterus; lack of a uterus together with breast development accounted for the third largest category (9); and those without breasts or a uterus were the least common (2) (Mashchak, 1981). This breakdown of the various accompanying conditions of primary amenorrhea reflects the referral pattern to the center and not necessarily the true incidence of each category. Other figures for the prevalence of various types of amenorrhea have been reported.

#### ***Breasts Absent and Uterus Present***

It would seem logical, as breast development is a biomarker of ovarian estrogen production, that individuals with no breast development and a uterus present have no estrogen production. This is either the result of a primary ovarian disorder or a CNS hypothalamic-pituitary abnormality, which provides the normal signal to the ovary. The phenotype of individuals with either of these causes of low estrogen status is similar.

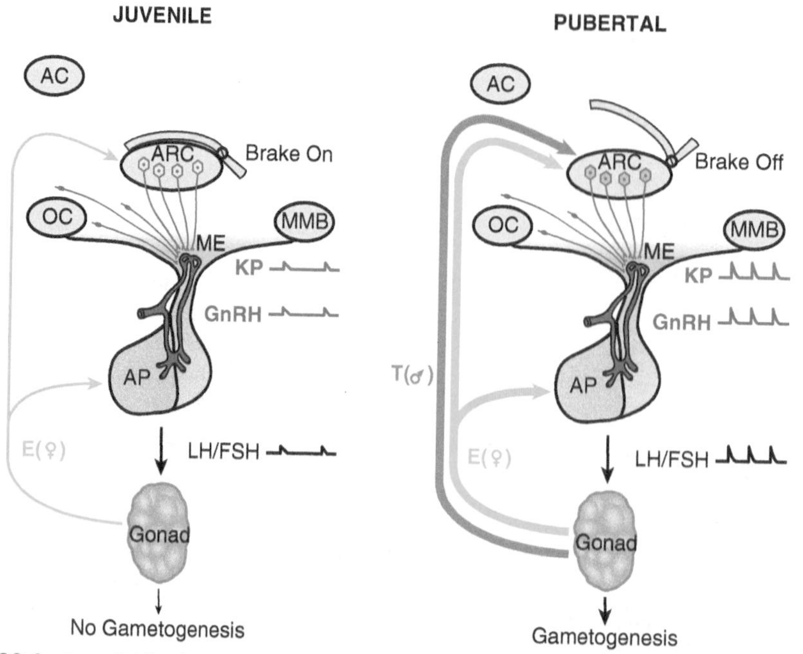


**Figure 38.4** A model for the control of the timing of puberty. The figure depicts the key role of kisspeptin (KP) signaling in generating GnRH release. In the juvenile state *(left panel)* a physiologic "brake " is operational, and in the pubertal state *(right panel)* the "brake" is off, allowing for kisspeptin and GnRH release and a fully integrated negative feedback system for testosterone *(blue)* in the male or estradiol *(gold)* in the female. (Modified from Terasawa E, Guerrier KA, Plant TM. Kisspeptin and puberty in mammals. In: Kauffman AS, Smith JT, eds. *Kisspeptin Signaling in Reproductive Biology.* New York: Springer; 2013:253.)

However, because the cause of the disorder and the prognosis for fertility differ, it is important to establish the specific diagnosis.

## Gonadal Failure (Hypergonadotropic Hypogonadism)

Failure of gonadal development is the most common cause of primary amenorrhea, occurring in almost 50% of those with this symptom. **Gonadal failure** is most frequently caused by a chromosomal disorder or deletion of all or part of an X chromosome, but it is sometimes caused by another genetic defect and, rarely, 17α-hydroxylase deficiency. The chromosomal disorders are usually caused by a random meiotic or mitotic abnormality (e.g., nondisjunction, anaphase lag) and thus are not inherited. However, if gonadal development is absent in the presence of a 46,XX (called **pure gonadal dysgenesis**), a gene disorder may be present, because it has been reported to occur in siblings. Reindollar reported that all individuals with gonadal failure and an X chromosome abnormality were shorter than 63 inches in height (Reindollar, 1981). Approximately one third also had major cardiovascular or renal anomalies.

Deletion of the entire X chromosome (as occurs in Turner syndrome) or of the short arm (p) of the X chromosome results in short stature. Deletions of only the long arm (q) usually do not affect height. In place of the ovary a band of fibrous tissue called a **gonadal streak** is present (Federman, 1967) (Fig. 38.6). When ovarian follicles are absent, synthesis of ovarian steroids and inhibin does not occur. Breast development does not occur because of the low circulating $E_2$ levels. Because the negative hypothalamic-pituitary action of estrogen and inhibin is not present, gonadotropin levels are markedly elevated, with FSH levels being higher than LH. Estrogen is not necessary for müllerian duct development or wolffian duct regression, so the internal and external genitalia are phenotypically female.

An occasional individual with mosaicism, an abnormal X chromosome, pure gonadal dysgenesis (46,XX), or even Turner syndrome (45,X) may have a few follicles that develop under endogenous gonadotropin stimulation early in puberty and may synthesize enough estrogen to induce breast development and a few episodes of uterine bleeding, resulting early in **premature ovarian failure**, usually before age 25. Rarely, ovulation and pregnancy can occur.

Goldenberg reported that all individuals with primary amenorrhea and plasma FSH levels higher than 40 mIU/mL have no functioning ovarian follicles in the gonadal tissue. Thus in women with primary amenorrhea, the diagnosis of gonadal failure can be established if the FSH levels are consistently elevated, without requiring ovarian tissue evaluation.

## 45,X Anomalies

Turner syndrome occurs in approximately 1 per 2000 to 3000 live births but is much more frequent in abortuses. In addition to primary amenorrhea and absent breast development, these individuals have other somatic abnormalities, the most prevalent being short stature (<60 inches in height), webbing of the neck, a short fourth metacarpal, and cubitus valgus. Cardiac abnormality, renal abnormalities, and hypothyroidism are also more prevalent. The diagnosis is usually made before puberty (see Chapter 2).

A wide variety of chromosomal mosaics are associated with primary amenorrhea and normal female external genitalia, the most common being X/XX. In addition, individuals with

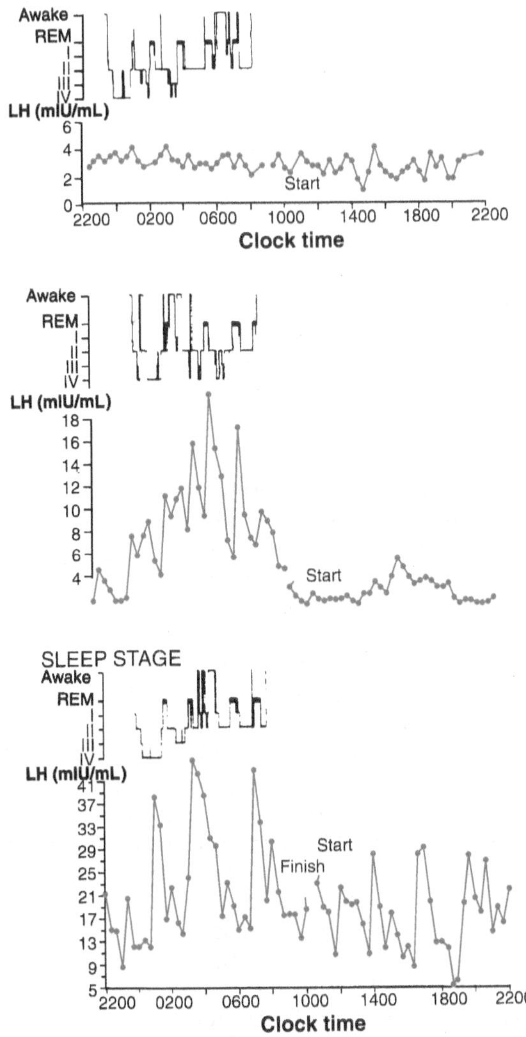


**Figure 38.5** Plasma luteinizing hormone (LH) concentration measured every 20 minutes for 24 hours in normal prepubertal girl *(upper panel)*, early pubertal girl *(center panel)*, and normal late pubertal girl *(lower panel)*. In top and center panels, sleep histogram is shown above period of nocturnal sleep. Sleep stages are awake, rapid eye movement (REM), and stages I to IV by depth of line graph. Plasma LH concentrations are expressed as mIU/mL. (Modified from Boyar RM, Katz J, Finkelstein JW, et al. Anorexia nervosa: immaturity of the 24-hour luteinizing hormone secretory pattern. *N Engl J Med.* 1974;291:861.)

**Box 38.1 Classification of Disorders with Primary Amenorrhea and Normal Female Genitalia**

**I. Absent breast development; uterus present**

A. Gonadal failure
   1. 45,X (Turner syndrome)
   2. 46,X, abnormal X (e.g., short- or long-arm deletion)
   3. Mosaicism (e.g., X/XX, X/XX,XXX)
   4. 46,XX or 46,XY pure gonadal dysgenesis
   5. 17α-hydroxylase deficiency with 46,XX

B. Hypothalamic failure secondary to inadequate GnRH release
   1. Insufficient GnRH secretion because of neurotransmitter defect
   2. Inadequate GnRH synthesis (Kallmann syndrome)
   3. Congenital anatomic defect in central nervous system
   4. CNS neoplasm (craniopharyngioma)

C. Pituitary failure
   1. Isolated gonadotrophin insufficiency (thalassemia major, retinitis pigmentosa)
   2. Pituitary neoplasia (chromophobe adenoma)
   3. Mumps, encephalitis
   4. Newborn kernicterus
   5. Prepubertal hypothyroidism

**II. Breast development; uterus absent**

A. Androgen resistance (testicular feminization)
B. Congenital absence of uterus (uterovaginal agenesis)

**III. Absent breast development; uterus absent**

A. 17,20-desmolase deficiency
B. Agonadism
C. 17α-hydroxylase deficiency with 46,XY karyotype

**IV. Breast development; uterus present**

A. Hypothalamic cause
B. Pituitary cause
C. Ovarian cause
D. Uterine cause

*CNS*, Central nervous system; *GnRH*, gonadotropin-releasing hormone.

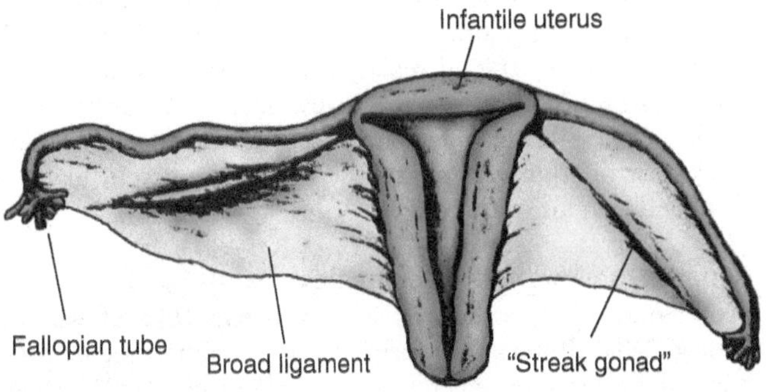


**Figure 38.6** Internal genitalia of patient with gonadal dysgenesis (Turner syndrome), featuring normal but infantile uterus, normal fallopian tubes, and pale, glistening streak gonads in both broad ligaments. (From Federman DD. Disorders of gonadal development: gonadal dysgenesis [Turner syndrome]. In: Federman DD, ed. *Abnormal Sexual Development: A Genetic and Endocrine Approach to Differential Diagnosis.* Philadelphia: WB Saunders; 1967.)

X/XXX and X/XX/XXX mosaicism have primary amenorrhea. These individuals are generally taller and have fewer anatomic abnormalities than individuals with a 45,X karyotype. In addition, some of them may have a few gonadal follicles and approximately 20% have sufficient estrogen production to menstruate. Occasionally, ovulation may occur, as stated earlier. Isolated phenotypic features of Turner syndrome (without gonadal failure) may also occur in males and is known as *Noonan syndrome.*

## Structurally Abnormal X Chromosome

Although individuals with this disorder have a 46,XX karyotype, part of one X chromosome is structurally abnormal. If there is deletion of the long arm of the X chromosome (Xq), normal height has been reported to occur but, in Reindollar's series, these individuals were all relatively short (Reindollar, 1981). They have no somatic abnormalities. However, if there is deletion of the short arm of the X chromosome (Xp), the individual will be short. A similar phenotype occurs in those with isochrome of the long arm of the X chromosome. Other X chromosome abnormalities include a ring X and minute fragmentation of the X chromosome.

**Pure Gonadal Dysgenesis (46,XX and 46,XY with Gonadal Streaks)**

As noted, this abnormality may have a familial/genetic association and has been reported in siblings. Abnormalities in genes involved in gonadal development are expected to be involved. These individuals have normal stature and phenotype, absence of secondary sexual characteristics, and primary amenorrhea. Some of these women have a few ovarian follicles, develop breasts, and may even menstruate spontaneously for a few years.

**46,XY gonadal dysgenesis** is the result of an abnormal testis in utero. There can be incomplete forms with some degree of testicular tissue, but in this context the "pure" form as a dysgenetic streak as in other forms of ovarian dysgenesis and previously has been referred to as **Swyer syndrome.**

If a Y chromosome is present (as in 46,XY gonadal dysgenesis) or is found as part of a mosaic karyotype, with or without any clinical signs of androgenization, gonadectomy should be performed.

**17α-Hydroxylase Deficiency with 46,XX Karyotype**

A rare gonadal cause of primary amenorrhea without breast development and normal female internal genitalia is deficiency of the enzyme 17α-hydroxylase (P450 C17) in an individual with a 46,XX karyotype (it can also occur in genetic males 46,XY) who may present in a similar fashion. Only a few such individuals have been described in the literature, but it is important for the clinician to be aware of this entity because, in contrast to those described earlier, these individuals have hypernatremia and hypokalemia. Because of decreased cortisol, ACTH levels are elevated. The mineralocorticoid levels are also elevated, because 17α-hydroxylase is not necessary for the conversion of progesterone to deoxycortisol or corticosterone. Thus there is excessive sodium retention and potassium excretion, leading to hypertension and hypokalemia. Serum progesterone levels are also elevated because progesterone is not converted to cortisol. In addition to sex steroid replacement, these individuals need cortisol administration. They usually have cystic ovaries and viable oocytes. Pregnancies have been documented following in vitro fertilization–embryo transfer (IVF-ET), despite low levels of endogenous sex steroids.

### Genetic Disorders with Hyperandrogenism

Hyperandrogenism occurs in approximately 10% of women with gonadal dysgenesis. Most have a Y chromosome or fragment of a Y chromosome, but some may only have a DNA fragment that contains the testes-determining gene (probably *SRY*) without a full Y chromosome. Those with hypergonadotropic hypogonadism and a female phenotype who have any clinical manifestation of hyperandrogenism, such as hirsutism, should have a gonadectomy, even if a Y chromosome is not present, because gonadal neoplasms are frequent.

### Central Nervous System–Hypothalamic–Pituitary Disorders

With CNS-hypothalamic-pituitary disorders, the low estrogen levels are caused by an abnormal or absent signal to the ovary, resulting in very low circulating gonadotropin levels. The cause of low gonadotropin production may be morphologic or endocrinologic.

**Central Nervous System Lesions**

Any anatomic lesion of the hypothalamus or pituitary can cause low gonadotropin production. These lesions can be congenital (e.g., stenosis of aqueduct, absence of sellar floor) or acquired (tumors). Many of these lesions, particularly pituitary adenomas, result in elevated prolactin levels (see Chapter 39).

However, non–prolactin-secreting pituitary tumors (**chromophobe adenomas**), as well as craniopharyngiomas, may not be associated with hyperprolactinemia and can rarely be the cause of primary amenorrhea with low gonadotropin levels. Thus all individuals with primary amenorrhea and low gonadotropin levels, with or without an elevated prolactin level, should have computed tomography (CT) scanning or magnetic resonance imaging (MRI) of the hypothalamic-pituitary region to rule out the presence of a lesion.

**Inadequate Gonadotropin-Releasing Hormone Release (Hypogonadotropic Hypogonadism)**

Those without a demonstrable lesion and a low gonadotropin level were previously thought to have primary pituitary failure (**hypogonadotropic hypogonadism**). However, when they are stimulated with GnRH, there is an increase in FSH and LH levels, indicating that the basic defect is either hypothalamic with insufficient GnRH synthesis or a CNS neurotransmitter defect, resulting in inadequate GnRH synthesis, release, or both. Although a single bolus of GnRH may not initially cause a rise in gonadotropin level in these individuals, after 4 days of GnRH administration (priming), the women will have a rise in gonadotropin levels after a single GnRH bolus. Because GnRH secretion occurs after migration of these specific cells from the olfactory lobe to the hypothesis during embryogenesis, anosmia may also occur in some patients with gonadotropin deficiency. This is caused by a specific defect of the *KAL* gene (Xp 22-3), which is responsible for neuronal migration. Other genetic defects resulting in gonadotropic deficiency may occur on the X chromosome or autosomes and include FGFR1, PROKR2, and GNRHR (Caronia, 2011) as well as loss of function mutations in the kisspeptin-1 receptor (Seminara, 2003).

Females with Kallmann syndrome and related forms of gonadotropic deficiency have normal height and an increase in growth of long bones, resulting in a greater wingspan-to-height ratio. Men affected by gonadotropic deficiency have hypogonadism, an increased wingspan-to-height ratio, and altered spatial orientation abilities. Anosmia in Kallmann syndrome must be tested for by blinded testing of certain characteristic smells, such as coffee, cocoa, or orange. Not all women in this category of GnRH deficiency states will have anosmia, which is specific for some patients with Kallmann syndrome.

There is a tendency for GnRH deficiency to be familial/inherited through a variety of mechanisms, although the majority of cases, over two thirds, are sporadic.

**Isolated Gonadotropin Deficiency (Pituitary Disease)**

Rarely, individuals with primary amenorrhea and low gonadotropin levels do not respond to GnRH, even after 4 days of administration. This is known as **isolated gonadotropin deficiency.** They almost always have an associated disorder such as thalassemia major (with iron deposits in the pituitary) or retinitis pigmentosa. Occasionally, this pituitary abnormality has been associated with prepubertal hypothyroidism, kernicterus, or mumps encephalitis.

**Estrogen Resistance**

This rare condition was first described in men and now has been described in a woman (breast absent, uterus present.) A mutation in ERα does not allow estrogen signaling and a biologic response to estrogen action. Endogenous estrogen levels are high, gonadotropins are higher than the normal range (to try to provoke an estrogen response), and the ovaries are cystic. Exogenous estrogen does not normally induce changes except minimal changes with very high pharmacologic doses (Quaynor, 2013).

### *Breast Development Present and Uterus Absent*

Two disorders present with primary amenorrhea are associated with normal breast development and an absence of a uterus: androgen resistance and congenital absence of the uterus. The former is a genetically inherited disorder, whereas the latter is an accident of development and does not have an established pattern of inheritance.

#### Androgen Resistance

**Androgen resistance syndrome**, originally termed **testicular feminization**, is a genetically transmitted disorder in which androgen receptor synthesis or action does not occur. It is rare, with an incidence of 1/60,000. The syndrome is caused by the absence of an X-chromosome gene responsible for cytoplasmic or nuclear testosterone receptor function. It is an X-linked recessive or sex-linked autosomal dominant disorder, with transmission through the mother. These individuals have an XY karyotype and normally functioning male gonads that produce normal male levels of testosterone and dihydrotestosterone. However, because of a lack of receptors in target organs, there is lack of male differentiation of the external and internal genitalia (Gustafson, 1994). The external genitalia remain feminine, as occurs in the absence of sex steroids. Wolffian duct development, which normally occurs as a result of testosterone stimulation, fails to take place. Because müllerian duct regression is induced by anti-müllerian hormone (AMH), also called *müllerian-inhibiting substance* (MIS, a glycoprotein synthesized by the Sertoli cells of the fetal testes), this process occurs normally in these individuals because steroid receptors are unnecessary for the action of glycoproteins. Thus women with this disorder have no female or male internal genitalia, normal female external genitalia, and a short or absent vagina. Pubic hair and axillary hair are absent or scanty as a result of a lack of androgenic receptors, but breast development is normal or enhanced. It is known that testosterone is responsible for inhibiting breast proliferation. Thus in androgen resistance, the absence of androgen action allows even low levels of estrogen to cause unabated breast stimulation. Estrogen levels here are in the normal male range, and LH is slightly elevated.

Testes that are intraabdominal or that occur in the inguinal canal have an increased risk of developing a malignancy (gonadoblastoma or dysgerminoma), with an incidence reported to be approximately 20%. However, these malignancies rarely occur before age 20. Therefore it is usually recommended that the gonads be left in place until after puberty is completed to allow full breast development and epiphyseal closure to occur. After these events occur, which is typically around age 18, the gonads should be removed. It is recommended that those with androgen resistance be informed that they have an abnormal sex chromosome, without specifically mentioning a Y chromosome, because it is widely known that an XY karyotype indicates maleness. Currently, however, some families choose to have full disclosure and a complete understanding of the abnormality. In addition, because psychologically and phenotypically these individuals are female and have been raised as such, the term *gonads* should be used instead of *testes*. These individuals should also be informed that they can never become pregnant because they do not have a uterus and that their gonads must be removed after age 18 because of their high potential for malignancy.

#### Congenital Absence of the Uterus (Uterine Agenesis, Uterovaginal Agenesis, Mayer-Rokitansky-Küster-Hauser Syndrome)

The *Hox* genes are important for uterine development, and mutations (e.g., in *Hox-A13*) have been found in genetic syndromes with uterine abnormalities (e.g., hand-foot-genital and Guttmacher syndromes) and also in cases of bicornuate uterus. To date, however, no abnormalities have been found in cases of congenital absence of the uterus.

This disorder is the second most frequent cause of primary amenorrhea. It occurs in 1 in 4000 to 5000 female births and accounts for approximately 15% of individuals with primary amenorrhea. Individuals with complete uterine agenesis have normal ovaries, with regular cyclic ovulation and normal endocrine function. Women with this disorder have normal breast and pubic and axillary hair development but have a shortened or absent vagina, in addition to absence of the uterus (Jones, 1971) (Fig. 38.7). Although often there are no bulbous structures, but merely streak-line tissue, in 7% to 10% of cases there are two nonfused rudimentary horns as in the figure. On occasion one or both horns may have some functioning endometrium. In this

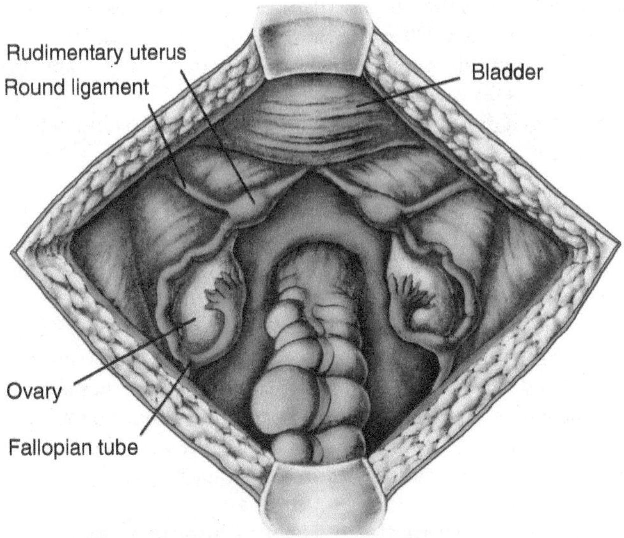


**Figure 38.7** Congenital absence of vagina. Laparotomy revealed rudimentary uterus that showed evidence of failure of fusion of Müllerian ducts. This is a common finding in this condition and indicates that the disorder is more extensive than simple anomaly of the vagina. (Modified from Jones HW Jr, Scott WW, eds. *Hermaphroditism, Genital Anomalies and Related Endocrine Disorders*. 2nd ed. Baltimore: Williams & Wilkins; 1971.)

setting of obstructed outflow, cyclic pelvic pain, which may be severe at times, may be encountered. Congenital renal abnormalities occur in approximately one third of these individuals and skeletal abnormalities in approximately 12%. Cardiac and other congenital abnormalities also occur with increased frequency. Occasional defects in the bones of the middle ear can also occur, resulting in some degree of deafness. The overwhelming majority of these disorders are caused by an isolated developmental defect, but on occasion the condition is genetically inherited. It is usually easy to differentiate these individuals from those with androgen resistance by the presence of normal pubic hair, but some with incomplete androgen resistance have some pubic hair. Because women with congenital absence of the uterus are endocrinologically normal females, and those with androgen resistance are endocrinologically male, with male testosterone levels and an XY karyotype, the differential diagnosis is easily made.

Women in this category are normal endocrinologically and have been able to have children using a surrogate or gestational carrier. Most recently a woman underwent a uterine transplantation from a donated postmenopausal uterus and was able to have a live birth (Brännström, 2015).

### Absent Breast and Uterine Development

Individuals with no breast or uterine development are rare. They usually have a male karyotype, elevated gonadotropin levels, and testosterone levels in the normal or below-normal female range. The differential diagnosis for this phenotype includes 17α-hydroxylase deficiency, 17,20-desmolase deficiency, and agonadism (Mashchak, 1981). Individuals with the first disorder have testes present but lack the enzyme necessary to synthesize sex steroids, and thus have female external genitalia. Because they have testes, AMH-MIS is produced and the female internal genitalia regress; with low testosterone levels, the male internal genitalia do not develop. Insufficient estrogen is synthesized to develop breasts. A similar lack of sex steroid synthesis occurs in males with a 17,20-desmolase deficiency. Individuals with agonadism, sometimes called the *vanishing testes syndrome,* have no gonads present, but because the female internal genitalia are also absent, it has been postulated that testicular AMH-MIS production occurred during fetal life but the gonadal tissue subsequently regressed.

### Secondary Sex Characteristics (Breast) Present and Female Internal Genitalia (Uterus) Present

This is the second largest category of individuals with primary amenorrhea, accounting for approximately one third of them. In the series reported by Mashchak, approximately 25% of these individuals had hyperprolactinemia and prolactinomas (Mashchak, 1981). The remaining women had profiles similar to those with secondary amenorrhea and thus should be subcategorized and treated similarly as women with secondary amenorrhea, which will be discussed in a separate section.

### Primary Amenorrhea with Absent Endometrium

This is a rare condition in this category of primary amenorrhea with uterus and breast present. Endocrine function is completely normal, as are the uterus, ovaries, and fallopian tubes. However, in two reported cases the endometrium was found to be absent, with repeated biopsies (Berker, 2008; Nigam, 2014). It is likely that some genetic defect is responsible for this rare finding, but the reported association of a translocation between chromosomes 4 and 20 (Nigam, 2014) is unlikely to be the cause.

## DIFFERENTIAL DIAGNOSIS AND MANAGEMENT

After a history is obtained and a physical examination performed, including measurement of height, span, and weight, those with primary amenorrhea can be grouped into one of the four general categories listed in Box 38.1, depending on the presence or absence of breasts and a uterus. If breasts are absent but a uterus is present, the diagnostic evaluation should differentiate between CNS-hypothalamic-pituitary disorders and failure of normal gonadal development. Although individuals with both of these disorders have similar phenotypes because of low $E_2$ levels, a single serum FSH assay can differentiate between these two major diagnostic categories (Mashchak, 1981) (Fig. 38.8). Women with hypergonadotropic hypogonadism (FSH >30 mIU/mL), not those with hypogonadotropic hypogonadism, should have a peripheral white blood cell karyotype obtained to determine whether a Y chromosome is present. If a Y chromosome is present, the streak gonads should be excised, because the incidence of subsequent malignancy, mainly gonadoblastomas, is relatively high. If a Y chromosome is absent, it is unnecessary to remove the gonads unless there are signs of hyperandrogenism. It is also unnecessary to perform a karyotype on the gonadal tissue to detect possible mosaicism with a Y chromosome in the gonad unless there is some evidence of hyperandrogenism.

All women with an elevated FSH level and an XX karyotype should have electrolyte and serum progesterone levels measured to rule out 17α-hydroxylase deficiency; a clue is if the patient is hypertensive. In addition to hypernatremia and hypokalemia, individuals with 17α-hydroxylase deficiency have an elevated serum progesterone level (>3 ng/mL), a low 17α-hydroxyprogesterone level (<0.2 ng/mL), and an elevated serum deoxycorticosterone level (>17 ng/100 mL) and usually have hypertension. Doses of conjugated equine estrogen (CEE) in the range of 0.625 mg or its equivalent are usually sufficient to cause breast proliferation. These rare individuals with 17α-hydroxylase deficiency need to have adequate cortisol replacement in addition to sex steroid treatment.

Women with ovarian failure or hypergonadotropic hypogonadism who wish to become pregnant may undergo egg donation. As long as the uterus is normal, which is usually the case, high pregnancy rates in the range of 60% to 70% per cycle may be expected.

If the FSH level is low, the underlying disorder is in the CNS-hypothalamic-pituitary region, and the serum PRL level should be determined. Even if the PRL level is not elevated, all women with hypogonadotropic hypogonadism should have a head CT scan or MRI to rule out a lesion. It is unnecessary to perform a karyotype, because all those with hypogonadotropic hypogonadism are expected to be 46,XX. The use of GnRH testing is optional but is usually clinically unnecessary unless GnRH is going to be used for ovulation induction. Ovulation can be induced in women with this disorder because their ovaries are normal. Initially, they should receive estrogen-progestogen treatment to induce breast development and cause epiphyseal closure. When fertility is desired, human menopausal gonadotropins or pulsatile GnRH should be administered. Clomiphene citrate will be ineffective because of low endogenous $E_2$ levels.

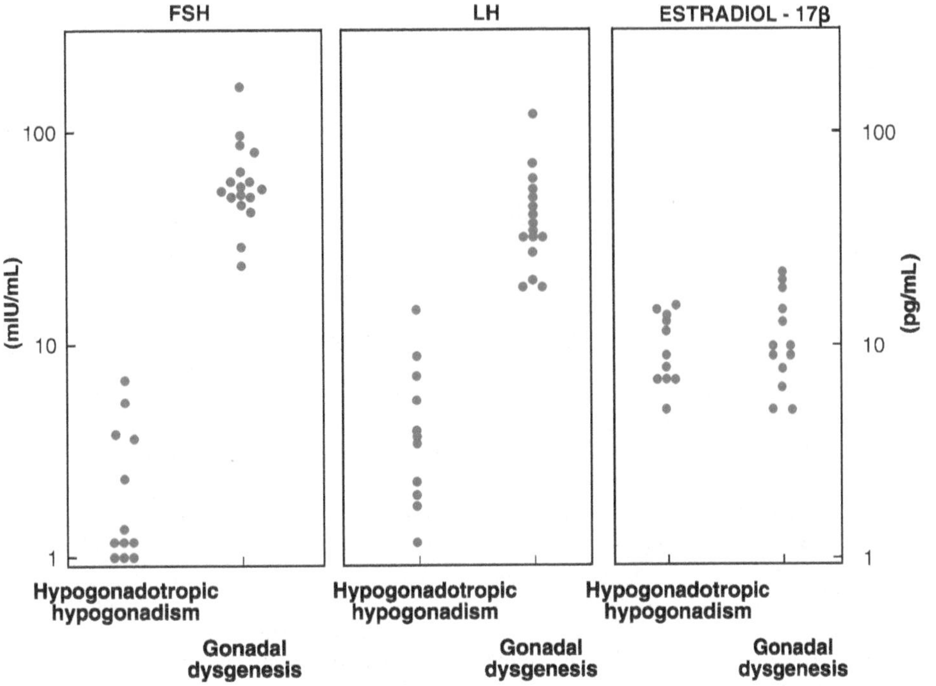


**Figure 38.8** Levels of serum FSH, LH, and estradiol in patients with primary amenorrhea who have an intact uterus and no breast development. *FSH*, Follicle-stimulating hormone; *LH*, luteinizing hormone. (From Mashchak CA, Kletzky OA, Davajan V, et al. Clinical and laboratory evaluation of patients with primary amenorrhea. *Obstet Gynecol.* 1981;57:715.)

The differential diagnosis of androgen resistance from uterine agenesis can easily be made by the presence in the latter condition of normal body hair, ovulatory and premenstrual-type symptoms, biphasic basal temperature, and a normal female testosterone level. Because women with uterine agenesis have normal female endocrine function, they do not require hormone therapy. A renal scan should be performed because of the high incidence of renal abnormalities. They may need surgical reconstruction of an absent vagina (McIndoe procedure), but progressive mechanical dilation with plastic dilators, as described by Frank, should be tried first and is usually successful in motivated individuals, particularly when using pressure from body weight, as with a bicycle seat. These women can now have their own genetic children. After ovarian stimulation and follicle aspiration, fertilized oocytes can be placed in the uterus of a surrogate recipient (gestational carrier). As noted earlier, a case report of a woman having a live birth after uterus transplantation has been reported (Brännström, 2015).

Individuals with androgen resistance have an XY karyotype and male levels of testosterone. After full breast development is attained and epiphyseal closure occurs, the gonads should be removed because of their malignant potential. Thereafter, estrogen therapy should be administered. They do not need progestogen therapy in the absence of a uterus, and lower doses of estrogen are sufficient (see Chapter 14).

The rare individuals without breast development and no internal genitalia should be referred to an endocrine center for the extensive evaluation necessary to establish the diagnosis. If gonads are present, they should be removed, because a Y chromosome is present. Hormone therapy should be administered to these individuals.

## SECONDARY AMENORRHEA

### *CAUSES*

The symptom of amenorrhea associated with hyperprolactinemia or excessive androgen or cortisol production will not be considered in this chapter because these disorders are discussed in Chapter 39 and Chapter 40. If amenorrhea is present without galactorrhea, hyperprolactinemia, or hirsutism, the symptom can result from disorders in the CNS-hypothalamic-pituitary axis, ovary, or uterus. In a review of 262 patients presenting with secondary amenorrhea during a 20-year period at a tertiary medical center, Reindollar reported that 12% of cases resulted from a primary ovarian problem, 62% from a hypothalamic disorder, 16% from a pituitary problem (including prolactinomas), and 7% from a uterine disorder. The uterine cause of secondary amenorrhea is the only one in which normal endocrine function is present and will be discussed first.

#### *Uterine Factor*

**Intrauterine adhesions** (IUAs) or **synechiae** (Asherman syndrome) can obliterate the endometrial cavity and produce secondary amenorrhea. Rarely, a missed abortion or endometrial tuberculosis can also cause endometrial destruction. The most frequent antecedent factor of IUAs is endometrial curettage associated with pregnancy—either evacuation of a live or dead fetus by mechanical means or postpartum or postabortal curettage. Curettage for a missed abortion results in a high incidence of IUA formation (30%). IUAs may also occur after diagnostic dilation and curettage (D&C) in a nonpregnant woman, so this procedure should be performed only when indicated and not routinely at the time of other surgical procedures (e.g., diagnostic laparoscopy). A less common cause of IUA is severe endometritis or fibrosis following a myomectomy, metroplasty, or cesarean delivery. This cause of amenorrhea should be considered most likely if a temporal relationship exists between the onset of symptoms and uterine curettage.

Confirmation of the diagnosis is usually made by a hysterosalpingogram (Fig. 38.9) or another form of imaging including hysteroscopy. Although it has been suggested that sequential administration of estrogen-progestogen be used as the initial diagnostic procedure when IUA is suspected, withdrawal bleeding occurs following administration of the estrogen/progestogen in many women with IUA and should not be relied upon.

### Central Nervous System and Hypothalamic Causes

#### Central Nervous System Structural Abnormalities

The same anatomic lesions in the brain stem or hypothalamus, which have been discussed as causing primary amenorrhea (by interfering with GnRH release), can also cause secondary amenorrhea. Hypothalamic lesions include craniopharyngiomas, granulomatous disease (e.g., tuberculosis, sarcoidosis), and sequelae of encephalitis. When such uncommon lesions are present, circulating gonadotropins and $E_2$ levels are low, and withdrawal uterine bleeding will not occur after progestogen administration.

#### Drugs

Phenothiazine derivatives, certain antihypertensive agents, and other drugs listed in Chapter 39 can also produce amenorrhea without hyperprolactinemia, although usually the PRL level is elevated. Therefore every individual with secondary amenorrhea should have a detailed medication history obtained, even if galactorrhea is not present. Oral contraceptive steroids inhibit ovulation by acting on the hypothalamus to suppress GnRH and directly on the pituitary to suppress FSH and LH. Occasionally, this hypothalamic-pituitary suppression persists for several months after oral contraceptives are discontinued, producing the syndrome termed *postpill amenorrhea.* This oral contraception–induced suppression should not last longer than 6 months. It has been reported that the incidence of amenorrhea persisting more than 6 months after discontinuation of oral contraceptives (0.8%) is approximately the same as the incidence of secondary amenorrhea in the general population (0.7%). Thus the reason for amenorrhea persisting more than 6 months after discontinuation of oral contraceptives is probably unrelated to their use, except that the regular withdrawal bleeding produced by oral contraceptives masks the development of this symptom.

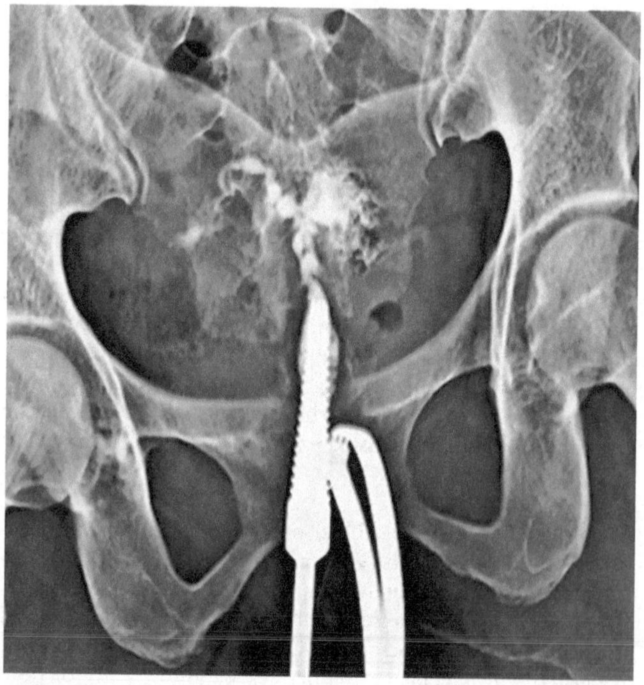

**Figure 38.9** Hysterosalpingogram from an infertile woman who had previously undergone a dilation and curettage procedure. Filling defects are noted throughout the cavity. (Courtesy of Dr. MGK Murthy, Dr. Sumer Sethi, Dr. Srujana, and Mr. Verkat. From Sethi S. Asherman syndrome-HSG. In: Sumer's Radiology Blog, 2013. www.sumerdoc.blogspot.com.)

#### Stress and Exercise

Stressful situations, including a sudden change in environment (e.g., going away to school), death in the family, or divorce, can produce amenorrhea. A high percentage of women who had been placed in concentration camps or those sentenced for execution also became amenorrheic as a result of stress.

Feicht and colleagues reported that the incidence of secondary amenorrhea in runners has a positive correlation with the number of miles run per week (Feicht, 1978) (Fig. 38.10). In a comparison of amenorrheic and eumenorrheic athletes, they reported that physical parameters such as age, weight, lean body mass, and body fat were similar. The only significant difference between the two groups was the fact that the amenorrheic athletes ran more miles weekly. McArthur and associates have also reported there is no significant difference in the percentage of body fat in amenorrheic runners compared with runners who were menstruating. Both stress and exercise can increase brain-derived factors that can inhibit GnRH release (CRH, opioid peptides etc.) In a longitudinal study of competitive swimmers, it has been suggested that inhibition of the GnRH axis is characterized by higher levels of catechol estrogens and opioid peptides (particularly β-endorphin [β-EP]). Adashi showed that catechol estrogen infusion can suppress the release of GnRH and LH; and Reid demonstrated the inhibition of LH by β-EP. It is probable that emotionally stressful situations such as divorce or a sudden change

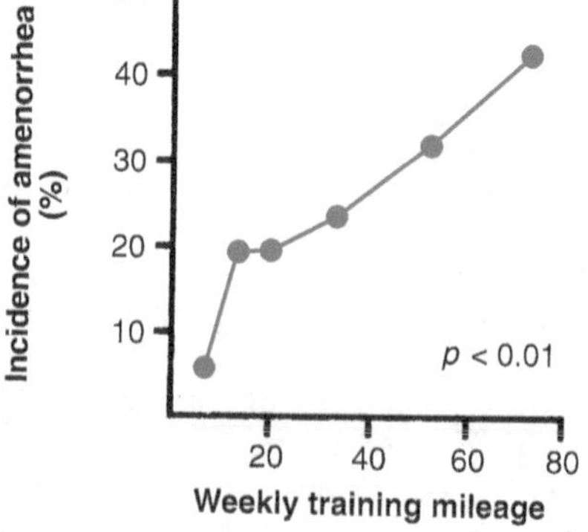


**Figure 38.10** Correlation between training mileage and amenorrhea. Each point represents an average of 21 respondents. Statistical significance of relationship was obtained from point-biserial correlation (1 mile [1.6 km]). (From Feicht CB, Johnson TS, Martin BJ. Secondary amenorrhoea in athletes. *Lancet.* 1978;2:1145.)

in environment can also alter brain chemistry. When the stressful situation abates, whether emotional in origin or related to strenuous exercise, normal cyclic ovarian function and regular menses usually resume in a few months.

## Weight Loss

Both male and female animals that are malnourished have decreased reproductive capacity. Weight loss is also associated with amenorrhea in women and has been classified into two groups: the moderately underweight group, which includes individuals whose weight is 15% to 25% below ideal body weight, and severely underweight women, whose weight loss is more than 25% of ideal body weight. Weight loss can occur from excessive dietary restrictions as well as malnutrition. Vigersky demonstrated that women with amenorrhea associated with simple weight loss have direct and indirect evidence of **hypothalamic dysfunction**, but pituitary and end organ function is normal. Mason showed that in contrast to women with normal cycles, a group of women with weight loss amenorrhea had similar mean levels of LH as well as LH pulse amplitude, but they had a decreased frequency of LH pulses. Thus the amenorrhea associated with weight loss appears to be caused mainly by failure of normal GnRH release, with the lack of a pituitary response under extreme conditions. Hypoleptinemia, alterations in ghrelin, as well as GH and thyroid dysfunction contribute to these findings.

A severe psychiatric disorder called anorexia nervosa is also associated with severe weight loss and amenorrhea. This condition is covered in Chapter 9.

## Polycystic Ovary Syndrome

**Polycystic ovary syndrome** (PCOS) is a heterogenous disorder that may present with prolonged periods of amenorrhea, although the more typical menstrual pattern is one of irregularity or oligomenorrhea. Women need not be overweight or obese, or have symptoms and signs of hyperandrogenism, which typically occurs. Although most women will have an elevated serum LH level, this level may be normal, and measurement of LH is not required as a diagnostic criterion. Nevertheless, the diagnosis of PCOS may be confirmed by visualizing polycystic ovaries on ultrasound, particularly in the absence of classic findings such as hyperandrogenism. According to the European Society of Human Reproduction and Embryology–American Society for Reproductive Medicine (ESHRE-ASRM) criteria for the diagnosis of PCOS, women may be diagnosed as having PCOS with only the menstrual disturbance (in this case amenorrhea) and polycystic ovaries seen with ultrasound. This subject is discussed in detail in Chapter 41.

## Functional Hypothalamic Amenorrhea

Women with secondary amenorrhea who do not ingest drugs, do not engage in strenuous exercise, are not undergoing environmental stress, have not lost weight, and who have no pituitary, ovarian, or uterine abnormalities have an entity called **functional hypothalamic amenorrhea** (FHA). During normal ovulatory cycles, LH is secreted in a pulsatile manner that varies in frequency and amplitude at different times of the cycle, being more rapid in the follicular phase than in the luteal phase (Reame, 1984) (Fig. 38.11). Women with amenorrhea caused

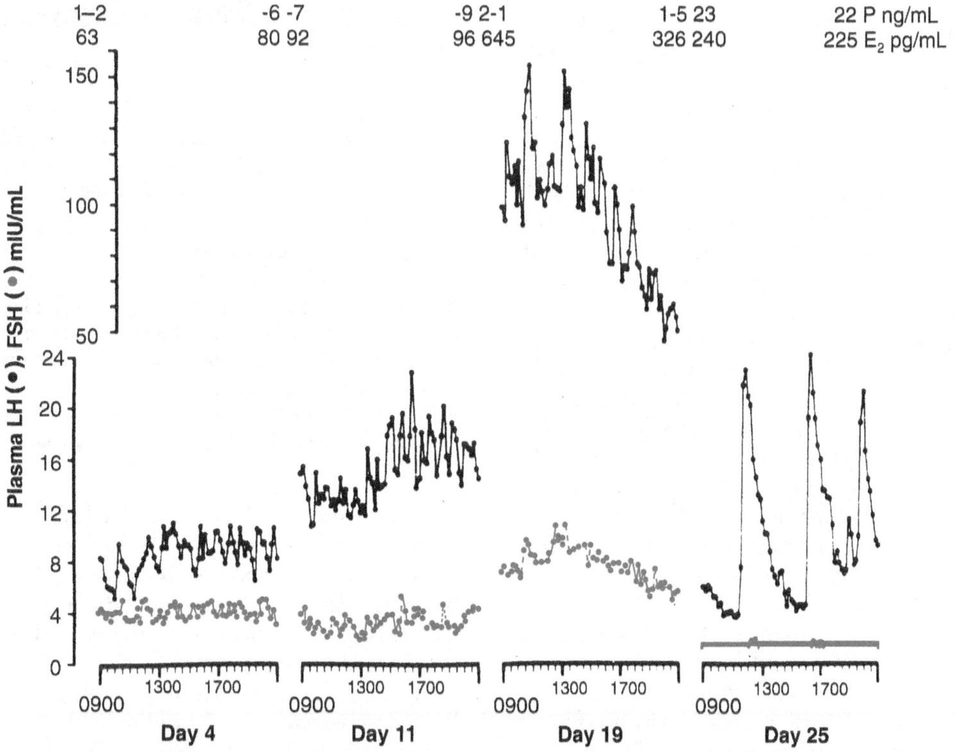


**Figure 38.11** Serial measurements of plasma LH and FSH in two subjects sampled every 10 minutes at weekly intervals during cycles in which LH surge was observed on one of the sampling days. *E*$_2$, Estradiol; *FSH*, follicle-stimulating hormone; *LH*, luteinizing hormone; *P*, pregnanediol. (From Reame NE, Sauder SE, Kelch RP, et al. Pulsatile gonadotropin secretion during the human menstrual cycle: evidence for altered frequency of gonadotropin-releasing hormone secretion. *J Clin Endocrinol Metab.* 1984;59:328.)

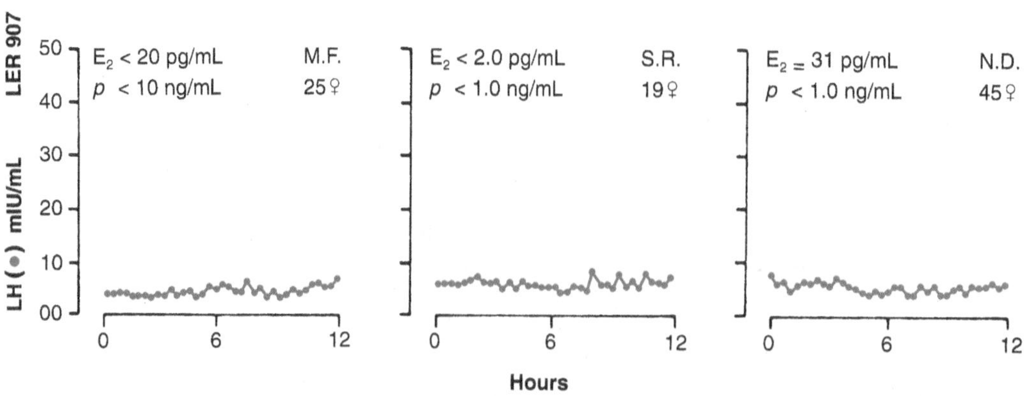


**Figure 38.12** Pulsatile pattern of LH secretion in women with hypogonadotropic hypogonadism and hypothalamic amenorrhea. *$E_2$*, Estradiol; *LH*, luteinizing hormone; M.F., S.R., and N.D. are the three patients' initials. (From Crowley WF Jr, Filicori M, Spratt DI, et al. The physiology of gonadotropin-releasing hormone [GnRH] secretion in men and women. *Rec Prog Hormone Res.* 1985;41:473.)

by hypothalamic dysfunction do not exhibit these characteristic cyclic alterations in LH pulsatility. They either have no pulses (Crowley, 1985) (Fig. 38.12) or have a persistent pattern of pulsatility that is normally found in only one portion of the ovulatory cycle, usually the slow frequency normally found in the luteal phase, despite having a steroid milieu similar to that in the follicular phase (see Fig. 38.12). Because each LH pulse represents a response to a pulse of GnRH, it appears that those with FHA have an abnormality in the normal cyclic variations of GnRH pulsatility, probably because of an abnormality in the CNS neurotransmitters and possibly produced by increased opioid activity. As reported by Ferin and colleagues, administration of the opioid antagonists naloxone and naltrexone to women with FHA is followed by an increase in frequency of LH pulses, as well as by induction of ovulation (Ferin, 1984).

Berga and associates measured several pituitary hormones at frequent intervals in a 24-hour period in 10 women with FHA and 10 women with normal cycles (Berga, 1989). As also reported by others, they found a 53% reduction in LH pulse frequency among the women with FHA; however, the LH pulse amplitude was similar in the two groups. In addition to reduced secretion of LH, there was reduced secretion of FSH, PRL, and thyroid-stimulating hormone (TSH), as well as altered rhythms of growth hormone (GH) and cortisol with elevated cortisol levels. However, the pituitary response to releasing hormones was unchanged. Thus a number of hormonal alterations occur in FHA as an adaptive central neuroendocrine event. Some data from Tschugguel and Berga have suggested that in stress-induced hypothalamic amenorrhea, hypnotherapy and cognitive behavior therapy may be able to restore ovarian activity (Tschugguel, 2003). Although this is a difficult approach that is not easy to duplicate, it is a logical approach from a physiologic perspective. Also, this method may be beneficial in that chronic stress reduction is generally beneficial for general health and can prevent cardiovascular problems and immune compromise. In a controlled study over 20 weeks, normal ovarian activity was restored in approximately 80% of women (Berga, 2003) (Fig. 38.13).

When sufficient GnRH is produced to facilitate gonadotropin stimulation of the ovaries producing $E_2$ levels sufficient to proliferate the endometrium (usually about 30 pg/mL), the term *hypothalamic-pituitary "dysfunction"* is used to characterize this disorder. However, when the $E_2$ levels fall below 40 pg/mL, the term *hypothalamic-pituitary "failure"* has been used, although these terms are arbitrary. There is not a marked distinction between women with dysfunction and failure, and this designation is merely a matter of severity of the hypothalamic suppression. Also, $E_2$ levels may fluctuate in this narrow range, and many clinical laboratories are not often able to measure these lower levels accurately. Accordingly, the functional or biologic estrogen status of these patients can be suggested by administering a progestogen. If endogenous $E_2$ has been sufficient to allow the endometrium to proliferate, then progestogen administration will result in withdrawal bleeding. This can also be determined by visualizing the endometrial stripe by ultrasound scan.

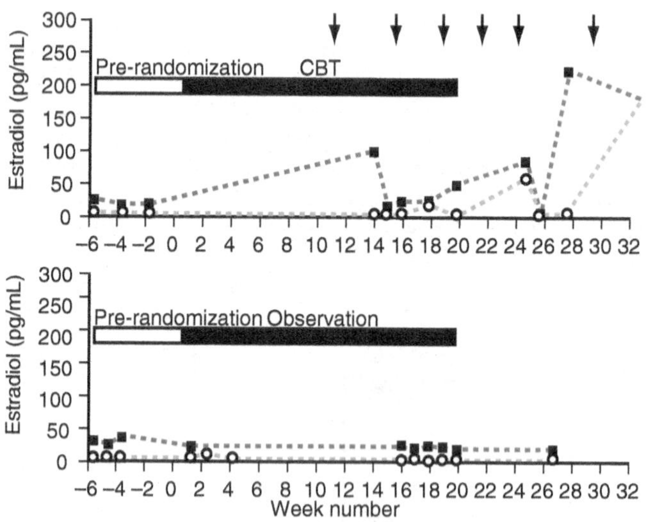


**Figure 38.13** Estradiol *(dot)* and progesterone levels *(square)* in a woman with functional hypothalamic amenorrhea (FHA) who had a return of ovulatory menstrual cycles while undergoing cognitive behavioral therapy (CBT) *(top panel)*, and estradiol and progesterone levels in a woman with FHA who remained anovulatory and amenorrheic during observation for 20 weeks *(bottom panel)*. (From Berga, SL, Marcus MD, Loucks, et al. Recovery of ovarian activity in women with functional hypothalamic amenorrhea who were treated with cognitive behavior therapy. *Fertil Steril.* 2003;80:976.)

If the thickness is less than 4 mm, hypoestrogenism is clearly present. The importance of knowing the estrogen status of these patients is that with the severe hypoestrogenism of hypothalamic "failure," bone loss occurs in these young women at a critical time, when attainment of peak bone mass should be occurring (up to age 30).

### *Pituitary Causes (Hypoestrogenic Amenorrhea)*

#### Neoplasms

Although most pituitary tumors secrete prolactin, some do not and may be associated with the onset of secondary amenorrhea without hyperprolactinemia. Chromophobe adenomas are the most common non–prolactin-secreting pituitary tumors; however, basophilic (ACTH-secreting) and acidophilic (GH-secreting) adenomas may not secrete prolactin. Individuals with the latter types of tumor, although having secondary amenorrhea, frequently have other symptoms produced by these lesions and present to the clinician with symptoms of acromegaly or Cushing disease.

#### Nonneoplastic Lesions

Pituitary cells can also become damaged or necrotic as a result of anoxia, thrombosis, or hemorrhage. When pituitary cell destruction occurs as a result of a hypotensive episode during pregnancy, the disorder is called *Sheehan syndrome.* When the disorder is unrelated to pregnancy, it is called *Simmonds disease.* It is important to diagnose this cause of secondary amenorrhea because, in contrast to the hypothalamic disorders, pituitary damage can be associated with decreased secretion of other pituitary hormones, particularly ACTH and TSH, in addition to LH and FSH. Specific stimulation studies are needed to characterize the different possible deficiencies. Thus these women may have secondary hypothyroidism or adrenal insufficiency that may seriously impair their health, in addition to their decreased estrogen levels.

### *Ovarian Causes (Hypergonadotropic Hypogonadism)*

The ovaries may fail to secrete sufficient estrogen to produce endometrial growth if the follicles are damaged as a result of infection, interference with blood supply, or depletion of follicles caused by bilateral cystectomies. These women may become amenorrheic after a variable period of time has elapsed following medical treatment of a bilateral tubo-ovarian abscess, after bilateral cystectomy for benign ovarian neoplasms, or sometimes after a hysterectomy during which the vascular supply to the ovaries is compromised (also called *cystic degeneration of the ovaries*).

Occasionally, the ovaries cease to produce sufficient estrogen to stimulate endometrial growth several years before the age of physiologic menopause. When this condition occurs before the age of 40, the term *premature ovarian failure (POF)* or *premature ovarian insufficiency (POI)* (Cooper, 2011) is used instead of premature menopause to best describe the clinical entity. A more in-depth discussion of POI may also be found in Chapter 14.

Coulam estimated that as many as 1% of women younger than 40 years have hypergonadotropic amenorrhea, with the incidence steadily increasing from ages 15 to 39. Frequently, the condition of POI is transient before permanent ovarian failure occurs; occasionally, women with a diagnosis of POI may ovulate and conceive during this transition period. POI frequently occurs after gonadal irradiation or systemic chemotherapy and has also been reported in women with steroid hormonal enzyme deficiencies who menstruate temporarily and then have secondary amenorrhea. Approximately 16% of women who carry the premutation for Fragile X may experience POI (Allingham-Hawkins, 1999). Other genetic susceptibilities are also known to exist and are discussed in Chapter 14.

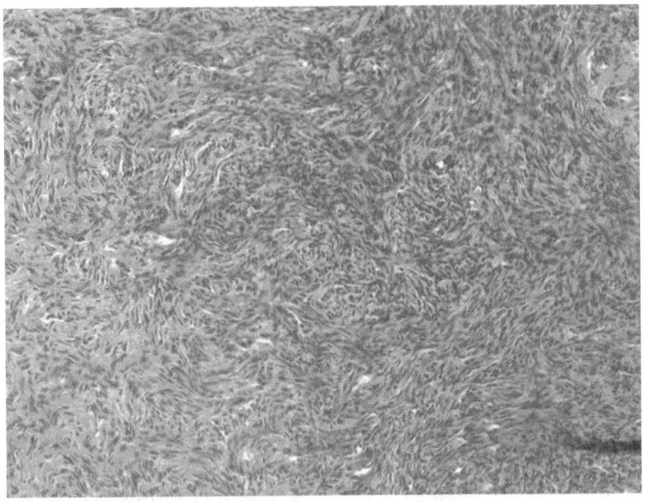

**Figure 38.14** Histology of an ovarian section from a woman with premature ovarian insufficiency, devoid of follicles. (From Ramnani D. Ovarian failure. WebPathology.com, 2015.)

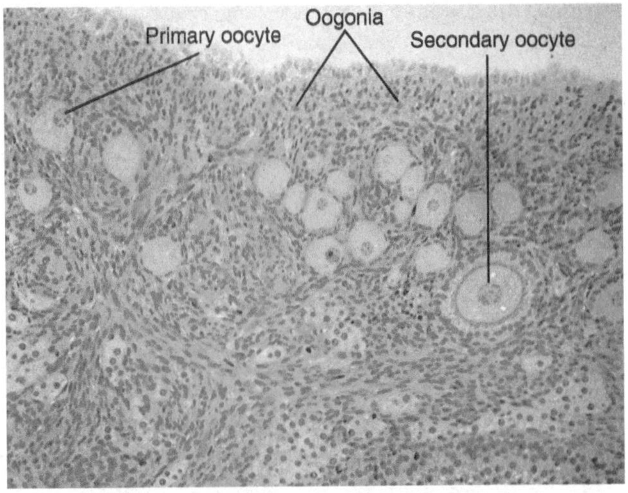


**Figure 38.15** Histologic section of an ovary showing follicles up to the preantral stage, which is typical of a woman presenting with insensitive or "resistant" ovary syndrome. (From Shaco-Levy R, Robboy SJ. Normal ovaries, inflammatory and non-neoplastic conditions. In: Mutter GL, Prat J. *Pathology of the Female Reproductive Tract.* 3rd ed. Philadelphia: Elsevier; 2014.)

Histologically, women with POI have two types of ovarian pathologic findings. In most of them, there is generalized sclerosis similar to the findings of a normal postmenopausal ovary (Fig. 38.14), whereas in up to 30%, numerous primordial follicles with no progression past the early antrum stage are seen, which looks identical to a normal ovary (Fig. 38.15). The latter condition is due either to an **autoimmune state,** which is more common (discussed later), or to a gonadotropin receptor defect and is called **gonadotropin-resistant ovary syndrome.** Women with ovarian resistance syndrome often have primary amenorrhea, but usually sufficient estrogen is produced so that they menstruate for several months or even years. More common are those individuals who have an autoimmune process with autoimmune diseases such as hypoparathyroidism, Hashimoto thyroiditis, or Addison disease. Many women with POI who do not have clinical evidence of an autoimmune disease have antibodies to gonadotropins as well as to several other endocrine organs, such as the thyroid and adrenal glands, suggesting an autoimmune origin. Although it is not recommended to do ovarian biopsies (which requires a full-thickness section) to make this diagnosis, the histologic findings often show lymphocytic infiltration along with the normal histology as shown in Figure 38.15.

Alper estimated that approximately 30% to 50% of women with chromosomally normal POI without a history of irradiation or chemotherapy have an associated autoimmune disease, most commonly thyroid disease, which was present in 85% of the group with an autoimmune disorder (Alper, 1985). Using sophisticated immunofluorescence techniques, Mignot demonstrated that 92% of women with POI have laboratory evidence of autosensitization (Mignot, 1989). Approximately two thirds of these were positive for non–organ-specific antibodies, mainly antinuclear antibodies and rheumatoid factors, and 50% had organ-specific antibodies. Although most of these women had no evidence of autoimmune disease, it is recommended that immunologic screening be performed in young women with POF. In the absence of symptoms, such as weakness, lethargy, or pain, which may suggest systemic disease, it is probably sufficient to obtain a complete blood count (CBC) and comprehensive metabolic panel, as well as TSH and antithyroid antibody levels. If adrenal failure (e.g., weakness) is suspected, adrenal antibodies (against 21-hydroxylase) and cortisol may be obtained; rarely, an ACTH stimulation test is warranted. It may be sufficient to obtain a general screen for adrenal function by obtaining levels of dehydroepiandrosterone sulfate (DHEA-S). Nevertheless some data point to slightly lower (age-specific) levels of DHEA-S in women with POI. Although available clinically, measurements of antiovarian antibodies have not been properly validated.

## DIAGNOSTIC EVALUATION AND MANAGEMENT

All women who consult a clinician for the symptom of **secondary amenorrhea** should have a diagnostic evaluation. The clinician should first take a detailed history and perform a physical examination to rule out pregnancy as a cause of the amenorrhea. The possibility of IUAs should be entertained initially. Any instrumentation of the endometrial cavity, particularly temporally related to pregnancy, should alert the clinician to the possibility of IUAs. If IUAs are ruled out, the history should disclose whether medications are currently being used or if oral contraceptives have been recently discontinued. In addition, questions regarding diet, weight loss, stress, and strenuous exercise are pertinent. A history of hot flushes, decreasing breast size, or vaginal dryness and physical examination are helpful in estimating the degree of estrogen deficiency. If the history and physical examination fail to reveal the cause of the amenorrhea, a CBC, urinalysis, and serum chemistries should be carried out to rule out systemic disease. A sensitive thyroid-stimulating hormone (TSH) assay should also be performed to rule out the uncommon asymptomatic thyroid disorders that produce secondary amenorrhea, and serum $E_2$, FSH, and prolactin levels should be measured (Fig. 38.16). If prolactin levels are elevated, a diagnostic

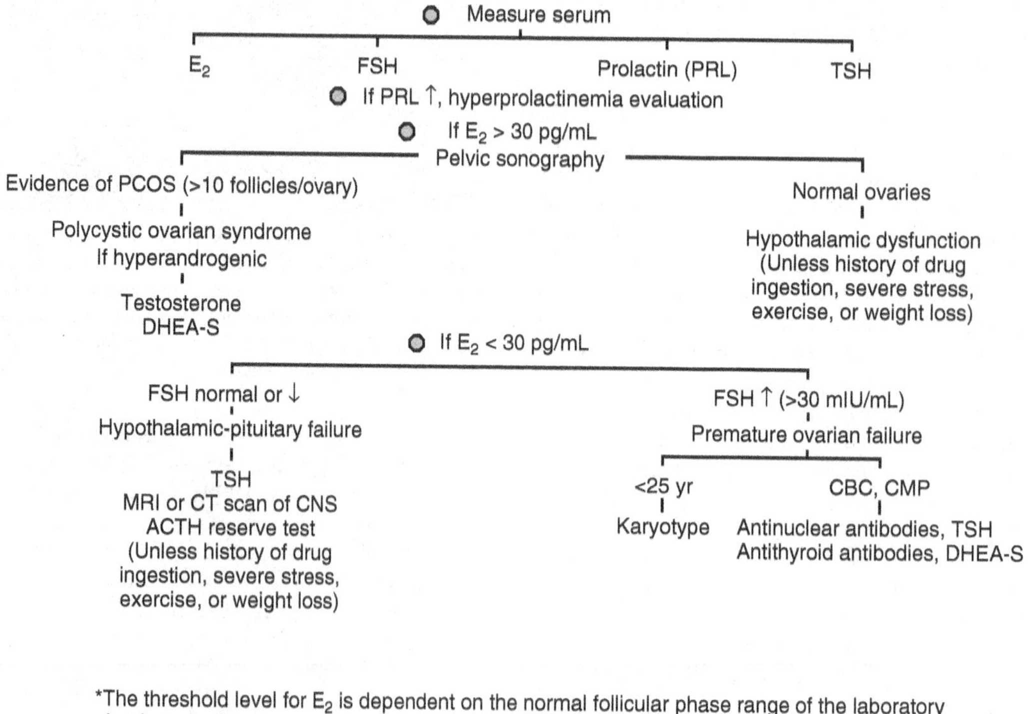


*The threshold level for $E_2$ is dependent on the normal follicular phase range of the laboratory but is typically around 30 pg/mL.

**Figure 38.16** Diagnostic evaluation of secondary amenorrhea. *ACTH*, Adrenocorticotropic hormone; *CBC*, complete blood count; *CMP*, comprehensive metabolic panel; *CNS*, central nervous system; *CT*, computed tomography; *DHEA-S*, dehydroepiandrosterone sulfate; *E₂*, estradiol; *FSH*, follicle-stimulating hormone; *MRI*, magnetic resonance imaging; *PCOS*, polycystic ovary syndrome; *TSH*, thyroid-stimulating hormone.

evaluation for the cause of this problem should be undertaken (see Chapter 39). Administration of injectable progesterone or oral progestogen is an indirect means of determining whether sufficient estrogen is present to produce endometrial growth that will slough after the progesterone levels fall (progesterone challenge test). However, it is preferable to order a sensitive $E_2$ assay, with organic solvent extraction, to determine the true estrogen status. As noted, the thickness of the endometrial stripe on ultrasound is also beneficial.

Women who exercise or who have PCOS, moderate stress, weight loss, or hypothalamic-pituitary dysfunction will usually have $E_2$ levels of at least 30 pg/mL and withdrawal bleeding after progestogens usually occur. Those with pituitary tumors, ovarian failure, severe dietary weight loss or anorexia nervosa, severe stress, or the rare hypothalamic lesion will usually have very low $E_2$ levels, typically in the postmenopausal range.

If a sensitive serum $E_2$ value is above 30 pg/mL, and ultrasound confirms the presence of polycystic ovaries, the diagnosis of PCOS may be considered (see Chapter 41). If there is no sonographic evidence of polycystic ovaries and the woman has a history of drug ingestion, stress, weight loss, or strenuous exercise, she should be told that hypothalamic-pituitary dysfunction is present and the exact cause cannot be determined with current technology because frequent LH sampling is costly and impractical. She should also be informed that hypothalamic-pituitary dysfunction is usually a self-limiting disorder and not a serious threat to health or a cause of untreatable infertility.

Women with low $E_2$ and low FSH levels have a CNS lesion or hypothalamic-pituitary failure. Women with low $E_2$ and elevated FSH levels (>30 mIU/mL) have POI. If severe weight loss, strenuous exercise, or severe stress is not present, and FSH and $E_2$ levels are low, CT or MRI of the hypothalamic-pituitary region should be performed to rule out a lesion, even if the prolactin level is normal. If a lesion is seen or if there is a history compatible with possible **pituitary destruction** (hypotension during pregnancy), a test of ACTH reserve should be performed. An **insulin tolerance test** in which hypoglycemia is induced should normally cause a cortisol increase of 7 μg/100 mL within 120 minutes and is a satisfactory test of ACTH function. An alternative test is administration of CRH. If no lesion is identified, the term *hypothalamic-pituitary failure* may be used as a nonspecific diagnosis. Frequently, individuals with this diagnosis resume normal ovarian function without treatment.

If POI is diagnosed because of an elevated FSH level and no cause of ovarian destruction is elicited, the possibility of autoimmune disease should be considered, particularly in younger women. Therefore antithyroid and antinuclear antibody levels should be measured and other screening tests should be performed, as noted previously. Although commercially available tests for antiovarian and antiadrenal antibodies are available, they are not measured routinely.

To rule out mosaicism or a dysgenetic gonad, including the possibility of a Y cell line, a karyotype should be obtained in women with POF who are 25 years of age or younger. Biopsy of the gonads by laparoscopy or laparotomy is not indicated. Suppression of gonadotropin levels with estrogen, oral contraceptives, and GnRH analogues has been advocated to induce rebound ovulation following their withdrawal. Although these agents suppress gonadotropins, these techniques are usually ineffective for inducing ovulation. If ovulation occurs following such treatment, it is a sporadic event and not a result of the therapy. Most cases of spontaneous pregnancy have occurred during estrogen replacement.

The appropriate treatment depends on the diagnosis and on whether conception is desired. Non–prolactin-secreting pituitary tumors should be surgically excised, if possible. Those who have lost weight should be advised to gain weight. If strenuous exercise results in low estrogen levels (<30 pg/mL), the amount of exercise should be reduced or estrogen supplementation administered to prevent possible development of osteoporosis. Several investigators have shown that amenorrheic and oligomenorrheic athletes with decreased $E_2$ levels have decreased density of trabecular bone in the lumbar spine (Lloyd, 1988) (Fig. 38.17).

Klibanski showed that women with low $E_2$ levels caused by hypothalamic amenorrhea who have normal nutrition and activity levels have a profound reduction in spinal bone mineral density. The reduction in bone loss is independent of whether the PRL level is elevated or not. Bone loss has been found to be similar in hyperprolactinemic amenorrheic women with low estrogen levels and women with normal prolactin and low estrogen levels (Fig. 38.18). A group of women with hyperprolactinemia and regular menses did not have bone loss.

If women with PCOS or hypothalamic-pituitary dysfunction desire conception, clomiphene citrate or letrozole administration is successful in inducing ovulation. If pregnancy is not desired, periodic progestogen administration (medroxyprogesterone acetate, 10 mg/day, for 10 to 12 days) should be given to reduce the increased risk of endometrial cancer associated with unopposed estrogen. It may be sufficient to administer the progestogen every 3 months. If a woman with hypothalamic-pituitary "failure" (low estrogen levels) desires fertility, ovulation can be induced with exogenous gonadotropins or pulsatile GnRH. Clomiphene is not successful if the estrogen

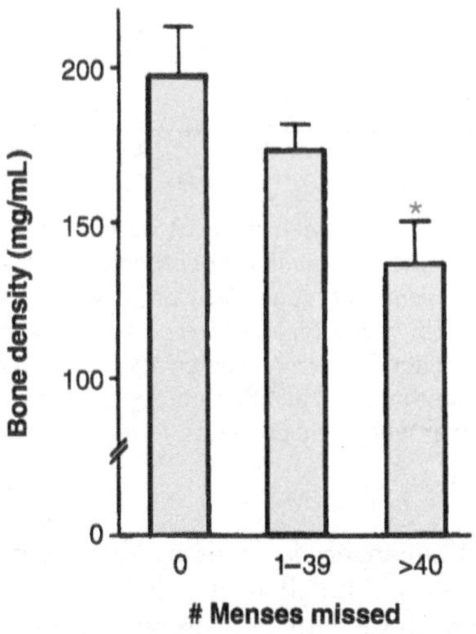


**Figure 38.17** Relationship between bone density and number of missed menses in collegiate women athletes. For each subject, number of missed menses was determined from her menarche to age 19. *Asterisk* indicates a significant difference from the control group. (From Lloyd T, Myers C, Buchanan JR, et al. Collegiate women athletes with irregular menses during adolescence have decreased bone density. *Obstet Gynecol.* 1988;72:639.)

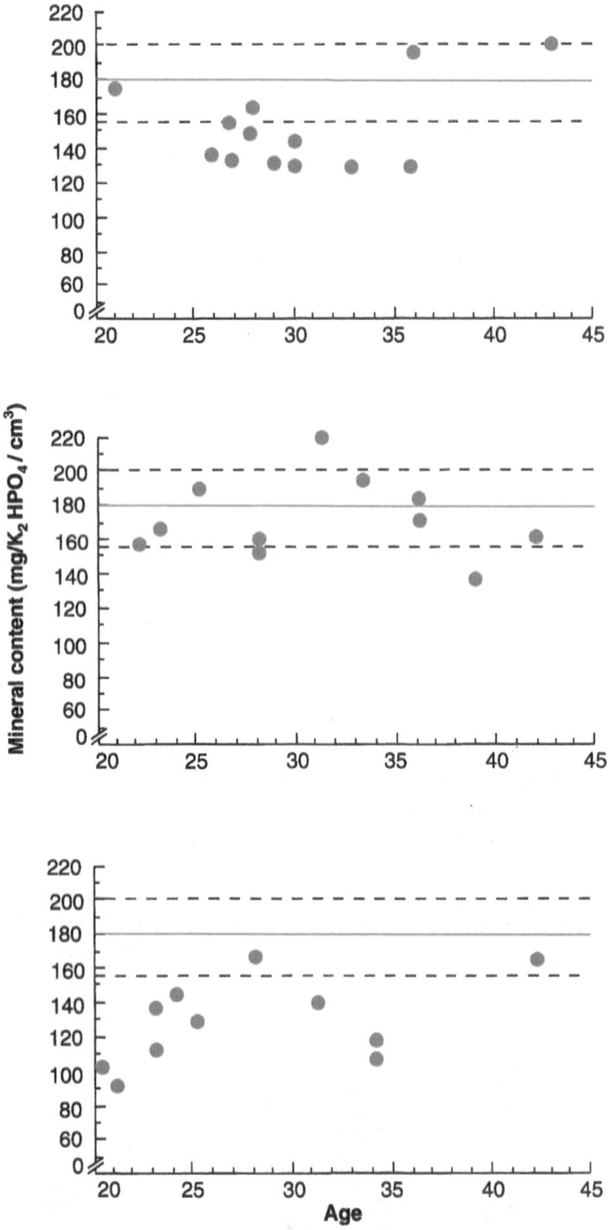


**Figure 38.18** Spinal bone density in 13 women with hyperprolactinemic amenorrhea *(top panel)*, 12 eumenorrheic hyperprolactinemic women *(middle panel)*, and 11 women with hypothalamic amenorrhea *(bottom panel)*. Mean *(solid lines)* and standard deviation (± SD, *dashed lines*) for 19 normal women are shown. (From Klibanski A, Biller BM, Rosenthal DI, et al. Effects of prolactin and estrogen deficiency in amenorrheic bone loss. *J Clin Endocrinol Metab.* 1988;67:124.)

levels are low. If pregnancy is not desired, estrogen-progestogen treatment is indicated for all amenorrheic women with low $E_2$ levels, including those with POI, to reduce the risk of osteoporosis. Young women with POI and chronic hypothalamic hypoestrogenic status are also vulnerable to accelerated atherosclerosis. There is no increased cardiovascular risk in prescribing estrogen to these women. Women with POI may become pregnant with the use of donor oocytes and the priming of their endometrium with estrogen and progesterone for embryo transfer.

## PRECOCIOUS PUBERTY

Puberty in the female is the process of biologic changes and physical development, after which sexual reproduction becomes possible. This is a time of accelerated linear skeletal growth and development of secondary sexual characteristics, such as breast development and the appearance of axillary and pubic hair. The usual sequence of the physiologic events of puberty begins with breast development and the subsequent appearance of pubic and axillary hair, followed by the period of maximal growth velocity and, finally, menarche. Menarche may occur before the appearance of axillary or pubic hair in 10% of normal females. Normal puberty occurs over a wide range of ages. Figure 38.19 gives the mean and ranges for pubertal onset and types of development in girls (Lee, 2003). The rate of growth is also of interest. Prior to breast development the growth velocity is close to 6 cm/year. At peak height velocity, around age 12, the velocity is around 8 cm/year; and by the completion of puberty, around age 14, the velocity is down to 1 cm/year, explained by closure of the epiphyses (Biro, 2006).

**Precocious puberty** is arbitrarily defined as the appearance of any signs of secondary sexual maturation at an early age. Puberty in girls is now recognized to be occurring earlier than in previous studies (Table 38.4). In an article by Kaplowitz and associates, it was suggested that girls with breast development or pubic hair should be evaluated when these signs occur before age 7 in whites and age 6 in black girls (Kaplowitz, 1999). This has been somewhat controversial, and others have suggested that an evaluation is not warranted until age 8 in girls, because suggesting a diagnosis earlier may mask the ability to identify other diseases (Midyett, 2003). Accordingly, we favor carrying out a complete evaluation of precocious puberty at 8 years of age.

Precocious puberty is associated with a wide range of disorders. It should be emphasized that regardless of the cause, precocious puberty is a rare disorder. The incidence of this condition in the United States is estimated to be approximately 1 in 10,000 young girls. When it is diagnosed, the physician should undertake a detailed investigation of the cause of the condition so as not to overlook a potentially correctable pathologic lesion. The two primary concerns of parents of children with precocious puberty are the social stigma associated with the child being physically different from her peers and the diminished ultimate height caused by the premature closure of epiphyseal growth centers.

Puberty is a time of accelerated growth, skeletal maturation, and resulting epiphyseal closure. Although precocious puberty may occur early in a child's life, it usually develops in the normal sequence. Early in the course of the disease the girls are taller and heavier than their chronologic peers who have not experienced the growth spurt (Fig. 38.20). However, although the patient is tall as a child, her eventual adult height will be shorter than normal because of premature closure of the epiphyses. Without therapy, approximately 50% of girls with precocious puberty will not reach the height of 5 feet.

### *TYPES OF DISORDERS*

Precocious puberty is subdivided into GnRH dependent (complete, true) and GnRH independent (incomplete, pseudo), and these causes have been subcategorized as feminizing (previously termed isosexual) or virilizing (previously termed heterosexual) disorders. These categories are of clinical value only after the eventual diagnosis has been established. The pathophysiology

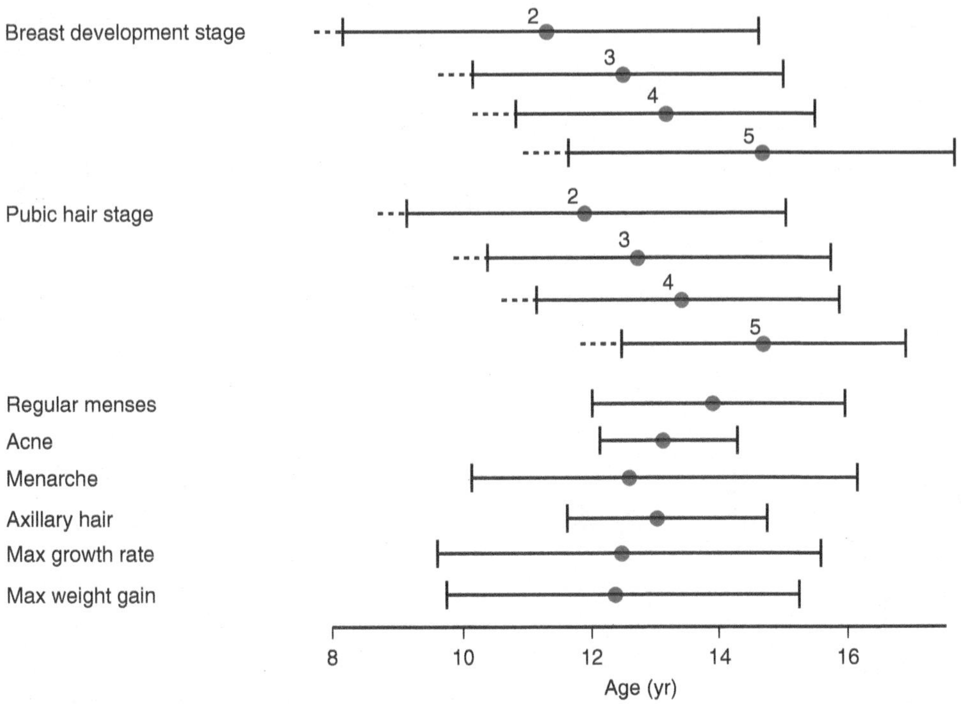


**Figure 38.19** Mean ages *(dots)* and ranges *(horizontal lines)* of pubertal onset and development in girls. Dashed lines show the earlier limit for African-American girls. Max, maximum. (From Lee PA. Puberty and its disorders. In: Lifshitz F, ed. *Pediatric Endocrinology.* 4th ed. New York: Marcel Dekker; 2003:212.)

**Table 38.4** Prevalence of Breast and Pubic Hair Development in White and Black Girls*

| | Age Range (yr) | | | | |
|---|---|---|---|---|---|
| **Parameter** | **5.00-5.99** | **6.00-6.99** | **7.00-7.99** | **8.00-8.99** | **9.00-9.99** |
| Prevalence of breast development at Tanner stage 2 or higher (%) | | | | | |
| White girl | 1.6 | 2.9 | 5.0 | 10.5 | 32.1 |
| Black girl | 2.4 | 6.4 | 15.4 | 37.8 | 62.6 |
| Prevalence of pubic hair development at Tanner stage 2 or higher (%) | | | | | |
| White | 0.4 | 1.4 | 2.8 | 7.7 | 20.0 |
| African American | 3.4 | 9.5 | 17.7 | 34.3 | 62.6 |

From Kaplowitz PB, Oberfield SE. Reexamination of the age limit for determining when puberty is precocious in girls in the United States: Implications for evaluation and treatment. Drug and Therapeutics and Executive Committees of the Lawson Wilkins Pediatric Endocrine Society. *Pediatrics.* 1999;104:937.
*Between 5 and 10 years of age.

and corresponding categories of precocious puberty may change during the course of the disease; for example, congenital adrenal hyperplasia initially is GnRH independent but subsequently, over many months, eventually becomes a GnRH dependent form of precocious puberty.

The pathophysiology of precocious puberty is divided into two distinct categories: a normal physiologic process involving GnRH secretion with an integrated hypothalamic–pituitary axis, which occurs at an abnormal time, or an abnormal physiologic process independent of an integrated hypothalamic-pituitary-ovarian axis.

GnRH dependent precocious puberty involves premature maturation of the hypothalamic-pituitary-ovarian axis and includes normal menses, ovulation, and the possibility of pregnancy. GnRH independent precocious puberty involves premature female sexual maturation, which may lead to estrogen-induced uterine stimulation and bleeding without any normal ovarian follicular activity. Both categories have increased circulating levels of estrogen. In the latter syndrome, however, secretion of estrogens is independent of hypothalamic-pituitary control. Depending on when the patient is first seen in relationship to the natural history of her disease, it may be necessary to observe her at regular intervals (for 2 to 3 years) to distinguish one syndrome from another (Table 38.5). Prolonged follow-up is sometimes necessary to rule out subtle, slow-growing lesions of the brain, ovary, or adrenal gland.

The majority of girls with precocious puberty (70%) develop a GnRH-dependent process. Figure 38.4 depicts the normal maturation of the HPO axis, with the integral role of kisspeptin facilitating GnRH release with puberty occurring when the physiologic "brake" is off. The exact cause of most cases of GnRH dependent precocious puberty is unknown (constitutional); however, approximately 30% are secondary to CNS disease. Kisspeptin, a hypothalamic peptide that stimulates the release of GnRH, is involved in the initiation of puberty. Two activating mutations of the kisspeptin receptor have been described in girls with central precocious puberty (Teles, 2008; Silveira, 2010). Another genetic mutation (MKRN3) has been found in a number of affected families (Abreu, 2013).

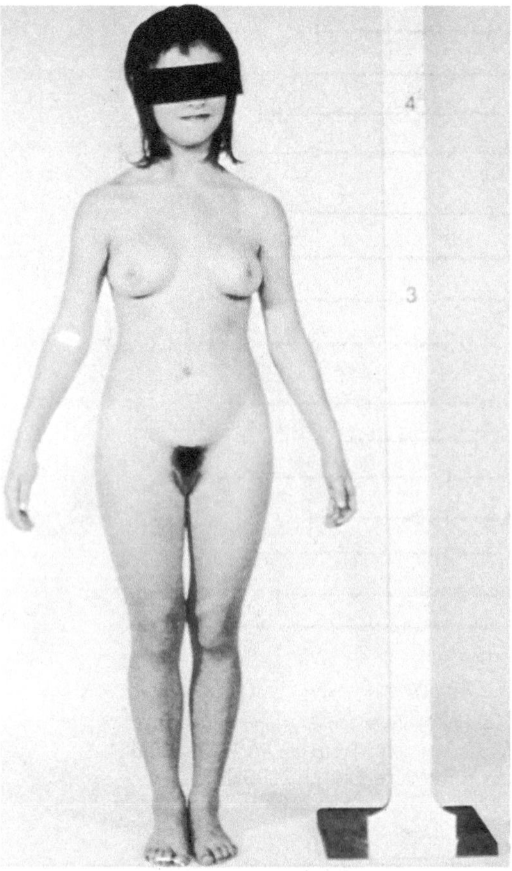

**Figure 38.20** Child age 7 years with constitutional precocious puberty. Note increased height for age. (From Dewhurst CJ. *Practical Pediatric and Adolescent Gynecology*. New York: Marcel Dekker; 1980.)

A definitive diagnosis is established more often for pseudoprecocious puberty, which is usually related to an ovarian or adrenal disorder. If the secondary sex characteristics are discordant with the genetic and phenotypic gender, the condition is termed *heterosexual* or *virilizing precocious puberty.* This is premature virilization in a female child and includes development of masculine secondary sexual characteristics. The androgens that cause heterosexual precocious puberty usually come from the adrenal gland.

### Premature Thelarche

Premature thelarche is defined as isolated unilateral or bilateral breast development as the only sign of secondary sexual maturation. It is not accompanied by other associated evidence of pubertal development, such as axillary or pubic hair or changes in vaginal epithelium. Estrogen levels are normal (prepubertal) as shown in the Figure 38.21 together with estrogen levels in pubertal girls, those with precocious puberty and adults (Escobar, 1976). Breast hyperplasia is a normal physiologic phenomenon in the neonatal period and may persist until the child is up to 6 months of age. Premature thelarche usually occurs in 2 waves: within the first 2 years, and between ages 6 and 8. The breast buds enlarge to 2 to 4 cm, and sometimes this process is asymmetric. Nipple development is absent. This is a benign self-limiting condition that does not require treatment. Often, the breast enlargement spontaneously regresses. It is important to observe these children closely for other signs of precocious puberty. It is associated with normal linear growth and a normal bone age. The cause of premature thelarche is not understood. It has been postulated to be related to a slight increase in estrogen-like activity, either due to transient low circulating estrogen levels (from transient ovarian follicular activity) or from exogenous sources including the possibility of exposure to environmental or dietary estrogen mimics. This disorder may be associated with female infants who had extremely low birth weights.

Table 38.5 Physical Findings among Patients with Various Precocious Puberty Syndromes

| | | | GnRH-Dependent and GnRH-Independent Syndromes | | | |
|---|---|---|---|---|---|---|
| **Findings** | **Premature Thelarche** | **Premature Adrenarche** | **Idiopathic** | **McCune-Albright Syndrome** | **Central Nervous System Tumor** | **Hypothyroid** |
| Breast enlargement | Yes | No | Yes | Yes | Yes | Yes |
| Pubic hair | No | Yes | Yes | Yes | Yes | Unusual |
| Vaginal bleeding | No | No | Yes | Yes | Yes | Yes |
| Virilizing signs | No | No | No | No | No | No |
| Bone age | Normal | Normal to minimally advanced | Advanced | Advanced | Advanced | Normal or retarded |
| Neurologic deficit | No | No | No | Yes | Yes | No |
| Abdominopelvic mass | No | No | Occasional | No | No | Occasional |
| | **Isosexual (Feminizing)** | | | **Heterosexual (Virilizing)** | | |
| **Findings** | **Ovarian Tumors** | **Adrenal Tumors** | **Factitious** | **Ovarian Tumors** | **Adrenal Tumors** | **Adrenal Hyperplasia** |
| Breast enlargement | Yes | Yes | Yes | Yes | Yes | Yes |
| Pubic hair | Yes | Yes | Yes | Yes | Yes | Yes |
| Vaginal bleeding | Yes | Yes | Yes | Yes | Yes | Yes |
| Virilizing signs | No | Yes | No | Yes | Yes | Yes |
| Bone age | Advanced | Advanced | Advanced | Advanced | Advanced | Advanced |
| Neurologic deficit | No | No | No | No | No | No |
| Abdominopelvic mass | Usually | No | No | Occasional | No | No |

From Ross GT. Disorders of the ovary and female reproductive tract. In: Wilson JD, Foster DW (eds). *Williams Textbook of Endocrinology*. 7th ed. Philadelphia: WB Saunders; 1985.
*GnRH*, Gonadotropin-releasing hormone.

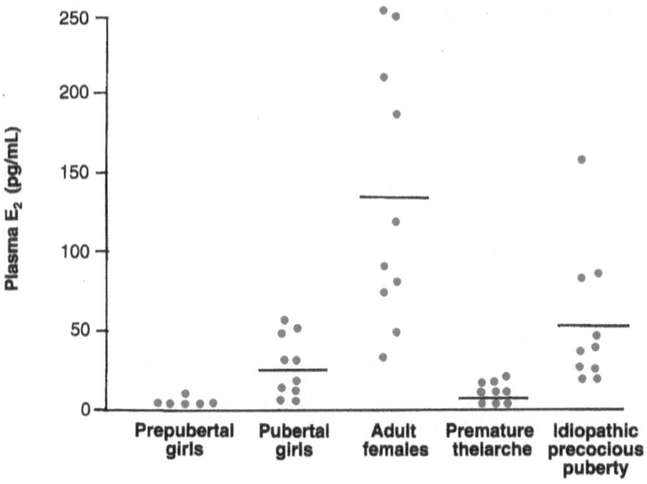


**Figure 38.21** Estradiol values in normal females and in patients with premature thelarche and idiopathic precocious puberty. *Horizontal lines* depict mean levels. (Modified from Escobar ME, Rivarola MA, Bergada C. Plasma concentration of oestradiol-17beta in premature thelarche and in different types of sexual precocity. *Acta Endocrinol.* 1976;81:351.)

### *Premature Pubarche or Adrenarche*

Premature pubarche is early isolated development of pubic hair without other signs of secondary sexual maturation. Premature adrenarche is isolated early development of axillary hair. Neither of these conditions is progressive, and the girls do not have clitoral hypertrophy. However, it is important to differentiate premature pubarche from the virilization produced by congenital adrenal hyperplasia. Some children with premature pubarche have abnormal electroencephalograms (EEGs) without significant neurologic disease. The bone age should not be advanced in this disorder. The cause is poorly understood but is believed to be related to increased androgen production by the adrenal glands (DHEA and DHEA-S). Similar to premature thelarche, the child should have periodic follow-up visits to confirm that the condition is not progressive. Many cases of premature adrenarche evolve into PCOS. Measurements of testosterone and 17-OH progesterone should also be carried out to rule out other conditions.

### *Gonadotropin-Releasing Hormone-Dependent Precocious Puberty*

#### Idiopathic

Idiopathic development is responsible for approximately 80% of the cases of GnRH dependent precocious puberty. Some of these children are simply at the earliest limits of the normal distribution of the biologic curve (see Tables 38.4 and 38.5). Most idiopathic cases are sporadic in distribution; however, some may be familial.

A high incidence of abnormal EEGs in children with idiopathic precocious puberty has raised the question of potential CNS disease. With the increasing use of high-resolution imaging techniques, such as brain CT scanning and MRI, the number of truly idiopathic cases is declining.

These girls have no genital abnormality except for early development. Occasionally, follicular cysts of the ovary may form secondary to increased pituitary gonadotropin levels (see Fig. 38.20). In these cases, the cysts are the result, not the cause, of precocious puberty. Gonadotropin levels, sex steroid levels, and response of LH after administration of GnRH are similar to those in normal puberty. The diagnosis is usually confirmed by measurements of LH and FSH and a pubertal response to GnRH. If basal levels of LH are 5 mIU/mL or greater, the diagnosis is usually made, but otherwise will need a GnRH stimulation test. Because of the lack of availability of GnRH, a GnRH agonist (usually leuprolide acetate 20 μg/kg subcutaneous) is given with LH and FSH measurements measured after 3 hours (Kandemir, 2011). LH responses suggesting GnRH dependency are >5 mIU/mL.

Most of the cases of premature maturation of the hypothalamic-pituitary-ovarian axis do not have a defined cause. The syndrome may appear as early as age 3 to 4 years. When observed for several decades, these women have normal menopausal ages. Emotional problems are a cause for concern because the young girls suffer from extreme social pressures. The intellectual, behavioral, and psychosocial development of girls with precocious puberty is appropriate for their chronologic age, but many are shy and withdraw from their peers.

#### Central Nervous System Lesions

A wide range of inflammatory, degenerative, neoplastic, or congenital defects that involve the CNS may produce GnRH dependent precocious puberty. This occurs in up to 20% of cases and warrants a careful evaluation by imaging. Usually, symptoms of a neurologic disease, especially headaches and visual disturbances, precede the manifestations of precocious puberty.

A most unusual neurologic symptom that may be associated with precocious puberty is seizures with inappropriate laughter (gelastic seizures). Anatomically, most CNS lesions are located near the hypothalamus in the region of the third ventricle, tuber cinereum, or mammillary bodies. Major CNS diseases associated with true precocious puberty include tuberculosis, encephalitis, trauma, secondary hydrocephalus, neurofibromatosis, granulomas, hamartomas of the hypothalamus, teratomas, craniopharyngiomas, cranial irradiation, and congenital brain defects, such as hydrocephalus and cysts in the area of the third ventricle. These children have markedly fluctuating estrogen levels and low gonadotropin concentrations that are independent of GnRH stimulation. These CNS space-occupying masses are most difficult to treat successfully by surgical means. The pathophysiology whereby CNS disease produces precocious puberty is poorly understood. It is known that hamartomas may secrete GnRH; this secretion is not subject to the normal physiologic inhibition that occurs during childhood.

#### Primary Hypothyroidism

Hypothyroidism is usually associated with delayed pubertal development. However, in rare cases, untreated hypothyroidism results in GnRH dependent precocious puberty. The hypothyroidism associated with precocious puberty is caused by primary thyroid insufficiency, usually Hashimoto thyroiditis, and not by a deficiency in pituitary TSH. The pathophysiology of this syndrome is a result of the diminished negative feedback of thyroxine, resulting in an increased production of TSH, which may be accompanied by an increase in production of gonadotropins. This has sometimes been referred to as the *Van Wyk–Grumbach syndrome* (Bhansali, 2000). Another possible mechanism is the stimulation of the FSH receptor by high levels of TSH (Anasti, 1995).

Interestingly, hypothyroidism is the only cause of precocious puberty in which the bone age is retarded. This syndrome is usually observed in girls between the ages of 6 and 8 years.

### *Gonadotropin-Releasing Hormone-Independent Precocious Puberty*

The most common cause of pseudo or feminizing precocious puberty is an estrogen-secreting ovarian cyst or large functioning follicle. Granulosa cell tumors are the most common type of solid ovarian tumor resulting in precocious puberty. These tumors are usually larger than 8 cm in diameter when associated with precocious puberty; 80% can be palpated abdominally. Other ovarian tumors that may be associated with precocious puberty include thecomas, luteomas, teratomas, Sertoli-Leydig tumors, choriocarcinomas, and benign follicular cysts. Usually, thecomas and luteomas are much smaller than granulosa cell tumors and cannot be palpated. Overall, these tumors are rare during childhood, with only 5% of granulosa cell tumors and 1% of thecomas occurring before puberty. The ability of many tumors, including teratomas, choriocarcinomas, and dysgerminomas, to secrete estrogen, human chorionic gonadotropin (hCG), α-fetoprotein, and other markers has been established.

Adrenocortical neoplasms may produce isosexual (feminizing) or heterosexual (virilizing) precocious puberty. The relationship between congenital adrenal hyperplasia and puberty depends on the time of initial diagnosis and therapy. If the disease is diagnosed in the neonatal period and treated, normal puberty ensues. If the disease is untreated, the girl usually develops heterosexual precocious puberty (signs of androgen excess) from the adrenal androgens over time. However, if congenital adrenal hyperplasia is diagnosed late in childhood, isosexual precocious puberty may follow initial treatment of the adrenal disease. In this category, apart from adrenal imaging, measurements of steroids to rule out the various forms of adrenal hyperplasia due to enzymatic deficiencies (e.g., 21- or 11β-hydroxylase or 3 β-ol dehydrogenase) have to be carried out.

**McCune-Albright syndrome** (MAS) is a rare condition caused by a mutation in the G3 protein leading to activation of adenylate cyclase (Shenker, 1993). This leads to a constant stimulation of pituitary hormones, including FSH, LH, TSH, and GH. It presents as precocious puberty with the first sign usually being vaginal bleeding. Clinically there is a triad of café-au-lait spots, polyostotic fibrous dysplasia, and cysts of the skull and long bones (Fig. 38.22). These patients also have facial asymmetry. Apart from vaginal bleeding due to high levels of estrogen from ovarian cysts that develop from constant stimulation, there are bony defects and a lifetime increased risk of malignancy.

**Iatrogenic or factitious precocious puberty** results when a young female has used hormone cream or ingested adult medications such as oral estrogen or birth control pills. The secondary sexual characteristics regress after discontinuation of the medication.

## *DIAGNOSIS*

The diagnostic workup of a young child with precocious puberty begins with a meticulous history and physical examination. The primary emphasis should be to rule out life-threatening neoplasms of the ovary, adrenal gland, or CNS. The secondary emphasis is to delineate the speed of the maturation process, because this is crucial in making decisions concerning therapy. The height of the girl and exact stage of pubertal development, including Tanner stage, should be recorded. Similar to other syndromes with a long list of causes, a number of tests, including imaging studies of the brain, serum estradiol level, FSH level, and thyroid function tests, may have to be carried out to establish the diagnosis. With the acceleration of development, the sex steroid and adrenal androgen (DHEA-S) levels are elevated, regardless of the cause. Acceleration of growth is one of the

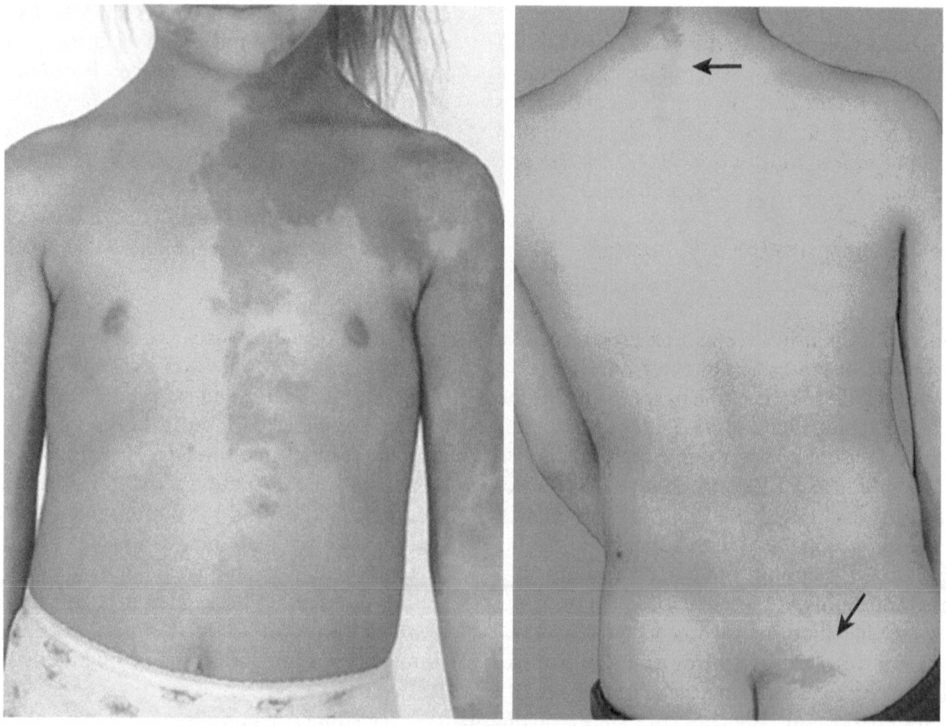

**Figure 38.22** A 5-year-old girl with precocious puberty and McCune-Albright syndrome. Note the breast development and the typical café-au-lait spots, the pattern of which is referred to as "the coast of Maine." (From Dumitrescu CE, Collins MT. McCune-Albright syndrome. *Orphanet J Rare Dis.* 2008;3:12.)

earliest clinical features of precocious puberty. Thus bone age should be determined by hand-wrist films and compared with standards for a patient's age (Fig. 38.23). Usually, these films are repeated at 6-month intervals to evaluate the rate of skeletal maturation and the corresponding need for active treatment of the disease. Advancement of bone age more than 95% of the norm for the child's chronologic age indicates an estrogen effect.

Diseases of the CNS are suggested by symptoms such as headaches, seizures, trauma to the head, and encephalitis. These conditions are confirmed or excluded by a series of tests, including neurologic and ophthalmologic examinations, EEGs, and brain imaging.

Hypothalamic hamartomas can be categorized based on the tumor topology on MRI. This classification has been shown to correlate with the clinical manifestations of precocious puberty. Ultrasound, CT, or MRI of the abdomen and pelvis should be performed to evaluate enlargement of the ovaries (ovarian volume), uterus, or adrenal glands.

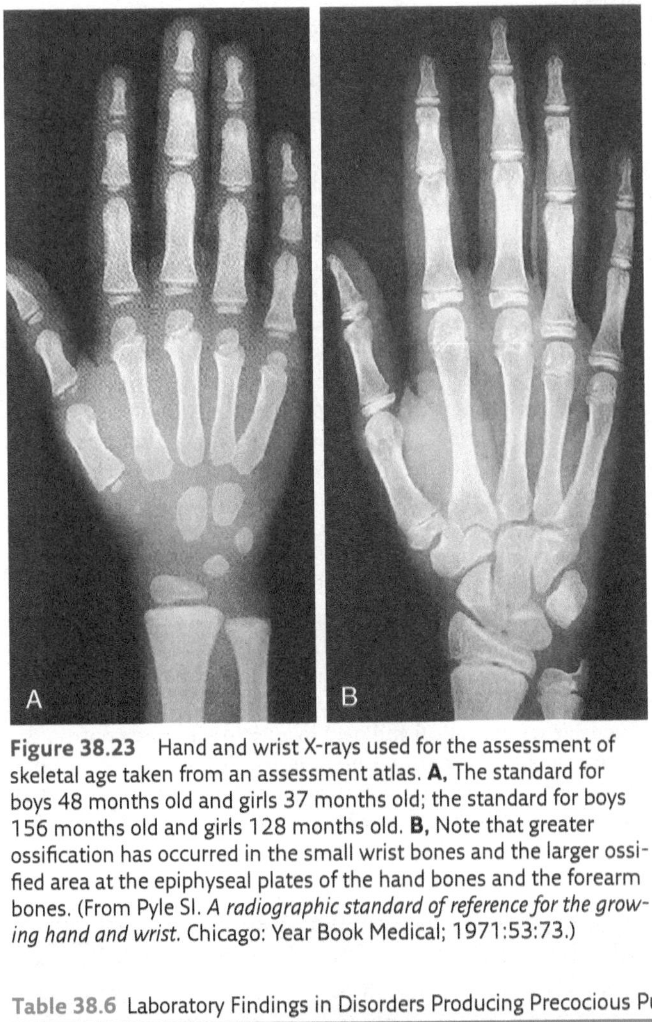


**Figure 38.23** Hand and wrist X-rays used for the assessment of skeletal age taken from an assessment atlas. **A,** The standard for boys 48 months old and girls 37 months old; the standard for boys 156 months old and girls 128 months old. **B,** Note that greater ossification has occurred in the small wrist bones and the larger ossified area at the epiphyseal plates of the hand bones and the forearm bones. (From Pyle SI. *A radiographic standard of reference for the growing hand and wrist.* Chicago: Year Book Medical; 1971:53:73.)

Serum levels of FSH, LH, prolactin, TSH, $E_2$, testosterone, DHEA-S, hCG, androstenedione, 17-hydroxyprogesterone, triiodothyronine ($T_3$), and thyroxine ($T_4$) may be of value in establishing the differential diagnosis.

A GnRH agonist stimulation test is diagnostic in differentiating incomplete from true precocious puberty as described previously, but it does not specifically identify children with CNS lesions. See Table 38.6 for summary.

## TREATMENT

The treatment of precocious puberty depends on the cause, extent, and progression of precocious signs and whether the cause may be removed operatively. For example, removal of a granulosa cell tumor and subtotal removal of a hypothalamic hamartoma are successful treatments because they remove the hormonal force. Because most cases involve premature maturation of the hypothalamic-pituitary-ovarian axis without a lesion, this discussion will focus on the medical management of this condition. Girls with menarche before age 8 years, progressive thelarche and pubarche, and bone age 2 years more than their chronologic age definitely should be treated. The goals of therapy are to reduce gonadotropin secretions and reduce or counteract the peripheral actions of the sex steroids, decrease the growth rate to normal, and slow skeletal maturation to allow development of maximal adult height.

The present drug of choice for GnRH dependent precocious puberty is one of the potent GnRH agonists, which have been studied extensively (Tanaka, 2005; Badaru, 2006). These drugs are typically given by monthly or trimonthly injections or, rarely, intranasally. GnRH agonists are safe and effective treatments for children with the disease secondary to disturbances in the hypothalamic-pituitary-ovarian axis. Therapy should be initiated as soon as possible after the diagnosis is established so that the child can achieve maximal adult height. The effect on adult height depends on the chronologic age at which therapy is initiated. Therapy is most effective in 4- to 6-year-olds. Continuous chronic administration of the drug is maintained until the median age of puberty. The optimal dosage of medication may be confirmed by determining that peripheral $E_2$ levels are in a normal prepubertal range. Medical treatment produces involution of secondary sexual characteristics, with amenorrhea and regression of breast development and amount of pubic hair. LH and FSH pulsations are abolished. Most important, the drug

**Table 38.6** Laboratory Findings in Disorders Producing Precocious Puberty

| | FINDINGS | | | | |
|---|---|---|---|---|---|
| **Disorder** | **Gonadal Size** | **Basal FSH, LH** | **Estradiol or Testosterone** | **DHAS** | **GnRH Response** |
| Idiopathic | Increased | Increased | Increased | Increased | Pubertal |
| Cerebral | Increased | Increased | Increased | Increased | Pubertal |
| Gonadal | Unilaterally increased | Decreased | Increased | Increased | Flat |
| Albright | Increased | Decreased | Increased | Increased | Flat |
| Adrenal | Small | Decreased | Increased | Increased | Flat |

Modified from Speroff L, Glass RH, Kase NG. *Clinical Gynecology Endocrinology and Infertility.* 6th ed. Baltimore: Lippincott Williams & Wilkins; 1999:396.
*DHAS*, Dehydroepiandrosterone sulfate; *GnRH*, gonadotropin-releasing hormone; *FSH*, follicle-stimulating hormone, *LH*, luteinizing hormone.

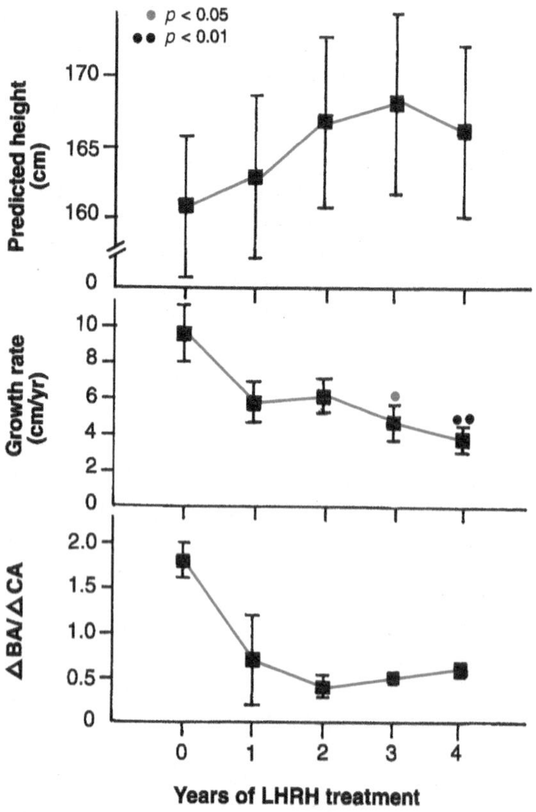


**Figure 38.24** Predicted height, growth rate, and rate of bone age advancement in six children with central precocious puberty who received 4 years of therapy with the long-acting analogue of luteinizing hormone-releasing hormone (LHRH). *Asterisks* indicate significant differences compared with pretreatment value. *ΔBA/ΔCA*, Change in bone age/change in chronologic age. (Modified from Comite F, Cassorla F, Barnes KM, et al. Luteinizing hormone-releasing hormone analogue therapy for central precocious puberty: long-term effect on somatic growth, bone maturation, and predicted height. *JAMA*. 1986;255:2615.)

not only reverses the ovarian cycle but definitely changes the growth pattern. Growth velocity is usually decreased by approximately 50% (Fig. 38.24). In one series, the predicted adult height increased a mean of 6.5 cm in girls who were 6 years of age or younger when therapy was initiated.

A number of studies have documented that agonist therapy decreases gonadotropin levels within 1 week and decreases sex steroid levels to the prepubertal range within the first 2 weeks of therapy. Serial ultrasound examinations have documented that the size of the ovaries and uterus regresses to a normal prepubertal shape and size. The most commonly observed side effect to agonists was a cutaneous reaction at the site of injection. However, approximately one in four girls experienced recurrent and sometimes prolonged vaginal bleeding while receiving GnRH agonists. The effects of these drugs are reversible when the agonists are discontinued after normal height has been achieved.

Although 3-month regimens are available, therapy usually begins with a once-per-month preparation at a dose of 0.3 mg/kg of leuprolide or its equivalent. Leuprolide acetate can be administered at doses of 7.5 mg, 11.25 mg, and 15 mg; the larger dose can be used if there is evidence for pubertal progression despite treatment. Treatment usually continues until around age 11.

It has been suggested that rare forms of GnRH-independent precocious puberty that do not respond to agonist therapy may be successfully treated using a GnRH antagonist. Here, there may be a direct antagonist effect on the ovary mediated through gonadotropin receptors. Small studies have suggested a minimal benefit from adding growth hormone to GnRH agonist therapy in girls with suboptimal growth (Walvoord, 1999). The initial observations of combination therapy have been encouraging, but the clinical data were from small series and of a preliminary nature.

McCune-Albright syndrome is caused by an activating mutation of a G protein that is coupled with gonadotropin receptors, resulting in the ovaries being stimulated autonomously. Girls may be treated with aromatase inhibitors (anastrozole, letrozole), which prevent the conversion to biologically active estrogens. Unfortunately this treatment has had limited success, as has the use of tamoxifen (Shulman, 2008). The most promising treatment appears to be the use of the "pure" estrogen receptor antagonist, fulvestrant. In early studies, monthly injections of fulvestrant have shown benefit (Sims, 2012).

The child with precocious puberty and her family need intensive counseling. The child will have the psychosocial and behavioral maturation of children of her chronologic age, not the age reflected by her physical appearance. She may be exposed to ridicule by her peers and to sexual exploitation. Thus the child needs extensive sex education and help in anticipating and confronting various social experiences. Often, it is possible to dress the child in clothes that diminish the recognition of her advanced sexual maturation until the effects of her disease have been inhibited by drug therapy.

## KEY POINTS

- Primary amenorrhea is diagnosed if no menstrual function has occurred by age 15, or 5 years after initial breast development.
- The incidence of secondary amenorrhea of more than 6 months' duration in the general population is approximately 0.7%.
- The incidence of amenorrhea lasting more than 6 months after discontinuation of oral contraceptives is 0.8%.
- The most important and probably most common cause of amenorrhea in adolescent girls is anorexia nervosa.
- An adolescent 13 years of age or older without any breast development has estrogen deficiency caused by an abnormality, which needs diagnostic evaluation.
- Menarche is delayed approximately 0.4 year for each year of premenarchal athletic training.
- Gonadal failure is the most common cause of primary amenorrhea, accounting for almost 50% of patients with this disorder.
- Individuals with gonadal failure and an X chromosome abnormality are shorter than 63 inches in height.

## KEY POINTS—cont'd

- The testes of individuals with androgen resistance have approximately a 20% chance of becoming malignant after the age of 20 years.
- Uterovaginal agenesis is the second most common cause of primary amenorrhea, with an incidence of approximately 15% of individuals with this symptom.
- Approximately one third of individuals with gonadal failure have major cardiovascular or renal abnormalities.
- Congenital renal abnormalities occur in approximately one third of women with congenital absence of the uterus.
- The differential diagnosis between estrogen deficiency caused by gonadal failure and hypogonadotropic hypogonadism is best established with measurement of serum FSH.
- The diagnosis of gonadal failure, or hypergonadotropic hypogonadism, can be established if the FSH level exceeds 30 mIU/mL.
- Individuals with gonadal failure should have a peripheral karyotype obtained to determine whether a Y chromosome is present. If it is present, or if there are signs of hyperandrogenism, the gonads should be excised to prevent the development of malignancy, mainly a gonadoblastoma.
- Individuals with primary amenorrhea and hypogonadotropic hypogonadism do not need karyotyping but need a cranial CT scan to rule out a CNS tumor.
- The most frequent cause of IUAs is curettage performed during pregnancy or shortly thereafter.
- When women experience weight loss to 15% or more below ideal body weight, amenorrhea can occur because of CNS-hypothalamic dysfunction. The normal cyclic pattern of LH pulsatility is not present in individuals with functional hypothalamic amenorrhea. Either there is no LH pulse activity or there are pulses of slow frequency, similar to those in the normal luteal phase.
- The GnRH alterations, as reflected in LH pulsatility, in persons with severe weight loss and anorexia nervosa are similar to those seen in normal prepubertal girls. When they regain weight, GnRH changes similar to those occurring during puberty take place.
- When uterine bleeding fails to occur after progestin is administered, $E_2$ levels are usually lower than 30 pg/mL.
- In contrast to hypothalamic disorders, pituitary causes of amenorrhea can be associated with ACTH and TSH deficiency.
- Individuals with premature ovarian failure or insufficiency have two different histologic findings: generalized sclerosis or primordial follicles scattered through the stroma.
- Women with premature ovarian failure or insufficiency may have antibodies to gonadotropins and other endocrine organs, indicating an autoimmune origin.
- A karyotype should be obtained in women with premature ovarian failure or insufficiency who are younger than 25 years but is not necessary in those who are older.
- Amenorrhea with low estrogen levels is associated with decreased bone density.
- The most frequent cause of secondary amenorrhea is hypothalamic dysfunction.
- Physiologic development in females with precocious puberty usually follows the normal sequence of changes of secondary sexual characteristics.
- If signs of pubertal progression (precocious puberty) are present in a girl, a workup is warranted by the age of 8 years.
- The two primary concerns of parents of children with precocious puberty are the social stigma associated with the child being physically different from her peers and the diminished ultimate height caused by the premature closure of epiphyseal growth centers.
- The exact cause of the majority of cases of GnRH-dependent (true or complete) precocious puberty is unknown; however, approximately 30% of cases are secondary to CNS disease.
- A definitive diagnosis is established more often for GnRH-independent (pseudoprecocious or incomplete) puberty and is usually related to an ovarian or adrenal disorder.
- Breast hyperplasia is a normal phenomenon in neonates and may persist until up to 6 months of age.
- The most common cause of GnRH independent precocious puberty is a functioning ovarian tumor. Granulosa cell tumors are the most common type, accounting for approximately 60% of neoplasms.
- The primary emphasis of the diagnostic workup of a child with precocious puberty should be to rule out life-threatening neoplasms of the ovary, adrenal glands, or CNS. The secondary emphasis is to delineate the speed of the maturation process, because this is critical when making a decision about therapy.
- The goals of therapy for precocious puberty are to reduce gonadotropin secretion, reduce or counteract the peripheral actions of sex steroids, and decrease the growth rate to normal and thus slow skeletal maturation. This is best accomplished with the use of GnRH agonists.
- The effect on adult height depends on the chronologic age at which GnRH therapy is initiated, with greater success if initiated at a younger age. The child with precocious puberty and her family need intensive counseling.

## KEY REFERENCES


Abreu AP, Dauber A, Macedo DB, et al. Central precocious puberty caused by mutations in the imprinted gene MKRN3. *N Engl J Med.* 2013;368:2467.

Allingham-Hawkins DJ, Babul-Hirji R, Chitayat D, et al. Fragile X permutation is a significant risk factor for premature ovarian failure: the International Collaboarative POF in Fragile X study-preliminary data. *Am J Med Genet.* 1999;83:322.

Alper MM, Garner PR. Premature ovarian failure: Its relationship to autoimmune disease. *Obstet Gynecol.* 1985;66:27.

Anasti JN, Flack MR, Froehlich J, et al. A potential novel mechanism for precocious puberty in juvenile hypothyroidism. *J Clin Endocinol Metab.* 1995;80:276.

Badaru A, Wilson DM, Bachrach LK, et al. Sequential comparisons of one-month and three-month depot leuprolide regimens in central precocious puberty. *J Clin Endocrinol Metab.* 2006;91:1862.

Berga SL, Marcus MD, Loucks TL, et al. Recovery of ovarian activity in women with functional hypothalamic amenorrhea who were treated with cognitive behavior therapy. *Fertil Steril.* 2003;80:976.

Berga SL, Mortola JF, Girton BS, et al. Neuroendocrine aberrations in women with functional hypothalamic amenorrhea. *J Clin Endocrinol Metab.* 1989;68:301.

Berker B, Taskin S, Taskin EA. Absence of endometrium as a cuase of primary amenorrhea. *Fertil Steril.* 2008;89:723.

Bhansali A, Kashyap A, Lodha S, et al. Isosexual precocity: uncommon presentation of a common disorder. *Postgrad Med J.* 2000;76:177.

Biro FM, Huang B, Lucky AW, et al. Pubertal correlatesin black and white girls. *J Pediatr.* 2006;148:234.

Brännström M, Johannesson L, Bokström H, et al. Livebirth after uterus transplantation. *Lancet.* 2015;385:607–616.

Boyar RM, Katz J, Finkelstein JW, et al. Anorexia nervosa: immaturity of the 24-hour luteinizing hormone secretory pattern. *N Engl J Med.* 1974;291:861. 1974.

Carel JC, Léger J. Clinical practice. Precocious puberty. *N Eng J Med.* 2008;358:2366.

Caronia LM, Marin C, Welt CK, et al. A genetic basis for functional hypothalamic amenorrhea. *N Engl J Med.* 2011;364:215.

Cooper AR, Baker VL, Sterling EW, et al. The time is now for a new approach to primary ovarian insufficiency. *Fertil Steril.* 1890;95:2011.

Crowley Jr WF, Filicori M, Spratt DL, et al. The physiology of gonadotropin-releasing hormone (GnRH) secretion in men and women. *Rec Prog Hormone Res.* 1985;41:473.

Escobar ME, Rivarola MA, Bergada C. Plasma concentration of oestradiol-17beta in premature thelarche and in different types of sexual precocity. *Acta Endocrinol.* 1976;81:351.

Federman DD. Disorders of gonadal development: Gonadal dysgenesis (Turner syndrome). In: Federman DD, ed. *Abnormal Sexual Development: A genetic and Endocrine Approach to Differential Diagnosis.* Philadephia: WB Saunders; 1967.

Feicht CB, Johnson TS, Matrin BJ. Secondary amenorrheain athletes. *Lancet.* 1978;1:1145.

Ferin M, Van Vugt D, Wardlaw S. The hypothalamic control of the menstrual cycle and the role of endogenous opioid peptides. *Recent Prog Horm Res.* 1984;40:441.

Frisch RE, Revelle R. Height and weight at menarche and a hypothesis of menarche. *Arch Dis Child.* 1971;46:695.

Gustafson ML, Donahoe PK. Male sex determination: current concepts of male sexual differentiation. *Annu Rev Med.* 1994;45:505.

Jones Jr HW, Scott WW, eds. *Hermaphroditism, Genital Anomalies and Related Endocrine Disorders.* 2nd ed. Baltimore: Williams & Wilkins; 1971.

Kandemir N, Demirbilek H, Ozon ZA, et al. GnRH stimulation test in precocious puberty: single sample is adequate for diagnosis and dose adjustment. *J Clin Res Pediatr Endocrinol.* 2011;3:12.

Kaplowitz PB, Oberfield SE. Reexamination of the age limit for defining when puberty is precocious in girls in the United States: Implications for evaluation and treatment. Drug and Therapeutics and Executive Committees of the Lawson Wilkins Pediatric Endocrine Society. *Pediatrics.* 1999;104:936.

Laughlin GA, Yen SSC. Hypoleptinemia in women athletes: absence of a diurnal rhythm with amenorrhea. *J Clin Endocrinol Metab.* 1997;82:318.

Lee PA. Puberty and its disorders. In: Lifshitz F, ed. *Pediatric Endocrinology.* 4th ed. New York: Marcel Dekker; 2003:p 213.

Lloyd T, Myers C, Buchanan JR, et al. Collegiate women athletes with irregular menses during adolescence have decreased bone density. *Obstet Gynecol.* 1988;72:639.

Marshall WA, Tanner JM. Variations in [attern of pubertal changes in girls. *Arch Dis Child.* 1969;44:291.

Mashchak CA, Kletzky OA, Davajan V, et al. Clinical and laboratory evaluation of patients with primary amenorrhea. *Obstet Gynecol.* 1981;57:715.

Midyett LK, Morre WV, Jacobson JD. Are pubertal changes in girls before age 8 benign? *Pediatrics.* 2003;111:47.

Mignot MH, Schoemaker J, Kleingeld M, et al. Premature ovarian failure. I. The association with autoimmunity. *Eur J Obstet Gynecol Reprod Biol.* 1989;30:59.

Nigam A, Ahmad A, Batra S. Absent endometrium due to balanced translocation (t(4;20)) presenting as primary amenorrhea. *J Hum Reprod Sci.* 2014;7:63.

Practice Committee of the American Society for Reproductive Medicine: Current evaluation of amenorrhea. *Fertil Steril.* 2008;90(Suppl):S219.

Quaynor SD, Stradtman Jr EW, Kim HG, et al. Delayed puberty and estrogen resistance in a woman with estrogen receptor α variant. *N Engl J Med.* 2013;369:164.

Reame NE, Sauder SE, Kelch RP, et al. Pulsatile gonadotropin secretion during the human menstrual cycle: Evidence for altered frequency of gonadotropin-releasing hormone secretion. *J Clin Endocrinol Metab.* 1984;59:328.

Reindollar RH, Byrd JR, McDonough PG. Delayed sexual development: A study of 252 patients. *Am J Obstet Gynecol.* 1981;140:371.

Schneider LF, Warren MP. Functional hypothalamic amenorrhea is associated with elevated ghrelin and disordered eating. *Fertil Steril.* 2006;86:1744.

Seminara SB, Messager S, Chatzidaki EE, et al. The GPR54 gene as a regulator of puberty. *N Engl J Med.* 2003;349:1614.

Shenker A, Weinstein LS, Moran A, et al. Severe endocrine and nonendocrine manifestations of the McCune-Albright syndrome associated with activating mutations of stimulatory G protein GS. *J Pediatr.* 1993;123:509.

Shulman DI, Francis GL, Palmert MR, et al. Use of aromatase inhibitors in children and adolescents with disorders of growth and adolescent development. *Pediatrics.* 2008;121:e975.

Silveira LG, Noel SD, Silveira-Neto AP, et al. Mutations of the KISSI gene in disorders of puberty. *J Clin Endocrinol Metab.* 2010;95:2276.

Sims EK, Garnett S, Guzman F, et al. Fuvestrant treatment of precocious puberty in girls with McCune-Albright syndrome. *Int J Pediatr Endocrinol.* 2012;26:2012.

Tanaka T, Niimi H, Matsuo N, et al. Results oflong-term follow-up after treatment of central precocious puberty with leuprorelin acetate: evaluation of effectiveness of treatment and recovery of gonadal function. The TAP-144-SR Japanese Study Group on Central Precocious Puberty. *J Clin Endocrinol Metab.* 2005;90:1371.

Teles MG, Bianco SD, Brito VN, et al. A GPR54-activating mutation in a patient with centroal precocious puberty. *N Engl J Med.* 2008;358:709.

Terasawa E, Guerrier KA, Plant TM. Kisspeptin andpuberty in mammals. In: Kauffman AS Smith JT, ed. *Kisspeptin Signaling in Reproductive Biology.* New York: Springer; 2013:252.

Tschugguel W, Berga SL. Treatment of functional hupothalamic amenorrhea with hypnotherapy. *Fertil Steril.* 2003;80:982.

Walvoord EC, Pescovitz OH. Combined use of growth hormone and gonadotropin-releasing hormone analogues in precocious puberty: theoretic and practical considerations. *Pediatrics.* 1999;104:1010.

Warren MP. The effects of exercise on pubertal progression and reproductive function in girls. *J Clin Endocrinol Metab.* 1980;51:1150.

Welt CK, Chan JL, Bullen J, et al. Recombinant human leptin in women with hypothalamic amenorrhea. *N Engl J Med.* 2004;351:987.


Suggested Readings can be found on ExpertConsult.com.

# 39

# Hyperprolactinemia, Galactorrhea, and Pituitary Adenomas

## Etiology, Differential Diagnosis, Natural History, Management

*Roger A. Lobo*

**Prolactin** (PRL) is a polypeptide hormone containing 198 amino acids and with a molecular weight (MW) of 22 kDa. It circulates in different molecular sizes: a monomeric (small) form (MW = 22 kDa), a polymeric (big) form (MW = 50 kDa), and an even larger polymeric (big-big) form (MW >100 kDa). Big PRL is presumed to be a dimer, and big-big PRL may represent an aggregation of monomeric molecules. The larger forms also contain added sugar moieties (glycosylation), which decreases biologic activity. The small form is biologically active and approximately 80% of the hormone is secreted in this form. Most immunoassays measure the small and large forms of PRL. The polymeric forms have reduced biologic activity and reduced binding to mammary tissue membranes. Women have been identified with high levels of PRL on routine immunoassay and who are completely normal clinically. This is because of "clumping" of abnormal forms of PRL, and if this unusual situation arises, where there is no reason to suspect a PRL elevation, the assay should be repeated, as will be described later.

PRL is synthesized and stored in the pituitary gland in chromophobe cells called *lactotrophs,* which are located mainly in the lateral areas of the gland. PRL is encoded by its gene (10 kb) on chromosome 6. At the molecular level, it is stimulated and suppressed by a number of factors. The principal stimulating factor is thyroid-releasing hormone (TRH), and the major inhibiting factor is dopamine, which has been suggested to be the prolactin-inhibiting factor (PIF). Estrogen also improves PRL secretion by enhancing the effects of TRH and inhibiting the effects of dopamine. A potential direct effect may also be mediated via galanin. The principal receptor with which dopamine interacts is D2, which is the target for various dopamine agonists used in the treatment of **hyperprolactinemia.**

In addition, PRL is synthesized in decidualized stroma of endometrial tissue. From these tissues, PRL is secreted into the circulation and, in the event of pregnancy, into the amniotic fluid. The control of decidual PRL is different from that of the pituitary and does not respond to dopamine. PRL is normally present in measurable amounts in serum, with mean levels of approximately 8 ng/mL in adult women. It circulates in an unbound form, has a 20-minute half-life, and is cleared by the liver and kidney. The main function of PRL is to stimulate the growth of mammary tissue as well as to produce and secrete milk into the alveoli; thus it has mammogenic and lactogenic functions. Specific receptors for PRL are present in the plasma membrane of mammary cells, as well as in many other tissues.

## PHYSIOLOGY

PRL synthesis and release from the lactotrophs are controlled by central nervous system neurotransmitters, which act on the pituitary via the hypothalamus. The major control mechanism is inhibition, because pituitary stalk section results in increased PRL secretion. It appears that the major physiologic inhibitor of PRL release is the neurotransmitter dopamine (PIF), which acts directly on the pituitary gland. There are specific dopamine receptors on the lactotrophs, and dopamine inhibits PRL synthesis and release in pituitary cell cultures. Although a hypothalamic prolactin-releasing factor (PRF) has not been isolated, it is known that the neurotransmitter serotonin and thyrotropin-releasing factor stimulate PRL release. Because the latter stimulates PRL release only minimally unless infused, it appears that serotonin is a PRF or is responsible for its secretion. The rise in PRL levels during sleep appears to be controlled by serotonin.

PRL is secreted episodically and serum levels fluctuate throughout the day and throughout the menstrual cycle, with peak levels occurring at midcycle. Although changes in PRL levels are not as marked as the pulsatile episodes of luteinizing hormone (LH), estrogen stimulates PRL production and release. Under the influence of estrogen, PRL levels increase in females at the time of puberty; there is a slight decline in levels after menopause.

During pregnancy, as estrogen levels increase, there is a concomitant hypertrophy and hyperplasia of the lactotrophs. The maternal increase in PRL levels occurs soon after implantation, concomitant with the increase in circulating estrogen. Circulating levels of PRL steadily increase throughout pregnancy, reaching approximately 200 ng/mL in the third trimester; the rise is directly related to the increase in circulating levels of estrogen.

However, there is a wide range of values of PRL in pregnancy, and values as high as 400 ng/mL can be found in normal pregnancy. Despite the elevated PRL levels during pregnancy, lactation does not occur because estrogen inhibits the action of PRL on the breast, most likely blocking PRL's interaction with its receptor. A day or two following delivery of the placenta, estrogen and PRL levels decline rapidly and lactation is initiated. PRL levels reach basal levels in nonnursing women in 2 to 3 weeks. Although basal levels of circulating PRL decline to the nonpregnant range approximately 6 months after parturition in nursing women, following each act of suckling, PRL levels increase markedly and stimulate milk production for the next feeding.

Nipple and breast stimulation also increase PRL levels in the nonpregnant female, as does trauma to the chest wall. Other physiologic stimuli that increase PRL release are exercise, sleep, and stress. In addition, PRL levels normally rise following ingestion of the midday meal. Thus PRL levels normally fluctuate throughout the day, with maximal levels observed during the night while asleep and a smaller increase occurring in the early afternoon. When the amount measured in the circulation in the nonpregnant woman exceeds a certain level, usually 20 to 25 ng/mL, the condition is called *hyperprolactinemia*. The optimal time to obtain a blood sample for assay to diagnose hyperprolactinemia is in the fasting state and, ideally, during the midmorning hours. Increases in PRL levels above the normal range can occur without a pathologic condition if the serum sample is drawn from a woman who has recently awakened, has exercised, or has had recent breast stimulation (such as breast palpation) during a physical examination.

The most frequent cause of slightly elevated PRL levels is stress, particularly the stress caused by visiting the physician's office. All women with initial PRL levels lower than 50 ng/mL should have subsequent samples drawn 60 minutes after resting in a quiet room to determine whether true pathologic hyperprolactinemia is present. Figure 39.1 depicts normalization of PRL only in those with stress-related elevations, which occurred during a 60-minute rest period (referred to in the study as a "test").

Hyperprolactinemia can produce disorders of gonadotropin sex steroid function, resulting in menstrual cycle derangement (oligomenorrhea and amenorrhea) and anovulation, as well as inappropriate lactation, or **galactorrhea**. The mechanism whereby elevated PRL levels interfere with gonadotropin release appears to be related to abnormal gonadotropin-releasing hormone (GnRH) release. Women with hyperprolactinemia have abnormalities in the frequency and amplitude of LH pulsations, with a normal or increased gonadotropin response following GnRH infusion.

This abnormality of GnRH cyclicity thus inhibits gonadotropin release but not its synthesis. The reason for this abnormal secretion of GnRH is an inhibitory effect of dopamine and opioid peptides at the level of the hypothalamus. In addition, elevated PRL levels have been shown to interfere with the positive estrogen effect on midcycle LH release. It has also been shown that elevated levels of PRL directly inhibit basal and gonadotropin-stimulated ovarian secretion of estradiol and progesterone. However, this mechanism is probably not the primary cause of anovulation, because women with hyperprolactinemia can have ovulation induced with various agents, including pulsatile GnRH. Some women with moderate hyperprolactinemia, as determined by radioimmunoassay, have a greater than normal

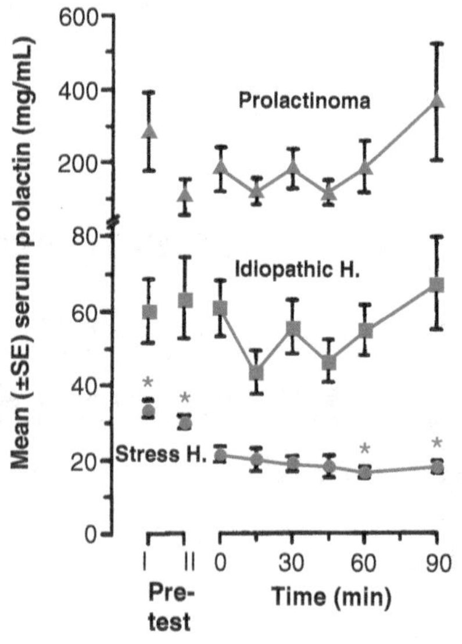


**Figure 39.1** Serum prolactin levels (mean plus or minus standard error [±SE]) in women with prolactinoma ($N = 20$) and idiopathic ($N = 30$) and stress-related ($N = 20$) hyperprolactinemia before (pretest I and II) and during hyperprolactinemia test. Differences (*$P < .01$) are in relation to time zero values. (Mean prolactin values among groups were also significantly different [$P < .01$] at all times.) (From Muneyyirci-Delale O, Goldstein D, Reyes FI, et al. Diagnosis of stress-related hyperprolactinemia: evaluation of the hyperprolactinemia rest test. *NY State J Med.* 1989;89[4]:205-208.)

proportion of the big-big forms. Because of the reduced bioactivity of this form of PRL, they can have normal pituitary and ovarian function.

The clinician should measure serum PRL levels in all women with galactorrhea, as well as those with oligomenorrhea and amenorrhea not explained by another reason such as ovarian failure (elevated level of follicle-stimulating hormone [FSH]). Hyperprolactinemia has been reported to be present in 15% to 20% of women who present with menstrual disturbances.

## SPECIAL CASES IN THE MEASUREMENT OF PROLACTIN

Because of possible aggregation of molecular forms of PRL when levels are high, if a tumor (adenoma) is suspected and values of PRL are only mildly elevated, the test should be repeated in a diluted sample. This has been called the "hook" effect and is explained by high endogenous levels of PRL binding up all the assay antibody, leaving an inadequate quantity for the assay (St-Jean, 1996).

The opposite occurrence was mentioned earlier, when PRL is found to be elevated in a woman who is normal clinically. This is due to "clumping" of glycosylated PRL with immunoglobulin and can be corrected by gel electrophoresis or merely by adding polyethylene glycol to the serum, which precipitates the abnormal forms (Leslie, 2001).

## GALACTORRHEA

Galactorrhea is defined as the nonpuerperal secretion of watery or milky fluid from the breast that contains neither pus nor blood. The fluid may appear spontaneously or after palpation.

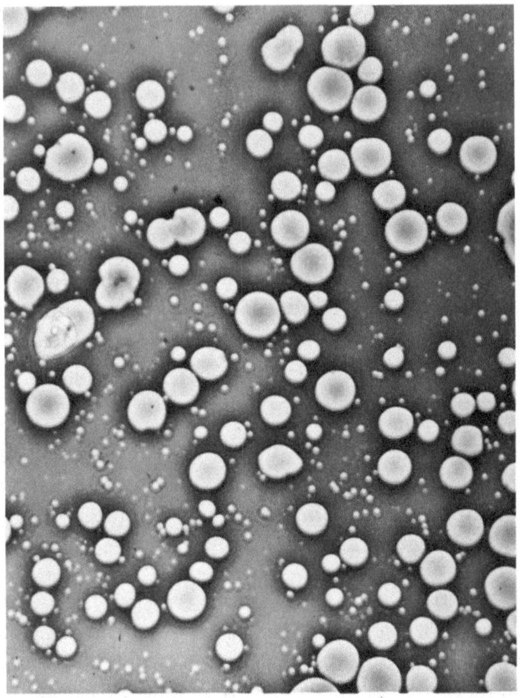

**Figure 39.2** Fat droplets seen under microscope from a patient with galactorrhea. (From Kletzky OA, Davajan V. Hyperprolactinemia: diagnosis and treatment. In: Mishell DR, Davajan V, Lobo RA, eds. *Infertility, Contraception and Reproductive Endocrinology.* 3rd ed. Cambridge, MA: Blackwell Scientific; 1991.)

To determine whether galactorrhea is present, the clinician should palpate the breast, moving from the periphery toward the nipple in an attempt to express any secretion. The diagnosis of galactorrhea can be confirmed by observing multiple fat droplets in the fluid when examined under low-power magnification (Fig. 39.2). The incidence of galactorrhea in women with hyperprolactinemia has been reported to range from 30% to 80%, and these differences probably reflect variations in the techniques used to detect mammary excretion. Unless there has been continued breast stimulation after a pregnancy, the presence of galactorrhea serves as a biologic indicator that the PRL level is abnormally elevated.

## CAUSES OF HYPERPROLACTINEMIA

Pathologic causes of hyperprolactinemia, in addition to a PRL-secreting pituitary adenoma (**prolactinoma**) and other pituitary tumors that produce acromegaly and Cushing disease, include hypothalamic disease, various pharmacologic agents, hypothyroidism, chronic renal disease, or any chronic type of breast nerve stimulation, such as may occur with thoracic operation, herpes zoster, or chest trauma. Box 39.1 lists the causes of hyperprolactinemia.

One of the most frequent causes of galactorrhea and hyperprolactinemia is the ingestion of pharmacologic agents, particularly tranquilizers, narcotics, and antihypertensive agents (Box 39.2). Of the tranquilizers, the phenothiazines and diazepam can produce hyperprolactinemia by depleting the hypothalamic circulation of dopamine or by blocking its binding sites and thus decreasing dopamine action.

**Box 39.1 Causes of Hyperprolactinemia**

**Pituitary Disease**
Prolactinomas
Acromegaly
Empty sella syndrome
Lymphocytic hypophysitis
Cushing disease

**Hypothalamic Disease**
Craniopharyngiomas
Meningiomas
Dysgerminomas
Nonsecreting pituitary adenomas
Other tumors
Sarcoidosis
Eosinophilic granuloma
Neuraxis irradiation
Vascular
Pituitary stalk section

**Medications**
See Box 39.2.

**Neurogenic**
Chest wall lesions
Spinal cord lesions
Breast stimulation

**Other**
Pregnancy
Hypothyroidism
Chronic renal failure
Cirrhosis
Pseudocyesis
Adrenal insufficiency
Ectopic
Polycystic ovary syndrome
Idiopathic

From Molitch ME. Prolactinoma. In: Melmed S, ed. *The Pituitary.* 2nd ed. Malden, MA: Blackwell; 2002:455-495.

The tricyclic antidepressants block dopamine uptake and propranolol, haloperidol, phentolamine, and cyproheptadine block hypothalamic dopamine receptors. The antihypertensive agent reserpine depletes catecholamines, and methyldopa blocks the conversion of tyrosine to dihydroxyphenylalanine (dopa). Ingestion of oral contraceptive steroids can also mildly increase PRL levels, with a greater incidence of hyperprolactinemia occurring with older higher estrogen formulations. Nevertheless, galactorrhea does not usually occur during oral contraceptive ingestion because the exogenous estrogen blocks the binding of PRL to its receptors.

Women who develop galactorrhea while ingesting oral contraceptives or any of the other drugs listed in Box 39.2 should ideally discontinue the medication, and the PRL level should be measured 1 month thereafter to determine if the level has returned to normal. If the medication cannot be discontinued, the PRL level should be measured and, if elevated above 100 ng/mL, imaging of the sella turcica should be performed to determine whether a **macroadenoma** is present.

Primary hypothyroidism can also produce hyperprolactinemia and galactorrhea because of decreased negative feedback of thyroxine ($T_4$) on the hypothalamic-pituitary axis. The resulting increase in TRH stimulates PRL secretion and

**Box 39.2 Pharmacologic Agents Affecting Prolactin Concentrations**

**Stimulators**
Anesthetics, including cocaine
Psychoactive drugs
Phenothiazines
Tricyclic antidepressants
Opiates
Chlordiazepoxide
Amphetamines
Diazepam
Haloperidol
Fluphenazine
Chlorpromazine
SSRIs

**Hormones**
Estrogen
Oral-steroid contraceptives
Thyrotropin-releasing hormone

**Antihypertensives**
α-Methyldopa
Reserpine
Verapamil

**Dopamine receptor antagonists**
Metoclopramide

**Antiemetics**
Sulpiride
Promazine
Perphenazine

**Others**
Cimetidine
Cyproheptadine
Protease inhibitors

**Inhibitors**
L-Dopa
Dopamine
Bromocriptine
Pergolide
Cabergoline
Depot bromocriptine

From Shoupe D, Mishell DR Jr. Hyperprolactinemia: diagnosis and treatment. In: Lobo RA, Mishell DR Jr, Paulson RJ, Shoupe D, eds. *Mishell's Textbook of Infertility, Contraception and Reproductive Endocrinology.* 4th ed. Cambridge, MA: Blackwell Scientific; 1997.
*SSRIs*, Selective serotonin reuptake inhibitors.

thyroid-stimulating hormone (TSH) secretion from the pituitary. Approximately 3% to 5% of individuals with hyperprolactinemia have hypothyroidism. Therefore TSH, the most sensitive indicator of hypothyroidism, should be measured in all individuals with hyperprolactinemia. If the TSH level is elevated, triiodothyronine ($T_3$) and $T_4$ should be measured to confirm the diagnosis of primary hypothyroidism, because a TSH-secreting pituitary adenoma will occasionally be present. Treatment with appropriate thyroid replacement usually returns the TSH and PRL levels to normal within a short time.

Hyperprolactinemia can occur in those with abnormal renal disease resulting from decreased metabolic clearance and increased production rate. The cause of the latter is unknown.

Mild hyperprolactinemia (30 to 50 ng/mL) may occur in women with polycystic ovary syndrome (PCOS). This occurs in up to 30% of women and may be related to the chronic state of unopposed estrogen stimulation.

## CENTRAL NERVOUS SYSTEM DISORDERS

### Hypothalamic Causes

Diseases of the hypothalamus that produce alterations in the normal portal circulation of dopamine can result in hyperprolactinemia. These include **craniopharyngioma** and infiltration of the hypothalamus by sarcoidosis, histiocytosis, leukemia, or carcinoma. All these conditions are rare, with craniopharyngioma being the most common. These tumors arise from remnants of Rathke's pouch along the pituitary stalk. Grossly, they can be cystic, solid, or mixed, and calcification is usually visible on a radiograph. They are most frequently diagnosed during the second and third decades of life and usually result in impairment of secretion of several pituitary hormones.

### Pituitary Causes

Various types of pituitary tumors, lactotroph hyperplasia, and the **empty sella syndrome** can be associated with hyperprolactinemia. It has been estimated that as many as 80% of all pituitary adenomas secrete PRL. The most common pituitary tumor associated with hyperprolactinemia is the prolactinoma, arbitrarily defined as a **microadenoma** if its diameter is less than 1 cm and as a macroadenoma if it is larger (Fig. 39.3). Hyperprolactinemia has been reported to occur in approximately 25% of those with acromegaly and 10% of those with Cushing disease, indicating that these pituitary adenomas, which mainly secrete growth hormone (GH) and adrenocorticotropic hormone (ACTH), frequently also secrete PRL. Hyperplasia of lactotrophs has been reported to occur in approximately 8% of pituitary glands examined at autopsy. Individuals with hyperplasia of the lactotrophs cannot be distinguished from those having a microadenoma by any clinical, laboratory, or radiologic method. The diagnosis can be made only at the time of surgical exploration of the pituitary gland. Pituitary enlargement with suprasellar extension caused by lactotroph hyperplasia has been reported. *Functional hyperprolactinemia* is the term used for the clinical diagnosis of cases of elevated PRL levels without imaging evidence of an adenoma.

Another cause of hyperprolactinemia is the primary empty sella syndrome. The term *primary empty sella syndrome* describes a clinical situation in which an intrasellar extension of the subarachnoid space results in compression of the pituitary gland and an enlarged sella turcica. The cause is believed to result from a congenital or acquired (by radiation or surgery) defect in the sella diaphragm that allows the subarachnoid membrane to herniate into the sella turcica (Fig. 39.4). The syndrome is usually associated with normal pituitary function, except for hyperprolactinemia. Although some with primary empty sella syndrome have a coexistent prolactinoma, Gharib and colleagues have reported a series of 11 patients with an empty sella and hyperprolactinemia who had no histologic evidence of a prolactinoma or hyperplasia of the lactotrophs (Gharib, 1983). They stated that approximately 5% of those with the empty sella have hyperprolactinemia, amenorrhea-galactorrhea, or both. It is theorized that with this syndrome, distortion of the infundibular stalk results in decreased levels of dopamine reaching the pituitary to inhibit

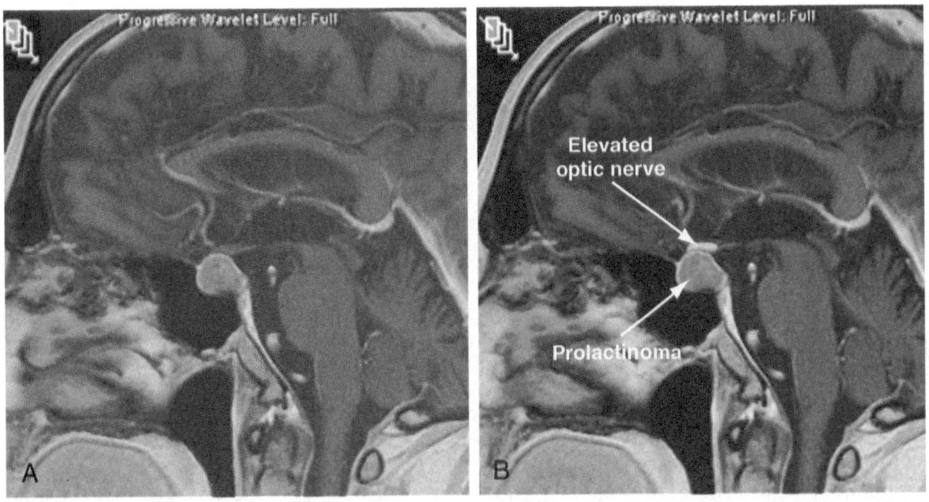


**Figure 39.3** **A,** Magnetic resonance imaging scan of the side view of the head (midway through the brain) showing a prolactinoma. **B,** Same image, colorized, showing that the top part of the tumor (shown in red) elevates the optic nerve (actually, the optic chiasm). (From UCLA Health System, *Neurosurgery,* issue 3: 31, 2010.)

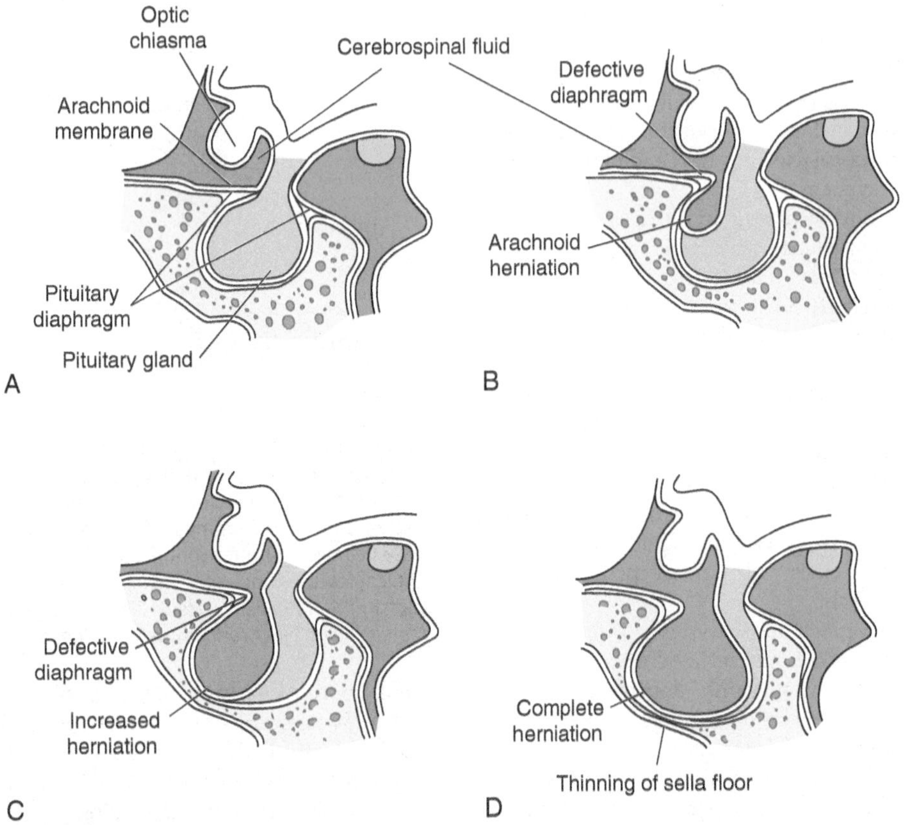


**Figure 39.4** Diagrammatic representation of empty sella syndrome. **A,** Normal anatomic relationship. **B-D,** Progression in development of empty sella syndrome. Note thinning of the floor and symmetrical enlargement of the sella turcica. (From Kletzky OA, Davajan V. Hyperprolactinemia: diagnosis and treatment. In: Mishell DR, Davajan V, Lobo RA, eds. *Infertility, Contraception and Reproductive Endocrinology.* 3rd ed. Cambridge, MA: Blackwell Scientific; 1991.)

PRL. Serum PRL levels are usually less than 100 ng/mL with the empty sella syndrome, and some women with this syndrome have normal PRL levels, with or without galactorrhea. Kleinberg and coworkers have reported that approximately 10% of all individuals with an enlarged sella turcica have the empty sella syndrome (Kleinberg, 1977). The best modality for diagnosing this condition is magnetic resonance imaging (MRI). It is important to establish the diagnosis because the syndrome has a benign course.

## PROLACTINOMAS

In an unselected series of 120 autopsies of individuals with no clinical evidence of pituitary disease, Burrow and associates found pituitary microadenomas to be present in 32 (27%) (Burrow, 1981). Molitch has noted that PRL incidentalomas occur in 11% of subjects at autopsy (Molitch, 1997). It has also been reported that adenomas were found in 78 of 486 (16%) of pituitary glands examined after unselected autopsies. In all series, PRL was found in approximately 50% of the glands, indicating that more than 10% of those in the general population have an undiagnosed prolactinoma.

Overall, approximately 50% of women with hyperprolactinemia have a prolactinoma. The incidence is higher when the PRL levels exceed 100 ng/mL, and almost all individuals with PRL levels greater than 200 ng/mL have a prolactinoma. There is an approximate positive correlation between the size of the adenoma and the PRL level. The majority of prolactinomas in women are microadenomas (<1 cm). Kleinberg and coworkers have reported that 20% of those with galactorrhea and 35% of women with amenorrhea-galactorrhea have radiologic evidence of pituitary tumors (Kleinberg, 1977).

Galactorrhea need not be present in all cases of adenoma. In approximately 20% of women with hyperprolactinemia and menstrual irregularities without galactorrhea, an adenoma may be found. Approximately 70% of women with hyperprolactinemia and galactorrhea, and secondary amenorrhea with low estrogen levels, have radiologic evidence of a pituitary adenoma. There is a correlation between the degree of suppression of the hypothalamic-pituitary-ovarian axis (resulting in hypoestrogenism) and the presence of an adenoma. However, an adenoma may be present in 20% to 30% of women with hyperprolactinemia and normal menses, oligomenorrhea, or secondary amenorrhea with normal estrogen status. No adenoma is found characteristically in individuals with normal menses, galactorrhea, and normal PRL levels.

Figure 39.5 depicts various possible causes of prolactinoma formation. In the past, it was firmly believed that adenomas or hyperplasia resulted from hypothalamic dopamine dysregulation, which was a functional defect or the result of altered blood supply. It is now believed that adenomas arise from single cell mutations, with clonal proliferation occurring subsequently. However, a search for mutations in oncogenes, the dopamine D2 or TRH receptor, signal transduction mechanisms, or transcription factors has not been rewarding to date. Prolactinomas that occur in 20% of patients with multiple endocrine neoplasia type 1 (MEN-1) may be caused by an inactivating mutation of the *MENIN* gene (Burgess, 1996), although this special case is clearly different from the usual type of prolactinomas.

It is also important to note that prolactinomas may also secrete other hormones with GH being the most common

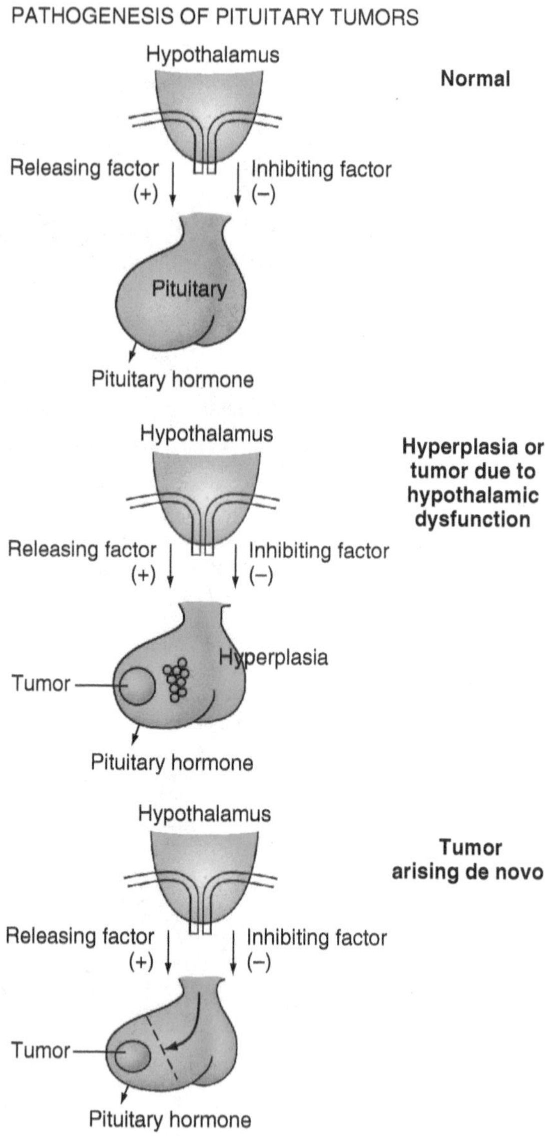


**Figure 39.5** Possible mechanisms leading to the formation of a prolactinoma. *Top,* Normal regulation. *Middle,* Tumors could arise because of an increase in prolactinreleasing factor (PRF) or a decrease in PRL-inhibiting factor (dopamine). *Bottom,* Tumors could arise de novo without hypothalamic influence. (From Molitch ME. Clinical features and epidemiology of prolactinomas in women. In: Olefsky JM, Robbins RJ, eds. *Prolactinomas: Practical Diagnosis and Management.* New York: Churchill Livingstone; 1986:67-95.)

companion. Also, up to 40% of primarily GH-secreting adenomas also secrete PRL. Combinations of PRL and ACTH, PRL and TSH, and PRL and FSH have been described. Indeed even "nonfunctioning" adenomas have been found to secrete isolated α and β subunits of gonadotropins.

Long-term studies of individuals with microadenomas have demonstrated that enlargement is uncommon and that many of these tumors regress spontaneously. The natural progression from micro- to macroadenoma has been estimated to be less than 7%. In a longitudinal retrospective study of women with hyperprolactinemia and a radiologic diagnosis of microadenoma, March and colleagues found that only 2 of 43 women had evidence of enlargement of the adenoma, with a mean duration of follow-up of 5 years (March, 1981). Of these 43 women, three had spontaneous regression of their hyperprolactinemia and resumption of normal menses. Koppelman and associates have reported similar results. Of 25 women with prolactinomas (18 with microadenomas and 7 with minimally enlarged sella) followed up for a mean duration of 11 years without treatment, only 1 woman had slight progression of a sella abnormality. None had visual field or other pituitary function changes, seven resumed normal menses spontaneously, and galactorrhea spontaneously resolved in six (Koppelman, 1984).

The results of these retrospective studies have been confirmed by two prospective studies of untreated microprolactinomas. In a 3- to 7-year prospective longitudinal study of 30 hyperprolactinemic women, Schlechte and coworkers found that of 13 women with initially abnormal radiographic findings, 4 became normal, 7 did not change, and 2 had evidence of progressive growth. Of 17 women with initially normal radiographic findings, the radiographic findings of 4 became minimally abnormal. None of the 30 developed a macroadenoma or pituitary hypofunction (Schlechte, 1989). In this study, as in the two retrospective studies reported earlier, more sensitive radiographic techniques (e.g., tomography, followed by computed tomography [CT]) were used as the study progressed and could account for the minimal evidence of tumor growth. Martin and coworkers followed the natural history of 41 women with idiopathic hyperprolactinemia and amenorrhea-galactorrhea for up to 11 years. During this time, 9 women conceived spontaneously and 16 resumed spontaneous menses with cessation of galactorrhea. Only one woman developed a microadenoma (Martin, 1985). Thus hyperprolactinemia with or without a microadenoma follows a benign clinical course in most women, and therapy is unnecessary unless pregnancy is desired or estrogen levels are low.

Several studies have reported that pregnancy is beneficial for women with functional hyperprolactinemia or PRL-secreting microadenomas. Following pregnancy, PRL levels decrease in approximately 50% of women. Crosignani and associates have reported that PRL levels normalized in approximately 30% of 176 hyperprolactinemic women after pregnancy. PRL levels decreased to normal in 36% of women with functional hyperprolactinemia and 17% of those with adenomas (Crosignani, 1992). Therefore if women with hyperprolactinemia desire to become pregnant, they should be encouraged to do so, because pregnancy is likely to result in normal or lowered PRL levels.

## DIAGNOSTIC TECHNIQUES

### *IMAGING STUDIES*

Current recommended techniques are to obtain a CT scan with intravenous contrast or an MRI with gadolinium enhancement. The latter provides better soft tissue definition, without radiation (23 rad; 0.03 Gy), and the CT scan is principally beneficial for bony structural abnormalities. The MRI provides 1-mm resolution and thus should be able to detect all microadenomas; it is currently the recommended imaging study to obtain.

### *RECOMMENDED DIAGNOSTIC EVALUATION*

It is recommended that PRL levels be measured in all women with galactorrhea, oligomenorrhea, or amenorrhea who do not have an elevated FSH level. PRL is also frequently measured in the workup of infertility. If the PRL level is elevated, a TSH assay should be performed to rule out the presence of primary hypothyroidism. If the TSH level is elevated, $T_3$ and $T_4$ should be measured to rule out the rare possibility of a TSH-secreting pituitary adenoma. If the TSH level is elevated and hypothyroidism is present, appropriate thyroid replacement should begin and the PRL level will usually return to normal. If the TSH level is normal and the woman has a normal PRL level with galactorrhea, no further tests are necessary if she has regular menses.

If PRL levels are elevated and the TSH level is normal, an MRI (preferably) or CT scan should be obtained to detect a microadenoma or macroadenoma. Macroadenomas are uncommon and rarely present with a PRL level less than 100 ng/mL. If the PRL level is more than 100 ng/mL or the woman complains of headaches or visual changes, the likelihood of a tumor extending beyond the sella turcica is increased. Microadenomas are a common cause of hyperprolactinemia and remain stable in most cases. Neither pregnancy, oral contraceptives, nor hormone therapy stimulates the growth of these small tumors; therapy is unnecessary unless ovulation induction is desired or hypoestrogenism is present.

Routine visual field testing and measurements of ACTH, GH, and thyroid function are not necessary unless warranted clinically. However, these evaluations, particularly visual field testing, should be performed in women with macroadenomas because suprasellar extension of the tumor may exert pressure on the optic chiasm, resulting in bitemporal visual field defects and interference with vision. The size of these tumors may also affect other aspects of pituitary function. With a macroadenoma, dynamic tests of pituitary function should be performed.

## TREATMENT

### *EXPECTANT TREATMENT*

Women with radiologic evidence of a microadenoma or functional hyperprolactinemia who do not wish to conceive may be followed without treatment by measuring PRL levels once annually. However, if estrogen is deficient, low estrogen levels in combination with hyperprolactinemia has been shown to be associated with the early onset of osteoporosis; thus exogenous estrogen should be administered. Hormonal therapy, as is used for postmenopausal women, or oral contraceptives may be used. Corenblum and Donovan have reported that a group of women with functional hyperprolactinemia and PRL-secreting pituitary microadenomas who were treated with cyclic estrogen and progestogen or oral contraceptives for several years did not have an increase in the size of the adenomas or increased PRL levels. Mean PRL levels actually declined with both treatment regimens (Corenblum, 1983). Testa also reported that 2 years of oral contraception use in a group of women with hyperprolactinemia with microadenoma did not alter the size of the adenoma (Testa, 1998). Because side effects and cost are less and compliance is better with exogenous estrogen than with dopamine agonist therapy, it is not necessary to use the latter unless ovulation and pregnancy are desired. Those with hyperprolactinemia, with or without microadenomas, who have adequate estrogen levels and who do not wish to conceive should be treated with periodic progestogen withdrawal (e.g., medroxyprogesterone acetate, 5 to 10 mg/day for 10 days each month) or with combination oral contraceptives to prevent endometrial hyperplasia.

## MEDICAL TREATMENT OF PROLACTINOMAS

The initial treatment for women with macroadenomas, as well as for those women with hyperprolactinemia who are anovulatory and wish to conceive, should be the administration of a dopamine receptor agonist. Cabergoline, **bromocriptine**, and pergolide have been used successfully; pergolide is currently not available.

### Bromocriptine

The greatest amount of clinical experience has been with the use of bromocriptine. This semisynthetic ergot alkaloid was developed in 1967 to inhibit PRL secretion. It directly stimulates dopamine 2 receptors and, as a dopamine receptor agonist, it inhibits PRL secretion in vitro and in vivo. After ingestion, bromocriptine is rapidly absorbed, with blood levels reaching a peak 1 to 3 hours later. Serum PRL levels remain depressed for approximately 14 hours after ingestion of a single dose, after which time the drug is not detectable in the circulation. Therefore the drug is usually given at least twice daily, with initial therapy being started at half of the 2.5-mg tablet to minimize side effects. The most frequent side effects are orthostatic hypotension, with an incidence of 15%, which can produce fainting and dizziness as well as nausea and vomiting. To minimize these symptoms, the initial dose should be taken in bed and with food at night. Less frequent adverse symptoms include headache, nasal congestion, fatigue, constipation, and diarrhea. Most of these reactions are mild, occur early in the course of treatment, and are transient. To reduce the adverse symptoms, the dose should be gradually increased every 1 to 2 weeks until PRL levels fall to normal. The greatest decrease in PRL occurs in the first 2 to 4 weeks. The therapeutic dose is usually titrated to normalize PRL. Figure 39.6 shows the rapid decline in PRL with

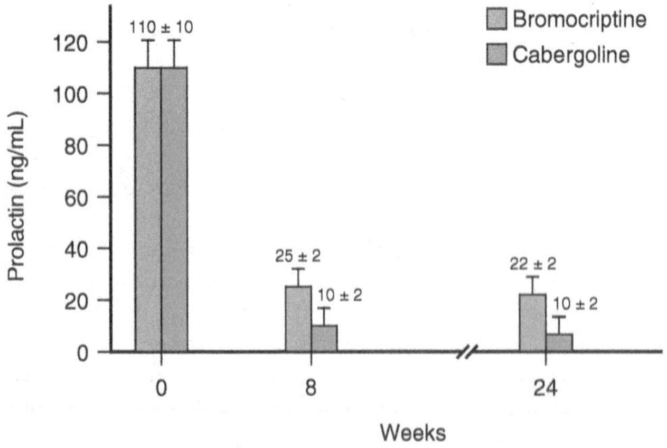


**Figure 39.6** Serum prolactin in women with hyperprolactinemic amenorrhea randomized to treatment with cabergoline or bromocriptine and followed for 24 weeks. (Data from Webster J Piscitelli MD, Polli A, et al. A comparison of cabergoline and bromocriptine in the treatment of hyperprolactinemic amenorrhea. Cabergoline Study Group. *N Engl J Med.* 1994;331[14]:904-909.)

bromocriptine as well as cabergoline in this randomized comparison study (Webster, 1994). Adverse effects of bromocriptine such as nausea, vomiting, and nasal congestion occur in approximately 50% of women and may cause them to discontinue treatment. Vermesh and colleagues have reported that the drug is well absorbed vaginally, without side effects. Furthermore, when a single tablet is placed deep into the posterior vaginal fornix, therapeutic blood levels persist for more than 24 hours, during which time PRL levels remain suppressed (Vermesh, 1988). Ginsburg and coworkers subsequently reported that this method of bromocriptine administration is well accepted and effective. The tablet was digitally placed deep into the vagina nightly at bedtime. A single 2.5-mg dose reduced PRL concentrations in 90% of patients treated and brought the levels to normal in one third of the women. Higher doses did not appear to be more effective (Ginsburg, 1992). In women wishing to conceive, sperm function is not adversely affected (Chenette, 1991).

### Cabergoline

Cabergoline is a long-acting dopamine receptor agonist and is currently preferred over bromocriptine for primary therapy, because of greater efficacy and fewer side effects (Ferrari, 1992; Wang, 2012). This agent directly inhibits pituitary lactotrophs, thereby decreasing PRL secretion. It is given orally in doses of 0.25 to 1 mg twice weekly. The initial dose is half a 0.5-mg tablet twice a week. Peak plasma levels occur in 2 to 3 hours, and the drug has a half-life of 65 hours. Its slow elimination and long half-life produce a prolonged PRL-lowering effect. The initial dose is 0.25 mg twice weekly, and the dosage may be increased at intervals of 4 weeks to achieve a satisfactory response (see Fig. 39.6). In a randomized trial with bromocriptine, cabergoline lowered PRL levels to normal in 83% of women, and only in 59% with bromocriptine. Cabergoline induced ovulation in 72% and eliminated galactorrhea in 90%. The effectiveness of cabergoline was greater than that of bromocriptine (Webster, 1994). Adverse effects, particularly nausea, headaches, and dizziness, occurred with both agents but were less frequent, less severe, and of shorter duration with cabergoline. In patients with pituitary adenoma who had been unsuccessfully treated previously with bromocriptine, cabergoline has been found to be effective (Table 39.1).

In Table 39.1, cabergoline has been compared with other agents in regard to effectiveness for reducing tumor size. It may be concluded that in women who have never been treated,

**Table 39.1** Comparison of Efficacy of Dopamine Agonists in Affecting Tumor Size Reduction*

| Dopamine Agonist | No. of Cases | Tumor Size Reduction (%) | | | |
|---|---|---|---|---|---|
| | | >50 | 25-50 | <25 | No Change |
| Bromocriptine | 112 | 40.2 | 28.6 | 12.5 | 18.7 |
| Pergolide* | 61 | 75.4 | 9.8 | 8.2 | 6.5 |
| Quinagolide* | 105 | 48.1 | 20.2 | 17.3 | 14.4 |
| Cabergoline* | 130 | 25.4 | 46.9 | 6.9 | 21.5 |

Modified from Molitch ME. Prolactin in human reproduction. In: Strauss JF III, Barbieri R,eds. *Yen and Jaffe's Reproductive Endocrinology*. Philadelphia: Elsevier; 2004:109.

*It should be noted that in many of the studies of pergolide, quinagolide, and cabergoline, many patients had previously been found to be resistant to or intolerant of bromocriptine.

cabergoline is the agent of choice for reducing PRL levels and effecting tumor shrinkage (Wang, 2012). It is recommended that after serum PRL levels have remained normal for 6 months, cabergoline be discontinued to determine whether the PRL levels will stay low without therapy. A potential concern with cabergoline and pergolide (now not available) is the development of cardiac valvular lesions. However, this has only been observed with large doses, as used for Parkinson disease, and has not been reported with lower doses (Drake, 2013; Caputo, 2014). It has been suggested that cardiac ultrasound be performed every 2 years in patients on chronic therapy of cabergoline at doses of less than 2 mg per week.

### *Outcomes of Treatment in Women with Prolactinomas*

Although cabergoline is currently the dopamine agonist of choice, bromocriptine is preferred if use is required in pregnancy because of its longer experience of use during pregnancy. Various incidence reports of use of bromocriptine or cabergoline in the first trimester have not shown any fetal defects or pregnancy complications. If pregnancy occurs after ovulation is induced with a dopamine agonist, therapy is usually discontinued, although there is no evidence that the drug is teratogenic or adversely affects pregnancy outcome.

When bromocriptine or cabergoline is used to treat hyperprolactinemia, therapy is usually continued for at least 12 months, after which it should be discontinued for a few weeks. Most women with microadenomas have recurrence of hyperprolactinemia, amenorrhea, and galactorrhea, although approximately 10% to 20% have permanent remission after discontinuation.

Moriondo and associates have reported that after 1 year of bromocriptine treatment, 11% of women with microadenomas have persistent normalization of PRL levels, with return of regular menses after the drug is discontinued (Moriondo, 1985) (Fig. 39.7). This incidence of permanent remission reached 22% after 2 years of treatment.

For macroadenoma, Kharlip and coworkers have suggested that the recurrence rate after cabergoline for macroadenomas was 50% to 60% within the first 18 months (Kharlip, 2009). The reduction in size of macroadenomas usually occurs rapidly. Figure 39.8 shows the reduction in size during bromocriptine therapy. Within a few weeks after starting treatment, size reduction occurs, but following withdrawal of drug the tumor size may increase just as rapidly. Thus the drug should be withdrawn cautiously. In contrast to the frequent occurrence of pituitary insufficiency, including diabetes insipidus, after surgical or radiologic treatment of large tumors, dopamine agonist treatment is not accompanied by any pituitary insufficiency.

Because permanent remission rarely occurs following withdrawal of treatment from individuals with large tumors, long-term treatment is usually necessary. Drug therapy has been maintained for over 10 years in many patients without any long-term sequelae or loss of efficacy.

Because of the excellent results of medical therapy and the poor initial results of surgery, particularly for large tumors with the high recurrence rates, it may be concluded that dopamine agonist therapy, specifically cabergoline, should be used as the initial management of those with PRL-secreting macroadenomas. After maximal shrinkage of tumor, medical therapy can be continued or operative treatment initiated. If surgery is elected medical therapy should be continued until the time of operation to prevent tumor expansion. The rates of success after operation are no different in those who received or did not receive medication prior to surgery.

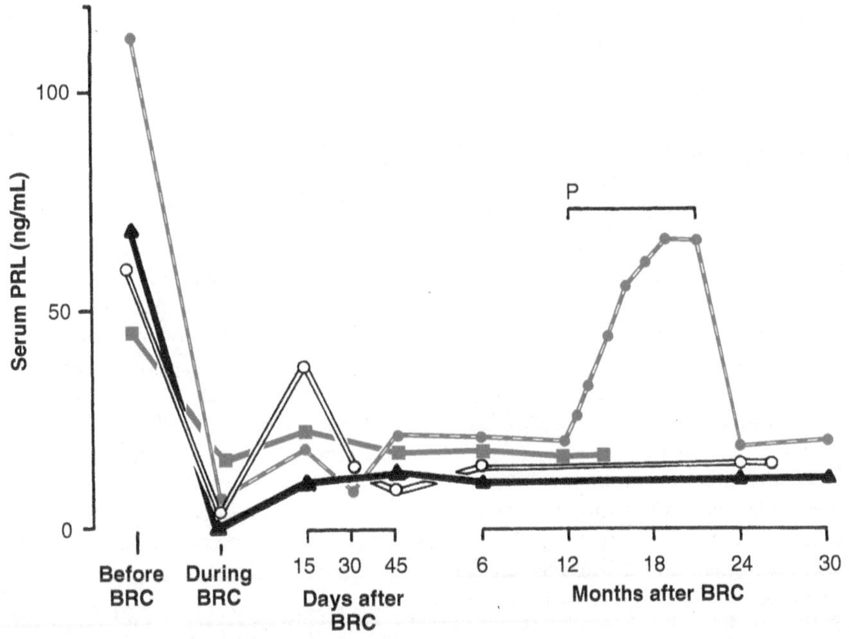


**Figure 39.7** Serum prolactin levels in four patients who had persistently normal prolactin levels (PRL) after bromocriptine (BRC) treatment for 12 months. *P*, Pregnancy. (From Moriondo P, Travaglini P, Nissim M, et al. Bromocriptine treatment of microprolactinomas: evidence of stable prolactin decrease after drug withdrawal. *J Clin Endocrinol Metab.* 1985;60[4]:764-772.)

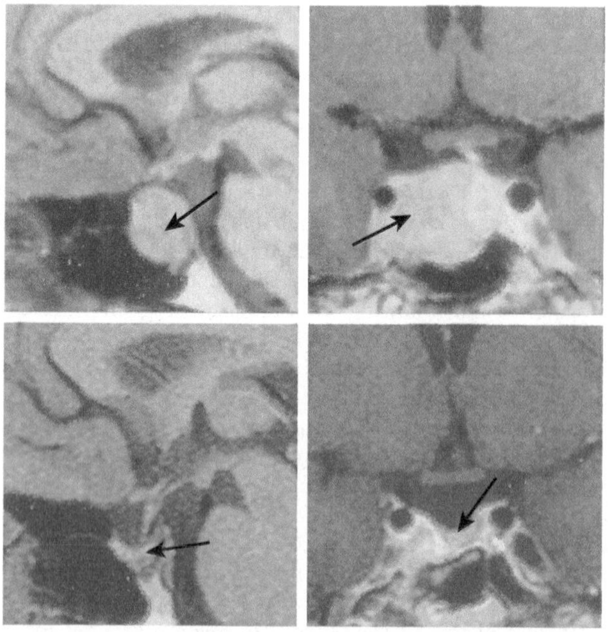

Figure 39.8 MRI scans of a patient with macroadenoma before *(above)* and during *(below)* bromocriptine treatment. *Left*, sagittal view; *Right*, coronal view. Note the marked decrease in tumor size. (From Molitch ME. Prolactin in human reproduction. In: *Yen & Jaffe's Reproductive Endocrinology*. 7th ed. Philadelphia: Elsevier; 2014.)

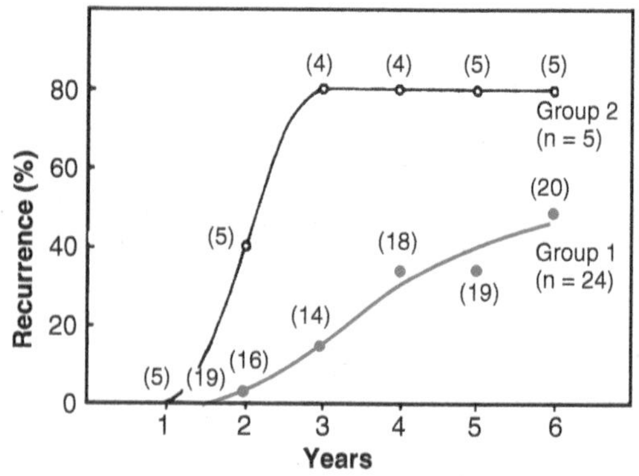


**Figure 39.9** Cumulative recurrence rate in patients with microprolactinoma (group 1) or macroprolactinoma (group 2) after initially successful operation. Figures in parentheses indicate the number of patients who were seen at each yearly interval. (From Serri O, Rasio E, Beauregard H, et al. Recurrence of hyperprolactinemia after selective transsphenoidal adenomectomy in women with prolactinoma. *N Engl J Med.* 1983;309[5]:280-283.)

## OPERATIVE APPROACHES FOR PROLACTINOMA

Trans-sphenoidal microsurgical resection of prolactinoma has been widely used for therapy, and numerous reports of large series of individuals treated by this technique have been published. In general, trans-sphenoidal operations have minimal risk, with a mortality of less than 0.5%. However, most deaths have been reported to occur after treatment of macroadenomas. The risk of temporary postoperative diabetes insipidus is 10% to 40%, but the risk of permanent diabetes insipidus and iatrogenic hypopituitarism is less than 2%. The initial cure rate, with normalization of PRL levels and return of ovulation, is relatively high for microadenomas (65% to 85%) but less so with macroadenomas (20% to 40%). Vision can return to normal in 85% of patients with loss of acuity and visual field defects.

The initial cure rate is related to the pretreatment PRL levels. Those tumors with PRL levels less than 100 ng/mL have an excellent prognosis (85%), and those with levels higher than 200 ng/mL have a poor prognosis (35%). Operative treatment of tumors in individuals older than 26 years with amenorrhea for longer than 6 months carries a poorer prognosis than tumors in younger women with a shorter duration of amenorrhea. Nevertheless, long-term follow-up of patients after operation has indicated that late recurrence of hyperprolactinemia is common. Serri and colleagues followed 28 women with microadenomas and 16 with macroadenomas for 6 years after operation. PRL levels normalized and menses resumed in 24 (85%) of those with microadenomas and 5 (31%) of those with macroadenomas. However, hyperprolactinemia recurred in 50% of those with microadenoma and 4 of 5 with macroadenomas after a mean period of 4 and 2.5 years, respectively (Serri, 1983) (Fig. 39.9). There was no significant difference in recurrence rates for those who conceived and those who did not. Rodman and coworkers have reported a lower postoperative recurrence rate (~20% for both microadenomas and macroadenomas) following initial cure rates of 85% and 37%, respectively (Rodman, 1984). The risk of recurrence in both series appeared to be related to the immediate postoperative PRL levels being greater in those with a PRL level >10 ng/mL.

Overall, it can be concluded that after surgery, recurrence rates for microadenomas or macroadenomas are similar (21% and 19.8%, respectively). Long-term surgical cure rates are 58% for microadenomas but only 26% for macroadenomas using a normal PRL level as a criterion.

Because of the good results with medical therapy, surgery is recommended only for women with macroadenoma who fail to respond to medical therapy or have poor compliance with this regimen. It is best to reduce the size of macroadenomas maximally with bromocriptine before surgical removal of these extrasellar tumors.

## RADIATION THERAPY FOR MACROADENOMAS

External radiation with cobalt, proton beam, or heavy particle therapy and brachytherapy with yttrium-90 rods implanted in the pituitary have all been used to treat macroadenomas but are not the primary mode of treatment. The current method of choice is probably the gamma knife and linear accelerator. Results have been inconsistent, and damage to normal pituitary tissue may occur, leading to abnormal anterior pituitary function and diabetes insipidus. Damage to the optic nerves may also occur, which led to the more precise technique of the gamma knife. Thus radiation therapy should be used only as adjunctive management following incomplete operative removal of large tumors.

## PREGNANCY AND TREATMENT OF PROLACTINOMAS

Many women with hyperprolactinemia, with or without adenomas, wish to become pregnant. A small percentage of these

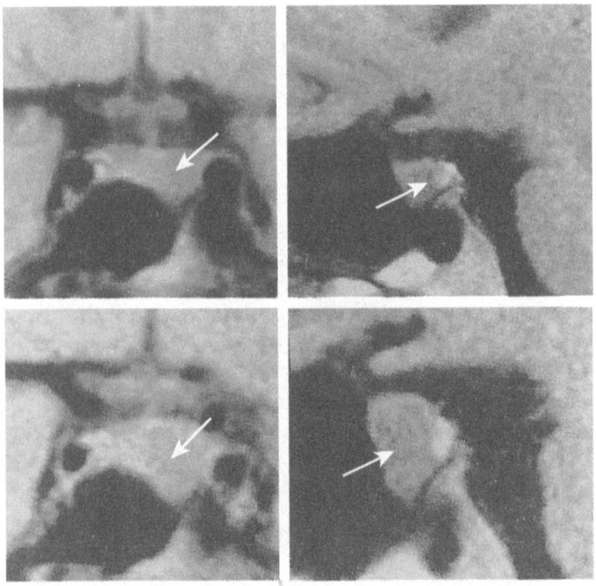

**Figure 39.10** Coronal and sagittal magnetic resonance imaging scans of an intrasellar prolactin secreting macroadenoma in a woman prior to conception *(above)* and at 7 months of gestation *(below)*. Note the marked tumor enlargement at the latter point, at which time the patient was complaining of headaches. (From Molitch ME. Medical treatment of prolactinomas. *Endocrinol Metab Clin North Am.* 1999;28[1]:143-169.)

women conceive spontaneously, but most require treatment to induce ovulation. Barbieri and Ryan have compiled a literature review of the pregnancy courses of 275 women with adenomas, most of whose conceptions had been induced by bromocriptine (Barbieri, 1983). They reported that of 215 women with microprolactinomas, less than 1% had changes in visual fields, radiologic evidence of tumor enlargement, or neurologic signs. Approximately 5% developed headaches during pregnancy. Of 60 women with macroprolactinomas, 20% developed adverse changes in their visual field and polytomographic or neurologic signs during pregnancy, and some of them required bromocriptine or operative treatment during pregnancy or shortly postpartum. The pituitary gland normally increases in size during pregnancy, and macroadenomas are at risk for enlarging to the point of causing symptoms (Fig. 39.10), particularly if they did not receive treatment prior to pregnancy. Molitch reported that if no treatment occurred before pregnancy, 2.7% of women with a microadenoma became symptomatic, whereas 22.9% of women with a macroadenoma were symptomatic (Molitch, 2011). However, with prepregnancy treatment, only 4.8% of women with a macroadenoma became symptomatic during pregnancy.

Women with a microadenoma do not require treatment during pregnancy, whereas women with macroadenoma only require treatment if they become symptomatic. Testing of visual fields every 3 months should be carried out in all women with a macroadenoma. Routine measurements of PRL during pregnancy have been controversial because of the wide range of values in pregnancy. However, it has been suggested that if PRL exceeds 400 ng/mL, this level should prompt visual field testing in women with an adenoma.

Although cabergoline is the dopamine agonist of choice for hyperprolactinemia, bromocriptine is used in pregnancy because there is a greater experience with bromocriptine, whereas there is no evidence of an adverse effect with cabergoline (Glezer, 2014). Using bromocriptine, Turkalj found there was a spontaneous abortion rate of 11%, an ectopic pregnancy rate of 0.7%, and a twin pregnancy rate of 1.8%. The incidence of minor (2.5%) and major (1%) congenital defects was similar to pregnancy outcomes in untreated populations of women (Turkalj, 1982). The mean amount of drug ingested and duration of postconception treatment were similar in mothers who had normal children and those who had children with defects. Thus ingestion of bromocriptine during pregnancy does not appear to increase the risk of congenital abnormalities, spontaneous abortion, or multiple gestations. Postnatal surveillance of more than 200 children born in this series has revealed no adverse effects to date.

Ruiz-Velasco compiled the obstetric histories of almost 2000 pregnancies occurring in hyperprolactinemic women that have been reported in the literature. Most of these pregnancies were induced with bromocriptine. There was a full-term delivery rate of 85%, an abortion rate of 11%, a prematurity rate of 2%, and a multiple pregnancy rate of 1.2% (Ruiz-Velasco, 1984). Although PRL levels increased during pregnancy, after delivery the levels returned to pretreatment values in approximately 85% of these women. A postpartum increase over pretreatment levels was uncommon (3%), and PRL levels returned to normal in 13%. Similarly, among women who had a postpartum radiologic examination, 84% showed no change, 9% improved, and 7% worsened. Thus stopping treatment during pregnancy only occasionally results in tumor growth.

*Breastfeeding may be initiated without adverse effects on the tumors and may be initiated after delivery unless there have been visual field defects during pregnancy* (Auriemma, 2013; Domingue, 2014). Treatment before conception and during pregnancy does not affect the incidence of persistent lactation following discontinuation of nursing. The incidence of menstrual abnormalities and degree of galactorrhea appear to be similar to the state that existed before starting medical therapy.

### Women with Hyperprolactinemia Who Do Not Wish to Conceive

For women who do not wish to conceive and for whom galactorrhea is not a problem, no therapy is necessary unless estrogen levels are low. Thus to prevent osteoporosis in this clinical situation, estrogen-progestogen hormone replacement or oral contraceptives should be given, regardless of whether an adenoma is present (Corenblum B, 1993). Long-term evaluation of all women with hyperprolactinemia should be carried out. Unless a macroadenoma is present, measurement of PRL levels once a year is advisable. Repeat imaging studies are unnecessary unless symptoms of headaches or visual disturbances occur or PRL levels increase substantially.

During medical treatment of macroadenomas, MRI or CT and occasional visual field examination should be performed to determine the effect of medication on the tumor. At these intervals, a decision can be made about whether to continue long-term treatment or to remove the tumor surgically.

## KEY POINTS

- The main symptoms of hyperprolactinemia are galactorrhea and amenorrhea, the latter caused by alterations in normal GnRH release.
- Pathologic causes of hyperprolactinemia include pharmacologic agents (e.g., tranquilizers, narcotics, antihypertensive drugs), hypothyroidism, chronic renal disease, chronic neurostimulation of the breast, hypothalamic disease, and pituitary tumors (e.g., prolactinoma, acromegaly, Cushing disease).
- Autopsy studies reveal that prolactinomas are present in approximately 10% of the population.
- Approximately 70% of women with hyperprolactinemia, galactorrhea, and amenorrhea with low estrogen levels will have a prolactinoma.
- Most macroadenomas enlarge with time; almost all microadenomas do not.
- The initial operative cure rate for microadenomas is approximately 80% and 30% for macroadenomas, but the long-term recurrence rate is at least 20% for each.
- In women with hyperprolactinemia and no macroadenoma, bromocriptine or cabergoline treatment returns PRL levels to normal in 90%, induces ovulatory cycles in 80%, and eradicates galactorrhea in 60%.
- The dopamine agonist of choice is cabergoline, because of increased efficacy and fewer side effects.
- Without prior treatment, 2.7% of women with microadenomas develop symptoms, whereas 22.9% of women with a macroadenoma will develop symptoms. Estrogen therapy or oral contraceptives will not stimulate the growth of PRL-secreting microadenomas and can be used for treatment of hyperprolactinemia and hypoestrogenism.
- Surgical treatment of prolactinomas is recommended only for patients who fail to respond or do not comply with medical management.

## KEY REFERENCES


Auriemma RS, Perone Y, Sarno Di, et al. Results of a single center observational 10-year survey study on recurrence of hyperprolactinemia after pregnancy and lactation. *J Clin Endocrinol Metab*. 2013;98:372-379.

Burgess JR, Shepherd JJ, Parameswaran V, et al. Prolactinomas in a large kindred with multiple endocrine neoplasia Type 1: clinical features and inheritance pattern. *J Clin Endocrinol Metab*. 1996;81:1841-1845.

Caputo C, Prior D, Inder WJ. The need for annual echocardiography to detect cabergoline-associated valvulopathy in patients with prolactinoma: a systematic review and additional clinical data. *Lancet Diabetes Endocrinol*. 2014;S2213-8587(14):70212-70218. [Epub ahead of print].

Chenette PE, Siegel MS, Vermesh M. Effect of bromocriptine on sperm function in vitro and in vivo. *Obstet Gynecol*. 1991;77:935-938.

Corenblum B, Donovan L. The safety of physiological estrogen plus progestin replacement therapy and with oral contraceptive therapy in women with pathological hyperprolactinemia. *Fertil Steril*. 1993;59:671.

Drake WM, Stiles CE, Howlett TA, et al. A cross-sectional study of the prevalence of cardiac valvular abnormalities in hyperprolactinemic patients treated with ergot-derived dopamine agonists. *J Clin Endocrinol Metab*. 2013;99(1):90-96.

Domingue ME, Devuyst F, Alexopoulou O, et al. Outcome of prolactinoma after pregnancy and lactation: a study on 73 patients. *Clin Endocrinol (Oxf)*. 2014;80:642-648.

Ferrari C, Paracchi A, Mattei AM, et al. Cabergoline in the long-term therapy of hyperprolactinemic disorders. *Acta Endocrinol*. 1992;126:489-494.

Glezer A, Bronstein MD. Prolactinomas, cabergoline in pregnancy. *Endocrine*. 2014;47:64-69.

Leslie H, Courtney CH, Bell PM, et al. Laboratory and clinical experience in 55 patients with macroprolactinemia identified with a simple polyethylene glycol precipitation method. *J Clin Endocrinol Metab*. 2001;86:2743-2746.

Molitch ME. Prolactinomas in pregnancy. *Best Prac Res Clin Endocrinol Metab*. 2011;25:885-896.

St-Jean E, Blain F. Comtois: High prolactin levels may be missed by immunoradiometric assay in patients with macroprolactinomas. *Clin Endocrinol*. 1996;44:305-309.

Vermesh ME, Fossum GT, Kletzky OA. Vaginal bromocriptine: pharmacology and effect on serum prolactin in normal women. *Obstet Gynecol*. 1988;72:693-698.

Wang AT, Mullan RJ, Lane MA, et al. Treatment of hyperprolactinemia: a systematic review and meta-analysis. *Syst Rev*. 2012;1:33.


Suggested Readings can be found on ExpertConsult.com.

# 40

# Hyperandrogenism and Androgen Excess

## Physiology, Etiology, Differential Diagnosis, Management

*Roger A. Lobo*

Hyperandrogenism in women is often referred to as ***androgen excess***. Although most women with hyperandrogenism will have hyperandrogenemia (elevated androgen levels in blood) as well as skin manifestations (e.g., **acne, hirsutism,** or **alopecia**), many women exhibit only skin manifestations without demonstrable findings in blood, and women can have no clinical signs of hyperandrogenism despite hyperandrogenemia. This chapter begins with a discussion of physiology, which will help explain this paradox.

The clinical signs associated with excessive androgen production in women are related to findings in skin and include acne, hirsutism, alopecia and, rarely, **virilization**. It is these complaints that warrant an evaluation and possible treatment. Hyperandrogenemia, per se, should not be the target of any treatment.

These skin disorders may be understood by understanding the **pilosebaceous unit (PSU)**. The PSU is composed of a sebaceous component and pilary component from which the hair shaft arises. Abnormalities of the sebaceous component lead to acne, and abnormalities of the pilary unit lead to excessive growth (hirsutism) or excessive shedding (alopecia). There are two types of hair; vellus hair is soft, fine, and unpigmented, whereas terminal hair is coarse, thick, pigmented, and undergoes cyclic changes. Anagen is the growth phase of hair. It is followed by the transitional catagen phase and, finally, by a resting, or telogen, phase, after which the hair sheds (Ebling, 1988). Androgen is necessary to produce development of terminal hair, and the duration of the anagen phase is directly related to the levels of circulating androgen (Rosenfield, 2005b). The duration of anagen also determines the length of hair, which varies in different parts of the body. For facial hair it is approximately 4 months, which has implications for the treatment of facial hirsutism, described later.

There are several steroidogenic enzymes in the hair follicle, but the activity level of the enzyme **5α-reductase** most directly influences the degree of androgenic effect on hair growth. With elevated levels of circulating androgen or increased activity of 5α-reductase, terminal hair appears where normally only vellus hair is present. With these alterations, the length of the anagen phase is prolonged and the hair becomes thicker. Excessive 5α-reductase activity also may lead to acne as well as scalp hair loss (alopecia).

The presence of hirsutism without other signs of virilization is associated with a milder increase in androgenic activity, compared to what is observed with virilization, and it has a longer, more gradual onset. The amount and location of hair growth found in women with hirsutism varies. In the milder forms, hair is found only on the upper lip and chin, whereas with increasing severity it appears on the cheeks, chest (intermammary), abdomen (superior to the umbilicus), inner aspects of the thighs, lower back, and intergluteal areas. The severity of the hirsutism can be roughly quantified by a modified scoring system of Ferriman and Gallwey (Ferriman, 1961; Hatch, 1981) (Fig. 40.1, Table 40.1). Examples of this scoring system may be found in Figure 40.2. Although a score greater than 7 or 8 has generally been considered to be consistent with hirsutism, this only pertains to the Caucasian or African-American population. In Asian women the threshold for an abnormal score is much lower at >3 (Escobar-Morreale, 2012). Increased hair growth only on the extremities or in isolated areas is called **hypertrichosis** and should not be confused with hirsutism.

Virilization is a relatively uncommon clinical finding and its presence is usually associated with markedly elevated levels of circulating testosterone (≥2 ng/mL). In contrast to the gradual development of hirsutism, signs of virilization usually occur over a relatively short period. These signs are caused by the masculinizing and defeminizing (antiestrogenic) actions of testosterone and include temporal balding, clitoral hypertrophy, decreased breast size, dryness of the vagina, and increased muscle mass. Women with virilization are almost always amenorrheic. The presence of androgen-secreting neoplasms should always be suspected in any woman who develops signs of virilization, particularly if the onset is rapid.

## PHYSIOLOGY OF ANDROGENS IN WOMEN

Androgen production in women is best understood by the concept of production from glandular tissues, namely the ovaries and adrenals, and from nonglandular tissues. This third compartment of production and modification of androgens includes many peripheral tissues and, for our discussion of hyperandrogenism, principally means the PSU itself, which not only responds to androgen but can modify it by enzymatic modifications. From a quantitative perspective, the major androgen produced by the ovaries is **testosterone** and that of the adrenal glands is **dehydroepiandrosterone sulfate (DHEAS)**. Measurement of the amount of these two steroids in the circulation provides clinically relevant information regarding the presence and source of increased androgen

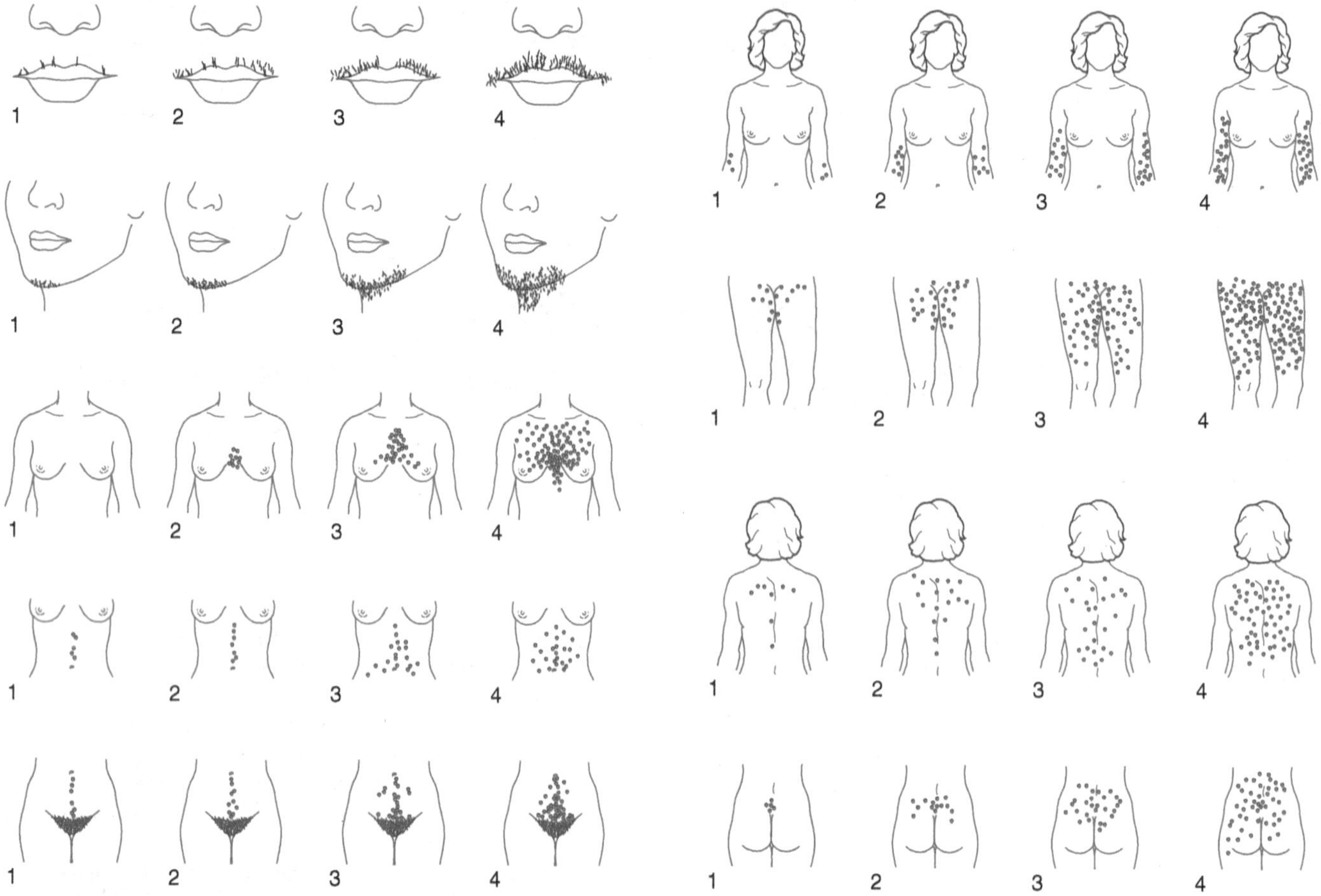

**Figure 40.1** Modified Ferriman Gallwey score. (Modified from Hatch R, Rosenfield RL, Kim MH, et al. Hirsutism: implications, etiology and management. *Am J Obstet Gynecol.* 1981;140[7]:815-830.)

**Table 40.1** Definition of Hair Gradings at 11 Sites*

| Site | Grade | Definition |
|---|---|---|
| Upper lip | 1 | Few hairs at outer margin |
| | 2 | Small mustache at outer margin |
| | 3 | Mustache extending halfway from outer margin |
| | 4 | Mustache extending to midline |
| Chin | 1 | Few scattered hairs |
| | 2 | Scattered hairs with small concentrations |
| | 3, 4 | Complete cover, light and heavy |
| Chest | 1 | Circumareolar hairs |
| | 2 | With midline hair in addition |
| | 3 | Fusion of these areas, with 75% cover |
| | 4 | Complete cover |
| Upper back | 1 | Few scattered hairs |
| | 2 | Rather more, still scattered |
| | 3, 4 | Complete cover, light and heavy |
| Lower back | 1 | Sacral tuft of hair |
| | 2 | With some lateral extension |
| | 3 | 75% cover |
| | 4 | Complete cover |
| Upper abdomen | 1 | Few midline hairs |
| | 2 | Rather more, still midline |
| | 3, 4 | Half- and full cover |
| Lower abdomen | 1 | Few midline hairs |
| | 2 | Midline streak of hair |
| | 3 | Midline band of hair |
| | 4 | Inverted V-shaped growth |
| Arm | 1 | Sparse growth affecting not more than 25% of limb surface |
| | 2 | More than this; cover still incomplete |
| | 3, 4 | Complete cover, light and heavy |
| Forearm | 1-4 | Complete cover of dorsal surface; two grades of light and two of heavy growth |
| Thigh | 1-4 | As for arm |
| Leg | 1-4 | As for arm |

From Ferriman D, Gallwey JD. Clinical assessment of body hair growth in women. *J Clin Endocrinol Metab.* 1961;21:1440-1447.

*Grade 0 at all sites indicates absence of terminal hair.

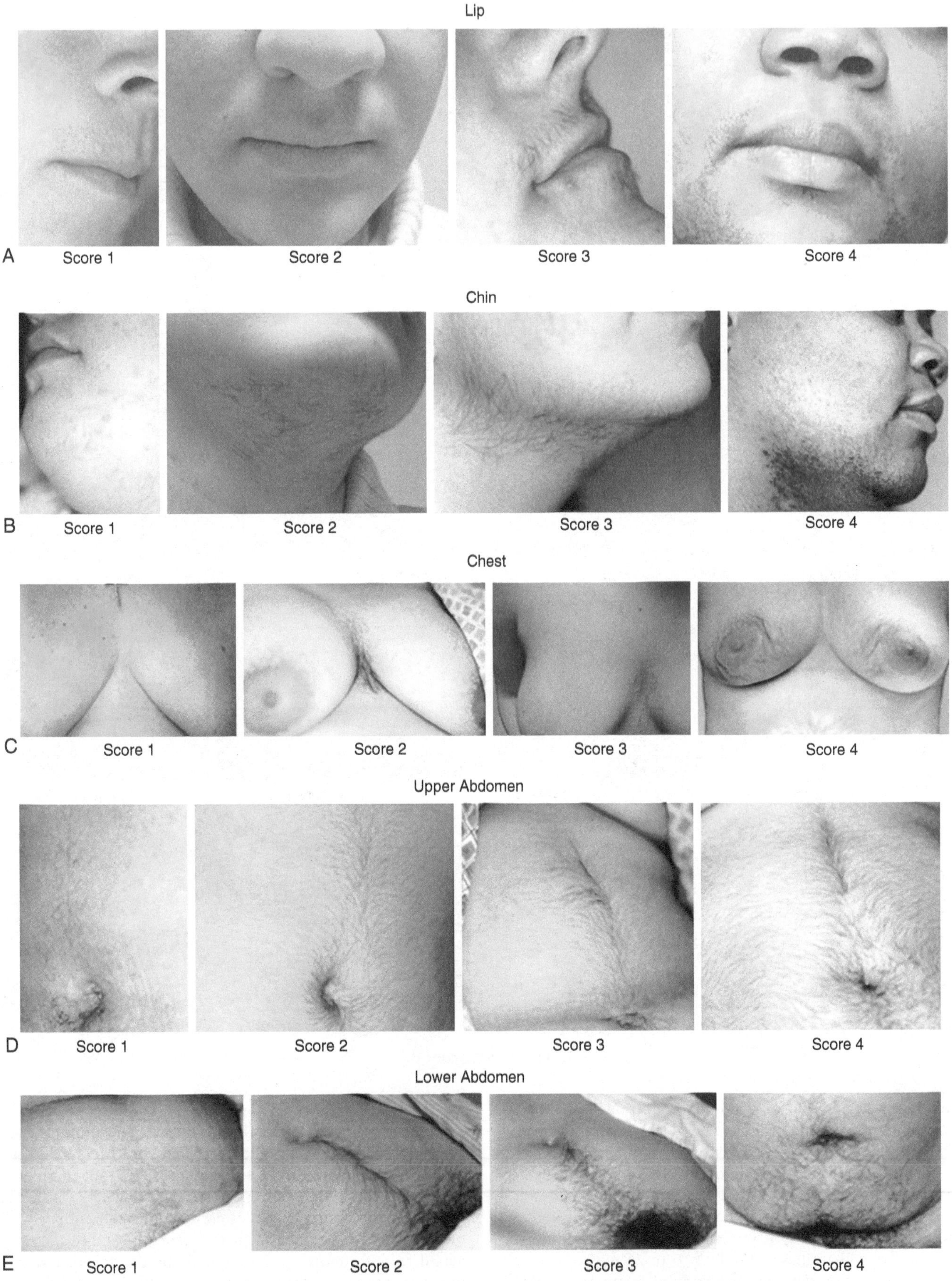


**Figure 40.2** Examples of scoring for hirsutism using the Ferriman Gallwey method in Figure 40.1. (Photographs of women without use of any method to remove body hair; obtained with personal confidentiality and institutional review board permission.) Panels **A-I** depict the 9 different body areas as listed on each panel. (Modified from Yildiz BO, Bolour S, Woods K, et al. Visually scoring hirsutism. *Hum Reprod Update*. 2010;16[1]:51-64.)

*Continued*

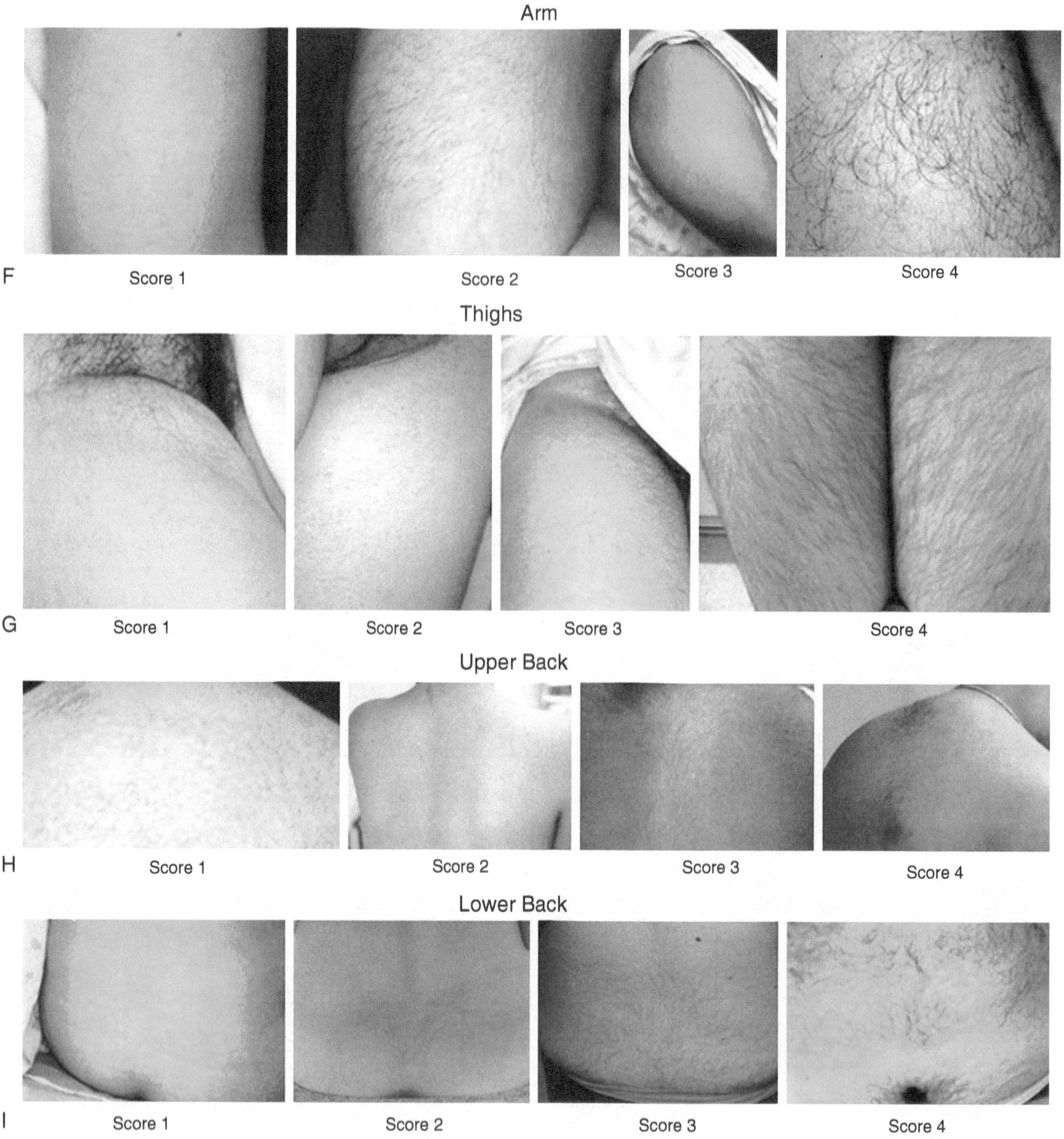


**Figure 40.2, cont'd**

production. In addition to glandular production of androgens, conversion of androstenedione and Dehydroepiandrosterone (DHEA) to testosterone occurs in peripheral tissues.

The ovaries secrete only approximately 0.1 mg of testosterone/day, mainly from the thecal and stroma cells. Other androgens secreted by the ovary are androstenedione (1 to 2 mg/day) and DHEA (<1 mg/day). The adrenal glands, in addition to secreting large quantities of DHEAS (6 to 24 mg/day), secrete approximately the same daily amount of androstenedione (1 mg/day) as the ovaries and less than 1 mg of DHEA/day. The normal adrenal gland secretes little testosterone, although some adrenal tumors have the ability to produce testosterone directly.

Androstenedione and DHEA do not have strong androgenic activity but are peripherally converted at a slow rate to the biologically active androgen, testosterone. Only approximately 5% of androstenedione and a smaller percentage of DHEA are converted to testosterone. The total daily production of testosterone in women is normally approximately 0.35 mg. Of this, 0.1

Table 40.2 Origin of Testosterone in Women

| Origin | Amount (mg/day) |
|---|---|
| Ovarian secretion | 0-1 |
| Peripheral conversion | |
| Androstenedione → testosterone | 0.2 |
| Dehydroepiandrosterone → testosterone | 0.05 |
| Total testosterone production | 0.35 |

From Lobo RA. Androgen excess. In: Mishell DR Jr, Davajan V, Lobo RA, eds. *Infertility, Contraception and Reproductive Endocrinology*. 3rd ed. Cambridge, MA: Blackwell Scientific; 1991.

Table 40.3 Plasma Concentrations of Androgens During Menstrual Cycle Same

| Steroid Hormone | Phase of Cycle | Plasma Concentration | |
|---|---|---|---|
| | | Mean | Range |
| Androstenedione (ng/mL) | * | 1.4 | 0.7-3.1 |
| Testosterone (ng/mL) | * | 0.35 | 0.15-0.55 |
| Dehydroepiandrosterone (ng/mL) | * | 4.2 | 2.7-7.8 |
| Dehydroepiandrosterone sulfate (μg/mL) | * | 1.6 | 0.8-3.4 |

From Goebelsmann U. Steroid hormones. In: Mishell DR Jr, Davajan V, eds. *Infertility, Contraception and Reproductive Endocrinology*. 2nd ed. Oradell, NJ: Medical Economics Books; 1986.

*Unspecified; no major changes during menstrual cycle.

mg comes from direct ovarian secretion, 0.2 mg from peripheral conversion of androstenedione, and 0.05 mg from peripheral conversion of DHEA (Table 40.2). Because the ovaries and adrenal gland secrete approximately equal amounts of androstenedione and DHEA, approximately two thirds (0.22 mg) of the daily testosterone produced in a woman originates from the ovaries. Thus increased circulating levels of testosterone usually indicate abnormal ovarian androgen production. Normal circulating levels of these androgens in women of reproductive age are shown in Table 40.3. For practical purposes, circulatory levels of DHEAS reflect an adrenal source of production, and in women more than 95% is adrenal derived. Occasionally, in women who have increased production of ovarian DHEA, such as some with polycystic ovary syndrome (PCOS), the elevated levels of DHEAS might have an ovarian component because DHEA may be converted to DHEAS in the circulation. Another specific marker of adrenal androgen production, used for research purposes, is 11β-hydroxyandrostenedione (Stanczyk, 1991), because the adrenal primarily has the ability to 11-hydroxylate androstenedione, whereas the ovary has a limited ability to do so.

Although DHEAS serves as a good marker of adrenal hyperandrogenism, several guidelines for the evaluation of hyperandrogenism in women omit this measurement, because DHEAS itself is a "weak" androgen and may not contribute much to the overall androgenicity. Nevertheless it is our perspective that the measurement of DHEAS gives a more complete picture of androgen production.

Most testosterone in the circulation (≈85%) is tightly bound to sex hormone-binding globulin (SHBG) and is believed to be biologically inactive. An additional 10% to 15% is loosely bound to albumin, with only approximately 1% to 2% not bound to any protein (**free testosterone**). Both the free and albumin-bound

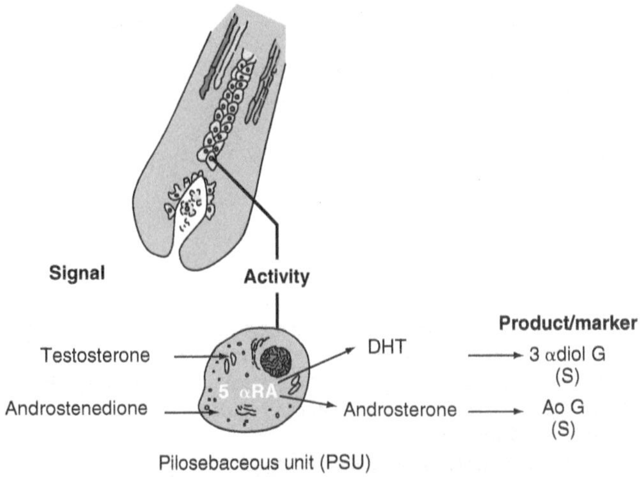


**Figure 40.3** Peripheral androgen metabolism and markers of this activity. *Ao G*, Androsterone glucuronide; *DHT*, dihydrotestosterone; 3 αdiol G, 3α-androstanediol glucuronide; *(S)*, serum. (From Lobo RA. Androgen excess. In: Mishell DR Jr, Davajan V, Lobo RA, eds. *Infertility, Contraception and Reproductive Endocrinology*. 3rd ed. Cambridge, MA: Blackwell Scientific; 1991.)

fractions (often called *unbound*) are biologically active. Serum testosterone can be measured as the total amount, the amount that is believed to be biologically active (unbound, or non-SHBG bound), and as the free form. As discussed later, because commercial laboratory measurements of "free" testosterone are not accurate, it may be useful to measure the ratio of testosterone and SHBG.

To exert a biologic effect, testosterone is metabolized peripherally in target tissues to the more potent androgen **5α-dihydrotestosterone** (**DHT**) by the enzyme **5α-reductase**. 5α-reductase activity is important for testosterone action peripherally (as in the PSU) as well as in the genitalia (Serafini, 1985a). It is not necessary for testosterone action in other areas such as in muscle or bone. After further 3-keto reduction, DHT is converted to another metabolite, 5α-androstane-3α,17β-diol (3α-diol). 3α-Diol is conjugated to the sulfate or glucuronide. The glucuronide, **5α-androstane-3α,17β-diol glucuronide** (**3α-diol-G**), is a stable, irreversible product of intracellular 5α-reductase activity and reflects this activity in blood (Fig. 40.3).

Even with normal circulatory levels of androgen, increased 5α-reductase activity in the PSU results in increased androgenic activity, producing hirsutism (Serafini, 1985a; Paulson, 1986) (Fig. 40.4). Measurements of 5α-reductase activity in skin biopsies have found that the level of activity correlated well with the degree of hirsutism present (Serafini, 1985b). The degree of 5α-reductase activity can be measured in skin biopsies by a variety of methods. This technique is only used for investigational purposes; if necessary for diagnostic reasons, 3α-diol-G levels can be directly measured in serum. We have found that the measurement of this metabolite is the most accurate indicator of the degree of peripheral androgen metabolism in women, as long as the level of glandular production (testosterone) is appreciated. Although serum levels of total testosterone are similar in normal and hirsute women, there are significant differences in 3α-diol-G (Lobo, 1983) (Fig. 40.5). In general, whereas non–SHBG-bound testosterone has been found to be

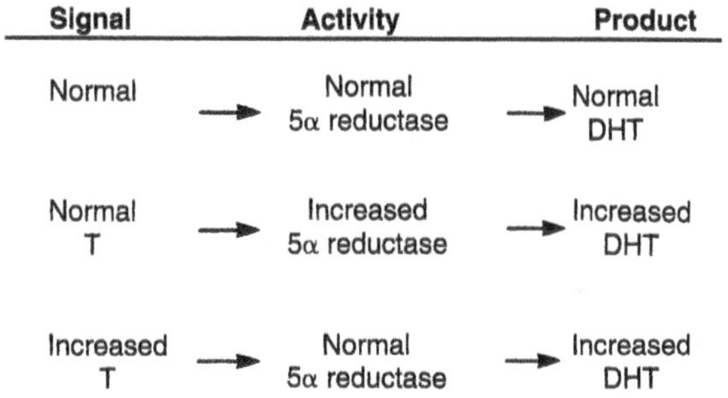

Signal
Activity
Product
Normal
Normal 5α reductase
Normal DHT
Normal T
Increased 5α reductase
Increased DHT
Increased T
Normal 5α reductase
Increased DHT


**Figure 40.4** Influence of androgen substrate (signal; e.g., testosterone or androstenedione) and 5α-reductase activity (in pilosebaceous units) on local production of biologically active androgens. *T*, Testosterone; *DHT*, dihydrotestosterone. (From Lobo RA. Androgen excess. In: Mishell DR Jr, Davajan V, Lobo RA, eds. *Infertility, Contraception and Reproductive Endocrinology*. 3rd ed. Cambridge, MA: Blackwell Scientific; 1991.)

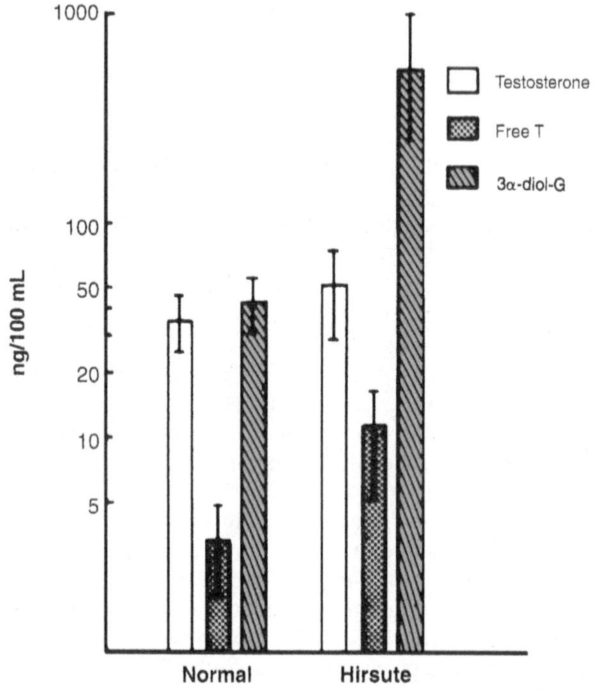


**Figure 40.5** Plasma total testosterone, unbound testosterone (free T) and 5α-androstane-3α,17β-diol glucuronide (3α-diol-G) in normal and hirsute women. Note insignificant elevation with overlap for testosterone and free T testosterone and highly significant increase in 3α-diol-G without overlap between two groups of women. (From Horton R, Hawks D, Lobo RA. 3α,17β-androstanediol glucuronide in plasma: a marker of androgen action in idiopathic hirsutism. *J Clin Invest.* 1982;69:1203-1206.)

elevated in approximately 60% to 70% of hirsute women, levels of 3α-diol-G have been found to be elevated in more than 80% of women in this setting.

In summary, there are three markers of androgen production in serum, one for each compartment in which androgens are produced (Table 40.4). These measurements best reflect the area of interest, although it is clear that each compartment also produces other hormones. Interpretation of levels of 3α-diol-G is controversial because these levels are highly dependent on circulating levels of precursor androgens, such as testosterone and also androstenedione. A reasonable argument may be that if testosterone and DHEAS are normal but there is significant hirsutism, then measuring 3α-diol-G may not be necessary and one may merely assume a peripheral source of androgen excess.

Table 40.4 Markers of Androgen Production

| Source | Marker |
|---|---|
| Ovary | Testosterone |
| Adrenal gland | DHEAS |
| Periphery | 3α-diol-G |

From Lobo RA. Androgen excess. In: Mishell DR Jr, Davajan V, Lobo RA, eds. *Infertility, Contraception and Reproductive Endocrinology*. 3rd ed. Cambridge, MA: Blackwell Scientific; 1991.
*DHEAS*, Dehydroepiandrosterone sulfate; *3α-diol-G*, 5α-androstane-3α,17β-diol glucuronide.

## CAUSES OF ANDROGEN EXCESS OR HYPERANDROGENISM

Although most causes will result in hirsutism, each of the diagnostic categories can lead to any of the manifestations of androgen excess: acne, hirsutism, or alopecia. One frequent causative factor of signs of androgen excess is the administration of androgenic medication. In addition to testosterone itself, various anabolic steroids, 19-norprogestogens, and danazol have androgenic effects. Thus a careful history of medication intake is important for all women with hirsutism.

Hirsutism or virilization can also be associated with some forms of abnormal gonadal development. With this cause, individuals have signs of external sexual ambiguity or primary amenorrhea, in addition to findings of androgen excess, and a Y chromosome is often present. These conditions are discussed further in Chapter 38.

Signs of androgen excess during pregnancy can be caused by increased ovarian testosterone production. This is usually caused by a luteoma of pregnancy or hyperreactio luteinalis. The former is a unilateral or bilateral solid ovarian enlargement; the latter is bilateral cystic ovarian enlargement. After pregnancy is completed, the excessive ovarian androgenic production resolves spontaneously and the androgenic signs regress.

A diagnosis of these three causes of androgen excess can usually easily be made by means of a careful history and physical examination. The remaining causes of androgen excess, together with the origin of hyperandrogenism, are listed in Table 40.5. Details of each of these causes will be described. Idiopathic hirsutism and PCOS are the most common disorders, together making up more than 90% of cases. PCOS is the most frequent disorder, and because of its overall prevalence and importance among reproductive women, it is covered in detail in a separate chapter.

### *IDIOPATHIC HIRSUTISM (PERIPHERAL DISORDER OF ANDROGEN METABOLISM)*

Idiopathic hirsutism is diagnosed when there are signs of hirsutism and regular menstrual cycles in conjunction with normal circulating levels of androgens (both testosterone and DHEAS). Because this type of disorder is frequently present in several individuals in

Table 40.5 Differential Diagnosis of Hirsutism and Virilization*

| Source | Diagnosis |
|---|---|
| Nonspecific | Exogenous, iatrogenic<br>Abnormal gonadal or sexual development |
| Pregnancy | Androgen excess in pregnancy, luteoma or hyperreactio luteinalis |
| Periphery | Idiopathic hirsutism |
| Ovary | Polycystic ovary syndrome†<br>Functional or idiopathic hyperandrogenism‡<br>Stromal hyperthecosis<br>Ovarian tumors |
| Adrenal gland | Adrenal tumors<br>Cushing syndrome<br>Adult-onset congenital adrenal hyperplasia |

*Idiopathic hirsutism and polycystic ovary syndrome do not present with virilization.
†The hyperandrogenism in PCOS can also be of adrenal origin, at least in part.
‡Functional hyperandrogenism may well be a type of PCOS, but without clearly defined polycystic ovaries on ultrasound, and can also have an adrenal source of hyperandrogenism.

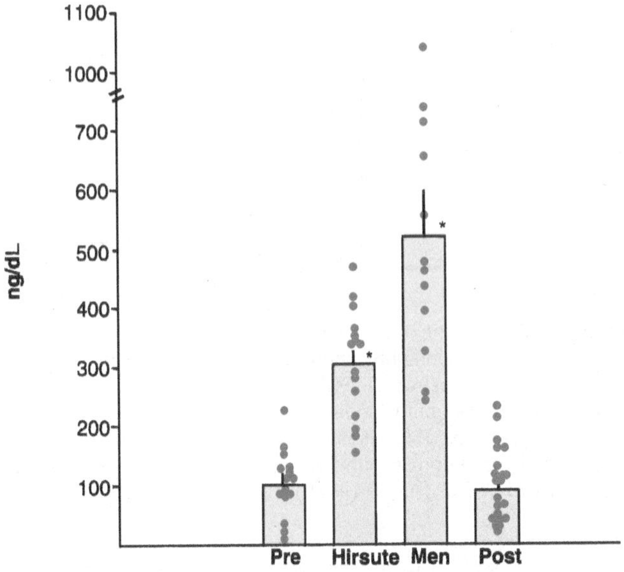


**Figure 40.6** Serum 3β-diol-G in premenopausal nonhirsute women (Pre), hirsute women, normal men, and postmenopausal nonhirsute women (Post). The *asterisks* denote $P < .05$, as compared with Pre. (From Paulson RJ, Serafini PC, Catalino JA, Lobo RA. Measurements of 3α,17β-androstanediol glucuronide in serum and urine and the correlation with skin 5α-reductase activity. *Fertil Steril.* 1986;46:222-226.)

the same family, particularly those of Mediterranean descent, it has also been called *familial*, or *constitutional, hirsutism*. Because neither ovarian nor adrenal androgen production is increased, the cause of the androgen excess has been called *idiopathic hirsutism.* Several studies have been done, where it has been documented that some women so diagnosed have subtle increases in androgen production and metabolism. However, the more important way to characterize this disorder, where androgens are normal or very slightly increased, is that there is an enhancement of androgen action in the PSU (i.e., an increased androgen sensitivity), which also has a familial predisposition. We have found that approximately 80% of these women have increased levels of 3α-diol-G, indirectly indicating that the cause of hirsutism is largely the result of increased 5α-reductase activity (Paulson, 1986) (Fig. 40.6). Also, we have directly measured the percentage conversion of testosterone to DHT in genital skin as an assessment of the 5α-RA level in the skin of women with idiopathic hirsutism. The amount of 5α-RA was increased in hirsute women as compared with normal women and correlated well with the degree of hirsutism and levels of serum 3α-diol-G (Serafini, 1985b). Thus idiopathic hirsutism is actually a disorder of the peripheral compartment and is possibly genetically determined, although it is also possible that early exposure to androgens can program increased 5α-RA. Antiandrogens that block peripheral testosterone action or interfere with 5α-RA are effective therapeutic agents for this disorder.

## POLYCYSTIC OVARY SYNDROME

Polycystic ovary syndrome (PCOS) is the most common disorder diagnosed in women presenting with symptoms and signs of androgen excess. A survey taken in 2012 suggested that it accounts for 71% of women presenting with hirsutism (Escobar-Morreale, 2012).

PCOS was originally described in 1935 by Stein and Leventhal as a syndrome consisting of amenorrhea, hirsutism, and obesity in association with enlarged polycystic ovaries (Stein, 1935). The classic definition of PCOS includes women who are anovulatory and have irregular periods as well as hyperandrogenism, as determined by signs such as hirsutism or elevated blood levels of androgens, testosterone, or DHEAS. The diagnosis should only be made in the absence of other known disorders, including enzymatic disorders (e.g., 21-hydroxylase deficiency), Cushing syndrome, or tumors (The Rotterdam ESHRE/ASRM-sponsored PCOS consensus workshop group, 2004; Azziz, 2006).

As will be discussed in Chapter 41, PCOS is also diagnosed in women with normal menstrual cycles, who are presumably ovulating, and in its widest spectrum of diagnostic categories is the most common reproductive disorder, occurring in 5% to 20% of all women of reproductive age (Fauser, 2012).

For the purposes of understanding the interaction of androgen excess and PCOS, it should be appreciated that the most important feature of PCOS is that it is a hyperandrogenic disorder (Azziz, 2006). Although the majority of women will have an ovarian source of hyperandrogenism (i.e., an elevation in testosterone), adrenal hyperandrogenism (elevations in DHEAS) may be found in up to 50% of women (Carmina, 1992). In some women with PCOS and signs of hyperandrogenism (acne, hirsutism, or alopecia), blood levels of androgens may be "normal." This most likely relates to the lack of sensitivity of current assays.

Because there are important aspects of PCOS that are prevalent (metabolic disease, fertility concerns, cancer risk, etc.) and because this disorder is extremely common in women of reproductive age, even though it may not be accurately diagnosed, a separate chapter (Chapter 41) is devoted to this discussion.

Serum testosterone levels usually range from 0.7 to 1.2 ng/mL, and androstenedione levels are usually from 3 to 5 ng/mL. In addition, approximately 50% of women with this syndrome have elevated levels of DHEAS, suggesting adrenal androgen involvement. However, in some countries, the prevalence of this putative adrenal involvement is lower. Evidence also exists for adrenal hyperactivity to stimulation in at least one third of women with PCOS. Because of the hyperandrogenic state, and the frequent hyperinsulinemia and overweight status in PCOS (discussed in Chapter 41), sex hormone binding globulin (SHBG)

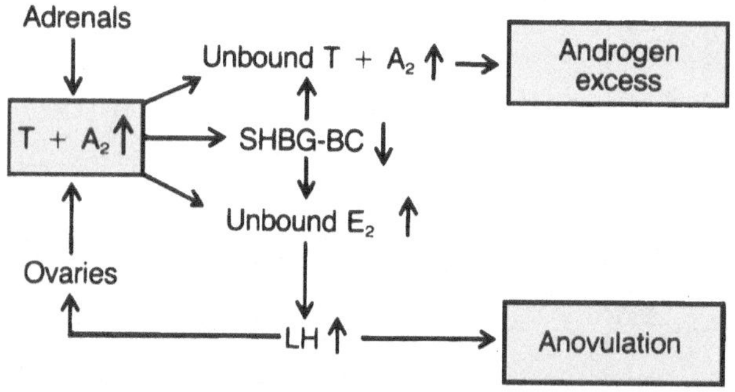


**Figure 40.7** Scheme depicting the possible role of adrenal-derived androgen in initiating androgen excess and anovulation. $A_2$, Androstanediol; $E_2$, estradiol; *LH,* luteinizing hormone; *SHBG-BC,* sex hormone-binding globulin binding capacity; *T,* testosterone. (From Lobo RA, Goebelsmann U. Effect of androgen excess on inappropriate gonadotropin secretion as found in polycystic ovary syndrome. *Am J Obstet Gynecol.* 1982;142:394-401.)

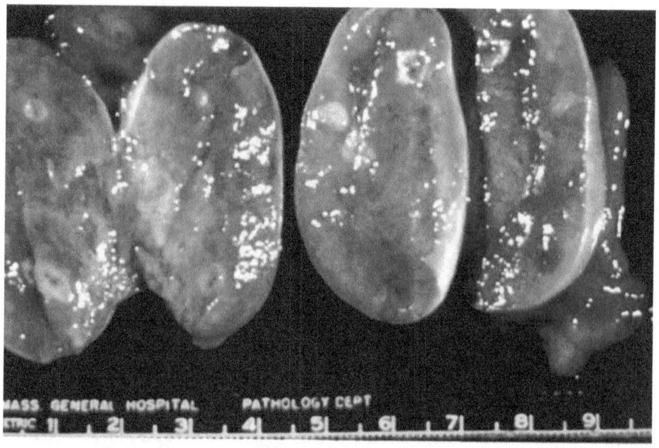


**Figure 40.8** Surgical specimen of ovarian stromal hyperthecosis. Note fleshy appearance, without cystic activity.

is decreased, leading to an increase in the unbound fraction of testosterone, thus heightening the androgenicity (Lobo, 1982) (Fig. 40.7). Although almost all women with PCOS have elevated levels of circulating androgens, the presence or absence of hirsutism depends on whether those androgens are converted peripherally by 5α-reductase to the more potent androgen DHT, as reflected by increased circulating levels of 3α-diol-G. Nonhirsute women with PCOS have elevated circulatory levels of testosterone, unbound testosterone, or DHEAS, but not 3α-diol-G (Lobo, 1983).

## FUNCTIONAL OR IDIOPATHIC HYPERANDROGENISM

This category is included because it may be found in other reviews in the literature and is more commonly diagnosed by European clinicians; it is considered to occur in up to 15% of women presenting with hirsutism (Escobar-Morreale, 2012). It is diagnosed when androgens are elevated (either ovarian or adrenal) and menstrual cycles are regular and ovulatory. There is also no evidence on ultrasound for polycystic ovaries, making this an "idiopathic" state. However, it is our view that this category is really a variant of PCOS, in which women may be ovulatory. Because ovarian morphology in women with PCOS is variable, this category may essentially be merged with PCOS.

## STROMAL HYPERTHECOSIS

**Stromal hyperthecosis** is an uncommon benign ovarian disorder in which the ovaries are typically bilaterally enlarged to approximately 5 to 7 cm in diameter. Histologically, there are nests of luteinized theca cells within the stroma (Fig. 40.8). The capsules of these ovaries are thick, similar to those found in PCOS but, unlike PCOS, subcapsular cysts are uncommon. The theca cells produce large amounts of testosterone, as determined by retrograde ovarian vein catheterization. The ultrasound picture of stromal hyperthecosis may be variable (Brown, 2009). Like PCOS, this disorder has a gradual onset and is initially associated with anovulation or amenorrhea and hirsutism. However, unlike PCOS, with increasing age the ovaries secrete steadily increasing amounts of testosterone. Thus when women with this disorder reach the fourth decade of life, the severity of the hirsutism increases and signs of **virilization**, such as temporal balding, clitoral enlargement, deepening of the voice, and decreased breast size, appear and gradually increase in severity. By this time, serum testosterone levels are usually higher than 2 ng/mL, similar to levels found in ovarian and adrenal testosterone-producing tumors. However, with the latter conditions, the symptoms of virilization appear and progress much more rapidly than with ovarian hyperthecosis, in which symptoms progress gradually over many years.

## ANDROGEN-PRODUCING TUMORS

Tumors are rare, occurring less than 1% of the time in women presenting with hyperandrogenism, but they represent the most important reason for evaluating women with androgen excess in order to rule out the diagnosis.

### Ovarian Neoplasms

It is possible for almost every type of ovarian neoplasm to have stromal cells that secrete excessive amounts of testosterone and cause signs of androgen excess. Thus on rare occasions, excess testosterone produced by benign and malignant cystadenomas, Brenner tumors, and Krukenberg tumors have caused hirsutism, virilization, or both. Certain germ cell tumors contain many testosterone-producing cells. The testosterone produced by two of these neoplasms, **Sertoli-Leydig cell tumors** and **hilus cell tumors**, almost always causes virilization. In addition, lipoid cell (adrenal rest) tumors can produce increased amounts of testosterone, DHEAS, or both. Rarely, granulosa/theca cell tumors can also produce testosterone in addition to increased levels of estradiol.

Androgen-producing ovarian tumors usually produce rapidly progressive signs of virilization. Sertoli-Leydig cell tumors usually develop during the reproductive years (second to fourth decades) and, by the time they produce detectable signs of androgen excess, the tumor is almost always (>85% of the time) palpable during bimanual examination. These tumors are uncommon. Less than 1% of solid ovarian neoplasms are Sertoli-Leydig cell tumors. Hilus cell tumors usually occur after menopause. They are usually small and not palpable during bimanual examination; however, the history of rapid development of signs of virilization and the presence of markedly elevated levels of testosterone (more than 2.5 times the upper limits of the normal range), with normal levels of DHEAS, usually facilitate the diagnosis.

### *Adrenal Tumors*

Almost all the androgen-producing adrenal tumors are adenomas or carcinomas that generate large amounts of the C19 steroids normally produced by the adrenal gland—DHEAS, DHEA, and androstenedione. Although these tumors do not usually secrete testosterone directly, testosterone is produced by extraglandular conversion of DHEA and androstenedione. Women with these tumors usually have markedly elevated serum levels of DHEAS (>8 μg/mL). Women with these laboratory findings and a history of rapid onset of signs of androgen excess should undergo a computed tomography (CT) scan or magnetic resonance imaging (MRI) of the adrenal glands to confirm the diagnosis. In addition to these uncommon tumors, a few testosterone-producing adrenal adenomas have been reported. The cellular patterns of these tumors resemble those of ovarian hilus cells, and the tumors secrete large amounts of testosterone. Because adrenal adenomas also secrete DHEAS, an adrenal adenoma is highly likely when DHEAS levels are greater than 8 μg/mL and testosterone levels are more than 1.5 ng/mL.

## *LATE-ONSET 21-HYDROXYLASE DEFICIENCY*

Congenital adrenal hyperplasia (CAH) is an inherited disorder caused by an enzymatic defect (usually 21-hydroxylase [21-OHase] or, less often, 11β-hydroxylase), resulting in decreased cortisol biosynthesis. As a consequence, adrenocorticotropic hormone (ACTH) secretion increases and adrenal cortisol precursors produced proximal to the enzymatic block accumulate. These are converted mainly to 17-hydroxyprogesterone and androstenedione, and androstenedione in turn is converted to testosterone, which produces signs of androgen excess. Late or adult onset CAH occurs in no more than 3% of women presenting with hirsutism (Escobar-Morreale, 2012).

Because the enzymatic defects are congenital, the classic severe form (complete block) usually becomes clinically apparent in fetal life by producing masculinization of the female external genitalia. The severe form of CAH is the most common cause of sexual ambiguity in the newborn. The more attenuated (mild) block of 21-hydroxylase activity usually does not produce the physical signs associated with increased androgen production until after puberty. Thus this condition, known as **late-onset 21-hydroxylase deficiency (LOHD)** or late-onset congenital adrenal hyperplasia (LOCAH), is associated with the development of signs of hyperandrogenism in a woman in the second or early third decade of life.

Although the incidence of classic CAH is only 1 in 14,500 live births worldwide, Speiser and coworkers, using histocompatibility locus antigen (HLA)-B genotyping of families with LOHD-affected individuals, have concluded that the incidence of LOHD varies among different ethnic groups but, overall, is probably the most frequent autosomal genetic disorder in humans. The incidence of LOCAH was estimated to be 0.1% in a diverse white population; in Yugoslavians, Hispanics, and Ashkenazi Jews, however, the incidence was 1.6%, 1.9%, and 3.7%, respectively (Speiser, 1985) (Fig. 40.9). Both classic CAH and LOCAH are transmitted in an autosomal recessive manner at the *CYP21B* locus and are linked to the HLA-B locus.

The molecular basis of the disease is complex. The gene for *CYP21* is located on 6p near the HLA complex. In proximity to this

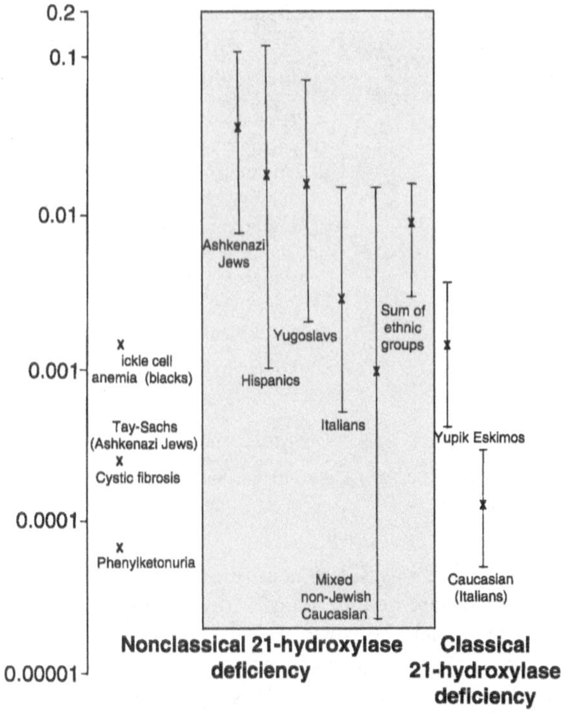


**Figure 40.9** Relative frequencies of Nonclassical 21-hydroxylase deficiency, classical 21-hydroxylase deficiency, and other autosomal recessive disorders. (From Speiser PW, Dupont B, Rubenstein P, et al. High frequency of nonclassical steroid 21-hydroxylase deficiency. *Am J Hum Genet.* 1985;37:650-657.)

gene is a nonfunctional or pseudogene *(CYP21P)*. Depending on the population, 20% to 25% of individuals with classic CAH have a deletion of the *CYP21* locus or a rearrangement between *CYP21* and *CYP21P*. Current molecular techniques of genotyping can pick up well over 95% of these abnormalities, with most cases being 1 of 10 common mutations. A spectrum of mutations results in the enzymatic defects and clinical presentations shown in Table 40.6.

LOCAH is a phenotype that is symptomatic after adolescence and does not define the genotype. Affected individuals may be homozygous for alleles, yielding mildly abnormal enzymatic activity, or compound heterozygotes with a combination of defective alleles. The so-called *cryptic 21-hydroxylase deficiency*, on the other hand, represents mild or asymptomatic individuals with biochemically identified defects that, with the advent of molecular diagnostic techniques, have been redefined as belonging to several different clinical presentations.

New and coworkers have proposed a schema for identifying and classifying the clinical spectrum of disease shown in Table 40.6. Because there are three possible manifestations of *CYP21Y* alleles (normal, mildly defective, or severely defective), there are six possible genotypes representing three clinical phenotypes (asymptomatic, LOCAH, and classic CAH). Individuals with LOCAH may be compound heterozygotes, with one mildly and one severely defective allele, or homozygous, with two mildly defective alleles. There is no perfect correlation between genotypes and phenotypes and—because the genetics are complex, with many possible abnormalities, particularly in diverse populations—it has been recommended that for clinical purposes, diagnosis and treatment of CAH should be based on

Table 40.6 Genotypic Characterization of the Forms of 21-Hydroxylase Deficiency

| Form of 21-Hydroxylase Deficiency | Clinical Phenotype | Hormonal Phenotype (in Response to ACTH) | Genotype |
|---|---|---|---|
| Classic (CAH) | Prenatal virilization, fully symptomatic | Marked elevation of precursors (serum 17-hydroxyprogesterone and $\Delta$-androstenedione) | 21-OH-def$^{severe}$ / 21-OH-def$^{severe}$ |
| Nonclassic (LOHD) | Symptomatic: later development of virilization; milder symptoms | Moderate elevation of precursors | 21-OH-def$^{severe}$ / 21-OH-def$^{mild}$ |
| | Asymptomatic: no virilization or other symptoms | | 21-OH-def$^{mild}$ / 21-OH-def$^{mild}$ |
| Carrier | Asymptomatic | Precursor level greater than normal | 21-OH-def$^{severe}$ / 21-OHase (normal) |
| | | | 21-OH-def$^{mild}$ / 21-OHase (normal) |
| Normal | Asymptomatic | Lowest levels—some overlap seen with carriers | 21-OHase (normal) / 21-OHase (normal) |

From New MI, White PC, Pang S, et al. The adrenal hyperplasias. In: Scriver CR, Beaudet AL, Sly S, Valle D, eds. *Metabolic Basis of Inherited Diseases*. 6th ed. New York: McGraw-Hill; 1989.

biochemical findings. Carriers can be identified among family members who are heterozygous, with one normal allele. They have normal basal 17-hydroxyprogesterone levels, a mild degree of hirsutism, if present, and smaller increases of 17-hydroxyprogesterone after ACTH stimulation, usually between 3.5 and 10 ng/mL. Molecular genotyping is primarily used for prenatal testing when there is a known severe mutation to determine the risk of having a severely affected child.

LOCAH is also usually associated with menstrual irregularity. It has been hypothesized that the mechanism for anovulation is similar to that which occurs with PCOS. The increased levels of androgen lower SHBG levels, thus increasing the amount of biologically active circulating estradiol. The increased estradiol stimulates tonic LH release, which increases ovarian androgen production and locally inhibits follicular growth and ovulation. Thus women with this disorder present with postpubertal onset of hirsutism and oligomenorrhea or amenorrhea, similar to women with PCOS. However, women with LOCAH, unlike those with PCOS, commonly have a history of prepubertal accelerated growth (at 6 to 8 years of age), with later decreased growth and a short ultimate height. A history of this growth pattern, a family history of postpubertal onset of hirsutism, and findings of mild virilization are indicators of the presence of CAH.

To differentiate LOCAH from PCOS, measurement of basal (early morning) serum 17-hydroxyprogesterone levels should be performed. If basal levels are greater than 8 ng/mL, the diagnosis of LOCAH is established. If 17-hydroxyprogesterone is above normal (2.5 to 3.3 ng/mL) but less than 8 ng/mL, an ACTH stimulation test should be performed. A baseline 17-hydroxyprogesterone level should be measured and 0.25 mg of synthetic ACTH infused as a single bolus. One hour later, another serum sample of 17-hydroxyprogesterone should be measured. If the level increases more than 10 ng/mL, the diagnosis of LOCAH is established (Baskin, 1987) (Fig. 40.10).

Corticosteroid treatment is normally reserved for patients wishing to conceive to restore ovulatory function. In other women, treatment is more efficient and safer using oral contraception (OC) pills, as in PCOS and other functional states described later.

It is important to measure 11-desoxycortisol during the ACTH stimulation when the diagnosis is being evaluated, because of the possibility of 11-hydroxylase deficiency. This

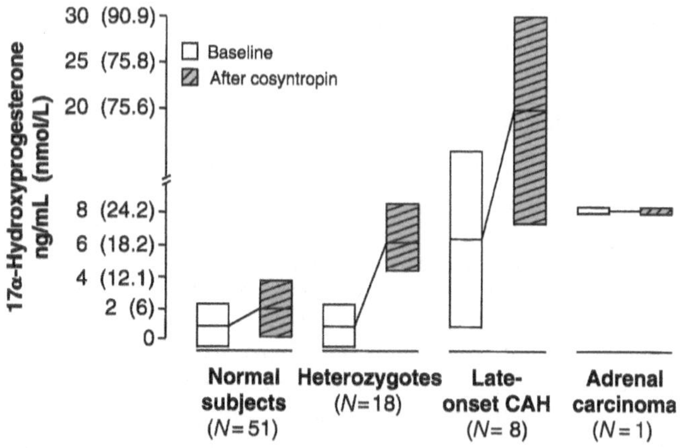


**Figure 40.10** Means and ranges of 17α-hydroxyprogesterone levels before and after cosyntropin administered intramuscularly in normal subjects, suspected heterozygotes, patients with late-onset congenital adrenal hyperplasia (CAH), and one patient with adrenal carcinoma. (From Baskin HJ. Screening for late-onset congenital adrenal hyperplasia in hirsutism or amenorrhea. *Arch Intern Med*. 1987;147:847-848.)

disorder is much more rare, but it also has an incomplete, adult form and may also be associated with hypertension. Women with this incomplete form also have increases in 17-hydroxyprogesterone and thus require the measurement of 11-desoxycortisol to differentiate it from 21-hydroxylase deficiency.

## *CUSHING SYNDROME*

Excessive adrenal production of glucocorticoids caused by increased ACTH secretion (Cushing disease) or adrenal tumors produces the signs and symptoms of Cushing syndrome. These findings include hirsutism and menstrual irregularity in addition to the classic findings of central obesity, dorsal neck fat pads, abdominal striae, and muscle wasting and weakness. The latter catabolic effect of glucocorticoid excess differs from the anabolic effects of testosterone excess, but some women with PCOS may have other clinical findings similar to those found with Cushing syndrome. Women with Cushing syndrome are more likely to present with other symptoms and signs of glucocorticoid excess, rather than because of hirsutism; but this has been found to occur in fewer than1% of cases.

Cushing syndrome can be easily excluded by performing an overnight dexamethasone suppression test. To perform this test, 1 mg of dexamethasone is ingested at 11 PM, and the plasma cortisol level is measured the following morning, at 8 AM. If the cortisol level is less than 5 μg/100 mL, Cushing syndrome is ruled out. If the cortisol level fails to suppress to this degree, the diagnosis of Cushing syndrome is not established. It is necessary to perform a complete dexamethasone suppression test (Liddle test) or measure the urinary free cortisol and plasma ACTH levels to determine whether Cushing syndrome exists.

Depression and other conditions can cause failure to suppress with the dexamethasone screening test just described. Accordingly, many endocrinologists prefer to depend on measurement of the 24-hour urinary free cortisol level or salivary cortisol. A creatinine level is also measured to gauge completeness of urine collection. Values above 100 μg/24 hours in urine are abnormal, and values greater than 240 μg are almost diagnostic of Cushing syndrome. Late night salivary cortisol is now considered to be the most accurate method. Samples are usually obtained on two separate nights; values above 0.4 μg/dL are diagnostic for Cushing syndrome (Sakihara, 2010).

Cushing syndrome may result from a pituitary tumor producing ACTH (Cushing disease), an ectopic tumor in the body, adrenal neoplasms, or hyperplasia. Various algorithms have been developed for this differential diagnosis.

## DIFFERENTIAL DIAGNOSIS

Women with androgen excess/hyperandrogenism will present with acne, hirsutism or alopecia, and some women will have more than one of these three complaints. All women with these complaints should have a careful history encompassing a physical exam, laboratory assessment of circulating androgens, and often some sort of imaging.

Measurements of total testosterone, free (unbound) testosterone, or the free androgen index have all been advocated to assist in the diagnosis of hyperandrogenism. In a clinical setting, commercial assays for testosterone are insensitive and cannot discriminate reliably between normal and abnormal values, unless values are very high (tumor or male range). Several organizations are addressing this factor, including the Endocrine Society, Centers for Disease Control and Prevention (CDC), Androgen Excess and PCOS Society (AE-PCOS) Society, American Society for Reproductive Medicine (ASRM), and American Congress of Obstetricians and Gynecologists (ACOG), and accurate assays will be soon been standardized (Rosner, 2010). Increasingly laboratories are using a chromatography/mass spectrometry analysis, and clinicians should make themselves familiar with the particular lab assays they use, and their normal ranges. Although the free androgen index or non–SHBG-bound testosterone level is a better discriminator of hyperandrogenism than total testosterone, an accurate measurement of total testosterone may be all that is necessary. It is not clinically important whether a hirsute woman has a total testosterone level in the highest portion of the normal range or a mildly elevated level of non–SHBG-bound testosterone. Thus to determine the magnitude of elevated androgens, as well as their source, measurement of total testosterone is more cost effective than the other assays and provides the clinician with the information necessary to establish the diagnosis. *To summarize, the laboratory workup should include an accurate measure of testosterone (unbound testosterone or the free androgen index [testosterone/SHBG is optional]), DHEAS, and 17 hydroxyprogesterone when LOCAH is suspected (younger individuals, family history of androgen excess, and in high prevalent ethnic groups).*

As noted, androgen excess caused by iatrogenic causes, sexual ambiguity, or pregnancy-associated ovarian tumors can usually be easily determined by the history and physical examination. Masculinizing ovarian or adrenal tumors are associated with rapidly progressive signs of hirsutism and virilization. Serum testosterone levels higher than 2 ng/mL, with normal DHEAS levels, indicate the probable presence of an ovarian tumor. The diagnosis can be confirmed by bimanual pelvic examination and ultrasonography, CT, or MRI. Women with a rapid progression of virilization and DHEAS levels greater than 8 μg/mL most likely have an androgen-producing adrenal adenoma; CT or MRI can confirm the diagnosis. A long history of gradually increasing hirsutism, even if accompanied by virilization, is not consistent with the diagnosis of adrenal or ovarian tumors. The diagnosis of ovarian stromal hyperthecosis should be suspected for women with these signs and testosterone levels greater than 1.5 ng/mL. Women with physical findings consistent with Cushing syndrome should have the diagnosis ruled out. PCOS, LOHD, and idiopathic hirsutism or those women diagnosed with functional hyperandrogenism may be associated with a similar history and findings at physical examination. Women with LOHD commonly have a family history of androgen excess and often belong to an ethnic group with a higher gene frequency for an abnormality. The diagnosis of LOHD is established by measurement of 17-hydroxyprogesterone, either by testing of an early morning serum sample or following ACTH stimulation.

Apart from tumors (requiring surgery), LOCAH, and Cushing syndrome (all of these being relatively rare disorders), the other disorders causing the androgen excess are functional disorders, in which the treatment is the same as discussed later. Women presenting with only acne or alopecia should still be evaluated as described previously, but each disorder will be discussed separately as well because of some of their unique features.

## TREATMENT OF ANDROGEN EXCESS/ HYPERANDROGENISM

The success of treatment of hyperandrogenic disorders requires patience and persistence. The nature of the PSU and the hair cycle requires a longer time for improvement to be witnessed. In general, among the disorders, the most successful disorder to treat is acne with approximately 90% of women showing benefit; this is followed by hirsutism with an approximate 70% response rate, and finally alopecia, which only has a 30% response rate.

### SPECIFIC DISORDERS

#### Ovarian and Adrenal Tumors

Tumors are best identified by high-grade imaging techniques. In the past, selective vein catheterization has been used, but this is seldom necessary today. Suppression/stimulation tests have not been beneficial because many tumors are LH responsive and androgens will be suppressed somewhat with oral contraceptives or GnRH agonists.

Almost all Sertoli-Leydig cell tumors are unilateral. If the woman has not completed her family and these tumors are well differentiated and confined to one ovary, the tumors may be treated by unilateral salpingo-oophorectomy. Because most hilus cell tumors occur after menopause, they are best treated by bilateral salpingo-oophorectomy and total abdominal hysterectomy. Adrenal adenomas and carcinomas should also be treated by operative removal. Adrenal carcinomas frequently have metastasized to the liver by the time the androgenic signs have developed. Despite chemotherapy, the prognosis is poor after metastases have occurred. Stromal hyperthecosis is also best treated by bilateral salpingo-oophorectomy. After removal of the ovaries of women with stromal hyperthecosis or any of the androgen-producing tumors, the acne and oiliness of the skin disappear, breast size increases, and clitoral size decreases. The excess central hair becomes finer and grows less rapidly but does not disappear. Electrolysis or laser treatment can remove the body hair more effectively once the source of PSU stimulation has been removed.

### *Late-Onset 21-Hydroxylase Deficiency (Congenital Adrenal Hyperplasia)*

The treatment of women with LOCAH depends on their primary complaint. The androgen excess and menstrual irregularity can be treated as in women with PCOS, usually with an oral contraceptive. However, if women wish to conceive, it is preferable to use glucocorticoids such as hydrocortisone (15 to 20 mg), prednisone (5 to 7.5 mg), or dexamethasone (0.5 to 0.75 mg) in divided doses. Doses as low as 2.5 mg of prednisone or 0.25 mg dexamethasone may be used initially. The aim of treatment is to suppress androstenedione and bring 17-hydroxyprogesterone and progesterone levels into the normal range. Ovulation usually resumes rapidly.

### *Polycystic Ovary Syndrome*

As is discussed in Chapter 41, because of the metabolic and other concerns in women with PCOS, lifestyle management has an important role in any treatment plan. It has been established that lifestyle measures and weight loss will assist in the treatment of hyperandrogenism in PCOS (Moran, 2011).

#### Treatment of Skin Manifestations of Androgen Excess

Although ovarian or adrenal androgen excess increases the likelihood of these complaints, enhancement of these effects because of increased 5α-reductase activity largely explains the abnormalities. Thus a successful strategy usually requires an antiandrogen added to suppression therapy, usually with an OC. Although it is reasonable to begin with monotherapy (OC), particularly if the disorder is relatively mild, in women with more significant complaints and findings, an antiandrogen can be used initially. It is important to use antiandrogens in conjunction with an OC because of the concerns of exposure during pregnancy.

In women who have "idiopathic" hirsutism and very mild and localized complaints, it is also reasonable not to use medical therapy and to use hair removal alone, as described later.

**Oral Contraceptive Steroids**

Oral contraceptive steroids (usually prescribed orally, but the effect would be similar with transdermal or vaginal preparations) suppress ovarian androgens by inhibiting LH stimulation of the ovary. They also decrease adrenal androgens (DHEAS) by about 30% (Klove, 1984); and inhibit 5α-reductase activity (Cassidenti, 1991). In addition, the potency of ethinyl estradiol in contraceptives increases SHBG, which results in lower free or unbound testosterone.

Among the various preparations, it would seem logical to use a less androgenic progestogen (norgestimate, desogestrel, drospirenone) than more potent ones (levonorgestrel). However, there are no randomized trial data to support this assertion. There are some data to support the superiority of cyproterone acetate (CPA), which has significant antiandrogen activity, but CPA is not available in the United States. Randomized data have shown, however, that there is no difference in efficacy in using a 20 μg or 30/35 μg preparation (Zimmerman, 2014) and therefore lower estrogen dose contraceptives should be used. Some evidence has suggested that the newer progestogens, which are less androgenic, as well as CPA, may increase the risk of thrombosis, compared to contraceptives containing levonorgestrel or norethindrone. If true, this effect is relatively small, and the absolute risk of thrombosis in young women is small and less than that of normal pregnancy. It is important, however, to use lower-dose estrogen products (20 μg). Also obesity is an additional risk factor for thrombosis, and thus lifestyle management is important, particularly in women with PCOS, who may be at greater risk for thrombosis.

**Antiandrogens**

Peripheral androgen blockade with antiandrogens is dose related. Receptor blockade with **spironolactone** and **flutamide** and a specific 5α-2 inhibitor, **finasteride**, are the agents most commonly used. Cyproterone acetate (2 mg), which is a progestogen is most frequently used in combination with ethinyl estradiol as an OC, although larger doses have been used as well. Drospirenone in the doses used in contraceptives (3 mg) does not have appreciable antiandrogenic activity.

Spironolactone has been used and studied extensively and should be considered the treatment of choice in the United States for women with idiopathic hirsutism, as well as many with PCOS (Lobo, 1985; Swiglo, 2008; Martin, 2008). In addition to being an androgen receptor blocker, it also decreases ovarian testosterone production and inhibits 5α-RA. Various dosages, from 50 to 200 mg daily, have been used. We have found that a dose of 200 mg/day of spironolactone is more effective than 100 mg/day (Lobo, 1985). Barth and associates have found a clinically evident response of decreased hair after 3 months of spironolactone, 200 mg/day (Barth, 1989). After 1 year of treatment, a 15% to 25% reduction was seen in hair shaft diameter and linear growth rate at all body sites. With the higher dose of spironolactone, liver function test results and plasma electrolyte levels are usually unchanged, and side effects occur infrequently, except for irregular uterine bleeding. The latter can be controlled with concomitant use of OCs. Electrolytes and blood pressure should be monitored for the first few weeks of therapy to ensure that hypotension and hyperkalemia do not occur.

Flutamide is a pure androgen blocker that has shown efficacy in the treatment of hirsutism. There is a dose-response relationship (250 to 750 mg/day), and even lower doses have some efficacy (Cusan, 1994; Inal, 2005). However, the major concern is hepatic toxicity (Bruni, 2012). which may lead to death. Most guidelines have advised against the use of flutamide for this reason (Martin, 2008). and if it is used it should be used with caution at lower doses and with close monitoring of hepatic function. As with other antiandrogens, contraception should be used.

Finasteride, a 5α-reductase inhibitor (5 mg/day), is an effective treatment for hirsutism, and 5 mg has similar efficacy as 100 mg of spironolactone (Wong, 1995; Bayram, 2002). Because finasteride is a specific 5α-2 inhibitor (there are two isoenzymes for 5α reductase: 1 and 2) and hirsutism is likely a combination of both types 1 and 2, a better inhibitor may be preferable, but it is unavailable at present. Finasteride is used currently as a second-line treatment when there are side effects or problems with using spironolactone.

**Other Agents for Treatment**

In severe cases, use of a **GnRH agonist** with estrogen or an OC add-back has been shown to be successful (Andreyko, 1986; Bayhan, 2000). However, this is expensive and cannot be used for long-term therapy. It has been used in women with high levels of circulating androgens.

**Ketoconazole**, which blocks adrenal and gonadal steroidogenesis by inhibiting cytochrome P450–dependent enzyme pathways, has been used in dosages of 200 mg, twice daily, to treat hyperandrogenism associated with PCOS and idiopathic hirsutism. This potent drug effectively decreases hair growth and acne, but major side effects and complications (including hepatitis) occur in most women so treated. These problems limit the use of ketoconazole to select women, who require careful monitoring. In these severe cases, it is probably preferable to use a GnRH agonist.

**Glucocorticoids** have been used for the treatment of androgen excess for many years. Although it is logical to suppress the adrenal gland in women who have adrenal androgen excess, and low doses have been used with some degree of success, the benefit is relatively modest (Carmina, 1998) compared with other agents such as antiandrogens. Because of its potential for serious side effects, glucocorticoids are not recommended for treating androgen excess but may be considered as an adjunct to ovulation induction in some women.

**Insulin sensitizers** have been proposed as agents to treat androgen excess and have been used in women with PCOS. Although some agents have shown some minor beneficial effects, they are not recommended as a primary therapy for manifestations of androgen excess (Cosma, 2008).

**Eflornithine cream 13.9%** is a topical treatment that has been approved by the U.S. Food and Drug Administration (FDA) for facial hirsutism. Eflornithine is an inhibitor of ornithine decarboxylase, which is an enzyme necessary for the growth and development of the hair follicle. It was originally developed for the treatment of trypanosomal sleeping sickness. It is approved only for facial hirsutism and its mechanism is such that it affects all hair follicles and is not specific for hirsutism; it has been used for older women with nonterminal hair growth (Wolf, 2007). Its application twice a day results in a modest improvement in about 8 weeks. Thus for isolated facial hirsutism it may have an adjunctive role in that it can hasten the overall response, which takes much longer with traditional suppressive therapy. Side effects are minimal and include some local irritation; it is also expensive.

**Follow-up for Treatment of Hirsutism**

Because of the length of the hair growth cycle, responses to treatment should not be expected to occur within the first 3 months of therapy, and it usually takes about 6 months to see a response. Objective methods of assessing changes of hair growth, such as photographs, are useful. With the use of various therapies, a successful response for hirsutism should occur in approximately 70% of women within 1 year of therapy. Remaining excess hair can be removed by electrolysis or laser techniques. Treatment should be continued for 3 years and then stopped to determine whether hirsutism recurs. If so, therapy can be reinitiated.

**Hair Removal Techniques**

These cosmetic measures can be used as a primary treatment for mild isolated hirsutism or should be initiated after adequate suppressive therapy to remove unwanted hair once the growth rate has been inhibited by therapy.

Many depilatory methods have been used, but more definitive therapies are available such as the use of electrolysis and lasers, although these therapies may be expensive.

**Electrolysis** uses electrical energy through a wire electrode. Destruction of hair follicles results in its permanent removal. A "blended" technique has been thought to be more effective (Richards, 1995) although electrolysis is somewhat painful and can only be used for small areas at a given time.

**Photoepilation** uses lasers that apply heat to pigmented hair follicles. There are four types of lasers: Nd:Yag, diode, alexandrite, and ruby, and a meta-analysis suggested superiority of the diode laser (Sadighha, 2009). In general, long wavelength, long pulse duration lasers such as the Nd:Yag or diode are recommended for pigmented darker hair. For women with light or blond hair, electrolysis is recommended (Harris, 2014).

**Acne**

Acne vulgaris is considered to be a manifestation of androgen excess, although it need not be, and particularly in adolescents it merely reflects the physiologic responses of the PSU to the changing hormonal status and alterations in the bacteriologic flora. In general, however, androgens stimulate sebum production, and high doses of estrogen can inhibit it. There are many scoring systems for acne vulgaris, and the most common is the method presented by Cook, although it is primarily used for research purposes (Cook, 1979). Among hyperandrogenic disorders, acne vulgaris is the disorder that is most successfully treated, with response rates of close to 90%.

Among women who present with acne, 52% can be found to have androgen excess, with increases in unbound testosterone being the most frequently encountered (Lucky, 1983). Thus in women who present with significant acne, particularly if they have not responded to routine dermatologic measures, an evaluation of androgen excess is warranted. An enhancement of 5α-reductase, mostly type 1, is a large part of the androgen abnormalities in acne (Carmina, 1991).

Treatment is usually with combination oral contraceptives (Arowojola, 2012), which is at least as effective as chronic antibiotic therapy (Koo, 2014). Among oral contraceptives, less androgenic progestogens have been preferred (Jaisamrarn, 2014), although there is limited evidence for superiority over androgenic progestogens (Kelly, 2010). The estrogen component of the contraceptive pill is particularly important for inhibiting sebum production, although it usually does not require increasing ethynyl estradiol above the 35 μg dose. Although most antiandrogenic agents are effective (Fig. 40.11), oral contraceptives and pure antiandrogens are superior to finasteride (Carmina, 2002a). If oral contraceptives alone are not completely successful, as with hirsutism, the addition of antiandrogens are beneficial (Carmina, 2002b; Zouboulis, 2010).

**Alopecia**

Alopecia in women is a major source of stress and fear. Previously called androgenic alopecia, the preferred term currently is **female pattern hair loss (FPHL)**. This may or may not be associated with androgen excess. Hair loss is usually on the frontal scalp and vertex, with relative sparing of the occipital scalp. It is important to rule out dermatologic diseases such as alopecia areata and specific scalp dermatologic diseases. Absent this, although it is important to rule out androgen excess, with hormonal evaluation as suggested previously, the prevalence of

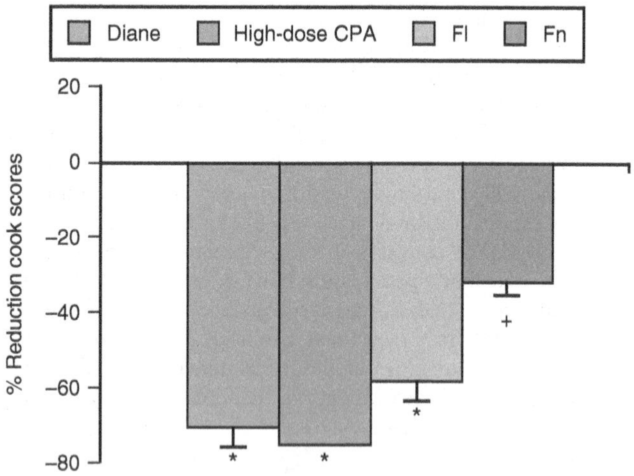


**Figure 40.11** Percentage reduction in Cook scores after 1 year of treatment with either Diane (contraceptive pill with CPA/EE2), high-dose CPA, flutamide 250 mg/day, finasteride 5 mg/day. The asterisk signifies reduction at $P < .01$; the cross at $P < .05$. (Modified from Carmina E, Lobo RA. A comparison of the relative efficacy of antiandrogens for the treatment of acne in hyperandrogenic women. *Clin Endocrinol [Oxf]*. 2002;57[2]:231-234.)

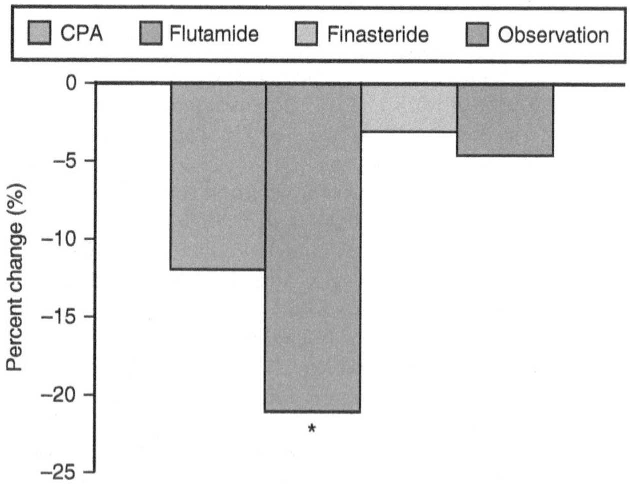


**Figure 40.12** Percentage decrease in Ludwig scores in four groups of women with hyperandrogenic alopecia. Only flutamide (−21%) showed a significant decrease in scores, $P < .05$. (Modified from Carmina E, Lobo RA. Treatment of hyperandrogenic alopecia in women. *Fertil Steril*. 2003;79[1]:91-95.)

androgen abnormalities is low, with elevations occurring in only 39% of women (Futterweit, 1988). Androgen excess, perhaps estrogen abnormalities, and genetics play into the etiology. With androgen excess, exaggerated 5α-reductase activity has been implicated in women with alopecia (Legro, 1994). There are several scoring systems for FHPL, with the method presented by Ludwig being the most commonly used, but mainly for research purposes (Ludwig, 1977).

Antiandrogen therapy is the mainstay of treatment. In women, spironolactone and flutamide (to be used with caution) have efficacy (Carmina, 2003) and of importance, finasteride, which is used widely in men, is not effective in women (Price, 2000; Carmina, 2003) (Fig. 40.12). Many dermatologists advocate local injections and applications of various products to the scalp, but there are few data to support this strategy. Minoxidil is also used to stimulate hair growth with limited effectiveness. In general the response rate to all treatments does not exceed 30%. Ultimately genetic manipulations and stem cell therapy may prove to be beneficial.

## KEY POINTS

- The major androgen produced by the ovaries is testosterone and that of the adrenal glands is DHEAS.
- There are three markers of androgen production, one for each compartment in which androgens are produced. In the ovary, it is testosterone; in the adrenal gland, DHEAS; and in the periphery, 3α-diol-G.
- Approximately 85% of testosterone is bound to SHBG and is biologically inactive, 10% to 15% is bound to albumin, and 1% to 2% is unbound. Both of the latter fractions are biologically active.
- Commercial assays for testosterone and unbound testosterone in women may be inaccurate; more detailed assays should be requested, and unbound testosterone is best assessed by the ratio of testosterone and SHBG.
- Women with idiopathic hirsutism have increased 5α-RA.
- There are three criteria to diagnose PCOS; the diagnosis is based on clinical criteria, not laboratory values.
- The most frequently used diagnostic criteria for PCOS (called the *Rotterdam criteria*) require finding any two of the following: menstrual irregularity, hyperandrogenism, or polycystic ovaries on ultrasound.
- Women with ovarian neoplasms have testosterone levels more than 2.5 times the upper limits of the normal range.
- The diagnosis of LOHD is established if the basal (early morning) serum 17-hydroxyprogesterone levels are greater than 2 to 3 ng/mL or if the level 1 hour after infusion of 0.25 µg ACTH is more than 10 ng/mL.
- Women with LOHD have a block in cortisol biosynthesis of 11β-hydroxylase or 21-hydroxylase, resulting in increased circulating levels of 17-hydroxyprogesterone.
- Because of the length of the hair growth cycle, response should not be expected until after 3 months of therapy.
- The best treatment for hirsutism is with an oral contraceptive, often together with an antiandrogen, with spironolactone being the preferred agent. Response rates are approximately 70%.
- Acne vulgaris is often a manifestation of androgen excess and may be effectively treated with oral contraceptives and sometimes with the addition of an antiandrogen. The response rate is approximately 90%.
- Female pattern hair loss (androgenic alopecia) may be due to enhanced scalp androgen action (5α-reductase activity). It is best treated with antiandrogen therapy, but the response rate is poor at ~30%.
- Excessive hair removal should be carried out once excessive androgen action (if present) has been suppressed. Laser treatment is more effective than electrolysis, although the latter is preferred for light-colored hair.

## KEY REFERENCES


Andreyko JL, Monroe SE, Jaffe RB. Treatment of hirsutism with a gonadotropin-releasing hormone agonist (nafarelin). *J Cin Endocrinol Metab.* 1986;63:854-859.

Arowojola AD, Gallo MF, Lopez LM, et al. Combined oral contraceptive pills for treatment of acne. *Cochrane Database Syst Rev.* 2012. CD004425.

Azziz R, Carmina E, Dewailly D, et al. Position statement: criteria for defining polycystic ovary syndrome as a predominantly hyperandrogenic syndrome: an Androgen Excess Society guideline. *J Clin Endocrinol Metab.* 2006;91:4237-4245.

Barth JH, Cherry CA, Wojnarowska F, et al. Spironolactone is an effective and well-tolerated systematic antiandrogen therapy for hirsute women. *J Clin Endocrinol Metab.* 1989;68:966-970.

Baskin HJ. Screening for late onset congenital adrenal hyperplasia in hirsutism or amenorrhea. *Arch Intern Med.* 1987;147:847-848.

Bayhan G, Bahceci M, Demirkol, et al. A comparative study of a gonadotropin releasing hormone agonist and finasteride on idiopathic hirsutism. *Clin Exp Obstet Gynecol.* 2000;27:203-206.

Bayram F, Muderris II , Guven M, et al. Comparison of high-dose finasteride (5 mg/day) versus low-dose finasteride (2.5 mg/day) in the treatment of hirsutism. *Eur J Endocrinol.* 2002;147:467-471.

Brown DL, Henrichsen TL, Clayton AC, et al. Ovarian stromal hyperthecosis: sonographic features and histologic associations. *J Ultrasound Med.* 2009;28(5):587-593.

Bruni V, Peruzzi E, Dei, et al. Hepatotoxicity with low and ultralow dose flutamide: a surveillance study on 203 hyperandrogenic young females. *Fertil Steril.* 2012;98:1047-1052.

Carmina E, Godwin AJ, Stanczyk FZ, et al. The association of serum androsterone glucuronide with inflammatory lesions in women with adult acne. *J Endocrinol Invest.* 2002b;25(9):765-768.

Carmina E, Koyama T, Chang L, et al. Does ethnicity influence the prevalence of adrenal hyperandrogenism and insulin resistance in polycystic ovary syndrome? *Am J Obstet Gynecol.* 1992;167:1807-1812.

Carmina E, Lobo RA. Peripheral androgen blockade versus glandular androgen suppression in the treatment of hirsutism. *Obstet Gynecol.* 1991;78:845-849.

Carmina E, Lobo RA. The addition of dexamethasone to antiandrogen therapy for hirsutism prolongs the duration of remission. *Fertil Steril.* 1998;69: 1975-1979.

Carmina E, Lobo RA. A comparison of the relative efficacy of antiandrogens for the treatment of acne in hyperandrogenic women. *Clin Endocrinology.* 2002a;57:231-234.

Carmina E, Lobo RA. Treatment of hyperandrogenic alopecia in women. *Fertil Steril.* 2003;79(1):91-94.

Cassidenti DL, Paulson RJ, Serafini P, et al. Effects of sex steroids on skin 5α-reductase activity in vitro. *Obstet Gynecol.* 1991;78:103-107.

Cook CH, Centner RL, Michaels SE. An acne grading method using photographic standards. *Arch Dermatol.* 1979;115(5):571-575.

Cosma M, Swiglo BA, Flynn DN, et al. Insulin sensitizers for the treatment of hirsutism: a systematic review and meta-analyses of randomized controlled trials. *J Clin Endocrinol Metab.* 2008;93(4):1135-1142.

Cusan L, Dupont A, Gomez JL, et al. Comparison of flutamide and spironolactone in the treatment of hirsutism: a randomized controlled trial. (see comment). *Fertil Steril.* 1994;61:281-287.

Ebling FJ. The hair cycle and its regulation. *Clin Dermatol.* 1988;6:67-73.

Escobar-Morreale HF, Carmina E, Dewailly D, et al. Epidemiology, diagnosis and management of hirsutism: a consensus statement by the Androgen Excess and Polycystic Ovary Syndrome Society. *Hum Reprod Update.* 2012;18(2):146-170.

Fauser BC, Tarlatzis BC, Rebar RW, et al. Consensus on women's health aspects of polycystic ovary syndrome (PCOS): the Amsterdam ESHRE/ASRM-Sponsored 3rd PCOS Consensus Workshop Group. *Fertil Steril.* 2012;97(1):28-38.

Ferriman D, Gallwey JD. Clinical assessment of body hair growth in women. *J Clin Endocrinol Metab.* 1961;21:1440-1447.

Futterweit W, Dunaif A, Yeh HC, et al. The prevalence of hyperandrogenism in 109 consecutive female patients with diffuse alopecia. *J Am Acad Dermatol.* 1988;19:831-836.

Harris K, Ferguson J, Hills S. A comparative study of hair removal at an NHS hospital: luminette intense pulsed light versus electrolysis. *J Dermatolog Treat.* 2014;25(2):169-173.

Hatch R, Rosenfield RL, Kim MH, et al. Hirsutism: implications, etiology, and management. *Am J Obstet Gynecol.* 1981;140:815-830.

Inal MM, Yildirim Y, Taner CE. Comparison of the clinical efficacy of flutamide and spironolactone plus Diane 35 in the treatment of idiopathic hirsutism: a randomized controlled study. *Fertil Steril.* 2005;84:1693-1697.

Jaisamrarn U, Chaovisitsaree S, Angsuwathana S, et al. A comparison of multiphasic oral contraceptives containing norgestimate or desogestrel in acne treatment: a randomized trial. *Contraception.* 2014;90(5):535-541.

S Davies E, Fearns S, et al. Effects of oral contraceptives containing ethinylestradiol with either drospirenone or levonorgestrel on various parameters associated with well-being in healthy women: a randomized, single-blind, parallel-group, multicentre study. *Clin Drug Investig.* 2010;30: 325-336.

Klove KL, Roy S, Lobo RA. The effect of different contraceptive treatments on the serum concentration of dehydroepiandrosterone sulfate. *Contraception.* 1984;29:319-324.

Koo EB, Petersen TD, Kimball AB. Meta-analysis comparing efficacy of antibiotics versus oral contraceptives in acne vulgaris. *J Am Acad Dermatology.* 2014;71(3):450-459.

Legro RS, Carmina E, Stanczyk FZ, et al. Alterations in androgen conjugate levels in women and men with alopecia. *Fertil Steril.* 1994;62:744-750.

Lobo RA, Goebelsmann U. Effect of androgen excess on inappropriate gonadotropin secretion as found in the polycystic ovary syndrome. *Am J Obstet Gynecol.* 1982;142:394-401.

Lobo RA, Goebelsmann U, Horton R. Evidence for the importance of peripheral tissue events in the development of hirsutism in polycystic ovary syndrome. *J Clin Endocrinol Metab.* 1983;57:393-397.

Lobo RA, Shoupe D, Serafini P, et al. The effects of two doses of spironolactone on serum androgens and anagen hair in hirsute women. *Fertil Steril.* 1985;43:200-205.

Lucky AW, McGuire J, Rosenfield RL, et al. Plasma androgens in women with acne vulgaris. *J Invest Dermatol.* 1983;81(1):70-74.

Ludwig E. Classification of the types of androgenic alopecia (common baldness occurring in the female sex). *Br J Dermatol.* 1977;97:247-254.

Martin KA, Chang RJ, Ehrmann DA, et al. Evaluation and treatment of hirsutism in premenopausal women: An Endocrine Society Clinical Practice Guideline. *J Clin Endocrinol Metab.* 2008;93:1105-1120.

Moran LJ, Hutchison SK, Norman RJ, et al. Lifestyle changes in women with polycystic ovary syndrome. *Cochrane Database Syst Rev.* 2011;(7). CD007506.

Paulson RJ, Serafini PC, Catalino JA, et al. Measurements of 3α, 17β- androstanediol glucuronide in serum and urine and the correlation with skin 5α-reductase activity. *Fertil Steril.* 1986;46:222-226.

Price VH, Roberts JL, Hordinsky M, et al. Lack of efficacy of finasteride in postmenopausal women with androgenic alopecia. *J Am Acad Dermatol.* 2000;43:768-776.

Richards RN, Meharg GE. Electrolysis: observations from 13 years and 140,000 hours of experience. *J Am Acad Dermatol.* 1995;33(4):662-666.

Rosenfield RL. Hirsutism and the variable response of the pilosebaceous unit to androgen. *J Investig Dermatol Symp Proc.* 2005(b);10:205-208.

Rosner W, Vesper H. Toward excellence in testosterone testing: a consensus statement. *J Clin Endocrinol Metab.* 2010;95:4542-4548.

Sadighha A, Mohaghegh Zahed G. Meta-analysis of hair removal laser trials. *Lasers Med Sci.* 2009;24(1):21-25.

Sakihara S, Kageyama K, Oki Y, et al. Evaluation of plasma, salivary, and urinary cortisol levels for diagnosis of Cushing's syndrome. *Endocr J.* 2010;57(4): 331-337.

Serafini P, Ablan F, Lobo RA. 5α-Reductase activity in the genital skin of hirsute women. *J Clin Endocrinol Metab.* 1985a;60:349-355.

Serafini P, Lobo RA. Increased 5α-reductase activity in idiopathic hirsutism. *Fertil Steril.* 1985b;43:74-78.

Speiser PW, Dupont B, Rubenstein P, et al. High frequency of nonclassical steroid 21-hydroxylase deficiency. *Am J Hum Genet.* 1985;37:650-667.

Stanczyk FZ, Chang L, Carmina E, et al. Is 11β-hydroxyandrostenedione a better marker of adrenal androgen excess than dehydroepiandrosterone sulfate? *Am J Obstet Gynecol.* 1991;166:1837-1842.

Stein IF, Leventhal ML. Amenorrhea associated with bilateral polycystic ovaries. *Am J Obstet Gynecol.* 1935;29:181.

Swiglo BA, Cosma M, Flynn DN, et al. Antiandrogens for the treatment of hirsutism: a systematic review and meta-analysis of randomized controlled trials. *J Clin Endocrinol Metab.* 2008;93(4):1153-1160.

The Rotterdam ESHRE/ASRM-sponsored PCOS consensus workshop group. Revised 2003 consensus on diagnostic criteria and long-term health risks related to polycystic ovary syndrome (PCOS). *Hum Reprod.* 2004;19:41-47.

Wolf Jr JE, Shander D, Huber F, et al. Randomized, double-blind clinical evaluation of the efficacy and safety of topical eflornithine HCI 13.9% cream in the treatment of women with facial hair. *Int J Dermatol.* 2007;46:94-98.
Wong IL, Morris RS, Chang L, et al. A prospective randomized trial comparing finasteride to spironolactone in the treatment of hirsute women. *J Clin Endocrinol Metab.* 1995;80:233-238.
Zimmerman Y, Eijkemans MJC, Coelingh Bennink HJT, et al. The effect of combined oral contraception on testosterone levels in healthy women: a systematic review and meta-analysis. *Hum Reprod U.* 2014;20:76-105.
Zouboulis CC, Rabe T. Hormonal antiandrogens in acne treatment. *J Dtsch Dermatol Ges Suppl.* 2010;1:S60-S74. Review.

Suggested Readings can be found on ExpertConsult.com.

# 41 Polycystic Ovary Syndrome

*Roger A. Lobo*

## POLYCYSTIC OVARY SYNDROME DEFINITION

Polycystic ovary syndrome (PCOS)—originally described in 1935 by Stein and Leventhal as a syndrome consisting of amenorrhea, hirsutism, and obesity in association with enlarged polycystic ovaries (Stein, 1935)—is the most common hormonal disorder in reproductive-aged women. The "classic" features occur in 3% to 7% of the population and with its broadest definition may occur in 15% to 20% of women (Fauser, 2012). The classic definition of PCOS includes women who are anovulatory and have irregular periods as well as hyperandrogenism, as determined by signs such as hirsutism or elevated blood levels of androgens. This should occur in the absence of enzymatic disorders (e.g., 21-hydroxylase deficiency), Cushing syndrome, or tumors. Usually, in the United States, the diagnosis does not require findings on ultrasound (US) of characteristic polycystic ovaries. This U.S.-based definition has been referred to as the National Institutes of Health (NIH) consensus definition because it followed an NIH conference in 1989, but this was not a consensus conference, and there was no true consensus among attendees (Zawadzki, 1992). However, there have been two other definitions used for PCOS, and a conference convened at NIH attempted to reconcile all these definitions (NIH Evidence-based Methodology Workshop, 2012) (Table 41.1).

In recognition that some women with PCOS may *not* have menstrual irregularity, and stressing the importance of the U.S. findings, the "Rotterdam" criteria emerged following a European Society for Human Reproduction and Embryology/American Society for Reproductive Medicine (ESHRE/ASRM) conference in 2004 (Rotterdam ESHRE/ASRM-Sponsored PCOS Consensus Workshop Group, 2004). Menstrual irregularity, symptoms or findings of hyperandrogenism, and polycystic ovaries on US are the three criteria used in the definition; but only two of these three criteria are required for the definition. Thus several phenotypes are possible, including hyperandrogenism and polycystic ovaries in ovulatory women (so-called *phenotype C*) and irregular cycles and polycystic ovaries in the absence of documented hyperandrogenism (phenotype D). The latter is the most controversial phenotype, which some investigators in the field have rejected.

Because hyperandrogenism is deemed to be an important feature of PCOS, the Androgen Excess and Polycystic Ovary Syndrome (AEPCOS) Society has offered a third definition of PCOS, which stresses hyperandrogenism as a key feature and then recognizes that women with PCOS can have polycystic ovaries on US or menstrual irregularity (anovulation) (Azziz, 2006).

A workshop at NIH in December 2012 attempted to draw consensus among the various definitions. It was concluded among independent panelists that the Rotterdam criteria should be adopted for convention and familiarity (it is the most commonly used definition worldwide) but that it is not ideal, and investigators should strive to find a more appropriate name for the disorder (NIH Evidence-based Methodology Workshop, 2012). Table 41.1 lists the four definitions with various phenotypes.

## OVARIAN MORPHOLOGY

As discussed previously, ultrasound morphology has become an important parameter in the diagnosis of PCOS. Figures 41.1 and 41.2 depict the typical appearance of the polycystic ovary (gross specimen) and by US in a sagittal plane. However, there is heterogeneity in ovarian morphology in women with PCOS and the lack of standard criteria for the minimum requirements for the US diagnosis of polycystic ovaries. According to Rotterdam criteria, any one ovary having 12 or more cystic structures (2 to 8 mm) or an ovarian volume >10 cc is sufficient. Although originally thought to be important, according to Rotterdam the orientation of the cysts is not important; these are typically peripherally oriented around a dense stroma, thus showing an increased stromal/peripheral area ratio. Others have found that the stromal/peripheral area ratio is the most important diagnostic criterion and correlates well with the androgen status of the woman (Fulghesu, 2007) (Fig. 41.3). Most recently, Christ has suggested that the cutoff should be 26 follicles throughout the ovary, or a volume >10 cc. The stromal/peripheral ratio was considered important, but it was second in diagnostic accuracy to the finding of 26 follicles, which eliminated the overlap in ovarian findings between normal women and those with PCOS (Christ, 2014). Although the criterion of 26 follicles represents the visualization of the entire ovary (and requires high-grade imaging capabilities), most have used the number of small follicles (2 to 8 mm) in a single sonographic plane that adequately depicts the increased cystic activity within the ovary. *Thus, although the US diagnosis is rather subjective and is in the "eyes of the beholder" with many US units not being able to make a specific diagnosis, in our view, bilateral cystic ovaries (10 or more in a single sonographic plane of an ovary, arranged peripherally) with a volume >10 cc should provide a practical way to make the US diagnosis.*

It is also important to note that 10% to 25% of the normal reproductive age population (no symptoms or signs of PCOS)

Table 41.1 Criteria for Diagnosis of Polycystic Ovary Syndrome

| Study* | Criteria |
|---|---|
| National Institute of Child Health and Human Development 1990 | Menstrual irregularity<br>Hyperandrogenism (clinical or biochemical) |
| ESHRE-ASRM 2003 "Rotterdam criteria" | Menstrual irregularity<br>Hyperandrogenism (clinical or biochemical)<br>Polycystic ovaries on ultrasound (two of three required) |
| AEPCOS 2006 | Hyperandrogenism (clinical or biochemical) and menstrual irregularity<br>Polycystic ovaries on ultrasound (either or both of the latter two) |
| NIH Workshop 2012 | Endorsement of Rotterdam criteria, acknowledging its limitations, and suggesting the name PCOS should be changed |

*All required the exclusion of other underlying hormonal disorders or tumors.

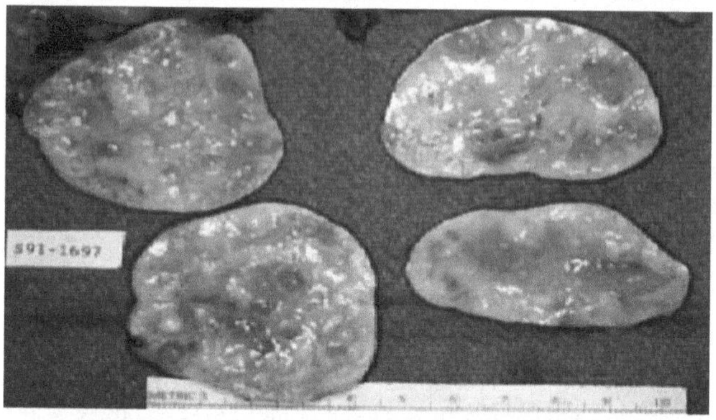

**Figure 41.1** Surgical specimen of polycystic ovaries.

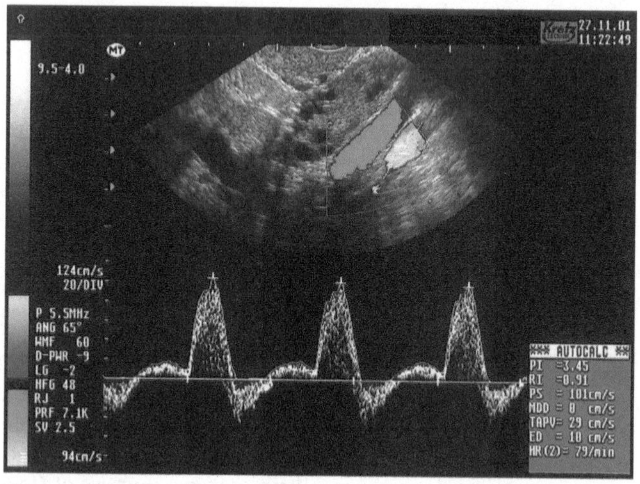


**Figure 41.2** Typical color Doppler ultrasound of a polycystic ovary showing increased blood flow. (From Strauss JF, Barbieri RL, eds. *Yen and Jaffe's Reproductive Endocrinology.* 6th ed. Philadelphia: Elsevier; 2009:822.)

may have polycystic ovaries found on US. These ovaries have been called *polycystic-appearing ovaries (PAO)* or *polycystic ovarian morphology (PCOM)* in the literature (Wong, 1995). This isolated finding should not be confused with the diagnosis of PCOS, but it may be a risk factor for other features of PCOS (e.g., insulin resistance, cardiovascular risk factors) discussed later.

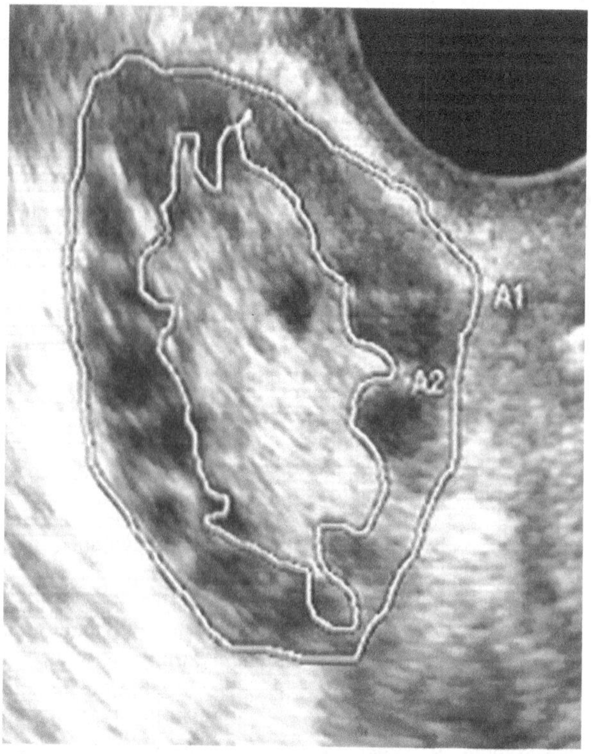


**Figure 41.3** Example of calculating the ovarian cystic area *(A1)* and the stromal area *(A2)*. (Modified from Fulghesu AM, Angioni S, Frau E, et al. Ultrasound in polycystic ovary syndrome—the measuring of ovarian stroma and relationship with circulating androgens: results of a multicentric study. *Hum Reprod.* 2007;22[9]:2501-2508.)

## MENSTRUAL IRREGULARITY

Menstrual irregularity includes oligomenorrhea (cycles over 35 days) as well as a menstrual frequency of every few months and frank amenorrhea (over 6 months missed). Though the majority of women with PCOS have irregular cycles, signifying problems with ovulation, the ovulatory phenotype ("C") reporting regular cycles occurs with variable frequencies in different populations: from 3% in Korea to 30% in Italy among women diagnosed with PCOS (Chae, 2008; Carmina, 2007). The ovulatory phenotype has less metabolic and cardiovascular risks as will be discussed later. It has been reported that menstrual irregularity is the best correlate of having insulin resistance in women with PCOS (Chae, 2008; Carmina, 2007). Additionally, although the subfertility of women with PCOS is predominantly due to problems of anovulation, many women with PCOS with ovulatory function will present with subfertility as well.

## HYPERANDROGENISM/ANDROGEN EXCESS

Often considered to be the cardinal feature of women with PCOS, androgen excess may be difficult to diagnose. As discussed in Chapter 40, production of androgens in excess may emanate from the ovary, adrenal, or the periphery. Although symptoms of androgen excess, particularly of hirsutism, is sufficient for the inclusion of this parameter in the diagnosis of PCOS, blood measurements of testosterone may not always be accurate and often are "normal" in women with symptoms.

The androgen excess has been implicated in contributing to abnormalities in LH secretion, weight gain and adipose deposition, and the metabolic derangements of PCOS, discussed later.

## DIAGNOSIS OF POLYCYSTIC OVARY SYNDROME IN ADOLESCENTS

An early diagnosis of PCOS in a teenager is not easy and should be made with caution. This is because in using Rotterdam criteria, all parameters for the diagnosis (menstrual irregularity, findings of androgen excess, and ovarian morphology) change and evolve during the postpubertal years. We have argued that a firm diagnosis of PCOS should only be made if all three Rotterdam criteria are present at least 3 years postmenarche (persistence of irregular menstruation, hirsutism and elevated testosterone, ovarian volume >10 cc) (Carmina, 2010). Adolescents for whom a firm diagnosis cannot be made are considered to be at risk and should be followed and merely treated for their specific complaint, if warranted. This prevents the burden of unnecessarily labeling an adolescent at an early age with a diagnosis that may not be correct.

## CHARACTERISTIC ENDOCRINE FINDINGS IN POLYCYSTIC OVARY SYNDROME

Characteristic endocrinologic features include abnormal gonadotropin secretion caused by increased gonadotropin-releasing hormone (GnRH) pulse amplitude or increased pituitary sensitivity to GnRH. These abnormalities result in tonically elevated levels of luteinizing hormone (LH) in approximately two thirds of the women with this syndrome (Fig. 41.4). After a bolus of GnRH, there is usually an exaggerated response of LH, but not of follicle-stimulating hormone (FSH; see Fig. 41.4). Because of issues of metabolic clearance, typically the more obese women with PCOS will be found to have normal LH levels, while thin women with PCOS often have elevated levels. The high tonic levels of LH, often referred to as "inappropriate gonadotropin secretion" is due to elevated androgen and unbound estradiol or hypothalamic/pituitary functional abnormalities related to neurotransmitters such as dopamine.

Because FSH levels in women with PCOS are normal or low, an elevated LH/FSH ratio has been used to diagnose PCOS. However, only 70% of women with a clinical diagnosis of PCOS have an elevated level of immunoreactive LH or an immunologic LH/FSH ratio greater than 3, although almost all women with PCOS had elevated serum levels of biologically active LH (Lobo, 1983) (Fig. 41.5). *However, an elevated LH level or an elevated LH/FSH ratio is neither specific for, nor required for, the diagnosis of PCOS.*

In addition to increased levels of circulatory androgens, women with PCOS have increased levels of biologically active (non–sex hormone-binding globulin [SHBG]–bound) estradiol, although total circulating levels of estradiol are not increased (Fig. 41.6). The increased amount of non–SHBG-bound estradiol is caused by a decrease in SHBG levels, which is brought about by the increased levels of androgens and obesity, with high insulin levels present in many of these women. Estrone is also increased because of increased peripheral (adipose) conversion of androgen. The tonically increased levels of biologically active estradiol may

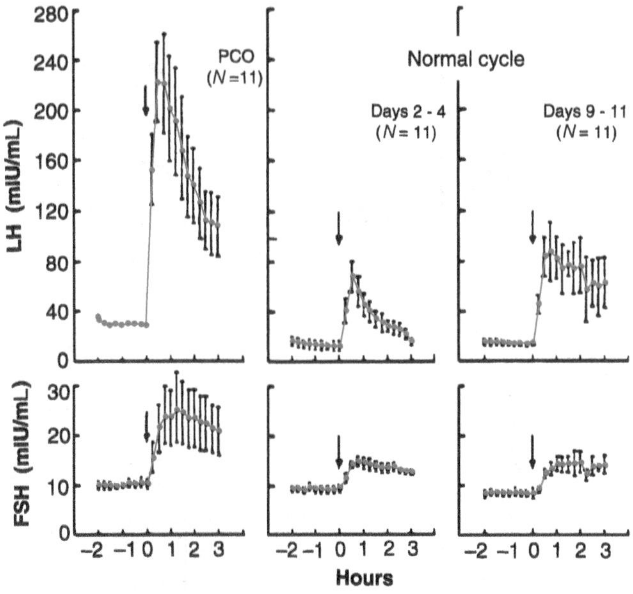


**Figure 41.4** Comparison of quantitative luteinizing hormone (LH) and follicle-stimulating hormone (FSH) release in response to a single bolus of 150 μg of gonadotropin-releasing hormone (GnRH) in patients with polycystic ovarian syndrome (PCO) and in normal women during low-estrogen (early follicular) and high-estrogen (late follicular) phases of their cycles. (From Rebar R, Judd HL, Yen SSC, et al. Characterization of the inappropriate gonadotropin secretion in polycystic ovary syndrome. *J Clin Invest.* 1976;57[5]:1320-1329.)

stimulate increased GnRH pulsatility and produce tonically elevated LH levels and anovulation. In addition, the lowered SHBG level increases the biologically active fractions of androgens in the circulation. The importance of the decreased levels of SHBG is shown schematically in Figure 41.7 (Lobo, 1982). This relative hyperestrogenism (elevated levels of estrone and non–SHBG-bound estradiol), which is unopposed by progesterone because of anovulation, increases the risk of endometrial hyperplasia.

Androgens from a variety of sources are elevated in women with PCOS (Fig. 41.8). Serum testosterone levels usually range from 0.7 to 1.2 ng/mL, and androstenedione levels are usually from 3 to 5 ng/mL. In addition, approximately 50% of women with this syndrome have elevated levels of dehydroepiandrosterone sulfate (DHEAS), suggesting adrenal androgen involvement. However, in some countries, this prevalence of putative adrenal involvement is lower. Evidence also exists for adrenal hyperactivity to stimulation in at least one third of women with PCOS. Although almost all women with PCOS have elevated levels of circulating androgens, the presence or absence of hirsutism depends on whether those androgens are converted peripherally by 5α-reductase to the more potent androgen dihydrotestosterone (DHT), as reflected by increased circulating levels of 3α-androstanediol glucuronide (3α-diol-G) (see Chapter 40). Nonhirsute women with PCOS have elevated circulatory levels of testosterone, DHEAS, or both, but not 3α-diol-G (Lobo, 1983).

Approximately 20% to 30% of women with PCOS also have mildly elevated levels of prolactin (20 to 35 ng/mL), possibly related to the increased pulsatility of GnRH, due to a relative dopamine deficiency or to tonic stimulation from unopposed estrogen. In this setting, if the diagnosis of PCOS is clear, these mild elevations in prolactin level only should be followed.

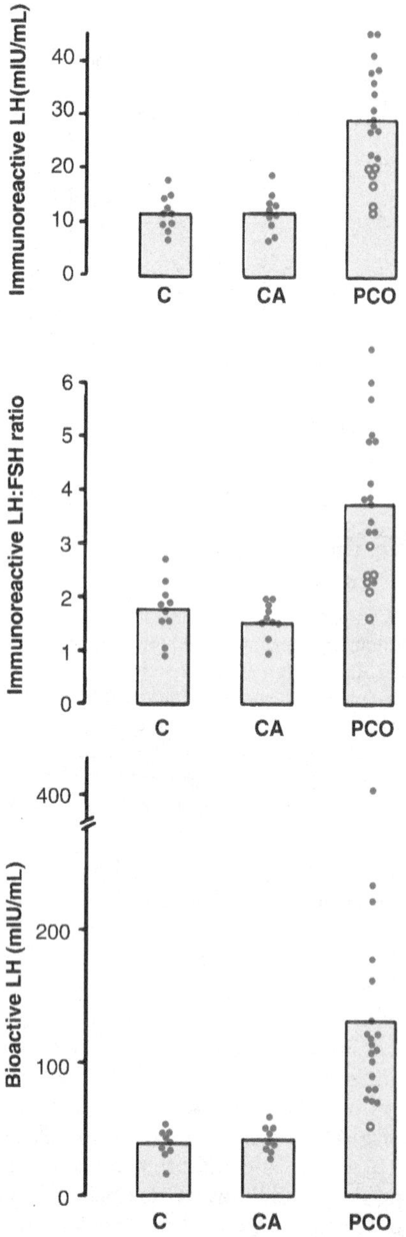


**Figure 41.5** Serum measurements of immunoreactive luteinizing hormone (LH), immunoreactive LH-to-follicle-stimulating hormone (FSH) ratios, and bioactive LH in control subjects *(C)*, women with chronic anovulation *(CA)*, and women with polycystic ovary syndrome *(PCO)*. Boxes represent the mean ±3 standard deviation (SD) of control levels. (From Lobo RA, Kletzky OA, Campeau JD, et al. Elevated bioactive luteinizing hormone in women with the polycystic ovary syndrome. *Fertil Steril.* 1983;39[5]:674-678.)

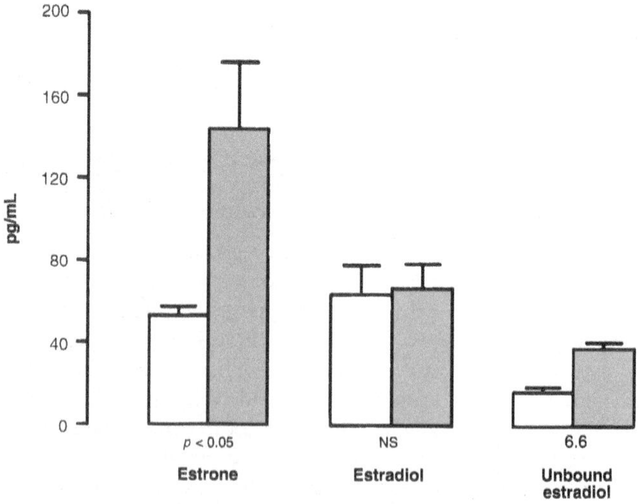


**Figure 41.6** Serum estrogen concentrations in 13 non-PCOS patients and 22 PCOS patients *(shaded areas)*. (From Lobo RA, Granger L, Goebelsmann U, et al. Elevation in unbound serum estradiol as a possible mechanism for inappropriate gonadotropin secretion in women with PCOS. *J Clin Endocrinol Metab.* 1981;52[1]:156-158.)

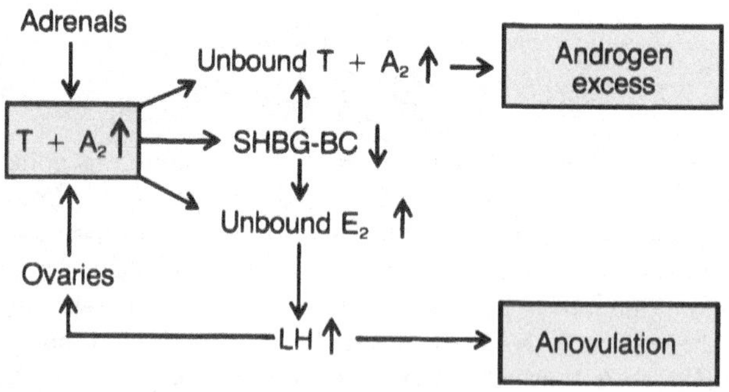


**Figure 41.7** Scheme depicting the possible role of adrenal-derived androgen in initiating androgen excess and anovulation. *A2*, Androstanediol; *E2*, estradiol; *LH*, luteinizing hormone; *SHBG-BC*, sex hormone-binding globulin binding capacity; *T*, testosterone. (From Lobo RA, Goebelsmann U. Effect of androgen excess on inappropriate gonadotropin secretion as found in polycystic ovary syndrome. *Am J Obstet Gynecol.* 1982;142[4]:394-401.)

## INSULIN RESISTANCE

It is well established that some degree of insulin resistance (IR) occurs in most women with PCOS, even in those of normal weight. Insulin and insulin-like growth factor 1 (IGF-1) enhance ovarian androgen production by potentiating the stimulatory action of LH on ovarian androstenedione and testosterone secretion. High levels of insulin bind to the receptor for IGF-1 as a result of the significant homology of the IGF-1 receptor with the insulin receptor. The granulosa cells also produce IGF-1 and IGF-binding proteins (IGFBPs). This local production of IGF-1 and IGFBP may result in paracrine control and enhancement of LH stimulation and production of androgens by the theca cells in women with PCOS. Because IGFBP levels are lower in women with PCOS, there is increased bioavailable IGF-1, which increases stimulation of the theca cells in combination with LH to produce higher levels of androgen production. In addition, elevated insulin levels (as well as androgen) stimulate adipocyte production of adipokines (adipocytokines), which interfere with the metabolism and breakdown of adipose tissue and further enhance IR (Fig. 41.9). IR in PCOS is primarily characterized by an insulin resistance in peripheral tissues, manifest primarily in muscle and adipose and minimally at the level of ovary or adrenal (Sam, 2003). Figure 41.10 reflects these events with the less efficient serine phosphorylation (rather than tyrosine phosphorylation) resulting in less efficient insulin action (metabolic

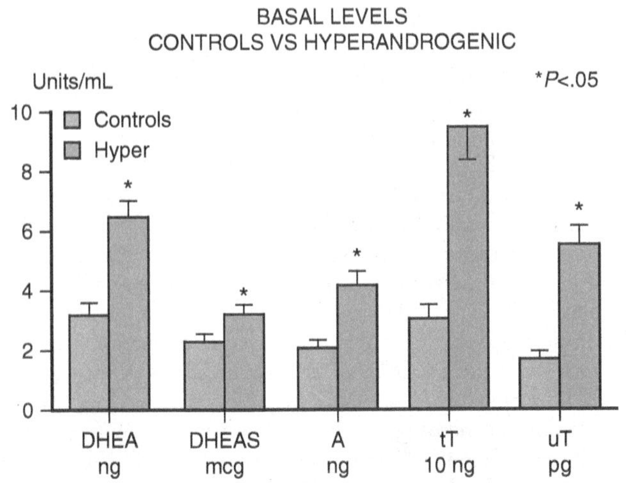


**Figure 41.8** Basal levels of various androgens in hyperandrogenic women with polycystic ovary syndrome (PCOS) versus matched controls. All androgens, dehydroepiandrosterone *(DHEA)*, DHEA sulfate *(DHEAS)*, androstenedione *(A)*, total testosterone *(tT)*, and unbound testosterone *(uT)*, are significantly elevated.

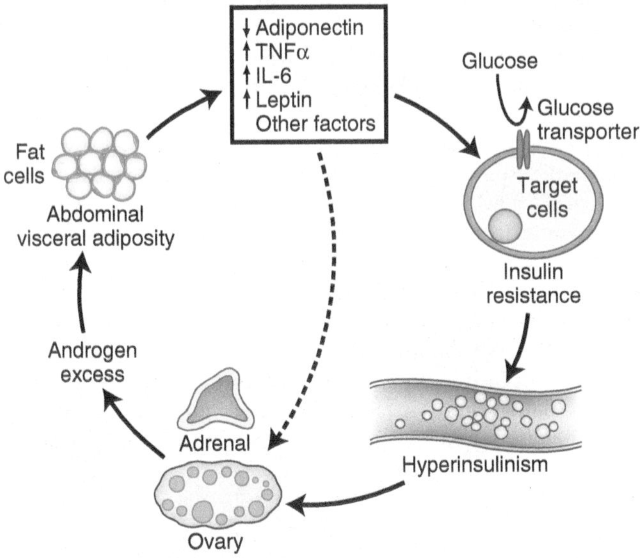


**Figure 41.9** Diagrammatic depiction of the relationship among androgens, insulin, and body fat (release of adipokines). (From Escobar-Morreale HF, San Milan JL. Abdominal adiposity and the polycystic ovary syndrome. *Trends Endocrinol Metab.* 2007;18[7]:266-272.)

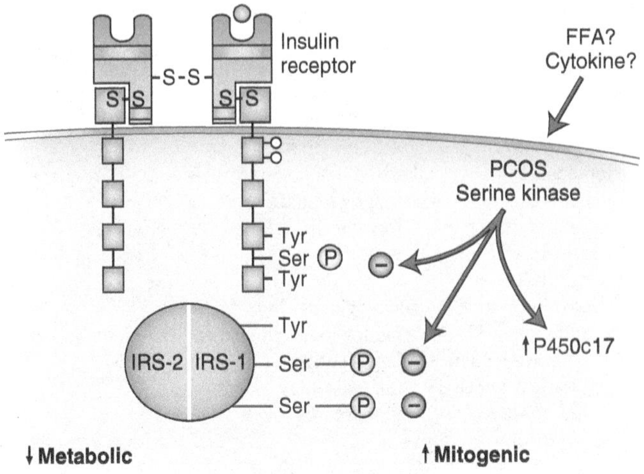


**Figure 41.10** Mechanism of insulin resistance (IR) in women with polycystic ovary syndrome. At specific sites, IR is due to serine phosphorylation affecting metabolic, but not mitogenic, actions of insulin. (From Sam S, Dunaif A. Polycystic ovary syndrome: syndrome XX? *Trends Endocrinol Metab.* 2003;14[8]:365-370.)

effect), but with no effects on the production of androgens (intact mitogenic effect) (Sam, 2003).

The cause of IR in PCOS is unknown; it is not caused by insulin receptor defects but by signaling abnormalities as noted previously. It is likely that genetic factors contribute to these findings. Most women with PCOS will be found to have euglycemia with peripheral IR; in more severe cases, there is also evidence of beta cell (secretory) dysfunction, which increases the risk of type 2 diabetes. In a prospective evaluation of 254 women with PCOS who had an oral glucose tolerance test, it was found that 31% had impaired glucose tolerance and 7.5% had undiagnosed diabetes. In nonobese women with PCOS, 10% had impaired glucose tolerance and 1.5% had diabetes (Legro, 1999). Norman and coworkers have shown that over a mean follow-up period of 6.2 years, 9% of women with PCOS in Australia progressed to having impaired glucose tolerance and 8% became diabetic (Norman, 2001). Thus the negative effects of obesity and PCOS on insulin resistance are additive. Although clinicians may assume most women with PCOS have some degree of IR, particularly those who are older and who are overweight or obese, it is recommended that testing should be directed at ruling out diabetes and glucose intolerance, rather than diagnosing IR (Fauser, 2012).

Fasting glucose levels are a poor predictor of diabetes in PCOS. More recently, it has been suggested that measuring the level of hemoglobin A1C (HbA1C; normal <6%) is the most efficient means of ruling out glucose intolerance or frank diabetes, but there is still disagreement about its role as a screening test.

Various techniques have been used to diagnose IR in women with PCOS. These include fairly complicated but more accurate measures used only in a research setting, such as the clamp test, intravenous frequent sampling glucose tolerance test, or the insulin tolerance test. Using fasting glucose and insulin measurements and calculating the quantitative insulin sensitivity check index (QUICKI) or homeostasis model assessment of insulin resistance (HOMA) have been useful and correlate well with the more invasive techniques (Table 41.2). However, as stated earlier, from a treatment standpoint, it may not be necessary to compute these parameters in routine practice; clinicians should assume that overweight or obese women with PCOS are insulin resistant and should be treated as such. An oral glucose tolerance test should be carried out to rule out impaired glucose tolerance or diabetes, which cannot be assumed or discounted. Figure 41.11 depicts the prevalence of abnormal testing parameters in women with PCOS (Carmina, 2004).

**Acanthosis nigricans** (AN) has been found in approximately 30% of hyperandrogenic women. Approximately 50% of the hyperandrogenic women who had PCOS and were obese had AN. Although it has been suggested that the presence of ***h***yper***an***drogenism, ***IR***, and ***AN*** constitutes a special syndrome (the HAIR-AN syndrome), most investigators believe that many women with PCOS have some degree of AN, particularly when obese, and do

Table 41.2 Measurements of Insulin Sensitivity

| Test | Measurement | Normal Value* |
|---|---|---|
| Hyperinsulinemic clamp | M/1 (mean glucose use/ mean plasma insulin concentration) | $>1.12 \times 10^{-4}$ |
| Homeostasis model assessment of insulin resistance (HOMAIR) | [Fasting insulin (μU/mL) × fasting glucose (mmol/L)]/22.5 | <2.77 |
| Glucose-to-insulin ratio | Fasting glucose (mg/dL)/ fasting insulin (μU/mL) | >4.5 |
| Quantitative insulin sensitivity check index (QUICKI) | 1/[log fasting insulin (μU/mL) + log + fasting glucose (mg/dL) ] | >0.357 |
| Fasting insulin | — | Assay dependent |

*Normal values may vary depending on the insulin assay used.

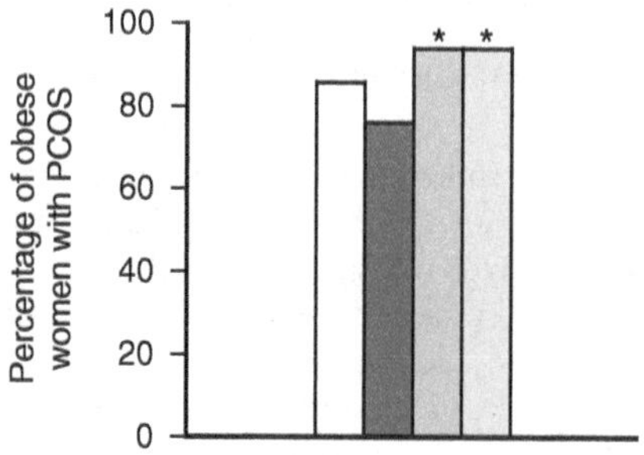


**Figure 41.11** Percentage of 129 obese women with polycystic ovary syndrome (PCOS) with insulin resistance (IR) based on fasting basal insulin (white), glucose/insulin (G/I) ratio (red), homeostasis model assessment of insulin resistance (HOMA) (yellow), or quantitative insulin sensitivity check index (QUICKI) (light blue). *$P < .01$ compared with G/I ratio. (From Carmina E, Lobo RA. The use of fasting blood to assess the prevalence of insulin resistance in women with polycystic ovary syndrome. *Fertil Steril.* 2004;82[3]:661-665.)

not have another distinct endocrine disorder. The combination of increased insulin and IGF-1 enhances the development of AN.

Müllerian-inhibiting substance (MIS) or anti-müllerian hormone (AMH) is a glycoprotein produced by the granulosa cells of preantral follicles. Because of the larger number of preantral follicles in PCOS, the MIS or AMH level is significantly elevated in women with PCOS (Dewailly, 2014). Physiologically, AMH or MIS attenuates a sensitivity of FSH in stimulating granulosa cells; the levels are higher in clomiphene-resistant women and in those who are chronically anovulatory compared to those with more regular cycles, even as they age (Fig. 41.12) (Carmina, 2012a). It has been suggested that AMH is involved in the pathophysiology of anovulation in PCOS and, because it reflects at least in part ovarian morphology, that AMH may be used as a blood test for PCOS without needing to perform US. One review suggested a cutoff value of about 4.7 ng/mL, (Iliodromiti, 2013); although the degree of overlap in values of AMH between PCOS and normal women precludes its routine use (Casadei, 2013).

## *PATHOPHYSIOLOGIC CONSIDERATIONS*

It is clear that there is a genetic predisposition to PCOS. However, it is likely that several genes are involved, and these are **susceptibility genes** that predispose the women affected to develop PCOS. A review by Kosova and Urbanek pointed out the many difficulties in finding a direct genetic linkage, which are related to the nature of the disorder, its heterogeneity, and the large sample size required to find meaningful associations (Kosova, 2013). There are also multiple family studies of sisters, brothers, and daughters of affected women all showing some traits associated with aspects of PCOS.

Environmental factors are clearly involved as well, based on twin studies, in which PCOS is not always concordant on a genetic basis (Vink, 2006). Maternal exposure to androgen has been shown in a monkey model to contribute to the development of PCOS (Abbott, 2005).

Most recently, genome-wide association studies in Han Chinese and European families have pointed out certain susceptibility genes with some consistency. These include loci at

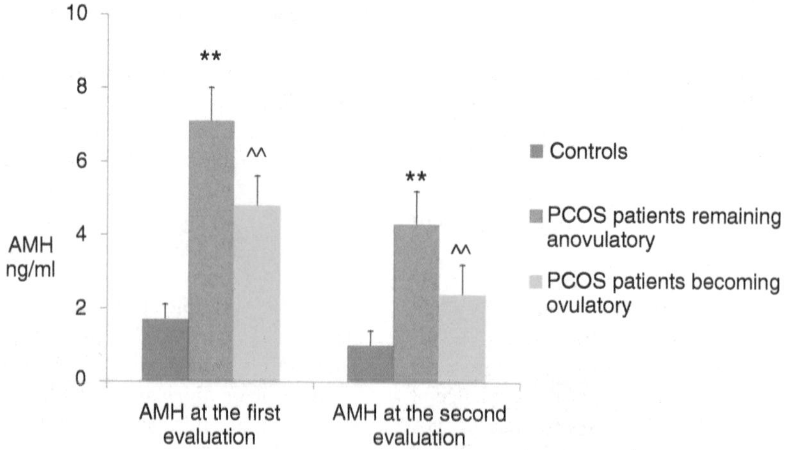


**Figure 41.12** Elevated levels of anti-müllerian hormone (AMH) in women with polycystic ovary syndrome (PCOS) decrease with time, and levels are lower in ovulatory women. Data from a 20-year longitudinal study in women with PCOS. (From Carmina E, Campagna AM, Mansuet P, et al. Does the level of serum antimullerian hormone predict ovulatory function in women with polycystic ovary syndrome with aging? *Fertil Steril.* 2012;98[4]:1043-1046.)

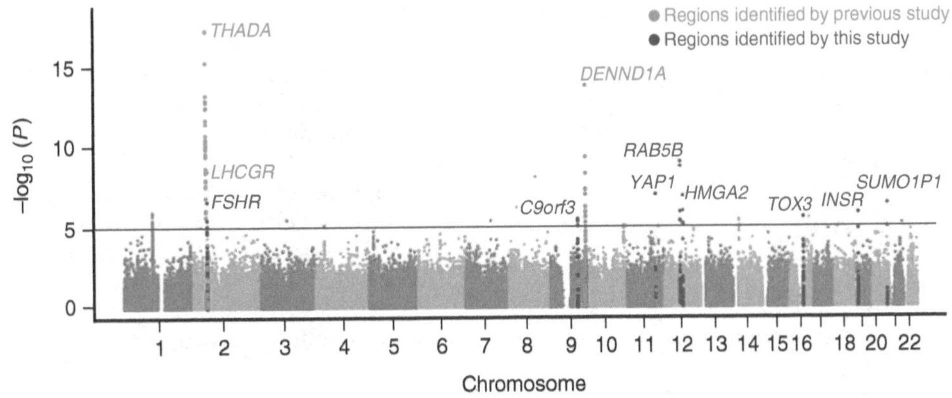


**Figure 41.13** Genome-wide association studies in 8226 women with polycystic ovary syndrome (PCOS) diagnosed by Rotterdam criteria and 7578 controls, with several loci identified for susceptibility genes of interest. (From Shi Y, Zhao H, Shi Y, et al. Genome-wide association study identifies eight new risk loci for polycystic ovary syndrome. *Nat Genet.* 2012;44[9]:1020-1027.)

2p16.3, 2p21, and 9q 33.3, involving the LH/human chorionic gonadotropin (hCG) receptor, a thyroid adenoma locus, and DENND1A, potentially affecting function of the endoplasmic reticulum (Chen, 2010). This was confirmed in subsequent studies with the addition of other potential loci (Shi, 2012; Zhao, 2012) (Fig. 41.13). The 2p16.3 locus was confirmed in a U.S. study (Mutharasan, 2013). It has been long established that a vicious cycle propagates the disorder in PCOS, regardless of how it begins (Strauss, 2009) (Fig. 41.14). Thus it was attractive to postulate that dopamine deficiency in the hypothalamus might give rise to the exaggerated LH responses in PCOS, and there are several similar hypotheses. However, it has been observed that morphologically identifiable polycystic ovaries are seen in children (Bridges, 1993). This occurrence predicts puberty and other normal endocrinologic events, suggesting a central role for altered polycystic ovarian morphology in the disorder.

Furthermore, not all women with isolated polycystic ovaries have PCOS as stated earlier. Thus a pathophysiologic model can be put together as follows. An ovary is polycystic in up to 20% of girls, according to data from Bridges and colleagues. Thus the ovary transitions early in life from normal to polycystic-appearing (PAO). This influence occurs in a specific way by genetic factors or environmental factors, or it is induced by other endocrine disturbances (Lobo, 1996) (Fig. 41.15). The woman who develops PAO may have normal menses, normal androgen levels, and normal ovulatory function and parity. However, if subjected to various susceptibility factors (likely genetic) or environmental or other challenges or insults, with varying degrees of severity, women with PAO may develop a full-blown syndrome (PCOS) (see Fig. 41.15). The syndrome, if full-blown, exhibits the full extent of hyperandrogenism and anovulation, with the most extreme form of this menstrual disturbance being amenorrhea (the type A or B phenotype according to Rotterdam criteria). However, in this spectrum of disorders, the androgen disturbances may also be near normal. Similarly, the menstrual disturbance may be mild.

This model requires that normal homeostatic factors may be able to ward off stressors or insults in some women who can go through life without PCOS but have PAO, which does not change morphologically. Alternatively, with varying degrees of success, a woman's homeostatic mechanisms may at any time, early or later

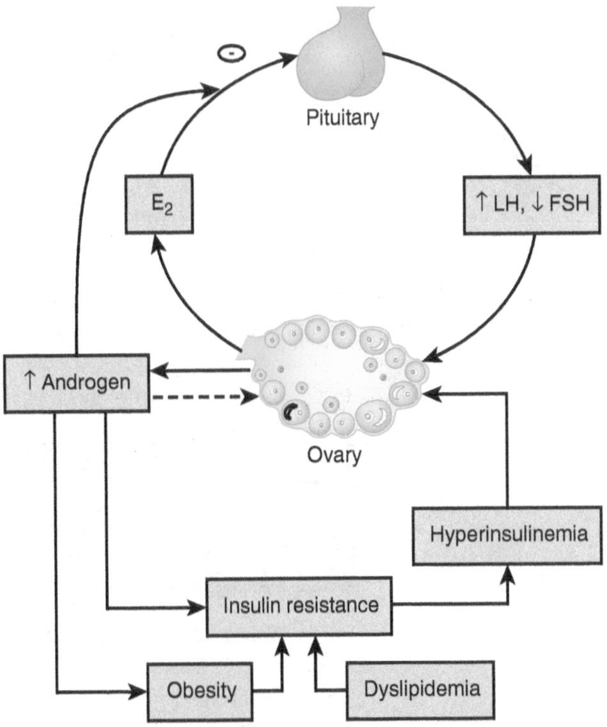


**Figure 41.14** Pathophysiologic concept of polycystic ovary syndrome (PCOS). Increased luteinizing hormone (LH) secretion, together with enhanced theca cell responsiveness, drives the production of excess ovarian androgen. Increased androgen production may inhibit steroid negative feedback effects on hypothalamic gonadotropin-releasing hormone pulse generation to account for the rapid LH pulse frequency observed in women with PCOS. In addition, increased androgen levels are associated with android obesity, visceral fat deposition, and dyslipidemia, all of which may contribute to insulin resistance. Independently, hyperandrogenemia, obesity, and hyperinsulinemia may decrease sex hormone-binding globulin, thereby increasing bioactive testosterone. Finally, increased androgen may have direct effects on the ovary to increase follicle number and follicle size and possibly enhance granulosa cell responsiveness to follicle-stimulating hormone (FSH). *E2*, Estradiol. (From Strauss JF, Barbieri RL, eds. *Yen and Jaffe's Reproductive Endocrinology.* 6th ed. Philadelphia: WB Saunders; 2009:509.)

in reproductive life, allow symptoms of PCOS to emerge with varying degrees of severity. Two of the major insults are thought to be weight gain and psychological stress. Therefore the typical teenager born with PAO may develop PCOS fairly quickly, but a PCOS picture may only develop later in life in some women, even after having children, with weight gain, for example.

## CONSEQUENCES OF POLYCYSTIC OVARY SYNDROME

The importance of diagnosing PCOS is that there are known long-term consequences of the diagnosis warranting lifelong surveillance. These include metabolic and cardiovascular risks as well as the risk of certain cancers with aging.

There have been several consensus meetings for the diagnosis and treatment of PCOS as mentioned earlier. The first two dealt with the diagnosis of PCOS (Rotterdam ESHRE/ASRM Sponsored PCOS Consensus Workshop Group, 2004) and the treatment of infertility (Thessaloniki ESHRE/ASRM-Sponsored PCOS Consensus Workshop Group, 2008). The third and most recent of these was held in Amsterdam and addressed the "long-term" consequences of PCOS (Fauser, 2012). Figure 41.16 depicts the shift in emphasis with aging, requiring a multidisciplinary approach. With aging, concerns

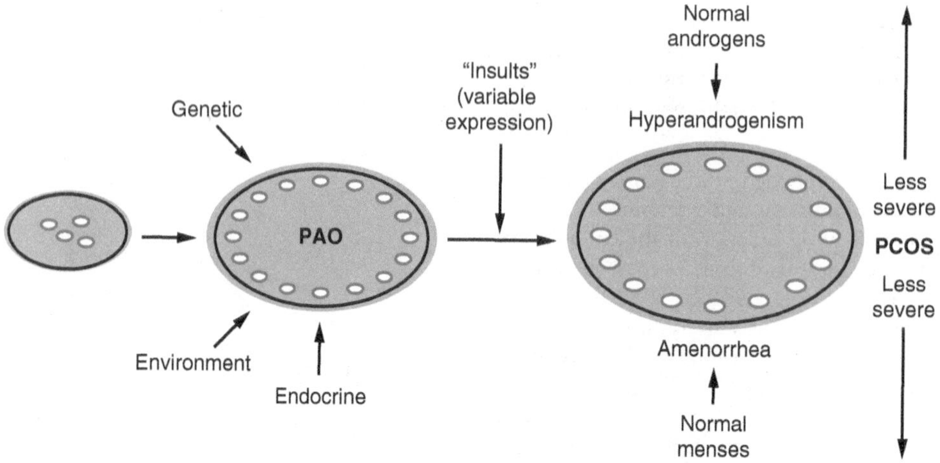


**Figure 41.15** Pathophysiology of polycystic ovary syndrome (PCOS) showing differences in presentation. *PAO*, Polycystic-appearing ovaries.

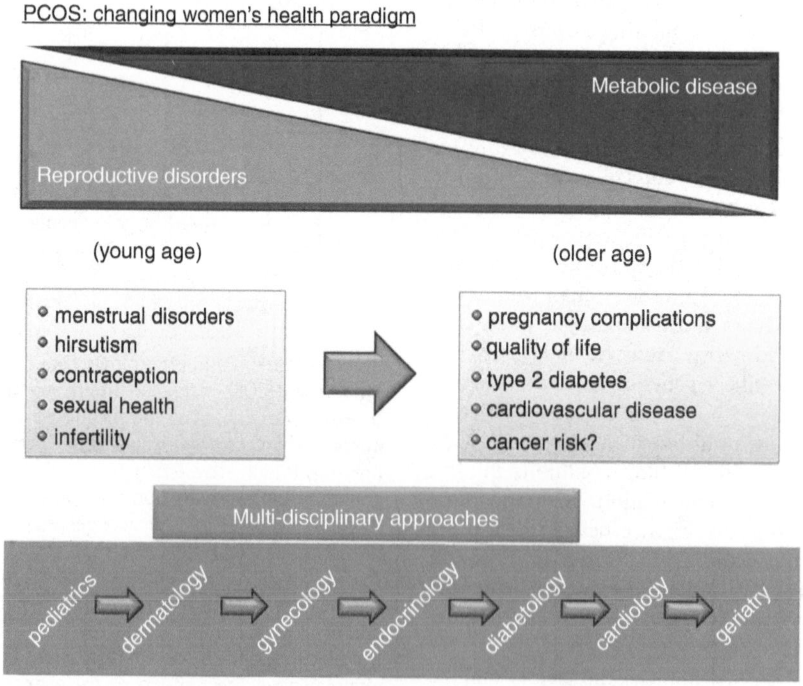


**Figure 41.16** Schematic representation of the change in emphasis from early age reproductive disorders to long-term metabolic and cardiovascular health. (From Fauser B, Tarlatzis B, Rebar RW, et al. Consensus on women's health aspects of polycystic ovary syndrome [PCOS]: the Amsterdam ESHRE/ASRM-sponsored 3rd PCOS Consensus Workshop Group. *Fertil Steril*. 2012;97[1]:28-38.e25.)

for cardiovascular disease including hypertension, metabolic syndrome, diabetes, and cancer (endometrial and ovarian) become more prominent.

## WEIGHT GAIN/OBESITY AND METABOLIC SYNDROME

Weight gain as women age is a major predictor of abnormal metabolic findings and the emergence of cardiovascular (CV) disease risks; indeed all the symptoms of PCOS are worse with increasing body weight. The prevalence of obesity varies widely in different countries. It is lowest in countries such as China and Japan (<10%) and highest in the United States and some other Western countries (~70%). There is increased abdominal and visceral fat in women with PCOS, and this has been correlated to IR and metabolic dysfunction (Lord, 2006). Therefore lifestyle management has to be a priority for women with PCOS and must be maintained lifelong.

Metabolic syndrome, which is largely driven by obesity and leads to diabetes and CVD, has a prevalence during the reproductive years. The prevalence of metabolic syndrome in the United States is approximately 60% in young (20 to 39 years) obese women with PCOS (Apridonidze, 2005). The diagnosis is made using Adult Treatment Panel III criteria (three of five of the following: waist circumference >88 cm, high-density lipoprotein <50 mg/dL, triglycerides >150 mg/dL; blood pressure >130/85 mm Hg, fasting blood sugar >110 mg/dL). In other countries in which obesity is less prevalent, the prevalence of metabolic syndrome in PCOS is still increased but is much lower (5% to 9%) (Carmina, 2006). The constellation of risk factors that make up metabolic syndrome will place women with PCOS at increased risk for CV disease and diabetes, but there is nothing specific of more significance regarding metabolic syndrome in PCOS.

## DIABETES

Type 2 diabetes mellitus is more prevalent (two to three times higher) in women with PCOS of reproductive age (Legro, 1999). This is driven by IR, which in turn is worsened by overweight status and menstrual irregularity. In prospective follow-up studies, there is a high conversion rate in women with PCOS from euglycemia toward impaired glucose tolerance, and in women followed for 6 years who had impaired glucose tolerance the conversion rate to frank diabetes was 54% (Norman, 2001). Thus it is extremely important to screen for diabetes in the overweight population with PCOS. It has been suggested that this is best done with an oral glucose tolerance test (Fauser, 2012). Lack of precision in the screening for diabetes with hemoglobin A1C measurements has precluded the recommendation of using hemoglobin A1C as a screening tool, although it has proven to be useful in the follow-up of women as they are being treated. Diet and exercise remain the mainstays of treatment, and metformin has a significant role to play. In at risk women and those with glucose intolerance and prediabetes, metformin is often used with doses of 1500 mg per day. Doses are often higher in the presence of diabetes.

## QUALITY-OF-LIFE ISSUES

Although the data are not completely consistent, it is generally stated that there is poor quality of life among women with PCOS. This is most likely related to their burden of being overweight, having irregular cycles, decreased fertility, and skin concerns such as acne and hirsutism, albeit not all women have the same number or degree of these symptoms. Depression is a factor, which may play a major role in women with PCOS seeking care and being compliant with diet, lifestyle, and various treatments. In a meta-analysis, Dokras found a fourfold increase in the prevalence of depression among women with PCOS (Dokras, 2011). A strong argument has been made for screening women with PCOS for depression. It has also been found that interventions, such as weight loss, are able to improve quality of life (Thomson, 2010).

## CARDIOVASCULAR CONCERNS

Women with PCOS have characteristic lipid and lipoprotein abnormalities (Wild, 1988) (Fig. 41.17), including the presence of abnormal lipoprotein particles, which adds to a long list of abnormalities that tend to increase cardiovascular (CV) risk. Table 41.3 depicts several CV risk factors, including the development of hypertension and diabetes as women approach menopause. Figure 41.18 depicts data that have been generated from retrospective observations, and although it is yet not definitively established that these risks pertain to all women with PCOS, it provides evidence suggesting concern. (Dahlgren, 1992). It is unlikely that these risks occur in women with "milder" phenotypes. Data have largely been obtained from women with more classic features of PCOS, particularly obesity. There is evidence that the milder phenotypes diagnosed using the Rotterdam criteria have fewer CV risk factors. Figure 41.19 depicts a hypothetical scheme for increasing CV risk in women with PCOS with various phenotypes (Jovanovic, 2010).

It is important to note, however, that there are no definitive data on whether PCOS increases CV mortality (Fauser, 2012). Although multiple risk factors are present (IR, lipids, adipocytokines, inflammatory markers, surrogate markers of atherosclerosis on imaging), (Fauser, 2012), retrospective analyses have shown no increase in mortality, except among diabetic women (Pierpoint, 1998; Wild, 2000; Fauser, 2012). There has been some consideration that the older retrospective studies focused on a younger population of women and may not have been sufficiently rigorous to establish whether there is, or is not, an increased CV risk in PCOS. However, a more recent study following a postmenopausal cohort presumed to have PCOS earlier in life has shown a lower CV event-free survival with time (greater CV mortality) in PCOS (Shaw, 2008) (Fig. 41.20). Although the conclusions are as yet unclear, women with PCOS should be counseled regarding CV risk factors and preventing hypertension, dyslipidemias, and diabetes by lifestyle modification and other means, as reviewed by the AEPCOS Society (Wild, 2010).

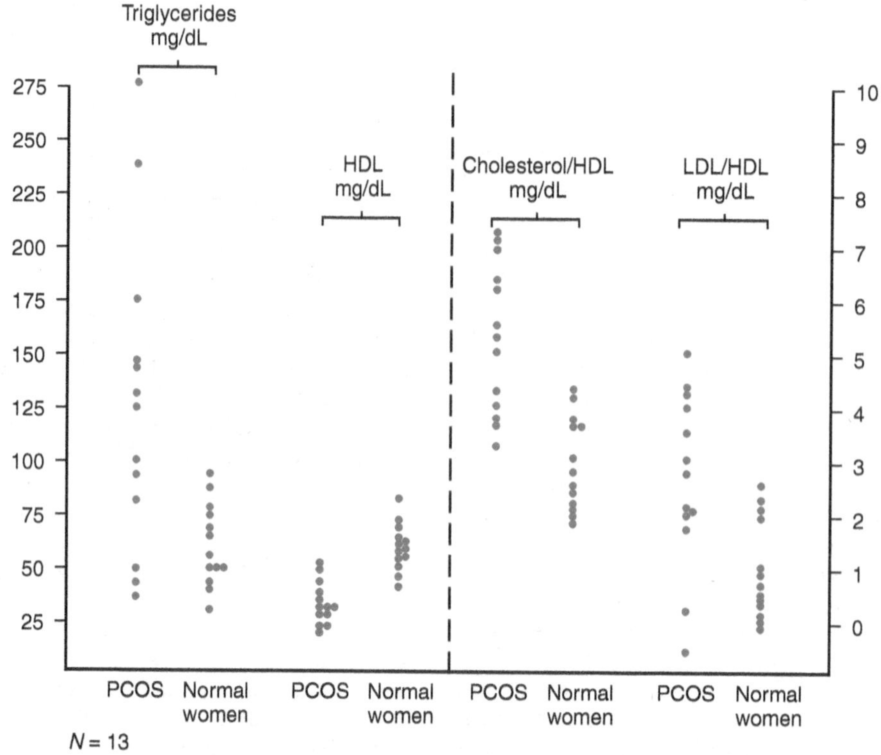


**Figure 41.17** Lipid and lipoprotein profiles in 13 women with polycystic ovary syndrome (PCOS) versus control group when matched for percent ideal body weight. Differences are evident in all measures ($P < .01$). *HDL,* High-density lipoprotein; *LDL,* low-density lipoprotein; *PCOS,* polycystic ovary syndrome . (From Wild RA, Bartholomew MJ. The influence of body weight on lipoprotein lipids in patients with polycystic ovary syndrome. *Am J Obstet Gynecol.* 1988;159[2]:423-427.)

**Table 41.3** Cardiovascular Risk Factors in Polycystic Ovary Syndrome

| Risk Factor | Features |
|---|---|
| Traditional risk factors | Obesity, insulin resistance, dyslipidemia, abnormal homocysteine, C-reactive protein, plasminogen activator inhibitor-1, increase in inflammatory adipocytokines such as TNF-α, decrease in adiponectin; higher prevalence of diabetes, hypertension |
| Atherosclerosis | Coronary catheterization studies, increase in carotid intima-media thickness, coronary calcium |
| Endothelial dysfunction by blood flow studies | All increased in classic PCOS; less of a concern with milder phenotypes using Rotterdam criteria |

*PCOS,* Polycystic ovary syndrome; *TNF-α,* tumor necrosis factor-α.

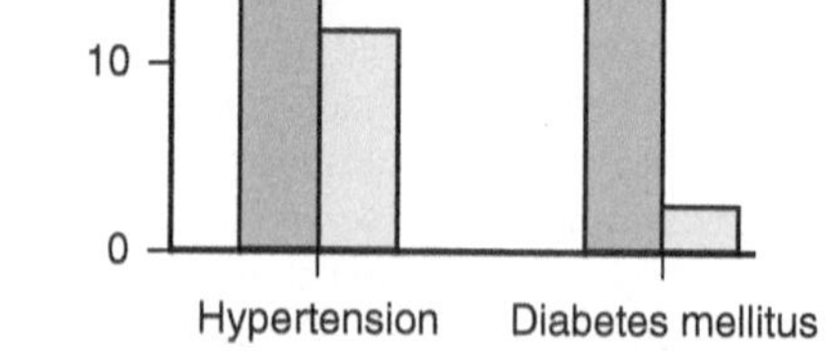

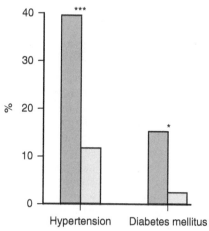


**Figure 41.18** Prevalence of hypertension (medically treated) and manifest diabetes mellitus in 33 polycystic ovary syndrome (PCOS) subjects and 132 referents. The *dark-shaded bars* indicate the PCOS subjects. The *light-shaded bars* indicate the referents. Statistical comparisons were made between the women with PCOS and referents. Differences were considered significant at $*P = .05$ and $***P = .001$. (From Dahlgren E, Janson PO, Johansson S, et al. Women with polycystic ovary syndrome wedge resected in 1956 to 1965: a long-term follow-up focusing on natural history and circulating hormones. *Fertil Steril.* 199;57[3]:505.)

**Evolving Cardio-Metabolic risks with various phenotypes relating to PCOS**

| | | IH | "PCOS" - D | OV-PCOS | "NIH" | Classic PCOS |
|---|---|---|---|---|---|---|
| Androgens NORMAL | NORMAL | ELEVATED | NORMAL | ELEVATED | ELEVATED | ELEVATED |
| Cycles NORMAL | NORMAL | NORMAL | IRREG (ANOV) | NORMAL (OVULAT) | IRREG (ANOV) | IRREG (ANOV) |
| Ovaries NORMAL | PAO/PCO | NORMAL | PAO/PCO | PAO/PCO | "NORMAL" | PAO/PCO |
| CV/Metab Risk NORMAL | NORMAL (+/-) | NORMAL-SMALL INCREASE | SMALL INCREASE | SOME INCREASE | INCREASE | INCREASE |
| Spectrum of risk modified by weight and familial/genetic profile | | | | | | |

**Figure 41.19** Evolving cardiometabolic risks with various phenotypes relating to polycystic ovary syndrome (PCOS). The spectrum of risk is modified by weight and familial and genetic profile. Anov, anovulatory; CV/Metab, cardiovascular/metabolic; IH, idiopathic hirsutism; NIH, National Institutes of Health; OV-PCOS, ovulatory PCOS; Ovulat, ovulatory; PAO/PCO, polycystic appearing ovary/polycystic ovary; PCOS-D, polycystic ovary syndrome phenotype D. (From Jovanovic VP, Carmina E, Lobo RA. Not all women diagnosed with PCOS share the same cardiovascular risk profiles. *Fertil Steril.* 2010;94[3]:826-832.)

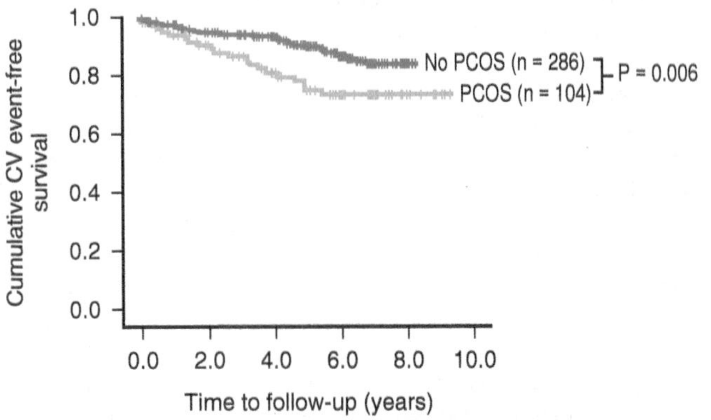


**Figure 41.20** Cumulative unadjusted cardiovascular (CV) death or myocardial infarction (MI)-free survival in postmenopausal women with or without clinical features of polycystic ovary syndrome (PCOS) ($P$ = .006). (From Shaw LJ, Merz CNB, Azziz R, et al. Postmenopausal women with a history of irregular menses and elevated androgen measurements at high risk for worsening cardiovascular event-free survival: results from the National Institutes of Health National Heart, Lung, and Blood Institute Sponsored Women's Ischemia Syndrome Evaluation. *J Clin Endocrinol Metab.* 2008;93[4]:1276-1284.)

## CANCERS IN POLYCYSTIC OVARY SYNDROME

As depicted in Figure 41.21, there is an age-specific onset for some of the consequences of PCOS. All cancers increase with aging, but endometrial cancer can begin at a younger age because of long-term anovulation and unopposed estrogen stimulation of the endometrium. It is likely that there are other susceptibilities as well, which contribute to the diagnosis of cancer at a younger age. Although breast cancer does not seem to be increased in women with PCOS (Chittenden, 2009), both endometrial and ovarian cancer are increased (Fauser, 2012; Chittenden, 2009). The data for these reports are negatively affected by the heterogeneity of the patient population and their retrospective nature. Most of the data pertain to women diagnosed with "classic" PCOS. It is likely that women with milder phenotypes may have little or no increased risk.

Endometrial cancer is increased at least two- to threefold, even when controlling for weight. Apart from unopposed estrogen being a risk factor, there may also be a defect in progesterone signaling in the endometrium among cancer patients (Savaris, 2011). The data are less strong for ovarian cancer, but the risk is thought to be about 2.5 times increased (Chittenden, 2009).

This level of risk for endometrial and ovarian cancer can be brought down to a normal rate with the use of oral contraceptives (OCs). The decreased risk of these cancers with the use of OCs for about 5 years is well known (Grimbizis, 2010) and translates into a good strategy for normalizing cancer risk in women with PCOS, particularly because many women normally would be treated with OCs in any event for other symptoms. Also of interest, is that there is a growing body of evidence that metformin, which may also be used for women with PCOS, has inhibitory effects on various cancers; the data are strongest for endometrial and breast cancer (Col, 2012; Tan, 2011).

## OVARIAN AGING: POLYCYSTIC OVARY SYNDROME AND MENOPAUSE

As all women age, the ovaries decrease in size and androgen levels decrease; this is true for those with PCOS as well. It is logical to assume therefore that at some juncture in time, the phenotype of PCOS may change or disappear. An interesting phenomenon, which has been well documented, is that as women with PCOS age, their menstrual cycles, if irregular when younger, become more regular and ovulatory (Elting, 2003; Carmina, 2012b).

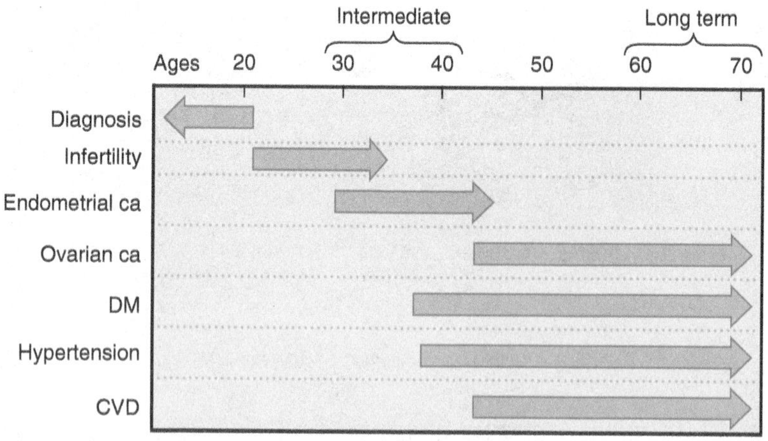


**Figure 41.21** Consequences of polycystic ovary syndrome (PCOS) as a function of age. *ca*, Cancer; *CVD*, cardiovascular disease; *DM*, diabetes mellitus.

This is because of a decrease in the total follicular cohort and subsequently lower levels of AMH (Carmina, 2012a). In our longitudinal studies of women with PCOS, followed for 20 years, by the fourth decade nearly half of the women had evidence of ovulatory function, and in 8% the diagnosis of PCOS could no longer be made (Carmina, 2012b).

Although with aging the follicular cohort is decreased, compared to other women of the same age, there are still more follicles, and typically higher levels of AMH. This leads to the notion that there may be preserved fertility in women with PCOS as they age. This has been confirmed in one retrospective study in an IVF model, in which the live birth rate was higher at an older age compared to women with tubal disease (Mellembakken, 2011). As women enter menopause, which is likely to be at a later age (although not well documented [Fauser, 2012]), despite lowered androgen levels, hirsutism may still be prevalent (Schmidt, 2011). There is also evidence that there is a persistence of the metabolic issues that existed at an earlier age (Puurunen, 2011), thus requiring continued vigilance in managing and following these women.

## ISOLATED POLYCYSTIC OVARIES

We have found that normal ovulatory women with PAO or PCOM have a subtle form of ovarian hyperandrogenism when stimulated with gonadotropins or human chorionic gonadotropin (hCG) (Wong, 1995). We have also found subtle changes in insulin sensitivity and altered lipoproteins (Chang, 2000). Therefore, although many women with isolated PAO or PCOM may not have any problems, this finding may be considered as a risk factor for developing the consequences of PCOS.

## TREATMENT OF POLYCYSTIC OVARY SYNDROME

Treatment of women with PCOS should be directed at the specific complaint. These concerns fall into three main categories: androgen excess and symptoms of hyperandrogenism; irregular bleeding (in this setting often called dysfunctional uterine bleeding) and risks of endometrial disease due to unopposed estrogen stimulation from anovulation; fertility concerns and subfertility, mostly due to anovulation. In addition, a common complaint is weight gain or the inability to lose weight. This is also related to IR and metabolic concerns discussed previously. Accordingly, regardless of the complaint, lifestyle management is an extremely important component of any treatment regimen.

Androgen excess (acne, hirsutism, and alopecia) occurs in the majority of women with PCOS, but not in all women. At times the symptoms are sufficiently mild that the treatment focus is on other concerns such as subfertility. Specific treatment for androgen excess symptoms is covered in Chapter 40 and usually involves the use of an OC, with or without an anti androgen.

Treatment of irregular bleeding should be directed at supplying the missing progesterone in anovulatory women. This potentially can lead to endometrial hyperplasia or cancer if not treated. Women who are overweight and older are a higher risk group, and endometrial biopsy may be indicated, although there are no validated guidelines as to when a biopsy should be carried out (Fauser, 2012). It is important to remember that it is the women with PCOS along with menstrual irregularity who have IR and are more likely to have metabolic dysfunction. OCs are the most logical and effective treatment, particularly because it is known that they reduce the risk of endometrial cancer. OCs may also be indicated for treatment of symptoms of androgen excess. In other women, progestogen therapy alone may be used at 2- to 3-month intervals to shed the endometrium in chronically anovulatory women. Medroxyprogesterone acetate (5 to 10 mg) or norethindrone acetate (2.5 to 10 mg) may be used in this setting. More complicated cases of menometrorrhagia are treated, as would other patients, as discussed in Chapter 26.

Treatment of subfertility in PCOS is predominantly due to anovulation. Even women with the ovulatory phenotype "C" may have subtle ovulatory disturbances, and it is known that some women have endometrial defects in progesterone and insulin signaling (DuQuesnay, 2009). Prior to treatment with ovulation induction, it is important to rule out other fertility factors, specifically male factors by obtaining a semen analysis (see Chapter 42).

## TREATMENT OF SUBFERTILITY IN POLYCYSTIC OVARY SYNDROME

Before ovulation induction, it is necessary to normalize overt abnormalities in glucose tolerance and to encourage weight loss for overweight women. Ovulation induction may be accomplished by a variety of agents, including metformin, clomiphene,

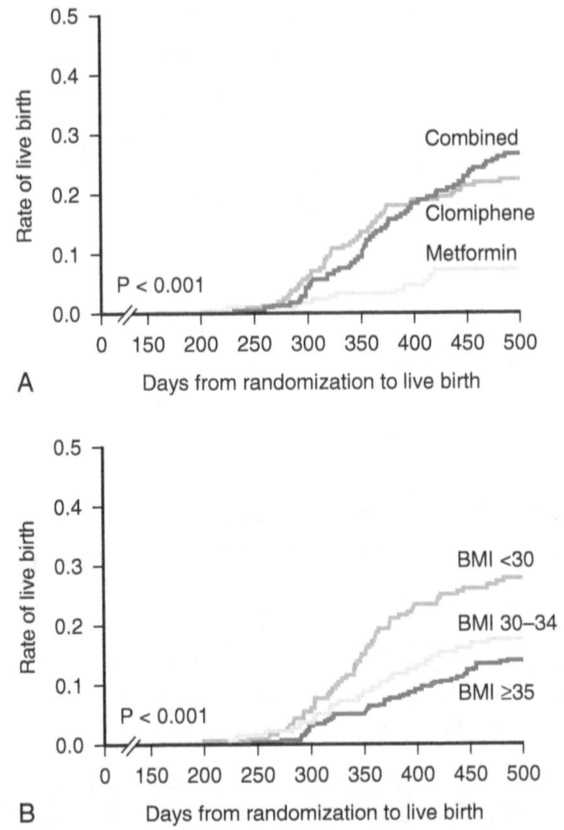


**Figure 41.22** Kaplan-Meier curves for live birth, according to study group (**A**) or by BMI, body mass index (**B**) (From Legro RS, Barnhart HX, Schlaff WD, et al. Clomiphene, metformin, or both for infertility in the polycystic ovary syndrome. *N Engl J Med.* 2007;356[6]:551-566.)

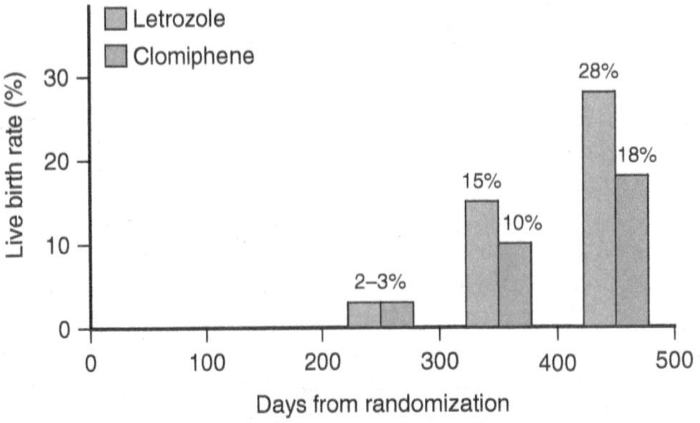


**Figure 41.23** Results of a prospective randomized trial in women with polycystic ovary syndrome (PCOS) comparing the live-birth rates of the administration of letrozole versus clomiphene (Kaplan-Meier curves). Letrozole performed significantly better. (Data from Legro RS, Brzyski RG, Diamond MP, et al. Letrozole versus clomiphene for infertility in the polycystic ovary syndrome. *N Engl J Med.* 2014;371[2]:119-129.)

letrozole, gonadotropins, and pulsatile GnRH, as well as ovarian diathermy or drilling. Adjunctive measures include the use of dexamethasone, dopamine agonists, thiazolidinediones, and various combinations of these options, although today, these agents are rarely used. In vitro fertilization (IVF; stimulated or unstimulated) may be indicated in difficult-to-manage cases or if other in fertility factors are present (Thessaloniki ESHRE/ASRM-Sponsored PCOS Consensus Workshop Group, 2008).

Although metformin had been used as a first-line treatment for infertility, with supportive evidence for some effectiveness including data from a Cochrane review (Tang, 2013), more recent randomized trials with a focus on live births as an end point have suggested that clomiphene is superior to metformin for first-line therapy (Legro, 2007) (Fig. 41.22). Metformin should be used for overweight and obese women to achieve better metabolic control prior to pregnancy and for those who may have a more casual approach to their fertility, in that metformin takes longer to become effective and may not induce ovulation in some women. Even when metformin cannot induce ovulation, its continued use may be beneficial when combined with clomiphene or gonadotropins. An improvement in oocyte quality with metformin has been suggested, but the effect has not been proved. It may decrease the risk of ovarian hyperstimulation syndrome (OHSS) in women with PCOS undergoing IVF (Tso, 2009; Palomba, 2011).

Clomiphene has been the mainstay for ovulation induction. Most pregnancies occur within the first few cycles. Accordingly, it is reasonable to use clomiphene, with or without metformin, as an initial approach, after obtaining a semen analysis, but not for more than three or four ovulatory cycles before a more comprehensive workup is undertaken. Letrozole (2.5 to 5 mg/day, 5 days) has proved to be efficacious as an alternative to clomiphene, and it is particularly suited for women who have side effects with clomiphene. In a randomized head-to head comparison of clomiphene and letrozole in women with PCOS, letrozole was found to be superior (Legro, 2014) (Fig. 41.23). This was also confirmed in a Cochrane review (Franik, 2015), and a cost analysis has also shown letrozole to be more cost effective as a first-line treatment, thus establishing its place as first-line treatment for women with PCOS. Low-dose gonadotropin therapy is highly effective as a second-line treatment (for failure with oral agents and for the occasional patient who may have transitory low estrogen status); there is no evidence that any one gonadotropin preparation is better than another (Thessaloniki ESHRE/ASRM-sponsored PCOS Workshop Group, 2008).

Currently, pulsatile GnRH therapy is rarely used, primarily because its use is cumbersome and less effective in PCOS compared with its use for hypothalamic amenorrhea. Ovarian drilling (diathermy) is a reasonable second-line therapy, particularly in clomiphene failures and when gonadotropin therapy has proved difficult. In randomized trials against standard gonadotropin therapy, ovarian drilling resulted in similar pregnancy rates but with a lower rate of multiple pregnancies (Thessaloniki ESHRE/ASRM-sponsored PCOS Workshop Group, 2008). However, in the United States, ovarian "drilling" or "diathermy" is rarely carried out, in part because of cost concerns.

For women who fail to conceive with ovulation induction over six cycles and in those with other infertility factors, IVF is the next step. Details of this treatment may be found in Chapter 43. *The only caveat to IVF treatment in women with PCOS is the higher-than-normal risk of OHSS.* This should always be kept in mind in treating women with PCOS, with significant dose adjustments in the treatment regimen, and using antagonist cycles, possibly metformin (when indicated) and the GnRH agonist trigger (see Chapter 43).

## METABOLIC AND WEIGHT CONCERNS

The key management strategy should be directed at altering lifestyle variables. Exercise regimens, particularly when coordinated with a group of similar women, have been shown to be beneficial. Details of these approaches may be found elsewhere. However, this approach should be part of all therapies for PCOS, acknowledging that some thin and normal-weight women with PCOS probably already have a healthy lifestyle.

Metabolic syndrome (MBS), driven largely by weight in the United States, is usually treated by a combination of diet and metformin. Six- to 12-month therapy has been shown to reduce weight by 5% to 7%, as well as to reduce insulin resistance and improve metabolic parameters. Positive results also have been reported with the use of bariatric surgery in obese women with PCOS, where most of the symptoms of PCOS were found to disappear after surgery (Escobar-Morreale, 2005). Nevertheless, this approach carries risks and should not be considered as first-line therapy.

Some data suggest that the use of antiandrogens (specifically flutamide) may also be efficacious for reducing body weight and visceral fat in women with PCOS (Gambineri, 2006). A combination of drospirenone and 17α-ethinylestradiol ($EE_2$) with flutamide and metformin also has been used successfully in adolescents (Ibanez, 2005). However, this multidrug regimen has not been tested in an adult population. Although therapy for women with PCOS should be directed at a woman's specific complaint, improvement of lifestyle variables, including weight reduction and fitness, should be the mainstay of all treatments. Metformin has an important role for metabolic concerns, particularly when MBS is present, and may aid in cases of subfertility.

A summary of various treatments for specific complaints in PCOS is provided in Table 41.4. Resources for patients may be found at Australia AEPCOS (jeanhailes.org.au/health-a-z/pcos), Endo Society (www.ae-society.org), and American Society for Reproductive Medicine (www.asrm.org).

**Table 41.4** Treatment for Women with Polycystic Ovary Syndrome

| Complaint | Treatment Options |
|---|---|
| Infertility | Letrozole, clomiphene, with or without metformin, gonadotropins, ovarian cautery ("drilling") |
| Skin manifestations | Oral contraceptive + antiandrogen (spironolactone, finasteride), GnRH agonists |
| Abnormal bleeding | Cyclic progestogen, oral contraceptives |
| Weight, metabolic concerns | Diet/lifestyle management, metformin |

*GnRH*, Gonadotropin-releasing hormone.

## KEY POINTS

- There are three criteria to diagnose PCOS; the diagnosis is based on clinical criteria, not laboratory values.
- The most frequently used diagnostic criteria for PCOS (called the *Rotterdam criteria*) require finding any two of the following: menstrual irregularity, hyperandrogenism, or polycystic ovaries on ultrasound.
- The disorder is heterogeneous and is not a single gene disorder, although several susceptibility genes have been identified; environmental influences are most likely involved as well.
- If untreated, women with PCOS have an increased risk of developing diabetes mellitus and hypertension after menopause; women with the disorder may have increased cardiovascular disease, although whether cardiovascular mortality is increased has not been confirmed.
- Treatment of women with PCOS should be directed at the specific complaint: menstrual function, skin disorders of androgen excess, or subfertility. Typically, more than one complaint exists and can be dealt with concomitantly unless the woman is trying to conceive.
- Weight gain and metabolic concerns (particularly insulin resistance, prediabetes, etc.) are extremely common and should be treated aggressively (usually with lifestyle management), particularly before pregnancy.
- Long-term consequences of PCOS include cardiovascular and metabolic concerns and the increased risks of endometrial and ovarian cancer, unless OCs have been used. With ovarian aging, cycles may become more regular, and some but not all the symptoms of PCOS may disappear as women approach menopause. The age of menopause may be later.
- Women with PCOS who desire fertility should be treated with agents that stimulate ovulation. Letrozole and clomiphene are first-line agents, with the former being more successful. Gonadotropins and ovarian "drilling" are second-line treatments, which are less commonly used today in the United States, with an approach of progressing women to IVF more quickly.

## KEY REFERENCES

Abbott DH, Barnett DK, Bruns CM, et al. Androgen excess fetal programming of female reproduction: a developmental aetiology for polycystic ovary syndrome? *Hum Reprod Update.* 2005;11:357–374.

Apridonidze T, Essah PA, Luorno MJ, et al. Prevalence and characteristics of the metabolic syndrome in women with polycystic ovary syndrome. *J Clin Edocrinol Metab.* 2005;90:1929–1935.

Azziz R, Carmina E, Dewailly D, et al. Positions statement: criteria for defining polycystic ovary syndrome. *Fertil Steril.* 2006;81:19–25.

Bridges NA, Cooke A, Healy MJ, et al. Standards for ovarian volume in childhood and puberty. *Fertil Steril.* 1993;60:456–460.

Carmina E, Campagna AM, Lobo RA. A 20-year follow-up of young women with polycystic ovary syndrome. *Obstet Gyn.* 2012b;119(2):263–269. Part 1.

Carmina E, Campagna AM, Mansuet P, et al. Does the level of serum antimullerian hormone predict ovulatory function in women with polycystic ovary syndrome with aging? *Fertil Steril.* 2012a;98(4):1043–1046.

Carmina E, Lobo RA. The use of fasting blood to assess the prevalence of insulin resistance in Polycystic Ovary Syndrome (PCOS). *Fertil Steril.* 2004; 82(3):661–665.

Carmina E, Lobo RA. Prevalence and metabolic characteristics of adrenal androgen excess in hyperandrogenic women with different phenotypes. *J Endocrinol Invest.* 2007;30(2):111–116.

Carmina E, Napoli N, Longo RA, et al. Metabolic syndrome in polycystic ovary syndrome (PCOS): lower prevalence in southern Italy than in the USA and the influence of criteria for the diagnosis of PCOS. *Eur J Endocrinol.* 2006;154(1):141–145.

Carmina E, Oberfield SE, Lobo RA. The diagnosis of polycystic ovary syndrome in adolescents. *Am J Obstet Gynecol.* 2010;203:201–205.

Casadei L, Madrigale A, Puca F, et al. The role of serum anti-Mullerian hormone (AMH) in the hormonal diagnosis of polycystic ovary syndrome. *Gynecol Endocrinol.* 2013;29(6):545–550.

Chae SJ, Kim JJ, Choi YM, et al. Clinical and biochemical characteristics of polycystic ovary syndrome in Korean women. *Hum Reprod.* 2008;23(8):1924–1931.

Chang PL, Lindheim SR, Lowre C, et al. Normal ovulatory women with polycystic ovaries have hyperandrogenic pituitary-ovarian responses to gonadotropin-releasing hormone-agonist testing. *J Clin Endocrinol Metab.* 2000;85(3):995–1000.

Chen Zi-Jiang, Zhao Han, He Lin, et al. Genome-wide association study identifies susceptibility loci for polycystic ovary syndrome on chromosome 2p16.3, 2p21 and 9q33.3. *Nat Genet.* 2010;43(1):55–60.

Chittenden BG, Fullerton G, Maheshwari A, et al. Polycystic ovary syndrome and the risk of gynaecological cancer: a systematic review. *Reprod BioMed Online.* 2009;19:398–405.

Christ JP, Willis AD, Brooks ED, et al. Follicle number, not assessments of the ovarian stroma, represents the best ultrasonographic marker of polycystic ovary syndrome. *Fertil Steril.* 2014;101(1):280–287.

Col NF, Ochs L, Spingmann V, et al. Metformin and breast cancer risk: a meta-analysis and critical literature review. *Breast Cancer Res Treat.* 2012; 135(3):P639–P646.

Dahlgren E, Janson PO, Johansson S, et al. Women with polycystic ovary syndrome wedge resected in 1956 to 1965: a long-term follow-up focusing on natural history and circulating hormones. *Fertil Steril.* 1992;57:505–513.

Dewailly D, Andersen CY, Balen A, et al: "http://www.ncbi.nlm.nih.gov/pubmed/24430863" The physiology and clinical utility of anti-Mullerian hormone in women. *Hum Reprod Update.* 2014;20:370–385.

Dokras A, Clifton S, Futterweit W, et al. Increased risk for abnormal depression scores in women with polycystic ovary syndrome: a systematic review and meta-analysis. *Obstet Gynecol.* 2011;117(1):145–152.

DuQuesnay R, Wright C, Azziz AA, et al. Infertile women with isolated polycystic ovaries are deficient in endometrial expression of osteopontin but not alphavbeta3 integrin during the implantation window. *Fertil Steril.* 2009;91(2):489–499.

Elting MW, Kwee J, Korsen TJ, et al. Aging women with polycystic ovary syndrome who achieve regular menstrual cycles have a smaller follicle cohort than those who continue to have irregular cycles. *Fertil Steril.* 2003;79:1154–1160.

Escobar-Morreale HF, Botella-Carretero JI, Alvarez-Blasco F, et al. The polycystic ovary syndrome associated with morbid obesity may resolve after weight loss induced by bariatric surgery. *J Clin Endocrinol Metab.* 2005;90: 6364–6369.

Fauser B, Tarlatzis B, Rebar RW, et al. Consensus on women's health aspects of polycystic ovary syndrome (PCOS): the Amsterdam ESHRE/ASRM-sponsored 3rd PCOS Consensus Workshop Group. *Fertil Steril.* 2012;97(1): 28–38e25.

Franik S, Kremer JA, Nelen WL, et al. Aromatase inhibitors for subfertile women with polycystic ovary syndrome: summary of a Cochrane review. *Fertil Steril.* 2015;103(2):353–355.

Fulghesu AM, Angioni S, Frau E, et al. Ultrasound in polycystic ovary syndrome—the measuring of ovarian stroma and relationship with circulating androgens: results of a multicentric study. *Hum Reprod.* 2007;22(9): 2501–2508.

Gambineri AA, Patton L, Vaccina A, et al. Treatment with flutamide, metformin and their combination added to a hypo caloric diet in overweight-obese women with polycystic ovary syndrome: a randomized, 12 month, placebo-controlled study. *J Clin Endocrinol Metab.* 2006;91:3970–3980.

Grimbizis GF, Tarlatzis BC. The use of hormonal contraception and its protective role against endometrial and ovarian cancer. *Best Pract Res Clin Obstet Gynaecol.* 2010;24(1):29–38.

Ibanez L, deZegher F. Flutamide-metformin plus ethinylestradiol-drospirenone for lipolysis and antiatherogenesis in young women with ovarian hyperandrogenism: the key role of metformin at the start and after more than one year of therapy. *J Clin Endocrinol Metab.* 2005;90(1). 39–34.

Iliodromiti S, Kelsey TW, Anderson RA, et al. Can anti-mullerian hormone predict the diagnosis of polycystic ovary syndrome? A systematic review and meta-analysis of extracted data. *J Clin Endocrinol Metab.* 2013;98(8): 3332–3340.

Jovanovic VP, Carmina E, Lobo RA. Not all women diagnosed with PCOS share the same cardiovascular risk profiles. *Fertil Steril.* 2010;94(3):826–832.

Kosova G, Urbanek M. Genetics of the polycystic ovary syndrome. *Mol Cell Endocrinol.* 2013;373(l-2):29–38.

Legro RS, Barnhart HX, Schlaff WD, et al. Clomiphene, metformin, or both for infertility in the polycystic ovary syndrome. *N Engl J Med.* 2007;356:551–566.

Legro RS, Brzyski RG, Diamond MP, et al. Letrozole versus clomiphene for infertility in the polycystic ovary syndrome. *N Engl J Med.* 2014;371(2): 119–129.

Legro RS, Kunselman AR, Dodson WC, et al. Prevalence and predictors of risk for type 2 diabetes mellitus and impaired glucose tolerance in polycystic ovary syndrome: a prospective, controlled study in 254 affected women. *J Clin Endocrinol Metab.* 1999;84:165–169.

Lobo RA. A unifying concept for polycystic ovary syndrome. In: Jeffrey Chang R, ed. *Polycystic Ovary Syndrome.* Serono Symposia USA: Springer; 1996.

Lobo RA, Goebelsmann U. Effect of androgen excess on inappropriate gonadotropin secretion as found in polycystic ovary syndrome. *Am J Obstet Gynecol.* 1982;142:394–401.

Lobo RA, Goebelsmann U, Horton R. Evidence for the importance of peripheral tissue events in the development of hirsutism in polycystic ovary syndrome. *J Clin Endocrinol Metab.* 1983;57:393–397.

Lord J, Thomas R, Fox B, et al. The central issue? Visceral fat mass is a good marker of insulin resistance and metabolic disturbance in women with polycystic ovary syndrome. *BJOG.* 2006;113:1203–1209.

Mellembakken JR, Berga SL, Kilen M, et al. Sustained fertility from 22 to 41 years of age in women with polycystic ovarian syndrome. *Hum Reprod.* 2011;26(9):2499–2504.

Mutharasan P, Galdones E, Penalver Bernabe B, et al. Evidence for chromosome 2p16.3 polycystic ovary syndrome susceptibility locus in affected women of European ancestry. *J Clin Endocrinol Metab.* 2013;98(1):E185–E190.

*NIH Evidence-based Methodology Workshop on Polycystic Ovary Syndrome (PCOS) Summary.* December, 2012. Full report available at. https://prevention.nih.gov/docs/programs/pcos/FinalReport.pdf.

Norman RJ, Masters L, Milner CR, et al. Relative risk of conversion from normoglycaemia to impaired glucose tolerance or non-insulin dependent diabetes mellitus in polycystic ovarian syndrome. *Hum Reprod.* 2001;16:1995–1998.

Palomba S, Falbo A, Carrillo L, et al. Metformin reduces risk of ovarian hyperstimulation syndrome in patients with polycystic ovary syndrome during gonadotropin-stimulated in vitro fertilization cycles: a randomized, controlled trial. *Fertil Steril.* 2011;96(6):1384–1390.

Panidis D, Tziomalos K, Misichronis G, et al. Insulin resistance and endocrine characteristics of the different phenotypes of polycystic ovary syndrome: a prospective study. *Hum Reprod.* 2012;27(2):541–549.

Pierpoint T, McKeigue PM, Isaacs AJ, et al. Mortality of women with polycystic ovary syndrome at long-term follow-up. *J Clin Epidemiol.* 1998;51:581–586.

Puurunen J, Piltonen T, Morin-Papunen L, et al. Unfavorable hormonal metabolic, and inflammatory alterations persist after menopause in women with PCOS. *J Clin Endocrinol Metab.* 2011;96:1827–1834.

Robinson S, Kiddy D, Gelding SV, et al. The relationship of insulin insensitivity to menstrual pattern in women with hyperandrogenism and polycystic ovaries. *Clin Endocrinol (Oxf).* 1993;39(3):351–355.

Rotterdam ESHRE/AS RM-Sponsored PCOS Consensus Workshop Group: Revised 2003 consensus on diagnostic criteria and long-term health risks related to polycystic ovary syndrome. *Fertil Steril.* 2004;81:19–25.

Sam S, Dunaif A. Polycystic ovary syndrome: syndrome XX? *Trends Endocrinol Metab14.* 2003:365–370.

Savaris RF, Groll JM, Young SL, et al. Progesterone resistance in PCOS endometrium: a microarray analysis in clomiphene citrate-treated and artificial menstrual cycles. *J Clin Endocrinol Metab.* 2011;96:1737–1746.

Schmidt J, Brannstrom M, Landin-Wilhelmsen K, et al. Reproductive hormone levels and anthropometry in postmenopausal women with polycystic ovary syndrome (PCOS): a 212-year follow-up study of women diagnosed with PCOS around 50 years ago and their age-matched controls. *J Clin Endocrinol Metab.* 2011;96:2178–2185.

Shaw LJ, Bairey Merz CN, Azziz R, et al. Postmenopausal women with a history of irregular menses and elevated androgen measurements at high risk for worsening cardiovascular event-free survival: results from the National Institutes of Health – National Heart, Lung, and Blood Institute sponsored Women's Ischemia Syndrome Evaluation. *J Clin Endocrinol Metab.* 2008;93:1276–1284.

Shi Y, Zhao H, Shi Y, et al. Genome-wide association study identifies eight new risk loci for polycystic ovary syndrome. *Nat Genet.* 2012;44(9):1020–1027.

Stein IF, Leventhal ML. Amenorrhea associated with bilateral polycystic ovaries. *Am J Obstet Gynecol.* 1935;29:181.

Strauss JF, Barbieri RL, eds. *Yen and Jaffe's Reproductive Endocrinology.* 6th ed. Philadelphia: WB Saunders; 2009:509.

Tan BK, Adya R, Chen JU, et al. Metformin treatment exerts antiinvasive and antimetastatic effects in human endometrial carcinoma cells. *J Clin Endocrinol Metab.* 2011;96(3):808–816.

Tang T, Balen AH. Use of metformin for women with polycystic ovary syndrome. *Hum Reprod Update.* 2013;19(1):1.

Thessaloniki ESHRE/ASRM-Sponsored PCOS Consensus Workshop Group. Consensus on infertility treatment related to polycystic ovary syndrome. *Fertile Steril.* 2008;89:505–522.

Thomson RL, Buckley JD, Lim SS, et al. Lifestyle management improves quality of life and depression in overweight and obese women with polycystic ovary syndrome. *Fertil Steril.* 2010;94:1812–1816.

Tso LOI, Costello MF, Albuquerque LE, et al. Metformin treatment before and during IVF or ICSI in women with polycystic ovary syndrome. *Cochrane Database Syst Rev.* 2009;(2):CD006105.

Vink JM, Sadrzadeh S, Lambalk CB, et al. Heritability of polycystic ovary syndrome in a Dutch twin-family study. *J Clin Endocrinol Metab.* 2006;91:2100–2104.

Wild RA, Bartholomew MJ. The influence of body weight on lipoprotein lipids in patients with polycystic ovary syndrome. *Am J Obstet Gynecol.* 1988;159: 423–427.

Wild RA, Carmina E, Diamanti-Kandarakis E, et al. Assessment of cardiovascular risk and prevention of cardiovascular disease in women with the polycystic ovary syndrome: a position statement by the Androgen Excess & Polycystic Ovary Syndrome (AE-PCOS) Society. *J Clin Endocrinol Metab.* 2010;95(5):1830–1832.

Wild S, Pierpoint T, McKeigue P, et al. Cardiovascular disease in women with polycystic ovary syndrome at long-term follow-up: a retrospective cohort study. *Clin Endocrinol (Oxf).* 2000;52:595–600.

Wong L, Morris RS, Lobo RA, et al. Isolated polycystic morphology in ovum donors predicts response to ovarian stimulation. *Hum Reprod.* 1995;10: 524–528.

Zawadzki JK, Dunaif A. Diagnostic criteria for polycystic ovary syndrome: towards a rational approach. In: Dunaif A, Merriam G, Haseltine F, eds. *Polycystic Ovary Syndrome.* Cambridge, MA: Blackwell Scientific; 1992:377–381.

Zhao Han, Su Xinghua, Xing Xiue, et al. Family-based analysis of susceptibility loci for polycystic ovary syndrome on chromosome 2p16.3, 2p21 and 90q33.3. *Hum Reprod.* 2012;27(1):294–298.

Suggested Readings can be found on ExpertConsult.com.

# 42

# Infertility

## Etiology, Diagnostic Evaluation, Management, Prognosis

*Roger A. Lobo*

The term *infertility* is generally used to indicate that a couple has a reduced capacity to conceive as compared with the mean capacity of the general population. In a group of normal fertile couples, the monthly ability to get pregnant, or *fecundability,* is approximately 20%. This figure is important for all couples seeking fertility to know, because it will alleviate unrealistic expectations of immediate success with various therapies, which can only approach 20%/cycle (with the exception of *in vitro fertilization–embryo transfer* [IVF-ET]). For most couples, the correct term should be *subfertility*, suggesting a decreased capacity for pregnancy but not an impossible feat.

The Centers for Disease Control and Prevention (CDC) also distinguishes between *infertility,* which uses a more strict definition of only married couples having trouble getting pregnant, and *impaired fecundity,* which is a more general term applying to all women who have difficulty conceiving or carrying a pregnancy to term (CDC, 2015).

The definition of infertility is the inability of a couple to conceive after one year of trying. This timeline is relevant to help determine when an infertility investigation should begin. In women older than 35 years, this timeline should be after 6 months of trying. An early investigation is also warranted if any of the following is present: oligo/amenorrhea; known tubal obstruction, uterine disease, or severe endometriosis; or known male factor (Practice Committee ASRM, 2012a).

The World Health Organization (WHO) has defined infertility as a disease and a significant cause of disability (warranting evaluation and treatment) (www.who.int/reproductivehealth/topics/infertility/definitions). Clearly, infertility is a cause of major distress for couples and should be assessed thoroughly and not neglected; and as with other disorders, counseling and support groups should be available in the clinical setting.

## INCIDENCE OF SUBFERTILITY AND INFERTILITY

Results from the three U.S. National Surveys of Family Growth performed under the direction of U.S. government agencies have provided information about infertility in this country. Analyses of the data obtained from the surveys performed in 1982, 1988, and 1995 have indicated that the proportion of U.S. women ages 15 to 44 years with impaired fecundity increased from 8% in 1982 and 1988 to 10% in 1995, a 20% rise. It was estimated that the number of women with impaired fecundity in the United States increased from 4.6 million to 6.2 million between 1982 and 1995, a 35% rise. Most of this increase occurred among nulliparous women in the oldest age group (35 to 44) because women of the Baby Boom generation were reaching this age. Many in this group had delayed childbearing. According to data from the CDC, in 2002, 7.4% of all women aged 15 to 44 in the United States had infertility, using the CDC's strict definition; and in the latest 2006-2010 survey, this occurred in 6% of the population. Impaired fecundity occurred in 10.9% of the reproductive age group in the 2006-2010 survey. The number of women in the reproductive age group who have ever received any infertility services has remained constant between the 2002 and 2006-2010 surveys: 7.4 million women, or 11.9% of the population (CDC, 2015).

## INFERTILITY AND AGE

Data from both older and more recent studies have indicated that the percentage of infertile couples increases with increasing age of the female partner. Analysis of data from three national surveys in the United States has revealed that the percentage of presumably fertile married women not using contraception who failed to conceive after 1 year of trying steadily increased from ages 25 to 44 years (Menken, 1986) (Table 42.1). Data from a study of presumably fertile nulliparous women married to husbands with azoospermia who underwent donor artificial insemination revealed that the percentage who conceived after 12 cycles of insemination declined substantially after age 30 (Schwartz, 1982) (Table 42.2). This older, classic study used fresh semen; currently, only frozen donor sperm is used, which does not achieve as favorable pregnancy rates. Decreasing fecundability with age is even more pressing in this context. With IVF, data from the Society for Assisted Reproductive Technology (SART) in the United States providing information on 165,172 cycles in 2012 has shown that the percentage of deliveries per oocyte retrieval procedure is 43.4% in women younger than 35, 25.4% by ages 38 to 40, and 14% by ages 41 to 42 years, and only 5% in women over 42 years (www.sart.org/find_frm.html).

In general terms, approximately one in seven couples are infertile if the wife is 30 to 34, one in five is infertile if she is 35 to 40, and one in four is infertile if she is 40 to 44 years of age. Another way to interpret these data is to state that as compared with women aged 20 to 24 years, fertility is reduced by 6% in the next 5 years, by 14% between ages 30 and 34, by 31% between ages 35 and 39, and to a much greater extent after age 40. Of interest is the finding that the most common diagnostic category among women undergoing IVF in the United States in the most recent survey (2012) cited previously is diminished ovarian reserve: 17% of cycles; which is a characteristic of older women undergoing treatment (www.sart.org/find_frm.html).

Table 42.1 Married Women Who Are Infertile, by Age*

| Age (yr) | Infertile (%) |
|---|---|
| 20-24 | 7.0 |
| 25-29 | 8.9 |
| 30-34 | 14.6 |
| 35-39 | 21.9 |
| 40-44 | 28.7 |

From Menken J, Trussell J, Larsen U. Age and infertility. *Science*. 1986;233:1389-1394.
*From three national U.S. surveys.

Table 42.2 Pregnancy Rates by Age at 1 Year in Normal Women with Azoospermatic Husbands after Donor Insemination

| Age (yr) | Pregnancy Rate (%) |
|---|---|
| <25 | 73.0 |
| 26-30 | 74.1 |
| 31-35 | 61.5 |
| 36-40 | 55.8 |

From Schwartz D, Mayaux MJ. Female fecundity as a function of age: results of artificial insemination in 2193 nulliparous women with azoospermic husbands. *N Engl J Med*. 1982;306(7):404-406.

## FECUNDABILITY: THE ABILITY TO CONCEIVE

Analysis of data from presumably fertile couples who stop using contraception to conceive has shown that approximately only 50% of the couples will conceive in 3 months, 75% will conceive in 6 months, and by 1 year approximately 90% will have conceived (Hull, 1985) (Fig. 42.1). Statistical analysis of these data indicates that the normal monthly fecundability is approximately 0.2 (20%).

This information is extremely important when analyzing data concerning the results of various treatment methods applied to a group of infertile couples. This group includes those with hypofertility from presumed causes (e.g., mild endometriosis) as well as those with idiopathic (unexplained) infertility. For example, it has been estimated that if the mean fecundability of the population is 0.2 (a 20% monthly rate), this rate decreases over time (Leridon, 1984) (Table 42.3). Analysis of these statistical tables reveals that after 2 years of trying to conceive, approximately 4% of these couples will not have conceived. Their mean monthly fecundability is approximately 0.08, and 57% will conceive in the next year. Of the 2% still not pregnant at this time, after 3 years after trying to conceive, the monthly fecundability drops to approximately 0.06, 0.05, and 0.04 in the next 3 years, respectively. Thus in the fourth, fifth, and sixth years of attempting to conceive, only 48%, 42%, and 37% of nonpregnant women should conceive without treatment.

Several studies have reported the incidence of spontaneous conception among infertile couples without a specifically diagnosed cause of infertility (unexplained infertility). A live birth rate among 873 infertile couples in several Canadian centers has been observed without treatment. The cumulative live conception rate at 3 years was 38.2% and was 45% after 7 years (Collins, 1995b) (Fig. 42.2). Among the total group with the diagnosis of unexplained infertility who received no treatment, one third had a live birth during the first 3 years of observation without treatment.

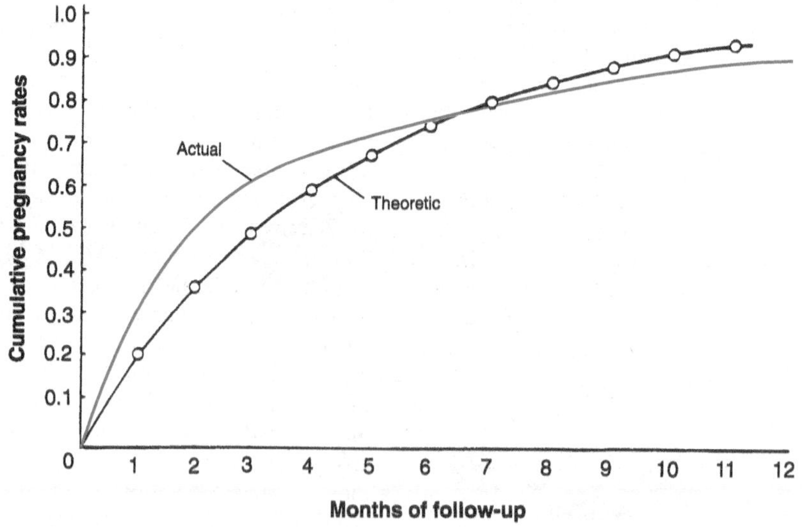


**Figure 42.1** Curve of theoretic time to pregnancy in women with a monthly fecundability of 0.2 *(open circles)* and curve of actual time to pregnancy in fertile women discontinuing contraception *(solid line)*. (Open circle data from Hull MG, Glazener CM, Kelly NJ, et al. Population study of causes, treatment, and outcome of infertility. *Br Med J*. 1985;291[6510]:1693-1697. Solid line data from Murray DL, Reich L, Adashi EY. Oral clomiphene citrate and vaginal progesterone suppositories in the treatment of luteal phase dysfunction: a comparative study. *Fertil Steril*. 1989;51[1]:35-41.)

Thus in order to determine that any method of treatment for infertility is superior to no treatment, the treatment results on the incidence of pregnancy over time must be statistically analyzed. Ideally, these results should be compared with an untreated control group. At the least, these pregnancy rates should be compared with the rates of the untreated women with a normal diagnostic evaluation (discussed later). Various statistical formulas for performing these analyses based on a life table analysis have been described. This statistical approach is necessary to determine whether treatment methods are beneficial.

## CAUSES OF INFERTILITY

The exact incidence of the various factors causing infertility varies among different populations and cannot be precisely determined. Collins reported that among 14,141 couples in 21 publications, ovulatory disorders occurred 27% of the time; male factors, 25%; tubal disorders, 22%; endometriosis, 5%; other, 4%; and unexplained factors, 17% (Collins, 1995a). It has not been shown that other abnormalities, such as antisperm antibodies, luteal phase deficiency, subclinical genital infection, or subclinical endocrine abnormalities such as hypothyroidism or hyperprolactinemia in ovulatory women are true causes of infertility. No prospective randomized studies have demonstrated that treatment of these latter entities results in greater fecundability than without treatment. If any of these do cause infertility, they do so infrequently. With current techniques of investigation, it is impossible to diagnose the cause of infertility in up to 20% of couples, and they are considered to have unexplained infertility. After a rigorous investigation, other reports have suggested this figure to be as low as 10%. However, it is unclear if subtle abnormalities, as noted, have much to do with infertility. Also, most couples with unexplained infertility are hypofertile (subfertile), and some are able to conceive without treatment, although it may take several years and with a diminishing probability of this occurrence over time.

Table 42.3 Incidence of Conception Over Time among Nonsterile Couples with Mean Fecundability of 0.2

| | Couples Not Yet Having Conceived | | |
|---|---|---|---|
| Months without Conception | Proportion (%) | Mean Fecundability | Proportion (%) of Couples Who Will Conceive (within 12 mo) |
| 0 | 100.0 | 0.20 | 86.0 |
| 6 | 31.9 | 0.14 | 77.0 |
| 12 | 14.0 | 0.11 | 69.2 |
| 24 | 4.3 | 0.08 | 57.0 |
| 36 | 1.9 | 0.06 | 48.2 |
| 48 | 1.0 | 0.05 | 41.7 |
| 60 | 0.6 | 0.04 | 36.7 |

Modified from Leridon H, Spira A. Problems in measuring the effectiveness of infertility therapy. *Fertil Steril.* 1984;41(4):580-586.

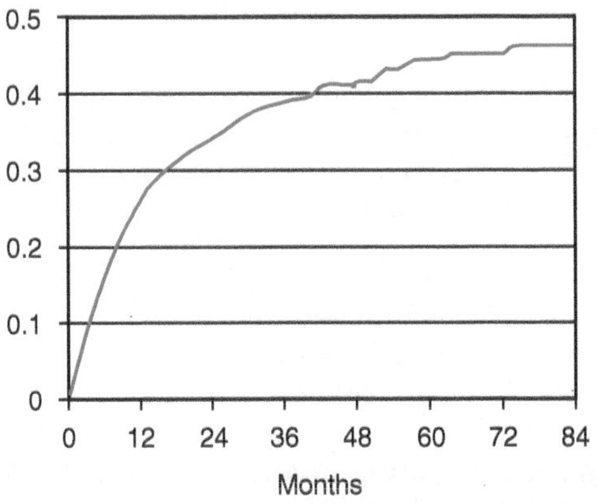


**Figure 42.2** Cumulative rate of conceptions leading to live birth. Couples (873) who remained untreated throughout follow-up; cumulative rate of live birth conception at 36 months was 38.2% (95% CI, 34.2-42.3). (Modified from Collins JA, Burrows EA, Wilan AR. The prognosis for live birth among untreated infertile couples. *Fertil Steril.* 1995;64[1]:22-28.)

## DIAGNOSTIC EVALUATION

The diagnostic evaluation of infertility should be thorough and completed as rapidly as possible. During the initial interview, the couple should be informed about normal human fecundity and how these probabilities decrease with increasing age of the female partner and with the duration of infertility. The various tests in the diagnostic evaluation and why they are performed should be thoroughly explained. The available therapies and prognosis for treatment of the various causes of infertility should also be included in the dialogue. The couple should be informed that after a complete diagnostic infertility evaluation, the cause for infertility cannot be determined in a large group of couples. For many couples, the reduced fecundability can be suggested to be age related. Methods to increase the fecundity of couples with a normal diagnostic evaluation, such as *controlled ovarian stimulation* (COS) and intrauterine insemination, as well as the possibility of *in vitro fertilization* (IVF) should also be covered.

Each couple should be instructed about the optimal time in the cycle for conception to occur and should be encouraged to have intercourse on the day before ovulation. Unless the husband has oligozoospermia (oligospermia), daily intercourse for 3 consecutive days at midcycle should be encouraged. When ovulation is more precisely determined, as with luteinizing hormone (LH) monitoring (discussed later), intercourse should occur for 2 consecutive days around the LH surge. Because the egg disintegrates less than 1 day after it reaches the ampulla of the oviduct, it is best that sperm be present in this area when the egg arrives so that fertilization can occur. Because normal sperm retain their fertilizing ability for up to 72 hours, it is preferable to have sperm in the oviduct prior to the arrival of the oocyte.

A study was performed by Wilcox and coworkers of fertile couples who stopped contraception to conceive and recorded the cycle day when they had sexual intercourse. Hormone analysis was performed to determine the day of ovulation. None of the women became pregnant in the group of couples who had intercourse after ovulation occurred. The pregnancy rate was approximately 30% if intercourse occurred on the day of ovulation, as well as 1 and 2 days prior to ovulation. The pregnancy rate was approximately 10% if coitus occurred 3, 4, or 5 days before ovulation. No pregnancies occurred when intercourse took place 6 days or more before ovulation (Wilcox, 1995)

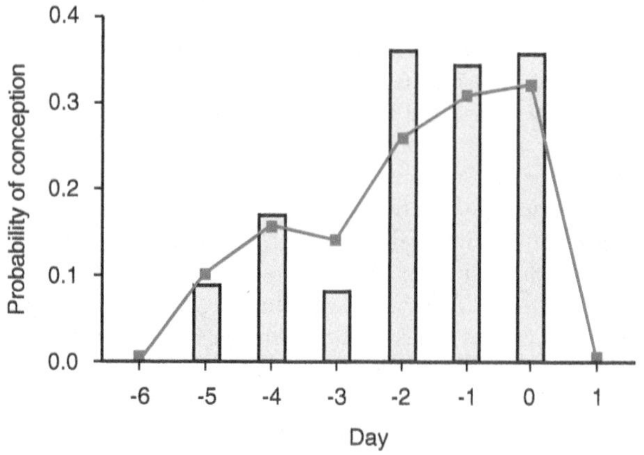


**Figure 42.3** Probability of conception on specific days near the day of ovulation. The *bars* represent probabilities calculated from data on 129 menstrual cycles in which sexual intercourse was recorded to have occurred on only a single day during the 6-day interval ending on the day of ovulation (day 0). The *solid line* shows daily probabilities based on all 625 cycles, as estimated by the statistical model. (From Wilcox AJ, Weinberg CR, Baird DD. Timing of sexual intercourse in relation to ovulation: effects on the probability of conception, survival of the pregnancy, and sex of the baby. *N Engl J Med.* 1995;333:1517-1521.)

(Fig. 42.3). It is therefore considered optimal to perform insemination or have sexual intercourse on the day before ovulation.

Because peak levels of LH occur 1 day before ovulation, measurement of LH by urinary LH immunoassays is the best way to determine the optimal time to have intercourse or an insemination. Tests that measure LH in a random daily urine specimen are usually more convenient for planning natural or artificial insemination than tests that detect LH in the first morning urine specimen. Ovulation most commonly occurs on the day following the detection of LH in a random specimen (12 to 24 hours later), and it occurs on the day when LH is detected in the first morning specimen, which contains urine formed during the prior night. Several types of commercial kits are available for determining peak LH, so women who find it difficult to determine a hormone change using one type can try another system or kit. Basal body temperature (BBT) charts are not as precise for determining ovulation, with ovulation occurring over a span of several days of the thermogenic shift.

In some cases, women produce less than adequate amounts of vaginal lubricant. Various vaginal lubricants and chemicals, as well as saliva, used to improve coital satisfaction may interfere with sperm transport. Some men experience midcycle impotence because of the pressure of performing intercourse on demand. In such cases, the intercourse schedule should be less rigorous. The couple should also be told that among fertile couples, there is only approximately a 20% chance of conceiving in each ovulatory cycle, even with optimally timed coitus, and that it takes time to become pregnant. Thus the terms *time* and *timing* should be emphasized during the initial counseling session. Couples should also be advised to cease smoking cigarettes and drinking caffeinated beverages in excess. Cigarette smoking and caffeine consumption have been shown independently in several studies to decrease the chances of conception. The common practice of vaginal douching also reduces the chance of conception by approximately 30%.

All couples should have a complete history taken, including a sexual history, and a physical examination. After this initial evaluation, tests should be undertaken to determine if the woman is ovulating and has patent fallopian tubes and if a semen sample of the male partner is normal.

## DOCUMENTATION OF OVULATION

Preliminary information that the woman is ovulatory is provided by a history of regular menstrual cycles. If the woman has regular menstrual cycles, a serum progesterone level should be measured in the midluteal phase to provide indirect evidence of ovulation as well as normal luteal function. Although serum progesterone levels vary in the normal luteal phase in a pulsatile manner, a serum progesterone level above 3 to 5 ng/mL suggests some ovulatory function, but it cannot indicate the adequacy of normal ovulation. Progesterone levels of 10 ng/mL or higher are found during at least 1 day of the luteal phase of normal ovulatory cycles in which conception occurred (Hull, 1982). Measurement of the daily BBT provides indirect evidence that ovulation has taken place but does not give as precise information about ovulation timing as the LH kit, or the quality of ovulation, by progesterone. The BBT graph also provides information about the approximate day of ovulation and duration of the luteal phase. The BBT should be taken shortly after awakening, only after at least 6 hours of sleep and prior to ambulating, with sublingual placement of a special thermometer with gradients between 96° and 100° F.

Women with oligomenorrhea (menses at intervals of 35 days or longer) or amenorrhea who wish to conceive should be treated with agents that induce ovulation, regardless of whether they have occasional ovulatory cycles. Therefore for these women, direct or indirect measurement of progesterone is unnecessary until after therapy is initiated.

The endometrial biopsy is sometimes considered as a diagnostic method for the adequacy of ovulation and luteal function. *We feel that an endometrial biopsy is not indicated in this setting.* It is invasive and painful, and it does not provide accurate information in terms of "endometrial dating" of the luteal phase, as was carried out in the past (Coutifaris, 2004).

## SEMEN ANALYSIS

Although information about ovulation is being obtained, the male partner's reproductive system should be evaluated by means of a semen analysis. Abnormalities in the semen analysis (male factor) occurs in approximately 20% of couples with infertility as the sole factor and may be involved in 30% to 40% of cases overall. The male partner should be advised to abstain from ejaculation for 2 to 3 days before collection of the semen sample. It is best to collect the specimen in a clean (not necessarily sterile) wide-mouthed jar after masturbation. It is important that the entire specimen be collected, because the initial fraction contains the greatest density of sperm. Ideally, collection should take place in the location where the analysis will be performed. The degree of sperm motility should be determined as soon as possible after liquefaction, which usually occurs 15 to 20 minutes after ejaculation. Sperm motility begins to decline 2 hours after ejaculation, and it is best to examine the specimen within this period. Semen should not be exposed to marked changes in temperature and, if collected at home during cold weather, the specimen should be kept warm during transport to the laboratory.

Parameters used to evaluate the semen include volume, viscosity, sperm density, sperm morphology, and sperm motility. The last parameter should be evaluated in terms of percentage of total motile sperm as well as quality of motility (rapidity of movement and amount of progressive motility). Sperm morphology is an extremely important parameter, which is correlated to fertilizing ability. Using strict criteria (Kruger), only approximately 4% or more of the sperm in an ejaculate may be considered normal according to the most recent WHO criteria (WHO, 2010). It should be remembered that the sperm analysis is a subjective test and that there is a fair degree of variability from test to test in the same man. Also, the semen profile reflects sperm production that occurred 3 months earlier, which is important to note if there were illness at that time. Table 42.4 lists the parameters that are generally considered normal for a semen analysis, according to the latest WHO study. It is beyond our scope here to discuss fully the causes and diagnostic evaluation of semen abnormalities. In broad terms, the various causes of semen abnormalities are cited in Table 42.5.

When semen analyses were performed on a group of men whose wives had conceived within the past 4 months, approximately 75% had at least one abnormal characteristic and 25% had two abnormalities. These results confirm that there is normally a wide variability in the parameters used to characterize semen. Because the characteristics of semen may vary over time and undergo normal biologic variability, it is best to repeat the test at least once if an abnormality is found. If abnormalities persist, the male should have a urologic exam. It is important not to miss a rare abnormality, such as a testicular tumor; in addition it has been appreciated that male factor infertility is associated with other medical conditions and subsequent problems (Eisenberg, 2015).

The comprehensive evaluation should include a history of physical exam (occasionally with ultrasound); hormonal evaluation (LH, follicle-stimulating hormone [FSH], testosterone, estradiol, prolactin [PRL], and thyroid-stimulating hormone [TSH]); and genetic abnormalities (karyotype, and defects such as cystic fibrosis mutations and Y-chromosome microdeletions), particularly with severe sperm abnormalities (Practice Committee ASRM, 2012a).

## EVALUATION AND LABORATORY TESTS

Aspects of the woman's medical history that should be highlighted include the following: any pregnancy complications if previously pregnant; previous pelvic surgery of any type; significant dysmenorrhea; dyspareunia or sexual dysfunction; abnormal cervical cytology or procedures to treat cervical abnormalities; and use of medication, drugs, and tobacco. Family history should be explored for genetically related illnesses, birth defects and, most importantly, the history of age of menopause in female family members. Finally, any symptoms suggestive of endocrine disorders should be solicited (e.g., weight changes, skin changes).

The physical examination should focus on extremes of body mass, skin changes, thyroid abnormalities, breast secretion, abnormal pain on abdominal or pelvic examination, and assessment of the vagina and cervix. In addition, if available, vaginal ultrasound performed at the same time may be extremely

**Table 42.4** Lower Fifth Percentile Values in Fertile Men*

| Parameter | Value |
|---|---|
| Semen volume (mL) | 1.5 |
| Sperm concentration (million/mL) | 15 |
| Total number (million/ejaculate) | 39 |
| Total motility (%) | 40 |
| Progressive motility (%) | 32 |
| Normal forms (%) | 4 |

Modified from Cooper TG, Noonan E, von Eckardstein S, et al. World Health Organization reference values for human semen characteristics. *Hum Reprod Update*. 2010;16(3):231-245.
*With time to pregnancy ≤12 months.

**Table 42.5** Causes of Semen Abnormalities

| Finding | Cause |
|---|---|
| **Abnormal Count** | |
| Azoospermia | Klinefelter's syndrome or other genetic disorder |
| | Sertoli-cell-only syndrome |
| | Seminiferous tubule or Leydig cell failure |
| | Hypogonadotropic hypogonadism |
| | Ductal obstruction, including Young syndrome |
| | Varicocele |
| | Exogenous factors |
| Oligozoospermia | Genetic disorder |
| | Endocrinopathies, including androgen receptor defects |
| | Varicocele and other anatomic disorders |
| | Maturation arrest |
| | Hypospermatogenesis |
| | Exogenous factors |
| **Abnormal Volume** | |
| No ejaculate | Ductal obstruction |
| | Retrograde ejaculation |
| | Ejaculatory failure |
| | Hypogonadism |
| Low volume | Obstruction of ejaculatory ducts |
| | Absence of seminal vesicles and vas deferens |
| | Partial retrograde ejaculation |
| | Infection |
| High volume | Unknown factors |
| Abnormal motility | Immunologic factors |
| | Infection |
| | Varicocele |
| | Defects in sperm structure |
| | Metabolic or anatomic abnormalities of sperm |
| | Poor liquefaction of semen |
| Abnormal viscosity | Cause unknown |
| Abnormal morphology | Varicocele |
| | Stress |
| | Infection |
| | Exogenous factors |
| | Unknown factors |
| Extraneous cells | Infection or inflammation |
| | Shedding of immature sperm |

From Bernstein GS, Siegel MS. Male factor in infertility. In: Mishell DR Jr, Davajan V, Lobo RA, eds. *Infertility, Contraception and Reproductive Endocrinology*. 3rd ed. Cambridge, MA: Blackwell Scientific; 1991:629.

valuable in picking up abnormalities of the uterus (e.g., fibroids) endometrial thickness, pelvic masses, and ovarian morphology (e.g., polycystic appearance, unusually small). These may provide a guide for further testing.

In a healthy asymptomatic woman, only a complete blood count (CBC), blood type, Rh factor, and rubella status are needed, together with a Pap smear obtained within 12 months of the previous test.

Increasingly it is recommended (although not mandatory) to screen for genetic carrier status. Comprehensive screening for carrier status including Fragile X and other abnormalities such as cystic fibrosis is easily carried out at the time of routine blood testing. There are several laboratories that can do such screening. We use the Family Prep Screen offered by Counsyl (www.counsyl.com), in which more than 100 diseases may be screened for free; Counsyl also offers follow-up consultation.

Infectious disease screening (for chlamydia and gonorrhea) is carried out routinely in most practices at the time of the Pap smear. Further infectious disease screening (e.g., syphilis, HIV, hepatitis) is warranted, particularly for couples undergoing insemination or IVF.

In most women, and particularly in women older than 35 years, serum follicle-stimulating hormone (FSH) and estradiol ($E_2$) levels should be obtained on cycle day 2 or 3. Elevated FSH values (>10 mIU/mL), suggest decreased ovarian reserve, which reflects the pool of viable oocytes remaining in the ovary. Levels over 20 mIU/mL afford a particularly poor prognosis. However, although FSH levels tend to fluctuate from cycle to cycle, once the FSH level has been elevated in a given cycle, the overall prognosis is reduced. $E_2$ levels, if elevated on days 2 and 3 (>70 pg/mL), do not allow for a valid interpretation of FSH values and may independently suggest a decreased prognosis regarding ovarian reserve (Evers, 1998).

Antimüllerian hormone (AMH) or müllerian-inhibiting substance (MIS) has become a valuable standard for assessing ovarian reserve. MIS, which is produced by the granulosa cells of small growing follicles, physiologically suppresses FSH stimulation of sustained follicular growth. Levels are highest in young women and lower with reproductive aging; various nomograms by age have been established (Seifer, 2011) (Fig. 42.4). Serum AMH/MIS decreases with aging, and when levels reach 0.05 ng/mL (essentially undetectable levels), menopause occurs within 4 to 5 years (Sowers, 2008). Levels are higher in women with polycystic ovary syndrome (PCOS) (Iliodromiti, 2013). In terms of ovarian reserve, higher levels (>2 ng/mL) suggest a larger cohort of small available follicles and low levels (<0.5 ng/mL) suggest a decreased ovarian reserve, with the levels of AMH reflecting the sensitivity of the ovary to gonadotropic stimulation, and thus the choice of treatment when ovarian stimulation is desired (La Marca, 2014).

Unlike FSH, AMH/MIS values are fairly constant and stable throughout the menstrual cycle, particularly in the low ranges. Higher values, however, exhibit more variability in the early to midfollicular phase. It is now established that use of oral contraceptive pills decreases values by 15% to 20%.

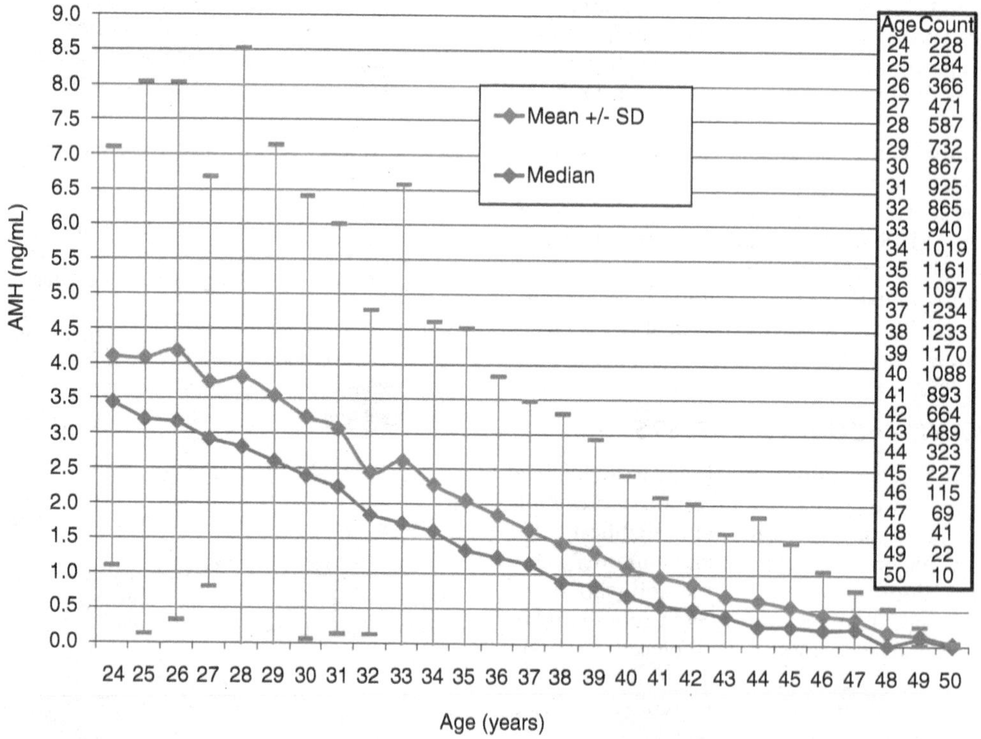


**Figure 42.4** AMH age-specific median values with mean ± standard deviation values for women ages 24 to 50, n = 17120, obtained at 1-year intervals. Note values are from a single laboratory using reagents from the older Beckman/Diagnostic Systems Laboratories (DSL) Generation 1 assay; thus assays systems will vary for the absolute numbers but not for the trend of declining values with age. (From Seifer D, Baker VL, Leader B. Age specific serum AMH values for 17120 women presenting to fertility centers within the United States. *Fertil Steril.* 2011;95[2]:747-750.)

From a clinical perspective, assays for AMH and MIS have not been standardized (several different assays have been used), requiring each clinician to establish his or her own normative data and receiver operating characteristic (ROC) curves, as our group has done, reflecting the values quoted earlier.

### *Use of Ultrasound in the Diagnostic Evaluation*

It is most common to carry out a pelvic ultrasound evaluation as part of the investigation. By so doing, significant pathology such as fibroids, endometriosis, and other pathology can be uncovered. In addition polycystic ovaries, which are prevalent, can be appreciated; and finally an antral follicle count (AFC) can be obtained, which is similar in value to the measurement of AMH, in the assessment of ovarian reserve. An age-related nomogram for AFCs has also been reported (Almog, 2011) (Fig. 42.5). For standardization it has been suggested that the AFC be obtained on cycle days 2 to 4 (Broekmans, 2010).

### *Other Blood Testing*

Some specialists obtain antibody titers for *Chlamydia trachomatis*, which if elevated may signify the possibility of tubal disease. It has been suggested that if the immunoglobulin G (IgG) antibody titer is greater than 1:32, 35% of patients have evidence of tubal damage. Whether this type of evaluation is routinely warranted as a focus for the infertility investigation continues to be debated.

Although not proven to be of major benefit in normal ovulatory women, most clinicians will measure TSH and prolactin at the screening visit. TSH values in the normal range (<4.4 μU/mL), but higher than 2.5 mIU/mL are often considered to be abnormal in women presenting with infertility. This is because normal values in the first trimester of pregnancy should be <2.5 μU/mL. However, there is no evidence that values between 2.5 to 4 μU/mL affect fertility status or outcomes of pregnancy (Practice Committee ASRM, 2015).

If an abnormality is found in one of the first two noninvasive diagnostic procedures (documentation of ovulation and semen analysis), it should be treated before proceeding with the more costly and invasive procedures, unless there is a history or findings suggestive of tubal disease. For example, if the woman has oligomenorrhea and does not ovulate each month, after a normal semen analysis is observed, ovulation should be induced with clomiphene citrate for two to three cycles before performing the other diagnostic measures. Provided that no other infertility factors are present, most anovulatory women (80%) conceive after induction of ovulation with therapeutic agents, and half the couples will conceive during the first three ovulatory cycles (Gysler, 1982).

If these initial diagnostic tests are normal, the more uncomfortable and costly hysterosalpingography (HSG) should be performed in the follicular phase of the next cycle.

### *Hysterosalpingography*

It is best to schedule the HSG during the week following the end of menses to avoid a possible pregnancy and also get better definition of the uterine cavity when the endometrium is still thin. The HSG should be avoided if there has been a history of salpingitis in the recent past or if there is tenderness on pelvic examination. As noted, most practices routinely screen for chlamydia and gonorrhea during the initial examination. However, we routinely prescribe prophylactic antibiotics at the time of HSG: doxycycline (100 mg twice daily for 3 days, starting 1 day before the procedure), but this recommendation is not universally followed. If a hydrosalpinx is seen with HSG, doxycycline should be continued for 1 week. The examination should be performed with use of a water-soluble contrast medium and

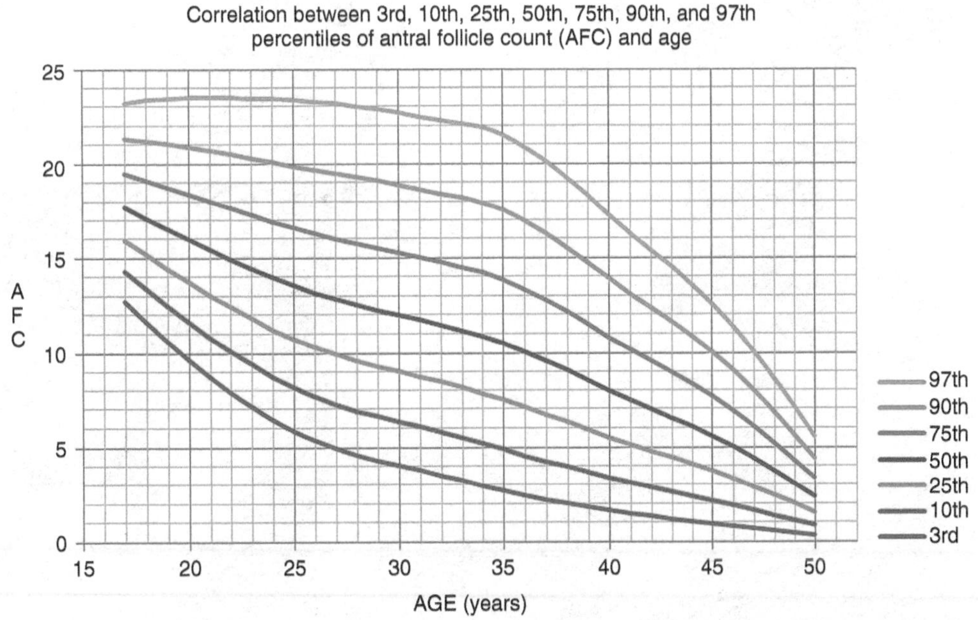


**Figure 42.5** Age-related nomogram for antral follicle count depicted by various percentiles showing a biphasic decline and with a poor antral follicle count defined by a value under eight. (From Almog B, Shehata F, Shalom-Paz E, et al. Age-related nomogram for antral follicle count: McGill reference guide. *Fertil Steril.* 2011; 95[2]:663-666.)

image-intensified fluoroscopy. A water-soluble contrast medium enables better visualization of the tubal mucosal folds and vaginal markings than an oil-based medium. It is important to be able to evaluate the appearance of the intratubal architecture to determine the extent of damage to the tube (Fig. 42.6, *A* and *B*). A meta-analysis, including four randomized trials, has indicated that a therapeutic benefit is more likely to occur when oil-soluble contrast media are used in an HSG performed for the diagnostic evaluation of infertility (Watson, 1994). The odds of pregnancy occurring after the procedure were twofold higher when oil-soluble media were used compared with water-soluble media. These results differ from those of a large randomized trial by Spring and colleagues that found no difference in pregnancy rates when the HSG was performed with oil-soluble or water-soluble contrast media (Spring, 2000). Thus the therapeutic benefit of oil-soluble contrast media remains inconclusive.

Because oil-soluble contrast media have more complications than water-soluble media, including pain resulting from peritoneal irritation and formation of granulomas, it is probably best to perform routine HSGs with water-based media. The diagnostic HSG will not only determine whether the tubes are patent but also, if disease is present, will help determine the magnitude of the disease process and provide information about the lining of the oviduct, and uterine cavity in particular, that cannot be obtained by laparoscopic visualization. The procedure can also determine whether salpingitis isthmica nodosa is present in the interstitial portion of the oviduct (Fig. 42.6, *C*). When an HSG shows lack of patency in one tube, this has been shown to be falsely positive, approximately 50% of the time at laparoscopy. Therefore it is not necessary to perform tubal reconstructive surgery on a woman with one patent tube. However, a diagnostic laparoscopy may be considered to detect the presence of peritubal adhesions. The finding of a normal endometrial cavity at the time of HSG obviates the need for hysteroscopy. If severe tubal disease, such as a large hydrosalpinx, is found at the time of HSG (Fig. 42.6, *D*), based on success rates, it is preferable for the couple to undergo IVF-ET than for the woman to have tubal surgery. If the hydrosalpinx is large and clearly visible on ultrasound, it is preferable to perform laparoscopic salpingectomy prior to IVF-ET because the pregnancy rate with IVF-ET may be decreased by as much as 40% (Zeyneloglu, 1998).

Quite frequently one or both tubes may show proximal obstruction. This may be the result of uterine spasm (contractions) due to the discomfort of the procedure, or due to true obstruction; the latter may be only a mild obstruction due to tubal debris. It has become common to attempt fluoroscopic-controlled

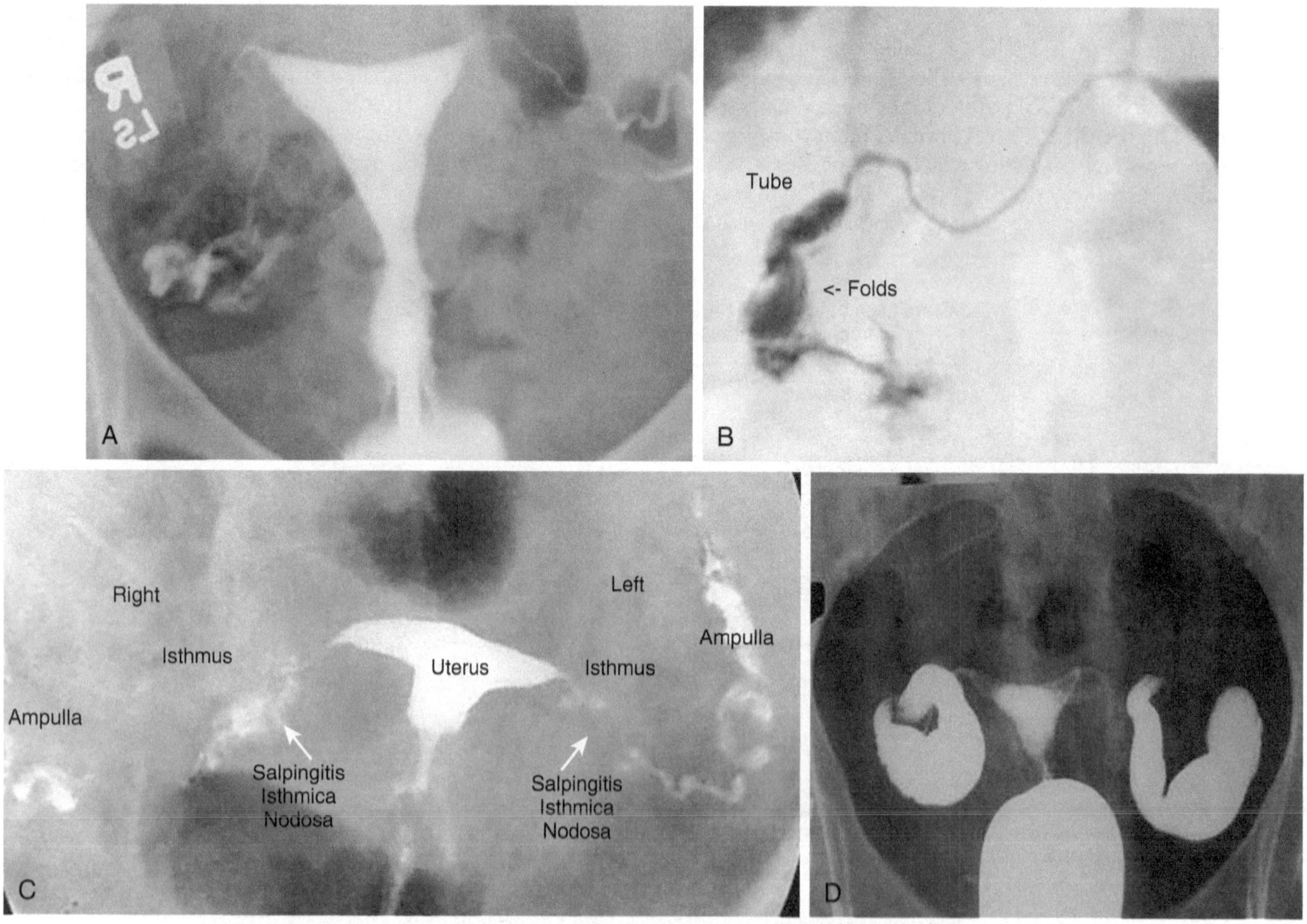


**Figure 42.6** Representative hysterosalpingograms showing a normal study (**A**), normal ampullary folds (**B**), bilateral salpingitis isthmica nodosa (proximal disease) (**C**), and bilateral hydrosalpinges (distal disease) (**D**).

selective cannulation of the proximal tube, either immediately or at a subsequent visit (Thurmond, 2008) (Fig. 42.7). This can be successful in up to 90% of cases, and if successful it alleviates either unnecessary concern or the need for laparoscopy or IVF.

When the extent of tubal disease is unclear or the couple prefers not to undergo IVF-ET, diagnostic laparoscopy should be carried out in the follicular phase of the cycle. In general, the goal should be to have all tubal reconstruction carried out laparoscopically (discussed later).

### *Postcoital Test (No Longer Routine)*

Although important from a physiologic standpoint (cervical mucus being important for sperm transport), the postcoital test (PCT) is now rarely indicated as a necessary part of the infertility investigation. It is a very subjective test. A normal PCT is one in which at least five motile sperm are visible in normal cervical mucus obtained from the upper canal just prior to ovulation. A suboptimal test can be the result of technique, timing of the test, and problems with cervical mucus or with sperm. Although a good PCT has been correlated with a better prognosis for pregnancy, sperm have been recovered at laparoscopy when there was a poor PCT. Moreover, because the suggested treatment for a poor PCT is intrauterine insemination after ovarian stimulation, this is the exact next step taken, even if the PCT is normal, in the setting of unexplained infertility. Occasionally, as may happen with an orthodox Jewish couple, a semen analysis cannot be obtained. Here, a PCT provides a surrogate for visualizing motile, normal-appearing sperm.

### *Laparoscopy: Is It a Routine Part of the Investigation?*

In the past, this was an obligatory final step in the infertility investigation when all other test results were normal. Data have shown that in 20% to 40% of cases, some minor abnormalities may be found (e.g., endometriosis, adhesions), which may have a bearing on fecundability. Obviously, if there is something suspicious on ultrasound or examination, there has been prior pelvic surgery or appendicitis, or there is pelvic pain or dyspareunia, the index of suspicion is increased. The probability that peritubal adhesions of sufficient severity to cause infertility will be found at the time of laparoscopy is less than 5% in a woman with no history of salpingitis or symptoms of dysmenorrhea, a normal bimanual pelvic examination, and normal antibody titers (if obtained) (Fatum, 2002). Provided the woman is younger than 40 years and is having ovulatory cycles, and there is an acceptable semen analysis and an age-appropriate maker of ovarian reserve such as AMH, several cycles of controlled ovarian stimulation and intrauterine insemination may be undertaken before performing diagnostic laparoscopy or going directly to IVF-ET. At this juncture, a decision can be revisited about whether performing a laparoscopy should be considered, although many couples usually prefer to proceed with IVF-ET, particularly if they have insurance coverage for IVF.

## *ADDITIONAL TESTING FOR COUPLES PRESENTING WITH INFERTILITY?*

### *Significance of a Diagnosis of Luteal Deficiency (Is This a True Diagnosis?)*

Although suggested for many years, it has never been established that luteal phase defects cause infertility. The diagnosis of luteal deficiency used to be made upon finding serum progesterone levels consistently below 10 ng/mL 1 week before menses or finding consistent evidence for a histologic delay (>3 days) in the pattern of the normal secretory endometrium, indicating an inadequate effect of progesterone on the endometrium. This endometrial defect had to be found in two consecutive cycles. Erroneous diagnoses of this

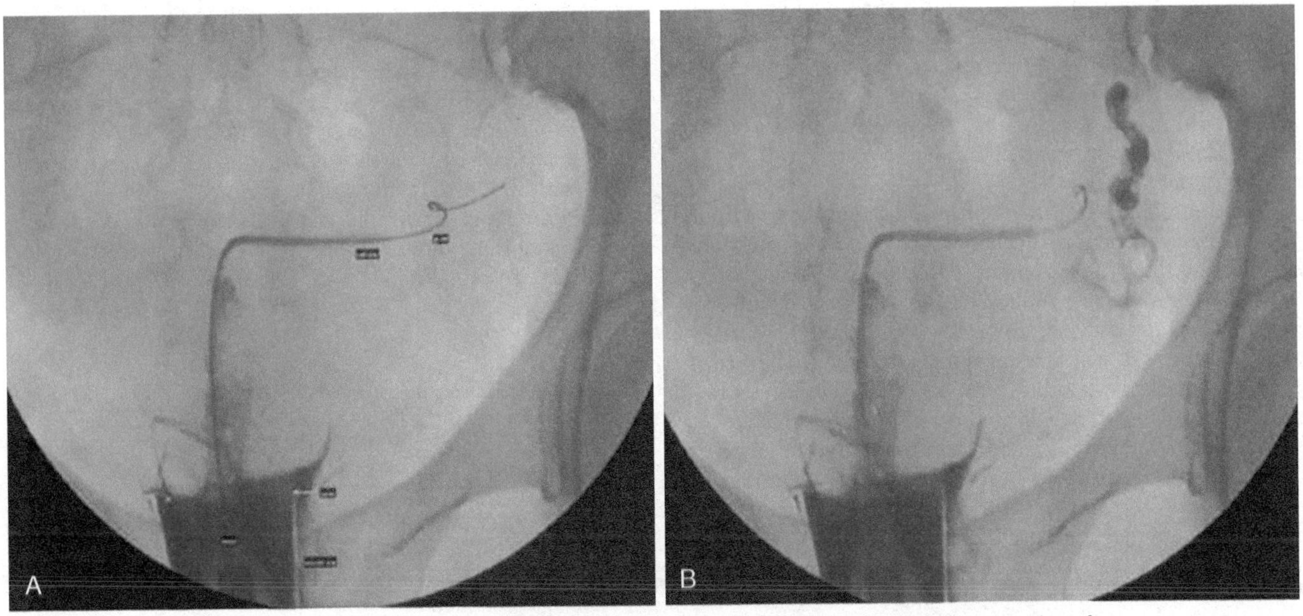


**Figure 42.7** Technique of tubal cannulation using a vacuum cup on the cervix, the introduction of a 5.5-French catheter into the tubal ostium under fluoroscopy; followed by a 0.015-inch guidewire into the fallopian tube for dislodgement of debris (**A**). **B** shows injection of contrast through a 3-French catheter into the tube confirming successful cannulation and a normal-appearing patent tube. (From Thurmond AS. Fallopian tube catheterization. *Semin Intervent Radiol.* 2008;25[4]:425-431.)

entity occur because of cycle variability and the subjective interpretation of histologic dating criteria. There is at least a 10% disagreement of more than 2 days when the same observer dated the specimens on two separate occasions, and even more interobserver variability. As noted earlier, more recent studies have confirmed the lack of efficacy of the endometrial biopsy (Coutifaris, 2004). *Routine endometrial biopsies for the diagnosis of infertility should not be carried out.*

As noted regarding the PCT, ovarian stimulation with intrauterine insemination (IUI) is often the first empirical treatment for unexplained infertility. This essentially treats the luteal inadequacy, if it exists, preempting the need for invasive and imprecise endometrial biopsies.

### Immunologic Factors in Subfertility?

Substantial evidence from animal studies has indicated that antibodies can be induced in females from antigens obtained from organs in the male reproductive tract, and that these antibodies interfere with normal reproduction. Both sperm-agglutinating and sperm-immobilizing antibodies have been found in the serum of some infertile women, but also in the serum of fertile control subjects. Agglutinating antibodies are found more frequently than immobilizing antibodies in most series and, in some reports, the incidence of sperm-agglutinating antibodies in infertile women is similar to that in the control group. Even with the finding of sperm agglutination or immobilization in interactions with serum (in vitro), it has not been demonstrated that a similar degree of sperm inactivation occurs in the lower genital tract. Thus there is no definitive evidence that sperm agglutination or immobilization in the serum of infertile women is the cause of their infertility. One of the reasons for this discrepancy is that both serum assays measure mainly IgM and IgG antibodies, whereas the antibodies locally produced in the genital tract are mainly IgA. Thus some investigators have measured antisperm antibodies in cervical mucus and found a correlation between their presence and infertility. However, no data have shown that the finding of antibodies against sperm in the male or female partner is a cause of infertility. In addition, corticosteroid treatment of the male or female partner does not significantly increase the pregnancy rate compared with no therapy.

Autoimmunity to sperm in semen and serum has been found in some infertile men, particularly those who have had testicular infection, injury, or a surgical procedure such as vasectomy reversal. Men with these antibodies have been treated with corticosteroid therapy and sperm-washing techniques. Nevertheless, the effectiveness of such treatment remains to be established.

Four prospective studies have reported the incidence of fertility occurring after a diagnostic infertility evaluation was performed in which the presence of antisperm antibodies was documented (Collins, 1993). These studies were performed in four different laboratories in three different countries. Several different techniques were used for the antibody tests. All four studies showed no correlation between the presence of antisperm antibodies in either member of the couple and the chance of conception. Pregnancy rates over time were similar in couples who had or did not have antisperm antibodies. Therefore tests to detect these antibodies as part of the diagnostic infertility evaluation are not justified because their presence does not affect fecundity.

### Significance of Infectious Diseases in Subfertility

Some researchers have suggested that asymptomatic, or occult, infection of the upper female genital tract and male genital tract is a cause of infertility. As early as 1973, it was suggested that infection with what was then called *T-mycoplasma* in the male could interfere with normal sperm function, and infection of the female reproductive tract could interfere with normal sperm transport. The current name now used for these organisms is *Ureaplasma urealyticum*. Two other microorganisms found in the female genital tract are *Mycoplasma hominis* and *M. fermentans*. Although it has been reported that treatment of infertile couples with antibiotics, such as tetracycline or doxycycline, that eradicate these organisms result in high pregnancy rates, controlled studies have reported no difference in pregnancy rates between couples treated with antibiotics and those not treated. Harrison and colleagues have studied 88 infertile couples with no demonstrable cause of infertility. One third were treated with doxycycline, one third received placebo, and one third received no treatment. T-mycoplasma was isolated from approximately two thirds of the couples in each group and was eradicated only in the group treated with doxycycline. Nevertheless, conception rates were similar in each group (Harrison, 1975) as was also reported by Matthews and coworkers (Matthews, 1978) (Table 42.6). Other investigators have suggested that asymptomatic *Chlamydia trachomatis* infection may also cause infertility, but the dosage of doxycycline used in the randomized studies cited earlier would also have eradicated these organisms. Thus there is no evidence that asymptomatic infection of the genital tract of the human male or female causes infertility.

### Are Other Tests of Sperm Function Indicated?

In that the semen analysis is subjective and variable, it has long been suggested that other more functional tests would improve the evaluation of the male partner (Oehninger, 2014).The zona-free hamster egg penetration test originally described by Yanagimachi and associates was a test developed to predict the fertilizing ability of sperm and provides an additional, perhaps more sensitive, parameter for assessing sperm function than routine semen analysis. However, many variables factors affect the test results. It has been shown that this test does not correlate well with IVF of human eggs. The sensitivity and specificity of the hamster egg penetration assay (sperm penetration assay) is considered to be too low to justify its routine use as part of the infertility investigation.

**Table 42.6** Controlled Studies of Outcome of Therapy of Couples with Unexplained Infertility and *Urea urealyticum* Infections

| Study* | Treatment | No. of Couples | No. of Pregnancies | Conceptions (%) |
|---|---|---|---|---|
| Harrison et al | Doxycycline | 30 | 5 | 17 |
| | Placebo | 28 | 4 | 14 |
| | None | 30 | 5 | 17 |
| Matthews et al | Treated | 51 | 10 | 20 |
| | None | 18 | 4 | 22 |

From Bernstein GS. Occult genital infection and infertility. In: Mishell DR Jr, Davajan V, Lobo RA, eds. *Infertility, Contraception and Reproductive Endocrinology*. 3rd ed. Cambridge, MA: Blackwell Scientific; 1991.
*From original source.

Other functional tests of sperm (such as the hypo-osmotic swelling test) assess the integrity of the sperm cell membrane, and others (the zona pellucida binding test, acrosome reaction, and the hyaluronan binding assay) assess maturity and viability (Oehninger, 2014). However, there is no evidence, at present, that these tests add information to the infertility investigation or affects treatment. The DNA fragmentation test in sperm has become popular. This test, which is carried out by flow cytometry or direct microscopy, determines the rate of DNA fragments; a DNA fragmentation index of more than 30% has been suggested to indicate a poorer rate of fertilization and therefore suggests the need for IVF with intracytoplasmic sperm injection (ICSI). However, at present, there is no evidence that this correlates with the success of IVF, and it cannot be advocated as a routine test (Practice Committee ASRM, 2014).

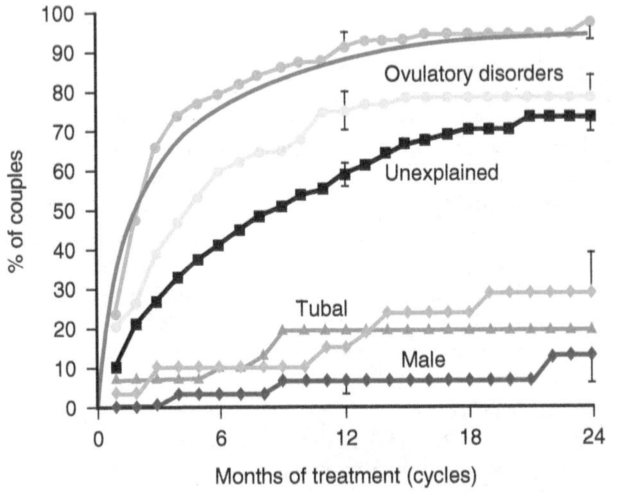


**Figure 42.8** Effect of various treatments on fecundability: ovulatory, tubal, and male factors. (Modified from Hull MG, Glazener CM, Kelly NJ, et al. Population study of causes, treatment, and outcome of infertility. *Br Med J.* 1985;291[6510]:1693-1697.)

## PROGNOSIS OF VARIOUS DIAGNOSES UNCOVERED BY THE INFERTILITY INVESTIGATION

Before discussing the specific treatments for abnormalities uncovered by the investigation, it is useful to frame a prognosis for the couple depending on what factor(s) have been found.

The highest probability of conception with treatment other than with IVF-ET occurs among couples in whom anovulation is the only abnormality, with substantially lower probabilities of pregnancy in couples with tubal disease and sperm abnormalities (Hull, 1985) (Fig. 42.8). Although these data are older, this information from Hull still provides the best available comparisons. Among a group of infertile couples with unexplained infertility who were followed for 2 years without treatment after the evaluation was completed, it was found that the chances of becoming pregnant were greater in women younger than 35 years (~75%) than in women older than 35 (50%) (Hull, 1985) (Fig. 42.9). The cumulative conception rate at the end of 2 years without therapy for those couples was much greater for those who had tried to conceive for less than 3 years before evaluation (~75%)

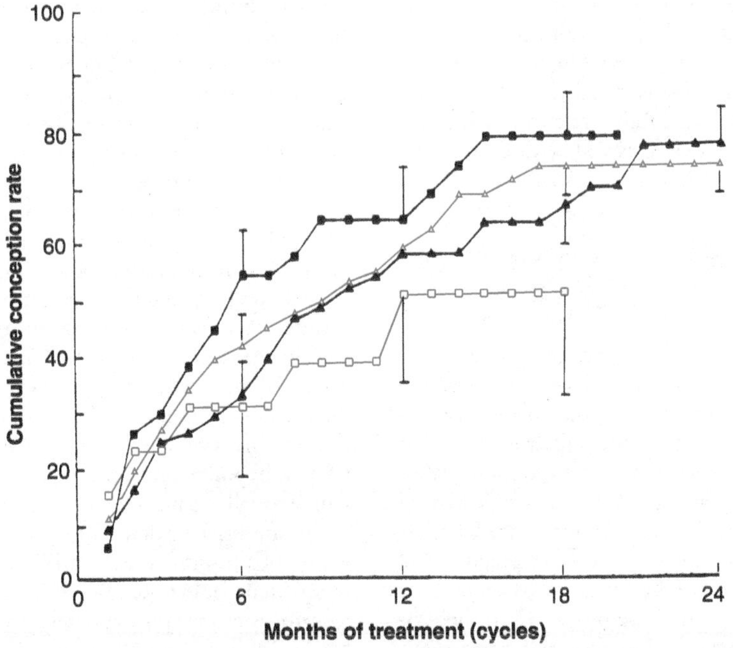


**Figure 42.9** Cumulative rates of conception from first attendance at clinic in couples with unexplained infertility related to age of woman. Rates for each age group are shown as solid squares, <25 years; blue triangles, 25 to 29 years; solid triangles, 30 to 34 years; blue squares, >35 years. Standard errors of proportions are given at 6, 12, 18, and 24 months. (From Hull MG, Glazener CM, Kelly NJ, et al. Population study of causes, treatment, and outcome of infertility. *Br Med J.* 1985;291[6510]:1693-1697.)

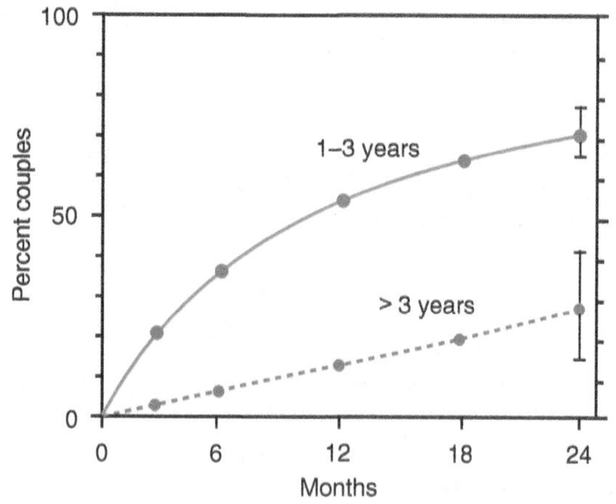


**Figure 42.10** Cumulative pregnancy rates in unexplained infertility without treatment related to duration of infertility. (From Hull MG. Effectiveness of infertility treatments: choice and comparative analysis. *Int J Gynaecol Obstet.* 1994;47[2]:99-108.)

than those who had tried to conceive for more than 3 years (~30%) (Hull, 1994) (Fig. 42.10). In three of the four studies of infertile couples who received no therapy mentioned earlier, more than 50% of the couples who eventually conceived did so in the first year after completing the infertility evaluation. It has been suggested that certain couples have a better prognosis for spontaneous conception after the initial investigation, based on age and the time of trying to conceive. This has been defined as >30% within a year of the evaluation (Hunault, 2004), and it has been suggested that in these couples, it may not be necessary to start empiric treatment (discussed later). Generally, for couples presenting with the inability to conceive, even if no factors have been found (unexplained infertility), in order to increase their chances of conception or to shorten the time interval until conception takes place, various empiric treatments have been advocated. This generally increases the fecundity rate from a baseline of around 4% to 9% to 10% per cycle as will be discussed later in the Unexplained Infertility section.

## OUTCOMES OF PREGNANCY IN WOMEN UNDERGOING VARIOUS TREATMENTS

Ovulation-inducing drugs and reconstructive tubal surgery have independently been shown to be associated with an *increased incidence of ectopic pregnancy* compared with the normal population (see Chapter 17). Use of ovulation-inducing drugs alone has been shown to increase the incidence of multiple gestations. With IVF the chances of multiple gestations is better controlled based on the decision to transfer one or more embryos (see Chapter 43). However, IVF does increase the risk of ectopic pregnancies, with a higher rate based on the number of embryos transferred (Perkins, 2015). There is also an increase in the risk of heterotopic pregnancies. Therefore if conception occurs after treatment with ovulation induction or tubal reconstructive surgery, monitoring of early gestation with serial human chorionic gonadotropin (HCG) levels and ultrasonography assists in determining whether the pregnancy is intrauterine and how many gestational sacs are present. However, infertile couples who conceive do not have a higher rate of spontaneous abortion or perinatal mortality than normal couples. In older women, nevertheless, there is a higher loss rate because of aneuploidy.

## TREATMENT OF THE CAUSES OF INFERTILITY

The management of the various causes of infertility will be presented here in the order generally followed in an infertility investigation.

### *MEDICAL TREATMENT FOR ANOVULATION*

Therapeutic agents currently available to induce ovulation are clomiphene citrate, letrozole, and urinary and recombinant gonadotropins. Adjunctive treatments include gonadotropin-releasing hormone (GnRH) agonist and antagonists, as well as HCG, which is used to trigger ovulation. In addition, as discussed in Chapter 39, if anovulation is caused by hyperprolactinemia, dopamine agonists are an effective means of inducing ovulation. As noted in Chapter 40, ovulation may be induced by corticosteroid therapy in women with congenital adrenal hyperplasia.

#### *Clomiphene Citrate*

Clomiphene citrate (CC) is the usual first-line pharmacologic agent for treating women with oligomenorrhea and those with amenorrhea who have sufficient ovarian estrogen production. CC is a racemic mixture of en- and zu-clomiphene, which act as estrogen antagonists. The former has a shorter half-life and is more active than the zu-clomiphene isomer, which has a much longer half-life and is more estrogen agonistic than antagonistic. CC acts by competing with endogenous circulating estrogens for estrogen-binding sites on the hypothalamus, thereby blocking the negative feedback of endogenous estrogen. GnRH is then released in a normal manner, stimulating FSH and LH, which in turn cause oocyte maturation, with increased $E_2$ production. The drug is usually given daily for 5 days, beginning 3 to 5 days after the onset of spontaneous menses or withdrawal bleeding induced with a progestogen.

During the days when the drug is ingested, serum levels of LH and FSH rise, accompanied by a steady increase in serum $E_2$ level. After ingestion of CC is discontinued, $E_2$ levels continue to increase and the negative feedback on the hypothalamic-pituitary axis causes a decrease in FSH and LH levels, similar to the change seen in the late follicular phase of a normal ovulatory cycle. Approximately 5 to 9 days (mean, 7 days) after the last CC tablet has been ingested, the exponentially rising level of $E_2$ from the dominant follicle has a positive feedback effect on the pituitary or hypothalamus, producing a surge in LH and FSH levels, which usually results in ovulation and luteinization of the follicle.

Presumptive evidence of ovulation can be obtained by observation of a sustained rise in BBT or measurement of an elevation of serum progesterone level. It is best to obtain the serum sample for progesterone approximately 2 weeks after the last CC tablet, because this will usually be in the middle of the luteal phase, approximately 1 week after ovulation. A rise in serum progesterone level above 3 ng/mL correlates well with the finding of a secretory endometrium, but it has been reported that the maximal midluteal progesterone levels in CC-induced ovulatory conception cycles are consistently above 15 ng/mL (Hammond, 1983).

These levels are higher than the 10 ng/mL level, which is the minimum concentration of progesterone found in spontaneous ovulatory conception cycles (Hull, 1982) because following ovulation induction with CC, more than one follicle usually matures and undergoes luteinization.

Various treatment regimens have been advocated for the use of CC. Most start with an initial dosage of 50 mg/day for 5 days, beginning on the fifth day of spontaneous or induced menses. If presumptive evidence of ovulation occurs with this dosage, the same dosage of clomiphene citrate is taken in subsequent cycles until conception occurs. If ovulation fails to occur with the initial dosage, a sequential, graduated, increasing dosage regimen has proven to be effective, with a minimum of side effects. With this regime, if ovulation does not occur with the 50-mg dose, the dosage of drug is increased in the next treatment cycle to 100 mg/day for 5 days. If ovulation does not occur with 100 mg/day in subsequent cycles, the dosage is sequentially increased to 150 mg. In the past, we have used doses up to 250 mg, with and without HCG (Lobo, 1982). In the 10 years' experience with this treatment regimen as reported by Gysler and associates, approximately half of the women who ovulated and half of those who conceived did so following treatment with the 50-mg/day regimen, and an additional 20% ovulated with the 100-mg/day dosage (Gysler, 1982). However, approximately 25% of all women who ovulated or conceived did so following treatment with a higher dosage regimen, indicating the value of the individualized sequential treatment regimen. However, from a practical standpoint, it is unusual to use doses higher than 150 mg, particularly when adjuncts are available, such as metformin in overweight women with PCOS or switching to letrozole.

A more recently used regimen, the stair-step regimen, does not wait for menses after a failed response before moving to the next dose (Hurst, 2009). Thus if there is no follicular development on ultrasound 5 days after the last clomiphene tablet, the patient is immediately placed on 100 mg for 5 days and subsequently to 150 mg for 5 days in the same cycle if follicular development does not occur. Although preliminary retrospective reports have shown that this is a reasonable approach to hasten therapy, prospective randomized trials are still in progress.

With the dosage regimen of CC up to 250 mg, more than 90% of women with oligomenorrhea and 66% with secondary amenorrhea and normal estrogen status will have presumptive evidence of ovulation. Although only approximately 50% of patients who ovulate with this treatment will conceive, Gysler and associates have reported that 85% of those with no other causes of infertility conceive after such treatment (Gysler, 1982). The fecundability during several months of treatment with CC, if no other causes of infertility are present, are similar to those of a normal fertile population. Using life table analysis, the monthly pregnancy rate (fecundability) of women treated with CC who had no other infertility factor was 22% compared with a rate of 25% for women discontinuing diaphragm use (Messinis, 1997). The monthly fecundability remained constant throughout almost 1 year of treatment. Almost all the anovulatory women without other infertility factors in this series, as well as other women with correctable infertility factors, had conceived after 10 cycles of treatment. This rate is also similar to the use of gonadotropins (Messinis, 1997) (Fig. 42.11).

These data indicate that discontinuation of therapy is the major reason for the reported difference in ovulation and

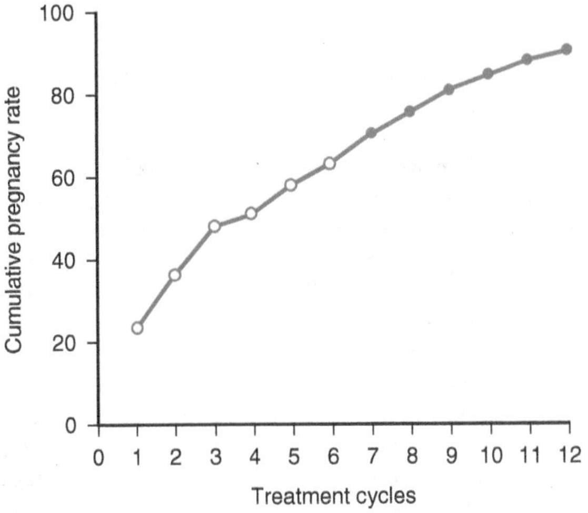


**Figure 42.11** Cumulative pregnancy rate of 60% at 6 months with clomiphene. (From Messinis IE, Milingos SD. Current and future status of ovulation induction in polycystic ovary syndrome. *Hum Reprod Update*. 1997;3[3]:235-253.)

conception rates in anovulatory women treated with CC. However, despite these data, many investigators believe that pregnancy rates are lower with CC than might be expected based on ovulation rates, and other factors (in some women), such as cervical mucus and endometrial problems, explain this discrepancy. In ovulatory women who respond to CC, HSG should be performed if a pregnancy does not occur after 3 months. A semen analysis should be done before starting CC. When conception occurs after ovulation has been induced with CC, the incidence of multiple gestation is increased to approximately 8%, with almost all being twin gestations. However, when the drug is used in normally ovulating women with unexplained infertility, the rate increases to almost 20%. The incidence of clinical spontaneous abortion ranges between 15% and 20%, similar to the rate in the general population. The rates of intrauterine fetal death and congenital malformation are also not significantly increased. Animal data have shown that if the drug is given in high dosages during the time of embryogenesis, there is an increased incidence of fetal anomalies. However, limited human data have indicated that if the drug is ingested during the first 6 weeks after conception has occurred, the incidence of fetal malformation, although higher (5.1%) than in the normal noninfertility population, it is not significantly increased. Although no definitive data have shown that the drug is teratogenic in humans, it is best that the woman be tested for pregnancy before each course of treatment. It is also important to determine that the ovaries have not become enlarged, because formation of ovarian cysts is the major side effect of CC treatment. If cysts are present, they will regress spontaneously without therapy, but if additional CC is given and further gonadotropin release is induced, stimulation and further enlargement of the cyst may occur. Clinically palpable ovarian cysts occur in approximately 5% of women treated with CC but in less than 1% of treatment cycles. The cysts usually range in size from 5 to 10 cm and do not require surgical excision, because they almost always regress spontaneously. Cysts can occur in any treatment cycle with any dosage, and the incidence is not increased with the higher dosages of drug.

Recurrence of cyst formation with the same dosage is uncommon. Other side effects, which occur in less than 10% of women treated with this drug, include vasomotor flushes, blurring of vision, abdominal pain or bloating, urticaria, and a slight degree of hair loss.

Up to 10% of women treated with CC fail to ovulate with the highest dosage. Older data have suggested that this so-called resistance is not caused by the inability of the hypothalamic-pituitary axis to respond, but to the lack of the ovarian response to raised gonadotropin levels. Contributors of CC resistance include body mass index, free androgen and insulin; higher values all contributing to this resistance (Imani, 2002). Although various prediction models have been generated to determine the CC response, none has proven to be useful prospectively. Findings in women with PCOS also suggest that higher levels of AMH may contribute to CC resistance as well as the dosage required for gonadotropins in women with PCOS; AMH inhibits FSH action in the ovary (Mahran, 2013).

Some data suggest that in women with elevated levels of androgen, particularly dehydroepiandrosterone sulfate (DHEAS), the use of low doses of dexamethasone may enhance the ovulation-inducing effect of CC. This approach is less frequently used today. Other adjuncts that have been tested, but that lack validation, include adding a dopamine agonist such as bromocriptine and antiandrogens. Metformin and insulin sensitizers have also been used as adjunctive treatments.

### *Metformin and Other Insulin Sensitizers*

Metformin, a biguanide used to control blood sugar in diabetics, has a role in ovulation induction in women with PCOS and has been shown to be superior to placebo. Although not a true insulin sensitizer, it decreases hepatic glucose production and has some minor peripheral action, leading to some decrease in insulin resistance. It also has a direct role in inhibiting ovarian androgen steroidogenesis and acts on the endometrium, which are probably the major mechanisms that help with ovulation and pregnancy.

Studies have confirmed the efficacy of metformin over placebo in inducing ovulation in women with PCOS. However, in direct comparisons with clomiphene, it was inferior to clomiphene in terms of live birth rates in women with PCOS (Legro, 2007) (Fig. 42.12). Therefore although not necessarily a first-line choice in women with PCOS, it is clearly an adjunct and may be helpful in women who exhibit some degree of insulin resistance. However, it should be considered as a preliminary option in heavy or obese women and for those with impaired glucose tolerance or significant insulin resistance prior to ovulation induction with other agents.

The typical dosage of metformin is 1500 mg/day. It is preferable to use long-acting tablets (extended release or extra strength) available in 500- and 750-mg tablet form and to ingest them all at the same time during a meal, preferably at dinner. However, it should be initiated only at 500 mg and titrated up over several weeks. This is because of gastrointestinal effects (e.g., nausea, vomiting, and diarrhea), which is the primary concern with metformin and precludes its use in up to 20% of women.

Lactic acidosis is a rare complication that occurs primarily in older individuals. However, checking blood levels after 3 months of metformin is good practice, and women also should be reminded not to drink alcohol heavily, although the occasional drink is acceptable. Many endocrinologists advocate a dose of 2000 mg/day for heavier women.

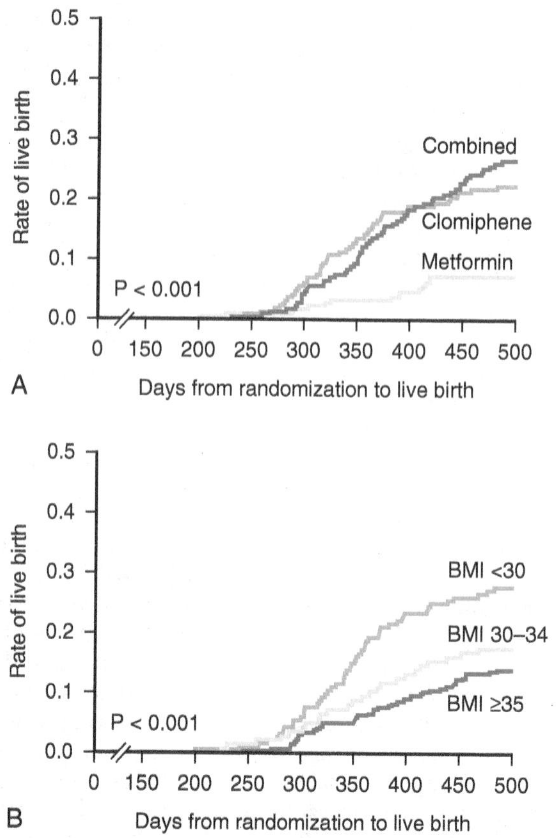


**Figure 42.12** Kaplan-Meier curves for live birth, according to study group Panel **A**: all three groups; Panel **B**: groups divided by BMI. (From Legro RS, Barnhart HX, Schlaff WD, et al. Clomiphene, metformin, or both for infertility in the polycystic ovary syndrome. *N Engl J Med.* 2007;356[6]:551-566.)

When metformin alone is prescribed for anovulatory women who wish to conceive, the ovulation rate is approximately 60% in adherent women. In CC-resistant patients, those who fail to ovulate with 150 mg/day (although the data are mixed), approximately 25% of women will respond to CC with metformin. Metformin is a category B substance for pregnancy and has been continued through the first trimester and beyond in select patients (see Chapter 41).

### *Letrozole*

Aromatase inhibitors are efficacious as primary agents for ovulation induction. Most of the experience is with letrozole. The mechanism of action is that of inhibition of $E_2$ production during the 5 days of administration, with a negative feedback causing an increase in FSH levels, much like the response to CC. Intraovarian androgen levels are also increased, which may enhance FSH sensitivity. Letrozole (2.5 or 5 mg; there is no good evidence for a dose difference) is administered for 5 days like clomiphene, beginning on cycle days 3 to 5.

Because letrozole is short acting, the problems of thick cervical mucus or a thin endometrium associated with clomiphene have not been reported with letrozole. However, $E_2$ levels are usually lower at ovulation. Pregnancy rates are comparable to those with

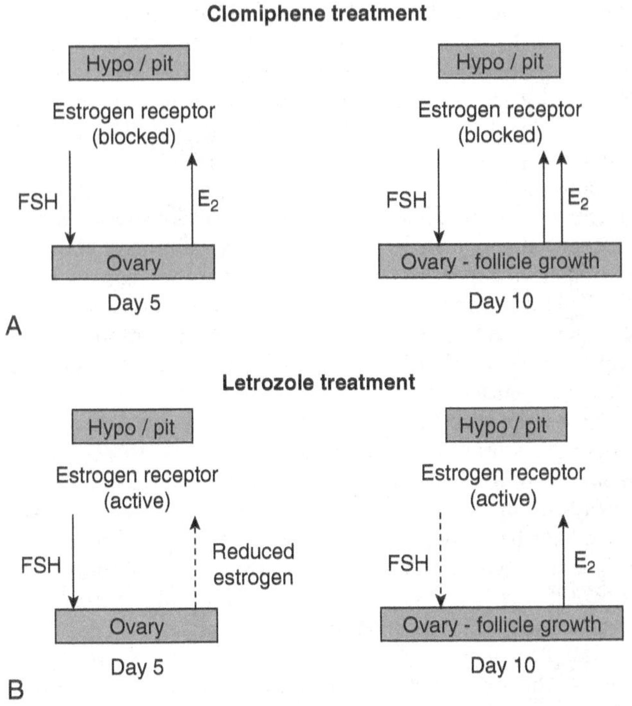


**Figure 42.13** Clomiphene citrate (Panel **A**) and letrozole treatment (Panel **B**). (From Casper RF, Mitwally MF. Review: aromatase inhibitors for ovulation induction. *J Clin Endocrinol Metab.* 2006;91[3]:760-771.)

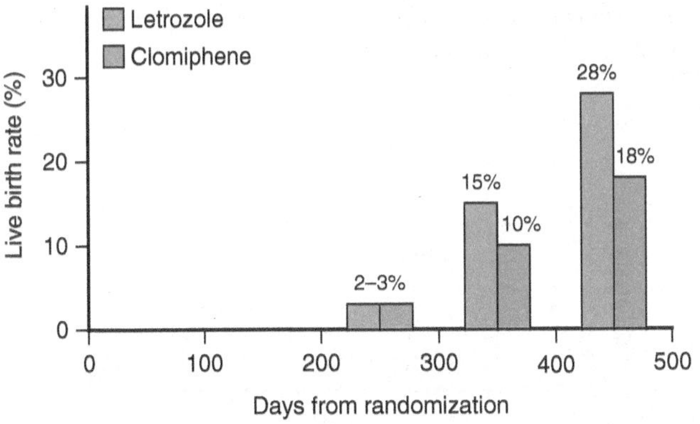


**Figure 42.14** Live birth rates in a randomized trial of letrozole versus clomiphene in women with polycystic ovary syndrome. (Data from Legro RS, Brzyski RG, Diamond MP, et al. Letrozole versus clomiphene for infertility in the polycystic ovary syndrome. *N Engl J Med.* 2014;371[2]:119-129.)

CC alone, and there has been a suggestion for a reduced incidence of multiple pregnancies because of its shorter half-life and lack of stimulation of gonadotropins beyond the early follicular phase (Casper, 2006) (Fig. 42.13). A randomized trial comparing letrozole and CC in women with PCOS showed the superiority of letrozole in terms of live births (Legro, 2014) (Fig. 42.14). In this trial there were no differences in adverse effects or congenital anomalies, and the multiple rates were comparable. Including this trial, a meta-analysis from Cochrane also confirmed the superiority of letrozole (Franik, 2014). In that it has also been deemed to be cost effective, letrozole should be considered the first-line treatment (over CC) in women with PCOS, although to date it still has not been approved by the U.S. Food and Drug Administration (FDA) for ovulation induction.

There is little information about the effects of letrozole in CC-resistant patients, but anecdotally it has been found to be effective in this regard in many women. Letrozole with gonadotropins has also been used for COS. It has been suggested that it can reduce the gonadotropin dose needed when used as a sequential regimen (letrozole priming followed by gonadotropins), and it may be used in combination with gonadotropins in poor responders for IVF.

### *Gonadotropins*

Gonadotropin therapy is indicated for ovulation induction when estrogen levels are low and when there is no repose to CC or letrozole. Low serum $E_2$ levels (usually <30 pg/mL) or lack of withdrawal bleeding after progestogen administration signifies a state that will be unresponsive to oral therapies (CC, letrozole) that are dependent on a negative feedback system. Apart from this indication in usually amenorrheic women, it is appropriate to use gonadotropins when there is resistance to CC or letrozole. Gonadotropins have also been used when there has been the inability to conceive after several (four to six) cycles of CC or letrozole, although this indication is not as frequently applied today.

The original gonadotropin preparations were extracts of postmenopausal urine. Although purified, they contained large amounts of protein contaminants. These preparations are used less often today but are still available worldwide (Pergonal, Humegon). More recent preparations with additional purification have allowed them to be administered subcutaneously (SC) rather than intramuscularly (IM). These preparations are titrated to provide an equal quantity of LH (75 IU) and FSH (75 IU) in one ampule.

Further modifications of these urinary products have eliminated most of the LH activity and provided a relatively pure FSH urinary preparation (Bravelle, Metrodin, containing 75 IU FSH/ampule). All nonrecombinant preparations, because they are extracted from human sources, have batch to batch variability in terms of biologic activity.

Recombinant pure FSH preparations (from Chinese hamster ovarian cells) are currently available for SC administration (Gonal-F, Follistim, 75 IU FSH). Recombinant pure LH has also become available as a supplement (Luveris, 75 IU LH), although it is unclear if the addition of LH is really necessary in most cases.

Because each woman responds individually to the dosage of gonadotropins, even the same woman in different treatment cycles, it is essential to monitor treatment carefully with frequent measurements of estrogen levels and ovarian ultrasonography. Close monitoring (US and $E_2$) is important to assess the adequacy of the response and to avoid ovarian hyperstimulation.

There is a different concept regarding induction of ovulation with gonadotropins when the problem is anovulation or when gonadotropins are used in the setting of unexplained infertility or for the purposes of IVF (discussed later). Many practitioners often lose this concept, which then leads to a high rate of hyperstimulation and multiple pregnancies. It is for these reasons that gonadotropins are often avoided in the setting of failure to conceive after several ovulatory cycles of CC or letrozole, favoring an approach of going directly to IVF.

The goal of therapy in anovulatory women is to produce one mature follicle, sometimes two. In women with low estrogen status, cycle fecundability approaches the ideal (~20%/cycle) if there are no other infertility factors. It is a little lower, however, in women who are CC failures or have PCOS (Lunenfeld, 1995) (Fig. 42.15). In these patients, the risk of hyperstimulation is greatest, and great care has to be used when monitoring these women (discussed later).

By injecting gonadotropins, the physiology behind this approach is to increase the serum FSH level above a critical threshold level, which is an unknown at the outset. The window for this therapeutic threshold is fairly wide in normal and hypoestrogenic women, but it is extremely narrow in PCOS, increasing the risk of hyperstimulation. A starting dose of 150 IU with FSH is used (as a recombinant preparation of pure FSH or a combination of LH and FSH in a urinary preparation). The $E_2$ level is determined and ultrasound is performed after approximately 5 days and then approximately every other day until a follicle reaches a diameter of at least 18 mm. The serum $E_2$ level should be at least in the range of 200 pg/mL for a mature follicle. At this point, 5000 to 10,000 IU of HCG is administered IM (or pure recombinant HCG, 250 μg SC) to trigger ovulation. Timed intercourse is usually advised if there is a normal semen analysis and good cervical mucus. Ovulation should occur between 36 and 48 hours after the trigger of HCG. Particularly in women with hypothalamic amenorrhea and low estrogen status, vaginal progesterone supplementation (100 mg/day) is usually prescribed, although this addition is not completely evidence based.

In women with PCOS in whom the ovary is extremely sensitive to gonadotropin, a starting dose of only 50 to 75 IU is used. A slow step-up regimen is usually preferred, increasing the dose slowly only after 7 days (Macklon, 2009) (Fig. 42.16). Although there have been advocates for the use of a step-down approach (higher initial dose and then a rapid decrease), randomized trials in PCOS have suggested the preference for using the traditional step-up approach, which has better outcomes.

The pregnancy rate per cycle should be similar to that following CC therapy (~20%). With sufficient duration of treatment and no other infertility factors, cumulative pregnancy rates are excellent. It has been reported that the cumulative pregnancy rate after nine cycles of gonadotropin therapy is approximately 77%. These effects are influenced by age and type of anovulation as noted previously (see Fig. 42.15). The incidence of spontaneous abortion after gonadotropin therapy is higher than the normal rate (25% to 35%), and the overall multiple pregnancy

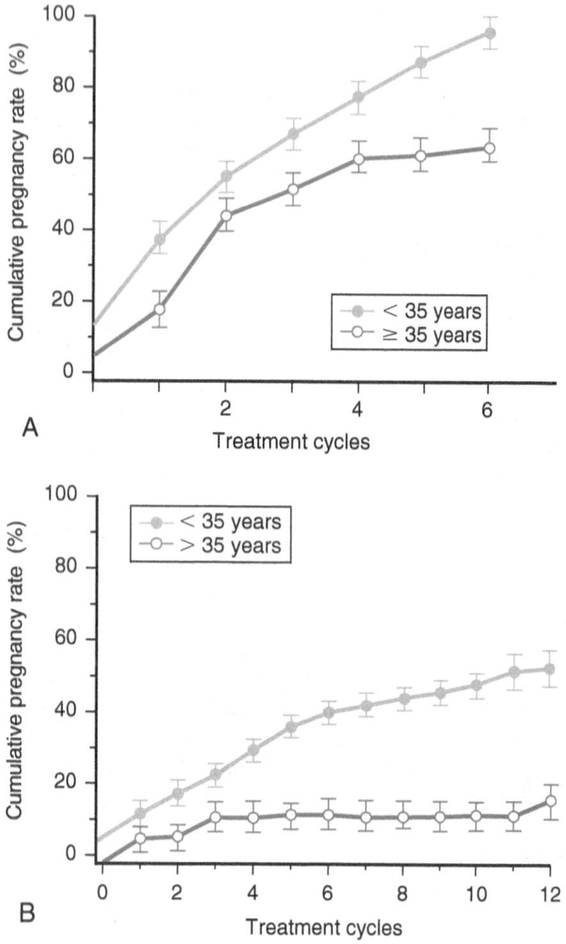


**Figure 42.15** **A,** Cumulative pregnancy rates for hypogonadotropic anovulatory women (WHO group I) treated with gonadotropins. *Solid circles* represent the cumulative pregnancy rate in women younger than 35 years. *Open circles* represent the cumulative pregnancy rate in women older than 35 years. **B,** Cumulative pregnancy rates following gonadotropin treatment for anovulatory women who did not respond to clomiphene induction of ovulation (WHO group II). *Solid circles* represent the cumulative pregnancy rate in women younger than 35 years. *Open circles* represent the cumulative pregnancy rate in women older than 35 years. (From Lunenfeld B, Insler V. Human gonadotropins. In: Wallach EE, Zacur HA, eds. *Reproductive Medicine and Surgery.* St. Louis: Mosby; 1995:617.)

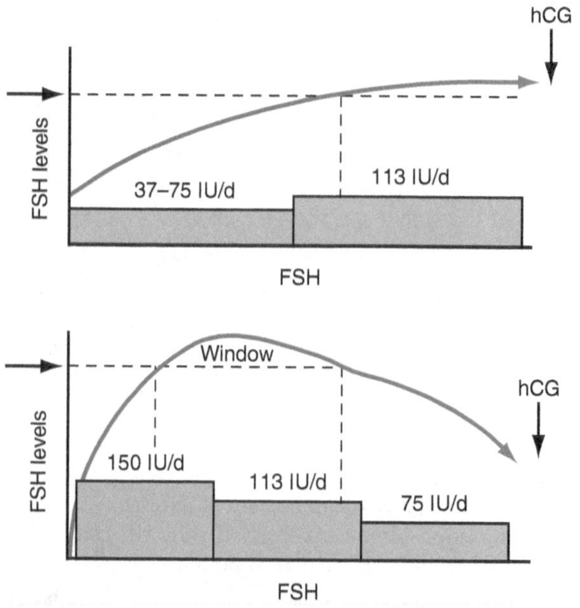


**Figure 42.16** Schematic representation of serum follicle-stimulating hormone (FSH) levels and daily dose of exogenous FSH during low-dose step-up or step-down regimens for ovulation induction. (From Macklon NS, Bart CJ. Medical approaches to ovarian stimulation for infertility. In: Strauss JF, Barbieri RL, eds. *Yen and Jaffe's Reproductive Endocrinology.* 6th ed. Philadelphia: WB Saunders; 2009:701.)

rate (usually twins) is in the range of 15%, but there is a risk of this being much higher.

### Ovarian Hyperstimulation Syndrome

Although enlarged ovaries are frequently encountered after gonadotropin administration, significant ovarian hyperstimulation syndrome (OHSS) occurs in approximately 0.5% of women receiving gonadotropins. OHSS can be life threatening, causing massive fluid shifts, ascites, pleural effusion, electrolyte disturbances, and thromboembolism (Tan, 2013). The cause has not been completely elucidated but is related to the large cystic ovaries, high $E_2$ levels, and the ovarian elaboration of substances such as vascular endothelial growth factor (VEGF), which increase vascularity and vascular permeability. Several investigators have classified OHSS into mild, moderate, and severe forms. A representative categorization may be found in Box 42.1(Navot, 1992). HCG triggers the syndrome, and blood levels of HCG continue to stimulate the ovaries in OHSS. Therefore the syndrome is worse if pregnancy occurs and abates within 1 week in the absence of pregnancy. For this reason, if severe OHSS is anticipated, HCG injection should be withheld. In IVF cycles, the embryos may be frozen rather than replaced to avoid pregnancy.

Treatment of OHSS is largely supportive, with judicious use of fluids and prevention of thrombosis. Correction of electrolyte disturbances and maintenance of urine output are of greatest importance. Occasionally, admission for intensive care unit (ICU) monitoring is necessary.

**Box 42.1 Classification of Ovarian Hyperstimulation Syndrome**

**Mild**
Ovarian enlargement (5 cm or less)
Abdominal discomfort

**Moderate**
Ovarian enlargement (6-10 cm)
Nausea or gastrointestinal symptoms
Abdominal discomfort
Normal laboratory evaluation
Mild ascites, not clinically evident

**Severe**
Symptoms as above and other symptoms, such as respiratory distress
Ovarian enlargement
Severe ascites (clinically evident)
Hydrothorax
Elevated hematocrit (>45%)
Elevated WBC count (>15,000/μL)
Elevated creatinine
Electrolyte abnormalities (hyponatremia, hyperkalemia)
Elevated liver function tests

**Critical (as a subcategory of severe)**
Severe end-organ dysfunction
- Oliguria, creatinine >1.6 mg/dL
- Severe respiratory distress

Thrombotic complications
Infection
Severe hemoconcentration
- Hematocrit >55%
- WBC count >25,000/μL

Modified from Navot D, Bergh PA, Laufer N. Ovarian hyperstimulation syndrome in novel reproductive technologies: prevention and treatment. *Fertil Steril.* 1992;58(2):249-261.

Avoidance of excessive stimulation is the primary approach for preventing OHSS. Lowering or withholding the dose of HCG is also advisable. An alternative approach is to use a GnRH agonist instead of HCG to trigger ovulation (as long as there is a normal pituitary able to release LH) because LH is much shorter acting and will clear from the circulation soon after ovulation, unlike HCG. An experimental approach being studied to treat OHSS is the use of a dopamine agonist such as cabergoline, which interferes with the action of VEGF.

The majority of studies and meta-analyses have not shown a statistically significant increased risk of ovarian or breast cancer in women receiving gonadotropin therapy (Diergaarde, 2014).

### *Gonadotropin-Releasing Hormone*

An alternative to the administration of gonadotropins is gonadotrophin-releasing hormone (GnRH) treatment, particularly in estrogen-deficient women. Because continuous administration of GnRH will saturate the receptors and thus inhibit gonadotropin release to induce ovulation, GnRH must be administered in a pulsatile manner at intervals of 1 to 2 hours. GnRH is a peptide, so it cannot be administered orally; the two methods of administration in current use are the IV and SC routes. More drugs must be administered by the SC route than by the IV route; however, the SC route avoids use of an IV catheter, with its accompanying problems. The success rates, however, are better with IV delivery. The medication is given by means of a small portable pump, which is usually worn attached to an article of clothing. Ovulation rates of approximately 75% to 85% per treatment cycle have been reported. However, this approach is cumbersome, requiring a continuous line and a portable pump 24 hours a day. Currently, it is not frequently used.

## *OTHER THERAPEUTIC MODALITIES*

### *Weight and Lifestyle Management*

Particularly in women who are clomiphene-resistant, weight loss will often ameliorate the situation. In overweight women, it is important to ensure that abnormalities in glucose and lipid metabolism are normalized as much as possible, before induction of ovulation. There is evidence that lifestyle changes in diet and exercise may improve overall fitness and metabolic parameters, as well as ovulatory responses, even in the absence of true weight loss, although there could be a redistribution of body fat with lifestyle changes.

### *Ovarian Electrocauterization*

At an ESRE/Adolescent Sexual and Reproductive Health (ASRH) consensus meeting for the treatment of infertility in PCOS, it was concluded that a possible alternative to gonadotropin therapy in clomiphene-resistant women with PCOS is the use of ovarian electrocautery, which has similar efficacy (Thessaloniki European Society for Human Reproduction and Embryology/American Society for Reproductive Medicine consensus meeting, 2008) (Fig. 42.17).

Laparoscopic electrical or laser-generated burn holes through the ovarian cortex have been associated with improving ovulation rates, as was described many years ago with ovarian wedge resection, which is no longer performed. The major advantage of this more invasive method of ovarian electrocauterization is that it

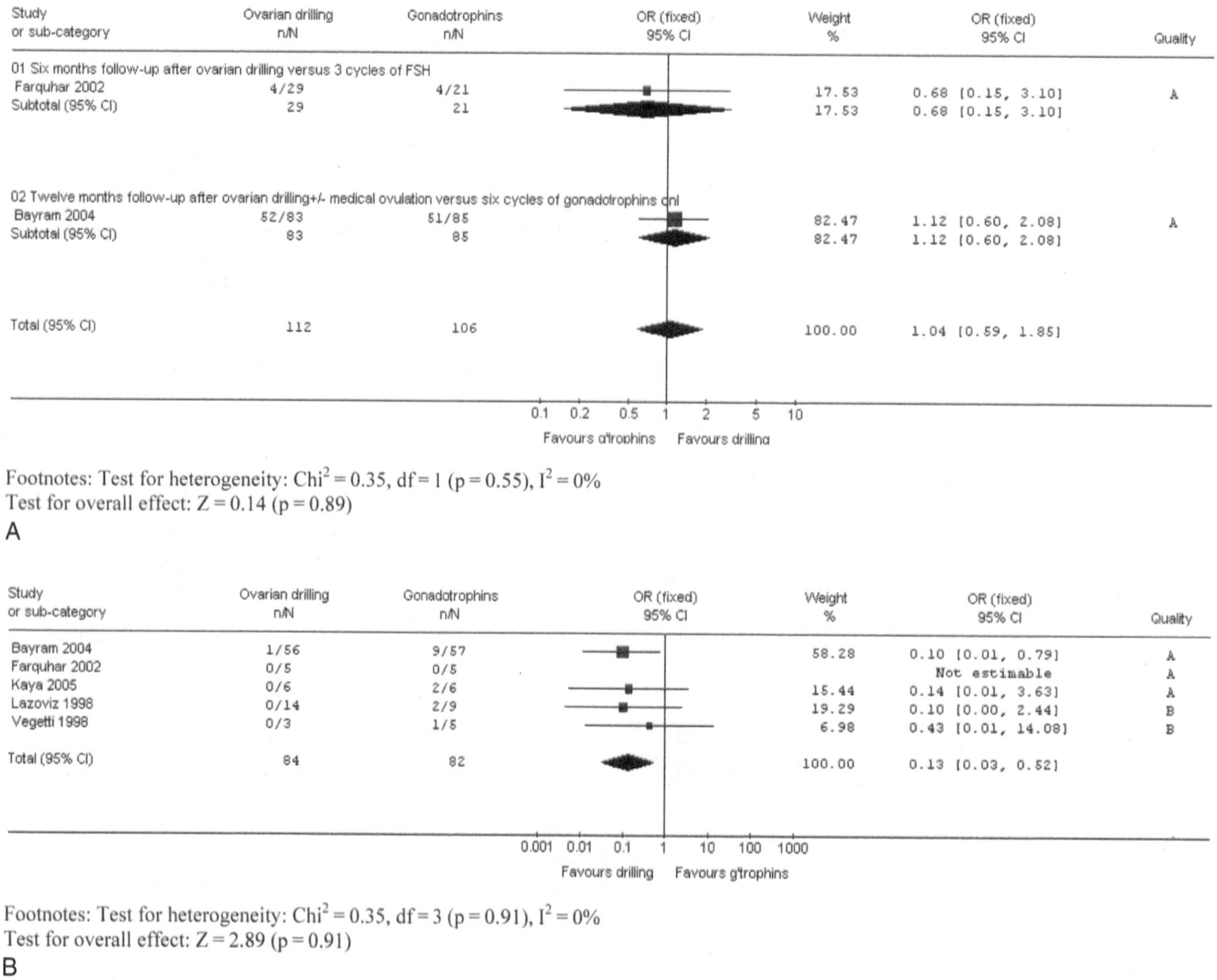


**Figure 42.17** Results from the meta-analysis of the randomized control trial of laparoscopic ovarian surgery versus gonadotropins for live birth rate (**A**) and multiple pregnancy rate (**B**). (From Thessaloniki ESHRE/ASRM-Sponsored PCOS Consensus Workshop Group. Consensus on infertility in PCOS. *Fertil Steril.* 2008;89:505-522.)

decreases the risk of hyperstimulation and multiple pregnancies. In addition to a concern of surgical complications, excessive destruction of the ovarian cortex can lead to premature ovarian failure. Only a limited number of burn holes (~10) should be made.

Figure 42.17 compares the pregnancy rates after electrocauterization and gonadotropin therapy. It has been reported that the endocrine changes may persist for at least 10 years (Gjonnaess, 1998). A Cochrane review has also reported an overall term pregnancy rate of 50% after surgery and a low multiple pregnancy rate (Farquhar, 2005).

Nevertheless, ovulation induction in women with PCOS should still be a medical treatment, particularly with the use of adjuncts, if necessary. In our view, ovarian electrocauterization should be reserved for patients who have difficulties with gonadotropin stimulation (failure of dominant follicle selection or hyperstimulation risk) even in the setting of IVF, which is usually the next step in women who tend to have hyperstimulation with gonadotropin induction of ovulation.

## DEALING WITH A MALE CAUSE OF INFERTILITY

All gynecologists who care for infertile couples should understand how to interpret a semen analysis and how to offer a prognosis for a disorder of abnormal semen. Although gynecologists usually do not perform a diagnostic evaluation or treat the man with a reproductive disorder, they should be able to provide counsel regarding the use of intrauterine insemination with the husband's or donor's semen, as well as with treatment by ICSI, testicular sperm extraction (TESE), or microsurgical epididymal serum aspiration (MESA).

### Male Partner Evaluation

If the semen analysis is abnormal and has been repeated, it is important that the man be evaluated by an andrologist, usually a urologist. Important medical conditions must be ruled out, and occasionally an abnormality is found that can be treated. Blood should be obtained for hormone and other testing, as needed, and a careful urologic examination can diagnose problems such

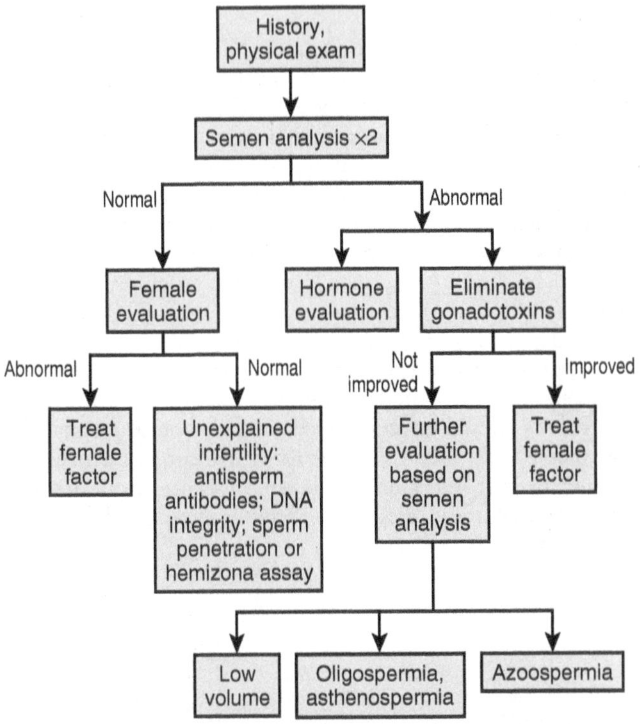


**Figure 42.18** General algorithm for the diagnostic evaluation of male infertility. (From Turek PJ. Practical approaches to the diagnosis and management of male infertility. *Nat Clin Pract Urol.* 2005;2:226-238.)

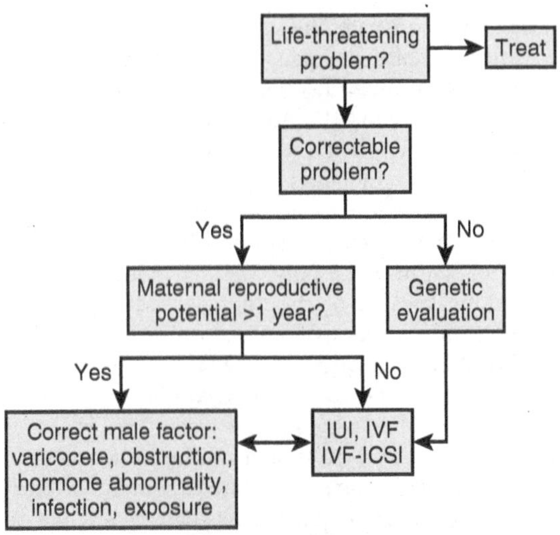


**Figure 42.19** General algorithm for treatment of male infertility. *ICSI*, Intracytoplasmic sperm injections; *IUI*, intrauterine insemination; *IVF*, in vitro fertilization. (From Turek PJ. Practical approaches to the diagnosis and management of male infertility. *Nat Clin Pract Urol.* 2005;2:226-238.)

as testicular abnormalities and infection (Fig. 42.18). The more treatable conditions are hormonal abnormalities (apart from an elevated FSH level, signifying end-organ seminiferous failure), as well as infection. Varicocele repair remains somewhat controversial, and the decision must be individualized based on the ages of the couple, other factors that may be involved, and whether the *varicocele is symptomatic, or at least clinically detected (palpable).* Although a varicocele has been shown to correlate with poor sperm characteristics, there is often a variable response to surgery. It is important to note that improvement may not be evident for 6 months, given that the cycle of spermatogenesis is approximately 3 months in length (Practice Committee ASRM, 2014).

If the evaluation is nondiagnostic or if no treatment is possible or indicated, the best therapy should be directed at improving the ejaculate for intrauterine insemination or to carry out IVF with ICSI. A general algorithm for treatment is shown in Figure 42.19.

Intrauterine insemination has been used to treat oligospermia and abnormalities of semen volume or viscosity to enhance fecundability. The limitation of successful IUI is when there is significant oligospermia or motility problems (<5 million motile sperm available) or with very poor morphology. Data, however, have suggested that abnormal morphology alone may not affect the success of IUI treatment (Deveneau, 2014).

The procedure of IUI (after washing and centrifugation of the ejaculate) is associated with higher pregnancy rates if combined with COS than when used in natural ovulatory cycles. IUI is also of benefit to women with variable degrees of cervical stenosis. Ideally, insemination should take place on the day of, or just prior to ovulation. It is advisable to use a urinary LH enzyme-linked immunosorbent assay (ELISA) kit to determine the optimal date to perform insemination because the urinary LH peak occurs on the day prior to ovulation. Insemination should be scheduled for the morning after LH is initially detected in an afternoon urine specimen. In women who have difficulty with LH kits, ovulation may be "triggered" with HCG injection (typically 250 μg of recombinant HCG subcutaneously), as long as follicular development is adequate (typically at least a 20-mm follicle on ultrasound).

Separation of sperm from the seminal fluid by double centrifugation, the swim-up technique, or use of a density gradient should be performed before IUI. This enhances sperm motility and is thought to increase capacitation (membrane changes in sperm that facilitate fertilization). IUI of unwashed seminal fluid should not be used because it may cause infection and can produce severe uterine cramps as a result of prostaglandin content in seminal fluid.

Until rather recently, if there were severe abnormalities in the semen analysis, the prognosis for fertility was less than that for any other cause of infertility (see Fig. 42.8), even with the use of IVF techniques. Attempts to enhance fertilization rates of aspirated oocytes with the technique of subzonal insemination of sperm were unsuccessful because fertilization rates remained low, approximately 15%. After Van Steirteghem and associates developed the technique of ICSI, fertilization rates of oocytes injected with a single normal sperm obtained from men with severe abnormalities in their semen analysis increased above 50% (Van Steirteghem, 1993). Pregnancy rates per embryo transfer are now similar after ICSI compared with other indications for IVF. When there is very low or no sperm in the ejaculate, IVF/ICSI can be carried out using testicular sperm (see Chapter 43).

Some couples, particularly those whose male partner has azoospermia, may choose to use donor sperm insemination. If they choose this option, the attitudes of both partners regarding the use of donor semen and the stability of the marriage must be thoroughly discussed before the procedure is performed. Donors from sperm banks are carefully screened for infectious diseases, and all semen samples are quarantined for at least 6 months because of the long time it takes for positive antibodies to HIV to appear after infection. The American Society for Reproductive Medicine has published a set of guidelines for semen donor insemination. These guidelines provide information regarding indications for donor insemination, as well as suggested procedures for selection and screening of possible semen donors.

Freezing of sperm is the only way that donor insemination should be done because of the time necessary to quarantine samples to rule out infectious diseases, but freezing sperm affects fecundability. A cumulative pregnancy rate after insemination of approximately 50%, and a monthly fecundity rate of only 9% has been reported after 6 months of treatment. However, the range is variable and may be as high as a fecundity rate of 18%, with a 45% cumulative pregnancy rate at 3 months. There is a known variability of semen quality after thawing, even in normal fertile sperm donors.

## UTERINE CAUSES OF INFERTILITY

In the evaluation of the uterus by HSG, a number of "filling defects" may be appreciated. These are usually polyps, submucous fibroids, or intrauterine adhesions. Each of these may affect the woman's ability to get pregnant or lead to miscarriage and should be corrected.

### Intrauterine Adhesions

In addition to menstrual abnormalities and recurrent abortion, some women may not be able to conceive because of the presence of intrauterine adhesions (IUAs). As noted in Chapter 16, most women with IUAs have had a previous curettage of the uterine cavity, usually during or shortly following a pregnancy. If the only abnormal finding in the infertility investigation is the presence of IUAs, the prognosis for conception after hysteroscopic lysis of the adhesions is good. March and Israel have reported that of 69 infertile women with IUAs and no other infertility factors, 52 (75%) conceived after hysteroscopic treatment.

### Leiomyoma

Congenital uterine defects rarely cause infertility, and the uterine anomalies associated with maternal ingestion of diethylstilbestrol (DES) have not been shown in randomized studies to be a cause of infertility. It is also difficult to assess the effect of leiomyomas on conception, because many women with leiomyomas have no difficulty conceiving. However, depending on their location, fibroids may decrease the chance of conception or increase the miscarriage rate. Data indicate a global change in endometrial receptivity, even with intramural fibroids (Rackow, 2010). If no other cause of infertility is found and myomas of moderate size and position are present, a myomectomy is justified. More recent data from the IVF literature point to a decreased pregnancy rate with submucous fibroids, and larger intramural fibroids (>4 cm), but in those (intramural and subserosal fibroids) that do not distort the cavity the pregnancy rate is not affected (Sunkara, 2010). *The overall pregnancy rate after myomectomy in women with no other causes of infertility has been found to be significantly improved in retrospective studies; surprisingly there are no prospective studies showing a benefit of myomectomy.*

### Tuberculosis

Although rare in the United States, genital tuberculosis should be kept in mind. If HSG reveals findings consistent with pelvic tuberculosis, endometrial biopsy and culture should be performed to confirm the diagnosis. The radiographic features of pelvic tuberculosis that are almost diagnostic include the following: (1) calcified lymph nodes or granulomas in the pelvis; (2) tubal obstruction in the distal isthmus or proximal ampulla, sometimes resulting in a pipe stem configuration of the tube proximal to the obstruction; (3) multiple strictures along the course of the tube; (4) irregularity to the contour of the ampulla; and (5) deformity or obliteration of the endometrial cavity without a previous curettage (Fig. 42.20). Appropriate antituberculosis medication should be initiated, but women with pelvic tuberculosis should be considered sterile, because pregnancies after therapy are rare. Tubal reconstructive surgical procedures are therefore not indicated. If tuberculosis is present in the tube but not in the uterus, pregnancies have been reported following IVF (Parikh, 1997).

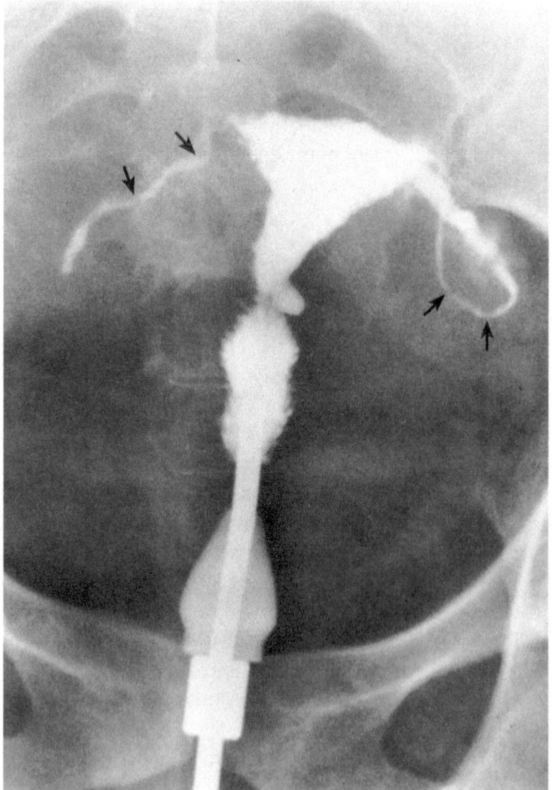

**Figure 42.20** Tuberculous salpingitis in 37-year-old nulligravida with primary infertility for 15 years. Right tube is obstructed in the zone of transition between the isthmus and the ampulla. *Arrows* indicate multiple strictures in both tubes. Nodular contour of endometrial cavity may also be related to tuberculosis and is analogous to the pattern found in the ampulla in other cases. Small diverticulum near internal os probably represents adenomyosis. Diagnosis of tuberculosis was confirmed by endometrial culture. (From Richmond JA. Hysterosalpingography. In: Mishell DR Jr, Davajan V, Lobo RA, eds. *Infertility, Contraception and Reproductive Endocrinology.* 3rd ed. Cambridge, MA: Blackwell Scientific; 1991.)

### *Tubal Causes of Infertility*

Since the 1980s, the incidence of infertility caused by damage to the fallopian tube has increased because of an increased incidence of salpingitis. Obstructions occur at the distal or proximal portion of the tube and sometimes in both regions. Distal obstruction, leading to a hydrosalpinx (Fig. 42.21) is much more common than proximal obstruction. The prognosis for fertility after surgical tubal reconstruction depends on the amount of damage to the tube, as well as the location of the obstruction. If there is extensive damage, the chances for conception after tubal reconstruction are unlikely. Women with extensive tubal disease have a greater chance of conceiving with an IVF procedure, so the extent and location of the intrinsic and extrinsic tubal disease should be ascertained by HSG and possibly laparoscopy in an effort to determine whether tubal reconstruction or IVF offers the better prognosis (Practice Committee ASRM, 2012b). As noted, if a large hydrosalpinx is seen at the time of HSG, it is best to suggest that the woman have IVF rather than undergo tubal reconstructive surgery. It is recommended that the hydrosalpinx be excised before IVF if it is large and visible by ultrasound. If proximal and distal obstructions of the tube exist, the damage to the tube is usually so extensive that the tube cannot function normally. Therefore although it is possible to achieve tubal patency after surgical repair with proximal and distal blockage, subsequent intrauterine pregnancy is uncommon and surgical reconstruction should not be performed in such cases. In general, infertility surgery for tubal disease is a dying art—the pregnancy rates with IVF are far superior, and most women would prefer to avoid surgery as long as they have insurance coverage for IVF.

### *Distal Tubal Disease*

HSG can help to determine whether the tubal obstruction is complete or partial, the size of the distal sacculation, and the appearance of the mucosal folds and rugal pattern of the endosalpinx (see Fig. 42.21). Laparoscopy will assist in determining the size of the hydrosalpinx, amount of muscularis, and thickness of the wall of the tube after distention with dye. Laparoscopic examination will determine whether pelvic adhesions are present and the extent of these adhesions. Women with fimbrial obstruction are not a homogeneous group, and the prognosis for intrauterine pregnancy following distal tubal reconstruction is related to the extent of the disease process. Therefore it is important to perform HSG and laparoscopy before surgical reconstruction to provide an individualized prognosis.

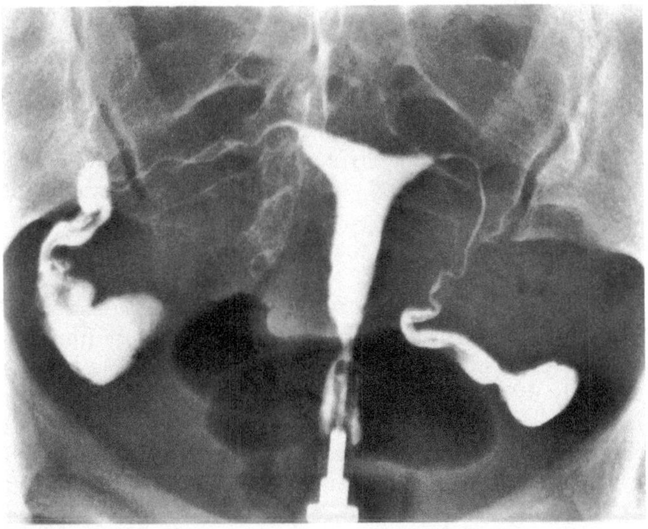

**Figure 42.21** Hysterosalpingography showing bilateral hydrosalpinges with dilation, clubbing, and obstruction at fimbriated ends. Patient was 32-year-old woman with 10-year history of primary infertility. (From Richmond JA. Hysterosalpingography. In: Mishell DR Jr, Davajan V, Lobo RA, eds. *Infertility, Contraception and Reproductive Endocrinology*. 3rd ed. Cambridge, MA: Blackwell Scientific; 1991.)

If the fimbriae of the distal end of the tube are relatively normal, with only partial occlusion by adhesions or fimbrial bridges, removal of these adhesions by means of a fimbrioplasty procedure will result in higher conception rates (~60%) than if the distal end is completely occluded and a cuff salpingostomy procedure is required. Overall conception rates following salpingostomy are in the 30% range, with a high percentage (~25%) being tubal pregnancies. Although microsurgical techniques had been used for all tubal infertility surgery, all procedures are currently carried out via laparoscopy. The incidence of ectopic pregnancy after surgical reconstruction for distal tubal disease is directly related to the amount of tubal damage existing before the operative procedure.

The results of tubal reconstruction correlate with the degree of tubal damage according to the severity of five factors: (1) extent of adhesions, (2) nature of adhesions, (3) diameter of the hydrosalpinx, (4) appearance of the endosalpinx, and (5) thickness of the tubal wall. Using these criteria, prognostic categories have been identified: good, with a cumulative pregnancy rate of approximately 75%; intermediate, approximately 20%; and poor, less than 5%. In the good category, only 1 of 22 pregnancies may be ectopic, but in the intermediate group 50% of the pregnancies may be expected to be tubal. In the poor prognostic group, most of the pregnancies will be ectopic. Accordingly, in women with fixed adhesions, with absent rugal folds and a thick, fixed tubal wall, distal tubal reconstructive surgery probably should not be performed.

The degree of distal tubal occlusion can be divided into four categories on the basis HSG findings (Donnez, 1986) (Fig. 42.22). Following microscopic tubal reconstruction, the cumulative pregnancy rate is directly related to the degree of occlusion. If the distal tubal ostium is completely normal but peritubal adhesions are present, lyses of these adhesions by salpingolysis have resulted in a 64% intrauterine pregnancy rate, similar to that obtained with a fimbrioplasty for partial obstruction. Approximately 50% of women who underwent salpingostomy for degree II occlusion conceived, with no ectopic pregnancies, but only approximately 25% of those with degree III or IV occlusions had subsequent intrauterine pregnancies, and the ectopic pregnancy rate was approximately 10% (Donnez, 1986) (Fig. 42.23; Table 42.7). Thus following operation for more extensive distal tubal disease, almost one third of the pregnancies that occurred were ectopic.

In all studies, the best prognostic factor was the thickness of the tubal wall. If there was a hydrosalpinx more than 2 cm in diameter, with a thick tubal wall, the prognosis for a term pregnancy following distal tubal reconstruction was extremely poor.

Rock and coworkers have classified women with distal fimbrial occlusion into three categories based on the extent of tubal disease (Rock, 1978) (Box 42.2). A life table analysis of couples in these three categories with no other causes of infertility was performed after the female partner underwent neosalpingostomy

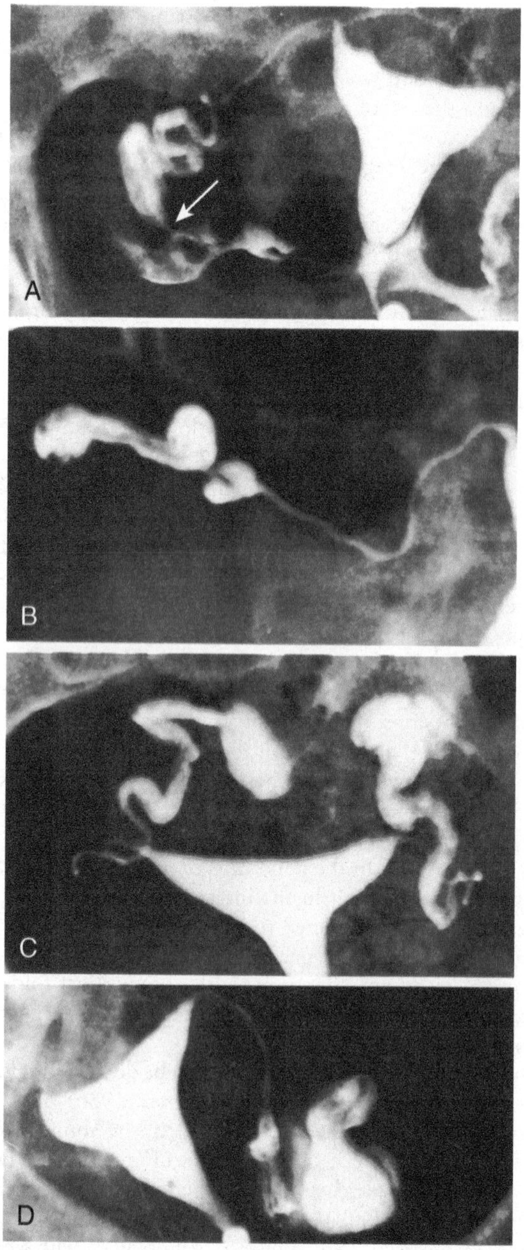


**Figure 42.22** Classification of distal tubal occlusion based on degree of dilation seen on hysterosalpingography. **A,** Degree I, conglutination of the fimbrial folds *(arrow)* with tubal patency. **B,** Degree II, complete distal occlusion with normal ampullary diameter. **C,** Degree III, complete distal occlusion with ampullary dilation of 15 to 25 mm in diameter. **D,** Degree IV, occlusion with ampullary distention greater than 25 mm. (From Donnez J, Casanas-Roux F. Prognostic factors of fimbrial microsurgery. *Fertil Steril.* 1986;46[2]:200-204.)

(Hassiakos, 1990). Of those women, 80% with mild tubal disease conceived, whereas only 31% of those with moderate disease and 16% of those with severe disease conceived (Fig. 42.24). The ectopic pregnancy rate was higher in the latter two categories. This information should be given to the woman when she is counseled, and if the prognosis for term pregnancy is poor, she should be advised to undergo IVF instead of surgical tubal reconstruction. Distal tubal reconstructive surgery should be carried out by operative laparoscopy. The results of a series of 65 consecutive distal tuboplasties, both fimbrioplasties and neosalpingostomies performed endoscopically, have shown that the intrauterine pregnancy rate is 26% after fimbrioplasty and 29% after neosalpingostomy, similar to the historical success rate after microsurgery. The prognoses for fertility after salpingostomy is correlated more with the extent of disease than with the type of surgical procedure. Basically, it can be expected that one third of the patients will have intrauterine pregnancies within 2 to 3 years if they have mild or moderate disease.

### Proximal Tubal Blockage

If no dye enters the tube during HSG, the diagnosis of proximal tubal blockage is likely. However, because spasm of the uterus during the procedure may occlude the intrauterine portion of the tube, the diagnosis cannot be confirmed. Here, at least half of the time, the tube will be found to be patent on subsequent testing or at laparoscopy. Laparoscopy also allows examination of the distal portion of the tube, which cannot be visualized radiographically if there is proximal blockage.

*Currently, it is preferred to attempt selective catheterization of the proximal portion of a tube at HSG under fluoroscopy if it does not fill with dye* (Thurmond, 2008) (see Fig. 42.7). Cannulation of the proximal portion is also possible under direct guidance at hysteroscopy. Cannulation to open the putative obstruction is possible as long as there is no gross disease visible, such as salpingitis isthmica nodosa (SIN). Proximal tubal blockage may be caused by debris or endometriosis, but a significant occlusion is usually explained by prior infection or SIN.

In the past, proximal obstructions were best handled by microsurgical cornual tubal reanastomosis, with pregnancy rates in the range of 50% and ectopic rates of only 10%. Although this approach may still be considered on a selective basis, *most cases of obstruction not relieved by fluoroscopic or hysteroscopic selective cannulation are now treated by IVF.*

### Adjunctive Therapy

Adjunctive procedures for surgical tubal reconstruction previously included prophylactic antibiotics, intraperitoneal corticosteroids, postoperative hydrotubation, and placement of tubal stents. Prospective studies have not demonstrated postoperative hydrotubation to have any benefit, and tubal stents should not be used because they may cause mucosal damage. Data from several studies have shown that intraperitoneal adjuncts are not effective.

It is important to stress surgical technique, attention to hemostasis, and irrigation of blood and debris away from the surgical site with Ringer's lactate solution. The only barriers currently used with some efficacy are an absorbable adhesion barrier (Gynecare Interceed, Ethicon), to be used only in areas that are dry and not bleeding, and barriers impregnated with hyaluronic acid (Seprafilm, Genzyme). The latter can be used as a slurry at the end of laparoscopy. Gore-Tex requires suturing and removal; therefore it is rarely used and is not applicable for tubal disease.

If pregnancy does not occur within 6 to 12 months after tubal reconstruction, HSG should be performed. If tubal obstruction has recurred, a repeat surgical procedure is not advised. In this setting, the pregnancy rates are less than 10%.

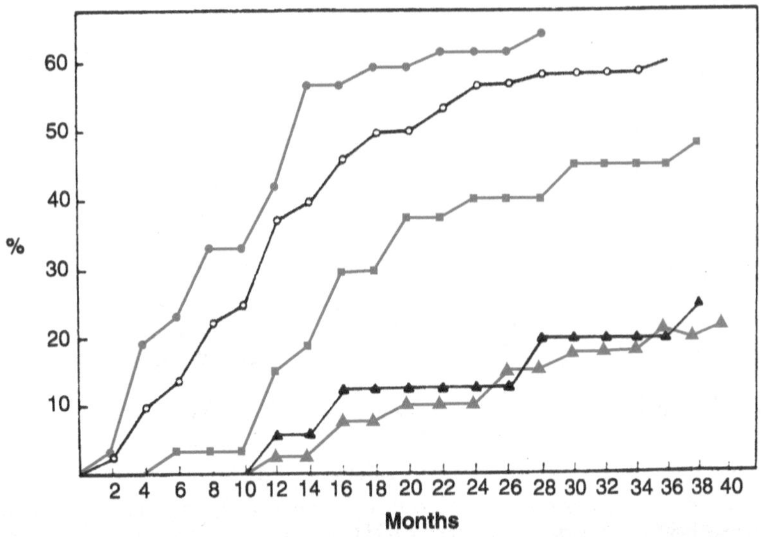


**Figure 42.23** Cumulative pregnancy rates following microsurgical repair of these lesions. *Solid circles*, salpingolysis; *open circles*, fimbrioplasty; *squares*, salpingostomy (degree II); *black triangles*, salpingostomy (degree III); *blue triangles*, salpingostomy (degree IV). (From Donnez J, Casanas-Roux F. Prognostic factors of fimbrial microsurgery. *Fertil Steril*. 1986;46[2]:200-204.)

**Table 42.7** Pregnancy Rate after Microsurgery and Ciliated Cell Percentage in Cases of Distal Tubal Occlusion

| Type of Operation | No. of Patients | No. of Intrauterine Pregnancies | Ectopic Pregnancies |
|---|---|---|---|
| Fimbrioplasty | | | |
| Occlusion of degree I | 132 | 79 (60%) | 2 (2%) |
| Salpingostomy | | | |
| Occlusion of degree II | 27 | 13 (48%) | 0 |
| Occlusion of degree III | 16 | 4 (25%) | 1 (6%) |
| Occlusion of degree IV | 40 | 9 (22%) | 5 (12%) |
| Total | 83 | 26 (31%) | 6 (7%) |
| Salpingolysis | 42 | 27 (64%) | 1 (2%) |

Modified from Donnez J, Casanas-Roux F. Prognostic factors influencing the pregnancy rate after microsurgical cornual anastomosis. *Fertil Steril*. 1986;46(6):1089-1092.

**Box 42.2 Classification of the Extent of Tubal Disease with Distal Fimbrial Obstruction**

**Mild**
Absent or small hydrosalpinx <15 mm diameter
Inverted fimbriae easily recognized when patency is achieved
No significant peritubal or periovarian adhesions
Preoperative hysterogram reveals rugal pattern

**Moderate**
Hydrosalpinx = 15-30 mm in diameter
Fragments of fimbriae not readily identified
Periovarian or peritubular adhesions without fixation, minimal cul-de-sac adhesions
Absence of a rugal pattern on preoperative hysterogram

**Severe**
Large hydrosalpinx >30 mm diameter
No fimbriae
Dense pelvic or adnexal adhesions with fixation of the ovary and tube to the broad ligament, pelvic sidewall, omentum, or bowel
Obliteration of the cul-de-sac
Frozen pelvis (adhesion formation so dense that limits of organs are difficult to define)

From Rock JA, Katayama P, Martin EJ, et al. Factors influencing the success of salpingostomy techniques for distal fimbrial obstruction. *Obstet Gynecol*. 1978;52(5):591-596.

## ENDOMETRIOSIS

Some investigators have estimated that as many as 40% of infertile women have endometriosis. If endometriosis is found at the time of laparoscopy, the extent of the disease should be documented. The causes, diagnosis, and treatment of endometriosis are presented in detail in Chapter 19.

Although endometriosis is frequently encountered in an infertility population (20% to 40%), the diagnosis may be subtle and may only be realized if a laparoscopy is carried out. As noted, laparoscopy is often currently bypassed in the investigative workup. Thus unless there is a strong component of pain as a presenting complaint, or a large endometrioma is seen on ultrasound, the diagnosis may not be appreciated. The treatment for pain is somewhat different and is reviewed in Chapter 19.

If laparoscopy is carried out and mild lesions are seen, it makes sense to ablate them surgically by electrocauterization or laser. Although this may not have a major therapeutic value, the current thinking is that peritoneal endometriosis may release substances that could impair fertilization at various levels.

A new classification of endometriosis has been developed, with fertility as the hard end point (see Chapter 19). The components of this classification scheme are based on structured factors that contribute to the infertility of endometriosis. In general, women with endometriosis have a reduced fecundity in relation to the extensiveness of the disease, and women with extensive disease usually have a mechanical (obstructive) cause of infertility as well.

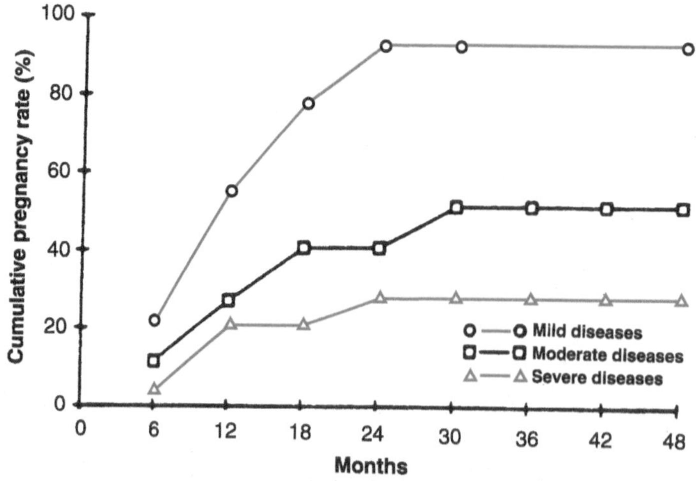


**Figure 42.24** Life table analysis of pregnancy outcome after neosalpingostomy by extent of disease. (From Schlaff WD, Hassiakos DK, Damewood MD, et al. Neosalpingostomy for distal tubal obstruction: prognostic factors and impact of surgical technique. *Fertil Steril.* 1990;54[6]:984-990.)

Surgery in the setting of infertility is reserved for those patients with pain and if large endometriomas are present. Smaller, 2- to 4-cm endometriomas may be observed, particularly in older women, because of the concern of compromising ovarian reserve by ovarian cystectomy. Otherwise, women should be treated as if they have unexplained infertility (discussed later). Many women with unexplained infertility may have endometriosis that has not been diagnosed because laparoscopy was not performed. The lowered cycle of fecundity in endometriosis is similar to that of women with unexplained infertility (~4%). COS, generally with IUI, is the usual initial treatment. If pregnancy does not occur in three to six cycles, IVF is offered as the next step. When surgery has been offered as the primary treatment for moderate to severe disease, which is easily diagnosed, pregnancy rates of approximately 50% have been recorded with operative laparoscopy. This rate is similar to the rate after laparotomy (Chapter 19).

IVF pregnancy rates have been suggested to be reduced, but this mainly occurs with severe disease. In select cases, prior suppression of known causes of endometriosis (e.g., using a GnRH agonist for 2 to 3 months) has been shown to improve IVF pregnancy rates.

## UNEXPLAINED INFERTILITY

This diagnostic category is relatively arbitrary and is probably never truly unexplained. Unexplained infertility is defined in couples with normal ovulation and pelvic evaluation with a normal uterus and patent tubes on hysterosalpingogram, as well as a normal semen analysis. In the past, the diagnosis also required a normal postcoital test and a laparoscopy. Laparoscopy is no longer carried out routinely unless there are clues to significant pelvic abnormalities. The rationale for omitting laparoscopy in the required diagnostic workup is that it is invasive and costly, and it is unlikely that the subtle abnormalities will change the outcome of treatment. Some studies have included couples into the category of unexplained infertility with mild abnormalities in the semen analysis and the suggestion of mild endometriosis.

Using the broad definition of unexplained infertility, approximately 20% of all couples will fall into this category. If exhaustive meticulous testing is carried out, including laparoscopy, this figure has been reported to be less than 5%. Additional testing for defects in sperm function and for endometrial histologic and biochemical variables has not been validated for routine use in making the diagnosis. Subtle defects may be overcome by standard empirical treatment for unexplained infertility.

**Table 42.8** Randomized Trial of Treatments for Unexplained Infertility

| Number of Initiated Cycles | CC/IUI | FSH/IUI | IVF |
|---|---|---|---|
| All subjects | 1294 | 700 | 622 |
| Live births per initiated cycle | 7.6% (6.2-9.2) | 9.8% (6.8-14) | 30.7% (27.1-34.5) |

Data from Reindollar RH, Regan MM, Neumann PJ, et al. A randomized clinical trial to evaluate optimal treatment for unexplained infertility: the fast track and standard treatment (FASTT) trial. *Fertil Steril.* 2010;94(3):888-899.
*CC,* Clomiphene; *IUI,* intrauterine insemination; *FSH,* follicle-stimulating hormone; *IVF,* in vitro fertilization.

The routine empirical treatment of unexplained infertility is ovarian stimulation with CC or gonadotropins, coupled with IUI. Prospective studies have shown that CC alone or IUI alone is not efficacious (Bhattacharya, 2008). Several European studies have also suggested that good prognosis patients, based on age and shorter duration of infertility, should undergo "expectant management," meaning continued timed intercourse for another 6 months before proceeding to treatment. This scenario is usually unacceptable for the U.S. population for social and economic reasons. Also in Europe, the standard management of unexplained infertility with CC/IUI results in a lower pregnancy rate per cycle (closer to an expectant group) because of a more conservative approach to ovarian stimulation (Custers, 2012). The efficiency of COS/IUI is highly age dependent. In women in their 30s, the expected fecundity rate is 8% to 9% and is not much different with the use of CC or gonadotropins, a conclusion that has been based on prospective data (Reindollar, 2010) (Table 42.8).

In 1998, Guzick and associates published a review of data from 45 published studies of various therapies of unexplained infertility, including mild endometriosis. After adjustment for study quality, pregnancy rates per initiated treatment cycle were 1.3% to 4.1% for no treatment, 8.3% for CC plus IUI, 17.1% for gonadotropins plus IUI, and 20.7% for IVF. Although the pregnancy rate in this analysis of nonrandomized studies was higher with gonadotropins/IUI than with CC/IUI, prospective data have shown that the rates are similar as noted previously (Reindollar, 2010). Although the rate of approximately 9% per cycle may seem low, the background rate for unexplained infertility is no more than 4%, thus the fecundity is more than doubled. In terms of the choice of CC/IUI, whereas in a non-PCOS patient with unexplained infertility, letrozole/IUI may also be used, it appears that CC/IUI may be more effective (National Institutes of Health Reproductive network: data in preparation).

*Unfortunately, even with monitoring, 20% or more of the pregnancies that occurred with the use of gonadotropins were multiple gestations, with approximately 8% being higher-order multiples (triplets or more).* For this reason, gonadotropin/IUI is less frequently used in couples with unexplained infertility.

A large prospective trial was carried out by Reindollar and colleagues to assess whether it was reasonable to skip gonadotropin-IUI therapy and proceed to IVF after three cycles of CC/IUI (called *fast track*). The logical next step after CC or gonadotropin/IUI therapy is still proceeding to IVF. One of the concerns with unexplained infertility is that there may be failure to fertilize, even if there are normal ovulation and semen characteristics. IVF also has a higher cycle fecundity rate (discussed later). In the prospective trial, as shown in Figure 42.25, there was an increased pregnancy rate in the accelerated arm (100% to 156%; hazard ratio, 1.25). The median time to pregnancy was also shorter, 8 versus 11 months, and average charges per delivery were $9800 lower. Individual per cycle pregnancy rates for CC/IUI, gonadotropin/IUI, and IVF were 7.6%, 9.8%, and 30%, respectively (Reindollar, 2010). The conclusion of these authors was that the gonadotropin/IUI step in the usual algorithm for unexplained infertility may be omitted. Age is a significant factor in terms of efficacy of treatment. Table 42.9 shows the results of a large retrospective study of the success of CC/IUI according to age (Dovey, 2008). It is clear that in older women, because of reduced efficacy (after age 42, cumulative pregnancy rates over 3 to 9 months are approximately 1.8%), couples should consider going directly to IVF. In a follow-up study by Reindollar in a slightly older population (38 to 42 years), it was concluded that in this group, going directly to IVF is probably a better option (Goldman, 2014).

Cycle fecundity may be reduced substantially, even in women younger than 40 years who have a low ovarian reserve. Accordingly, it is important to measure day 2 to 3 FSH levels as well as MIS/AMH and an antral follicle count. Low parameters will help dictate how aggressive treatment should be, with many couples being directed toward IVF as a primary treatment. Because of the importance of IVF as a treatment option in current infertility management, a separate chapter is devoted to IVF and newer therapies (Chapter 43).

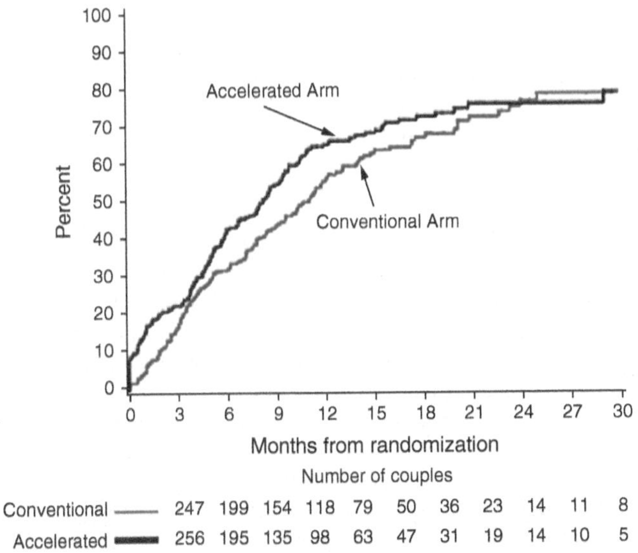


| Time Period (m) | Hazard Ratio | 95% CI | | P-value |
|---|---|---|---|---|
| ≤3 | 1.52 | 1.02 | 2.28 | 0.04 |
| >3 to 11 | 1.40 | 1.03 | 1.90 | 0.03 |
| >11 | 0.60 | 0.34 | 1.06 | 0.08 |

**Figure 42.25** Randomized clinical trial to evaluate optimal treatment for unexplained infertility: the fast track and standard treatment (FASTT) trial. (From Reindollar RH, Regan MM, Neumann PJ, et al. A randomized clinical trial to evaluate optimal treatment for unexplained infertility: the fast track and standard treatment [FASTT] trial. *Fertil Steril.* 2010;94[3]:888-899.)

**Table 42.9** Realistic Chances of Pregnancy with Intrauterine Insemination: Age Dependency*

| Age of Woman (yr) | Pregnancy Rate per Cycle (%) |
|---|---|
| <35 | ≈10-11.5 |
| 35-37 | ≈8.2-9.2 |
| 38-40 | ≈6.5-7.3 |
| 40-41 | ≈3.6-4.3 |
| >42† | ≈0.8-1.0 |

From Dovey S, Sneeringer RM, Penzias AS. Clomiphene citrate and intrauterine insemination: analysis of more than 4100 cycles. *Fertil Steril.* 2008;90(6): 2281-2286.

*Large cohort of 4100 cycles of CC IUI.†In women >42 years, cumulative pregnancy rates = 1.8% (1 in 55).

## COUNSELING AND EMOTIONAL SUPPORT

The diagnosis of infertility can be a devastating and life-altering event that affects many aspects of a woman's life. Infertility and its treatment can affect a woman and her spouse or partner medically, financially, socially, emotionally, and psychologically. Feelings of anxiety, depression, isolation, and helplessness are not uncommon in women undergoing infertility treatment. Strained and stressful relationships with spouses, partners, and other loved ones occur among patients undergoing infertility treatment as treatment gets under-way and progresses.

It is important that every program address the emotional and social needs of couples undergoing treatment. Individual counseling and support groups, as well as patient information sessions, should be part of every infertility practice. National support groups such as the National Infertility Association (RESOLVE, www.resolve.org) and the American Fertility Association (www.theafa.org) are also available to provide assistance and information. The American Society for Reproductive Medicine (ASRM) also has many educational resources, specifically designed for patients with a separate portal available at the society's website (www.asrm.org.) Patient-oriented videos are available regarding various aspects of infertility at www.reproductivefacts.org.

## KEY POINTS

- Approximately 10% of all U.S. couples with women of reproductive age are infertile, approximately more than 7 million women, and the incidence of infertility steadily increases in women after age 30.
- Among fertile couples who have coitus in the week before ovulation, approximately 20% (monthly fecundability, 0.2) have a chance of developing a clinical pregnancy.
- In the United States, approximately 20% of cases of infertility are caused by anovulation, 30% to 40% by an abnormality of semen production, 30% to 40% by pelvic disease, and approximately 10% to 20% of cases are unexplained.
- A systematic evaluation of factors involved in infertility should be carried out rapidly, along with markers of ovarian reserve (antral follicle count, AMH); this will help frame the discussion with couples as to how best to proceed with treatment.
- Of all the causes of infertility, treatment of anovulation results in the greatest success with ovulation induction, if no other causes of infertility are present; conception rates over time are close to those of a normal fertile population.
- Letrozole for ovulation induction in women with polycystic ovary syndrome may be superior to the use of clomiphene.
- When conception occurs after clomiphene treatment in anovulatory women, the incidence of multiple gestation is increased to approximately 8%; almost all of them being twin pregnancies. The incidences of clinical spontaneous abortion, ectopic gestation, intrauterine fetal death, and congenital malformation are not significantly increased, although ectopic pregnancies are more common following assisted reproductive technology.
- The prognosis for fertility after tubal reconstruction depends on the amount of damage to the tube as well as the location of the obstruction. Mild abnormalities of the proximal tube may be treated with selective catheterization/cannulation under fluoroscopy. Large hydrosalpinges (distal disease) are best treated by salpingectomy and IVF.
- If both proximal and distal obstructions of the tube exist, intrauterine pregnancy is uncommon, and operative reconstruction should not be performed; IVF is the best therapy.
- In women with unexplained infertility, the use of COS and IUI with clomiphene/IUI or gonadotropins/IUI yields monthly fecundity rates of approximately 8% to 10% (at least doubling the baseline rate) and should be the initial treatment for unexplained infertility. Use of gonadotropins does not offer a major advantage over clomiphene and carries more risks in terms of hyperstimulation and multiple pregnancies.
- After three to six cycles of COS/IUI, IVF should be offered as the next step, and IVF should be the primary therapy in women around age 40.

## KEY REFERENCES


Almog B, Shehata F, Suissa S, et al. Age-related normograms of serum antimullerian hormone levels in a population of infertile women: a multicenter study. *Fertil Steril.* 2011;95(7):2359-2363.

Bhattacharya S, Harrild K, Mollison J, et al. Clomiphene citrate or unstimulated intrauterine insemination compared with expectant management for unexplained infertility: pragmatic randomised controlled trial. *BMJ.* 2008;337:a716.

Broekmans FJ, de Ziegler D, Howles CM, et al. The antral follicle count: practical recommendations for better standardization. *Fertil Steril.* 2010;94(3):1044-1051.

Casper RF, Mitwally MF. Review: aromatase inhibitors for ovulation induction. *J Clin Endocrinol Metab.* 2006;91(3):760-771.

Centers for Disease Control and Prevention (CDC). *Infertility FAQs*; 2015. Available at www.cdc.gov/reproductivehealth/infertility/. Accessed August 27, 2015.

Collins JA. Unexplained infertility. In: Keye WR, Chang RJ, Rebar RW, Soules MR, eds. *Infertility: Evaluation and Treatment.* Philadelphia: WB Saunders; 1995b:249-262.

Collins JA, Burrows EA, Wilan AR. The prognosis for live birth among untreated infertile couples. *Fertil Steril.* 1995a;64:22-28.

Collins JA, Burrows EA, Yeo J, et al. Frequency and predictive value of antisperm antibodies among infertile couples. *Hum Reprod.* 1993;8:592-598.

Coutifaris C, Myers ER, Guzick DS, et al. Histological dating of timed endometrial biopsy tissue is not related to fertility status. *Fertil Steril.* 2004;82:1264-1272.

Custers IM, van Rumste MM, van der Steeg JW, et al. Long-term outcome in couples with unexplained subfertility and an intermediate prognosis initially randomized between expectant management and immediate treatment. *Hum Reprod.* 2012;27(2):444-450.

Deveneau NE, Sinno O, Krause M, et al. Impact of sperm morphology on the likelihood of pregnancy after intrauterine insemination. *Fertil Steril.* 2014;102(6):1584-1590.

Diergaarde B, Jurta ML. Use of fertility drugs and risk of ovarian cancer. *Curr Opin Obstet Gynecol.* 2014;26:125-129.

Donnez J, Casanas-Roux F. Prognostic factors of fimbrial microsurgery. *Fertil Steril.* 1986;46:200-204.

Dovey S, Sneeringer RM, Penzias AS. Clomiphene citrate and intrauterine insemination: analysis of more than 4100 cycles. *Fertil Steril.* 2008;90:2281-2286.

Eisenberg ML, Shufeng Li, Behr B, et al. Relationship between semen production and medical comorbidity. *Fertil Steril.* 2015;103(1):66-71.

Evers JL, Slaats P, Land JA, et al. Elevated levels of basal estradiol-17beta predict poor response in patients with normal basal levels of follicle-stimulating hormone undergoing in vitro fertilization. *Fertil Steril.* 1998;69:1010-1014.

Farquhar C, Lilford RJ, Marjoribanks J, et al. Laparoscopic "drilling" by diathermy or laser for ovulation induction in anovulatory polycystic ovary syndrome. *Cochrane Database Syst Rev*. 2005;(3). CD001122.

Fatum M, Laufer N, Simon A. Investigation of the infertile couple: Should diagnostic laparoscopy be performed after normal hysterosalpingography in treating infertility suspected to be of unknown origin? *Hum Reprod*. 2002;17:1-3.

Franik S, Kremer JA, Nelen WL, et al. Aromatase inhibitors for subfertile women with polycystic ovary syndrome. *Cochrane Database Syst Rev*. 2014;(2). CD010287.

Gjonnaess H. Late endocrine effects of ovarian electrocautery in women with polycystic ovary syndrome. *Fertil Steril*. 1998;69:697-701.

Goldman MB, Thornton K, Ryley D, et al. A randomized clinical trial to determine optimal infertility treatment in older couples: the forty and over treatment trial (FORT-T). *Fertil Steril*. 2014;101:1574-1581.

Gysler M, March CM, Mishell Jr DR, et al. A decade's experience with an individualized clomiphene treatment regimen including its effect on the postcoital test. *Fertil Steril*. 1982;37:161-167.

Hammond MG, Halme JK, Talbert LM. Factors affecting the pregnancy rate in clomiphene citrate induction of ovulation. *Obstet Gynecol*. 1983;62:196-202.

Harrison RF, DeLouvois J, Blades M, et al. Doxycycline treatment and human infertility. *Lancet*. 1975;1:605-607.

Hull MG. Effectiveness of infertility treatments: choice and comparative analysis. *Int J Gynaecol Obstet*. 1994;47:99-108.

Hull MG, Glazener CM, Kelly NJ, et al. Population study of causes, treatment, and outcome of infertility. *Br Med J (Clin Res Ed)*. 1985;291:1693-1697.

Hull MG, Savage PE, Bromham DR, et al. The value of a single serum progesterone measurement in the midluteal phase as a criterion of a potentially fertile cycle ("ovulation") derived from treated and untreated conception cycles. *Fertil Steril*. 1982;37(3):355-360.

Hunault CC, Habbema JD, Eijkemans MJ, et al. Two new prediction rules for spontaneous pregnancy leading to live birth among subfertile couples, based on the synthesis of three previous models. *Hum Reprod*. 2004;19(9):2019-2026.

Hurst BS, Hickman JM, Matthews ML, et al. Novel clomiphene "stair-step" protocol reduces time to ovulation in women with polycystic ovarian syndrome. *Am J Obstet Gynecol*. 2009;200(5):510.e1-510.e4.

Iliodromiti S, Kelsey T, Anderson RA, et al. Can anti-mullerian hormone predict the diagnosis of polycystic ovary syndrome? A systematic review and meta-analysis of extracted data. *J Clin Endocrinol Metab*. 2013;98(8):3332-3340.

Imani B, Eijkemans MJ, te Velde ER, et al. A nomogram to predict the probability of live birth after clomiphene citrate induction of ovulation in normogonadotropic oligoamenorrheic infertility. *Fertil Steril*. 2002;77(1):91-97.

La Marca A, Sunkara S. Individualization of controlled ovarian stimulation in IVF using ovarian reserve markers: from theory to practice. *Hum Reprod Update*. 2014;20(1):124-140.

Legro RS, Barnhart HX, Schlaff WD, et al. Clomiphene, metformin, or both for infertility in the polycystic ovary syndrome. *N Engl J Med*. 2007;356(6):551-566.

Legro RS, Brzyski RG, Diamond MP, et al. Letrozole versus clomiphene for infertility in the polycystic ovary syndrome. *N Engl J Med*. 2014;371(2):119-129.

Leridon H, Spira A. Problems in measuring the effectiveness of infertility therapy. *Fertil Steril*. 1984;41:580-586.

Lobo RA, Granger LR, Davajan V, et al. An extended regimen of clomiphene citrate in women unresponsive to standard therapy. *Fertil Steril*. 1982;37:762-766.

Lunenfeld B, Insler V. Human gonadotropins. In: Wallach EE, Zacur HA, eds. *Reproductive Medicine and Surgery*. St. Louis: Mosby; 1995:617.

Macklon NSK, Bart CJM. Medical approaches to ovarian stimulation for infertility. In: Strauss JF, Barbieri RL, eds. *Yen and Jaffe's Reproductive Endocrinology*. 6th ed. Philadelphia: Elsevier; 2009:701.

Mahran A, Abdelmeged A, El-Asawy AR, et al. The predictive value of circulating anti-mullerian hormone in women with polycystic ovarian syndrome receiving clomiphene citrate: a prospective observational study. *J Clin Endocrin Metab*. 2013;98(10):4170-4175.

Matthews CD, Clapp KH, Tansing JA, et al. T-mycoplasma genital infection: The effect of doxycycline therapy on human unexplained infertility. *Fertil Steril*. 1978;30:98-99.

Menken J, Trussell J, Larsen U. Age and infertility. *Science*. 1986;233:1389-1394.

Messinis IE, Milingos SD. Current and future status of ovulation induction in polycystic ovary syndrome. *Hum Reprod Update*. 1997;3:235-253.

Navot D, Bergh PA, Laufer N. Ovarian hyperstimulation syndrome in novel reproductive technologies: prevention and treatment. *Fertil Steril*. 1992;58(2):249-261.

Oehninger S, Franken DR, Ombelet W. Sperm functional tests. *Fertil Steril*. 2014;102(6):1528-1533.

Parikh FR, Nadkarni SG, Kamat SA, et al. Genital tuberculosis—a major pelvic factor causing infertility in Indian women. *Fertil Steril*. 1997;67(3):497-500.

Perkins KM, Boulet SL, Kissin DM, et al. Risk of ectopic pregnancy associated with assisted reproductive technology in the United States, 2001-2011. *Obstet Gynecol*. 2015;125(1):70-78.

Practice Committee of the American Society for Reproductive Medicine. Diagnostic evaluation of the infertile female: a committee opinion. *Fertil Steril*. 2012a;98:302-307.

Practice Committee of American Society for Reproductive Medicine. Role of tubal reconstructive surgery in the era of assisted reproductive technology: a committee opinion. *Fertil Steril*. 2012b;97:539-545.

Practice Committee of the American Society for Reproductive Medicine and the Society for Male Reproduction and Urology. Report on varicocele and infertility: a committee opinion. *Fertil Steril*. 2014;102(6):1556-1560.

Practice Committee of the American Society for Reproductive Medicine. Subclinical hypothyroidism: a committee opinion. *Fertil Steril*. 2015 (in press).

Rackow BW, Taylor HS. Submucosal uterine leiomyomas have a global effect on molecular determinants of endometrial receptivity. *Fertil Steril*. 2010;93(6):2027-2034.

Reindollar RH, Regan MM, Neumann PJ, et al. A randomized clinical trial to evaluate optimal treatment for unexplained infertility: the fast track and standard treatment (FASTT) trial. *Fertil Steril*. 2010;94:888-899.

Rock JA, Katayama P, Martin EJ, et al. Factors influencing the success of salpingostomy techniques for distal fimbrial obstruction. *Obstet Gynecol*. 1978;52:591-596.

Schwartz D, Mayaux MJ. Female fecundity as a function of age: results of artificial insemination in 2193 nulliparous women with azoospermic husbands. Federation CECOS. *N Engl J Med*. 1982;306:404-406.

Seifer DB, Baker VL, Leader B. Age-specific serum antiMullerian hormone values for 17,120 women presenting to fertility centers within the United States. *Fertil Steril*. 2011;95(2):747-750.

Sowers MR, Eyvazzadeh AD, McConnell D, et al. Anti-mullerian hormone and inhibin B in the definition of ovarian aging and the menopause transition. *J Clin Endocrinol Metab*. 2008;93(9):3478-3483.

Spring DB, Barka HE, Pruyn SC. Potential therapeutic effects of contrast materials in hysterosalpingography: a prospective randomized clinical trial. *Radiology*. 2000;214:53-57.

Sunkara SK, Khairy M, El-Toukhy T, et al. The effect of intramural fibroids without uterine cavity involvement on the outcome of IVF treatment: a systematic review and meta-analysis. *Hum Reprod*. 2010;25(2):418-429.

Tan BK, Mathur R. Management of ovarian hyperstimulation syndrome. Produced on behalf of the BFS Policy and Practice Committee. *Hum Fertil (Camb)*. 2013;16(3):151-159.

Thessaloniki ESHRE/ASRM-Sponsored PCOS Consensus Workshop Group. Consensus on infertility in PCOS. *Fertil Steril*. 2008;89:505-522.

Thurmond AS. Fallopian tube catheterization. *Semin Intervent Radiol*. 2008;25(4):425-431.

Van Steirteghem AC, Liu J, Joris H, et al. Higher success rate by intracytoplasmic sperm injection than by subzonal insemination: report of a second series of 300 consecutive treatment cycles. *Hum Reprod*. 1993;8:1055-1060.

Watson A, Vail A, Vandekerckhove P, et al. A meta-analysis of the therapeutic role of oil- soluble contrast media at hystersalpingography: a surprising result? *Fertil Steril*. 1994;61:470-477.

Wilcox AJ, Weinberg CR, Baird DD. Timing of sexual intercourse in relation to ovulation. Effects on the probability of conception, survival of the pregnancy, and sex of the baby. *N Engl J Med*. 1995;333:1517-1521.

World Health Organization (WHO). *Department of Reproductive Health and Research: WHO laboratory manual for the examination and processing of human semen*. 5th edition. WHO; 2010. Available at http://www.who.int/reproductivehealth/publications/infertility/9789241547789/en/index.html.

Zeyneloglu HB, Arici A, Olive DL, et al. Comparison of intrauterine insemination with timed intercourse in superovulated cycles with gonadotropins: a meta-analysis. *Fertil Steril*. 1998;69:486-491.

Suggested Readings can be found on ExpertConsult.com.

# 43
# In Vitro Fertilization

*Janet Choi, Roger A. Lobo*

Because of the central importance of in vitro fertilization (IVF) in the treatment of infertility as well as its potential to answer fundamental questions in reproductive biology, a separate chapter has been devoted to this topic. IVF is often used interchangeably with the term *assisted reproductive technologies* (ART), which the American Society for Reproductive Medicine (ASRM) has defined as the manipulation of sperm and egg outside of the body. However, some clinicians include ovarian stimulation cycles with the use of intrauterine insemination (IUI) in the definition of ART.

In 2010, Bob Edwards was awarded the Nobel Prize for physiology and medicine for his pioneering work in making IVF a reality (Steptoe, 1978). IVF has revolutionized the field of reproduction. Not only has it opened many avenues of research and broadened our understanding of basic human reproductive physiology, but its successful clinical use has allowed millions of couples to conceive who might otherwise have been unable to do so. IVF has provided the ability to diagnose significant genetic defects before implantation and has led to the possibility of embryonic stem cell research. IVF has also opened possibilities for fertility preservation (Lobo, 2005). Reproductive-aged patients newly diagnosed with cancer can undergo ART to cryopreserve oocytes or embryos prior to embarking on their cancer therapy. More recently, healthy reproductive-aged women not yet ready to conceive but concerned about the normal age effect on their fecundity may pursue elective fertility preservation. Indications for IVF are listed in Box 43.1.

IVF was originally carried out for women with tubal disease. This is still a major indication for IVF, and over time with the success of IVF, reconstructive tubal surgery is much less frequently carried out in favor of a direct approach of IVF. As discussed in Chapter 42, a significantly dilated tube (hydrosalpinx) on ultrasound is an indication for salpingectomy before carrying out IVF. Endometriosis is also a major indication for IVF.

## SPECIFIC INDICATIONS FOR IN VITRO FERTILIZATION

### *MALE FACTOR INFERTILITY*

In the past, if there were severe abnormalities in the semen analysis, the prognosis for fertility was less than that for any other cause of infertility, even with the use of IVF. Attempts to enhance fertilization rates of aspirated oocytes with the technique of subzonal insemination of sperm were unsuccessful because fertilization rates remained low at approximately 15%. After Van Steirteghem and associates developed the technique of intracytoplasmic sperm injection (ICSI) (Palermo, 1992), fertilization rates of oocytes injected with a single normal sperm obtained from men with severe abnormalities in their semen analysis increased above 50%. Pregnancy rates per embryo transfer are now similar after ICSI compared with other indications for IVF. Fertilization rates of approximately 60% of the oocytes injected may be achieved with sperm from semen samples containing no motile sperm, few motile sperm, and high numbers of motile sperm (Tsirgotis, 1994). In addition, a fertilization rate of approximately 60% was attained whether the sperm were freshly obtained by masturbation, by electro-ejaculation, or were previously frozen. A fertilization rate of oocytes of almost 50% was also achieved when the sperm were aspirated directly from the epididymal fluid.

The excellent results obtained with ICSI by the group that originally described the technique have been replicated in other centers. By using this technique, the pregnancy rate of couples whose male partner has an extremely low concentration of motile sperm in the semen samples (<100,000/mL) can reach a normal pregnancy rate for IVF, based on the age of the woman (discussed later). Studies of pregnancies resulting from ICSI and standard IVF have revealed a similar rate of pregnancy loss and multiple gestation. Therefore ICSI is now the treatment of choice for all causes of male infertility, as well as for couples with no known cause of infertility for whom fertilization has failed with standard IVF procedures. At present, ICSI is utilized in 60% to 70% of all cases of IVF. The number of ICSI cases has increased because ICSI has been used even for minor sperm abnormalities and in other cases such as unexplained infertility and in older women where there is a concern about the rate of fertilization (Fig. 43.1). (Also see the video of an ICSI procedure [Video 43.1].)

The clinical pregnancy rate is higher when testicular or epididymal sperm is retrieved from men with obstruction of the vas deferens (obstructive azoospermia) than when testicular sperm is retrieved from men with azoospermia without reproductive tract obstruction (nonobstructive azoospermia) (Palermo, 1999). Even if the sperm retrieved from the testes remain immotile, the pregnancy rate after ICSI is acceptable at 15% or higher. The likelihood of retrieval of spermatozoa from testicular tissue of men with azoospermia and normal follicle-stimulating hormone (FSH) levels is almost 100%.

**Box 43.1 Indications for In Vitro Fertilization**

Blocked or absent fallopian tubes
Low sperm counts or absent sperm (azoospermia requiring TESE)
Advanced reproductive age
Endometriosis
Unexplained infertility unresponsive to IUI therapy
Screening for aneuploid embryos and/or genetic disease
Fertility preservation

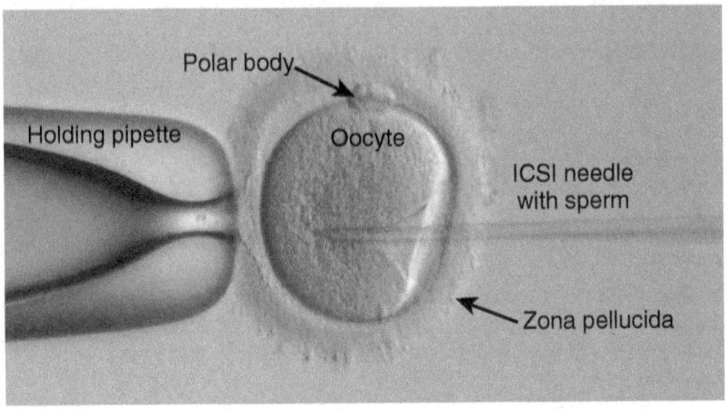


**Figure 43.1** ICSI-intracytoplasmic sperm injection. (Courtesy of Center for Women's Reproductive Care at Columbia University.)

Even if the man's FSH levels are markedly elevated, there is at least a 50% likelihood that spermatozoa can be retrieved from the testes and used to perform an ICSI procedure (Jezek, 1998). Thus the presence of a combination of azoospermia and an elevated FSH level is not a contraindication for performing a testicular sperm extraction (TESE) procedure, although it is advantageous to carry out a diagnostic TESE prior to an IVF cycle. Diligence is required with the aid of microscopy to select the best sperm for use in ICSI, and several groups have advocated a surgical microdissection of the testicular tubules in order to obtain viable sperm (Schlegel, 1999).

## UNEXPLAINED INFERTILITY/ADVANCED REPRODUCTIVE AGING

Patients with unexplained infertility may consider IVF treatment particularly if they fail to conceive following a few treatments with controlled ovarian stimulation and IUI. In fact, women of advanced reproductive age and infertility may be advised to consider moving directly to IVF, by-passing IUI therapy altogether (Donderwinkel, 2000).

A large prospective trial was carried out by Reindollar and colleagues to assess whether it was reasonable to skip gonadotropin-IUI therapy and proceed to IVF after three cycles of clomiphene-IUI (called "fast track") in women with unexplained infertility (Reindollar, 2010). The logical next step after clomiphene or gonadotropin-IUI therapy is still IVF. One of the concerns with unexplained infertility is that there may be failure to fertilize, even if there are normal ovulation and semen characteristics. IVF also has a higher cycle fecundity rate than IUI. In the prospective trial, which also included a cost analysis, conventional therapy included three months of clomiphene-IUI followed by three cycles of gonadotropin-IUI and then up to six cycles of IVF. The other arm of this randomized trial omitted the gonadotropin-IUI step and proceeded directly to IVF after clomiphene-IUI (Fig. 43.2).

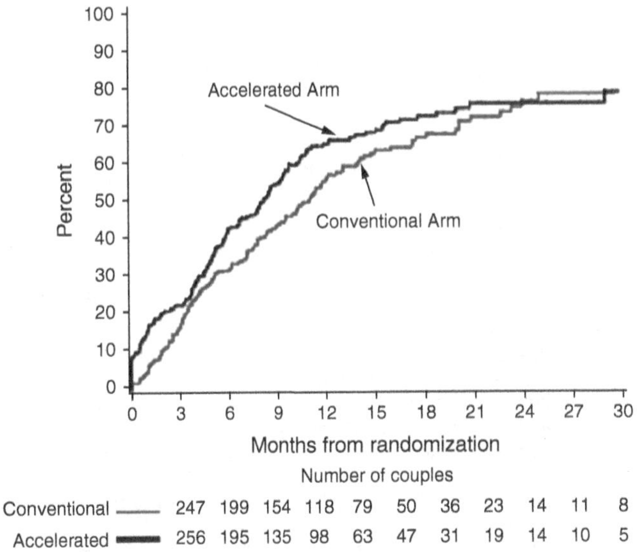


| Time Period (m) | Hazard Ratio | 95% CI | | P-value |
|---|---|---|---|---|
| ≤3 | 1.52 | 1.02 | 2.28 | 0.04 |
| >3 to 11 | 1.40 | 1.03 | 1.90 | 0.03 |
| >11 | 0.60 | 0.34 | 1.06 | 0.08 |

**Figure 43.2** Randomized clinical trial to evaluate optimal treatment for unexplained infertility: the fast track and standard treatment (FASTT) trial. (From Reindollar RH, Regan MM, Neumann PJ, et al. A randomized clinical trial to evaluate optimal treatment for unexplained infertility: the fast track and standard treatment [FASTT] trial. *Fertil Steril*. 2010;94[3]:888-899.)

As shown in Figure 43.2, there was an increased pregnancy rate in the accelerated arm (100% to 156%; hazard ratio, 1.25). The median time to pregnancy was also shorter, 8 versus 11 months, and average charges per delivery were $9800 lower. Individual per cycle pregnancy rates for clomiphene-IUI, gonadotropin-IUI, and IVF were 7.6%, 9.8%, and 30%, respectively. The authors concluded that the gonadotropin-IUI step in the usual algorithm for unexplained infertility may be omitted. However, this remains an area of controversy and may not be applicable to couples who do not have insurance coverage for IVF, unlike in Massachusetts (where the study was carried out) where IVF coverage is mandated.

The extension of this study (the Forty and Over Treatment Trial [FORT-T]) in older women, 38 to 42 years, strongly suggested that infertile women in this age category should consider going directly to IVF (Goldman, 2014). In this study, patients who proceeded directly to IVF achieved significantly higher clinical pregnancy rates as compared with patients who tried two cycles of IUI treatment (with either clomiphene citrate or gonadotropin therapy). Additionally, the ratio of treatment cycles to live birth rates was significantly lower in patients who went straight to IVF versus patients who started with conservative treatment (Table 43.1).

Table 43.2 shows the results of a large retrospective study of the success of clomiphene-IUI (Dovey, 2008). Because of the age-related decline in Clomid/IUI pregnancy rates (after age 42, cumulative pregnancy rates over 3 to 9 months are approximately

Table 43.1 Clinical Pregnancy and Live Birth Rates per Couple, by Randomization Assignment for the First Two Treatment Cycles and at the End of All Treatment

| Randomized Treatment Arm | No. of Couples (%) | First Two Treatment Cycles: No. of Clinical Pregnancies*† (%, 97.5% CI) | First Two Treatment Cycles: No. of Live Births‡ (%, 97.5% CI) | Duration of Study: No. of Clinical Pregnancies§ (%, 97.5% CI) | Duration of Study: No. of Live Births§ (%, 97.5% CI) |
|---|---|---|---|---|---|
| CC/IUI | 51 (33.1) | 11 (21.6, 10.2-37.3) | 8 (15.7, 6.2-30.5) | 38 (74.5, 58.4-86.9) | 25 (49.0, 32.9-65.2) |
| Gonadotropin (FSH)/IUI | 52 (33.8) | 9 (17.3, 7.3-32.2) | 7 (13.5, 4.9-27.6) | 34 (65.4, 49.0-79.5) | 22 (42.3, 27.1-58.7) |
| Immediate IVF | 51 (33.1) | 25 (49.0, 32.9-65.2) | 16 (31.4, 17.7-47.9) | 38 (74.5, 58.4-86.9) | 24 (47.1, 31.2-63.4) |
| Total¶ | 154 | 45 (29.2, 21.3-38.2) | 31 (20.1, 13.4-28.4) | 110 (71.4, 62.5-79.3) | 71 (46.1, 37.0-55.4) |

From Goldman MB, Thornton KL, Ryley D, et al. A randomized clinical trial to determine optimal infertility treatment in older couples: the Forty and Over Treatment Trial (FORT-T). *Fertil Steril*. 2014;101(6):1574-1581.

Note: Includes treatment-dependent pregnancies.

*CC*, Clomiphene citrate; *CI*, confidence interval; *FSH*, follicle-stimulating hormone; *IUI*, intrauterine insemination; *IVF*, in vitro fertilization.

*Number of clinical pregnancies includes all ultrasound confirmed pregnancies, including pregnancy losses.

†For clinical pregnancy rate after first two treatment cycles. P=.0067 for comparison between CC/IUI and immediate IVF; P=.0007 for comparison between FSH/IUI and immediate IVF.

‡For live-birth rate after first two treatment cycles. P=.101 for comparison between CC/IUI and immediate IVF; P=.035 for comparison between FSH/IUI and immediate IVF.

§For clinical pregnancy and live-birth rates after all treatment, there are no statistically significant differences, reflecting subsequent IVF, treatment in all arms.

¶Of these, there were 5, 2, and 4 clinical pregnancies and 5, 1, and 3 live births in the CC/IUI, FSH/IUI and immediate IVF arms, respectively, that occurred before treatment was initiated or between treatment cycles one and two. Over the duration of the study there were 11, 3, and 9 clinical pregnancies and 7, 1, and 6 live births in the CC/IUI, FSH, IUI, and immediate IVF arms, respectively, that occurred outside of treatment cycles.

1.8%), couples in which the female partner is older should consider going directly to IVF. This recommendation is particularly suited for women age 40 or older, those with a borderline elevated day 2 to day 3 FSH level, and women with decreased antral follicle counts and antimüllerian hormone levels.

### OOCYTE/EMBRYO CRYOPRESERVATION FOR FERTILITY PRESERVATION

This indication for pursuing ART procedures has been growing. Not only is it an important method to preserve fertility in young women with cancer about to undergo chemotherapy, but increasingly it is being used in healthy young women who electively wish to delay childbearing with the knowledge of the detrimental effects of aging on reproductive capacity. If the woman has a male partner and either is married or is in a stable relationship, use of sperm to fertilize the oocytes and then freeze embryos rather than oocytes is more successful in terms of ultimate pregnancy rates and therefore remains an option. This topic is discussed in more detail later in the chapter.

### PRECONCEPTION GENETIC SCREENING AND DIAGNOSIS

Another indication for IVF is to screen embryos for aneuploidy or genetic disease (see "Preimplantation Genetic Diagnosis/Screening" presented later in the chapter). Couples suffering recurrent aneuploid pregnancy loss (due to a balanced translocation in a partner, for example) may consider IVF/preconception genetic screening (PGS) as a means of screening their embryos prior to conceiving again and potentially suffering another miscarriage. However, the most recent studies have not been able to demonstrate a statistical benefit, in part because of a relatively high rate of success with natural conception after two to three losses (Stray-Pedersen, 1984).

Couples who are found to carry mutations in life-threatening diseases (e.g., cystic fibrosis, Tay-Sachs disease, Huntington disease) may opt to do IVF with preconception genetic diagnosis

Table 43.2 Realistic Chances of Pregnancy with Intrauterine Insemination: Age Dependency*

| Age of Woman (years) | Pregnancy Rate per Cycle (%) |
|---|---|
| <35 | ≈10-11.5 |
| 35-37 | ≈8.2-9.2 |
| 38-40 | ≈6.5-7.3 |
| 40-41 | ≈3.6-4.3 |
| >42† | ≈0.8-1.0 |

From Dovey S, Sneeringer RM, Penzias AS. Clomiphene citrate and intrauterine insemination: analysis of more than 100 cycles. *Fertil Steril*. 2008;90(6):2281-2286.

*Large cohort of 4100 cycles of CC IUI.

†In women >42 years, cumulative pregnancy rates = 1.8% (1 in 55).

(PGD) to eliminate the transmission of these diseases by excluding affected embryos using specific probes. Although controversial for ethical reasons, couples may also opt to undergo IVF/PGS for gender selection or "family balancing."

## IN VITRO FERTILIZATION PROCEDURE

The goal of a successful IVF treatment is the generation of good-quality embryos. IVF can be carried out in a natural cycle, which was the original approach used by Steptoe and Edwards that led to the birth of Louise Brown. However, here usually only one oocyte and one embryo can be expected, and the success rate is far lower than with conventional IVF, in which gonadotropins are administered to increase the number of oocytes retrieved. Although unstimulated IVF remains an option on an individual basis, its use is currently limited because of the lower pregnancy rates and the expectations of couples to become pregnant as efficiently as possible.

With conventional IVF, gonadotropin stimulation (75 IU to 600 IU of FSH or hMG) is administered, usually subcutaneously, for approximately 10 days. The starting daily dose typically ranges from 75 to 600 IU of FSH or hMG (human menopausal gonadotropin—i.e., preparations containing both 75 IU of FSH and 75 IU of LH). The starting dose is chiefly determined by

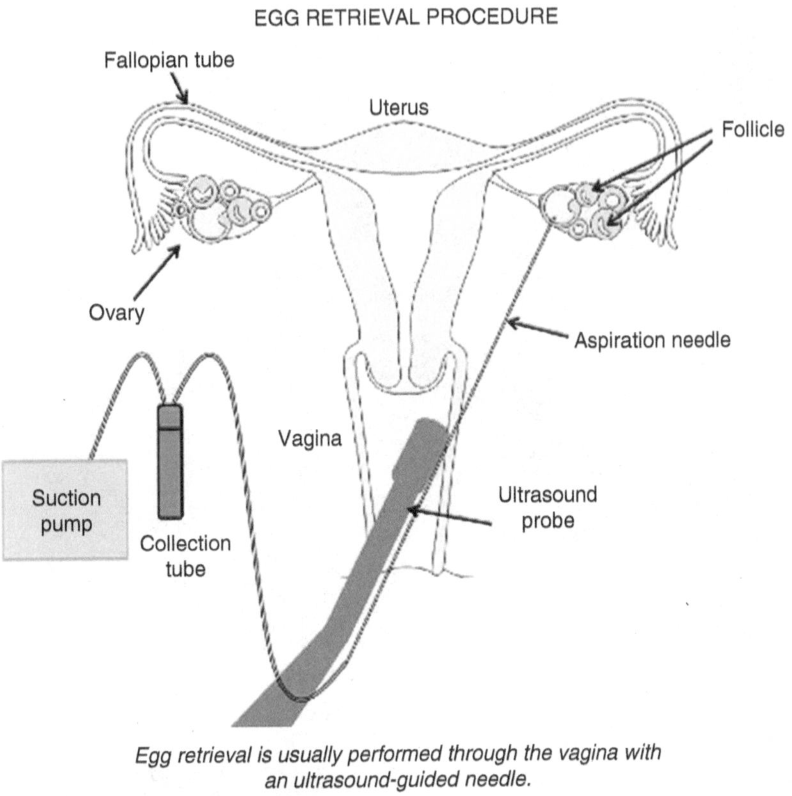


**Figure 43.3** Diagram of oocyte retrieval. (Modified from American Society for Reproductive Medicine: *Assisted reproductive technologies: a guide for patients.* American Society for Reproductive Medicine, Birmingham, AL: 2015.)

the patient's ovarian reserve and age, with higher doses used for older patients with decreased ovarian reserve and lower doses for patients with a more robust reserve and for women with PCOS. The traditional long cycle protocol begins with down-regulation using a gonadotropin-releasing hormone (GnRH) agonist for two weeks prior to gonadotropin administration. Once down-regulation is evidenced with estradiol levels <50 pg/mL, the patient is then started on gonadotropin stimulation while maintaining ovulation suppression with the daily use of the GnRH agonist. Increasingly, however, a GnRH antagonist is used to block spontaneous ovulation from occurring once follicular development occurs. With this "short protocol," gonadotropins are begun on cycle day 2, without prior down-regulation, and the antagonist is added around day 6 of stimulation. Data support an equal efficacy of the two approaches (Al-Inany, 2011).

When at least three mature follicles are seen on ultrasound (≈18 mm) with an appropriate rise of serum $E_2$, human chorionic gonadotropin (HCG) is administered (5,000 to 10,000 IU). Vaginal ultrasound aspiration of the follicles is typically carried out 34 to 36 hours later (Fig. 43.3). This procedure is usually performed with the patient sedated, although it can be performed with local anesthetic use. Complications include infection, torsion, and internal bleeding, though rates are low (<0.25%) (Roest, 1996).

The harvested oocytes are then combined with a sperm sample from a male partner or from donor sperm. One of two methods is used to fertilize the oocytes: insemination (where a high concentration of sperm is placed into a dish with an oocyte) or intracytoplasmic sperm injection (ICSI). On average, about 60%

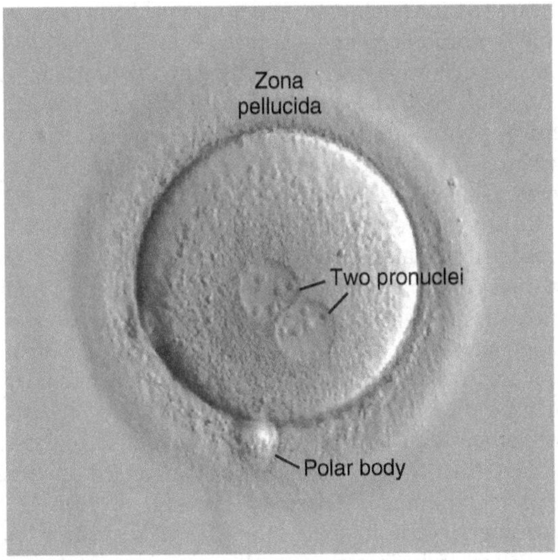


**Figure 43.4** Evidence of normal fertilization:2pn (pronuclei). (Courtesy of Center for Women's Reproductive Care at Columbia University.)

to 70% of the mature oocytes should fertilize with insemination and normal-functioning sperm/oocytes. With ICSI, embryologists can select individual sperm and microinject a sperm into each mature (MII) oocyte. Approximately 12 to 18 hours later the oocytes are inspected for evidence of fertilization (Fig. 43.4). ICSI does not yield "better" fertilization rates than in the normal

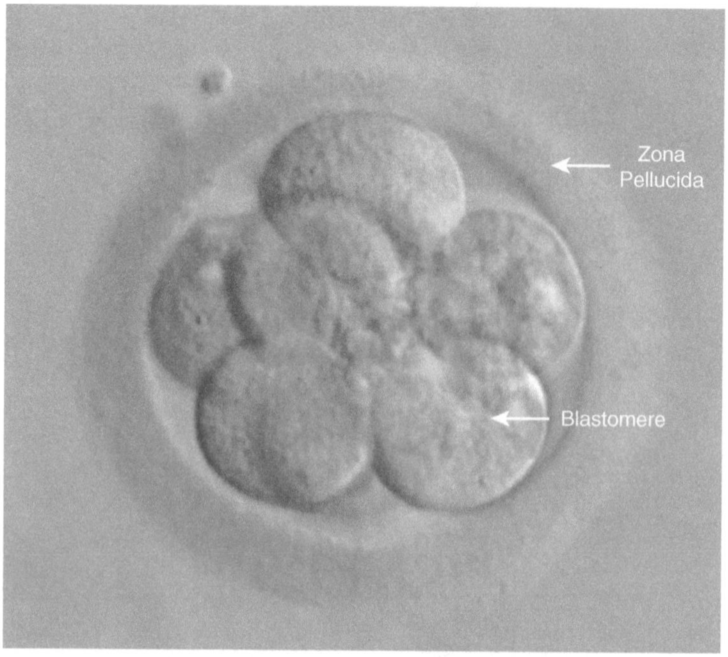


Figure 43.5 Day 3 embryo.

situation; rather, it helps to produce "normal" fertilization rates in situations where fertilization may not occur or will occur at a low rate.

The embryology laboratory environment is the key factor in the success of IVF. Typically, 3 days after aspiration, six to eight cell cleavage stage embryos are obtained. Three-day-old embryos can be assessed for potential transfer using criteria assessing the blastomere morphology and symmetry as well as the degree of embryo fragmentation (Fig. 43.5). Fragmentation is felt to be the extracellular debris created by the dividing embryonic cells, and embryos with a high degree of fragmentation (i.e., >10% of the embryo) are associated with lower implantation and pregnancy rates (Luke, 2014).

At the time of a day 3 transfer, the embryologist may opt to utilize assisted hatching (AH). Using acid or a laser, the embryologist can drill a small hole in the zona pellucida of the embryo. A meta-analysis suggested improved implantation and clinical pregnancy rates with AH use but concluded that live birth rates were not improved (Carney, 2012). The authors concluded that AH may be most useful in older women (i.e., >37 years old) and in women with previously unexplained IVF failures. One downside to the use of AH is the slightly increased potential for monozygotic twinning (1% to 2%) (Hershlag, 1999).

Increasingly, with improved quality of sequential culture media, embryo culture is continued to days 5 to 6, when a blastocyst has developed (Fig. 43.6).

Fertilized oocytes that can be cultured on day 5/6 are usually of better quality and afford a higher pregnancy rate over day 3 embryos (Glujovsky, 2012). Typically, patients are awake for the embryo transfer, which is carried out with one of several specialized catheters (similar to those used for IUI) under ultrasound guidance (Fig. 43.7).

The decision regarding the number of embryos to transfer is key to optimizing success and reducing the chance of multiple pregnancies. The American Society for Reproductive Medicine (ASRM) has published firm guidelines to assist in this decision-making process (Practice Committee ASRM, 2013) (Table 43.3). Implementation of these guidelines has proved to be successful in reducing the rate of high-order multiple pregnancies, although the rate of twins has not decreased substantially. In 2013, the Society for Assisted Reproductive Technologies (SART) reported a nearly 30% twin rate in patients under 35. In women with a good overall prognosis for pregnancy—such as women under the age of 35 or women with a history of a prior live pregnancy—elective single embryo transfer (eSET) can still lead to an acceptable pregnancy rate while minimizing the risk of multiples (Luke, 2015). Single embryo transfer does not totally eliminate the

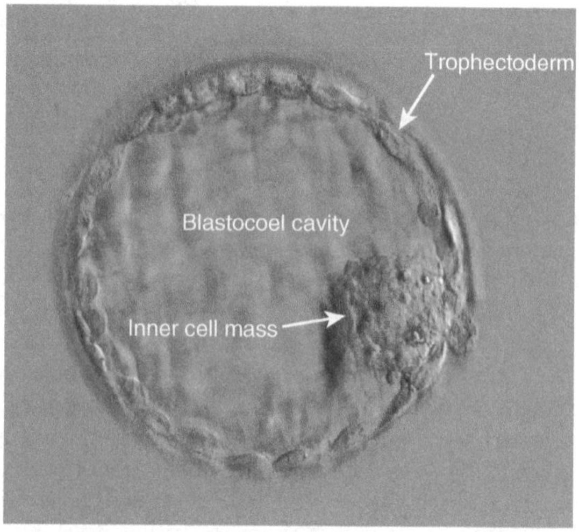


Figure 43.6 Blastocyst (day 5 or 6 embryo).

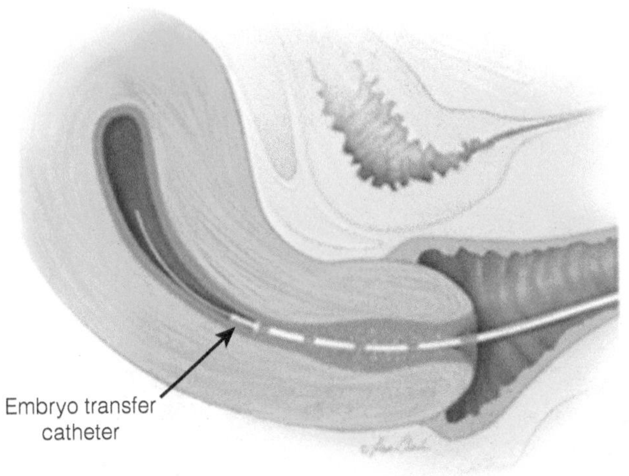


**Figure 43.7** Embryo transfer with catheter. (Copyright Lisa Clark, courtesy of Cook Medical, 2010.)

Table 43.3 American Society for Reproductive Medicine's Recommended Limits on the Numbers of Embryos to Transfer

| | Age (years) | | | |
|---|---|---|---|---|
| **Prognosis** | **<35** | **35-37** | **38-40** | **41-42** |
| **Cleavage-Stage Embryos*** | | | | |
| Favorable† | 1-2 | 2 | 3 | 5 |
| All others | 2 | 3 | 4 | 5 |
| **Blastocysts*** | | | | |
| Favorable† | 1 | 2 | 2 | 3 |
| All others | 2 | 2 | 3 | 3 |

From Practice Committees of the American Society for Reproductive Medicine and the Practice Committee of the Society for Assisted Reproductive Technology. Criteria for number of embryos to transfer: a committee opinion. *Fertil Steril.* 2013;99(1):44-46.

*See text for more complete explanations. Justification for transferring one additional embryo more than the recommended limit should be clearly documented in the patient's medical record.

†Favorable ¼ first cycle of IVF, good embryo quality, excess embryos available for cryopreservation, or previous successful IVF cycle.

risk for multiples, as there is a nearly 2% risk for monozygotic twinning following blastocyst transfer (Kanter, 2015). Transferring embryos on day 5 when the embryos are more developed and proportionately more "normal," is becoming the trend for all IVF cycles. This means, however, that some women who have poor embryo quality may not have any good-quality embryos for transfer.

Several methods have been suggested to help in the selection of a normal embryo for transfer. This includes an analysis of the culture media for metabolic parameters and secreted proteins, as well as an analysis of time-lapse videos of the cultured embryos for normal developmental parameters (Krisher, 2015; Kirkegaard, 2015). However, none of these methods is currently the standard of practice in IVF.

Excess embryos of good quality that are not transferred may be cryopreserved by the use of several validated techniques, typically slow cooling or vitrification, with the latter being the preferred technique. The pregnancy rates from thawed, good-quality embryos are almost equal to the rate of fresh cycles. No known increased fetal risks are associated with embryo cryopreservation.

## IN VITRO FERTILIZATION SUCCESS RATES

What is important to couples is their overall chance of pregnancy resulting in a live birth. Clinical data published by SART may be found in Table 43.4. These rates are influenced by age and far less so by diagnosis of treatment. Live birth rates per cycle range from 40.1% in women <35 years to 4.5% at age >42. When a larger number of cycles have been studied over time, the overall optimistic chance of pregnancy after six cycles of IVF is 72% (95% confidence interval [CI], 70%-74%) (Dor, 1996).

*Optimistic* means continuous treatment without any dropouts; the conservative cumulative pregnancy rate, which includes some dropouts, is 51% (CI: 49%-52%) (Malizia, 2009) (Fig. 43.8). However, this is influenced by age, as noted previously (Fig. 43.9).

Pregnancy rates over six cycles are fairly constant over time and may continue to increase at the same rate, although some data suggest a plateau effect after six cycles (Fig. 43.10). This latter point is unclear because few IVF patients (<10%) exceed six cycles of treatment.

Most recently, patients can estimate their chance for IVF success using SART's interactive calculator—"Predict My Success"—found on the organization's home page (www.sart.org). This patient predictor is based on data obtained from nearly 500,000 treatment cycles performed in the United States and is based on the experience of all SART clinics. This calculator therefore gives an average expectation for success with cycles one, two, and so on, and for the number of embryos replaced. Patients merely enter demographic data and their infertility diagnosis in order to calculate their chance for IVF pregnancy.

## GAMETE INTRAFALLOPIAN TRANSFER AND OTHER ALTERNATIVES TO "TRADITIONAL" IN VITRO FERTILIZATION

A modification of IVF, called *gamete intrafallopian transfer (GIFT),* can be used if the infertile woman has functional fallopian tubes. With this technique, both oocytes and sperm are placed into the tube through a catheter at the time of laparoscopy. Although IVF, embryo culturing, and embryo transfer into the uterus are avoided by this technique, controlled ovarian hyperstimulation and laparoscopy are still required. Because this technique requires a laparoscopy, GIFT is rarely done at present because pregnancy rates are similar or lower to those of routine in vitro fertilization and embryo transfer (IVF-ET) when matched for age and diagnosis (Leeton, 1987; Ranieri, 1995). Modifications of GIFT include pronuclear stage tubal transfer (PROST), or zygote intrafallopian transfer (ZIFT), and tubal embryo stage transfer (TEST). With ZIFT, the oocytes are fertilized in vitro and transferred 24 hours later. Tubal embryo transfer (TET) is similar to ZIFT except that the embryos are transferred 8 to 72 hours after fertilization. Again, because laparoscopy is required, these procedures are rarely performed today.

Another option for IVF is to aspirate immature eggs in a natural cycle, usually in anovulatory women with PCOS. No

Table 43.4 Society for Assisted Reproductive Technologies (SART)–Clinic Outcome Reporting System (CORS) IVF Clinic Success Rate, 2013

| Treatment Type | | Procedure Frequency | | Diagnosis Frequency | |
|---|---|---|---|---|---|
| IVF | >99% | ICSI | 67% | Tubal factor | 6% |
| GIFT | <1% | Unstimulated | 1% | Ovulatory dysfunction | 7% |
| ZIFT | <1% | PGD | 6% | Diminished ovarian reserve | 18% |
| | | | | Endometriosis | 3% |
| | | | | Uterine factor | 1% |
| | | | | Male factor | 16% |
| | | | | Other factor | 7% |
| | | | | Unknown factor | 13% |
| | | | | Multiple female factor | 12% |
| | | | | Female and male factor | 17% |

**Fresh Embryos from Nondonor Oocytes**

| | Age of Woman (Years) | | | | |
|---|---|---|---|---|---|
| | <35 | 35-37 | 38-40 | 41-42 | >42 |
| Number of cycles | 36958 | 18508 | 16853 | 9026 | 5744 |
| % of cycles resulting in pregnancies | 46.0 | 37.8 | 28.6 | 18.8 | 8.9 |
| % of cycles resulting in live births | 40.1 | 31.4 | 21.2 | 11.2 | 4.5 |
| Reliability range | (39.6-40.6) | (30.7-32.0) | (20.6-21.8) | (10.5-11.8) | (3.9-5.0) |
| % of retrievals resulting in live births | 42.5 | 34.5 | 24.2 | 13.3 | 5.6 |
| % of transfers resulting in live births | 47.7 | 39.2 | 28.5 | 16.3 | 7.3 |
| % of cycles with elective single embryo transfer | 22.5 | 13.9 | 6.6 | 4.1 | 5.3 |
| % of cancellations | 5.8 | 9.1 | 12.6 | 15.8 | 20.2 |
| Implantation rate | 39.5 | 30.0 | 19.3 | 10.2 | 4.5 |
| Average number of embryos transferred | 1.8 | 1.9 | 2.3 | 2.7 | 2.8 |
| % of live births with twins | 28.3 | 25.5 | 19.9 | 13.5 | 8.2 |
| % of live births with triplets or more | 0.9 | 1.0 | 1.0 | 0.2 | 0.4 |

**Thawed Embryos from Nondonor Oocytes**

| | Age of Woman (Years) | | | | |
|---|---|---|---|---|---|
| | <35 | 35-37 | 38-40 | 41-42 | >42 |
| Number of transfers | 18801 | 9602 | 7116 | 2731 | 1765 |
| % of transfers resulting in live births | 44.4 | 40.6 | 36.1 | 31.6 | 21.2 |
| Average number of embryos transferred | 1.7 | 1.6 | 1.7 | 1.8 | 1.9 |
| Number of cycles | 19970 | 10328 | 7727 | 3062 | 1994 |
| % of cycles where thaw was attempted that resulted in live birth | 43.9 | 39.9 | 35.4 | 30.6 | 20.7 |

**Donor Oocytes (All Ages)**

| | Fresh Embryos | Banked Donor Eggs | Thawed Embryos | Donated Embryos |
|---|---|---|---|---|
| Number of cycles | 8921 | 2227 | 8172 | 1201 |
| % of recipient starts resulting in live births | 49.6 | 43.2 | 37.5 | 37.1 |
| Number of transfers | 7875 | 2038 | 7553 | 1084 |
| % of transfers resulting in live births | 56.1 | 47.1 | 40.5 | 41.0 |
| Average number of embryos transferred | 1.7 | 1.6 | 1.6 | 1.9 |

Data from Society for Assisted Reproductive Technology. SART national summary: clinic summary report: all SART member clinics, 2013. Available at www.sart.org. Data are for all treatment types, all diagnoses. Total cycles: 174,962.

or minimal gonadotropin stimulation is used prior to oocyte aspiration. In vitro maturation (IVM) of the oocytes is then carried out, followed by ICSI. IVM may be most reasonable in women with PCOS, as their larger ovaries with multiple small follicles allow for easier aspiration of immature oocytes (vs. women with decreased ovarian reserve, for instance) (Walls, 2015). The main advantage of IVM is the elimination of hyperstimulation risk. However, even in specialized centers, the success rate for IVM is significantly lower than the rates seen with conventional IVF-ET, and it is currently not recommended for routine use (Practice Committees ASRM and SART, 2013a; Chian, 2009).

## RISKS OF IN VITRO FERTILIZATION

### *OVARIAN HYPERSTIMULATION SYNDROME*

Ovarian hyperstimulation syndrome (OHSS) is typically an iatrogenic complication of gonadotropin stimulation. Patients at highest risk of OHSS are those with polycystic ovary syndrome, normo-ovulatory patients with a high ovarian reserve, and patients who previously experienced OHSS in a prior IVF cycle. OHSS was discussed in Chapter 42.

Avoidance of excessive stimulation is the primary approach for preventing OHSS. However, even with careful monitoring of gonadotropin dosage and follicular response, OHSS can still

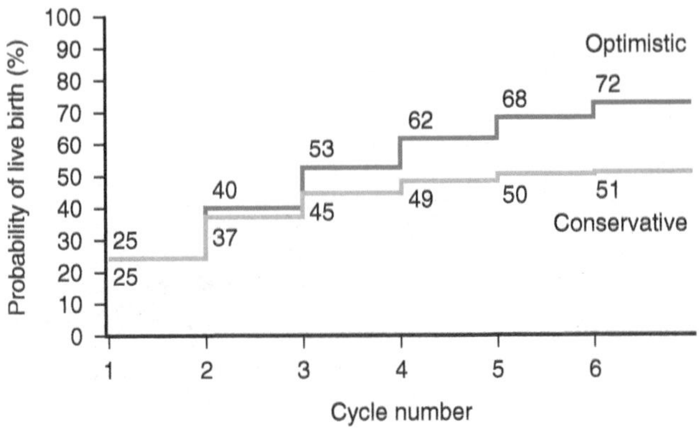


**Figure 43.8** Expectations of live birth with IVF-ET. (From Malizia BA, Hacker MR, Penzias AS. Cumulative live-birth rates after in vitro fertilization. *N Engl J Med.* 2009;360[3]:236-243.)

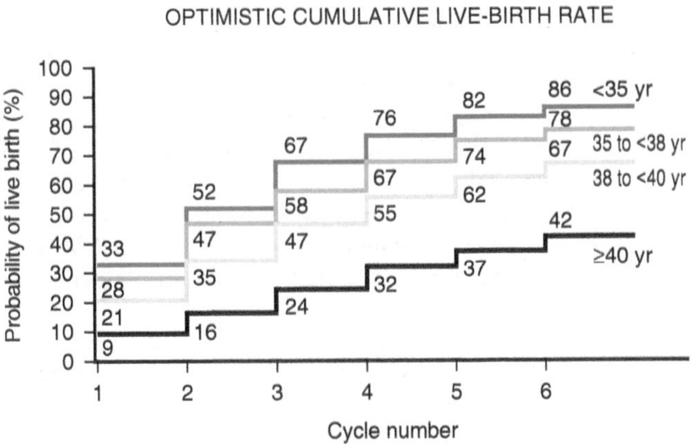


**Figure 43.9** Expectations of live birth with IVF-ET by age. (From Malizia BA, Hacker MR, Penzias AS. Cumulative live-birth rates after in vitro fertilization. *N Engl J Med.* 2009;360[3]:236-243.)

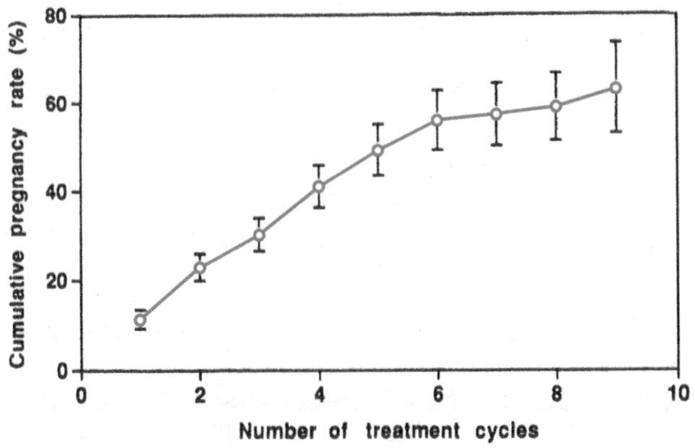


**Figure 43.10** Overall cumulative pregnancy rate in IVF treatment (95% CI). (From Dor J, Seidman DS, Ben-Shlomo I, et al. Cumulative pregnancy rate following in vitro fertilization: the significance of age and infertility aetiology. *Hum Reprod.* 1996;11[2]:425-428.)

develop. Coasting (withholding daily gonadotropin treatment while monitoring follicular development toward the end of the IVF cycle) may help decrease OHSS risk, although suboptimal pregnancy rates have been noted with more than 3 days of coasting (Nardo, 2006). GnRH antagonist cycles have been associated with lower OHSS rates as opposed to GnRH agonist "long" cycles (Xiao, 2014). Deferring embryo transfer immediately post retrieval and cryopreserving the embryos for a future frozen embryo transfer cycle helps decrease the duration of OHSS by (temporarily) avoiding pregnancy.

Administration of a daily dopamine agonist for starting immediately post-hCG trigger administration for up to 8 days following the hCG trigger has been shown in some studies to decrease OHSS development (Leitao, 2014).

To date the most effective means of decreasing OHSS risks with conventional IVF is using a GnRH agonist trigger. Using doses of 1 to 4 mg of GnRH agonist in lieu of hCG has dramatically (though not entirely) reduced OHSS development in the most high-risk patients. Lower pregnancy rates likely due to luteal phase insufficiency limited the use of this method until recent years. This defect likely occurs for the same reason that the GnRH agonist trigger successfully limits OHSS risks—the shorter half-life of the GnRH agonist versus hCG minimizes the cascade of events leading to prolonged OHSS. By combining the agonist trigger with a greatly reduced dose of hCG (i.e., 1000 IU or 1500 IU) and with the addition of supplemental estrogen/progesterone in the luteal phase, pregnancy rates are similar to those found with the conventional hCG trigger (Griffin, 2012).

## *IN VITRO FERTILIZATION PREGNANCY COMPLICATIONS*

The major pregnancy concerns after IVF are related to multiple gestations resulting in prematurity and other sequelae (Schieve, 1999). Because of the risks of prematurity with high-order multiples, couples may elect to undergo selective fetal reduction early in pregnancy. This is considered a safe procedure but carries an overall risk of pregnancy loss of approximately 1%.

However, there are some pregnancy-related risks that occur, even with singletons (Table 43.5). Therefore careful obstetric care is extremely important. Congenital anomaly risks in IVF pregnancies may be slightly increased (3% to 4%) compared with the natural rate of birth defects in the normal population (2% to 3%) but not when compared with an infertility population not undergoing IVF.

Although controversial, there may be a slightly increased risk of chromosomal structural defects in children born after ICSI. In a study of 8319 live births, Van Steirteghem and coworkers found a rate of sex chromosomal aneuploidy of 0.6% in the ICSI offspring versus 0.2% in the general neonatal population and structural autosomal abnormalities in 0.4% versus 0.07%, as well as an increase in structural aberrations related to the infertile fathers (Van Steirteghem, 2002). Increasingly data have suggested that although there may be a slightly increased rate of birth defects with IVF compared with the general population, it is not increased when compared with an infertile population that did not use IVF to conceive (Rimm, 2011). Similarly the latest meta-analysis to date has suggested no difference in risk between IVF with and without ICSI (Wen, 2012). Also there

**Table 43.5** Potential Risks in Singleton In Vitro Fertilization Pregnancies

| Perinatal Risks | Absolute Risk in IVF Pregnancies (%) | Relative Risk (vs. Non-IVF Pregnancies) |
|---|---|---|
| Preterm birth | 11.5 | 2.0 (1.7-2.2) |
| Low birth weight (<2500 g) | 9.5 | 1.8 (1.4-2.2) |
| Very low birth weight (<1500 g) | 2.5 | 2.7 (2.3-3.1) |
| Small for gestational age | 14.6 | 1.6 (1.3-2.0) |
| Neonatal ICU admission | 17.8 | 1.6 (1.3-2.0) |
| Stillbirth | 1.2 | 2.6 (1.8-3.6) |
| Neonatal mortality | 0.6 | 2.0 (1.2-3.4) |
| Cerebral palsy | 0.4 | 2.8 (1.3-5.8) |
| **Genetic Risks** | | |
| Imprinting disorder | 0.03 | 17.8 (1.8-432.9) |
| Major birth defect | 4.3 | 1.5% (1.3-1.8) |
| **Chromosomal Abnormalities (after ICSI)** | | |
| Of a sex chromosome | 0.6 | 3.0 |
| Of another chromosome | 0.4 | 5.7 |

Modified from Reddy UM, Wapner RJ, Rebar RW, et al. Infertility, assisted reproductive technology, and adverse pregnancy outcomes. Executive Summary of a National Institute of Child Health and Human Development Workshop. *Obstet Gynecol*. 2007;109(4):967-977.

In this table, the absolute risk is the percentage of IVF pregnancies in which the risk occurred. The relative risk is the risk in IVF versus the risk in non-IVF pregnancies; for example, a relative risk of 2.0 indicates that twice as many IVF pregnancies experience this risk as compared with non-IVF pregnancies. The numbers in parentheses (confidence interval) indicate the range in which the actual relative risk lies.

is no direct evidence of ICSI increasing the risk of imprinting disorders, which was suggested previously (Vermeiden, 2013). Follow-up of the children, however, does suggest an increased rate of urogenital abnormalities, which may be related to the male subfertility. Counseling of patients before ICSI about these findings is important. The uncertainty surrounding these issues is that it is likely that the infertile population also carries some risks (independent of IVF) when compared with the normal fertile population (Simpson, 2014).

## OVARIAN AND BREAST CANCER RISKS AFTER IN VITRO FERTILIZATION

Most studies do not show an increased risk for ovarian and breast cancer in patients previously exposed to IVF treatment (Brinton, 2013).Overall, IVF complication rates are low, with the most recent survey of ART complications (i.e., OHSS, hospitalizations, infections, maternal deaths) in the United States revealing rates far below 1% (Kawwass, 2015).

## PREIMPLANTATION GENETIC DIAGNOSIS/ SCREENING

A variety of genetic tests can help clinicians screen for heritable diseases or aneuploidy prior to embryo transfer. Preimplantation genetic diagnosis (PGD) identifies specific genetic mutations that are known to cause disease. A common use of PGD is to screen for the presence of autosomal recessive diseases such as cystic fibrosis (CF). If both potential parents are CF carriers, PGD can identify embryos that are homozygous for CF genes. Parents may elect to use PGD to avoid implanting these embryos. Preimplantation genetic selection (PGS) refers to screening embryos for aneuploidy. Because aneuploid pregnancy rates increase with maternal age, PGS may be offered to older women (above age 37 to 38) to select for euploid embryos. This may increase the chance for a live birth with IVF (Forman, 2014). Although ethically controversial (ASRM Ethics Committee, 2004), PGS can be used for gender selection and family balancing.

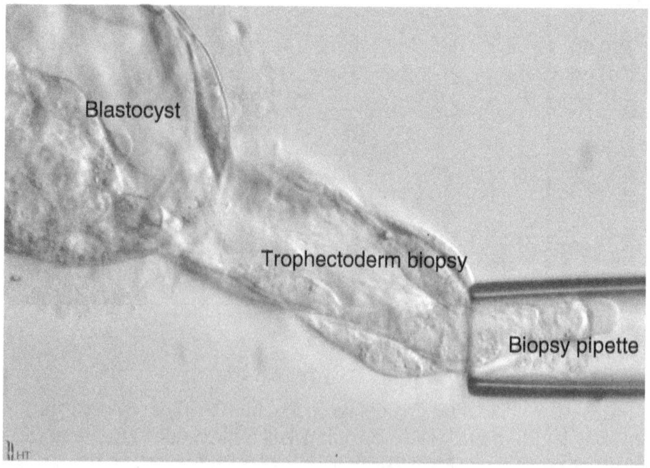


**Figure 43.11** Trophectoderm biopsy. (Courtesy of Center for Women's Reproductive Care at Columbia University.)

PGD/PGS can be conducted on the polar body of unfertilized oocyte, blastomeres from cleavage-stage (day 3) embryos or the trophectoderm of day 5/6 blastocysts. Because polar body biopsy cannot detect genetic errors occurring postfertilization, PGD/PGS is most commonly conducted on embryos. Until recently, PGD/PGS most commonly occurred with day 3 embryos with the removal of one to two blastomeres per embryo. Fluorescence in situ hybridization (FISH) was then conducted on the biopsied cells. Results could return within 24 to 48 hours at which point only the euploid embryos could be selected for transfer on blastocyst (embryo day 5 or 6). Because of false-positive and false-negative test risks (Hanson, 2009) as well as the risk of embryonic mosaicism leading to incomplete biopsy results, researchers sought more sensitive screening tests. With the development of array comprehensive genetic hybridization (aCGH) and blastocyst biopsy techniques, more accurate results could be obtained with trophectoderm biopsy of day 5/6 blastocysts (Fig. 43.11). Biopsy at the later blastocyst stage does not seem to impair embryonic survival in contrast to embryos biopsied on day 3 (Scott, 2013).

A variety of genetic screening techniques can be used to test embryonic cells: FISH (fluorescence in situ hybridization), single nucleotide polymorphism microarray, aCGH, real-time polymerase chain reaction, and next-generation sequencing. Currently, aCGH is most commonly used, as it allows analysis of all 23 chromosome pairs (unlike FISH, which can only screen a few chromosomal pairs at a time). However, comparative genomic hybridization cannot detect certain chromosomal issues such as balanced translocations, uniparental disomy, polyploidy, or point mutations. Eventually, next-generation sequencing, which allows for aneuploidy and genetic mutations at the same time, may become the screening tool of choice for PGS/PGD.

Studies (Franasiak, 2014) have shown that PGS for aneuploidy screening of embryos may help maintain consistently high live birth rates for those patients fortunate enough to undergo embryo transfer post-PGS even with advancing reproductive age. Compared with age-matched controls undergoing IVF without PGS, women who underwent IVF/PGS and embryo transfer were found to achieve higher live birth rates. However, fewer patients undergo transfer, as PGS leads to the diagnosis of abnormal embryos, which are not transferred.

## *RISKS OF PREIMPLANTATION GENETIC DIAGNOSIS/SCREENING*

False-positive results may stem from mosaicism within the biopsied embryo leading to the discard of a potentially normal embryo. False-negative results can lead to the transfer of an affected embryo and the conception of a disease-affected pregnancy. Because of this small risk (1% to 2%), patients are still advised to undergo antenatal genetic testing (i.e., chorionic villus sampling or amniocentesis) even post-PGS. Compared with standard IVF, PGD/PGS does not seem to be associated with an increased risk for obstetrical complications or congenital anomalies in resultant offspring (Eldar-Geva, 2014; Beukers, 2013).

## *DONOR IN VITRO FERTILIZATION*

Donor IVF enables fertilization in patients who are unable to conceive using their own oocytes due to decreased ovarian reserve or menopausal changes occurring naturally or post gonadotoxic therapy for cancer. A known or anonymous oocyte donor undergoes controlled ovarian stimulation. Once her oocytes are retrieved, they can then be fertilized with sperm (patient's partner or donor sperm). Resultant embryos are then transferred into the "recipient" patient's uterus following estrogen/progesterone priming to promote endometrial receptivity (see the "Frozen Embryo Transfer" section). Because of age-related effects on declining oocyte quality, pregnancy rates using oocytes from younger age oocyte donors (20 to 30) are typically in the 60% to 70% rate. The rate is relatively independent of the age of the recipient as long as her uterus is normal. Egg donation cycles can safely be carried out in healthy women into their 50s. Pregnancy rates may slightly decline in recipients over the age of 40, but live birth rates of close to 50% per donor cycle can be expected in women into their 50s. Obstetrical complication rates increase, however, in the extremes of advanced maternal age with higher incidences of gestational diabetes and preeclampsia (Paulson, 2002; Kort, 2012).

## *FROZEN EMBRYO TRANSFER*

Estrogen therapy (administered via oral, transdermal, or intramuscular routes) is administered typically over a 2-week period to "prime" the endometrium, readying it for embryo transfer. Monitoring of patient response to the hormone therapy can be done with vaginal ultrasound measurement of endometrial thickness as well as blood measurements of estradiol. Once an endometrial thickness of 6 to 8 mm or more is attained, progesterone supplementation (via either vaginal or intramuscular injection route) is begun 4 to 6 days before the scheduled embryo transfer.

Embryos are thawed on the day of the scheduled transfer. Survival rates of frozen embryos vary from clinic to clinic. The freezing method (most commonly vitrification at the present time) as well as the baseline quality of the embryos prior to cryopreservation impact embryo survival rates. Thawed embryos are then transferred into the patient's uterus.

The number of thawed embryos to transfer depends on the age of the woman at the time of freezing and on ASRM guidelines. Because implantation/pregnancy rates decline with female age and oocyte quality, the recommended number to transfer will increase with the age of the woman at the time of freeze. For instance, women who froze embryos prior to turning age 35 would be counseled to transfer just one to two embryos. Women freezing embryos at age 40 and above might be advised to transfer three or more. As with fresh IVF transfer, there is an increasing trend toward transferring exclusively at the blastocyst (day 5/6) stage over the day 3 stage.

Some studies now suggest improved pregnancy rates with the use of frozen embryo transfer versus a fresh cycle in certain patient populations. Proponents of frozen embryo transfer over fresh point to better endometrial receptivity and synchronization with the implantation window in programmed frozen cycles (Roque, 2013). Because not all frozen embryos survive the thawing process, however, some women may not be able to undergo a frozen embryo transfer.

## *FERTILITY PRESERVATION*

Patients at risk for future infertility due to gonadotoxic therapy for cancer or an immunologic disorder have several fertility preservation (FP) options. ART to harvest and cryopreserve mature oocytes or embryos is the most well-established method of fertility preservation. Oocyte biology leads to generally lower pregnancy rates with cryopreserved oocytes over embryos. Improvements in oocyte cryopreservation methods have led to improved freeze/thaw survival rates of oocytes and hence pregnancy rates. Nevertheless, even in younger (i.e., <37 years old) women, the pregnancy rate per frozen oocyte has ranged from 4% to 12% with a rapid decline occurring with older patients (Practice Committee ASRM, 2013). To date, only a few thousand live births have been reported from cryopreserved/thawed oocytes, whereas millions of pregnancies have resulted from cryopreserved embryos (Noyes, 2009).

ASRM has long stated that FP should be discussed with any reproductive-aged woman at risk for iatrogenic premature ovarian failure. However, it was not until 2013 that ASRM finally reversed its opinion that elective fertility preservation be considered "experimental." However, ASRM has still not endorsed its routine use for storing or "banking" embryos for the purpose of delaying pregnancy (Practice Committee ASRM, 2013). Although IVF and embryo cryopreservation has led to millions of pregnancies in infertile populations of women, few studies exist demonstrating cryopreservation pregnancy rates in women undergoing FP electively. Concern that the ART process may endanger a woman's future fertility potential—for instance, due to a postprocedure infection leading to pelvic adhesions—is an area of concern and for discussion when counseling women seeking to electively freeze oocytes/embryos. Additionally, concern remains that a woman might receive false hope through a FP cycle, leading her to further delay child-bearing to an age when ART may no longer be able to assist her should she develop infertility.

### OVARIAN TISSUE CRYOPRESERVATION

Research is ongoing in the area of ovarian tissue cryopreservation. For patients unable to go through an ART procedure, surgical removal of a whole or part of an ovary for cryopreservation may offer another way to preserve future fertility potential. The frozen tissue can then be thawed and orthotopically or heterotopically transplanted back into the patient's body at a future date if the need arises. To date, few live births (Donnez, 2013) have been reported following this process. Ovarian tissue cryopreservation is currently available at a limited number of centers in the United States and requires Institutional Review Board (IRB) approval. Ovarian tissue cryopreservation is not advised for patients suffering from hematologic cancers such as leukemia. Metastatic sites have been found in ovarian tissue harvested from patients with leukemia, leading to concern that transplantation of such tissue may lead to reseeding of malignant cells (Bastings, 2013).

GnRH agonist use may confer some ovarian protection against the gonadotoxic effect of certain chemotherapeutic agents (Del Mastro, 2014). GnRH agonists may work in one of several possible ways to protect the ovaries: suppression of the hypothalamic-pituitary gonadal axis leading to decreased blood flow to the ovaries, thereby minimizing ovarian exposure to chemotherapy; suppression of FSH-driven follicular recruitment; and activation of factors within the ovaries that might work directly to protect ovarian reserve (Blumenfeld, 2007). GnRH agonist administration initially leads to a transient increase in endogenous gonadotropin secretion, potentially stimulating the maturation of a "wave" of oocytes and thereby exposing more oocytes to the gonadotoxic agent. Because of this flare effect, it is important to administer the agonist 7to10 days prechemotherapy exposure. This sequence allows for the flare effect to fade and the agonist's suppressive/protective effect to come to the forefront. A study in reproductive-age breast cancer patients showed that GnRH agonist administration before and during chemotherapy significantly improved ovarian function as well as pregnancy potential following cancer therapy when compared with the control patients who received no agonist (Moore, 2015).

Patients facing impending pelvic radiation therapy may consider ovarian transposition via laparoscopy or laparotomy; the ovaries can be lifted above the pelvic brim and fixed to the anterior abdominal wall. Fixing the ovaries out of the field of radiation may help shield them from injury, thus helping patients to maintain their ovarian function (Gubbala, 2014).

## FUTURE DEVELOPMENTS

IVF and PGS have opened opportunities for stem cell research. Somatic cell nuclear transfer into oocytes has led to the development of pluripotent stem cell lines. Research into inducing somatic cells transformation into pluripotent stem cells may allow for tissue development for organ transplantation and repair of injured tissue. This technology may translate into repairing injured cardiac myocytes following an infarction, repairing damaged retinal tissue, or possibly generating oocytes for patients diagnosed with ovarian failure. Nuclear transfer into an enucleated donor cell has paved the way for treating rare mitochondrial diseases (Paull, 2013). All of these areas are still experimental, conducted under IRB approval where appropriate (Trounson, 2013).

To date, more than 5 million babies have resulted from IVF since Louise Brown was conceived via IVF in 1978. In the United States, 1% of babies are conceived via IVF, whereas in Europe, up to 3% are conceived with IVF. With improvements in PGS and IVF technology, goals include improving pregnancy rates particularly in women of advanced reproductive age while minimizing the risk for multiple pregnancies. In the future, advances in stem cell research may allow for innovative treatments for rare genetic and more common medical disorders while also offering possibilities for extending reproductive opportunities for patients with gonadal failure.

## KEY POINTS

- For IVF with and without ICSI, the delivery rate per cycle in which ova are retrieved is as high as 50%, depending on the age of the woman. The rate of pregnancy following IVF is directly related to the number of embryos placed in the uterine cavity. The rate of pregnancy is inversely related to the age of the female patient.
- Strict guidelines set forth by ASRM, which limit the number of embryos transferred, has reduced the rate of high-order multiple pregnancies in the United States.
- Preimplantation genetic selection and diagnosis allow for screening of embryos for aneuploidy or genetic disease prior to embryo transfer. Because advancing reproductive age is associated with higher rates of aneuploid embryos, PGS may help improve pregnancy rates in older women.
- Donor in vitro fertilization offers women who cannot conceive with their own oocytes the opportunity to experience pregnancy.
- Oocyte and embryo cryopreservation gives women the possibility of maintaining their future fertility potential even when faced with the possibility of premature menopause due to gonadotoxic medical treatments. Though still experimental, ovarian tissue freezing is another possible method of fertility preservation. Oocyte cryopreservation is available for healthy females who are interested in elective fertility preservation, but they need to be carefully counseled about the low pregnancy rates associated with cryopreserved oocytes.
- IVF technology has helped to expand research into stem cell therapy, which may further improve treatments for infertility as well as other medical conditions in the near future.

## KEY REFERENCES


Al-Inany HG, Youssef MA, Aboulghar M, et al. Gonadotropin-releasing hormone antagonists for assisted reproductive technology. *Cochrane Database Syst Rev*. 2011;(5). CD001750.

Bastings L, Beerendonk CC, Westphal JR, et al. Autotransplantation of cryopreserved ovarian tissue in cancer survivors and the risk of reintroducing malignancy: a systematic review. *Hum Reprod Update*. 2013;19(5):483-506.

Beukers F, van der Heide M, Middelburg KJ, et al. Morphologic abnormalities in 2-year-old children born after in vitro fertilization/intracytoplasmic sperm injection with preimplantation genetic screening: follow-up of a randomized controlled trial. *Fertil Steril*. 2013;99(2):408-413.

Blumenfeld Z. How to preserve fertility in young women exposed to chemotherapy? The role of GnRH agonist cotreatment in addition to cryopreservation of embryos, oocytes, or ovaries. *Oncologist*. 2007;12:1044-1054.

Brinton LA, Trabert B, Shalev V, et al. In vitro fertilization and risk of breast and gynecologic cancers: a retrospective cohort study within the Israeli Maccabi Healthcare Services. *Fertil Steril*. 2013;99(5):1189-1196.

Carney SK, Das S, Blake D, et al. Assisted hatching on assisted conception (in vitro fertilisation (IVF) and intracytoplasmic sperm injection (ICSI). *Cochrane Database Syst Rev*. 2012;(12). CD001894.

Chian RC, Huang JY, Gilbert L, et al. Obstetric outcomes following vitrification of in vitro and in vivo matured oocytes. *Fertil Steril*. 2009;91(6):2391-2398.

Del Mastro L, Ceppi M, Poggio F, et al. Gonadotropin-releasing hormone analogues for the prevention of chemotherapy-induced premature ovarian failure in cancer women: systematic review and meta-analysis of randomized trials. *Cancer Treat Rev*. 2014;40(5):675-683.

Donderwinkel PF, van der Vaart H, Wolters VM, et al. Treatment of patients with long-standing unexplained subfertility with in vitro fertilization. *Fertil Steril*. 2000;73(2):334-337.

Donnez J, Dolmans MM, Pellicer A, et al. Restoration of ovarian activity and pregnancy after transplantation of cryopreserved ovarian tissue: a review of 60 cases of reimplantation. *Fertil Steril*. 2013;99(6):1503-1513.

Dor J, Seidman DS, Ben-Shlomo I, et al. Cumulative pregnancy rate following in vitro fertilization: the significance of age and infertility aetiology. *Hum Reprod*. 1996;11(2):425-428.

Dovey S, Sneeringer RM, Penzias AS. Clomiphene citrate and intrauterine insemination: analysis of more than 100 cycles. *Fertil Steril*. 2008;90(6):2281-2286.

Eldar-Geva T, Srebnik N, Altarescu G, et al. Neonatal outcome after preimplantation genetic diagnosis. *Fertil Steril*. 2014;102(4):1016-1021.

Forman EJ, Hong KH, Franasiak JM, et al. Obstetrical and neonatal outcomes from the BEST Trial: single embryo transfer with aneuploidy screening improves outcomes after in vitro fertilization without compromising delivery rates. *Am J Obstet Gynecol*. 2014;210(2):157.e1-157.e6.

Franasiak JM, Forman EJ, Hong KH. The nature of aneuploidy with increasing age of the female partner: a review of 15,169 consecutive trophectoderm biopsies evaluated with comprehensive chromosomal screening. *Fertil Steril*. 2014;101(3):656-663.

Glujovsky D, Blake D, Farquhar C, et al. Cleavage stage versus blastocyst stage embryo transfer in assisted reproductive technology. *Cochrane Database Syst Rev*. 2012;(7). CD002118.

Goldman MB, Thornton KL, Ryley D, et al. A randomized clinical trial to determine optimal infertility treatment in older couples: the Forty and Over Treatment Trial (FORT-T). *Fertil Steril*. 2014;101(6):1574-1581.

Griffin D, Benadiva C, Kummer N, et al. Dual trigger of oocyte maturation with gonadotropin-releasing hormone agonist and low-dose human chorionic gonadotropin to optimize live birth rates in high responders. *Fertil Steril*. 2012;97(6):1316-1320.

Gubbala K, Laios A, Gallos I, et al. Outcomes of ovarian transposition in gynaecological cancers; a systematic review and meta-analysis. *J Ovarian Res*. 2014;7:69.

Hanson C, Hardarson T, Lundin K, et al. Re-analysis of 166 embryos not transferred after PGS with advanced reproductive maternal age as indication. *Hum Reprod*. 2009;24(11):2960-2964.

Hershlag A, Paine T, Cooper GW, et al. Monozygotic twinning associated with mechanical assisted hatching. *Fertil Steril*. 1999;71(1):144-146.

Jezek D, Knuth UA, Schulze W. Successful testicular sperm extraction (TESE) in spite of high serum follicle stimulating hormone and azoospermia: correlation between testicular morphology, TESE results, semen analysis and serum hormone values in 103 infertile men. *Hum Reprod*. 1998;13(5):1230-1234.

Kanter JR, Boulet SL, Kawwass JF, et al. Trends and correlates of monozygotic twinning after single embryo transfer. *Obstet Gynecol*. 2015;125(1):111-117.

Kawwass JF, Kissin DM, Kulkarni AD, et al. Safety of assisted reproductive technology in the United States, 2000-2011. *JAMA*. 2015;313(1):88-90.

Kirkegaard K, Ahlstrom A, Infersley HJ, et al. Choosing the best embryo by time lapse versus standard morphology. *Fertil Steril*. 2015;103(2):323-332.

Kort DH, Gosselin J, Choi JM, et al. Pregnancy after age 50: defining risks for mother and child. *Am J Perinatol*. 2012;29(4):245-250.

Krisher RL, Schoolcraft WB, Katz-Jaffe MG. Omics as a window to view embryo viability. *Fertil Steril*. 2015;103(2):333-341.

Leeton J, Rogers P, Caro C, et al. A controlled study between the use of gamete intrafallopian transfer (GIFT) and in vitro fertilization and embryo transfer in the management of idiopathic and male infertility. *Fertil Steril*. 1987;48(4):605-607.

Leitao VM, Moroni RM, Seko LM, et al. Cabergoline for the prevention of OHSS: systematic review and meta-analysis of randomized controlled trials. *Fertil Steril*. 2014;101(3):664-675.

Lobo RA. Potential options for preservation of fertility in women. *N Engl J Med*. 2005;353(1):64-73.

Luke B, Brown MB, Stern JE, et al. Using the Society for Assisted Reproductive Technology Clinic Outcome System morphological measures to predict live birth after assisted reproductive technology. *Fertil Steril*. 2014;102(5):1338-1344.

Luke B, Brown MB, Wantman E, et al. Application of a validated prediction model for in vitro fertilization: comparison of live birth rates and multiple birth rates with 1 embryo transferred over 2 cycles vs 2 embryos in 1 cycle. *Am J Obstet Gynecol*. 2015;212(5):676.e1-676.e7.

Malizia BA, Hacker MR, Penzias AS. Cumulative live-birth rates after in vitro fertilization. *N Engl J Med*. 2009;360(3):236-243.

Moore HC, Unger JM, Phillips KA, et al. Goserelin for ovarian protection during breast-cancer adjuvant chemotherapy. *N Engl J Med*. 2015;372(10):923-932.

Nardo LG, Cheema P, Gelbaya TA, et al. The optimal length of 'coasting protocol' in women at risk of ovarian hyperstimulation syndrome undergoing in vitro fertilization. *Hum Fertil*. 2006;9(3):175-180.

Noyes N, Porcu E, Borini A. Over 900 oocyte cryopreservation babies born with no apparent increase in congenital anomalies. *Reprod Biomed Online*. 2009;18(6):769-776.

Palermo G, Joris H, Devroey P, Van Steirteghem AC. Pregnancies after intracytoplasmic injection of single spermatozoon into an oocyte. *Lancet*. 1992;340(8810):17-18.

Palermo GD, Schlegel PN, Hariprashad JJ, et al. Fertilization and pregnancy outcome with intracytoplasmic sperm injection for azoospermic men. *Hum Reprod*. 1999;14(3):741-748.

Paull D, Emmanuele V, Weiss KA, et al. Nuclear genome transfer in human oocytes eliminates mitochondrial DNA variants. *Nature*. 2013;493(7434):632-637.

Paulson RJ, Boostanfar R, Saadat P, et al. Pregnancy in the sixth decade of life: obstetrical outcomes in women of advanced reproductive age. *JAMA*. 2002;288(18):2320-2323.

Practice Committee of American Society for Reproductive Medicine. Fertility preservation in patients undergoing gonadotoxic therapy or gonadectomy: a committee opinion. *Fertil Steril*. 2013;100(5):1214-1223.

Practice Committees of the American Society for Reproductive Medicine and the Society for Assisted Reproductive Technology. In vitro maturation: a committee opinion. *Fertil Steril*. 2013a;99(3):663-666.

Practice Committees of the American Society for Reproductive Medicine and the Society for Assisted Reproductive Technology. Mature oocyte cryopreservation: a guideline. *Fertil Steril*. 2013;99:37-43.

Ranieri M, Beckett VA, Marchant S, et al. Gamete intra-fallopian transfer or in-vitro fertilization after failed ovarian stimulation and intrauterine insemination in unexplained infertility? *Hum Reprod*. 1995;10(8):2023-2026.

Reindollar RH, Regan MM, Neumann PJ, et al. A randomized clinical trial to evaluate optimal treatment for unexplained infertility: the fast track and standard treatment (FASTT) trial. *Fertil Steril*. 2010;94(3):888-899.

Rimm AA, Katayama AC, Katayama KP. A meta-analysis of the impact of IVF and ICSI on major malformations after adjusting for the effect of subfertility. *J Assist Reprod Genet*. 2011;28:699-705.

Roest J, Mous HV, Zeilmaker GH, et al. The incidence of major clinical complications in a Dutch transport IVF programme. *Hum Reprod Update*. 1996;2(4):345-353.

Roque M, Lattes K, Serra S, et al. Fresh embryo transfer versus frozen embryo transfer in in vitro fertilization cycles: a systematic review and meta-analysis. *Fertil Steril*. 2013;99(1):156-162.

Schieve LA, Peterson HB, Meikle SF, et al. Live-birth rates and multiple-birth risk using in vitro fertilization. *JAMA*. 1999;282(19):1832-1838.

Schlegel PN. Testicular sperm extraction: microdissection improves sperms yield with minimal tissue excision. *Hum Reprod*. 1999;14:131-135.

Scott RT, Upham KM, Forman EJ, et al. Cleavage-stage biopsy significantly impairs human embryonic implantation potential while blastocyst biopsy does not: a randomized and paired clinical trial. *Fertil Steril.* 2013;100(3):624-630.

Simpson JL. Birth defects and assisted reproductive technologies. *Semin Fetal Neonatal Med.* 2014;19(3):177-182.

Steptoe PC, Edwards RG. Birth after the reimplantation of a human embryo. *Lancet.* 1978;2(8085):366.

Stray-Pedersen B, Stray-Pedersen S. Etiologic factors and subsequent reproductive performance in 195 couples with a prior history of habitual abortion. *Am J Obstet Gynecol.* 1984;148(2):140-146.

The Ethics Committee of the American Society of Reproductive Medicine. Sex selection and preimplantation genetic diagnosis. *Fertil Steril.* 2004;82(Suppl 1):S245-S248.

Trounson A. A rapidly evolving revolution in stem cell biology and medicine. *Reprod Biomed Online.* 2013;27(6):756-764.

Tsirgotis M, Nicholson N, Yang D, et al. Assisted fertilization with intracytoplasmic sperm injection. *Fertil Steril.* 1994;62(4):781-785.

Van Steirteghem A, Bonduelle M, Devroey P, et al. Follow-up of children born after ICSI. *Hum Reprod.* 2002;8(2):111-116.

Vermeiden JP, Bernardus RE. Are imprinting disorders more prevalent after human in vitro fertilization or intracytoplasmic sperm injection? *Fertil Steril.* 2013;99(3):642-651.

Walls ML, Hunter T, Ryan JP, et al. In vitro maturation as an alternative to standard in vitro fertilization for patients diagnosed with polycystic ovaries: a comparative analysis of fresh, frozen and cumulative cycle outcomes. *Hum Reprod.* 2015;30(1):88-96.

Wen J, Jiang J, Ding C, et al. Birth defects in children conceived by in vitro fertilization and intracytoplasmic sperm injection: a meta-analysis. *Fertil Steril.* 2012;97(6):1331-1337.

Xiao JS, Su CM, Zeng XT. Comparisons of GnRH antagonist versus GnRH agonist in supposed normal ovarian responders undergoing IVF: a systematic review and meta-analysis. *PLoS One.* 2014;9(9):e106854.

# Index



*Note:* Page numbers followed by *f* indicate figures, *t* indicate tables and *b* indicate boxes.

**H**

## I

J



K



L

**Q**



**R**

## T